Evidence-Based Orthopedics

Evidence-Based Orthopedics

CHIEF EDITOR

Mohit Bhandari MD, PhD, FRCSC

Professor and Academic Chair
Canada Research Chair
Division of Orthopaedic Surgery
Department of Surgery
McMaster University
Hamilton, ON
Canada

ASSOCIATE EDITORS

Rajiv Gandhi
Brad A. Petrisor
Marc Swiontkowski

MANAGING EDITOR

Sheila Sprague

SECTION EDITORS
Anthony Adili
Dianne Bryant
Jason W. Busse
Thomas A. Einhorn
Michelle Ghert
Mininder Kocher
Joy C. MacDermid
Rudolf W. Poolman
Emil H. Schemitsch
Andrew H. Schmidt
Robert M. Szabo
Achilleas Thoma

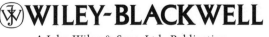

WILEY-BLACKWELL
A John Wiley & Sons, Ltd., Publication

BMJ|Books

This edition first published 2012, © 2012 by Blackwell Publishing Ltd

BMJ Books is an imprint of BMJ Publishing Group Limited, used under licence by Blackwell Publishing which was acquired by John Wiley & Sons in February 2007. Blackwell's publishing programme has been merged with Wiley's global Scientific, Technical and Medical business to form Wiley-Blackwell.

Registered office: John Wiley & Sons, Ltd, The Atrium, Southern Gate, Chichester, West Sussex, PO19 8SQ, UK

Editorial offices: 9600 Garsington Road, Oxford, OX4 2DQ, UK

The Atrium, Southern Gate, Chichester, West Sussex, PO19 8SQ, UK

111 River Street, Hoboken, NJ 07030-5774, USA

For details of our global editorial offices, for customer services and for information about how to apply for permission to reuse the copyright material in this book please see our website at www.wiley.com/wiley-blackwell

The right of the author to be identified as the author of this work has been asserted in accordance with the UK Copyright, Designs and Patents Act 1988.

Library of Congress Cataloging-in-Publication Data

Evidence-based orthopedics / chief editor, Mohit Bhandari ; section editors, Anthony Adili ... [et al.].

p. ; cm.

Includes bibliographical references and index.

ISBN-13: 978-1-4051-8476-2 (hardcover : alk. paper)

ISBN-10: 1-4051-8476-0 (hardcover : alk. paper)   1. Orthopedic surgery.   2. Musculoskeletal system–Wounds and injuries.   3. Evidence-based medicine.   I. Bhandari, Mohit.   II. Adili, Anthony.

[DNLM: 1. Bone and Bones--surgery.   2. Evidence-Based Medicine.   3. Fractures, Bone--surgery.   4. Joints--surgery.   5. Orthopedic Procedures. WE 168]

RD732.E96 2011

617.4'7–dc22

2011007202

A catalogue record for this book is available from the British Library.

This book is published in the following electronic formats: ePDF 9781444345070; Wiley Online Library 9781444345100; ePub 9781444345087; Mobi 9781444345094

Set in 9.25/12 pt Palatino by Toppan Best-set Premedia Limited
Printed and bound in Malaysia by Vivar Printing Sdn Bhd

1   2012

Contents

Contributors, x

Foreword, xx

Preface, xxii

Abbreviations, xxiii

Section I Methodology of Evidence-Based Orthopedics

1 Principles of Evidence-Based Orthopedics, 3
Simrit Bains, Mohit Bhandari, and Paul Tornetta III

2 Understanding Hierarchies of Evidence and Grades of Recommendation, 7
Raman Mundi and Brad A. Petrisor

3 Critical Appraisal Tools for Surgeons 12
Farrah Hussain, Sheila Sprague, and Harry E. Rubash

4 Understanding Diagnosis, Therapy, and Prognosis, 17
Helena Viveiros, Sarah Resendes, Tania A. Ferguson, Mohit Bhandari, and Joel Matta

5 Systematic Reviews and Meta-Analysis, 25
Nasir Hussain, Farrah Hussain, Mohit Bhandari, and Saam Morshed

6 Economic Analysis, 30
Laura Quigley, Sheila Sprague, and Theodore Miclau III

Section II Orthopedic Medicine

7 Osteoporosis and Metabolic Disorders, 37
Celeste J. Hamilton, Sophie A. Jamal, and Earl R. Bogoch

8 Thromboprophylaxis in Orthopedic Practice, 56
Ernest Kwek and Richard E. Buckley

9 Blood Transfusion, 72
David W. Sanders and Jeffrey L. Carson

10 Wound Infections, 78
Wesley G. Lackey, Kyle J. Jeray, Atul F. Kamath, John G. Horneff III, and John L. Esterhai, Jr

11 Gouty Arthritis, 86
Jasvinder A. Singh

12 Perioperative Medical Management, 93
Daniel A. Mendelson, Susan M. Friedman, and Joseph A. Nicholas

13 Orthobiologics, 100
T. William Axelrad and Thomas A. Einhorn

Section III Joint Reconstruction

III.I Hip and Pelvic Reconstruction/Arthroplasty

14 The Role of Computer Navigation in Total Hip Arthroplasty, 119
Jonathan M. Loughead and Richard W. McCalden

15 Highly Crosslinked Polyethylene in Total Hip Arthroplasty, 131
Glen Richardson, Michael J. Dunbar, and Joseph P. Corkum

16 Hip Resurfacing vs. Metal-on-Metal Total Hip Arthroplasty, 137
Sanket R. Diwanji, Pascal-André Vendittoli, and Martin Lavigne

17 The Role of Ceramic in Total Hip Arthroplasty, 153
Peter M. Lewis and James P. Waddell

18 Minimally Invasive Techniques in Total Hip Arthroplasty, 164
Amre Hamdi and Paul E. Beaulé

III.II Hip Revision Surgery

19 Management of Femoral Periprosthetic Fractures After Hip Replacement, 171
Tamim Umran, Donald S. Garbuz, Bassam A. Masri, and Clive P. Duncan

20 Evaluation of the Painful Total Hip Replacement, 178
Matthew Oliver and James N. Powell

21 Revision of the Femoral Components: Role of Structural Bulk Allografts and Impaction Grafting, 186
Christopher R. Gooding, Bassam A. Masri, Donald S. Garbuz, and Clive P. Duncan

22 Revision of the Acetabular Components: Role of Structural Bulk Allografts and Porous Tantalum Implants, 205
John Antoniou, Alan J. Walsh, and Vassilios S. Nikolaou

III.III Knee Reconstruction/Arthroplasty

23 Antibiotic Cement in Total Knee Arthroplasty, 212
Philip A. O'Connor and Steven J. MacDonald

24 Cemented vs. Uncemented Fixation in Total Knee Arthroplasty, 220
Eric R. Bohm, Ili Slobodian, Thomas R. Turgeon, and Martin Petrak

25 High-Flexion Implants vs. Conventional Design Implants, 228
Nicholas Paterson, Robert J. Orec, and Douglas D.R. Naudie

26 The Neuropathic/Charcot Joint, 236
Rajrishi Sharma and Mitchell J. Winemaker

III.IV Knee Revision Surgery

27 Cemented vs. Uncemented Stems in Revision Knee Arthroplasty: Indications, Technique, and Outcomes, 242
Gerard M.J. March and Paul R. Kim

28 Management of Structural Defects in Revision Knee Arthroplasty: Femoral Side, 249
Sandor Gyomorey, Paul T.H. Lee, and David J. Backstein

29 Patellar Options in Revision Knee Arthroplasty, 257
Hatem Al-Harbi and Paul Zalzal

III.V Shoulder Reconstruction/Arthroplasty

30 Total Shoulder Replacement vs. Hemiarthroplasty in the Treatment of Shoulder Osteoarthritis, 263
Olivia Y.Y. Cheng and Michael D. McKee

31 Cemented vs. Uncemented Fixation in Shoulder Arthroplasty, 270
Shahryar Ahmadi and Christian Veillette

32 Reverse Total Shoulder Arthroplasty, 278
Ryan T. Bicknell

33 Glenoid Fixation in Total Shoulder Arthroplasty: What Type of Glenoid Component Should We Use?, 284
Eric C. Benson, Kenneth J. Faber, and George S. Athwal

III.VI Foot and Ankle Reconstruction/Arthroplasty

34 Fusion vs. Arthroplasty in the Treatment of Ankle Arthritis, 294
Timothy R. Daniels, Mark Glazebrook, Terence Chin, and Roger A. Haene

35 Fusion vs. Arthroplasty in the Treatment of 1st MTP Arthritis, 307
Jeffrey G.M. Tan, Gilbert Yee, and Johnny T.C. Lau

36 Charcot–Marie–Tooth Disease and the Treatment of the Cavo-Varus Foot, 317
David N. Townshend and Alastair S.E. Younger

Section IV Trauma

IV.I Upper Extremity

IV.I.I Shoulder Girdle

37 Acromioclavicular Joint, 325
Bill Ristevski and Michael D. McKee

38 Clavicle, 332
Bill Ristevski and Michael D. McKee

39 Scapula, 341
Peter A. Cole and Lisa K. Schroder

40 Post-Traumatic Avascular Necrosis of the Proximal Humerus, 351
Ilia Elkinson and Darren S. Drosdowech

IV.I.II Humerus

41 Proximal Humerus Fractures, 360
Job N. Doornberg and David Ring

42 Humeral Shaft Fractures, 366
Amy Hoang-Kim, Jörg Goldhahn, and David J. Hak

43 Distal Humerus Fractures, 374
Aaron Nauth and Emil H. Schemitsch

IV.I.III Elbow and Forearm

44 Fracture-Dislocations of the Elbow, 383
Reyhan A. Chaudhary, Maurice Tompack, and J. Whitcomb Pollock

45 Radial Head Fractures, 397
Andrea S. Bauer and David Ring

46 Monteggia Fracture-Dislocations, 403
Bryce T. Gillespie and Jesse B. Jupiter

47 Olecranon Fractures, 409
Bryce T. Gillespie and Jesse B. Jupiter

48 Forearm Fractures, Including Galeazzi Fractures, 416
S. John Ham, Matthijs R. Krijnen, and Rudolf W. Poolman

IV.I.IV Wrist and Hand

49 Distal Radius Fractures, 425
Boris A. Zelle and Michael Zlowodzki

50 Perilunate Dislocations, 437
Geert A. Buijze, Job N. Doornberg, and David Ring

51 Carpal Fractures, 443
Bertrand H. Perey, Anne-Marie Bedard, and Fay Leung

52 Metacarpal Fractures, 462
Brent Graham

IV.II Lower Extremity

IV.II.I Hip

53 Hip Dislocations, 468
Gregory J. Della Rocca, Brett D. Crist, and Yvonne M. Murtha

54 Femoral Head Fractures, 474
Chad P. Coles

55 Intracapsular Fractures, 480
Jennifer A. Klok, Marc Swiontkowski, and Mohit Bhandari

56 Intertrochanteric Fractures, 491
Ole Brink and Lars C. Borris

IV.II.II Femur

57 Subtrochanteric Fractures, 497
Steven Papp, Wade Gofton, and Allan S.L. Liew

58 Femoral Shaft Fractures, 504
Costas Papakostidis and Peter V. Giannoudis

59 Distal Femur Fractures, 522
Matthijs R. Krijnen, J. Carel Goslings, and Rudolf W. Poolman

IV.II.III Knee

60 Knee Dislocations, 527
James P. Stannard and Allan Hammond

IV.II.IV Tibia

61 Proximal Tibia, 534
Richard J. Jenkinson and Hans J. Kreder

62 Tibial Shaft, 541
Jennifer A. Klok

63 Distal Tibia/Plafond, 549
Hossein Pakzad and Peter J. O'Brien

IV.II.V Foot and Ankle

64 Malleolar Fractures, 561
David W. Sanders and Ajay Manjoo

65 Talus Fractures, 567
Gregory K. Berry

66 Calcaneus Fractures, 574
Stephen J. McChesney and Richard E. Buckley

67 Midfoot/Metatarsal Fractures, 583
Robin R. Elliot and Terence S. Saxby

IV.III Pelvis and Acetabulum

68 Pelvis, 593
G. Yves Laflamme, Stephane Leduc, and Dominique M. Rouleau

69 Acetabulum, 602
Kelly A. Lefaivre and Adam J. Starr

IV.IV General

70 Open Fractures, 617
Atul F. Kamath, John G. Horneff, John L. Esterhai, Jr., Wesley G. Lackey, Kyle J. Jeray, and J. Scott Broderick

71 Acute Compartment Syndrome, 627
Andrew H. Schmidt

72 Noninvasive Technologies for Fracture Repair, 636
Yoshinobu Watanabe, Makoto Kobayashi, and Takashi Matsushita

73 Calcium Phosphate Cements in Fracture Repair, 642
Ross K. Leighton, Kelly Trask, Thomas A. Russell, Mohit Bhandari, and Richard E. Buckley

74 Damage Control Orthopedics, 649
Philipp Kobbe and Hans-Christoph Pape

75 Mangled Extremity, 655
Ted V. Tufescu

Section V Adult Spine

V.I Cervical Spine

76 Mechanical Neck Pain, 663
Gabrielle van der Velde

77 Whiplash, 669
Gabrielle van der Velde

V.II Mechanical Low Back Pain without Neuropathy

78 Mechanical Low Back Pain: Operative Treatment—Fusion, 675
Rahul Basho, Alex Gitelman, and Jeffrey C. Wang

79 Mechanical Low Back Pain: Nonoperative Management, 678
Andrea D. Furlan, Victoria Pennick, Jill A. Hayden, and Carlo Ammendolia

V.III Low Back Pain with Neuropathy

80 Neurogenic Claudication—Operative Management (Decompression and Fusion), 686
Hormuzdiyar H. Dasenbrock, Reza Yassari, and Timothy F. Witham

Contents

81 Neurogenic Claudication: Nonoperative
Management, 694
Carlo Ammendolia

82 Adolescent Idiopathic Scoliosis—Nonoperative
Management, 702
Calvin T. Hu and James O. Sanders

83 Adolescent Idiopathic Scoliosis—Operative
Management, 710
Calvin T. Hu and James O. Sanders

84 Metastatic/Myeloma Disease—Operative
Management, 721
Harsha Malempati, Erion Qamirani, and Albert J.M. Yee

85 Metastatic/Myeloma Disease—Nonoperative
Management, 728
*Harsha Malempati, Erion Qamirani, and
Albert J.M. Yee*

Section VI Sports Medicine

VI.I Shoulder

86 Treatment of the First Shoulder Dislocation, 737
Charles L. Cox, and John E. Kuhn

87 Chronic Shoulder Instability, 744
Joost I.P. Willems and W. Jaap Willems

88 Rotator Cuff Injury, 752
John E. Kuhn

89 Shoulder Impingement Syndrome, 763
Ron L. Diercks and Oscar Dorrestijn

90 Pathology of the Long Head of the Biceps, 772
Paul W.L. ten Berg, Luke S. Oh, and David Ring

VI.II Elbow

91 Ulnar Collateral Ligament Injury, 781
Denise Eygendaal and Laurens Kaas

92 Tennis Elbow, 787
*Peter A.A. Struijs, Rachelle Buchbinder,
and Sally E. Green*

VI.III Knee

93 Initial Management of the Sports Injured Knee, 796
*Jaskarndip Chahal, Christopher Peskun,
and Daniel B. Whelan*

94 Meniscal Tears (Meniscectomy, Meniscopexy,
Meniscal Transplants/Scaffolds), 803
*Nicola Maffulli, Umile Giuseppe Longo, Stefano Campi,
and Vincenzo Denaro*

95 Anterior Cruciate Ligament Injury, 812
*Verena M. Schreiber, Kenneth D. Illingworth,
Hector A. Mejia, and Freddie H. Fu*

96 Posterior Cruciate Ligament Injury, 822
Rune Bruhn Jakobsen and Bent Wulff Jakobsen

97 Operative vs. Nonoperative Treatment of Combined
Anterior Cruciate Ligament and Medial Collateral
Ligament Injuries, 832
*Rocco Papalia, Sebastiano Vasta, Vincenzo Denaro, and
Nicola Maffulli*

98 Posterolateral Corner Injury, 841
Pankaj Sharma and Daniel B. Whelan

99 Cartilage Injury, 847
*Joris E.J. Bekkers, Anika I. Tsuchida, and Daniël
B.F. Saris*

100 Runner's Knee, 853
Ella W. Yeung and Simon S. Yeung

VI.IV Foot and Ankle

101 Ankle Ligament Injury, 862
*Michel P.J. van den Bekerom, Rover Krips, and
Gino M.M.J. Kerkhoffs*

102 Achilles Tendinopathy, 872
*Nicola Maffulli, Umile Giuseppe Longo, Stefano Campi,
and Vincenzo Denaro*

VI.V Hip

103 Labral Tears, 879
Sanaz Hariri, Henk Eijer, and Marc R. Safran

104 Hip Impingement, 892
Marc J. Philippon and Karen K. Briggs

105 Snapping Hip, 898
Bas van Ooij and Matthias U. Schafroth

VI.VI Other Injuries

106 Ergogenic Aids: Creatine Supplementation as a
Popular Ergogenic Aid in Young Adults, 905
Michael J. O'Brien

Section VII Wrist and Hand Surgery

VII.I Wrist Surgery

107 Acute Management of Distal Radius Fractures, 913
Ruby Grewal

108 Prognosis: Pain and Disability After Distal Radius
Fracture, 923
Joy C. MacDermid and Ruby Grewal

109 Reconstruction of Malunited Distal Radius
Fracture, 930
James T. Monica and David Ring

110 Scaphoid Fractures, 938
Ruby Grewal

111 Nonunions of the Scaphoid, 946
     Nina Suh and Ruby Grewal

112 Trapeziometacarpal Arthritis of the Thumb, 954
     *Anne Wajon, Emma Carr, Louise Ada, and
     Ian A. Edmunds*

113 Salvage Procedures for the Treatment of Wrists with
     Scapholunate Advanced Collapse, 962
     *Jonathan Mulford, Paul K. Della Torre, and
     Stuart J.D. Myers*

114 Wrist Arthroscopy, 969
     *Aaron M. Freilich, Bryan S. Dudoussat,
     Fiesky A. Nunez Jr, Thomas Sarlikiotis,
     and Ethan R. Wiesler*

115 Rheumatoid Wrist Reconstruction (Arthrodesis and
     Arthroplasty), 979
     Warren C. Hammert and Kevin C. Chung

VII.II Hand Surgery

116 Management of Finger Fractures, 987
     Kristin B. de Haseth and David Ring

117 Prevention of Adhesion in Flexor Tendon
     Surgery, 993
     Filippo Spiezia, Vincenzo Denaro, and Nicola Maffulli

118 Therapy: Flexor Tendon Rehabilitation, 998
     B. Jane Freure and Mike Szekeres

119 Carpal Tunnel Syndrome—Conservative
     Management, 1012
     Jean-Sébastien Roy and Jessica Collins

120 Carpal Tunnel Syndrome—Surgical Management, 1021
     *Jessica Collins, Jean-Sébastien Roy, Leslie L. McKnight,
     and Achilleas Thoma*

121 Dupuytren's Disease, 1029
     *Larisa Kristine Vartija, Leslie L. McKnight,
     and Achilleas Thoma*

122 Extensor Tendon Surgery, 1039
     Carolyn M. Levis and Monica Alderson

123 Rheumatoid Hand Reconstruction, 1046
     Oluseyi Aliu and Kevin C. Chung

124 Flexor Tendon Surgery, 1057
     Shima C. Sokol and Robert M. Szabo

125 Replantation, 1072
     *Stephanie Ma, Leslie L. McKnight, and
     Achilleas Thoma*

Section VIII Orthopedic Oncology

126 Radiation in Soft Tissue Sarcoma: Pre- or
     Postoperative, 1083
     *Kurt R. Weiss, Rej Bhumbra, Peter C. Ferguson,
     Brian O'Sullivan, and Jay S. Wunder*

127 Soft Tissue Sarcoma: Does the Evidence Support the
     Administration of Chemotherapy?, 1088
     *Jennifer L. Halpern, Jill Gilbert, Ginger E. Holt,
     Vicki L. Keedy, and Herbert S. Schwartz*

128 Surgery in Bone Sarcoma: Allograft vs.
     Megaprosthesis, 1097
     *Kelly C. Homlar, Jennifer L. Halpern,
     Herbert S. Schwartz, and Ginger E. Holt*

129 Biopsy of Soft Tissue Masses, 1108
     *Bruce T. Rougraff, Albert J. Aboulafia, J. Sybil Biermann,
     and John Healey*

130 Surgical Margins in Soft Tissue Sarcoma: What Is a
     Negative Margin?, 1112
     Bruce T. Rougraff

Index, 1121

Contributors

Albert J. Aboulafia MD FACS MBA
Director Sarcoma Services
Sinai Hospital and University of Maryland, Baltimore, MD, USA

Louise Ada PhD
Associate Professor of Physiotherapy
University of Sydney, Sydney, NSW, Australia

Anthony Adili PEng MD FRCSC
Associate Professor
McMaster University
Chief of Surgery, Chief of Orthopaedics St. Joseph's Healthcare, Hamilton, ON, Canada

Shahryar Ahmadi MD FRCSC
Assistant Professor of Orthopaedics
Director
Shoulder and Elbow Surgery, Department of Orthopaedics, University of Arkansas for Medical Sciences, Fayetteville, AR, USA

Monica Alderson BSc(OT) OT Reg.(Ont.)
Clinical Leader and Manager
St. Joseph's Healthcare, Hamilton, ON, Canada

Hatem Al-Harbi MB ChB FRCSC
Clinical Fellow in Adult Reconstruction
McMaster University, Hamilton, ON, Canada

Oluseyi Aliu MD
Surgical Resident
University of Michigan, Ann Arbor, MI, USA

Carlo Ammendolia DC PhD
Clinical Researcher
Mount Sinai Hospital
Assistant Professor
University of Toronto
Associate Scientist, Institute for Work & Health, Toronto, ON, Canada

John Antoniou MD PhD FRCSC
Associate Professor
McGill University, Montreal, QC, Canada

George S. Athwal MD FRCSC
Associate Professor of Surgery
St. Joseph's Health Care, University of Western Ontario, London, ON, Canada

T. William Axelrad MD PhD
Director
Orthopaedic Trauma and Limb Reconstruction
Lake Charles Memorial Hospital, Lake Charles, LA, USA

David J. Backstein MEd MD FRCSC
Associate Professor
University of Toronto, Mount Sinai Hospital, Toronto, ON, Canada

Simrit Bains HBSc, MA MD(Cand)
McMaster University, Hamilton and University of Western Ontario, London, ON, Canada

Rahul Basho MD
UCLA Spine Center Fellow
UCLA Medical Center, Santa Monica, CA, USA

Andrea S. Bauer MD
Fellow in Hand Surgery
Massachusetts General Hospital, Boston, MA, USA

Paul E. Beaulé MD FRCSC
Associate Professor and Head, Adult Reconstruction Service
University of Ottawa, Ottawa Hospital, Ottawa, ON, Canada

Anne-Marie Bedard MD FRCSC
Upper Extremity Fellow
Laval University, Centre Hospitalier Universitaire de Quebec, Quebec, QC, Canada

Joris E.J. Bekkers MD
PhD Student
University Medical Center Utrecht, Utrecht, The Netherlands

Eric C. Benson MD
Assistant Professor
University of New Mexico, Albuquerque, NM, USA

Gregory K. Berry MDCM FRCSC
Staff Orthopaedic Surgeon and Associate Director Surgical Services
McGill University, Montreal, QC, Canada

Mohit Bhandari MD PhD FRCSC
Professor and Academic Chair
Canada Research Chair
Division of Orthopaedic Surgery
Department of Surgery
McMaster University, Hamilton, ON, Canada

Rej Bhumbra MBBS PhD (Orth), FRCS (Tr & Orth)
Senior Register
London Sarcoma Service
Royal National Orthopaedic Hospital
London, UK

Ryan T. Bicknell MSc MD FRCSC
Assistant Professor of Orthopaedic Surgery
Queen's University, Kingston, ON, Canada

J. Sybil Biermann MD
Associate Professor Orthopaedic Surgery
University of Michigan Hospital and Health Systems, Ann Arbor, MI, USA

Earl R. Bogoch MSc MD FRCSC
Medical Director, Mobility Program, St. Michael's Hospital
Professor, Department of Surgery, University of Toronto, Toronto, ON, Canada

Eric R. Bohm BEng MD MSc FRCSC
Associate Professor
Director of Arthroplasty Research
University of Manitoba and Concordia Joint
    Replacement Group, Winnipeg, MB, Canada

Lars C. Borris MD
Consultant Surgeon
Århus University Hospital, Århus, Denmark

Karen K. Briggs MPH
Director of Clinical Research
Steadman Philippon Research Institute, Vail,
    CO, USA

Ole Brink MD PhD MPA
Associate Professor and Consultant Surgeon
Århus University Hospital, Århus, Denmark

J. Scott Broderick MD
Associate Professor
Director of Orthopaedic Trauma
Greenville Hospital System University
    Medical Center
GHS-Associate Professor
University of South Carolina School of
    Medicine-Greenville, Greenville, SC, USA

Dianne Bryant MSc PhD
Associate Professor
Division of Orthopaedic Surgery, University
    of Western Ontario
Associate Professor
School of Physical Therapy and Schulich
    School of Medicine & Dentistry
Associate Professor
Clinical Epidemiology & Biostatistics,
    McMaster University, Hamilton, ON,
    Canada

Rachelle Buchbinder MB BS (Hons) MSc PhD FRACP
Director
Monash Department of Clinical
    Epidemiology, Cabrini Institute, Malvern
Department of Epidemiology and
    Preventive Medicine
School of Public Health and Preventive
    Medicine, Monash University, Melbourne
Joint Coordinating Editor, Cochrane
    Musculoskeletal Group, Malvern, VIC,
    Australia

Richard E. Buckley MD FRCSC
Professor and Head of Orthopaedic Trauma
Foothills Medical Centre, University of
    Calgary, Calgary, AB, Canada

Geert A. Buijze MD
PhD Research Fellow
Orthopaedic Research Center Amsterdam,
    Academic Medical Center, Amsterdam,
    The Netherlands

Jason W. Busse DC PhD
Scientist
Institute for Work & Health, Toronto
Assistant Professor
Department of Clinical Epidemiology
    & Biostatistics, McMaster University,
    Hamilton, ON, Canada

Stefano Campi MD
Resident
Campus Bio-Medico University, Rome, Italy

Emma Carr PT MHSc CHT
Senior Hand Therapist
Pacific Hand Therapy Services, Dee Why,
    NSW, Australia

Jeffrey L. Carson MD
Professor and Chief, Division of General
    Internal Medicine
University of Medicine and Dentistry of
    New Jersey, New Brunswick, NJ, USA

Jaskarndip Chahal MD
Orthopaedic Sport Medicine and
    Arthroscopy Fellow
University of Toronto, Toronto, ON, Canada

Reyhan A. Chaudhary MBA MD FRCSC
Shoulder and Elbow Clinical Fellow
University of Ottawa, Ottawa, ON, Canada

Olivia Y.Y. Cheng MD FRCSC
Clinical Fellow
St. Michael's Hospital, University of
    Toronto, Toronto, ON, Canada

Terence Chin MB BS FRACS
Fellow
Queen Elizabeth II Health Sciences Centre,
    Halifax, NS, Canada

Kevin C. Chung MS MD
Professor of Surgery, Section of Plastic
    Surgery, Department of Surgery
Assistant Dean for Faculty Affairs
University of Michigan Medical School, Ann
    Arbor, MI, USA

Peter A. Cole MD
Chief, Regions Hospital
Professor, Department of Orthopaedic
    Surgery, University of Minnesota, Saint
    Paul, MN, USA

Chad P. Coles MD FRCSC
Associate Professor
Dalhousie University, Halifax, NS, Canada

Jessica Collins MD
Plastic Surgery Resident
McMaster University, Hamilton, ON,
    Canada

Joseph P. Corkum BEng
Orthopaedic Researcher
Dalhousie University, Halifax, NS, Canada

Charles L. Cox MD
Assistant Professor
Vanderbilt University School of Medicine,
    Nashville, TN, USA

Brett D. Crist MD FACS
Assistant Professor and Co-director,
    Orthopaedic Trauma Service
University of Missouri, Columbia, MO, USA

Timothy R. Daniels MD FRCSC
Associate Professor
St. Michael's Hospital, University of
    Toronto, Toronto, ON, Canada

Hormuzdiyar H. Dasenbrock BA
Medical Student
Johns Hopkins University School of
    Medicine, Baltimore, MD, USA

Kristin B. de Haseth MD
Research Fellow
Massachusetts General Hospital, Boston,
    MA, USA

Gregory J. Della Rocca MD PhD FACS
Assistant Professor and Co-director,
    Orthopaedic Trauma Service
University of Missouri, Columbia, MO, USA

Paul K. Della Torre MB BS (Hons) BSc (Hons)
Orthopaedic Registrar
Concord Hospital, Concord, NSW, Australia

Vincenzo Denaro MD
Professor and Head of Department of
    Orthopaedic and Trauma Surgery,
    Campus Bio-Medico University, Rome,
    Italy

Contributors

Ron L. Diercks MD PhD
Professor of Clinical Sports Medicine and Chief, Sports Medicine Center
University Medical Center Groningen, University of Groningen, Groningen, The Netherlands

Sanket R. Diwanji MS
Clinical Fellow
Hospital Maisonneuve Rosemont, Montreal, QC, Canada

Job N. Doornberg MD PhD
Postdoctoral Research Fellow
Orthotrauma Research Center Amsterdam
Resident
Orthopaedic Surgery, Academic Medical Centre, St. Lucas Andreas Hospital, Amsterdam, The Netherlands

Oscar Dorrestijn MD PhD
Orthopaedic Resident
University Medical Center Groningen, University of Groningen, Groningen, The Netherlands

Darren S. Drosdowech MD FRCSC
Associate Professor
St Joseph's Health Care, University of Western Ontario, London, ON, Canada

Bryan S. Dudoussat MD
Fellow
Wake Forest University School of Medicine, Winston-Salem, NC, USA

Michael J. Dunbar MD FRCSC PhD
Professor
Dalhousie University, Halifax, NS, Canada

Clive P. Duncan MSc MD FRCSC
Professor
University of British Columbia
Consultant Orthopaedic Surgeon
Vancouver Hospital and Health Sciences Centre, Vancouver, BC, Canada

Ian A. Edmunds MB BS FRACS (Orth)
Head of Orthopaedic Department
Hornsby Ku–ring–gai Hospital
Hand Surgeon, Hornsby Hand Centre
Hornsby, NSW, Australia

Henk Eijer MBA MD PhD
Orthopedic Surgeon
Regionalspital Emmental, Burgdorf, Switzerland

Thomas A. Einhorn MD
Professor and Chairman, Department of Orthopaedic Surgery, Boston University Medical Center, Boston, MA, USA

Ilia Elkinson BHB MB ChB FRACS
Clinical Fellow
St Joseph's Health Care, London, ON, Canada

Robin R. Elliot MB BS MA FRCS
Orthopaedic Fellow
Brisbane Foot and Ankle Centre, Brisbane, QLD, Australia

John L. Esterhai, Jr. MD
Professor of Orthopaedic Surgery
Hospital of the University of Pennsylvania, and Veterans Affairs Hospital, Philadelphia, PA, USA

Denise Eygendaal MD PhD
Orthopedic Surgeon
Amphia Hospital, Breda, The Netherlands

Kenneth J. Faber MD MHPE FRCSC
Associate Professor of Surgery
St. Joseph's Health Care, University of Western Ontario, London, ON, Canada

Peter C. Ferguson MD MSc FRCSC
Associate Professor
University Musculoskeletal Oncology Unit, Mount Sinai Hospital, University of Toronto, Toronto, ON, Canada

Tania A. Ferguson MD
Assistant Professor
University of California Davis Medical Center, Sacramento, CA, USA

Aaron M. Freilich MD
Assistant Professor
University of Virginia, Charlottesville, VA, USA

B. Jane Freure BSc (PT) MManipTher (AU) CAMT Diploma in Sport PT
Physiotherapist
St Joseph's Health Care, London, ON, Canada

Susan M. Friedman MD MPH AGSF
Associate Professor, Geriatrics
University of Rochester School of Medicine and Dentistry
Research Director
Geriatric Fracture Center, Highland Hospital, Rochester, NY, USA

Freddie H. Fu MD DSc(Hon) DPs(Hon)
David Silver Professor and Chairman
Department of Orthopaedic Surgery
University of Pittsburgh School of Medicine, Pittsburgh, PA, USA

Andrea D. Furlan MD PhD
Associate Scientist, Institute for Work & Health
Physiatrist, Toronto Rehabilitation Institute
Assistant Professor
University of Toronto, Toronto, ON, Canada

Rajiv Gandhi MD MS FRCSC
Assistant Professor
University of Toronto, Division of Orthopedic Surgery, University Health Network, Toronto Western Hospital, Toronto, ON, Canada

Donald S. Garbuz MHSc MD FRCSC
Associate Professor and Head
Division of Lower Limb Reconstruction and Oncology, University of British Columbia, Vancouver, BC, Canada

Michelle Ghert
Associate Professor
Division of Orthopaedic Surgery, McMaster University, Hamilton, ON, Canada

Peter V. Giannoudis BSc MB MD FRCS
Professor
University of Leeds, Leeds General Infirmary, Leeds, UK

Jill Gilbert MD
Associate Professor of Medicine
Section Chief, Solid Tumor Oncology
Director, Hematology Oncology Fellowship Program
Vanderbilt University Medical Center, Nashville, TN, USA

Bryce T. Gillespie MD
Orthopedic Surgery Resident
Massachusetts General Hospital, Boston, MA, USA

Alex Gitelman MD
Spine Surgery Fellow
UCLA Medical Center, Santa Monica, CA, USA

Mark Glazebrook MSc MD PhD FRCSC
Associate Professor
Dalhousie University Orthopaedic Surgery
Orthopaedic Surgeon
Queen Elizabeth II Health Sciences Centre, Halifax, NS, Canada

Wade Gofton BScH MD MEd FRCSC
Assistant Professor
University of Ottawa, Ottawa Civic Hospital, Ottawa, ON, Canada

Jörg Goldhahn MD MAS
Schulthess Clinic, Zurich, Switzerland

Christopher R. Gooding BSc MD FRCS (Tr & Orth)
Orthopaedic Sport Medicine and Arthroscopy Fellow
Fellow in Lower Limb Reconstructive Orthopaedic Surgery
University of British Columbia, Vancouver, BC, Canada

J. Carel Goslings MD PhD
Director, Trauma Unit
Academic Medical Center, Amsterdam, The Netherlands

Brent Graham MSc MD FRCSC
University Health Network
Toronto Western Hospital, Toronto, ON, Canada

Sally E. Green PhD
Professor
Monash Institute of Health Services Research, Clayton, VIC, Australia

Ruby Grewal MD MSc FRCSC
Assistant Professor
Hand and Upper Limb Centre, St. Joseph's Health Centre, University of Western Ontario, London, ON, Canada

Sandor Gyomorey MSc MD FRCSC
Associate Staff
William Osler Health Center, Etobicoke General Hospital, Toronto, ON, Canada

Roger A. Haene MB BCh FRCS (Tr & Orth)
Fellow
St. Michael's Hospital, University of Toronto, Toronto, ON, Canada

David J. Hak MBA MD
Professor
Denver Health, University of Colorado, Denver, CO, USA

Jennifer L. Halpern MD
Assistant Professor
Vanderbilt University Medical Center, Nashville, TN, USA

S. John Ham MD PhD
Orthopaedic Surgeon
Onze Lieve Vrouwe Gasthuis, Amsterdam, The Netherlands

Amre Hamdi MB BS MD FRCSC
University of Ottawa, Ottawa, ON, Canada

Celeste J. Hamilton BHK MSc
Research Associate
Multidisciplinary Osteoporosis Research Program, Women's College Hospital
PhD Candidate
University of Toronto, Toronto, ON, Canada

Warren C. Hammert MD
Associate Professor
University of Rochester Medical Center, Rochester, NY, USA

Allan Hammond MD
Assistant Professor
University of Manitoba Health Science Centre, Winnipeg, MB, Canada

Sanaz Hariri MD
Fellow in Sports Medicine
Stanford University, Redwood City, CA, USA

Jill A. Hayden DC PhD
Assistant Professor
Dalhousie University, Halifax, NS, Canada

John Healey MD FACS
Attending Orthopaedic Surgeon
Hospital for Special Surgery, Weill Cornell Medical College and Memorial Sloan-Kettering Cancer Center, New York, NY, USA

Amy Hoang-Kim MSc
PhD Candidate
St. Michael's Hospital, University of Toronto, Toronto, ON, Canada

Ginger E. Holt MD
Associate Professor
Vanderbilt University Medical Center, Nashville, TN, USA

Kelly C. Homlar MD
Fellow
Vanderbilt University Medical Center, Nashville, TN, USA

John G. Horneff III BA MD
Instructor
Hospital of the University of Pennsylvania, Philadelphia, PA, USA

Calvin T. Hu MD
Resident
University of Rochester Medical Center, Rochester, NY, USA

Farrah Hussain BSc (Hons) MD(Cand)
Research Assistant
McMaster University, Hamilton, ON, Canada

Nasir Hussain HBSc, MSc(Cand)
McMaster University, Hamilton, ON, Canada

Kenneth D. Illingworth MD
Post-doctoral Research Associate
Department of Orthopaedic Surgery
University of Pittsburgh Medical Center, Pittsburgh, PA, USA

Bent Wulff Jakobsen MD
Medical Director
Hamlet Private Hospital, Science Center Skejby, Åarhus, Denmark

Rune Bruhn Jakobsen MD
Researcher
Oslo Sports Trauma Research Center, Norwegian School of Sport Sciences
Norway Institute of Basic Medical Sciences, Faculty of Medicine, University of Oslo, Oslo, Norway

Sophie A. Jamal MD PhD FRCPC
Director, Multidisciplinary Osteoporosis
Research Program, Women's College
Hospital
Associate Professor
University of Toronto, Toronto, ON, Canada

Richard J. Jenkinson MD FRCSC
Orthopaedic Surgeon
Sunnybrook Health Sciences
Lecturer
University of Toronto, Toronto, ON, Canada

Kyle J. Jeray MD
Vice-Chair and Program Director,
Department of Orthopaedic Surgery
Greenville Hospital System University
Medical Center
GHS-Associate Professor
University of South Carolina School of
Medicine-Greenville, Greenville, SC, USA

Jesse B. Jupiter MD
Hansjorg Wyss/AO Professor
Harvard Medical School
Chief, Hand and Upper Extremity Service
Massachusetts General Hospital, Boston,
MA, USA

Laurens Kaas MD
Resident in Orthopaedic Surgery
Orthopaedic Research Center Amsterdam,
Academic Medical Center, Amsterdam,
The Netherlands

Atul F. Kamath MD
Clinical Instructor
Hospital of the University of Pennsylvania,
Philadelphia, PA, USA

Vicki L. Keedy MSci MD
Assistant Professor
Vanderbilt University Medical Center,
Nashville, TN, USA

Gino M.M.J. Kerkhoffs MD PhD
Orthopedic Surgeon
Academic Medical Centre, Amsterdam, The
Netherlands

Paul R. Kim MD FRCSC
Associate Professor
University of Ottawa, Ottawa, ON, Canada

Jennifer A. Klok MSc MD
Surgery Resident
University of Ottawa, Ottawa, ON, Canada

Makoto Kobayashi MD PhD
Associate Professor
Teikyo University School of Medicine,
Tokyo, Japan

Philipp Kobbe MD
Attending Surgeon and Associate Professor
University Hospital, Aachen, Germany

Mininder S. Kocher MD MPH
Associate Director
Division of Sports Medicine, Childrens
Hospital Boston
Associate Professor of Orthopaedic Surgery,
Harvard Medical School, Boston, MA,
USA

Hans J. Kreder MPH MD FRCSC
Professor
University of Toronto
Chief, Holland Musculoskeletal Program
MT Chair & Chief, Division of Orthopaedic
Surgery
Toronto, ON, Canada

Matthijs R. Krijnen MD PhD
Chief Resident in Orthopaedic Surgery
Onze Lieve Vrouwe Gasthuis, Amsterdam,
The Netherlands

Rover Krips MD PhD
Orthopedic Surgeon
Diaconessenhuis, Leiden, The Netherlands

John E. Kuhn MD
Associate Professor and Chief of Shoulder
Surgery
Vanderbilt University School of Medicine,
Nashville, TN, USA

Ernest Kwek MB BS FRCSEd
Clinical Fellow
University of Calgary, Calgary, AB, Canada

Wesley G. Lackey MD
Orthopaedic Resident
Greenville Hospital System University
Medical Center, Greenville, SC, USA

G. Yves Laflamme MD FRCSC
Assistant Professor, Head of Ortho-Trauma
Sacre-Coeur Hospital, University of
Montreal, Montreal, QC, Canada

Johnny T.C. Lau MD MSC FRCSC
Assistant Professor
University of Toronto, Toronto, ON, Canada

Martin Lavigne MSc MD FRCSC
Associate Professor
University of Montreal
Hospital Maisonneuve Rosemont, Montreal,
QC, Canada

Stephane Leduc MD FRCSC
Assistant Professor
University of Montreal
Trauma Coordinator
Sacré-Coeur Hospital, Montreal, QC,
Canada

Paul T.H. Lee MB BCh, MA, FRCS(Eng) FRCS(T& O)
Senior Clinical Fellow
The Royal Orthopaedic Hospital,
Birmingham, UK

Kelly A. Lefaivre MSc MD FRCSC
Assistant Professor
University of British Columbia, Vancouver,
BC, Canada

Ross K. Leighton MD FRCSC FACS
Professor of Surgery
Queen Elizabeth II Health Sciences Centre,
Halifax Infirmary Site, Dalhousie
University, Halifax, NS, Canada

Fay Leung MD, FRCSC
Orthopedic Fellow
University of British Columbia, Vancouver,
BC, Canada

Carolyn M. Levis MD MSc FRCSC
Associate Professor of Surgery, Division
of Plastic and Reconstructive Surgery,
McMaster University
Head of Service, St. Joseph's Healthcare,
Hamilton, ON, Canada

Peter M. Lewis MB BCh FRCS(Orth)
Consultant Orthopaedic Surgeon
Prince Charles Hospital and Royal
Glamorgan Hospital, South Wales, UK

Allan S.L. Liew MD FRCSC
Assistant Professor
University of Ottawa
Director of Orthopaedic Trauma
The Ottawa Hospital, Ottawa, ON, Canada

Umile Giuseppe Longo MD MSc
Specialist in Orthopaedic and Trauma
    Surgery
Campus Bio-Medico University, Rome, Italy

Jonathan M. Loughead MB BS MSc FRCS (Tr & Orth)
Consultant Orthopaedics and Trauma
Queen Elizabeth Hospital, Gateshead, UK

Stephanie Ma BSc(PT) MD MDCM
Plastic and Reconstructive Surgery Resident
McMaster University, Hamilton, ON,
    Canada

Joy C. MacDermid PhD
Professor
McMaster University, Hamilton
Co-director of Clinical Research
Hand and Upper Limb Centre, London, ON,
    Canada

Steven J. MacDonald MD FRCSC
Professor
University of Western Ontario
Chief of Surgery, Chief of Orthopaedics
University Hospital, London, ON, Canada

Nicola Maffulli MS PhD MD FRCS(Orth)
Centre Lead and Professor of Sports and
    Exercise Medicine
Consultant Trauma and Orthopedic Surgeon
Barts and The London School of Medicine
    and Dentistry, London, UK

Harsha Malempati MD
University of Toronto, Toronto, ON, Canada

Ajay Manjoo MD FRCSC
Clinical and Research Trauma Fellow
London Health Sciences Centre
and The University of Western Ontario,
    London, ON, Canada

Gerard M.J. March MD FRCSC
Fellow
University of Ottawa, Ottawa, ON, Canada

Bassam A. Masri MD FRCSC
Professor and Head, Department of
    Orthopaedics
University of British Columbia, Vancouver,
    BC, Canada

Takashi Matsushita MD DMSc
Professor and Director of Department of
    Orthopaedic Surgery
Teikyo University School of Medicine,
    Tokyo, Japan

Joel Matta MD
Director, Hip and Pelvis Institute
St. John's Health Center, Santa Monica, CA,
    USA

Richard W. McCalden MPhil MD FRCSC
Associate Professor
University of Western Ontario, London
    Health Sciences Centre, London, ON,
    Canada

Stephen J. McChesney MB ChB, FRACS (Orth)
Clinical Fellow
University of Calgary, Calgary, AB, Canada

Michael D. McKee MD FRCSC
Professor
St. Michael's Hospital, University of
    Toronto, Toronto, ON, Canada

Leslie L. McKnight MSc
Research Assistant, Department of Surgery,
    McMaster University, Hamilton, ON,
    Canada

Hector A. Mejia MD
Tallahassee Orthopedic Clinic
Clinical Instructor
Florida State University Medical School
Tallahassee, FL, USA

Daniel A. Mendelson MS MD FACP AGSF
Associate Professor, Geriatrics
University of Rochester School of Medicine
    and Dentistry
Director, Consultative Services
Highland Hospital, Rochester, NY, USA

Theodore Miclau III MD
Professor and Vice Chairman, Department
    of Orthopaedic Surgery
University of California
Director, Orthopaedic Trauma Institute
Chief, Orthopaedic Surgery
San Francisco General Hospital, San
    Francisco, CA, USA

James T. Monica MD
Fellow
Massachusetts General Hospital and
    Harvard Medical School, Boston, MA,
    USA

Saam Morshed MD MPH
Assistant Professor
Orthopaedic Trauma Institute, San Francisco
    General Hospital and the University of
    California, San Francisco, CA, USA

Jonathan Mulford MBBS (Hons) FRACS Dip Clinical Trials
Orthopaedic Surgeon
Prince of Wales Hospital, Sydney, NSW,
    Australia

Raman Mundi BHSc MD(Cand)
Medical Student
McMaster University, Hamilton, ON,
    Canada

Yvonne M. Murtha MD
Assistant Professor
University of Missouri, Columbia, MO, USA

Stuart J.D. Myers MB BS(Hons), FRACS (Orth), FAOrthA
Hand Surgeon
Prince of Wales Hospital, Sydney, NSW,
    Australia

Douglas D.R. Naudie MD FRCSC
Assistant Professor
University of Western Ontario, London, ON,
    Canada

Aaron Nauth MD
Clinical Fellow
St. Michael's Hospital, University of
    Toronto, Toronto, ON, Canada

Contributors

Joseph A. Nicholas MD MPH
Assistant Professor, Geriatrics
University of Rochester School of Medicine
and Dentistry
Attending Physician
Highland Hospital, Rochester, NY, USA

Vassilios S. Nikolaou MD
Clinical Fellow
McGill University, Montreal, QC, Canada

Fiesky A. Nunez Jr. MD
Postdoctoral Research Fellow
Wake Forest University School of Medicine,
Winston-Salem, NC, USA

Michael J. O'Brien MD
Instructor in Sports Medicine
Harvard Medical School, Children's
Hospital Boston, Boston, MA, USA

Peter J. O'Brien MD FRCSC
Associate Professor
Head of the Division of Orthopaedic
Trauma, University of British Columbia,
Vancouver, BC, Canada

**Philip A. O'Connor FRCSI
(Orth)**
Clinical Fellow
University of Western Ontario and London
Health Sciences Centre, London, ON,
Canada

Luke S. Oh MD
Sports Medicine Orthopaedic Surgeon
Department of Orthopaedic Surgery,
Massachusetts General Hospital
Instructor of Orthopaedic Surgery, Harvard
Medical School, Boston, MA, USA

**Matthew Oliver MB BS FRCS
(Tr & Orth)**
Joint Reconstruction Fellow
University of Calgary, Calgary, AB, Canada

Robert J. Orec MB ChB FRACS
Orthopaedic Surgeon
Middlemore Hospital, Otahuhu, Manukau,
New Zealand

**Brian O'Sullivan MB FRCPI
FRCPC FFRRCSI(Hon)**
Professor and Consultant Radiation
Oncologist
Princess Margaret Hospital, University of
Toronto, Toronto, ON, Canada

Hossein Pakzad MD FRCSC
Trauma Fellow
University of British Columbia, Vancouver,
BC, Canada

Costas Papakostidis MD
Orthopaedic Consultant
Research Collaborator
University of Leeds, Leeds General
Infirmary, Leeds, UK

Rocco Papalia MD PhD
Staff Surgeon
Campus Bio-Medico University, Rome, Italy

**Hans-Christoph Pape MD
FACS**
Professor and Chairman
Department of Trauma and Orthopaedic
Surgery, Aachen University Medical Center,
Aachen, Germany

Steven Papp MSc MD FRCSC
Assistant Professor
University of Ottawa, Ottawa Civic
Hospital, Ottawa, ON, Canada

Nicholas Paterson BScH
Research Assistant
University of Western Ontario, London,
ON, Canada

Victoria Pennick RN MHSc
Managing Editor, Cochrane Back Review
Group
Institute for Work & Health
University of Toronto, Toronto, ON, Canada

Bertrand H. Perey MD FRCSC
Clinical Assistant Professor
University of British Columbia, Port Moody,
BC, Canada

Christopher Peskun MD
Orthopaedic Sport Medicine and
Arthroscopy Fellow
University of Toronto, Toronto, ON, Canada

Martin Petrak BEng MSc PEng
Concordia Hip and Knee Institute
Winnipeg, MB, Canada

**Brad A. Petrisor MSc MD
FRCSC**
Assistant Professor
McMaster University, Hamilton, ON,
Canada

Marc J. Philippon MD
Orthopaedic Surgeon
Steadman Clinic
Director of Hip Research
Steadman Philippon Research Institute, Vail,
CO, USA
Associate Clinical Professor
McMaster University, Hamilton, ON,
Canada

**J. Whitcomb Pollock MSc MD
FRCSC**
Assistant Professor
University of Ottawa, Ottawa, ON, Canada

Rudolf W. Poolman MD PhD
Director of Clinical Research
Onze Lieve Vrouwe Gasthuis, Amsterdam,
The Netherlands

James N. Powell MD FRCSC
Clinical Associate Professor in Orthopaedics
University of Calgary, Calgary, AB, Canada

Erion Qamirani MD PhD
Resident
University of Toronto, Toronto, ON, Canada

Laura Quigley MSc
University of Toronto, Toronto, ON, Canada

**Sarah Resendes BSc
MPH(Cand)**
Research Associate
University of Guelph, Guelph, ON, Canada

Glen Richardson MD FRCSC
Assistant Professor
Dalhousie University, Halifax, NS, Canada

David Ring MD PhD
Director of Research
Harvard Medical School and Massachusetts
General Hospital, Boston, MA, USA

Bill Ristevski MSc MD FRCSC
Fellow
St. Michael's Hospital, University of
Toronto, Toronto, ON, Canada

Bruce T. Rougraff MD
Orthopaedic Surgeon
OrthoIndy, Indianapolis, IN, USA

Dominique M. Rouleau MSc MD FRCSC
Assistant Professor
Sacré-Coeur Hospital, University of Montreal, Montreal, QC, Canada

Jean-Sébastien Roy PT PhD
Associate Professor and Researcher
Laval University, Quebec, QC, Canada

Harry E. Rubash MD
Chief, Department of Orthopaedic Surgery
Massachusetts General Hospital, Boston, MA, USA

Thomas A. Russell MD
Professor
Campbell Clinic, University of Tennessee and Center for the Health Sciences, Memphis, TN, USA

Marc R. Safran MD
Professor, Orthopedic Surgery
Associate Director, Sports Medicine
Stanford University, Redwood City, CA, USA

David W. Sanders MSc MD FRCSC
Associate Professor
London Health Sciences Centre and the University of Western Ontario, London, ON, Canada

James O. Sanders MD
Professor and Chief of Pediatric Orthopaedics
University of Rochester Medical Center, Rochester, NY, USA

Daniël B.F. Saris MD PhD
Professor of Reconstructive Medicine, MIRA Institute, Univeristy of Twente, Enschede
Orthopedic Surgeon
University Medical Center Utrecht, Utrecht, The Netherlands

Thomas Sarlikiotis MD
Postdoctoral Fellow
Wake Forest University School of Medicine, Winston-Salem, NC, USA

Terence S. Saxby MB BS FRACS
Orthopaedic Surgeon
Brisbane Foot and Ankle Centre, Brisbane, QLD, Australia

Matthias U. Schafroth MD
Academic Medical Center and Orthopedic Research Center Amsterdam, Amsterdam, The Netherlands

Emil H. Schemitsch MD
Professor of Surgery
University of Toronto
Head, Division of Orthopaedic Surgery, St. Michael's Hospital, Toronto, ON, Canada

Andrew H. Schmidt MD
Professor
University of Minnesota
Faculty
Hennepin County Medical Center, Minneapolis, MN, USA

Verena M. Schreiber MD
Resident
Department of Orthopaedic Surgery
University of Pittsburgh Medical Center, Pittsburgh, PA, USA

Lisa K. Schroder BS MBA
Director, Orthopaedic Trauma Academic Programs
University of Minnesota—Regions Hospital, Saint Paul, MN, USA

Herbert S. Schwartz MD
Professor
Vanderbilt University Medical Center, Nashville, TN, USA

Pankaj Sharma MB BS FRCS (Tr & Orth)
Orthopaedic Sport Medicine and Arthroscopy Fellow
University of Toronto, Toronto, ON, Canada

Rajrishi Sharma MD FRCSC
Arthroplasty Fellow
Hip and Knee Adult Reconstruction
University of Western Ontario, London, ON, Canada

Jasvinder A. Singh MB BS MD MPH
Associate Professor
University of Alabama at Birmingham
Staff Physician
Birmingham Veterans Affairs Medical Center, Birmingham, AL, USA

Ili Slobodian BSc MSc
Research Coordinator, Concordia Joint Replacement Group
University of Manitoba, Winnipeg, MB, Canada

Shima C. Sokol MD
Physician, Prohealth Care Associates
Lake Success, NY, USA

Filippo Spiezia MD
Resident in Trauma and Orthopaedic Surgery
Campus Bio-Medico University, Rome, Italy

Sheila Sprague MSc PhD(Cand)
McMaster University, Hamilton, ON, Canada

James P. Stannard MD
J Vernon Luck Distinguished Professor and Chairman, Orthopaedic Surgery
University of Missouri Hospital, Columbia, MO, USA

Adam J. Starr MD
Associate Professor
University of Texas Southwestern Medical Center, Dallas, TX, USA

Peter A.A. Struijs MD PhD
Orthopaedic Surgeon
Academic Medical Centre, Amsterdam, The Netherlands

Nina Suh MD
Orthopedic Resident
University of Western Ontario, London, ON, Canada

Marc Swiontkowski MD
Professor
University of Minnesota
Chief Executive Officer
TRIA Orthopaedic Center
Minneapolis, MN, USA

Robert M. Szabo MD MPH
Professor and Chief, Hand and Upper Extremity Service
University of California—Davis, Sacramento, CA, USA

Mike Szekeres OT Reg (Ont.) CHT
Occupational Therapist
St Joseph's Health Care, London, ON, Canada

Jeffrey G.M. Tan MD MRCS (Edin) FRCS (Edin)
Clinical Fellow
Toronto Western Hospital, University of Toronto, Toronto, ON, Canada

Paul W.L. ten Berg MSc
Research Fellow
Orthopaedic Hand and Upper Extremity Service
Massachusetts General Hospital, Boston, MA, USA

Achilleas Thoma MD MSc FRCSC FACS
Clinical Professor and Head, Division of Plastic Surgery
McMaster University, Hamilton, ON, Canada

Maurice Tompack MD
Resident
University of Ottawa, Ottawa, ON, Canada

Paul Tornetta III MD
Professor
Director of Orthopaedic Trauma
Boston University Medical Center
Boston, MA, USA

David N. Townshend MBBS FRCS(Orth)
Foot and Ankle Surgery Fellow
University of British Columbia, Vancouver, BC, Canada

Kelly Trask BEng MSc CCRP
Research Manager
Queen Elizabeth II Health Sciences Centre, Halifax, NS, Canada

Anika I. Tsuchida MD
PhD Student
University Medical Center Utrecht, Utrecht, The Netherlands

Ted V. Tufescu BSc MD FRCSC
Assistant Professor
University of Manitoba, Winnipeg, MB, Canada

Thomas R. Turgeon BSc MD MPH FRCSC
Assistant Professor
University of Manitoba and Concordia Joint Replacement Group, Winnipeg, MB, Canada

Tamim Umran MD FRCSC
Clinical and Research Fellow
University of British Columbia, Vancouver, BC, Canada

Michel P. J. van den Bekerom MD
Resident in Orthopedic Surgery
Academic Medical Centre, Amsterdam, The Netherlands

Gabrielle van der Velde DC PhD
Scientific Associate
Toronto Health Economics and Technology Assessment (THETA) Collaborative, University of Toronto
Adjunct Scientist
Institute for Work & Health, Toronto, ON, Canada

Bas van Ooij MD
PhD Fellow
Academic Medical Center and Orthopedic Research Center Amsterdam, Amsterdam, The Netherlands

Larisa Kristine Vartija MD BHSc
Resident in Plastic Surgery
McMaster University, Hamilton, ON, Canada

Sebastiano Vasta MS
House Surgeon
Campus Bio-Medico University, Rome, Italy

Christian Veillette MD MSc FRCSC
Shoulder and Elbow Reconstructive Surgery
Toronto Western Hospital
University Health Network
Assistant Professor
Department of Surgery, University of Toronto, Toronto, ON, Canada

Pascal-André Vendittoli MSc MD FRCSC
Associate Professor and Director of Research for the Orthopaedic Division
Hospital Maisonneuve Rosemont, Montreal, QC, Canada

Helena Viveiros BSc BA MSc(Cand)
Research Coordinator
McMaster University, Hamilton, ON, Canada

James P. Waddell MD FRCSC
Professor
St Michael's Hospital, University of Toronto, Toronto, ON, Canada

Anne Wajon PT PhD CHT
Director and Senior Hand Therapist
Macquarie Hand Therapy, Macquarie University, Sydney, NSW, Australia

Alan J. Walsh FRCSI (Tr & Orth)
Clinical Fellow
McGill University, Montreal, QC, Canada

Jeffrey C. Wang MD
Professor of Orthopaedic Surgery and Neurosurgery
UCLA Spine Center, UCLA School of Medicine, Santa Monica, CA, USA

Yoshinobu Watanabe MD PhD
Associate Professor
Teikyo University School of Medicine, Tokyo, Japan

Kurt R. Weiss MD
Assistant Professor
Division of Musculoskeletal Oncology, Department of Orthopaedic Surgery, University of Pittsburg, Pittsburg, PA, USA

Daniel B. Whelan MSc MD FRCSC
Assistant Professor
St. Michael's Hospital, University of Toronto, Toronto, ON, Canada

Ethan R. Wiesler MD
Associate Professor
Wake Forest University School of Medicine, Winston-Salem, NC, USA

Joost I.P. Willems BSc
Medical Student
Free University, Amsterdam, The Netherlands

W. Jaap Willems MD PhD
Orthopaedic Surgeon and Chief Department of Orthopedics
Onze Lieve Vrouwe Gasthuis, Amsterdam, The Netherlands

Mitchell J. Winemaker MD FRCSC
Associate Clinical Professor
McMaster University, Hamilton, ON, Canada

Timothy F. Witham MD FACS
Associate Professor and Director, The Johns
  Hopkins Bayview Spine Program
Johns Hopkins University, Baltimore, MD,
  USA

Jay S. Wunder MD MSc FRCSC
Professor
University Musculoskeletal Oncology Unit
Mount Sinai Hospital, University of Toronto,
  Toronto, ON, Canada

Reza Yassari MD
Instructor in Neurosurgery
Johns Hopkins University, Baltimore, MD,
  USA

Albert J.M. Yee MD MSc FRCSC
Active Staff
Division of Orthopaedic Surgery
Associate Scientist
Holland Musculoskeletal Program
Consultant in Surgical Oncology
Odette Cancer Centre
Sunnybrook Health Sciences Centre,
  Toronto, ON, Canada

**Gilbert Yee MEd MBA MD
FRCSC**
Consultant
The Scarborough Hospital, Scarborough,
  ON, Canada

Ella W. Yeung PT PhD
Associate Professor
Department of Rehabilitation Sciences,
  Hong Kong Polytechnic University,
  Kowloon, Hong Kong

Simon S. Yeung PT PhD
Associate Professor
Department of Rehabilitation Sciences,
  Hong Kong Polytechnic University,
  Kowloon, Hong Kong

**Alastair S.E. Younger MB ChB
MSc FRCSC ChM**
Associate Professor, Head of Division of
  Extremity Surgery
University of British Columbia, Vancouver,
  BC, Canada

Paul Zalzal MASc MD FRCSC
Assistant Clinical Professor
McMaster University, Hamilton
Staff Orthopedic Surgeon
Oakville Trafalgar Memorial Hospital
Oakville, ON, Canada

Boris A. Zelle MD
Assistant Professor
Department of Orthopaedic Surgery
Division of Orthopaedic Trauma Surgery
University of Texas Health Science Center at
  San Antonio
San Antonio, TX, USA

Michael Zlowodzki MD
Resident
University of Minnesota, Minneapolis, MN,
  USA

Foreword

Evidence-based medicine (EBM)—or evidence-based surgery, or evidence-based orthopedics (EBO)—is about solving clinical problems. In particular, EBO provides tools for using the medical and surgical literature to determine the benefits and risks of alternative patient management strategies, and to weigh those benefits and risks in the context of an individual patient's experiences, values and preferences.

The term evidence-based medicine first appeared in the medical literature in 1991; it rapidly became something of a mantra. EBM is sometimes perceived as a blinkered adherence to randomized trials, or a health care managers' tool for controlling and constraining recalcitrant physicians. In fact, EBM and EBO involve informed and effective use of all types of evidence, but particularly evidence from the medical literature, in patient care.

EBM's evolution has included outward expansion—we now realize that optimal health care delivery must include evidence-based nursing, physiotherapy, occupational therapy, and podiatry—and specialization. We need evidence-based obstetrics, gynecology, internal medicine and surgery and, indeed, urology and neurosurgery. And of course, we need evidence-based orthopedics.

Applying EBO to management decisions in individual patients involves use of a hierarchy of study design, with high-quality randomized trials showing definitive results directly applicable to an individual patient at the apex, to relying on physiological rationale or previous experience with a small number of similar patients near the bottom rung. Ideally, systematic reviews and meta-analyses summarize the highest quality available evidence. The hallmark of evidence-based practitioners is that, for particular clinical decisions, they know the quality of the evidence, and therefore the degree of uncertainty.

What is required to practice EBO? Practitioners must know how to frame a clinical quandary to facilitate use of the literature in its resolution. Evidence-based orthopedic surgeons must know how to search the literature efficiently to obtain the best available evidence bearing on their question, to evaluate the strength of the methods of the studies

they find, extract the clinical message, apply it back to the patient, and store it for retrieval when faced with similar patients in the future.

Traditionally, neither medical schools nor postgraduate programs have taught these skills. Although this situation has changed dramatically in the last decade, the biggest influence on how trainees will practice is their clinical role models, few of whom are currently accomplished EBO practitioners. The situation is even more challenging for those looking to acquire the requisite skills after completing their clinical training.

This text primarily addresses the needs of both trainees and of this last group, practicing orthopedic surgeons. Appearing 20 years after the term EBM was coined, the text represents a landmark in a number of ways. It is the first comprehensive EBO text. The book represents a successful effort to comprehensively address the EBO-related learning needs of the orthopedic community, and summarize the key areas of orthopedic practice.

To achieve its goals of facilitating evidence-based orthopedic practice, the text begins with chapters that introduce the tools for evaluating the original orthopedic literature. Those interested in delving deeper into issues of how to evaluate the literature, and apply it to patient care, can consult a definitive text, the *Users' Guides to the Medical Literature*.

The bulk of the current text, however, provides evidence summaries to guide each of the key common problems of orthopedic practice. Thorough and up to date at the time of writing, they provide a definitive guide to evidence-based orthopedic practice today. That evidence will, of course, change—and in some areas change quickly. Clinicians must therefore use *Evidence-Based Orthopedics* not only as a text for the present, but as a guide for updating their knowledge in the future. That future will hopefully hold the advent of an evidence-based secondary journal similar to those that have been developed in other areas including *Evidence-Based Mental Health*, *Evidence-Based Nursing*, and the *ACP Journal Club*, which does the job for internal medicine. These survey a large number of journals relevant to their area and choose individual studies and systematic reviews that meet both relevance and validity screening criteria. These journals present the results of these studies in structured abstracts that provide clinicians with the key information they need to judge their applicability to their own practices. Fame and fortune await the enterprising group that applies this methodology to produce *Evidence-Based Orthopedics*.

Whatever the future holds for the increasing efficiency of evidence-based practice, the current text provides an introduction to a system of clinical problem-solving that is becoming a prerequisite for modern orthopedic practice.

Gordon H. Guyatt, MD
Professor
Department of Clinical Epidemiology and Biostatistics
McMaster University, Hamilton, ON, Canada

Preface

Evidence-based orthopedics, in principle, is simple. It aims to empower health care providers and patients with valid and reliable information on which to base important decisions about a therapy, a prognosis, or even a diagnostic test. But there is a fundamental requisite to finding the best evidence—finding the time to do it! Evidence-based practitioners begin with a clinical question, conduct a comprehensive search to identify high-quality publications, critically evaluate and appraise the content of the resultant publications, assimilate the findings across the literature, and use this new knowledge (or evidence) to plan their next action. The challenge in medicine is not the theory of the evidence cycle, but its practicality to busy clinicians, health care providers and students alike. The solution has come in the form of pre-appraised resources in medicine. These resources have been targeted to clinicians who need answers to clinically important questions but simply lack the expertise or time to feel confident acquiring and appraising orthopedic evidence. Resources for the surgical community, specifically our orthopedic surgical community, are deficient and often limited in scope.

A desire to create a practical, evidence-based compendium of orthopedic questions and answers fueled the conception and development of *Evidence-Based Orthopedics*. This book is a critical evidence resource in the field of orthopedics, spanning a wide spectrum of topics including orthopedic medicine, arthroplasty, trauma, spinal disorders, sports, upper extremity and hand, foot and ankle and oncology. Our approach is simple. Using the principle, "evidence cycle begins and ends with the patient," we begin all our chapters with clinical cases and formulate a series of 5–10 top questions about the scenario. Each chapter follows the evidence cycle for each question towards an evidence-based recommendation for action. Transparency is the key to our recommendations. All chapters contain our key search strategies, a summary of studies we identified and our appraisal of this evidence. A trusted resource for best evidence, readers can quickly review the recommendations sections in each chapter to gain the evidence-based summary of the topic.

The uniqueness of *Evidence-Based Orthopedics* has as much to do with our global family of expert contributors as our innovative, standardized format. With over 260 contributors, this book was an enormous undertaking of commitment and purpose. I personally thank each and every individual, from Associate Editors to Section Editors to Chapter Contributors for aligning their chapters into the most comprehensive summary of orthopedics in our field. A special thank you to our administrative staff, Ngan Pham, Teresa Chien, Kim Madden, and Ivanna Ramnath, for all of their diligent work. A heartfelt thanks to our publishing partners and friends. To Mary Banks, with whom this idea developed and flourished, this is a testament to the desire for evidence in the orthopedic community. And to Cathryn Gates, Jon Peacock, Simone Dudziak, Ruth Swan, and Brenda Sibbald for all your support in moving our written words to a beautiful resource for the orthopedic community at large.

Finally, this book is as much for me as I hope it is for you. I have learned from so many of our contributors about streamlining evidence into palatable segments, with the overriding goal of making evidence accessible and simply put, fun! While this book in its publication represents the best evidence in our field, evidence is not static—and we will provide online updates to ensure you are always armed with nothing else but the best evidence.

Mohit Bhandari MD, PhD, FRCSC
McMaster University
Hamilton, ON, Canada

Abbreviations

AA	arachidonic acid	BMP	bone morphogenetic protein
AAOS	American Academy of Orthopaedic Surgeons	CAROC	Canadian Association of Radiologists/Osteoporosis Canada
AAV	adeno-associated viral	CBA	cost-benefit analyses
ACCP	American College of Chest Physicians	CBC	complete blood cell count
ACI	autologous chondrocyte implantation	CC	ceramic-on-ceramic
ACL	anterior cruciate ligament	CC	coracoclavicular
ADL	activities of daily living	CCI	characterized chondrocyte implantation
AFA	arthroscopic and fluoroscopic-assisted	CD	Cotrel–Dubousset
AIDS	acquired immunodeficiency syndrome	CDC	Centers for Disease Control
AIS	adolescent idiopathic scoliosis	CEA	cost-effectiveness analysis
AJCC	American Joint Committee on Cancer	CHMP	Committee for Human Medicinal Products
AJRR	Australian Joint Replacement Registry	CI	confidence interval
AL	annular ligament	CJRR	Canadian Joint Replacement Registry
ALBC	antibiotic laden bone cement	CKC	closed kinetic chain
ALI	acute lung injury	CM	ceramic-on-metal
ALIF	anterior lumbar interbody fusion	CMA	cost-minimization analysis
ALPSA	anterior labro-periosteal sleeve avulsion	COTS	Canadian Orthopaedic Trauma Society
AMC	anteromedial coronoid	CP	ceramic-on-polyethylene
AOFAS	American Orthopaedic Foot and Ankle Score	CR	cruciate retaining
AORI	Anderson Orthopaedic Research Institute	CRP	C-reactive protein
AOS	ankle osteoarthritis score	CRPS	complex regional pain syndrome
APP	anterior pelvic plane	CS	compartment syndrome
ARDS	acute respiratory distress syndrome	CSF	cerebrospinal fluid
AROM	active range of motion	CSVL	center sacral vertical line
ARR	absolute risk reduction	CT	computed tomography
ASBMR	American Society for Bone and Mineral Research	CTA	CT arthrography
		CTS	carpal tunnel syndrome
ASCO	American Society of Clinical Oncology	CUA	cost-utility analysis
ASES	American Shoulder and Elbow Surgeons (score)	DALY	disability-adjusted life-years
		DaPP	Danish Prolonged Prophylaxis
ASIS	anterior superior iliac spine	DASH	Disabilities of the Arm, Shoulder, and Hand (score)
AT	Achilles tendinopathy		
ATFL	anterior talofibular ligament	DBM	demineralized bone matrix
AVN	avascular necrosis	DCO	damage control orthopedics
BHR	Birmingham Hip Resurfacing	DD	Dupuytren disease
BMD	bone mineral density	DEXA	dual energy X-ray absorptiometry
BMI	body mass index		

DIPJ	distal interphalangeal joint	IKDC	International Knee Documentation Committee
DMARD	disease-modifying antirheumatic drugs	IMN	intramedullary nail
DRF	distal radius fracture	ISS	injury severity score
DRUJ	distal radioulnar joint	IUAC	International Union Against Cancer
DSS	disease-specific survival	IVC	inferior vena cava
DVT	deep vein thrombosis	JSN	joint space narrowing
EBM	evidence-based medicine	KOOS	Knee Injury and Osteoarthritis Outcome Score
ECU	extensor carpi ulnaris	LBP	low back pain
EF	external fixation	LCL	lateral collateral ligament
EHB	extensor hallucis brevis	LDH	large-diameter head
ELISA	enzyme-linked immunosorbant assay	LDUH	low-dose unfractionated heparin
EMA	European Medicines Agency	LEAS	Lower Extremity Activity Scale
EORTC	European Organization for Research and Treatment of Cancer	LF	limited fasciectomy
EPC	endothelial precursor cells	LFCN	lateral femoral cutaneous nerve
EPL	extensor pollicis longus	LHB	long head of biceps brachii
EPM	early protective motion	LIPUS	low-intensity pulsed ultrasound
ESR	erythrocyte sedimentation rate	LISS	less invasive stabilization system
ESWT	extracorporeal shockwave treatment	LLLT	low-level laser therapy
EU	European Union	LM	lateral medial
EV	end vertebra	LMWH	low molecular weight heparin
FA	fluoroscopic-assisted	LR	likelihood ratio
FARES	fast, reliable, and safe (reduction of shoulder dislocation)	LRTI	ligament reconstruction and tendon interposition
FBI	foreign-body infection	LSS	lumbar spinal stenosis
FDA	Food and Drug Administration	LUCL	lateral ulnar collateral ligament
FDP	flexor digitorum profundus	LVST	laxity valgus stress test
FDS	flexor digitorum superficialis	MACI	matrix-induced autologous chondrocyte implantation
FIT	fracture intervention trial	MCID	minimal clinically important difference
FKB	functional knee bracing	MCL	medial collateral ligament
FNA	fine needle aspiration	MD	mean difference
FPL	flexor pollicis longus	MEP	motor evoked potentials
FSG	French Sarcoma Group	MEPI	Mayo Elbow Performance Index
FT	fracture table	MESCC	metastatic epidural spinal cord compression
GCS	Glasgow Coma Scale	MHHS	modified Harris hip score
GDP	gross domestic product	MHQ	Michigan Hand Questionnaire
GT	greater trochanter	MIAMI	marrow-isolated adult multilineage inducible
HA	hyalouronic acid	MID	minimum important difference
HAF	human amniotic fluid	MIPO	minimally invasive plate osteosynthesis
HAGL	humeral avulsion of the glenohumeral ligaments	MIS	minimally invasive
HDE	Humanitarian Device Exemption	MM	metal-on-metal
HF	high-flexion	MODEMS	Musculoskeletal Outcomes Data Evaluation and Management Systems
HHR	humeral head replacement	MOF	multiple organ failure
HHS	Harris hip score	MP	metal-on-polyethylene
HO	heterotopic ossification	MRA	magnetic resonance arthography
HR	hazard ratio	MRSA	meticillin-resistant *Staphylococcus aureus*
HR	hip resurfacing	MSC	mesenchymal stems cells
HRT	hormone replacement therapy	MT	manual traction
ICBG	iliac crest bone graft	NCS	nerve conduction studies
ICER	incremental cost-effectiveness ratio	NIS	national inpatient sample
ICRS	International Cartilage Repair Society		
ICU	intensive care unit		
ICUR	incremental cost-utility ratio		

NNIS	National Nosocomial Infections Surveillance		SAE	serious adverse events
NNT	number needed to treat		SARI	Surface Arthroplasty Risk Index
NOS	not otherwise specified		SB	single bundle
NPV	negative predictive value		SBRN	superficial branch of radial nerve
NPWCT	negative-pressure wound closure therapy		SD	standard deviation
NR	not reported		SEAS	Scientific Exercises Approach to Scoliosis
NS	not significant		SFDA	State Food and Drug Administration
NSAID	nonsteroidal anti-inflammatory drugs		SFMA	Short Musculoskeletal Function Assessment
NSCLC	non-small-cell lung cancer		SG	standard gamble
NV	neutrally rotated vertebra		SHS	sliding hip screw
NWI	notch width index		SI	standard incision
OAT	Osteochondral autologous transplantation		SIR	scoliosis in-patient rehabilitation
ODI	Oswestry Disability Index		SIS	shoulder impingement syndrome
OKC	open kinetic chain		SL	scapholunate ligament
ORIF	open reduction and internal fixation		SLAC	scapholunate advanced collapse
PA	palmar aponeurosis		SMD	standardized mean differences
PBC	plain bone cement		SMFA	Short Musculoskeletal Function Assessment
PCL	posterior cruciate ligament		SmPC	summary of product characteristics
PCR	polymerase chain reaction		SNAC	scaphoid nonunion advanced collapse
PDGF	platelet derived growth factor		SOB	shortness of breath
PE	pulmonary embolism		SP	syringe pressurization
PEP	Pulmonary Embolism Prevention		SPORT	Spine Patient Outcomes Research Trial
PET	positron emission tomography		SRS	Scoliosis Research Society
PF	piriformis fossa		SS	synovial sarcoma
PFH	pain and function of the hip		SSEP	somatosensory evoked potentials
PFPS	patellofemoral pain syndrome		SSI	surgical site infection
PFT	pulmonary function test		SSSC	superior shoulder suspensory complex
PLC	posterolateral corner		STAR	Scandinavian Total Ankle Replacement
PMA	premarket approval		STAR	Study of the Treatment of Articular Repair
PMC	posteromedial corner		STS	soft tissue sarcoma
PNF	percutaneous needle fasciotomy		STT	scapho-trapezial-trapezoid
PPV	positive predictive value		SV	stable vertebra
PRC	proximal row carpectomy		TA	tendo achilles
PROM	passive range of motion		TAA	total ankle arthroplasty
PRP	platelet-rich plasma		TAM	total active motion
PRUJ	proximal radioulnar joint		TAW	traction-absorbing wiring
PRWE	Patient Rated Wrist Evaluation		TBF	tension band fixation
PS	plate and screw		TBL	total blood loss
PS	posterior stabilizing		TBW	tension band wire
PTFL	posterior talofibular ligament		TEA	total elbow arthroplasty
PVST	pain valgus stress test		TENS	transcutaneous electrical nerve stimulation
QALY	quality-adjusted life years		TFCC	triangular fibrocartilage complex
QUOROM	Quality of Reports of Meta-analysis		THA	total hip arthroplasty
RA	rheumatoid arthritis		THR	total hip replacement
RCL	radial collateral ligament		TILT	transverse intraosseous loop technique
RCT	randomized controlled trials		TKA	total knee arthroplasties
RF	rheumatoid factor		TKA	total knee arthroplasty
ROM	range of motion		TKR	total knee replacement
RR	relative rate		TNS	transcutaneous neural stimulation
RR	relative risk		TOW	time off work
RRR	relative risk reduction		TPBS	triple-phase isotope bone scan
RSD	reflex sympathetic dystrophy		TPED	total passive extension deficit
RTSA	reverse total shoulder arthroplasty		TRALI	transfusion-related acute lung injury
RVU	resource value unit		TRAP	triceps-reflecting anconeus pedicle

Abbreviations

TROPOS	Treatment of Peripheral Osteoporosis	VAS	visual analog scale
TS	total stabilizing	VC	vital capacity
TSA	total shoulder arthroplasty	VEGF	vascular endothelial growth factor
TSS	total Sharp score	VKA	vitamin K antagonists
TTO	time trade-off	VL	vastus lateralis
UCL	ulnar collateral ligament	VMO	vastus medialis obliquus
UD	ulnar deviation	VRE	vancomycin-resistant enterococci
UFH	unfractionated heparin	WHI	Women's Health Initiative
UHMPE	ultra-high-molecular-weight polyethylene	WHO	World Health Organization
USS	Universal Spine System	WMD	weighted mean difference
VA	Veterans Affairs	WOOS	Western Ontario Osteoarthritis of the Shoulder (score)
VAC	vacuum-assisted closure		

Methodology of Evidence-Based Orthopedics

1 Principles of Evidence-Based Orthopedics

Simrit Bains[1], Mohit Bhandari[1], and Paul Tornetta III[2]

[1]McMaster University, Hamilton, ON, Canada
[2]Boston University Medical Center, Boston, MA, USA

Introduction

The traditional approach to solving clinical problems involves a great emphasis on professional authority, with the approach being dictated almost exclusively by the experience and rationale of the clinician.[1] This approach was dictated largely by the opinions of practitioners, which is problematic because there are a wide variety of opinions and it is reasonable to suggest that not all of these opinions can be correct. Evidence-based orthopedics is a contrast to this paradigm and has arisen from a need of effectively solving clinical problems.[1] Evidence-based orthopedics is part of a broader movement known as evidence-based medicine, a term first used at McMaster University during an informal residency training program. Since that time, evidence-based medicine has entered the vocabulary of every medical field and has steadily gained prominence.[2] Although orthopedic surgeons have been generally slow to adopt this new approach, it is becoming increasingly accepted as a positive alternative in patient care.[3] Evidence-based orthopedics does not accept the traditional paradigm as being adequate to address clinical problems, especially when considering the large quantity of valuable information available to clinicians to help them in their problem-solving process. Less emphasis is placed on the clinician's own professional authority.[1] His or her experiences, beliefs, and observations alone are not enough to make satisfactory decisions with respect to patient care. Evidence-based orthopedics promotes the need to evaluate the evidence available in the medical literature from published research and integrate it into clinical practice. As such, critical appraisal of studies is of paramount importance.[3]

The importance of evidence-based orthopedics

To fully appreciate the principles of evidence-based orthopedics, it is helpful to have an understanding of the importance and value of this approach. The ultimate goal of a clinician is to provide the best clinical care for his or her patient.[4] To that end, the clinician's own experiences and training are important assets. However, there is a wealth of information available in the literature that can assist the clinician in numerous ways, from assessing the efficacy of a certain treatment to recommending lifestyle changes that may help prevent illness.[5] As such, it is important for the clinician to evaluate and incorporate this evidence into his or her own reasoning and judgment when considering the best approach to patient care. A failure to consider such evidence while adopting a clinical approach may result in patients being denied the best possible care.[4] There is a greater risk of applying an inappropriate treatment or not applying an appropriate treatment.

Top four questions

1. What are the most important principles of evidence-based orthopedics?
2. How do you apply these principles to a clinical approach?
3. What is an example of applying these principles to a clinical approach?
4. What are some common misconceptions about evidence-based orthopedics?

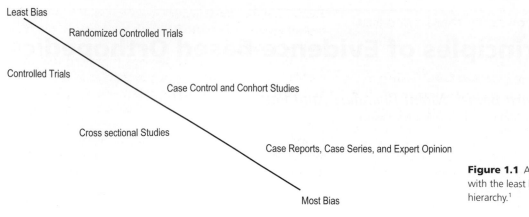

Least Bias

Randomized Controlled Trials

Controlled Trials

Case Control and Conhort Studies

Cross sectional Studies

Case Reports, Case Series, and Expert Opinion

Most Bias

Figure 1.1 A general hierarchy of evidence, with the least bias present at the top of the hierarchy.[1]

Question 1: What are the most important principles of evidence-based orthopedics?

Patient values

This principle is fundamental to any clinician. The key goal of good clinical practice is to deliver the highest quality care to patients, and this can only be done if there is a thorough understanding of the patient and his or her problem.[1] This includes knowledge of the patient's values, demographics, and circumstances. Consideration of the patient's desires based on their values or preferences is paramount in evidence-based orthopedics and it must be considered an important factor when a clinician decides which course to pursue in order to treat the patient.[3] Evidence-based orthopedics therefore stresses patient involvement and understanding. This is positive for ethical reasons and also for improving patient satisfaction and care.

The need for evidence

Once the clinician has a thorough understanding of the problem, he or she can begin to seek evidence to supplement their judgment. The intuition, experience, and rationale of a trained clinician are all immensely valuable and essential to delivering high-quality care. However, evidence-based orthopedics seeks to supplement the skills and judgment of the clinician with the relevant information that has been gathered about the particular problem.[6] Such evidence can assist a clinician with comparing the efficacy of different types of surgery, an operative vs. a nonoperative approach, and more. This is especially true now because of the sheer quantity of easily accessible evidence available to clinicians.[5]

The evidence is unequal

The large quantity of available data is of benefit to clinicians looking for the best clinical approach, but it is easy to be inundated with such large amounts of information.[7]

Integrating questionable evidence into a clinical approach may cause more harm than benefit to the patient.[3] Therefore, evidence-based orthopedics is specific in its emphasis on evidence published in the literature and careful assessment of this evidence.[7] Clinicians must therefore be adept at understanding study design and critically appraising the literature.[5] The various study designs are typically represented in a hierarchy of evidence (Figure 1.1), where they are ranked according to the validity of their results. Expert opinion is at the bottom, being the most susceptible to bias and producing the most questionable evidence.[8] At the top of the hierarchy are randomized controlled trials and meta-analyses, which are the least vulnerable to bias. Randomization is an important feature of a study because of the random allocation of patients to treatment and control groups, which balances known and unknown prognostic factors between the two groups.[9] However, the clinician must still determine if the study is methodologically sound. A poorly designed randomized trial, for example, would no longer qualify as producing evidence of high validity.[5]

Integrating evidence and clinical expertise

The clinician must appropriately apply the relevant evaluated evidence to the clinical problem. This must be done with the full context of the situation taken into consideration, which is dependent upon the clinician's expertise and experience.[3] He or she must consider the evidence in light of the patient's characteristics: values, preferences, demographics, medical history and more. The clinician also knows the specific details of a patient's condition and medical problem, which may differ slightly but importantly from what is discussed in the literature. It is therefore up to the clinician to use his or her best judgment and skill, in consultation with the patient, to pursue the best possible course of action. In other words, that which is indicated by the evidence as the best course of action will not always dictate the clinical approach.[7]

Question 2: How do you apply these principles to a clinical approach?

The evidence cycle

With the key principles of evidence-based orthopedics having been presented, a general clinical approach that employs these principles can be shown. This approach is called the *evidence cycle*.[4]

1. *Assess:* The first step for the clinician is to thoroughly understand the patient and his or her problem.

2. *Ask:* With the patient's problem in mind, the clinician must next formulate a research question that seeks a solution to the problem and lays the foundation for a search of the literature.

3. *Acquire:* This step involves obtaining evidence from databases.

4. *Appraise:* Next, the clinician must critically appraise the evidence. It must be determined where the study fits on the hierarchy of evidence, whether the methodology is sound, relevance of the results, and so on.

5. *Apply:* The evidence that the clinician has obtained and evaluated must now be applied to the patient, but only with the full context of the situation in mind. The patient's values and the circumstances of the problem must be considered when applying the evidence.

Question 3: What is an example of applying these principles to a clinical approach?

Case scenario

A patient presents in clinic with a vertebral fracture. He is compromised with respect to daily function and also experiences a high degree of pain from this fracture. The goal here is to relieve the patient's pain, allow him to at least partially return to his daily activities and heal the fracture. A typical procedure for a case like this is vertebroplasty, a stabilizing surgery that involves injection of a "cement" substance into the spine. It is widely believed that this surgery helps to heal such fractures, reduces pain, and improves daily functioning of the patient.[10] However, the patient asks you if this surgery is absolutely necessary as it is a procedure that he is uncomfortable with. With knowledge of the patient and their condition established, you can now begin to search the literature with a specific question in mind: What is the evidence for the efficacy of vertebroplasty?

Vertebroplasty is a common procedure and therefore numerous studies have been published about this type of surgery. Many of the studies show dramatic positive effects of this surgery on patients. Healing was found to be accelerated, pain reduced, and daily function improved—all goals of the clinician. However, when it comes time to evaluate the evidence you have obtained, you notice significant flaws in these studies. Not only do they lack randomization, but there is also no comparison to a placebo control group.[11] These studies rank quite low on the hierarchy of evidence.[8]

On the other hand, a randomized controlled trial from the Mayo Clinic compared two groups of compression fracture patients.[10] One group had the vertebroplasty performed while the control group had a placebo surgery performed. The result was a lack of significant difference between the vertebroplasty and the placebo surgery with respect to pain relief and returning the patient to daily function.[10] Another randomized trial from Australia reached the same conclusions.[11] The studies are methodologically sound, the results are highly relevant, and, as a randomized trial, it ranks high on the hierarchy of evidence. The evidence generated by this study is therefore of high validity.

At this point you can return to your patient and inform him with a high degree of confidence that if he is uncomfortable with the surgery, he may choose to forego it without risking detrimental effects to his recovery.

Question 4: What are some common misconceptions about evidence-based orthopedics?

There are many common misconceptions regarding evidence-based orthopedics.

Evidence-based orthopedics replaces the judgment of the clinician

As previously mentioned, the judgment of the clinician that arises from professional training and experience is highly valuable in clinical practice and is irreplaceable. Evidence-based orthopedics seeks to supplement rather than replace the authority of the clinician by expanding the tools he or she uses to achieve the best possible care for their patients.[6]

Only randomized controlled trials are acceptable evidence

Although randomized controlled trials may be of the highest quality, evidence-based orthopedics does not suggest that they are to be used as the exclusive source of information.[7] Due to ethical and technical considerations, randomized controlled trials are not always a feasible way to generate the desired information, so the clinician must turn to the information provided from other studies.[8] Alternatively, a randomized controlled trial available on the issue of interest may have serious design flaws that bring the validity of the evidence into question. To approach clinical problems with the most effectiveness and to improve patient outcomes, it is important to consider all types of evidence and apply it if appropriate.[5]

The clinician is bound to a certain course of action by the evidence

The evidence is to serve as a guide, not as a dictate. It is up to the clinician to use the evidence as he or she believes appropriate given the circumstances of the situation.[3]

Conclusion

A vast amount of information is available to clinicians to use in an effort to improve patient care. The paradigm of evidence-based orthopedics stresses the importance of using this evidence to achieve the best possible outcome for patients, but only by critically appraising the evidence and integrating it with the clinician's own judgment and knowledge of the specific circumstances of the patient's case. It is a practice growing in popularity but also continues to be hampered by misconceptions, so being familiar with the principles of evidence-based orthopedics is important to any clinician seeking to get the most out of this alternative approach to patient care.

References

1. Schunemann HJ, Bone L. Evidence-based orthopaedics: a primer. Clin Orthop Relat Res 2003;413:117–32.
2. Spindler KP, Kuhn JE, Dunn W, Matthews CE, Harrell FE, Dittus RS. Reading and reviewing the orthopaedic literature: a systematic, evidence-based medicine approach. J Am Acad Orthop Surg 2005;13(4):220–9.
3. Narayanan UG, Wright JG. Evidence-based medicine: a prescription to change the culture of pediatric orthopaedics. J Pediatr Orthop 2002;22(3):277–8.
4. Poolman RW, Kerkhoffs GM, Struijs PAA, Bhandari M. Don't be misled by the orthopaedic literature: tips for critical appraisal. Acta Orthop 2007;78(2):162–71.
5. Bhandari M, Tornetta P. Issues in the design, analysis, and critical appraisal of orthopaedic clinical research. Clin Orthop Relat Res 2003;413:9–10.
6. Wright JG, Swiontkowski MF. Introducing a new journal section: evidence-based orthopaedics. J Bone Joint Surg Am 2000;82:759.
7. Guyatt GH, Rennie D. Users' Guides to the Medical Literature: A Manual for Evidenced Based Clinical Practice. American Medical Association, Chicago, 2002.
8. Brighton B, Bhandari M, Tornetta P, Felson DT. Hierarchy of evidence: from case reports to randomized controlled trials. Clin Orthop Relat Res 2003;413:19–24.
9. Bhandari M, Tornetta P, Guyatt GH. Glossary of evidence-based orthopaedic terminology. Clin Orthop Relat Res 2003;413:158–63.
10. Kallmes DF, Comstock BA, Heagerty PJ, Turner JA, Wilson DJ, Diamond TH, et al. A randomized trial of vertebroplasty for osteoporotic spinal fractures. New Engl J Med 2009;361(6):569–79.
11. Buchbinder R, Osborne RH, Ebeling PR, Wark JD, Mitchell P, Wriedt C, et al. A randomized trial of vertebroplasty for painful osteoporotic vertebral fractures. New Engl J Med 2009;361(6):557–68.

2 Understanding Hierarchies of Evidence and Grades of Recommendation

Raman Mundi and Brad A. Petrisor
McMaster University, Hamilton, ON, Canada

Case scenario

As an attending orthopedic surgeon at a teaching hospital, you are approached by a medical resident new to the specialty and eager to learn. As a proponent of evidence-based medicine, you had asked this resident the day earlier to "search the literature for recent best evidence on the management of displaced femoral neck fractures in patients less than 60 years of age."

Excited to present his findings, the young resident tells you, "According to this study I found on a series of 50 patients all treated with internal fixation, the best surgical management appears to be internal fixation."

Slightly disappointed, but not surprised, you ask, "But is this the 'best available' evidence?"

Introduction

In making treatment decisions, the practice of evidence-based medicine mandates the integration of the best available evidence, patient preferences and values, and clinical expertise.[1] Although eliciting patient values and being mindful of the clinical setting (i.e., surgeon experience, funding, etc.) are reasonable requests for the busy clinician, routinely sifting through a myriad of literature, appraising all relevant articles, and synthesizing findings to ascertain the "best available evidence" can at times seem overwhelming.[2] Nevertheless, clinicians must be aware of the evidence that exists so as to provide their patients with optimal care.

Hierarchies of evidence have been established to assist clinicians in approaching the medical literature by providing a measure of quality.[3] In general, such hierarchies rank-order research studies from the most methodologically sound, to those with less methodological rigor and a higher propensity for biased results. In addition to providing readers with a direct grading system, these hierarchies also allow journals to monitor the quality of the orthopedic literature.[3] Furthermore, it is from these hierarchies that conclusions can be drawn to set out grades of recommendation and clinical practice guidelines.[4]

This chapter begins with a discussion of study designs and examples of hierarchies of evidence for therapeutic trials. We conclude with a discussion of the grades of recommendation as put forward by the GRADE Working Group.

Understanding hierarchies of evidence: therapeutic studies

As mentioned, hierarchies of evidence are important in helping readers discriminate higher-quality studies from lower-quality studies, tracking the overall quality of the orthopedic literature, and knowing the quality of evidence that is incorporated into reviews that inform clinical practice guidelines.[2,3] Because of its importance, orthopedic journals such as the *Journal of Bone and Joint Surgery* and *Clinical Orthopaedics and Related Research* have started reporting the level of evidence of individual studies.[3,5]

In the orthopedic literature, several classes of studies exist including studies of therapy, prognosis, diagnosis, and economic analysis. These different classes of studies all have their individual hierarchies of evidence.[5] Given that most of the orthopedic literature consists of therapeutic studies, this section focuses on levels of evidence for this specific class.[6,7]

Evidence-Based Orthopedics, First Edition. Edited by Mohit Bhandari.
© 2012 Blackwell Publishing Ltd. Published 2012 by Blackwell Publishing Ltd.

Therapeutic studies are those that investigate the effect of a treatment or intervention.[5] Several organizations and groups have developed systems of hierarchy for therapeutic studies, some of which are presented later in this section. Despite subtle differences, the general principles behind these hierarchies are the same. They all place those studies which best minimize bias and are more likely to yield an accurate estimate of the truth at the top or as highest quality. In order to understand these hierarchies then, it is important to discuss which factors favor and diminish bias. Specifically, this merits a discussion of both study design and study quality.

Top six questions

1. What are randomized controlled trials?
2. What are systematic reviews and meta-analyses?
3. What are observational studies?
4. What are case series and case reports?
5. What are systems of hierarchies?
6. What are grades of recommendation?

Question 1: What are randomized controlled trials?

Studies of an intervention can be either observational in nature or have a randomized experimental design.[2,6] The randomized controlled trial (RCT), in which patients are randomly allocated to the different treatment arms of the study, is considered the highest level of evidence. By the power of randomization, these trials attempt to control for both known and unknown prognostic factors by distributing these prognostic variables among all treatment arms. In this way, the RCT strives to eliminate variation between treatment arms and in turn, a biased outcome which could either over- or under-represent the true treatment effect.[8]

However, the process of randomization in itself does not make RCTs immune to other methodological flaws that can compromise study quality and introduce bias into the trial. For instance, allocation concealment entails that the individuals responsible for recruiting and allocating patients into the trial are unaware of which group the next patient will be randomized to. Methods that fail to uphold allocation concealment include randomization using chart numbers, unsealed envelopes, and odd vs. even days.[6] It has been shown that failure to uphold allocation concealment in an RCT can result in an overestimation of the treatment effect.[9] Other methodological parameters that safeguard RCTs from bias include blinding, ensuring equivalent surgical experience and skill for all treatment groups, minimizing loss to follow-up, and using the intention-to-treat principle (assessing patients based on the groups they were originally assigned to, regardless of which treatment was actually received).

Question 2: What are systematic reviews and meta-analyses?

Systematic reviews and meta-analyses of RCTs are also considered high-level evidence. Systematic reviews rank highly because they employ a systematic approach in collecting, appraising, and synthesizing data. Meta-analyses are an extension of systematic reviews, in that they pool the data across all studies to effectively increase the sample size and produce a single estimate of the treatment effect.[10]

As for RCTs, there are quality issues that, if unmet, can shift systematic reviews and meta-analyses lower in the hierarchy. These studies are only as good as their component parts. That is, their quality is directly contingent upon the quality of studies included in the review. First and foremost, systematic reviews and meta-analyses that exclusively include RCTs are of higher quality and provide more compelling evidence than those that include nonrandomized studies.[11,12] Secondly, even among those meta-analyses that include only RCTs, the strength of the single estimate of the treatment effect is dependent on the homogeneity of the RCTs. If the included trials have precise and consistent results, the results of the meta-analyses are strong, whereas heterogeneous trials with inconsistent results and large confidence intervals make the statistical pooling less trustworthy.[6]

Question 3: What are observational studies?

Not all questions surrounding interventions can be answered with a randomized trial. Although lower in the hierarchy of evidence, observational studies remain important in answering questions surrounding interventions that RCTs cannot.

In *cohort studies*, patients who are exposed to a risk factor or treatment are compared to unexposed patients. The patients are followed to determine the rate of occurrence of the outcome of interest.[13] This study design works well for issues of harm, in which randomizing patients to a harmful exposure or intervention would be unethical. For instance, an RCT investigating the effect of smoking on nonunion rates in patients with tibial shaft fractures would be inappropriate, as forcing a patient to smoke is unethical.[6] Among the observational studies, the cohort study ranks highest on the levels of evidence. The primary reason is that these studies are often prospective, and thus ensure more rigorous data collection and more thorough patient follow-up.[6] Furthermore, investigators can attempt to match patients in the different treatment arms for known prognostic variables, although unknown prognostic variables may still bias the trial outcome.

Below cohort studies in the hierarchy of evidence is the *case-control study* design. In effect, this study design is the reverse of the cohort design. A group of patients that have already developed the outcome of interest are compared to a similar group of patients who have not developed the outcome. These groups are then assessed retrospectively for differences in exposures to risk factors that may be associated with developing the outcome.[13] Case-control studies are valuable when dealing with rare disease entities, or for those outcomes that develop over a long time (for instance, lung cancer due to smoking), and when multiple risk factors need to be assessed.[13] In addition to the inability to control groups for unknown prognostic factors, the primary limitation of this study design is its retrospective nature which makes it more prone to bias.

Question 4: What are case series and case reports?

Lower in the hierarchy of evidence are case series and case reports, the former being a description of a series of patients and the latter being a description of individual patients. Because these studies have no control group, conclusions should not be made regarding cause-and-effect relationships.[13] Often these studies are prone to bias due to their retrospective nature and have limited generalizability as they usually depict the experience of a single center or surgeon. These studies are valuable, however, for describing rare diseases or complications of interventions, and for generating hypotheses that can be investigated by higher-quality research methods.[6] The young resident described in the scenario at the beginning of this chapter was indeed referring to a case series.

Question 5: What are systems of hierarchies?

As mentioned, several organizations and groups have developed systems for rank-ordering evidence into levels.[2] The hierarchy proposed by Guyatt and Rennie[1] is: (I) N of 1 randomized controlled trial; (II) systematic review of randomized trials; (III) single randomized trial, (IV) systematic review of observational studies addressing patient-important outcomes; (V) single observational study addressing patient-important outcomes, (VI) physiologic studies; and (VII) unsystematic clinical observation. There are two aspects of this system that merit discussion. First, at the top of the hierarchy is the "N of 1" randomized trial in which the patient alternates between a period of target treatment and control treatment. The order is randomized, both the patient and clinician are blind as to whether target treatment or control is being received, and the patient continues alternating until it is concluded that an effect exists or does not exist. This study ranks highly because the patient of interest is directly involved in the trial and the results are definitive as no generalizations are being made from a separate population of patients. Secondly, the authors recognize that both RCTs and observational studies can upgrade or downgrade levels on this hierarchy, depending in part on the methodological quality of the trial. Large observational studies with consistent results can provide more compelling evidence than RCTs; however, it must be kept in mind that RCTs have also been shown to contradict the results of large observational studies with consistent results.[1]

In the system used by the Centre for Evidence-Based Medicine at Oxford University,[12] not only are there five levels of evidence, but sublevels within them. Furthermore, the study design in itself does not determine level of evidence as study quality is also taken into consideration by this system. For instance, high-quality RCTs with precise estimates of treatment effect are considered level I evidence, whereas lower-quality RCTs with less methodological rigor are considered level II evidence.[12] The Oxford levels of evidence have also been developed for other classes of study, such as studies regarding prognosis, diagnosis, and economic analyses. These levels of evidence are easily accessible at the Oxford Centre for Evidence-Based Medicine website, www.cebm.net.[12] In a review of the orthopedic literature in 2003, it was demonstrated that only 11.3% of studies (therapy, prognostic, diagnostic, and economic) qualify as level I according to the Oxford levels of evidence.[7]

These evidence scales do have certain drawbacks: they are mostly developed by expert opinion and lack validation; studies are ranked inconsistently across the different systems making universal communication difficult; and agreement in which level to assign a study in a given system is sometimes low (i.e., low inter-rater reliability).[2,4]

Question 6: What are grades of recommendation?

In order to establish a grade of recommendation for an intervention or treatment, a full systematic review of all similar studies in terms of the intervention, outcomes, and patient population, must be carried out.[4] Furthermore, discussions with content experts also prove helpful in establishing grades of recommendation.[6]

The GRADE Working Group has proposed a grading system in which they outline four factors that need be considered when giving an intervention one of four possible grades of recommendation.

• *The overall quality of the evidence.* Each study included in the systematic review needs to be assessed for its quality. It is suggested that the "overall" quality of evidence should be based on the lowest quality of evidence for outcomes that are critical in making a decision. This includes both outcomes regarding benefits and harms associated with the

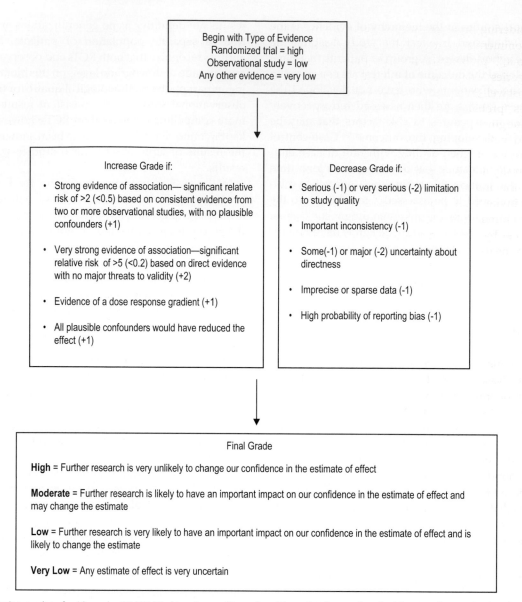

Begin with Type of Evidence
Randomized trial = high
Observational study = low
Any other evidence = very low

Increase Grade if:

- Strong evidence of association— significant relative risk of >2 (<0.5) based on consistent evidence from two or more observational studies, with no plausible confounders (+1)

- Very strong evidence of association—significant relative risk of >5 (<0.2) based on direct evidence with no major threats to validity (+2)

- Evidence of a dose response gradient (+1)

- All plausible confounders would have reduced the effect (+1)

Decrease Grade if:

- Serious (-1) or very serious (-2) limitation to study quality

- Important inconsistency (-1)

- Some(-1) or major (-2) uncertainty about directness

- Imprecise or sparse data (-1)

- High probability of reporting bias (-1)

Final Grade

High = Further research is very unlikely to change our confidence in the estimate of effect

Moderate = Further research is likely to have an important impact on our confidence in the estimate of effect and may change the estimate

Low = Further research is very likely to have an important impact on our confidence in the estimate of effect and is likely to change the estimate

Very Low = Any estimate of effect is very uncertain

Figure 2.1 Assigning grades of evidence by GRADE Working Group. (Reproduced from Grading quality of evidence and strength of recommendations, Atkins D, Best D, Briss PA, et al, 328, 1490, 2004 with permission from BMJ Publishing Group Ltd.)

intervention.[2] In grading studies, this system combines four elements of the trial: study design, study quality, consistency, and directness. *Consistency* refers to similarity in results across other studies addressing the same issue. If an inconsistency is present—for example, differences in direction of treatment effect—than the grade of recommendation is considered lower quality as we are less confident about the results. *Directness* refers to how well the study can be generalized to the patients of interest. It takes into account how similar the study patients, interventions, and outcome measures are to those of interest to the clinician, patient, and clinical setting. In placing a study within this hierarchy, this system first assigns a grade of either "high," "low," or "very low", based solely on study design. From

there, study quality, consistency, and directness influence the final grade of the study which will be either "high," "moderate," "low," or "very low" (Figure 2.1).[2]

- *The benefits vs. harms (i.e. trade-offs).* This necessitates placing a value judgment on each outcome. It is important to consider the setting and the values of the patient population of interest.[2]

- *Translating the evidence into a specific setting.* Practical issues that may influence the size of the treatment effect also need to be considered. For instance, if the success of an intervention depends on a surgeon's level of training, then the availability of the necessary expertise must be considered.[2]

- *Baseline risk for population of interest.*

After considering these four factors, there are four categories of recommendation to place an intervention in: "do it," "don't do it," "probably do it," and "probably don't do it." The categories "do it" and "don't do it" indicate a judgment that most well-informed people would make, whereas the categories "probably do it" and "probably don't do it" indicate a judgment that a majority of well-informed people would make, but a substantial minority would not.[2]

A recommendation for an intervention does not always apply universally across all patients. It remains important to consider the individual patient, inform them of all options, and invite them into the decision-making process. Grades of recommendation facilitate and aid this decision-making process by taking into account the best available evidence and the general values of the population of interest. It is important to remember that it facilitates, but does not replace, the decision-making process.[2]

Conclusion

Various hierarchies of evidence have been developed for the different classes of studies (therapeutic, prognostic, diagnostic, economic) and, within the therapeutic class alone, several systems have emerged. The majority of these hierarchies take into account study design and study quality to place studies into levels. Those with a more sound study design (RCTs, meta-analyses) and methodological rigor (blinding, allocation concealment) are less vulnerable to biased results and rank highly in the hierarchy. Those studies that are more subject to biased results (observational studies) are less likely to provide an accurate estimation of the true treatment effect and thus rank lower in the hierarchy.

These hierarchies not only aid readers in gauging the validity of studies, but are crucial for establishing grades of recommendation. The overall quality of evidence surrounding an intervention, along with the benefits vs. harms, practical issues for the clinical setting, and baseline population risk, all govern how strongly an intervention will be recommended. Thus, the hierarchies of evidence and grades of recommendation together provide clinicians with a method for finding the "best available" evidence, and in turn, facilitate evidence-based decision making.

References

1. Guyatt G, Haynes RB, Jaeschke R, et al. Introduction: The philosophy of evidence-based medicine. In: Guyatt GH, Rennie D, eds. Users' guides to the medical literature: A manual for evidence-based clinical practice, 5th printing, pp. 3–12. AMA Press, Chicago, 2005.
2. Atkins D, Best D, Briss PA, et al. Grading quality of evidence and strength of recommendations. BMJ 2004;328:1490.
3. Wright JG, Swiontkowski MF, Heckman JD. Introducing levels of evidence to the journal. J Bone Joint Surg Am 2003;85:1–3.
4. Petrisor BA, Keating J, Schemitsch E. Grading the evidence: levels of evidence and grades of recommendation. Injury 2006; 37:321–7.
5. Bhandari M, Joensson A, eds. Hierarchy of research studies: from case series to meta-analyses. In: Clinical research for surgeons, pp. 37–43. Thieme, New York, 2009.
6. Petrisor BA, Bhandari M. The hierarchy of evidence: levels and grades of recommendation. Indian J Orthop 2007;41:11–15.
7. Obremskey WT, Pappas N, Attallah-Wasif E, et al. Level of evidence in orthopaedic journals. J Bone Joint Surg Am 2005;87: 2632–8.
8. Guyatt G, Cook D, Devereaux PJ, et al. Therapy. In: Guyatt G, Rennie D, eds. Users' guides to the medical literature: A manual for evidence-based clinical practice, 5th printing, pp. 55–79. AMA Press, Chicago, 2005.
9. Schulz KF, Chalmers I, Hayes RJ, et al. Empirical evidence of bias. Dimensions of methodological quality associated with estimates of treatment effects in controlled trials. JAMA 1995;273: 408–12.
10. Oxman A, Guyatt G, Cook D, et al. Summarizing the evidence. In: Guyatt GH, Rennie D, eds. Users' guides to the medical literature: A manual for evidence-based clinical practice, 5th printing, pp. 155–173. AMA Press, Chicago, 2005.
11. Audigé L, Bhandari M, Griffin D, et al. Systematic reviews of nonrandomized clinical studies in the orthopaedic literature. Clin Orthop Relat Res 2004;427:249–57.
12. Centre for Evidence-Based Medicine. Oxford Centre for Evidence-Based Medicine—levels of evidence (March 2009). [cited on August 12, 2009]. Available from: http://www.cebm.net
13. Levine M, Haslam D, Walter S, et al. Harm. In: Guyatt GH, Rennie D, eds. Users' guides to the medical literature: A manual for evidence-based clinical practice, 5th printing, pp. 81–100. AMA Press, Chicago, 2005.

3 Critical Appraisal Tools for Surgeons

Farrah Hussain[1], Sheila Sprague[1], and Harry E. Rubash[2]

[1]McMaster University, Hamilton, ON, Canada
[2]Massachusetts General Hospital, Boston, MA, USA

Introduction

Surgical innovation is the core of orthopedic surgical practice. However, many surgical procedures are innovations that are brought into practice with a degree of uncertainty. Therefore, critical appraisal skills are necessary to make informed decisions about patient care based on the evidence available.

Evidence-based orthopedic surgery makes use of a clear definition of relevant clinical questions through a literature search pertaining to the questions, a critical appraisal of available evidence and its applicability to the clinical situation, and a balanced application of the evidence to the clinical problem. Critical appraisal involves a judgment on how much confidence can be placed in the evidence and recommendations provided by a study.[1] However, what is the "best available" evidence? Randomized controlled trials (RCTs) are considered to be the highest level of evidence, as randomization is the optimal method to balance known and unknown prognostic factors in treatment and control groups in therapeutic studies. However, RCTs cannot answer all clinical questions.[2] Randomized controlled trials compose 14% of published articles in the medical literature.[3] In some cases, it is unethical to randomize patients to certain prognostic or risk factors. Moreover, due to sample size and follow-up requirements, RCTs may not always be feasible. Therefore, in orthopedic surgery, lower forms of evidence often provide valuable insights that RCTs cannot. The most important idea to keep in mind is that evidence-based orthopedic surgery makes effective use of the all types of available evidence in clinical decision-making, whether it be an RCT or a case review.[2] The tools for critical appraisal discussed in this chapter will help orthopedic surgeons successfully bring evidence into practice.

Top three questions

1. What are the criteria for determining level of evidence?
2. What are the steps involved in critical appraisal?
3. What are some other examples of tools for critical appraisal?

Question 1: What are the criteria for determining level of evidence?

Guidelines, or recommendations, have been developed systematically by panels of people with access to the available evidence and an understanding of the clinical problem and research methods. However, different organizations use a variety of systems to grade the quality of evidence and the strength of recommendations, thus creating confusion and hindering effective communication.[1] Recently, the GRADE (Grading of Recommendations Assessment, Development and Evaluation) working group, interested in the shortcomings of varied grading systems in health care, devised a new rating system to address such inadequacies (Table 3.1). The advantages of this system over others are that it makes clear what each of the grades indicates, as well as what to consider when assigning these grades. Furthermore, it ensures the proper consideration of the key components of quality of evidence (e.g., study design, quality, consistency, and directness of evidence), relative importance of outcomes, trade-offs between important benefits and harms, as well as other factors affecting the quality of evidence (e.g., imprecise or sparse data, reporting bias, strength of association, and confounding variables).[1,4]

Evidence-Based Orthopedics, First Edition. Edited by Mohit Bhandari.
© 2012 Blackwell Publishing Ltd. Published 2012 by Blackwell Publishing Ltd.

Table 3.1 GRADE criteria for assigning grade of evidence, which consists of a quality assessment and a summary of findings[1] (Reproduced from Grading quality of evidence and strength of recommendations, Atkins D, Best D, Briss PA et al , 328,1490–1497, 2004 with permission from BMJ Publishing Group Ltd.)

Type of evidence

Randomized trial = high quality

Quasi-randomized trial = moderate quality

Observational study = low quality

Any other evidence = very low quality

Decrease grade(s) if:

Serious (–1) or very serious (–2) limitation to study quality

Important inconsistency (–1)

Some (–1) or major (–2) uncertainty about directness

Imprecise or sparse data (–1)

High probability of reporting bias (–1)

Increase grade(s) if:

Strong evidence of association—significant relative risk of >2 (<0.5) based on consistent evidence from two or more observational studies, with no plausible confounders (+1)

Very strong evidence of association—significant relative risk of >5 (<0.2) based on direct evidence with no major threats to validity (+2)

Evidence of a dose response gradient (+1)

All plausible confounders would have reduced the effect (+1)

Question 2: What are the steps involved in critical appraisal?

Surgical interventions often have inherent benefits and associated risks. A three-step approach can be helpful in appraising surgical interventions:

1. *Are the results of the study valid?* The validity of a study concerns the credibility of the results. In this step, one should examine the degree to which the reported estimate of the treatment effect represents the underlying true effect, or whether the results represent an unbiased estimate of the treatment effect. *Systematic error* or *bias* is the first factor that can impact confidence in research results. Bias is directly linked to the design and execution of a study, and thus, the first step in critically appraising a study is to question its validity as well as the extent to which bias is present.[5] Bias is particularly undesirable when the conclusions influence medical decisions.[6] If the results are indeed valid, it may be feasible to examine the results further.[5]

2. *What are the results?* In this step, one should examine the size and precision of the treatment's effect, which may be superior in larger studies, such as multicenter trials.[5]

3. *How can these results be applied to practice?* This final step involves two parts: *generalizability* of the results and

the *net impact* of the treatment. Generalizability is concerned with how similar or dissimilar the patient in question is in comparison to those who participated in the trial. The net impact of the treatment is dependent on the benefits and risks of the treatment, as well as the consequences of withholding treatment.[5]

Although this chapter focuses on the evaluation of studies investigating therapy, it is also important to consider other study designs because of their inherent differences in bias. The hierarchy of evidence ranks literature on the basis of how accurately it provides an estimate of the truth, or how rigorous the study design is. There are three steps in classifying a clinical study.

• First, one must determine whether a study is investigating the results of a treatment, the outcome of a disease, or a diagnostic test, or developing a decision analysis.

• Then, one must place the study in the hierarchy between level I and level V evidence (see Chapter 2).

• Finally, the study needs to be subclassified within the level of evidence.[7]

Using this three-step approach, this chapter discusses how to critically appraise studies investigating therapy, diagnostic tests, and prognosis. For an in-depth look at selecting the appropriate diagnostic tests and therapies, and determining the most likely prognoses for patients, see Chapter 4.

Studies investigating therapy

• Step 1: Are the results of the study valid?

When assessing the validity of a study investigating a therapeutic approach, one must ask if the patients were randomized. The goal of surgical treatment studies is to determine the impact of an intervention on the trial's target outcomes or events such as reoperations, infections, and death. Prognostic factors determine the frequency with which a trial's target outcome occurs. Bias can occur when prognostic factors are unbalanced between the treatment and control groups. The randomization of participants eliminates this bias by enabling an equal distribution of prognostic factors between the two groups.[7] Randomization should also be concealed, as unconcealed randomization may cause surgeons to selectively enroll sicker or less sick patients to either treatment or control groups, leading to a biased result.[7]

One must also ask if patients were analyzed in the groups to which they were randomized. Analyzing patients to the group to which they were randomized is known as the "intention-to-treat" principle.[7] For example, a patient may be assigned to receive a procedure, A, but due to a technical difficulty (e.g., bleeding), the surgeon may decide to carry out the alternative procedure, B. If this occurred with every patient with a poor prognosis, only those with a good prognosis would receive procedure A, resulting in an overestimation of its treatment effect.[8]

Patients in the treatment and control groups should also be similar with respect to known prognostic factors. If the treatment groups are not similar at baseline, statistical techniques can allow for the adjustment of the study result for baseline differences. A small sample size can result in an unbalance in prognostic factors and can also be statistically neutralized.[7]

The sources of blinding in the study must also be determined. By blinding patients, investigators are able to avoid the effects of patient awareness of allocation (placebo effects) and therefore add credibility to the results of their study. However, in some surgical trials, it may be unethical or impossible to blind patients, especially if the trial is comparing surgical with medical treatments. Those who are assessing outcome, such as those interpreting the data, the adjudication committee, and study personnel, should also be blinded to ensure that the outcome is assessed in a uniform manner in both experimental and control groups. Blinding becomes especially important when a judgment is necessary to determine whether a patient has suffered a target outcome, such as a nonunion.[7]

Finally, one must ask whether follow-up of patients was complete. Patients whose status is unknown or lost to follow-up can result from the patient not returning to the clinic for assessment, due to either suffering adverse outcomes or doing well.[7,9] It is a threat to the validity of a study, because patients who are lost commonly have different prognoses from those who are not lost. A study's validity is not compromised if the inferences following a study's conclusions are not altered by assuming the worst-case scenario (i.e., all patients lost to follow-up had the worst outcome). The rule of thumb to use when assessing loss to follow-up is that a study that loses 20% of its patients to follow-up has poor follow-up procedures.[7]

• Step 2: What are the results?

Outcomes in RCTs can be continuous (e.g., blood pressure, points in a functional outcome measure) or dichotomous (e.g., reoperation, death, infection). Dichotomous measures are more frequently used in RCTs to monitor how often patients experience an adverse event or outcome.[7,8] Results can be presented as the *absolute risk reduction, absolute risk difference*, or more simply, the difference between the proportion who suffered an adverse event in the control group and the proportion who suffered an adverse event in the treatment group. The impact of the treatment can also be presented as a *relative risk*, or the risk of an adverse event in patients in the treatment group relative to those in the control group. Dichotomous treatment effects are most commonly reported as the complement of the relative risk, or the *relative risk reduction*. The relative risk reduction is expressed as a percentage. A greater relative risk reduction indicates a more effective therapy. Therefore, a relative risk reduction of 70% means that the treatment under study reduced the risk of patients experiencing an adverse event by 70% relative to the risk among control patients. Investigators may also calculate the *hazard ratio* or the relative risk over a period of time in a *survival analysis*.[7,8]

The precision of the estimate of treatment effect should also be discerned. Greater precision allows for greater confidence to be placed in the results. The precision can be determined in a rudimentary manner through the *p value*, which demonstrates how often an apparent estimate of a treatment effect will occur in a long run of identical trials if, in reality, no true effect exists. The p value does *not* assist clinicians in determining the range within which the treatment effect estimate resides. This job is reserved for the confidence interval.[8]

The *confidence interval* is a set of values in which one can be confident that the true value of the point of estimate resides. This is an arbitrarily chosen breadth; 95% is commonly used. A confidence interval of 95% means that if the study is repeated 100 times, the point of estimate will be found within the range of the confidence interval 95 times. The greater the sample size, generally, the narrower the confidence interval, and the greater the precision and confidence.[8]

• Step 3: How can these results be applied to practice?

The patients one sees in surgical practice frequently differ from those enrolled in the trial. If a patient meets all the inclusion criteria and does not violate any of the exclusion criteria, one can apply the results directly to that patient with substantial confidence.[6,7] Treatments are not uniformly effective, however, and RCTs estimate an average treatment effect.[7] This proves to be a limitation and applying these effects could mean that some patients benefit while others may not. An additional problem arises when a patient's characteristics fit within a subgroup of a study in which the investigators performed a subgroup analysis showing a benefit for that particular subgroup. It is common for investigators to test multiple subgroups, seeking any significant effect after the data becomes available.[8] Since they are not planned ahead of time, subgroup analyses should be assessed rigorously and met with a degree of uncertainty.[7]

When asking how the results of a study could be applied to practice, one also needs to determine whether all clinically important outcomes were considered. Treatments should result in improved outcomes that are important to patients, such as preventing reoperations, improving function, or survival.[7] Moreover, because conventional RCTs estimate *average* treatment effects, one must remember that few real patients will fit perfectly within a subgroup. Keep in mind that patients have their own values and beliefs, and often have other problems with their health. Therefore, all treatments are not uniformly effective; some patients may be exposed to the risks of treatment without achieving any benefit.[7]

Studies investigating diagnostic tests Most tests can separate healthy persons from those who have a severe condition. However, this is not indicative of the clinical utility of a test. The true value of diagnostic test studies lies in its resemblance to clinical practice and the ability of the tests to distinguish between conditions that might otherwise be confused. Therefore, when assessing the validity of a diagnostic test study, readers must ask if clinicians face diagnostic uncertainty. Readers must also ask whether an appropriate and independent reference standard (e.g., biopsy, surgery, autopsy, etc.) has been applied in a blind comparison of the accuracy of the diagnostic test in both treatment and control groups. The diagnostic test under study must not be part of the gold standard. Finally, when assessing the validity of such studies, one must ask whether the results of the diagnostic test influence the decision to perform the reference standard. This is also called *verification bias* or *workup bias.*[10]

When assessing the results of diagnostic test studies, readers need to ask what *likelihood ratios* were associated with the range of possible test results. A likelihood ratio indicates the degree to which a specific diagnostic test result will increase or decrease the pretest probability of the target disorder. In other words, it is a ratio of two likelihoods: (1) how likely is it that patients with the condition will have positive test results? and (2) how often is the same test result is found among people in which a condition was suspected but has been ruled out? In general, if the likelihood ratio is greater than 1, there is an increased probability that the target disorder is present, while likelihood ratios of less than 1 decrease this probability. Sensitivity and specificity can also be used to interpret the results of diagnostic test studies; however, the likelihood ratio approach is recommended because of its simplicity and efficiency.[10]

When seeking to apply the results of a diagnostic test study to patient care, one should ask if the reproducibility of the test result and its interpretation will be satisfactory in their clinical setting, whether the results are applicable to the patient in question, whether the results will change their management strategy, and finally, whether patients will be better off as a result of the test.[10]

Studies investigating prognosis Having an idea of a patient's prognosis is valuable in making the right diagnostic and treatment decisions. If a patient is at a low risk for adverse outcomes, high-risk, expensive, or toxic procedures are probably not the best idea. Similarly, a patient may be destined to experience adverse outcomes no matter the treatment offered. Aggressive therapy in such patients will prolong suffering and waste resources. Prognosis is also useful in the resolution of issues that are broader than the care of the patient in question, such as using outcomes to compare the quality of care across clinicians and institu-

tions. To assess the validity of such studies, readers should ask whether the sample of patients was representative, whether patients were sufficiently homogenous with respect to prognostic risk, whether follow-up was sufficiently complete, and whether objective and unbiased outcome criteria were used. To assess the results of studies investigating prognosis, one should ask how likely the outcomes are over time, and how precise are the estimates of likelihood. When applying the results to patient care, one should examine whether study participants are similar to those in their practice. One should also take into account the sufficiency of the length of follow-up and whether the results can be applied to manage patients in their practice.[11]

Question 3: What are some other examples of tools for critical appraisal?

Although this chapter focuses on one tool for critical appraisal, others do exist and are commonly used. There has been much progress internationally in the development of guidelines for critical appraisal, and these guidelines may be the most suitable for the local circumstances in which they were developed. The National Guideline Clearinghouse is a publicly accessible resource for evidence-based clinical practice guidelines (http://www.guideline.gov) from institutions, professional societies, and government agencies worldwide.[12]

Many international groups have created guidelines to ensure that different types of studies contain all of the necessary information to ensure readers can adequately evaluate the study. Each of these guidelines has their own benefits and limitations.[13] One of these guidelines includes the CONSORT (Consolidated Standards of Reporting Trials) statement for RCTs.[14] This statement or set of guidelines provides a 25-item checklist pertaining to the content of the title, abstract, introduction, methods, results, discussion, trial registration, protocol, and funding. It also provides a flow diagram which depicts information from the enrolment, intervention allocation, follow-up, and analysis stages of an RCT. The statement is flexible and continuously evolving, as the checklist and flow diagram can be modified to incorporate new evidence required to properly evaluate a trial. In this way, the guideline is developed using an evidence-based approach. Limitations of the CONSORT statement include its specificity to two groups, parallel randomized controlled trials and meta-analyses, and the absence of recommendations for designing and conducting RCTs.[14,15]

Not only are there guidelines to assess the quality of evidence provided by clinical research, there are also guidelines which have been developed to appraise the quality of other clinical guidelines. The AGREE (Appraisal of Guidelines, REsearch, and Evaluation) statement is designed to evaluate the quality of clinical practice guideline development and how well the process of development is reported. The instrument is the first of its kind to be developed and tested internationally and consists of six quality domains: scope and purpose, stakeholder involvement, rigor of development, clarity and presentation, applicability, and editorial independence. The statement can be used by a wide range of professionals in European and non-European countries and provides standards for the planning, execution, and monitoring of guideline programs.[16] Because it uses a numerical scoring scale, it also facilitates the comparison of different guidelines internationally.[16,17] However, the instrument is not without its limitations. First, it is difficult to classify a clinical practice guideline as "good" or "bad" because it is impossible to set thresholds for the domain scores. In addition, the instrument does not address the clinical content or the quality of evidence supporting the recommendations of clinical practice guidelines. This is also a common problem with other existing tools for critical appraisal.[17]

Conclusion

There has been a shift in practice from an approach involving anecdotes, previous experiences, and expert opinions, to one that attempts to incorporate the best and most current available evidence into clinical practice.[7,9] Orthopedic surgeons today are faced with the challenge of providing medical care that stems from valid and current evidence. As the credibility of clinical results varies from study to study, it is imperative that surgeons adopt an approach that selects only for valid results to be applied to practice.[6] Critical appraisal of the orthopedic literature achieves this goal in an objective and structured manner.[6,18]

References

1. Atkins D, Best D, Briss PA, et al.Grading quality of evidence and strength of recommendations. BMJ 2004;328:1490–7.
2. Bhandari M, Joensson A, eds. Myths and misconceptions about evidence-based medicine. In: Clinical Research for Surgeons, p. 13. Thieme, New York, 2009.
3. Bhandari M, Giannoudis PV. Evidence-based medicine: what it is and what it is not. Injury 2006;37:302–6.
4. Petrisor BA, Keating J, Schemitsch E. Grading the evidence: Levels of evidence and grades of recommendation. Injury 2006;37:321–7.
5. Schünemann HJ, Bone L. Evidence-based orthopaedics: A primer. Clin Orthop Relat Res 2003;413:117–32.
6. Raslich MA, Onady GM. Evidence-based medicine: Critical appraisal of the literature (critical appraisal tools). Pediatr Rev 2007;28:132–8.
7. Bhandari M, Haynes RB. How to appraise the effectiveness of treatment. World J Surg 2005;29:570–5.
8. Bajammal S, Bhandari M, Dahm P. What every urologist should know about surgical trials Part I: Are the results valid? Indian J Urol 2009;24:281–8.
9. Busse JW, Heetveld MJ. Critical appraisal of the orthopaedic literature: Therapeutic and economic analysis. Injury 2006;37:312–20.
10. Jaeschke R, Guyatt G, Lijmer J. Diagnostic tests. In: Guyatt G, Rennie D, eds. Users' Guide to the Medical Literature, pp. 49–52, 121–137. McGraw Hill, New York, 2002.
11. Randolph A, Cook DJ, Guyatt G. Prognosis. In: Guyatt G, Rennie D, Meade MO, Cook DJ, eds. Users' Guide to the Medical Literature, 2nd edn, p. 513. McGraw Hill, New York, 2008.
12. Poolman RW, Verheyen C, Kerkhoffs GM et al. From evidence to action Acta Orthop 2009;80:113–18.
13. Brand RA. Standards of reporting: the CONSORT, QUORUM, and STROBE guidelines. Clin Orthop Relat Res 2009;467:1393–4.
14. Moher D, Schulz KF, Altman DG. The CONSORT statement: revised recommendations for improving the quality of reports of parallel group randomized trials. BMC Med Res Methodol 2001;1:2.
15. Schulz KF, Altman DG, Moher D. CONSORT 2010 statement: updated guidelines for reporting parallel group randomized trials. PLoS Med 2010;7;1–7.
16. AGREE Collaboration. Development and validation of an international appraisal instrument for assessing the quality of clinical practice guidelines: the AGREE project. Qual Saf Health Care 2003;12:18–23.
17. Vlayen J, Aertgeerts B, Hannes K, Sermeus W, Ramaekers D. A systematic review of appraisal tools for clinical practice guidelines: multiple similarities and one common deficit. Internat J Qual Health Care 2005;17:235–42.
18. Dziri C, Fingerhut A. What should surgeons know about evidence-based surgery. World J Surg 2005;29:545–6.

4 Understanding Diagnosis, Therapy, and Prognosis

Helena Viveiros[1], Sarah Resendes[2], Tania A. Ferguson[3], Mohit Bhandari[1], and Joel Matta[4]

[1]McMaster University, Hamilton, ON, Canada
[2]University of Guelph, Guelph, ON, Canada
[3]University of California—Davis Medical Center, Sacramento, CA, USA
[4]St John's Health Center, Santa Monica, CA, USA

Introduction

In order to make the best patient care decisions, advocates of evidence-based medicine (EBM) promote a methodological approach that integrates the best available evidence from the medical community, the surgeon's experience, and the patient's personal goals and values (Figure 4.1).[1,2] Many branches of medicine have embraced the principles of EBM, and orthopedic surgeons are among its strong advocates.[3,4] Orthopedic surgeons help patients through three interrelated processes: first, by selecting the best diagnostic test for making a sound diagnosis (i.e., determining the disorder or disease from its signs and symptoms); second by administering appropriate therapy (i.e., a treatment that is intended to restore health); and third, by providing the most likely prognosis (i.e., indicating the likely outcomes for patients within the near future).

Hierarchies of evidence

Orthopedic surgeons wishing to integrate the best research evidence into their practice should understand what constitutes higher levels of evidence, as well as what constitutes higher quality evidence. A fundamental principle of EBM is the hierarchy of research study design with the randomized controlled trial (RCT) and systematic reviews at the apex.[5,6] While many surgeons are aware that RCTs provide the best evidence for therapeutic studies, many do not realize RCTs are not the best sources of evidence for either diagnostic or prognostic studies.

In this chapter we provide three tables listing the hierarchy of study design as it applies to studies relating to diagnosis, therapy, and prognosis.[5] For each of these types of studies, systematic reviews are indicated at the pinnacle as level I evidence, but this space is not shared by RCTs in each case. For diagnostic studies the best evidence is retrieved from testing of previously developed diagnostic criteria in series of consecutive patients (Table 4.1). For therapeutic studies the best evidence is actually found in ideal RCTs with narrow confidence intervals (Table 4.2). For prognostic studies the best evidence is derived from high-quality prospective studies that enrolled all patients at the same point in their disease and maintained 80% or greater follow-up of enrolled patients (Table 4.3).

Critical appraisal for validity, results, and applicability

In this chapter we discuss the relevance of each of these processes within the context of EBM principles for critical appraisal of research studies. Five steps are involved in progressing from a clinical patient presentation to developing a plan towards a clinical resolution (Figure 4.2).[2] When presented with a problem we need to develop a structured question, and investigate this question by conducting a literature search for the available evidence. Knowing the hierarchies of evidence, as they apply to the three different

Evidence-Based Orthopedics, First Edition. Edited by Mohit Bhandari.
© 2012 Blackwell Publishing Ltd. Published 2012 by Blackwell Publishing Ltd.

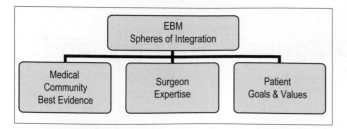

Figure 4.1 Three spheres of integration for evidence-based medicine.

Table 4.1 Levels of evidence for diagnostic studies

Level	Diagnostic studies investigating a diagnostic test
I	Testing of previously developed diagnostic criteria in series of consecutive patients (with universally applied reference gold standard) Systematic review of level I studies
II	Development of diagnostic criteria on basis of consecutive patients (with universally applied reference gold standard) Systematic review of level II studies
III	Study of nonconsecutive patients (without consistently applied reference gold standard) Systematic review of level III studies
IV	Case-control study Poor reference standard
V	Expert opinion

Table 4.2 Levels of evidence for therapeutic studies

Level	Therapeutic studies investigating the results of treatment
I	High-quality randomized controlled trial with statistically significant differences or no statistically significant difference, but narrow confidence intervals Systematic review of level I randomized controlled trials (and study results were homogeneous)
II	Lesser-quality randomized controlled trials (e.g., <80% follow-up, no blinding, or improper randomization) Prospective comparative study Systematic review of level II studies or level I studies with inconsistent results
III	Case-control study Retrospective comparative study Systematic review of level III studies
IV	Case series
V	Expert opinion

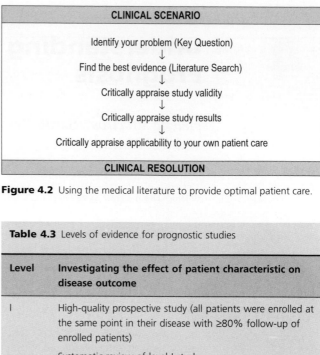

Figure 4.2 Using the medical literature to provide optimal patient care.

Table 4.3 Levels of evidence for prognostic studies

Level	Investigating the effect of patient characteristic on disease outcome
I	High-quality prospective study (all patients were enrolled at the same point in their disease with ≥80% follow-up of enrolled patients) Systematic review of level I study
II	Retrospective study Untreated controls from a randomized controlled trial Lesser-quality prospective study (e.g., patients enrolled at different points in their disease or <80% follow-up) Systematic review of level II studies
III	Case-control study
IV	Case series
V	Expert opinion

types of studies, helps us select the best available study articles. We can best progress to critical appraisal of these articles when guided by three overarching questions about validity (i.e., Are the results valid?), results (i.e., What are the study results?), and applicability (i.e., How are the results applicable to patient care?).[2] These three overarching questions lead us to eight to nine key subquestions for consideration for understanding diagnosis, therapy, and prognosis.

In this chapter we provide three tables to function as users' guides for navigating these three questions when assessing studies of diagnosis (Table 4.4), therapy (Table 4.5), and prognosis (Table 4.6). These tables are based on two EBM resources. The first is the seminal work, *Users' Guide to the Medical Literature*, first presented by the EBM Working Group in a series of articles and later compiled into a book.[2] The second is a related series of articles published in the *Journal of Bone and Joint Surgery*, developed by a group of orthopedic surgeons who have adopted the

Table 4.4 User's guide for an article about diagnostic tests

I	**Are the results valid?**
	Q1: Did clinicians face diagnostic uncertainty?
	Q2: Was there an independent, blind comparison with a reference standard?
	Q3: Did the test results influence the decision to perform the reference standard?
	Q4: Were methods for performing the test described in detail to permit replication?
II	**What are the results?**
	Q5: Are the test likelihood ratios, or data necessary for their calculation, provided
III	**How can I apply the results to patient care?**
	Q6: Will reproducibility and interpretation of the test result be satisfactory in my setting?
	Q7: Are the results applicable to my patient?
	Q8: Will the results change my management of the patient?
	Q9: Will patients be better off as a result of the test?

Table 4.6 User's guide for an article about prognosis

I	**Validity: Are the results valid?**
	Q1: Was the patient sample representative?
	Q2: Were the patients sufficiently homogeneous with respect to prognostic risk?
	Q3: Was follow-up sufficiently complete?
	Q4: Were outcome criteria objective and unbiased?
II	**Results: What are the results?**
	Q5: How likely are the outcomes over time?
	Q6: How precise are the estimates of likelihood?
III	**Applicability: How can I apply the results to patient care?**
	Q7: Were the study patients and their management similar to those in my practice?
	Q8: Was the follow-up sufficiently long?
	Q9: Can I use the results in the management of patients in my practice?

Table 4.5 User's guide for an article about therapy

I	**Validity: Are the results valid?**
	Q1: Did intervention and control groups start with the same prognosis?
	Were patients randomized?
	Was randomization concealed?
	Were patients in the study groups similar with respect to known prognostic factors?
	Q2: Was prognostic balance maintained as the study progressed?
	To what extent was the study blinded?
	Q3: Were the groups prognostically balanced at the study's completion?
	Was follow-up complete?
	Were patients analyzed in the groups to which they were randomized?
	Was the trial stopped early?
II	**Results: What are the results?**
	Q4: How large was the treatment effect?
	Q5: How precise was the estimate of the effect?
III	**Applicability: How can I apply the results to patient care?**
	Q6: Were the study patients similar to my patient?
	Q7: Were all patient-important outcomes considered?
	Q8: Are the likely treatment benefits worth the potential harm and costs?

principles of EBM.[6-9] The following overview is comprehensive but brief. For more detailed discussions, often accompanied by informative clinical case studies and examples of study articles, we recommend the *Journal of Bone and Joint Surgery* articles. Additionally, for a useful review of statistics in orthopedic papers we recommend the review article by Petrie.[10]

Diagnosis

For diagnostic studies the best evidence is retrieved from testing of previously developed diagnostic criteria in series of consecutive patients (Table 4.1).[7] Surgeons make a diagnosis by assessing the signs and symptoms of disease or disorder presented by their patients. Diagnostic decisions are made by integrating the surgeon's experienced clinical judgment and using previously validated diagnostic tests. Diagnostic tests can be very useful, but only if the correct tests are used.[11,12] Accurate tests can help the surgeon rule in, or rule out, a patient condition. This is the first step in helping us to best direct therapy and determine the most likely prognosis.

Investigators conducting a diagnostic test study hope to establish the test's power to differentiate between those patients who have the target condition and those who do not. In these studies the main issues to consider in determining the validity of a diagnostic test study are how the authors assembled their patients and whether or not they used an appropriate reference standard for each of these patients.[7]

Validity: are the study results valid?

Question 1: Did clinicians face diagnostic uncertainty?

Using tests to distinguish between severely affected and healthy patients is easy because there is minimal overlap between the two groups of patients. It is when test results for patients with the target condition are similar to results for those free of the condition that clinicians will want to apply diagnostic tests.[7]

Question 2: Was there an independent, blind comparison with a reference standard?

Readers should check that investigators applied independently the test under investigation and an appropriate reference standard (e.g., biopsy, surgery) to all patients. That is, the assessors of the test results should be blinded to the reference standard, and the assessor reference standard should remain blinded to the test results. When blinding is not used there is a significant danger of overestimating test performance.[2,7,11]

Question 3: Did test results influence the decision to perform the reference standard?

If the results of a test influence the decision to carry out the reference standard, the properties of the diagnostic test will be distorted. This is called *verification bias* or *workup bias*. To avoid this bias, be wary of studies in which different reference standards were used for patients with and without the target condition.[7]

Question 4: Were methods for performing the test described in detail to permit replication?

The question to consider when assessing the validity of a study is whether or not sufficient detail was reported for performing the tests. Unless tests are applied in a homogeneous manner, there is too great a risk for variability in results.

Results: what are the results?

Question 5: Are test likelihood ratios, or data necessary for their calculation, provided?

The first step in the process of diagnosis starts with determining the probability that the target disease is present in a given patient group before the next test is performed—the *pretest probability*. This is determined by the integration of the evidence on disease presentation coupled with the surgeon's clinical experience and judgment. The second step in the process of diagnosis is to examine the characteristic of the test that indicates the direction magnitude of this change in probability, the *likelihood ratio* (LR). The LR represents the likelihood that a given test result will be expected in a patient with the target disorder compared with the likelihood that the same test result would be expected in a patient without the target disorder. Many studies will present the properties of diagnostic tests in terms of sensitivity and specificity. Although less clinically useful than LRs, these terms can still be used for its calculation.[2,7]

Applicability: how can I apply the results to my patient care?

Orthopedic surgeons rely heavily on radiographs for diagnosis, so it is important that some mention of the image acquisition protocol, or lack thereof, should be documented in well-reported studies. So much of orthopedic diagnosis is radiographic, and the way/orientation of the image beam changes the radiographic image so greatly that the acquisition protocol should be standardized and well described to the reader. If the images are not obtained in a precisely defined way, the study's repeatability and reproducibility will be compromised, as will the study findings.

Question 6: Will reproducibility and interpretation of the test result be satisfactory in my setting?

The value of a diagnostic test often depends on its reproducibility when applied within your own clinical setting. Highly reproducible tests are often simple and easily applied, or were conducted by highly skilled investigators.[2] If the latter is true, caution is warranted if you are in a setting in which only unskilled interpretation is available.

Question 7: Are the results applicable to my patient?

In general, if your patient meets the study eligibility criteria and your clinical practice setting is similar to that described in the study, you may be confident that the results are applicable to your own patient. Do take into consideration that test properties may be sensitive to the stages of disease severity and to different distributions of competing conditions.[2,7]

Question 8: Will the results change my management of the patient?

When making management decisions, it is useful to link them explicitly with the probability of the target disorder. For most disorders we can speak of probabilities between the test threshold and the treatment threshold.[2,7] It is when the probability of the target disorder lies between these two thresholds that you should adopt testing in the management of your patients.

Question 9: Will patients be better off as a result of the test?

The most important criterion for the usefulness of a diagnostic test is whether or not the benefits to patients outweigh the associated risks.[2,7] In general, a test is particularly valuable when the risks of test are minimal, the target disorder has major consequences if left untreated, or the disorder is readily treated once diagnosed.

Therapy

For therapeutic studies the best evidence is found in the research design known as the RCT, and ideally in ideal RCTs with narrow confidence intervals (Table 4.2). In RCTs patients are allocated by chance to an intervention or a control group. Often in therapeutic studies researchers compare the outcome of two or more types of interventions in order to determine which is more effective and so the treatment that surgeons should employ in their practice.[8]

Validity: are the results valid?

Question 1: Did the intervention and control groups start with the same prognosis?

When evaluating the literature, surgeons should value studies that employ random allocation by chance, a tactic that ensures no method has been used in order to allocate patients to experimental or control groups, therefore ensuring that each group has the same baseline prognoses and characteristics.[13] Other important items that a surgeon should assess when evaluating the literature are whether or not blinding was used, i.e., whether allocation concealment was employed that help to eliminate bias.[2,8] Patients in both groups should be similar with respect to known prognostic factors. Differences in prognosis between the two study groups will result in bias either for or against the treatment being investigated.

Question 2: Was prognostic balance maintained as the study progressed?

When possible, blinding is the optimal strategy for maintaining prognostic balance.[2,8,10] In surgical trials it is not possible to keep surgeons blinded. Although patients may be blinded to what treatment group they were allocated, keeping them blinded after surgery is challenging and unlikely. At the very least outcome assessors can be kept blinded when adjudicating patient outcomes should and can remain blinded.[8]

Question 3: Were groups prognostically balanced at the study's completion?

Even with concealed randomization conducted at patient enrolment, with effective blinding maintained during monitoring, the quality of follow-up completion is essential for ensuring study groups remained prognostically balanced at study close-out. Ideally, at the study conclusion you should know the status of every patient enrolled with respect to target outcome, and the proportion of patients

lost within each group should be none to minimal. Additionally, all patients should be analyzed in the groups into which they were randomized, and the trial should not be stopped early but continue until planned follow-up.[2,8]

Results: what are the results?

Question 4: How large was the treatment effect?

In surgical trials patients either do or do not have an event such as reoperation or deep infection. One way to report the proportion of patients who have such an event can be as the absolute difference (i.e., *absolute risk reduction* (ARR) or risk difference) between the proportions of those having the event in both treatment groups. Another way to express the treatment effect would be as *relative risk* (RR), the risk of the event among patient treatment groups. The most commonly reported measure of treatment effect is the complement of relative risk, *relative risk reduction* (RRR). A discussion of statistics is beyond the scope of this chapter, but a general rule is that the greater the RRR the more effective the therapy.[2,8,10]

Question 5: How precise was the estimate of the treatment effect?

The range within which the true effect likely lies is calculated with *confidence intervals* (CI). The accepted general rule is to use the 95% CI. Assuming the study was well conducted and has minimal bias, we can consider the 95% CI as defining the range that includes the true RRR 95% of the time. The true RRR will generally lie beyond these extremes only 5% of the time, a property of the CI that relates closely to the statistical significance of $p < 0.05$. A further discussion of statistical significance is beyond this chapter, but another general rule is that the larger the sample size, the narrower the CI.[10]

When reviewing the results of a study, it is important to take the sample size of the study into consideration. The size of a sample needs to be large enough to ensure that the study has adequate *power*. Power refers to the likelihood that a difference between two interventions will be detected if one is present. For instance, a study with a sample size that is too small may result in no difference being found between two treatments when one truly exists (*beta error*) or a difference being found between two treatments when there is no difference in actuality (*alpha error*). A study by Bhandari and colleagues notes that the conventionally accepted standard for study power is 80%.[14]

Applicability: how can I apply the results to my patient care?

Question 6: Can the results be applied to my patient?

Lastly, we must consider if and how the results can be applied to patients in our own practice. We can determine this by asking three questions about patient similarity, important outcomes, and overall benefits. First, consider whether your patient would be included in the study group. Given that the inclusion and exclusion criteria are clearly delineated, is there something about your own patient that would lead to his or her exclusion from the study? If so, the results may not apply to your patient. Second, consider whether your patient fits into a group whose benefit was demonstrated with a subgroup analysis. If the investigation benefits were identified from a post-hoc subgroup analysis, those findings are suspect due to poor design and caution should be taken if a therapeutic recommendation is made due to a subgroup analysis. Third, you must consider whether your surgical skills are comparable to the skills of the investigating surgeon(s).

Question 7: Were all clinically important outcomes considered?

One must also think about whether or not all outcomes of the treatment were reported (e.g., adverse events, etc.).[2] Surgical treatments are indicated if they provide benefits, but only if these benefits include outcomes that are important to your patient (i.e., are in line with their own goals and values).

Question 8: Are the likely treatment benefits worth the potential harm and costs?

For the safety and benefit of patients, it is critical that the potential benefits of the treatment outweigh any potential harm to the patient, or any unreasonable costs.[2,8]

Prognosis

Although RCTs are the gold standard for evaluating new drugs and medical or surgical procedures, they are not commonly used for assessing prognostic factors. In practice it is not ethical to assign patients to potential risk factors. Generally, surgical studies investigating prognostic factors are observational studies, and the best such design is a cohort study. Ideally, the highest level of evidence for prognosis comes from high-quality prospective studies in which all subjects were enrolled at the same point in their disease or treatment and an 80% or greater follow-up rate was maintained (Table 4.3).[5,9,15]

These cohort studies may be either prospective or retrospective. A *prospective cohort study* identifies potential prognostic factors and follows the study group forward in time to determine if any factors have a significant impact on outcomes. Unfortunately, these studies demand substantial planning in advance and require considerable time and resources to complete.[2,9] Furthermore, new prognostic markers are continuously reported and may not have been identified at the inception of the data collection.

An alternative observational study is a *retrospective cohort study* or a *retrospective case-control study*. In case-control studies one starts with the outcome of interest and then looks backward to examine potential causal factors by comparing those who have the outcome (i.e., cases) with those who do not have the outcome (i.e., controls). The major drawback of retrospective studies is that the data quality is based mainly on patient records, and these records may not be sufficiently accurate. Another drawback of retrospective studies is that they are prone to *recall bias*, and this decreases the validity of results.[2,9]

In studies of prognosis researchers examine prognostic variables to determine their relationship to possible outcomes, disease, therapeutic treatment, and predictions of the probability associated with their effect (i.e., the probability with which those outcomes can be expected to occur).[2,9] It is possible to refine the prognosis by looking at subgroups defined by demographic variables (e.g., gender, age, comorbidity factors, socioeconomic status, disease stage). In the best-designed studies investigators will distinguish subgroups of patients based on prognostic variables.[9] When variables or factors predict which patients do better or worse, we call them *prognostic factors*. Prognostic factors should not be confused with *risk factors* (i.e., those patient characteristics that are associated with disease in the first place).

Validity: are study results valid?

Question 1: Was the patient sample representative?

In well-designed prognostic studies, the patient sample enrolled must match the target population under study.[9] A patient sample is not representative when it differs systematically from the population of interest. Differences may result in a systematic over- or underestimation of the likelihood of adverse outcomes; i.e., the sample patients will have a worse or better prognosis respectively than the target population. A prognostic study is biased when it yields such differences from the truth about adverse outcomes.[2,10]

Question 2: Were patients sufficiently homogeneous with respect to prognostic risk?

To estimate patient prognosis we examine outcomes in groups of patients with similar clinical presentation. The best-designed studies would have all enrolled patients similar enough for prognostic risk for the outcome of interest to be applicable to each and every one of them. Such similarity could include age, disease stage, smoking history, gender, and socioeconomic status. Ideally, prognostic factors should be validated in several studies to ensure that they are related to the outcome of interest. If patients enrolled were not sufficiently homogeneous, investigators should at least provide estimates for all clinically relevant subgroups in the study.[9]

Question 3: Was follow-up sufficiently complete?

We can only be confident in the validity of a cohort study of prognosis if the majority of the patients enrolled have completed follow-up. The proportion of loss to follow-up that threatens validity is related to the proportion of patients who had an adverse outcome. Generally, the larger the proportion of lost patients in relation to the proportion of patients with adverse outcomes, the less likely the study results are valid.[2,9]

Question 4: Were outcome criteria objective and unbiased?

In well-designed studies investigators should define their target outcomes before study start-up, and they should base their criteria on the most clinically relevant measures. Furthermore, investigators should describe the type of patient monitoring and the frequency of follow-up. In orthopedic studies outcomes are objective when they are obvious to measure, such as reoperations or death. Some outcomes, such as fracture healing or nonunion, require more clinical judgment to assess. For the study to remain unbiased, it is very important that adjudicators remain blinded to all prognostic factors. Other outcomes, such as functional ability or quality of life, are subjective and challenging to measure. For these most difficult outcomes investigators should use previously validated and reliable measurement scales.[15]

Results: what are the results?

Question 5: How likely are the outcomes over time?

Quantitative results from studies of prognosis or risk are the number of events that occur over time. These events must be of a discrete nature and linked to a precise time. In orthopedic studies these events typically include reoperations, serious adverse events (SAEs), or death. A common and informative way to depict these quantitative results is as a *survival curve*. A survival curve may be understood as either the number of events over time, or conversely as the change of freedom from results over time.[2] For example, if the chance of outcome is much later after initial surgical treatment, this is typically represented by a curve that starts out flat and then becomes steep.

Question 6: How precise are the estimates of likelihood?

Investigators usually report risks of adverse outcomes with their associated 95% CI. If the study is valid, the 95% CI defines the range of risks within which it is likely that the true risk lies. The more precise the estimate of prognosis a study provides, the less uncertainty about the estimated prognosis and the more useful the study is for us. In most survival curves, results are derived from more patients during the early follow-up periods rather than the later

periods. This results from losses to follow-up and because study patients are rarely enrolled at the same time. This means that survival curves are more precise during the earlier periods of follow-up.

Applicability: how can I apply the results to my patient care?

Question 7: Were study patients and their management similar to those in my practice?

In well-written articles, investigators describe the study sample in sufficient detail for readers to make a comparison with their own patients. This should include patient characteristics, and how these are defined. Oddly enough, while therapy is one factor that could strongly influence outcome it is rarely mentioned in prognostic studies. Therapeutic strategies can vary markedly among institutions, and change over time as new treatments become available or old treatments regain popularity. To the extent that treatments are beneficial or detrimental, overall patient outcome might improve or become worse. Studies that do not provide sufficient details about therapeutic strategies limit your ability to assess applicability. Given the rapid pace of evolving therapies in orthopedics, authors should detail the variety of implants, technologies, and surgical techniques used for long-term outcome studies in order for readers to assess the generalizability of the results to their own patients.[9]

Question 8: Was follow-up sufficiently long?

Because the presence of illness often precedes the development of an outcome event by a long period of time, investigators should follow patients for long enough to detect the outcomes of interest. A prognostic study may provide an unbiased assessment of outcome during a short period of time, but only if it meets certain validity criteria. Such a study may be of little use for patients who are interested in their prognosis over a longer period of time.

Question 9: Can I use the results in the management of patients in my practice?

Prognostic data often provide the basis for practical decisions about surgical treatments. Knowing the expected clinical course of your patient's condition can help you judge whether or not a specific treatment is warranted. For example, for patients at very low risk of adverse outcomes even potentially beneficial therapies may not be justified. Specifically, for patients who are most likely to get well, clinicians should not recommend treatments that are potentially toxic or exorbitantly expensive. For those patients at high risk of poor outcomes, regardless of therapy course, aggressive therapy may only serve to prolong suffering and waste costly resources. Even in cases where the prognostic results do not help with selecting an effective therapy, they may help you in counseling a concerned patient or relative about appropriate next steps in care.[2,9]

Conclusion

Orthopedic surgeons wishing to apply the principles of EBM should learn to integrate the best available evidence from the medical community, and their own surgical experience, as well as their patients' own goals and values. In this chapter we provide users' guides for the best studies of diagnosis, therapy, and prognosis. Each of these guides is based on the three-step process of critical appraisal of study validity, results, and applicability to your own patients. By following these steps for critical appraisal, orthopedic surgeons can select the most appropriate tests to make a sound diagnosis, choose the most appropriate therapies available, and determine the most likely prognosis for their patients.

References

1. Sackett DL, Rosenberg WM, Gray JA, Haynes RB, Richardson WS. Evidence-based medicine: what it is and what it isn't. BMJ 1996;312:71–2.
2. Guyatt G, Rennie D, Meade MO, Cook DJ. Users' Guide to the Medical Literature: A Manual for Evidence-Based Clinical Practice (2nd ed). American Medical Association Press, Chicago, 2008.
3. Kreder HJ. Evidence-based surgical practice: what is it and do we need it? World J Surg 1999;23:1232–5.
4. Bhandari M, Tornetta III P. Evidence-based orthopaedics: a paradigm shift. Clin Orthop Relat Res 2003;413:9–10.
5. Centre for Evidence-Based Medicine home page. Available at www.cebm.net. Accessed August 2009.
6. Bhandari M, Guyatt GH, Montori V, Devereaux PJ, Swionkkowski MF. User's guide to the orthopaedic literature: how to use a systematic literature review. J Bone Joint Surg Am 2002;84:1672–82.
7. Bhandari M, Montori VM, Swiontkowski MF, Guyatt GH. User's guide to the surgical literature: how to use an article about a diagnostic test. J Bone Joint Surg Am 2003;85:1133–40.
8. Bhandari M, Guyatt GH, Swiontkowski MF. User's guide to the orthopaedic literature: how to use an article about a surgical therapy. J Bone Joint Surg Am 2001;83:916–26.
9. Bhandari M, Guyatt GH, Swiontkowski MF. User's guide to the orthopaedic literature: how to use an article about prognosis. J Bone Joint Surg Am 2001;83:1555–64.
10. Petrie A. Statistics in orthopaedic papers. J Bone Joint Surg Br 2006;88:1121–36.
11. Graham B. Diagnosis, diagnostic criteria, and consensus. Hand Clin 2009;25:43–8.
12. Roy, JS, Michlovitz S. Using evidence-based practice to select diagnostic tests. Hand Clin 2009;25:49–57.
13. Sibbald B, Roland M. Understanding controlled trials: why are randomized controlled trials important? BMJ 1998;316:201.
14. Bhandari M, Richards RR, Sprague S, Schemitsch EH. The quality of reporting of randomized trials in the Journal of Bone and Joint Surgery from 1988 through 2000. J Bone Joint Surg Am 2002;4(3):388–96.
15. Degen RM, Hoppe DJ, Petrisor BA, Bhandari M. Making decisions about prognosis in evidence-based practice. Hand Clin 2009;25:59–66.

5 Systematic Reviews and Meta-Analysis

Nasir Hussain[1], Farrah Hussain[1], Mohit Bhandari[1], and Saam Morshed[2]

[1]McMaster University, Hamilton, ON, Canada
[2]San Francisco General Hospital and the University of California, San Francisco, CA, USA

Introduction

Over 3 million new articles are published in scientific journals each year.[1,2] Consequently, a researcher would be required to read close to 20 articles every day to keep current with research.[1] Obviously this is a daunting and impossible task for most healthcare professionals. Therefore, the accumulation of new evidence makes it easy to lose past findings and forget about them. The use of reviews has become an invaluable tool in orthopedic medicine to help keep up to date with the best available evidence. There are three types of reviews: narrative reviews, systematic reviews, and meta-analysis.[1,2] Each of these is discussed in detail in this chapter.

Top six questions

1. What is a narrative review?
2. What is a systematic review?
3. What are the differences between a systematic review and a narrative review?
4. What is a meta-analysis?
5. Where do narrative reviews, systematic reviews, and meta-analyses rank on the hierarchy of evidence?
6. How are systematic reviews and meta-analyses critically appraised?

Question 1: What is a narrative review?

A narrative review summarizes different primary studies from which a broad perspective can be formulated. Interpretations contributed by the reviewers' own experience, and existing theories and models are often included in narrative reviews.[3,4] For example, a narrative review may review the broad topic of femoral fractures.[3]

Current concepts are also a form of narrative review. They frequently describe the approach used by a group of surgeons to treat a situation, often discussing multiple treatment options.[3] The literature used in the narrative review is summarized, but the methods used to locate and select the studies for inclusion are not systematic. In addition, the studies included are not formally critically appraised. For this reason, a narrative review may miss relevant studies, or the authors may have selected studies on the basis of their own preferences and opinions.[3,4] Narrative reviews are also helpful in answering background questions, as these types of questions are broad in scope and are used to help understand the principle or problem. An example of a background question would be: "What are the epidemiology, prognosis, and screening approaches following a femoral fracture in adults?"

The strengths of this type of review lie in its ability to understand the diversity of ideologies surrounding scholarly research topics.[3] As well, it provides the author of the

Evidence-Based Orthopedics, First Edition. Edited by Mohit Bhandari.
© 2012 Blackwell Publishing Ltd. Published 2012 by Blackwell Publishing Ltd.

review with the opportunity to contribute their own knowledge and insight into this shared educational phenomenon.[3] However, narrative reviews do not necessarily state the rules for inclusion of studies, nor do they state the rules used to determine to relevance and validity of included studies.[3,4]

Example from literature: narrative review

Source
Doherty T, MacDermid JC. Clinical and electrodiagnostic testing of carpel tunnel syndrome: a narrative review. Orthop Sports Phys Ther 2004;34(10):565–88.

Abstract
Carpal tunnel syndrome (CTS) is a pressure-induced neuropathy that causes sensorimotor disturbances of the median nerve, which impair functional ability. A clear history that elicits relevant personal and work exposures and the nature of symptoms can lead to a high probability of a correct diagnosis. Hand diagrams and diagnostic questionnaires are available to provide structure to this process. A variety of provocative tests have been described and have variable accuracy. The Phalen's wrist flexion and the carpal compression tests have the highest overall accuracy, while Tinel's nerve percussion test is more specific to axonal damage that may occur as a result of moderate to severe CTS. Sensory evaluation of light touch, vibration, or current perception thresholds can detect early sensory changes, whereas 2-point discrimination changes and thenaratrophy indicate loss of nerve fibers occurring with more severe disease. Electrodiagnosis can encompass a variety of tests and is commonly used to assess the presence/severity of neuropathic changes and to preclude alternative diagnoses that overlap with CTS in presentation. The pathophysiologic changes occurring with different stages of nerve compression must be considered when interpreting diagnostic test results and predicting response to physical therapy management.

Question 2: What is a systematic review?

Unlike a narrative review, a systematic review addresses a specific question and uses a planned and systematic approach.[4] This type of review is appropriate for answering foreground questions.[4,5] An example of this type of question would be "In a patient with an acute rupture of the lateral ankle ligament, is cast immobilization or functional taping a better treatment option if the patient wants to return to work as soon as possible?"[4] After this question has been asked, a systematic and rigorous literature search is performed followed by the critical analysis of the studies to be included.[3,4] Lastly, the results are summarized and discussed.[4]

This type of review has various strengths, some of which include a narrow research question, a comprehensive and exhaustive search for evidence, a criterion for assessing relevant literature for validity, the objective summary provided, and the implication for evidence-based medicine.[3] However, the primary problem with systematic reviews is that the narrow focus may not allow for comprehensive coverage.[3] The strict criteria used by systematic reviews may limit studies which are relevant, thus information may be lost.

Example from literature: systematic review

Source
Struijs PA, Smidt N, Arola H, Dijk CN, Buchbinder R, Assendelft WJ. Orthotic devices for the treatment of tennis elbow. Cochrane Database Syst Rev 2002;CD001821(1):1–18.

Abstract
Lateral epicondylitis (tennis elbow) is a frequently reported condition. A wide variety of treatment strategies has been described. As of yet, no optimal strategy has been identified. The objective of our study was to assess the effectiveness of orthotic devices for the treatment of tennis elbow. We searched Medline, Embase, CINAHL, the Cochrane Controlled Trial Register, Current Contents up to May 1999 and reference lists from all retrieved articles. Experts on the subjects were approached for additional trials. All randomized clinical trials (RCT) describing individuals with diagnosed lateral epicondylitis and comparing the use of an orthotic device as a treatment strategy were evaluated for inclusion. Two reviewers independently assessed the validity of the included trials and extracted data on relevant outcome measures. Dichotomous outcomes were expressed as Relative Risks (RRs) and continuous outcomes as Standardised Mean Differences (SMD), both with corresponding 95% confidence intervals (95% CI). Five RCTs (N per group 7–49) were included. Validity score ranged from 3–9 positive items out of 11. Subgroup analyses were not performed due to the small number of trials. The limited number of included trials present few outcome measures and limited longterm results. Pooling was not possible due to large heterogeneity amongst trials. No definitive conclusions can be drawn concerning effectiveness of orthotic devices for lateral epicondylitis. More well-designed and well-conducted RCTs of sufficient power are warranted.

Question 3: What is a meta-analysis?

Often confused with systematic reviews, meta-analyses are the statistical analysis of results from multiple separate studies.[1,4] Usually this statistical analysis is included in systematic reviews that use quantitative methods, but this may not always be the case.[1] Like a systematic review, a meta-analysis typically answers a foreground question.[4] A meta-analysis is conducted to determine the significance of the results from multiple research studies pertaining to the same research question.[3,4] It can therefore increase the statistical power of the primary research by pooling the data and thus allows for the results to be more generalized.[3,4]

Meta-analyses are performed using a concise, stepwise method. The steps include: (1) defining the research question, (2) performing the literature search, (3) selecting the studies, (4) extracting the data, (5) analyzing the data, and (6) reporting the results. Numerous protocols have been developed, such as the Quality of Reports of Meta-analysis (QUOROM), that provide detail on how to properly conduct each step.[2]

A meta-analysis is very beneficial in assessing effective treatment options. For example, a meta-analysis of clinical trials may help to increase the precision of estimates of treatment effects, thus decreasing the probability of false-negative results.[2] Therefore, by statistically pooling results from relevant studies, a meta-analysis allows for accurate and precise analysis, and increases the statistical power of the primary research by pooling the data and allowing the results to be more generalized.[2] However, the quality of a meta-analysis can be compromised if the included data is flawed due to poor methodological quality.[2] As well, various biases such as *publication bias* can be associated with a meta-analysis.[2]

Example from literature: meta-analysis

Source

Kerkhoffs GM, Struijs PA, Marti RK, Blankevoort L, Assendelft WJ, van Dijk CN. Functional treatments for acute ruptures of the lateral ankle ligament: a systematic review. Acta Orthop Scand 2003;74(1):69–77.

Abstract

Our aim with this systematic review was to assess the effectiveness of various functional treatments for acute ruptures of the lateral ankle ligament in adults. We performed an electronic database search using MEDLINE, EMBASE, COCHRANE CONTROLLED TRIAL REGISTER and CURRENT CONTENTS. We evaluated randomized clinical trials describing skeletally mature subjects with an acute rupture of the lateral ankle ligament and compared functional treatments for inclusion in this study. 9 trials met our inclusion criteria. Two reviewers independently assessed the quality of these trials and extracted relevant data on treatment outcome. Where appropriate, results of comparable studies were pooled. Individual and pooled statistics are reported as relative risks (RR) for dichotomous outcome and (weighted) mean differences ((W)MD) for continuous outcome measures with 95% confidence intervals (95% CI). Heterogeneity between the trials was tested using a standard chi-square test. Persistent swelling at short-term follow-up was less with lace-up ankle support than with semi-rigid ankle support (RR 4.2; 95% CI 1.3–14), an elastic bandage (RR 5.5; 95% CI 1.7–18) and tape (RR 4.1; 95% CI 1.2–14). A semi-rigid ankle support required a shorter period for return to work than an elastic bandage (WMD 4.2; 95% CI 2.4–6.1) (p = 0.7). One trial reported better results for subjective instability using the semi-rigid ankle support than the elastic bandage (RR 8.0; 95% CI 1.0–62). Treatment with tape resulted in more complications, mostly skin problems, than that with an elastic bandage (RR 0.1; 95% CI 0.0–0.8). We found no other statistically significant differences. We conclude that an elastic bandage is a less effective functional treatment. Lace-up supports seem better, but the data are insufficient as a basis for definite conclusions.

Question 4: Where do narrative reviews, systematic reviews, and meta-analyses rank on the hierarchy of evidence?

Systematic reviews and meta-analysis of randomized controlled trials are considered to be the highest quality of evidence and are commonly ranked as level I evidence.[4-6] A meta-analysis pools the data from all relevant studies found for a specific research question. This pooling allows for the results to be generalized then they normally would be from the results of a single trial.[3,4] As well, due to the systematic and rigorous approach used in conducting a systematic review or meta-analysis, the level of bias is greatly reduced.[3]

Ultimately, the quality of the systematic review and meta-analysis depends on the quality of the included studies.[5] Poorly conducted trials compromise the quality of the meta-analysis.[5] In essence, one should aim for homogeneity amongst the included studies. This occurs when similar studies are arriving at the same outcome, thus leading to a strong meta-analysis.[4] On the contrary, heterogeneity occurs when studies analyzing the same outcome arrive at different results, which leads to a weak meta-analysis.[4]

Question 5: What are the differences between a systematic review, meta-analysis and a narrative review?

Various differences exist between a narrative review, systematic review, and a meta-analysis. The first major difference is at the level of the research question. Systematic reviews and meta-analyses pose a concise and specific research question which is called a *foreground question*.[7,8] This allows for a greater insight into the research of interest and also helps make the search for relevant published literature much easier. A good example of a foreground question is, "In a patient with an acute rupture of the lateral ankle ligament, is cast immobilization or functional taping a better treatment option if the patient wants to return to work as soon as possible?"[4] This foreground question should be answered in depth with many sources of information, criteria-based selection of patients/trials, and critical appraisal and synthesis of all relevant studies.[7,8] On the other hand, the question raised by a narrative review is often much more generalized and is known as a *background question*. An example of this type of question is, "How do bones heal after all treatments of humeral shaft fractures?" [8] Since this question is very broad, large numbers of studies can be included in the analysis, some of which may now be relevant to the research question.

Another difference between these types of studies is the amount of *bias*. The studies which are commonly included in a narrative review are selectively chosen by the author, thus creating a *selection bias*.[8,9] As well, narrative reviews often mix expert opinion with evidence, and this may cause inconsistencies in the reported findings.[8,10] On the other hand, a systematic review and meta-analysis utilize an exclusive stepwise approach for the selection and methodological validity of the studies included.[4,9] This in turn helps provide a safeguard against many common biases, such as publication bias and *citation bias*. The factors affecting the inclusion of studies are predefined by the researcher in order to ensure consistency.[4] Some of these factors include study design, population characteristics, type of treatment/exposure, and outcome measures.[11]

Differences between a narrative review and systematic review also exist in the quality of the literature search. A systematic review uses a comprehensive, specific search in order to obtain maximal results.[7] In contrast, a narrative review uses a generalized search in which many different studies are found, some of which may not be relevant to the research question.[7,11] After the search is completed, there are also differences in the inclusion and exclusion criteria. In a systematic review, studies are included on the basis of many different factors such as validity of the results, research methodology, type of treatments, and the outcome measures used.[12] Various tools such as the Jadad score, T.C. Chalmers score, and QUOROM checklist are regularly used to determine the quality of the study.[12] Thus, the inclusion criteria for a systematic review are specified and exhaustive whereas a narrative review adopts a more open-ended approach which incorporates the author's opinion in the selection of included studies.[12] A summary on questions to consider when reviewing and evaluating included articles can be found in Chapter 3 on critical appraisal.

Question 6: What is a critical appraisal of systematic reviews and meta-analyses?

As already discussed in Chapter 3, it is important to carefully evaluate the studies included in a systematic review. Various characteristics of the studies are assessed such as the participants, outcome measures used, completeness of study, follow-up, and appropriateness of statistical meas-

Table 5.1 Oxman and Guyatt index

1. Were the search methods used to find evidence stated?

2. Was the search for evidence reasonable comprehensive?

3. Were the criteria for deciding which studies to include in the overview reported?

4. Was bias in the selection of studies avoided?

5. Were the criteria used for assessing the validity of the included studies reported?

6. Was the validity of all studies referred to in the text assessed using appropriate criteria?

7. Were the methods used to combine the findings of the relevant studies reported?

8. Were the findings of the relevant studies combined appropriately relative to the primary question the overview addresses?

9. Were the conclusions made by the author(s) supported by the data and/or analysis reported in the overview?

Question 10 summarized the previous ones, and, specifically, asks to rate the scientific quality of the review from 1 (being extensively flawed) to 3 (carrying major flaws) to 5 (carrying minor flaws) to 7 (minimally flawed). The developers of the index specify that if the "partially/can't tell" answer is used one or more times in questions 2, 4, 6, or 8, a review is likely to have minor flaws at best and is difficult to rule out major flaws (i.e., a score ≤4). If the "no" option is used on question 2,4,6, or 8, the review is likely to have major flaws (i.e., a score ≤3).

Reprinted from Journal of Clinical Epidemiology, 44, Oxman AD, Guyatt GH, Validation of an index of the quality of review articles, 1271–1278, 1991, with permission from Elsevier.

ures.[4] Tools such as the Oxman and Guyatt Index are used to critically evaluate the scientific quality of a systematic review (Table 5.1).[4]

One may also encounter overlapping systematic reviews which address the same clinical question but are conducted by different groups of authors.[4] These conflicting studies can also have conflicting results. To help resolve this problem an algorithm was developed by Jaded et al. to help analyze and evaluate the conflicting systematic reviews to determine which is the most appropriate.[4] In this algorithm aspects such as the methodological quality are assessed.[4]

Conclusion

Systematic reviews are becoming increasingly important in modern-day clinical research because of the vast amount of literature published every year. If they are conducted appropriately, they can effectively provide an accurate, descriptive, and concise summary of the available literature. Thus, when properly conducted using high quality primary studies, systematic reviews can provide the highest level of current evidence to answer specific clinical questions.

References

1. Shea B, Grimshaw J, Wells G, et al. Development of AMSTAR: a measurement tool to assess the methodological quality of systematic reviews. BMC Med Res Methodol 2007;7:10.
2. Chung KC, Burns PB, Kim MH. A practical guide to meta-analysis. J Hand Surg 2006;31:1671–8.
3. Yuan Y, Hunt RH. Systematic reviews: the good, the bad, and the ugly. Am J Gastroenterol 2009;104:1086–92.
4. Meta-analysis. In: Bhandari M, Joensson A, eds. Clinical Research for Surgeons. Thieme, New York, 2009.
5. Zlowodzki M, Poolman RW, Kerkhoffs GM, Tornetta P, Bhandari M. How to interpret a meta-analysis and judge its clinical value as a guide for clinical practice. Acta Orthop 2007;78:598–609.
6. Zwahlen M, Renehan A, Egger M. Meta-analysis in medical research: Potentials and limitations. Urol Oncol 2008;26:320–9.
7. De Sousa MR, Ribeiro AL. Systematic review and meta-analysis of diagnostic and prognostic studies: a tutorial. Arq Bras Cardiol 2008;92:229–38.
8. Bhandari M, Devereaux PJ, Montori V, Cina C. Users' guide to the surgical literature: how to use a systematic literature review and meta-analysis. Can J Surgery 2004;47:60–7.
9. Cook DJ, Mulrow CD, Haynes BR. Systematic reviews: synthesis of best evidence for clinical decisions. Am Coll Phys 1997;126:376–80.
10. Montori VM, Smieja M, Guyatt GH. Publication bias: a brief review for clinicians. Mayo Clin Proc 2000;75:1284–8.
11. Chan KS, Morton SC, Shekelle PG. Systematic reviews for evidence-based management: how to find them and what to do with them. Am J Managed Care 2004;10:806–12.
12. McAuley L, Pham B, Tugwell P, Moher D. Does the inclusion of grey literature Influence estimates of intervention effectiveness reported in meta-analysis? Lancet 2000;356:1228–31.

Economic Analysis

6

Laura Quigley[1], Sheila Sprague[2], and Theodore Miclau III[3]

[1]University of Toronto, Toronto, ON, Canada
[2]McMaster University, Hamilton, ON, Canada
[3]University of California, San Francisco, CA, USA

Importance of economic analyses

With rising healthcare costs, it is important for decision-makers to efficiently allocate resources. Between 1970 and 2008, the percentage of the United States gross domestic product (GDP) spent on health care has increased from 7.1% to 16%.[1] Economic evaluations are important because people, time, facilities, equipment, and knowledge are scarce resources, and choices need to be made in order to determine optimal utilization.[2,3] Economic analyses identify, measure, value, and compare alternative courses of action in terms of costs and consequences.[2,3] They provide standardized, quantitative estimates of the likely cost per unit of health benefit achieved by a given procedure, which help reach the primary goal of identifying procedures that produce the greatest health benefit for a given cost.[1] The breadth of outcomes considered varies according to the type of economic analysis performed. Furthermore, the costs and benefits considered vary depending on the viewpoint adopted in the analysis. Thus, economic analyses vary in scope, perspective, applicability, and complexity.[4] Economic analyses in orthopedic surgery are particularly important, as this field has experienced tremendous growth and innovation over the past two decades.[4]

Top six questions

1. What are the different types of economic analyses?
2. Which costs are included in an economic analysis?
3. What perspective is adopted in an economic analysis and how does this affect the costs included?
4. What is the time horizon adopted in an economic analysis?
5. What are sensitivity analyses?
6. How are economic evaluations interpreted?

Question 1: What are the different types of economic analyses?

The four types of economic analyses most commonly reported in the literature are cost-minimization, cost-effectiveness analysis, cost-utility analysis, and cost-benefit analysis. Each of these analyses involves the systematic identification and valuation of the relevant costs and consequences of healthcare interventions.[4]

Cost-minimization analysis

A cost-minimization analysis (CMA) is used to compare cost differences among competing alternative procedures when these treatments produce equivalent outcomes.[3,4] Only the costs of each alternative procedure, which are selected based on the chosen perspective, are considered and the least costly alternative is supported. While CMAs may provide useful information by identifying all of the costs associated with a particular treatment, they can be used to compare treatments only when there is strong clinical evidence that patient outcomes are the same or similar. Otherwise, inclusion of only costs can lead to misleading results.[4]

An example of an appropriate use for a CMA is a comparison of absorbable internal fixation devices (N = 994) and conventional metallic devices (N = 1173) in fracture patients.[5] Several randomized controlled trials (RCTs) comparing these devices have shown no significant difference in outcomes, therefore a CMA is an appropriate analysis

Evidence-Based Orthopedics, First Edition. Edited by Mohit Bhandari.
© 2012 Blackwell Publishing Ltd. Published 2012 by Blackwell Publishing Ltd.

to conduct. The costs included in the CMA resulted from the patients' medical care and their time lost from work. When the costs for an implant removal procedure after metallic fixation were included, the average cost saved per patient by using absorbable implants in fractures of the olecranon was $410. Due to this cost saving, the authors concluded that absorbable implants should be the standard treatment.[5]

Cost-effectiveness analysis

In cost-effectiveness analysis (CEA), both the costs and consequences of health programs are examined.[2] A CEA compares procedures in terms of their monetary value per natural unit of health outcome (i.e., cost per life saved, cost per limb salvaged, etc.).[6] When conducting a CEA, a perspective is selected to identify which costs are included, and the measure of effectiveness is established. It is important to provide a thorough description of the categories of costs included and how the effectiveness data are to be obtained. The medical literature is an important source of effectiveness data; however, an appraisal of the quality of the data is important. In situations where limited or no clinical evidence exists, the CEA may proceed by making assumptions about the clinical evidence, and then undertake *sensitivity analyses* of the economic results with differing assumptions. A sensitivity analysis is a statistical method used to account for uncertainty in an economic analysis.[7] If such analyses reveal that the final result is not sensitive to the estimate used for a given variable, then the inferences made using these data are more robust.[8]

Cost-effectiveness is typically expressed as an *incremental cost-effectiveness ratio (ICER)*. An ICER is an estimate of the additional cost per additional unit of effectiveness of using one treatment in preference to another. In estimating an ICER, the numerator of the ICER is the difference of the mean cost of each procedure, and the denominator is the mean difference of the effectiveness.[3,4,6] The equation for the ICER is:

$$ICER = [Cost_{(Treatment A)} - Cost_{(Treatment B)}]/$$
$$[Effect_{(Treatment A)} - Effect_{(Treatment B)}]$$

Cost-effectiveness studies do not consider subjective factors such as patient preferences and the value of a particular treatment or health state to a patient. One advantage of this technique is that, with a common unit of outcome or effectiveness, different procedures can be compared and can be expressed in terms of cost per unit of outcome. However, CEAs are not helpful for choosing between treatments that have different outcomes or for which the outcomes were measured with different techniques.[4] For example, a study which uses the outcome of life-years saved cannot be easily compared to a study where the outcome is disability days avoided, as these are not common units of effect.

An example of an appropriate cost-effectiveness study would be an evaluation of the cost per successful union in the treatment of open tibial fractures. The first treatment option of intramedullary nailing without reaming may cost $25,000 per patient, whereas treatment by external fixation may cost $20,000. Recent studies report that intramedullary nailing yielded a much lower rate of nonunion (15%) than did external fixation (42%). Thus, even though intramedullary nailing is more costly, it is more cost-effective for the treatment of open tibial fractures because of the lower cost per successful union.[4]

Cost-utility analysis

The cost-utility analysis (CUA) is a form of evaluation that focuses on the quality of the health outcome produced or forgone by health programs.[2] A CUA differs from a CEA because the incremental cost of a program from a particular perspective is compared to the incremental health improvement attributable to the program expressed in terms of a single *utility-based* unit of measurement and not natural units as in a CEA. Examples of utilities include *quality-adjusted life-years (QALYs)* gained and *disability-adjusted life-years (DALYs)* gained, thus the results are expressed as a cost per QALY or DALY gained.[2] An *incremental cost-utility ratio (ICUR)* can be calculated, which is similar to the ICER in a CEA.[2] To value health utility, or benefit, a variety of approaches are adopted, including the *standard gamble (SG), time trade-off (TTO)*, and *visual analog scales (VAS)*. All are based on the value individuals place on not having a particular disease.[5] The consideration of quality recognizes that individuals have different preferences for certain states of health.[5]

Definitions

- **QALY:** Quality-adjusted life-years is a measure of life expectancy weighted by the quality of life.[3] A QALY is computed as a year of life gained, multiplied by the utility score during that year, which is expressed on a scale of 0 to 1.[6]
- **Standard gamble:** Respondents considering a particular health state find the balance between a chance of returning to perfect health and a risk of possibly dying in the process.[6]
- **Time trade-off:** Respondents find the point of balance between a shorter life in perfect health vs. a longer life in the health state under investigation.[6]
- **Utility:** A term used by health economists for the strength of preference for a state of health, attribute, or procedure.[3,4,6] A higher value is placed on time spent in good health and a lower value is placed on time spent with impaired physical and emotional function.[4] The values range from 0 to 1 (perfect health).[3,7]
- **Visual analog scale:** Respondents indicate the desirability of a health state on a line with well-defined endpoints, usually from 0 to 1.21.[6]

By converting effectiveness data (i.e., Harris hip score) to a common unit of measure (i.e., QALYs gained) a CUA is able to incorporate simultaneously both the changes in the quantity of life (mortality) and the changes in the quality of life (morbidity).[2] Also, the measurement of utilities allows for valid comparisons among multiple treatment options, particularly when alternative treatments produce different outcomes or when longer survival is acquired at the expense of reduced quality of life.[4]

Haentjens et al. provide a practical example of a CUA in which they compare the costs and health outcomes of standard versus prolonged prophylaxis with low molecular weight heparin (LMWH), among patients undergoing elective total hip or knee replacement.[6] The study adopted the perspective of a societal healthcare payer, in this case the Belgian Federal Ministry of Health. Costs were obtained from a panel of orthopedic surgeons and from the Federal Ministry of Health, while QALYs were based on utility scores found in the literature. The authors found that prolonged prophylaxis with LMWH was associated with a cost-utility ratio of €6,964/QALY after total hip replacement and €64,907/QALY after total knee replacement.[9] According to European guidelines, an intervention costing less than €20,000/QALY exhibits strong evidence for adoption while one costing €20,000–100,000/QALY exhibits moderate evidence for adoption.[9] The authors therefore concluded that there is strong evidence for adoption of prolonged enoxaparin prophylaxis among total hip replacement patients, but only moderate evidence for adoption among total knee replacement patients.[9]

Cost-benefit analysis

Cost-benefit analyses (CBA) provide an estimate of the monetary resources consumed by each procedure under study compared to the value of resources the procedure might save.[8] In a CBA both the costs and health outcomes are valued in monetary units.[2–4,6] One method of assigning values to health consequences is by determining a patient's willingness to pay.[4] In practice, it is difficult to quantify health consequences in monetary terms, and ethical issues exist in assigning an amount of money to the value of human life, pain, and suffering.[6] After the costs and consequences are quantified in monetary terms, a direct comparison can be made between the program's incremental costs and its incremental consequences in equal units of measurement.[2] To compare treatment options CBA commonly uses two comparators, the *net present value* and the *cost-benefit ratio*. The net present value is the value of health benefits minus costs, and the cost-benefit ratio is the ratio between the two.[6] CBA has the advantage of allowing direct comparisons across programs. Also, the analysis of a single program can determine whether it is economically worthwhile.[4,6]

Vasen et al. provide an example of a CBA.[10] They compared the total cost of open vs. endoscopic technique for the surgical treatment of carpal tunnel syndrome, from a societal perspective. The costs included those incurred from medical procedures and complications as well as from lost wages. The authors hypothesized the two procedures could have different complication rates and different amounts of time off work. For this study design, outcomes were given a dollar value. Outcomes such as infection and nerve injury were translated as a cost in dollars. All complications except nerve laceration were assigned a cost of the operative correction of the complication plus 1 year's wages, because it is assumed that patients with complications would not return to work for 1 year. Patients with nerve lacerations were assigned the present value of their wage replacement throughout the remainder of their life expectancy in addition to cost of the operative procedure. In the base case, the cost (including surgery, complications, and wages) of the open technique was found to be $6,315 and that of the endoscopic technique was found to be $5,896, indicating that the endoscopic technique is the less costly alternative.[10]

Question 2: Which costs are included in an economic analysis?

The costs included in an economic analysis will vary on the basis of the time frame and perspective being considered in the study. Ideally, a thorough economic analysis measures direct, indirect, and intangible costs. Direct medical costs include all costs that are directly related to the procedure, including those for personnel, supplies, and the facility involved in the treatment. Direct nonmedical costs include costs borne by patients and their families in the course of treatment (i.e., transportation).[4] Indirect costs include costs associated with lost productivity, usually valued as lost wages or a monetary value of time. For determination of intangible costs, an attempt is made to assign a dollar value to reductions in quality of life. Those costs are often included in the measurement of QALYs. It is also important to consider the downstream costs of resources that will be consumed in the future but are still attributable to the procedure.[4] An allowance for the differential timing of costs and consequences due to time preference is also required. Thus, economic analyses should discount costs, and the rates of three and five percent are recommended.[2]

Question 3: Which perspective is adopted in an economic analysis and how does this affect the costs included?

Before beginning any economic analysis, the perspective of the analysis needs to be determined and explicitly stated.

Perspectives that can be adopted include that of the government, the hospital, the primary payer, or society.[7] If the economic analysis is completed from a governmental perspective, an interest in identifying the employment costs may be apparent.[8] The hospital perspective includes only costs that are incurred by the hospital, such as the costs of the surgery, costs of diagnostic tests, the cost of the medical device, the cost of the medications the patient takes during their hospital stay, and the cost of staying in the hospital ward. In contrast, the perspective of the primary payer includes all medical costs that are covered by the primary payer, in addition to those incurred in the hospital. For example, both in-hospital costs and costs after the patient has been discharged are included (e.g., home care and medications).[7] The societal perspective includes all costs related to the treatments and is not limited to medical costs. Examples of additional costs include time lost from employment and all patient expenses.[7] The societal perspective is generally recommended, especially if the analysis will otherwise overlook an important financial burden to the patient, their family, and society in general.[7]

Question 4: What is the time horizon adopted in an economic analysis?

The time horizon of a healthcare economic evaluation is the period of time for which the costs and outcomes are measured. The time horizon should be specified and justified as being appropriate for the clinical condition being studied. Other time-sensitive issues that should be considered include technological improvements and overall societal well-being that occur over time, as well as the learning curve effect that follows the introduction of a new technology.[4]

Question 5: What are sensitivity analyses?

Sensitivity analyses are a method of accounting for uncertainty in an economic analysis.[7] Sensitivity analyses are utilized to assess the impacts of various model parameters or assumptions on the study results.[2,4] There are three key elements to consider when conducting a sensitivity analysis: (1) how the uncertain parameters are identified; (2) how the plausible ranges for the variables are specified; and (3) whether an appropriate form of sensitivity analysis is used.[2]

There are five different forms of sensitivity analyses. The simplest is the *one-way analysis*. Estimates for each parameter are varied one at a time in order to investigate the impact on study results.[2] A *multi-way analysis* recognizes that more than one parameter is uncertain and that each could vary within its specified range.[2] In a *scenario analysis*, a series of scenarios is constructed to represent a subset of the potential multi-way analyses. The scenarios typically include the most realistic (best guess), optimistic (best case), and pessimistic (worst case). The analyst may also include scenarios that they feel are applicable.[2] A *threshold analysis* identifies the critical value(s) of a parameter or parameters central to the decision. The analyst can then assess which combinations of parameter estimates could cause the threshold to be exceeded.[2] Alternatively, the threshold values for key parameters that would cause the program to be too costly or not cost-effective could be identified.[2] The fifth form of sensitivity analysis is the *probabilistic sensitivity analysis*. In this type of analysis, probability distributions are applied to the specified ranges for the key parameters. Samples are then drawn randomly from these distributions to generate an empirical distribution of the cost-effectiveness ratio.[2] If the sensitivity analysis for an economic evaluation reveals that the final result is not sensitive to the estimate of a given variable, then the inference made using these data are stronger.[8]

Question 6: How are economic evaluations interpreted?

The goal of an economic evaluation is generally to compare two treatment options in order to select the one that provides the maximum health benefit for a given increment of cost. There are nine possible outcomes when comparing one procedure to another in a CEA (Figure 6.1).[2] In particular, cell 1 in Figure 6.1 shows that the new procedure is less expensive and more effective than the standard treatment, and should be adopted. In cell 2, the new procedure costs more and is less effective than the standard treatment, and should not be adopted. The most common case is when a new procedure is both more effective and more costly (cell 7). In this case, the hospital administration, surgeon, and patient need to determine if the increased effectiveness is worth the additional cost.[2] When the result falls into a nondominance cell (cells 7–9) it may be useful to calculate the ICER or ICUR of the new procedure.[4] Additionally, guidelines exist to recommend whether to adopt or reject a new procedure. For example, in North America US$50,000/QALY is often recommended as a threshold for a cost-effectiveness procedure. Procedures which have an incremental cost higher than this are likely to be rejected.[7] For example, in the study by Haentjens et al. described previously,[9] the European guidelines for CUAs indicate that a procedure costing less than €20,000/QALY exhibits strong evidence for adoption, whereas one costing €20,000–100,000/QALY exhibits moderate evidence for adoption. Thus, according to these standards, the authors found strong evidence for adoption of prolonged prophylaxis among total hip replacement patients, and moderate evidence for adoption among total knee replacement patients. Sensitivity analyses incorporating 20% changes from the base-case analysis showed this outcome to be robust.[9]

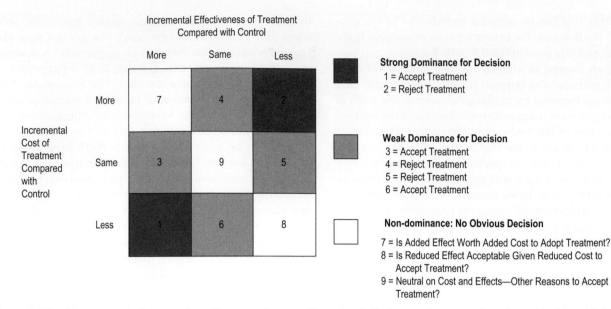

Figure 6.1 Possible outcomes in the comparison of incremental costs and incremental effectiveness of two procedures. (Reproduced from Methods for the Economic Evaluation of Health Care Programmes (Third Edition) by Michael F. Drummond, Mark J. Sculpher, George W. Torrance, Bernie J. O'Brien and Greg L. Stoddart (2005), Figure: Box 2.2, p. 13. By permission of Oxford University Press.)

Lastly, it is important to assess whether the conclusions of another study are applicable to the clinician's own practice (i.e., in terms of patient population, practice patterns, level of resource consumption, and relative costs).[4]

Conclusions

In view of rising healthcare spending, it is becoming increasingly important to use the most cost-effective health program that fits within the available budget. The use of economic analyses can help determine which health program provides the greatest effect at lowest cost. It is important to carefully consider the perspective, time horizon, discount rate, and sensitivity analyses when interpreting economic analyses. High-quality economic analyses are important for orthopedic research.

References

1. Organisation for Economic Co-operation and Development. OECD Health Data 2010—Selected data: Health Expenditure. Accessed from: http://stats.oecd.org/Index.aspx?DataSetCode=SOCX_AGG

2. Drummond MF, Sculpher MJ, Torrance GW, O'Brien BJ, Stoddart GL. Methods for the Economic Evaluation of Health Care Programmes, 3rd edn. Oxford University Press, New York, 2005.

3. Myers J, McCabe S, Gohmann S. Economic analysis in hand surgery. J Hand Surg Am 2006;31(4):664–8.

4. Bozic KJ, Rosenberg AG, Huckman RS, Herndon JH. Economic evaluation in orthopaedics. J Bone Joint Surg Am 2003;85:129–42.

5. Bostman OM. Metallic or absorbable fracture fixation devices. A cost minimization analysis. Clin Orthop 1996;329:233–9.

6. Haentjens P, Annemans L. Health economics and the orthopaedic surgeon. J Bone Joint Surg Br 2003;85(8):1093–9.

7. Sprague S, Quigley L, Adili A, Bhandari M. Understanding cost effectiveness: money matters? J Long Term Eff Med Implants 2007;17(2):145–52.

8. Busse JW, Heetveld MJ. Critical appraisal of the orthopaedic literature: Therapeutic and economic analysis. Injury 2006;37(4):312–20.

9. Haentjens P, De Groote K, Annemans L. Prolonged enoxaparin therapy to prevent venous thromboembolism after primary hip or knee replacement. A cost-utility analysis. Arch Orthop Trauma Surg 2004;124(8):507–17.

10. Vasen AP, Kuntz KM, Simmons BP, Katz JN. Open versus endoscopic carpal tunnel release: a decision analysis. J Hand Surg Am 1999;24(5):1109–17.

Orthopedic Medicine

7 Osteoporosis and Metabolic Disorders

Celeste J. Hamilton[1,2], Sophie A. Jamal[1,2], and Earl R. Bogoch[2,3]

[1]Women's College Hospital, Toronto, ON, Canada
[2]University of Toronto, Toronto, ON, Canada
[3]St. Michael's Hospital, Toronto, ON, Canada

Case scenario

A 70 year old ambulatory white woman who is living independently is brought to the Emergency Department after slipping and falling in her bathtub. She is unable to weight bear and is complaining of pain in the right groin area. Radiography reveals a right femoral neck fracture and she is subsequently sent to surgery for fracture repair.

Relevant anatomy

Hip fractures are anatomically classified as *intracapsular* or *extracapsular* depending on the site of the fracture in relation to the insertion of the capsule of the hip joint on to the proximal femur. Femoral neck (*intracapsular*) and intertrochanteric (*extracapsular*) fractures are the most common types of hip fractures in patients with osteoporosis.[1] Biomechanically, osteoporotic fractures occur due to skeletal fragility (from decreased bone quantity or impaired bone quality) and/or from falling.[2] The greater trochanter is generally the point of impact in a fall, making the femoral neck particularly vulnerable to fractures.[3]

Importance of the problem

Osteoporosis is characterized by a reduction in bone mass and a disruption of skeletal microarchitecture leading to an increased susceptibility to fracture with minimal trauma.[4] Over 200 million people worldwide suffer from osteoporosis[5] and osteoporotic fractures account for 0.83% of the global burden of noncommunicable disease.[6] In the year 2000, there were an estimated 9 million osteoporotic fractures worldwide, of which 1.6 million were hip fractures, 1.7 million were forearm fractures, and 1.4 million were vertebral fractures.[6] The lifetime risk of any osteoporotic fracture is 40–50% in women and 13–22% in men.[7]

Hip fractures are the most severe type of osteoporotic fracture as they require hospital admission and are associated with significant morbidity and mortality.[7] At 1 year post hip fracture, mortality (in part due to other comorbidities) ranges from 12% to 20%,[7] with the majority of deaths occurring within the first few months after fracture. An excess risk of death may persist for at least 5 years afterwards.[8] Globally, there are approximately 740,000 deaths per year due to hip fracture and resulting complications.[9] Loss of function and independence among survivors is also profound, with 40% of patients unable to walk independently and 60% requiring assistance a year later.[10] Hip fracture risk rises exponentially with age[11] and as populations age, annual numbers of hip fractures are expected to escalate. The long-term costs associated with hip fractures are also devastating. By the year 2041, annual economic implications of hip fracture are expected to reach $9.8 billion in the United States and $650 million in Canada.[12]

Top five questions

Diagnosis

1. Are hip fracture patients receiving appropriate evaluation and treatment for osteoporosis?
2. How do I decide which fragility fracture patients are at high risk for future fracture and which patients to treat pharmacologically?

Evidence-Based Orthopedics, First Edition. Edited by Mohit Bhandari.
© 2012 Blackwell Publishing Ltd. Published 2012 by Blackwell Publishing Ltd.

Therapy

3. What medications reduce the risk of hip fracture?

4. Does starting bisphosphonate therapy interfere with fracture healing?

Harm

5. What are the side effects associated with long-term bisphosphonate therapy?

Question 1: Are hip fracture patients receiving appropriate evaluation and treatment for osteoporosis?

Case clarification

After fracture repair, the patient is sent for bone mineral density (BMD) testing by dual-energy X-ray absorptiometry (DXA) and has blood tests to rule out secondary causes of osteoporosis.

> The diagnosis of osteoporosis is determined by measuring a patient's BMD [the average concentration of bone mineral (g) per unit of bone area (cm^2)]. BMD is measured using DXA, the gold standard method of measurement.

Relevance

The presence of a hip or other fragility fracture is a major risk factor for osteoporosis, especially in patients aged 50 years or older, and is an important indicator for osteoporosis diagnosis and treatment.[13] Orthopedic surgeons are in an ideal position either individually or collaboratively with colleagues to initiate and provide osteoporosis care for patients with fragility fractures, as they are the first physicians to make contact with the patient following fracture.

Current opinion

Current opinion suggests that many patients who sustain hip or other fragility fractures do not receive appropriate evaluation or treatment for osteoporosis.

Finding the evidence

- Cochrane Database with search terms: "osteoporosis care gap"
- MEDLINE (1996 to August Week 1 2009) and Embase (1980 to 2009 Week 33) search strategy:
  1 exp Osteoporosis/ or osteoporosis.mp.
  2 exp Physician's Practice Patterns/ or osteoporosis care gap.mp.
  3 1 and 2
  4 limit 3 to (English language and humans)

- A review of reference lists of relevant articles for additional published trials

Quality of the evidence

Level I
- 3 systematic reviews or meta-analyses
- 6 randomized controlled trials

Findings

A recent systematic review of 35 studies that evaluated practice patterns relating to osteoporosis management after fragility fracture found that recognition and treatment of osteoporosis in these patients remained inadequate,[14] confirming the persistence of an earlier identified global osteoporosis care gap.[15] In this review, a clinical diagnosis of osteoporosis was reported in less than 30% of patients in the majority of studies. Further, DXA scans were performed in less than 15% of patients in studies that reported on BMD testing. More than half of the studies reported that no more than 30% of fracture patients were taking calcium and vitamin D and less than 15% of patients were receiving bisphosphonate therapy.

Despite these alarming statistics, over the past decade international awareness has grown regarding the need for effective osteoporosis management in high-risk patient groups, such as those with hip and other fragility fractures. While there are evident barriers to osteoporosis care in the orthopedic environment,[16] the initiation and development of various intervention programs has facilitated a consistent improvement in osteoporosis diagnosis and treatment rates. A summary of randomized controlled trials that have piloted various interventions to improve the diagnosis and treatment of osteoporosis in patients with hip fractures is outlined in Table 7.1. A total of six randomized controlled trials were identified,[17–22] all of which demonstrated significant improvements in osteoporosis diagnosis and treatment rates among patients randomized to an intervention vs. those receiving usual care. Several different intervention models proved to be effective including: (1) direct evaluation and management of osteoporosis by an orthopedic surgeon within a specialized osteoporosis clinic;[22] (2) use of a clinical coordinator to identify, educate, and refer patients for treatment with their primary care physician;[18,20,21] and (3) mail-outs or e-mail notifications to patients or primary care physicians about guidelines and recommendations for osteoporosis management.[17,19] The common thread among these models was the establishment of effective communication between the orthopedic surgeon, patient, and primary care physician.

The most successful model to date appears to be the *clinical coordinator model*. In addition to evidence from randomized trials, there is a substantial body of literature from nonrandomized data supporting this program type in reference to hip as well as other fragility fractures.[23–25] In the

Table 7.1 Summary of randomized controlled trials to improve the diagnosis and treatment of osteoporosis in patients with hip fracture

Reference	Population	Fracture site and etiology	Intervention	Results
Miki et al. 2008[22]	INT: n = 26 CON: n = 24 Mean age 79.2 yrs 71% female	Hip Low trauma	INT: In hospital OP evaluation including BMD scans of the hip and spine and blood work. Started 1500 mg calcium and 800 IU vitamin D daily and were booked for a follow-up appointment in the orthopaedic OP clinic up to 1 month post-operatively. At follow-up, clinic team reviewed results of the BMD scans and lab work and prescribed risedronate 35 mg. Follow-up visits and/or phone calls at 2 months and 6 months. Care transferred to primary physician at 6 months. CON: Started 1500 mg calcium and 800 IU vitamin D daily. Asked to approach family physician for an osteoporosis evaluation. Follow-up phone call at 6 months.	The percentage of patients (58%) who were on pharmacologic treatment for OP at 6 mo postfracture was significantly greater when the evaluation was initiated by the orthopaedic surgeon and was managed in a specialized orthopaedic OP clinic vs. treatment managed by a primary care physician (29%) (p = 0.04)
Gardener et al. 2005[20]	INT: n = 36 CON: n = 36 Mean age 82 yrs 78% female	Hip Low trauma	INT: Prior to discharge received a 15 min discussion from clinical coordinator about the association between OP and hip fractures, the efficacy of DXA scans in the diagnosis of OP and bisphosphonates in its treatment, and the importance of medical follow-up for OP management. Received 5 questions regarding OP treatment to be given to their primary care physician. Follow-up call 6 weeks later to remind them about the questions and at 6 months to determine if OP had been addressed. CON: At discharge received a 2-page pamphlet on fall prevention. Follow-up phone call at 6 months to determine if OP had been addressed.	A greater percentage of patients in the intervention group (42% vs. 19%) had their OP assessed by their primary physician (p = 0.036)
Davis et al. 2007[18]	INT: n = 28 Mean age 80.4 yrs 75% female CON: n = 20 Mean age 82.6yrs 65% female	Hip Low trauma	INT (PEPA): (a) Usual care for the fracture including surgical treatment (b) OP information and a letter for the patients that encouraged them to return to their primary care physicians for further investigation (c) A request for patients to take a letter from the orthopedic surgeon to their primary care physician alerting that physician to the hip fracture and encouraging OP investigation (d) A telephone call at 3 months and 6 months to determine whether OP investigation and treatment had occurred. CON: (a) Usual care for the fracture including surgical treatment (b) A telephone call at 3 months (general health inquiry) and 6 months to determine whether OP investigation and treatment had occurred.	PEPA group 68% were offered one or more components of best practice care compared with 35% in the usual care group (p < 0.05) 54% PEPA prescribed bisphosphonate therapy vs. 0% CON (p < 0.01) 29% PEPA had a BMD scan vs. 0% CON (p < 0.01) 39% PEPA prescribed calcium and vitamin d vs. 30% CON (p = 0.32) 32% PEPA were prescribed exercise vs. 0% CON (p < 0.01)
Bliuc et al. 2006[17]	INT1: n = 75 47% <50 yrs; 53% ≥ 50 yrs 51% female INT2: n = 79 54% <50 yrs; 46% ≥50 yrs 59% female	Any site Minimal or moderate trauma	Intervention initiated 3 months postfracture if patients had not been investigated or treated for OP by their primary care physician. INT1: Patients sent a personalized letter that outlined their risk factors for OP and recommended follow-up with their primary care physician. Follow-up phone call at 6 months. INT2: Same personalized letter plus an offer of a free BMD assessment. Follow-up telephone call at 6 months.	Significant increase in the number of people investigated for OP in the group receiving the letter plus BMD offer: 38%(letter + BMD) vs 7% (letter only); p = 0.001 Rates of treatment in both groups were very low (6%)

(Continued)

Table 7.1 (Continued)

Reference	Population	Fracture site and etiology	Intervention	Results
Majumdar et al. 2007[21]	INT: n = 110 CON: n = 110 Median age 74 yrs 60% female	Hip Any etiology	INT: Case manager provided one-on-one counseling about importance of BMD testing and the ability of bisphosphonate therapy and other treatments to reduce the risk of future fractures and arranged for a BMD test. Based on BMD results, case manager discussed risks and benefits of bisphosphonate therapy and arranged treatment for appropriate patients. All results and treatment plans communicated to the patient's primary care physician. CON: Study personnel provided counseling on fall prevention and the need for additional intake of calcium and vitamin D. Patients given educational materials on OP and were asked to discuss the materials with their primary care physician. 6 month follow-up	At 6 months postfracture 51% of patients in INT were receiving bisphosphonate therapy compared with 22% in CON group (adjusted odds ratio, 4.7; 95% CI, 2.4–8.9; p < 0.001) BMD tests performed in 80% of patients in INT group vs 29% in CON (p < 0.001)
Feldstein et al. 2006[19]	INT1: n = 101 34.6% 50–69 yrs 65.4% 70–89 yrs INT2: n = 109 37.6% 50–69 yrs 62.4% 10–89 yrs CON: n = 101 36.6% 50–69 yrs 63.4% 70–89 yrs	Any site No open fractures	INT1: Primary care physician sent a patient-specific EMR providing clinical guideline advice on OP. 3 months later another EMR sent to physicians who had not ordered a BMD or prescribed pharmacological treatment for enrolled study patients. INT2: Same as INT1 plus patients received a single mailing of an advisory letter identifying their risk, discussing clinical guideline recommendations and requesting that they discuss OP management options with a primary care physician. Educational materials were also included. CON: Usual care 6 month follow-up	At 6 months, provider reminder resulted in 51.5% of patients receiving BMD measurement or OP meds, provider reminder plus patient education resulted in 43.1% and usual care resulted in 5.9% (p < 0.001) Effect of provider advice combined with patient education was not significantly different from provider advice alone (p = 0.88)

BMD, bone mineral density; CON, control; DXA, dual-energy x-ray absorptiometry; EMR, electronic medical record; INT intervention; IU, international units; OP, osteoporosis; PEPA patient empowerment and physician alerting.

coordinator model, a staff member in the fracture clinic (termed the coordinator) is assigned the task of identifying patients with probable fragility fractures. The coordinator then works with the orthopedic surgeon and other health professionals to educate the patient and ensure appropriate treatment and follow-up with the family physician. The coordinator program has been shown to be both effective[23] and cost-effective,[26] and the challenge today is to allocate systems and resources to facilitate this kind of care. A similar model that has been effective in Glasgow (UK) is termed a fracture liaison service.[25]

Recommendations

In patients aged 50 years or older who have sustained a hip or other fragility fracture, evidence suggests that:
• Many patients are not receiving appropriate evaluation and treatment for osteoporosis postfracture [overall quality: high]

• Significant progress has been made towards developing and implementing programs to address this care gap [overall quality: high]

Question 2: How do I decide which fragility fracture patients are at high risk for future fracture and which patients to treat pharmacologically?

Case clarification

The DXA scan reveals that the patient has a T-score of −2.0 at the lumbar spine (L1–L4), a T-score of −3.9 at the left femoral neck and a T-score of −4.1 at the left total hip. On further questioning, the patient discloses that she has had a prior wrist fracture at age 55 and that her mother had a hip fracture. She is not taking oral steroids, does not have rheumatoid arthritis, does not smoke, and drinks less than one drink per month. Blood tests to identify secondary causes of osteoporosis were negative.

> A T-score is the number of standard deviations (SD) above or below the mean value of BMD for young adults (20–30 years old). The World Health Organization (WHO) defines osteoporosis as a T-score of –2.5 or less at the hip or lumbar spine.

Relevance

Many patients who sustain a fragility fracture do not receive appropriate pharmacologic treatment for underlying osteoporosis.[14] It is important to identify those at high risk for future fracture and those who would benefit from pharmacologic treatment in order to prevent future fractures.

Current opinion

Current opinion suggests that lack of education and training about osteoporosis is an important barrier to orthopedic postfracture care. Opinion is divergent among orthopedic surgeons on which patients should be considered for pharmacologic treatment.

Finding the evidence

- Cochrane Database with search terms: "osteoporosis and treatment guidelines"
- MEDLINE (1996 to August Week 1 2009) and Embase (1980 to 2009 Week 33) search strategy:
  1 exp Osteoporosis/di [Diagnosis]
  2 exp Practice Guideline/
  3 2 and 1
  4 limit 3 to (English language and humans)
- A review of reference lists of relevant articles for additional published trials

Quality of the evidence

Level I
- 8 systematic reviews or meta-analyses
- 3 clinical practice guidelines

Findings

Until recently, decisions about osteoporosis therapy were made based on the presence or absence of fractures and on T-score values ≤ –2.5 SD from DXA measurements of BMD. Although low BMD is a strong and independent risk factor for fracture,[27,28] it is not the only one. Indeed, most fractures occur in women with osteopenia (T-score between –1.0 and –2.5 SD) and not osteoporosis.[29] The main reason for this observation is that BMD measures bone quantity and does not take into account bone quality. Bone quality represents essentially all of the other characteristics of bone tissue other than BMD that contribute to the strength of a bone such as geometry, microarchitecture, remodeling, mineralization and damage accumulation.[30] It is the interplay between both quantitative and qualitative factors that ultimately determines the fragility of a bone and its susceptibility to fracture.[31] For this reason, recent treatment guidelines have focused on evaluating a patient's absolute fracture risk, which considers BMD as well as other clinical risk factors for fracture that are thought to capture some aspects of bone quality.

The World Health Organization (WHO) has developed an international Fracture Risk Assessment Tool (FRAX®), that can be used to compute the 10-year probability of fractures in men and women based on clinical risk factors for fracture (which represent bone quality), with or without the measurement of femoral neck BMD.[32] The algorithms used in the FRAX model are based on a series of meta-analyses using primary data from population-based cohorts that have identified several clinical risk factors for fracture.[33] The performance characteristics of the clinical risk factors have been validated in independent, population-based prospectively studied cohorts with over a million person years of observation.[33] The FRAX tool calculates the 10-year probability of a major osteoporotic fracture (clinical spine, hip, forearm, or proximal humerus) and hip fracture calibrated to the fracture and death hazard of several countries.[34]

The FRAX calculation tool is available for public use online at http://www.shef.ac.uk/FRAX/index.htm. After selecting an appropriate country of origin, a patient's 10-year fracture risk probability can be determined by answering a simple set of 12 questions pertaining to the patient's clinical risk factors for fracture (Table 7.2). Current fracture risk cutoffs for the tool are based on cost effectiveness. For example, low bone mass (T-score between –1.0 and –2.5 at the femoral neck or spine) and a 10-year probability of a hip fracture ≥ 3% or a 10-year probability of a major osteoporosis-related fracture ≥ 20% was shown to be cost-effective in the USA.[35] In a study from the UK, the fracture risk in women with a history of osteoporotic fracture was selected as the treatment cutoff, corresponding to a risk level of 7.5%.[32] It should be noted that cutoffs have not been established for all countries that can utilize the FRAX tool.

While the FRAX tool facilitates the determination of who is at high risk for fracture, by assessing quantity and indirectly quality, it does have several limitations. Although FRAX is an international tool, it is suitable for use only in those countries for which epidemiological data are available.[36] The set of clinical risk factors used in the FRAX tool also has limitations. For instance, several risk factors can be indicated only as present or absent ("yes" or "no") in the question set, such as glucocorticoid therapy or previous fracture. However, there is evidence that the risk associated with the use of glucocorticoids is dose responsive.[37,38] In

Table 7.2 List of clinical risk factors included in the WHO Fracture Risk Assessment Model (FRAX)

Clinical risk factor
Geographic region
Race
Sex
Weight
Height
Prior fragility fracture
Parent with hip fracture
Glucocorticoid use (≥5 mg/day of prednisone for ≥3 mo ever)
Rheumatoid arthritis
Secondary osteoporosis
Current smoking
Alcohol intake (≥3 or more drinks/day)

WHO, World Health Organization.

addition, the risk of future fracture increases progressively with the number of prior fractures.[39] Further, only femoral neck BMD is taken into account by FRAX, as it was the only site for which BMD data was available for all of the study cohorts. BMD measurement by DXA at the femoral neck site is difficult as accurate measurements require correct rotation of the femur and positioning of the region of interest by the technician. As a result, considerable variability in femoral neck BMD may occur. However, it should be noted that a patient's fracture risk probability can be obtained without entering BMD data into the FRAX tool, emphasizing again the importance of factors other than BMD on future fracture risk. Additionally, the FRAX tool can only be used to assess previously untreated patients.

Although the FRAX tool is available for use internationally, it is not incorporated into all sets of treatment guidelines for osteoporosis worldwide. Treatment guidelines for osteoporosis vary by country, and only some countries recommend the use of the FRAX tool. A summary of North American and European guidelines for fracture risk assessment and treatment of osteoporosis is presented in Table 7.3. The US National Osteoporosis Foundation (NOF)[40] and the European Society for Clinical and Economic Aspects of Osteoporosis and Osteoarthritis (ESCEO)[41] both recommend the use of the FRAX tool to calculate absolute fracture risk in their treatment guidelines for osteoporosis. The Osteoporosis Canada 2010 Guidelines[42] suggest the use of one of two closely related tools for estimating 10-year risk of major osteoporotic fracture: the FRAX tool or the Canadian Association of Radiologists/Osteoporosis Canada (CAROC) tool. Both were calibrated using the same Canadian fracture data and were validated in Canadians.[43–45] The CAROC tool stratifies men and women over age 50 into three 10-year major osteoporotic

fracture risk zones (low, moderate, and high). An initial risk category is obtained from age, sex, and T-score at the femoral neck. Clinical risk factors—the presence of a prior fragility fracture after age 40 or recent prolonged systemic glucocorticoid use—increase fracture risk independent of BMD.

Recommendations

In patients aged 50 years or older who have sustained a fragility fracture, and have not received prior pharmacologic treatment, evidence suggests that:

- The FRAX tool can be used to calculate the 10-year probability of a major osteoporotic fracture (clinical spine, hip, forearm, or proximal humerus) and hip fracture [overall quality: high]
- Alternative methods are also available to determine absolute fracture risk [overall quality: high]
- Treatment decisions should be patient specific and guidelines developed by the appropriate country of origin should be considered [overall quality: high]

Question 3: What medications reduce the risk of hip fracture?

Case clarification

A complete dietary history reveals that the patient consumes 1 glass of milk (350 mg dietary calcium), 1000 mg of elemental calcium in the form of supplements, and 800 IU of vitamin D per day. She is not currently taking any prescription medications.

Recommended daily calcium and vitamin D intakes for populations vary by country. The Institute of Medicine (IOM) recommends a daily calcium intake of 1000 mg for men 51–70 years and 1200 mg for women. For men and women 71 years of age and older the recommendation is 1200 mg per day. Vitamin D recommendations are 600 IUs a day for men and women 51–70 years of age and 800 IUs per day for men and women 71 years of age and older

Relevance

A number of different pharmacologic agents are available for the treatment of osteoporosis.[46] Opinion among orthopedic surgeons is divergent on which pharmacologic agents are best to reduce the relative risk of hip fractures in postmenopausal women who present with low BMD or a prior fragility fracture.

Current opinion

Current opinion suggests that orthopedic surgeons prescribe a variety of different pharmacologic agents for the treatment of fragility fractures.

Table 7.3 North American and European guidelines for fracture risk assessment and treatment of osteoporosis

Continent	Fracture risk assessment	Treatment guidelines
North America (USA)[a]	WHO Fracture Risk Assessment Tool (FRAX)	Postmenopausal women and men age 50 and older presenting with the following should be considered for treatment: • A hip or vertebral (clinical or morphometric) fracture. • T-score ≤–2.5 at the femoral neck or spine after appropriate evaluation to exclude secondary causes • Low bone mass (T-score between –1.0 and –2.5 at the femoral neck or spine) and a 10-year probability of a hip fracture ≥3% or a 10-year probability of a major osteoporosis-related fracture ≥20% based on the US-adapted WHO algorithm
North America (Canada)[b]	Approach 1: WHO FRAX Approach 2: Canadian Association of Radiologists/Osteoporosis Canada (CAROC) 1 Select the table appropriate for the patient's sex 2 Identify the row that is closest to the patient's age 3 Determine the patient's absolute fracture risk category by using the lowest T-score from the recommended skeletal sites (lumbar spine, total hip, femoral neck, and trochanter, with forearm 1/3 radius if either spine or hip is not valid) 4 Evaluate clinical factors that may move the patient into a higher fracture risk category (fragility fractures after 40 yrs of age and current systemic glucocorticoid therapy >3 mo raise the patient to the next higher risk category; if both factors are present, move to high risk) Determine the patient's absolute fracture risk category	Approach 1 Determine fracture risk category using the WHO FRAX® tool Approach 2 Absolute fracture risk categories: • Low risk (<10%, 10-yr fracture risk) • Moderate risk (10–20%, 10-yr fracture risk) • High risk (>20%, 10-yr fracture risk) In both approaches, a patient's fracture risk category is the basis for deciding on treatment and frequency of BMD monitoring
Europe[c]	No universally accepted policy for population screening in Europe to identify patients with osteoporosis or those at high risk of fracture Patients are identified opportunistically using a case-finding strategy on the finding of a previous fragility fracture or the presence of significant risk factors Approach 1: BMD as intervention threshold Approach 2: WHO FRAX	Approach 1 • Postmenopausal women with a previous fracture can be considered for treatment without the need for a BMD test • Postmenopausal women with other clinical risk factors should be considered for BMD testing, and treatment should be considered where the T-score for BMD at the femoral neck is –1.0 SD or lower for postmenopausal women with a parental history of hip fracture, –2.0 SDs in women committed to long-term oral glucocorticoids, and –2.5 SD or lower for women with rheumatoid arthritis, who smoke or who drink 3 units of alcohol or more daily Approach 2 • Postmenopausal women with prior fragility fracture should be considered for treatment • FRAX probability determines whether the patient is above or below the intervention threshold for treatment. The intervention threshold at each age is set at a risk equivalent to that associated with a prior fracture and therefore rises with age

BMD, bone mineral density; SD, standard deviation; WHO, World Health Organization.
[a] US National Osteoporosis Foundation Guidelines[40].
[b] Canadian Association of Radiologist/Osteoporosis Canada Guidelines[42].
[c] European Society for Clinical and Economic Aspects of Osteoporosis and Osteoarthritis Guidelines[41].

Finding the evidence

- Cochrane Database with search terms: "osteoporosis and treatment and hip fracture"
- MEDLINE (1996 to August Week 1 2009) and Embase (1980 to 2009 Week 33) search strategy:
  1 exp Bone Density Conservation Agents/tu [Therapeutic Use]
  2 exp Hip Fractures/
  3 1 and 2
  4 limit 3 to (English language and humans)
- A review of reference lists of relevant articles for additional published trials

Quality of the evidence
Level I
- 8 systematic reviews or meta-analyses
- 18 randomized controlled trials

Findings

The majority of pharmacologic agents available for the treatment of osteoporosis are antiresorptive agents, which include bisphosphonates (oral or intravenous), hormone replacement therapy (HRT), raloxifene, denosumab, and calcitonin. Other available agents are parathyroid hormone (an anabolic agent) and strontium ranelate (a combination antiresorptive and anabolic agent).[46] A summary of the efficacy of pharmacologic agents on the relative risk reduction of hip fractures is presented in Table 7.4. As the majority of pivotal clinical trials were in postmenopausal women, data in men is limited and will not be reviewed.

A recent review article[47] summarized the efficacy results from pivotal clinical trials of four commonly prescribed bisphosphonates—alendronate, risedronate, ibandronate and zoledronic acid—for the treatment of postmenopausal osteoporosis. A total of 11 randomized placebo-controlled trials were identified (3 for alendronate,[48–50] 4 for risedronate,[51–54] 2 for ibandronate,[55,56] and 2 for zoledronic acid[57,58]). Compared with placebo controls, alendronate, risedronate, and zoledronic acid but not ibandronate (no available hip data) were found to reduce the relative risk of hip fractures in postmenopausal women with low BMD and/or prior vertebral fracture by 30% to 51%. Similarly, two randomized placebo-controlled trials looking at the fracture efficacy of HRT in postmenopausal women with[59] and without[60] hysterectomy demonstrated that HRT could reduce the relative risk of hip fracture by 39% and 30% respectively. The clinical trial of denosumab reported a relative risk reduction of hip fracture with denosumab of 40%.[61] In contrast, randomized placebo-controlled trials with raloxifene[62] and calcitonin[63] have failed to demonstrate successful relative risk reductions of hip fracture in postmenopausal women. Two pivotal trials[64–71] have examined the effects of hPTH(1–34) and hPTH(1–84) on fracture risk reduction in postmenopausal women. hPTH(1–34) was shown to reduce the relative risk of nonvertebral fractures;[71] however, the number of women with hip fractures was too small to estimate the incidence of hip fracture, and thus the specific relative risk reduction at the hip site. Similarly, the hPTH(1–84) trial[72] did not report on the specific relative risk reduction of hip fractures, but the difference in the number of reported nonvertebral fractures was not statistically significant between treated and untreated groups. Finally, four randomized placebo-controlled trials have evaluated the effects of strontium ranelate on fracture risk reduction in postmenopausal women.[73–76] Only one of these trials specifically assessed the efficacy of the drug on the relative risk reduction of hip fractures,[76] and failed to show a significant relative risk reduction.

Recommendation

In patients aged 50 years or older with low BMD or prior fragility fractures, evidence suggests that:
- Alendronate, risedronate, zoledronic acid, denosumab, and HRT are all effective pharmacologic agents for reducing the relative risk of hip fracture [overall quality: high]

Question 4: Does starting bisphosphonate therapy interfere with fracture healing?

Case clarification
After 1 week in hospital for hip fracture repair, the patient is discharged to a long-term care facility. Before discharge, she is prescribed an oral bisphosphonate.

Relevance
Bisphosphonates are antiresorptive agents used to treat osteoporosis and other bone diseases characterized by increased osteoclast-mediated bone resorption. As bone formation and resorption are coupled,[76] and hard callus remodeling during fracture repair is osteoclast-mediated,[77] a common concern of orthopedic surgeons is whether or not bisphosphonates interfere with the fracture healing process.

Current opinion
Current opinion suggests that the majority of orthopedic surgeons do not feel that bisphosphonate therapy interferes with clinical fracture healing.

Finding the evidence
- Cochrane Database with search terms: "bisphosphonates and fracture healing"
- MEDLINE (1996 to August Week 1 2009) and Embase (1980 to 2009 Week 33) search strategy:
  1 bisphosphonates.mp. or exp Diphosphonates/
  2 fracture healing.mp. or exp Fracture Healing/
  3 1 and 2
  4 limit 3 to English language

Table 7.4 Efficacy of pharmacologic agents on the relative risk reduction of hip fractures in postmenopausal women

Drug	Description of clinical trial	% relative risk reduction for hip fracture
Oral bisphosphonates		
Alendronate[48–50]	FIT-1; n = 2027; postmenopausal women with low femoral neck BMD and ≥1 vertebral fracture; alendronate 5 mg/d (then increased to 10 mg/d at 24 months) or placebo; 3 yrs	51%
	FIT-2; n = 4432; postmenopausal women with low femoral neck BMD but no vertebral fracture; alendronate 5 mg/d (then increased to 10 mg/d at 24 months) or placebo; 4 yrs	NS
	FLEX; n = 1099; postmenopausal women from FIT-1 and FIT-2 trials; alendronate 5 mg/d or alendronate 10 mg/d or placebo; 5 yrs	NR
Risedronate[51–54]	VERT-NA; n = 2458; postmenopausal women with ≥2 vertebral fractures or 1 vertebral fracture and low lumbar spine BMD; risedronate 2.5 mg/d (discontinued partway through trial) or risedronate 5 mg/d or placebo; 3 yrs	NR
	VERT-MN; n = 1226; postmenopausal women with ≥2 vertebral fractures; risedronate 2.5 mg/d (discontinued partway through trial) or risedronate 5 mg/d or placebo; 3 yrs	NR
	VERT-MN Extension; n = 265; risedronate 5 mg/d or placebo; 2 yrs	NR
	HIP; n = 9331; postmenopausal women with osteoporosis at femoral neck and/or with ≥1 nonskeletal risk factor for hip fracture; risedronate 2 mg/d or risedronate 5 mg/d or placebo; 3 yrs	30%
Ibandronate[55]	BONE; n = 2946; postmenopausal women with 1 to 4 vertebral fractures and osteoporosis in ≥1 vertebra; ibandronate 2.5 mg/d or ibandronate 20 mg every other day for 12 doses every 3 months or placebo; 3 yrs	NR
Intravenous bisphosphonates		
Ibandronate[56]	DIVA; n = 1395; postmenopausal women with osteoporosis; 2 mg ibandronate injections every 2 months plus oral placebo or 3 mg ibandronate injections every 3 months plus oral placebo or 1 of 2 groups receiving oral ibanronate 2.5 mg/day plus placebo injections every 2 or every 3 months; 1 yr	NR
Zoledronic acid[57,58]	HORIZON—Pivotal Fracture Trial; n = 7765; postmenopausal women with osteoporosis at femoral neck with or without vertebral fracture or osteopenia with radiologic evidence of ≥2 mild vertebral fractures or 1 moderate vertebral fracture; single 5 mg infusion of zoledronic acid every 12 months or placebo; 3 yrs	41%
	HORIZON—Recurrent Fracture Trial; n = 2127 men and women ≥50 yrs who had undergone recent surgical repair of a low trauma hip fracture; single 5 mg infusion of zoledronic acid every year; 2 yrs	30%
Other		
Raloxifene[62]	MORE; n = 7705; postmenopausal women with osteoporosis; raloxifene 60 mg/d or raloxifene 120 mg/d or placebo; 3 yrs	NS
Denosumab[61]	FREEDOM; n = 7868; postmenopausal women with osteoporosis; denosumab 60 mg subcutaneously every 6 months or placebo; 3 years	40%
Calcitonin[63]	PROOF; n = 1255; postmenopausal women with osteoporosis; calcitonin 100 IU/d or calcitonin 200 IU/d or calcitonin 400 IU/d or placebo; 5 yrs	NS

(Continued)

Table 7.4 (Continued)

Drug	Description of clinical trial	% relative risk reduction for hip fracture
HRT[59,60]	WHI:	
	(a) n = 16608; postmenopausal women with intact uterus; conjugated equine estrogen 0.625 mg/d + medroxyprogesterone acetate 2.5 mg/d or placebo; 5.6 yrs	33%
	(b) n = 10739;postmenopausal women who had undergone hysterectomy; conjugated equine estrogen 0.625 mg/d or placebo; 6.8 yrs	39%
Anabolic agents		
Teriparatide (parathyroid hormone 1–34)[71]	Neer et al. ; n = 1637; postmenopausal women with prior vertebral fractures; PTH(1–34) 20 μg/d or PTH(1–34) 40 μg/day of or placebo; 1.8 yrs	NR
Parathyroid hormone (1–84)[72]	TOP; n = 2679 ; postmenopausal women with low BMD at hip or spine; recombinant human PTH(1–84) 100 μg/d or placebo; 1.5 yrs	NR
Antiresorptive/anabolic agents		
Strontium ranelate[76]	TROPOS; n = 5091; postmenopausal women with osteoporosis; strontium ranelate 2 g/d or placebo; 3 yrs	NS

BMD, bone mineral density; BONE, Oral Ibandronate Osteoporosis Vertebral Fracture Trial in North America and Europe; DIVA, Dosing Intravenous Administration Trial; FIT, Fracture Intervention Trial; FLEX, Fracture Intervention Trial Long-Term Extension; FREEDOM, Fracture Reduction Evaluation of Denosumab in Osteoporosis Every 6 Months; HIP, Hip Intervention Program Trial; HORIZON, Health Outcomes and Reduced Incidence with Zoledronic Acid Once Yearly; HRT, hormone replacement therapy; IU, international units; MN, multinational; MORE, Multiple Outcomes of Raloxifene Evaluation; n, total number of participants randomized; NA, North America; NR, (separate hip data) not reported; NS, not statistically significant; PROOF, Prevent Recurrence of Osteoporotic Fractures Study; PTH, parathyroid hormone; TOP, Treatment of Osteoporosis Study; TROPOS, Treatment of Peripheral Osteoporosis Study; VERT, Vertebral Efficacy with Risedronate Therapy; WHI, Women's Health Initiative.

• A review of reference lists of relevant articles for additional published trials

Quality of the evidence

Level I
• 2 randomized controlled trials

Level IV
• 1 case series

No classification
• 14 trials in animals

Findings

The majority of studies examining the effects of bisphosphonates on fracture healing have been in animal models. Very few studies have examined this relationship in humans.

Animal studies Fourteen animal studies have documented the effects of bisphosphonate therapy on fracture healing[78–91]: 1 in sheep, 3 in dogs, 1 in rabbits and 9 in rats (Table 7.5). Several studies in both rat and dog models demonstrate that long-term continuous administration of bisphosphonates can delay hard callus remodeling.[81,82,85,86,89,90] However, the mechanical integrity of the callus is generally not compromised.[85,86,90] In fact, further studies of continuous bisphosphonate administration in rat and sheep models suggest that treatment can improve the bone mineral content of the callus.[81,82,87,91] The most promising results, however, have been seen with single-dosing regimens of bisphosphonates. When bisphosphonates such as zoledronate are given in a single dose, the delays in hard callus remodeling appear to be reduced[89] and improvements are seen in both tissue volume and strength,[78,79,88,89] suggesting that bisphosphonates may even assist the healing process.[92]

Human studies Despite the large number of patients treated annually with bisphosphonates, only two studies have examined the effects of these drugs on fracture healing in human models.[93–95] One randomized placebo-controlled prospective trial examined BMD in the fracture callus of 32 postmenopausal women with a distal radial fracture treated with cast immobilization.[93] At 2 months postfracture, women treated with clodronate had a 20% increase in

Table 7.5 Summary of animal studies examining the effects of bisphosphonates on fracture healing

Reference	Model	Agent and mode of administration	Effects on fracture healing
Goodship et al. 1994[82]	Sheep	Pamidronate; A	More prolific callus formation with an associated rise in the rate of BMC as well as improved torsional strength; Callus remodeling was reduced but not arrested
Bauss et al. 2004[80]	Dog	Ibandronate; B and A	No impairment in BMD, bone structure, bone repair, coupling nor serum parameters for bone formation and turnover after long-term administration
Peter et al. 1996[90]	Dog	Alendronate; B and A	Treatment before or during fracture healing or both increased fracture callus size and delayed callus remodeling but had no adverse effects on the union, strength or mineralization of bone
Lenehan et al. 1985[84]	Dog	EHDP; A	Dose-dependent and reversible inhibitory effects on fracture healing
Matos et al. 2007[88]	Rabbit	Zoledronate; A	Improved bone formation resulting in larger trabecular bone volume and little fibrosis volume
McDonald et al. 2008[89]	Rat	Zoledronate; A	Weekly dosing delayed hard callus remodeling
Yang et al. 2007[91]	Rat	Pamidronate; B and A	Callus ultimate load to failure was decreased (NS)
Amanat et al. 2007[79]	Rat	Zoledronate; A	Greater callus BMD, volume and strength; Delayed drug administration produced a larger and stronger callus
Amanat et al. 2005[78]	Rat	Pamidronate; A	Greater callus BMC, volume and strength
Koivukangas et al. 2003[83]	Rat	Clodronate; B and A	Increased size of the fracture callus but fracture healing process not prolonged even with administration of the drug on a long-term basis before fracture
Cao et al. 2002[81]	Rat	Alendronate; B and A	Suppressed remodeling of the callus leading to higher woven bone content, lower lamellar bone content and persistent visibility of the original fracture line
Li et al. 2001[85]	Rat	Incadronate; B and A	Long-term continuous treatment delayed fracture healing particularly with high-dose treatment, but without impairing the mechanical integrity of the callus
Li et al. 1999[86]	Rat	Incadronate; B and A	Pretreatment did not affect fracture healing; Continuous treatment led to a larger callus and delayed bone remodeling especially with high-dose treatment
Madsen et al. 1998[87]	Rat	Clodronate; B and A	Increased BMC and BMD when drug given before and after fracture, but no adverse effects on fracture healing

A, after fracture; B, before fracture; BMC, bone mineral content; BMD, bone mineral density; NS, not statistically significant.

BMD at the fracture site compared with the placebo group; however, the difference between groups diminished over time. A double-blind randomized placebo-controlled trial in a comparable population also showed similar effects on BMD postfracture after the administration of alendronate.[95] Greater BMD was observed in the treated group compared with the placebo group up to 1 year postfracture. Finally, it is also noteworthy to mention that data from the pivotal clinical trials of bisphosphonates in patients with osteoporosis (see Question 3) have not indicated that fracture healing is impaired, nor has return of fractures been reported with long-term bisphosphonate therapy.[96]

Recommendations

On the basis of evidence available from preclinical investigations, it is evident that:

• Continuous administration of a bisphosphonate in the presence of a fracture may modestly delay hard callus remodeling, but generally does not compromise the mechanical integrity of the fracture callus [overall quality: very low]

• Single-dosing of bisphosphonates in the presence of a fracture can reduce delays in hard callus remodeling and improve bone strength [overall quality: very low]

On the basis of evidence from clinical investigations, it is evident that:

• Administration of a bisphosphonate in the presence of a fracture can improve BMD in the short-term at the site of fracture [overall quality: moderate]

Question 5: What are the side effects associated with long-term bisphosphonate therapy?

Case clarification

The patient is scheduled to have dental implants next month.

Relevance

Bisphosphonates are the most frequently prescribed drugs for the treatment of osteoporosis.[97] Long-term safety information about these agents is therefore clinically important. A concern of many orthopedic surgeons is whether or not long-term treatment with bisphosphonate therapy is safe for patients aged 50 years or older who have sustained a hip or other fragility fracture.

Current opinion

Current opinion suggests that orthopedic surgeons are concerned about the potential adverse effects of long-term bisphosphonate use.

Finding the evidence

• Cochrane Database with search terms: "bisphosphonates and side effects," "bisphosponates and adverse effects"
• MEDLINE (1996 to August Week 1 2009) and Embase (1980 to 2009 Week 33) search strategy:
  1 bisphosphonates.mp. or exp Diphosphonates/
  2 exp Bone Density Conservation Agents/ae [Adverse Effects]
  3 1 and 2
  4 limit 3 to (english language and humans)
• A review of reference lists of relevant articles for additional published trials

Quality of the evidence

Level I
• 5 systematic reviews or meta-analyses
• 5 randomized controlled trials

Level II
• 1 cohort study

Level III
• 2 case-controlled studies

Level IV
• 5 case series

Level V
• 1 expert opinion

Findings

Atrial fibrillation In 2007, the US Food and Drug Administration (FDA) announced an ongoing safety review of a potential link between bisphosphonate use and "serious" atrial fibrillation[98] based on data from two randomized trials: the HORIZON Pivotal Fracture Trial and the FIT Trial (Table 7.4).[50,57] In the HORIZON Pivotal Fracture Trial,[57] more patients in the zoledronic acid group developed arrhythmia (6.9% vs. 5.3%, p < 0.003) compared to the placebo group. The incidence of serious atrial fibrillation (defined as life-threatening or resulting in hospitalization or disability) was also significantly higher among those using zoledronic acid. In the FIT Trial,[99] a trend towards a higher incidence of serious atrial fibrillation was seen in the alendronate group (relative hazard 1.51; 95% CI 0.97–2.40; p = 0.07) compared to the placebo group, however, no increase in the overall occurrence of atrial fibrillation (relative hazard, 1.14; 95% CI, 0.83 to 1.57; p = 0.42) was observed.

A recent meta-analysis[100] evaluated the risk of atrial fibrillation with bisphosphonate therapy in all studies to date that have reported on atrial fibrillation events. Bisphosphonate exposure was found to be significantly associated with the risk of serious atrial fibrillation events (OR 1.47; 95% CI 1.01–2.14; p = 0.04; $I^2 = 46\%$) based on data from four pivotal randomized controlled trial data sets.[50,57,58,99,101] However, meta-analysis of all atrial fibrillation events (serious and nonserious) from the same data sets yielded a pooled OR of 1.14; 95% CI 0.96–1.36; p = 0.15; $I^2 = 0\%$). The two case-controlled studies included in the meta-analysis showed different results. One found a significant association between any bisphosphonate exposure (ever users) and atrial fibrillation[102] (adjusted OR 1.86; 95% CI 1.09–3.15), whereas the other study found no association[103] (adjusted OR 0.99; 95% CI 0.90–1.10). In both studies, however, the association was not statistically significant when restricted to current users. Another register-based restricted cohort study[104] comparing fracture patients beginning bisphosphonates (n = 15,795) with unexposed patients of the same age, sex and fracture type (n = 31,590), reported incidence rates of atrial fibrillation to be 16.5/1000 person years for untreated fracture patients and 20.6/1000 person years in bisphosphonate users, corresponding to an age- and sex-adjusted hazard ratio of 1.29 (1.17–1.41). The effect size was further reduced to 1.18 (1.08–1.29) by adjustment for comedications and comorbidity. The study also found that bisphosphonate users were at increased risk of hospital-treated atrial fibrillation (adjusted HR 1.13 (1.01–1.26)), but the risk among bisphosphonate users was inversely proportional to adherence. Based on the current evidence to date, the FDA has communicated that there is no clear association between bisphosphonate use and the rate of serious or nonserious atrial fibrillation, regardless of dose or duration of bisphosphonate therapy. Further, the FDA maintains that the current indications for bisphosphonate use should remain unchanged.[105]

Osteonecrosis of the jaw Since 2003, there have been several case reports of osteonecrosis of the jaw (ONJ) associated with the use of bisphosphonates, primarily in patients with cancer,[106,107] although a consensus on diagnostic criteria for ONJ is vague. The American Society for Bone and Mineral Research (ASBMR) task force on ONJ,[108] a multidisciplinary expert group assembled to address key questions related to the disorder, developed the following definition of ONJ to help future investigations of the condition:

> an area of exposed bone in the maxillofacial region that has not healed within 8 weeks after identification by a healthcare provider in a patient who is receiving or has been exposed to a bisphosphonate and has not had radiation therapy to the craniofacial region.

The clinical severity of ONJ has led to a number of investigations examining the incidence and prevalence of ONJ among bisphosphonate users.[109] Current evidence from case reports suggests that the risk for ONJ associated with oral bisphosphonate therapy for osteoporosis is very low.[108,110] The ASBMR task force on ONJ recently reviewed published and unpublished case reports of ONJ,[108] and identified 57 cases of ONJ in patients treated with bisphosphonates for osteoporosis, the majority of which were associated with alendronate. The review concluded that the risk for ONJ in this patient group was very low (between 1 in 10,000 and <1 in 100,000 patient-treatment years). The ASBMR task force on ONJ also developed a number of clinical management recommendations regarding ONJ for patients initiating or already receiving bisphosphonate therapy, which are outlined in Table 7.6. Woo et al.[110] also conducted a systematic review of all potential cases of ONJ reported between 1966 and 2006 and came to a similar conclusion as the ASBMR task force on ONJ. Only 15 of 368 reported cases of ONJ were in patients using oral bisphosphonates for osteoporosis.

In data from randomized clinical trials of the bisphosphonates marketed in the US for the treatment of osteoporosis, no cases of ONJ have been reported, out of over 17,000 patients exposed to alendronate, more than 44 000 patient-years of exposure to risedronate and over 12,000 patients exposed to ibandronate.[109] However, none of these trials included the reporting of dental adverse events, nor was there an adjudication of suspicious dental findings. These findings were documented in a recent review paper

Table 7.6 ASBMR Task Force on ONJ recommendations and precautions for patients with osteoporosis or other nonmalignant bone disease initiating or already receiving bisphosphonate therapy[108]

Patient Group	Recommendations and precautions
Inititating bisphosphonate therapy	Patients should be informed that the risk of developing bisphosphonate-associated ONJ with routine oral therapy for osteoporosis or Paget's disease seems to be low, ranging between 1/10,000 and 1/100,000
	Patients who express concern about ONJ should be encouraged to seek additional information from a dentist or dental specialist
	Healthcare providers should encourage patients who are starting to take bisphosphonates to practice good oral hygiene and have regular dental visits
	Because the risk of developing bisphosphonate-associated ONJ seems to be related to longer duration of bisphosphonate exposure and the risk is low, it is not necessary to recommend a dental examination before beginning oral bisphosphonate therapy or to otherwise alter routine dental management
Receiving bisphosphonate therapy	Healthcare providers should encourage patients to practice good oral hygiene and have regular dental visits
	Patients with periodontal disease should receive appropriate nonsurgical therapy. If surgical treatment is necessary, it should be aimed primarily at reducing or eliminating periodontal disease. Modest bone recontouring may be considered when necessary
	Current information indicates that taking bisphosphonates for osteoporosis is not a contraindication for dental implant placement. However, if dental implants are considered, appropriate informed consent is recommended and should be documented
	Endodontic treatment is preferable to extraction or periapical surgery when possible
	If an invasive dental procedure is anticipated, some experts suggest stopping the bisphosphonate for a period before and after the procedure. There are no data to suggest stopping the bisphosphonate will improve dental outcomes, however, given the long retention of bisphosphonates in the skeleton, temporary discontinuation of bisphosphonate therapy is unlikely to have an adverse effect on the patient's skeletal condition

Adapted from Khosla et al. Bisphosphonate-associated osteonecrosis of the jaw: Report of a Task Force of the American Society for Bone and Mineral Research. J Bone Miner Res 2007;22(10)1479–89.

by Silverman et al.[109] and were based on personal communications between the authors and the corresponding drug companies. In a recently completed trial entitled the Health Outcomes and Reduced Incidence with Zoledronic Acid Once Yearly (HORIZON) Pivotal Fracture Trial[57]—a major randomized clinical trial that evaluated yearly zoledronic acid 5 mg for the treatment of postmenopausal osteoporosis in 7,736 postmenopausal women—an adverse event review process was established to assess maxillofacial adverse events objectively and independently. This is the largest trial to date in which ONJ has been examined in a systematic fashion with adjudication of all potential cases.[111] In the HORIZON Pivotal Fracture Trial there were no spontaneous reports of ONJ; however, after a thorough review of all maxillofacial adverse events, two potential cases of ONJ were found to meet predefined adjudication criteria (exposed bone in the oral cavity present >6 weeks): one case in the treatment group and one in the placebo group, making incidence rates similar between groups. In both patients, the condition resolved after antibiotic therapy and debridement.

Atypical fractures Several case reports[94,112–115] have documented atypical fractures linked to long-term bisphosphonate use. Atypical fractures are those occurring at sites that are uncommon (but not absolutely unlikely) for osteoporosis such as the midshaft femur, pelvis, and tibia, as well as those that have exhibited impaired healing. Recently, a multidisciplinary expert group (task force), similar to the one discussed previously for the issue of ONJ, was established by the ASBMR to address key questions related to these fractures. A report put out by this task force[116] developed a formal case definition for the condition, reviewed available published and unpublished data, and provided a set of recommendations for orthopedic and medical management (Table 7.7). The report reviewed 310 cases of atypical femoral fractures and found that 291 patients (94 %) with this condition had taken a bisphosphonate; however, a causal association was not established. The report concluded that the incidence of atypical femoral fractures associated with bisphosphonate therapy for osteoporosis is very low (~3–10 per 10,000 patients), particularly in comparison to the number of vertebral, hip and other fractures that are prevented by bisphosphonates. However, the findings suggested that the risk increases with increasing duration of exposure, thus there was concern that a lack of awareness and under-reporting may currently mask the true incidence of the problem. Given the rarity of atypical femoral fractures, the task force recommended that specific diagnostic and procedural codes be created and that an international registry be established to facilitate studies of the clinical and genetic risk factors and optimal surgical and medical management of these fractures. Physicians and patients will also be made aware of the possibility of atypical femoral fractures through a change in labeling of bisphosphonates.

Recommendations

In patients aged 50 years or older who use long-term bisphosphonate therapy for osteoporosis, evidence suggests that:

• There is no clear association between bisphosphonate use and the rate of serious or nonserious atrial fibrillation, regardless of dose or duration of bisphosphonate therapy [overall quality: high]

• The risk of developing bisphosphonate-associated ONJ with routine oral therapy for osteoporosis is very low [overall quality: high]

• The benefits of bisphosphonates in preventing hip and other osteoporotic fractures outweigh the risk of developing atypical femoral fractures. [overall quality: low]

Summary of recommendations

• Many patients who have sustained a hip or other fragility fracture are not receiving appropriate evaluation and treatment for osteoporosis postfracture

• Significant progress has been made towards developing and implementing programs to address the osteoporosis care gap

• The FRAX tool can be used to calculate the 10-year probability of a major osteoporotic fracture (clinical spine, hip, forearm or proximal humerus) and hip fracture

• Alternative methods are also available to determine absolute fracture risk

• Treatment decisions should be patient specific and guidelines developed by the appropriate country of origin should be considered

• Alendronate, risedronate, zoledronic acid, denosumab and HRT are all effective pharmacologic agents for reducing the relative risk of hip fracture in patients with low BMD or prior fragility fractures

• Continuous administration of a bisphosphonate in the presence of a fracture may modestly delay hard callus remodeling in animals, but generally does not compromise the mechanical integrity of the fracture callus

• Single-dosing of bisphosphonates in the presence of a fracture can reduce delays in hard callus remodeling and improve bone strength in animals

• Administration of a bisphosphonate in the presence of a fracture can improve BMD in the short-term at the site of fracture

• There is no clear association between bisphosphonate use and the rate of serious or nonserious atrial fibrillation, regardless of dose or duration of bisphosphonate therapy

• The risk of developing bisphosphonate-associated ONJ with routine oral therapy for osteoporosis is very low

Table 7.7 ASBMR Task Force on Atypical Femoral Fractures recommendations for orthopedic and medical management of atypical femoral fractures[116]

Issue	Recommendations
Surgical management	
History of thigh or groin pain in a patient on bisphosphonate therapy	Rule out femoral fracture. AP and lateral plain radiographs of the hip, including the full diaphysis of the femur should be performed. If the radiograph is negative and the level of clinical suspicion is high, a technetium bone scan or MRI of the femur should be performed to detect a periosteal stress reaction
Complete subtrochanteric/ diaphyseal femoral fracture	Orthopedic management includes stabilizing the fracture and addressing the medical management (below). Endochondral fracture repair is the preferred method of treatment since bisphosphonates inhibit osteoclast remodeling. Intramedullary reconstruction full-length nails accomplish this goal and protect the femur. Locking plates preclude endochondral repair, have a high failure rate, and are not recommended as the method of fixation. The medullary canal should be overreamed to compensate for the narrow intramedullary diameter, facilitate insertion of the reconstruction nail and prevent fracture of the remaining shaft. The proximal fragment may require additional reaming to permit passage of the nail and avoid malalignment. The contralateral femur must be evaluated radiographically whether or not symptoms are present
Incomplete subtrochanteric/ femoral shaft fractures	Prophylactic reconstruction nail fixation is recommended if pain is present. If there is minimal pain, a trial of conservative therapy in which weight bearing is limited through the use of crutches or a walker may be considered. However, if there is no symptomatic and radiographic improvement after 2–3 months of conservative therapy, prophylactic nail fixation should be strongly considered because of the possibility of complete fracture. For patients with no pain, weight bearing may be continued but should be limited and vigorous activity avoided. Reduced activity should be continued until there is no bone edema on MRI
Medical management	
Prevention	Decisions to initiate pharmacologic treatment including bisphosphonates to manage patients with osteoporosis should be made based on an assessment of benefits and risks. Patients who are deemed to be a low risk of osteoporosis-related fractures should not be started on bisphosphonates. Physicians need to be wary of thigh or groin pain in patients on bisphosphonates. Complaints of thigh or groin pain in a patient on bisphosphonates require urgent radiographic evaluation of both femurs even if pain is unilateral
Treatment	For patients with a stress reaction, stress fracture, or incomplete or complete subtrochanteric femoral shaft fracture, potent antiresorptive agents should be discontinued. Dietary calcium and vitamin D status should be assessed and adequate supplementation should be prescribed. Teriparatide should be considered in patients who suffer these fractures, particularly if there is little evidence of healing by 4 to 6 weeks after surgical intervention

Adapted from Shane et al. Atypical subtrochanteric and diaphyseal femoral fractures: Report of a Task Force of the American Society for Bone and Mineral Research. J Bone Miner Res 2010; 25:2267–94.

- The benefits of bisphosphonates in preventing hip and other osteoporotic fractures outweigh the risk of developing atypical femoral fractures

Conclusion

This chapter reviewed orthopedic issues relating to osteoporosis including: (1) the identification of osteoporosis in patients with fractures, (2) treatment guidelines for patients with osteoporosis, (3) effective pharmacologic therapies for reducing fracture risk, (4) bisphosphonate therapy and fracture healing and (5) adverse effects associated with pharmacologic therapies for osteoporosis. Clinical evidence confirms that osteoporosis is an important orthopedic concern and necessitates continued evaluation and attention.

References

1. Brien E, Healey J. Treatment of common osteoporotic fractures. In: Sartoris DJ, ed. Osteoporosis Diagnosis and Treatment, pp. 97–146. Informa Health Care, London, 1996.
2. Cumming RG, Nevitt MC, Cummings SR. Epidemiology of hip fractures. Epidemiol Rev 1997;19(2):244–57.
3. Keyak JH, Skinner HB, Fleming JA. Effect of force direction on femoral fracture load for two types of loading conditions. J Orthop Res 2001;19(4):539–44.
4. Osteoporosis prevention, diagnosis, and therapy. JAMA 2001; 285(6):785–95.

5. Cooper C, Campion G, Melton LJ, 3rd. Hip fractures in the elderly: a world-wide projection. Osteoporos Int 1992;2(6): 285–9.

6. Johnell O, Kanis JA. An estimate of the worldwide prevalence and disability associated with osteoporotic fractures. Osteoporos Int 2006;17(12):1726–33.

7. Johnell O, Kanis J. Epidemiology of osteoporotic fractures. Osteoporos Int 2005;16 Suppl 2:S3–7.

8. Magaziner J, Lydick E, Hawkes W, Fox KM, Zimmerman SI, Epstein RS, et al. Excess mortality attributable to hip fracture in white women aged 70 years and older. Am J Public Health 1997;87(10):1630–6.

9. Johnell O, Kanis JA. An estimate of the worldwide prevalence, mortality and disability associated with hip fracture. Osteoporos Int 2004;15(11):897–902.

10. Magaziner J, Simonsick EM, Kashner TM, Hebel JR, Kenzora JE. Predictors of functional recovery one year following hospital discharge for hip fracture: a prospective study. J. Gerontol1 990;45(3):M101–7.

11. Riggs BL, Melton LJ, 3rd. Involutional osteoporosis. New Engl J Med 1986;314(26):1676–86.

12. Papadimitropoulos EA, Coyte PC, Josse RG, Greenwood CE. Current and projected rates of hip fracture in Canada. CMAJ 1997;157(10):1357–63.

13. Papaioannou A, Giangregorio L, Kvern B, Boulos P, Ioannidis G, Adachi JD. The osteoporosis care gap in Canada. BMC Musculoskelet Disord 2004;5:11.

14. Giangregorio L, Papaioannou A, Cranney A, Zytaruk N, Adachi JD. Fragility fractures and the osteoporosis care gap: an international phenomenon. Semin Arthritis Rheum 2006;35(5): 293–305.

15. Elliot-Gibson V, Bogoch ER, Jamal SA, Beaton DE. Practice patterns in the diagnosis and treatment of osteoporosis after a fragility fracture: a systematic review. Osteoporos Int 2004;15(10):767–78.

16. Kaufman JD, Bolander ME, Bunta AD, Edwards BJ, Fitzpatrick LA, Simonelli C. Barriers and solutions to osteoporosis care in patients with a hip fracture. Journal Bone Joint Surg Am 2003;85-A(9):1837–43.

17. Bliuc D, Eisman JA, Center JR. A randomized study of two different information-based interventions on the management of osteoporosis in minimal and moderate trauma fractures. Osteoporos Int 2006;17(9):1309–17.

18. Davis JC, Guy P, Ashe MC, Liu-Ambrose T, Khan K. HipWatch: osteoporosis investigation and treatment after a hip fracture: a 6-month randomized controlled trial. J Gerontol 2007;62(8): 888–91.

19. Feldstein A, Elmer PJ, Smith DH, Herson M, Orwoll E, Chen C, et al. Electronic medical record reminder improves osteoporosis management after a fracture: a randomized, controlled trial. J Am Geriatr Soc 2006;54(3):450–7.

20. Gardner MJ, Brophy RH, Demetrakopoulos D, Koob J, Hong R, Rana A, et al. Interventions to improve osteoporosis treatment following hip fracture. A prospective, randomized trial. The Journal of bone and joint surgery. 2005 Jan;87(1):3–7.

21. Majumdar SR, Beaupre LA, Harley CH, Hanley DA, Lier DA, Juby AG, et al. Use of a case manager to improve osteoporosis treatment after hip fracture: results of a randomized controlled trial. Arch Intern Med 2007;167(19):2110–15.

22. Miki RA, Oetgen ME, Kirk J, Insogna KL, Lindskog DM. Orthopaedic management improves the rate of early osteoporosis treatment after hip fracture. A randomized clinical trial. J Bone Joint Surg 2008;90(11):2346–53.

23. Bogoch ER, Elliot-Gibson V, Beaton DE, Jamal SA, Josse RG, Murray TM. Effective initiation of osteoporosis diagnosis and treatment for patients with a fragility fracture in an orthopaedic environment. J Bone Joint Surg 2006;88(1):25–34.

24. Chevalley T, Hoffmeyer P, Bonjour JP, Rizzoli R. An osteoporosis clinical pathway for the medical management of patients with low-trauma fracture. Osteoporos Int 2002;13(6):450–5.

25. McLellan AR, Gallacher SJ, Fraser M, McQuillian C. The fracture liaison service: success of a program for the evaluation and management of patients with osteoporotic fracture. Osteoporos Int 2003;14(12):1028–34.

26. Sander B, Elliot-Gibson V, Beaton D, et al. Targeting fragility fractures in an orthopaedic treatment unit: cost-effectiveness of a dedicated coordinator. J Bone Miner Res Br Proc 2004;87 (Suppl 3):361.

27. Cummings SR, Bates D, Black DM. Clinical use of bone densitometry: scientific review. JAMA 2002;288(15):1889–97.

28. Cummings SR, Nevitt MC, Browner WS, Stone K, Fox KM, Ensrud KE, et al. Risk factors for hip fracture in white women. Study of Osteoporotic Fractures Research Group. New Engl J Med 1995;332(12):767–73.

29. Siris ES, Chen YT, Abbott TA, Barrett-Connor E, Miller PD, Wehren LE, et al. Bone mineral density thresholds for pharmacological intervention to prevent fractures. Arch Intern Med 2004;164(10):1108–12.

30. Dempster D, Mark S, Watts N. Determinants of bone strength and impact of antiresorptive therapy. Clin Cour 2006;24(3): 1–8.

31. Turner CH. Biomechanics of bone: determinants of skeletal fragility and bone quality. Osteoporos Int 2002;13(2):97–104.

32. Kanis JA, McCloskey EV, Johansson H, Strom O, Borgstrom F, Oden A. Case finding for the management of osteoporosis with FRAX–assessment and intervention thresholds for the UK. Osteoporos Int 2008;19(10):1395–408.

33. Kanis JA, Borgstrom F, De Laet C, Johansson H, Johnell O, Jonsson B, et al. Assessment of fracture risk. Osteoporos Int 2005 Jun;16(6):581–9.

34. Kanis JA, Johnell O, Oden A, Johansson H, McCloskey E. FRAX and the assessment of fracture probability in men and women from the UK. Osteoporos Int 2008;19(4):385–97.

35. Tosteson AN, Melton LJ, 3rd, Dawson-Hughes B, Baim S, Favus MJ, Khosla S, et al. Cost-effective osteoporosis treatment thresholds: the United States perspective. Osteoporos Int 2008; 19(4):437–47.

36. Roux C, Thomas T. Optimal use of FRAX. Joint Bone Spine 2009;76(1):1–3.

37. Kanis JA, Johansson H, Oden A, Johnell O, de Laet C, Melton IL, et al. A meta-analysis of prior corticosteroid use and fracture risk. J Bone Miner Res 2004;19(6):893–9.

38. van Staa TP, Leufkens HG, Abenhaim L, Zhang B, Cooper C. Oral corticosteroids and fracture risk: relationship to daily and cumulative doses. Rheumatology (Oxford, England) 2000; 39(12):1383–9.

39. Delmas PD, Genant HK, Crans GG, Stock JL, Wong M, Siris E, et al. Severity of prevalent vertebral fractures and the risk of

subsequent vertebral and nonvertebral fractures: results from the MORE trial. Bone 2003;33(4):522–32.

40. National Osteoporosis Foundation. Clinician's Guide to Prevention and Treatment of Osteoporosis. National Osteoporosis Foundation, Washington, DC, 2008.

41. Kanis JA, Burlet N, Cooper C, Delmas PD, Reginster JY, Borgstrom F, et al. European guidance for the diagnosis and management of osteoporosis in postmenopausal women. Osteoporos Int 2008;19(4):399–428.

42. Papaioannou A, Morin S, Cheung AM, Atkinson S, Brown JP, Feldman S, et al. 2010 clinical practice guidelines for the diagnosis and management of osteoporosis in Canada: summary. CMAJ 182(17):1864–73.

43. Fraser LA, Langsetmo L, Berger C, Ioannidis G, Goltzman D, Adachi JD, et al. Fracture prediction and calibration of a Canadian FRAX® tool: a population-based report from CaMos. Osteoporos Int 2011;22(3):829–37.

44. Leslie WD, Lix LM, Johansson H, Oden A, McCloskey E, Kanis JA. Independent clinical validation of a Canadian FRAX tool: fracture prediction and model calibration. J Bone Miner Res 2010;25(11):2350–8.

45. Leslie WD, Tsang JF, Lix LM. Simplified system for absolute fracture risk assessment: clinical validation in Canadian women. J Bone Miner Res. 2009;24(2):353–60.

46. Bonura F. Prevention, screening, and management of osteoporosis: an overview of the current strategies. Postgrad Med 2009;121(4):5–17.

47. Bilezikian JP. Efficacy of bisphosphonates in reducing fracture risk in postmenopausal osteoporosis. Am J Med 2009;122(2 Suppl):S14–21.

48. Black DM, Cummings SR, Karpf DB, Cauley JA, Thompson DE, Nevitt MC, et al. Randomised trial of effect of alendronate on risk of fracture in women with existing vertebral fractures. Fracture Intervention Trial Research Group. Lancet 1996; 348(9041):1535–41.

49. Black DM, Schwartz AV, Ensrud KE, Cauley JA, Levis S, Quandt SA, et al. Effects of continuing or stopping alendronate after 5 years of treatment: the Fracture Intervention Trial Long-term Extension (FLEX): a randomized trial. JAMA 2006; 296(24):2927–38.

50. Cummings SR, Black DM, Thompson DE, Applegate WB, Barrett-Connor E, Musliner TA, et al. Effect of alendronate on risk of fracture in women with low bone density but without vertebral fractures: results from the Fracture Intervention Trial. JAMA 1998;280(24):2077–82.

51. Harris ST, Watts NB, Genant HK, McKeever CD, Hangartner T, Keller M, et al. Effects of risedronate treatment on vertebral and nonvertebral fractures in women with postmenopausal osteoporosis: a randomized controlled trial. Vertebral Efficacy With Risedronate Therapy (VERT) Study Group. JAMA 1999 Oct 13;282(14):1344–52.

52. McClung MR, Geusens P, Miller PD, Zippel H, Bensen WG, Roux C, et al. Effect of risedronate on the risk of hip fracture in elderly women. Hip Intervention Program Study Group. New Engl J Med 2001;344(5):333–40.

53. Reginster J, Minne HW, Sorensen OH, Hooper M, Roux C, Brandi ML, et al. Randomized trial of the effects of risedronate on vertebral fractures in women with established postmenopausal osteoporosis. Vertebral Efficacy with Risedronate Therapy (VERT) Study Group. Osteoporos Int 2000;11(1): 83–91.

54. Sorensen OH, Crawford GM, Mulder H, Hosking DJ, Gennari C, Mellstrom D, et al. Long-term efficacy of risedronate: a 5-year placebo-controlled clinical experience. Bone 2003; 32(2):120–6.

55. Chesnut IC, Skag A, Christiansen C, Recker R, Stakkestad JA, Hoiseth A, et al. Effects of oral ibandronate administered daily or intermittently on fracture risk in postmenopausal osteoporosis. J Bone Miner Res 2004;19(8):1241–9.

56. Delmas PD, Adami S, Strugala C, Stakkestad JA, Reginster JY, Felsenberg D, et al. Intravenous ibandronate injections in postmenopausal women with osteoporosis: one-year results from the dosing intravenous administration study. Arthritis Rheum 2006 Jun;54(6):1838–46.

57. Black DM, Delmas PD, Eastell R, Reid IR, Boonen S, Cauley JA, et al. Once-yearly zoledronic acid for treatment of postmenopausal osteoporosis. New Engl J Med 2007;356(18):1809–22.

58. Lyles KW, Colon-Emeric CS, Magaziner JS, Adachi JD, Pieper CF, Mautalen C, et al. Zoledronic acid and clinical fractures and mortality after hip fracture. New Engl J Med 2007;357(18): 1799–809.

59. Anderson GL, Limacher M, Assaf AR, Bassford T, Beresford SA, Black H, et al. Effects of conjugated equine estrogen in postmenopausal women with hysterectomy: the Women's Health Initiative randomized controlled trial. JAMA 2004;291(14): 1701–12.

60. Cauley JA, Robbins J, Chen Z, Cummings SR, Jackson RD, LaCroix AZ, et al. Effects of estrogen plus progestin on risk of fracture and bone mineral density: the Women's Health Initiative randomized trial. JAMA 2003 Oct 1;290(13):1729–38.

61. Cummings SR, San Martin J, McClung MR, Siris ES, Eastell R, Reid IR, et al. Denosumab for prevention of fractures in postmenopausal women with osteoporosis. New Engl J Med 2009;361(8):756–65.

62. Ettinger B, Black DM, Mitlak BH, Knickerbocker RK, Nickelsen T, Genant HK, et al. Reduction of vertebral fracture risk in postmenopausal women with osteoporosis treated with raloxifene: results from a 3-year randomized clinical trial. Multiple Outcomes of Raloxifene Evaluation (MORE) Investigators. JAMA 1999;282(7):637–45.

63. Chesnut CH, 3rd, Silverman S, Andriano K, Genant H, Gimona A, Harris S, et al. A randomized trial of nasal spray salmon calcitonin in postmenopausal women with established osteoporosis: the prevent recurrence of osteoporotic fractures study. PROOF Study Group. Am J Med 2000;109(4):267–76.

64. Black DM, Greenspan SL, Ensrud KE, Palermo L, McGowan JA, Lang TF, et al. The effects of parathyroid hormone and alendronate alone or in combination in postmenopausal osteoporosis. New Engl J Med 2003;349(13):1207–15.

65. Body JJ, Gaich GA, Scheele WH, Kulkarni PM, Miller PD, Peretz A, et al. A randomized double-blind trial to compare the efficacy of teriparatide [recombinant human parathyroid hormone (1–34)] with alendronate in postmenopausal women with osteoporosis. J Clin Endocrinol Metab 2002;87(10): 4528–35.

66. Cosman F, Nieves J, Woelfert L, Formica C, Gordon S, Shen V, et al. Parathyroid hormone added to established hormone therapy: effects on vertebral fracture and maintenance of bone

mass after parathyroid hormone withdrawal. J Bone Miner Res 2001;16(5):925–31.

67. Cosman F, Nieves J, Zion M, Woelfert L, Luckey M, Lindsay R. Daily and cyclic parathyroid hormone in women receiving alendronate. New Engl J Med 2005;353(6):566–75.

68. Hodsman AB, Fraher LJ, Watson PH, Ostbye T, Stitt LW, Adachi JD, et al. A randomized controlled trial to compare the efficacy of cyclical parathyroid hormone vs. cyclical parathyroid hormone and sequential calcitonin to improve bone mass in postmenopausal women with osteoporosis. J Clin Endocrinol Metab 1997;82(2):620–8.

69. Hodsman AB, Hanley DA, Ettinger MP, Bolognese MA, Fox J, Metcalfe AJ, et al. Efficacy and safety of human parathyroid hormone-(1–84) in increasing bone mineral density in post-menopausal osteoporosis. J Clin Endocrinol Metab 2003;88(11):5212–20.

70. McClung MR, San Martin J, Miller PD, Civitelli R, Bandeira F, Omizo M, et al. Opposite bone remodeling effects of teri-paratide and alendronate in increasing bone mass. Arch Intern Med 2005;165(15):1762–8.

71. Neer RM, Arnaud CD, Zanchetta JR, Prince R, Gaich GA, Reginster JY, et al. Effect of parathyroid hormone (1–34) on fractures and bone mineral density in postmenopausal women with osteoporosis. New Engl J Med 2001;344(19):1434–41.

72. Greenspan SL, Bone HG, Ettinger MP, Hanley DA, Lindsay R, Zanchetta JR, et al. Effect of recombinant human parathyroid hormone (1–84) on vertebral fracture and bone mineral density in postmenopausal women with osteoporosis: a randomized trial. Ann Intern Med 2007;146(5):326–39.

73. Meunier PJ, Roux C, Seeman E, Ortolani S, Badurski JE, Spector TD, et al. The effects of strontium ranelate on the risk of verte-bral fracture in women with postmenopausal osteoporosis. New Engl J Med 2004;350(5):459–68.

74. Meunier PJ, Slosman DO, Delmas PD, Sebert JL, Brandi ML, Albanese C, et al. Strontium ranelate: dose-dependent effects in established postmenopausal vertebral osteoporosis–a 2-year randomized placebo controlled trial. J Clin Endocrinol Metab 2002;87(5):2060–6.

75. Reginster JY, Deroisy R, Dougados M, Jupsin I, Colette J, Roux C. Prevention of early postmenopausal bone loss by strontium ranelate: the randomized, two-year, double-masked, dose-ranging, placebo-controlled PREVOS trial. Osteoporos Int 2002;13(12):925–31.

76. Reginster JY, Seeman E, De Vernejoul MC, Adami S, Compston J, Phenekos C, et al. Strontium ranelate reduces the risk of nonvertebral fractures in postmenopausal women with oste-oporosis: Treatment of Peripheral Osteoporosis (TROPOS) study. J Clin Endocrinol Metab 2005;90(5):2816–22.

77. Einhorn TA. The cell and molecular biology of fracture healing. Clin Orthop Relat Res 1998;355(Suppl):S7–21.

78. Amanat N, Brown R, Bilston LE, Little DG. A single systemic dose of pamidronate improves bone mineral content and accel-erates restoration of strength in a rat model of fracture repair. J Orthop Res 2005;23(5):1029–34.

79. Amanat N, McDonald M, Godfrey C, Bilston L, Little D. Optimal timing of a single dose of zoledronic acid to increase strength in rat fracture repair. J Bone Miner Res 2007;22(6):867–76.

80. Bauss F, Schenk RK, Hort S, Muller-Beckmann B, Sponer G. New model for simulation of fracture repair in full-grown beagle dogs: model characterization and results from a long-term study with ibandronate. J Pharmacol Toxicol Methods 2004;50(1):25–34.

81. Cao Y, Mori S, Mashiba T, Westmore MS, Ma L, Sato M, et al. Raloxifene, estrogen, and alendronate affect the processes of fracture repair differently in ovariectomized rats. J Bone Miner Res 2002;17(12):2237–46.

82. Goodship AE, Walker PC, McNally D, Chambers T, Green JR. Use of a bisphosphonate (pamidronate) to modulate fracture repair in ovine bone. Ann Oncol 1994;5 Suppl 7:S53–5.

83. Koivukangas A, Tuukkanen J, Kippo K, Jamsa T, Hannuniemi R, Pasanen I, et al. Long-term administration of clodronate does not prevent fracture healing in rats. Clinical Orthop Related Res 2003;408:268–78.

84. Lenehan TM, Balligand M, Nunamaker DM, Wood FE, Jr. Effect of EHDP on fracture healing in dogs. J Orthop Res 1985;3(4):499–507.

85. Li C, Mori S, Li J, Kaji Y, Akiyama T, Kawanishi J, et al. Long-term effect of incadronate disodium (YM-175) on fracture healing of femoral shaft in growing rats. J Bone Miner Res 2001;16(3):429–36.

86. Li J, Mori S, Kaji Y, Mashiba T, Kawanishi J, Norimatsu H. Effect of bisphosphonate (incadronate) on fracture healing of long bones in rats. J Bone Miner Res 1999;14(6):969–79.

87. Madsen JE, Berg-Larsen T, Kirkeby OJ, Falch JA, Nordsletten L. No adverse effects of clodronate on fracture healing in rats. Acta Orthop Scand 1998;69(5):532–6.

88. Matos MA, Araujo FP, Paixao FB. The effect of zoledronate on bone remodeling during the healing process. Acta Cirurg Bras/Soc Bras Desenvolv Pesqui Cirurg 2007;22(2):115–9.

89. McDonald MM, Dulai S, Godfrey C, Amanat N, Sztynda T, Little DG. Bolus or weekly zoledronic acid administration does not delay endochondral fracture repair but weekly dosing enhances delays in hard callus remodeling. Bone 2008;43(4):653–62.

90. Peter CP, Cook WO, Nunamaker DM, Provost MT, Seedor JG, Rodan GA. Effect of alendronate on fracture healing and bone remodeling in dogs. J Orthop Res 1996;14(1):74–9.

91. Yang KH, Won JH, Yoon HK, Ryu JH, Choo KS, Kim JS. High concentrations of pamidronate in bone weaken the mechanical properties of intact femora in a rat model. Yonsei Med J 2007;48(4):653–8.

92. Little DG, Ramachandran M, Schindeler A. The anabolic and catabolic responses in bone repair. J Bone Joint Surg Br 2007;89(4):425–33.

93. Adolphson P, Abbaszadegan H, Boden H, Salemyr M, Henriques T. Clodronate increases mineralization of callus after Colles' fracture: a randomized, double-blind, placebo-control-led, prospective trial in 32 patients. Acta Orthop Scand 2000;71(2):195–200.

94. Odvina CV, Zerwekh JE, Rao DS, Maalouf N, Gottschalk FA, Pak CY. Severely suppressed bone turnover: a potential com-plication of alendronate therapy. J Clin Endocrinol Metab 2005;90(3):1294–301.

95. van der Poest Clement E, Patka P, Vandormael K, Haarman H, Lips P. The effect of alendronate on bone mass after distal forearm fracture. J Bone Miner Res 2000;15(3):586–93.

96. Bone HG, Hosking D, Devogelaer JP, Tucci JR, Emkey RD, Tonino RP, et al. Ten years' experience with alendronate for osteoporosis in postmenopausal women. New Engl J Med 2004;350(12):1189–99.

97. Recker RR, Lewiecki EM, Miller PD, Reiffel J. Safety of bisphosphonates in the treatment of osteoporosis. Am J Med 2009;122(2 Suppl):S22–32.

98. US FDA. Early communication of an ongoing safety review of bisphosphonates. [cited July 21, 2009]; Available from: http://www.fda.gov/cder/drug/early_comm/bisphosphonates.htm

99. Cummings SR, Schwartz AV, Black DM. Alendronate and atrial fibrillation. New Engl J Med 2007;356(18):1895–6.

100. Loke YK, Jeevanantham V, Singh S. Bisphosphonates and atrial fibrillation: systematic review and meta-analysis. Drug Saf 2009;32(3):219–28.

101. Karam R, Camm J, McClung M. Yearly zoledronic acid in postmenopausal osteoporosis. New Engl J Med 2007;357(7):712–3; author reply 4–5.

102. Heckbert SR, Li G, Cummings SR, Smith NL, Psaty BM. Use of alendronate and risk of incident atrial fibrillation in women. Arch Intern Med 2008;168(8):826–31.

103. Merck. Statement by Merck & Co., Inc., regarding the fracture intervention trial (FIT) with FOSOMAX(R) (alendronate sodium) and incidence of atrial fibrillation [online]. [cited July 15, 2009]; Available from: http://www.merck.com/newsroom/press_releases/product/2007_0502.html

104. Abrahamsen B, Eiken P, Brixen K. Atrial fibrillation in fracture patients treated with oral bisphosphonates. J Intern Med 2009;265(5):581–92.

105. US FDA. Update of safety review follow-up to the October 1, 2007 early communication about the ongoing safety review of bisphosphonates, 2008 [cited September 3, 2009]; Available from: http://www.fda.gov/Drugs/DrugSafety/Postmarket DrugSafetyInformationforPatientsandProviders/DrugSafety InformationforHeathcareProfessionals/ucm136201.htm

106. Marx RE. Pamidronate (Aredia) and zoledronate (Zometa) induced avascular necrosis of the jaws: a growing epidemic. J Oral Maxillofac Surg 2003;61(9):1115–7.

107. Ruggiero SL, Mehrotra B, Rosenberg TJ, Engroff SL. Osteonecrosis of the jaws associated with the use of bisphosphonates: a review of 63 cases. J Oral Maxillofac Surg 2004;62(5):527–34.

108. Khosla S, Burr D, Cauley J, Dempster DW, Ebeling PR, Felsenberg D, et al. Bisphosphonate-associated osteonecrosis of the jaw: report of a task force of the American Society for Bone and Mineral Research. J Bone Miner Res 2007;22(10):1479–91.

109. Silverman SL, Landesberg R. Osteonecrosis of the jaw and the role of bisphosphonates: a critical review. Am J Med 2009;122(2 Suppl):S33–45.

110. Woo SB, Hellstein JW, Kalmar JR. Systematic review: bisphosphonates and osteonecrosis of the jaws. Ann Intern Med 2006;144:753–61.

111. Grbic JT, Landesberg R, Lin SQ, Mesenbrink P, Reid IR, Leung PC, et al. Incidence of osteonecrosis of the jaw in women with postmenopausal osteoporosis in the health outcomes and reduced incidence with zoledronic acid once yearly pivotal fracture trial. J Am Dental Assoc 2008;139(1):32–40.

112. Goh SK, Yang KY, Koh JS, Wong MK, Chua SY, Chua DT, et al. Subtrochanteric insufficiency fractures in patients on alendronate therapy: a caution. J Bone Joint Surg Br 2007;89(3):349–53.

113. Kwek EB, Goh SK, Koh JS, Png MA, Howe TS. An emerging pattern of subtrochanteric stress fractures: a long-term complication of alendronate therapy? Injury 2008;39(2):224–31.

114. Lenart BA, Lorich DG, Lane JM. Atypical fractures of the femoral diaphysis in postmenopausal women taking alendronate. New Engl J Med 2008;358(12):1304–6.

115. Neviaser AS, Lane JM, Lenart BA, Edobor-Osula F, Lorich DG. Low-energy femoral shaft fractures associated with alendronate use. J Orthop Trauma 2008;22(5):346–50.

116. Shane E, Burr D, Ebeling PR, Abrahamsen B, Adler RA, Brown TD, et al. Atypical subtrochanteric and diaphyseal femoral fractures: report of a task force of the American Society for Bone and Mineral Research. J Bone Miner Res 2010;25(11):2267–94.

8

Thromboprophylaxis in Orthopedic Practice

Ernest Kwek and Richard E. Buckley
Foothills Medical Center, University of Calgary, Calgary, AB, Canada

Case scenario

A 52 year old healthy man was involved in a low-energy ski collision. He sustained bilateral proximal humeral fractures and a right distal tibia fracture. He was initially assessed and treated in a local hospital before being sent to the regional trauma center 12 hours later. Due to resource constraints, surgery was delayed for a further 38 hours during which time the patient did not receive any thromboprophylaxis. Simultaneous successful fracture surgery was performed on the left shoulder and right ankle, but the patient desaturated acutely after the tourniquet on the right lower limb was released. He became hypotensive and required cardiac massage and inotropic support. A transesophageal echocardiogram was performed in the operating room and a large clot was found in the right atrium. The patient underwent immediate open cardiac surgery to remove the clot, but continued complications resulted in an intraoperative stroke and brain death. He eventually succumbed to complications 3 days later.

Relevant anatomy

Venous thromboembolism (VTE) is a significant complication of major orthopedic surgery, and can manifest as deep venous thrombosis (DVT) or pulmonary embolism (PE). DVT typically occurs in the lower extremities, with distal DVT involving the deep calf veins, and proximal DVT defined as thrombosis at or above the popliteal vein. PE results when a piece of thrombus is detached from a vein wall and lodges within the pulmonary arteries. This is the most serious and life-threatening complication of DVT.

Importance of the problem

The global incidence of VTE is unknown, because of its silent nature in asymptomatic patients, as well as significant differences in incidence depending on race/ethnicity. However, in studies involving predominantly white populations, the incidence of first-time, symptomatic VTE, standardized for age and sex to the United States population, ranged from 71 to 117 cases per 100,000 population.[1-5] This incidence rate cannot be extrapolated to nonwhites because of the 2.5–4-fold lowered risk in Asians/Pacific Islanders and Hispanics, and the slightly higher risk in African-Americans.[6-8] Clinical studies (that do not include autopsy data) report the incidence of clinically diagnosed DVT to be approximately twice that of PE.[1,9] When autopsy data is included, studies generally report a higher proportion of PE (~55% PE, 45% DVT), possibly due to the detection of asymptomatic cases of PE at autopsy.[2,10] Proximal extension of symptomatic calf vein thrombosis occurs in 40 to 50% of cases,[11] with an estimated 30% of these cases resulting in fatal PE.[2,12]

Evidence-Based Orthopedics, First Edition. Edited by Mohit Bhandari.
© 2012 Blackwell Publishing Ltd. Published 2012 by Blackwell Publishing Ltd.

Almost all hospitalized patients have at least one risk factor for VTE, with 40% having three or more risk factors.[12–16] The incidence of hospital-acquired DVT is approximately 40–60% following major orthopedic surgery.[17] In American acute care hospitals, VTE is the second most common medical complication, the second most common cause of prolonged length of stay, and the third most common cause of excess charges.[18] PE is the most common preventable cause of hospital death.[19] With an estimated 1 million individuals affected each year by symptomatic VTE, the management of VTE incurs a significant healthcare cost of approximately $1.5 billion/year.[20] Moreover, the burden of VTE extends beyond the initial event to include long-term complications like recurrent VTE, post-thrombotic syndrome, and chronic pulmonary hypertension.

Top ten questions

Diagnosis

1. What is the diagnostic modality of choice to detect DVT?

Therapy

2. Which patients require thromboprophylaxis?
3. Which orthopedic procedures require thromboprophylaxis?
4. Are mechanical thromboprophylactic measures effective?
5. What is the role of inferior vena caval filters?
6. What is the ideal anticoagulant agent?
7. What about aspirin or warfarin?
8. When should anticoagulant treatment be initiated?
9. What should the duration of anticoagulant treatment be?

Harm

10. What is the risk of bleeding with anticoagulants?

Question 1: What is the diagnostic modality of choice to detect DVT?

Relevance

The basis of the diagnosis of DVT or PE has evolved from invasive to noninvasive tests over the past 15 years. Ultrasonography (US) has replaced venography for the diagnosis of deep vein thrombosis, and CT pulmonary angiography has replaced pulmonary angiography and ventilation/perfusion (V/Q) lung scans for detection of PE. Recent evidence also supports the use of clinical prediction rules and D-dimer assays for assessing pretest probability of DVT or PE before ordering more definitive tests.

Current opinion

Venography remains the gold standard for DVT diagnosis, whereas spiral CT angiography is now the diagnostic tool of choice for PE. The need for such definitive testing can be reduced by using clinical prediction rules and D-dimer assays.

Finding the evidence

- Cochrane Database, with keywords "diagnosis" and "venous thromboembolism," "pulmonary embolism," or "deep vein thrombosis"
- PubMed clinical queries search: "diagnosis" and "venous thromboembolism," "pulmonary embolism," or "deep vein thrombosis"
- PubMed sensitivity search using keywords "ultrasonography," "D-dimer," "clinical predictor rule," "helical CT" with "deep vein thrombosis" and "pulmonary embolism"

Quality of the evidence

Level II

- 3 systematic reviews/meta-analyses of cohort studies
- 21 cohort studies

Findings

Clinical prediction rules combined with rapid D-dimer assays In a systematic review of 12 studies (N = 5431 patients),[21–33] outpatients who had a low clinical probability of DVT using the Wells clinical prediction rule (Table 8.1)[34] and a normal D-dimer assay (using the less sensitive SimpliRED assay) had a 3 month VTE incidence of 0.5% (95% CI 0.07–1.1%). When a highly sensitive D-dimer assay was used, the 3 month incidence of VTE was 0.4% (95% CI 0.04–1.1%) among patients with low or moderate clinical probability and a normal D-dimer assay.

Ultrasonography for DVT A meta-analysis of 100 cohort studies (N = 10323 patients)[35] compared US to venography in patients with suspected DVT. Duplex US (combined compression and color Doppler US) had pooled sensitivity of 96.5% (95% CI 95.1–97.6) for proximal DVT and 71.2% (95% CI 64.6–77.2) for distal DVT, and specificity of 94.0% (95% CI 92.8–95.1). Compression US alone had pooled sensitivity of 93.8% (95% CI 92.0–95.3%) for proximal DVT, 56.8% (95% CI 49.0–66.4) for distal DVT and specificity of 97.8% (95% CI 97.0–98.4).

Spiral CT angiography for PE A meta-analysis of 9 studies (N = 520 patients)[36–45] reported a pooled sensitivity for single- or double-row helical CT of 86.0% (95% CI 80.2–92.1%), and specificity of 93.7% (95% CI 91.1–96.3%). The reliability of multislice CT angiography may be enhanced by clinical assessment (pretest probability) and CT venography, but this has yet to be borne out in large prospective trials.

Table 8.1 Wells prediction rule for deep venous thrombosis: clinical evaluation table for predicting pretest probability of deep vein thrombosis

Clinical characteristic	Score
Active cancer (treatment ongoing, within previous 6 months or palliative)	1
Paralysis, paresis or recent plaster immobilization of the lower extremities	1
Recently bedridden >3 days, or major surgery within 12 weeks requiring general or regional anesthesia	1
Localized tenderness along the distribution of the deep venous system	1
Entire leg swollen	1
Calf swelling 3 cm larger than asymptomatic side (measured 10 cm below tibial tuberosity)	1
Pitting edema confined to the symptomatic leg	1
Collateral superficial veins (nonvaricose)	1
Alternative diagnosis at least as likely as deep venous thrombosis	−2

Note: A score of 3 or higher indicates a high probability of deep vein thrombosis; 1 or 2, a moderate probability; and 0 or lower, a low probability. In patients with symptoms in both legs, the more symptomatic leg is used.

Table 8.2 Risk factors for venous thromboembolism

Surgery

Trauma (major trauma or lower-extremity injury)

Immobility, lower-extremity paresis

Cancer (active or occult)

Cancer therapy (hormonal, chemotherapy, angiogenesis inhibitors, radiotherapy)

Venous compression (tumor, hematoma, arterial abnormality)

Previous VTE

Increasing age

Pregnancy and the postpartum period

Estrogen-containing oral contraceptives or hormone replacement therapy

Selective estrogen receptor modulators

Erythropoiesis-stimulating agents

Acute medical illness

Inflammatory bowel disease

Nephrotic syndrome

Myeloproliferative disorders

Paroxysmal nocturnal hemoglobinuria

Obesity

Central venous catheterization

Inherited or acquired thrombophilia (activated protein C resistance, antithrombin III deficiency, protein C/S deficiency, heparin cofactor II deficiency, factor V Leiden mutation, prothrombin mutation 20210 ga, hyperhomocysteinemia, lupus anticoagulant, anticardiolipin antibodies)

Recommendations

• The use of a D-dimer assay combined with a clinical prediction rule has a very high negative predictive value. Less sensitive D-dimer assays can be used to exclude VTE in patients with low clinical probability of VTE, while more sensitive assays can be applied to patients with low or moderate probability of VTE. D-dimer assays have no role in patients with high probability of VTE [overall quality: moderate]

• Ultrasonography has high sensitivity for proximal DVT, modest sensitivity for distal DVT and high specificity for all locations. Optimal sensitivity, particularly for distal DVT, is achieved by using duplex or triplex US, while compression US alone has optimal specificity for proximal DVT. Ultrasonography also has other benefits including wide availability, noninvasiveness and the ability to exclude alternative diagnoses. Despite this, venography has higher sensitivity for detecting distal DVT and remains the gold standard [overall quality: moderate]

• With modern, multidetector row CT scanners, the sensitivity and specificity of spiral CTs are approaching the gold standard set by the pulmonary angiogram, and many consider CT angiograms to be the new gold standard. Despite the apparent lack of sensitivity, it is safe to withhold anti-coagulation after a negative good-quality CT scan [overall quality: moderate]

Question 2: Which patients require thromboprophylaxis?

Relevance

Every patient undergoing surgery should be stratified for VTE risk to assist in the surgeon's decision-making process. There are several approaches to doing this: one is to determine the VTE risk in each patient based on predisposing factors (Table 8.2).[17] Risk assessment models for DVT have been devised for medical and surgical patients.[46] A second approach is to assign patients to one of four VTE risk levels based on several factors (Table 8.3).[46] A final approach involves group-specific thromboprophylaxis as recommended by the American College of Chest Physicians (Table 8.4).[47]

Current opinion

Current risk assessment models are not comprehensive and have not been validated in orthopedic surgery. Controversy exists as to whether all the commonly cited risk factors are relevant for postoperative VTE.

Table 8.3 Stratification of venous thromboembolism risk level

Low	Moderate	High	Highest
Uncomplicated minor surgery in patients <40 years old	Surgery in patients 40–60 years old without risk factors	Major surgery in patients >60 years old without risk factors	Major surgery in patients >60 years old
			With:
No risk factors	Major surgery in patients <40 years old and no risk factors	Major surgery in patients >40 years old with risk factors	Previous VTE Malignancy
	Minor surgery in any age group with risk factors		Orthopedic surgery Thrombophilia Stroke/spinal injury Hip fracture

Table 8.4 Group-specific stratification of thromboembolism risk level

Levels of risk	Approximate DVT risk without thromboprophylaxis (%)	Suggested thromboprophylaxis options
Low risk Minor surgery in mobile patients Medical patients who are fully mobile	<10	No specific thromboprophylaxis Early and aggressive ambulation
Moderate risk Most general, open gynaecologic or urologic surgery patients Medical patients, bed rest or sick Moderate VTE risk plus high bleeding risk	10–40	LMWH (at recommended doses), LDUH bid or tid, fondaparinux Mechanical thromboprophylaxis
High risk Hip or knee arthroplasty Hip fracture surgery Major trauma, spinal cord injury High VTE risk plus high bleeding risk	40–80	LMWH (at recommended doses), fondaparinux, oral vitamin K antagonist (INR 2–3) Mechanical thromboprophylaxis

Finding the evidence

- Cochrane Database, with keywords "risk stratification," "risk factors," "risk assessment models" and "venous thromboembolism"
- PubMed sensitivity search using keywords "risk stratification," "risk factors," "risk assessment models" and "venous thromboembolism"

Quality of the evidence

Level II
- 1 systematic review/meta-analysis

Findings

Risk assessment models No validated risk assessment models that are specific to orthopedic surgery are currently available.

Validity of common risk factors A systematic review was performed to determine the evidence base behind commonly cited risk factors, and found good evidence associating postoperative DVT with increased age, obesity, previous thromboembolism, varicose veins, the oral contraceptive pill, malignancy, factor V Leiden gene mutation, general anesthesia and orthopedic surgery.[48] There is a paucity of strong evidence, however, with regards to the suggested risk factors of hormone replacement therapy, gender, ethnicity or race, chemotherapy, other thrombophilias, cardiovascular factors, smoking, and blood type.

Recommendation

- A group-specific approach as recommended by the ACCP (American College of Chest Physicians) is the best approach to VTE risk stratification in patients. Currently, there is very little evidence recommending individualized risk factor assessment or the relationship of such factors to postoperative VTE risk [overall quality: low]

Question 3: Which orthopedic patients require thromboprophylaxis?

Relevance

It is widely accepted that major orthopedic procedures including hip and knee arthroplasty and hip fracture surgery confer the highest risk for venous thromboembolic events. More controversial are the indications for thromboprophylaxis in spine patients, knee arthroscopy patients, pelvic and acetabular fractures, and isolated lower extremity fractures.

Current opinion

There is a lack of consensus regarding the need for prophylaxis in patients other than those undergoing hip/knee arthroplasty or hip fracture surgery, stemming from the scarcity of evidence currently available.

Finding the evidence

- Cochrane Database, with keywords "venous thromboembolism" and "spinal surgery," "spinal cord injury," "arthroscopy," or "fractures"
- PubMed sensitivity search using keywords "venous thromboembolism" and "spinal surgery," "spinal cord injury," "arthroscopy," or "fractures"

Quality of the evidence

Level I

- 3 systematic reviews/meta-analyses
- 6 randomized trials

Level II

- 1 systematic review of cohort studies
- 1 randomized trials with methodological limitations
- 2 cohort studies

Findings

Spine surgery In a systematic review of 25 cohort studies (N = 9991 patients),[49] the pooled DVT rate for patients undergoing elective spine surgery without prophylaxis was 2.7% and the PE rate was 0.2%. The DVT/PE rate was 2.7%/0.6% in patients who received prophylaxis with graduated compression stockings, 4.6%/1.1% with pneumatic compression devices, 1.3%/1% with compression devices and compression stockings, 0.6%/0.3% with chemical anticoagulation, and 22%/1% with inferior vena cava (IVC) filters or other methods of prophylaxis.

Spinal cord injury The incidence of DVT in patients with acute spinal cord injury has been reported to be more than 50%, with the incidence of fatal PE estimated to be as high as 5%. In a systematic review of 23 studies examining various interventions for VTE prevention,[50] the best evidence available (2 RCTs, N = 148 patients),[51,52] suggests that low molecular weight heparin (LMWH), in particular enoxaparin, is more effective than standard subcutaneous heparin at reducing venous thromboembolic events. Moreover, the incidence of bleeding complications appears to be less with LMWH.

Knee arthroscopy A meta-analysis of 4 studies (N = 527 patients) included predominantly male patients (age range 31–44 years) undergoing various knee arthroscopic interventions.[53–57] The relative risk of thrombotic events was 0.16 (95% CI 0.05–0.52) comparing any type of LMWH vs. placebo. All thrombotic events but one (PE in the LMWH group) were distal venous thrombosis. The number needed to benefit was 17. Adverse events were most common in the intervention group than in the control group (relative risk = 2.04, 95% CI 1.21–3.44). The number needed to harm was 20 for any adverse events.

Pelvic/acetabular trauma A systematic review of 11 studies included 1760 patients with pelvic and acetabular fractures.[58] Most studies were observational designs with minimal control data and quantitative pooling was not possible based on significant study heterogeneity. In one prospective cohort study the proximal DVT rate was 10%, with a symptomatic PE incidence of 5%.[59] No practical guidelines could be made based on the lack of strong evidence.

Lower extremity trauma In a prospective cohort study examining patients with lower extremity fractures distal to the hip (N = 102 patients),[60] the overall incidence of DVT was 28% (95% CI 19.9–38.2%), of which only 12% were proximal DVT. Risk of embolization was low. Another randomized controlled trial (N = 238 patients) studied the effect of LMWH on patients with surgically fixed fractures below the knee.[61] The incidence of venographically proven DVT between patients receiving LMWH and placebo was similar (8.7% vs. 12.6%, p = 0.22), suggesting that thromboprophylaxis is not necessary for patients with fractures below the knee.

Recommendations

- As the VTE rate after elective spinal surgery is low, anticoagulation as the primary method of prophylaxis cannot be recommended. A combination of graduated compression stockings and intermittent pneumatic compression should suffice [overall quality: moderate]
- Spinal cord injury patients have a high rate of VTE. The best available evidence suggests LMWH as the thromboprophylactic of choice [overall quality: low]
- There is no strong evidence to suggest the routine use of thromboprophylaxis for patients undergoing knee arthroscopy is beneficial or safe [overall quality: low]
- There is inadequate evidence to suggest that any particular thromboprophylaxis regime is superior for patients with pelvic and acetabular fractures. Existing guidelines

recommend the use of LMWH in these high-risk patients [overall quality: low]

• Current available evidence suggests that lower extremity fractures below the knee do not require chemical thromboprophylaxis [overall quality: low]

• Patients with more proximal lower extremity fractures (above the knee) are more likely to develop DVT, and thus prophylaxis is recommended [overall quality: low]

Question 4: Are mechanical thromboprophylactic measures effective?

Relevance
Mechanical compression methods, including graduated compression stockings, intermittent pneumatic compression and foot pumps, are widely available, inexpensive, and have very few contraindications. These measures can be employed as monotherapy in patients with contraindications to anticoagulant therapy, or in conjunction with anticoagulants in higher-risk patients. Evidence regarding the effectiveness of mechanical thromboprophylaxis has been contradictory.

Current opinion
Mechanical measures effectively reduce the risk of venous thromboembolism, and are a useful adjuvant to anticoagulation agents.

Finding the evidence
• Cochrane Database, with keywords "mechanical thromboprophylaxis"
• PubMed clinical queries search: "mechanical thromboprophylaxis"
• PubMed sensitivity search using keywords "mechanical thromboprophylaxis"

Quality of the evidence
Level I
• 3 systematic reviews/meta-analyses
• 12 randomized trials

Level II
• 2 randomized trials with methodological limitations

Findings
Graduated compression stockings Seven studies (N = 1027 patients) reported on the incidence of DVT in a mixed population of surgical and medical patients.[62–69] Patients who were treated with compression stockings developed a lower rate of DVT compared to the control group (relative risk = 0.36, 95% CI 0.26–0.49, p < 0.00001).

Intermittent pneumatic compression Three studies (N = 302 patients) reported on the use of cyclical compression

devices in patients undergoing hip fracture surgery.[70–74] These devices significantly reduced the incidence of DVT and PE when compared to the control group (relative risk = 0.27, p = 0.00085).

Foot pumps Two studies (N = 147 patients) reported on the use of arteriovenous foot impulse systems in patients undergoing hip fracture surgery.[75,76] These devices significantly reduced the incidence of DVT and PE when compared to the control group (relative risk = 0.20, p = 0.000068).

Combined therapy Two studies (N = 1934 patients) reported on the incidence of DVT in high-risk patients.[77–79] Patients who were treated with compression modalities and anticoagulants had a significantly lower incidence of DVT compared to patients who were given anticoagulants alone (relative risk = 0.13, 95% CI 0.05–0.35).

Recommendation
• All the various methods of mechanical thromboprophylaxis have been shown to significantly reduce the incidence of DVT, whether provided as monotherapy or in combination with anticoagulant therapy. Judicious use is recommended, especially in patients with contraindications to anticoagulant therapy [Overall Quality: Moderate]

Question 5: What is the role of IVC filters?

Relevance
IVC filters were historically used for patients with proven VTE but developed complications on anticoagulation, had contraindications to systemic anticoagulation, or had recurrent VTE despite adequate anticoagulation. However, these indications have expanded in the last two decades despite the lack of evidence-based guidelines (Table 8.5).[80,81]

Current opinion
There has been increasing use of IVC filters, particularly with the advent of retrievable filters. Relative indications other than those recommended are not based on any existing clinical evidence.

Finding the evidence
• Cochrane Database, with keywords "inferior vena caval filters"
• PubMed sensitivity search using keywords "inferior vena caval filters"

Quality of the evidence
Level I
• 1 systematic review

Level II
• 1 randomized trial with methodological limitations
• 1 cohort study

Table 8.5 Indications for IVC filter use

Recommended use according to evidence-based guidelines

Proven VTE with contraindication for anticoagulation

Proven VTE with complications of anticoagulation treatment

Recurrent VTE despite anticoagulation treatment (failure of anticoagulation)

Expanded use (not guideline recommended)

Recurrent PE complicated by pulmonary hypertension

Patients with DVT and limited cardiopulmonary reserve or chronic obstructive pulmonary

disease

Patients with large, free-floating ileofemoral thrombus

Following thrombectomy, embolectomy, or thrombolysis of DVT

High-risk trauma patients (head and spinal cord injury, pelvic or lower extremity fractures) with a contraindication for anticoagulation

High-risk surgical patients with a contraindication for anticoagulation

Patients with DVT who have cancer, burns, or are pregnant

Contraindications for filter placement

Chronically thrombosed IVC

Anatomical abnormalities preventing access to the IVC for filter placement

Findings

Permanent IVC filters Only one randomized controlled trial has been published in the literature (n = 400 patients).[82,83] This study was flawed because it excluded patients with contraindications to anticoagulation or who had failed anticoagulation. It compared patients with permanent filters to a control group without filters, although both groups received anticoagulation concurrently.[84] At 8 years, the rate of symptomatic PE in the filter group was significantly reduced (hazard ratio = 0.37, 95% CI 0.17–0.79, p = 0.008), although the risk of recurrent DVT was increased with prolonged filter use (hazard ratio = 1.52, 95% CI 1.02–2.27, p = 0.042).

Temporary/retrievable IVC filters One prospective study (n = 47 patients) evaluated the use of temporary or retrievable filters.[85] Some contraindications to anticoagulation listed in this study include major trauma with pelvic fracture, planned operation, and childbirth. Twelve patients also received filters as a prophylactic measure, without any evidence of VTE. Two patients developed PE during or after filter removal; two filters migrated, requiring repositioning or replacement; and two patients required surgical filter removal due to trapped thrombi.

Recommendation

• There is a distinct lack of clinical evidence guiding the current use of IVC filters. In the absence of evidence, the current accepted indication for filters remains "the contraindication to anticoagulation." Clinical judgment should be exercised for the use of temporary or retrievable filters, or use of filters in nonrecommended situations [overall quality: low]

Question 6: What is the ideal anticoagulant agent?

Relevance

The 2008 ACCP guidelines recommend the use of several anticoagulants for orthopedic surgery.[17] These include low-dose unfractionated heparin (LDUH), LMWH, subcutaneous pentasaccharide fondaparinux, and vitamin K antagonists (VKAs), exemplified by warfarin. The ideal anticoagulant should have high efficacy, safety, low levels of bleeding, rapid onset of action, fixed dosing, and no requirement for therapeutic monitoring. In this section, the evidence for the injectable anticoagulants is presented. Warfarin is discussed in the next section.

Current opinion

LDUH has largely been surpassed by LMWH. The factor Xa inhibitor fondaparinux has even greater thromboprophylactic efficacy, but this is balanced by a higher rate of bleeding events.

Finding the evidence

• Cochrane Database, with keywords "heparin" or "anticoagulant" and "venous thromboembolism"
• PubMed sensitivity search using keywords "heparin" or "anticoagulant" and "venous thromboembolism"
• Preference was given to orthopedically relevant studies

Quality of the evidence

Level I

• 1 systematic review/meta-analyse
• 21 randomized trials

Level II

• 1 cohort study

Findings

Efficacy of injectable anticoagulants A retrospective cohort study analysed 144,806 patients undergoing major orthopedic surgery using dalteparin, enoxaparin, fondaparinux, and LDUH.[86] VTE was less frequent in the fondaparinux group (1.5%). Patients receiving LDUH were most likely to have a VTE (odds ratio = 1.98, 95% CI 1.67–2.34, p < 0.0001), while patients in the enoxaparin and dalteparin groups were 40% (odds radio = 1.39, 95% CI 1.19–1.62, p < 0.0001) and 20% (odds ratio = 1.22, 95% CI 1.01–1.46, p = 0.0370) more likely to have VTE than the fondaparinux group.

Bleeding rates In a meta-analysis of 21 studies (N = 20,523 patients) comparing the use of warfarin, unfractionated heparin (UFH), LMWH, and fondaparinux in patients undergoing major orthopedic surgery, LMWH resulted in fewer major bleeding episodes than UFH (relative risk = 1.52, 95% CI 1.04–2.23) and fondaparinux (relative risk = 1.52, 95% CI 1.11–2.09) but more than warfarin (relative risk = 0.59, 95% CI0.44–0.80).[87–109]

Cost In the same large cohort study mentioned above, patients who received fondaparinux had significantly lower adjusted mean costs than patients on LMWH or LDUH (p < 0.01), compared to LDUH which had the highest adjusted mean cost per patient.[86] This takes into account that patients who had an episode of VTE or major bleeding would incur greater costs.

Recommendations
• LMWH remains the best anticoagulation agent currently available for thromboprophylaxis in orthopedic patients. It is effective, safe, and relatively inexpensive [overall quality: moderate]
• Fondaparinux has the strongest thromboprophylactic efficacy and overall costs for treatment per patient is lower. However, the significantly higher risk of bleeding compared to LMWH limits fondaparinux use in postoperative orthopedic patients [overall quality: high]

Question 7: What about aspirin or warfarin?

Relevance
As a VKA, warfarin has been the only oral anticoagulant available for the past 65 years, and has historically been used for thromboprophylaxis in total hip arthroplasty patients. However, warfarin has numerous limitations, including its narrow therapeutic window, slow onset of action, multiple food and drug interactions, and genetic metabolic variations.[110] Newer oral anticoagulants are being developed that are free from warfarin's drawbacks.

There has also been much interest in aspirin as a prophylactic agent in VTE, especially in its potential for use as an oral agent in extended-duration, out-of-hospital prophylaxis. It is believed that aspirin's overwhelming benefit in arterial occlusive disease may similarly have an effect on venous thrombus formation.

Current opinion
Warfarin remains a viable alternative to heparin in VTE prophylaxis. Aspirin, although effective, does not have an established role in VTE prophylaxis and its routine use is not recommended.

Finding the evidence
• Cochrane Database, with keywords "warfarin" or "aspirin" and "thromboprophylaxis" or "venous thromboembolism"

• PubMed sensitivity search using keywords "warfarin" or "aspirin" and "thromboprophylaxis" or "venous thromboembolism"

Quality of the evidence
Level I
• 1 systematic review/meta-analysis
• 21 randomized trials

Findings
Warfarin A meta-analysis of 20 randomized controlled trials (N = 6,900 patients) assessed LMWH, UFH, and warfarin as prophylaxis in orthopedic surgery patients.[111] The relative risk of DVT for LMWH vs. warfarin was 0.78 (95% CI 0.69—0.87, p<0.05). The relative risk of PE for LMWH vs. warfarin was 1.00 (95% CI 0.10—9.94). Significantly more minor bleeding was found with LMWH vs. warfarin (relative risk = 3.28, 95% CI 2.21–4.70, p < 0.05).

Aspirin In a large randomized controlled trial involving 13,356 patients undergoing hip fracture surgery, low-dose aspirin was administered preoperatively and continued for 35 days after surgery.[112] Aspirin produced proportional reductions in pulmonary embolism of 43% (95% CI 18–60, p = 0.002) and in symptomatic DVT of 29% (95% CI 3–48, p = 0.03). In the same study, similar reduced rates of VTE were seen in 4088 patients who underwent elective hip arthroplasty. However, excess episodes of postoperative transfused bleeding were noted with its use (p = 0.04).

Recommendations
• Warfarin is less effective than LMWH in the prevention of VTE. However, it remains a feasible option because of its cost-benefit ratio and relative ease of administration [overall quality: moderate]
• While there is good evidence that aspirin does effectively reduce VTE, its use as a monotherapy agent in VTE prophylaxis is not clearly defined. First-line agents like LMWH and warfarin have suggested superior efficacy and safety profiles [overall quality: moderate]
• Newer oral anticoagulants that target either thrombin or factor Xa have the potential to surpass warfarin as the oral anticoagulant of choice. Drugs like dabigatran etexilate, rivaroxaban, and apixaban are currently undergoing phase III clinical trials and/or seeking US Food and Drug Administration approval for use in the orthopedic population [overall quality: low]

Question 8: When should anticoagulant treatment be initiated?

Relevance
Much controversy exists regarding the optimal time to initiate thromboprophylaxis. On one hand, the belief that

venous thrombi are formed perioperatively[113] has directed the European practice of providing antithrombotic therapy preoperatively to maximize antithrombotic effectiveness. On the other hand, the North American practice is to start anticoagulation postoperatively to allow hemostasis of the wound and reduce the risk of bleeding complications.[114] In addition, the administration of preoperative anticoagulation may preclude the use of neuraxial anesthesia for fear of developing spinal hematomas with catastrophic consequences.

Current opinion

Current opinion suggests that there is no significant difference in VTE incidence whether thromboprophylaxis is initiated pre- or postoperatively.

Finding the evidence

- Cochrane Database, with keywords "timing" and "anticoagulation" or "thromboprophylaxis"
- PubMed sensitivity search using keywords "timing" and "anticoagulation" or "thromboprophylaxis"

Quality of the evidence

Level I
- 2 systematic reviews/meta-analyses
- 7 randomized trials

Findings

No large-scale randomized controlled trials exist which address the relative efficacy and safety of preoperative vs. postoperative initiation of VTE prophylaxis

Antithrombotic efficacy Six studies (N = 987 patients) evaluated the use of enoxaparin in patients undergoing elective hip replacement.[115-121] When comparing the preoperative regimen (initiated 10–12 hours before surgery) to the postoperative regimen (initiated within 24 hours after surgery), there was no significant difference in the incidence of all DVT (10% vs. 15.3%, p = 0.02, 95% CI −9.58 to −1.06) or proximal vein thrombosis (p = 0.38, 95% CI −1.67 to 4.71).

Bleeding risk Six studies (N = 1219) compared the incidence of major and minor bleeding episodes between the preoperative and postoperative regimens in patients undergoing hip arthroplasty using enoxaparin prophylaxis.[115-121] The frequency of major bleeding was surprisingly less for the preoperative group than for the postoperative group (0.9% vs. 3.5%, p = 0.01, 95% CI −4.24 to −1.10).

Perioperative regimens One study (N = 1501 patients) randomized patients undergoing hip arthroplasty into three groups: dalteparin within 2 hours before surgery, dalteparin at least 4 hours postsurgery, and oral anticoagulation with warfarin.[122] Both dalteparin regimens administered in this "close proximity" or "just-in-time" fashion showed significant reduction in DVT rates compared to the warfarin group (p < 0.001, relative risk reduction = 50%). However, increased major bleeding was observed for the preoperative dalteparin group compared to the warfarin group (p = 0.01).

Recommendations

- Thromboprophylaxis started 12 hours before surgery has not been shown to be more effective than prophylaxis initiated 12–24 hours after surgery [overall quality: moderate]
- Close-proximity perioperative regimens may provide the optimal effectiveness in thromboprophylaxis, but this has to be balanced against a higher risk for bleeding complications [overall quality: moderate]

Question 9: What should the duration of anticoagulant treatment be?

Relevance

Thromboprophylaxis is commonly administered for the duration of the hospital stay, which can range from 4 to 14 days. However, recent evidence shows that patients are still at risk of developing symptomatic thromboembolism after discharge from hospital. New guidelines now recommend the use of extended, out-of-hospital prophylaxis but this has to be balanced against the cost-effectiveness and risk-benefit ratio of such regimens.

Current opinion

The optimal duration of prophylaxis after major orthopedic surgery is still controversial.

Finding the evidence

- Cochrane Database, with keywords "extended" and "thromboprophylaxis"
- PubMed sensitivity search using keywords "extended" or "out-of-hospital" and "thromboprophylaxis"

Quality of the evidence

Level I
- 2 systematic reviews/meta-analyses
- 9 randomized trials

Findings

Efficacy of extended-duration prophylaxis In a meta-analysis of nine randomized controlled trials (N = 3999 patients), it was found that extended-duration prophylaxis for 30–42 days with LMWH or UFH reduced the rate of symptomatic VTE (1.3% vs. 3.3%, odds ratio = 0.38, 95% CI 0.24–0.61).[123-132] Risk reduction was greater in patients undergoing hip arthroplasty (1·4% vs. 4·3%, odds ratio = 0.33, 95% CI 0.19–0.56) compared with knee arthroplasty (1.0% vs. 1.4%, odds ratio = 0.74, 95% CI 0.26–2.15).

Safety of extended-duration prophylaxis In the same meta-analysis, there was no increase in major bleeding but extended-duration prophylaxis was associated with excessive minor bleeding (3.7% vs. 2.5%, odds ratio 1.56, 95% CI 1.08–2.26, number needed to harm = 83).

Cost-effectiveness of extended-duration prophylaxis In a meta-analysis of eight studies using LMWH and warfarin prophylaxis for hip arthroplasty patients, primary economic analysis found that the cost-effectiveness of LMWH relative to no further prophylaxis ($106,454 per quality-adjusted life year gained) was unattractive, with the primary cost driver being the proportion of patients who required home nursing services for drug injection.[133]

Recommendations

• Extended-duration prophylaxis is an effective and safe means to reduce the rate of symptomatic out-of-hospital venous thromboembolic events in arthroplasty patients, although knee arthroplasty patients may benefit less from it [overall quality: moderate]
• Cost-effectiveness of routine out-of-hospital prophylaxis with LMWH remains an issue. Less costly alternatives should be considered and evaluated [overall quality: moderate]

Question 10: What is the risk of bleeding with anticoagulants?

Relevance

Many orthopedic surgeons are averse to thromboprophylaxis because of the perceived risk of postoperative bleeding when using anticoagulant agents. Bleeding, when it does occur, is more acute than VTE itself, and potentially compromises the result of the procedure. This misperception remains one of the major barriers to routine thromboprophylaxis within the orthopedic community.

Current opinion

There is no good evidence that anticoagulant agents produce significant postoperative bleeding, or that it compromises operative outcomes.

Finding the evidence

• Cochrane Database, with keywords "bleeding risk" or "postoperative bleeding" and "anticoagulation" or "thromboprophylaxis"
• PubMed sensitivity search using keywords "postoperative bleeding" and "anticoagulation" or "thromboprophylaxis"
• Preference was given to orthopedically relevant studies

Quality of the evidence

Level I
• 1 systematic review/meta-analysis
• 4 randomized trials

Level II
• 1 randomized trials with methodological limitations

Findings

Wound hematoma Two studies (N = 81 patients) reported on the postoperative development of wound hematomas.[70–72,134] Patients who were given perioperative heparin (LDUH or LMWH) thromboprophylaxis for hip fracture surgery did not have a higher risk of developing wound hematomas when compared to a placebo group (relative risk = 1.10, p = 0.90).

Blood loss Two studies (N = 90 patients) reported on estimated blood loss after hip fracture surgery and did not find any significantly increased blood loss after perioperative heparin (LDUH or LMWH) thromboprophylaxis (weighted mean difference = 47.21 mL, p = 0.25).[70,134,135]

Transfusion requirements One study (N = 31 patients)[71,72] reported on postoperative transfusion amount, and three studies (N = 249)[71,72,136,137] reported the number of patients receiving transfusion after hip fracture surgery. There was no difference in transfusion amount (weighted mean difference = 83.82 mL, p = 0.54), or number of patients requiring transfusions between the heparin group and the placebo group (relative risk = 0.90, p = 0.48)

Recommendation

• The use of anticoagulants for thromboprophylaxis does not increase the risk of blood loss, wound hematoma formation, or transfusion requirements. The surgeon should realize that postoperative bleeding is a multifactorial problem and careful hemostatic techniques should be observed [overall quality: moderate]

Summary of recommendations

• The use of a D-dimer assay combined with a clinical prediction rule has a very high negative predictive value. Less sensitive D-dimer assays can be used to exclude VTE in patients with low clinical probability of VTE, while more sensitive assays can be applied to patients with low or moderate probability of VTE. D-dimer assays have no role in patients with high probability of VTE
• Ultrasonography has high sensitivity for proximal DVT, modest sensitivity for distal DVT and high specificity for all locations. Optimal sensitivity, particularly for distal DVT, is achieved by using duplex or triplex US, while compression US alone has optimal specificity. Ultrasonography also has other benefits of wide availability, noninvasiveness and the ability to exclude alternative diagnoses. Despite this, venography has higher sensitivity for detecting distal DVT and remains the gold standard

- With modern, multidetector row CT scanners, the sensitivity and specificity of spiral CTs are approaching the gold standard set by the pulmonary angiogram, and many consider CT angiograms to be the new gold standard. Despite the apparent lack of sensitivity, it is safe to withhold anticoagulation after a negative good-quality CT scan
- A group-specific approach as recommended by the ACCP is the best approach to VTE risk stratification in patients. There is very little evidence behind individualized risk factor assessment or the relationship of such factors to postoperative VTE
- As the VTE rate after elective spinal surgery is low, anticoagulation as the primary method of prophylaxis cannot be recommended. A combination of graduated compression stockings and intermittent pneumatic compression should suffice
- Spinal cord injury patients are associated with a high rate of VTE. The best available evidence suggests LMWH as the thromboprophylactic of choice
- There is no strong evidence to suggest the routine use of thromboprophylaxis for patients undergoing knee arthroscopy is beneficial or safe
- There is inadequate evidence to suggest that any particular thromboprophylaxis regime is superior for patients with pelvic and acetabular fractures. Existing guidelines recommend the use of LMWH in these high-risk patients
- Current available evidence suggests that lower extremity fractures below the knee do not require chemical thromboprophylaxis
- Patients with more proximal lower extremity fractures (above the knee) are more likely to develop DVT, although this tends to be below the popliteal fossa, with less likelihood of embolization
- All the various methods of mechanical thromboprophylaxis have been shown to significantly reduce the incidence of DVT, whether provided as monotherapy or in combination with anticoagulant therapy. Judicious use is recommended, especially in patients with contraindications to anticoagulant therapy
- There is a distinct lack of clinical evidence guiding the current use of IVC filters. In the absence of evidence, the current accepted indications for filters remain as failure of, or contraindication to anticoagulation. Clinical judgment should be exercised for the use of temporary or retrievable filters, or use of filters in nonrecommended situations
- LMWH remains the best anticoagulation agent currently available for thromboprophylaxis in orthopedic patients. It is effective, safe, and relatively inexpensive
- Fondaparinux has the strongest thromboprophylactic efficacy and overall costs for treatment per patient is lower. However, the significantly higher risk of bleeding compared to LMWH limits fondaparinux use in postoperative orthopedic patients

- Warfarin is less effective than LMWH in the prevention of VTE. However it remains a feasible option because of its cost-benefit ratio and relative ease of administration
- While there is good evidence that aspirin does effectively reduce VTE, its use as a monotherapy agent in VTE prophylaxis is not recommended. First-line agents like LMWH and warfarin have suggested superior efficacy and safety profiles
- Newer oral anticoagulants that target either thrombin or factor Xa have the potential to surpass warfarin as the oral anticoagulant of choice. Drugs such asdabigatran etexilate, rivaroxaban, and apixaban are currently undergoing phase III clinical trials and/or seeking US Food and Drug Administration approval for use in the orthopedic population
- Thromboprophylaxis started 12 hours before surgery has not been shown to be more effective than prophylaxis initiated 12–24 hours after surgery
- Close-proximity perioperative regimens may provide the optimal effectiveness in thromboprophylaxis, but this has to be balanced against a higher risk for bleeding complications
- Extended-duration prophylaxis is an effective and safe means to reduce the rate of symptomatic out-of-hospital VTE events in arthroplasty patients, although knee arthroplasty patients may benefit less from it
- Cost-effectiveness of routine out-of-hospital prophylaxis with LMWH remains an issue. Less costly alternatives should be considered and evaluated
- The use of anticoagulants for thromboprophylaxis does not increase the risk of blood loss, wound hematoma formation, or transfusion requirements. The surgeon should realize that postoperative bleeding is a multifactorial problem and careful hemostatic techniques should be observed

References

1. Anderson FA Jr., Wheeler HB, Goldberg RJ, et al. A population-based perspective of the hospital incidence and case-fatality rates of deep vein thrombosis and pulmonary embolism. The Worcester DVT Study. Arch Intern Med 1991;151:933–8.
2. Silverstein MD, Heit JA, Mohr DN, et al. Trends in the incidence of deep vein thrombosis and pulmonary embolism: a 25-year population-based study. Arch Intern Med 1998;158:585–93.
3. White RH. The epidemiology of venous thromboembolism. Circulation 2003;107, I4–8.
4. Coon WW. Epidemiology of venous thromboembolism. Ann Surg 1977;186:149–4.
5. Gillum RF. Pulmonary embolism and thrombophlebitis in the United States, 1970–1985. Am Heart J 1987;114:1262–4.
6. White RH, Zhou H, Romano PS. Incidence of idiopathic deep venous thrombosis and secondary thromboembolism among ethnic groups in California. Ann Intern Med 1998;128:737–40.

7. Hirst AE, Gore I, Tanaka K, et al. Myocardial infarction and pulmonary embolism. Arch Pathol 1965;80:365–70.

8. Klatsky AL, Armstrong MA, Poggi J. Risk of pulmonary embolism and/or deep venous thrombosis in Asian-Americans. Am J Cardiol 2000;85:1334–7.

9. Murin S, Romano PS, White RH. Comparison of outcomes after hospitalization for deep venous thrombosis or pulmonary embolism. Thromb Haemost 2002;88:407–14.

10. Hansson PO, Welin L, Tibblin G, et al. Deep vein thrombosis and pulmonary embolism in the general population. "The Study of Men Born in 1913." Arch Intern Med 1997;157: 1665–70.

11. Kakkar VV, Howe CT, Flanc C, Clarke MB. Natural history of postoperative deep-vein thrombosis. Lancet1969;ii, 230–2.

12. Heit JA, Cohen AT, Anderson FA, VTE Impact Assessment Group. Estimated annual number of incident and recurrent, non-fatal and fatal venous thromboembolism (VTE) events in the U.S. Blood 2005;106:267a.

13. Rosendaal FR. Risk factors for venous thrombotic disease. Thromb Haemost 1999;82:610–19.

14. Rosendaal FR. Venous thrombosis: a multicausal disease. Lancet 1999;353:1167–73.

15. Anderson FA, Spencer FA. Risk factors for venous thromboembolism. Circulation 2003;107:I9–16.

16. Edmonds MJ, Crichton TJ, Runciman WB. Evidence-based risk factors for postoperative deep vein thrombosis. ANZ J Surg 2004;74:1082–97.

17. Geerts WH, Bergqvist D, Graham F, et al. Prevention of venous thromboembolism: American College of Chest Physicians Evidence-Based Clinical Practice Guidelines (8th edition). Chest 2008;133:318–453S.

18. Zhan C, Miller MR. Excess length of stay, charges, and mortality attributable to medical injuries during hospitalization. JAMA 2003;290:1868–74.

19. Cohen AT, Tapson VF, Bergmann JF, et al. Venous thromboembolism risk and prophylaxis in the acute hospital care setting (ENDORSE study): a multinational cross-sectional study. Lancet 2008;371:387–94.

20. Spyropoulos AC, Hurley JS, Ciesla GN, de Lissovoy G. Management of acute proximal deep vein thrombosis: pharmacoeconomic evaluation of outpatient treatment with enoxaparin vs inpatient treatment with unfractionated heparin. Chest 2002;122:108–14.

21. Fancher TL, White RH, Kravitz RL. Combined use of rapid D-dimer testing and estimation of clinical probability in the diagnosis of deep vein thrombosis: systematic review. BMJ 2004;329:821–8.

22. Anderson DR, Wells PS, Stiell I, MacLeod B, Simms M, Gray L, et al. Management of patients with suspected deep vein thrombosis in the emergency department: combining use of a clinical diagnosis model with d-dimer testing. J Emerg Med 2000;19: 225–30.

23. Perrier A, Desmarais S, Miron MJ, de Moerloose P, Lepage R, Slosman D, et al. Non-invasive diagnosis of venous thromboembolism in outpatients. Lancet 1999;353:190–5.

24. Bucek RA, Koca N, Reiter M, Haumer M, Zontsich T, Minar E. Algorithms for the diagnosis of deep-vein thrombosis in patients with low clinical pretest probability. Thromb Res 2002; 105:43–7.

25. Kraaijenhagen RA, Piovella F, Bernardi E, Verlato F, Beckers EA, Koopman MM, et al. Simplification of the diagnostic management of suspected deep vein thrombosis. Arch Intern Med 2002;162:907–11.

26. Shields GP, Turnipseed S, Panacek EA, Melnikoff N, Gosselin R, White RH. Validation of the Canadian clinical probability model for acute venous thrombosis. Acad Emerg Med 2002;9: 561–6.

27. Wells PS, Anderson DR, Bormanis J, Guy F, Mitchell M, Lewandowski B. SimpliRED d-dimer can reduce the diagnostic tests in suspected deep vein thrombosis. Lancet 1998;351:1405–6.

28. Ginsberg JS, Kearon C, Douketis J, Turpie AG, Brill-Edwards P, Stevens P, et al. The use of D-dimer testing and impedance plethysmographic examination in patients with clinical indications of deep vein thrombosis. Arch Intern Med 1997;157: 1077–81.

29. Bates SM, Kearon C, Crowther M, Linkins L, O'Donnell M, Douketis J, et al. A diagnostic strategy involving a quantitative latex d-dimer assay reliably excludes deep venous thrombosis. Ann Intern Med 2003;138:787–94.

30. Kearon C, Ginsberg JS, Douketis J, Crowther M, Brill-Edwards P, Weitz JI, et al. Management of suspected deep venous thrombosis in outpatients by using clinical assessment and D-dimer testing. Ann Intern Med 2001;135:108–11.

31. Schutgens RE, Ackermark P, Haas FJ, Nieuwenhuis HK, Peltenburg HG, Pijlman AH, et al. Combination of a normal D-dimer concentration and a non-high pretest clinical probability score is a safe strategy to exclude deep venous thrombosis. Circulation 2003;107:593–7.

32. Tick LW, Ton E, van Voorthuizen T, Hovens MM, Leeuwenburgh I, Lobatto S, et al. Practical diagnostic management of patients with clinically suspected deep vein thrombosis by clinical probability test, compression ultrasonography, and d-dimer test. Am J Med 2002;113:630–5.

33. Aguilar C, Martinez A, Del Rio C, Vazquez M, Rodriguez FJ. Diagnostic value of D-dimer in patients with a moderate pretest probability of deep venous thrombosis. Br J Haematol 2002;118:275–7.

34. Wells PS, Owen C, Doucette S, et al. Does this patient have deep vein thrombosis? JAMA 2006; 295:199–207.

35. Goodacre S, Sampson F, Thomas S, et al. Systematic review and meta-analysis of the diagnostic accuracy of ultrasonography for deep vein thrombosis. BMC Med Imaging 2005;5:6.

36. Segal JB, Eng J, Tamariz LJ, Bass EB. Review of the evidence on diagnosis of deep venous thrombosis and pulmonary embolism. Ann Fam Med 2007;5:63–73.

37. Winer-Muram HT, Rydberg J, Johnson MS, et al. Suspected acute pulmonary embolism: evaluation with multi-detector row CT versus digital subtraction pulmonary arteriography. Radiology 2004;233:806–15.

38. Remy-Jardin M, Remy J, Wattinne L, Giraud F. Central pulmonary thromboembolism: diagnosis with spiral volumetric CT with the single-breath-hold technique—comparison with pulmonary angiography. Radiology 1992;185:381–7.

39. Blum AG, Delfau F, Grignon B, et al. Spiral-computed tomography versus pulmonary angiography in the diagnosis of acute massive pulmonary embolism. Am J Cardiol 1994;74:96–8.

40. Goodman LR, Curtin JJ, Mewissen MW, et al. Detection of pulmonary embolism in patients with unresolved clinical and

scintigraphic diagnosis: helical CT versus angiography. AJR Am J Roentgenol 1995;164:1369–74.

41. Remy-Jardin M, Remy J, Deschildre F, et al. Diagnosis of pulmonary embolism with spiral CT: comparison with pulmonary angiography and scintigraphy. Radiology 1996;200:699–706.

42. Christiansen F. Diagnostic imaging of acute pulmonary embolism. Acta Radiol Suppl 1997;410:1–33.

43. Drucker EA, Rivitz SM, Shepard JA, et al. Acute pulmonary embolism: assessment of helical CT for diagnosis. Radiology 1998;209:235–41.

44. Qanadli SD, Hajjam ME, Mesurolle B, et al. Pulmonary embolism detection: prospective evaluation of dual-section helical CT versus selective pulmonary arteriography in 157 patients. Radiology 2000;217:447–55.

45. Velmahos GC, Vassiliu P, Wilcox A, et al. Spiral computed tomography for the diagnosis of pulmonary embolism in critically ill surgical patients: a comparison with pulmonary angiography. Arch Surg 2001;136:505–11.

46. Arcelus JI, Caprini JA, Reyna JJ. Finding the right fit: effective thrombosis risk stratification in orthopedic patients. Orthopedics 2000;23:633S–8S.

47. Clagett GP, Anderson FA Jr, Geerts W, et al. Prevention of venous thromboembolism. Fifth ACCP Consensus Conference on Antithrombotic Therapy. Chest 1998;114:531–60S.

48. Edmonds MJR, Crichton TJH, Runciman WB, Pradhan M. Evidence-based risk factors for postoperative deep vein thrombosis. ANZ J Surg 2004;74:1082–97.

49. Glotzbecker MP, Bono CM, Wood KB, Harris MB. Thromboembolic disease in spinal surgery. Spine 2009;34: 291–303.

50. Teasell RW, Hsieh JT, Aubut JA, Eng JJ, Krassioukov A, Tu L; Spinal Cord Injury Rehabilitation Evidence Review Research Team. Venous thromboembolism after spinal cord injury. Arch Phys Med Rehabil 2009;90:232–45.

51. Spinal Cord Injury Thromboprophylaxis Investigators. Prevention of venous thromboembolism in the rehabilitation phase after spinal cord injury: prophylaxis with low-dose heparin or enoxaparin. J Trauma 2003;54:1111–15.

52. Green D, Lee MY, Lim AC, et al. Prevention of thromboembolism after spinal cord injury using low-molecular-weight heparin. Ann Intern Med 1990;113:571–4.

53. Ramos J, Perrotta C, Badariotti G, Berenstein G. Interventions for preventing venous thromboembolism in adults undergoing knee arthroscopy. Cochrane Database Syst Rev 2008;4:CD005259.

54. Canata GL, Chiey A. Prevention of venous thromboembolism after ACL reconstruction: a prospective, randomized study. ISAKOS (International Society of Arthroscopy, Knee Surgery and Orthopaedic Sports Medicine) 2003, Poster 71-2003.

55. Michot M, Conen D, Holtz D, Erni D, Zumstein MD, Ruflin GB, et al. Prevention of deep-vein thrombosis in ambulatory arthroscopic knee surgery: A randomized trial of prophylaxis with low-molecular weight heparin. Arthroscopy 2002;18:257–63.

56. Roth P. Prophylaxis of deepvein thrombosis in outpatients undergoing arthroscopic meniscus operation [Thromboembolieprophylaxe bei ambulant durchgefürten arthroskopischen Meniskusoperationen]. Orthop Praxis 1995;5:345–8.

57. Wirth T, Schneider B, Misselwitz F, Lomb M, Tüylü H, Egbring R, et al. Prevention of venous thromboembolism after knee arthroscopy with low-molecular weight heparin (Reviparin): Results of a randomized controlled trial. Arthroscopy 2001;17: 393–9.

58. Slobogean GP, Lefaivre KA, Nicolaou S, O'Brien PJ. A systematic review of thromboprophylaxis for pelvic and acetabular fractures. J Orthop Trauma 2009;23:379–384.

59. Steele N, Dodenhoff RM, Ward AJ, et al. Thromboprophylaxis in pelvic and acetabular trauma surgery. The role of early treatment with low molecular-weight heparin. J Bone Joint Surg Br 2005;87:209–212.

60. Abelseth G, Buckley RE, Pineo GR, Hull R, Rose MS. Incidence of deep-vein thrombosis in patients with fractures of the lower extremity distal to the hip. J Orthop Trauma 1996;10:230–5.

61. Goel DP, Buckley RE, deVries G, Abelseth G, et al. Prophylaxis of deep-vein thrombosis in fractures below the knee: a prospective randomized controlled trial. J Bone Joint Surg Br 2009;91: 388–94.

62. Amaragiri SV, Lees T. Elastic compression stockings for prevention of deep vein thrombosis. Cochrane Database Syst Rev 2000;1:CD001484.

63. Allan A,Williams JT, Bolton JP, LeQuesne LP. The use of graduated compression stockings in the prevention of postoperative deep vein thrombosis. Br J Surg 1983;70:172–4.

64. Holford CP. Graded compression stockings for preventing deep vein thrombosis. Br Med J 1976;ii:969–70.

65. Hui AC, Heras-Palou C, Dunn I, Triffitt PD, Crozier A, Imeson J, et al. Graded compression stockings for prevention of deep-vein thrombosis after hip and knee replacement. J Bone Joint Surg Br 1996;78:550–4.

66. Scurr JH, Ibrahim SZ, Faber RG, Le Quesne LP. The efficacy of graduated compression stockings in the prevention of deep vein thrombosis. Br J Surg 1977;64:371–3.

67. Tsapogas MJ, Goussous M, Peabody RA, Karmody AM, Eckert C. Postoperative venous thrombosis and the effectiveness of prophylactic measures. Arch Surg 1971;103:561–7.

68. Turner GM, Cole SE, Brooks JH. The efficacy of graduated compression stockings in the prevention of deep vein thrombosis after major gynaecological surgery. Br J Obstet Gynaecol 1984;91:588–91.

69. Turpie AGG, Hirsh J, Gent M, Julian D, Johnson J. Prevention of deep vein thrombosis in potential neurosurgical patients: A randomized trial comparing graduated compression stockings alone or graduated compression stockings plus intermittent pneumatic compression with control. Arch Intern Med 1989; 149:679–81.

70. Handoll HH, Farrar MJ, McBirnie J, et al. Heparin, low molecular weight heparin and physical methods for preventing deep vein thrombosis and pulmonary embolism following surgery for hip fractures. Cochrane Database Syst Rev 2002;4:CD000305.

71. Araujo A, Atallah A. Individual patient data (as supplied 4 July 1998). Data tables. Atallah A., personal communication, May 26, 1998.

72. Silvestre JMS. Randomised controlled trial with low molecular weight heparin and intermittent pneumatic compression in the prevention of deep venous thrombosis in patients submitted to a surgical treatment of lower limb fractures (dissertation). Escola Paulista de Medicina, Sao Paulo (SP), 1994.

73. Fisher CG, Blachut PA, Salvian AJ, Meek RN, O'Brien PJ. Effectiveness of pneumatic leg compression devices for the prevention of thromboembolic disease in orthopaedic trauma

patients: A prospective, randomized study of compression alone versus no prophylaxis. J Orthop Trauma 1995;9:1–7.

74. Hartman JT, Pugh JL, Smith RD, Robertson WW, Yost RP, Janssen HF. Cyclic sequential compression of the lower limb in prevention of deep venous thrombosis. J Bone Joint Surg Am 1982;64:1059–62.

75. Gargan MF, Lawrence J, Thomas H, Trundle H, Fairbank JTC. Thromboembolic prophylaxis following hip fracture using a foot pump (A-V impulse system). Unpublished trial (abstract).

76. Stranks GJ, MacKenzie NA, Grover ML, Fail T. The A-V impulse system reduces deep-vein thrombosis and swelling after hemiarthroplasty for hip fracture. J Bone Joint Surg Br 1992;74:775–8.

77. Kakkos SK, Caprini JA, Geroulakos G, Nicolaides AN, Stansby GP, Reddy DJ. Combined intermittent pneumatic leg compression and pharmacological prophylaxis for prevention of venous thromboembolismin high-risk patients. Cochrane Database Syst Rev 2008;4:CD005258.

78. Turpie AGG, Bauer KA, Caprini JA, Comp PC, Gent M, Muntz JE, on behalf of the APOLLO Investigators. Fondaparinux combined with intermittent pneumatic compression vs. intermittent pneumatic compression alone for prevention of venous thromboembolism after abdominal surgery: a randomized, double-blind comparison. J Thromb Haemost 2007;5:1854–61.

79. Woolson ST, Watt JM. Intermittent pneumatic compression to prevent proximal deep venous thrombosis during and after total hip replacement. A prospective, randomized study of compression alone, compression and aspirin, and compression and low-dose warfarin. J Bone Joint Surg Am 1991;73:507–12.

80. Crowther MA. Inferior vena cava filters in the management of venous thromboembolism. Am J Med 2007;120, S13–17.

81. Weichman K, Ansell JE. Inferior vena cava filters in venous thromboembolism. Prog Cardiovasc Dis 2006;49:98–105.

82. Decousus H, Leizorovicz A, Parent F, et al. A clinical trial of vena caval filters in the prevention of pulmonary embolism in patients with proximal deep venous thrombosis. Prévention du Risque d'Embolie Pulmonaire par Interruption Cave Study Group. N Engl J Med 1998;338:409–415.

83. PREPIC Study Group. Eight-year follow-up of patients with permanent vena cava filters in the prevention of pulmonary embolism: the PREPIC randomized study. Circulation 2005;112:416–422.

84. Young T, Tang H, Aukes J, Hughes R. Vena caval filters for the prevention of pulmonary embolism. Cochrane Database Syst Rev 2007;4:CD006212.

85. Linsenmaier U, Rieger J, Schenk F, Rock C, Mangel E, Pfeifer KJ. Indications, management, and complications of temporary inferior vena cava filters. Cardiovasc Intervent Radiol 1998;21:464–9.

86. Shorr AF, Kwong LM, Sarnes M, et al. Venous thromboembolism after orthopedic surgery: Implications of the choice of prophylaxis. Thromb Res 2007;121:17–24.

87. Muntz J, Scott DA, Lloyd A, Egger M. Major bleeding rates after prophylaxis against venous thromboembolism: Systematic review, meta-analysis, and cost implications. Int J Technol Assess Health Care 2004;20:405–14.

88. Bauer KA, Eriksson BI, LassenMR, et al. Fondaparinux compared with enoxaparin for the prevention of venous throm-

boembolism after elective major knee surgery. N Engl J Med 2001;345:1305–10.

89. Colwell CW, Collis DK, Paulson R, et al. Comparison of enoxaparin and warfarin for the prevention of venous thromboembolic disease after total hip arthroplasty. Evaluation during hospitalization and three months after discharge. J Bone Joint Surg Am 1999;81:932–40.

90. Colwell CW, Spiro TE, Trowbridge AA, et al. Use of enoxaparin, a low-molecular-weight heparin, and unfractionated heparin for the prevention of deep venous thrombosis after elective hip replacement. A clinical trial comparing efficacy and safety. Enoxaparin Clinical Trial Group. J Bone Joint Surg Am 1994;76:3–14.

91. Colwell CW, Spiro TE, Trowbridge AA, et al. Efficacy and safety of enoxaparin versus unfractionated heparin for prevention of deep venous thrombosis after elective knee arthroplasty. Enoxaparin Clinical Trial Group. Clin Orthop 1995;321:19–27.

92. Eriksson BI, Bauer KA, Lassen MR, et al. Fondaparinux compared with enoxaparin for the prevention of venous thromboembolism after hip-fracture surgery. N Engl J Med 2001;345:1298–304.

93. Fauno P, Suomalainen O, Rehnberg V, et al. Prophylaxis for the prevention of venous thromboembolism after total knee arthroplasty. A comparison between unfractionated and low-molecular-weight heparin. J Bone Joint Surg Am 1994;76:1814–18.

94. Fitzgerald RHJ, Spiro TE, Trowbridge AA, et al. Prevention of venous thromboembolic disease following primary total knee arthroplasty. A randomized, multicenter, open-label, parallel group comparison of enoxaparin and warfarin. J Bone Joint Surg Am 2001;83:900–6.

95. Francis CW, Pellegrini VD, Totterman S, et al. Prevention of deep-vein thrombosis after total hip arthroplasty. Comparison of warfarin and dalteparin. J Bone Joint Surg Am 1997;79:1365–72.

96. Freick H, Haas S. Prevention of deep vein thrombosis by low molecular-weight heparin and dihydroergotamine in patients undergoing total hip replacement. Thromb Res 1991;63:133–43.

97. Haas S, Fareed J, Breyer HG, et al. Prevention of severe venous thromboembolism after hip and knee replacement surgery—A randomized comparison of low-molecular weight heparin with unfractionated heparin. Presented to ASH, December 7–11, 2001, Orlando. Abstract 2957. Blood 2001;98.

98. Hamulyak K, Lensing AW, van derMeer J, et al. Subcutaneous low-molecular weight heparin or oral anticoagulants for the prevention of deep-vein thrombosis in elective hip and knee replacement? Fraxiparine Oral Anticoagulant Study Group. Thromb Haemost 1995;74:1428–31.

99. Hull R, Raskob G, Pineo G, et al. A comparison of subcutaneous low-molecular-weight heparin with warfarin sodium for prophylaxis against deep-vein thrombosis after hip or knee implantation. N Engl J Med 1993;329:1370–6.

100. Hull RD, Pineo GF, Francis C, et al. Low-molecular-weight heparin prophylaxis using dalteparin in close proximity to surgery vs warfarin in hip arthroplasty patients: A double blind, randomized comparison. The North American Fragmin Trial Investigators. Arch Intern Med 2000;160:2199–207.

101. Hull RD, Raskob GE, Pineo GF, et al. Subcutaneous low molecular-weight heparin vs warfarin for prophylaxis of deep

vein thrombosis after hip or knee implantation. An economic perspective. Arch Intern Med 1997;157:298–303.

102. Kakkar VV, Howes J, Sharma V, Kadziola Z. A comparative double-blind, randomised trial of a new second generation LMWH (bemiparin) and UFH in the prevention of postoperative venous thromboembolism. The Bemiparin Assessment group. Thromb Haemost 2000;83:523–9.

103. Lassen MR, Bauer KA, Eriksson BI, et al. Postoperative fondaparinux versus preoperative enoxaparin for prevention of venous thromboembolism in elective hip-replacement surgery: A randomised double-blind comparison. Lancet 2002;359: 1715–20.

104. Lassen MR, Borris LC, Christiansen HM, et al. Heparin/dihydroergotamine for venous thrombosis prophylaxis: Comparison of low-dose heparin and low molecular weight heparin in hip surgery. Br J Surg 1988;75:686–9.

105. Leclerc JR, Geerts WH, Desjardins L, et al. Prevention of venous thromboembolism after knee arthroplasty. A randomized, double-blind trial comparing enoxaparin with warfarin. Ann Intern Med 1996;124:619–26.

106. Levine MN, Hirsh J, Gent M, et al. Prevention of deep vein thrombosis after elective hip surgery. A randomized trial comparing low molecular weight heparin with standard unfractionated heparin. Ann Intern Med 1991;114:545–51.

107. Planes A, Vochelle N, Mazas F, et al. Prevention of postoperative venous thrombosis: A randomized trial comparing unfractionated heparin with low molecular weight heparin in patients undergoing total hip replacement. Thromb Haemost 1988; 60:407–10.

108. The German Hip Arthroplasty Trial (GHAT) Group. Prevention of deep vein thrombosis with low molecular-weight heparin in patients undergoing total hip replacement: A randomized trial. Arch Orthop Trauma Surg 1992;111:110–20.

109. Turpie AGG, Bauer KA, Eriksson BI, et al. Postoperative fondaparinux versus postoperative enoxaparin for prevention of venous thromboembolism after elective hip-replacement surgery: A randomised double-blind trial. Lancet 2002;359: 1726.

110. Weitz JI. Unanswered questions in venous thromboembolism. Thromb Res 2009;123, S2–10.

111. Palmer A J, Koppenhagen K, Kirchhof B, Weber U, Bergemann R. Efficacy and safety of low molecular weight heparin, unfractionated heparin and warfarin for thrombo-embolism prophylaxis in orthopaedic surgery: a meta-analysis of randomised clinical trials. Haemostasis 1997;27:75–84.

112. Pulmonary Embolism Prevention (PEP) Trial Collaborative Group. Prevention of pulmonary embolism and deep vein thrombosis with low dose aspirin: Pulmonary Embolism Prevention (PEP) Trial. Lancet 2000;355:1295–302.

113. Sharrock NE, Go G, Harpel PC, Ranawat CS, Sculco TP, Salvati EA. Thrombogenesis during total hip arthroplasty. Clin Orthop 1995;319:16–27.

114. Raskob GE, Hirsh J. Controversies in timing of the first dose of anticoagulant prophylaxis against venous thromboembolism after major orthopedic surgery. Chest 2003;124:379–385S.

115. Hull RD, Brant RF, Pineo GF, et al. Preoperative vs postoperative initiation of low-molecular-weight heparin prophylaxis against venous thromboembolism in patients undergoing elective hip replacement. Arch Intern Med 1999;159:137–41.

116. Turpie AGG, Levine MN, Hirsh J, et al. A randomized controlled trial of a low-molecular-weight heparin (enoxaparin) to prevent deep-vein thrombosis in patients undergoing elective hip surgery. N Engl J Med 1986;315:925–9.

117. Planes A, Vochelle N, Mazar F, et al. Prevention of postoperative venous thrombosis: a randomized trial comparing unfractionated heparin with low molecular weight heparin in patients undergoing total hip replacement. Thromb Haemost 1988; 60:407–10.

118. Levine MN, Hirsh J, Gent M. Prevention of deep vein thrombosis after elective hip surgery: a randomized trial comparing low molecular weight heparin with standard unfractionated heparin. Ann Intern Med 1991;114:545–51.

119. Planes A, Chastang CL, Vochelle N, et al. Comparison of antithrombotic efficacy and haemorrhagic side effects of reviparin-sodium versus enoxaparin in patients undergoing total hip replacement surgery. Blood Coagul Fibrinolysis 1993;4, S33–8.

120. Spiro TE, Johnson CJ, Christie MJ, et al. Efficacy and safety of enoxaparin to prevent deep venous thrombosis after hip replacement surgery. Ann Intern Med 1994; 121:81–9.

121. Samama CM, Clergue F, Barre J, et al. Low molecular weight heparin associated with spinal anaesthesia and gradual compression stockings in total hip replacement surgery. Br J Anaesth 1997;78:660–5.

122. Hull RD, Pineo GF, Francis C, Bergqvist D, et al. Low-molecular-weight heparin prophylaxis using dalteparin in close proximity to surgery vs warfarin in hip arthroplasty patients. Arch Intern Med 2000;160:2199–207.

123. Eikelboom JW, Quinlan DJ, Douketis JD. Extended-duration prophylaxis against venous thromboembolism after total hip or knee replacement: a meta-analysis of the randomized trials. Lancet 2001;358:9–15.

124. Planes A, Vochelle N, Darmon JY, Fagola M, Bellaud M, Huet Y. Risk of deep-venous thrombosis after hospital discharge in patients having undergone total hip replacement: double-blind randomised comparison of enoxaparin versus placebo. Lancet 1996;348(9022):224–8.

125. Dahl OE, Andreassen G, Aspelin T, et al. Prolonged thromboprophylaxis following total hip replacement surgery—results of a double-blind, prospective, randomised, placebo-controlled study with dalteparin (Fragmin). Thromb Haemost 1997;77: 26–31.

126. Hull RD, Pineo GF, Francis C, et al. Low-molecular-weight heparin prophylaxis using dalteparin extended out-of-hospital vs in-hospital warfarin/out-of-hospital placebo in hip arthroplasty patients: a double blind, randomized comparison. North American Fragmin Trial Investigators. Arch Intern Med 2000; 160:2208–15.

127. Heit JA, Elliott CG, Trowbridge AA, Morrey BF, Gent M, Hirsh J, for the Ardeparin Arthroplasty Study Group. Ardeparin sodium for extended out-of-hospital prophylaxis against venous thromboembolism after total hip or knee replacement. A randomized, double-blind, placebo-controlled trial. Ann Intern Med 2000;132:853–61.

128. Comp PC, Spiro TE, Friedman RJ, et al. Prolonged enoxaparin therapy to prevent venous thromboembolism after primary hip or knee replacement. J Bone Joint Surg Am 2001;83:336–45.

129. Bergqvist D, Benoni G, Bjorgell O, et al. Low-molecular-weight heparin (enoxaparin) as prophylaxis against venous throm-

boembolism after total hip replacement. N Engl J Med 1996; 335:696–700.

130. Lassen MR, Borris LC, Anderson BS, et al. Efficacy and safety of prolonged thromboprophylaxis with a low molecular weight heparin (dalteparin) after total hip arthroplasty—the Danish Prolonged Prophylaxis (DaPP) Study. Thromb Res 1998;89: 281–7.

131. Manganelli D, Pazzagli M, Mazzantini D, et al. Prolonged prophylaxis with unfractionated heparin is effective to reduce delayed deep vein thrombosis in total hip replacement. Respiration 1998;65:369–74.

132. Haentjens P. Venous thromboembolism after total hip arthroplasty: a review of incidence and prevention during hospitalization and after hospital discharge. Acta Orthop Belg 2000; 66:1–8.

133. Skedgel C, Goeree R, Pleasance S, et al. The cost-effectiveness of extended-duration antithrombotic prophylaxis after total hip arthroplasty. J Bone Joint Surg Am 2007;89:819–28.

134. Xabregas A, Gray L, Ham JM. Heparin prophylaxis of deep vein thrombosis in patients with a fractured neck of the femur. Med J Aust 1978;1:620–2.

135. Bergqvist D, Efsing HO, Hallbook T, Hedlund T. Thromboembolism after elective and post-traumatic hip surgery—a controlled prophylactic trial with dextran 70 and low-dose heparin. Acta Chir Scand 1979;145:213–18.

136. Jorgensen PS, Knudsen JB, Broeng L, Josephsen L, Bjerregaard P, Hagen K, et al. The thromboprophylactic effect of a low-molecular weight heparin (Fragmin) in hip fracture surgery. A placebo-controlled study. Clin Orthop Related Res 1992;278: 95–100.

137. Kiviluoto O, Julkunen H, Honkonen K. Prevention of venous thromboemboli with low doses of heparin in patients with proximal femur fractures. Zentralbl Chir 1980;105:460–4.

9

Blood Transfusion

David W. Sanders[1] and Jeffrey L. Carson[2]

[1]University of Western Ontario, London, ON, Canada
[2]University of Medicine and Dentistry of New Jersey, New Brunswick, NJ, USA

Case scenario

An 84 year old woman is admitted to hospital with an intertrochanteric hip fracture. Her medical history is significant for coronary artery disease, hypertension, and chronic renal failure. Surgery is performed using an intramedullary device for this independent, active community ambulator. On the second postoperative day, the patient is having difficulty ambulating due to fatigue. Vital signs are stable; Blood pressure is 115/75; ECG is unchanged. Postoperative blood work reveals a hemoglobin concentration of 8.2 g/dL.

Relevant physiology

The hemoglobin molecule includes four globin components, each of which includes an oxygen-binding heme ring. As the partial pressure of oxygen increases, the oxygen-binding affinity of hemoglobin increases. This allows oxygen loading in the lung and unloading in the tissues. Hypoxia occurs when oxygen delivery is insufficient to meet metabolic needs.

The physiologic reserves of the healthy human body are substantial. Oxygen delivery is related to hemoglobin concentration, hemoglobin saturation, and cardiac output, all of which adapt to an increasing need for oxygen delivery. In health, a decrease in hemoglobin to 5 g/dL decreases oxygen delivery to the critical threshold, at which point oxygen delivery equals consumption.

Adaptive mechanisms that occur to protect tissue oxygenation in anemia include a shift in the oxyhemoglobin dissociation curve to increase oxygen delivery, due to 2,3-diphosphoglycerate or decreased pH; increases in cardiac output; increased sympathetic tone to protect the coronary and cerebral circulation; and reduced blood viscosity. In the microcirculation, capillary recruitment and flow increases and oxygen extraction is increased.

The ability of the body to adapt to anemia relies upon healthy adaptive mechanisms. Age, coincident heart, lung, and cerebrovascular disease, severe illness, and certain medications (beta-blockers) decrease the adaptive response. The heart is most prone to adverse events as the myocardium requires high oxygen extraction, and coronary perfusion is restricted during systole due to left ventricular pressures.

Importance of the problem

Seventy-five million units of blood are collected worldwide annually. Transfusion is one of the only therapeutic interventions available to increase oxygen delivery to tissues. However, transfusion is expensive and not without risk. The cost of a unit of allogeneic blood ranges from US$185 to US$250, plus costs related to storage and administration. Blood transfusion safety is continuously improving, but

Evidence-Based Orthopedics, First Edition. Edited by Mohit Bhandari.
© 2012 Blackwell Publishing Ltd. Published 2012 by Blackwell Publishing Ltd.

adverse events including transfusion-related acute lung injury (TRALI), cardiac overload, hemolysis, and infection do occur.

Top five questions

Diagnosis

1. How common are anemia and blood transfusion in orthopedic surgery, and what strategies reduce transfusion rate?

Therapy

2. What is an appropriate hemoglobin level to act as a transfusion trigger?

Prognosis

3. What is the effect of anemia on morbidity and mortality?
4. What is the effect of anemia and blood transfusion on function?

Harm

5. What are the risks of blood transfusion?

Question 1: How common are anemia and blood transfusion in orthopedic surgery, and what strategies reduce transfusion rate?

Case clarification

The patient had a hemoglobin of 11.2 g/dL on presentation to the Emergency Department. A repeat blood count done in the recovery room indicated a hemoglobin level of 10.4. On the second postoperative day, the hemoglobin level has dropped to 8.4 g/dL. Her family is concerned.

Relevance

Anemia is common in perioperative and elderly patients. In some studies, anemia is associated with increased short-term mortality.

Current opinion

Perioperative anemia follows major orthopedic interventions such as spinal surgery, hip fracture repair, and total joint arthroplasty. Assessing for anemia is an essential part of good clinical care.

Finding the evidence

• Cochrane Database, with search term "perioperative anemia"

• PubMed (www.ncbi.nlm.nih.gov/pubmed/) clinical queries search/ systematic reviews: "blood transfusion incidence" AND "orthopedic surgery"

Quality of the evidence

Level I
• 3 systematic reviews/meta-analyses
• 4 randomized controlled trials

Level II
• 8 randomized trials with methodological limitations

Findings

Orthopedic procedures associated with a high rate of transfusion include major spinal surgery, total joint arthroplasty, and hip fracture surgery. Transfusion rates for these procedures exceed 80% of patients in some studies. Variables such as closed suction wound drainage devices, antifibrinolytic therapy, autologous blood donation, and use of erythropoietin may affect transfusion rates.

A recent Cochrane Database meta-analysis compared transfusion rates with and without closed suction wound drainage. For total hip replacement, transfusion was required in 168/417 (40.3%) patients with drains vs. 132/421 (31.4%) in patients without drains (RR 1.28, 95% CI 1.07–1.52). Similar results were reported for total knee replacement.[1]

Antifibrinolytic therapy is still investigational, but may reduce transfusion rates. A systematic review of randomized trials describing perioperative tranexamic acid, epsilon-aminocaproic acid, or aprotinin administration reported that patients receiving antifibrinolytic agents had reduced transfusion need (RR 0.52; 95% CI 0.42–0.64; p < 0.00001).[2] However, aprotinin is associated with increased mortality in cardiac surgery, and some antifibrinolytics raise concerns related to risk of thromboembolic events.

Red blood cell salvage and autologous blood donation reduce rates of allogeneic blood transfusion. Meta-analysis of clinical trials confirm a 40% reduction of allogeneic blood transfusion using autologous blood.[3] However, autologous predonation is associated with a 30% increased blood transfusion rate (allogeneic or autologous). In one randomized controlled trial of nonanemic patients (hemoglobin >12.0 g/dL), autologous blood donation was associated with an additional cost of $758 per patient with no alteration in allogeneic transfusion rate.[4]

Preoperative erythropoietin administration may decrease the need for allogeneic transfusion in elective procedures. In a randomized controlled trial of 200 patients undergoing major orthopedic procedures, allogeneic transfusion rates were 54% in patients treated with placebo compared to 17% in patients treated with high dose erythropoietin (p < 0.001).[5] Perioperative erythropoietin can minimize the need for allogeneic red blood cell transfusion but is very expensive.

Recommendations

• Closed suction drainage devices increase transfusion requirements after orthopedic surgery [overall quality: high]
• Antifibrinolytic drugs hold promise, but concerns surrounding adverse side effects limit routine use [overall quality: moderate]
• Autologous blood predonation and perioperative erythropoietin may both reduce the need for allogeneic transfusion, but cost concerns remain [overall quality: moderate]

Question 2. What is an appropriate hemoglobin level to act as a transfusion trigger?

Case clarification
The patient now has a hemoglobin level of 8.2 g/dL and has mild symptoms of anemia (fatigue). She has a history of coronary artery disease, hypertension, and renal failure, and may be at risk of complications such as myocardial infarction as a result of her anemia.

Relevance
The decision to transfuse is based upon clinical findings and hemoglobin level. The specific hemoglobin level that should be used to trigger transfusion is controversial.

Current opinion
Healthy patients can tolerate anemia. Older patients, and those with cardiac disease or risk factors, may be less tolerant. However, the hemoglobin level which determines a positive risk/benefit balance for transfusion is unknown.

Finding the evidence
• Cochrane Database, with search term "transfusion trigger"
• PubMed search for randomized trials/systematic reviews using terms "transfusion trigger"

Quality of the evidence
Level I
• 1 meta-analysis of randomized trials
• 10 randomized controlled trials

Findings
Ten randomized trials compares transfusion thresholds. Three trials included over 100 patients each. The Transfusion Requirements In Critical Care (TRICC) trial[6] randomly assigned over 800 ICU patients to a restrictive transfusion threshold of 7 g/dL or a liberal transfusion threshold of 10 g/dL. The number of units transfused was lower in the restrictive group (2.6 vs 5.6 units). Overall 30 day mortality did not differ between the groups. However, mortality was lower in the restrictive group for patients under 55 years of age (p < 0.02) and less ill patients (p < 0.02). In another

trial, 127 knee arthroplasty patients were assigned to receive autologous blood immediately after surgery (liberal group) compared to receiving autologous blood only for a hemoglobin value less than 9 g/dL.[7] Transfusion rates were 100% vs. 27%, with no differences in outcome. Eighty-four patients with hip fractures were randomized to a transfusion threshold of 10 g/dL, vs. transfusion for symptoms or hemoglobin of less than 8 g/dL.[8] There were no differences in outcomes including functional recovery, morbidity, and mortality. In a meta-analysis of trials, use of a restrictive transfusion threshold decreased transfusion rate by 42% with no negative effects on mortality, cardiac events, or length of hospital stay.[9]

Nonrandomized trials offer additional evidence. A study of 1958 patients who refused blood transfusion suggested that anemia is substantially less well tolerated in the presence of cardiovascular disease.[10] The FOCUS trial studied over 2000 patients with hip fracture, all of whom have coexistent cardiovascular disease or risk factors. Morbidity, mortality, and functional outcome were compared between patients treated with a liberal transfusion threshold (10 g/dL) or a restrictive threshold (symptoms of anemia or 8 g/dL). This study will provide the best current evidence related to transfusion threshold.[11]

Recommendation
• Transfusion thresholds are controversial, and may vary dependent upon comorbidities such as cardiac disease. Current evidence supports a restrictive transfusion threshold of 7.0–8.0 g/dL for healthy patients [overall quality: high].

Question 3. What is the effect of anemia on morbidity and mortality?

Case clarification
The patient has cardiovascular disease. Moderate anemia could be a risk for cardiac events and even mortality.

Relevance
Patients with known cardiac disease may be the most likely to benefit from blood transfusion. Although controversial, a more liberal transfusion threshold may benefit these individuals.

Current opinion
This issue is highly controversial, with advocates for and against transfusion in this population.

Finding the evidence
• Cochrane Database, with search terms "transfusion and mortality"
• PubMed search of clinical trials, randomized trials, and systematic reviews using keywords "erythrocyte transfusion" and "mortality"

Quality of the evidence
Level I
- 2 meta-analyses of controlled trials
- 1 systematic review
- 8 randomized trials (including subanalyses)

Findings
Data supporting the use of red blood cell transfusion in moderate anemia remains limited, even in the presence of cardiovascular disease. Meta-analyses of transfusion thresholds[12] note no improvement in mortality with transfusion. One randomized trial tested the rates of silent myocardial ischemia related to hemoglobin concentration in a population of patients undergoing arthroplasty. Holter monitoring was used to assess the rates of silent myocardial ischemia. A postoperative episode of ischemia was experienced by 19% of patients in the restrictive transfusion group, compared with 24% of patients in the liberal transfusion group (95% CI −15.5% to 6%).[13] The TRICC trial included 257 patients with severe ischemic heart disease. The restrictive transfusion group had lower (but nonsignificant) survival rates compared to the patients in the liberal group.[14] There is limited evidence related to morbidity and mortality surrounding transfusion in the setting of moderate anemia.

Recommendation
- Although anemia is a known risk factor for cardiac events in the presence of pre-existing cardiovascular disease, current clinical evidence does not support a more aggressive transfusion protocol in this population [overall quality: moderate]

Question 4. What is the effect of anemia and blood transfusion on function?

Case clarification
This patient is a previously vital community ambulator. Currently, she is having difficulty ambulating due to fatigue. Early ambulation, a primary goal of hip fracture surgery, is not being accomplished.

Relevance
Elderly patients following hip surgery are at risk of complications of sustained recumbency such as thromboembolic events and infection.

Current opinion
Transfusion is performed to increase oxygen carrying capacity of blood to tissues. Many patients appear to "perk up" with increased energy, vitality, and ambulatory capacity following transfusion. It is unclear whether this apparent benefit is in fact substantial and sustained.

Finding the evidence
- Cochrane Database, with search term "perioperative anemia"

- PubMed clinical queries search/ systematic reviews: "blood transfusion and function and orthopedic surgery"

Quality of the evidence
Level I
- 2 randomized controlled trials

Level II
- 8 nonrandomized trials or trials with methodological limitations

Findings
Blood transfusion increases tissue oxygenation in the presence of anemia. Less evidence is available to confirm that the benefits of transfusion extend to function. Foss et al., in a randomized study of 120 patients with hip fracture, compared functional recovery in patients transfused at a restrictive (8.0 g/dL) or liberal (10.0 g/dL) transfusion threshold. There were no differences in a postoperative ambulation score.[15] In an observational study of 551 hip fracture patients, Halm et al. suggested that overall mobility scores were improved with transfusion only when the transfusion threshold exceeded 10.0 g/dL.[16] These authors suggested that only patients in whom transfusion restored a normal hemoglobin level achieved the functional benefit. Carson et al. compared 84 patients with hip fracture randomly assigned to transfusion thresholds of 10.0 g/dL or transfusion for symptoms. No differences in functional recovery were detected comparing the two groups.[17] In cancer patients, quality of life might be closely tied to energy and mobility, and therefore potentially related to hemoglobin level. In a recent study comparing erythropoietin therapy with placebo, improved hemoglobin levels in the treatment group did not seem to achieve the desired improvements in quality of life.[18]

Recommendation
- Limited evidence suggests a higher transfusion threshold does not improve function after orthopedic surgery [overall quality: low-moderate]

Question 5. What are the risks of blood transfusion?

Case clarification
Before considering a blood transfusion, the patient and family request information on the risks of blood transfusion.

Relevance
Transfusion risks are constantly evolving. Infection risk, for example, was substantial prior to routine high-quality screening and testing programs. Other risks, such as acute hemolytic reactions, require urgent intervention to reduce ill effects.

Finding the evidence

- PubMed clinical queries search/ systematic reviews: "red blood cell transfusion and risks and orthopedic surgery"

Quality of the evidence
Level II

- 2 randomized trials

Findings

Acute hemolytic reactions are the most immediate of the adverse events associated with red blood cell transfusion. Reaction rates are 1 per 18,000, and mortality approximately 1 per 1,000,000. Accidental transfusion of ABO-incompatible blood is the leading cause of fatal reactions. Delayed hemolytic reactions can occur secondary to red blood cell alloantibodies in 1 per 5,000 units. Febrile non-hemolytic reactions occur in about 3% of patients, but are usually self-limited. Leukoreduction reduces the incidence of febrile reaction. TRALI (transfusion-related acute lung injury) is a severe reaction to donor leukocyte antibodies. Estimated risk of this potentially serious reaction is 1 in 5,000 transfusions.[19]

Infection risk from transfused blood appears to be decreasing. Current estimates suggest the risk of HIV transmission of under 1 in 2,000,000; hepatitis B 1 in 100,000; and hepatitis C, 1 in 1,000,000. The risk of other pathogens such as Creutzfeldt–Jakob disease is unknown.[20]

Perioperative blood transfusion may increase the risk of surgical-site infection or infection at remote sites such as pneumonia or urinary tract infection. Transfusion-mediated immune modulation may result in a reduced host response to pathologic organisms. In a meta-analysis of 20 studies relating transfusion and bacterial infection, the authors quote an increased risk of infection after transfusion of 3.45 (CI 1.43–15.15) and even higher in the trauma patient (RR 5.26, CI 5.03–5.43).[21]

Recommendation

- The risks of transfusion include hemolytic and non-hemolytic reactions, infection, and immune modulation [overall quality: high]

Summary of recommendations

- Closed suction drainage devices increase transfusion requirements after orthopedic surgery
- Antifibrinolytic drugs hold promise, but concerns surrounding adverse side effects limit routine use
- Autologous blood predonation and perioperative erythropoietin may both reduce the need for allogeneic transfusion, but cost concerns remain
- Transfusion thresholds are controversial, and may vary dependent upon comorbidities such as cardiac disease.

Current evidence supports a restrictive transfusion threshold of 7.0–8.0 g/dL for healthy patients
- Although anemia is a known risk factor for cardiac events in the presence of pre-existing cardiovascular disease, current clinical evidence does not support a more aggressive transfusion protocol in this population
- Limited evidence suggests a higher transfusion threshold does not improve function after orthopedic surgery
- The risks of transfusion include hemolytic and non-hemolytic reactions, infection, and immune modulation

---

References

1. Parker MJ, Livingstone V, Clifton R, McKee A. Closed suction surgical wound drainage after orthopaedic surgery. Cochrane Database Syst Rev 2006;1:CD001825.
2. Kagoma YK, Crowther MA, Douketis J, Bhandari M, Eikelboom J, Lim W. Use of antifibrinolytic therapy to reduce transfusion in patients undergoing orthopedic surgery: a systematic review of randomized trials. Thromb Res 2009;123(5):687–96.
3. Henry DA, Carless PA, Moxey AJ, O'Connell D, Forgie MA, Wells PS, et al. Pre-operative autologous donation for minimising perioperative allogeneic blood transfusion. Cochrane Database Syst Rev 2002;2:CD003602.
4. Billote DB, Glisson SN, Green D, Wixson RL. A prospective, randomized study of preoperative autologous donation for hip replacement surgery. J Bone Joint Surg Am. 2002;84-A(8): 1299–304.
5. Faris PM, Ritter MA, Abels RI. The effects of recombinant human erythropoietin on perioperative transfusion requirements in patients having a major orthopaedic operation. The American Erythropoietin Study Group. J Bone Joint Surg Am 1996;78(1): 62–72.
6. Hebert, P, Wells G, Blajchman M, etal. A multicenter, randomized, controlled clinical trial of transfusion requirements in critical care. Transfusion Requirements in Critical Care Investigators, Canadian Critical Care Trials Group. N Engl J Med 1999;340:409–17.
7. Lotke P, Barth P, Garino J, Cook E. Predonated autologous blood transfusions after total knee arthroplasty: Immediate versus delayed administration. J Arthroplasty 199•;14:647–50.
8. Carson J, Terrin M, Barton F, et al. A pilot randomized trial comparing symptomatic vs. hemoglobin-level-driven red blood cell transfusions following hip fracture. Transfusion 1998;38: 522–9.
9. Carson J, Hill S, Carless P, et al. Transfusion triggers: A systematic review of the literature. Transfus Med Rev 2002;16:187–99.
10. Carson J, Duff A, Poses R, et al. Effect of anaemia and cardiovascular disease on surgical mortality and morbidity. Lancet 1996;348:1055–60.
11. Carson J, Terrin M, Magaziner J, et al. Transfusion trigger trial for functional outcomes in cardiovascular patients undergoing surgical hip fracture repair (FOCUS). Transfusion 2006;46: 2192–206.
12. Hill S, Carless PA, Henry DA, Carson JL, Hebert PPC, Henderson KM, McClelland B. Transfusion thresholds and other strategies

for guiding allogeneic red blood cell transfusion. Cochrane Database Syst Rev 2000;1:CD002042.

13. Grover M, Talwalkar S, Casbard A, Boralessa H, Contreras M, et al. Silent myocardial ischaemia and haemoglobin concentration: a randomized controlled trial of transfusion strategy in lower limb arthroplasty. Vox Sang 2006;90:105–12.

14. Hébert PC, Yetisir E, Martin C, Blajchman MA, Wells G, Marshall J, et al. Transfusion Requirements in Critical Care Investigators for the Canadian Critical Care Trials Group. Is a low transfusion threshold safe in critically ill patients with cardiovascular diseases? Crit Care Med 2001;29:227–34.

15. Foss NB, Kristensen MT, Jensen PS, Palm H, Krasheninnikoff M, Kehlet H. The effects of liberal versus restrictive transfusion thresholds on ambulation after hip fracture surgery. Transfusion 2009;49:227–234.

16. Halm EA, Wang JJ, Boockvar K, Penrod J, Silberzweig SB, Magaziner J, et al. Effects of blood transfusion on clinical and functional outcomes in patients with hip fracture. Transfusion 2003;43:1258–365.

17. Carson J, Terrin M, Barton F, et al. A pilot randomized trial comparing symptomatic vs. hemoglobin-level-driven red blood cell transfusions following hip fracture. Transfusion 1998;38: 522–9.

18. Christodoulou C, Dafni U, Aravantinos G, Koutras A, Samantas E, Karina M, et al. Effects of epoetin-alpha on quality of life of cancer patients with solid tumors receiving chemotherapy. Anti Cancer Res 2009;29(2):693–702.

19. Klein HG, Spahn DR, Carson JL. Red blood cell transfusion in clinical practice. Lancet 2007;370:415–26.

20. Pineda AA, Vamvakas EC, Gorden LD, Winters JL, Moore SB. Trends in the incidence of delayed hemolytic and delayed serologic transfusion reactions. Transfusion 1999;39:1097–103.

21. Hill GE, Frawley WH, Griffith KE, et al. Allogeneic blood transfusion increases the risk of postoperative bacterial infection: a meta-analysis. J Trauma 2003;54:908–14.

10 Wound Infections

Wesley G. Lackey[1], Kyle J. Jeray[1], Atul F. Kamath[2], John G. Horneff III[2], and John L. Esterhai, Jr[2,3]

[1]Greenville Hospital System University Medical Center, Greenville, SC, USA
[2]Hospital of the University of Pennsylvania, Philadelphia, PA, USA
[3]Veterans Affairs Hospital, Philadelphia, PA, USA

Case scenario

A 28-year-old man is brought to the Emergency Department after falling 8 feet (2.5 m) from a ladder. Examination and radiographs reveal a closed split-depression tibial plateau fracture. The soft tissue envelope allows primary open reduction and internal fixation of the fracture with a lateral buttress plate. At the 2 week follow-up, there is drainage from the wound with surrounding erythema.

Importance of the problem

Surgeons perform over 27 million operations yearly in the United States,[1] with almost 500,000 of these procedures resulting in a surgical site infection (SSI),[2] implying that infection complicates nearly 2% of all surgical wounds. Open fractures, which occur at a rate of 250,000 per year in the US,[3] have an increased rate of infection; although the risk varies depending on the severity of injury, the rate of infection can be as great as 50% in contaminated fracture wounds.[4,5] These wound infections may require multiple subsequent operative procedures and prolonged antibiotic treatment courses, and result in complications such as delayed fracture union and possible amputation.

Wound infections cost an estimated $1.5 billion per year in the US, with an estimated $3,000–$30,000 spent per infectious event.[6] According to epidemiologic hospital data, a patient who develops an SSI is five times more likely to be readmitted to the hospital and has mortality rates twice that of a patient without an SSI.[7] The National Surgical Infection Prevention Project was initiated in the US in August 2002 by Medicare and Medicaid to better characterize the nature of SSI and to formulate better strategies to prevent and combat these infections.[8] Although access to care and advances in technology and sanitation have improved health-related outcomes, infections and wound complications are still major factors relating to morbidity and mortality.

The risk of infection has also been strongly correlated with medical comorbidities[9,10] and other host factors.[11] The additional treatment required to treat infections, as well as wound and bone healing complications, leads to a significant increase in healthcare costs and significantly impacts the patient's quality of life.

Despite aggressive medical and surgical management and evolving diagnostic and treatment modalities, orthopedic infections remain a challenging problem for both patients and clinicians. Where possible, a summary of the best available literature has been provided; due to the lack of homogeneity, well-controlled human clinical trials (level I and level II evidence) and suitable meta-analyses do not exist for most topics.

Relevant anatomy

Wound infections may occur in any anatomic location, and multiple factors contribute to their occurrence. For example, a contaminated open tibia fracture has a higher risk of infection than a clean, elective hand surgery case. Associated orthopedic hardware influences the risk of infection and hampers its treatment because of the persistent nature of bacterial biofilms. Efforts have been made to categorize infections in order to better guide treatment as well as improve surveillance and standardize reporting of SSIs.

The US Centers for Disease Control (CDC) has developed criteria for defining SSIs in an attempt to create a national standard for diagnosis,[12] as summarized in the box below.

Surgical site infection: definitions

- *Superficial incisional SSI:* Infection, within 30 days of operation, that involves only skin and subcutaneous tissue.
- *Deep incisional SSI:* Infection occurs within 30 days after the operation if no implant is left in place, or within 1 year if implant is in place and infection appears to be related to the operation. Infection involves deep soft tissues (within the fascia or muscle).
- *Organ/space SSI:* Infection occurs within 30 days after the operation if no implant is left in place, or within 1 year if implant is in place and infection appears to be related to the operation. Infection involves any part of the anatomy (e.g., organs or spaces), other than the incision, which was opened or manipulated during an operation.

In the case of orthopedic wound infections, the infected organ/space is most often bone. Osteomyelitis has been further categorized by Cierny et al. in a clinical staging system (Table 10.1), which combines 4 anatomic types of osteomyelitis with 3 physiologic classifications to define 12 clinical stages of osteomyelitis.[13] The purpose is to define the influential variables associated with osteomyelitis in order to better study the efficacy of treatment methods and to guide treatment.

Top five questions

Prophylaxis

1. What are the current recommendations regarding prophylactic antibiotic administration in the prevention of wound infections in orthopedic surgery?
2. What are the current recommendations regarding screening for meticillin-resistant *Staphylococcus aureus* (MRSA), treatment of carriers, and antibiotic prophylaxis?

Diagnosis

3. What is the optimal diagnostic approach in a patient with a suspected wound infection?

Table 10.1 The UTMB staging system for adult osteomyelitis

Anatomic type	
Type I	Medullary osteomyelitis
Type II	Superficial osteomyelitis
Type III	Localized osteomyelitis
Type IV	Diffuse osteomyelitis
Physiologic class	
A-Host	Good immune system and delivery
B-Host	Compromised locally (BL) or systemically (BS)
C-Host	Requires suppressive or no treatment; minimal disability; treatment worse than disease; not a surgical candidate
Clinical stage	
Type + class = clinical stage	Example: Stage IVBS osteomyelitis = a diffuse lesion in a systemically compromised host

4. What is the role of wound culture in diagnosing and treating orthopedic infections?

Therapy

5. What is the management of infected hardware?

Question 1: What are the current recommendations regarding prophylactic antibiotic administration in the prevention of wound infections in orthopedic surgery?

Case clarification

At the time of the initial surgery, the wound was "prepped and draped in the usual sterile fashion." Cefazolin was given intravenously within 30 minutes of surgery and stopped at 24 hours postoperatively.

Relevance

Despite guidelines established for SSI prevention based on studies demonstrating decreased rates of perioperative infections with prophylactic antibiotics, studies show that antibiotic prophylaxis is not always correctly administered.[14,15] A pay-for-performance study found that 13% of patients did not receive timely antibiotic prophylaxis.[16] Furthermore, the inappropriate use of antibiotics contributes to antibiotic resistance, increased risk of adverse reactions, and increased healthcare costs.[17]

Current opinion

Factors determining appropriate antibiotic prophylaxis include wound location, type of procedure, initial level of contamination, and host immune status. A systematic and evidence-based approach must be taken, and adequate preoperative checks must be used to ensure the effective and timely administration of prophylactic antibiotics.

Finding the evidence
- Cochrane Database (http://www.cochrane.org/reviews): "prophylactic antibiotic orthopedic infection"
  ° 9 results
- PubMed (www.ncbi.nlm.nih.gov/pubmed/): "prophylactic antibiotic orthopedic infection"
  ° Limits: English
  ° 62 results, 22 reviews
- Embase (www.embase.com; excluding Medline duplicates): "prophylactic antibiotic orthopedic infection"
  ° Limits: English, Embase only
  ° 55 results

Quality of the evidence (best available)
- Level I: 19
- Level II: 3
- Level III: 5
- Level IV: 7
- Level V: 13

Findings
In larger studies of infection epidemiology, *Staphylococcus aureus*, coagulase-negative *Staphylococci*, *Enterococcus* species, and *Escherichia coli* are the most frequently isolated pathogens.[18] An increasing proportion of SSIs are caused by antimicrobial-resistant pathogens, such as MRSA or vancomycin-resistant enterococci (VRE).

The 1 hour window to administer preoperative antibiotics has its roots in studies by Burke in 1961 in a *Staphylococcus aureus* infection model in guinea-pigs.[19] When antibiotics were given within 1 hour before bacterial inoculation, there was no inflammatory response. Guinea-pigs that received antibiotics 3 hours or more after inoculation received no more benefit than those animals not receiving antibiotics.

The shortest effective duration of antimicrobial administration for preventing postoperative infection is not known.[14,20] Studies comparing single-dose prophylaxis with multiple-dose prophylaxis have shown conflicting benefits in terms of SSI rate with the additional doses.[21,22] Continuing antibiotic prophylaxis longer than 24 hours after wound closure has not proven to be beneficial; indeed, it may contribute to the development of antimicrobial resistance.[20,21] A Cochrane review from 2001 examined the rates of SSI associated with either the use of single- or multiple-dose antibiotic prophylaxis in proximal femur and closed long bone fractures. They demonstrated the need to redose antibiotics in order to maintain tissue levels above the minimum inhibitory concentration throughout the duration of the surgical procedure.[23] Antibiotics should be redosed at one to two times the half-life of the antibi-

otic[22,24,25] or when there is significant intraoperative blood loss.[26–28]

Slobogean et al. conducted a meta-analysis of antibiotic prophylaxis in 7 trials encompassing 3,808 patients with closed long bone fractures.[29] When compared to a regimen of multiple doses of prophylactic antibiotics, administration of a single preoperative dose has a risk ratio of 1.24 (95% CI 0.60–2.60) with no statistical significance. Pooled results failed to demonstrate superiority of multiple-dose prophylaxis over a single-dose strategy in the management of closed long bone fractures.[29]

Recommendations
The proportion of antibiotic-resistant surgical wound pathogens in the subsequent decade will be an important factor in directing future recommendations for surgical antibiotic prophylaxis. Local bacterial flora and resistance profiles are important to tailoring hospital-specific protocols.[30]

To maximize the beneficial effect of prophylactic antibiotics while minimizing adverse effects, recommendations include the following [overall quality: high]:
- Antibiotic administered prior to incision
- Perioperative antibiotic course should not exceed 24 hours
- Antibiotics should be redosed when the duration of the procedure exceeds one to two times the antibiotic half-life[22,24,25] or with significant intraoperative blood loss[26–28]
- Verification of prophylactic antibiotic administration at the time of the "Time-Out" protocol may increase compliance rate[6]

Question 2: What are the current recommendations regarding MRSA screening, treatment of carriers, and antibiotic prophylaxis?

Case clarification
This patient has no known history of MRSA infection, but his sister did have a peculiar "spider bite" on her hip 1 year ago that was culture-positive for MRSA.

Relevance
MRSA infections represent a particularly prevalent and challenging issue in wound infection, especially now that community-acquired MRSA often represents the predominant organism of skin and soft tissue infections in many communities.[31] Although MRSA is prevalent, the institution of prophylactic vancomycin for all surgical cases could theoretically yield to increasing resistance. Therefore, there has been a movement to study MRSA screening and treatment prior to elective surgery or even hospital-wide, but general recommendations for MRSA screening and prophylaxis have been varied.

Current opinion

Cephalosporins remain the standard prophylactic antibiotic. MRSA screening and treatment of carriers is not universal. Vancomycin is not routinely used for surgical prophylaxis, but may be used in patients with known or suspected MRSA infection or carriage.

Finding the evidence

- Cochrane Database (http://www.cochrane.org/reviews): "MRSA screening orthopedic surgery"
  - 1 relevant review
- PubMed (www.ncbi.nlm.nih.gov/pubmed/): "MRSA screening orthopedic surgery"
  - Limits: English
  - 56 results, 17 relevant, 3 reviews

Quality of the evidence

- Level I: 1
- Level II: 6
- Level III: 4
- Level IV: 3
- Level V: 1

Findings

Currently, many institutions screen for MRSA by using a polymerase chain reaction (PCR) test for gene sequencing and identification of the nasal carriage of MRSA. This testing is available in a point-of care testing device (a small machine which runs a PCR test result at the bedside) that has proven its accuracy as well as its convenience.[32] Of 2,473 patients studied by Shukla et al., 3.2% were MRSA carriers upon admission.[33] Those carrying MRSA at the time of admission were more likely to develop SSI with MRSA (8.8% vs. 2.2% infection rate; $p < 0.001$).[33]

Some data exist regarding the use of mupirocin to reduce nasal carriage of *Staphylococcus aureus* and rates of SSI in elective orthopedic surgery.[34–36] A prospective study of MRSA surveillance using PCR-based testing, including 5,094 patients undergoing Surgical Infection Prevention Project procedures, showed a reduction of MRSA SSI from 0.23% to 0.09% with preoperative treatment including mupirocin.[37]

In 2007 and 2008, a Texas Veterans Affairs (VA) hospital implemented a "MRSA prevention bundle" including MRSA nasal screening of patients upon admission, transfer, and discharge; contact isolation of positive patients; standardized hand hygiene; a cultural transformation education campaign; and ongoing monitoring of process and outcome measures. They reported significant decreases in MRSA transmissions, SSIs, and overall MRSA nosocomial infections.[38] In contrast, a randomized, double-blind, placebo controlled trial in nonorthopedic surgical patients failed to show a decrease in the overall incidence of SSIs, but the study did show a decrease in *Staphylococcus aureus* infections in treated carriers.[39]

Despite the rise in bacterial strains resistant to common prophylactic antibiotics, such as cefazolin (not only MRSA but also strains of the ubiquitous *Staphylococcus epidermidis*),[40] recommendations for prophylactic vancomycin are conservative. The American Academy of Orthopaedic Surgeons (AAOS) recommends that vancomycin use be limited to patients with known colonization with MRSA or in facilities with recent MRSA outbreaks.[25,41]

Recommendations

Current recommendations for MRSA screening include the following [overall quality: moderate]:

- Routine MRSA screening and treatment with mupirocin may reduce the prevalence of MRSA colonization and incidence of postoperative infections
- Point-of-care screening for MRSA using PCR is available and is as effective as the laboratory test
- No threshold exists for prevalence rates justifying routine vancomycin use in prophylaxis, though it is recommended for colonized patients and in institutions with perceived high rates or outbreaks of MRSA infection

Question 3: What is the optimal diagnostic approach in a patient with a suspected wound infection?

Case clarification

The patient presents for routine follow-up and suture removal at 2 weeks. He complied with his nonweightbearing status. Purulent discharge is noted on the dressing. The wound is not healed. There is some dehiscence over the proximal 20% of the incision with surrounding erythema. The hardware is not exposed.

Relevance

Diagnosis of a wound infection, particularly the extent of the infection, is important for guiding treatment. Laboratory values can be used for diagnostic purposes as well as for following improvement. Radiographic changes are rarely present in acute infection.

Current opinion

The evaluation of a suspected wound infection is largely clinically based. Laboratory values such as C-reactive protein (CRP) and erythrocyte sedimentation rate (ESR) can be useful for diagnosis and for following treatment response.

Finding the evidence

- Cochrane Database (http://www.cochrane.org/reviews): "ESR CRP orthopedic wound infection diagnosis"
  - 0 relevant reviews

- PubMed (www.ncbi.nlm.nih.gov/pubmed/): "ESR CRP wound infection"
  - ° Limits: English

Quality of the evidence (best available)
- Level I: 1
- Level II: 1
- Level III: 7
- Level IV: 1
- Level V: 1

Findings
New or persistent drainage, induration, or erythema around a wound, may signify a deep infection. However, the diagnosis of a deep wound infection is made in the operating room,[42] as SSIs are defined by their anatomic depth as discussed in the relevant anatomy section above.

Leukocyte count and ESR were originally used together for laboratory evaluation of infection, but CRP has gained attention as a better barometer of a clinical process due to its more prompt elevation (6–8 hours) and faster resolution (50% decline per day).[42] In any case, ESR and CRP are best used together, with a sensitivity of 98% in a study of 265 children with culture-positive osteoarticular infections.[43]

Although neither value is routinely followed after elective surgery, CRP was shown to be more "applicable, predictable, and responsive in the early postoperative period compared with ESR," in terms of monitoring for postoperative infection when drawn daily.[44] In this study, the CRP value demonstrated a half-life of 2.6 days, while the ESR showed no reproducible pattern. A similar study attempted to quantify the CRP levels with postoperative infections in elective fracture surgeries. The authors noted that CRP peaked 2 days postoperatively and began to decline thereafter. When the values remained above 96 mg/L after the fourth postoperative day, the authors noted a sensitivity and specificity for deep infection of 92% and 93%, respectively.[45]

It is often appropriate to draw these labs around the time of irrigation and debridement, even in the case of an obvious infection, in order to establish peak reference value. While lab values are inconsistent between patients and diagnoses, falling values can help confirm effective treatment and be used for screening in suspected recurrent infections.

Recommendations
Current recommendations for the diagnostic approach of wound infections include the following [overall quality: moderate]:
- The diagnosis of a wound infection is made in the operating room
- Increased pain, drainage, erythema, or dehiscence may suggest a wound infection

- CRP and ESR should be used together to support or help rule out a suspected wound infection

Question 4: What is the role of wound culture in diagnosing orthopedic infections?

Case clarification
The patient is admitted to the hospital for irrigation and debridement of the wound in the operating room. At the time of surgery, a wound culture is obtained in the operating room and submitted for microbiologic analysis.

Relevance
Isolating a culture of the causative bacteria is important for directed antibiotic therapy. An *intraoperative* wound infection specimen is the best chance to isolate an organism to facilitate directed antibiotic therapy.

Current opinion
Superficial wound culture in the outpatient setting is of limited value for diagnosis and treatment of a wound infection. Though routine intraoperative wound culture is not often used in clean or elective orthopedic surgery, deep culture at the time of surgical debridement of a wound infection is used to guide antibiotic therapy.

Finding the evidence
- Cochrane Database (http://www.cochrane.org/reviews) and PubMed (www.ncbi.nlm.nih.gov/pubmed/) were searched using combinations of keywords "wound culture, orthopedic infection"

Quality of the evidence (best available)
- Level I: 1
- Level II: 3
- Level III: 4
- Level IV: 2
- Level V: 2

Findings
Studies have shown that intraoperative cultures in a non-infected wound, whether surgical or traumatic, clean or contaminated, are not advisable. Lee et al. studied pre- and postdebridement cultures of open wounds.[46] Only 8% of organisms cultured eventually caused infection; conversely, 7% of patients with negative cultures eventually became infected. Postdebridement cultures had similar results: only 25% of organisms cultured caused ultimate infection; 12% of patients with negative cultures became infected.[46] The poor predictive value of initial wound cultures has been demonstrated in other reports.[47]

In a study of wound infections after open fractures by Carsenti-Etesse et al., 92% of infections were caused by nosocomial (hospital-acquired) bacteria, rather than by the initially cultured organism.[48] In one prospective trial with relatively small sample size, only 18% of infections in open fracture wounds were caused by initially cultured organism.[49]

Bernard et al. examined 1,256 subfascial cultures in 1,102 patients undergoing elective/ "clean" orthopedic surgery.[50] Wound cultures demonstrated 38% sensitivity, 92% specificity, 7% positive predictive value, and 99% negative predictive value.[50] The study's literature review found only four of nine studies showing predictive benefit from intraoperative wound cultures in clean orthopedic surgery. The utility of wound cultures must be gauged against the timing, type of procedure, and clinical history of the patient.

Obtaining a specimen for culture is appropriate at the time of irrigation and debridement for a presumed wound infection in order to guide antibiotic therapy. A retrospective review of 800 image-guided bone biopsies for osteomyelitis showed that laboratory values, fever, and previous administration of antibiotics, could not be used to predict the success of growing positive cultures, but obtaining an aspirate of ≥2 ml of purulent fluid was significantly correlated (5 of 6 positive cultures, 83%).[51] Increased sensitivity of wound cultures has been shown with the inoculation of blood culture bottles, because of the rich culture medium.[52]

Recommendations

Recommendations for wound cultures in orthopedic surgery [overall quality: moderate]:
• Routine cultures of traumatic or clean surgical wounds are not recommended
• Superficial wound swab cultures of a suspected wound infection are of little value
• Intraoperative deep cultures if positive can help guide antibiotic therapy if an organism is isolated
• Sensitivity of cultures is increased if some of the specimen is placed in a blood culture bottle

Question 5: What is the management of infected internal fixation hardware?

Case clarification

The patient is 2 weeks from surgery and has a deep infection. His hardware is in good position but the fracture is clearly not healed.

Relevance

Infection rates are low in arthroscopy and hand surgery, while many SSIs occur in the presence of hardware, particularly when that hardware was introduced in the cases of open fractures. How to deal with this infected hardware may vary from case to case.

Current opinion

The surgeon must balance the goal of eradication of infection with the goal of fracture healing, which usually requires the hardware to remain in place.

Finding the evidence

• Cochrane Database (http://www.cochrane.org/reviews): "infected hardware orthopedic fracture stability"
  ° 0 relevant reviews
• PubMed (www.ncbi.nlm.nih.gov/pubmed/): "orthopedic infected hardware"
  ° Limits: English

Quality of the evidence

• Level I: 1
• Level II: 2
• Level IV: 6

Findings

In 1998, Zimmerli et al. had success with eradication of infection with retained hardware, reporting 12/12 cure rate with a prolonged course of ciprofloxacin-rifampin in patients with acute infections after open reduction and internal fixation (ORIF).[53] On the contrary, Rightmire et al. found lower success rates in 2008 when they reviewed 69 cases of infected internal fixation hardware treated with irrigation and debridement, antibiotics, and hardware retention, and found a 32% failure rate, defined as hardware removal prior to healing.[54]

Many authors contest that infected fractures will heal if the fracture is stable.[55] Simultaneously, it has long been accepted that an infection cannot be eradicated in the presence of infected hardware.[56] The principles of treatment should include adequate debridement, obliteration of dead space, and specific antimicrobial therapy.[57] It is reasonable to conclude that hardware should be retained until healing or at least relative fracture stability is achieved.

Recommendations

Current recommendations on managing infected hardware include the following [overall quality: low]:
• Prompt irrigation and debridement is recommended for deep infections, but hardware removal should be delayed until fracture stability is achieved
• Removal of infected hardware is probably necessary for complete eradication of infection

Summary of recommendations

• Prophylactic antibiotics should be administered prior to incision and should be continued for a maximum of 24 hours postoperatively. Antibiotics should be redosed at recommended intervals during surgery
• Screening and treatment for MRSA nasal carriage may reduce MRSA SSIs in MRSA carriers. Vancomycin should not be routinely used for prophylaxis, but is appropriate for patients who are MRSA carriers or in settings of MRSA outbreaks

- The diagnosis of a wound infection is made in the operating room
- Increased pain, drainage, erythema, or dehiscence may suggest a wound infection
- ESR and CRP should be used together as part of the workup for a wound infection and as a monitor of treatment effectiveness
- Superficial wound swab cultures of a suspected wound infection are of little value
- Wound culture should only be used at the initial irrigation and debridement of a wound infection. Increased sensitivity of deep wound cultures is associated with larger volumes of specimen in a blood culture bottle medium
- Infected hardware may prevent complete eradication of a wound infection, but the timing of hardware removal must be balanced with the need for fracture stability in treating a wound infection. Thus, in the majority of cases the hardware is retained in the acute infection period and removed after fracture stability/healing is achieved

Conclusion

Orthopedic wound infections represent a complex interplay among host factors and surgical interventions. Prevention will continue to be the best way to treat wound/surgical site infections in order to improve outcomes and reduce the economic burden of infection. Further well-designed clinical investigations are needed to guide the future of prevention and management of wound infections in the face of ever-changing bacterial resistance profiles in order to allow the surgeon to continue the practice of evidence-based orthopedics.

References

1. Centers for Disease Control and Prevention, National Center for Health Statistics: Detailed Diagnoses and Procedures, National Hospital Discharge Survey, 1994. Vital Health Statistics, Series 13, vol 127. US Department of Health and Human Services, Hyattsville, MD, 1997.
2. Wong ES. Surgical site infections. In: Mayhall DG, ed. Hospital Epidemiology and Infection Control, 2nd ed., pp. 189–210. Lippincott, Williams & Wilkins, Philadelphia, PA, 1999.
3. Anglen JO. Wound irrigation in musculoskeletal injury. J Am Acad Orthop Surg 2001;9:219–26.
4. Bhandari M, Adili A, Schemitsch EH. The efficacy of low-pressure lavage with different irrigating solutions to remove adherent bacteria from bone. J Bone Joint Surg Am 2001;83:412–19A.
5. Tsukayama DT, Schmidt AH. Open fractures. Curr Treat Opt Infect Dis 2001;3:301–7.
6. Rosenberg AD, Wambold D, Kraemer L, et al. Ensuring appropriate timing of antimicrobial prophylaxis. J Bone Joint Surg Am 2008;90(2):226–32.
7. Kirkland KB, Briggs JP, Trivette SL, Wilkinson WE, Sexton DJ. The impact of surgical site infections in the 1990s: Attributable mortality, excess length of hospitalization, and extra costs. Infect Control Hosp Epidemiol 1999;20:725–30.
8. Bratzler DW, Hunt DR. The Surgical Infection Prevention and Surgical Care Improvement Projects: national initiatives to improve outcomes for patients having surgery. Clin Infect Dis 2006;43:322–30.
9. Olsen MA, Nepple JJ, Riew KD, Lenke LG, Bridwell KH, Mayfield J, Fraser VJ. Risk factors for surgical site infection following orthopaedic spinal operations. J Bone Joint Surg Am 2008;90(1):62–9.
10. Fascia DT, Singanayagam A, Keating JF. Methicillin-resistant *Staphylococcus aureus* in orthopaedic trauma: identification of risk factors as a strategy for control of infection. J Bone Joint Surg Br 2009;91(2):249–52.
11. Bowen TR, Widmaier JC. Host classification predicts infection after open fracture. Clin Orthop Relat Res 2005;433:205–11.
12. Mangram AJ, Horan TC, Pearson ML. Guideline for Prevention of Surgical Site Infection, 1999. Centers for Disease Control and Prevention (CDC) Hospital Infection Control Practices Advisory Committee. Am J Infect Control 2009;27(2):97–132; quiz 133–4; discussion 96.
13. Cierny G 3rd, Mader JT, Penninck JJ. A clinical staging system for adult osteomyelitis. Clin Orthop Relat Res. 2003;414:7–24.
14. Bratzler DW, Houck PM, Richards C, et al. Use of antimicrobial prophylaxis for major surgery: Baseline results from the National Surgical Infection Prevention Project. Arch Surg 2005;140:174–82.
15. Classen DC, Evans RS, Pestotnik SL, Horn SD, Menlove RL, Burke JP. The timing of prophylactic administration of antibiotics and the risk of surgical-wound infection. N Engl J Med 1992;326:281–6.
16. Bhattacharyya T, Hooper DC. Antibiotic dosing before primary hip and knee replacement as a pay-for-performance measure. J Bone Joint Surg Am 2007;89:287–91.
17. Prokuski L. Prophylactic antibiotics in orthopaedic surgery. J Am Acad Orthop Surg 2008;16(5):283–93.
18. National Nosocomial Infections Surveillance (NNIS) report, data summary from October 1986–April 1996, issued May 1996. A report from the National Nosocomial Infections Surveillance (NNIS) System. Am J Infect Control 1996;24:380–8.
19. Burke JF. The effective period of preventive antibiotic action in experimental incisions and dermal lesions. Surgery 1961;50:161–8.
20. Li JT, Markus PJ, Osmon DR, Estes L, Gosselin VA, Hanssen AD. Reduction of vancomycin use in orthopaedic patients with a history of antibiotic allergy. Mayo Clin Proc 2000;75:902–6.
21. Bratzler DW, Houck PM, Surgical Infection Prevention Guidelines Writers Workgroup, et al. Antimicrobial prophylaxis for surgery: An advisory statement from the National Surgical Infection Prevention Project. Clin Infect Dis 2004;38:1706–15.
22. Dellinger EP, Gross PA, Barrett TL, et al. Quality standard for antimicrobial prophylaxis in surgical procedures. Clin Infect Dis 1994;18:422–427.
23. Gillespie WJ, Walenkamp G. Antibiotic prophylaxis for surgery for proximal femoral and other closed long bone fractures. Cochrane Database Syst Rev 2001;1:CD000244.
24. Finkelstein R, Rabino G, Mashiah T, et al. Vancomycin versus cefazolin prophylaxis for cardiac surgery in the setting of a high

prevalence of methicillin-resistant staphylococcal infections. J Thorac Cardiovasc Surg 2002;123:326–32.

25. American Academy of Orthopaedic Surgeons Advisory Statement: Recommendations for the use of intravenous antibiotic prophylaxis in primary total joint arthroplasty. c2004 [accessed March 19, 2010]. Available from: http://www.aaos.org/about/papers/advistmt/1027.asp.

26. Medical Letter: Antimicrobial prophylaxis in surgery. Med Lett Drugs Ther 2001;43:92–7.

27. Swoboda SM, Merz C, Kostuik J, Trentler B, Lipsett PA. Does intraoperative blood loss affect antibiotic serum and tissue concentrations? Arch Surg 1996;131:1165–71.

28. Deacon JS, Wertheimer SJ, Washington JA. Antibiotic prophylaxis and tourniquet application in podiatric surgery. J Foot Ankle Surg 1996;35:344–9.

29. Slobogean GP, Kennedy SA, Davidson D, O'Brien PJ. Single- versus multiple-dose antibiotic prophylaxis in the surgical treatment of closed fractures: a meta-analysis. J Orthop Trauma 2008;22(4):264–9.

30. Raymond DP, Kuehnert MJ, Sawyer RG. Preventing antimicrobial- resistant bacterial infections in surgical patients. Surg Infect (Larchmt) 2002;3:375–85.

31. Fridkin SK, Hageman JC, Morrison M, et al. Active bacterial core surveillance program of the emerging infections program network. Methicillin-resistant *Staphylococcus aureus* disease in three communities. N Engl J Med 2005;352:1436–44.

32. Brenwald NP, Baker N, Oppenheim B. Feasibility study of a real-time PCR test for methicillin-resistant *Staphylococcus aureus* in a point of care setting. J Hosp Infect. 2010;74(3):245–9.

33. Shukla S, Nixon M, Acharya M, Korim MT, Pandey R. Incidence of MRSA surgical-site infection in MRSA carriers in an orthopaedic trauma unit. J Bone Joint Surg Br 2009;91(2):225–8.

34. Gernaat-van der Sluis AJ, Hoogenboom-Verdegaal AM, Edixhoven PJ, Spies-van Rooijen NH. Prophylactic mupirocin could reduce orthopaedic wound infections: 1,044 patients treated with mupirocin compared with 1,260 historical controls. Acta Orthop Scand 1998;69:412–14.

35. Kalmeijer MD, van Nieuwland-Bollen E, Gogaers-Hofman D, de Baere GA. Nasal carriage of Staphylococcus aureus is a major risk factor for surgical-site infections in orthopaedic surgery. Infect Control Hosp Epidemiol 2000;21:319–23.

36. Wilcox MH, Hall J, Pike H, et al. Use of perioperative mupirocin to prevent methicillin-resistant *Staphylococcus aureus* (MRSA) orthopedic surgical site infections. J Hosp Infect. 2003;54: 196–201.

37. Pofahl WE, Goettler CE, Ramsey KM, et al. Active surveillance screening of MRSA and eradication of the carrier state decreases surgical-site infections caused by MRSA. J Am Coll Surg. 2009;208(5):981–6; discussion 986–8.

38. Awad SS, Palacio CH, Subramanian A, et al. Implementation of a methicillin-resistant *Staphylococcus aureus* (MRSA) prevention bundle results in decreased MRSA surgical site infections. Am J Surg. 2009;198(5):607–10.

39. Perl TM, Cullen JJ, Wenzel RP, et al. Mupirocin and the risk of Staphylococcus aureus study team. Intranasal mupirocin to prevent postoperative *Staphylococcus aureus* infections. N Engl J Med. 2002;34:1871–7.

40. Meehan J, Jamali AA, Nguyen H. Prophylactic antibiotics in hip and knee arthroplasty. J Bone Joint Surg Am. 2009;91(10): 2480–90.

41. American Society of Health-System Pharmacists ASHP Therapeutic Guidelines on Antimicrobial Prophylaxis in Surgery. American Society of Health-System Pharmacists. Am J Health Syst Pharm 1999;56(18):1839–88.

42. Prokuski L. Treatment of acute infection. J Am Acad Orthop Surg 2006;14:S101–4.

43. Pääkkönen M, Kallio MJ, Kallio PE, Peltola H. Sensitivity of erythrocyte sedimentation rate and C-reactive protein in child- hood bone and joint infections. Clin Orthop Relat Res 2010;468(3): 861–6.

44. Mok JM, Pekmezci M, Murat MD, et al. Use of C-reactive protein after spinal surgery: comparison with erythrocyte sedimentation rate as predictor of early postoperative infectious complications. Spine 2008;33(4):415–21.

45. Neumaier M, Scherer MA. C-reactive protein levels for early detection of post-operative infection after fracture surgery in 787 patients. Acta Orthop 2008;79(3):428–32.

46. Lee J. Efficacy of cultures in the management of open fractures. Clin Orthop Relat Res 1997;339:71–5.

47. Valenziano CP, Chattar-Cora D, O'Neill A, et al. Efficacy of primary wound cultures in long bone open extremity fractures: are they of any value? Arch Orthop Trauma Surg 2002;122:259–61.

48. Carsenti-Etesse H, Doyon F, Desplaces N, et al. Epidemiology of bacterial infection during management of open leg fractures. Eur J Clin Microbiol Infect Dis 1999;18:315–23.

49. Patzakis MJ, Bains RS, Lee J, et al. Prospective, randomized, double-blind study comparing single-agent antibiotic therapy, ciprofloxacin, to combination antibiotic therapy in open fracture wounds. J Orthop Trauma 2000;14:529–33.

50. Bernard L, Sadowski C, Monin D, et al. The value of bacterial culture during clean orthopedic surgery: a prospective study of 1,036 patients. Infect Control Hosp Epidemiol. 2004;25(6):512–14.

51. Wu JS, Gorbbachova T, Morrison WB, Haims AH. Imaging- guided bone biopsy for osteomyelitis: are there factors associ- ated with positive or negative cultures? AJR Am J Roentgenol. 2007;188:1529–34.

52. Ngan PG, O'Neill JK, Goodwin-Walters A. Increased culture sensitivity with direct inoculation of seroma fluid in blood culture bottles. J Plast Reconstr Aesthet Surg. 2010;63:e428–9.

53. Zimmerli W, Widmer AF, Blatter M, et al. Role of rifampin for treatment of orthopedic implant-related staphylococcal infec- tions: a randomized controlled trial. Foreign-Body Infection (FBI) Study Group. JAMA 1998;279:1573–41.

54. Rightmire E, Zurakowski D, Vrahas M. Acute infections after fracture repair: management with hardware in place. Clin Orthop Relat Res. 2008;466:466–72.

55. Worlock P, Slack R, Harvey L, Mawhinney R. The prevention of infection in open fractures: an experimental study of the effect of fracture stability. Injury 1994;25:31–8.

56. Waldvogel FA, Medoff G, Swartz MN. Osteomyelitis: a review of clinical features, therapeutic considerations, and unusual aspects. N Engl J Med 1970;282:198–206.

57. Mader JT, Cripps MW, Calhoun JH. Adult post-traumatic osteo- myelitis of the tibia. Clin Orthop Relat Res 1999;360:14–21.

Gouty Arthritis

Jasvinder A. Singh

University of Alabama at Birmingham, Birmingham, AL, USA

Case scenario

A 75 year old man who is currently ambulatory and living independently came to the Emergency Department complaining of pain for 1 day in his left great toe. He has a history of coronary artery disease status post angioplasty, hypertension, diabetes, and peptic ulcer disease with major gastrointestinal bleeding 10 years ago. He has had increasing frequency of lower extremity joint pain and swelling involving the great toe, ankles, and knees in the last 2–3 years, now with acute attacks of arthritis occurring every 3–4 months, lasting 7–14 days. He is currently unable to step with his left foot. On examination, his left first metatarsophalangeal (MTP) joint is moderately swollen, erythematous, and very tender to palpation. Examination of the ankle, knees, opposite foot, and other joints is unremarkable. The patient is requesting some medication to relieve the excruciating pain.

Relevant anatomy and pathophysiology

Arthritis of the foot can be due to inflammatory causes (rheumatoid arthritis, spondyloarthritis or crystalline arthritis such as gout, pseudogout or calcium oxalate disease) or noninflammatory causes (osteoarthritis, metabolic/endocrine arthropathies). This chapter focuses on management options for gout, a common type of inflammatory arthritis with a predilection for involvement of lower extremity joints. Gout is the commonest inflammatory arthritis in older men and can present either as acute intermittent monarticular or polyarticular arthritis. It is characterized by hyperuricemia (serum urate above the solubility level of 6.8 mg/dl), which leads to formation of urate crystals in the joints and bursae leading to acute inflammation in one or multiple joints (acute gout). Untreated hyperuricemia in gout patients leads to chronic gouty arthritis characterized by chronic inflammation in the joints associated with chronic pain, swelling, joint destruction as well as formation of subcutaneous deposits of urate—the tophi.

Importance of the problem

It is estimated that approximately 5 million Americans have gout.[1] A recent study estimated that $27 million are spent annually for care of new acute gout cases in the United States.[2] Gout accounted for 1.4 million outpatient visits in 2002.[3] In two studies of large U.S. employer databases, compared to patients without gout, those with gout had $3,000 higher annual medical costs.[4-5] Over 31,400,000 hits appear on Google when the search term "gout" is entered. A PubMed search revealed 10,948 results for "gout."

Evidence-Based Orthopedics, First Edition. Edited by Mohit Bhandari.

Top four questions

Diagnosis

1. How accurate is clinical examination for the diagnosis of acute gout and what role does joint aspiration for documentation of urate crystals have in the diagnosis of gout?

Therapy

2. What is the role of oral colchicine in treatment of acute gout?

3. How effective are other treatments including nonsteroidal anti-inflammatory drugs (NSAIDs), corticosteroids, and adrenocorticotropic hormone (ACTH) in the management of acute gout as compared to placebo and each other?

4. What is the role for use of chronic anti-inflammatory therapy (colchicine, NSAIDs, etc.) in patients with gout?

Question 1: How accurate is clinical examination for the diagnosis of acute gout and what role does joint aspiration for documentation of urate crystals have in the diagnosis of gout?

Case clarification

The patient has had multiple attacks of lower extremity arthritis without any diagnosis. Radiography of the feet shows mild joint space narrowing of bilateral MTP joints. The patient is presented with two options—to undergo joint aspiration for a definitive diagnosis or have a presumptive diagnosis based on clinical features.

A typical X-ray finding in patients with gout is a "punched out erosion with overhanging margin", but it may not be present in every patient with gout, many of whom may have no radiographic abnormality or joint space narrowing only.

Relevance

Making a definitive diagnosis of gout as the underlying cause of patient's inflammatory arthritis is critical to institution of appropriate, effective treatment. Current opinion is divergent among practitioners on whether to aspirate the joint. However, joint aspiration is rarely done in emergent or outpatient settings for most patients, primarily due to lack of training (joint aspiration) among internists and family practitioners and/or lack of perceived value for a definitive diagnosis.

Current opinion

Current practice pattern suggests that the majority of practitioners use the clinical features based on preliminary American Rheumatism Association (ARA) criteria to diagnose gout, rather than joint fluid aspiration.

Finding the evidence

- Cochrane Database, with search term "gout diagnostic criteria"
- PubMed (www.ncbi.nlm.nih.gov/PubMed/) clinical queries search/ systematic reviews: "gout AND diagnostic criteria"
- PubMed (www.ncbi.nlm.nih.gov/PubMed/) -sensitivity search using keywords "gout" AND "diagnostic criteria" as well as "gout" AND "classification criteria"

Quality of the evidence

Level III
- 2 observational studies

Findings

Two studies (n = 142 patients) provide data regarding the accuracy of clinical classification/diagnostic criteria and of radiographic features for gout. Malik et al. compared the clinical criteria with the gold standard of synovial fluid analysis for gout.[6] In 82 patients with suspected gout who underwent joint fluid aspiration and examination for urate crystals (gold standard), the sensitivity of the ARA (now American College of Rheumatism (ACR)) preliminary classification criteria was 70%, specificity 79%, and positive predictive value, 66%. For two other clinical criteria for gout, the New York criteria and the Rome criteria, the sensitivity was 70% and 67% and specificity was 83% and 89%, respectively. Barthelemy et al. performed a prospective study of the radiographic features of 60 patients with gouty arthritis; the diagnosis was made based on crystal-documentation or satisfying 6 of the 12 ARA classification criteria. In this study 60% (36/60) patients had radiographic findings diagnostic of gouty arthritis in one or more joints; 32% (19/60) had features indistinguishable from osteoarthritis and 8% (5/60) had normal radiographs.[7] In a literature synthesis of studies of quality control for examination of urate and other crystals in synovial fluid, moderate evidence for quality control was found.[8]

Recommendations

In patients with suspected gout, evidence suggests:
- Clinical criteria have moderate accuracy in the diagnosis of gouty arthritis [overall quality: low]
- Radiographic features typical of gout may be present in up to 60% of the patients with gout and assist in making the diagnosis of gout [overall quality: low]
- The gold standard for diagnosis of gout is documentation of urate crystals in joint fluid/material aspirated from joint, bursa, or tophaceous deposit using polarized microscopy [overall quality: low]

Question 2: What is the role of oral colchicine in treatment of acute gout?

Case clarification
The patient has a history of gastrointestinal bleeding, contraindicating the use of NSAIDs.

Relevance
Selecting the appropriate treatment for acute gout is important, since adverse events sometimes occur even with short-term medication use. The onset of pain relief may be rapid with NSAIDs or corticosteroids; however, one must be aware of potential adverse events and drug interactions of these medications. The pain relief achieved with colchicine may take longer to occur and one must be aware of associated gastrointestinal adverse events, including diarrhea, with this drug.

Current opinion
Current practice patterns suggest that the majority of practitioners avoid NSAIDs for treatment in such a patient and may use oral colchicine or oral or intra-articular corticosteroids.

Finding the evidence
• Cochrane Database, with search terms "gout," "colchicine," "randomized"
• PubMed (www.ncbi.nlm.nih.gov/PubMed/) clinical queries search/ systematic reviews: "gout colchicine randomized"
• PubMed (www.ncbi.nlm.nih.gov/PubMed/)—sensitivity search using keywords "gout," "colchicine," "randomized"

Quality of the evidence
Level I
• 1 systematic review/meta-analysis
• 2 randomized trials

Findings
A Cochrane systematic review found only one randomized study comparing colchicine to placebo for the treatment of acute gout.[9] The single study included in this review by Ahern et al.[10] is discussed in detail in the following paragraph. Since the publication of the review, another much larger randomized placebo-controlled trial has been published. Therefore, instead of presenting results from the Cochrane review, we provide updated forest plots (Figure 11.1 and Figure 11.2).

Two studies (n = 229 patients) provide data regarding the use of colchicine for treatment of acute gout. In a randomized study of 45 patients, 22 patients with gout were randomized to colchicine 1 g followed by 0.5 mg every 2 hours until complete response or toxicity occurred, and 21 patients received placebo;[10] 2 patients were excluded because they were unable to understand the visual analog scale used for reporting pain. A significantly higher proportion of patients had at least a 50% reduction in pain score (73%) in the colchicine group compared to the placebo group (36%) (p < 0.01). Terkeltaub et al. compared low-dose (1.8 mg total over 1 hour) and high-dose colchicine

Study or Subgroup	Colchicine Events	Total	Placebo Events	Total	Weight	Risk Ratio M-H, Random, 95% CI	Risk Ratio M-H, Random, 95% CI
1.2.2 High dose Colchicine versus placebo							
Ahern 1987	16	22	7	21	49.5%	2.18 [1.13, 4.21]	
Terkeltaub 2010	17	52	5	29	27.1%	1.90 [0.78, 4.61]	
Subtotal (95% CI)		74		50	76.6%	2.08 [1.22, 3.52]	
Total events	33		12				
Heterogeneity: Tau^2 = 0.00; Chi^2 = 0.06, df = 1 (P = 0.80); I^2 = 0%							
Test for overall effect: Z = 3.71 (P = 0.007)							
1.2.3 Low Dose Colchicine versus placebo							
Terkeltaub 2010	28	74	4	29	23.4%	2.74 [1.05, 7.13]	
Subtotal (95% CI)		74		29	23.4%	2.74 [1.05, 7.13]	
Total events	28		4				
Heterogeneity: Not applicable							
Test for overall effect: Z = 2.07 (P = 0.04)							
Total (95% CI)		148		79	100.0%	2.22 [1.40, 3.52]	
Total events	61		16				
Heterogeneity: Tau^2 = 0.00; Chi^2 = 0.32, df = 2 (P = 0.85); I^2 = 0%							
Test for overall effect: Z = 3.37 (P = 0.0007)							

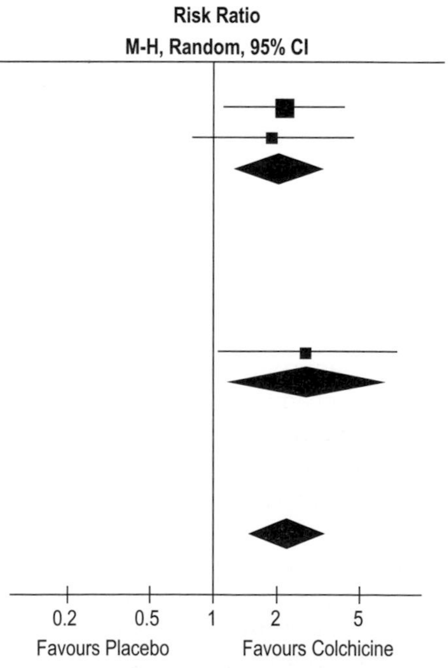

0.2 0.5 1 2 5
Favours Placebo   Favours Colchicine

Figure 11.1 Efficacy of colchicine vs. placebo in 50% pain reduction.

Study or Subgroup	Colchicine Events	Colchicine Total	Placebo Events	Placebo Total	Weight	Risk Ratio M-H, Random, 95% CI	Risk Ratio M-H, Random, 95% CI
1.2.1 High dose Colchicine versus placebo							
Ahern 1987	22	22	6	21	34.4%	3.91 [1.89, 8.09]	
Terkeltaub 2010	40	52	6	29	34.3%	3.72 [1.80, 7.70]	
Subtotal (95% CI)		74		50	68.7%	3.81 [2.28, 6.38]	
Total events	62		11				
Heterogeneity: Tau^2 = 0.00; Chi^2 = 0.01, df = 1 (P = 0.92); I^2 = 0%							
Test for overall effect: Z = 5.10 (P = 0.00001)							
1.2.2 Low Dose Colchicine versus placebo							
Terkeltaub 2010	19	74	6	30	31.3%	1.28 [0.57, 2.90]	
Subtotal (95% CI)		74		30	31.3%	1.28 [0.57, 2.90]	
Total events	19		6				
Heterogeneity: Not applicable							
Test for overall effect: Z = 0.60 (P = 0.55)							
Total (95% CI)		148		80	100.0%	2.71 [1.37, 5.38]	
Total events	81		17				
Heterogeneity: Tau^2 = 0.22; Chi^2 = 4.93, df = 2 (P = 0.09); I^2 = 59%							
Test for overall effect: Z = 2.86 (P = 0.004)							

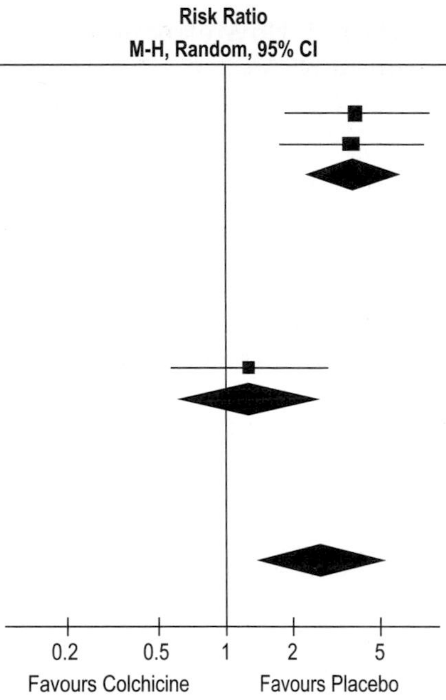

0.2　0.5　1　2　5
Favours Colchicine　　Favours Placebo

Figure 11.2 Gastrointestinal adverse events in colchicine vs. placebo.

(4.8 mg total over 6 hours) to placebo in 575 patients with acute gout.[11] Of these, 185 patients had a qualifying acute gout flare (52 in high-dose colchicine, 74 in low-dose colchicine, and 59 in placebo group), of whom 184 were included in the efficacy analyses (1 patient in placebo group did not provide data/flare confirmation) and all 185 were included in safety analyses. A 50% reduction in joint pain at 24 hours was noted in a significantly greater proportion of patients in the high-dose colchicine group (17/52, 32.7%) and the low-dose colchicine group (28/74, 37.8%) compared to the placebo group (9/58, 15.5%; p = 0.034 and 0.005, respectively).

A combined analysis of the two randomized controlled trials showed that high-dose colchicine was significantly more likely than placebo to be associated with 50% pain relief at 24–36 hours with a relative risk of 2.08 favoring colchicine (95% CI 1.22–3.52). The absolute risk reduction was 25% (95% CI 2–28%), relative risk reduction was 108% (95% CI 22–252%) and number needed to treat to benefit (NNT-B) was 4 (95% CI 2–50). Low-dose colchicine was significantly more likely than placebo (RR 2.74; 95% CI 1.05–7.13) to provide 50% pain relief at 24–36 hours. The absolute risk reduction was 24% (95% CI 7–41%), relative risk reduction was and NNT-B was 4 (95% CI 2–14).

Two studies provided data for gastrointestinal toxicity of colchicine. Compared to placebo, gastrointestinal adverse events were significantly more common in high-dose colchicine with relative risk of 3.81 (95% CI 2.28–6.38). Low-

dose colchicine did not lead to more gastrointestinal adverse effects compared to placebo with relative risk of 1.28 (95% CI 0.57–2.90). The number needed to treat to harm (NNT-H) for gastrointestinal toxicity was 2 (95% CI 2–3) for high-dose colchicine and not applicable for low-dose colchicine (no significant differences compared to placebo). Any adverse event (RR 2.79; 95% CI, 1.52–5.12) and diarrhea (RR 5.58; 95% CI, 2.22–14.02) were reported by significantly more patients in the high-dose colchicine vs. placebo group. The low-dose colchicine group did not differ significantly compared to placebo for any adverse event (RR 1.37; 95% CI 0.70–2.66) or diarrhea (RR 1.72; 95% CI 0.63–4.70). For any adverse event, the NNT-H for high-dose colchicine was 3 (95% CI 2–4) and for diarrhea the NNT-H was 2 (95% CI 2–3).

Recommendations

In patients with acute gout, evidence suggests:
- Colchicine is better than placebo in improving pain in the first 24–48 hours [overall quality: high]
- Low-dose colchicine is as effective as high-dose colchicine for treatment of acute gout, which are both better than placebo [overall quality: moderate]
- Colchicine is associated with significantly more gastrointestinal adverse events than placebo; high-dose colchicine is associated with more gastrointestinal adverse events than placebo; and low-dose colchicine was not statistically significantly different than placebo [overall quality: moderate]

Question 3: How effective are other treatments including NSAIDs, corticosteroids, and ACTH in the management of acute gout as compared to placebo and each other?

The case clarification, relevance and current opinion relating to this question have already been presented in the context of Question 2.

Finding the evidence
- Cochrane Database, with search terms "gout," "Nonsteroidal anti-inflammatory drugs," "NSAID," "steroid," "randomized"
- PubMed (www.ncbi.nlm.nih.gov/PubMed/) clinical queries search/ systematic reviews: "gout," "Nonsteroidal anti-inflammatory drugs," "NSAID". "steroid"
- PubMed (www.ncbi.nlm.nih.gov/PubMed/) -sensitivity search using keywords "gout," "Nonsteroidal anti-inflammatory drugs," "NSAID," "steroid," and "randomized"

Quality of the evidence
Level I
- 2 systematic reviews/meta-analyses
- 2 randomized trials

Findings
In a systematic review, use of NSAIDs, corticosteroids, and ACTH in acute gout was reviewed.[12] The systematic review identified one placebo-controlled trial comparing tenoxicam (an NSAID) to placebo,[13] but no placebo-controlled trials of steroids or ACTH use in acute gout. One randomized controlled trial compared tenoxicam 30 mg/day to placebo (n = 30). In this study 67% of tenoxicam-treated vs. 26% of placebo-treated patients had 50% or more reduction in pain at 24 hours, but no difference at the end of treatment at 4 days. A report in the Cochrane Database notes that there are no placebo-controlled trials of corticosteroids in gout.[14] Of the nine studies that compared NSAIDs to each other, seven low-quality studies found no differences in efficacy of NSAIDs compared to each other. Only two were high-quality studies.[15,16] A combined analysis showed that when comparing etoricoxib to indomethacin, there were significantly lower relative risks of any adverse event (0.77; 95% CI 0.63–0.95) and drug-related adverse events (0.47; 95% CI 0.33–0.66) in favor of etoricoxib. No differences were noted in the relative risk of serious adverse events (0.56; 95% CI, 0.03 to 9.40) or withdrawals due to adverse events (0.50; 95% CI 0.15–1.62).

One study compared ACTH to intramuscular triamcinolone (a corticosteroid) and found similar efficacy of the two with respect to the time required for complete resolution of acute gout.[17] No placebo-controlled trials compared steroids or ACTH to placebo.

Two studies compared NSAIDs to prednisone in patients with acute gout, but there are no studies comparing colchicine or ACTH to NSAIDs or prednisone. In one study of 90 patients, an oral prednisolone/acetaminophen combination was found to be as effective as oral indomethacin/acetaminophen combination in relieving pain and was associated with fewer adverse effects.[18] In an equivalence study of prednisolone and naproxen for acute gout, no significant differences were noted between treatment arms for pain reduction at 90 hours.[19] Adverse events were similar between groups.

Recommendations
- NSAIDs may relieve symptoms of acute gout including pain and a variety of NSAIDs have similar efficacy in this regard [overall quality: low].
- Corticosteroids can also relieve pain during acute gouty arthritis [overall quality: low]

Question 4: What is the role of colchicine in prophylaxis during initial urate-lowering therapy?

The case clarification, relevance and current opinion relating to this question have already been presented in the context of Question 2.

Finding the evidence
- Cochrane Database, with search terms "gout" "colchicine" "randomized"
- PubMed (www.ncbi.nlm.nih.gov/PubMed/) clinical queries search/ systematic reviews: "gout colchicine randomized"
- PubMed (www.ncbi.nlm.nih.gov/PubMed/)—sensitivity search using keywords "gout colchicine randomized" AND as well as "gout colchicine randomized".

Quality of the evidence
Level II
- 2 randomized trials with methodological limitations

Findings
There were no systematic reviews on this topic. Two randomized controlled studies with methodological limitations (n = 95 patients) provided data regarding the use of colchicine for prophylaxis of acute flares when initiating urate-lowering therapy. In a randomized double-blind study, 51 patients with crystal-proven gouty arthritis with high serum urate and frequent gout attacks/tophi were enrolled, 8 of whom were excluded since they did not participate beyond the initial enrollment and did not receive study drug. Of the 43 patients analyzed, 21 patients with gout were randomized to colchicine 0.6 mg twice a day orally and 21 to placebo twice a day orally for 3 months beyond

attaining a serum urate of less than 6.5 mg/dL.[20] All patients received allopurinol starting at 100 mg orally and escalated by 100 mg increments (in renal failure, 50 mg increments) until the target serum urate was achieved. Patients treated with colchicine experienced fewer flares during the entire study (0.52 vs. 2.91, p = 0.008), and less severe flares as reported on a visual analog scale (3.64 vs. 5.08, p = 0.018). Overall, fewer patients in the colchicine (33%) vs. placebo (77%) group reported any gout flares (p = 0.008) or recurrent gout flares: 14% vs. 63%, respectively (p = 0.004). Comparing the safety profile of colchicine to placebo, similar proportions had overall withdrawals (14% vs. 18%) or any adverse event (43% vs. 38%, p = 0.76). A significantly higher proportion had diarrhea as an adverse event in colchicine (38%) vs. the placebo group (4.5%) (p = 0.009).

In a two-center randomized double-blind study, Paulus et al. compared two regimens in 52 patients with hyperuricemia and history of typical attacks of acute arthritis:[21] 500 mg of probenecid tablet orally three time a day vs. 500 mg of probenecid + 0.5 mg of colchicine tablet three time a day. They analyzed 38 patients after excluding 18 as a result of noncompliance or loss to follow-up. Mean gout flares/month/patient were significantly less frequent in the colchicine vs. the placebo group, 0.19 vs. 0.48 (p < 0.05). Diarrhea was reported by 9/20 in colchicine and 6/18 in placebo group. Gastrointestinal adverse events were reported by 15/20 patients in the colchicine group and 8/18 in the placebo group.

The data from the two trials described above could be pooled for two outcomes: adverse event and diarrhea. Analyses showed that relative risk of any adverse effect (1.47 [0.94, 2.32]) or diarrhea (2.75 [0.41, 18.28]) was slightly higher in the colchicine vs. the placebo group, but the difference was not statistically significant.

Recommendations

• Prophylaxis with colchicine is effective in preventing acute gout flares during the initial urate-lowering therapy [overall quality: moderate]
• Adverse events with prophylactic colchicine during initial urate-lowering therapy are not significantly different from placebo [overall quality: low to moderate]

Summary of recommendations

• Clinical criteria have moderate accuracy in helping with the diagnosis of gouty arthritis
• Radiographic features typical of gout may be present in up to 60% of the patients with gout and assist in making diagnosis of gout
• The gold standard for diagnosis of gout is documentation of urate crystals in joint fluid/material aspirated

from joint, bursa or tophaceous deposit using polarized microscopy
• Colchicine is better than placebo in improving pain in the first 24–48 hours
• Low-dose colchicine is as effective as high-dose colchicine for treatment of acute gout, and both high and low dose colchicine are better than placebo
• Colchicine is associated with significantly more gastrointestinal adverse events than placebo; high-dose colchicine is associated with more gastrointestinal adverse events than placebo and low-dose colchicine was not statistically significantly different than placebo
• NSAIDs may relieve symptoms of acute gout including pain and variety of NSAIDs have similar efficacy in this regard
• Corticosteroids relieve pain during acute gouty arthritis
• Prophylaxis with colchicine is effective in preventing acute gout flares during the initial urate-lowering therapy
• Adverse events with prophylactic colchicine during initial urate-lowering therapy are not significantly different from placebo

Conclusions

The most common methods used in clinical practice to diagnose gout, including the clinical/classification criteria and radiographic criteria, do not have high specificity or sensitivity. Documentation of urate or other crystals in synovial fluid or tophaceous subcutaneous deposits is highly recommended to differentiate gout from pseudogout and osteoarthritis. Colchicine is effective in reducing pain associated with acute gouty arthritis, with low-dose (1.8 mg) being as effective as the high-dose hourly colchicine (4.8 mg) regimen. Other effective options for treatment of acute gouty arthritis include NSAIDs, corticosteroids (oral and intra-articular) and ACTH. Anti-inflammatory prophylaxis with colchicine or NSAID is indicated at initiation of urate-lowering therapy in patients with gout, to be continued for a few months to prevent acute flares. Colchicine seems to be well tolerated when used as prophylactic therapy at the time of urate-lowering therapy initiation.

References

1. Kramer HM, Curhan G. The association between gout and nephrolithiasis: the National Health and Nutrition Examination Survey III, 1988–1994. Am J Kidney Dis 2002;40(1):37–42.
2. Kim KY, Ralph Schumacher H, Hunsche E, Wertheimer AI, Kong SX. A literature review of the epidemiology and treatment of acute gout. Clin Ther 2003;25(6):1593–617.
3. Krishnan E, Griffith C, Kwoh K. Burden of illness from gout in ambulatory care in the United States. Arthritis Rheum 2005;52(9)(suppl):S656.

4. Brook RA, Kleinman NL, Patel PA, Melkonian AK, Brizee TJ, Smeeding JE, et al. The economic burden of gout on an employed population. Curr Med Res Opin 2006;22(7):1381–9.

5. Wu EQ, Patel PA, Yu AP, Mody RR, Cahill KE, Tang J, et al. Disease-related and all-cause health care costs of elderly patients with gout. J Manag Care Pharm 2008;14(2):164–75.

6. Malik A, Schumacher HR, Dinnella JE, Clayburne GM. Clinical diagnostic criteria for gout: comparison with the gold standard of synovial fluid crystal analysis. J Clin Rheumatol 2009;15(1):22–4.

7. Barthelemy CR, Nakayama DA, Carrera GF, Lightfoot RW, Jr., Wortmann RL. Gouty arthritis: a prospective radiographic evaluation of sixty patients. Skeletal Radiol 1984;11(1):1–8.

8. Swan A, Amer H, Dieppe P. The value of synovial fluid assays in the diagnosis of joint disease: a literature survey. Ann Rheum Dis 2002;61(6):493–8.

9. Schlesinger N, Schumacher R, Catton M, Maxwell L. Colchicine for acute gout. Cochrane Database Syst Rev 2006;4:CD006190.

10. Ahern MJ, Reid C, Gordon TP, McCredie M, Brooks PM, Jones M. Does colchicine work? The results of the first controlled study in acute gout. Aust N Z J Med 1987;17(3):301–4.

11. Terkeltaub RA, Furst DE, Bennett K, Kook KA, Crockett RS, Davis MW. High versus low dosing of oral colchicine for early acute gout flare: Twenty-four hour outcome results of the first randomized, placebo-controlled, dose comparison colchicine trial. Arthritis Rheum 2010;62(4):1060–8.

12. Sutaria S, Katbamna R, Underwood M. Effectiveness of interventions for the treatment of acute and prevention of recurrent gout—a systematic review. Rheumatology (Oxford) 2006;45(11):1422–31.

13. de la Torre IG. [Parallel double-blind study comparing tenoxicam to placebo in acute gouty arthritis]. Invet Med Int 1987;14:92–7.

14. Janssens HJ, Lucassen PL, Van de Laar FA, Janssen M, Van de Lisdonk EH. Systemic corticosteroids for acute gout. Cochrane Database Syst Rev 2008;2:CD005521.

15. Rubin BR, Burton R, Navarra S, Antigua J, Londono J, Pryhuber KG, et al. Efficacy and safety profile of treatment with etoricoxib 120 mg once daily compared with indomethacin 50 mg three times daily in acute gout: a randomized controlled trial. Arthritis Rheum 2004;50(2):598–606.

16. Schumacher HR, Jr., Boice JA, Daikh DI, Mukhopadhyay S, Malmstrom K, Ng J, et al. Randomised double blind trial of etoricoxib and indometacin in treatment of acute gouty arthritis. BMJ 2002;324(7352):1488–92.

17. Siegel LB, Alloway JA, Nashel DJ. Comparison of adrenocorticotropic hormone and triamcinolone acetonide in the treatment of acute gouty arthritis. J Rheumatol 1994;21(7):1325–7.

18. Man CY, Cheung IT, Cameron PA, Rainer TH. Comparison of oral prednisolone/paracetamol and oral indomethacin/paracetamol combination therapy in the treatment of acute gout-like arthritis: a double-blind, randomized, controlled trial. Ann Emerg Med. 2007;49(5):670–7.

19. Janssens HJ, Janssen M, van de Lisdonk EH, van Riel PL, van Weel C. Use of oral prednisolone or naproxen for the treatment of gout arthritis: a double-blind, randomised equivalence trial. Lancet 2008;371(9627):1854–60.

20. Borstad GC, Bryant LR, Abel MP, Scroggie DA, Harris MD, Alloway JA. Colchicine for prophylaxis of acute flares when initiating allopurinol for chronic gouty arthritis. J Rheumatol 2004;31(12):2429–32.

21. Paulus HE, Schlosstein LH, Godfrey RG, Klinenberg JR, Bluestone R. Prophylactic colchicine therapy of intercritical gout. A placebo-controlled study of probenecid-treated patients. Arthritis Rheum 1974;17(5):609–14.

12 Perioperative Medical Management

Daniel A. Mendelson, Susan M. Friedman, and Joseph A. Nicholas

Highland Hospital, University of Rochester School of Medicine and Dentistry, Rochester, NY, USA

Case scenario

An 84 year old woman with heart failure, hypertension, hyperlipidemia, asthma, and diabetes trips on a rug at home. She is unable to bear weight, and is brought to the hospital. She is found to have a right intertrochanteric hip fracture.

Relevant anatomy

Hip fractures can be classified in relation to the hip capsule as intracapsular (femoral neck) fractures or extracapsular fractures, which includes both intertrochanteric and subtrochanteric fractures.

Importance of the problem

Since most patients who sustain hip fractures undergo surgery, optimizing the perioperative management of these patients is essential. Perioperative mortality is approximately 4%, with 1 year mortality ranging from 10% to 35%. Complications sustained during hospitalization may lead to a delay in rehabilitation, further functional decline, poor quality of life, and death.

Optimizing perioperative medical management has been shown to reduce complication rates, including cardiac complications, thromboembolism, infection, and delirium. Length of hospital stay is also reduced. This reduction in complications translates to a reduction in healthcare costs.

Top five questions

Diagnosis

1. Is preoperative echocardiography indicated for asymptomatic patients?

Therapy

2. Which approaches to delirium prevention work?
3. Does comanagement improve processes and outcomes?
4. Are beta-blockers useful in perioperative management?

Harm

5. What is the harm associated with delay to surgery?

Question 1: Is preoperative echocardiography indicated for asymptomatic patients?

Case clarification

Because the patient has a history of heart failure and cardiac risk factors, the anesthesiologist requests clarification of the patient's cardiac status. The patient has no new cardiac symptoms or findings.

Relevance

Echocardiography adds costs and often delays definitive care, which may result in worse outcomes. Recent studies suggest that proceeding to surgery quickly may result in lower hospital mortality, lower length of stay, and lower

Evidence-Based Orthopedics, First Edition. Edited by Mohit Bhandari.
© 2012 Blackwell Publishing Ltd. Published 2012 by Blackwell Publishing Ltd.

30 day rehospitalization. Avoiding unnecessary echocardiography may produce better outcomes at lower cost.

Current opinion

There is no clear consensus upon obtaining preoperative echocardiograms for asymptomatic patients. There are wide practice variations.[1]

Finding the evidence

- Cochrane Database (http://www.cochrane.org/reviews): with search terms: "hip fracture" and "echocardiogram"
   ° Returned 1 results
- PubMed (www.ncbi.nlm.nih.gov/PubMed/): with search terms: "hip fracture" and "preoperative cardiac evaluation"
   ° Returned 9 references
- MEDLINE (1990 to March 31, 2010) with search strategy:
   1 exp Hip Fractures
   2 exp Echocardiography
   3 1 and 2
   ° Returned 16 references
- A review of reference lists of relevant articles for additional published trials

Quality of the evidence

- Level III: case series

Findings

Although physicians caring for hip fracture patients may feel more comfortable obtaining an echocardiogram prior to surgery, such evaluation rarely changes management when there are no new signs or symptoms of cardiac dysfunction. For the majority of patients, thoughtful fluid management, timely surgery, and appropriate medical management results in best outcomes without the cost or delay associated with obtaining additional cardiac testing.[1,2]

Recommendation

- Echocardiography should not be obtained in patients without signs or symptoms of new cardiac conditions [overall quality: low]

Question 2: Which approaches to delirium prevention work?

Case clarification

At baseline, the patient is cognitively intact, pleasant, and interactive. On postoperative day 2, she screams at the nurse, accusing her of trying to poison her, and pulls out her intravenous line and urinary catheter. She is agitated, appears uncomfortable, and either does not answer questions at all, or responds inappropriately.

Relevance

Delirium is the most common postoperative complication following hip fracture surgery, with incidence estimates up to 60%.[3,4] Delirium occurs more commonly in this population than in other hospitalized older adults. The occurrence of delirium is associated with increased risk of complications, increased length of stay, decline in activities of daily living, decline in ambulation, admission to nursing home, and death.[5-7] Furthermore, although delirium is considered to be an acute condition, about 40% of those who develop delirium still have symptoms on hospital discharge,[6] which can in turn impact their ability to participate in rehabilitation.[8] Patients who are admitted to rehabilitation with delirium are more likely to suffer further complications, more likely to be rehospitalized, and less than half as likely to be discharged to the community as those who are not delirious.[9]

Current opinion

Although delirium is extremely common following surgical repair of hip fractures, few centers have standardized, comprehensive approaches to delirium prevention. Optimizing medical and surgical treatment will help reduce the incidence and severity of delirium.

Finding the evidence

- Cochrane Database (http://www.cochrane.org/reviews): with search terms: "hip fracture" and "delirium"
   ° Returned 15 results
- PubMed (www.ncbi.nlm.nih.gov/PubMed/): with search terms: "hip fracture" and "delirium," limited to clinical trial, meta-analysis, randomized controlled trial or review, AND English
   ° Returned 18 references
- MEDLINE (1990 to December 14, 2009) with search strategy:
   ° exp Hip Fractures
   ° Delirium: prevention & control
   ° Returned 22 references
- A review of reference lists of relevant articles for additional published trials

Quality of the evidence

Level I
- 2 systematic reviews or meta-analyses
- 4 randomized controlled trials

Level II
- 3 cohort studies

Findings

Interventions to reduce delirium have included comprehensive programs and specific medications.[10] A randomized controlled trial of proactive geriatric assessment was completed on 126 hip fracture patients. The geriatrician visited daily and made recommendations based on a structured protocol. Recommendations focused on 10 topics, including fluid management, treatment of pain, medication management, bowel and bladder function, nutrition, and mobilization. Incidence of delirium was lower (32% vs. 50%, RR = 0.64, with 95% CI = 0.37–0.98). Severe delirium incidence was 12% vs. 29% (RR = 0.4, with 95% CI = 0.19–0.89). For those who developed delirium, there was no difference in number of hospital days with delirium.[11] An intervention of pre- and postoperative geriatric assessment, early surgery, oxygen, prevention of blood pressure falls, and treatment of complications led to a rate of delirium of 47.6% vs. 61.3% in historic controls.[12] Incidence of severe delirium and length of stay were also reduced. A pre-post study of nurse education, systematic cognitive screening, consultation, and a scheduled pain protocol showed a reduction in delirium severity and duration but not overall incidence.[13]

Haloperidol prophylaxis (0.5 mg three times daily) was studied in a randomized controlled trial of 430 hip fracture patients aged 70 and over. There was no difference in the primary endpoint of postoperative delirium incidence (15.1% vs. 16.5%, with RR = 0.91, 95% CI = 0.6–1.3). However, for those who developed delirium, severity was less (p < 0.001), duration was shorter (5.4 vs. 11.8 days, 95% CI for difference = 4.0–8.0, p < 0.001), and mean length of stay was lower (17.1 vs. 22.6 days, p < 0.001).[14] Overall incidence of delirium in this population was low, which may be a result of all patients receiving proactive geriatric consultation. Randomized trials of donepazil[15] and of citicoline[16] did not affect delirium incidence.

There is observational evidence that delirium is associated with experiencing severe pain (RR = 9.0, 95% CI = 1.8–45.2), receiving less than 10 mg of parenteral morphine daily (RR = 5.4, 95% CI = 2.4–12.3), or receiving meperidine (RR = 2.4, 95% CI = 1.3–4.5).[17]

Recommendations

• Proactive, standardized geriatric assessment reduces delirium incidence and severity [overall quality: high]
• Low-dose haloperidol prophylaxis in a high-risk population may reduce delirium severity and duration [overall quality: moderate]
• Poorly treated pain may increase risk of delirium [overall quality: low]

Question 3: Does comanagement improve processes and outcomes?

Case clarification

The patient was admitted to the orthopedic surgery service and was comanaged by a geriatrics hospitalist. Medication, pain, and fluid management were primarily monitored by the geriatrician. The patient had surgery within 12 hours of admission and was discharged for rehabilitation at a skilled nursing facility on the third postoperative day.

Relevance

Patients admitted for fragility fractures frequently have comorbidities that warrant careful management by experts. The complexity of these patients is beyond what an orthopedic surgeon should be expected to manage on their own. Surgeons are busy in the operating room and often do not have the time to manage medical problems and coordinate care with the patient, family, and care team during regular working hours.[18]

Current opinion

There is a growing trend for geriatricians or hospitalists to specialize in the comanagement of geriatric fractures in order to improve outcomes including morbidity, mortality, length of stay, and costs.[19]

Finding the evidence

• Cochrane Database (http://www.cochrane.org/reviews): with search terms: "hip fracture" and "comanagement" or "co-management"
  ◦ Returned 0 results
• PubMed (www.ncbi.nlm.nih.gov/PubMed/): with search terms: "hip fracture" and "comanagement" or "co-management"
  ◦ Returned 4 references
• MEDLINE (1990 to March 31, 2010) with search strategy:
  1 exp Hip Fractures
  2 comanagement.mp
  3 co-mangement.mp
  4 2 or 3
  5 1 and 4
  ◦ Returned 4 references
• A review of reference lists of relevant articles for additional published trials

Quality of the evidence

• Level II: cohort studies, consensus

Findings

Comanagement of fragility fractures by geriatricians has been shown to improve in hospital mortality (1.5 vs. 3.2 %), length of stay (4.6 vs. 5.2 days), and 30 day readmission rates (9.7 vs. 19.4%). Comanagement compared with usual care is associated with shorter time to surgery (24.1 vs. 37.4 hours), fewer postoperative infections (2.3 vs. 19.8 %), less complications overall (30.6 vs. 46.3 %), and less use of restraints (0 vs. 14.1 %).[20,21]

Recommendation

• Comanagement should be considered for fragility fractures [overall quality: moderate]

Question 4: Are beta-blockers useful in perioperative management?

Case clarification

The patient has a history of congestive heart failure, hypertension, hyperlipidemia, asthma, and diabetes mellitus. Her preoperative blood pressure is recorded as 108/62, with a pulse of 88 beats/minute.

Relevance

Despite an initial enthusiasm for the widespread use of beta-blockers in the perioperative setting, more recent studies have highlighted risks from beta-blocker therapy for some patients. Dose, timing and patient selection are likely important factors to consider.

Current opinion

Recommended practice has moved to limited beta-blocker use in patients with known coronary heart disease or who are already on a beta-blocker. Reduced risk for myocardial ischemia and infarction need to be weighed against risk for acute stroke. There is debate over the recommended dosing of beta-blockers, target population, target heart rate.

Finding the evidence

- Cochrane Database (http://www.cochrane.org/reviews/index.htm): with search terms "beta-blocker" and "surgery"
  - ° No relevant reviews; 2 relevant protocols
- PubMed (www.ncbi.nlm.nih.gov/PubMed/): with search terms "beta-blocker" and "perioperative," limited to clinical trial, meta-analysis, or randomized controlled trial, AND English
  - ° 91 references
- A review of reference lists of relevant articles for additional published trials.

Quality of the evidence

Level I
- 1 systemic review or meta-analysis
- 5 randomized controlled trials

Level II
- 1 cohort study

Findings

Since the initial publication of data galvanizing the widespread use of beta-blockers in the perioperative setting, a number of subsequent studies have suggested a more nuanced approach in patients undergoing noncardiac surgery, with many studies failing to confirm benefit.[22–24]

The most recent published meta-analysis found reductions in nonfatal myocardial ischemia were offset by non-fatal strokes and significant perioperative bradycardia and hypotension, with no effect on all-cause mortality.[25] The meta-analysis was dominated by the recently completed POISE trial,[26] which found increased mortality and strokes in patients started 2–4 hours preoperatively on a target dose of 200 mg/day extended-release metoprolol. More recently, the DECREASE-IV trial of bisoprolol 2.5 mg/day, started 30 days before surgery, did find a significant reduction 30-day cardiac death or infarction rates, without an associated increase in strokes, heart failure, bradycardia, or hypotension.[27] The protocols of these two major trials differed in many plausibly important ways, including study drug, dose, timing of drug initiation, and heart rate targets. DECREASE-IV enrolled a younger population than POISE and had a higher bradycardia threshold for holding the study drug .

There are no trials dedicated to studying the risk-benefit of perioperative beta-blockade in patients older than 75 years. There are no large, high-quality trials of lower-dose beta-blockade (less than metoprolol 50 mg/day) initiated just prior to surgery. In older patients with diminished physiologic reserve, requiring acute, noncardiac surgery, the risk-benefit of modest-dose beta-blockade remains unclear. Observational data suggests that a perioperative protocol for frail, elderly patients with hip fractures that includes low-dose metoprolol may be associated with significantly improved outcomes, including low myocardial ischemia and stroke rates.[20] After review of the POISE trial, the American College of Cardiology and American Heart Association have revised their guidelines, advising against perioperative initiation of high fixed-dose regimens in beta-blocker-naive patients undergoing intermediate-risk procedures.[28] Less aggressive or slowly titrated beta-blockade, and continuing chronic beta-blockade, is likely less harmful, and may be associated with improved outcomes.

Recommendations

- For patients on chronic beta-blocker therapy undergoing nonvascular surgery, continue beta-blockers in the perioperative period [overall quality: low]
- Consider the initiation of low-dose beta-blocker (equivalent to metoprolol 25–50 mg/day) therapy in patients at increased risk for perioperative cardiac events; consider starting days to weeks in advance of surgery if possible [overall quality: moderate]
- Titrate beta-blockers carefully, to avoid hypotension and/or bradycardia [overall quality: high]
- Do not routinely use perioperative beta-blockade in patients at low risk for perioperative cardiac events [overall quality: moderate]
- Do not initiate high-dose beta-blockers in naive patients in the immediate perioperative period [overall quality: high]

Question 5: What is the harm associated with delay to surgery?

Case clarification

The patient is admitted early Friday evening. Although she is medically stable, operating room time is limited over the weekend. On Monday, she is added to the surgical schedule at the end of the day, after more "urgent" cases are completed.

Relevance

Length of hospitalization for hip fracture repair varies tremendously depending on the healthcare system. The demand for urgent surgery often exceeds available resources. Guidance is needed to determine whether delays in surgery in medically stable patients will lead to poorer outcomes.

Current opinion

In many centers, surgical repair of a hip fracture is not viewed as urgent care.

Finding the evidence

- Cochrane Database (http://www.cochrane.org/reviews): with search terms: "hip fracture" AND "surgical delay" or "time to surgery" or "surgery timing"
  ° Returned 21 results (0 related to topic)
- PubMed (www.ncbi.nlm.nih.gov/PubMed/): with search terms: "hip fracture" and "surgery timing," limited to English
  ° Returned 84 references (19 relevant)
- A review of reference lists of relevant articles for additional published trials

Quality of the evidence

Level I
- 1 systematic reviews or meta-analyses

Level II
- 18 cohort studies

Findings

Because of the ethical nature of this question, a randomized trial to address it is not feasible. In a recent systematic review of 52 studies involving 291,413 patients,[29] 3 studies involving 6,954 patients were prospective, excluded unfit patients, and adjusted for confounders. In one of these studies,[30] a delay of 4 or more days in medically stable patients increased mortality at 90 days (HR 2.25, 95% CI = 1.2–4.3, p = 0.01) and at 1 year (HR 2.4, 95% CI = 1.45–3.99, p = 0.001). Patients who were delayed due to acute medical comorbidities on admission had a higher mortality at 30 days (HR = 2.3, 95% CI = 1.62–3.33), 90 days (HR 2.1, 95% CI = 1.6–2.7, p < 0.001), and 1 year (HR 1.72, 95%

CI = 1.38–2.15, p < 0.001), and there was no significant difference in mortality in this subgroup relating to surgical timing. In the second study, patients undergoing surgery within 24 hours had lower mean pain scores, fewer days of severe and very severe pain, shorter length of stay, and improved self-care at 6 months than those who had surgery after 24 hours, but did not have improved mortality.[31] In a subanalysis restricted to individuals who did not have marked abnormal clinical findings on presentation and did not need further preoperative evaluation, early surgery was associated with a reduction in major postoperative complications (OR 0.26, 95% CI = 0.07–0.95). A third study showed no difference in discharge destination or mortality after adjusting for baseline characteristics, but did note an increase in length of stay.[32]

Recommendations

- Delay in surgery more than 4 days in stable patients may increase mortality [overall quality: low]
- Surgery within 24 hours lowers overall pain and duration of severe pain [overall quality: moderate]
- Hip fracture patients who also have acute medical comorbidities are at increased risk of death due to those comorbidities, regardless of timing of surgery [overall quality: moderate]

Summary of recommendations

- Echocardiography should not be obtained in patients without signs or symptoms of new cardiac conditions
- Proactive, standardized geriatric assessment reduces delirium incidence and severity
- Low-dose haloperidol prophylaxis in a high-risk population may reduce delirium severity and duration
- Poorly treated pain may increase risk of delirium
- Comanagement should be considered for fragility fractures
- For patients on chronic beta-blocker therapy undergoing nonvascular surgery, continue beta-blockers in the perioperative period
- Consider the initiation of low-dose beta-blocker (equivalent to metoprolol 25–50 mg/day) therapy in patients at increased risk for perioperative cardiac events; consider starting days to weeks in advance of surgery if possible
- Titrate beta-blockers carefully, to avoid hypotension and/or bradycardia
- Do not routinely use perioperative beta-blockade in patients at low risk for perioperative cardiac events
- Do not initiate high-dose beta-blockers in naive patients in the immediate perioperative period
- Delay in surgery more than 4 days in stable patients may increase mortality

• Surgery within 24 hours lowers overall pain and duration of severe pain
• Hip fracture patients who also have acute medical comorbidities are at increased risk of death due to those comorbidities, regardless of timing of surgery

References

1. Sandby-Thomas M, Sullivan G, Hall JE. A national survey into the peri-operative anaesthetic management of patients presenting for surgical correction of a fractured neck of femur. Anaesthesia 2008;63(3):250–8.
2. Ricci WM, Della Rocca GJ, Combs C, Borrelli J. The medical and economic impact of preoperative cardiac testing in elderly patients with hip fractures. Injury 2007;38 Suppl 3: S49–52.
3. Robertson BD, Robertson TJ. Postoperative delirium after hip fracture. J Bone Joint Surg Am 2006;88(9):2060–8.
4. Bitsch M, Foss N, Kristensen B, Kehlet H. Pathogenesis of and management strategies for postoperative delirium after hip fracture: a review. Acta Orthop Scand 2004;75(4):378–89.
5. Rockwood K. Delays in the discharge of elderly patients. J Clin Epidemiol 1990;43(9):971–5.
6. Marcantonio ER, Flacker JM, Michaels M, Resnick NM. Delirium is independently associated with poor functional recovery after hip fracture. J Am Geriatr Soc. 2000;48(6):618–24.
7. Edelstein DM, Aharonoff GB, Karp A, Capla EL, Zuckerman JD, Koval KJ. Effect of postoperative delirium on outcome after hip fracture. Clin Orthop Relat Res 2004;422:195–200.
8. Olofsson B, Lundstrom M, Borssen B, Nyberg L, Gustafson Y. Delirium is associated with poor rehabilitation outcome in elderly patients treated for femoral neck fractures. Scand J Caring Sci 2005;19(2):119–27.
9. Marcantonio ER, Kiely DK, Simon SE, John Orav E, Jones RN, Murphy KM, et al. Outcomes of older people admitted to postacute facilities with delirium. J Am Geriatr Soc 2005;53(6): 963–9.
10. Siddiqi N, Stockdale R, Britton AM, Holmes J. Interventions for preventing delirium in hospitalised patients. Cochrane Database Syst Rev 2007;2:CD005563.
11. Marcantonio ER, Flacker JM, Wright RJ, Resnick NM. Reducing delirium after hip fracture: a randomized trial. J Am Geriatr Soc 2001;49(5):516–22.
12. Gustafson Y, Brannstrom B, Berggren D, Ragnarsson JI, Sigaard J, Bucht G, et al. A geriatric-anesthesiologic program to reduce acute confusional states in elderly patients treated for femoral neck fractures. J Am Geriatr Soc 1991;39(7):655–62.
13. Milisen K, Foreman MD, Abraham IL, De Geest S, Godderis J, Vandermeulen E, et al. A nurse-led interdisciplinary intervention program for delirium in elderly hip-fracture patients. J Am Geriatr Soc 2001;49(5):523–32.
14. Kalisvaart KJ, de Jonghe JF, Bogaards MJ, Vreeswijk R, Egberts TC, Burger BJ, et al. Haloperidol prophylaxis for elderly hip-surgery patients at risk for delirium: a randomized placebo-controlled study. J Am Geriatr Soc 2005;53(10): 1658–66.
15. Liptzin B, Laki A, Garb JL, Fingeroth R, Krushell R. Donepezil in the prevention and treatment of post-surgical delirium. Am J Geriatr Psychiatry 2005;13(12):1100–6.
16. Diaz V, Rodriguez J, Barrientos P, Serra M, Salinas H, Toledo C, et al. [Use of procholinergics in the prevention of postoperative delirium in hip fracture surgery in the elderly. A randomized controlled trial]. Rev Neurol 2001;33(8):716–9.
17. Morrison RS, Magaziner J, Gilbert M, Koval KJ, McLaughlin MA, Orosz G, et al. Relationship between pain and opioid analgesics on the development of delirium following hip fracture. J Gerontol A Biol Sci Med Sci 2003;58(1):76–81.
18. Sharma G, Kuo YF, Freeman J, Zhang DD, Goodwin JS. Comanagement of hospitalized surgical patients by medicine physicians in the United States. Arch Intern Med 2010;170(4): 363–8.
19. Auron-Gomez M, Michota F. Medical management of hip fracture. Clin Geriatr Med 2008;24(4):701–19, ix.
20. Friedman SM, Mendelson DA, Bingham KW, Kates SL. Impact of a comanaged Geriatric Fracture Center on short-term hip fracture outcomes. Arch Intern Med 2009;169(18):1712–7.
21. Friedman SM, Mendelson DA, Kates SL, McCann RM. Geriatric co-management of proximal femur fractures: total quality management and protocol-driven care result in better outcomes for a frail patient population. J Am Geriatr Soc 2008; 56(7):1349–56.
22. Yang H, Raymer K, Butler R, Parlow J, Roberts R. The effects of perioperative beta-blockade: results of the Metoprolol after Vascular Surgery (MaVS) study, a randomized controlled trial. Am Heart J 2006;152(5):983–90.
23. Juul AB, Wetterslev J, Gluud C, Kofoed-Enevoldsen A, Jensen G, Callesen T, et al. Effect of perioperative beta blockade in patients with diabetes undergoing major non-cardiac surgery: randomised placebo controlled, blinded multicentre trial. BMJ 2006;332(7556):1482.
24. Brady AR, Gibbs JS, Greenhalgh RM, Powell JT, Sydes MR. Perioperative beta-blockade (POBBLE) for patients undergoing infrarenal vascular surgery: results of a randomized double-blind controlled trial. J Vasc Surg 2005;41(4):602–9.
25. Bangalore S, Wetterslev J, Pranesh S, Sawhney S, Gluud C, Messerli FH. Perioperative beta blockers in patients having non-cardiac surgery: a meta-analysis. Lancet 2008;372(9654): 1962–76.
26. Devereaux PJ, Yang H, Yusuf S, Guyatt G, Leslie K, Villar JC, et al. Effects of extended-release metoprolol succinate in patients undergoing non-cardiac surgery (POISE trial): a randomised controlled trial. Lancet 2008;371(9627):1839–47.
27. Dunkelgrun M, Boersma E, Schouten O, Koopman-van Gemert AW, van Poorten F, Bax JJ, et al. Bisoprolol and fluvastatin for the reduction of perioperative cardiac mortality and myocardial infarction in intermediate-risk patients undergoing noncardiovascular surgery: a randomized controlled trial (DECREASE-IV). Ann Surg 2009;249(6):921–6.
28. Fleischmann KE, Beckman JA, Buller CE, Calkins H, Fleisher LA, Freeman WK, et al. 2009 ACCF/AHA focused update on perioperative beta blockade: a report of the American college of cardiology foundation/American heart association task force on practice guidelines. Circulation 2009;120(21): 2123–51.

29. Khan SK, Kalra S, Khanna A, Thiruvengada MM, Parker MJ. Timing of surgery for hip fractures: a systematic review of 52 published studies involving 291,413 patients. Injury 2009;40(7): 692–7.

30. Moran CG, Wenn RT, Sikand M, Taylor AM. Early mortality after hip fracture: is delay before surgery important? J Bone Joint Surg Am 2005;87(3):483–9.

31. Orosz GM, Magaziner J, Hannan EL, Morrison RS, Koval K, Gilbert M, et al. Association of timing of surgery for hip fracture and patient outcomes. JAMA 2004;291(14):1738–43.

32. Siegmeth AW, Gurusamy K, Parker MJ. Delay to surgery prolongs hospital stay in patients with fractures of the proximal femur. J Bone Joint Surg Br 2005;87(8):1123–6.

13 Orthobiologics

T. William Axelrad[1] and Thomas A. Einhorn[2]

[1]Lake Charles Memorial Hospital, Lake Charles, LA, USA
[2]Boston University Medical Center, Boston, MA, USA

Case scenarios

Case 1

A 64 year old man presents 2 years after sustaining a Gustilo–Anderson type II distal-third tibia fracture treated with a statically locked intramedullary nail. He has type 1 diabetes and has smoked a pack of cigarettes a day for over 40 years. The patient had a small residual gap at the fracture site, and did not develop significant bridging callus. His fracture was treated with dynamization of the nail at 9 months with removal of the proximal interlocking screws, and then revision intramedullary nailing 6 months later for continued lack of healing. He continues to have pain at the fracture site and shows no evidence of cortical bridging on plain radiographs.

Case 2

A 55 year old woman is seen for debilitating low back and neck pain for over 8 months. She has failed 3 months of physical therapy as well as having had two epidural steroid injections approximately 2 months ago. MRI shows degenerative disc disease at L3–4 and L4–5 as well as C5–6.

Relevant anatomy

Fracture healing is affected by a variety of conditions as well as the anatomic location of the injury. Smoking, comorbidities such as diabetes, open fractures, and advanced age all have negative effects on the healing of fractures. Several anatomic regions have a higher rate of nonunion, such as the proximal metaphysis of the 5th metatarsal, the scaphoid, the femoral neck, and the subtrochanteric region of the femur.[1–3] It is presumed that the tenuous nature of the local blood supply is largely responsible for the resistance to union at these sites.

Open tibia fractures have been the subject of intense research with regard to improving clinical outcomes related to bone healing and reducing the risk of infection. The blood supply to the tibia is predominately supplied by the posterior tibial artery.[4] Fractures that have soft tissue stripping (which devitalizes the bone) or an associated vascular injury are at increased risk for delayed union and nonunion. Dickson et al. obtained angiograms in 114 patients treated for an open tibia fracture.[5] They found that open fractures with documented arterial disruption had a rate of delayed and nonunion of 46% compared to a rate of 16% in similar injuries with a normal angiographic study. Others have achieved union in both distal femur and tibial nonunions after revascularization procedures alone.[6,7] Anatomic studies of the vascular supply of the tibia have shown that the proximal tibia is richly vascularized, while the diaphysis contains few extraosseous vessels.[8] Disruption of these vessels after fracture results in rapid revascularization. Delayed union and nonunion are characterized by an avascular area at the fracture site; in these cases restoration of stability and possibly bone grafting can result in healing.[9]

Several bones, when fractured, are resistant to union because their intraosseous vascular supply is provided by

Evidence-Based Orthopedics, First Edition. Edited by Mohit Bhandari.
© 2012 Blackwell Publishing Ltd. Published 2012 by Blackwell Publishing Ltd.

a single vessel that is typically disrupted by the fracture. For example, fracture of the proximal 5th metatarsal diaphysis, also known as a Jones fracture, occurs in a vascular watershed, which likely contributes to the higher rate of nonunion in this region.[10] The scaphoid is also prone to nonunion, as the proximal pole receives its blood supply proximally. Successful treatment has been accomplished with vascularized grafts,[11] further emphasizing the importance of the vascular supply in fracture healing.

Importance of the problem

In general, fractures heal, although the healing process can be impaired at specific anatomic sites, in fractures associated with soft tissue injuries, and in fractures occurring in patients with specific risk factors. With an aging population it is predicted by the World Health Organization that by 2050 there will be 6.3 million hip fractures worldwide, a significant increase from the estimated 1.66 million that occurred in 1990. Currently the highest rates of hip fractures are seen in North America and Europe, although by 2050 more than half of all hip fractures may occur in Asia.[12] A 2008 study on the incidence of all fracture types in England found that lifetime prevalence in middle-aged men was over 50% and it was 40% for women who lived past age 75.[13] While some countries have reported a recent decline in the age-adjusted rate of hip fractures,[14] studies from Finland, Canada, and Germany show that the absolute number of osteoporotic fractures continues to rise.[15–19] Regardless of the change in rates, Kannus et al. note that the burden of osteoporotic fractures in Finland, for example, will continue to rise along with the rapidly aging population.[20] A separate review of perimenopausal and postmenopausal women from 2000 to 2005 found a significant increase in rates of distal radius, hip, and pelvic fractures.[21] It is clear that with the increasing population worldwide, we will continue to experience the burden of both nonunions and delayed unions. Without appropriate interventions, this will likely result in significant increases in costs to both the patient and society. Not only will direct hospital and other medical costs increase, but the lost time from work by the patient and family members who become care givers will negatively impact society's productivity overall. Certain modalities, if used in targeted patients, may decrease the risk of nonunion or delayed union and thus decrease the overall cost of care for a given injury.

It appears that the incidence of clinically significant spine pathology is also increasing rapidly. From 1997 to 2006 the number of patients seeking medical attention for back complaints increased from 14.8 million to 21.9 million.[22] This increase is consistent with the 77% increase in the number of spinal fusions that were performed during the five year period from 1996 to 2001.[23] Degenerative disk disease that

fails conservative management has been treated with decompression and fusion with or without instrumentation. The risk of pseudoarthrosis in patients undergoing spine fusion with iliac crest bone graft is estimated to be as high as 12%, with advancing age being a risk factor for this complication.[24] Chronic pain at the operative site is another complication that has been found to occur in nearly 40% of patients,[25] with both major and minor complications occurring in 10% and 39% respectively.[26]

Top five questions

Risk factors

1. What patient and injury-related factors negatively affect bone healing?

Treatment

2. When should orthobiologics be used in the acute setting?
3. What orthobiologics are recommended for healing of recalcitrant nonunions?

Government regulations

4. What rules govern the use of orthobiologics?

Complications

5. What are the reported risk factors with the use of the various FDA (Food and Drug Aadinistration)/EMEA approved orthobiologics?

Question 1: What factors negatively affect bone healing?

Case 1 clarification
Our patient has several perceived risk factors for impaired fracture healing. Smoking and diabetes are known risk factors for impaired bone healing. Aging might also be a risk factor for nonunion of a fracture, since the pool of available mesenchymal stem cells declines with age. Our patient is a candidate for revision intramedullary nailing with autograft or with an orthobiologic agent.

Relevance
There are a number of issues that can affect a patient's health and potentially affect bone healing after trauma or during elective procedures such as spinal fusion or correction of malunion. It is well established that diabetes and malnutrition can negatively affect wound healing and other factors, either in combination or alone, may help predict the likelihood of delayed union or nonunion following fracture.

Current opinion

It is a common belief that multiple factors affect bone healing negatively. This includes patient-specific factors such as age, diabetes, malnutrition, and immune compromise. Smoking and alcohol abuse are also thought to have a negative impact on bone remodeling. The need to use orthobiologics in patients considered to be at risk for impaired healing has not been validated with randomized clinical trials, but remains an available option for the treating surgeon, although in many cases such use is "off-label" and appropriate discussion with the patient is required preoperatively (see Question 4).

Finding the evidence: aging and bone healing

• PubMed (www.ncbi.nlm.nih.gov/pubmed/): "aging bone marrow stromal changes" and "aging osteogenic potential"

Quality of the evidence (best available)

• Basic science: 19 animal studies, 11 human studies

Findings

Bone healing occurs in part through the recruitment of osteoprogenitor cells. This occurs through the release of local and circulating growth factors that induce an inflammatory response under relatively hypoxic conditions, which in turn results in early recruitment of mesenchymal stems cells (MSCs) to the site of injury.[27] The higher rate of nonunion reported in elderly patients, such as those older than 75 years of age, has been postulated to be the result of various factors. Some have suggested that the increase in incidence in nonunion is the result of a delay or decrease in the initial angiogenic response at the fracture site. This has been confirmed in animal models in which there is an age-related decline in blood vessel formation after fracture.[28] Street et al. studied 32 patients undergoing emergent fracture repair.[29] They obtained samples of fracture hematoma at the time of surgery, as well as plasma samples from venipuncture at a distant site. The test subjects evenly divided into two groups: half of the patients were less than 40 years of age and the remaining group was older than 75 years of age. Circulating factors known to be involved in angiogenesis, including vascular endothelial growth factor (VEGF) and platelet derived growth factor (PDGF), were quantified using enzyme-linked immunosorbant assay (ELISA). The absolute amount of VEGF in the samples from the older cohort was significantly reduced when compared to the controls (31.4 vs. 68.4 pg/mL); however, the relative increase in the injured patients compared to age- and gender-matched uninjured control was nearly tenfold for the older group, while only a fivefold increase was seen in the controls. No significant differences were seen with regards to PDGF. In-vitro endothelial cell proliferation and

blood vessel tube formation on Matrigel was also increased comparably when treated with plasma from each group. Finally, fracture hematoma and plasma from both groups induced robust new blood vessel formation in a murine subcutaneous wound pocket assay. One issue with this study is that the cells studied were isolated from human umbilical veins, and others have shown that the response of the cells involved in new blood vessel formation, the endothelial precursor cells (EPCs), is attenuated in elderly individuals.[30] Overall, the available studies indicate that the inflammatory response is maintained in the elderly population, although the angiogenic response may be attenuated secondary to age-related changes in the cellular response.

Conflicting data has been published on the number and health of MSCs in elderly individuals, although this may be related to the methods used in harvesting and assaying the cells in culture.[31] It is likely that aging results in a decrease in both the absolute numbers and health of MSCs. Most studies in animals have found changes in MSCs associated with aging.[32–34] Several investigators have shown a decrease in the osteogenic potential and growth rate in MSCs taken from long bones in aged mice,[35,36] while Bellows et al. found that cells isolated from the vertebral column responded similarly to treatments regardless of age.[37] Although the anatomic origin of the cells could be one reason for the differences seen in the various studies,[38] experiments in strains of mice that age at different rates suggest that variations in growth and differentiation may also be the result of differences in local growth factors and matrix composition of the donor.[39] D'Ippolito et al. studied the ability of MSCs from vertebral marrow aspirates to form colonies in vitro that expressed alkaline phosphatase, a marker of osteoblastic differentiation. Their results found that osteogenic potential declined with age up to approximately 40 years of age.[40] This same group isolated MSCs that they termed marrow-isolated adult multilineage inducible (MIAMI) cells, which also demonstrated an age-related decline from 0.01% of total marrow nucleated cells at 3 years of age, to 0.0018% by age 45.[41] Similar to their previous study on MSCs, they found that the decline stabilized at this time and it appears that these cells are resistant to the effects of aging seen in other MSCs, with the exception of an increase in the doubling time by 30%.[41,42] Stolzing et al. compared human MSCs from three age groups.[43] They found an age-related decline in the number of stems cells isolated from iliac crest bone marrow aspirates up to the age of 40. Cells isolated from patients over 40 years of age displayed an increase in the expression of the apoptosis markers p53 and, to a lesser extent, p21, with a significant increase in the rate of apoptosis. When the investigators assessed the ability of MSCs to differentiate into osteoblastic cells, the aged population showed a significant decline in alkaline phosphatase activity, and this decline was evident in patients beginning after 18 years of age, with a 40% decline occurring in 19–40 year old group. Bidula et al. found a decline in relation to age in the number of marrow cells isolated from the anterior iliac crest.[44] However, they found no difference in the prevalence of alkaline phosphatase-positive cultures between subjects.

Recommendation

Although the debate continues, it appears that evidence favors an age-related change in MSC activity and health. However, what role this plays in bone repair as the population continues to age throughout the world remains to be determined with larger controlled trials.

• The current evidence does not support treating elderly patients with fractures differently than any other group of patients with regards to the use of orthobiologics to stimulate fracture healing [overall quality: moderate-high]

Finding the evidence: diabetes

• PubMed (www.ncbi.nlm.nih.gov/pubmed/): "diabetes fracture healing," "diabetic fracture"

Quality of the evidence (best available)

• Basic science: 2 animal studies, 1 human study
• Level III: 2
• Level IV: 1

Findings

Several medical conditions affect bone health and are related to an increase in fracture risk and possibly a higher rate of healing complications. Diabetes has many effects on cellular health and increased rates of fractures have been seen in both type 1 and type 2 diabetics. This increase in fracture risk may be multifactorial and includes a decreased bone strength as well as an increase in the rate of falls secondary to poor vision, peripheral neuropathy, and episodes of hypoglycemia.[45] Complications related to diabetes include delayed wound healing and difficulties with achieving bony union.[46–48] Animal models of diabetic fracture healing indicate that in type 1 diabetes, the fracture callus is negatively affected by an upregulation of inflammatory markers, with an associated increase in osteoclast activity and cartilage breakdown.[49] There are, however, few clinical studies showing that diabetics have difficulties with fracture healing. Cozen reported on nine consecutive diabetic patients with delayed union or nonunion when compared to matched case controls.[50] Loder retrospectively reviewed 31 closed fractures in diabetic patients.[51] These authors compared healing time, as measured by radiographic parameters and time to full weightbearing, with accepted healing times obtained from literature review. They determined that overall healing time was increased in the diabetic patients with an odds ratio of 1.63. Furthermore,

there was an increased incidence of delayed union in non-insulin-dependent diabetics, patients treated operatively, and those older than 50 years of age.[48] In a separate retrospective review of 84 patients with diabetes and operatively managed ankle fractures, Costigan et al. failed to show a difference in the rate of union.[52] They did, however, note that 10 patients developed complications such as infection. These problems occurred in patients with absent pedal pulses and in those patients with peripheral neuropathy.

Two animal studies have been published examining the effect of approved orthobiologics on fracture healing in a diabetic model. Kidder et al. studied OP-1 (Stryker Biotech, Hopkinton, MA) in 54 streptozotocin-induced diabetic rats that were subjected to a traumatic femoral fracture.[53] The fractures were fixed acutely with an intramedullary pin and either 25 µg of OP-1 in a collagen carrier, carrier alone, or nothing. At both the 2 week and 4 week time points, the radiographic area of callus was significantly greater in the OP-1 treated animals. This increased callus did not result in a change in the torque to failure between any of the tested groups, including a nondiabetic control group. In a similar study, rhBMP-2 (Medtronic, Minneapolis, MN) was evaluated in diabetic Wistar rats.[54] The diabetic state in these rats was induced by an autoimmune reaction as opposed to chemical induction. Femoral fractures were created and stabilized in both diabetic and nondiabetic rats and either rhBMP-2 or vehicle alone was applied. There was no significant increase in new bone at the fracture site for the rhBMP-2 treated animals, however, there was an increase in the number of blood vessels in the diabetic animals. Interestingly, at both the 3 week and 6 week time points, no difference in the amount of new bone between the diabetic and nondiabetic animals was detected.

Recommendations

The available data are limited, although it appears that diabetic patients are at a higher risk for wound complications and infection. The results in the single animal study reviewed showed a positive effect of OP-1 on fracture callus mineralization, although it had no effect on the strength of the fracture callus. This study in isolation does not indicate a dramatic potential for OP-1 use in the acute fracture setting.

• Until larger and prospective human studies are available, diabetic patients deserve special attention with regards to management of lower extremity fractures, with particular attention to wound care, peripheral vascular disease, peripheral neuropathy, and renal disease [overall quality: moderate-low]

Finding the evidence: endocrine/nutritional deficits

• PubMed (www.ncbi.nlm.nih.gov/pubmed/): "endocrine nonunion," "nutrition fracture healing"

Quality of the evidence (best available)
- Level I: 1
- Level IV: 1

Findings

Endocrine abnormalities other than diabetes may also play a role in fracture healing. Brinker et al. created an algorithm by which patients who suffered a nonunion that could not be explained by technical error, had sustained a previous low-energy fracture with at least one nonunion, or had a nonunion of a nondisplaced pubic rami or sacral ala fracture, were referred to an endocrinologist.[55] The investigators identified 37 patients out of a consecutive series of 683 nonunions, of which 31 were diagnosed with a new endocrine or metabolic abnormality. Medical management resulted in union in 30 of the 31 patients, with one patient treated with a hip arthroplasty for subtrochanteric nonunion. Eight of these 31 patients had no further operative treatment to achieve union. The most common abnormality identified was related to calcium homeostasis and vitamin D deficiency. Vitamin D deficiency is a significant health concern worldwide, with seasonal variations occurring in conjunction with variations in available sunlight. Studies in Australia found that the incidence of vitamin D insufficiency was as high as 74% in healthy middle-aged women during the winter months.[56] Similar differences were not seen in comparable male subjects,[57] although studies in Europe found rates of deficiency in 36% of elderly men and 47% of elderly women.[58] Doetsh et al. randomized 30 patients with proximal humerus fractures and a diagnosis of osteopenia or osteoporosis into two groups.[59] Each group was managed nonoperatively, with the treatment group receiving daily supplementation of 1g of calcium and 800IU of vitamin D3. Over a 12 week period the investigators observed an increase in the bone mineral density (BMD) of both groups, with the greatest increase seen at 6 weeks. The treated patients showed significantly higher BMD when compared to placebo (0.623 vs. $0.570\,g/cm^2$, p = 0.006). Clinical differences were not reported, but the results suggest that fracture healing can be modulated by medical management.

Recommendation

- The prevalence of endocrine abnormalities, as well as the need to treat these conditions regardless of their effect on bone healing, should alert the treating physician to recognize patients at risk early in the treatment of fractures. In this way the appropriate tests can be administered and appropriate treatments can be implemented [overall quality: moderate-high]

Finding the evidence: HIV/AIDS
- PubMed (www.ncbi.nlm.nih.gov/pubmed/): "HIV fracture healing"

Quality of the evidence (best available)
- Basic science: 1 human study
- Level I: 3

Findings

Increasing rates of infection with HIV and increased rates of AIDS worldwide, particularly in the aging population, has implications for both the incidence and treatment of fractures.[60–63] It has been shown that HIV infection is associated with an increased risk for osteopenia and osteoporosis, as well as an increase in the serum levels of the inflammatory cytokine TNF-α.[64] Delayed wound healing and infection after fracture treatment may be increased in patients with HIV,[65,66] specifically in relation to open fractures.[67,68] Only one study has demonstrated an increased risk of fracture nonunion in individuals affected by HIV, but the difference in union rate only approached significance (p = 0.059) in this small cohort of patients with open fractures.[68]

Recommendation

- With regard to HIV-infected patients, the available evidence suggests a trend that Gustilo–Anderson type II and III fractures are at an increased risk of infection and possibly nonunion, although larger randomized controlled trials are needed to better answer this question [overall quality: moderate]

Finding the evidence: obesity
- PubMed (www.ncbi.nlm.nih.gov/pubmed/): "obesity fracture healing," "obesity fracture complications"

Quality of the evidence (best available)
- Level I: 1
- Level IV: 1

Findings

Obesity, and particularly morbid obesity, is a common problem that has reached epidemic rates in many parts of the world.[69,70] Although obesity has not been shown to be a predictor of delayed fracture healing,[71] obese patients are at a higher risk for wound and other perioperative complications.[72,73] Nonunion is a difficult problem when it occurs, and complications, such as early hardware failure, have been shown.[74]

Recommendation

In obese patients, methods that could promote faster healing could potentially reduce the rate of reoperation in this group that is at high risk of complications, although this hypothesis has not been adequately tested.

- Obesity alone is not an indication for the use of an orthobiologic agent [overall quality: moderate-low]

Finding the evidence: alcohol and tobacco abuse

- PubMed (www.ncbi.nlm.nih.gov/pubmed/): "alcohol fracture healing" alcohol nonunion" "tobacco fracture healing" "nicotine fracture nonunion"

Quality of the evidence (best available)

- Basic science: 9 animal studies, 1 human study
- Level I: 3
- Level II: 6
- Level IV: 1

Findings

Addictive behaviors can have a major impact on the incidence and recovery of patients sustaining orthopedic injuries.[75–77] Alcohol abuse can affect patient compliance and can be associated with tobacco use and malnutrition.[78] Animal studies suggest that alcohol abuse itself has a negative effect on bone remodeling,[79–81] and specifically osteoblast activity, although one study proposed that there was no effect on the healing of tibia fractures in rats.[82] In this study, animals were fed increasing concentrations of ethanol for 8 days, at which time the tibial shafts were fractured and fixed with an intramedullary pin. The animals were killed at 6 weeks and both the injured and uninjured limbs were tested for mechanical strength. The results indicated that ethanol-fed animals had significantly lower total body BMD and bone calcium content when compared to control animals. Energy to refracture was also less in the animals treated with ethanol. Histologic or radiographic analysis was not done, and the conclusion that fracture healing was equivalent in the two groups was not supported by the reported findings. Studies on the effects of alcohol abuse on the rate of fracture healing in the clinical setting are scarce. Kristensson et al. reviewed the records of 107 chronic alcoholics and determined that the incidence of fracture in this group, when compared to age-matched controls, was increased by nearly fourfold.[83] They did not comment on the time to union or the incidence of complications related to the fracture treatment. Nyquist et al. reviewed tibial fractures in 49 alcoholics and compared rates of healing and complications with 150 patients who did not have a history of alcohol abuse.[84] Interestingly, there was no difference in complications or an increased incidence of nonunion. In the subset of patients who sustained a transverse tibial fracture, a statistical difference in the time to achieve union was present.

Smoking has long been regarded as a risk factor for wound healing and postoperative complications.[85,86] Recent data from animal studies, however, suggest that nicotine may have positive effects on angiogenesis and wound healing but these effects may be countered by vasoconstriction resulting in decreased perfusion.[87,88] Jacobi et al. found an endogenous cholinergic pathway that was involved in angiogenesis.[87] This pathway is activated by nicotine through endothelial nicotine acetylcholine receptors. When the investigators treated wounds in diabetic mice with topical nicotine they noted healing rates that were similar to those treated with basic fibroblast growth factor. Fracture healing has also been extensively studied in animal models and, similar to the findings with regards to alcohol, not all studies have demonstrated a negative effect of tobacco use.[89–92] Skott et al. studied femoral fracture healing in rates treated with an intramedullary pin.[93] Animals were pretreated for 7 days with either subcutaneous nicotine, tobacco extract with or without nicotine, or placebo. Mechanical testing of the fracture at 21 days demonstrated a significant decrease in ultimate torque and torque at yield point for the tobacco extract group when compared to both groups. The addition of nicotine to the tobacco extract treated group did not have an effect on mechanical strength. Interestingly, no difference was seen in ultimate stiffness, energy absorption, or callus BMD within any of the groups.

Human studies on the effects of tobacco and nicotine have also had conflicting results. Analysis of marrow aspirates from the anterior iliac crest of 62 patients who were either nonsmokers, previous smokers, or current smokers, found no difference in the number of MSCs or the ability of these cells to undergo osteogenic differentiation.[94] Weresh et al. found no association between smoking and the need for multiple revision surgeries for femoral nonunions.[95] A review of 24,774 patients who had undergone spinal decompression and fusion found an overall infection rate of 3.04%, with tobacco use associated with an increased risk of infection (RR 1.19, p = 0.09), although the results only approached significance and the increased risk was relatively small.[96] A significant decrease in the time to union in tibial osteotomies was found in patients who used smokeless tobacco when compared to both smokers and nonsmokers.[97] The difference between union times in smokers and nonsmokers was only 1 week, and was reported as statistically significant (p = 0.03). With regard to the rate of nonunion and delayed union, no difference was seen between smokers and nonsmokers. The same group had previously reported an increase of 2 weeks to union in smokers when compared to nonsmokers, with smokers having a 2.5-fold increased risk for complications.[98] McKee et al. reviewed a series of patients treated with Ilizarov reconstruction for malunion, nonunion, and leg length discrepancy.[99] They found that the relative risk for nonunion in the smoking group was 5.8. Preoperatively, there was a trend towards significance (p = 0.14) in the rate of infections in the group of smokers. The authors also failed to mention the number of nonunions in each group preoperatively, a factor that could have preselected patients that had difficulty with achieving union and influenced the final outcome. Bhandari et al. found an association between smoking and secondary procedures after treatment of open tibial fractures with intramedullary nail with or without rhBMP-2 supplementation.[100] They defined these outcomes as "all procedures with the potential of promoting fracture healing (or events such as inadvertent screw breakage associated with unlocking of the intramedullary nail, resulting in self-dynamization)" and the rate in smokers was 33% higher than in nonsmokers. The rate was significantly reduced for smokers who received 1.5 mg/mL rhBMP-2 (30% vs. 52%, p = 0.0138).

The most extensive research on the correlation between smoking and bone healing has occurred in spinal surgery. Hilibrand et al. evaluated the impact of smoking on the rate of pseudoarthrosis in anterior cervical spine fusion.[102] The effect of smoking on fusion was variable in this series, with no differences seen in patients who had undergone corpectomy and strut graft with either fibular allograft or iliac crest autograft. In a larger series of patients who had multilevel interbody grafting, the rate of solid fusion at all levels was significantly less in smokers (62%) when compared to nonsmokers (76%). It should be noted that the rate of follow-up in this study was only 75%. In a retrospective review of 375 patients who underwent instrumented lumbar fusion, the rate of pseudoarthrosis in smokers was shown to be 26.5% compared to 14.2% for nonsmokers. In a third group that had quit smoking for at least 6 months, the rate of nonunion remained significantly higher.[102] Finally, Mok et al. retrospectively reviewed 89 consecutive patients undergoing initial fusion of at least five levels.[103] While reoperation for any reason was high in smokers (RR 2.59), the investigators did not find a correlation with infection, implant failure, or rate of pseudoarthrosis. The higher rate of reoperation appears to result from the high incidence of pain in spinal segments adjacent to that of the index procedure in smokers when compared to nonsmokers (18.1% vs. 0%).

Recommendation
- The physician should counsel patients on smoking cessation and reducing or eliminating other risky behavior such as drug and alcohol abuse, as these interventions will promote the overall health of the patient and will likely decrease the risk of complications in those treated both operatively and nonoperatively [overall quality: moderate-high]

Question 2: When should orthobiologics be used in the acute setting?

Case 1 clarification
When examining our patient we noticed a small irregular scar approximately 3 cm in length over the site of the fracture. The patient informs us that at the time of the injury he had a bleeding wound at that site.

Case 2 clarification
Our patient decides to have anterior cervical discectomy and fusion at C5–6 with a staged fusion of L3–4 and L4–5

through either a combined anterior and posterior approach or through a posterior only approach.

Finding the evidence: fracture of the appendicular skeleton
- PubMed (www.ncbi.nlm.nih.gov/pubmed/): "fracture rhBMP-2," "bone healing rhBMP-2," "bone healing OP-1"

Quality of the evidence (best available)
- Basic science: 11 animal studies
- Level I: 4
- Level II: 1

Findings
Extensive research using rhBMP-2 in both rodents and larger mammals indicates that it stimulates faster and more robust fracture healing.[104–106] However, there are only a couple of clinical trials of rhBMP-2 use in human fractures. Govender et al. conducted a large prospective randomized study using rhBMP-2 that include 450 patients who had sustained an open tibial shaft fracture.[107] Treatments were standardized in that each patient had their fracture managed with standard soft tissue management and the fractures were definitively treated with an intramedullary nail. Patients were then randomized to receive a type 1 collagen sponge containing either 0.75 mg/mL or 1.50 mg/mL of rhBMP-2 or nothing at the time of definitive wound closure. The primary outcome measure was return to the operating room for a subsequent procedure within 12 months of the operation. Patients treated with 1.5 mg/ml of rhBMP-2 had a significantly decreased need for reoperation. Secondary outcome measures of wound healing and infection rates were also significantly improved in this group. After the completion of this study, a subgroup analysis of Gustilo–Anderson type III open fractures, combined with results of a concurrent and similar randomized trial of 60 patients, found that initial treatment of an open tibia fracture with rhBMP-2 and either reamed or unreamed intramedullary nailing reduced the rate of secondary procedures, including bone grafting, and reduced the risk for infection by 48% (95% CI 8–70%).[108] There are several concerns with regard to the methods and outcomes in these studies. In the larger group, the randomization process was centralized, and resulted in heterogeneity between the control and treatment groups. Patients treated with 1.5 mg of rhBMP-2 were more likely to have reaming of the intramedullary canal prior to insertion of the nail (41% vs. 27%). This may have favored the treatment group, as recent randomized trial of reamed and unreamed nails in tibial fractures found that in the subgroup of open fractures there was a trend towards an increase in the use of dynamization and drainage of hematomas when reaming was used (RR 1.16, p = 0.16).[100] A more recent study has called into question some of the findings in the original. Aro et al. con-

ducted a randomized study of 277 patients treated with reamed intramedullary nailing with or without rhBMP-2.1.[109] The study had planned to enrol 300 patients but was suspended after a higher rate of deep infection was noted in the rhBMP-2 group (12 [9%] vs 3 [2%]). This increase in deep infections was particularly prevalent in Gustilo-Anderson type III injuries (7 [16%] vs 1 [2%]).

Jones et al. studied rhBMP-2 in combination with allograft as a substitute for autograft in the treatment of tibia fractures with critical-sized defects.[110] They defined these defects as being 1–5 cm in length and at least 50% of the circumference of the diaphysis. Patients were initially stabilized with either an intramedullary nail or external fixation. They randomized 30 patients and followed them for 12 months and measured the rate of union and patient satisfaction using the Short Musculoskeletal Function Assessment (SMFA). They found no difference in the rate of union or satisfaction among the 24 patients (80%) who were available at the final follow-up.

OP-1 (Stryker Biotech, Hopkinton, MA) has been studied in both animal and human models and has been shown to positively affect the healing of nonunions.[130–133] However, these positive findings were not confirmed in a randomized trial of the treatment of distal radius malunions.[111] In the study, 20 patients were randomized to treatment with either OP-1 or autograft after corrective osteotomy of the distal radius and dorsal plating. There was no difference in the clinical outcomes at the final follow-up, although the investigators did find that OP-1 use resulted in a significantly longer time to union (18 vs. 7 weeks) and a higher rate of partial union. In the autograft group, all 10 patients had complete osseous union, while only 4 patients in the OP-1 treated group had similar results. These findings highlight the risk of using orthobiologics for indications that have not yet been tested, as the response in different anatomic areas cannot be predicted based on previous studies.

Recommendation

The results of the available randomized controlled trials indicate that rhBMP-2 is effective at achieving bony union in human subjects. The significant cost associated with the use of bone morphogenetic protein (BMP) is a concern and should prohibit its use in routine, closed fractures at this time.

- On the basis of the existing literature, use of rhBMP-2 in open fractures can only be recommended in high-energy open tibia fractures treated with unreamed nails; there is no data in other long bones or with other modes of fracture stabilization [overall quality: high]

Finding the evidence: primary spinal fusion

- PubMed (www.ncbi.nlm.nih.gov/pubmed/): "spine fusion rhBMP-2," "lumbar fusion rhBMP-2," "spine fusion OP-1"

Quality of the evidence (best available)

- Basic science: 12 animal studies
- Level I: 7
- Level II: 2
- Level IV: 2

Findings

Pain and disability from degenerative spine disease, particularly low back pain, is a tremendous burden on both patients and society.[112] Treatment of this disorder is typically conservative, although fusion of the spine is an option for patients who have failed conservative management. This can be accomplished from an anterior, posterior, or combined approach, and stability and fusion can be accomplished with or without the use of instrumentation. The gold standard to enhance fusion is autograft in the form of iliac crest bone graft (ICBG), although there is reported morbidity associated with harvesting it, and the additional operative time, blood loss, and postoperative pain make an "off-the-shelf" bone-graft substitute product very attractive.[113] In an effort to decrease the need for autologous graft, orthobiologics and allografts have been used with increasing frequency.

Animal studies have demonstrated the efficacy of rhBMP-2 in spinal fusion.[114–119] Human studies have shown similar benefits. One of the earliest published studies was a pilot study for posterolateral spinal fusion. In this study 25 patients were randomized to either instrumented posterior fusion supplemented with either autograft or BMP-2 or BMP-2 alone without instrumentation.[120] The rate of fusion at 1 year follow-up was only 40% in the patients treated with autograft, while 100% of the patients who were treated with BMP-2 had achieved fusion. A larger randomized study compared rhBMP-2 in an absorbable collagen sponge carrier or ICBG in combination with a structural allograft dowel for anterior lumbar interbody fusion (ALIF).[121] The patients were followed for 2 years, and at the final follow-up fusion was significantly greater in the rhBMP-2 treated patients (98.5 vs. 76.1, p < 0.001). Revision procedures were also more common in the control group, with eight patients returning to the operating room as compared to only two patients in the rhBMP-2 group.

Dawson et al. randomized 46 patients who underwent posterolateral spinal fusion with instrumentation to receive either rhBMP-2 on an absorbable collagen sponge with a ceramic granule bulking agent or autogenous ICBG. Their results showed a trend towards improvements in clinical outcomes and a higher rate of fusion in the rhBMP-2 group.[122] A modification of the rhBMP-2 carrier to include a matrix that contained 15% hydroxyapatite and 85% beta-tricalcium phosphate particles was developed, with the evidence demonstrating that the new carrier would have improved properties with respect to bone remodeling.[123] Dimar et al. studied this new formulation in 463 patients who underwent posterolateral instrumented fusion who were randomized to receive either autogenous ICBG or rhBMP-2.[124] With regard to the index procedure, patients in the ICBG group had longer operative times and greater blood loss, although the length of hospital stay was comparable with the BMP-treated group. Follow-up at 2 years was 89% and included both clinical and radiographic outcomes. The rates of fusion were higher for rhBMP-2 at all time points, with 96% achieving fusion by radiographic parameters compared to 89% at 2 years (p = 0.014).

A cost analysis was performed in conjunction with a randomized controlled trial of patients over 60 years of age who underwent posterolateral lumbar fusion.[125] The investigators found the final costs at 2 years were over $2000 higher per patient for those treated with autogenous ICBG. It was suggested by the authors that the increased costs in the ICBG group may have been related to the insignificant increased rate of nonunion and subsequent revision operations. Other nonrandomized or retrospective studies have also found high rates of fusion with the use of rhBMP-2 in lumbar fusions that were comparable to autogenous ICBG.[126–128]

Initial studies in spinal fusion surgery using OP-1 were for posterolateral fusion in patients with degenerative spondylolisthesis. Results were comparable to historical controls and complications were minimal.[129,130] These reports were followed by a randomized controlled trial that included 335 patients treated with posterolateral fusion for degenerative spondylolisthesis.[131] The patients were randomized in a 2:1 fashion to receive either OP-1 putty or autogenous ICBG as the sole means of fusion. The use of OP-1 was associated with shorter operative times as well as less intraoperative blood loss. When the investigators analyzed patients with more than 36 months of follow-up they found that clinical and dynamic radiographic parameters were comparable. What was seen was a significant difference in the presence of new bone in the intertransverse process region as measured by CT scan, with only 56% of the OP-1 putty group showing bridging bone compared to 83% of the autograft group. This difference did not translate into a clinical difference, particularly in relation to revision procedures. The authors also noted a transient increase in OP-1 antibodies, although they reported no evidence of systemic toxicity from this.

Recommendations

The large numbers of randomized studies indicate that rhBMP-2 is effective in achieving fusion and this rate of fusion is superior, or at least equivalent to, that achieved with ICBG.
• While clinical outcomes appear equivalent, the cost analysis reported by Carreon et al. supports the use of rhBMP-2 as a potential cost-saving measure in lumbar fusion [overall quality: moderate-high][132]
• The trials have shown equivalent clinical outcomes when OP-1 is used as an adjunct to posterolateral fusion,

and although they did show shorter operative times and a decrease in blood loss in comparison to use of ICBG, the magnitude of these differences and the costs associated with the use of OP-1 do not warrant its use as a standard treatment at this time [overall quality: moderate-high]

Question 3: What orthobiologics are recommended for healing of recalcitrant nonunions?

Case 1 clarification
Our patient has persistent pain at the site of the fracture. Imaging shows an atrophic nonunion at the site of injury.

Case 2 clarification
Our patient returns for the 2 year follow-up with continued pain in the lumbar spine. Imaging confirms a pseudoarthrosis of both operative levels.

Finding the evidence: nonunion of long bones
• PubMed (www.ncbi.nlm.nih.gov/pubmed/): "nonunion OP-1," "fracture nonunion rhBMP-2"

Quality of the evidence (best available)
• Basic science: 6 animal studies
• Level I: 1
• Level IV: 4

Findings
BMP-7, also known as osteogenic protein-1 (OP-1), is a member of the TGF-β superfamily that has been shown to be involved in fracture healing. This molecule shows an increase in expression during enchondral ossification, and has been shown to strongly induce osteoblastic differentiation.[133,134] The strong association between fracture healing and OP-1 expression led to human clinical studies to rescue nonunions, potentially through the stimulation of local osteoprogenitor cells. The first randomized study using OP-1 was conducted by Friedlander et al. in which 124 patients were randomized to receive either autograft or a type 1 collagen sponge containing rhOP-1 (OP-1) at the site of nonunion.[135] During the initial 9 months, 81% of the OP-1 treated patients and 85% of the autograft treated patients were able to bear full weight, an indicator for clinical union. Giannoudis et al. retrospectively reviewed a prospectively collected database of 45 patients treated with a combination of autologous bone graft and OP-1.[136] This study included a mix of fracture locations, including 19 tibia fractures and 7 humeral and 19 femoral nonunions. Each of the patients had failed at least one previous attempt to achieve union. In this series of recalcitrant nonunions, all of the patients proceeded to unite at an average of 6.8 months (range 4–16). Pelvic pain from the donor site was the most common complication and was seen in six patients, followed by superficial wound infections in three patients

that resolved with a short course of antibiotic treatment. They also noted an absence of deep infections, which is usually high in revision fracture fixation.[135]

There has been an increase in the published reports of patients treated with OP-1 for nonunions in areas other than the tibia. In an industry-sponsored study of 23 patients treated for humeral atrophic nonunion, Bong et al. found that supplementation with 3.5 mg of OP-1 resulted in union in all patients after revision surgery.[137] There were several problems with the design of this study, including the large variation in the type of bone graft used and the type of fixation employed. Pelvic nonunions and instability can be a source of significant pain. OP-1 was tested as a potential adjuvant in the treatment in these patients. A series of nine patients—four post traumatic nonunions, four patients with postpartum pelvic instability, and one patient with a significant bone defect after sacroilliitis—were treated surgically and supplemented with OP-1.[138] Overall, this group of patients had undergone an average of 1.6 procedures and had to have a preoperative bone defect of at least 2 cm. Three of the patients with postpartum instability had failed autogenous bone grafting. Union was achieved in eight cases at a minimum follow-up of 12 months.

Recommendation

The limited numbers of randomized studies showing a significant difference in the rate of union with the use of OP-1 make it difficult to recommend it for use in long bones, when other alternatives are available. Reports from our experience[139] and others[140] in the upper extremity give concern when considering using OP-1.
• There is a need for more randomized studies, particularly in the upper extremity, to elucidate the safety and efficacy of OP-1 before expanded use can be recommended [overall quality: moderate-low]

Finding the evidence: spinal pseudoarthrosis

• PubMed (www.ncbi.nlm.nih.gov/pubmed/): "nonunion spine rhBMP-2," "pseudoarthrosis spine rhBMP-2," "nonunion spine OP-1," "pseudoarthrosis spine OP-1"

Quality of the evidence (best available)

• Basic science: 1 animal study
• Level I: 1
• Level IV: 4

Findings

Fusion of the spine can result in pseudarthrosis, and when pain is present, revision fixation is usually indicated. Grauer et al. developed a spinal pseudoarthrosis model in New Zealand white rabbits.[141] The investigators compared OP-1 to autograft in these animals and found an 82% rate of fusion for OP-1 compared to 42% for autograft. Furlan et al.[142] prospectively enrolled 30 patients scheduled for posterior spinal fusion to evaluate OP-1 as an adjuvant to

autograft in patients who had a previous spinal pseudoarthrosis and/or were at high risk for nonunion. They were able to show an 80% rate of union at the 2 year follow-up. There were no significant events relating to OP-1 use, although they did note asymptomatic linear opacification in the soft tissues, resembling heterotopic ossification.

rhBMP-2 has also been tested in the spine as an alternative to autologous bone graft. It has been used in combination with MasterGraft™, a medical grade combination of 15% hydroxypatite and 85% beta-tricalcium phosphate.[143] The graft must be used in combination with supplemental posterior fixation and can be used for two or more levels. Two studies[144,145] as well as a pilot clinical trial[146] were the impetus for the approval of this product by the U.S. Food and Drug Administration (FDA) . In the clinical trial, 25 patients received INFUSE/MasterGraft and 21 control patients receiving autograft. The rate of pseudoarthrosis was found to be 4% in the patients treated with INFUSE/MasterGraft while 9.5% of patients in the control groups suffered from this complication. Adverse events were similar between each group.

Recommendation

Spinal pseudoarthrosis is a difficult problem to address. The available evidence suggests that both OP-1 and rhBMP-2 may have benefits in patients at risk for continued nonunion after revision.
• In patients at risk for continued nonunion after revision, and when ICBG is not a reasonable option, then the use of either OP-1 or rhBMP-2 can be recommended, in light of the lack of other alternatives [overall quality: moderate-high]

Question 4: What rules govern the use of orthobiologics?

Cases 1 and 2 clarification

Neither patient wants to have autograft taken from their "hip" as they have heard that the pain after this procedure can be permanent and debilitating.

Regulatory process

The approval process for new drugs and medical devices is an expensive proposition for pharmaceutical companies, estimated to cost $0.8–1.7 billion.[147] Separate agencies regulate this process in each country. In the United States, the FDA is responsible for reviewing and approving new medical treatments. The European Medicines Agency (EMA) is the FDA equivalent in for the European Union (EU), while China regulates new drugs through the State Food and Drug Administration (SFDA). In the case of rhBMP-2, marketed as Infuse™ in the US and InductOs in Europe (Medtronic Sofamor Danek. Inc, Minneapolis, MN), it was first granted a community market authorization for use for open tibia fractures treated with an intramedullary nail in Europe after a centralized application was reviewed by the Committee for Human Medicinal Products (CHMP). This committee is made up of delegates from each EU member state and a network of over 3,500 experts.[147] Two other processes, the mutual recognition procedure and the decentralized procedure, are available for achieving approval, although all biotechnology substances must use the centralized procedure. Once a drug or substance receives approval, a summary of product characteristics (SmPC) is published and includes such information as therapeutic indications, dosing, and any warnings. This information is updated as new information is published or new indications are granted.

In the US, the approval process proceeds in one of two ways, depending on the results of the clinical trial and the perceived and known risks and benefits, and results in the product receiving one of two designations. The different mechanisms for approval have important implications on how a drug can be used and marketed. Infuse was granted a pre-market approval (PMA) by the FDA shortly after its approval in Europe for a similar indication with regards to open tibia fractures. It has also received PMAs for anterior single-level lumbar spinal fusion and certain oral maxillofacial and dental regeneration procedures.[148–150] The PMA allows the device to be used as the surgeon deems appropriate but sets regulations on how the company can market the product.

The other designation that a device or drug may receive is a Humanitarian Device Exemption (HDE). This is a much more complicated designation, and is used when safety has been established in clinical trials but efficacy remains in question. The FDA uses this as a way to approve products quickly for use in patients in whom there are few, if any, feasible alternatives. rhBMP-7 (OP-1™, Stryker Biotech, Hopkinton, MA) has received an HDE for two indications. These include "use as an alternative to autograft in recalcitrant long bone nonunions where use of autograft is unfeasible and alternative treatments have failed"[151] and in spinal fusion surgery in patients who "have failed a previous spinal fusion surgery, and are not able to provide their own bone or bone marrow for grafting because of a condition such as osteoporosis, diabetes, or smoking."[152] The approval is further limiting in that the use of OP-1 is restricted to only 4,000 cases per year in the US.

Question 5: What are the reported risk factors with the use of the various FDA/EMEA approved orthobiologics?

Case 1 clarification
The patient is treated with revision intramedullary nailing and OP-1 with allograft.

Finding the evidence
• PubMed (www.ncbi.nlm.nih.gov/pubmed/): "rhBMP-2 complications," "OP-1 complications"

Quality of the evidence (best available)
• Level IV: 11

Findings
Complications have been reported with the use of both BMP-2 and OP-1. These have ranged from case reports of heterotopic ossification[139] to increased risk of postoperative swelling.[153] Some have suggested that the use of BMPs should be restricted to patients who are older than 18 years of age and who are not pregnant or expecting to be pregnant in 1 year, based on the supposition that its involvement in growth and development could negatively affect a developing child or fetus.[154] There is no clinical evidence to support the concern in younger patients, and in fact two groups have used BMP-2 in the repair of oral and maxillofacial surgery in at total of 53 patients less than 18 years of age (range 6–14) without short-term complications, other than transient increased swelling of the gums during the first postoperative week.[155,156] With regard to the restrictions in women of childbearing age, there is evidence from in-vitro studies on both mice and humans that BMP-2 expression, through activation of a Wnt4 signaling pathway, is involved in the early development of the fetus and particularly the process of decidualization.[157] BMP-2 has also been shown to be involved in stimulating vascularization of tumors[158,159] as well as preventing apoptosis in breast cancer cells[160] and thus there is a theoretical reason to avoid use in patients with active malignancy or in areas of resected tumor.

Each of the BMPs in clinical use has been associated with the formation of heterotopic bone. Wysocki and Cohen reported on a single case of triceps ossification after application of OP-1 for nonunion of a distal humerus fracture.[161] A similar report of four cases in the upper extremity was reported by Axelrad et al.[139] OP-1 was used in three of the cases, while BMP-2 was involved in one case, and all cases involved the humerus. The radiographic appearance of the heterotopic ossification (HO) indicated that it was following the fascial planes, similar to the plane of surgical dissection. In a series of 23 humeral nonunions treated with OP-1, one patient suffered from development of HO around the shoulder that was reported as painful and restrictive.[137] Boraiah et al. retrospectively reviewed 40 patients treated for tibial plateau fractures.[140] Each patient underwent open reduction and internal fixation with metaphyseal defects treated with freeze-dried fibular allograft supplemented with BMP-2 in a collagen sponge carrier or bone void filler. The relative risk of developing HO was 14 (p < 0.001) in patients treated with BMP-2. Four patients treated with BMP-2 required surgical removal of the HO. Similar findings have been seen in spine surgery, although none of the reported cases have resulted in removal of the new bone or long-term sequelae.[162,163]

The two approved BMPs are members of the TGF-β family, and part of the mechanism of action is through stimulation of the inflammatory process. Crawford et al. reviewed rhBMP-2 use in posterior cervical fusion procedures and found an increased rate of wound complications, although the number only approached significance (p = 0.113).[164] They proposed that this finding was related to a local inflammatory reaction induced by rhBMP-2. It is not surprising that there are several reports of postoperative swelling associated with its use.[155,165–167] Sheilds et al. reported a 18.5% complication rate related to postoperative swelling after ACDF with INFUSE® graft.[165] This included 15 (8.6%) patients with hematoma, 8 of whom required a return to the operating room for evacuation. A similar review of 234 patients found a clinically significant increase in the rate of swelling, with only a 3.6% rate seen in the patients treated with autograft or allograft alone.[167]

Summary of recommendations

• With regards to the use of orthobiologics to stimulate fracture healing, the current evidence does not support treating elderly patients with fractures differently than any other group of patients
• Diabetic patients deserve special attention with regards to management of lower extremity fractures, with particular attention to wound care, peripheral vascular disease, peripheral neuropathy, and renal disease
• The prevalence of endocrine abnormalities, as well as the need to treat these conditions regardless of their effect on bone healing, should alert the treating physician to recognize patients at risk early in the treatment of fractures
• For HIV-infected patients, the available evidence suggests a trend that Gustilo–Anderson type II and III fractures are at an increased risk of infection and possibly nonunion
• Obesity alone is not an indication for the use of an orthobiologic agent
• The physician should counsel patients on smoking cessation and reducing or eliminating other risky behavior such as drug and alcohol abuse, as these interventions will promote the overall health of the patient and will likely decrease the risk of complications in those treated both operatively and nonoperatively
• Use of rhBMP-2 in open fractures can only be recommended in high-energy open tibia fractures treated with nails; there is no data in other long bones or with other modes of fracture stabilization
• Cost analysis supports the use of rhBMP-2 as a potential cost-saving measure in lumbar fusion
• The use of OP-1 as a standard treatment is not warranted at this time

• There is a need for more randomized studies, particularly in the upper extremity, to elucidate the safety and efficacy of OP-1 before expanded use can be recommended.
• In patients at risk for continued nonunion after revision, and when ICBG is not a reasonable option, then the use of either OP-1 or rhBMP-2 can be recommended, in light of the lack of other alternatives

Conclusion

The evidence regarding the use of orthobiologics is slowly evolving. Currently, the expanding use of these products is reflected in an increasing number of case reports and series that evaluate the treatment of nonunions in areas of the body for which the product has not been tested. Long-term follow-up and larger-scale randomized trials will need to be conducted to confirm the safety and efficacy of these procedures, as well as the cost benefits when compared to current practice standards.

References

1. Jackson M, Learmonth ID. The treatment of nonunion after intracapsular fracture of the proximal femur. Clin Orthop Relat Res 2002;339;119–28.
2. Bedi A, Toan LT. Subtrochanteric femur fractures. Orthop Clin North Am 2004;35:473–483.
3. Freedman DM, Botte MJ, Gelberman RH. Vascularity of the carpus. Clin Orthop Relat Res 2001;394:47–59.
4. Brinker MR, Bailey DE, Jr. Fracture healing in tibia fractures with an associated vascular injury. J Trauma 1997; 42:11–19.
5. Dickson K, Katzman S, Delgado E, et al. Delayed unions and nonunions of open tibial fractures. Correlation with arteriography results. Clin Orthop Relat Res 1994;302:189–93.
6. Graves ML, Ryan JE, Mast JW. Supracondylar femur nonunion associated with previous vascular repair: importance of vascular exam in preoperative planning of nonunion repair. J Orthop Trauma 2005;19:574–7.
7. Pretre R, Peter RE, Kursteiner K. Limb revascularization to stimulate bone fracture healing. Am Surg 1997;63:836–8.
8. Borrelli J, Jr., Prickett W, Song E, et al. Extraosseous blood supply of the tibia and the effects of different plating techniques: a human cadaveric study. J Orthop Trauma 2002;16:691–5.
9. Rhinelander FW. Tibial blood supply in relation to fracture healing. Clin Orthop Relat Res 1974;105:34–81.
10. Smith JW, Arnoczky SP, Hersh A. The intraosseous blood supply of the fifth metatarsal: implications for proximal fracture healing. Foot Ankle 1992;13:143–52.
11. Jones DB, Jr., Burger H, Bishop AT, et al. Treatment of scaphoid waist nonunions with an avascular proximal pole and carpal collapse. A comparison of two vascularized bone grafts. J Bone Joint Surg Am 2008;90:2616–25.

12. Woolf AD, Pfleger B. Burden of major musculoskeletal conditions. Bull World Health Organ 2003;81:646–56.

13. Donaldson LJ, Reckless IP, Scholes S, et al. The epidemiology of fractures in England. J Epidemiol Community Health 2008; 62:174–80.

14. Kannus P, Niemi S, Parkkari J, et al. Nationwide decline in incidence of hip fracture. J Bone Miner Res 2006;21:1836–8.

15. Lonnroos E, Kautiainen H, Karppi P, et al. Increased incidence of hip fractures. A population based-study in Finland. Bone 2006;39:623–7.

16. Leslie WD, O'Donnell S, Jean S, et al. Trends in hip fracture rates in Canada. JAMA 2009;302:883–9.

17. Kannus P, Niemi S, Palvanen M, et al. Rising incidence of low-trauma fractures of the calcaneus and foot among Finnish older adults. J Gerontol A Biol Sci Med Sci 2008; 63:642–5.

18. Kannus P, Palvanen M, Niemi S, et al. Rate of proximal humeral fractures in older Finnish women between 1970 and 2007. Bone 2009;44:656–9.

19. Icks A, Haastert B, Wildner M, et al. Trend of hip fracture incidence in Germany 1995–2004: a population-based study. Osteoporos Int 2008;19:1139–45.

20. Kannus P, Palvanen M, Niemi S, et al. Stabilizing incidence of low-trauma ankle fractures in elderly people Finnish statistics in 1970–2006 and prediction for the future. Bone 2008;43: 340–2.

21. Islam S, Liu Q, Chines A, et al. Trend in incidence of osteoporosis-related fractures among 40- to 69-year-old women: analysis of a large insurance claims database, 2000–2005. Menopause 2009;16:77–83.

22. Martin BI, Turner JA, Mirza SK, et al. Trends in health care expenditures, utilization, and health status among US adults with spine problems, 1997–2006. Spine 2009;34:2077–84.

23. Cahill KS, Chi JH, Day A, et al. Prevalence, complications, and hospital charges associated with use of bone-morphogenetic proteins in spinal fusion procedures. JAMA 2009;302:58–66.

24. Glassman SD, Polly DW, Bono CM, et al. Outcome of lumbar arthrodesis in patients sixty-five years of age or older. J Bone Joint Surg Am 2009;91:783–90.

25. Fernyhough JC, Schimandle JJ, Weigel MC, et al. Chronic donor site pain complicating bone graft harvesting from the posterior iliac crest for spinal fusion. Spine 1992;17:1474–80.

26. Banwart JC, Asher MA, Hassanein RS. Iliac crest bone graft harvest donor site morbidity. A statistical evaluation. Spine 1995;20:1055–60.

27. Raheja LF, Genetos DC, Yellowley CE. Hypoxic osteocytes recruit human MSCs through an OPN/CD44-mediated pathway. Biochem Biophys Res Commun 2008;366:1061–6.

28. Lu C, Hansen E, Sapozhnikova A, et al. Effect of age on vascularization during fracture repair. J Orthop Res 2008;26: 1384–9.

29. Street JT, Wang JH, Wu QD, et al. The angiogenic response to skeletal injury is preserved in the elderly. J Orthop Res 2001; 19:1057–66.

30. Thum T, Hoeber S, Froese S, et al. Age-dependent impairment of endothelial progenitor cells is corrected by growth-hormone-mediated increase of insulin-like growth-factor-1. Circ Res 2007;100:434–43.

31. Zhou S, Greenberger JS, Epperly MW, et al. Age-related intrinsic changes in human bone-marrow-derived mesenchymal stem cells and their differentiation to osteoblasts. Aging Cell 2008;7:335–43.

32. Becerra J, Andrades JA, Ertl DC, et al. Demineralized bone matrix mediates differentiation of bone marrow stromal cells in vitro: effect of age of cell donor. J Bone Miner Res 1996;11: 1703–14.

33. Tsuji T, Hughes FJ, McCulloch CA, et al. Effects of donor age on osteogenic cells of rat bone marrow in vitro. Mech Ageing Dev 1990;51:121–32.

34. Bergman RJ, Gazit D, Kahn AJ, et al. Age-related changes in osteogenic stem cells in mice. J Bone Miner Res 1996;11: 568–77.

35. Kretlow JD, Jin YQ, Liu W, et al. Donor age and cell passage affects differentiation potential of murine bone marrow-derived stem cells. BMC Cell Biol 2008;9:60.

36. Chen TL. Inhibition of growth and differentiation of osteoprogenitors in mouse bone marrow stromal cell cultures by increased donor age and glucocorticoid treatment. Bone 2004; 35:83–95.

37. Bellows CG, Pei W, Jia Y, et al. Proliferation, differentiation and self-renewal of osteoprogenitors in vertebral cell populations from aged and young female rats. Mech Ageing Dev 2003;124: 747–57.

38. Martinez ME, del Campo MT, Medina S, et al. Influence of skeletal site of origin and donor age on osteoblastic cell growth and differentiation. Calcif Tissue Int 1999;64:280–6.

39. Fehrer C, Laschober G, Lepperdinger G. Aging of murine mesenchymal stem cells. Ann N Y Acad Sci 2006;1067:235–42.

40. D'Ippolito G, Schiller PC, Ricordi C, et al. Age-related osteogenic potential of mesenchymal stromal stem cells from human vertebral bone marrow. J Bone Miner Res 1999;14:1115–22.

41. D'Ippolito G, Howard GA, Roos BA, et al. Sustained stromal stem cell self-renewal and osteoblastic differentiation during aging. Rejuvenation Res 2006;9:10–19.

42. D'Ippolito G, Diabira S, Howard GA, et al. Marrow-isolated adult multilineage inducible (MIAMI) cells, a unique population of postnatal young and old human cells with extensive expansion and differentiation potential. J Cell Sci 2004;117: 2971–81.

43. Stolzing A, Jones E, McGonagle D, et al. Age-related changes in human bone marrow-derived mesenchymal stem cells: consequences for cell therapies. Mech Ageing Dev 2008;129: 163–73.

44. Bidula J, Boehm C, Powell K, et al. Osteogenic progenitors in bone marrow aspirates from smokers and nonsmokers. Clin Orthop Relat Res 2006;442:252–9.

45. Vestergaard P, Rejnmark L, Mosekilde L. Diabetes and its complications and their relationship with risk of fractures in type 1 and 2 diabetes. Calcif Tissue Int 2009;84:45–55.

46. Herskind AM, Christensen K, Norgaard-Andersen K, et al. Diabetes mellitus and healing of closed fractures. Diabete Metab 1992;18:63–4.

47. Wukich DK, Kline AJ. The management of ankle fractures in patients with diabetes. J Bone Joint Surg Am 2008;90:1570–8.

48. Loder RT. The influence of diabetes mellitus on the healing of closed fractures. Clin Orthop Relat Res 1988;232:210–16.

49. Alblowi J, Kayal RA, Siqueria M, et al. High levels of tumor necrosis factor-α contribute to accelerated loss of cartilage in diabetic fracture healing. Am J Pathol 2009;175(4):1574–85.

50. Cozen L. Does diabetes delay fracture healing? Clin Orthop Relat Res 1972;82:134–40.

51. Loder RT. The influence of diabetes mellitus on the healing of closed fractures. Clin Orthop Relat Res 1988;232:210–16.

52. Costigan W, Thordarson DB, Debnath UK. Operative management of ankle fractures in patients with diabetes mellitus. Foot Ankle Int 2007;28:32–7.

53. Kidder LS, Chen X, Schmidt AH, et al. Osteogenic protein-1 overcomes inhibition of fracture healing in the diabetic rat: a pilot study. Clin Orthop Relat Res 2009;467(12):3249–56.

54. Azad V, Breitbart E, Al-Zube L, et al. rhBMP-2 enhances the bone healing response in a diabetic rat segmental defect model. J Orthop Trauma 2009; 23:267–76.

55. Brinker MR, O'Connor DP, Monla YT, et al. Metabolic and endocrine abnormalities in patients with nonunions. J Orthop Trauma 2007; 21:557–70.

56. Lucas JA, Bolland MJ, Grey AB, et al. Determinants of vitamin D status in older women living in a subtropical climate. Osteoporos Int 2005; 16:1641–8.

57. Bolland MJ, Grey AB, Ames RW, et al. Determinants of vitamin D status in older men living in a subtropical climate. Osteoporos Int 2006;17:1742–8.

58. van der Wielen RP, Lowik MR, van den BH, et al. Serum vitamin D concentrations among elderly people in Europe. Lancet 1995;346:207–10.

59. Doetsch AM, Faber J, Lynnerup N, et al. The effect of calcium and vitamin D3 supplementation on the healing of the proximal humerus fracture: a randomized placebo-controlled study. Calcif Tissue Int 2004;75:183–8.

60. Amiel C, Ostertag A, Slama L, et al. BMD is reduced in HIV-infected men irrespective of treatment. J Bone Miner Res 2004;19:402–9.

61. Dolan SE, Huang JS, Killilea KM, et al. Reduced bone density in HIV-infected women. AIDS 2004;18:475–83.

62. Kilmarx PH. Global epidemiology of HIV. Curr Opin HIV AIDS 2009;4:240–6.

63. van GF, de Lind van Wijngaarden JW, Baral S, et al. The global epidemic of HIV infection among men who have sex with men. Curr Opin HIV AIDS 2009;4:300–7.

64. Richardson J, Hill AM, Johnston CJ, et al. Fracture healing in HIV-positive populations. J Bone Joint Surg Br 2008;90:988–94.

65. Paiement GD, Hymes RA, LaDouceur MS, et al. 1994; Postoperative infections in asymptomatic HIV-seropositive orthopedic trauma patients. J Trauma 37:545–50.

66. Norrish AR, Lewis CP, Harrison WJ. Pin-track infection in HIV-positive and HIV-negative patients with open fractures treated by external fixation: a prospective, blinded, case-controlled study. J Bone Joint Surg Br 2007;89:790–3.

67. Harrison WJ, Lewis CP, Lavy CB. 2002; Wound healing after implant surgery in HIV-positive patients. J Bone Joint Surg Br 84:802–6.

68. Harrison WJ, Lewis CP, Lavy CB. Open fractures of the tibia in HIV positive patients: a prospective controlled single-blind study. Injury 2004;35:852–6.

69. Kemper HC, Stasse-Wolthuis M, Bosman W. The prevention and treatment of overweight and obesity. Summary of the advisory report by the Health Council of The Netherlands. Neth J Med 2004;62:10–17.

70. Burkhauser RV, Cawley J, Schmeiser MD. The timing of the rise in U.S. obesity varies with measure of fatness. Econ Hum Biol 2009;7(3):307–18.

71. Tucker MC, Schwappach JR, Leighton RK, et al. Results of femoral intramedullary nailing in patients who are obese versus those who are not obese: a prospective multicenter comparison study. J Orthop Trauma 2007;21:523–9.

72. Jupiter JB, Ring D, Rosen H. The complications and difficulties of management of nonunion in the severely obese. J Orthop Trauma 1995;9:363–70.

73. Abidi NA, Dhawan S, Gruen GS, et al. Wound-healing risk factors after open reduction and internal fixation of calcaneal fractures. Foot Ankle Int 1998;19:856–61.

74. Porter SE, Russell GV, Dews RC, et al. Complications of acetabular fracture surgery in morbidly obese patients. J Orthop Trauma 2008;22:589–94.

75. Levy RS, Hebert CK, Munn BG, et al. Drug and alcohol use in orthopedic trauma patients: a prospective study. J Orthop Trauma 1996;10:21–7.

76. Blake RB, Brinker MR, Ursic CM, et al. Alcohol and drug use in adult patients with musculoskeletal injuries. Am J Orthop 26:1997;704–9.

77. Brainard BJ, Slauterbeck J, Benjamin JB, et al. Injury profiles in pedestrian motor vehicle trauma. Ann Emerg Med 18:1989;881–3.

78. Chakkalakal DA. Alcohol-induced bone loss and deficient bone repair 1. Alcohol Clin Exp Res 2005;29:2077–90.

79. Peng TC, Garner SC, Frye GD, et al. Evidence of a toxic effect of ethanol on bone in rats. Alcohol Clin Exp Res 1982;6:96–9.

80. Hefferan TE, Kennedy AM, Evans GL, et al. Disuse exaggerates the detrimental effects of alcohol on cortical bone. Alcohol Clin Exp Res 2003;27:111–17.

81. Elmali N, Ertem K, Ozen S, et al. Fracture healing and bone mass in rats fed on liquid diet containing ethanol. Alcohol Clin Exp Res 2002;26:509–13.

82. Nyquist F, Halvorsen V, Madsen JE, et al. Ethanol and its effects on fracture healing and bone mass in male rats. Acta Orthop Scand 1999;70:212–16.

83. Kristensson H, Lunden A, Nilsson BE. Fracture incidence and diagnostic roentgen in alcoholics. Acta Orthop Scand 1980;51:205–7.

84. Nyquist F, Berglund M, Nilsson BE, et al. Nature and healing of tibial shaft fractures in alcohol abusers. Alcohol Alcohol 1997;32:91–5.

85. Silverstein P. Smoking and wound healing. Am J Med 1992;93:22–4S.

86. Capen DA, Calderone RR, Green A. Perioperative risk factors for wound infections after lower back fusions. Orthop Clin North Am 1996;27:83–86.

87. Jacobi J, Jang JJ, Sundram U, et al. Nicotine accelerates angiogenesis and wound healing in genetically diabetic mice. Am J Pathol 2002;161:97–104.

88. Zheng LW, Ma L, Cheung LK. Changes in blood perfusion and bone healing induced by nicotine during distraction osteogenesis. Bone 2008;43:355–61.

89. Riebel GD, Boden SD, Whitesides TE, et al. The effect of nicotine on incorporation of cancellous bone graft in an animal model. Spine 1995;20:2198–202.

90. Raikin SM, Landsman JC, Alexander VA, et al. Effect of nicotine on the rate and strength of long bone fracture healing. Clin Orthop Relat Res 1998;353:231–7.

91. Akhter MP, Iwaniec UT, Haynatzki GR, et al. Effects of nicotine on bone mass and strength in aged female rats. J Orthop Res 2003;21:14–19.

92. Iwaniec UT, Fung YK, Akhter MP, et al. Effects of nicotine on bone mass, turnover, and strength in adult female rats. Calcif Tissue Int 2001;68:358–64.

93. Skott M, Andreassen TT, Ulrich-Vinther M, et al. Tobacco extract but not nicotine impairs the mechanical strength of fracture healing in rats. J Orthop Res 2006;24:1472–9.

94. Bidula J, Boehm C, Powell K, et al. Osteogenic progenitors in bone marrow aspirates from smokers and nonsmokers. Clin Orthop Relat Res 2006;442:252–9.

95. Weresh MJ, Hakanson R, Stover MD, et al. Failure of exchange reamed intramedullary nails for ununited femoral shaft fractures. J Orthop Trauma 2000;14:335–8.

96. Veeravagu A, Patil CG, Lad SP, et al. Risk factors for postoperative spinal wound infections after spinal decompression and fusion surgeries. Spine 2009;34:1869–72.

97. Dahl A, Toksvig-Larsen S. No delayed bone healing in Swedish male oral snuffers operated on by the hemicallotasis technique: a cohort study of 175 patients. Acta Orthop 2007;78:791–4.

98. Dahl A, Toksvig-Larsen S. Cigarette smoking delays bone healing: a prospective study of 200 patients operated on by the hemicallotasis technique. Acta Orthop Scand 2004;75:347–51.

99. McKee MD, DiPasquale DJ, Wild LM, et al. The effect of smoking on clinical outcome and complication rates following Ilizarov reconstruction. J Orthop Trauma 2003;17:663–7.

100. Bhandari M, Guyatt G, Tornetta P, III, et al. Randomized trial of reamed and unreamed intramedullary nailing of tibial shaft fractures. J Bone Joint Surg Am 2008;90:2567–78.

101. Hilibrand AS, Fye MA, Emery SE, et al. Impact of smoking on the outcome of anterior cervical arthrodesis with interbody or strut-grafting. J Bone Joint Surg Am 2001;83:668–73.

102. Glassman SD, Anagnost SC, Parker A, et al. The effect of cigarette smoking and smoking cessation on spinal fusion. Spine 2000;25:2608–15.

103. Mok JM, Cloyd JM, Bradford DS, et al. Reoperation after primary fusion for adult spinal deformity: rate, reason, and timing. Spine 2009;34:832–9.

104. Einhorn TA, Majeska RJ, Mohaideen A, et al. A single percutaneous injection of recombinant human bone morphogenetic protein-2 accelerates fracture repair. J Bone Joint Surg Am 2003; 85: 1425–35.

105. Wang EA, Rosen V, D'Alessandro JS, et al. Recombinant human bone morphogenetic protein induces bone formation. Proc Natl Acad Sci U S A 1990;87:2220–4.

106. Sciadini MF, Johnson KD. Evaluation of recombinant human bone morphogenetic protein-2 as a bone-graft substitute in a canine segmental defect model. J Orthop Res 2000;18:289–302.

107. Govender S, Csimma C, Genant HK, et al. Recombinant human bone morphogenetic protein-2 for treatment of open tibial fractures: a prospective, controlled, randomized study of four hundred and fifty patients. J Bone Joint Surg Am 2002;84: 2123–34.

108. Swiontkowski MF, Aro HT, Donell S, et al. Recombinant human bone morphogenetic protein-2 in open tibial fractures. A sub-group analysis of data combined from two prospective randomized studies. J Bone Joint Surg Am 2006;88:1258–65.

109. Aro HT, Govender S, Patel AD, et al. Recombinant human bone morphogenetic protein-2: a randomized trial in open tibial fractures treated with reamed nail fixation. J Bone Joint Surg Am 2011;93:801–8.

110. Jones AL, Bucholz RW, Bosse MJ, et al. Recombinant human BMP-2 and allograft compared with autogenous bone graft for reconstruction of diaphyseal tibial fractures with cortical defects. A randomized, controlled trial. J Bone Joint Surg Am 2006; 88:1431–41.

111. Ekrol I, Hajducka C, Court-Brown, et al. A comparison of RhBMP-7 (OP-1) and autogenous graft for metaphyseal defects after osteotomy of the distal radius. Injury 2008;39(Suppl 2):S73–82.

112. Jensen MC, Brant-Zawadzki MN, Obuchowski N, et al. Magnetic resonance imaging of the lumbar spine in people without back pain. N Engl J Med 1994;331:69–73.

113. Kim DH, Rhim R, Li L, et al. Prospective study of iliac crest bone graft harvest site pain and morbidity. Spine J 2009;9(11): 886–92.

114. Sandhu HS, Kanim LE, Kabo JM, et al. Evaluation of rhBMP-2 with an OPLA carrier in a canine posterolateral (transverse process) spinal fusion model. Spine 1995;20:2669–82.

115. Sandhu HS, Toth JM, Diwan AD, et al. Histologic evaluation of the efficacy of rhBMP-2 compared with autograft bone in sheep spinal anterior interbody fusion. Spine 2002;27:567–75.

116. Abbah SA, Lam CX, Hutmacher DW, et al. Biological performance of a polycaprolactone-based scaffold used as fusion cage device in a large animal model of spinal reconstructive surgery. Biomaterials 2009;30:5086–93.

117. Sandhu HS, Kanim LE, Kabo JM, et al. Effective doses of recombinant human bone morphogenetic protein-2 in experimental spinal fusion. Spine 1996;21:2115–122.

118. Boden SD, Martin GJ, Jr., Morone MA, et al. Posterolateral lumbar intertransverse process spine arthrodesis with recombinant human bone morphogenetic protein 2/hydroxyapatite-tricalcium phosphate after laminectomy in the nonhuman primate. Spine 1999;24:1179–85.

119. Fischgrund JS, James SB, Chabot MC, et al. Augmentation of autograft using rhBMP-2 and different carrier media in the canine spinal fusion model. J Spinal Disord 1997;10:467–72.

120. Boden SD, Kang J, Sandhu H, et al. Use of recombinant human bone morphogenetic protein-2 to achieve posterolateral lumbar spine fusion in humans: a prospective, randomized clinical pilot trial: 2002 Volvo Award in clinical studies. Spine 2002;27: 2662–73.

121. Burkus JK, Sandhu HS, Gornet MF, et al. Use of rhBMP-2 in combination with structural cortical allografts: clinical and radiographic outcomes in anterior lumbar spinal surgery. J Bone Joint Surg Am 2005;87:1205–12.

122. Dawson E, Bae HW, Burkus JK, et al. Recombinant human bone morphogenetic protein-2 on an absorbable collagen sponge with an osteoconductive bulking agent in posterolateral arthrodesis with instrumentation. A prospective randomized trial. J Bone Joint Surg Am 2009;91:1604–13.

123. Suh DY, Boden SD, Louis-Ugbo J, et al. Delivery of recombinant human bone morphogenetic protein-2 using a compression-resistant matrix in posterolateral spine fusion in the rabbit and in the non-human primate. Spine 2002;27:353–60.

124. Dimar JR, Glassman SD, Burkus JK, et al. Clinical and radiographic analysis of an optimized rhBMP-2 formulation as an autograft replacement in posterolateral lumbar spine arthrodesis. J Bone Joint Surg Am 2009;91:1377–86.

125. Carreon LY, Glassman SD, Djurasovic M, et al. RhBMP-2 versus iliac crest bone graft for lumbar spine fusion in patients over 60 years of age: a cost-utility study. Spine 2009;34:238–43.

126. Maeda T, Buchowski JM, Kim YJ, et al. Long adult spinal deformity fusion to the sacrum using rhBMP-2 versus autogenous iliac crest bone graft. Spine 2009;34:2205–12.

127. Acosta FL, Cloyd JM, Aryan HE, et al. Patient satisfaction and radiographic outcomes after lumbar spinal fusion without iliac crest bone graft or transverse process fusion. J Clin Neurosci 2009;16(9):1184–7.

128. Haid RW, Jr., Branch CL, Jr., Alexander JT, et al. Posterior lumbar interbody fusion using recombinant human bone morphogenetic protein type 2 with cylindrical interbody cages. Spine J 2004;4:527–38.

129. Vaccaro AR, Patel T, Fischgrund J, et al. A pilot study evaluating the safety and efficacy of OP-1 Putty (rhBMP-7) as a replacement for iliac crest autograft in posterolateral lumbar arthrodesis for degenerative spondylolisthesis. Spine 2004;29:1885–92.

130. Vaccaro AR, Patel T, Fischgrund J, et al. A 2-year follow-up pilot study evaluating the safety and efficacy of op-1 putty (rhbmp-7) as an adjunct to iliac crest autograft in posterolateral lumbar fusions. Eur Spine J 2005;14:623–9.

131. Vaccaro AR, Lawrence JP, Patel T, et al. The safety and efficacy of OP-1 (rhBMP-7) as a replacement for iliac crest autograft in posterolateral lumbar arthrodesis: a long-term (>4 years) pivotal study. Spine 2008;33:2850–62.

132. Carreon LY, Glassman SD, Djurasovic M, et al. RhBMP-2 versus iliac crest bone graft for lumbar spine fusion in patients over 60 years of age: a cost-utility study. Spine 2009;34:238–43.

133. Onishi T, Ishidou Y, Nagamine T, et al. Distinct and overlapping patterns of localization of bone morphogenetic protein (BMP) family members and a BMP type II receptor during fracture healing in rats. Bone 1998;22:605–12.

134. Kloen P, Di PM, Borens O, et al. BMP signaling components are expressed in human fracture callus. Bone 2003;33:362–71.

135. Friedlaender GE, Perry CR, Cole JD, et al. Osteogenic protein-1 (bone morphogenetic protein-7) in the treatment of tibial nonunions. J Bone Joint Surg Am 2001;83(Suppl 1):S151–8.

136. Giannoudis PV, Kanakaris NK, Dimitriou R, et al. The synergistic effect of autograft and BMP-7 in the treatment of atrophic nonunions. Clin Orthop Relat Res 2009;467(12): 3239–48.

137. Bong MR, Capla EL, Egol KA, et al. Osteogenic protein-1 (bone morphogenic protein-7) combined with various adjuncts in the treatment of humeral diaphyseal nonunions. Bull Hosp Jt Dis 2005;63:20–3.

138. Giannoudis PV, Psarakis S, Kanakaris NK, et al. Biological enhancement of bone healing with Bone Morphogenetic Protein-7 at the clinical setting of pelvic girdle non-unions. Injury 2007;38(Suppl 4), S43–8.

139. Axelrad TW, Steen B, Lowenberg DW, et al. Heterotopic ossification after the use of commercially available recombinant human bone morphogenetic proteins in four patients. J Bone Joint Surg Br 2008;90:1617–22.

140. Boraiah S, Paul O, Hawkes D, et al. Complications of recombinant human BMP-2 for treating complex tibial plateau fractures: a preliminary report. Clin Orthop Relat Res 2009;467(12): 3257–62.

141. Grauer JN, Vaccaro AR, Kato M, et al. Development of a New Zealand white rabbit model of spinal pseudarthrosis repair and evaluation of the potential role of OP-1 to overcome pseudarthrosis. Spine 2004;29:1405–12.

142. Furlan JC, Perrin RG, Govender PV, et al. Use of osteogenic protein-1 in patients at high risk for spinal pseudarthrosis: a prospective cohort study assessing safety, health-related quality of life, and radiographic fusion. Invited submission from the Joint Section on Disorders of the Spine and Peripheral Nerves, March 2007. J Neurosurg Spine 2007;7:486–95.

143. Tillman D. HDE H040004 Letter of Approval. 2008. Department of Health and Human Services, Center for Devices and Radiological Health. 8-4-0009.

144. Boden SD, Kang J, Sandhu H, et al. Use of recombinant human bone morphogenetic protein-2 to achieve posterolateral lumbar spine fusion in humans: a prospective, randomized clinical pilot trial: 2002 Volvo Award in clinical studies. Spine 2002;27:2662–73.

145. Burkus JK, Sandhu HS, Gornet MF, et al. Use of rhBMP-2 in combination with structural cortical allografts: clinical and radiographic outcomes in anterior lumbar spinal surgery. J Bone Joint Surg Am 2005;87:1205–12.

146. HDE H040004 FDA Summary of Safety and Probable Benefit. 2009. Department of Health and Human Services, Center for Devices and Radiological Health. 8-4-0009.

147. San Miguel MT, Vargas E. Drug evaluation and approval process in the European Union. Arthritis Rheum 2006;55:12–14.

148. Schultz DG. P000054 Letter of Approval. 4-30-2004. Department of Health and Human Services, Center for Devices and Radiological Health. 8-4-2009.

149. Schultz DG. P000058 Letter of Approval. 7-2-2002. Department of Health and Human Services, Center for Devices and Radiological Health. 8–4-0009.

150. Schultz DG. P050053 Letter of Approval. 3-9-2007. Department of Health and Human Services, Center for Devices and Radiological Health. 8-4-0009.

151. Schultz DG. HDE H010002 Letter of Approval. 11-17-2001. Department of Health and Human Services, Center for Devices and Radiological Health. 8-4-0009.

152. Schultz DG. HDE H020008 Letter of Approval. 5-7-2004. Department of Health and Human Services, Center for Devices and Radiological Health. 8-4-2009.

153. Shields LB, Raque GH, Glassman SD, et al. Adverse effects associated with high-dose recombinant human bone morphogenetic protein-2 use in anterior cervical spine fusion. Spine 2006;31:542–7.

154. Carter TG, Brar PS, Tolas A, et al. Off-label use of recombinant human bone morphogenetic protein-2 (rhBMP-2) for reconstruction of mandibular bone defects in humans. J Oral Maxillofac Surg 2008; 66:1417–25.

155. Herford AS, Boyne PJ, Rawson R, et al. Bone morphogenetic protein-induced repair of the premaxillary cleft. J Oral Maxillofac Surg 2007;65:2136–41.

156. Chin M, Ng T, Tom WK, et al. Repair of alveolar clefts with recombinant human bone morphogenetic protein (rhBMP-2) in patients with clefts. J Craniofac Surg 2005;16:778–89.

157. Li Q, Kannan A, Wang W, et al. Bone morphogenetic protein 2 functions via a conserved signaling pathway involving Wnt4 to regulate uterine decidualization in the mouse and the human. J Biol Chem 2007;282:31725–32.

158. Langenfeld EM, Bojnowski J, Perone J, et al. Expression of bone morphogenetic proteins in human lung carcinomas. Ann Thorac Surg 2005;80:1028–32.

159. Raida M, Clement JH, Leek RD, et al. Bone morphogenetic protein 2 (BMP-2) and induction of tumor angiogenesis. J Cancer Res Clin Oncol 2005;131:741–50.

160. Raida M, Clement JH, Ameri K, et al. Expression of bone morphogenetic protein 2 in breast cancer cells inhibits hypoxic cell death. Int J Oncol 2005;26:1465–70.

161. Wysocki RW, Cohen MS. Ectopic ossification of the triceps muscle after application of bone morphogenetic protein-7 to the distal humerus for recalcitrant nonunion: a case report. J Hand Surg Am 2007;32:647–50.

162. Joseph V, Rampersaud YR. Heterotopic bone formation with the use of rhBMP2 in posterior minimal access interbody fusion: a CT analysis. Spine 2007;32:2885–90.

163. Brower RS, Vickroy NM. A case of psoas ossification from the use of BMP-2 for posterolateral fusion at L4-L5. Spine 2008;33: E653–5.

164. Crawford CH, III, Carreon LY, McGinnis MD, et al. Perioperative complications of recombinant human bone morphogenetic protein-2 on an absorbable collagen sponge versus iliac crest bone graft for posterior cervical arthrodesis. Spine 2009;34: 1390–4.

165. Shields LB, Raque GH, Glassman SD, et al. Adverse effects associated with high-dose recombinant human bone morphogenetic protein-2 use in anterior cervical spine fusion. Spine 2006;31:542–7.

166. Vaidya R, Carp J, Sethi A, et al. Complications of anterior cervical discectomy and fusion using recombinant human bone morphogenetic protein-2. Eur Spine J 2007;16:1257–65.

167. Smucker JD, Rhee JM, Singh K, et al. Increased swelling complications associated with off-label usage of rhBMP-2 in the anterior cervical spine. Spine 2006;31:2813–19.

Joint Reconstruction

14 The Role of Computer Navigation in Total Hip Arthroplasty

Jonathan M. Loughead[1] and Richard W. McCalden[2]

[1]Queen Elizabeth Hospital, Gateshead, UK
[2]London Health Sciences Centre, London, ON, Canada

Case scenario

A 54 year old woman, who works as an accountant and is normally active and independent, complains of increasing pain in her right groin. She can no longer play golf, and is having difficulty sleeping. Radiographs show significant loss of joint space as a result of osteoarthritis, and she has restricted flexion and internal rotation of her hip. She has made the decision, alongside her surgeon, to proceed with total hip arthroplasty.

Relevant anatomy

Alignment of total hip arthroplasty is important to reduce the risk of dislocation of the implant, and also to minimize edge loading and accelerated wear of the bearing surfaces. This chapter focuses on the role of navigated surgery to improve the alignment of hip arthroplasty or hip resurfacing. The orientation of the acetabulum is best described in operative terms as *inclination* in the coronal plane (rotation around the AP or sagittal axis), and *anteversion* (rotation around the transverse axis).

Importance of the problem

A large number of total hip replacements (THR) are performed annually in many developed countries. In Canada (2006–2007)[1] 24,000 were performed, and data in the from the UK joint registry recorded 71,000 THRs in 2008.[2] There is a trend towards increasing number of both primary and revision THRs. Extrapolation of data from the USA suggests that number of primary THRs will increase from 202,500 in 2003 to at least 572,000 by 2030.[3] This increase in numbers of THRs is the result of a trend for operating on younger patients earlier in the disease, population expansion, and ageing of the population. In the UK the percentage of the population over the age of 65 years is increasing from 16% in 2008 to a projected 23% by 2033.[4] In the USA in 2004 there were 36.3 million people aged over 65, and by 2050 this figure is projected to reach 86.7 million.[5]

Dislocation

Orientation of THR, in particular of the acetabular component, correlates with the risk of dislocation. Original work by Lewinnek et al.[6] demonstrated a "safe zone" where the acetabular component could be inserted with a lower risk of dislocation. This zone was 40° abduction ±10° and 15° anteversion ±10°. Subsequent work supports a lower angle of abduction, resulting in a lower rate of dislocation.[7] Dislocation following total hip replacement varies widely between publications but in most series is between 1–3%. Data from the New Zealand joint registry highlights dislocation as the most common reason for revision THR between 1999 and 2006.[8]

Wear

In addition to the increased risk of dislocation with poor acetabular component orientation, considerable evidence exists for an increase in wear of the joint surfaces and osteolysis. A number of studies have demonstrated lower polyethylene wear rates when the abduction angle is less than 45°.[9–11] Additionally, a higher cup inclination angle has been associated with pelvic osteolysis.[7,12] As we move towards alternative bearing surfaces the same trend for greater wear (as measured by metal ion concentration) has

Evidence-Based Orthopedics, First Edition. Edited by Mohit Bhandari.
© 2012 Blackwell Publishing Ltd. Published 2012 by Blackwell Publishing Ltd.

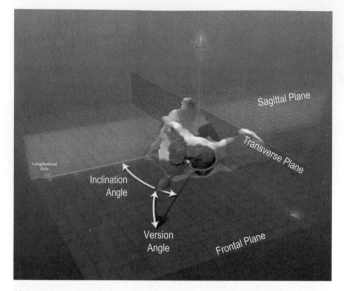

Figure 14.1 Acetabular inclination and anteversion (operative).

been demonstrated with a higher abduction angle,[13,14] and in one study by a higher anteversion angle.[14] Since significant osteolysis may lead to revision, acetabular orientation can be correlated with a clinical outcome.

Defining acetabular component position

A multitude of terms are used to describe acetabular orientation, with inclination and anteversion being the most widely accepted (Figure 14.1). The orientation relates to the acetabular axis, which is perpendicular to the plane of the socket face. Most of the literature on acetabular orientation relates to measurements taken from a supine AP pelvic radiograph, but this measurement may differ to the position at the time of surgery when the pelvis may lie in a different plane, or the functional position when the patient is mobile.

When using navigation or CT, the orientation of the acetabulum is referenced to the anterior pelvic plane (the plane subtended by the pubic tubercles and the anterior superior iliac spines). It is important to note that this may not always be aligned with the coronal plane, and will therefore affect the measured anteversion of the cup.[15] Additionally, if CT is used to measure component position then it may be based on the anatomic definition of anteversion and inclination as described by Murray,[16] or it may use the radiographic definition. Using the anatomic definition of cup orientation will increase the measured inclination and anteversion.

As measured cup position on CT scan references off the anterior pelvic plane (APP), this correlates well with Lewineek's work as he attempted to standardize radiographs using a tripod level externally applied to the APP. Since conventional radiographs are normally aligned with

the coronal plane rather than the APP, any degree of pelvic tilt will affect the measurements taken on the AP radiograph. If the radiograph is centered on the pubic symphysis, rather than the hip, the anteversion is affected by divergence of the x-ray beam. Additionally, some investigators[14] have used standing AP pelvic radiographs (which will alter pelvic tilt compared to supine films), arguing that this represents a more functional position. The vast difference in terminology and radiographic techniques in determining acetabular component position is problematic and certainly confounds comparison between studies.

An extremely large body of information on hip surgery and navigation is available to surgeons and the general public over the internet: a Google search returns more than 489,000 hits when the search terms "navigation" and "hip surgery" are entered. The variability in quality of the available information necessitates reference to good-quality, evidence-based literature.

Top five questions

1. Does navigation improve component alignment following hip arthroplasty?
2. Which type of navigation should be used and how should the patient be positioned?
3. When should navigation be used?
4. Does navigation improve alignment in hip resurfacing?
5. Does navigation improve clinical outcomes following THR?

Question 1: Does navigation improve component alignment following hip arthroplasty?

Case clarification
The patient and surgeon in question are anxious to avoid complications following elective THR irrespective of time or costs involved. Would the use of navigation reduce the likelihood of poor alignment?

Relevance
If the acetabular component is poorly aligned then the patient may be predisposed to a higher risk of dislocation or increased wear.

Current opinion
Hip navigation is likely to reduce the number of cups placed at the extremes of alignment compared to conventional surgery.

Finding the evidence
• Cochrane Database: under the search terms "hip AND navigation OR computer"

- PubMed (www.ncbi.nlm.nih.gov/pubmed/) clinical queries search/systematic reviews: hip AND navigation OR computer
- MEDLINE search identifying the intervention (hip arthroplasty or hip replacement or hip resurfacing). We used the keywords "computer assisted" OR "navigation"
- The search was focused to exclude papers not directly related to alignment of hip replacement

Quality of the evidence

Level I
- 1 meta-analysis
- 3 randomized trials

Level II
- 1 randomized trials with methodologic limitations

Level III
- 4 case control studies

Level IV
- 3 case series

Findings

The articles from our search were narrowed down to those with the best quality of evidence. The main focus of concern is acetabular orientation, since this is technically the most error-prone step in THR. No Cochrane reviews were identified, but a single meta-analysis and three randomized con-

trolled trials (RCTs) exist. Additionally, there are four comparative series. The best evidence is summarized in Table 14.1. The remainder of the studies were either case series or based on model or cadaveric work and therefore represented a lower quality of evidence. We included all techniques of hip navigation (CT based, fluoroscopic, and imageless), and all hip approaches.

Evaluation of the final component position was performed using CT scan in the studies by Kalteiss et al.[18] and Parratte et al.[19] In contrast, the study by Leenders et al.[20] used standing AP pelvic radiographs centered on the pubic symphysis and only measured cup inclination, not cup anteversion. However, since cup inclination can be more reliably measured and the same technique was used in both groups, the results of their study are noteworthy. It should be remembered that measured cup anteversion on plain radiograph is affected by pelvic tilt and rotation and is more difficult to assess accurately. There is consistent reduction in outliers (as defined by Leewineek et al.[6]) using either CT or imageless navigation. Since we are interested in avoiding cups placed outside the "safe zone," this would appear to be more valid than looking at the mean cup inclination and anteversion. All of the studies have analyzed either variance of the measured values from the safe zone or absolute numbers outside the safe zone. The study by Leenders et al.[4] included three cohorts of patients, the first of which was performed freehand, while the subsequent two were randomized to either freehand

Table 14.1 Best evidence comparing hip navigation with free hand

Author	Type of study	Technique	N navigated	N control	Results	P value
Gandhi et al.[17]	Meta-analysis (3 studies)	?various	140	110	Odds ratio 0.285	<0.001
Kalteiss et al.[18]	RCT	CT/imageless/control	30 + 30	30	Outliers 53% vs. 17% (CT) vs. 7% (imageless)[a]	<0.001 vs. control
Leenders et al.[20]	RCT	CT/control	50	50	Reduction in outliers/reduced SD	NS
Parratte et al.[19]	RCT	Imageless/control	30	30	57% outliers vs. 20%	<0.002 χ^2 of outliers
Lazovic et al.[21]	Comparative series	Imageless/control	127	110	Outliers 2.7% vs. 0.8% (inclination) and 7.3% vs. 2.4% anteversion	Not given
Sugano et al.[22]	Comparative series	CT/control	59	111	Outliers 28% vs. 0%	<0.0001
Haaker et al.[23]	Comparative series	Imageless/control	98	69	Outliers (aneteversion) 28% vs. 7%	<0.0001
Najarian et al.[24]	Comparative series	Imageless/control	50 + 50	55	NS difference between control and 1st cohort nav. P = 0.025 between control and 2nd cohort	= 0.025

NS, not significant.

[a] P = 0.067 CT-based vs. imageless.

Table 14.2 Additional randomized controlled trial (Reproduced with kind permission from Springer Science+Business Media: Babisch J, Layher F, Sander K. Chapter 44: Imageless cup and stem navigation in dysplastic hips with the navitrack and vector vision systems.pp.344–51. Navigation and MIS in Orthopaedic Surgery: Springer Heidelberg 2007.)

	N cases	Outliers—inclination[a]	Outliers—anteversion	Dislocations	10° liner used
Freehand	37 (2 missing CT)	6	2	1	6
Navigated	37 (12 missing CT)	0	1	0	1

[a] >10° from optimum position.

technique or navigation. There was a reduction in outliers comparing groups 2 and 3, which did not reach statistical significance, while both groups 2 and 3 were significantly better than the first cohort.

An additional clinical study is that by Babisch et al.[25] Although this was a randomized trial of imageless navigation vs. control, unfortunately its quality is significantly reduced by having follow-up CT data for only 60 of the 74 patients. The results of this study are summarized in Table 14.2.

Once again this study shows a reduction in outliers in the navigated group, and additionally a lower use of lipped liners. Numerous other studies have validated the use of other navigation systems by performing a series of cases followed by postoperative CT, while a number of laboratory-based studies compare cup position with navigation and freehand methods. Almost universally these studies demonstrate improved alignment with the navigation. It is worthwhile mentioning some of the earliest work performed by DiGioia et al.[26] who demonstrated orientation outside the safe zone in 59 of 74 cups aligned using a conventional mechanical guide, using a CT-based navigation system as the control.

In summary, by reducing the number of outliers, navigation does appear to improve acetabular component position following THR. However, it is worth considering two further issues. First, although the studies demonstrate improved positioning of the cup (placed where the surgeon had planned), given our concerns about pelvic tilt and the change in orientation of the acetabulum in a functional position (standing, walking, etc.), we may be no further forward in placing the cup in the ideal position for each patient; secondly, radiographically measured alignment is a surrogate measure of success, but it remains unclear whether this leads to an improvement in clinical outcomes (discussed in Question 5).

Furthermore, since positioning the cup in a predetermined position may not be ideal for all patients, perhaps navigation should be used to assess the range of movement with cup and stem in situ, look for impingement, and confirm restoration of leg length and offset.[21,27–29]

Recommendation

For patients undergoing THR, evidence suggests:
• Navigation reduces the number of acetabular components placed outside the "safe zone" [overall quality: moderate]

Question 2: Which type of navigation should be used and how should the patient be positioned?

Case clarification

Having decided to proceed with a navigated hip replacement, the surgeon wants to establish what is the best position to have the patient in to optimize the navigation, and which navigation technique to employ. The surgeon normally operates with the patient in the lateral decubitus position.

Relevance

Changing the technique which a surgeon normally employs for THR may increase complications in the learning curve. There are three different navigation techniques which are widely available.

Current opinion

Hip navigation must be performed with the patient supine and is most accurate using a CT-based system.

Finding the evidence

The best-quality studies identified for question 1 were re-evaluated. Additionally, further Level IV evidence was evaluated:
• 8 case series

Findings

Navigation concepts Hip navigation systems have evolved from the early systems which were based on a preoperative CT scan which is then mapped into the navigation software to create a virtual pelvis. During the surgery a solid reference array must be placed in the ilium, and then, using a pointer imaged with an infrared camera, key points on the

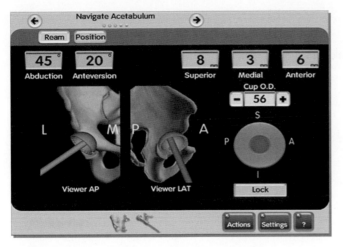

Figure 14.2 Use of navigation for component positioning.

pelvis are acquired. Eventually, through acquisition of sufficient points the navigation system software is able to correlate the pelvis mapped out on the surgery table with the virtual pelvis. The representation of the pelvis then appears animated on a screen, and with an array attached to the surgical instruments, the acetabular component can be reamed and seated (Figure 14.2). Greatest accuracy is obtained if the points acquired closely match the virtual pelvis and the points are obtained at maximum separation. Conventionally the frontal plane of the pelvis is therefore acquired together with additional points around the acetabulum.

In contrast, imageless systems do not require the use of specialized preoperative imaging or the use of ionizing radiation during the surgery. This system uses the same technique of acquiring bony landmarks from the frontal plane of the pelvis and the acetabulum, but does not match this to the patient's previously imaged virtual pelvis. Instead, fluoroscopic systems utilize calibrated image intensifier images obtained at the time of surgery to digitize bony landmarks around the pelvis, and otherwise acquire points within the surgical field in a similar fashion to an imageless system.

Patient position Crucial to almost all of the systems in use is to accurately map out the frontal plane of the pelvis. This involves acquiring points from the contralateral side to the surgical site; in particular, the contralateral anterior superior iliac spine (ASIS) and pubic tubercle must be acquired. This is difficult to do with the patient in the lateral decubitus position. The most straightforward solution is to perform the surgery with the patient supine, and include the contralateral pelvis in the surgical field. The added advantage of the supine position is that it can control pelvic tilt and pelvic rotation to some extent, and may therefore facilitate acetabular positioning even without navigation.

With increasing frequency, however, THR is performed in the lateral decubitus position. In particular, the posterior approach cannot be performed with the patient supine, which arguably may preclude the use of navigation. In response a number of techniques have evolved to allow acquisition of the frontal plane of the pelvis while operating on the patient in the lateral position. The simplest of these involves setting the patient up in the lateral position, performing surgery in a conventional manner and using fluoroscopy to acquire the pubic tubercles and contralateral ASIS. This technique has been employed by a number of surgeons.[30–34] Alternatively, the patient can be placed supine, have the reference array placed on the ipsilateral ilium percutaneously and remote to the surgical field, following which acquisition of the frontal plane is performed before final positioning and aseptic preparation of the patient. In future, it may be possible to use navigation without acquiring the frontal plane of the pelvis, and rather to utilize more points around the acetabulum and the transverse acetabular ligament.

Evidence for the techniques The best clinical studies identified (one meta-analysis, three randomized controlled trials, and four comparative series) have been stratified by the technique employed and the patient position (Table 14.3).

While all of the RCTs have positioned the patient supine and employed a lateral or anterolateral approach, there is supportive evidence for the CT-based and the imageless systems, although the imageless system in fact performs better. Two of the studies clearly specify the patient is positioned laterally and have used the posterior approach. Once again the findings are supportive of positioning the patient laterally and using either technique, although only the second cohort of patients having navigation in the series by Najarian et al. was significantly better than the historical controls.[24] Interestingly, Najarian et al. registered the contralateral ASIS having already positioned the patient in the lateral decubitus position, and it may be that this limits the accuracy of the system, particularly in obese patients. Additional support for the use of the lateral position with navigation is available from validated case series.[35–37]

None of the above studies used fluoroscopy, although this technique has been successfully employed by other authors,[30–34] and lends itself to registration of the contralateral pelvis when the patient is in the lateral position.

Summary
Good-quality evidence exists for the use of either CT-based or imageless navigation systems. Although the quality of evidence supporting the use of fluoroscopy is poorer there are still a number of case series of its use, and validation with postoperative CT.

Table 14.3 Evidence for navigation by patient position and approach

Study	Number of cases	Technique	Patient position	Surgical approach	Results	P value
Kalteiss et al.[18]	30 + 30	CT/imageless	Supine	Lateral	Outliers 53% vs. 17% (CT) vs. 7% (imageless)[a]	<0.001 vs. control
Leenders et al.[20]	50	CT	Supine	Anterolateral	Reduction in outliers/ reduced SD	NS
Parratte et al.[19]	30	Imageless	Supine	Anterolateral	57% outliers vs. 20%	<0.002
Lazovic et al.[21]	127	Imageless	Supine	Lateral (Hardinge)	Outliers 2.7% vs. 0.8% (inclination) and 7.3% vs. 2.4% anteversion	Not given
Sugano et al.[22]	59	CT	Lateral decubitus	Posterior	Outliers 28% vs. 0%	<0.0001
Haaker et al.[23]	98	CT	Not specified	Anterolateral	Outliers (anteversion) 28% vs. 7%	<0.0001
Najarian et al.[24]	50 + 50	Imageless	Lateral	MIS posterior	NS difference between control and 1st cohort nav. P = 0.025 between control and 2nd cohort	= 0.025

[a] P = 0.067 CT-based vs. imageless.

Clearly not all departments will readily have access to CT which can be transferred onto a navigation platform, and there is an issue about the use of ionizing radiation if it can be avoided. The imageless technique has the advantage that minimal additional equipment is required, and it is likely to appeal to those who are familiar with its use for knee replacement surgery. The system is most accurate if data is acquired with the patient supine or semilateral before final positioning. However, this will prolong surgery and for those who prefer to operate with the patient in the lateral position the option exists to utilize fluoroscopy to acquire the frontal plane of the pelvis.

Recommendation

For patients undergoing navigated THR, evidence suggests:
• CT based and imageless systems appear equally effective [overall quality: very low]

Question 3: When should navigation be used?

Case clarification

Having used the navigation system successfully for his first case, the surgeon is unsure whether he should incorporate navigation into all his cases or whether it should be used only in specific cases.

Relevance

Introducing navigation for THR will increase operative time and costs. As complication rates following THR are low, introducing it for all cases may not be cost-effective.

Current opinion

Hip navigation is time consuming and the benefit in introducing it for all patients would be marginal.

Finding the evidence

• Cochrane Database: under the search terms "hip AND navigation OR computer"
• PubMed (www.ncbi.nlm.nih.gov/pubmed/) clinical queries search/ systematic reviews: hip AND navigation OR computer
• MEDLINE search identifying the intervention (Hip arthroplasty OR hip replacement OR hip resurfacing. We used the keywords "computer assisted" OR "navigation"
• Search results were focused to evaluate clinical case series and clinical trials for length of surgery, and use of navigation in complex cases and minimally invasive surgery

Quality of the evidence

Level I
• 2 randomized trials

Level II
• 1 randomized trial with methodologic limitations

Level III
• 3 case control study

Level IV
- 4 case series

Level V
- 1 "bench" study
- 1 expert opinion

Findings

If navigation is to be used for all patients undergoing THR then one of the potential concerns is the surgical time. Studies that have compared surgery time with navigation and control are shown in Table 14.4. All studies demonstrate an increase in surgery time (ranging from 7 to 58 minutes per case), although one study comments on lengthy computing time which added to the length of the procedure.[22] The study by Leenders et al.[20] comments on an additional preoperative CT planning time of 20 minutes. Three studies document blood loss in navigated and conventional THR with no difference seen.[18,22,24]

Complex cases As a result of the increased surgical time with the use of hip navigation, it is arguably not a viable option for all cases; however, perhaps it has a role in more complex cases. The prospective randomized trial by Babisch et al.[25] employed navigation or control in a total of 74 patients with congenital hip dysplasia (CDH) (see Table 14.2). Although limited by not all patients having undergone postoperative CT to evaluate cup position, this study shows a considerable improvement in cup position, need for 10° lipped liner, and also more accurate restoration of planned leg length. There are other reports of the use of navigation in dysplasia by Jingushi[38] (imageless) and Ohashi[39] (CT-based). Where substantial deformity exists preoperatively, then logically a CT-based planning and subsequent navigation as described by Ohashi[39] would seem to have clinical merit.

Table 14.4 Operative time

Study	Study design	Increase in surgical time with navigation vs. control (mean)
Kalteiss et al.[18]	RCT	Imageless 7 min CT 17 min
Parratte et al.[19]	RCT	12 min
Lazovic et al.[21]	Comparative series	11 min
Sugano et al.[22]	Comparative series	58 min[a]
Najarian et al.[24]	Comparative series	23 mins (19 min in 2nd cohort)

[a] Authors comment on lengthy computing time.

In addition, navigation could also be considered for revision cases (where the anatomy of the acetabulum will be distorted) where reference could still be made to the anterior pelvic plane, perhaps leading to a decreased risk of dislocation, a problem more common in revision surgery.

Training Hip navigation could be used in the training of orthopedic residents. This may facilitate the transition from the resident relying on the consultant to make the decision about direction of reaming and final cup position, to learning to adjust the cup position independently with the use of the navigation feedback. From work done by Gofton et al.[40] there is evidence that hip navigation can improve accuracy of cup placement in early training and that this knowledge can be retained following delayed retesting without the navigation software.

Minimally invasive surgery Where a surgeon wishes to perform THR using a minimal approach and where the potential for incomplete visualization of the normal anatomic landmarks exists,[41] then navigation may well have a role in aligning not only the acetabulum but also the femur. The study by Najarian et al.[24] employs a minimally invasive single-incision posterior approach in both groups, and navigation has been reported by other proponents of minimally invasive hip surgery.[42–44]

Cost-effectiveness The main aim of using hip navigation is to reduce revision rates following surgery from recurrent dislocation or accelerated wear. Dislocation can result in considerable excess cost with multiple trips to the operating room for reduction of the hip, and then a subsequent revision surgical procedure.

Without good evidence clearly showing a reduction in the risk of dislocation with navigation, it is difficult to estimate the healthcare cost benefits. In order to be cost-effective, the additional equipment and running cost of the navigation, allied to the extended procedure time, would need to be counterbalanced by a saving in terms of revision surgery required. This calculation has been performed by Slover et al.[45] for the use of navigation in knee surgery. They have estimated that in larger centers, if a 2–2.5% reduction in annual revision rate was achieved with navigation, then over a 20 year period, computer navigation would be cost-effective. Unfortunately, even in total knee replacement (TKR), where navigation has been used for some time, sufficient data on relative risk of revision surgery for navigated and non-navigated TKR does not exist. Data from large joint registries may be necessary to demonstrate any true benefit to navigation.

Recommendations

For patients undergoing THR, evidence suggests:
- Operative surgical time is increased with the use of navigation [overall quality: moderate]

- Blood loss is equal with or without navigation [overall quality: very low]

Question 4: Does navigation improve alignment in hip resurfacing?

Case clarification

The patient and surgeon in question decide to proceed with hip resurfacing. This surgeon has performed limited numbers of this procedure and is anxious to reduce the error in placement of the femoral component. Would the use of navigation reduce the likelihood of misplacement of the femoral component?

Relevance

Both mechanical jigs and navigation are in use for guide wire placement in the femoral neck during hip resurfacing; there is no consensus amongst surgeons on the best technique.

Current opinion

Hip navigation could readily be applied to directing the guide wire for hip resurfacing, thus reducing the risk of notching, oversizing the femoral component, or malposition of the femoral component (excessive varus or valgus).

Finding the evidence

- Cochrane Database: under the search terms "hip AND navigation OR computer"
- PubMed (www.ncbi.nlm.nih.gov/pubmed/) clinical queries search/ systematic reviews: hip AND navigation OR computer
- MEDLINE search identifying the intervention (hip arthroplasty OR hip replacement OR hip resurfacing.

We used the keywords "computer assisted" OR "navigation"
- The search focused to include only papers relating to the use of navigation in hip resurfacing

Quality of the evidence

Level III
- 5 case control studies

Level IV
- 3 case series

Level V
- 4 "bench" studies

Findings

Hip resurfacing is gaining increasing popularity as an alternative to THR, but it is a technically demanding procedure to learn. In particular, acetabular exposure can be difficult as a result of the femoral head being left in situ, and, additionally, it requires careful placement of the femoral component in slight valgus to reduce the risk of femoral neck fracture while avoiding notching of the superior tension cortex. Upsizing of the femoral component reduces the likelihood of the above complications but may result in removal of more acetabular bone. Since resurfacing of the femoral head is technically demanding, and is a newer technique, it lends itself to computer navigation. Studies which have compared the use of navigation and freehand placement of the femoral guide pin are summarized in Table 14.5.

The larger series published by Ganapathi et al.[48] and Resubal et al.[49] show a significant improvement in guide

Table 14.5 Use of navigation in femoral head resurfacing

Author	Type of study	N navigated	N control	Results	P value	Additional time with navigation
Schnurr et al.[46]	Retrospective comparison	30	30	NS neck shaft angle, 3 cases <130 in conventional group		15 min
Kruger et al.[47]	Retrospective comparison	9	9	NS diff		0
Ganapathi et al.[48]	Retrospective comparison	51	88	38% 5° off planned stem shaft angle in control vs. 0%. 4 notches in control vs. 0.	<0.0001	6 min
Resubal et al.[49]	Retrospective comparison	45	131	24% outliers for SSA vs. 0 3 notches vs. 0.	0.001	n/a
Seyler et al.[50]	Retrospective comparison	47	49	Outliers of SSA reduced using navigation, NS difference in notching	n/a	n/a

NS, not significant; SSA, stem–shaft angle.

pin placement with the use of imageless navigation. The work by Seyler et al.[50] is limited by the fact that the planned preoperative stem–shaft angle (SSA) for the mechanical jig group was not recorded, and they were therefore unable to analyze variability in planned and achieved SSA for the conventional group. Their results did, however, graphically show a reduction in spread of SSA with the use of navigation and additionally acceptable results achieved by residents in training.

A number of studies[51–54] have performed comparison between mechanical techniques and navigated techniques (either imageless or CT-based), performed either on cadavers or CT-based models. They have universally shown an improvement in alignment with navigation compared to control. Additionally there are three good-quality case series in the literature demonstrating good results for imageless navigation in resurfacing: Olsen et al.[55] (100 cases), Bailey et al.[56] (37 cases), and Romanowski et al.[57] (71 cases).

Of note, there is no large prospective randomized trial to answer this question, although this seems highly justified as both conventional and computer-navigated techniques are currently being used. On the basis of the weaker evidence above, there appears to be an improvement in alignment in the coronal plane with the use of imageless navigation, associated with an increase in time for the procedure of between 0 and 15 minutes.

Recommendation

For patients undergoing hip resurfacing:
• Navigation improves the accuracy of femoral component position [overall quality: low]

Question 5: Does navigation improve clinical outcomes following THR?

Case clarification

The surgeon has been convinced of the evidence for improved alignment using hip navigation, but he wishes to know if there is any objective evidence of improved clinical outcomes with the use of navigation.

Relevance

Objectively reported improvements in clinical outcomes are the gold standard by which any new technique should be evaluated.

Current opinion

There is no clinical evidence of improved outcome with the use of navigation for total hip replacement.

Finding the evidence

• Cochrane Database: under the search terms "hip AND navigation OR computer"

• PubMed (www.ncbi.nlm.nih.gov/pubmed/) clinical queries search/systematic reviews: hip AND navigation OR computer
• MEDLINE search identifying the intervention (hip arthroplasty OR hip replacement OR hip resurfacing. We used the keywords "computer assisted" OR "navigation"
• All clinical studies were reviewed for clinical outcomes following navigated THR

Quality of the evidence

Level I
• 2 randomized trials

Level II
• 1 randomized trials with methodologic limitations

Level III
• 3 case control studies

Level V
• 1 "bench" study

Findings

Patient-reported clinical outcome measures are the current gold standard for assessing improvement with any new intervention. Although the radiographic analysis of a new procedure is important, it is arguably more critical that this adjuvant technique results in either a reduction in complications for the patient or an objective improvement in function. This so called "improvement" is difficult to demonstrate in THR, which is highly successful with a very low complication rate.

Clinical outcome measures Babisch et al.[25] compared Harris hip score (HHS), Merle d'Aubigné and Postel score, SF-36, and WOMAC between navigation and control groups in dysplastic cases. No statistically significant difference was seen in SF-36 or WOMAC, while the HHS and Merle d'Aubigné and Postel score were both significantly better in the navigated group. This study also reported on the reproduction of the planned leg length at the end of the procedure; as this was significantly improved in the navigated group, it may account for the improvement in outcomes above.

Other studies by Sugano et al.[22] (Merle d'Aubigné and Postel hip score), and by Kruger et al.[47] (WOMAC, satisfaction and HHS) both showed no significant difference between groups. It is not surprising that simply improving the alignment of the cup does not show a clear improvement in clinical outcomes. Patients who have either subluxation or frank dislocation of their THR may record a better score but, as clinical experience shows, even patients whose cup orientation is suboptimal frequently function well. One should recognize that restoration of leg length

Table 14.6 Dislocations

Authors	N dislocations (cases at risk)		
	Navigated	**Control**	
Babisch et al.[25]	0 (37)	1 (37)	
Kalteiss et al.[18]	0 (60)	1 (30)	
Parratte et al.[19]	0 (30)	0 (30)	
Lazovic et al.[21]	4.7% (1st cohort) 0.3% (2nd cohort)	6.4%	
Sugano et al.[22]	0 (59)	7 (111)	P = 0.049

and offset, rather than improved cup orientation, may well improve patient satisfaction and perhaps represents the greatest chance of clinical improvement associated with the use of navigation.

Rate of dislocation As a marker for success in hip navigation, episodes of dislocation are a rigid endpoint which can be evaluated. Those comparative studies in which there were any dislocations are summarized in Table 14.6.

For most of the studies the dislocation rate is too low to draw any meaningful conclusion. The dislocation rate in the study by Lazovic et al.[21] is high in both the navigated and control groups initially, but was considerably reduced in a subsequent second cohort of navigated patients. Sugano et al.[22] with a 6 year follow-up for the patients had a significantly higher dislocation rate in the non-navigated group. However, analysis of the acetabular position of these cases showed that two of the cases were outside Lewineek's safe zone and five cases were inside, emphasizing how other factors such as head size and soft tissue repair may influence dislocation. Sugano also noted evidence of femoral neck impingement as demonstrated by wear on follow up radiographs in five of the non-navigated cases, and two further cases in the non-navigated group had evidence of impingement after retrieval at revision surgery.

Unfortunately, as the dislocation rate following THR is low, it would take a large comparative study to convincingly show a reduction in dislocation with the use of acetabular navigation.

Restoration of kinematics As discussed above, Babisch[25] shows more accurate restoration of leg length with the use of navigation, and similarly Sugano et al.[22] quote correct restoration of leg length in 44 of the navigated cases and incorrect leg length in 11 of 83 non-navigated hips (p = 0.01). Unfortunately, Sugano does not explain the reason for

incomplete follow-up of all the patients and the method of assessment of leg length postoperatively. While the data may be lacking, if navigation is used to assess leg length and offset and to adjust it intraoperatively, one would expect it to be accurate, and relatively straightforward. It does not require insertion of a further array into the femur.

Petrella et al.[58] have published on computer prediction of impingment and range of movement based on digital acquisition of a patient's CT pelvis, and virtual planning of acetabular component position. By varying the orientation of the acetabulum, while keeping the center of rotation in the same place, they have predicted the point of impingement (either implant to implant or implant to bone) of inserting the cup in different orientations. They defined an acceptable range of movement (ROM) of the hip as: flexion 90°, external rotation 30°, extension 15°, abduction and adduction 30°. Using the variability in component position from previous published work,[19] they calculated that non-navigated hips would impinge in 3–5% of cases before achieving this ROM, but all of the navigated hips would achieve this ROM.

Other complications Other problems have been reported with navigation including loosening of the reference array, breakage of the reference pin, and technical failure. Most of the reported series noted an inability to complete the navigated procedure in a small number of cases and felt that this was part of the normal learning curve.

Recommendation
None.

Summary of recommendations

- Navigation reduces the number of acetabular components placed outside the "safe zone"
- Operative surgical time is increased with the use of navigation
- Blood loss is equal with or without navigation
- CT based and imageless systems appear equally effective
- For patients undergoing hip resurfacing, navigation improves the accuracy of femoral component position

Conclusion

Computer navigation has evolved from the early days of slow, CT-based systems into more surgeon-friendly imageless systems. Although it does add additional complexity to the case, there is evidence that navigation can reduce outliers compared to conventional acetabular preparation and seating. Imageless systems appear to have good accuracy and have the benefit of not requiring preoperative CT scanning and planning, and the patient can be positioned either supine or in the lateral decubitus position. There are outstanding issues about the cost-effectiveness of navigation applied to all cases, and it is not yet possible to quantify any benefits beyond radiographic positioning. While navigation appears to be helpful in positioning the guide wire in femoral head resurfacing, a good-quality clinical randomized trial is needed to confirm the clear benefit of navigation. For the future, it will be interesting to see how hip navigation is incorporated into training of orthopedic residents, and whether acceptable accuracy is obtained simply by referencing from the ipsilateral pelvis. At present the routine use of navigation for THR is not the standard of care.

References

1. Canadian Joint Replacement Registry. Hip and Knee Replacements in Canada 2008–9 Annual Report. Canadian Institute for Health Information, Ottawa, 2009.

2. National Joint Registry for England and Wales, 6th annual report for 2008–09.

3. Kurtz S, Ong K, Lau E, Mowat F, Halpern M. Projections of primary and revision hip and knee arthroplasty in the United States from 2005 to 2030. J Bone Joint Surg Am 2007;89:780–5.

4. UK Office for National Statistics. http://www.statistics.gov.uk/cci/nugget.asp?ID=949

5. US Government Info. http://usgovinfo.about.com/od/censusandstatistics/a/olderstats.htm

6. Lewinnek GE, Lewis JL, Tarr R, Compere CL, Zimmerman JR. Dislocations after total hip replacement arthroplasties. J Bone Joint Surg Am 1978;60(2):217–20.

7. Kennedy JK, Rogers WB, Soffe KE, Sullivan RJ, Griffen DG, Sheehan LJ. Effect of component orientation on recurrent dislocation, pelvic osteolysis, polyethylene wear and component migration. J Arthroplasty 1998;13(5):530–4.

8. Hooper GJ, Rothwell AG, Streinger M, Frampton C. Revision following cemented and uncemented primary total hip replacement a seven-year analysis from the New Zealand Joint Registry. J Bone Joint Surg Br 2009;91(4):451–8.

9. Udomkiat P, Dorr LD, Wan Z. Cementless hemispheric porous coated sockets implanted with press fit technique without screws: average ten year follow up. J Bone Joint Surg Am 2002; 84:1195–200.

10. Patil S, Bergula A, Chen PC, Colwell CW, D'Lima DD. Polyethylene wear and acetabular component orientation. J Bone Joint Surg Am 2003;85:56–63.

11. Wan Z, Boutary M, Dorr L. The influence of acetabular component position on wear in total hip arthroplasty. J Arthroplasty 2008;23(1):51–6.

12. Schmalzried TP, Guttmann D, Grecula M, Amstutz HC. The relationship between the design, position, and articular wear of acetabular components inserted without cement and the development of osteolysis. J Bone Joint Surg Am 1994;76: 677–88.

13. Brodner W, Grubl A, Jankovsky R, Meisinger V, Lehr S, Gottsauner-Wolf F. Cup inclination and serum concentration of cobalt and chromium after metal-on-metal total hip arthroplasty. J Arthroplasty 2004;19(8) Suppl 3:66–70.

14. Langton DJ, Jameson SS, Joyce TJ, Webb J, Nargol AVF. The effect of component size and orientation on the concentrations of metal ions after resurfacing arthroplasty of the hip. J Bone Joint Surg Br 2008;90(9):1143–51.

15. Wan Z, Malik A, Jaramaz B, Chao L, Dorr LD. Imaging and navigation measurement of acetabular component position in THA. Clin Orthop Relat Res 2009;467:32–42.

16. Murray DW. The definition and measurement of acetabular orientation. J Bone Joint Surg Br 1993;75:228–32.

17. Gandhi R, Marchie A, Farrokhyar F, Mahomed N. Computer navigation in total hip replacement: a meta-analysis. International Orthopaedics 2009;33:593–7.

18. Kalteis T, Handel M, Bäthis H, Perlick L, Tingart M, Grifka A. Imageless navigation for insertion of the acetabular component in total hip arthroplasty: is it as accurate as CT-based navigation? J Bone Joint Surg Br 2006;88(2):163–7.

19. Parratte S, Argenson JN. Validation and usefulness of a computer-assisted cup-positioning system in total hip arthroplasty. A prospective, randomized, controlled study. J Bone Joint Surg Am 2007;89:494–9.

20. Leenders T, Vandevelde D, Mahieu G, Nuyts R. Reduction in variability of acetabular cup abduction using computer assisted surgery: a prospective and randomized study. Comput Aided Surg 2002;7:99–106.

21. Lazovic D, Kaib N. Results with navigated bicontact total hip arthroplasty. Orthopedics 2005;28(10):1227.

22. Sugano N, Nishii T, Miki H, Yoshikawa H, Sato Y, Tamura S. Mid-term results of cementless total hip replacement using a ceramic-on-ceramic bearing with and without computer navigation. J Bone Joint Surg Br 2007;89(4):455–60.

23. Haaker RG, Tiedjen K, Ottersbach A, Rubenthaler F, Stockheim M, Stiehl JB. Comparison of conventional versus computer-navigated acetabular component insertion. J Arthroplasty 2007;22:151–9.

24. Najarian BC, Kilgore JE, Markel DC. Evaluation of component positioning in primary total hip arthroplasty using an imageless navigation device compared with traditional methods. J Arthroplasty 2009;24(1):15–21.

25. Babisch J, Layher F, Sander K. Imageless cup and stem navigation in dysplastic hips with the navitrack and vector vision systems. Chapter 44 in: Navigation and MIS in Orthopaedic Surgery, pp. 344–51. Springer, Heidelberg, 2007.

26. DiGioia AM, Jaramaz B, Plakseychuk AY, et al. Comparison of a mechanical acetabular alignment guide with computer placement of the socket. J Arthroplasty 2002;17:359–64.

27. Lazovic D. Cup and stem navigation with the orthopilot system. Chapter 48 in: Navigation and MIS in Orthopaedic Surgery, pp. 372–7. Springer, Heidelberg, 2007.

28. Miki H, Yamanashi W, Nishii T, Sato Y, Yoshikawa H, Sugano N. Anatomic range of motion after implantation during total hip arthroplasty as measured by a navigation system. J Arthroplasty 2007;22(7):946–52.

29. Widmer KH, Zurfluh B. Compliant positioning of total hip components for optimal range of motion. J Orthop Res 2004;22: 815–21.

30. Zheng G, Marx A, Langlotz U, Widmer KH, Buttaro M, Nolte LP. A hybrid CT free navigation system for total hip arthroplasty. Comput Aided Surg 2002;7:129–45.

31. Stiehl JB. Computer-guided total hip arthroplasty. Chapter 23 in: MIS Techniques in Orthopaedics, pp. 367–89. Springer, New York, 2006.

32. Langlotz U, Grutzner PA, Bernsmann K, Kowal JH, Tannast M, Caversaccio M, Nolte L-P. Accuracy considerations in navigated cup placement for total hip arthroplasty. Proc Inst Mech Eng [H] 2007;221(7):739–53.

33. Grutzner PA, Zheng G, Langlotz U, von Recum J, Nolte LP, Wentzensen A, et al. C-arm based navigation in total hip arthroplasty—background and clinical experience. Injury 2004; 35(Suppl 1):A90–5.

34. Hube R, Birke A, Hein W, Klima S. CT based and fluoroscopy based navigation for cup implantation in total hip arthroplasty. Surg Technol Internat 2003;11:275–80.

35. DiGioia AM, Jaramaz B, Plakseychuk AY, Moody JE, Nikou C, LaBarca RS, et al. Comparison of a mechanical acetabular alignment guide with computer placement of the socket. J Arthroplasty 2002;17(3):359–63.

36. Dorr LD, Hishiki Y, Wan Z, Newton D, Yun A. Development of imageless computer navigation for acetabular component position in total hip replacement. Iowa Orthop J 2005;25:1–9.

37. Fukunishi S, Fukui T, Imamura F, Nishio S, Shibanuma N, Yoshiya S. Assessment of accuracy of acetabular cup orientation in CT free navigated total hip arthroplasty. Orthopedics 2008; 31(10):1–4.

38. Jingushi S, Hideki M, Nakashima Y, Yamamoto T, Mawatari T, Iwamoto Y. Computed tomography-based navigation to determine the socket location in total hip arthroplasty of an osteoarthritis hip with a large leg length discrepancy due to severe acetabular dysplasia. J Arthroplasty 2007;22(7):1074–8.

39. Ohashi H, Matsuura M, Okamoto Y, Ebara T, Kakeda K, Takahashi S. Status of navigated total hip arthroplasty in dysplastic osteoarthritis. Orthopedics 2007;30(10):S117–20.

40. Gofton W, Dubrowski A, Tabloie F, Backstein D. The effect of computer navigation on trainee learning of surgical skills. J Bone Joint Surg Am 2007;89:2819–27.

41. DiGioia AM, Plakseychuk, Levison TJ, Jaramaz B. Mini-incision technique for total hip arthroplasty. J Arthroplasty 2003; 18(2):123–8.

42. Wixson RL, MacDonald MA. Total hip arthroplasty through minimal posterior approach using computer assisted hip navigation. J Arthroplasty 2005;20(7 Suppl3):51–6.

43. Judet H. Five years experience in hip navigation using a mini-invasive anterior approach. Orthopedics 2007;30(10):S141–143.

44. Walde HJ, Walde TA. Minimally invasive orthopaedic surgery: first results in navigated total hip arthroplasty. Orthopedics 2006;29(10):S139–141.

45. Slover JD, Tosteson ANA, Bozic KJ, Rubash HE, Malchau H. Impact of hospital volume on the economic value of computer navigation for total knee replacement. J Bone Joint Surg Am 2008;90:1492–500.

46. Schnurr C, Michael JWP, Eysel P, Konig DP. Imageless navigation of hip resurfacing arthroplasty increases the implant accuracy. Internat Orthop 2009;33:365–72.

47. Kruger BS, Zambelli PY, Leyvraz PF, Jolles BM. Computer assisted placement technique in hip resurfacing arthroplasty: improvement in accuracy? Internat Orthop 2009;33:27–33.

48. Ganapathi M, Vendittoli PA, Lavigne M, Gunther KP. Femoral component positioning in hip resurfacing with and without navigation. Clin Orthop Relat Res 2009;467:1341–7.

49. Resubal JRE, Morgan DAF. Computer assisted vs mechanical jig technique in hip resurfacing arthroplasty. J Arthroplasty 2009; 24(3):341–50.

50. Seyler TM, Lai LP, Sprinkle DI, Ward WG, Jinnah RH. Does computer assisted surgery improve accuracy and decrease the learning curve in hip resurfacing? A radiographic analysis. J Bone Joint Surg Am 2008;90(Suppl 3):71–80.

51. Hodgson AJ, Inkpen KB, Shekman M, Anglin C, Tonetti J, Masri BA, et al. Computer assisted femoral head resurfacing. Comput Aided Surg 2005;10(5/6):337–43.

52. Davis ET, Gallie P, Macgroarty K, Waddell JP, Schemitsch E. The accuracy of image free computer navigation in the placement of the femoral component of the Birmingham hip resurfacing. J Bone Joint Surg Br 2007;89;4:557–60.

53. Hodgson A, Helmy N, Masri BA, Greidanus NV, Inkpen KB, Duncan CP, et al. Comparative repeatability of guide pin axis positioning in computer assisted and manual femoral head resurfacing arthroplasty. Proc Inst Mech Eng [H] 2007; 221:713–24.

54. Cobb JP, Kannan V, Dandachli W, Iranpour F, Brust KU, Hart AJ. Learning how to resurface cam type femoral heads with acceptable accuracy and precision: the role of computed tomography-based navigation. J Bone Joint Surg Am 2008;90(Suppl 3): 57–64.

55. Olsen M, Davis ET, Waddell JP, Schemitsch EH. Imageless computer navigation for placement of the femoral component in resurfacing arthroplasty of the hip. J Bone Joint Surg Br 2009;91:310–15.

56. Bailey C, Gul R, Falworth M, Zadow S, Oakeshott R. Component alignment in hip resurfacing using computer navigation. Clin Orthop Relat Res 2009;467:917–22.

57. Romanowski JR, Swank ML. Imageless navigation in hip resurfacing: avoiding component malposition during the surgeon learning curve. J Bone Joint Surg Am 2008;90(Suppl 3):65–70.

58. Petrella AJ, Stowe JQ, D'Lima DD, Rullkoetter PJ, Laz PJ. Computer assisted versus manual alignment in THA. Clin Orthop Relat Res 2009;467:50–5.

15 Highly Crosslinked Polyethylene in Total Hip Arthroplasty

Glen Richardson, Michael J. Dunbar, and Joseph P. Corkum

Dalhousie University, Halifax, NS, Canada

Case scenario

A 55 year old woman presents to an orthopedic surgeon with advanced osteoarthritis in her right hip. She is able to bear weight, but her gait is poor and overall activity is extremely limited due to the pain in her hip. Conservative treatment options are exhausted, but her pain persists so she is scheduled for a total hip arthroplasty (THA).

Relevant anatomy

Endstage arthritis of the hip joint is often managed with THA. In a THA the proximal femur of the hip is replaced with a prosthesis, and the acetabular liner is placed inside the acetabular cup. There are a number of options to choose for this bearing interface, including highly crosslinked polyethylene (HCLPE).

Importance of the problem

One of the main limitations of THA has been the longevity of the bearing surface (Figure 15.1). Much work has been invested in attempts at improving the bearing championed by Charnley. Any change to the bearing surface raises the potential for adverse unexpected outcomes. HCLPE has been taken up broadly by the orthopedic community, just as short-term results are becoming available. Joint replacement registries have illustrated the extent of crosslinked polyethylene in THA. The Canadian Joint Replacement Registry (CJRR) reported the use of crosslinked polyethylene increased from 45% of hip replacements in 2002–2003

to 76% of hip replacements in 2006–2007.[1] Furthermore, surgeons reporting to the CJRR are using more 32mm heads, up from 13% in 2003–2004 to 31% of THAs in 2006–2007. Coupling this trend with a greater number of younger patients undergoing THA and there certainly is a concern for accelerated wear of THA.

Top four questions

Prognosis

1. Is HCLPE more resistant to wear than ultra-high molecular weight polyethylene (UHMWPE)?
2. Does the improved wear rate of HCLPE allow for the use of larger femoral head sizes in THA?
3. Has the advent of HCLPE resulted in a decrease in the prevalence of osteolysis after THA?

Harm

4. Can the use of HCLPE compromise mechanical properties??

Question 1: Is HCLPE more resistant to wear than UHMWPE?

Case clarification
The patient enjoys outside activities that may put high levels of stress on the implant. Will she be better off in terms of wear by having a HCLPE acetabular liner?

Relevance
UHMWPE that wears more than 0.1mm per year is at higher risk of osteolysis and early implant failure.[2]

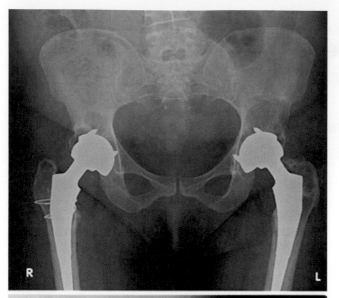

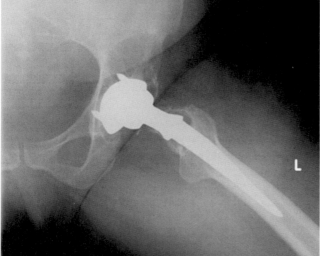

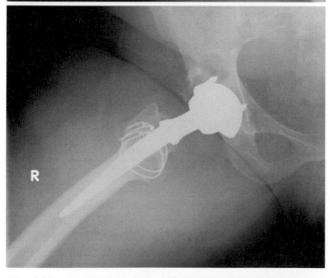

Figure 15.1 AP and lateral views of bilateral hip replacements with UHMWPE demonstrating advanced polyethylene wear and associated osteolysis 16 years postoperatively in a moderately active woman.

Current opinion

Both in-vivo and in-vitro studies have convincingly demonstrated a reduction in wear rates when comparing HCLPE with conventional polyethylene.

Finding the evidence

• Cochrane Database, with search term "cross linked polyethylene"
  ○ Revealed 0 hits
• PubMed (www.ncbi.nlm.nih.gov/pubmed/) clinical queries search/ systematic reviews: "crosslinked" OR "cross-linked" AND "polyethylene" AND "hip arthroplasty" AND "wear"
  ○ Found 28 articles
• PubMed (www.ncbi.nlm.nih.gov/pubmed/) -sensitivity search using keywords "crosslinked" OR "cross-linked" AND "polyethylene" AND "hip arthroplasty" AND "wear"
  ○ Retrieved 70 articles with 47 potentially relevant

Quality of the evidence

Level I
• 10 high-quality randomized controlled trials

Level II
• 5 prognostic studies

Level III
• 11 retrospective studies

Level IV
• 4 case series

Level V
• 10 case reports and expert opinion

Nonclinical
• 7 basic science

Findings

All the manufacturers report significant decreases in wear rates, reporting 85–100% reductions in wear from hip simulator data.[3] HCLPE was highly resistant to wear and performed better than conventional polyethylene (i.e., UHMWPE that is not crosslinked) in environments that are felt to increase wear such as the presence of third-body wear particles and roughened femoral heads.[4-6]

In order to interpret the substantial amount of reported data on HCLPE, a basic knowledge of the different methods of measuring in-vivo wear of polyethylene is necessary. There are manual techniques that rely on manual edge detection to calculate the migration of the femoral head.[7] To improve accuracy and reproducibility, computer-aided techniques have been developed.[8,9] The most accurate method of measuring wear is radiostereometry analysis (RSA).[10,11] Studies looking at wear rates require follow-up

Table 15.1 Summary of evidence for highly cross-linked polyethylene

Study	Year	Methods	Wear analysis	Femoral head size	Liner	Follow-up (years)	Outcome
Ayers et al.[29]	2009	RCT	RSA	28 mm	Longevity	2	Penetration rate 0.065 mm vs. 0.169 mm
Calvert et al.[23]	2009	RCT	Devane	28 mm	Marathon	4	Volumetric wear rate 13.741 mm³ vs. 60.24 mm³
McCalden et al.[30]	2009	RCT	Martell	28 mm	Longevity	6.8	Penetration rate 0.003 mm/yr vs. 0.051 mm/yr
Garcia-Rey et al.[25]	2008	RCT	Dorr with AutoCAD	28 mm	Durasul	5	Mean wear was 6 μm vs. 38 μm
Glyn-Jones et al.[26]	2008	RCT	RSA	28 mm	Longevity	2 yrs	Penetration rate 0.06 mm/yr vs. 0.1 mm/yr
Bragdon et al.[34]	2007	Prospective consecutive cases	RSA	28 mm vs. 36 mm	Longevity	2	No statistical difference in wear
Digas et al.[21]	2007	Bilateral THA control	RSA	28 mm	Longevity	5	Proximal head migration 0.08 mm vs. 0.34 mm
Digas et al.[21]	2007	RCT	RSA	28 mm	Durasul	5	Proximal head migration 0.1 mm vs. 0.29 mm
Rohrl et al.[33]	2007	Prospective cohort	RSA	28 mm	Crossfire	6	Total penetration 0.23 mm vs. 0.75 mm including creep
Triclot et al.[28]	2007	RCT	Martell	28 mm	Durasul	4.9	Penetration rate 0.025 mm/yr vs. 0.106 mm/yr
Engh Jr et al.[24]	2006	RCT	Martell	28 mm	Marathon	5.7	Mean wear rate 0.01 mm/yr vs. 0.19 mm/yr
Geerdink et al.[31]	2006	RCT	Martell	28 mm	Duration	5	Wear rate 0.083 mm/yr vs. 0.123 mm/yr
Martell et al.[27]	2003	RCT	Martell	28 mm	Crossfire	2	2-and 3-dimensional linear wear rate reductions of 42% and 50%

RCT, randomized controlled trial; RSA, radiostereometry analysis.

of at least 2 years, in order to get a true estimate of steady-state wear rate because of the effect of plastic deformation (otherwise known as bedding-in or creep).[12–14]

There are seven papers reporting on randomized controlled trials (RCTs) using cobalt chrome femoral heads on HCLPE and using some form of computer-assisted technique to measure the polyethylene wear.[15–21] Many of the major manufactures of HCLPE are represented in these articles. Marathon (5 Mrads), Durasul (9.5 Mrads), Longevity (10 Mrads), and Crossfire (7.5 Mrads) have all demonstrated significant reductions in steady-state wear rates compared to UHMWPE. The reduction in wear varies from 55% to 95% and is often is a function of the wear properties of the control group. Importantly, the follow-up was 4–5 years, but there are no long-term studies.

Five RSA studies on HCLPE have been reported in the literature[14,22–25]. Durasul, Longevity, and Crossfire HCLPE have all been demonstrated to significantly decrease wear rates compared to UHMWPE. The length of follow-up varied from 2 to 6 years.

A summary of the evidence for HCLPE, regardless of measurement technique, is presented in Table 15.1.

Recommendation
- HCLPE has been demonstrated to decrease wear rates in vitro and in vivo compared to UHMWPE [overall quality: high]

Question 2: Does the improved wear rate of HCLPE allow for the use of larger femoral head sizes in THA?

Case clarification
The surgeon must choose an optimal head size for the femoral component.

Relevance
Larger femoral head components are felt to increase range of motion and decrease dislocation rates of THA.

Current opinion

With UHMWPE, the chosen head size was limited as a result of increased volumetric wear with increasing ball diameter.

Finding the evidence

- PubMed (www.ncbi.nlm.nih.gov/pubmed/) clinical queries search/ systematic reviews: "crosslinked" OR "cross-linked" AND "polyethylene" AND "head size"
    - Found 2 articles
- PubMed (www.ncbi.nlm.nih.gov/pubmed/)—sensitivity search using keywords "crosslinked" OR "cross-linked" AND "polyethylene" AND "head size"
    - Retrieved 16 articles with 10 potentially relevant

Quality of the evidence

Level III
- 2 retrospective studies

Level IV
- 6 case series

Level V
- 2 case reports and expert opinion

Findings

Muratoglu et al. demonstrated no significant increase in wear associated with head sizes from 22 to 46 mm[3]. This was also replicated with 32 mm and 38 mm heads articulating against HCLPE treated with 9.5 Mrad.[26] In a case series with a 5–8 year follow-up Lachiewicz et al. found no correlation between linear wear rate and head size, but did find an association with volumetric wear.[27] Bragdon et al. found similar results when they retrospectively compared 28 and 32 mm heads in a case series involving 200 hips with a minimum follow-up of 6 years.[28] RSA has been used to compare 28 and 36 mm heads in a cohort study and no significant difference was found at 3 years.[22]

Recommendation

- The use of larger femoral head components with HCLPE does not appear to increase wear rates in short-term studies [overall quality: low]

Question 3: Has the advent of HCLPE resulted in a decrease in the prevalence of osteolysis after THA?

Case clarification

The 55 year old women receiving a THA can realistically expect to live another 20–25 years. Over this period of time the THA is more likely to fail due to osteolysis than any other failure mechanism.

Relevance

Periprosthetic osteolysis is the leading cause of long-term failure in THA.[29]

Current opinion

The use of UHMWPE in active THA patients will lead to osteolysis and aseptic loosening.

Finding the evidence

- PubMed (www.ncbi.nlm.nih.gov/pubmed/) clinical queries search/ systematic reviews: "crosslinked" OR "cross-linked" AND "polyethylene" AND "osteolysis"
    - Found 22 articles
- PubMed (www.ncbi.nlm.nih.gov/pubmed/) -sensitivity search using keywords "crosslinked" OR "cross-linked" AND "polyethylene" AND "osteolysis"
    - Retrieved 81 articles with 13 potentially relevant

Quality of the evidence

Level II
- 2 cohort studies/low-quality RCTs

Level III
- 8 systematic review of case-controlled studies, case-controlled and retrospective studies

Level V
- 3 expert opinion

Findings

In-vitro studies have demonstrated increased inflammatory response to HCLPE wear particles, but clinical studies utilizing CT scans to evaluating osteolysis demonstrate significant reductions in lytic lesions.[30–33] Others have shown that HCLPE generates a similar macrophage response to conventional polyethylene, and have made the logical conclusion that their lower wear rates should reduce osteolysis.[34]

Recommendation

- HCLPE reduces the risk of osteolysis at short-term follow up compared to UHMWPE [overall quality: moderate]

Question 4: Can the use of HCLPE compromise mechanical properties?

Case clarification

Should this active patient be concerned about the altered mechanical properties of HCLPE and the possibility of implant failure?

Relevance

In processing HCLPE the steps taken to increase the crosslinking worsen its mechanical properties and this could result in clinical failures.

Current opinion

Increasing the crosslinking in UHMWPE does have a measurable effect on mechanical properties; specifically, fatigue properties, crack propagation, and toughness are all decreased.

Finding the evidence

• PubMed (www.ncbi.nlm.nih.gov/pubmed/) clinical queries search/ systematic reviews: "crosslinked" OR "cross-linked" AND "polyethylene" AND "mechanical properties"
  ◦ Found 10 articles
• PubMed (www.ncbi.nlm.nih.gov/pubmed/) -sensitivity search using keywords "crosslinked" OR "cross-linked" AND "polyethylene" AND "mechanical properties"
  ◦ Retrieved 91 articles with 28 potentially relevant

Quality of the evidence

Level III
• 5 retrospective studies

Level IV
• 1 case series

Level V
• 4 case reports and expert opinion

Nonclinical
• 18 basic science

Findings

The creation of HCLPE results in unfavorable changes with ultimate tensile strength, ductility, modulus, toughness, and crack propagation resistance.[35,36] Cases of liner failures are reported in the literature, but some of the failures were likely related to implant design.[37]

Recommendations

• Mechanical properties of HCLPE are negatively affected by crosslinking [overall quality: high]
• Clinical reports of implant failure are rare [overall quality: moderate]

Summary of recommendations

• HCLPE has been demonstrated to decrease wear rates in vitro and in vivo compared to UHMWPE
• The use of larger femoral head components with HCLPE does not appear to increase wear rates in short-term studies
• HCLPE reduces the risk of osteolysis at short-term follow up compared to UHMWPE

• Mechanical properties of HCLPE are negatively affected by crosslinking
• Clinical reports of implant failure are rare

Conclusion

The exposure of UHMWPE to radiation creates a material that behaves differently both on the hip simulator and in the patient. In every study there has been a significant reduction in wear and—even more encouraging—there is a reduction in the number and size of osteolytic lesions. This is not the final story, as the longest follow-up in the best methodological studies is only 6 years. There remains the risk that wear rates could dramatically increase with longer follow-up. Despite the reported liner failures in case series,[37,38] there have been no liner-associated complications in any of the studies presented in this chapter. Caution must be exerted when using larger head sizes, as there is one RSA RCT that shows there is no effect after only 2 years.[22] At present, there is enough reported evidence to support the continued use of HCLPE in THA patients.

References

1. Canadian Institute for Health Information. Hip and Knee Replacements in Canada—Canadian Joint Replacement Registry 2008–2009 Annual Report. Canadian Institute for Health Information Ottawa, 2009)
2. Dumbleton JH, Manley MT, Edidin AA. A literature review of the association between wear rate and osteolysis in total hip arthroplasty. J Arthroplasty 2002;17(5):649–61.
3. Muratoglu OK, Bragdon CR, O'Connor DO, Jasty M, Harris WH. A novel method of cross-linking ultra-high-molecular-weight polyethylene to improve wear, reduce oxidation, and retain mechanical properties. Recipient of the 1999 HAP Paul Award. J Arthroplasty 2001;16(2):149–60.
4. Bragdon CR, Jasty M, Muratoglu OK, Harris WH. Third-body wear testing of a highly cross-linked acetabular liner: the effect of large femoral head size in the presence of particulate poly(methyl-methacrylate) debris. J Arthroplasty 2005;20(3): 379–85.
5. Laurent MP, Johnson TS, Crowninshield RD, Blanchard CR, Bhambri SK, Yao JQ. Characterization of a highly cross-linked ultrahigh molecular-weight polyethylene in clinical use in total hip arthroplasty. J Arthroplasty 2008;23(5):751–61.
6. Ito H, Maloney CM, Crowninshield RD, Clohisy JC, McDonald DJ, Maloney WJ. In vivo femoral head damage and its effect on polyethylene wear. J Arthroplasty 2009;25(2):302–8.
7. Livermore J, Ilstrup D, Morrey B. Effect of femoral head size on wear of the polyethylene acetabular component. J Bone Joint Surg Am 1990;72(4):518–28.
8. Devane PA, Bourne RB, Rorabeck CH, Hardie RM, Horne JG. Measurement of polyethylene wear in metal-backed acetabular cups. I. Three-dimensional technique. Clin Orthop Relat Res 1995;319:303–16.

9. Martell JM, Berdia S. Determination of polyethylene wear in total hip replacements with use of digital radiographs. J Bone Joint Surg Am 1997;79(11):1635–41.

10. Bragdon CR, Estok DM, Malchau H, Karrholm J, Yuan X, Bourne R, et al. Comparison of two digital radiostereometric analysis methods in the determination of femoral head penetration in a total hip replacement phantom. J Orthop Res 2004;22(3): 659–64.

11. Bragdon CR, Malchau H, Yuan X, Perinchief R, Karrholm J, Borlin N, et al. Experimental assessment of precision and accuracy of radiostereometric analysis for the determination of polyethylene wear in a total hip replacement model. J Orthop Res 2002;20(4):688–95.

12. Dorr LD, Wan Z, Shahrdar C, Sirianni L, Boutary M, Yun A. Clinical performance of a Durasul highly cross-linked polyethylene acetabular liner for total hip arthroplasty at five years. J Bone Joint Surg Am 2005;87(8):1816–21.

13. Manning DW, Chiang PP, Martell JM, Galante JO, Harris WH. In vivo comparative wear study of traditional and highly cross-linked polyethylene in total hip arthroplasty. J Arthroplasty 2005;20(7):880–6.

14. Digas G, Karrholm J, Thanner J, Herberts P. 5-year experience of highly cross-linked polyethylene in cemented and uncemented sockets: two randomized studies using radiostereometric analysis. Acta Orthop 2007;78(6):746–54.

15. Calvert GT, Devane PA, Fielden J, Adams K, Horne JG. A double-blind, prospective, randomized controlled trial comparing highly cross-linked and conventional polyethylene in primary total hip arthroplasty. J Arthroplasty 2009;24(4):505–10.

16. Engh CA, Jr., Stepniewski AS, Ginn SD, Beykirch SE, Sychterz-Terefenko CJ, Hopper RH, Jr., et al. A randomized prospective evaluation of outcomes after total hip arthroplasty using cross-linked marathon and non-cross-linked Enduron polyethylene liners. J Arthroplasty 2006;21(6 Suppl 2):17–25.

17. Garcia-Rey E, Garcia-Cimbrelo E, Cruz-Pardos A, Ortega-Chamarro J. New polyethylenes in total hip replacement: a prospective, comparative clinical study of two types of liner. J Bone Joint Surg Br 2008;90(2):149–53.

18. Martell JM, Verner JJ, Incavo SJ. Clinical performance of a highly cross-linked polyethylene at two years in total hip arthroplasty: a randomized prospective trial. J Arthroplasty 2003;18(7 Suppl 1):55–9.

19. Triclot P, Grosjean G, El Masri F, Courpied JP, Hamadouche M. A comparison of the penetration rate of two polyethylene acetabular liners of different levels of cross-linking. A prospective randomised trial. J Bone Joint Surg Br 2007;89(11):1439–45.

20. McCalden RW, MacDonald SJ, Rorabeck CH, Bourne RB, Chess DG, Charron KD. Wear rate of highly cross-linked polyethylene in total hip arthroplasty. A randomized controlled trial. J Bone Joint Surg Am 2009;91(4):773–82.

21. Geerdink CH, Grimm B, Ramakrishnan R, Rondhuis J, Verburg AJ, Tonino AJ. Crosslinked polyethylene compared to conventional polyethylene in total hip replacement: pre-clinical evaluation, in-vitro testing and prospective clinical follow-up study. Acta Orthop 2006;77(5):719–25.

22. Bragdon CR, Greene ME, Freiberg AA, Harris WH, Malchau H. Radiostereometric analysis comparison of wear of highly cross-linked polyethylene against 36- vs. 28-mm femoral heads. J Arthroplasty 2007;22(6 Suppl 2):125–9.

23. Glyn-Jones S, Isaac S, Hauptfleisch J, McLardy-Smith P, Murray DW, Gill HS. Does highly cross-linked polyethylene wear less than conventional polyethylene in total hip arthroplasty? A double-blind, randomized, and controlled trial using roentgen stereophotogrammetric analysis. J Arthroplasty 2008;23(3):337–43.

24. Ayers DC, Hays PL, Drew JM, Eskander MS, Osuch D, Bragdon CR. Two-year radiostereometric analysis evaluation of femoral head penetration in a challenging population of young total hip arthroplasty patients. J Arthroplasty 2009;24(6 Suppl):9–14.

25. Rohrl SM, Li MG, Nilsson KG, Nivbrant B. Very low wear of non-remelted highly cross-linked polyethylene cups: an RSA study lasting up to 6 years. Acta Orthop 2007;78(6):739–45.

26. Estok DM, 2nd, Burroughs BR, Muratoglu OK, Harris WH. Comparison of hip simulator wear of 2 different highly cross-linked ultra high molecular weight polyethylene acetabular components using both 32- and 38-mm femoral heads. J Arthroplasty 2007;22(4):581–9.

27. Lachiewicz PF, Heckman DS, Soileau ES, Mangla J, Martell JM. Femoral head size and wear of highly cross-linked polyethylene at 5 to 8 years. Clin.Orthop.Relat.Res 2009;467(12):3290–6.

28. Bragdon CR, Kwon YM, Geller JA, Greene ME, Freiberg AA, Harris WH, et al. Minimum 6-year followup of highly cross-linked polyethylene in THA. Clin.Orthop.Relat.Res. 2007;465:122–7.

29. Harris WH. The problem is osteolysis. Clin.Orthop.Relat.Res 1995; 311:46–53.

30. Engh CA, Jr, Stepniewski AS, Ginn SD, Beykirch SE, Sychterz-Terefenko CJ, Hopper RH, Jr, et al. A randomized prospective evaluation of outcomes after total hip arthroplasty using cross-linked marathon and non-cross-linked Enduron polyethylene liners. J.Arthroplasty 2006;21(6 Suppl 2):17–25.

31. Illgen RL,2nd, Forsythe TM, Pike JW, Laurent MP, Blanchard CR. Highly crosslinked vs. conventional polyethylene particles—an in vitro comparison of biologic activities. J Arthroplasty 2008;23(5):721–31.

32. Illgen RL, 2nd, Bauer LM, Hotujec BT, Kolpin SE, Bakhtiar A, Forsythe TM. Highly crosslinked vs. conventional polyethylene particles: relative in vivo inflammatory response. J Arthroplasty 2009;24(1):117–24.

33. Ries MD, Scott ML, Jani S. Relationship between gravimetric wear and particle generation in hip simulators: conventional compared with cross-linked polyethylene. J Bone Joint Surg Am 2001;83(Suppl 2 Pt 2):116–22.

34. Sethi RK, Neavyn MJ, Rubash HE, Shanbhag AS. Macrophage response to cross-linked and conventional UHMWPE. Biomaterials 2003;24(15):2561–73.

35. Pruitt LA. Deformation, yielding, fracture and fatigue behavior of conventional and highly cross-linked ultra high molecular weight polyethylene. Biomaterials 2005;26(8):905–15.

36. Bradford L, Baker D, Ries MD, Pruitt LA. Fatigue crack propagation resistance of highly crosslinked polyethylene. Clin Orthop Relat Res 2004; 429:68–72.

37. Tower SS, Currier JH, Currier BH, Lyford KA, Van Citters DW, Mayor MB. Rim cracking of the cross-linked longevity polyethylene acetabular liner after total hip arthroplasty. J Bone Joint Surg Am 2007;89(10):2212–17.

38. Bradford L, Kurland R, Sankaran M, Kim H, Pruitt LA, Ries MD. Early failure due to osteolysis associated with contemporary highly cross-linked ultra-high molecular weight polyethylene. A case report. J Bone Joint Surg Am 2004;86(5):1051–6.

16 Hip Resurfacing vs. Metal-on-Metal Total Hip Arthroplasty

Sanket R. Diwanji, Pascal-André Vendittoli, and Martin Lavigne

Hospital Maisonneuve Rosemont, Montreal, QC, Canada

Case scenario

A 40 year old active man with no past medical history presents to your clinic complaining of right groin pain of 6 months' duration. He has restricted right hip motion and a mild limp. Radiography of the pelvis shows advanced osteoarthritis in the right hip with cystic changes in the femoral head.

Relevant anatomy

Precise knowledge of the vascular supply of the femoral head is important when considering surgical procedures around the femoral head and neck junction. The blood supply to the femoral head epiphysis has been studied in the past, with emphasis on the critical role of the deep branch of the medial femoral circumflex artery (traveling under the short rotators) and the lateral retinacular vessels (traveling along the posterolateral femoral neck).[1-5] Since the femoral component of hip resurfacing is supported in part by the femoral head epiphysis, it seems intuitive that damage to the blood supply could eventually jeopardize component fixation. None the less, clinical evidence has not confirmed this assumption as most surgeons use a posterior surgical approach without significant occurrence of femoral head collapse/failure.

Clarke described the femoral neck shape as being not circular but more of an ovoid shape with its larger diameter oriented from 2 o'clock to 8 o'clock.[6] Thus, head–neck offset (distance between head equator and femoral neck surface) is not constant around the head/neck circumference. To replicate natural hip range of motion and avoid femoral neck impingement on the acetabular component, surgeons performing hip resurfacing must make every effort to reproduce or restore the natural femoral head/neck offset all around the femoral neck.[7,8] A detailed understanding of the relation between femoral neck diameter and femoral component diameter with the amount of acetabular bone resection and resultant range of motion is critical to optimize success of hip resurfacing.

Importance of the problem

Total hip arthroplasty (THA)* continues to be the gold standard for treatment of degenerative hip disorders. Although it has demonstrated satisfactory clinical outcome in elderly patients, concerns still exist regarding its longevity in young patients.[9] Among male patients receiving a primary hip arthroplasty in the last decade, the group of patients between 45–54 years of age has grown rapidly, at a rate of 140% compared to the 36% rate seen in older (65–74 years) age group.[10] The concern about the durability of hip arthroplasty in young adults, along with recent improvements in metal-on-metal bearing designs, has led to resurgence of metal-on-metal hip resurfacing (HR).

Since the introduction of metal-on-metal HR devices in the 1990s, over 300,000 procedures have been performed worldwide.[11] While HR is being performed with increasing frequency in the US, Canada and the UK,[10,12,13] it is not quite as popular in Scandinavia[14] and its use in Australia is on the decline.[15] HR accounted for 7.6% of all primary total

---

*Throughout this chapter, THA means 28 or 32 mm THA (where the diameter of the prosthetic femoral head is 28 or 32 mm). The term "LDH (large-diameter head)-THA" is specifically used for studies where diameter of the head is larger than 36 mm.

Evidence-Based Orthopedics, First Edition. Edited by Mohit Bhandari.
© 2012 Blackwell Publishing Ltd. Published 2012 by Blackwell Publishing Ltd.

hip replacements recorded by the Australian Joint Replacement Registry (AJRR) in 2008.[15] Most patients were male around 50 years old, suffering from osteoarthrosis of the hip. There has been a reduction in the number of female patients undergoing HR, from 27.7% in 2004 to 20.4% in 2008. HR accounted for 2.73% of all hip replacements in Canada in 2006–2007 and HR represented less than 0.5% of all hip arthroplasties in Nordik Hip Registry from 1995 to 2006.[10,14]

The current surge in patient interest for HR is partly driven by direct-to-consumer advertising over the internet. The search term "hip resurfacing" yields 216,000 results on Google. Furthermore, surgeons are attracted by HR despite benefits that have not yet been validated. Some purported advantages of HR over THA are improved function, femoral bone preservation, better restoration of hip biomechanics, enhanced stability, and easier conversion to THA if need arises.[16,17] On the other hand, femoral neck fracture, aseptic loosening of the femoral component, lack of long-term outcomes, and surgeon's learning curve have prevented widespread adoption of procedure.[18–20] In this scenario, it is imperative to define evidence-based guidelines for selection of the HR procedure over the gold standard THA.

Top ten questions

Perioperative parameters

1. What are the differences relating to surgical technique and hospitalization after HR and THA?
2. Is acetabular bone jeopardized in hip resurfacing?
3. How precise is biomechanical reconstruction of the hip joint after HR and THA?

Outcome of the procedures

4. Does HR provide better clinical outcomes and activity level than THA?
5. Does HR offer greater range of hip motion than THA?
6. Do patients have better gait and postural balance after HR?

Complications and survivorship

7. Is there any difference between procedures in the rate of complication?
8. What level of metal ion release is seen after HR and metal-on-metal THA?
9. Which procedure has higher failure rate: HR or THA?
10. Is HR revision surgery easier than revision of THA, and does it provide better outcomes?

Question 1: What are the differences relating to the surgical technique and hospitalization after HR and THA?

Case clarification

The patient's BMI is 32 and his hemoglobin level is 13 g%. You explain the patient about operative time, length of incision, approximate blood loss, intraoperative complications, and duration of hospitalization for both procedures.

Relevance

Acetabular cavity exposure is more difficult due to conservation of the femoral head, and femoral component positioning is technically more challenging; HR usually requires more extensive exposure, length of incision and is longer in duration. On the other hand, the femoral canal is not violated in HR, which should lead to reduced blood loss and marrow damage.

Current opinion

Current opinion is conflicting regarding intraoperative outcomes and duration of hospitalization for both procedures.

Finding the evidence

- Cochrane Database with search term "hip resurfacing OR surface replacement arthroplasty" AND "total hip arthroplasty OR total hip replacement"
- PubMed (www.ncbi.nlm.nih.gov/pubmed) sensitivity search using key words: "hip resurfacing OR surface replacement arthroplasty" AND "total hip arthroplasty OR total hip replacement"
- Embase with search term "hip resurfacing OR surface replacement arthroplasty" AND "total hip arthroplasty OR total hip replacement"

Quality of the evidence
Level I
- 2 randomized trials

Level III
- 3 retrospective comparative studies

Findings
Two randomized controlled trials (RCTs) and three retrospective studies compared perioperative outcomes of HR and THA.[12,21–25]

Vendittoli and coworkers found significantly longer surgical time in HR (mean 103 minutes) as compared to 85 minutes for THA (p < 0.001).[21,22] The differences in incision length (17.2 cm in HR vs. 14.5 cm in THA, p < 0.001) and length of hospital stay (5.0 days in HR and 6.1 days in THA, p = 0.01) were statistically significant, whereas total blood loss and transfusion rates were not. Regarding perioperative complications, two (1.94%) acetabular fissures were reported in the HR group and four (3.92%) intraoperative femoral fissures in THA, all without clinical consequences. The authors also reported that four (3.73%) patients randomized to the HR group were converted intraoperatively to THA for reasons such as extensive femoral head necrosis, severe femoral neck retroversion, acetabular component size not available for the particular system, and need for a supplementary screw fixation in a dysplastic acetabulum.

Three retrospective studies reported on perioperative outcome.[12,23,24] Fowble and colleagues reported less estimated surgical blood loss (p = 0.005) and less postoperative drain output (p = 0.05) resulting in 252 mL less total blood loss (p = 0.0005) and fewer blood transfusions (p < 0.0001) after HR as compared to THA.[12] Vail and colleagues did not find substantial differences in the duration of hospital stay or estimated blood loss, and reported three (3.2%) intraoperative calcar cracks in the THA group.[23] Mont et al. found no difference in the duration of surgery and duration of hospitalization between 54 patients with HR and 54 patients with THA.[24]

In an RCT comparing HR to large-diameter head THA (LDH-THA), Lavigne and colleagues reported three (12.5%) femoral calcar cracks in the LDH-THA group and one (4.16%) injury to the branch of the obturator artery in the HR group.[25]

Recommendations

• Length of incision is longer for HR than THA [overall quality: moderate]
• There is conflicting evidence regarding duration of surgery, blood loss and duration of hospitalization after HR and THA [overall quality: low]
• The rate of perioperative complication is similar, but the types of complication are different for HR and THA

Question 2: Is acetabular bone stock jeopardized in hip resurfacing?

Case clarification

The patient's radiographic evaluation shows a remodeled femoral neck which seems larger than the contralateral normal side. The surgeon discusses the possibility of using a larger acetabular component to accommodate the femoral component of HR.

Relevance

Compared to THA, HR clearly preserves more proximal femoral bone stock. In HR, the size of the acetabular component (and thus the amount of acetabular bone resection) is determined by the femoral component diameter. The size of the femoral component may not match the native head

diameter because of a particular patient's neck anatomy, femoral neck enlargement by remodeling or osteophytes, or fear of femoral neck notching. Consequently, there is an ongoing debate on whether more acetabular bone is resected during HR.

Current opinion

Current opinion suggests that hip resurfacing may require a larger acetabular component and thus more acetabular bone removal than conventional THA.

Finding the evidence

• Cochrane Database with search term "hip resurfacing" AND "surface replacement arthroplasty"
• PubMed (www.ncbi.nlm.nih.gov/pubmed) sensitivity search using key words: "hip resurfacing OR surface replacement arthroplasty" AND "acetabular bone"
• Embase with search term "hip resurfacing OR surface replacement arthroplasty" AND "acetabular bone"

Quality of the evidence

Level I
• 1 randomized trial

Level II
• 1 prospective comparative study

Level III
• 3 retrospective comparative studies

Findings

Vendittoli et al. prospectively randomized 210 hips to compare conservation of acetabular bone after HR (Durom, Zimmer, Warsaw, USA) and THA (Allofit cup, Zimmer, Warsaw, USA).[26] The size of the last reamer used before cup implantation served as a surrogate of acetabular bone resection. They did not find any significant difference in the mean or median diameters of the last acetabular reamer used or the mean size of the acetabular component (54.9 mm for HR and 54.7 mm for THA, p = 0.770). However, in 6.8% of HR procedures the size of the acetabular component had to be increased by 2 mm to accommodate the selected femoral component.

In a prospective study, Brennan et al. compared weight of dehydrated, defatted acetabular bone reamed during HR and THA.[27] The mean weights of reamed bone were 13.8 g and 11.7 g and the mean external diameters of the acetabulum were 58 mm and 54 mm in the HR and THA groups, respectively. Because their study groups had significant differences in covariates of acetabular size they used nonparametric analysis of covariance (ANCOVA); regression curves displayed no significant difference in the mean weight of acetabular bone removed between the two groups.

Three retrospective studies compared resection of acetabular bone in HR (Birmingham Hip Resurfacing (BHR), Smith & Nephew, UK and Durom, Zimmer Warsaw, USA) and THA (various designs).[28-30] Two of them reported increased acetabular bone resection for HR. Loughead and colleagues found significantly larger acetabular component size in an HR group (56.6 mm) as compared to a hybrid THA group (52.0 mm) (p < 0.001).[28] Naal et al. also reported that HR required larger cups than conventional THAs in women (52.0 mm vs. 49.9 mm; p = 000012) and in men (57.3 mm vs. 55.1 mm; p = 4.1E-14).[29] Conversely, the third study found a mean outside diameter of the BHR acetabular components of 2.03 mm less than that of the acetabular components in the uncemented THAs for the age-matched women, whereas in men no significant difference was found.[30]

Recommendations

• Removal of acetabular bone during HR may be comparable to, or slightly greater than, that of conventional THA [overall quality: moderate]
• Implant design (femoral head size increment and acetabular component thickness) and surgical technique play a crucial role in acetabular bone removal.

Question 3: How precise is biomechanical reconstruction of the hip joint after HR and THA?

Case clarification

The patient's AP pelvic radiograph shows limb length shortening of 1.5 cm and femoral offset of 34 mm on the affected side vs. 44 mm on the normal contralateral side. The patient expressed concerns about equalization of his leg lengths and resolution of his limp after HR.

Limb length is evaluated clinically by the spinomalleolar distance or the use of blocks under the affected limb, and radiographically by the perpendicular distance from the interteardrop line to the top of each lesser trochanter. The femoral offset is defined as the perpendicular distance from a line drawn in the center of the femoral canal to the center of rotation of the femoral head.

Relevance

Restoration of normal hip anatomy at hip arthroplasty is associated with improved outcome. Failure to restore the femoral offset is associated with a higher rate of impingement, dislocation, muscle weakness, limping, and bearing surfaces wear. Leg length discrepancy may lead to patient dissatisfaction, litigation, limp, and low back pain. HR should facilitate more precise biomechanical reconstruction of the hip.

Current opinion

Current opinion suggests that leg length equality and femoral offset restoration is more precise with HR.

Finding the evidence

• Cochrane Database with search term "hip resurfacing OR surface replacement arthroplasty" AND "total hip arthroplasty OR total hip replacement"
• PubMed (www.ncbi.nlm.nih.gov/pubmed) sensitivity search using key words: "hip resurfacing OR surface replacement arthroplasty" AND "biomechanical reconstruction OR femoral offset OR leg length"
• Embase with search term "hip resurfacing OR surface replacement arthroplasty" AND "biomechanical reconstruction OR femoral offset OR leg length"

Quality of the evidence

Level I
• 1 randomized trial

Level III
• 3 retrospective comparative studies

Findings

One RCT and two retrospective comparative studies described more precise biomechanical reconstruction after HR as compared to THA, whereas one retrospective study reported the opposite.[31-34]

Girard and colleagues studied 120 patients randomized for unilateral HR or THA.[31] When normal, the contralateral hip was used as a control. The postoperative femoral offset was restored within ±4 mm in 57% of those with HR and 25% of those with THA (p < 0.001). Leg length inequality was restored within ±4 mm in 86% of the HR and 60% of the THA patients (p = 0.002).

In a retrospective study comparing two groups of HR and hybrid THA, Ahmed and colleagues reported that HR restored the femoral offset more accurately and produced less change in leg length than THA.[32] The mean difference in femoral offset was −1.3 mm in the HR group and 3.5 mm in THA group (t 2.025, p < 0.05). The mean difference in leg length was 4.9 mm (95% CI 3.3–6.4 mm) in the HR group vs. 11.9 mm (95% CI 8.2–15.6 mm) in the THA group. (t 3.597, p < 0.001). Silva et al. compared 50 hips that had a HR with 40 THAs.[33] They concluded that restoration of leg length equality and femoral offset was more precise with HR provided that the preoperative difference was less than 1 cm.

Loughead and coworkers found significant reduction in femoral offset (from 49.4 mm preoperatively to 44.9 mm postoperatively) (p = 0.0004) and increase in length (3.7 mm preoperatively to 6.8 mm postoperatively) (p = 0.001) in 28 patients who had undergone HR, whereas femoral offset and overall hip length were accurately restored in 26 patients after hybrid THA.[34]

Recommendations

- HR has the potential to preserve femoral offset and leg length better than THA [overall quality: moderate]
- HR has less potential than THA for restoring normal biomechanics in subjects with significant preoperative deformed anatomy [overall quality: low]

Question 4: Does HR provide better clinical outcomes and activity level than THA?

Case clarification

The patient was told the choice of procedure was crucial as he would like to be able to perform martial arts and play competitive tennis after surgery.

Relevance

By preserving the proximal femoral anatomy (restoring precise hip biomechanics, using a large head diameter and providing more physiological mechanical loading), HR may potentially provide better clinical function than conventional THA.

Current opinion

Current opinion suggests that the level of activity after HR is higher than after THA.

Finding the evidence

- Cochrane Database with search term "hip resurfacing OR surface replacement arthroplasty" AND "total hip arthroplasty OR total hip replacement"
- PubMed (www.ncbi.nlm.nih.gov/pubmed) sensitivity search using key words: "hip resurfacing OR surface replacement arthroplasty" AND "total hip arthroplasty OR total hip replacement"
- Embase with search term "hip resurfacing OR surface replacement arthroplasty" AND "total hip arthroplasty OR total hip replacement"

Quality of the evidence

Level I
- 3 randomized trials

Level II
- 1 prospective comparative studies

Level III
- 6 retrospective comparative studies

Findings

Vendittoli et al. randomized 210 hips to receive a hybrid HR (109 hips) or 28 mm THA (100 hips).[21,22] A preliminary report showed no significant difference on the WOMAC and Merle d'Aubigné scores at 6 months.[35,36] In a recent follow-up evaluation, patients with HR achieved greater WOMAC functional scores by 3.3 points at 2 years follow-up (p = 0.007). However, the authors do not believe this difference to be clinically relevant.

With the same group of patients as Vendittoli's study, Lavigne and colleagues compared a subgroup of 81 HRs with 71 THAs to assess type, intensity, and frequency of sports activities performed after each procedure.[37] They did not find significant difference in the overall activity score and UCLA score between the groups at 1 year after surgery.[38] The degree and intensity of postoperative sporting activities were greater in the HR group although the difference was not significant.

In a prospective comparative study, Fowble and coworkers found higher function score (Harris Hip Score (HHS) minus the pain, deformity, and range of motion components), SF-12 physical activity score, and UCLA scores in HR patients.[12] However, the authors believed that patients undergoing resurfacing were younger, in better general health, and had higher preoperative UCLA scores than patients who underwent THA.

We found six retrospective studies comparing clinical outcomes after HR and THA. Five studies described similar clinical scores,[24,39–42] whereas one showed higher HHS in HR.[23] Four studies found higher activity levels after HR[23,24,39,42] while the other two could not demonstrate a difference.[40,41] (Table 16.1)

In a double-blind RCT of HR vs. LDH-THA, Lavigne and coworkers did not find any difference in the WOMAC and UCLA scores.[25] Similarly, Garbuz and colleagues prospectively randomized 104 patients to undergo either HR or LDH-THA.[43] At 1 year follow-up, they did not find any difference between two groups in the PAT-5D (Paper Adaptive Test in five domains of Quality of Life in Arthritis Questionnaire), WOMAC, and UCLA scores.

Recommendations

- Controversies persist regarding the clinical outcome and activity level after HR and conventional THA, although most studies favorable to HR included a bias in patient selection. The only RCT of HR and conventional THA found a difference in WOMAC score that was not clinically relevant and no difference in UCLA score [overall quality: low]
- Clinical outcomes and level of activity after HR and LDH-THA are similar [overall quality: moderate]

Question 5: Does HR offer greater range of hip motion than THA?

Case clarification

On clinical examination, the patient has hip flexion of 100°, abduction 15°, adduction 5°, external rotation 15°, and internal rotation 5°. Since the patient would like to perform

Table 16.1 Summary of clinical outcomes

Study	Level of evidence	Procedure	No. of patients (hips)	Follow-up (months)	Mean clinical scores in points (range)	Conclusion
Pollard et al. 2006	III	HR	54(54)	61	OHS(15.9 (12–42) UCLA 8.4 (4–10)	Similar Oxford hip scores. Resurfacing associated with higher activity levels
		THA	54 (54)	80	OHS: 18.5 (12–41) UCLA: 6.8 (3–10)	
Vail et al. 2006	III	HR	52(57))	36	HHS: 98 Activity subscore: 14	RHA associated with significantly higher HHS, ROM subscore, activity subscore, and function subscore
		THA	84(93	36	HHS: 93 Activity score: 12.7	
Vendittoli et al. 2006	I	HR	103 (hips)	12	WOMAC: 9.2 P-M: 16.7 UCLA: 7.1	Significantly higher activity level in HR group (p = 0.037)
		THA	102 (hips)	12	WOMAC: 11.7, P-M: 16.6, UCLA: 6.3	
Girard et al. 2008	II	HR	69		P-M: 17 ± 0.35 WOMAC: 9.2 ± 15.1	Similar clinical scores
		THA	79		P-M: 17 ± 0.4 WOMAC: 11.7 ± 11.4	
Lavigne et al. 2008	II	HR	81 (81)	12	Overall activity: 17.9 points WOMAC: 8.1 ± 13.1 points UCLA: 7.17 ± 2.8 points	Preoperative activity scores of the two groups were similar. RHA associated with more frequent and more intense sports activities postoperatively
		THA	71 (71)	12	Overall activity: 12.7 points WOMAC: 9.8 ±10.9 points UCLA: 6.75 ± 1.71 points	
Mont et al. 2009	III	HR	54 (54)	39	HHS: 90 (50–100) Satisfaction: 9.2 (2–10) Activity: 11.7 (0–32)	Midterm clinical outcomes and satisfaction scores similar. HR patients had higher activity scores, but also had higher preoperative activity scores
		THA	54 (54)	39	HHS: 91 (62–100) Satisfaction: 8.8 (0–10) Activity: 7 (0–20)	
Shrader et al. 2009	II	HR	7 (7)	3	LEAS: 12.6 HHS: 92.4 (better ROM scores with HR)	Better functional capability with HR. Greater improvements in hip extension and abduction moment after HR
		THA	7 (7)	3	LEAS: 11.5 HHS: 90.4	
Le Duff et al. 2009	III	HR	35(35)	88	UCLA pain score: 9 (7–10)	No difference in clinical scores
		THA	35(35)	96	UCLA pain score: 9 (4–10)	

Table 16.1 (*Continued*)

Study	Level of evidence	Procedure	No. of patients (hips)	Follow-up (months)	Mean clinical scores in points (range)	Conclusion
Fowble et al. 2009	II	HR	50(50)	24	HHS: 97 (81–100) UCLA: 8.2 (4–10) SF-12 Physical score 53.6(36.9–63) SF-12 Mental score 54.6 (26.7–61.7) Function: 46.4 (42–47) Pain: (Slight/Mild): 43%	HR patients had higher function (p = 0.007),SF-12 physical activity scores (p = 0.002) and UCLA activity scores (p = 0.0001), but also a higher incidence of slight or mild pain (p = 0.007)
		THA	35 (44)	24	HHS: 96 (66–100) UCLA: 5.9 (3–10) SF-12 Physical score 47 (15.2–57.6) SF-12 Mental score 52.5 (32.1–66.6) Function: 44.9 (36–47) Pain: (Slight/Mild): 20%	
Lavigne et al. 2009	I	HR	24(24)	12	WOMAC: 3 (0–12), P-M: 17.9 (16–18), UCLA: 8 (5–10) SF-36 Mental Score : 51.9 (45–60) SF-36 Physical score: 55.2 (48–62)	Clinical scores are similar
		THA	24(24)	12	WOMAC: 2.7 (0–16), P-M: 18 (18), UCLA: 8.3 (6–10) SF-36 Mental Score: 52.1 (36–65) SF-36 Physical score 53.3 (53–70)	
Garbuz et al. 2009	I	HR	48	12	WOMAC Pain: 91.51 Stiffness: 85.60 Function: 90.64 Global: 90.40 SF-36 Physical score 51.22 SF-36 Mental score 53.87	Clinical scores are similar. No difference in PAT-5D ambulation domain scores between two groups
		THA	56	12	WOMAC Pain: 90 Stiffness: 83 Function: 91.07 Global: 90.18 SF-36 Physical Score 51.28 SF-36 Mental Score 55.13	
Stulberg et al. 2009	III	HR	337	24	Total HHS (% of patients in excellent category): 91.3 HHS Pain score: (% of patients having no pain): 80.6	Early advantages in HHS observed in HR group, but all differences faded by 24 months. Ability to climb stair is the only subcomponent that is higher in HR group at 24 months
		THA	266	24	Total HHS (% of patients in excellent category): 91.1 HHS Pain score: (% of patients having no pain): 76.3	

(*Continued*)

Table 16.1 (*Continued*)

Study	Level of evidence	Procedure	No. of patients (hips)	Follow-up (months)	Mean clinical scores in points (range)	Conclusion
Zywiek et al. 2009	III	HR	33	42	Weighted Activity Score: 10.0 (1.0–27.5) HHS: 91 (32–100) Satisfaction Score: 9.1 (5–10) Pain Score: 1.3 (0–10)	Activity levels were significantly higher in the HR group(p < 0.001)
		THA	33	45	Weighted Activity Score: 5.3 (0–12.0) HHS: 90 (50–100) Satisfaction Score: 9.1 (2–10) Pain Score: 1.2 (0–5)	

martial arts after surgery, you explain him about expected improvement in range of motion (ROM) after HR vs. THA.

Relevance

ROM after hip arthroplasty is becoming an important issue, as patients present at a younger age and are willing to return to a high level of activity. The larger head diameter of HR is theoretically beneficial for improving hip ROM, although the larger neck diameter is unfavorable for the head to neck diameter ratio.

Current opinion

Current opinion suggests that the use of a larger head size in HR may provide greater clinical ROM compared to 28 mm THA.

Finding the evidence

- Cochrane Database with search term "hip resurfacing" or "surface replacement arthroplasty"
- PubMed (www.ncbi.nlm.nih.gov/pubmed) sensitivity search using key words: "hip resurfacing or surface replacement arthroplasty" AND "range of motion"
- Embase with search term "hip resurfacing or surface replacement arthroplasty" AND "range of motion"

Quality of the evidence

Level III

- 6 retrospective comparative studies

Findings

Six retrospective studies have compared ROM between HR and THA. LeDuff et al. reviewed 35 patients who had undergone bilateral surgery with HR on one side and THA on the other.[40] They found no difference in any of the ROM measurements even after separating the cohort into two groups based on femoral head size of the THA (<40 mm

and ≥40 mm). Fowble et al. compared 50 HR with 44 THA procedures at a minimum follow-up of 2 years, and found no significant difference in the postoperative range of motion between the two groups.[12] However, the patients undergoing THA started with less ROM and had greater postoperative improvements in flexion, extension, and abduction.

Stulberg et al. compared Harris hip ROM score in 337 HR arthroplasties with 266 ceramic-on-ceramic THAs and found that although the THA group demonstrated greater flexion value, the resurfacing group showed slightly better results in abduction, adduction and internal rotation.[41] Therefore, overall arc of motion at 24 months was similar between the two groups.

Li and colleagues measured ROM after HR and ceramic-on-ceramic THA in two groups of 21 patients, each with osteoarthritis secondary to hip dysplasia, and found significantly better ROM in the HR group (p < 0.05).[44]

In another study comparing clinical outcome of HR vs. THA, the HR group exhibited significantly greater total ROM at 2 years (99° vs. 97°, p < 0.001).[23] The authors believed that since the examiners were not blinded they may have been more reluctant to force extreme ROM in the THA group for fear of causing dislocation. It is important to note that a difference of 2° in ROM is clinically insignificant.

Lavigne et al. performed hip ROM measurements in 165 patients (LDH-THA, n = 55; THA, n = 50; and HR, n = 60) at minimum 1 year follow-up with a novel standardized method of hip ROM assessment.[45] They found similar hip ROM in THA and HR. LDH-THA demonstrated a significant 20° increase in the total arc of hip ROM (p = 0.001).

Recommendations

- There is no difference in the postoperative ROM between HR and THA [overall quality: low]

- A greater hip ROM was observed with LDH-THA compared to 28 mm THA or HR [overall quality: low]

Question 6: Do patients have better gait and postural balance after HR?

Case clarification

The patient now walks slowly with a mild lurch on the affected side. He inquires about improvement in gait after hip arthroplasty.

Relevance

Gait and postural balance analysis can detect subtle differences in functional outcome after hip arthroplasty.[46] By conserving parts of femoral head and neck, HR has been considered to better preserve hip anatomy. Whether or not this leads to better gait or postural balance parameters is a matter of debate.

Current opinion

Current opinion suggests that gait and postural balance after HR are better than after THA.

Finding the evidence

- Cochrane Database with search term "hip resurfacing OR surface replacement arthroplasty" AND "total hip arthroplasty OR total hip replacement"
- PubMed (www.ncbi.nlm.nih.gov/pubmed) sensitivity search using key words: "hip resurfacing OR surface replacement arthroplasty" AND "gait OR posture"
- Embase with search term "hip resurfacing OR surface replacement arthroplasty" AND "gait OR posture"

Quality of the evidence

Level I
- 1 randomized trial

Level II
- 1 prospective comparative study

Level III
- 1 systematic review of retrospective comparative studies
- 1 retrospective comparative study

Findings

Gait analysis In a prospective pilot study, Shrader et al. compared Lower Extremity Activity Scale (LEAS), gait parameters (maximum hip abduction, maximum hip abduction moment, step width, walking speed, and stride length) and HHS in 7 patients each with HR and THA (with 36 mm head).[47] At 3 months postoperatively, the HR group had greater improvements in hip extension and abduction moment, indicating a more normalized loading of the hip.

In a systematic review comparing HR vs. conventional THA, Marker et al. included three gait studies.[48] The first one was a retrospective gender-matched study by Mont and colleagues. The study found at a mean 13-month follow-up that patients in the HR group walked faster than patients in either THA or control groups. However, there were no significant differences in hip abductor and extensor moments of patients in those two groups. Lavigne and coworkers examined the distribution of energy generation and absorption in three groups of patients: HR, THA with large-diameter heads and THA with small-diameter heads. They found that patients who received HR and LDH-THA returned to more normal gait patterns than patients who had small-diameter femoral heads. Shimmin and associates compared HR and THA patients who had HHS of 100 to age-matched asymptomatic control patients. They reported no significant difference in gait speed at either fast walking or jogging paces among any of the groups.

Lavigne et al. analysed gait speed and postural balance after HR and LDH-THA in a prospectively randomized double-blind study of 48 patients.[25] A third group of 14 healthy subjects served as control. During normal and fast walking and for postural evaluation, both study groups showed similar postoperative results at 12 months. The time period needed for both groups of patients to reach the normal control subject's value for each functional test was 3 months, except for the normal walking speed of the HR group, which reached the control value at 6 months postoperatively.

The postural balance study by Nantel and colleagues reported that THA had greater medial to lateral centers of pressure and mass displacement during dual stance when compared to HR ($p < 0.05$).[49] The authors attributed the difference to better anatomical preservation, absence of femoral stem, and the larger bearing component in HR.

Recommendations

- Gait speed is greater and postural balance seems better after HR than after THA [overall quality: low]
- There is no difference in gait pattern and postural balance after HR and LDH-THA [overall quality: low]

Question 7: Is there any difference between procedures in the rate of complication?

Case clarification

The patient is concerned about neck fracture of HR and risk of dislocation of THA when performing martial arts.

Relevance

Complications such as femoral neck fracture and avascular necrosis of femoral head are unique to HR. The types and rate of complication seen after both procedures should be compared to assess the benefit of HR.

Current opinion

It is believed that HR has a higher rate of early complications than THA.

Finding the evidence

• Cochrane Database with search term "hip resurfacing" OR "surface replacement arthroplasty" AND " total hip arthroplasty OR total hip replacement"
• PubMed (www.ncbi.nlm.nih.gov/pubmed) sensitivity search using key words: "hip resurfacing" OR "surface replacement arthroplasty" AND "complications"
• Embase with search term "hip resurfacing" OR "surface replacement arthroplasty" AND "complications"

Quality of the evidence

Level I
• 2 randomized trials

Level III
• 5 retrospective comparative studies
• 1 cohort study

Findings

The findings are summarized in Table 16.2.

Postoperative femoral neck/shaft fracture Vendittoli et al. did not have any femoral neck fracture in an RCT comparing HR with THA.[21,22]

Three retrospective comparative studies reported the incidence of femoral neck fracture after HR and femoral shaft fracture after THA.[23,24,42] Pollard and colleagues described a 5.5% rate of femoral neck fracture after 54 HRs and no fracture after 54 THAs.[42] Vail and colleagues reported femoral neck fracture rate of 1.92% after HR and femoral shaft fracture in two patients after THA (2.4%).[23] In a series of 54 HRs, Mont et al. described one (1.9%) traumatic femoral neck fracture while no fracture occurred in a comparative group of 54 THA patients.[24]

A multisurgeon national audit of 3429 HRs performed in Australia over a 4 year period demonstrated a fracture rate of 1.46%:[18] 1.91% for women and 0.98% for men. The relative risk of fracture for women vs. men was 1.94961 and this was statistically significant (p < 0.01).

Dislocation In an RCT, Vendittoli and colleagues reported 0% dislocation rate in their HR group compared to 3% in the THA group.[21,22]

Three retrospective comparative studies compared dislocation rate after HR and THA. Pollard et al. reported a

dislocation rate of 7.4% amongst 54 patients post-THA while none occurred in 54 HR patients.[42] Vail and coworkers described similar findings; four dislocations (4.3%) in the THA group and none in the HR group.[23] Fowble and colleagues had one posterior dislocation in each group (44 THAs, 50 HRs).[12]

No dislocation was observed in two randomized studies comparing LDH-THA with HR (Lavigne, HR 24 vs. THA 24; Garbuz, HR 48 vs. THA 56).[25,43]

Heterotopic ossification One randomized study and three retrospective studies discussed heterotopic ossification (HO) after HR and. THA. Vendittoli and colleagues evaluated incidence and severity of HO as part of an RCT.[50] The incidence of HO was 43.7% in the HR group compared to 30.9% in the THA group (p = 0.057). The HR group had a significantly higher rate of severe HO (Brooker grades 3–4) than THA (12.6% vs. 2.1%, p = 0.02).[51] In a study by Fowble and colleagues, Brooker grade I or II HO occurred in 10 HR hips (20%) and four THAs (9.1%).[12] Two resurfaced hips had Grade III HO. There was no difference in the incidence of HO in two other retrospective studies of HR and THA.[24,40]

Other complications Aseptic loosening of the femoral component of HR was reported by three studies, but no loosening of femoral component of THA was found in any of those studies.[12,21,42] One randomized study and three retrospective studies reported incidence of infection after THA and HR. While three studies found no significant difference, Vendittoli observed five deep infections in THA and none in HR.[21,23,24,42] Differences were found in the incidences of venous thromboembolic events and nerve palsy, but without statistical significance.[12,21,23,42]

Recommendations

• The incidence of femoral neck fracture after HR is 0–5% with an average of 1.5% [overall quality: moderate]
• THA has a higher rate of dislocation than HR. The dislocation rates for HR and LDH-THA are similar [overall quality: moderate]
• The incidence of HO is higher after HR than after THA [overall quality: moderate]
• There seems to be no difference between HR and THA in the rate of infection, nerve injury, and thromboembolic events [overall quality: moderate]

Question 8: What level of metal ion release is seen after HR and metal-on-metal THA?

Case clarification

The patient wonders about possibility of metal ion release and its consequences after HR.

Table 16.2 Comparison of complications after HR and THA

Study	Procedure	No of patients (hips)	Follow-up (months)	Revision/ awaiting revision	Intraoperative fracture	Postop. femoral neck /shaft fracture	Infection	HO	Aseptic loosening (femur)	Nerve palsy	Dislocation	DVT/ PE	Other
Pollard et al. 2006	HR	54 (54)	61	4		3	1		1		0	2/1	1[a]
	THA	54 (54)	80	4			3			1	4	2/1	
Vail et al. 2006	HR	52 (57)	36	2		1	1					1	
	THA	84(93)	36	4	3[b]	2	0				4	3	
Vendittoli et al. 2006/	HR	103	12	2	2[d]		0	44	2	1		2	
Rama et al. 2008[c]	THA	102	12	1	4[b]		2	30		2	3	2	
Mont et al 2009	HR	54 (54)	39	2		1	0	1					1[e]
	THA	54 (54)	39	2		—	1	1					1[e]
LeDuff et al. 2009	HR	35 (35)	88	—		—	—	7					
	THA	35 (35)	96	—		—	—	9					
Fowble et al. 2009	HR	50 50	24	1		—	—	10	1	1	1		
	THA	35 (44)	24	0		—	—	4	—	—	1		
Lavigne et al. 2009	THA	24(24)	12	—	—	—	—	—	—	—	—		1[f]
	HR	24 (24)	12	—	3	—	—	—	—	—	—		1[g]

[a] Psoas impingement.
[b] Calcar cracks.
[c] These two papers are from a single randomized controlled trial.
[d] Intraoperative acetabular fissure.
[e] Acetabular cup loosening.
[f] Myocardial infarction.
[g] Obturator artery injury.

Relevance

> Currently available metal-on-metal articulations are made of cobalt and chromium alloys. Metal ions are released as a result of combined effect of bearing surfaces wear and implant corrosion. Normal serum levels are 0.1–0.2 µg/L for chromium and less than 0.1 µg/L for cobalt.[52,53]

Metal-on-metal bearing wear and implant corrosion generate insoluble metal particles and soluble metal ions, the later passing into the systemic circulation.[54] Concerns exist over metal hypersensitivity, osteolysis, chromosomal mutation, carcinogenicity, and fetal exposure to elevated ion levels.[55] This has prevented broader application of metal-on-metal arthroplasty to some extent.

Current opinion

Current opinion suggests the amount of metal ions released after HR is similar to THA.

Finding the evidence

- Cochrane Database with search term "hip resurfacing" AND "surface replacement arthroplasty"
- PubMed (www.ncbi.nlm.nih.gov/pubmed) sensitivity search using key words: "hip resurfacing OR surface replacement arthroplasty" AND "metal ions" as well as "total hip replacement AND metal ions"
- Embase with search term "hip resurfacing OR surface replacement arthroplasty" AND "metal ions" as well as "total hip replacement AND metal ions"

Quality of the evidence

Level I
- 2 randomized trials

Level II
- 2(?) prospective comparative studies

Level III
- 5 retrospective comparative studies

Findings

Hip resurfacing vs. 28 mm head THA Vendittoli et al. compared postoperative chromium, cobalt, and titanium concentrations in 117 patients THA with metal-on-metal articulation and HR.[56] Significantly higher chromium and cobalt levels were found at 3 months in the HR group than in the THA group. No significant difference was found at 2 year postoperative follow-up: THA = 1.62 µg/L and HR = 1.58 µg/L for chromium (p = 0.819) and THA = 0.94 µg/L and HR = 0.67 µg/L for cobalt (p = 0.207).

Antoniou and coworkers compared metal ion levels among patients with a metal-on-metal THA with either a 28 mm (Metasul, Zimmer, Warsaw, USA) or 36 mm (Ultamet Depuy Orthopaedics, Warsaw, IN) femoral head diameter and patients with HR prosthesis (ASR, Depuy Orthopaedics, Warsaw, USA).[57] Neither the median (whole blood) cobalt level nor the median chromium levels were significantly different among the three groups at 1 year.

In retrospective studies using various implants, Clarke et al. and Witzleb et al. found significantly higher serum levels of cobalt and chromium in the HR group.[58,59] Moroni et al. found no difference in ion levels between HR and THA patients.[60] Similarly, Daniel and colleagues found no significant difference in the values of cobalt and chromium in serum and urine of two groups.[61]

HR vs. LDH-THA Garbuz et al. measured chromium and cobalt ions in 26 of 107 patients randomized to a LDH-THA (Durom LDH system, Zimmer, Warsaw, IN) or HR (Durom system, Zimmer, Warsaw, IN).[43] At 1 year after surgery the median serum level for cobalt was 10-fold higher (p = 0.000) and median serum chromium level was 2.6 fold higher (p = 0.023) in the LDH-THA group than in the HR group.

Vendittoli et al. reported on chromium, cobalt, and titanium ion levels in whole blood in subjects with LDH-THA and HR (Durom LDH-THA and HR systems, Zimmer, Warsaw, IN).[62] They found significantly higher cobalt levels in LDH-THA (2.2 µg/L vs. 0.7 µg/L, p < 0.001) at 1 year follow-up. They demonstrated that the addition of a sleeve with modular junctions and an open femoral head design of LDH-THA were significant sources of ion release.

Recommendations

Comparison of the data reported in the literature is complicated by differences in sampling (whole blood, serum, erythrocytes or urine), measurements with various technologies in different laboratories, type of data reported (mean or median, different units of measurement, compared or not to preoperative levels), and different types of implant combinations.

- Durom LDH-THA showed significantly higher cobalt ion release as compared to the Durom HR [overall quality: good]
- The cobalt and chromium ion release after HR and 28 mm THA has shown contradictory results depending on the type of implants studied [overall quality: good]

Question 9: Which procedure has higher failure rate: HR or THA?

Case clarification

The patient's radiograph shows a 1.5 cm cyst in the femoral head and this, combined with his activity level, produces a Surface Arthroplasty Risk Index (SARI) of 3.

The Surface Arthroplasty Risk Index (SARI) was developed by Beaule and Antoniades.[63] It is based on a 6-point scoring system:
- Femoral head cyst >1 cm = 2 points
- Weight <82 kg = 2 points
- Previous hip surgery = 1 point
- University of California (UCLA) activity score >6 = 1 point
  A SARI score greater than 3 represents a 12-fold increase risk in early failure or adverse radiographic changes.

Relevance

With newer bearing surfaces and better fixation options, the results of modern cementless THA in young patients are quite encouraging.[20] At the same time, survival rates for HR are improving as surgeons have moved beyond their learning curves and refined their techniques.[24]

Current opinion

Current opinion suggests that HR has higher early failure rate than THA.

Finding the evidence

- Cochrane Database with search term "hip resurfacing OR surface replacement arthroplasty" AND "total hip arthroplasty OR total hip replacement"
- PubMed (www.ncbi.nlm.nih.gov/pubmed) sensitivity search using key words: "hip resurfacing OR surface replacement arthroplasty" AND "total hip arthroplasty OR total hip replacement"
- Embase with search term "hip resurfacing OR surface replacement arthroplasty" AND "total hip arthroplasty OR total hip replacement"

Quality of the evidence

Level I
- 1 randomized trial

Level II
- Report of the AJRR (2009)

Level III
- 5 retrospective comparative studies
- 1 meta-analysis

Findings

Springers and colleagues performed a meta-analysis of modern cementless femoral components in young patients (mean age < 55 years) having HR or THA.[20] Fifteen studies on HR (n = 3002; hips = 3269) and 22 studies (n = 5907; hips = 6408) on THA were included. At a mean of 3.9 years of follow-up, the pooled mechanical failure rate of the femoral component for HR was 2.6% (95% CI 2.0–3.4%); it accounted for 70% of all failures of HR. The most common

reasons were femoral neck fracture and aseptic loosening of the femoral component. The pooled failure rate for THA using femoral revision for mechanical failure as an endpoint was 1.3% (95% CI 1.0–1.7%) at a mean 8.4 years of follow-up. The pooled acetabular and overall failure rate (using failure for any reason as criteria) were respectively 2.8 % (2.0–3.9%) and 4.6% (95% CI 3.7–5.6) for HR at a mean average follow-up of 3.9 years and. 14.1% (95% CI 13.1–15.2%) and 16.1% (95% CI 14.9–17.3%) for THA at a mean average follow-up 8.5 years.

The annual report of the AJRR (2009) reported that HR had a significantly higher revision rate than THA (hazard ratio adjusted for age and sex) (adj HR) = 1.37; 95% CI (1.22, 1.55), p < 0.001).[15] At 8 years the cumulative revision is 5.3% for HR compared to 4% for THA. The most common type of revision in HR group was a "femoral component only revision" and was most often undertaken for femoral neck fracture. There was no significant difference in the risk of revision for THA with respect to gender, whereas for HR women had a significantly higher rate of revision. The risk of revision also increased with increasing age in HR population. The registry reported an inverse relationship between the femoral component head size and the risk of revision.

In a randomized study, Vendittoli et al. reported similar rate of reoperations in HR group (four revisions for femoral aseptic loosening, one excision of HO, and one osteoplasty for femoro-acetabular impingement) and THA (one revision for chronic deep infection, one revision for recurrent dislocation, four debridement for early deep infection, and one distal femoral shortening osteotomy for symptomatic leg length discrepancy).[22] Pollard et al. reported 4 revisions (out of 63 HR) for failure of femoral component and 4 in THA (3 for osteolysis and 1 for recurrent dislocation).[42] Vail and colleagues described two reoperations in the HR group (one for fracture of femoral neck and one for deep infection) and two in the THA group (reasons not specified).[23] Fowble also reported one revision in the HR group for femoral neck fracture and none in the THA group.[12] Mont and colleagues reported two revisions in the HR group (one for neck fracture and one for displaced acetabular socket) and two in the THA group (one for acetabular loosening and one for infection).[24]

Recommendations

- Aseptic loosening of femoral component and femoral neck fracture are the two common modes of failure of HR, which accounts for a higher failure rate of the femoral component of HR vs. THA [overall quality: high]
- Female gender and increasing age have higher risk of revision for HR as compared to males [overall quality: moderate]
- Rates of reoperation seem similar, but reasons for reoperation differ between HR and THA [overall quality: moderate]

Question 10: Is HR revision surgery easier than revision of THA, and does it provide better outcomes?

Case clarification

The patient is aware that revision surgery will likely occur eventually because he is relatively young. He wants to know how complicated the revision surgery will be after HR in comparison to THA.

Relevance

One likely advantage of HR is preservation of the proximal femur since failed femoral components can easily be revised with a primary femoral stem as the femoral canal is not violated during the index procedure.

Current opinion

Current opinion supports easier revisability of HR compared to THA.

Finding the evidence

• Cochrane Database with search term "hip resurfacing OR surface replacement arthroplasty" AND "total hip arthroplasty OR total hip replacement"
• PubMed (www.ncbi.nlm.nih.gov/pubmed) sensitivity search using key words: "hip resurfacing OR surface replacement arthroplasty" AND "revision"
• Embase with search term "hip resurfacing OR surface replacement arthroplasty" AND "revision"

Quality of the evidence

Level II
• Report of the AJRR (2009)

Level III
• 2 retrospective comparative studies

Findings

The Australian Joint Replacement Registry reported the risk of subsequent revision following the first revision of HR and primary conventional THA.[15] They report that 3 years after the first revision for THA and 5 years after for HR, the cumulative percentage for a major total (both femoral and acetabular) revision is 5.3% for HR and 9.2% for THA.

Two studies have compared the outcomes of failed HR procedures converted to conventional THAs with patients who had primary conventional THA.[64,65] Ball and colleagues compared revisions of 21 HR (in 20 patients) to a group of 58 hips (in 64 patients) who had undergone primary THA, all by the same surgeon.[64] They found no significant difference between the groups in terms of operative blood loss, operative time, or complication rate. At mean follow-up times of 46 months for the HR group and

57 months for the THA group, there were no significant differences in the HHS, UCLA pain, walking, or activity subscores, or the SF-12 scores.

McGrath and associates compared the perioperative factors, complications, and clinical and radiographic outcomes of 39 patients whose resurfacings were converted to THA to a group of THA patients matched by gender, age, BMI, and preoperative HHS, all performed by the same surgeon.[65] They found mean operative time for HR conversions were longer by 19 minutes, but all other perioperative measures were similar. At a mean follow-up of 45 months, the HHS of the two groups were similar.

Recommendations

• Clinical outcome of revision after a failed HR is comparable to that of a primary THA [overall quality: low]
• Re-revision rate after first revision seems lower for HR than for THA [overall quality: low]

Summary of recommendations

• HR requires more extensile exposure than THA but there is conflicting evidence regarding duration of surgery, blood loss, and duration of hospitalization after HR and THA
• The rate of perioperative complication is similar, but the types of complication are different for HR and THA
• Removal of acetabular bone during HR may be comparable, or slightly greater, to that of conventional THA
• Implant design (femoral head size increment and acetabular component thickness) and surgical technique play a crucial role in acetabular bone removal
• Hip resurfacing has the potential to better restore femoral offset and leg length as compared to THA, but has less capacity to correct severe deformities
• Controversy persists regarding clinical outcomes and level of activity after HR and THA, but was found to be similar after HR and LDH-THA
• No difference in hip ROM was found between HR and THA. A greater hip ROM has been observed with LDH-THA compared to HR or THA
• Gait speed is greater and postural balance seems better after HR when compared to THA; but is similar to LDH-THA
• Incidence of femoral neck fracture after HR is 0–5%; HR has higher rate of HO and lower rate of dislocation than conventional THA
• Durom LDH-THA showed significantly higher cobalt ion release as compared to the Durom HR
• The release of cobalt and chromium ion after HR and THA has shown contradictory results depending on the type of implants studied
• Higher rate of early femoral component failure has been found in HR as compared to THA

- Female gender and increasing age have higher risk of revision for HR as compared to males
- Rates of reoperation seem similar, but reasons for reoperation differ between HR and THA
- Clinical outcome of revision after a failed HR is comparable to that of a primary THA

Conclusions

The existing evidence does not clearly suggest that HR provide superior clinical outcomes to conventional THA. Preservation of proximal femoral bone can be a distinct advantage of HR, provided complications such as femoral neck fracture and avascular necrosis can be prevented. RCTs with long-term follow-up would be valuable to prove superiority of one procedure over the other.

References

1. Crock HV. An Atlas of Vascular Anatomy of the Skeleton and Spinal Cord. Martin Dunitz, London, 1996.
2. Chung SMK. The arterial supply of the developing proximal end of the human femur. J Bone Joint Surg Am 1976;58(7):961–70.
3. Notzli HP, Siebenrock KA, Hempfing A, et al. Perfusion of the femoral head during surgical dislocation of the hip. Monitoring by laser Doppler flowmetry. J Bone Joint Surg Br 2002;84(2):300–4.
4. Ogden JA. Changing patterns of proximal femoral vascularity. J Bone Joint Surg Am 1974;56(5):941–50.
5. Lavigne M, Kalhor M, Beck M, et al. Distribution of vascular foramina around the femoral head and neck junction: relevance for conservative intracapsular procedures of the hip. Orthop Clin N Am 2005;36:171–6.
6. Clarke, I.C. Symposium on Surface Replacement Arthroplasty of the Hip. Biomechanics: multifactorial design choices—an essential compromise? Orthop Clin North Am 1982;13:681–707.
7. Beaule, P.E., Harvey, N., Zaragoza, E et al. The femoral head/neck offset and hip resurfacing. J Bone Joint Surg Br 2007;89:9–15.
8. Vendittoli P-A, Ganpathi M, Nuno N, et al. Factors affecting hip range of motion in surface replacement arthroplasty. Clin Biomechanics 2007;22:1004–12.
9. Malchau H, Herberts P, Eisler T et al. The Swedish Total Hip Replacement Register. J Bone Joint Surg Am 2002;84 (suppl 2):S2–20.
10. Canadian Institute for Health Information. Hip and Knee Replacements in Canada. Canadian Joint Replacement Registry (CJRR) 2008–2009 Annual Report. CIHI, Ottawa, 2009.
11. Learmonth ID, Young C, Rorabeck C. The operation of the century: total hip replacement. Lancet 2007;370:1508–19.
12. Fowble VA, de la Rosa MA, Schmalzried TP. A comparison of total hip resurfacing and total hip arthroplasty—patients and outcomes. Bull N Y U Hosp Jt Dis 2009;67(2):108–12.
13. Loughead JM, Starks I, Chesney D, et al. Removal of acetabular bone in resurfacing arthroplasty of the hip: a comparison with hybrid total hip arthroplasty. J Bone Joint Surg Br 2006;88(1):31–4.
14. Havelin LI, Fenstad AM, Salomonsson R, et al. The Nordic Arthroplasty Register Association. Acta Orthop 2009;80(4):393–401.
15. Australian Orthopaedic Association National Joint Replacement Registry. Annual Report. AOA, Adelaide, 2010.
16. Thomas BJ, Amstutz HC. Revision surgery for failed surface arthroplasty of the hip. Clin Orthop Relat Res 1982;170:42–9.
17. Beaule PE, Dorey FJ, LeDuff M, et al. Risk factors affecting outcome of metal-on-metal surface arthroplasty of the hip. Clin Orthop Relat Res 2004;418:87–93.
18. Shimmin AJ, Back D. Femoral neck fractures following Birmingham hip resurfacing: a national review of 50 cases. J Bone Joint Surg Br 2005;87:463–4.
19. Morlock MM, Bishop N, Ruther W, et al. Biomechanical, morphological, and histological analysis of early failures in hip resurfacing arthroplasty. Proc Inst Mech Eng [H] 2006;220:333–44.
20. Springer BD, Connelly SE, Odum SM, et al. Cementless femoral component in young patients : review and meta-analysis of total hip arthroplasty and hip resurfacing. J Arthroplasty 2009;24(6 Suppl 1).
21. Vendittoli PA, Lavigne M, Roy AG et al. A prospective randomized clinical trial comparing metal-on-metal total hip arthroplasty and metal-on-metal total hip resurfacing in patients less than 65 years old. Hip Int 2006;16 (Suppl 4):73–81.
22. Vendittoli PA, Ganapathi M, Roy AG, Lusignan D, Lavigne M. A comparison of clinical results of hip resurfacing arthroplasty and 28 mm metal on metal total hip arthroplasty: a randomised trial with 3–6 years follow-up. Hip Int 2010;20(1):1–13.
23. Vail TP, Mina CA, Yergler JD, et al. Metal-on-metal hip resurfacing compares favorably with THA at 2 years follow-up. Clin Orthop Relat Res 2006;453:123–31.
24. Mont MA, Marker DR, Smith JM et al. Resurfacing is comparable to total hip arthroplasty at short-term follow-up. Clin Orthop Relat Res 2009;467:66–71.
25. Lavigne M, Therrien M, Nantel J, et al. The functional outcome of hip resurfacing and large-head THA is the same: a randomized, double-blind study. Clin Orthop Relat Res 2010;468(2):326–36.
26. Vendittoli PA, Lavigne M, Girard J, et al. A randomised study comparing resection of acetabular bone at resurfacing and total hip replacement. J Bone Joint Surg Br 2006;88(8):997–1002.
27. Brennan SA, Harty JA, Gormley C, et al. Comparison of acetabular reamings during hip resurfacing vs. uncemented total hip arthroplasty. J Orthop Surg (Hong Kong) 2009;17(1):42–6.
28. Loughead JM, Starks I, Chesney D, et al. Removal of acetabular bone in resurfacing arthroplasty of the hip: a comparison with hybrid total hip arthroplasty. J Bone Joint Surg Br 2006;88(1):31–4.
29. Naal FD, Kain MS, Hersche O, et al. Does hip resurfacing require larger acetabular cups than conventional THA? Clin Orthop Relat Res 2009;467(4):923–8.
30. Moonot P, Singh PJ, Cronin MD, et al. Birmingham hip resurfacing: is acetabular bone conserved? J Bone Joint Surg Br 2008;90(3):319–23.
31. Girard J, Lavigne M, Vendittoli PA, et al. Biomechanical reconstruction of the hip: a randomised study comparing total hip resurfacing and total hip arthroplasty. J Bone Joint Surg Br 2006;88(6):721–6.

32. Ahmad R, Gillespie G, Annamalai S, et al. Leg length and offset following hip resurfacing and hip replacement. Hip Int 2009;9(2):136–40.

33. Silva M, Lee KH, Heisel C, et al. The biomechanical results of total hip resurfacing arthroplasty. J Bone Joint Surg Am 2004;86: 40–6.

34. Loughead JM, Chesney D, Holland JP, et al. Comparison of offset in Birmingham hip resurfacing and hybrid total hip arthroplasty. J Bone Joint Surg Br 2005;87(2):163–6.

35. Bellamy N, Buchanan WW, Goldsmith CH, et al. Validation study of WOMAC: a health status instrument for measuring clinically important patient relevant outcomes to antirheumatic drug therapy in patients with osteoarthritis of the hip or knee. J Rheumatol 1988;15:1833–40.

36. Merle d'Aubigné R. Cotation chiffrée de la fonction de la hanche. Rev Chir Orthop 1990;76:371–4.

37. Lavigne M, Masse V, Girard J, et al. Return to sport after hip resurfacing or total hip arthroplasty: a randomized study. Rev Chir Orthop Repar Appar Mot 2008;94(4):361–7.

38. Amstutz HC, Thomas BJ, Jinnah R, et al. Treatment of primary osteoarthritis of the hip. A comparison of total joint and surface replacement arthroplasty. J Bone Joint Surg Am 1984;66:228–41.

39. Zywiel MG, Marker DR, McGrath MS, et al. Resurfacing matched to standard total hip arthroplasty by preoperative activity levels—a comparison of postoperative outcomes. Bull N Y U Hosp Jt Dis. 2009;67(2):116–19.

40. Le Duff MJ, Wisk LE, Amstutz HC. Range of motion after stemmed total hip arthroplasty and hip resurfacing—a clinical study. Bull N Y U Hosp Jt Dis 2009;67(2):177–81.

41. Stulberg BN, Fitts SM, Bowen AR, et al. Early return to function after hip resurfacing is it better than contemporary total hip arthroplasty? J Arthroplasty 2010;25(5):748–53.

42. Pollard TC, Baker RP, Eastaugh-Waring SJ, et al. Treatment of the young active patient with osteoarthritis of the hip. A five- to seven-year comparison of hybrid total hip arthroplasty and metal-on-metal resurfacing. J Bone Joint Surg Br 2006;88(5): 592–60.

43. Garbuz DS, Tanzer M, Greidanus NV, et al. Metal-on-metal hip resurfacing versus large-diameter head metal-on-metal total hip arthroplasty: a randomized clinical trial. Clin Orthop Relat Res 2010;468(2):318–25.

44. Li J, Xu W, Xu L, Liang Z. Hip resurfacing for the treatment of developmental dysplasia of the hip. Orthopedics 2008;31(12).

45. Lavigne M, Ganapathi M, Mottard S, Girard J, Vendittoli PA. Range of motion of large head total hip arthroplasty is greater than 28 mm total hip arthroplasty or hip resurfacing. Clin Biomech (Bristol, Avon) 2011;26(3):267–73.

46. Lindemann U, Becker C, Unnewehr I, et al. Gait analysis and WOMAC are complementary in assessing functional outcome in total hip replacement. Clin Rehabil 2006;20(5):413–20.

47. Shrader MW, Bhowmik-Stoker M, Jacofsky MC, et al. Gait and stair function in total and resurfacing hip arthroplasty: a pilot study. Clin Orthop Relat Res 2009;467(6):1476–84.

48. Marker DR, Strimbu K, McGrath MS, et al. Resurfacing vs. conventional total hip arthroplasty—review of comparative clinical and basic science studies. Bull N Y U Hosp Jt Dis 2009;67(2): 120–7.

49. Nantel J, Termoz N, Centomo H, et al. Postural balance during quiet standing in patients with total hip arthroplasty and surface replacement arthroplasty. Clin Biomechan 2008;23:402–7.

50. Rama KR, Vendittoli PA, Ganapathi M, et al. Heterotopic ossification after surface replacement arthroplasty and total hip arthroplasty: a randomized study. J Arthroplasty 2009;24(2): 256–62.

51. Brooker AF, Bowerman JW, Robinson RA, et al. Ectopic ossification following total hip replacement. Incidence and a method of classification J Bone Joint Surg Am 1973;55:1629–32.

52. Cornelis R, Heinzow B, Herber RFM, et al. Sample collection guidelines for trace elements in blood and urine. J Trace Elements Med Biol 1996;10:103–27.

53. Keegan GM, Learmonth ID, Case CP. A systematic comparison of the actual, potential, and theoretical health effects of cobalt and chromium exposures from industry and surgical implants. Crit Rev Toxicol 2008;38:645–74.

54. Jacobs JJ, Skipor AK, Patterson LM, et al. Metal release in patients who have had a primary total hip arthroplasty. A prospective controlled longitudinal study. J Bone Joint Surg Am 1998;80: 1447–58.

55. MacDonald SJ. Metal-on-metal total hip arthroplasty: the concerns. Clin Orthop Relat Res 2004;429:86–93.

56. Vendittoli P-A, Mottard S, Roy A, et al. Release from bearing wear and corrosion with 28 mm and large diameter metal-on-metal bearing articulations. J. Bone Joint Surg Br 2010;92(1): 12–19.

57. Antoniou J, Zukor DJ, Mwale F, et al. Metal ion levels in the blood of patients after hip resurfacing: a comparison between twenty-eight and thirty-six-millimeter-head metal-on-metal prostheses. J Bone Joint Surg Am 2008;90(3):142–8.

58. Clarke MT, Lee PT, Arora A, et al. Levels of metal ions after small- and large-diameter metal-on-metal hip arthroplasty. J Bone Joint Surg Br 2003;85(6):913–17.

59. Witzleb WC, Ziegler J, Krummenauer F, et al. Exposure to chromium, cobalt and molybdenum from metal-on-metal total hip replacement and hip resurfacing arthroplasty. Acta Orthop 2006;77(5):697–705.

60. Moroni A, Savarino L, Cadossi M, et al. Does ion release differ between hip resurfacing and metal-on-metal THA? Clin Orthop Relat Res 2008;466(3):700–7.

61. Daniel J, Ziaee H, Salama A, et al. The effect of the diameter of metal-on-metal bearings on systemic exposure to cobalt and chromium. J Bone Joint Surg Br 2006;88(4):443–8.

62. Vendittoli P-A, Amzica T, Roy A, et al. Metal ion release with large-diameter metal-on-metal hip arthroplasty. J Arthroplasty 2011;26(2):282–8.

63. Beaule PE, Antoniades J. Patient selection and surgical technique for surface arthroplasty of the hip. Orthop Clin N Am 2005;36 177–85.

64. Ball S T, Le Duff M J, Amstutz HC. Early results of conversion of a failed femoral component in hip resurfacing arthroplasty. J Bone Joint Surg Am 2007;89:735–41.

65. McGrath MS, Marker DR, Seyler TM, et al. Surface replacement is comparable to primary total hip arthroplasty. Clin Orthop Relat Res 2009;467:94–100.

17 The Role of Ceramic in Total Hip Arthroplasty

Peter M. Lewis[1] and James P. Waddell[2]
[1]Prince Charles Hospital and Royal Glamorgan Hospital, South Wales, UK
[2]St Michael's Hospital and University of Toronto, Toronto, ON, Canada

Case scenario

An active 57 year old woman has progressively developed severe pain in her right hip. She has exhausted conservative treatments and is keen to remain active with hobbies including golf and badminton. At present she has mild rest pain and occasional sleep disturbance, but walking is limited to half a mile and she is unable to perform any sporting activities. She is otherwise fit and well.

Importance of the problem

Total hip replacement surgery is one of the commonest procedures performed in Western societies and is considered one of the most effective orthopedic procedures.[1] It is a safe and reliable procedure with an excellent long-term survival in the elderly population. Conventional metal-on-polyethylene (MP) replacements are the traditionally implanted bearings, used initially by Charnley in the 1960s, and still recommended by many today. The long-term survival of this bearing combination is, however, limited by the risk of polyethylene wear and wear-related osteolysis.[2] In the younger patient, with a longer life expectancy and increased activity demands, there is an up to tenfold increase in the tribological demands of any replacement bearing.[3] Conventional MP may not therefore be the ideal option in this age group. In a long-term study of patients under the age of 51, a failure rate requiring revision arthroplasty of over 25% was identified at 20 years and almost 50% at 27 years.[4] Revision procedures are challenging to both surgeon and patient and are of considerable cost to healthcare providers.[5] Alternative bearings and joint replacements have therefore been developed. Options include ceramic bearings, metal-on-metal (MM) resurfacings and replacements, and highly cross-linked polyethylene, all aimed to prolong a joint replacement's survival, and prevent the occurrence of osteolysis and its consequences.

Over 4.5 million alumina ceramic components have been implanted worldwide over the last 35 years.[6] This chapter focuses on the efficacy of ceramic options available to the orthopedic hip surgeon.

Surgeons and patients are inundated with an ever-increasing easily accessible body of information about health, and specifically about total hip replacement surgery and its options. A Google search for "ceramic hip replacement" returns almost 600,000 hits. High-profile cases such as the article on squeaking ceramic hip replacements published on the front page of the *New York Times* in 1998,[7] the variable quality, and lack of filtering mandates the need for preappraised evidence-based guides.

Top seven questions

Therapy

1. What are the orthopedic generations of ceramic?
2. What bearing options are available when using ceramics in total hip arthroplasty?
3. Are the clinical outcomes of ceramic total hip replacements equal to those of more conventional articulations?

Prognosis

4. Does a ceramic articulation truly reduce the amount of wear and wear-related osteolysis?
5. What is the risk of fracture?

Evidence-Based Orthopedics, First Edition. Edited by Mohit Bhandari.
© 2012 Blackwell Publishing Ltd. Published 2012 by Blackwell Publishing Ltd.

6. What is the risk of squeaking for a patient considering a ceramic total hip replacement?

Harm

7. What is the risk of revision and what revision options are available if ceramic fails?

Question 1: What are the orthopedic generations of ceramic?

Case clarification
Your patient is intrigued to hear that a ceramic might provide her with an ideal orthopedic bearing. She is, however, interested to know that ceramics were initially related to a high level of failure. What improvements have been made to ceramics in order to limit failures?

Relevance
Optimizing a bearing surface at the expense of its safety is not a satisfactory solution to any initial presenting issue.

Current opinion
Modern ceramics are used with varying popularity around the world. The stigma of initial generations failing will remain of concern to the orthopedic community.

Finding the evidence
• PubMed (www.ncbi.nlm.nih.gov/pubmed/) search using keywords: "ceramic," "ceramic hip," and "ceramic bearings"
• MEDLINE search using keywords: "ceramic," "ceramic hip," and "ceramic bearings"

Quality of the evidence
• Historical review

Findings
Alumina has been continually improved over the years. First-generation alumina ceramics (1974–1988) were characterized by low density, high porosity, and a relatively large grain size. First-generation ceramics did not perform well. Early series reported high failure rates, although the majority of the failures were not due directly to the alumina itself. The main failures were due to aseptic loosening of the femoral stem[8,9] or of the monoblock acetabular system.[10] The alumina itself was, however, not ideal, with a reported fracture rate of 3–13%.[11] The aim with first-generation ceramics was to achieve full or nearly full density (no porosity), which required long sintering times.[12] This resulted in large grain or crystal sizes that translated into a reduction of strength and the high risk of fracture. Lessons were learned from these early series and became the driving force behind the development of second-generation ceramics in the 1980s.

Second- and third-generation alumina ceramics (1988–1994 and 1994–present respectively) are characterized by a reduction in grain size with increased alumina purity. Second-generation ceramics were developed with the addition of calcium oxide or magnesium oxide materials which would limit the increase in alumina grain size during the long sintering process,[12] resulting in a higher-strength product. With third-generation ceramics there have been further improvements with the introduction of processes of hot isostatic pressing, laser etching to avoid surface stress risers, and proof testing. The last of these has been described as the single most important development in improving the reliability of ceramics.[11] Before the advent of proof testing, ceramic components were subject to a finished product audit in which a certain number of components from each batch were subject to testing to destruction. If these tests showed values within an acceptable range then the batch was released for sale. Proof testing or "nondestructive stressing" involves subjecting each component to a substantial overload in a manner that ensures the part is not being damaged in any way yet eliminates the possibility of an internal flaw not being detected. One such method is to pressurize the taper portion of a ceramic head with fluid beyond the stresses expected from the metal trunnion. The problem with such techniques is that if an excessively low pressure is used not all flawed heads will be fractured, whereas if a pressure is too high, too many heads will fracture without reducing clinical failures or potentially damaging heads that were not defective.[13]

Advances during each generation resulted in grain size improvement from 4.2 μm to 3.2 μm to 1.8 μm over first, second and third generations with a resultant burst strength improvement of 46 kN, 58 kN and 65 kN respectively.[14]

Despite these improvements there persisted a search for a ceramic material to satisfy increasingly more challenging patient demands such as smaller components and additional sizes along with even greater reliability and longevity. It is for this reason that alumina matrix composite was developed. Known as fourth-generation ceramic or by the trade name BIOLOX® (CeramTec AG, Plochingen, Germany) it is a combination of both the major subsets of ceramic, an alumina matrix with zirconia particles homogenously dispersed and encapsulated. Using a principle that dates back to the early 1970s,[8] when any crack touches the zirconium it triggers transformation with the resultant volume increase of the particle impeding crack propagation. This process increases the fracture toughness of the material. With the subsequent addition of chromium oxide this restrains the progress of cracking through the formation of platelet-like crystal or whiskers, resulting in further significant gains in mechanical properties.[11]

Recommendation

With regard to ceramic used in orthopedic hip surgery, evidence suggests:

• There has been an improvement in the purity, production techniques and overall quality of ceramics between early-generation ceramics and current options [overall quality: moderate]

Question 2: What bearing options are available when using ceramics in total hip arthroplasty?

Case clarification

The patient has been reassured by the explanation of ceramic and its history. Having done some research on total hip replacement, she assumed she would receive a polyethylene liner.

Relevance

The aim of using ceramic components is to optimize the bearing for a young active patient. Although ceramic may be used against a conventional polyethylene liner it may also be used with both ceramic and metal liners.

Current opinion

A recent review of practices in the UK showed there was no clear consensus as to component choice or even fixation method in the younger patient.[15]

Finding the evidence

• PubMed (www.ncbi.nlm.nih.gov/pubmed/) search using keywords: "ceramic," "ceramic hip," and "ceramic bearings"
• MEDLINE search using keywords "ceramic," "ceramic hip," and "ceramic bearings"

Quality of the evidence

• Historical/industry review

Findings

The proposed advantages of ceramic can be utilized in a number of different bearing options. It may be used as an alternative to a metal head in a conventional hard-on-soft bearing against polyethylene. With a lower R_a and improved wettability it has the potential to provide a low-wear alternative to either stainless steel or cobalt–chrome. It may also be used as a more modern hard-on-hard bearing against either a ceramic liner or, as more recently introduced, ceramic-on-metal (CM) bearing couple. An advantage with hard-on-hard bearings is the potential for fluid film lubrication, an exceptionally low wear rate, and avoidance of osteolytic polyethylene debris. Using hard-on-hard bearings also allows the use of large heads, which, if used with a conventional polyethylene option, would create excessive volumetric wear. Ceramic-on-ceramic (CC) options also avoid the production of metal ions, which are released and may complicate MP and MM alternatives.[16]

No bearing option is perfect, however. A number of complications specific to ceramic, such as fracture and articular squeaking, are discussed in detail later in this chapter. A factor involved in all cases of CC hip replacement is the loss of head and liner option. Using a MP articulation a surgeon has access to multiple head sizes and modular neck lengths spanning 20 mm. On the acetabular side, in addition to multiple inner diameter options, there is also the availability of lateralized liners; elevated rims; and anteverted, eccentric, and constrained liners. In contrast, most CC systems have only one head size per cup diameter, with three or four head lengths spanning 10 mm or less. Ultimately this results in 20 times fewer options in the ceramic option compared with traditional MP. Equalizing leg lengths and maximizing stability are two crucial goals of total hip arthroplasty.[13] The availability of numerous liners and head options is one of the ways of achieving this goal. The aforementioned complications of squeak and fracture associated with ceramic articulations are related to design and technique, and apply to a relatively low percentage of patients in clinical practice.[13] Loss of all of these options may currently be the most substantial disadvantage of CC THA.

Recommendations

With regard to ceramic used in orthopedic hip surgery, evidence suggests:

• Ceramic may be used as a conventional hard-on-soft bearing with a ceramic femoral head articulating against polyethylene, or as a hard-on-hard CC or CM bearing.
• There is less modularity with ceramic bearings as compared to metal and polyethylene implants, limiting the available options to optimize leg lengths and stability.

Question 3: Are the clinical outcomes of ceramic total hip replacements equal to those of more conventional articulations?

Case clarification

On offering the patient a ceramic total hip replacement you need to assure her that her outcome will be at least as good as with conventional bearings.

Relevance

Any proposed benefit of the longevity of a ceramic bearing would be limited if the clinical outcome for the patient was below the standard expected with a conventional hip replacement.

Current opinion

Most would assume the outcome scores for a patient receiving a ceramic total hip replacement would be equivalent to a conventional replacement.

Finding the evidence

- Cochrane Database, with search: "ceramic hip"
- PubMed (www.ncbi.nlm.nih.gov/pubmed/) clinical queries search/systematic reviews/randomized control trials: "ceramic hip"
- MEDLINE search using keywords: "ceramic hip"

Quality of the evidence

- Level I: 7
- Level II: 1
- Level IV: 2

Findings

A randomized controlled trial (RCT) comparing 31 CC total hip replacements in 31 patients with 30 cobalt–chrome on highly cross-linked polyethylene in 30 patients revealed no difference in outcome scores between the two groups, looking at WOMAC and SF-36 scores at a follow-up of between 2 and 24 months.[17] An RCT comparing 30 CC replacements with 26 ceramic-on-polyethylene replacements reports no significant difference in joint specific outcome scores at a mean follow-up of 8 years.[18] With a mean follow-up of 35.2 months, an RCT comparing 346 alumina CC hip replacements with a 168 cobalt–chrome-on-polyethylene replacements reports equivalent Harris hip scores (HHS) and patient satisfaction.[14] The results of a mean 5 year RCT comparing 213 CC hips with 101 cobalt–chrome on conventional polyethylene hips concludes that CC articulations are at least equivalent in performance to the MP design:[19] The HHS was 96.6 in the ceramic group and 97 for the MP group. An extension of this series assessing a titanium-coated ceramic bearing again identified no difference in HHS with a mean of 96.6 with a mean of 4.2 years of follow-up.[20] Subsequent review of the same cohorts, now with mean follow-up of 8 years, again identified no difference in outcome scores.[21] Finally, a minimum 2 year follow-up RCT comparing 250 CC articulations with 250 conventional ceramic-on-polyethylene hips showed no difference in clinical outcome and concludes that ceramic hips "reflected the typical results of primary total hip replacements."[22]

A retrospective observational study reports a mean HHS of 90.4 in 107 hips at a minimum follow-up of 7 years.[23] A further retrospective review of 999 CC hips reports am improvement in HHS from 66.5 to 91.2 points and, interestingly, reports an improvement of HHS from 60.1 to 91.3 in the 2.7% of squeaking ceramic hips without significant difference between the groups.[24]

Recommendations

In terms of outcomes obtained by patients receiving a ceramic total hip replacement, evidence suggests:
- Patients obtain a significant improvement in disease-specific outcome and quality of life scores following a CC total hip replacement [overall quality: high]
- Patients can expect disease-specific and quality of life outcome score improvement at least equivalent to a conventional hard-on-soft total hip replacement at mid-term follow-up [overall quality: high]

Question 4: Does a ceramic articulation truly reduce the amount of wear and wear-related osteolysis?

Case clarification

Your patient is understandably keen to know what complications she might be prone to with a CC articulation.

Relevance

The reason to consider a ceramic bearing within a total hip replacement is to limit the amount of wear and wear-related osteolysis. Any advantage in using a low-wear ceramic bearing aiming to optimizing the long-term survival will clearly be lost if there is an unacceptably high rate of complications.

Current opinion

Most would consider a ceramic articulation to be a low-wear articulation, but its use continues to cause concern to the orthopedic community with concerns of dislocation through a lack of modularity and lip liners and catastrophic complications such as fracture and requiring potentially complex revision procedures.

Finding the evidence

- Cochrane Database, with search: "ceramic hip"
- PubMed (www.ncbi.nlm.nih.gov/pubmed/) clinical queries search/systematic reviews/randomized control trials: "ceramic hip" AND "revision"
- MEDLINE search using keywords: "wear" AND "ceramic hip"
- MEDLINE search using keywords: "ceramic hip" AND "osteolysis"
- PubMed (www.ncbi.nlm.nih.gov/pubmed/) search using keywords "ceramic hip" AND "osteolysis"

Quality of the evidence

- Level I: 7
- Level II: 1

Findings

In-vitro studies have shown very low wear rates for ceramic couples, with volumetric wear combinations from 2000 to 4000 times less than MP.[14,25] A clinical review of in-vivo studies supports wear properties of ceramic in a hybrid articulation with wear rates reduced by 1.5–4-fold in comparison to MP.[26]

An RCT comparing cobalt–chrome vs. zirconia femoral heads measured subsequent polyethylene wear with computer software at 51 months. It showed no difference in wear, with an annual head penetration of 0.06 mm/year in the cobalt–chrome articulation and 0.055 mm/year in the zirconia cohort.[27] This study was subsequently abandoned with concerns about the long-term stability of zirconia. A further RCT involving zirconia directly compared zirconia heads with cobalt–chrome heads in sequential randomized bilateral THAs in 52 patients. It revealed an annual wear rate of 0.17 mm/year in the cobalt–chrome group but a wear rate of 0.08 mm/year in the ceramic head.[28] Interestingly, two ceramic heads required revision as a result of aseptic femoral loosening. There had been little phase transformation of the surfaces, with R_a values of 15.87 and 17.35 nm. This compares to cobalt–chrome unimplanted heads with R_a values of up to 50 nm. Consistent with this zirconia ceramic wear rate, another RCT comparing alumina ceramic heads against two different conventional polyethylene liners reported polyethylene wear of 0.27 mm at 3 years.[29]

An RCT comparing migration of CC vs. ceramic on highly cross-linked polyethylene confirmed two factors: there was no increase in migration of the hard-on-hard cup compared to the more conventional hard-on-soft, but mean wear in the cross-linked polyethylene was 0.016 mm between 2 and 24 months. In a longer-term RCT comparing 30 CC with 26 ceramic-on-polyethylene reports, an attempt was made to measure the amount of wear in a ceramic articulation.[18] There was significantly greater wear in the polyethylene group, with a mean annual wear of 0.11 mm/year in that group but 0.02 mm in the ceramic group.

Ceramics are not immune to wear, however, and with hard-on-hard articulations component positioning is critical. Vertical cup positions increased wear with ceramic bearings—cups with angles greater than 60° had higher wear in vitro than cups at 45°.[30] This was confirmed with retrieval studies confirming greater wear with acetabular angles greater than 55°.

An issue unique to ceramic bearings is that of *stripe wear*. This is the description given to a localized crescent-shaped area of surface alteration of a ceramic femoral head.[13] Its cause is not fully understood, but proposed causes include microseparation, equatorial loading, abducted cup position, or loose bodies in the articulation causing eccentric stresses.[13] The resultant damage to the surface is in the form

of grain fracture or pullout with resultant loose bodies and a roughened surface (R_a 0.21 μm compared to 0.10 μm for the conventionally worn areas of the head). This roughened area may be the precursor of more extensive excessive wear.[13] With unknown etiology, stripe wear could be the occasional but random cause of severe wear in CC articulations.

With the resurgent interest in metal bearings with the success of second-generation MP hip replacements, there have been attempts to match an alumina head against a metal acetabulum. A limited number of studies are available, with only one identified RCT on the subject.[31] That paper reports lower overall wear and incidence of stripe wear in adverse conditions in vitro. Within the current short follow-up of 6 months, the randomized trial of 31 patients only reports on reduced metal ions in the CM compared to those with a MP articulation. In contrast to this study, an in vitro study reported significantly greater wear in the CM group than the CC articulation after 5 million cycles.[32]

A short-term RCT comparing CC and cobalt–chrome on cross-linked polyethylene reports no osteolysis at 24 months in either group.[17] This is not unexpected, as even with conventional polyethylene hips wear-related osteolysis is not a short-term or even mid-term complication. In a longer-term study, with mean follow-up of 8 years, cortical erosions were reported in 4 of 287 (1.4%) alumina ceramic hips and in 25 of 82 (30.5%) control MP hips.[21] Within this latter group, one patient required revision of cup and liner for osteolysis at 10.5 years and another had a liner exchange at 52 months for polyethylene wear and osteolysis at 8 years.[21] This report followed an earlier 5 year mean publication of the cohorts with osteolysis recorded in 1.4% of 213 alumina hips and 14% of the 101 control cobalt–chrome on polyethylene hips.[19] Linear wear was identified as higher in those hips with increased radiographic femoral scalloping, supporting the concept of wear-related osteolysis. A further mid- to long-term RCT (median 8 years), comparing 30 alumina CC with 26 ceramic-on-polyethylene articulations, reported significantly greater wear in the polyethylene group.[18] One hip showed radiolucency around the acetabular component, but without accelerated wear and no osteolysis reported in any of the patients.[18]

A retrospective review of 103 total hip arthroplasties with ceramic implants reported a rate of osteolysis far higher than that found in these RCTs. At a mean follow-up of 92 months femoral osteolysis was found in 23 hips (22%) with 10 hips going on to require revision for loosening.[33] Tissue retrieved at revision confirmed abundant wear particles with conclusion that ceramic particles can stimulate foreign body response and periprosthetic osteolysis. This was the first published series of patients with a CC articulation demonstrating such a high level of osteolysis. It does, however, report on a prosthesis that was subsequently withdrawn in the US due to high failure rates, and on a ceramic head that has a skirt leading to CC impingement.[34] In order to have an osteolytic environment appropriate-sized particulate matter must be present in an adequate quantity, whether metal, plastic, or ceramic. This failure is felt by a number of authors to be a component design failure.[34] A further case study from 1997 reported a case of massive osteolysis with debris confirmed to be neither polyethylene nor cement.[35] Although this incited correspondence from other units,[36] the authors felt justified in concluding ceramic debris may not be bioinert and not a solution to osteolysis.[36]

Reiterating the importance of avoidance of impingement, a further case report of two ceramic articulations revealed significant osteolysis.[37] Stripe wear of the ceramic head and neck impingement of the titanium shell was found, with periacetabular tissue revealing ceramic and titanium debris in both cases. It is unclear which caused the osteolysis, but this is a further demonstration of the risk that modern-generation alumina may be associated with osteolysis.

Numerous mid- and long-term retrospective studies and reviews have shown limited or no evidence of osteolysis in modern, well-functioning ceramic articulations.[25,38–41]

Recommendations

With ceramic used in total hip arthroplasty, evidence suggests:
- Wear with CC articulations is significantly reduced in comparison to conventional hard-on-soft polyethylene replacements [overall quality: high]
- Wear with a ceramic head on polyethylene gives less wear than a similar articulation with a metal head [overall quality: moderate]
- Stripe wear is an occasional cause of severe wear in CC articulations [overall quality: low]
- Using CM articulations may reduce the overall amount of wear and the incidence of stripe wear [overall quality: very low]
- Any articulation, including a ceramic type, which produces excessive particulate wear, is likely to cause osteolysis [overall quality: moderate]
- A modern well-fixed CC bearing, without impingement, reduces the risk of mid- to long-term osteolysis compared to a comparable MP articulation [overall quality: high]

Question 5: What is the risk of fracture?

Case clarification

When you explained the risks and benefits of a ceramic hip replacement your patient was concerned to know that fracture is a risk of the procedure.

Relevance

Fracture is a catastrophic complication of a ceramic articulation requiring immediate revision. Benefits of low-wear articulations need to outweigh specific risks associated with the bearing.

Current opinion

With modern ceramics fracture is recognized to be a relatively rare, although catastrophic, complication.

Finding the evidence

- Cochrane Database, with search: "ceramic hip"
- PubMed (www.ncbi.nlm.nih.gov/pubmed/) clinical queries search/systematic reviews/randomized control trials: "ceramic hip"
- MEDLINE search using keywords: "ceramic hip" AND "fracture"
- PubMed (www.ncbi.nlm.nih.gov/pubmed/) using keywords: "ceramic hip" AND "fracture"

Quality of the evidence

- Level I: 4
- Level II: 2
- Level III: 7
- Level IV: 1

Findings

Early in the production of ceramics, the fracture rate was as high as 13.4% for those manufactured before 1990, with catastrophic consequences.[42] The same paper reports the survival of ceramic BIOLOX femoral heads as 0.026% for first-generation alumina and 0.014% for second-generation alumina and 0.004% for femoral heads manufactured after 1994, based on data collected from over 2 million femoral heads. Sedel's review of the 30-year history of alumina suggests the risk of fracture is 1 in 2000 for a 10-year period.[38] A further historical review reports 80% of ceramic head fractures occur within the first 2 years and 90% within the first 3 years.[22] Barrack et al.'s "concerned" review of ceramic implants states that 1 in 10,000 ceramic revisions will be solely attributable to fracture[13] despite proof testing and improved properties.

Reviewing the level I evidence, an RCT comparing MP with a number of full ceramic options confirmed 2 fractures, at 6.5 years and at 9 years, in a total cohort of 380 ceramic hips with overall mean follow-up of 8 years.[21] There were also four ceramic chips on insertion of the liner, which were immediately changed to a new liner and shell, and none have required revision.[21] In order to address the issue of fracture on insertion, a titanium-cased alumina ceramic component was introduced as a fourth group within this study. In a separate publication,[20] this group showed no chips, fractures, or failures at a mean follow-up of 4.2 years in 209 hips. An RCT by Bierbaum et al. involving 514 hips in 458 patients compared cobalt–chrome-on-polyethylene articulations with alumina CC.[14] It revealed no fractures in the 346 in the ceramic group with a mean follow-up of 35.2 months. There was, however, an insertional chip rate of 2.6% (9 of 346 hips) each identified and replaced at the time of surgery with as yet no sequelae. A minimum of 2 year RCT reports on 236 CC and 224 ceramic-on-polyethylene (CP) hips, with 1 rim chip in the study group.[22] A large medium-term study involving 500 hips comparing an equal number of CC articulations with CP, at a minimum follow-up of 2 years, reports no ceramic fractures.[22] One liner chipped on insertion, requiring exchange (0.4%). Finally, a review of 56 hips at a mean follow-up of 8 years reported no ceramic fracture or liner chips in 30 CC articulations and 26 CP hips.[18]

As important with regard to prevalence of an issue are observational studies. No fractures are reported at a mean of 50.4 months in 103 hips in 97 patients in a retrospective review.[39] A further retrospective observational study reports 3 fractures in 107 hips (2%) at a minimum follow-up of 7 years, although each was associated with an extra-long neck, an option that is now no longer used.[23] Numerous case reports of fracture have been published, one of which from 1995 reviews the available data from 10 previous published fracture reports. The authors concluded that, including their own case, common characteristics included young age at surgery, heavy, and active, and 8 of the 10 were male.[43] Torán et al. in 2006 published a case of fracture and similarly reported risk of failure to be increased in the heavy and active patient.[44]

Recommendations

With regard to risk of fracture using ceramic bearings in total hip replacements, the evidence suggests:
• Care must be taken on insertion of ceramic liners to avoid the risk of insertional chips. This remains an issue even with modern materials and components [overall quality: high]
• Improvements in manufacturing and components have reduced the risk of fracture of ceramic components [overall quality: moderate]
• Risk of fracture may be increased in the young, heavier, active male [overall quality: very low]

Question 6: What is the risk of squeaking for a young active patient considering a ceramic total hip replacement?

Case clarification

Your patient recalls a newspaper article about a patient with a hip that squeaks. She asks if that was related to a ceramic hip. You need to explain the risk of squeaking with a ceramic articulation.

Relevance

Any hip replacement must improve not only the patient's physical quality of life but also their mental quality of life. An articulation that causes audible noises with every step will be difficult for any patient to tolerate.

Current opinion

Squeaking remains a significant concern with hard-on-hard CC usage.

Finding the evidence

• Cochrane Database, with search: "ceramic hip"
• PubMed (www.ncbi.nlm.nih.gov/pubmed/) clinical queries search/ systematic reviews/ randomized control trials: "ceramic hip" AND "squeak"
• MEDLINE search using keywords: "ceramic hip"
• PubMed (www.ncbi.nlm.nih.gov/pubmed/) using keywords: "squeak" AND "ceramic"

Quality of the evidence

• Level I: 1
• Level III: 5
• Level IV: 3

Findings

Squeaking from the site of total hip arthroplasty is a phenomenon unique to hard-on-hard bearings, whether MP or CC.[45–49] The cause is not fully understood, and a number of possible etiologies have been postulated including component mismatch and insufficient lubrication, stripe wear, and third-body metal debris.[45]

Squeak is reported in 3 hips of 380 in an RCT comparing a CC articulation with polyethylene with a minimum follow-up of 5 years and a mean of 8 years.[21] All were reported as transient in nature although one underwent revision for unexplained groin pain. A prospectively followed group of 159 arthroplasties in 143 patients with matched control group reported a 10.7% incidence of audible squeak during normal activities.[45] This was reproducible clinically in only four patients but, importantly, only one patient had complained of the squeak prior to direct questioning. This study showed no relationship between implant positioning and squeaking.

A recent retrospective review revealed 9 of 43 CC implants (20.9%) squeaking at a minimum 39.4 months (mean 47.3 months), and again suggests the incidence may in fact be under-reported.[50] No relationship was found with regard to cup inclination or anteversion, but shorter neck lengths were found to be associated with squeaking. No relationship was found with patient demographics. At a mean of 50.4 months in 103 hips in 97 patients, a retrospective review identified squeaking in 5 patients (4.9%).[39] The squeak was intermittent in nature and found only in active patients. No radiological abnormality was identified within the squeaking hips with stable implantation and no obvious etiology. Again, in this series hip abduction angles were found not to vary from the controls. In contrast, a review of 17 squeaking hips against matched controls by Walter et al. suggested association with high cup abduction angles.[51] In this series of ceramic hips 75% of 17 squeaking hips had an abduction angle outside 45±10°. The hips started squeaking after an average of 14 months, with patients with squeaking hips being younger, heavier, and taller than patients with silent hips.

A large retrospective review of 999 hips reports a squeak in 28 hips (2.7%).[24] A cohort was matched to analyze if cup position may be related to the onset of squeaking. No significant alteration was found in either cup inclination or version between the groups. In four hips that underwent revision, stripe wear was identified on the femoral heads and metal debris was found in the ceramic articulation.

Recommendations

In patients undergoing a CC total hip replacement, the evidence suggests:
- Squeaking is unique to hard-on-hard bearings [overall quality: high]
- The overall incidence squeaking may be under-reported [overall quality: moderate]
- Ideal component positioning may reduce the risk of squeaking [overall quality: very low]
- The risk of a squeaking articulation is increased in the younger, heavier, and taller patient [overall quality: very low]

Question 7: Is a CC articulation less likely to require revision than a conventional replacement? For any patient contemplating a ceramic hip replacement, what options are available should the bearings fail at any stage?

Case clarification

Because of her relatively young age, the patient has concerns about the need for further surgery in the future. She has read about squeaking and also fracture in ceramic hips. She asks what options are available to her should this occur.

Relevance

Although there are some undisputable advantages to ceramic bearings, consideration must be made of the potential for failure and need for revision within the lifetime of a younger patient.

Current opinion

The majority of surgeons would consider revision following a failed ceramic articulation to be one of the most challenging procedures in orthopedics, particularly if following ceramic fracture.

Finding the evidence

- Cochrane Database, with search: "ceramic hip"
- PubMed (www.ncbi.nlm.nih.gov/pubmed/) clinical queries search/ systematic reviews/ randomized control trials: "ceramic hip" AND "revision"
- MEDLINE search using keywords: "revision," "fracture," AND "ceramic hip"
- PubMed (www.ncbi.nlm.nih.gov/pubmed/) using keywords: "revision," "fracture," AND "ceramic hip"

Quality of the evidence

- Level I: 5
- Level III: 1
- Level IV: 4

Findings

Five trials[14,17,18,21,22] (N = 1511) report postoperative revision rates in comparative randomized studies involving CC alumina articulations. Three further trials were excluded from analysis as they were previous publications of the same cohort.[19,20,52] The results of pooled statistics are shown in Table 17.1. Two studies[18,22] compare CC articulations with CP articulations, with a reduced risk of revision identified in the CC group (RR 0.309, 95% CI 0.063–1.502). Follow-up in these studies varied between a minimum of 2 years (N = 460) to a median of 8 years (N = 55). Two hips required revision in the ceramic group due to recurrent dislocations, while in the control group seven revisions were performed, one for pain of unknown etiology, one loose acetabulum, and five for recurrent dislocation. Within the remaining three studies[14,17,19] comparison was made between CC and MP articulations in 1036 hips. Again a

Table 17.1 Revision surgery (values <1 favor ceramic-on-ceramic, >1 favor control)

	N	Events		RR	95% CI
		CC	Control		
CC vs. CP	475	2/226	7/249	0.309	0.063–1.502
CC vs. MP	1036	14/744	16/292	0.331	0.159–0.687
CC vs. all	1511	16/970	23/541	0.378	0.198–0.721

CC, ceramic-on-ceramic; CP, ceramic-on-polyethylene; MP, metal-on-polyethylene; RR, relative risk of revision with CC compared to alternatives.

reduced overall risk of revision was identified in the ceramic group (RR 0.331, 95% CI 0.159–0.687). Follow-up in these studies was 2 years (N = 61), mean 35.2 months (N = 500) and a mean of 8 years (N = 475). Taking all CC articulations and comparing with all of the controls reveals a relative risk of revision of 0.378 (N = 1511, 95% CI 0.198–0.721) for the CC option.

Revision of any hip replacement is a complex undertaking. Ideally the use of ceramic articulations during primary surgery would remove the need for a future revision hip replacement. If ultimately one is required, "the absence of osteolysis facilitates revision surgery"[41] avoiding the need for bone graft.[40] Unfortunately, however, the use of any bearing will produce wear. Although the quantity is reduced with a ceramic bearing, what is produced is exceptionally hard and a potentially damaging third body for any subsequent articulation. Worse, if revision is required following fracture there will be extensive third-body debris within the effective joint space, damaging exposed femoral trunnions and acetabular shells. Any delay will cause further damage and soft tissue contamination and revision is therefore an urgent undertaking. The revision will likely require exchange of all components due to this damage with subsequent bearings likely exposed to macro- and microscopic particles of ceramic, limiting longevity.

Level I evidence reviewing this issue is difficult to obtain, but observational and retrospective evidence is available. Allain has published a case report and a study on a large series of head fractures.[53,54] The case report was of a 54 year old patient who sustained a traumatic fracture of their femoral head 5 years after implantation.[53] This was revised to a stainless steel on polyethylene liner. Subsequently at 11 months the patient developed pain and then at 18 months required a second revision. Intraoperatively the stainless steel femoral head was deformed and severe metallosis was noted. Histologically, fragments of both stainless steel and alumina ceramic were noted in the soft tissue. A multicenter review by the same author[54] reviewed 105 revisions for ceramic head fractures: 31% went on to require at least one repeat revision with an overall 5 year survival rate of only 63%. This rate is worse than most revision series and in all likelihood due to retained ceramic particles.[13] Allain's review is the most extensive review available in the literature and makes a number of recommendations.[54] Factors influencing results included whether the cup was changed (57% required re-revision without, 21% with exchange), extent of synovectomy (re-revision in 67% with partial synovectomy, 19% with complete synovectomy) and patient age (54 years in those requiring revision and 63 in those who did not (p = 0.02)). Although definitive conclusions could not be made as to whether the femoral component required exchange, this paper does conclude that any revision following ceramic fracture should include cup exchange, total synovectomy, and a cobalt–chrome or ceramic head. A revision following fracture is not therefore a simple undertaking, requiring an extensive revision and not simply a head and liner exchange.[13] Even without previous fracture, revision of a previous ceramic articulation will be susceptible to retained ceramic wear particles, potentially limiting longevity.

Recommendations

With regard to revision for a failed ceramic hip replacement, evidence suggests:

• With maximum mean follow-up of 8 years CC hips have a lower risk of revision in comparison to alternatives in currently available level I studies [overall quality: high]
• Following ceramic fracture, revision total hip arthroplasty has a poorer survival than following conventional hip replacements [overall quality: low]
• Following ceramic fracture complete component revision is required due to damage to trunnions and cups by the exceptionally hard fragments [overall quality: low]
• Total synovectomy is required during any ceramic revision to reduce the amount of highly abrasive wear debris from the previous articulation [overall quality: low]
• Caution should be used before considering the use of any "soft" bearing such as polyethylene or stainless steel with risk of deformation, accelerated wear, and failure from retained abrasive third-body wear [overall quality: low]

Summary of recommendations

• Ceramics are exceptionally hard, wettable, and chemically inert, but they are brittle and, unlike metal components, prone to fracture
• Zirconia undergoes phase transformation, limiting its safety as an orthopedic device
• There has been an improvement in the purity, production techniques, and overall quality of ceramics between early-generation ceramics and current options
• Ceramic may be used as a conventional hard-on-soft bearing with a ceramic femoral head articulating against polyethylene, or as a hard-on-hard CC or CM bearing
• There is less modularity with ceramic bearings as compared to metal and polyethylene implants, limiting the available options for optimizing leg lengths and stability
• Patients can expect disease-specific and quality of life outcome score improvement at least equivalent to a conventional hard-on-soft total hip replacement at mid-term follow-up
• Wear with CC articulations is significantly reduced in comparison to conventional hard-on-soft polyethylene replacements

- Stripe wear is an occasional cause of severe wear in CC articulations
- With maximum mean follow-up of 8 years CC hips have a lower risk of revision in comparison to alternatives in currently available level I studies
- Using CM articulations may reduce the overall amount of wear and the incidence of stripe wear
- Any articulation, including a ceramic type, which produces excessive particulate wear, is likely to cause osteolysis
- A modern well-fixed CC bearing, without impingement, reduces the risk of mid to long-term osteolysis compared to a comparable MP articulation
- Improvements in manufacturing and components have reduced the risk of fracture of ceramic components
- Risk of fracture may be increased in the young, heavier, active male
- Care must be taken on insertion of ceramic liners to avoid the risk of insertional chips; this remains an issue even with modern materials and components
- Squeaking is unique to hard-on-hard bearings
- The overall incidence squeaking may be under-reported
- Ideal component positioning may reduce the risk of squeaking
- The risk of a squeaking articulation may be increased in the younger, heavier, and taller patient
- Following ceramic fracture, revision total hip arthroplasty has a poorer survival than following conventional hip replacements
- Following ceramic fracture, complete component revision is required due to damage to trunnions and cups by the exceptionally hard fragments
- Total synovectomy is required during any ceramic revision to reduce the amount of highly abrasive wear debris from the previous articulation
- Caution should be used before considering the use of any "soft" bearing such as polyethylene or stainless steel during a ceramic hip revision, with risk of deformation, accelerated wear and failure from retained abrasive third-body wear

Conclusions

The use of modern ceramic bearings has become significantly safer than when they were first introduced over 30 years ago. With improved manufacture and testing techniques, the risk of catastrophic failure through fracture has improved. A patient receiving a CC total hip arthroplasty can expect a low-wear articulation, outcome scores equivalent to a conventional hip replacement, and a low risk of long-term osteolysis. Fracture does, however, remain a risk, as does squeaking, which may be an under-reported issue. Revision procedures following failed ceramic hip replace-ments are challenging. Exceptionally hard retained wear and fracture debris often necessitates complete component revision with the potential to compromise the long-term survival of the revised hip.

References

1. NHS National Institute of Clinical Excellence: Guidance on the Selection of Prostheses for Primary Total Hip Replacement. NICE, London, 2000.
2. Wright T, Goodman S. Implant Wear: the Future Of Joint Replacement. American Academy of Orthopaedic Surgeons, Rosemont, IL, 1995.
3. Schmalzried TP, Szuszczewicz ES, Northfield MR, et al. Quantitative assessment of walking activity after total hip and knee replacement. J Bone Joint Surg Am 1998;80:54. 417.
4. Wrolbewski BM, Siney PD, Flemming PA. Charnley low-frictional torque arthroplasty in patients under the age of 51 years. Follow up to 33-years. J Bone Joint Surg Br 2002;84:540–3.
5. Bozic KJ, Kurtz SM, Lau E, Ong K, Vail TP, Berry DJ. The epidemiology of revision total hip arthroplasty in the United States. J Bone Joint Surg Am 2009;91:128–33.
6. Willmann G. Alumina ceramic components for total hip arthroplasty. Orthopaedics 1997;4:269–76.
7. Feder BJ. That must be Bob. I hear his new hip squeaking. New York Times, May 11, 2008.
8. Mittelmeier H. Report on the first decennium of clinical experience with a cementless ceramic total hip replacement. Acta Orthop Belg 1985;51(2–3):367–76.
9. Miller E. Self bearing, uncemented alumina ceramic total hip replacement arthroplasty. AAOS Instructional Course 1986;35: 188.
10. Nizard RS et al. Ten-year survivorship of cemented ceramic-ceramic total hip prosthesis. Clin Orthop Relat Res 1992;282: 53–63.
11. Ceramtec. Current perspective on the use of ceramics in total hip arthroplasty. Biolox. January 13, 2007.
12. Skinner HB. Ceramic bearing surfaces. Clin Orthop Relat Res. 1999;369:83–91.
13. Barrack RL, Burak C, Skinner HB. Concerns about ceramics in THA. Clin Orthop Relat Res 2004;429:73–9.
14. Bierbaum BE, Nairus J, Kuesis D, Morrison JC, Ward D. Ceramic-on-ceramic bearings in total hip arthroplasty. Clin Orthop Relat Res 2002;405:158–63.
15. Mundy GM, Esler CNA, Harper WM. Primary hip replacement in young osteoarthritic patients: current practices in one UK region. Hip 2005;15:159.
16. Pandit H, Glyn-Jones S, McLardy-Smith P, et al. Pseudotumours associated with metal-on-metal hip resurfacings. J Bone Joint Surg Br 2008;90:847–51.
17. Zhou ZK, Li MG, Börlin N, Wood DJ, Nivbrant B. No increased migration in cups with ceramic-on-ceramic bearing: an RSA study. Clin Orthop Relat Res 2006;448:39–45.
18. Lewis PM, Al-Belooshi A, Olsen M, Schemitsch EH, Waddell JP. Prospective randomised trial comparing alumina ceramic on ceramic with ceramic on conventional polyethylene bearings in total hip arthroplasty. J Arthroplasty 2010;25(3):392–7.

19. D'Antonio J, Capello W, Manley M, Naughton M, Sutton K. Alumina ceramic bearings for total hip arthroplasty: five-year results of a prospective randomized study. Clin Orthop Relat Res 2005;436:164–71.

20. D'Antonio JA, Capello WN, Manley MT, Naughton M, Sutton K. A titanium-encased alumina ceramic bearing for total hip arthroplasty: 3- to 5-year results. Clin Orthop Relat Res 2005;441: 151–8.

21. Capello WN, D'Antonio JA, Feinberg JR, Manley MT, Naughton M. Ceramic-on-ceramic total hip arthroplasty: update. J Arthroplasty 2008;23(7 Suppl):39–43.

22. Sonny Bal B, Aleto TJ, Garino JP, Toni A, Hendricks KJ. Ceramic-on-ceramic versus ceramic-on-polyethylene bearings in total hip arthroplasty: Results of a multicenter prospective randomized study and update of modern ceramic total hip trials in the United States. Hip Int 2005;15:129–35.

23. Aldrian S, Nau T, Gillesberger F, Petras N, Ehall R. Medium-term analysis of modern ceramic-on-ceramic bearing in THA. Hip Int 2009;19(1):36–40.

24. Restrepo C, Parvizi J, Kurtz SM, Sharkey PF, Hozack WJ, Rothman RH. The noisy ceramic hip: is component malpositioning the cause? J Arthroplasty 2008;23(5):643–9.

25. Nizard R, Sedel L, Hannouche D, Hamadouche M, Bizot P. Aspects of current management. Alumina pairing in total hip replacement. J Bone Joint Surg Br 2005;87:755–8.

26. Clarke I, Gustafson A. Clinical and hip simulator comparisons of ceramic on polyethylene and metal on polyethylene wear. Clin Orthop Relat Res 2000;379:34–40.

27. Kraay MJ, Thomas RD, Rimnac CM, Fitzgerald SJ, Goldberg VM. Zirconia versus Co-Cr femoral heads in total hip arthroplasty: early assessment of wear. Clin Orthop Relat Res 2006;453: 86–90.

28. Kim YH. Comparison of polyethylene wear associated with cobalt-chromium and zirconia heads after total hip replacement. A prospective, randomized study. J Bone Joint Surg Am 2005;87(8):1769–76.

29. Palm L, Olofsson J, Aström SE, Ivarsson I. No difference in migration or wear between cemented low-profile cups and standard cups : a randomized radiostereographic study of 53 patients over 3 years. Acta Orthop 2007;78(4):479–84.

30. Walter A. On the material and tribology of alumina-alumina couplings for hip joint prostheses. Clin Orthop 1992; 282: 31–4647.

31. Williams S, Schepers A, Isaac G, Hardaker C, Ingham E, van der Jagt D, et al. The 2007 Otto Aufranc Award. Ceramic-on-metal hip arthroplasties: a comparative in vitro and in vivo study. Clin Orthop Relat Res 2007;465:23–32.

32. Affatato S, Spinelli M, Squarzoni S, Traina F, Toni A. Mixing and matching in ceramic-on-metal hip arthroplasty: An in-vitro hip simulator study. J Biomech 2009;42(15):2439–46.

33. Yoon TR, Rowe SM, Jung ST, Seon KJ, Maloney WJ. Osteolysis in association with a total hip arthroplasty with ceramic bearing surfaces. J Bone Joint Surg Am 1998;80(10):1459–68.

34. Orthopaedic forum. Osteolysis and ceramic bearing surfaces. J Bone Joint Surg Am 2000;10:1518–21.

35. Wirganowicz, PZ, Thomas BJ. Massive osteolysis after ceramic on ceramic total hip arthroplasty: a case report. Clin Orthop Relat Res 1997;338:100–4.

36. Sedel L, Nizard R, Bizot P. Letters to the editor. Clin Orthop Relat Res 1998;349:273–4.

37. Murali R, Bonar SF, Kirsh G, Walter WK, Walter WL. Osteolysis in third-generation alumina ceramic-on-ceramic hip bearings with severe impingement and titanium metallosis. J Arthroplasty 2008;23(8):1240.

38. Sedel L. Total hip arthroplasty using a ceramic prosthesis. Clin Orthop Relat Res 2000;379:3–11.

39. Greene JW, Malkani AL, Kolisek FR, Jessup NM, Baker DL. Ceramic-on-ceramic total hip arthroplasty. J Arthroplasty 2009;24(6 Suppl):15–18.

40. Hannouche D, Hamadouche M, Nizard R, Bizot P, Meunier A, Sedel L. Ceramics in total hip replacement. Clin Orthop Relat Res 2005;430:62–71.

41. Sedel L. Evolution of alumina-on-alumina implants: a review. Clin Orthop Relat Res 2000;379:48–54.

42. Willmann G. Ceramic femoral head retrieval data. Clin Orthop 2000;379:22–8.

43. Higuchi F, Shiba N, Inoue A, Wakeve I. Case report. Fracture of an alumina ceramic head in total hip arthroplasty. J Arthroplasty 1995;10(6)851–4.

44. Torán MM, Cuenca J, Martinez AA, Herrera A, Thomas JV. Fracture of a ceramic femoral head after ceramic-on-ceramic total hip arthroplasty. J Arthroplasty 2006;21(7):1072–3.

45. Jarrett CA, Ranawat AS et al. The squeaking hip phenomenon of ceramic on ceramic total hip arthropplasty. J Bone Joint Surg Am 2009;91:1344–9.

46. Buchanan JM. Ceramic on ceramic bearings in total hip arthroplasty. Key Eng Mater 2003;240(2):793–6.

47. Ebied A, Journeaux SF, Pope JA. Hip resurfacing arthroplasty: the Liverpool experience. Read at the International Conference: Engineers and Surgeons—Joined at the Hip, June 13–15, 2002, London, UK.

48. Eickmann TH, Clarke IC, Gustafson GA. Squeaking in ceramic on ceramic total hip. In: Zippel H, Dietrich M, eds. Ceramics in Orthopaedics. Bioceramics in Joint Arthroplasty: 8th BIOLOX Symposium Proceedings, March 28–29, 2003, pp. 187–92. Steinkopf Verlag, Darmstadt, 2003.

49. Morlock M, Nassutt R, Janssen R, Willmann G, Honl M. Mismatched wear couple zirconium oxide and aluminum oxide in total hip arthroplasty. J Arthroplasty 2001;16:1071–4.

50. Keurentjes JC, Kuipers RM, Wever DJ, Schreurs BW. High incidence of squeaking in THAs with alumina ceramic-on-ceramic bearings. Clin Orthop Relat Res 2008; 466(6):1438–43.

51. Walter WL, O'Toole GC, Walter WK, Ellis A, Zicat BA. Squeaking in ceramic-on-ceramic hips: the importance of acetabular component orientation. J Arthroplasty 2007;22(4):496–503.

52. D'Antonio J, Capello W, Manley M, Bierbaum B. New experience with alumina-on-alumina ceramic bearings for total hip arthroplasty. J Arthroplasty 2002;17(4):390–7.

53. Allain J, Goutallier D, Voisin Mc, Lemouel S, Failure of a stainless-steel femoral head of a revision total hip arthroplasty performed after a fracture of a ceramic femoral head. A case report. J Bone Joint Surg Am 1998;80:1355–60.

54. Allain J, Roudot-Thoraval F, Delecrin J, Anract P, Migaud H, Goutallier D. Revision total hip arthroplasty performed after fracture of a ceramic femoral head. A multicenter survivorship study. J Bone Joint Surg Am 2003;85:825–30.

Minimally Invasive Techniques in Total Hip Arthroplasty

Amre Hamdi and Paul E. Beaulé
University of Ottawa, Ottawa, ON, Canada

Case scenario

A 53 year old woman who is otherwise healthy presents with left-sided groin pain that was first noticed 2 years ago and has been getting progressively worse over the last 3 months. Currently, she cannot walk for more than 30 minutes but does not use any walking aids. She has tried various anti-inflammatories and physiotherapy with no improvement. On clinical examination, she walks with an antalgic gait. Range of motion shows flexion of 100° with no internal and external rotation respectively in 90° of hip flexion. She has 5° of fixed flexion contracture, and leg lengths are equal . Motor power is 5/5 in flexion, abduction and extension. Her radiographs show a severely arthritic hip joint.

Importance

Total hip arthroplasty (THA) is one the most successful surgeries in modern era because of the overall marked improvement of the patient's function and quality of life.[1] Once a surgical intervention has achieved a certain standard of efficacy and reproducibility, further developments can be placed on minimizing the morbidity of the intervention. Less invasive surgical techniques as well as multimodal pain management have also evolved over the last decade in the field of joint replacements, especially THA, enabling patients to potentially recover faster as well as optimize their overall function by avoiding excessive muscle dissection.[2] As with any new surgical technique, initial enthusiasm was based on high patient expectations[3] as well as surgeon enthusiasm but, as is all too common in surgery, over enthusiasm lead to some serious complications.[4] In this chapter we review the current techniques as well as clinical results and future of minimally invasive (MIS) hip replacement surgery.

One of the reasons total hip replacement (THR) surgery has been so successful is the standardization as well as reproducibility of the surgical approaches. As one would expect, different areas of the world will favor certain approaches because of history as well as available instrumentation, with the classic approaches in the literature for primary THR being posterior, lateral, anterolateral, and anterior (Table 18.1). To discuss how each of them evolved as well and became part of daily practice is not the purpose of this chapter; however, certain basic principles are common to those approaches for performing a successful THR:

- proper visualization and access to bony interfaces
- low risk of neurovascular injury
- minimal to no significant compromise on patient function.

The two-incision technique is probably the approach that brought the new MIS THR surgical technique to the forefront, with its optimization of pain management protocols as well as a rapid discharge program.[2] This also led to decreasing the length of the skin incision (6–10 cm) compared to standard surgical approaches such as the posterior and lateral approaches.[5]

Anatomy and surgical approaches

With respect to surgical approaches, we now briefly discuss the different techniques based on patient positioning and identified in the literature as MIS.

Evidence-Based Orthopedics, First Edition. Edited by Mohit Bhandari.
© 2012 Blackwell Publishing Ltd. Published 2012 by Blackwell Publishing Ltd.

Table 18.1 Advantages and disadvantages of different MIS surgical approaches

	Posterior	Anterior	Lateral	Two-incision
Advantages	Excellent exposure	Excellent exposure to acetabulum	Very good exposure	Smaller incision
	Preserving the abductors	Internervous plane	Less risk of dislocation	
Disadvantages	Release of short external rotators	Difficult exposure to femur	Violating the abductors	Difficult exposure
	Increase risk of dislocation	Neuropraxia of lateral femoral cutaneous nerve	Chronic limp	Damage to abductors

Lateral decubitus position

For both posterior and lateral approaches the patient is placed in the lateral decubitus position with the hip flexed 45–60° and adducted 10°. For the posterior approach an oblique incision is placed near the tip of the trochanter. The deep dissection splits the fascia over the gluteus maximus muscle and proceeds posterior to the gluteus medius and minimus muscle into the hip joint .The posterior approach generally requires transection of the piriformis tendon and at least a portion of the short external rotators down to the quadratus femoris muscle.[6] Penenberg et al.[7] recently reported on a technique which uses percutaneous portals for acetabular preparation and component insertion permitting only release of the piriformis tendon.

For the lateral approach, the skin incision is similar to that described for the posterior approach, with the incision placed obliquely over the greater trochanter, generally starting 1–2 cm above the tip of the trochanter and proceeding distally. For the anterolateral approach(Roetinger/ Watson-Jones)[8,9] the superficial dissection is between the tensor and gluteus medius and deep dissection between gluteus minimus and rectus femoris. An alternative is the standard lateral approach is splitting the anterior portion of the gluteus medius tendon in a continuous sleeve with the vastus lateralis and gluteus minimus in one layer with the hip capsule.[8–10] The main downside to these approaches is that they are not truly intervnervous and damage to the gluteus minimus is common either during the exposure or femoral preparation.

Supine position

The direct anterior approach or Hueter approach represents the only truly internervous approach to the hip passing through the sheath of the tensor fascia lata muscle (superior gluteal nerve) with the sartorius muscle medially (femoral nerve).[11] The deeper plane is between rectus femoris and gluteus minimus.[12,13] In order to facilitate access to the femur the leg can be placed in a "figure 4" position or by using an orthopedic positioning table permitting extension of the leg without the need for an assist-

ant to hold it.[14] Recent multicenter data has shown this approach to be safe and reproducible.[15]

The two-incision approach for THA uses a small direct anterior approach for acetabular exposure and component placement, and a small posterior approach for femoral preparation and femoral implant insertion.[2] This approach is less and less used because of a high initial complication rate[16] as well as significant damage to the gluteus minimus muscle.[17]

Finding the evidence

Since the evidence in the literature is lacking, it is difficult to critically analyze and formulate well-founded answers to the key clinical questions. We therefore present all the available evidence within MIS THR first, followed by attempts to answer the clinical questions.

- Cochrane Database, with search term "minimally invasive total hip replacement," "minimally invasive total hip arthroplasty"
- PubMed (www.ncbi.nlm.nih.gov/pubmed/) clinical queries search/systematic reviews, "minimally invasive total hip replacement," "minimally invasive total hip arthroplasty"
  ◦ 8208 hits
- MEDLINE search identifying the population ("hip" AND "minimally invasive total hip replacement"
  ◦ 10,230 hits
- PubMed (www.ncbi.nlm.nih.gov/pubmed/), sensitivity search using keywords "minimally invasive total hip replacement"
  ◦ 10,300 hits and, after review, 230 potentially relevant articles

Quality of the evidence

- Level I: 30
- Level II: 50
- Level III: 34 retrospective studies
- Level V: 19 case reports and expert opinion

Top four questions

- Does a MIS technique lead to quicker recovery?
- Does a MIS technique lead to less blood loss?
- Does a MIS technique lead to better patient function?
- Does MIS THR have similar complication rates to standard approaches?

Question 1: Does a MIS technique lead to quicker recovery?

Findings

The main premise for the introduction of these less invasive approaches was that patients would experience less pain and less blood loss, leading to a shorter hospital stay as well as overall quicker recovery to normal activities. The proponents of these techniques felt that these new procedures represented a dramatic evolution in hip arthroplasty by minimizing injury to tissues while maintaining the efficacy and safety of the classic surgical approaches. However, because of the advent of new anesthetic techniques during the same time it remained unclear what was mainly responsible for this quicker recovery: the smaller incision or the anesthetic protocol. In the vast majority of the clinical series on MIS THR, the anesthetic protocol involved premedication with anti-inflammatory several days before surgery, an oral narcotic on the day of surgery, and regional anesthesia and multimodal pain protocol postoperatively which included oral narcotics and anti-inflammatories.[18]

In a detailed review of the literature, Chen and associates[19] illustrate well the difficulty in evaluating new surgical techniques in the field of orthopedics with no validated endpoint to establish the efficacy of the surgical technique, making it difficult to compare the different approaches and to interpret the conclusions. In terms of level I evidence, Ogonda et al.[20] compared 219 THR patients who were either randomized to a MIS posterior approach (≤10 cm) or standard incision (16 cm) posterior approach with a single surgeon performing all procedures with the same anesthetic protocol as well as postoperative physiotherapy regimen with all the allied health professionals blinded to the incision. They found no significant difference between the two groups in terms of hospital stay, blood loss, and complications as well as functional outcome at 6 weeks. In another randomized controlled trial (RCT) comparing the mini-posterior to the two-incision technique in 21 patients, Pagnano and associates[21] found that patients in the two-incision group tended to have a slower rate of recovery at 6 weeks based on gait parameters and muscle strength evaluations. These findings are consistent with the anatomical studies comparing these two approaches which showed greater damage to the glutei muscles in the two-incision group compared to the mini-posterior.[17] In nonran-

domized trials, four studies[22–25] comparing small-incision THR to standard incision posterior approach THR in which the comparison groups were similar in demographic parameters, especially body mass index, found no significant difference. Similarly, deBeer and associates[22] also found no beneficial effect to the smaller incision when used with the lateral approach to the hip.

Recommendation

- With similar anesthetic protocols, the length of the incision had little impact on patient recovery and length of stay. More importantly, the two-incision technique was actually inferior to the mini-posterior approach. Similarly, the use of narcotics postoperatively was not impacted by the length of the incision but dependent on multimodal analgesia [overall quality: strong]

Question 2: Does a MIS technique lead to less blood loss?

Findings

Ogonda et al.[26] found no significant difference in blood loss between THR patients that were either randomized to a MIS posterior approach (≤10 cm) or standard incision (16 cm) posterior approach. Similarly, in their meta-analysis of randomized trials on MIS THR Cheng et al.[27] found that the only significant improvements with MIS techniques were in the short term, i.e., less intraoperative blood loss and shortened hospital stay (Table 18.2) but because of the significant heterogeneity they could not reach firm conclusions regarding efficacy of the various MIS techniques. Two studies[22,28] reported lower average intraoperative blood losses of 43 and 67 mL in patients undergoing the mini-incision THRs; however, there was no difference in the transfusion rates in these patient groups.

Recommendation

- MIS hip surgery showed no difference in blood loss [overall quality: strong]

Question 3: Does a MIS technique lead to better patient function?

Findings

Bennett and associates[29] found no difference in regards to velocity, step length of the affected or unaffected leg, stride length, or stance phase duration between the two groups.

Dorr et al.[30] concluded that compared with conventional THR performed through a posterior incision, posterior MIS THR resulted in better early pain control, earlier discharge to home, and less use of assistive devices. Subsequent evaluations at 6 weeks and 3 months showed equivalency between the clinical results in the two groups. In another review looking specifically at matched cohort studies of

Table 18.2 Summary of clinical studies on MIS THR

Study	Methods	Participants	Interventions	Outcome
Zhang et al. (China)	RCT; FU = 11 weeks	FNF = 60 MI vs. 60 SI; similar DC; unilateral THA	MI anterolateral 8.2 cm vs. SI posterior 14 cm; similar DC; unilateral THA Versys cementless prosthesis	Operative time; blood loss; HHS; complications
Wright et al. (USA)	qRCT; presence of assistant; FU = 5 years	OA, ON, RA = 42 MI vs. 42 SI; similar DC; unilateral THA	MI posterolateral 8.8 ± 1.5 cm vs. SI posterolateral 23.0 ± 2.1 cm press-fit cup and cemented stem; a senior surgeon	Operative time; blood loss; HHS; complications; radiographic evaluation
Chung et al. (Australia)	qRCT; observer blinded; alternation; FU = 14 months	OA = 60 MI vs. 60 SI; similar DC; unilateral THA	MI postetolateral 9.2 cm vs. SI posterolateral 20.0 cm; porous-coated cup and uncemented stem	Operative time; blood loss; length of hospital stay; HHS; complications
Hart et al. (Czech Republic)	RCT; observer blinded; FU = 39 months	OA = 60 MI vs. 60 SI; similar DC; unilateral THA	MI posterolateral 9–10 cm vs. SI posterolateral 20 cm; cemented prosthesis; two experienced surgeons	Operative time; blood loss; complications; radiographic evaluation
Chimento et al. (USA)	RCT draw card observer blinded; FU = 2 years	OA = 28 MIS vs. 32 SIS; similar DC; unilateral THA	MI posterolateral 8 cm vs. SI posterolateral 15 cm; press-fit cup cemented, or press-fit stem; a senior surgeon	Operative time; blood loss; complications; radiographic evaluation
Yan et al. (China)	RCT; FU = 6 months	OA, ON, FNF = 15 MI vs. 15 SI; similar DC; unilateral THA	MI anterior two incisions 3.6 cm; 5.7 cm vs. SI posterolateral 12 cm; Versys cementless prosthesis; a senior surgeon	Operative time; blood loss; complications; radiographic evaluation
Ogonda et al. (UK)	RCT sealed envelope patient and observer blinded; FU = 6 weeks	OA, ON, RA = 109 MI vs. 110 SI; similar DC; unilateral THA	MI posterolateral 9.5 ± 0.95 cm vs. SI posterolateral 15.81 ± 0.93 cm cementless cup cemented stem; an experienced surgeon	Operative time; blood loss; HHS; complications; a radiographic evaluation
Zhang et al. (China)	RCT sealed envelope; FU = 20 months	OA, RA = 60 MIS vs. 60 SIS; similar DC; unilateral THA	MI anterior 6.9 cm vs. SI posterolateral 16.3 cm Versys hip prosthesis	Operative time; blood loss; HHS; complications; radiographic evaluation
Kim et al. (Korea)	RCT randomized number table observer blinded; FU = 26.4 months	ON, OA, AS = 70 MIS vs. 70 SIS; similar DC;	MI posterolateral 8.8 ± 1.5 cm vs. SI posterolateral 23.0 ± 2.1 cm; bilateral THA cementless cup and cementless stem: a senior surgeon	Operative time; blood loss; HHS; length of hospital stay; complications; radiographic evaluation
Dorr et al. (USA)	RCT patient and observer blinded; FU = 3 months	OA, PA, HD, ON = 30 MIS vs. 30 SIS; similar DC; unilateral THA	MI posterior 10 ± 2 cm vs. SI posterior 20 ± 2 cm; cementless cup noncemented stem; two experienced surgeons	Operative time: blood loss; HHS; complications; radiographic evaluation
Dutka et al. (Poland)	qRCT odd or even day observer blinded; FU = 9.5 months	OA, HD, ON = 60 MIS vs. 60 SIS; similar DC; unilateral THA	MI lateral 6–8 cm vs. SI direct lateral 20–25 cm	Operative time; blood loss; HHS; length of hospital stay; complications
Speranza et al. (Italy)	RCT draw; FU = 6 months	OA, ON, FNF = 50 MIS vs. 50 SIS; similar DC; unilateral THA	MI direct lateral 7.1 ± 1.1 cm vs. SI posterior 12.8 ± 2.3 cm; cementless cup cementless stem; a senior surgeon	Operative time; blood loss; HHS: length of hospital stay; complications

DC, demographic characteristics; FNF, femoral neck fracture; FU, follow-up; HD, hip dysplasia; HHS, Harris hip score; MI, mini-incision; OA, osteoarthritis; ON, osteonecrosis; PA, post-traumatic arthritis; RA, rheumatoid arthritis; SI, standard incision.
Reproduced from Cheng et al.[40]

Table 18.3 Summary of clinical studies on mini-incision THR

Study	Study type	Surgical approach	No. mini-incision/ standard	Mini-incision benefits / disadvantages	Mini-incision group BMI loss	Transfusion	LOS	Incidence of complications	Incidence of malposition
Ogonda et al. 2005	RP	Posterior	100 100	None			NS	NS	NS	NS
Wright et al. 2005	RP	Posterior	50 50	None			NS	NS	NS	NS
Chimento et al. 2005	RP	Posterior	28 32	EBL 43 mL TBL 126 mL Limp at 6 weeks			NS	NS	NS	NS
de Beer et al. 2005	M CC	Lateral	30 30	EBL 67 mL			NS	NS	NS	NS
DiGioia et al. 2005	M CC	Posterior	35 35	HHS at 3 and 6 months		0.7 units 1.1 units	NS	NS	NS
Woolson et al. 2004	CS CC	Posterior	50 57	None		Yes	NS	NS	Mini-incision with more wound complications	Mini-incision with more AC and FC
Wright at al. 2004	CC	Posterior	42 42	ST -7 minutes HHS -3 points		Yes	NS	NS	NS	NS
Howell et al. 2004	CS CC	Anterior-inter muscular	50 57	EBL 82 mL ST +13 min		Yes	NS	4 days 5 days	NS	NS
O'Brien and Rorabeck	CS CC	Lateral	34 53	ST -6 min		Yes	NS	5.4 days 6.2 days	IO fracture 6% 2% NS	NS

A, change; AC, acetabular component; BMI, body mass index; CC : case controlled; CS, consecutive series; EBL, estimated blood loss; FC, femoral component; HHS, Harris hip score; IO, intraoperative; LOS, length of hospital stay; M :matched; NS, not statistically significant; RP, randomized prospective; ST, surgical time; TBL, total blood loss.
Reproduced from Vail and Callaghan.[6]

mini-incision THRs, Vail and Callaghan[6] concluded that although these could be done safely in patients who are not obese there were no real differences in clinical outcome (Table 18.3). Having said that, Howell et al.[31] gave significant importance to the psychological impact of improved cosmesis on patient attitude, satisfaction, and motivation for recovery. They cautioned that this appeal should not be underestimated when evaluating less invasive THR surgeries, with most studies reporting improved cosmesis and patient satisfaction with these smaller-incision approaches.[32,33]

Recommendation

• No significant difference was found with regards to patient function, but the evidence is moderate as current tools to evaluate patient function may not be sufficiently sensitive. The positive impact on patient cosmesis is strong

Question 4: Does MIS THR have similar complication rates to standard approaches?

Findings

Finally, when assessing the overall clinical value of MIS THR it is critical to look at the overall incidence of complications as well as their severity. Mow et al. have shown evidence of more subcutaneous tissue necrosis and/or poor wound healing after the mini-incision procedures[34]. All two-incision cohort studies report relatively long surgical times compared with those of open techniques, thus confirming the high degree of difficulty of this procedure. Although Berger[33] reported a low risk of femoral fracture (1%), others reported fracture rates of 7–9%.[35,36] One author reported a 4% early revision rate for treatment of postoperative fractures that were assumed to have occurred intraoperatively but were not detected by fluoroscopy or by immediate postoperative radiographs.[37] Another report showed a high 10% early revision rate for fracture, dislocation, and infection in patients who had THR with the two-incision procedure.[38] Two other studies also showed a relatively high incidence of nerve injury at 2.5–3.2%[36,39] with the two-incision technique. Other less invasive approaches such as the mini-posterior as well as the anterior Hueter approach have not reported higher rates of complications. In a multicenter study of 9 surgeons and 1277 THRs examining the introduction of the anterior Hueter approach,[15] the overall rate of revision was 2.7% with an incidence of proximal fracture of 1.8% including calcar splits. Obviously, the higher rate of complications associated with the two-incision technique reflects the difficulty in surgical exposure as well as the lack of familiarity for the surgeon in terms of patient positioning and instrumentation.

Recommendation

• The integration of new surgical techniques and approaches such as MIS may have a higher initial complication rate [overall quality: strong.]
• In regards to reproducibility, if the surgical technique is sound then it can be safely reproducible [overall quality: moderate]

Summary of recommendations

• With similar anesthetic protocols the length of the incision had little impact on patient recovery and length of stay. More importantly, the two-incision technique was actually inferior to the mini-posterior approach. Similarly, the use of narcotics postoperatively was not affected by the length of the incision but dependent on multimodal analgesia
• MIS hip surgery showed no difference in blood loss
• No significant difference was found with regard to patient function, whereas the positive impact on cosmesis is strong
• The integration of new surgical techniques and approaches such as MIS may have a higher initial complication rate
• With regard to reproducibility, if the surgical technique is sound then it can be safely reproducible

References

1. Rorabeck CH, Bourne RB, Laupacis A, Feeny D, Wong C, Tugwell P, et al. A double-blind study of 250 cases comparing cemented with cementless total hip arthroplasty. Cost-effectiveness and its impact on health-related quality of life. Clin Orthop 1994;298:156–64.

2. Berry DJ, Berger RA, Callaghan JJ, Dorr LD, Duwelius PJ, Hartzband MA, et al. Symposium: minimally invasive total hip arthroplasty. development, early results, and a critical analysis. J Bone Joint Surg 2003;85:2235–46.

3. Pour AE, Parvizi J, Sharkey PF, Hozack WJ, Rothman RH. Minimally invasive hip arthroplasty: what role does patient pre-conditioning play? J Bone Joint Surg Am 2007;89:1920–7.

4. Fehring TK, Mason JB. Catastrophic complications of minimally invasive hip surgery. A series of three cases. J Bone Joint Surg Am 2005;87:711–14.

5. Sculco TP, Jordan LC. The mini-incision approach to total hip arthroplasty. Instr Course Lect 2004;53:141–7.

6. Vail TP, Callaghan JJ. Minimal incision total hip arthroplasty. J Am Acad Orthop Surg 2007;15:707–15.

7. Penenberg B, Bolling WS, Riley M. Percutaneously assisted total hip arthroplasty (PATH): a preliminary report. J Bone Joint Surg 2008;90:209–20.

8. Bertin KC, Rottinger D. Anterolateral mini-incision hip replacement surgery: a modified Watson-Jones approach. Clin Orthop Relat Res 2004;429:248–55.

9. Watson-Jones R. Fracture of the neck of the femur. Br J Surg 1935;23:787.

10. Hardinge K. The direct lateral approach to the hip. J Bone Joint Surg Br 1982;64:17–19.

11. Rachbauer F, Kain MSH, Leunig M. The history of the anterior approach to the hip. Orthop Clin North Am 2009;40(3):311–20.

12. Smith-Petersen MN. A new supra-articular subperiosteal approach to the hip joint. Am J Orthop Surg 1917;15:592–95.

13. Light TR, Keggi KJ. Anterior approach to hip arthroplasty. Clin Orthop Rel Res 1980;152:255–60.

14. Judet J, Judet R. The use of an artificial femoral head for arthroplasty of the hip joint. J Bone Joint Surg 1950;32B:166–73.

15. Anterior Total Hip Arthroplasty Collaborative Investigators. Outcomes following the single-incision anterior approach to total hip arthroplasty: a multicenter observational study. Orthop Clin North Am 2009;40:329–42.

16. Pagnano MW, Leone J, Lewallen DG, Hanssen AD. Two-incision THA had modest outcomes and some substantial complications. Clin Orthop Relat Res 2005;441:86–90.

17. Mardones RM, Pagnano MW, Nemanich JP, Trousdale RT. The Frank Stinchfield Award: muscle damage after total hip arthroplasty done with the two-incision and mini-posterior techniques. Clin Orthop Relat Res 2005;441:63–7.

18. Tang R, Evans H, Chaput A, Kim C. Multimodal analgesia for hip arthroplasty. Orthop Clin North Am 2009;40:377–87.

19. Chimento GF, Pavone V, Sharrock N, Kahn B, Cahill J, Sculco TP. Minimally invasive total hip arthroplasty: a prospective randomized study. J Arthroplasty 2005;20:139–44.

20. Ogonda L, Wilson R, Archbold P, Lawlor M, Humphreys P, O'Brien S, Beverland D. A minimal-incision technique in total hip arthroplasty does not improve early postoperative outcomes. A prospective, randomized, controlled trial. J Bone Joint Surg Am 2005;87:701–10.

21. Krych AJ, Pagnano MW, Wood KC, Meneghini RM, Kaufmann K. No benefit of the two-incision THA over mini-posterior THA: a pilot study of strength and gait. Clin Orthop Relat Res 2010;468:565–70.

22. de Beer J, Petruccelli D, Gandhi R, Winemaker M. Single-incision, minimally invasive total hip arthroplasty: length doesn't matter. J Arthroplasty 2004;19:945–50.

23. Ogonda L, Wilson R, Archbold P, Lawlor M, Humphreys P, O'Brien S, Beverland D. A minimal-incision technique in total hip arthroplasty does not improve early postoperative outcomes. A prospective, randomized, controlled trial. J Bone Joint Surg Am 2005;87:701–10.

24. Chimento GF, Pavone V, Sharrock N, Kahn B, Cahill J, Sculco TP. Minimally invasive total hip arthroplasty: a prospective randomized study. J Arthroplasty 2005;20:139–44.

25. DiGioia AM, Plakseychuk AY, Levison TJ, Jaramaz B. Mini-incision technique for total hip arthroplasty with navigation. J Arthroplasty 2003;18:123–28.

26. Ogonda L, Wilson R, Archbold P, Lawlor M, Humphreys P, O'Brien S, Beverland D. A minimal-incision technique in total hip arthroplasty does not improve early postoperative outcomes. A prospective, randomized, controlled trial. J Bone Joint Surg Am 2005;87:701–10.

27. Cheng T, Feng JG, Liu T, Zhang XL. Minimally invasive total hip arthroplasty: a systematic review. Int Orthop 2009;33:1473–81.

28. Chimento GF, Pavone V, Sharrock N, Kahn B, Cahill J, Sculco TP. Minimally invasive total hip arthroplasty: a prospective randomized study. J Arthroplasty 2005;20:139–44.

29. Bennett D, Ogonda L, Elliott D, Humphreys L, Beverland DE. Comparison of gait kinematics in patients receiving minimally invasive and traditional hip replacement surgery: a prospective blinded study. Gait Posture 2006;23:374–82.

30. Dorr LD, Maheshwari AV, Long WT, Wan Z, Sirianni LE. Early pain relief and function after posterior minimally invasive and conventional total hip arthroplasty. A prospective, randomized, blinded study. J Bone Joint Surg Am 2007;89:1153–60.

31. Howell JR, Masri BA, Duncan CP. Minimally invasive versus standard incision anterolateral hip replacement: a comparative study. Orthop Clin North Am 2004;35:153–62.

32. Wright JM, Crockett HC, Delgado S, Lyman S, Madsen M, Sculco TP. Mini-incision for total hip arthroplasty: a prospective, controlled investigation with 5-year follow-up evaluation. J Arthroplasty 2004;19:538–45.

33. Berger RA, Jacobs JJ, Meneghini RN, Della Valle CJ, Paprosky W, Rosenberg AG. Rapid rehabilitation and recovery with minimally invasive total hip arthroplasty. Clin Orthop Relat Res 2004;429:239–47.

34. Mow CS, Woolson ST, Ngarmukos SG, Park EH, Lorenz HP. Comparison of scars from total hip replacements done with a standard or a mini-incision. Clin Orthop Relat Res 2005;441: 80–5.

35. Pagnano MW, Leone J, Lewallen DG, Hanssen AD. Two-incision THA had modest outcomes and some substantial complications. Clin Orthop Relat Res 2005;441:86–90.

36. Archibeck MJ, White REJ. Learning curve for the two-incision total hip replacement. Clin Orthop Relat Res 2004;429:232–38.

37. Pagnano MW, Leone J, Lewallen DG, Hanssen AD. Two-incision THA had modest outcomes and some substantial complications. Clin Orthop Relat Res 2005;441:86–90.

38. Bal SB, Haltom D, Aleto T, Barrett M. Early complications of primary total hip replacement performed with a two-incision minimally invasive technique. J Bone Joint Surg 2005;87A: 2432–38.

39. Pagnano MW, Leone J, Lewallen DG, Hanssen AD. Two-incision THA had modest outcomes and some substantial complications. Clin Orthop Relat Res 2005;441:86–90.

40. Cheng T, Feng JG, Liu T, Zhang XL. Minimally invasive total hip arthroplasty: a systematic review. Int Orthop 2009;33:1473–81.

19 Management of Femoral Periprosthetic Fractures After Hip Replacement

Tamim Umran, Donald S. Garbuz, Bassam A. Masri, and Clive P. Duncan
University of British Columbia, Vancouver, BC, Canada

Case scenario

An 81 year old woman presents with severe thigh pain and inability to weight bear after a simple slip and fall. She had a previous total hip arthroplasty (THA). Examination reveals external rotation deformity of the leg, bony crepitus, and tenderness around the proximal and mid thigh. Neurovascular exam is normal. Radiographs demonstrate a displaced periprosthetic femur fracture.

Relevant anatomy and pathomechanics

It is useful, when considering treatment, to divide the femur into three regions with reference to the stem: trochanteric (A); around or just below the stem (B); and distal to that (C). Furthermore, to integrate this with treatment, it is useful to subdivide the B type into those with a well-fixed stem (B1), a loose stem (B2), and a loose stem with poor bone stock (B3).

Importance of the problem

The prevalence of periprosthetic fractures ranges between 0.4 and 3.9% for all arthroplasties depending on whether it occurs in the primary or the revision setting.[1-3] These numbers have been steadily increasing over time as a function of the advancing age of the population and the increasing use of total hip arthroplasty (THR). This chapter discusses risk factors, diagnosis, management options, and outcomes of postoperative periprosthetic femur fractures, as supported by current available literature.

Top five questions

Etiology

1. Are there patient factors that may be predictive of a periprosthetic femur fracture?

Diagnosis

2. What classification system is effective in guiding treatment?

Therapy

3. What is the optimal management and outcome of Vancouver type A fractures?
4. What is the optimal management and outcome of Vancouver type B fractures?
5. What is the optimal management of Vancouver type C fractures (intraoperative and postoperative)?

> Difficulty arises when comparing the results in these studies due to variability in length of follow-up, patient demographics, number of revision arthroplasties, types of implants used, technical methods employed to treat the fractures, and variable outcome measures used to assess patients.

Question 1: Are there patient factors that may be predictive of a periprosthetic femur fracture?

Case clarification

An 80 year old patient had a cemented THR 18 years ago. Recent follow-up visits have demonstrated progressive

Evidence-Based Orthopedics, First Edition. Edited by Mohit Bhandari.
© 2012 Blackwell Publishing Ltd. Published 2012 by Blackwell Publishing Ltd.

osteolysis and loosening of the femoral component. While on the waiting list for revision surgery, she falls and sustains a periprosthetic femur fracture.

Relevance

Recognition of features associated with periprosthetic fractures could allow for prophylactic measures to preclude a fracture in the at-risk patient.

Current opinion

Current opinion suggests that patients with poor bone stock, loose components, and advanced age may have increased risk of periprosthetic fracture.

Finding the evidence

- PubMed (Clinical queries) (etiology): "periprosthetic hip fracture"
- PubMed: "periprosthetic hip fracture" AND ("risk factor" OR "epidemiology")
- MEDLINE: "periprosthetic hip fracture" AND "risk factors" OR "epidemiology"

Quality of the evidence

Level IV

- Retrospective cohort studies

Findings

Gender There are 11 studies providing epidemiologic data regarding periprosthetic fracture and gender. In most case series the majority of fracture patients are female.[1,4–7] This was questioned by the report of Lindahl et al. in 2005, whose results from the Swedish Hip Registry described a nearly equal rate of periprosthetic fractures in men and women.[3] In agreement with this is a recent retrospective survivorship analysis by Cook et al.[8] that found no relationship with gender looking at 124 periprosthetic fractures. Although some studies are suggestive that female gender appears to be a risk factor, it is likely that a multitude of other features contribute to this complication.

Patient age and length of time from index procedure It is clear that increasing age results in progressive weakening of bone because of osteoporosis. This is aggravated by osteolysis, if it develops. Epidemiologic data from a subset of series demonstrates an average age of 73.5 years (1220 fractures).[3–5] In their survivorship analysis, Cook et al.[8] found that patients older than 70 years had a relative risk of 2.9 for sustaining a fracture. He also reports a 0.8% incidence of periprosthetic fracture at 5 years, and 3.5% incidence at 10 years following primary THA.[8]

The literature also shows that the incidence of late postoperative periprosthetic fracture is increasing.[1,9–13] The average time post-procedure for a fracture to occur is reported in a number of studies. Holley et al. report an average of 112 months in a series of 99 patients.[5] Lindahl et al. report an average of 7.4 years post primary THA (688 fractures), and 3.9 years post revision hip arthroplasty (361 fractures).[3] Notably, Lindahl et al. looked retrospectively at the mean age at the time of the index operation and found a statistically significant higher fracture rate in those patients who were younger when they had their original surgery ($p < 0.001$). They postulated that younger and more active patients have a higher risk for sustaining an implant-related fracture in the future than those receiving arthroplasty later in life.[3] This observation, that the younger the patient at the time of the primary arthroplasty the greater the risk for subsequent fracture, was confirmed in later studies.[14]

Rheumatoid arthritis Several authors have demonstrated a relationship between increased fracture risk and rheumatoid arthritis (RA).[3,9,15] In the Swedish National Register of 191,351 hip replacements, only 6% of these entire group were patients with RA. Rheumatoid patients, however, had an increased representation in the periprosthetic fracture group, with an incidence of 11% and 10% in the primary and revision population respectively ($p < 0.001$).[3]

Osteoporosis and prior fragility fracture The presence of osteoporosis is a risk factor for intraoperative periprosthetic fracture. Taylor reports a series where 80% of the patients with periprosthetic fractures had osteoporosis.[16] Wu et al. found that preoperative osteoporosis (according to the Singh index) was a significant predictor for fracture.[17] Using fracture as a hallmark for osteoporosis, Beals and Tower observed that 38% of patients in their study had prior fragility fractures, and therefore osteoporosis.[18] In a small case-control study, Sarvilanna reported a risk ratio of 4.4 for periprosthetic fracture if the primary diagnosis for arthroplasty was fracture, with confidence intervals of 1.4–14.[19] Thus, osteoporotic patients, or those patients who have already sustained a fracture are at increased risk of having a periprosthetic fracture, a finding supported by several studies.

Component loosening Loose femoral components appear to be at risk for periprosthetic fracture. In an in-vitro study, Harris et al. found that femoral component loosening was a risk factor for periprosthetic fracture in cemented hips.[20] Several authors have reported that 50–75% of patients demonstrated evidence of loosening prior to fracture.[21,22] This is in keeping with the Swedish Hip Registry findings indicating that 70% of the implants were loose prior to periprosthetic fracture.[3]

Recommendations

- Older female patients (>70 years) who have a history of RA, osteoporosis, or previous fragility fracture are at increased risk of periprosthetic hip fracture

• Patients exhibiting loosening of the femoral component on plain radiographs are at increased risk of periprosthetic fracture. Surgical intervention prior to fracture should be considered

Question 2: What classification system is effective in guiding treatment?

Case clarification
An 82 year old patient sustains a periprosthetic femur fracture. The fracture extends from the mid-stem region to the mid-diaphysis. The implant appears to be loose, and the bone stock is poor. The surgeon begins therapeutic planning based on an understanding of the classification of this fracture.

Relevance
Orthopedic surgery has classification systems intended to facilitate management. The variability of pathology seen in periprosthetic fractures of the femur necessitates an effective classification system to aid in the communication of diagnoses among surgical colleagues, and develop management plans. The ability to classify these fractures properly will assist in their management.

Current opinion
The classification method most commonly used is the Vancouver system, because of its relevance to the principles of management and to the measurement of outcomes.

Finding the evidence
• PubMed: "periprosthetic" AND "classification" AND "validation" OR "kappa"

Quality of the evidence
Level IV
• Retrospective cohort studies

Findings
A useful classification system incorporates clinical and radiographic information to guide management, allowing for appropriate treatment and comparison of similar fractures.

Early classification systems focused on the location of the fracture,[23] but became more sophisticated with time as surgeons recognized the implications of fracture pattern and implant stability on treatment.[21,24–26]

A formal inclusion of implant stability into periprosthetic classification scheme was presented by Beals and Tower. In their retrospective review of 102 periprosthetic fracture treatments, they increased the level of sophistication by considering both anatomic fracture location and stability of the implant (inferred by implant/cement or implant/bone interface disruption).[18]

In 1995 Duncan and Masri published the Vancouver classification in order to emphasize the significance in the therapeutic decision-making process not only of the quality of the prosthetic–bone interface (stability), but also of the host bone stock.[27,28] The Vancouver classification system has been subject to reliability and validity testing in both North America and Europe.[29–31] Brady demonstrated the reliability of the system when evaluated by experts and nonexperts alike, with intraobserver agreement ranging from 0.73 to 0.83, and interobserver agreement of 0.61–0.64 by kappa analysis, indicating substantial agreement between observers. Validity was also evaluated revealing substantial agreement (kappa value of 0.78).[29] Rayan revalidated the classification system in Europe, demonstrating its reliability and usability by experts and nonexperts, and its use across continents.[30]

As outlined earlier, the Vancouver system divides the femur into three regions with reference to the stem: the trochanteric (A); around or just below the stem (B); and distal to that (C). Furthermore, to integrate this with treatment, the B type is subdivided into those with a well-fixed stem (B1), a loose stem (B2), and a loose stem with poor bone stock (B3).

Recommendation
• The Vancouver classification for postoperative periprosthetic fractures of the femur is reliable and valid for both experts and nonexperts [overall quality: high].

Question 3: What is the optimal management and outcome of Vancouver type A fractures?

Case clarification
An 82 year old woman has radiographs that demonstrate an uncemented THA with a fully porous-coated stem. She has an undisplaced fracture of the greater trochanter. The stem appears to be stable.

Current opinion
Current opinion suggests that proximal femoral periprosthetic fractures (Vancouver A type) can be treated either nonoperatively or operatively, depending on the stability and displacement of the fracture, assuming the stem is stable.

Finding the evidence
• PubMed (Clinical queries) (etiology): "periprosthetic hip fracture"
• PubMed: "periprosthetic hip fracture" AND ("risk factor" OR "epidemiology")
• MEDLINE: "periprosthetic hip fracture" AND "risk factors" OR "epidemiology"

Quality of the evidence
Level IV
- Retrospective cohort studies

Findings
The fractures are classified as type A_G (involving the greater trochanter) or A_L (involving the lesser trochanter). Those of the greater trochanter are often stable, and can be treated nonoperatively if displaced less than 2 cm[32] including limitation of active abduction for 3 months. If displaced more than 2 cm they can be managed with open reduction and internal fixation (ORIF) using a trochanteric claw plate. Vancouver A_L fractures are rare, and do not generally require surgical management, unless the stability of the implant is impaired by substantial disruption of the proximal medial femur, such as fractures associated with a substantial tongue of cortical bone. These are technically a B2 type fracture and management should be along those principles. The presence of trochanteric fractures is usually related to osteolysis and polyethylene wear, and treatment should be directed towards the cause of the osteolysis.

Recommendations
- Vancouver type A_G fractures that are displaced greater than 2 cm can be managed with ORIF [overall quality: low]
- Vancouver type A_L do not require surgical intervention unless they are technically a B2 fracture

Question 4: What is the optimal management and outcome of Vancouver type B fractures?

Case clarification
A 70 year old woman with an uncemented THA has an oblique fracture around the stem from the subtrochanteric region to a point just distal to the tip of the stem.

Relevance
The treatment is based on the stability of the stem, as well as the quantity and quality of the bone stock available in that location.

Current opinion
Although there is variability between centers on many specific details, the guiding principles include revision of the stem, replenishment of bone stock unless its loss is so severe that segmental replacement is needed, and reduction of the fracture around the underlying reconstruction.

Finding the evidence
- PubMed (Clinical queries) (etiology): "periprosthetic hip fracture"
- PubMed: "periprosthetic hip fracture" AND ("risk factor" OR "epidemiology")
- MEDLINE: "periprosthetic hip fracture" AND "risk factors" OR "epidemiology"

Quality of the evidence
Level IV
- Retrospective cohort studies

Findings

Type B1 Type B1 fractures are located around or adjacent to a stable femoral implant. The guiding principles include reduction, stable fixation and when necessary, the addition of bone graft. The surgical approach may be standard or minimally invasive (MIPO).

Haddad demonstrated 98% union (39/40) when onlay allografts were used with, or without, a plate. In this series, there was only one nonunion and no malunions above 10°.[33] Similarly, Chandler's report on 19 B1 cases with a cortical onlay allograft revealed union in 17 and malunion in only one of these 19 fractures.[34] This treatment technique has been well documented.[35]

Ebraheim reports 13 consecutive B1 fractures treated with reversed distal femoral locking plates. All fracture healed, with only one delayed union.[36] Conversely, Buttaro reports on 14 B1 fractures treated with locked compression plating with unicortical screw fixation with or without additional strut allograft. Because of over 50% failure in the plate-only group, and only a 20% failure in the combination allograft/plate constructs, the authors favored the latter approach.[37] This is supported by other authors, including Holley who suggests that for the B1 fracture the plate and strut are superior to the plate alone.[5] Recent biomechanical studies by Zdero also support this finding. In this study a variety of fixation strategies were examined for a periprosthetic fracture just distal to the tip of a well-fixed stem. Among the fixation strategies used, the authors demonstrate that a non-locking plate with cabled allograft provides the stiffest construct in vivo.[38] This finding is in keeping with previous biomechanical studies.[39]

Ricci et al. advocate the use of the minimally invasive plate osteosynthesis technique (MIPO), with indirect reduction and minimal soft tissue stripping. A union rate of 100% in 41 fractures was reported, at a mean of 12 weeks using a variety of plates. Minor implant failure was observed in only three instances, without influencing union.[40] In contrast, Tadross reports on four failures in a small series of seven fractures treated with the Dall–Miles cable plate system, including two nonunions and two malunions. This outcome was attributed to varus malalignment of the femoral component, which caused distraction at the fracture site.[41]

It is clear from the literature that B1 fractures should be treated with open or minimally invasive reduction and internal fixation, with or without cortical strut allograft.

Type B2 and B3 Types B2 and B3 fractures are characterized by the presence of fracture around or just below the stem, with a loose femoral implant. The discriminating feature is the quality and quantity of the surrounding bone stock; adequate (B2) or poor (B3). Numerous surgical strategies have been successfully employed in managing both B2 and B3 fractures.

Tsiridis retrospectively reviewed the results of 106 patients with types B2 and B3 fractures; 89 treated with impaction allografting, and 17 treated with cemented revision stems alone. Fractures treated with impaction grafting and a long stem had increased union compared to impaction grafting with a short stem (odds ratio 5.5, 95% CI 1.54–19.6, p = 0.009). Also, in this setting, impaction allografting with a long stem achieved higher union rates than long-stem revision alone (odds ratio 4.07, 95% CI 1.10–15.0, p = 0.035).[13]

Some authors have advocated the use of allograft in the management of the B3 fracture.[42] In a 1999 study, Wong and Gross report successful outcomes on 15 patients with B3 fractures treated with proximal femoral circumferential allografts. In their series they report one nonunion of the host–allograft junction requiring plating and grafting and one revision due to aseptic loosening of the femoral implant. 13/15 had good results, with postoperative Charnley scores of 5.1 with satisfactory pain relief and returned to their preoperative level of function.[42]

Using another successful technique, Maury reports on his outcomes of 25 Vancouver B3 fractures treated with allograft prosthetic composites, with 20 hip scores at 2 years of 70.8.[43] The majority of their patients were ambulatory (23/24) and pain-free (21/24) at this time. Notably, patients who had died or who were lost to follow-up (n = 8) prior to the 2 year mark had lower 20 hip scores (62.5) and more pain (3/8 pain-free). Four of the 25 hips required repeat revision.

Park et al. recently reported encouraging results for treating B2 and B3 fractures with fluted modular titanium, with a 92.6 % (25 of 27) successful outcome.[44]

Finally, in elderly patients with B3 fractures, the use of proximal femoral replacement prostheses is advocated due to a reduced rehabilitation time and immediate weight-bearing capacity that these implants allow.[45] Proximal femoral replacements have been shown to be effective, and survivorship at 12 years is reported at 64%, which is adequate for elderly patients with a limited life expectancy.

As with most revision operations, complication rates are higher than in the primary setting. Data obtained from early series of surgically managed periprosthetic femoral fractures shows high complication rates and significant patient morbidity.[6,16] Variable rates of complications have been published in the literature for the B3 fracture, as high as 29–66%. Major complications include dislocations, deep-seated infections, nonunion, refracture, heterotopic ossifi-

cation, pulmonary embolism, and cerebrovascular incidents.[5,16,25] Lindahl noted an overall complication rate of 23%, including nonunion, refracture, aseptic loosening, recurrent dislocation, deep infection, and ORIF failure in 1049 surgically managed fractures. In spite of this finding, Lindahl reports 76% patient satisfaction following revision for periprosthetic fracture (407 respondees). In the same group, 30% had at least one reoperation, 39% had no pain, and 61% had variable rates of pain.[3]

Recommendations
- B1 fractures generally can be treated by ORIF with plate devices and/or the use of cortical strut allografts. Augmentation with strut allograft may be beneficial [overall quality: moderate]
- B2 and B3 fractures can be treated with revision to a long-stem femoral component, with or without the addition of plate or allograft augmentation. Cementless, cemented, or cemented within impaction allografting can be used to address the pathology [overall quality: moderate]
- B3 fractures can be treated with an allograft–prosthetic–composite revision, segmental prosthesis, or with modular titanium fluted stems with or without allograft struts [overall quality: moderate]
- In the presence of a loose femoral component, internal fixation alone is inadequate in managing the periprosthetic fracture [overall quality: moderate]

Question 5: What is the optimal management of Vancouver type C fractures (intraoperative and postoperative)?

Case clarification
An 82 year old woman has radiographs that demonstrate an uncemented THA, with a proximal porous-coated taper wedge stem. The stem is well fixed, and there is no fracture of the proximal femur. A fracture is seen in the metadiaphyseal region of the distal femur.

Current opinion
Vancouver type C fractures can be treated nonoperatively or operatively, and can be typically addressed independent of the proximal femoral implant. Operative options include locked plating, nonlocked plating, and combi-plating (cable and screw combination).

Finding the evidence
- PubMed (Clinical queries) (etiology): "periprosthetic hip fracture"
- PubMed: "periprosthetic hip fracture" AND ("risk factor" OR "epidemiology")
- MEDLINE: "periprosthetic hip fracture" AND "risk factors" OR "epidemiology"

Quality of the evidence

Level IV

- Retrospective cohort studies

Findings

Postoperative type C fractures are those that occur well distal to the tip of the stem. Their morphology is quite variable. Nonoperative management is not considered suitable except in the sickest of patients because of poor results (malunion, nonunions) with high morbidity to the patient (partly due to prolonged bed rest).[46] Operative management of these fractures entails reduction and fixation, independent of the proximally located stem,[4] and is beyond the scope of this chapter.

Recommendation

- Type C periprosthetic fractures (displaced fracture) can be treated with ORIF using traditional fixed-angle devices, or combination cable/screw-based implants. In addition they should be managed with touch weightbearing status for 6–8 weeks postoperatively, predicated on clinical and radiographic features of healing [overall level: low]

Summary of recommendations

- Patients with osteoporosis or otherwise weak bone (e.g., RA) and a loose femoral component are at higher risk of having a periprosthetic fracture
- The Vancouver Classification for postoperative periprosthetic fractures of the femur is reliable and valid for both experts and nonexperts
- Type A_G fractures do not require operative management unless displaced
- Type A_L fractures are rare and do not require operative management
- Type B fractures are managed based on the stability of the femoral implant and integrity of the host bone around the implant. B1 fractures are treated with open or minimally invasive reduction, and internal fixation, with consideration given to strut allograft. B2 and B3 fractures can be treated with a variety of techniques including impaction allograft, cemented or cementless revision stems for bypass fixation, allograft–prosthetic–composites, or proximal femoral replacement
- Type C fractures are treated independent of the femoral prosthesis, using current trauma techniques and strategies

---

References

1. Berry DJ. Epidemiology: hip and knee. Orthop Clin North Am 1999;30:183–90.

2. Lowenhielm GF, Hansson LI, Karrholm J. Fracture of the lower extremity after total hip replacement. Arch Orthop Trauma Surg 1989;108:141–3.

3. Lindahl H, Malchau H, Herberts P, Garellick G. Periprosthetic femoral fractures classification and demographics of 1049 periprosthetic femoral fractures from the Swedish National Hip Arthroplasty Register. J Arthroplasty 2005;20:857–65.

4. Mukundan C, Rayan F, Kheir E. Management of late periprosthetic femur fractures: a retrospective cohort of 72 patients. Int Orthop 2010;34(4):485–9.

5. Holley K, Zelken J, Padgett D, Chimento G, Yun A, Buly R. Periprosthetic fractures of the femur after hip arthroplasty: an analysis of 99 patients. HSS J 2007;3:190–7.

6. Khan MA, O'Driscoll M. Fractures of the femur during total hip replacement and their management. J Bone Joint Surg Br 197759:36–41.

7. Schwartz JT, Mayer JG, Engh CA. Femoral fracture during noncemented total hip arthroplasty. J Bone Joint Surg Am 1989;71:1135–42.

8. Cook RE, Jenkins PJ, Walmsley PJ, Patton JT, Robinson CM. Risk factors for periprosthetic fractures of the hip: a survivorship analysis. Clin Orthop Relat Res 2008;466:1652–6.

9. Berry DJ Periprosthetic fractures associated with osteolysis: a problem on the rise. J Arthoplasty 200318:107–11.

10. Malchau HF, Herberts PF, Eisler TF, Garellick GF, Soderman P. The Swedish Total Hip Replacement Register. J Bone Joint Surg Am 2002 84(Suppl 2):2–20.

11. Abendschein W. Periprosthetic femur fractures—a growing epidemic. Am J Orthop 2003;32:34–6.

12. Lewallen DG, Berry DJ. Periprosthetic fracture of the femur after total hip arthroplasty: treatment and results to date. Instr Course Lect 1998;47:243–9.

13. Tsiridis E, Haddad FS, Gie GA. The management of periprosthetic femoral fractures around hip replacements. Injury 2003;34:95–105.

14. Lindahl H, Garrelick G, Regner H, Herberts P, Malchau H. Three hundred and twenty-one periprosthetic femoral fractures. J. Bone Joint Surg Am 2006;88:1215–22.

15. Sarvilanna RF, Huhtala HS, Sovelius R, Halonen P, Nevalainen JK, Pajamaki KJ. Factors predisposing to periprosthetic fracture after hip arthroplasty: a case (n = 31) control study. Acta Orthop Scand 2004;75:16–20.

16. Taylor MM, Meyers MH, Harvey JP. Intraoperative femur fractures during total hip replacement. Clin Orthop Relat Res 1978;137:96–103.

17. Wu CC, Au MK, Wu SS, Lin LC. Risk factors for postoperative femoral fracture in cementless hip arthroplasty. J Formos Med Assoc 1999;98:190–4.

18. Beals RK, Tower SS. Periprosthetic fractures of the femur. An analysis of 93 fractures. Clin Orthop 1996;327:238–46.

19. Sarvilinna R, Huhtala HS, Sovelius RT, Halonen PJ, Nevalainen JK, Pajamäki KJ. Factors predisposing to periprosthetic fracture after hip arthroplasty: a case (n = 31)-control study. Acta Orthop Scand 2004;75(1):16–20.

20. Harris B, Owen JR, Wayne JS, Jiranek WA. Does femoral component loosening predispose to femoral fracture? An in vitro comparison of cemented hips. Clin Orthop Relat Res 2010;468(2):497–503.

21. Bethea JS, DeAndrade JR, Fleming LL, Lindenbaum SD, Welch RB. Proximal femoral fractures following total hip arthroplasty. Clin Orthop 1982;170:95–106.

22. Jensen JS, Barfod GF, Hansen DF, Larsen E, Menck HF. Femoral shaft fracture after hip arthroplasty. Acta Orthop Scand 1988;59:9–13.

23. Parrish TF, Jones JR. Fracture of the femur following prosthetic arthroplasty of the hip. J Bone Joint Surg Am 1964;46:241–8.

24. Whittaker RP, Sotos LN, Ralston EL. Fractures of the femur about endoprostheses. J Trauma 1974;14:675–94.

25. Johansson JE, McBroom R, Barrington TW, Hunter GA. Fractures of the ipsilateral femur in patients with total hip replacement. J Bone Joint Surg Am 1981;63:1435–42.

26. Cooke PH, Newman JH. Fractures of the femur in relation to cemented hip prostheses. J Bone Joint Surg Br 1988;70(3):386–9.

27. Duncan CP, Masri BA. Fracture of the femur after hip replacement. Instr Course Lect 1995;44:293–304.

28. Brady OH, Garbuz DS, Masri BA, Duncan CP. Classification of the hip. Orthop Clin North Am 1999;30(2): 215–20.

29. Brady OH, Garbuz DS, Masri BA, Duncan CP. The reliability and validity of the Vancouver classification of femoral fractures after hip replacement. J Arthroplasty 2000;15:59–62.

30. Rayan F, Dodd M, Haddad FS. European validation of the Vancouver classification of peri-prosthetic proximal femoral fractures. J Bone Joint Surg Br 2008;90:1576–9.

31. Landis JR, Koch GC. The measurement of observer agreement for categorical data. Biometics 1977;33:159–74.

32. Pritchett JW. Fracture of the greater trochanter after hip replacement. Clin Orthop Relat Res 2001;390:221–6.

33. Haddad FS, Duncan CP, Berry DJ, Lewallen DG, Gross AE, Chandler HP. Periprosthetic femoral fractures around well-fixed implants:use of cortical onlay allografts with or without a plate. J Bone Joint Surg Am 2002;84:945–50.

34. Chandler HP, King D, Limbird R, Hedley A, McCarthy J, Penenberg B, Danylchuk K. The use of cortical allograft struts for fixation of fractures associated with well-fixed total joint prostheses. Semin Arthroplasty 1993;4(2):99–107.

35. Haddad FS, Duncan CP. Cortical onlay allograft struts in the treatment of periprosthetic femoral fractures. Instr Course Lect 2003;52:291–300.

36. Ebraheim NA, Gomez C, Ramineni SK, Liu J. Fixation of periprosthetic femoral shaft fractures adjacent to a well-fixed femoral stem with reversed distal femoral locking plate. J Trauma 2009;66(4):1152–7.

37. Buttaro MA, Farfalli G, Nunez MP, Comba F, Piccaluga F. Locking compression plate fixation of Vancouver type-B1 periprosthetic femoral fractures. J Bone Joint Surg Am 2007;89:1964–9.

38. Zdero R, Walker R, Waddell JP, Schemitsch E. Biomechanical evaluation of periprosthetic femoral fracture fixation. Journal Bone Joint Surg Am 2008;90:1068–77.

39. Wilson D, Frei H, Masri BA, Oxland TR, Duncan CP. A biomechanical study comparing cortical onlay allograft struts and plates in the treatment of peri-prosthetic femoral fractures. Clin Biomech 2005;20:70–6.

40. Ricci WM, Bolhofner BR, Loftus T, Cox C, Mitchell S, Borrelli J, Jr. Indirect reduction and plate fixation, without grafting, for periprosthetic femoral shaft fractures about a stable intramedullary implant. J Bone Joint Surg Am 2005;87:2240–5.

41. Tadross TS, Nanu AM, Buchanan MJ, Checketts RG. Dall-Miles plating for periprosthetic B1 fractures of the femur. J Arthroplasty 2000;15:47–51.

42. Wong P, Gross AE. The use of structural allografts for treating periprosthetic fractures about the hip and knee. Orthop Clin North Am 1999;30(2):259–64.

43. Maury AC, Pressman A, Cayen B, Zalzal P, Backstein D, Gross A. Proximal femoral allograft treatment of Vancouver type-B3 periprosthetic femoral fractures after total hip arthroplasty. J Bone Joint Surg Am 2006;88(5):953–8.

44. Park MS, Lim YJ, Chung WC, Ham DH, Lee SH. Management of periprosthetic femur fractures treated with distal fixation using a modular femoral stem using an anterolateral approach. J Arthroplasty 2009;24(8):1270–6.

45. Masri BA, Meek RMD, Duncan CP. Periprosthetic fractures evaluation and treatment. Clin Orthop Relat Res 2004;420: 80–95.

46. Somers JF, Suy R, Stuyck J, Mulier M, Fabry G. Conservative treatment of femoral shaft fractures in patients with total hip arthroplasty. J Arthroplasty 1998;13:162–71.

20 Evaluation of the Painful Total Hip Replacement

Matthew Oliver and James N. Powell
University of Calgary, Calgary, AB, Canada

Case scenario

A 70 year old man, with no medical comorbidities, underwent a cementless total hip arthroplasty for osteoarthritis of the hip joint 3 years ago. He returned to an active lifestyle. He now presents with a 2 month history of thigh pain.

Importance of the problem

Total hip arthroplasty (THA) is undoubtedly one of the most successful innovations of the last millennium. In the United States, 231,000 THAs were performed in 2006 and it is projected that the number will reach in excess of 500,000/year by 2030.[1,2] The National Joint Registry of England and Wales recorded 71,367 total hip procedures in 2008, an increase of 3.6% compared to the previous year.[3]

THA provides excellent pain relief[4] and an improved level of function.[5] It has been shown to be one of the most cost-effective healthcare interventions as measured by cost per quality-adjusted life years gained.[6]

The rise in the number of arthroplasties being performed, especially in young and obese patients, coupled with an increase in life expectancy, will lead to patients outliving their prosthesis. In the US between 1990 and 2002 the number of revision hip procedures increased by 79%.[7] The average billed charges in the US for all types of revision hip surgery were estimated at $54,553.[8] The massive financial impact that revision hip surgery has upon healthcare resources can therefore be appreciated. It must not be forgotten that revision surgery is associated with significant morbidity. The goal of this chapter is to provide a modern evidence-based approach to the evaluation of a painful THA.

Top six questions

1. What important symptoms and signs can be elicited from the history and clinical examination?
2. What is the role of plain radiographs in the evaluation of a painful THA?
3. Which is the best preoperative test to diagnose infection?
4. What role do nuclear imaging investigations have in the evaluation of a painful THA?
5. What is the role of ultrasound, CT, and MRI in the evaluation of a painful THA?
6. Are metal ion levels useful in evaluating painful metal-on-metal bearings?

Finding the evidence

- PubMed (www.ncbi.nlm.nih.gov/pubmed/) clinical queries search/ systematic reviews: "topic of interest AND total hip replacement AND systematic reviews"
- PubMed (www.ncbi.nlm.nih.gov/pubmed/) broad sensitivity search, diagnosis category using keywords "topic of interest AND total hip replacement"
- General MEDLINE search identifying the population (total hip replacement), the intervention (diagnostic tests), and the methodology (clinical trial)
- Cross-referencing from clinical papers obtained by the above methods

Question 1: What important symptoms and signs can be elicited from the history and clinical examination?

A complete history from the patient combined with a thorough physical examination is critical to successful

Evidence-Based Orthopedics, First Edition. Edited by Mohit Bhandari.
© 2012 Blackwell Publishing Ltd. Published 2012 by Blackwell Publishing Ltd.

Table 20.1 Differential diagnosis of a painful total hip arthroplasty

Intrinsic etiology	Extrinsic etiology
Infection	Lumbar spine pathology
Aseptic loosening	Peripheral vascular disease
Distal stem pain (modulus mismatch)	Neurological injury
Periprosthetic fracture	Metabolic bone disease
Osteolysis	Malignancy
Recurrent instability/dislocation	Hernia
Bursitis	Complex regional pain syndrome
Tendonitis	Gynacological
	Urological

acquisition of any diagnosis in medicine. The differential diagnosis of a painful THA is extensive and has been categorized by various authors[9,10] into intrinsic (directly related to the hip) and extrinsic causes (Table 20.1).

Pain is the most important descriptor in the history. The natural history of pain after THA was studied in over 2000 patients by Britton et al.[11] It was noted that the pain level was the most informative outcome as a predictor of revision and correlated well with patients' opinions of their outcomes. Pain is a highly subjective outcome measure, however, and needs to be interpreted with caution.

It is crucial to elicit the temporal onset of pain. An initial pain-free time period would suggest an intrinsic etiology such as aseptic loosening. If the patient was never pain free postoperatively then emphasis on searching for causes such as infection, initial failure of the implant to stabilize, or occult fracture perioperatively would be appropriate.

The site of pain serves as a useful diagnostic aid.[12] Pain localized to the buttock is suggestive of neurogenic or vascular claudication. This pain can radiate down the leg, and nerve root entrapment will need to be distinguished from arterial disease. Pain felt in the groin may indicate acetabular loosening or osteolysis or iliopsoas impingement/tendinopathy, or it can be due to a variety of herniae.[13] Iliopsoas impingement should be considered in patients complaining of pain in the groin during activities that require active hip flexion.[14] Gynecological and urological causes must not be ignored.

Thigh pain is suggestive of a loose femoral implant. It is acknowledged that patients with well-fixed femoral implants, either cemented or cementless, can still have low-intensity thigh pain. A mismatch in the modulus of elasticity of the host bone and a stiffer femoral implant has been recognized as a possible pain generator in the thigh.[15,16] Persistent or resting pain felt should alert the clinician to an infective or malignant process. Pain exacerbated by activity suggests loosening of the implants.

It is imperative to question the patient about their early postoperative recovery. Any wound infection, persistent wound discharge, or any course of empirical antibiotics, strongly points towards an infection as the pain generator.

Recent infections of other body systems such as a dental abscess or a urinary tract infection need to be documented. It is important to quantify the patient's comorbidities such as obesity, ischemic heart disease, diabetes, or immunosuppression, as these have a bearing on the diagnosis as well as the definitive treatment plan.

A comprehensive examination of both hips, both knees, and the spine is obligatory. The patients gait must be observed for evidence of antalgia, limb length discrepancy, and muscle weakness. A Trendelenburg gait is indicative of abductor muscle dysfunction. Progressive limb shortening is suggestive of subsidence of the femoral component.

It is imperative to inspect the operative site to ensure it has healed without complication.

The active and passive range of motion of the hip must be assessed. Any apprehension by the patient during this assessment of motion, especially in extreme positions, may indicate hip instability. Anterior and posterior impingement tests should be performed. This is important in hip resurfacing patients due to a decreased head–neck diameter ratio.

A neurovascular examination of the lower extremities is mandatory.

Question 2: What is the role of plain radiographs in the evaluation of a painful THA?

Case clarification
The patient's AP pelvis radiograph revealed extensive reactive lines around the cementless femoral component.

Relevance
Plain radiographs are a cheap and noninvasive first line investigation. However, the radiographs are open to misinterpretation, which can lead to a wrong diagnosis.

Current opinion
Current opinion suggests that plain radiographs provide useful information, but, as a single investigation, rarely lead to a confirmed diagnosis.

Quality of the evidence
- Level I: 2 meta-analyses/systematic reviews
- Level II: 1
- Level III: 3
- Level IV: 1

Findings

A critical review of serial plain radiographs from the time of surgery to the present date is ideal. This enables the clinician to evaluate for signs of osteolysis, loosening, or migration of the implants.

The most recognized criteria for radiographic loosening of cemented femoral stems were proposed by O'Neill and Harris.[17] In their study, plain radiographs were found to be accurate in predicting loose cemented femoral stems with a sensitivity of 89% and specificity of 92%. This study reported less impressive results for predicting loose acetabular components, with a sensitivity of 37% and specificity of 63%.[17]

With regard to cementless femoral prostheses, Engh et al. have defined the major and minor radiographic signs of osseointegration.[18] Engh et al. also devised a fixation/ stability scoring system to help predict implant failure.[18]

A meta-analysis by Temmerman et al. reported on the accuracy of diagnostic imaging techniques in the diagnosis of aseptic loosening of femoral components. The meta-analysis stated that plain radiography had a mean sensitivity and specificity of 82% (95% CI 76–87) and 81% (95% CI 73–87) respectively in diagnosing aseptic loosening. The study concluded that the diagnostic performance of plain radiography, subtraction arthrography, nuclear arthrography, and bone scintigraphy was not significantly different. It recommended plain radiography, supplemented if necessary by bone scintigraphy, for the evaluation of suspected aseptic loosening of the femoral component because of their efficacy and lower risk of patient morbidity.[19] Of note, the meta-analysis commented that the methodological quality of the studies analyzed was limited, being either confounded by verification bias or an appropriate "gold standard" not being applied to all patients, leading to a possible overestimation of diagnostic accuracy.[19]

Temmerman et al. also published a systematic review assessing the diagnostic performance of the above modalities in determining a loose acetabular component.[20] This review stated the pooled sensitivity and specificity rates for plain radiography were 70% (95% CI 59–79%) and 80% (95% CI 73–86%), respectively. Bone scintigraphy had a sensitivity of 67% (95% CI 57–76%) and specificity of 75% (95% CI 64–83%). Subtraction arthrography had a sensitivity of 89% (95% CI 84–93%) and 76% (95% CI 68–82%). It was therefore recommended to use subtraction arthrography as an additional test when plain radiography was found to be inconclusive in determining a loose acetabular component.[20] However, the use of arthrography has declined in recent years, mainly because of problems with standardizing and interpreting the test.

Differentiation of septic from aseptic loosening on plain radiographs is difficult unless the infection is locally aggressive or advanced. In this case the radiographic signs are usually obvious and include endosteal scalloping, osteopenia, periosteal new bone formation, and extensive osteolysis.

Serial evaluation of plain radiographs can reveal eccentric wear of the polyethylene liner of an acetabular component and alert the clinician to look for associated osteolysis. Several methods have been described to quantify polyethylene wear rates.[21–23] Early osteolysis is often asymptomatic and therefore the patient should be carefully followed up with serial radiographs to prevent catastrophic failure and avoid a challenging revision operation at a later date.

Recommendations

The evidence suggests:
- Plain radiographs are an easily obtainable, relatively cheap, and noninvasive investigation with an acceptable level of diagnostic accuracy [overall quality: moderate]

Question 3: Which is the best preoperative test to diagnose infection?

Case clarification

A complete blood cell count (CBC), erythrocyte sedimentation rate (ESR), and C- reactive protein (CRP) were performed. The ESR and CRP were elevated above the normal range. This prompted a preoperative hip aspiration for bacterial culture.

Relevance

The clinician needs to exclude between septic and aseptic etiologies as the treatment plans of each differ considerably.

Current opinion

A CBC and nonspecific inflammatory markers (CRP and ESR) are routinely requested to rule out an infective etiology.

Quality of the evidence

- Level II: 3
- Level III: 1
- Level IV: 6

Findings

Serological white cell count Canner et al. stated that only 15% of patients with a confirmed periprosthetic infection had an abnormally elevated white cell count.[24] Spangehl et al. found that an elevated white cell count had a sensitivity of only 20% (95% CI 9–38%), a specificity of 96% (95% CI 91–98%), a positive predictive value (PPV) of 54% (95% CI 24–76%) and a negative predictive value (NPV) of 85% (95% CI 79–90%).[25]

ESR This test showed a sensitivity of 82% (95% CI 65–93%), a specificity of 85% (95% CI 78–91%).[25] Other studies have shown that patients with documented periprosthetic infections have significantly elevated ESRs (mean 60 mm/hour), whereas those with mechanical loosening or those that are asymptomatic have lower or normal levels (<20 mm/hour).[26]

CRP This test showed a sensitivity of 96% (95% CI 78–100%) and a specificity of 92% (95% CI 85–96%).[25] Four studies have stated that CRP is a more sensitive test than ESR in differentiating between septic and aseptic loosening.[25–29]

Combined CRP and ESR Both these tests may be elevated in patients with chronic diseases unrelated to the hip joint and thus these tests are often criticized for their lack of specificity. However, if the clinician has performed a detailed medical history and examination and taken into account any factors that could result in a falsely elevated test, these tests are valid screening tools for possible infection. In fact, Spangehl et al. stated that when ESR and CRP both reveal negative findings then the probability of infection is zero (95% CI 0–4%). If they both report a positive result then the probability of infection is 83% (95% CI 62–95%).[25] Sanzen and Carlsson reported similar results in a previous study.[29]

Preoperative hip aspiration, culture, and sensitivity It is recommended to perform this investigation only when there is a high index of suspicion for infection with positive CRP and ESR results. If routinely performed for all patients in pain this test has poor specificity.[30] The patient should not have taken antibiotics for a minimum of 2 weeks prior to aspiration. Such investigations have shown sensitivities ranging from 50% to 92% and specificities of 88–97%.[25,31,32,33] The variability in results is due to the difference in sampling technique, interpretation of positive findings, and the potential for unrecorded use of antibiotics. In the study by Spangehl et al., the preoperative aspiration had a sensitivity of 86% and a specificity of 96% when patients taking antibiotics were excluded.[25]

Combined CRP, ESR, and preoperative hip aspiration When all three tests have negative results, the probability for an infected hip arthroplasty has been calculated at zero (95% CI 0–4%). When all three tests are positive, the probability has been calculated at 89% (95% CI 52–100%).[25]

Recommendations

In the evaluation of periprosthetic infection:
- Normal levels of CRP and ESR reliably exclude periprosthetic infection [overall quality: moderate]
- The combined use of hip aspiration with ESR and CRP (when elevated) yields the highest diagnostic accuracy for infection [overall quality: moderate].

Question 4: What role do nuclear imaging investigations have in the evaluation of a painful THA?

Case clarification
The patient underwent a triple-phase isotope bone scan (TPBS) and a leukocyte labeled bone scan to confirm whether both implants were loose and infected.

Relevance
The clinician needs to exclude between septic and aseptic etiologies as the treatment plans of each differ considerably.

Current opinion
The isotope bone scan is a valuable screening tool but lacks specificity. However, it is readily available and relatively cheap. Clinicians commonly use leukocyte labeled scans to aid confirmation of periprosthetic infection.

Quality of the evidence
- Level I: 3 meta-analyses/systematic reviews
- Level III: 3
- Level IV: 3

Findings
Technetium-99 methylene diphosphonate (Tc-99 MDP) bone scintigraphy Clinicians find this test most useful when the result is negative as it means the hip implants are not likely to be involved in a pathological process. The problem is this test lacks specificity.[34] The test can be positive for up to 2 years in well-fixed cemented and cementless prostheses.[35] The meta-analysis by Temmerman et al. stated this test had an overall sensitivity of 85% (95% CI 79–89) and specificity of 72% (95% CI 64–79) in detecting aseptic loosening of the femoral component. Only one study analyzed cementless femoral components, reporting a sensitivity of 82% (95% CI 57–96) and a specificity of only 43% (95% CI 43–71).[19] The overall results for the acetabular component were a sensitivity and specificity of 67% (95% CI 57–76) and 75% (95% CI 64–83) respectively. Again, only one study analyzed cementless acetabular components, reporting a sensitivity of 75% (95% CI 61–85) and a specificity of 41% (95% CI 18–67).[20] Lieberman found that technetium bone scans had a lower sensitivity and specificity than serial plain radiographs for diagnosing component loosening, recommending the use of bone scans only if radiographs were inconclusive.[34]

When a Tc-99 MDP scan is positive, a gallium-67 scan can help increase the specificity for differentiating between aseptic and septic loosening.[36] When the two techniques are combined the sensitivity lowers considerably to 57%, thus limiting its usefulness.[37]

TPBS Nagoya et al. reported that TPBS had PPV and NPV for infection of 83% and 93%, respectively. This group also reported a diagnostic sensitivity of 88% and specificity of 90%. Their conclusion was that it was a cost-effective method of screening.[38] A systematic review analyzing the accuracy of TPBS, white cell imaging (WBC), and positron emission tomography (PET) reported that TPBS yielded the least favorable results, with an accuracy of 80% in diagnosing infection.[39] The systematic review concluded that TPBS still has a role, especially in units without facilities for PET scans and WBC scans, as it excels in simplicity and cost-effectiveness.[39]

Labeled leukocyte scan (WBC scan) A dual tracer technique has delivered vast improvements in diagnostic accuracy, namely with a leukocyte scan performed simultaneously with a Tc-99 MDP bone scan. The accuracy is further improved by performing bone marrow scintigraphy with Tc-99 sulfur colloid. The systematic review reported that the leukocyte labeled scan had the highest diagnostic accuracy when compared to TPBS and PET, yielding an accuracy of 91%. The accuracy was even higher in the studies using bone marrow scintigraphy and leukocyte labeled scans.[39] However, this imaging modality is invasive, labor intensive, and expensive, and requires delayed imaging after 24 hours.[39]

FDG-PET PET has shown great promise for diagnosing infection, with a sensitivity and specificity of 94% and 95% respectively. However, there are no consistent assessment criteria in the literature.[40] FDP-PET ranked second in the systematic review with an overall accuracy of 89%.[39] This test is expensive and limited to specialist centers.

Recommendations

In routine practice:
- TPBS is a useful and cost-effective screening tool for aseptic and septic loosening [overall quality: moderate]
- The leukocyte labeled scan combined with Tc-99 sulfur colloid bone marrow scintigraphy should be considered the gold standard nuclear imaging test for diagnosing periprosthetic infection [overall quality: moderate]

Question 5: What is the role of ultrasound, CT, and MRI in the evaluation of a painful THA?

Relevance

Further imaging modalities—ultrasound, CT, and MRI—can add important information when used appropriately to answer a specific question.

Current opinion

Ultrasound has both a diagnostic and therapeutic role. Modern MRI and CT scanners have metal artifact reduction capabilities, improving their diagnostic value.

Quality of the evidence

- Level II: 1
- Level III: 8
- Level IV: 4

Findings

Ultrasound Advantages of ultrasonography over other cross-sectional imaging modalities are that it is less expensive, employs no exposure to radiation, and it has dynamic real time assessment capabilities. It can be used to image the soft tissue envelope around the hip joint, enabling the diagnosis of joint effusions, soft tissue masses, and iliopsoas impingement.[41,42] It can also be used to guide aspiration of a joint effusion distinguishing between a superficial fluid collection, a fluid collection communicating with the joint, or an intra-articular effusion. In a therapeutic role, it can be used to guide local anesthetic and steroid injections into peritendinous regions such as the iliopsoas or trochanteric bursa.[41–44]

CT CT has been proven to demonstrate areas of osteolysis with greater sensitivity than plain radiographs and enables accurate quantification of volume of bone loss.[45,46] It can detect subtle fractures and has been regarded as the gold standard in the assessment of iliopsoas impingement.[14,42,47]

Hart et al. reported promising results using three dimensional (3-D) CT scans to assess failing hip resurfacings when mechanical symptoms were diagnosed clinically.[48] These 3-D CT scans are able to confirm a clinical diagnosis of impingement and identify components at risk of high wear by calculating the true version and inclination of the acetabular component.[48]

MRI If technical adjustments to counteract metal artifact are employed, the MRI scan is a sensitive and all-inclusive modality for evaluating a painful hip arthroplasty. It can detect periprosthetic fatigue fractures even before completion of the fracture, enabling the surgeon to intervene at an earlier stage.[49]

MRI is also able to diagnose periprosthetic collections and allows evaluation of neurovascular structures, particularly if there is concern about entrapment by heterotopic bone or extravasated cement,[50] and is able to diagnose abductor muscle detachment.[51]

Studies have shown that MRI can more accurately demonstrate the presence and extent of osteolysis than plain radiographs.[50] This was validated with a cadaveric model yielding a sensitivity, specificity, and accuracy of 95%, 98%, and 96% respectively when compared to plain radiographs including Judet views.[52]

Hart et al. used a metal artifact reduction sequence (MARS) MRI to assess 26 patients with unexplained pain following a metal-on-metal bearing hip arthroplasty. The MARS MRI revealed 16 periprosthetic lesions, 2 of which were solid masses.[48] These masses have been labeled "pseudo-tumors." A pseudo-tumor is a periprosthetic soft tissue mass that has occurred as a result of a hypersensitivity immune reaction to metal debris. It is highly destructive to the soft tissue envelope of the hip. Results of revision surgery for pseudo-tumors have been poor.[53]

Recommendations

In routine practice:
- Ultrasound should be considered before CT and MRI if there is a targeted clinical question to a specific area of interest (i.e., impingement) or if a diagnostic or therapeutic injection/aspiration is required [overall quality: moderate]
- MRI can diagnose intraosseous, intra-articular and peri-articular pathology and its use for evaluating nonspecific hip symptoms or a suspected regional nerve injury is valid [overall quality: moderate]

Question 6: Are metal ion levels useful in evaluating painful metal-on-metal bearings?

Relevance

The national joint registries indicate that hip resurfacing is failing earlier than conventional THA.[3,54] The main reason has been femoral neck fracture (25%), but failures due to unexplained pain (23%) are of concern.[3]

Current opinion

Hip resurfacings seem to have specific modes of failure that are not detectable using traditional work-up algorithms. The mechanisms of failure appear to be high wear rates with associated high metal ion concentrations and a local metal hypersensitivity reaction.

Quality of the evidence

- Level II: 4
- Level III: 2
- Level IV: 0

Findings

Metal ion levels and acetabular component orientation Excess chromium and cobalt ions are known to have potentially toxic effects in humans.[55] It has been postulated that high metal ion levels of chromium and cobalt in a patient indicate a failing bearing surface. In a study by De Smet et al. a highly significant correlation was found between the maximum wear scar depth on explanted femoral components and the metal ion concentrations in both serum and joint fluid. The study recommended routine metal ion measurement in patients with metal-on-metal hip arthroplasties. De Smet et al. found there was more likely to be

metallosis in the hip joint in patients with concentrations of serum chromium greater than $17 \mu g/L$ and serum cobalt greater than $19 \mu g/L$.[56]

Several studies have found a strong correlation between high metal ion levels and increased inclination of the acetabular component ($>50°$).[49,57-59] Hart et al. recommended using a low-dose 3-D CT protocol to more accurately calculate acetabular component position.[48]

Increased metal ion levels were seen in one study with acetabular components positioned with more than 20° of anteversion, less than 10° of anteversion and more than 55° of inclination.[60]

Recommendations

In routine practice:
- Symptomatic patients should have blood chromium and cobalt ion measurements [overall quality: moderate]
- There is no published data on its diagnostic accuracy due to some control subjects having raised ion levels and indecision on setting normal threshold values. The use of routine testing of every patient cannot be recommended at this stage [overall quality: low]

Summary of recommendations

- Plain radiographs are an easily obtainable, relatively cheap and noninvasive investigation with an acceptable level of diagnostic accuracy
- Normal levels of CRP and ESR reliably exclude periprosthetic infection
- The combined use of hip aspiration with ESR and CRP (when elevated) yields the highest diagnostic accuracy for infection
- The TPBS is a useful and cost-effective screening tool for aseptic and septic loosening
- The leukocyte labeled scan combined with Tc-99 sulfur colloid bone marrow scintigraphy should be considered the gold standard nuclear imaging test for diagnosing periprosthetic infection
- Ultrasound should be considered before CT and MRI if there is a targeted clinical question to a specific area of interest (i.e., impingement) or if a diagnostic or therapeutic injection/aspiration is required
- MRI can diagnose intraosseous, intra-articular, and peri-articular pathology and its use for evaluating nonspecific hip symptoms or a suspected regional nerve injury is valid
- Symptomatic patients with metal-on-metal bearings should have blood chromium and cobalt ion measurements
- There is no published data on its diagnostic accuracy due to some control subjects having raised ion levels and indecision on setting normal threshold values. The use of routine testing of every patient cannot be recommended at this stage

Conclusions

- Complete clinical assessment of the pain is mandatory
- Serial plain radiographs reveal useful diagnostic information
- Preoperative hip aspiration when ESR and CRP are elevated yields the highest diagnostic accuracy for infection
- Leukocyte labeled scan plus bone marrow scintigraphy is the best nuclear imaging test for diagnosing infection
- The MRI scan is an all-inclusive modality for evaluating a painful hip arthroplasty, especially for nonspecific pain
- Symptomatic patients with metal-on-metal bearings should have blood metal ion levels measured as well as assessment of the acetabular component version

References

1. National Health Statistics Reports, Number 5. July 30, 2008.
2. Kurtz SM, Lau E, et al. Infection burden for hip and knee arthroplasty in the United States. J Arthroplasty 2008;23:984–91.
3. National Joint Registry for England and Wales, 5th Annual Report, 2008.
4. Visuri T, Koskenvuo M, et al. The influence of total hip replacement on hip pain and the use of analgesics. Pain 1985;23:19–26.
5. Alonso J, Lamarca R, et al. The pain and function of the hip (PFH) scale: a patient-based instrument for measuring outcome after total hip replacement. Orthopedics 2000;23:1273–8.
6. Chang C, Pellisser J, et al. A cost-effective analysis of total hip arthroplasty for osteoarthritis of the hip. JAMA 1996;275:858–65.
7. Kurtz S, Mowat F, et al. Prevalence of primary and revision total hip and knee arthroplasty in the United States from 1990 through 2002. J Bone Joint Surg Am 2005;87(7):1487–97.
8. Bozic K, Kurtz S, et al. The epidemiology of revision total hip arthroplasty in the United States. J Bone Joint Surg Am 2009;91(1):128–33.
9. Bozic K, Rubash H. The painful total hip replacement. Clin Orthop Relat Res. 2004;420;18–24.
10. Duffy P, Masri B, et al. Evaluation of patients with pain following total hip replacement. J Bone Joint Surg Am 2005;87(11):2566–74.
11. Britton AR, Murray DW, et al. Pain levels after total hip replacement: their use as endpoints for survival analysis. J Bone Joint Surg Br 1997;79:93–8.
12. Pritchett JW. Fracture of the greater trochanter after hip replacement. Clin Orthop Relat Res 2001;390:221–6.
13. Gaunt ME, Tan SG, et al. Strangulated obturator hernia masquerading as pain from a total hip replacement. J Bone Joint Surg Br 1992;74:782–3.
14. Dora C, Houweling M, et al. Iliopsoas impingement after total hip replacement. J Bone Joint Surg Br 2007;89(8):1031–5.
15. Bourne RB, Rorabeck CH, et al. Pain in the thigh following total hip replacement with a porous-coated anatomic prosthesis for osteoarthrosis. J Bone Joint Surg Am 1994;74:1464–70.
16. Brown TE, Larson B, et al. Thigh pain after cementless total hip arthroplasty: evaluation and management. J Am Acad Orthop Surg 2002;10:385–92.
17. O'Neill D, Harris WH. Failed total hip replacement: Assessment by plain radiographs, arthrograms, and aspiration of the hip joint. J Bone Joint Surg Am 1984;66:540–6.
18. Engh CA, Massin P, et al. Roentgenographic assessment of the biologic fixation of porous-surfaced femoral components. Clin Orthop 1990;257:107–28.
19. Temmerman OP, Raijmakers P, et al. Accuracy of diagnostic imaging techniques in the diagnosis of aseptic loosening of the femoral component of a hip prosthesis. A meta-analysis. J Bone Joint Surg Br 2005;87:781–5.
20. Temmerman OP, Raijmakers P, et al. The use of plain radiography, subtraction arthrography, nuclear arthrography and bone scintigraphy in the diagnosis of a loose acetabular component of a total hip prosthesis: a systematic review. J Arthroplasty 2007;22(6):818–27.
21. Dowd JE, Sychterz C, et al. Characterization of long term femoral head penetration rates. Associations with and prediction of osteolysis. J Bone Joint Surg Am 2000;82:1102–7.
22. Hamaji H, Yamamoto S, et al. Novel method to evaluate femoral head penetration in the poly liner after total hip arthroplasty: 3-D evaluation on standing radiographs. J Orthop Sci 2008;13(5):425–32.
23. Claus AM, Walde TA, et al. Management of patients with acetabular socket wear and pelvic osteolysis. J Arthroplasty 2003;18(3 Suppl 1):112–17.
24. Canner GC, Steinberg ME, et al. The infected hip after total hip arthroplasty. J Bone Joint Surg 1984;66:1393–9.
25. Spangehl MJ, Masri BA, et al. Prospective analysis of preoperative and intraoperative investigations for the diagnosis of infection at the sites of two hundred and two revision total hip arthroplasties. J Bone Joint Surg 1999;81:672–83.
26. Forster IW, Crawford R. Sedimentation rate in infected and uninfected total hip arthroplasty. Clin Orthop 1982;168:48–52.
27. Aalto K, Osterman K, et al. Changes in erythrocyte sedimentation rate and C-reactive protein after total hip arthroplasty. Clin Orthop 1984;184:118–20.
28. Shih L-Y, Wu JJ, et al. Erythrocyte sedimentation rate and C-reactive protein values in patients with total hip arthroplasty. Clin Orthop 1987;225:238–46.
29. Sanzen L, Carlsson AS. The diagnostic value of C-reactive protein in infected total hip arthroplasties. J Bone Joint Surg Br 1989;71(4):638–41.
30. Barrack RL, Harris WH. The value of aspiration of the hip joint before revision total hip arthroplasty. J Bone Joint Surg Am 1993;75:66–76.
31. Lachiewicz PF, Rogers GD, et al. Aspiration of the hip joint before revision total hip arthroplasty: clinical and laboratory factors influencing attainment of a positive culture. J Bone Joint Surg Am 1996;78:749–54.
32. Fehring TK, Cohen B. Aspiration as a guide to sepsis in revision total hip arthroplasty. J Arthroplasty 1996;11:543–7.
33. Roberts P, Walters AJ. Diagnosing infection in hip replacements: the use of a fine needle aspiration and radiometric culture. J Bone Joint Surg Br 1992;74:265–9.
34. Lieberman JR, Huo MH, et al. Are technetium bone scans necessary? J Bone Joint Surg Br 1993;75:475–8.
35. Utz JA, Lull R, et al. Asymptomatic total hip prosthesis: natural history determined using Tc-99M MDP bone scans. Radiology 1986;161:509–12.

36. Merkel KD, Brown ML, et al. Sequential technetium-99 m HMDP-gallium-67 citrate imaging for the evaluation of infection in the painful prosthesis. J Nucl Med 1986;27:1413–17.

37. Kraemer WJ, Saplys R, et al. Bone scan, gallium scan, and hip aspiration in the diagnosis of infected total hip arthroplasty. J Arthroplasty 1993;8:611–15.

38. Nagoya S, Kaya M, et al. Diagnosis of peri-prosthetic infection at the hip using triple-phase bone scintigraphy. J Bone Joint Surg Br 2008;90:140–4.

39. Reinartz P. FDG-PET in patients with painful hip and knee arthroplasty: technical breakthrough or just more of the same. Q J Nucl Med Mol Imaging 2009;53(1):41–50.

40. Reinartz P, Mumme T, et al. Radionuclide imaging of the painful hip arthroplasty. Positron-emission tomography versus triple-phase bone scanning. J Bone Joint Surg Br 2005;87: 465–70.

41. Wank R, Miller TT, et al. Sonographically guided injection of anesthetic for iliopsoas tendinopathy after total hip arthroplasty. J Clin Ultrasound 2004;32(7):354–7.

42. Rezig R, Copercini M, et al. Ultrasound diagnosis of anterior iliopsoas impingement in total hip replacement. Skelet Radiol 2004;33:112–16.

43. Adler RS, Buly R, et al. Diagnostic and therapeutic use of sonography-guided iliopsoas peritendinous injections. AJR Am J Roentgenol 2005;185:940–3.

44. Blankenbaker DG, DeSmet AA, et al. Sonography of the iliopsoas tendon and injection of the iliopsoas bursa for diagnosis and management of the painful snapping hip. Skelet Radiol 2006;35:565–71.

45. Kitamura N, Pappedemos PC, et al. The value of anteroposterior radiographs in evaluating pelvic osteolysis. Clin Orthop 2006; 453:239–345.

46. Claus AM, Totterman SM, et al. Computed tomography to assess pelvic lysis after total hip replacement. Clin Orthop 2004; 422:167–74.

47. Jasani V, Richards P, et al. Pain related to the psoas muscle after total hip replacement. J Bone Joint Surg Br 2002;84:991–3.

48. Hart AJ, Sabah S, et al. The painful metal on metal hip resurfacing. J Bone Joint Surg Br 2009;91:738–44.

49. Cook SM, Pellicci PM, et al. Use of magnetic resonance imaging in the diagnosis of an occult fracture of the femoral component after total hip arthroplasty. J Bone Joint Surg Am 2004;86: 149–53.

50. Potter HG, Nestor BJ, et al. Magnetic resonance imaging after total hip arthroplasty: evaluation of periprosthetic soft tissues. J Bone Joint Surg Am 2004;86:1947–54.

51. Twair A, Ryan M, et al. MRI of the failed total hip replacement caused by abductor muscle avulsion. AJR Am J Roentgenol 2003;181:1547–50.

52. Weiland DE, Walde TA, et al. Magnetic resonance imaging in the evaluation of periprosthetic acetabular osteolysis: a cadaveric study. J Orthop Res 2005;23:713–19.

53. Grammatopolous G, Pandit H, et al. Hip resurfacings revised for inflammatory pseudotumour have a poor outcome. J Bone Joint Surg Br 2009;91:1019–24.

54. Australian Orthopaedic Association National Joint Replacement Registry Annual Report, 2008.

55. Keegan G, Learmonth I, et al. Orthopaedic metals and their potential toxicity in the arthroplasty patient. A review of current knowledge and future strategies. J Bone Joint Surg Br 2007; 89:567–73.

56. De Smet K, De Haan R, et al. Metal ion measurement as a diagnostic tool to identify problems with metal-on-metal hip resurfacing. J Bone Joint Surg Am 2008;90:202–8.

57. De Haan R, Pattyn C, et al. Correlation between inclination of the acetabular component and metal ion levels in metal on metal hip resurfacing replacement. J Bone Joint Surg Br 2008;90:1291–7.

58. Hart AJ, Buddhdev P, et al. Cup inclination angle of greater than 50 degrees increases whole blood concentrations of cobalt and chromium ions after metal on metal hip resurfacing. Hip Int 2008;18:212–19.

59. Langton DJ, Jameson SS, et al. The effect of component size and orientation on the concentrations of metal ions after resurfacing arthroplasty. J Bone Joint Surg Br 2008;90:1143–51.

60. Langton DJ, Sprowson AP, et al. Blood metal ion concentrations after hip resurfacing arthroplasty. A comparative study of Articular Surface Replacement and Birmingham Hip Resurfacing Arthroplasties. J Bone Joint Surg Br 2009;91:1287–95.

21 Revision of the Femoral Components: Role of Structural Bulk Allografts and Impaction Grafting

Christopher R. Gooding, Bassam A. Masri, Donald S. Garbuz, and Clive P. Duncan

University of British Columbia, Vancouver, BC, Canada

Case scenario

A 55 year old man presents to the clinic with a 12 month history of left groin pain. He had a total hip arthroplasty (THA) on that side 15 years ago. The pain is getting worse and he is now housebound. On examination, he walks with an antalgic gait and the surgical scar over the left hip is well healed with no clinical evidence of infection. He has equal leg lengths, a fixed flexion deformity of 15° and joint motion is limited in every direction because of pain. Examination of the spine, as well as the vascular and neurological status of the left lower limb, reveals no remarkable findings.

Relevant anatomy

Revision of the femoral component of a THA can be technically challenging. Careful analysis of bone loss, and planning, are key to success. With so many options available for reconstruction it is helpful to have a system for classifying the femoral defects to help the surgeon achieve a thorough understanding of the problem and to be appropriately prepared with the necessary implants and instruments.

The most widely used classification system is that proposed by Paprosky et al.,[1] the 2000 version is summarized here.

Classification of femoral defects[1]

- *Type I:* A well preserved metaphyseal cancellous bone with an intact diaphysis. This is often seen following the removal of a cementless femoral component without any ingrowth.
- *Type II:* Considerable loss of metaphyseal cancellous bone but with an intact diaphysis. This pattern is commonly seen following the removal of a cemented femoral component.
- *Type IIIA:* Severely damaged metaphysis that is unable to support an implant but more than 4 cm of intact diaphyseal bone is available for distal fixation. Paprosky gives the example of a loose femoral component that has been inserted with first-generation cementing techniques, i.e., poor cement pressurization.
- *Type IIIB:* A severely damaged metaphysis as for type IIIA but with less than 4 cm of diaphyseal bone available for distal fixation. Such a picture of bone destruction can be seen following a failed cemented stem, inserted with a cement restrictor. As well as osteolysis proximally in the metaphysis there is also considerable osteolysis surrounding the polyethylene cement restrictor. A similar pattern can also be seen with an uncemented femoral stem associated with distal osteolysis.
- *Type IV:* With this pattern of bone destruction there is considerable damage to both the metaphysis and diaphysis associated with a widened femoral canal as a result of which the isthmus is unable to support an implant.

Evidence-Based Orthopedics, First Edition. Edited by Mohit Bhandari.
© 2012 Blackwell Publishing Ltd. Published 2012 by Blackwell Publishing Ltd.

Importance of the problem

In 2000 it was estimated that 183,000 total hip replacements were performed in the United States and that 31,000 (17%) were revision procedures.[2] By 2003 these figures had increased to approximately 200,000 and 36,000 respectively.[3] In England and Wales the 2007 report from the National Joint Registry recorded 62,253 primary hip replacements and 6353 revision hip replacements.[4] This was a substantial increase compared to the figures for 2003–2004 when 3012 revisions were reported, representing more than double the number of revision procedures.[4] However, this may represent a degree of under-reporting, as the UK National Joint Registry was in its infancy in 2003–2004. Nonetheless it is clear that revision hip arthroplasty is becoming an increasing problem with an increasing number being done worldwide and an aging population who have had a THA. In 2006, Hootman et al. estimated that the number of revision hip procedures increased by 60% in the previous decade compared to an increase of 50% for primaries.[5]

Revision hip surgery places a greater financial burden on healthcare expenditure, as the majority of patients require longer hospital stays and generally have higher rates of morbidity.[6] The rate of readmission for any cause within 30 days from the date of surgery has been reported at 8.48% for revision hip surgery compared to 4.91% for primaries.[3]

Orthopedic surgeons and their patients have access to a large amount of information about revision hip surgery. The Google search engine finds over a quarter of a million hits when the search term "revision hip surgery" is entered. Even if the more specific search term "bone allografts in revision hip surgery" is used, there are more than 124,000 hits. Clearly, this type of review will yield a lot of information but of variable quality, highlighting the need for the development of an evidence-based approach.

Top ten questions

Basic science

1. How does morselized impaction graft and structural allograft become incorporated into the host bone?
2. What biomechanical factors contribute to long-term success?

Therapy

3. What are the technical aspects of impaction allografting for revision of a femoral component in THA?

4. What are the results of impaction allografting in femoral revision in revision THA?
5. What are the technical aspects in using a structural allograft in femoral revision in revision THA?
6. What choices of femoral implant are available when using a structural bone allograft?
7. What are the results of using a structural allograft in revision THA and what are its advantages and disadvantages?

Harm

8. What are the complications of impaction allografting for revision of a femoral component in THA?
9. What are the complications of using a structural bulk allograft for revision of a femoral component in THA?

Current practice and the future

10. What is the current state of the popularity of these techniques? Are there better alternatives?

Question 1: How does morselized impaction graft and structural allograft become incorporated into the host bone?

Allograft bone can be used to replace or reinforce the proximal femur,[7-9] as a cortical strut graft to reinforce the calcar or lateral cortex, or as morselized graft, as in impaction grafting.[10]

Bone graft can become incorporated within the host bone by different processes. These include osteoinduction and osteoconduction as well as osteogenesis. *Osteoinduction* refers to the ability of the graft to stimulate new bone formation by recruiting pluripotential stem cells from the surrounding host bone. This is mediated by a number of bone matrix proteins of which the bone morphogenic proteins (BMP) are the best characterized. *Osteoconduction* refers to the ability of bone graft to function as a scaffold for the ingrowth of new capillaries as well as the migration of osteoprogenitor cells from the host. This bone graft scaffold is gradually replaced over time with host bone by a process called *creeping substitution*. *Osteogenesis* refers to bone's ability to regenerate itself by producing new bone. This process is mediated by osteoblasts. Bone resorption is also a fundamental process by which bone grafts eventually become incorporated into the host bone, and is mediated by osteoclasts. Unlike autograft bone, which can become incorporated into the host bone via osteoinduction, osteoconduction, or osteogenesis, allograft bone becomes incorporated via osteoconduction alone.

In the context of femoral impaction grafting, morselized allograft is used as filler. The graft has a rich vascular bed provided by the endosteal blood supply. This type of construct will incorporate through a combination of revascularization, osteoconduction, and remodeling. It becomes incorporated with the host bone similar to autogenous cancellous bone graft, albeit at a slower rate, and necrotic bone graft may persist at the site of implantation.[11]

Histological studies of biopsies from patients who have had impaction allografting have shown incorporation.[12–14] Examination of a femur from a patient who had impaction grafting with cement 3.5 years before postmortem examination showed that the graft had organized into three zones: a zone of regenerated cortical bone, an interface between cement and bone, and nonviable bony trabeculae embedded in cement.[15] There were some islands of nonviable bone but more than 90% of the outer neocortex was viable.

Structural allograft incorporation has been extensively studied in animals; the results may not be directly applicable to humans but give us some idea of how allografts become incorporated in the host. Fresh allografts stimulate a rejection reaction, which may lead to graft resorption. Processing allografts by freezing or freeze-drying decreases the immunogenicity,[16–18] but the biologic activity is also reduced by removing all live cells.[19]

The structural allograft first incites an inflammatory response that brings in the pluripotential cells needed for new bone formation. The union and incorporation processes are initiated by osteoclasts which resorb the haversian systems of the allograft until the osteoblasts appear (derived from the endosteal lining of the host and from the surrounding soft tissues) and fill in this area. This process is slow and can take as much as eight times longer to heal than an autogenous bone graft.[20,21] Unlike morselized allografts, revascularization, creeping substitution, and remodeling occur only to a limited extent[21,22] and are usually limited to the periphery of the graft adjacent to the host–graft junction. Human retrieval studies have also shed some light on the behavior of frozen allografts.[23,24] Enneking showed that union at the cortical host–graft junction initially starts with callus formation. Less than 20% of the graft remodeled and this only took place at the superficial ends of the graft.[23] Soft tissues appeared to become firmly attached to the graft by a layer of new bone.

Union between the graft and host can be improved by placing autograft at the graft–host junction. This autograft can be obtained from the iliac crest, or from reamings from the host femur that can be wrapped around the graft–host junction as suggested by Gross.[25] Since autograft possesses osteoblasts it is capable of osteogenesis, as well as possessing osteoinductive substances.

It is clear that allograft incorporation is a somewhat complex process that is dependent on many factors. The complete incorporation of a graft, i.e., the removal of the donor bone and its replacement by new bone from the host, is not necessary in all clinical situations. The goal in cortical grafts is union at the graft–host junction together with some limited remodeling so that the graft can provide some mechanical support and is able to withstand physiologic weightbearing without pain or fracture.[22]

Question 2: What biomechanical factors contribute to long-term success?

Processed structural allograft can be described as biologically inert and therefore functions like an implant. The biomechanical consequence of this is that the allograft supported by internal fixation, such as a femoral stem, is as strong as living bone because it is the mineralized matrix of bone that gives it its strength. Therefore, an allograft–prosthesis construct can be considered a success when union has occurred at the graft–host junction. But, unlike living bone, it is unable to remodel in response to accumulated load and is therefore prone to fatigue failure with time. In addition, revascularization can lead to graft resorption.

The problems facing impaction allografting are different to those faced by structural allografting. Some reports have indicated a high prevalence of intra and postoperative fractures[26–29] and high levels of implant migration of more than 10 mm.[30–33] Inadequate compaction of the graft[34–37] and defects in the cement mantle[35,38] as well as resorption of the endosteal layer[39] are thought to play a role. Although studies have shown radiological evidence of remodeling of the impacted allograft,[40–42] histological reports have revealed that the graft does not fully remodel into viable bone even up to 8 years following the index procedure.[13,43] Additionally, there are some reports that the cement can penetrate all the way to the endosteal cortex.[39,44] It is uncertain whether this is desirable in terms of achieving initial composite stability, or undesirable by compromising bone graft remodeling. Reducing cement pressure or increasing its viscosity can reduce the amount of cement penetration which may enhance local vascularization around the graft and hence its ability to be remodeled.[45] However, this may have the deleterious result of reducing the shear strength of the endosteal interface, leading to excessive migration of the stem.[46] Albert et al.[47] used a cadaveric model to assess pressurization of the cement and its penetration through the impacted allograft. They observed that impaction grafting without cement pressurization led to a reduction of cement contact with the endosteal cortex; however, the migration and micromotion of the implant were significantly increased. The authors went on to conclude that longer-term stability of the implant is likely to be compromised if the cement is not pressurized.

Clearly a balance is desirable, but how to achieve that in the highly variable surgical setting is a challenge. If the cement reaches the endosteal bone then it will impede remodeling and integration of the impacted allograft.

However, a cement mantle which is less than 2mm thick will lead to excessive implant subsidence.[35,38] This conflict of biological and structural goals of impaction allografting has been highlighted by other studies which have shown that the strength of the endosteal surface with the graft/cement is proportional to the amount of cement contact.[44,46] Albert et al.[47] showed that with more than 50% of cement contact to the endosteal surface resulted in lower distal migration and micromotion than if there was less contact.

In summary, a number of biomechanical factors are implicated in the long-term success of structural and impaction allografting. With proximal structural allografts the femoral implant serves as an intramedullary fixation device, reducing the risk of fracture of the allograft as well as stabilizing it and so promoting union of the graft to the host.[48-50] For impaction allografting to be a success the graft has to be sufficiently compacted to be able to support a femoral implant and a balance has to be established between sufficient cement pressurization to ensure stability of the construct but not so much as to interfere with incorporation of the morselized allograft into the host bone.

Question 3: What are the technical aspects of impaction allografting for revision of a femoral component in THA?

Concerns have been raised about the incidence of massive (>10mm) early subsidence following impaction grafting with allograft. Eldridge et al.[31] reported on 79 consecutive cases of revision THA using morselized allograft, polymethylmethacrylate cement, and a double tapered, polished, collarless stem. Nine patients (11%) showed evidence of massive subsidence, with another nine patients subsiding to a lesser extent. Similar concerns have been raised in other studies.[38] This subsidence is significant as it subsequently leads to early implant failure.

The biomechanical factors which may have some influence whether a revision with impaction allografting is a success or failure have been discussed. In this section the surgical factors are outlined.

Nelissen et al.[35] reviewed 18 patients who underwent revision surgery with impaction grafting and a tapered, cemented stem. The femoral defects were classified according to the 1993 version of the Paprosky classification system:[50a] 1 type IIA (absent calcar extending just below the intertrochanteric level), 3 type IIB (anterolateral metaphyseal bone loss), 10 type IIC (absent calcar with posteromedial metaphyseal bone loss), and 4 type III (type II defects with additional diaphyseal bone loss). From this study two factors appeared to influence migration of the femoral stems. The first was the extent of the femoral defect and the second was the presence of cement mantle defects. However the difference of stem migration between the Paprosky groups was small and was discounted. The great-est increase in migration occurred during the first 3 months after surgery. Subsidence that occurs during the first few weeks can be attributed to additional graft compaction, as seen in other studies.[51] The pattern of stem migration was subsidence and varus rotation and antetorsion. This pattern could be due either to cement mantle defects at the medial Gruen zones or to less impacted allograft chips. All of the eight cases that showed continuous migration of the femoral implant had cement mantle defects (thickness of cement ≤2mm) in at least two Gruen zones. The cement mantle allows for a smooth transition of forces from the femoral implant to the adjacent bone. Since the bone graft deforms permanently during the process of creeping substitution, cement mantle defects may cause progressive migration and failure of the construct. This finding is similar to the findings from other studies which have concluded that the durability of a cemented stem albeit in the primary setting is related to the quality of the cement mantle.[52-57]

Masterson et al.[30,38] concluded that the cement mantle defects that they observed were due to poor instrumentation and that a good cementing technique was essential for impaction allografting to be successful. This finding has been further corroborated by other studies.[35] Another reasons for massive stem subsidence is poor packing of the allograft. Knight et al.[26] reported that this was a problem in 94% of their cases which resulted in varus or valgus alignment and a medial or lateral stem displacement. They attributed this to the technically demanding nature of the procedure, which was not helped by the lack of appropriate instruments to facilitate the technique.

More recently a variety of instrument systems have been introduced to help standardize the impaction technique. The difficulty is deciding when the construct has achieved adequate stability. In answer to this problem, one study has suggested the use of a torque wrench to assess rotational stability of the impactor.[58]

By the very nature of revising the femoral component of a THA there is a risk of fracture. Ornstein et al.[27] reported on 144 consecutive revision hip arthroplasties of which 108 involved revising the femoral component with impaction allografting. Thirty-nine femoral fractures occurred in 37 hips, 29 of which occurred intraoperatively and 10 within 5 months of surgery. Additionally they reported that in 7 cases they created a femoral cortical window and inadvertently perforated the femoral cortex in 14. Knight et al.[26] reported a 16% technique related fracture rate and Fetzer et al.[28] reported on 3 postoperative fractures out of a total of 26 femoral revisions with impaction allografting. Schreurs et al.[59] reported on 33 cases of femoral component revision with impaction allografting; there was 1 unrecognized intraoperative fracture and 3 postoperative femoral fractures which were all through cortical defects at the level of the tip of the prosthesis.

As mentioned earlier, tight packing of the morselized allograft is essential for the impaction grafting to be a success. However, this can lead to intraoperative fracture which can go unrecognized. The proponents of the technique quote a prevalence of only 4%, in contrast to the figures already mentioned.[60] However, it is apparent that the fractures occur through areas of weakened bone at the level of the tip of the prosthesis. As a result, the use of a longer stem would be expected to decrease the prevalence of fractures in patients with major femoral deficiencies. Sierra et al.[61] reported on 42 consecutive long-stem revisions (stems >220 mm) where a long stem was chosen to bypass an area of bony deficiency. This represented 7.4% of all femoral impaction grafting that occurred during the period of study. At a mean follow-up of 7.5 years only two postoperative fractures were reported. The authors recommended that cortical defects should be bypassed by the implant/cement/allograft construct by at least two diaphyseal diameters. Although they suggested that additional struts and plates can be used to augment fixation in the case of periprosthetic fractures, these were unnecessary in areas of smaller cortical defects that can be covered with a stainless steel mesh and then bypassed by a longer stem (Figure 21.1). They added that in many instances the fractures could be avoided by releasing the tight soft tissues around the proximal part of the femur, ensuring a good exposure of the entrance to the femoral canal and so avoiding any bending stresses and torque within the femur at the time of impaction. As with other revision techniques, fractures associated with cement removal, as well as debridement of the canal, were also seen. They acknowledged that an extended trochanteric osteotomy could facilitate cement removal although they only used this technique in

four cases. The use of a prophylactic cerclage wire prior to proximal impaction, in areas in which the calcar is still present and thin, would be prudent. Prophylactic cerclage wires or cables should also be placed around the diaphysis in areas of thin cortical bone.

Others have also confirmed that long stems as well as extramedullary augmentation have a role when revising a femoral stem with the impaction allografting technique. Barker et al.[62] demonstrated that both extramedullary augmentation and longer stems reduced the strain around a femoral defect by 31–50%.

Impaction allografting is a technically demanding procedure but with the appropriate instrumentation and an awareness of its pitfalls a successful outcome can be achieved (Figure 21.2).

Question 4: What are the results of impaction allografting in femoral revision in revision THR?

Case clarification
The patients' radiographs reveal a failed uncemented femoral component with a Paprosky type IIIB defect.

Relevance
As the indications for THA expand, including younger and more active patients, some may require two or more revisions during their lifetime. With implant failure, host bone is lost as a result of a combination of stress shielding, osteolysis, instability, implant failure, and/or infection. This

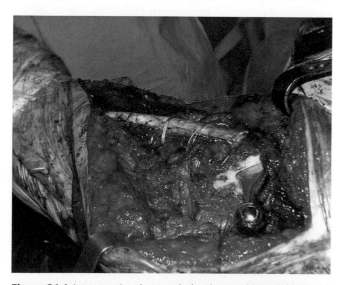

Figure 21.1 Intraoperative photograph showing a revision total hip arthroplasty with impaction allografting along with a cortical strut graft and mesh for a proximal femoral defect.

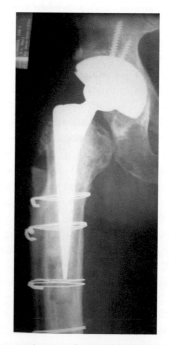

Figure 21.2 Postoperative AP radiograph of the proximal femur showing the revision of a failed total hip arthroplasty with impaction allografting and a cortical strut graft for a proximal femoral defect.

problem may be exacerbated by additional bone loss during the removal of the failed implant.

As well as choosing a suitable implant for revision of a failed femoral component it is also important, particularly in a younger patient, to minimize bone loss and restore bone stock. Of the many methods of reconstruction available to the surgeon performing a revision, there are only two techniques that have the aim of reconstituting bone stock: impaction bone grafting and the use of structural allograft. In the answer to this question, the results of impaction allografting will be considered and the results of structural allografts will be addressed in answer to Question 7.

Current opinion

Current opinion suggests that good results for impaction allografting can be achieved in specialist centers.

Finding the evidence

- Cochrane Database: no relevant reviews
- PubMed (www.ncbi.nlm.nih.gov/pubmed): single citation matcher: "impaction allografting"
- MEDLINE: searched under "impaction allografting"

Quality of the evidence

Level IV
- 13 case series

Findings

When it comes to reviewing the results for femoral revision with impaction grafting a number of problems are encountered. The first problem is the inconsistent use of inclusion criteria. A number of studies have limited their inclusion criteria to femurs with more advanced stages of bone los[38,42,63] whereas others, particularly in their early series, have specifically excluded some of those femurs[41] because of concerns about expanding the indications for impaction allografting to the most challenging cases.[64] Another difficulty encountered when reviewing the results is the large number of potential confounding factors that may affect the outcome of the technique. These may include differences regarding the type and viscosity of cement used as well as the technique of cementing; the source, consistency, and pretreatment of the allograft itself; the operative approach; and the postoperative care, to name but a few.

The majority of studies published to date using the impaction grafting technique have identified the polished, tapered femoral stem as the implant of choice. In Gie et al.'s[41] first authoritative report on the technique, 58 hips were revised by 11 different surgeons with a mean follow-up of 30 months. The average clinical scores for pain, function, and mobility had improved at the final follow-up. In 89% of the cases radiographic evidence of incorporation of the allograft or reconstitution of the cortical bone stock was

demonstrated. The exclusion criteria in this study were different from those quoted in other studies. Femurs which displayed "endosteal bone lysis associated with a large cortical diaphyseal defect" at the time of revision were excluded; however, more recent studies have identified this pattern of femoral bone deficiencies as a prime indication for impaction grafting. This may explain some of the differences in results between this group and other studies looking at impaction grafting.[38,42,63]

Elting et al.[65] reported on their early results of revision of the femoral component with impaction grafting and a CPT femoral stem. Of the 56 patients available for follow-up, 50 (89%) reported mild or no pain and only 8 (14%) needed a walking aid. However, similar to the study of Gie et al.,[41] the majority of patients had minimal bone loss.

Because of the initial concerns of subsidence with polished tapered stems[31,42] some have used a precoated, collared straight stem that has previously been proven to be a durable option in femoral reconstruction with cement.[66,67] Leopold et al.[63] reviewed 29 patients with a mean follow-up of 48 months, Harris hip scores (HHS) improved from a mean of 54 (out of 100) preoperatively to mean of 87 at the time of most the most recent follow-up. Kaplan–Meier survival analysis with aseptic radiographic failure or clinical failure as the endpoint suggested a survival rate of 92% at 6 years. Radiographic incorporation of allograft was seen in only 24% of patients, which is much lower than that reported in other studies with different femoral stems.[31,41,42,65] However, the authors of this study argued that more than 90% of the stems appeared radiographically stable at a mean of more than 5 years, which may suggest that bone remodeling may be occurring although not evident on plain radiographs. This has been supported by other studies which have identified patients where there is no evidence of allograft incorporation on plain radiographs but it is found on histological analysis of biopsy specimens.[13]

Van Biezen et al.[32] reviewed 21 hips with severe femoral defects after a mean follow-up of 60 months. The mean HHS improved by 39 to 78 points and none of the patients required a further revision.

Knight et al.[26] used a collarless polished tapered stem with impaction grafting to revise 31 femoral components. At a mean follow-up of 31 months the modified HHS improved from 41 points preoperatively to 86 points. No stem subsidence was seen in 50%, subsidence of less than 5 mm in 33%, subsidence of between 6 and 8 mm in 13%, and subsidence of more than 10 mm in 1 patient (4%). From a subjective view, 87% patients thought the procedure had improved their function with 97% saying that they would recommend it.

Fetzer et al.[28] reviewed 26 cases of cemented femoral revisions with impaction allografting but using a collared femoral implant in patients with severe femoral bone loss.

The mean follow-up was 6 years and 20 patients were available at final follow-up. None of the patients required a further revision and there was no radiographic evidence of loosening at final follow-up. In one of the cases the femoral component had subsided, but this was less than 5 mm.

Piccaluga et al.[33] used a Charnley stem with morselized impacted allograft to revise 59 loose femoral components. The mean clinical follow-up was 56.7 months and the mean radiographic follow-up was 54.4 months. The latest follow-up radiographs in 56 reconstructions showed evidence of a stable, well-fixed stem in 52 (93%) cases but evidence of loosening in 4 (7%). Of these 4, 2 required revision to give a re-revision rate of 3.5% and the other two were asymptomatic after follow-up at 120 months. Of the 52 successful revisions the mean subsidence was 0.38 mm (0–4 mm).

Ullmark et al.[68] reported on 57 hips in 56 patients who were revised using the Lubinus SP-II prosthesis or the Charnley prosthesis together with morselized impaction grafting. They reported a significant improvement of the Modified Merle d'Aubigné–Postel score in those patients with a mean follow-up of 64 months with radiographic evidence of remodeling of the graft.

Cabanela et al.[40] reviewed 57 femoral revisions in 54 patients using a collarless, tapered, polished stem and impaction grafting. Additionally, 40 hips required strut allografts for reinforcement of the femoral shaft. The clinical results after 6.3 years were judged excellent and radiographic evaluation did not show any evidence of loosening in any of the surviving 53 hips. Subsidence of 1–3 mm was seen in 40 hips and 4–6 mm in 2. Evidence of remodeling was seen in 42 hips.

Halliday et al.[60] reviewed 207 patients (a total of 226 hips) at one center involving 32 surgeons. The survivorship of the revisions with further surgery on the femur as the endpoint was 90.5%, whereas the survivorship based on femoral reoperation for symptomatic aseptic loosening alone was 99.1% at 10–11 years. From the authors' review of their own experience they concluded that long stems are indicated when the host bone around the tip of a short stem is compromised, such as patients with large femoral defects or when a femoral fracture occurs.

Arif et al.[69] reviewed eight patients who underwent a revision THA with an Exeter stem and impaction allografting as well as strut allografts. They used an anterior approach to gain exposure to the hip and an anterior cortical window to remove the old implant. The mean follow-up was 74 months. The strut allografts incorporated in all cases, there was one femoral implant that had subsided 2 mm within the cement mantle, two that subsided by 1 mm at the cement bone interface, and one that subsided 15 mm and required revision. The authors concluded that the use of an anterior cortical window did not predispose the construct to failure.

Schreurs et al.[59] reviewed 33 femoral revisions with the use of the impaction grafting technique and a cemented polished stem. None of the patients required revision at a mean of 10.4 years follow-up. The mean stem subsidence was 3 mm. The average HHS improved from 49 points preoperatively to 85 postoperatively with an 8–13 year follow-up. Kaplan–Meier analysis with an endpoint of femoral revision for whatever reason showed a survivorship of 100% at 10.4 years.

A more recent review by Ornstein et al.[70] from the Swedish Hip Registry identified 1188 patients who had femoral impaction allografting with follow-up between 5 and 18 years. Kaplan–Meier survivorship analysis for all causes of failure was 94% for women and 94.7% for men at 15 years. Survivorship for aseptic loosening was 99.1%, for infection 98.6%, for subsidence 99%, and for fracture 98.7% at 15 years. The authors also identified statistically significant predictors for failure which included the year in which the revision was conducted post index surgery and the number of previous revisions, which almost reached statistical significance (p = 0.056). Interestingly, the age of the patient, gender, length of the stem, and previous septic loosening were not predictors for failure.

Table 21.1 summarizes the results for impaction grafting

Recommendations

In patients requiring revision arthroplasty for loose femoral stems with considerable proximal bone loss, evidence suggests:

- Impaction allografting is not for the inexperienced surgeon [overall quality: high]
- Excellent preliminary results for impaction grafting in femurs without endosteal bone lysis and without large cortical diaphyseal defects can be achieved [overall quality: moderate]
- There is a significant risk of intraoperative fracture with impaction allografting [overall quality: high]
- Subsidence of the femoral implant is a concern with this technique [overall quality: moderate]
- The risk of postoperative fracture continues for months after the reconstruction [overall quality: moderate]

Question 5: What are the technical aspects in using a structural allograft in femoral revision in revision THA?

Before considering reconstruction of the proximal femur with a structural allograft, careful planning is essential to ensure the best possible outcome. This includes excluding infection as a cause for failure of the implant, detailed templating, and making sure that suitable allograft is available together with the necessary implants and instruments.

Table 21.1 Summary of the results of impaction allografting in femoral revision in revision total hip arthroplasty

Author	No. of cases	Mean follow-up	Results
Gie[41]	58 hips	30 months	89% demonstrated radiographic evidence of incorporation of allograft. Mean pain/function/mobility scores improved
Elting[65]	56 patients	31 months	89% (50 patients) mild/no pain, 14% (8 patients) needed walking aid
Leopold[63]	29 patients	48 months	HHS improved from a mean of 54 preoperatively to a mean of 87 postoperatively. 92% survivorship rate 6 years. Radiographic incorporation only 24%, but 90% radiographically stable at 5 years
Van Biezen[32]	21 hips	60 months	HHS improved by 39 points to 78 postoperatively
Knight[26]	31 hips	31 months	HHS improved from a mean of 41 points preoperatively to 86 points postoperatively
Fetzer[28]	20 hips at final follow-up	6 years	No further revisions and no radiographic evidence of loosening
Piccaluga[33]	59 cases	56.7 months	Of the 56 patients available for radiographic follow-up, 93% were stable
Ullmark[68]	57 hips	64 months	Significant improvement of the mean modified Merle d"Aubigné–Postel score following surgery
Cabanela[40]	57 hips	6.3 years	Excellent clinical results, with no radiographic evidence of loosening of the 53 surviving hips
Halliday[60]	226 hips	10–11 years	90.5% survivorship with further surgery on the femur as the endpoint
Arif[69]	8 patients	74 months	All patients had impaction grafting with an anterior cortical window and a large strut allograft. The strut allografts incorporated in all cases
Schreurs[59]	33 hips	10.4 years	HHS improved from 49 preoperatively to 85 postoperatively. 100% survivorship at 10.4 years with further surgery on the femur as the endpoint
Ornstein[70]	1188 patients 1305 hips	15 years	Survivorship analysis revealed 94% at 15 years for all causes of failure in women and 94.7% in men. Survivorship for aseptic loosening 99.1%, infection 98.6%, subsidence 99%, fracture 98.7%

HHS, Harris hip score.

Full circumferential allografts (proximal femoral allografts) are reserved for Paprosky type IIIB and IV defects, whereas noncircumferential allografts (cortical struts) are used in the less severe defects. Cortical struts also have a role in reinforcing cortical windows and in stabilizing periprosthetic fractures as well as osteotomy sites, and for augmenting the graft–host junction in proximal femoral allografts. For small defects whole fibular diaphyseal segments can be used, although their shape and size are awkward for the task. For larger defects segments of tibia, humerus, or femur can be utilized. The surgical technique for cortical strut grafts is relatively straightforward. The grafts are tailored to fit the femur and secured to the host femur with cerclage wires or cables. Additionally, some of the autogenous reamings from the femur can be placed along the allograft–host junction to facilitate union. Soft tissue stripping of the host femur should be kept to a

minimum to preserve as much of the periosteal blood supply as possible.

The surgical technique for proximal femoral allografts is technically more demanding. Possible surgical approaches that may be used include either a trochanteric slide[71,72] or a longitudinal trochanteric splitting approach. The advantage of the slide is that it very much reduces the risk of proximal migration of the trochanter[73] and its consequences as compared to classic trochanteric osteotomy. Once the proximal femur is exposed, an assessment of the length of allograft required is made by implanting the femoral prosthesis into the host femoral canal and reducing it into the cup. The length of allograft depends on the stability of the reduced hip and assessment of limb lengths.

The majority of allografts are processed to reduce the risk of disease transmission and to reduce the immunogenicity of the graft. The commonest methods of processing are freezing and freeze-drying. This enables long-term graft preservation, with bone frozen at −70 °C lasting for 5 years or more.[74] Additional processing with irradiation reduces the risk posed by viral transmission[75] and may further reduce immunogenicity. At the time of surgery when the allograft is brought into the operating room, specimens should be taken from it for culture and then it should be immersed in an antibiotic-containing solution.

Since the allograft is biologically inactive, bone ingrowth onto an implant cannot occur and therefore an uncemented prosthesis is likely to fail due to subsidence or fracture of the allograft.[71,76] For this reason the prosthesis should be fixed to the allograft with cement to which antibiotics have been added.[77] Another caveat is to avoid over-reaming of the allograft so as to maintain its strength and reduce the risk of fracture even when the host canal is larger, as is usually the case.[78] If there is a large discrepancy between the diameter of the host femur and the allograft and stabilization of the graft–host junction is proving difficult, then telescoping the graft inside the host femur is an option.

For this technique to be successful the graft–host junction must unite, which is by and large host-dependent. For union to occur, the junction between host and allograft must be stable. One technique that has been described is a step-cut or an oblique cut, which is then reinforced with cerclage wires or cables at the junction to attain rotational stability (Figure 21.3).[25,79–83] Other suggestions have included the use of two plates,[48,71] allograft struts,[84] and cementing of the prosthesis into the allograft and the allograft to the host.[85] There are some concerns that screws placed through a plate may disrupt the fixation of the stem and lead to stress risers which may fracture the allograft,[86] and struts may fail before union of the graft–host junction has been achieved.[71]

In summary, the chances of union are improved if the host femur is carefully exposed preserving as much of its soft tissue attachments and blood supply. The graft–host junction should be kept free of cement and augmented with autogenous bone graft. Additionally, a step or oblique cut should be used and augmented with an additional strut allograft with wires/cables if needed. Once initial fixation is achieved, any of the remaining proximal host femoral bone can be wrapped around the graft–host junction as additional autogenous bone graft. The risk of dislocation can be decreased by reattaching the greater trochanter remnant to the proximal femur with cerclage wires or with the use of a cable-grip system. If there is no greater trochanteric fragment available then reattaching the abductors to the fascia lata or allograft can also be worthwhile.

Question 6: What choices of femoral implant are available when using a structural bone allograft?

A wide range of femoral implants have been employed with no uniformity of methods of fixation either to the allograft or within the host femur. The options for distal fixation have included distal cementing, which is not recommended, a distal press-fit,[71,87] interlocking fixation,[88] the use of a step-cut and wires[79] to provide stability, or plates. Cementing has proved unpopular in this setting since although cadaveric biomechanical testing showed good stability with distal cementing,[89–91] there is a risk that some of the cement may get into the gap at the graft–host interface and prevent union. Additionally, rigid fixation distal to the junction may reduce the load at the junction and lead not only to nonunion of the junction but to potential resorption of the allograft. Also, should the implant/allograft construct need to be removed, e.g., because of infection, it would prove more of a challenge if the implant is cemented distally with the risk of causing additional damage to the remaining femur. For these reasons an uncemented component that can achieve fixation to the host bone by a press or wedge fit distally has been gaining popularity.[71] Gross et al.[92] cautioned against this, however, because of the risk of having to use a large implant to get a press fit distally, which reduces the amount of cement mantle between the allograft and prosthesis proximally and also increases the probability of having to ream the allograft to make room for the implant. They also argued that a tight distal fit may

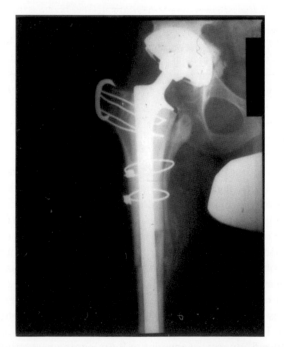

Figure 21.3 Postoperative AP radiograph of the proximal femur showing the revision of a failed total hip arthroplasty with a long-stemmed implant with a proximal femoral structural allograft. The implant has been cemented to the allograft but is uncemented distally to the host femur.

result in distraction at the graft–host junction and thereby increasing the risk of nonunion. In answer to some of these criticisms, some have advocated the use of a modular, long, thin uncemented femoral components, with the majority of the stability of the construct being achieved through the graft–host junction.

Question 7: What are the results of using a structural allograft in revision THA and what are its advantages and disadvantages?

Case clarification

Having obtained further radiographic views of the proximal femur it is concluded that there is insufficient bone stock for the patient to have a femoral reconstruction with impaction allografting. Instead, the decision is made to proceed with a proximal femoral allograft.

Current opinion

Current opinion suggests that very few centers today favor the use of circumferential segmental allograft as a preferred method of managing substantial proximal femoral bone loss during revision hip replacement.

Finding the evidence

- Cochrane Database: no relevant reviews
- PubMed (www.ncbi.nlm.nih.gov/pubmed): single citation matcher: "proximal femoral allografts," "bulk structural allografts and hip arthroplasty"
- MEDLINE: searched under "proximal femoral allografts," "structural allografts"

Quality of the evidence

Level IV
- 10 case series

Findings

Wong et al.[93] reviewed 52 patients who underwent revision THA with the use of cortical strut grafts derived from the fibula. In this study 33 patients had graft plus a porous-coated femoral implant without cement; 5 with a press-fit stem; 7 with a cemented component; and 7 in association with a proximal femoral allograft. Mean follow-up was 4.8 years. From review of the radiographs there was evidence of graft resorption in 45 of the 47 hips, with a mean decrease in length of the cortical strut of 8%. However, there were two patients whose grafts resorbed by more than 50%. There were two cases of nonunion of the struts but neither of them had fractured, therefore there was a rate of union of 96% and the average time to union was 10 months.

The authors commented that the majority of resorption occurred at the ends of the grafts and appeared to be part of the remodeling process, except in the two patients whose grafts resorbed by more than 50%. Although average time

for the grafts to unite was 10 months, the process of incorporation would continue for up to 2 years. The HHS improved from a mean of 39.4 points to 65.6 points. The rate of a further revision was 12% at 10 years. Some of the stems subsided, but the cortical graft was not being used to support the implant and was not considered a causative factor.

Chandler et al.[84] reviewed 29 patients (30 hips) who had a mean follow-up of 22 months. All patients were revised with a long-stemmed modular prosthesis which was fixed with cement to the proximal femoral allograft and secured to the host femur distally with a press-fit uncemented stem. The mean HHS improved from 35 preoperatively to 78 points postoperatively. There were two nonunions and one hip that had evidence of graft resorption on radiographic review. Four hips (13%) needed an additional operation.

Head et al.[94] reported their results of 22 patients who had a revision hip arthroplasty with a proximal femoral allograft with a mean follow-up of 28 months. Ten patients had cement fixation of the implant to the graft as well as cementing of the implant distally to the host; in three patients the implant was secured to the host distally with cement and the allograft was not cemented proximally; and nine patients had no cement fixation either proximally or distally. Sixteen patients (73%) had a significant functional improvement based on the HHS (mean preoperative score of 26 points and mean postoperative score of 65), and four patients had a poor result. Two hips went on to develop a nonunion with a stable implant and one had a nonunion with partial resorption of the graft.

Roberson[95] reviewed 21 patients (24 hips) who had a revision hip arthroplasty with a structural femoral allograft after a failed total hip replacement with a mean follow-up of 4 years. Based on the HHS, 12 patients had a good or excellent result, 6 had a fair result and 2 had a poor result, and for 1 patient no data was available. There were two nonunions and five hips showed evidence of graft resorption.

Zmolek et al.[76] reviewed 11 patients with a mean follow-up of 4 years who had an uncemented revision THA with a proximal femoral allograft. Nine hips had evidence of a radiographic union at a mean of 13 months and two failed because of nonunion.

Masri et al.[96] reviewed 58 reconstructions with a proximal femoral allograft–prosthetic composite; 41 were available for follow-up with a mean duration of 4 years. The mean HHS was 83 points. Four patients (10%) had a nonunion of the graft–host junction and severe graft resorption was reported in 10 patients (24%). Five patients (12%) required revision of the allograft for a fracture, nonunion, infection, or resorption.

Gross et al.[7] reviewed 168 hips that had been treated with a revision hip arthroplasty with a proximal femoral allograft with mean follow-up of 4.8 years. Of the 132 patients who were available for follow-up, the mean HHS increased from a preoperative score of 30 to 66 points postoperatively. Only 17 hips required further surgery, 5 hips had a nonunion, and 6 hips showed evidence of resorption of the graft. A further review by Gross et al.,[81] where 200 reconstructions were reviewed using a circumferential allograft that was more than 5 cm long, 25 patients (13%) required a further revision procedure. Of these revision procedures, two failed again and required an excision arthroplasty. Nonunion was seen in seven hips and were all treated successfully with the use of a plate and autogenous bone grafting and leaving the allograft construct in situ. Graft resorption was identified in six hips and observed to occur on the periosteal side of the graft. It was never full thickness and was less than 1 cm long, except in one hip in which it was 4 cm long. However, no revisions were indicated for graft resorption. Of the 130 patients, 111 (85%) had an increase of the HHS of 20 points, a stable implant, and no further operations related to the allograft at a mean follow-up of 4.8 years; they were deemed successful[7]. A further study by Hutchison and Gross presented at the American Academy of Orthopedic Surgeons with a longer mean follow-up of 9 years reported a similar success rate (55 out of 65 hips).[81]

Blackley et al.[97] performed a comprehensive review of 60 revision total hip arthroplasties done by Dr. A.E. Gross that involved a proximal femoral allograft. These patients had a circumferential proximal femoral deficiency of more than 5 cm in length and required a proximal femoral allograft of a minimum length of 10 cm with a mean length of 15 cm. The mean number of previous arthroplasties was 3.8, but one patient had had nine. At 9.3 years after surgery, 45 patients were available for follow-up. The mean HHS improved from 30 points preoperatively to 71 points at a mean follow-up of 11 years. Radiographically, four hips (6%) had a nonunion at the graft–host junction. Significant trochanteric escape of more than 1 cm occurred in 14 hips (22%). Graft resorption was seen in 33% of the surviving patients who had more than 9 years of follow-up. The resorption occurred around the cerclage wires in 9 of the 13 hips, but no revisions were performed for graft resorption. Kaplan–Meier survival analysis estimated a survival rate of 90% at 5 years and 86% at 10 years.

Haddad et al.[8] reviewed a consecutive series of 40 proximal femoral allografts with a mean follow-up of 8.8 years. In this study the stem was cemented into both the allograft and host femur in all patients. The mean HHS improved from 39 to 79. There were four cases of patients requiring further surgery, two for infection, one for nonunion of the graft–host junction, and one for allograft resorption which was noted at the time of revision of a failed acetabular component.

Graft resorption which was full thickness was seen in seven patients (17.5%) although none of these cases was associated with failure of the reconstructions.

Table 21.2 summarizes the results for structural allografts in revision hip surgery.

There remains some controversy regarding the use of structural allografts in revision hip arthroplasty. Nonetheless, they do present certain advantages. Allograft possesses a limited capacity to become incorporated into the host bone and also has the potential for soft tissues to attach to it. It provides a good interface for cementing, with the added advantage of not requiring cement fixation to the distal femur, and therefore should not compromise any revision in the future, if needed. Once the allograft incorporates into the host femur it potentially increases the surface area for distal fixation of the femoral implant and therefore reduces the risk of loosening. Although there is no exact consensus on the indications for a proximal femoral structural allograft, the majority would agree that the deficiency should be circumferential and of more than 5 cm long with grade III bone loss according to the system described by the American Academy of Orthopaedic Surgeons.[98]

Disadvantages include the fact that the construct itself is technically demanding and is expensive and difficult to obtain. It is a technique that is not without potential complications and requires careful follow-up to identify them early should they occur. The greatest concern to patients and surgeons alike is the risk of disease transmission, and this deters a number of patients from having the procedure. HIV and hepatitis virus are the agents that attract the greatest attention, but other viruses can also be implicated.[99,100] This risk can be reduced by adhering to well-established standards of donor selection such as that provided by the American Association of Tissue Banks which reduce the risk of transmission of HIV to less than 1 in a million.[101,102] Graft irradiation may reduce the risk further,[75] although it may also weaken the bone.[103] Other concerns include the risk of fracture, graft resorption and nonunion.

Recommendations

In patients requiring revision arthroplasty for loose femoral stems with considerable proximal bone loss, evidence suggests:

• In the short to medium term good results can be achieved with revision THA involving a proximal femoral allograft [overall quality: low to moderate]

• Although graft resorption is seen following revision THA with a proximal femoral allograft it is rarely an indication on its own for further surgery [overall quality: moderate]

• Nonunion is a significant problem following revision THA with a proximal femoral allograft leading to the

Table 21.2 Summary of the results of using a structural allograft in revision total hip arthroplasty

Author	No. of cases	Mean follow-up	Results
Wong[93] (cortical strut allografts)	52 patients	4.8 years	Graft resorption in 45 of 47 hips. Nonunion in 2 cases (union rate 96% at a mean of 10 months). HHS improved from a mean of 39.4 preoperatively to 65.6 postoperatively. Risk of further revision of 12% at 10 years
Chandler[84]	29 patients (30 hips)	22 months	HHS improved from 35 preoperatively to 78 postoperatively. 2 nonunions, 1 case of graft resorption, and 13% required further surgery
Head[94]	22 patients	28 months	73% had a significant functional improvement. HHS improved from 26 preoperatively to 65 postoperatively. 4 patients had a poor result. 2 hips had a nonunion but with a stable implant. 1 hip had a nonunion with graft resorption
Roberson[95]	21 patients (24 hips)	4 years	12 good/excellent results based on the HHS, 6 fair and 2 poor. 2 cases where the graft failed to unite and 5 where the graft appeared to resorb radiographically
Zmolek[76]	11 patients	4 years	9 hips showed radiographic evidence of union at 13 months. 2 cases of failure due to nonunion
Masri[96]	41 hips available for follow-up	4 years	Postoperative HHS of 83. 4 (10%) hips showed evidence of nonunion, 10 (24%) showed evidence of severe graft resorption. 5 (12%) patients required revision of the allograft for either fracture, nonunion, infection, or resorption
Gross[7]	132 hips available for follow-up	4.8 years	HHS improved from 30 preoperatively to 66 postoperatively. 17 hips required further surgery. 5 cases of nonunion and 6 of graft resorption
Gross[81]	200 hips	4.8 years	25 (13%) patients required an additional revision procedure. 7 cases of nonunion and 6 of graft resorption. Of the 130 patients available for follow-up, 111 (85%) had an increase in the HHS postoperatively of 20 points, a stable implant, and did not require any further surgery
Blackley[97]	45 hips available for follow-up	11 years	HHS improved from a preoperative score of 30 to a postoperative score of 71. 4 cases (6%) of nonunion and 13 (33%) of graft resorption. 90% survival rate at 5 years and 86% at 10 years
Haddad[8]	40 patients	8.8 years	HHS improved from a preoperative score of 39 to a postoperative score of 79. 4 cases requiring further surgery and 7 (17.5%) cases of severe graft resorption, although not associated with failure

HHS, Harris hip score.

failure of the construct in the medium to long term [overall quality: moderate]

Question 8: What are the complications of impaction allografting for revision of a femoral component in THA?

Impaction grafting is a technically demanding procedure as reflected by the early results of the technique and the incidence of reported complications. The majority of failures following impaction allografting have been due to periprosthetic fractures[38,41,42] requiring further surgery. The reported prevalence of fractures ranges from 5% to 24%.[27,38,41,42,60,63,65] Not surprisingly, those patients with the greatest proximal bone loss were associated with the higher rates of fracture.[38,42,63] Intraoperative fractures tend to occur during impaction of the allograft,[42] which can be partially avoided by adequate exposure, prophylactic cerclage fixation, and augmentation of the femoral shaft with cortical strut grafts.[42,65] Intraoperative perforation of the shaft usually occurs during cement removal and has been reported in up to 10% of cases of impaction allografting.[27] The key is to recognize this complication when it happens and augment with a cortical strut graft.[104] Postoperative fractures may be due to an unrecognized intraoperative fracture or perforation, or can occur through areas of osteolysis which have not been adequately addressed. In the first year after surgery Ornstein et al.[27] reported that 6% of their patients sustained a diaphyseal fracture. Fractures, whether they occur intra- or postoperatively, are associated with failure of the construct[41,42] and invariably lead to further surgery.[38,41,42,65]

Component subsidence of more than 1mm has been reported to be as high as 79% (44 out of 56 hips) following impaction allografting with a polished, tapered stem.[63] In the same study, subsidence at the interface between the graft–cement composite and host bone was 20% (11 out of 56 hips) and in 11% of patients (6 out of 56 hips) continued for more than 2 years.

Initially, subsidence of the implant was thought to be desirable. Gie et al.[41] suggested that the wedge-shaped stem facilitated the incorporation of the allograft by the compression it produced as it subsided. However, significant subsidence may be undesirable because it may imply mechanical failure of allograft–cement composite, and ultimate failure of the reconstruction. This has been supported by other studies on polished, tapered, cemented stems.[65,105] The implication of subsidence on the clinical result may be related to the type of femoral implant used. Subsidence of cemented implants that have a coating or roughened surface suggests aseptic loosening of the stem.[66,67,106] The difficulty with polished stems is defining when a subsiding stem is loose. Gie et al.[41] suggested that the implant can subside at either the stem–cement interface or the cement/

graft–host bone interface, with evidence of radiolucent lines, and still not necessarily be loose. Elting et al.[65] reported that almost 50% of the stems subsided at the implant–stem interface with nearly 20% demonstrating substantial subsidence of more than 2mm. With polished stems any subsidence that occurs is thought to allow the wedge-shaped stem to "self-tighten" because of the cold flow of the cement.[41,65,105] However, Masterson et al.[38] observed that there was a high prevalence of early cement fractures around stems that had subsided, which suggests some limitations to the cold flow theory. This observation has been further supported from data provided by a study using radiostereometric analysis.[107] Other associations with stem subsidence have been thigh pain,[31] particularly in those with subsidence of more than 10mm, and dislocation.[38] The implications of stem subsidence are still not fully known and further studies are needed to clarify its role in impaction allografting.

General complications such as dislocation have been reported of between 3%[65] and 6%,[27,38] with similar infection rates. Other reported complications have included trochanteric bursitis related to prominent metalwork[63] as well as heterotopic ossification.[41,42,63,65] Whether the presence of morselized allograft increases the risk of heterotopic ossification compared with other reconstructive techniques is not known, as no comparison studies have been performed to date. In those patients who have had an osteotomy of the greater trochanter there has been a high incidence of nonunion with reports of between 33%[63] and 50%;[42] this could be because of the poor proximal bone stock or because of the presence of cement at the osteotomy site preventing union.

Among the complications encountered following impaction allografting, intraoperative fractures are responsible for the majority of failures of this technique and can be partially avoided by augmenting the porotic femoral shaft with a cortical strut graft.

Question 9: What are the complications of using a structural bulk allograft for revision of a femoral component in THA?

The most commonly reported complications associated with the use of structural allografts in femoral revision after a failed THA are infection, instability, nonunion and fracture.

The prevalence of infection following a revision arthroplasty performed with the use of a structural allograft has been reported to be between 4% and 13%.[48,81,97,108–110]. The duration of the procedure, soft tissue dissection, contamination of the graft, and blood loss have all been associated with increased risk of infection.[79,110,111] Great care must be taken in preparation of the graft, and prophylactic antibiotics should be given both systemically and in the bone cement used to secure the graft.[77] Should the construct get infected then a standard two-stage procedure with reimplantation of a fresh allograft can be used.[7,108]

The rate of dislocation has been reported to be as high as 6% in some series.[97] Certainly, the risk of dislocation is higher if the femoral component alone is revised,[7] although we would not suggest revising a well-fixed acetabular component unless it is malpositioned. Undoubtedly, a significant proportion of the instability following reconstruction of the proximal femur with allograft is due to the lack of soft tissue stabilization.

The rate of nonunion has been reported between 4%[7] and 23%.[112] As pointed out earlier, a considerable number of these nonunions are related to the interposition of cement at the graft–host junction.[84] Additionally, insertion of cement into the distal host femur may distract the graft–host junction and affect bony union.[113] This problem can be successfully addressed with autogenous bone grafting and the use of a plate.[48,81] Trochanteric nonunion is only a problem should the trochanter escape and result in defunctioning of the abductors. Nonunion of the trochanter is common because of the fact that it is under distraction as opposed to compression, and also the blood supply to the junction of the trochanter and the graft comes from the trochanter alone. This problem can be avoided by performing a trochanteric slide rather than a transverse trochanteric osteotomy.

Fractures tend to occur between 2 and 3 years following reconstruction with a structural allograft.[81,112,114] This could be because the graft has fatigued after it has failed to unite to the host, or because of a stress riser such as a screw hole, or due to excessive reaming of the graft.

Graft resorption has also been a problem following reconstruction with a structural allograft, with some reports of up to 34%.[96] It is not clear whether this resorption is due to an immune phenomenon, the way the allograft is processed, or the bone cement. Others have concluded that the resorption is related to a local vascular phenomenon caused by the cerclage wires.[108]

In summary, infection and nonunion are responsible for the majority of complications following reconstruction with a proximal femoral allograft. Careful attention to surgical technique should help keep these complications to a minimum.

Question 10: What is the current state of the popularity of these techniques? Are there better alternatives?

Morselized allograft bone has many potential advantages, including the avoidance of morbidity associated with harvesting autogenous bone graft. However, the disadvantages include the immune response that is initiated by the host, the lack of osteogenic cells, decreased osteoinductive factors, and the risk of infection. Furthermore, the use of structural allografts in revision hip arthroplasty remains controversial since, although early results have been successful, the long-term results have been inconsistent.

An alternative to morselized allograft bone includes demineralized bone matrix (DBM) which is made by acid extraction of the mineralized phase of bone. The product of this process is composed of noncollagenous proteins and growth factors as well as collagen.[115] In animal studies DBM was thought to be capable of inducing osteogenesis by recruiting mesenchymal stem cells from the host tissues,[116–118] although more recent reports have suggested that DBMs have excellent osteoconductive potential but limited osteoinductive capacity.[119,120] However, adding bone marrow to DBM does seem to increase its osteogenic potential in certain clinical situations such as the grafting of contained bony defects.

Other alternatives to morselized allografts include ceramics. Ceramics provide an osteoconductive matrix usually consisting of hydroxyapatite, tricalcium phosphate, or calcium sulfate.[121] However, these ceramics have minimal tensile strength and so the surrounding bone must be stable or the defect must be contained for it to be successfully used. Although a number of ceramics are approved for the use in filling non-weight-bearing areas in hip revision,[122] the efficacy of these materials in this clinical scenario are not known.

Growth factors, specifically the BMPs and recombinant BMPs may be used in revision hip surgery to treat cavitary defects or as an adjunct in encouraging the healing and incorporation of allografts. In a canine model, osteogenic protein 1 (OP-1) combined with bovine type 1 collagen significantly improved the healing and incorporation of a cortical onlay strut allograft based on radiographic and histologic evidence.[123] However, this model does not accurately reproduce the clinical situation found in revision THA. Early results using OP-1 in revision THA in conjunction with a proximal femoral allograft, bulk femoral head allograft, cortical strut allograft, or morselized allograft have shown that new bone formed earlier and graft incorporation was more rapid than would be expected without OP-1.[124]

Other potential adjuncts in revision hip surgery include the use of autologous cells as bone graft substitutes, as well as gene therapy and tissue engineering, but further research is needed to assess their contribution in this field.

Current alternatives to reconstruction of the proximal femur using either impaction allografting or a proximal femoral structural allograft have been the use of an uncemented stem which is designed to gain fixation in the distal femur. The most popular methods at present of uncemented fixation in the diaphysis is by an extensively porous-coated stem or a fluted, tapered, grit-blasted stem.

Uncemented, extensively porous-coated stems have been considered the gold standard of uncemented revision femoral stems in North America for some years[125–137] and, although it has been successful in the revision setting,[126,136,137] stress shielding remains a concern because of the relative stiffness of the implant. An alternative method of uncemented diaphyseal stem fixation is the use of a modular, fluted, tapered, grit-blasted stem. These stems are able to gain axial and rotational stability in the diaphysis of the femur by their tapered design. The distal part of the implant, which is cone shaped, is wedged into the diaphysis to achieve primary stability. Limiting the contact zone between the implant and bone helps to reduce the stiffness of the construct. Stems with flutes enable the use of a less stiff implant and as a result will reduce the stress shielding seen with the fully porous-coated cylindrical implants. Additionally, using a modular stem allows the surgeon to implant the distal part of the stem in the diaphysis, ensuring a good wedge fit, with a number of options available for the proximal part that optimize leg length, femoral offset, femoral version, and stability. Good results have been reported with this implant design. McInnis et al.[138] retrospectively reviewed 70 patients with a mean follow-up of 47 months. Combined metaphyseal/diaphyseal bone loss was observed preoperatively in 36 (51%) of 70 hips. At the final review, restoration of the proximal bone was noted in 56% of patients. Park et al.[139] reviewed 62 patients who underwent a revision THA with a fluted, tapered, modular femoral stem. The mean HHS was 87.3 points postoperatively with a mean follow-up of 4.2 years. Similar results have been reported by other authors with survivorship of up to 97% at 9 years.[140,141]

A disadvantage of the modular, tapered, fluted stem design in the elderly patient is that normally patients are required to undergo a period of toe-touch weightbearing because of the poor cortical bone stock that is prevalent in this patient population. In some patients toe-touch weight-bearing is an unrealistic aim, and so the substitution of the proximal femur with a modular oncology prosthesis may be more appropriate and will enable the patient to fully weightbear from day 1 postoperatively.

Summary of recommendations

• Impaction allografting is not for the inexperienced surgeon
• Excellent preliminary results for impaction grafting in femurs without endosteal bone lysis associated or large cortical diaphyseal defects can be achieved
• There is a significant risk of intraoperative fracture with impaction allografting
• Subsidence of the femoral implant is a concern with impaction allografting

• The risk of postoperative fracture continues for months after the reconstruction
• In the short to medium term good results can be achieved with revision THA involving a proximal femoral allograft
• Nonunion is a significant problem following revision THA ,with a proximal femoral allograft leading to the failure of the construct in the medium to long term
• Although graft resorption is seen following revision THA with a proximal femoral allograft it is rarely an indication on its own for further surgery

Conclusions

Both impaction allografting and reconstruction of the proximal femur with a bulk structural allograft in revision hip surgery are technically demanding procedures. The current literature suggests that these techniques are best performed in specialist centers. However, newer implants such as the tapered, modular, fluted stem are showing encouraging preliminary results and may have a considerable contribution to make in the treatment of this challenging patient group.

References

1. Paprosky WG, Aribindi R. Hip replacement: treatment of femoral bone loss using distal bypass fixation. Instr Course Lect 2000;49:119–30.
2. Arthroplasty and Total Joint Replacement Procedures 1991 to 2000. American Academy of Orthopaedic Surgeons, 2009.
3. Zhan C, Kaczmarek R, Loyo-Berrios N, Sangl J, Bright RA. Incidence and short-term outcomes of primary and revision hip replacement in the United States. J Bone Joint Surg Am 2007;89:526–33.
4. National Joint Registry for England and Wales, 5th Annual Report. National Joint Registry, 2009.
5. Hootman JM, Helmick CG. Projections of US prevalence of arthritis and associated activity limitations. Arthritis Rheum 2006;54:226–9.
6. Barrack RL. The economics of revision arthroplasty. Orthopedics 1995;18:874–5.
7. Gross AE, Hutchison CR, Alexeeff M, Mahomed N, Leitch K, Morsi E. Proximal femoral allografts for reconstruction of bone stock in revision arthroplasty of the hip. Clin Orthop Relat Res 1995;151–8.
8. Haddad FS, Garbuz DS, Masri BA, Duncan CP. Structural proximal femoral allografts for failed total hip replacements: A minimum review of 5 years. J Bone Joint Surg Br 2000;82: 830–6.
9. Haddad FS, Garbuz DS, Masri BA, Duncan CP, Hutchison CR, Gross AE. Instructional course lectures, the American Academy of Orthopaedic Surgeons—Femoral bone loss in patients managed with revision hip replacement: results of circumferential allograft replacement. J Bone Joint Surg Am 1999;81:420–36.
10. Gie GA, Linder L, Ling RS, Simon JP, Slooff TJ, Timperley AJ. Contained morselized allograft in revision total hip arthro-

plasty. Surgical technique. Orthop Clin North Am 1993;24: 717–25.

11. Goldberg VM. Selection of bone grafts for revision total hip arthroplasty. Clin Orthop Relat Res 2000;68–76.

12. Buma P, Lamerigts N, Schreurs BW, Gardeniers J, Versleyen D, Slooff TJ. Impacted graft incorporation after cemented acetabular revision. Histological evaluation in 8 patients. Acta Orthop Scand 1996;67:536–40.

13. Nelissen RG, Bauer TW, Weidenhielm LR, LeGolvan DP, Mikhail WE. Revision hip arthroplasty with the use of cement and impaction grafting. Histological analysis of four cases. J Bone Joint Surg Am 1995;77:412–22.

14. van der Donk S, Buma P, Slooff TJ, Gardeniers JW, Schreurs BW. Incorporation of morselized bone grafts: a study of 24 acetabular biopsy specimens. Clin Orthop Relat Res 2002;131–41.

15. Ling RS, Timperley AJ, Linder L. Histology of cancellous impaction grafting in the femur. A case report. J Bone Joint Surg Br 1993;75:693–6.

16. Burwell RG. Studies in the transplantation of bone, V. The capacity of fresh and treated homografts of bone to evoke transplantation immunity. J Bone Joint Surg Br 1963;45: 386–401.

17. Cook SD, Baffes GC, Wolfe MW, Sampath TK, Rueger DC. Recombinant human bone morphogenetic protein-7 induces healing in a canine long-bone segmental defect model. Clin Orthop Relat Res 1994;302–12.

18. Friedlaender GE. The antigenicity of preserved allografts. Transplant Proc 1976;8:195–200.

19. Goldberg VM, Stevenson S. Natural history of autografts and allografts. Clin Orthop Relat Res 1987;7–16.

20. Burchardt H. The biology of bone graft repair. Clin Orthop Relat Res 1983;28–42.

21. Burchardt H. Biology of bone transplantation. Orthop Clin North Am 1987;18:187–96.

22. Stevenson S, Horowitz M. The response to bone allografts. J Bone Joint Surg Am 1992;74:939–50.

23. Enneking WF, Mindell ER. Observations on massive retrieved human allografts. J Bone Joint Surg Am 1991;73:1123–42.

24. Enneking WF, Campanacci DA. Retrieved human allografts : a clinicopathological study. J Bone Joint Surg Am 2001;83: 971–86.

25. Gross AE. Revision arthroplasty of the hip using allograft bone. In: Czitrom AA, Gross AE, eds. Allografts in Orthopaedic Practice, pp. 147–73. Williams & Wilkins, Baltimore, 1992.

26. Knight JL,,Helming C. Collarless polished tapered impaction grafting of the femur during revision total hip arthroplasty: pitfalls of the surgical technique and follow-up in 31 cases. J Arthroplasty 2000;15:159–65.

27. Ornstein E, Atroshi I, Franzén H, Johnsson R, Sandquist P, Sundberg M. Early Complications after one hundred and forty-four consecutive hip revisions with impacted morselized allograft bone and cement. J Bone Joint Surg Am 2002;84 :1323–8.

28. Fetzer GB, Callaghan JJ, Templeton JE, Goetz DD, Sullivan PM, Johnston RC. Impaction allografting with cement for extensive femoral bone loss in revision hip surgery: a 4- to 8-year follow-up study. J Arthroplasty 2001;16: 195–202.

29. Schreurs BW, Arts JJC, Verdonschot N, Buma P, Slooff TJJH, Gardeniers JWM. Femoral component revision with use of impaction bone-grafting and a cemented polished stem. J Bone Joint Surg Am 2005;87:2499–507.

30. Masterson EL, Duncan CP. Subsidence and the cement mantle in femoral impaction allografting. Orthopedics 1997;20: 821–2.

31. Eldridge JD, Smith EJ, Hubble MJ, Whitehouse SL, Learmonth ID. Massive early subsidence following femoral impaction grafting. J Arthroplasty 1997;12:535–40.

32. van Biezen FC, ten Have BL, Verhaar JA. Impaction bone-grafting of severely defective femora in revision total hip surgery: 21 hips followed for 41–85 months. Acta Orthop Scand 2000;71:135–42.

33. Piccaluga F, Valle AGD, Fernandez JCE, Pusso R. Revision of the femoral prosthesis with impaction allografting and a Charnley stem: A 2- to 12-year follow-up. J Bone Joint Surg Br 2002;84:544–9.

34. Karrholm J, Hultmark P, Carlsson L, Malchau H. Subsidence of a non-polished stem in revisions of the hip using impaction allograft: Evaluation with radiostereometry and dual-energy X-ray absorptiometry. J Bone Joint Surg Br 1999;81 :135–42.

35. Nelissen RG, Valstar ER, Poll RG, Garling EH, Brand R. Factors associated with excessive migration in bone impaction hip revision surgery: a radiostereometric analysis study. J Arthroplasty 2002;17:826–33.

36. Malkani AL, Voor MJ, Fee KA, Bates CS. Femoral component revision using impacted morsellised cancellous graft: A biomechanical study of implant stability. J Bone Joint Surg Br 1996;78:973–8.

37. Gokhale S, Soliman A, Dantas JP, Richardson JB, Cook F, Kuiper JH et al. Variables affecting initial stability of impaction grafting for hip revision. Clin Orthop Relat Res 2005;174–80.

38. Masterson EL, Masri BA, Duncan CP. The cement mantle in the Exeter impaction allografting technique. A cause for concern. J Arthroplasty 1997;12:759–64.

39. Frei H, O'Connell J, Masri BA, Duncan CP, Oxland TR. Biological and mechanical changes of the bone graft-cement interface after impaction allografting. J Orthop Res 2005;23: 1271–9.

40. Cabanela ME, Trousdale RT, Berry DJ. Impacted cancellous graft plus cement in hip revision. Clin Orthop Relat Res 2003;175–82.

41. Gie GA, Linder L, Ling RS, Simon JP, Slooff TJ, Timperley AJ. Impacted cancellous allografts and cement for revision total hip arthroplasty. J Bone Joint Surg Br 1993;75:14–21.

42. Meding JB, Ritter MA, Keating EM, Faris PM. Impaction bone-grafting before insertion of a femoral stem with cement in revision total hip arthroplasty. A minimum two-year follow-up study. J Bone Joint Surg Am 1997;79:1834–41.

43. Linder L. Cancellous impaction grafting in the human femur: histological and radiographic observations in 6 autopsy femurs and 8 biopsies. Acta Orthop Scand 2000;71:543–52.

44. Frei H, Mitchell P, Masri BA, Duncan CP, Oxland TR. Allograft impaction and cement penetration after revision hip replacement: a histomorphometric analysis in the cadaver femur. J Bone Joint Surg Br 2004;86:771–6.

45. Frei H, Gadala MS, Masri BA, Duncan CP, Oxland TR. Cement flow during impaction allografting: a finite element analysis. J Biomech 2006;39:493–502.

46. Frei H, Mitchell P, Masri BA, Duncan CP, Oxland TR. Mechanical characteristics of the bone-graft-cement interface after impaction allografting. J Orthop Res 2005;23:9–17.

47. Albert C, Patil S, Frei H, Masri B, Duncan C, Oxland T et al. Cement penetration and primary stability of the femoral component after impaction allografting: A biomechanical study in the cadaveric femur. J Bone Joint Surg Br 2007;89:962–70.

48. Mankin HJ, Doppelt S, Tomford W. Clinical experience with allograft implantation. The first ten years. Clin Orthop Relat Res 1983;69–86.

49. Parrish FF. Treatment of bone tumors by total excision and replacement with massive autologous and homologous grafts. J Bone Joint Surg Am 1966;48:968–90.

50. Parrish FF. Allograft replacement of all or part of the end of a long bone following excision of a tumor. J Bone Joint Surg Am 1973;55:1–22.

50a. Pak JH, Paprosky WG, Jablonsky WS, Lawrence JM. Femoral strut allografts in cementless revision total hip arthroplasty. Clin Orthop Relat Res 1993;298:172–8.

51. Ornstein E, Franzen H, Johnsson R, Sundberg M. Radiostereometric analysis in hip revision surgery-optimal time for index examination: 6 patients revised with impacted allografts and cement followed weekly for 6 weeks. Acta Orthop Scand 2000;71:360–4.

52. Ebramzadeh E, Sarmiento A, McKellop HA, Llinas A, Gogan W. The cement mantle in total hip arthroplasty. Analysis of long-term radiographic results. J Bone Joint Surg Am 1994;76:77–87.

53. Jasty M, Maloney WJ, Bragdon CR, O'Connor DO, Haire T, Harris WH. The initiation of failure in cemented femoral components of hip arthroplasties. J Bone Joint Surg Br 1991;73:551–8.

54. Alfaro-Adrian J, Gill HS, Murray DW. Cement migration after THR: A comparison of Charnley Elite and Exeter femoral stems using RSA. J Bone Joint Surg Br 1999;81:130–4.

55. Ballard WT, Callaghan JJ, Sullivan PM, Johnston RC. The results of improved cementing techniques for total hip arthroplasty in patients less than fifty years old. A ten-year follow-up study. J Bone Joint Surg Am 1994;76:959–64.

56. Barrack RL, Castro F, Guinn S. Cost of implanting a cemented versus cementless femoral stem. J Arthroplasty 1996;11:373–6.

57. Huiskes R. The various stress patterns of press-fit, ingrown, and cemented femoral stems. Clin Orthop Relat Res 1990;27–38.

58. Hostner J, Hultmark P, Karrholm J, Malchau H, Tveit M. Impaction technique and graft treatment in revisions of the femoral component: laboratory studies and clinical validation. J Arthroplasty 2001;16:76–82.

59. Schreurs BW, Arts JJC, Verdonschot N, Buma P, Slooff TJJH, Gardeniers JWM. Femoral component revision with use of impaction bone-grafting and a cemented polished stem. J Bone Joint Surg Am 2005;87:2499–507.

60. Halliday BR, English HW, Timperley AJ, Gie GA, Ling RSM. Femoral impaction grafting with cement in revision total hip replacement: Evolution of the technique and results. J Bone Joint Surg Br 2003;85:809–17.

61. Sierra RJ, Charity J, Tsiridis E, Timperley JA, Gie GA. The use of long cemented stems for femoral impaction grafting in revision total hip arthroplasty. J Bone Joint Surg Am 2008;90:1330–6.

62. Barker R, Takahashi T, Toms A, Gregson P, Kuiper JH. Reconstruction of femoral defects in revision hip surgery: Risk of frcature and stem migration after impaction bone grafting. J Bone Joint Surg Br 2006;88:832–6.

63. Leopold SS, Berger RA, Rosenberg AG, Jacobs JJ, Quigley LR, Galante JO. Impaction allografting with cement for revision of the femoral component. a minimum four-year follow-up study with use of a precoated femoral stem. J Bone Joint Surg Am 1999;81:1080–92.

64. Ling RSM. Femoral component revision using impacted morsellised cancellous graft. J Bone Joint Surg Br 1997;79:874.

65. Elting JJ, Mikhail WE, Zicat BA, Hubbell JC, Lane LE, House B. Preliminary report of impaction grafting for exchange femoral arthroplasty. Clin Orthop Relat Res 1995;159–67.

66. Berger RA, Kull LR, Rosenberg AG, Galante JO. Hybrid total hip arthroplasty: 7- to 10-year results. Clin Orthop Relat Res 1996;134–46.

67. Oishi CS, Walker RH, Colwell CW. The femoral component in total hip arthroplasty. Six to eight-year follow-up of one hundred consecutive patients after use of a third-generation cementing technique. J Bone Joint Surg Am 1994;76:1130–6.

68. Ullmark G, Hallin G, Nilsson O. Impacted corticocancellous allografts and cement for femoral revision of total hip arthroplasty using Lubinus and Charnley prostheses. J Arthroplasty 2002;17:325–34.

69. Arif M, Sivananthan S, Choon DS. Revision of total hip arthroplasty using an anterior cortical window, extensive strut allografts, and an impaction graft: follow-up study. J Orthop Surg (Hong Kong) 2004;12:25–30.

70. Ornstein E, Linder L, Ranstam J, Lewold S, Eisler T, Torper M. Femoral impaction bone grafting with the Exeter stem—the Swedish experience: survivorship analysis of 1305 revisions performed between 1989 and 2002. J Bone Joint Surg Br 2009;91:441–6.

71. Chandler H, Clark J, Murphy S, McCarthy J, Penenberg B, Danylchuk K et al. Reconstruction of major segmental loss of the proximal femur in revision total hip arthroplasty. Clin Orthop Relat Res 1994;67–74.

72. Masri BA, Campbell DG, Garbuz DS, Duncan CP. Seven specialized exposures for revision hip and knee replacement. Orthop Clin North Am 1998;29:229–40.

73. Glassman AH, Engh CA, Bobyn JD. A technique of extensile exposure for total hip arthroplasty. J Arthroplasty 1987;2:11–21.

74. Czitrom AA. Biology of bone grafting and principles of bone banking. In: Weinstein SL, ed. The Pediatric Spine: Principles and Practice, pp 1285–98. Raven Press, New York, 1994.

75. Fideler BM, Vangsness CT, Moore T, Li Z, Rasheed S. Effects of gamma irradiation on the human immunodeficiency virus. A study in frozen human bone-patellar ligament-bone grafts obtained from infected cadavera. J Bone Joint Surg Am 1994;76:1032–5.

76. Zmolek JC, Dorr LD. Revision total hip arthroplasty. The use of solid allograft. J Arthroplasty 1993;8:361–70.

77. Ozaki T, Hillmann A, Bettin D, Wuisman P, Winkelmann W. Intramedullary, antibiotic-loaded cemented, massive allografts for skeletal reconstruction. 26 cases compared with 19 uncemented allografts. Acta Orthop Scand 1997;68:387–91.

78. Incavo SJ, Ames SE. Allograft-host mismatch in revision total hip replacement. Orthop Rev 1994;23:832–6.

79. Gross AE, Allan DG, Lavoie GJ, Oakeshott RD. Revision arthroplasty of the proximal femur using allograft bone. Orthop Clin North Am 1993;24:705–15.

80. Gross AE, Allan DG, Leitch KK, Hutchison CR. Proximal femoral allografts for reconstruction of bone stock in revision arthroplasty of the hip. Instr Course Lect 1996;45:143–7.

81. Gross AE, Hutchison CR. Proximal femoral allografts for reconstruction of bone stock in revision arthroplasty of the hip. Orthop Clin North Am 1998;29:313–7.

82. Gruen TA, McNeice GM, Amstutz HC. "Modes of failure" of cemented stem-type femoral components: a radiographic analysis of loosening. Clin Orthop Relat Res 1979;17–27.

83. Markel MD, Wood SA, Bogdanske JJ, Rapoff AJ, Kalscheur VL, Bouvy BM, et al. Comparison of allograft/endoprosthetic composites with a step-cut or transverse osteotomy configuration. J Orthop Res 1995;13:639–41.

84. Chandler HP, Penenberg B. Bone Stock Deficiency in Total Hip Replacement: Classification and Management. Slack, New Jersey, 1989.

85. Head WC, Wagner RA, Emerson RH, Malinin TI. Restoration of femoral bone stock in revision total hip arthroplasty. Orthop Clin North Am 1993;24:697–703.

86. Thompson RC, Pickvance EA, Garry D. Fractures in large-segment allografts. J Bone Joint Surg Am 1993;75:1663–73.

87. Chandler HP. Reconstruction of major segmental loss of the proximal femur in revision total hip replacement. Orthopedics 1997;20:801–3.

88. Head WC, Malinin TI, Berklacich F. Freeze-dried proximal femur allografts in revision total hip arthroplasty. A preliminary report. Clin Orthop Relat Res 1987;109–21.

89. Markel MD, Gottsauner-Wolf F, Rock MG, Frassica FJ, Chao EY. Mechanical characteristics of proximal femoral reconstruction after 50% resection. J Orthop Res 1993;11:339–49.

90. Kohles SS, Markel MD, Rock MG, Chao EY, Vanderby R. Fixation of femoral allograft/prosthesis composites after 25%, 50% and 75% resection. Med Eng Phys 1996;18:115–21.

91. Kohles SS, Markel MD, Rock MG, Chao EY, Vanderby R. Mechanical evaluation of six types of reconstruction following 25, 50, and 75% resection of the proximal femur. J Orthop Res 1994;12:834–43.

92. Gross AE, Blackley H, Wong P, Saleh K, Woodgate I. The use of allografts in orthopaedic surgery—part II: the role of allografts in revision arthroplasty of the hip. J Bone Joint Surg Am 2002;84:655–67.

93. Wong PKC, King A, Hutchison CR, Gross AE. Cortical strut allograft in revision total hip arthroplasty. Hip Int 2001;186–90.

94. Head WC, Berklacich FM, Malinin TI, Emerson RH. Proximal femoral allografts in revision total hip arthroplasty. Clin Orthop Relat Res 1987;22–36.

95. Roberson JR. Proximal femoral bone loss after total hip arthroplasty. Orthop Clin North Am 1992;23:291–302.

96. Masri B, Spangehl MJ, Duncan CP, Beauchamp CP, Myerthal SL. Proximal femoral allografts in revision total hip arthroplasty: a critical review. J Bone Joint Surg Br 1995;77:306–7.

97. Blackley HRL, Davis AM, Hutchison CR, Gross AE. Proximal femoral allografts for reconstruction of bone stock in revision arthroplasty of the hip : a nine to fifteen-year follow-up. J Bone Joint Surg Am 2001;83:346.

98. D'Antonio J, McCarthy JC, Bargar WL, Borden LS, Cappelo WN, Collis DK, et al. Classification of femoral abnormalities in total hip arthroplasty. Clin Orthop Relat Res 1993;133–9.

99. Nemzek JA, Arnoczky SP, Swenson CL. Retroviral transmission by the transplantation of connective-tissue allografts. An experimental study. J Bone Joint Surg Am 1994;76:1036–41.

100. Nemzek JA, Arnoczky SP, Swenson CL. Retroviral transmission in bone allotransplantation. The effects of tissue processing. Clin Orthop Relat Res 1996;275–82.

101. Buck BE, Malinin TI, Brown MD. Bone transplantation and human immunodeficiency virus. An estimate of risk of acquired immunodeficiency syndrome (AIDS). Clin Orthop Relat Res 1989;129–36.

102. Buck BE, Resnick L, Shah SM, Malinin TI. Human immunodeficiency virus cultured from bone. Implications for transplantation. Clin Orthop Relat Res 1990;249–53.

103. Hamer AJ, Strachan JR, Black MM, Ibbotson CJ, Stockley I, Elson RA. Biomechanical properties of cortical allograft bone using a new method of bone strength measurement: A comparison of fresh-frozen and irradiated bone. J Bone Joint Surg Br 1996;78:363–8.

104. Duncan CP, Masterson EL, Masri BA. Impaction allografting with cement for the management of femoral bone loss. Orthop Clin North Am 1998;29:297–305.

105. Fowler JL, Gie GA, Lee AJ, Ling RS. Experience with the Exeter total hip replacement since 1970. Orthop Clin North Am 1988;19:477–89.

106. Harris WH, McCarthy JC, O'Neill DA. Femoral component loosening using contemporary techniques of femoral cement fixation. J Bone Joint Surg Am 1982;64:1063–7.

107. Franzen H, Toksvig-Larsen S, Lidgren L, Onnerfalt R. Early migration of femoral components revised with impacted cancellous allografts and cement. A preliminary report of five patients. J Bone Joint Surg Br 1995;77:862–4.

108. Hutchison CR, Mahomed N, Agnidis Z, Leitch K, Alexeeff M, Gross AE. Proximal femoral allografts in revision hip arthroplasty-minimum 5 year follow up. Orthop Trans 1996;20:94.

109. Loty B, Tomeno B, Evrard J, Postel M. Infection in massive bone allografts sterilised by radiation. Int Orthop 1994;18:164–71.

110. Tan MH, Mankin HJ. Blood transfusion and bone allografts. Effect on infection and outcome. Clin Orthop Relat Res 1997;207–14.

111. Tomford WW, Thongphasuk J, Mankin HJ, Ferraro MJ. Frozen musculoskeletal allografts. A study of the clinical incidence and causes of infection associated with their use. J Bone Joint Surg Am 1990;72:1137–43.

112. Martin WR, Sutherland CJ. Complications of proximal femoral allografts in revision total hip arthroplasty. Clin Orthop Relat Res 1993;161–7.

113. Hanson PD, Warner C, Kofroth R, Osmond C, Bogdanske JJ, Kalscheur VL, et al. Effect of intramedullary polymethylmethacrylate and autogenous cancellous bone on healing of frozen segmental allografts. J Orthop Res 1998;16:285–92.

114. Berrey BH, Lord CF, Gebhardt MC, Mankin HJ. Fractures of allografts. Frequency, treatment, and end-results. J Bone Joint Surg Am 1990;72:825–33.

115. Gazdag AR, Lane JM, Glaser D, Forster RA. Alternatives to autogenous bone graft: efficacy and indications. J Am Acad Orthop Surg 1995;3:1–8.

116. Urist MR. Bone: formation by autoinduction. Science 1965;150: 893–9.

117. Wang J, Glimcher MJ. Characterization of matrix-induced osteogenesis in rat calvarial bone defects: I. Differences in the cellular response to demineralized bone matrix implanted in calvarial defects and in subcutaneous sites. Calcif Tissue Int 1999;65:156–65.

118. Wang J, Glimcher MJ. Characterization of matrix-induced osteogenesis in rat calvarial bone defects: II. Origins of bone-forming cells. Calcif Tissue Int 1999;65:486–93.

119. Oakes DA, Lee CC, Lieberman JR. An evaluation of human demineralized bone matrices in a rat femoral defect model. Clin Orthop Relat Res 2003;281–90.

120. Schwartz Z, Mellonig JT, Carnes DL, de la Fontaine J, Cochran DL, Dean DD, et al. Ability of commercial demineralized freeze-dried bone allograft to induce new bone formation. J Periodontol 1996;67:918–26.

121. Bucholz RW. Nonallograft osteoconductive bone graft substitutes. Clin Orthop Relat Res 2002;44–52.

122. Bauer TW, Smith ST. Bioactive materials in orthopaedic surgery: overview and regulatory considerations. Clin Orthop Relat Res 2002;11–22.

123. Cook SD, Barrack RL, Santman M, Patron LP, Salkeld SL, Whitecloud TS. The Otto Aufranc Award. Strut allograft healing to the femur with recombinant human osteogenic protein-1. Clin Orthop Relat Res 2000;47–57.

124. Cook SD, Barrack RL, Shimmin A, Morgan D, Carvajal JP. The use of osteogenic protein-1 in reconstructive surgery of the hip. J Arthroplasty 2001;16:88–94.

125. Engh CA, Hopper RH. Extensively porous-coated stems: a choice for all seasons. Orthopedics 2000;23:951–2.

126. Engh CA, Ellis TJ, Koralewicz LM, McAuley JP, Engh CA. Extensively porous-coated femoral revision for severe femoral bone loss: minimum 10-year follow-up. J Arthroplasty 2002;17: 955–60.

127. Engh CA, Hopper RH. The odyssey of porous-coated fixation. J Arthroplasty 2002;17:102–7.

128. Engh CA, Fenwick JA. Extensively porous-coated stems: avoiding modularity. Orthopedics 2008;31:911–2.

129. Moreland JR, Bernstein ML. Femoral revision hip arthroplasty with uncemented, porous-coated stems. Clin Orthop Relat Res 1995;141–50.

130. Nourbash PS, Paprosky WG. Cementless femoral design concerns. Rationale for extensive porous coating. Clin Orthop Relat Res 1998;189–99.

131. Paprosky WG, Greidanus NV, Antoniou J. Minimum 10-year-results of extensively porous-coated stems in revision hip arthroplasty. Clin Orthop Relat Res 1999;230–42.

132. Paprosky WG, Weeden SH. Extensively porous-coated stems in femoral revision arthroplasty. Orthopedics 2001;24:871–2.

133. Paprosky WG, Burnett RS. Extensively porous-coated femoral stems in revision hip arthroplasty: rationale and results. Am J Orthop 2002;31:471–4.

134. Sporer SM, Paprosky WG. Extensively coated cementless femoral components in revision total hip arthoplasty: an update. Surg Technol Int 2005;14:265–74.

135. Sugimura T, Tohkura A. THA revision with extensively porous-coated stems. 32 hips followed 2–6.5 years. Acta Orthop Scand 1998;69:11–3.

136. Weeden SH, Paprosky WG. Minimal 11-year follow-up of extensively porous-coated stems in femoral revision total hip arthroplasty. J Arthroplasty 2002;17:134–7.

137. Wu LD, Xiong Y, Yan SG, Yang QS, Dai XS. Femoral component revision using extensively porous-coated cementless stem. Chin J Traumatol 2005;8:358–63.

138. McInnis DP, Horne GF, Devane PA. Femoral revision with a fluted, tapered, modular stem seventy patients followed for a mean of 3.9 years. J Arthroplasty 2006;21:372–80.

139. Park YS, Moon Y-W, Lim SJ. Revision total hip arthroplasty using a fluted and tapered modular distal fixation stem with and without extended trochanteric osteotomy. J Arthroplasty 2007;22:993–9.

140. Mumme TF, Muller-Rath RF, Andereya S, Wirtz DC. Uncemented femoral revision arthroplasty using the modular revision prosthesis MRP-TITAN revision stem. Oper Orthop Traumatol 2007;19:56–77.

141. Garbuz DS, Toms AF, Masri BA, Duncan CP. Improved outcome in femoral revision arthroplasty with tapered fluted modular titanium stems. Clin Orthop Relat Res 2006; 453:199–202.

22 Revision of the Acetabular Components: Role of Structural Bulk Allografts and Porous Tantalum Implants

John Antoniou, Alan J. Walsh, and Vassilios S. Nikolaou
McGill University, Montreal, QC, Canada

Case scenario

A 41 year old man presented with a 2 year history of progressive left groin pain on weightbearing. He had a total hip arthroplasty (THA) performed 15 years ago for osteoarthritis of his left hip secondary to a displaced fracture of the acetabular dome. Clinical examination of the left hip showed restricted motion and antalgia, but good abductor muscle function.

Relevant anatomy

The three-dimensional anatomy of the acetabulum is difficult to interpret from plain radiographs alone. CT can help define the topography of missing bone. The landmarks of the bony acetabulum relevant to the classification of bony defects prior to revision acetabular reconstruction are shown on a pelvic radiograph (Figure 22.1).

Importance of the problem

THA is one of the most widespread and successful surgical procedures performed worldwide. In the United States, over 168,000 primary and 30,000 revision hip arthroplasties are performed every year.[1] The rate of primary THA has recently increased and the number of revisions could more than double by 2030.[2] Nordic arthroplasty registers have reported failure of 7% of primary prostheses within 10 years.[3] Expanded indications for THA in younger patients and improved lifespans of all THA patients will lead to even more revision surgery. The acetabulum with significant bone loss is a major surgical challenge and there is debate concerning the surgical techniques most appropriate for such revisions. Surgical decision-making preoperatively is key to the longevity and re-revisability of revision hip arthroplasties.

Top three questions

1. Which classification systems quantify acetabular bone deficiency prior to revision hip arthroplasty?
2. What options has the orthopedic surgeon for reconstruction of acetabular bone loss?
3. What is the role of porous tantalum implants in revision acetabular arthroplasty?

Question 1: Which classification systems quantify acetabular bone deficiency prior to revision hip arthroplasty?

Case clarification

An AP view of both hips of our patient (Figure 22.2) and a lateral view of the left hip (Figure 22.3) are shown after a first-stage revision THA performed elsewhere for infection. A second-stage procedure was planned after a period of appropriate antibiotic therapy and normalization of inflammatory markers.

Relevance

Classification of the defect preoperatively is important to quantify the deficiency of acetabular bone stock. This facilitates surgical planning and highlights requirements for bone graft or particular reconstructive hardware.

Current opinion

The three classification systems for acetabular bone loss commonly used are those of D'Antoniou,[4] recommended by the American Academy of Orthopaedic Surgeons (AAOS), Paprosky et al.[5] and Gross et al.[6]

Evidence-Based Orthopedics, First Edition. Edited by Mohit Bhandari.
© 2012 Blackwell Publishing Ltd. Published 2012 by Blackwell Publishing Ltd.

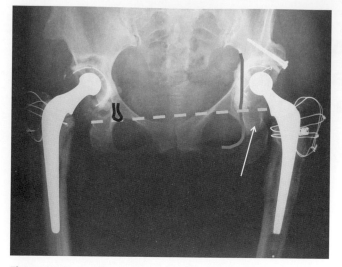

Figure 22.1 AP radiograph of a patient with bilateral cemented total hip arthroplasties showing cup loosening on the right side and a high hip center with a healed bulk femoral head allograft on the left side. The four main anatomic landmarks relevant to the Paprosky classification of acetabular bone loss are indicated (superior transverse obturator line, ilioischial line, teardrop, typical zone of ischial lysis).

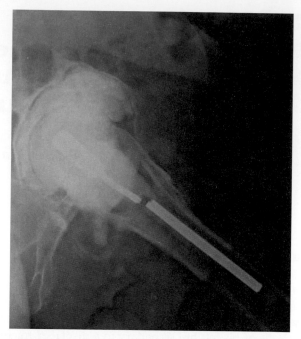

Figure 22.3 Lateral radiograph of the left hip of the clinical case showing a fractured cement spacer in situ after a first-stage revision left total hip arthroplasty.

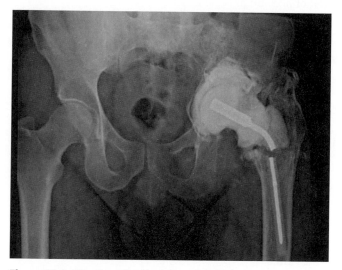

Figure 22.2 AP radiograph of both hips of the clinical case showing a fractured cement spacer in situ after a first-stage revision left total hip arthroplasty.

Table 22.1 AAOS classification

Type	Description of deficiency
IA	Segmental (peripheral)
IB	Segmental (central)
II	Cavitary
III	Combined
IV	Pelvic discontinuity
V	Arthrodesis

Finding the evidence

- PubMed (www.ncbi.nlm.nih.gov/pubmed/)—sensitivity search using keywords "bone loss" AND "acetabulum" AND "classification"

Quality of the evidence

- Level II: 1
- Level V: 3

Findings

The AAOS classification (Table 22.1) of D'Antoniou[4] is a descriptive classification. Cavitary defects are contained, whereas segmental defects involve the acetabular rim or columns. Pelvic discontinuity occurs when there is deficiency of both the acetabular columns.

The Paprosky classification[5] uses anatomical landmarks to classify the extent of bony deficiency (Table 22.2) and guides reconstruction based on available techniques. Defects can be graded as completely (type 1), partially (type 2), or non (type 3) supportive. Superior cup migration implies damage to the superior dome whereas medial migration implies medial wall deficiency. Lysis involving the teardrop or ischium represents damage to the anterior and posterior acetabular columns respectively. Gross et al.[6] devised a classification based on the type of bone graft

Table 22.2 Paprosky classification

Type of defect	Superior migration of hip center[a]	Medial migration of hip center[b]	Osteolysis of teardrop[c]	Osteolysis of ischium[d]
I	Minimum	None	None	None
2A	Minimum	Grade I	Mild	Mild
2B	Minimum to Marked	Grade II	Mild	Mild
2C	Minimum	Grade III	Moderate or Severe	Mild
3A	Marked	Grade II+ or III	Moderate	Moderate
3B	Marked	Grade III+	Severe	Severe

[a] Minimum is ≤3 cm proximal to the superior transverse obturator line, and marked is >3 cm proximal to the superior transverse obturator line.
[b] Grade I, lateral to Kohler's ilioischial line; grade II, to Kohler's line; grade II+, medial expansion of Kohler's line into the pelvis; grade III, violation of Kohler's line with some migration into the pelvis; grade III+, marked migration into the pelvis.
[c] Mild, minimum loss of the lateral border; moderate, complete loss of the lateral border; severe, loss of the lateral and medial borders.
[d] Mild, 0–7 mm distal to the superior transverse obturator line; moderate, 8–14 mm distal to the obturator line; severe, ≥15 mm distal to the obturator line.

Table 22.3 Gross classification

Type	Description of deficiency
I	Contained defect with intact rim and columns
IIA	Noncontained defect—minor column (>50% of host acetabulum in contact with cup
IIB	Noncontained defect—major column (<50% of host acetabulum in contact with cup

required for revision (Table 22.3). Campbell et al.[7] have critically evaluated the reliability of these three classification systems, showing inconsistency in both interobserver and intraobserver reliability.

Recommendation
• These classifications show limited reliability and should be considered a general guide to discern between simple and complex reconstructive scenarios [overall quality: low]

Question 2: What options has the orthopedic surgeon for reconstruction of acetabular bone loss?

Case clarification
The patient required reconstruction of his acetabular deficiency. After classification of preoperative bone loss, a decision was made on the appropriate reconstructive technique.

Relevance
There is no consensus regarding the optimal method of reconstruction in cases of revision hip arthroplasty with severe bone loss. The major decisions regarding surgical technique for complex acetabular revision concern the use of bone graft, cages and cemented vs. cementless components. The plethora of potential combinations of grafts and metallic devices has lead to a huge diversity of reconstructive options in revision acetabular arthroplasty. This creates significant difficulty for systematic analysis of clinical literature incorporating a very heterogenous mix of surgical techniques.

Current opinion
Acetabular bone loss can be compensated by placing a high hip center or by using asymmetrical or bilobed acetabular components. Cementless hemispherical cups provide durable survivorship in the revision setting if initial stability and contact with sufficient host bone is possible. Cemented fixation of a polyethylene cup or liner into a supporting cage has often been the construct of choice where allograft is required to support more than 50% of the new acetabular component. Supplementary acetabular fixation may be necessary to stabilize pelvic discontinuity and protect or support bone graft and/or cups. Trabecular metal shells can be used for severe acetabular defects where bone grafting has traditionally performed poorly.

Finding the evidence
• PubMed (www.ncbi.nlm.nih.gov/pubmed/): sensitivity search using keywords "treatment options revision hip" AND "revision hip acetabulum"

Quality of the evidence
• Level III: 2
• Level IV: 28
• Level V: 8

Findings
Contained or cavitary defects (Paprosky types 1 and 2, Gross type I) can be treated with impacted morsellized cancellous allograft bone chips. Satisfactory outcomes have been reported using cementless porous hemispherical acetabular components for these defects.[8–10] Noncontained, segmental defects are subdivided into those where host bone support for the implant is more than 50% (Paprosky 3A, Gross IIA) or less than 50% (Paprosky 3B, Gross IIB). Radiologically these defects produce significant superolateral and superomedial cup migration respectively. Sporer et al.[11] achieved 78% 10 year survival with cementless acetabular components

supported by distal femoral structural bulk allograft buttress for 3A defects. Others have shown either good medium-term survival with bulk grafts[12–14] or frequent loosening with graft resorption.[15,16] Options for 3B defects include placing the component high on remaining host bone, implanting a large cementless acetabular component, using structural bone graft or replacing lost bone with massive partial or total acetabular allograft, protected with an antiprotrusio cage, containing a cemented liner. Reconstructing the acetabulum with a high hip center has been associated with early loosening,[17] although 94% survival at 10.4 years is reported.[18] Treatment of type 3B defects with cemented polyethylene cups and large allografts alone has produced poor results.[19,20] The use of reconstruction cages improves their survival despite implantation difficulties and low potential for biological bone ingrowth.[21] Use of porous tantalum acetabular shells, cups, and augmentations can address these difficulties.[22–36] Brubaker et al.[37] proposed specific interventions for different grades of acetabular defect based on a modification of the classification of Gross et al.,[6] validated by Saleh et al.[38] They calculated a prognosis for each intervention based on the available literature (Table 22.4). Kosashvili et al.[32] reported good short term outcomes with the "component-cage technique," combining ilioischial cages with trabecular metal shells for pelvic discontinuity.

Recommendation

• There are no trials in the clinical literature to differentiate between treatment modalities for each grade of acetabular bone loss in revision hip arthroplasty. Evidence for different surgical techniques is limited to comparison of case series and expert reviews [overall quality: low]

Question 3: What is the role of porous tantalum implants in revision acetabular arthroplasty?

Case clarification

A large porous tantalum trabecular metal acetabular implant with supplementary screw fixation was chosen for reconstruction (Figure 22.4). Allograft reconstruction of the acetabulum was avoided in this patient to reduce the risk of recurrent infection.

Relevance

The advent[39] and validation[40] of porous tantalum trabecular metal shells signalled a new era in the management of severe acetabular defects. Tantalum is more porous, less stiff, and creates more friction with bone than conventional porous-coated acetabular implants.

Current opinion

Porous tantalum acetabular implants represent an improvement from conventional porous materials by achieving increased bone ingrowth and enhanced interface fixation strength for acetabular revision surgery with severe bone loss.

Finding the evidence

• PubMed (www.ncbi.nlm.nih.gov/pubmed/): sensitivity search using keywords "porous" AND "tantalum" AND "hip arthroplasty" as well as "trabecular metal" AND "hip arthroplasty"

Table 22.4 Modified Gross classification

Defect type	Bone loss	Treatment	Survival (min 5 years)
I	None	Primary component	As for primary THA
II	Contained	Morcelized allograft ± roof ring	84–95%
III	Segmental <50%	Minor column structural allograft + cage, or bilobed cup, or tantalum component	76–94%
IV	Segmental >50%	Major column or acetabular structural allograft with cage, or custom implant	77–100%
V	Discontinuity	As for type IV + fixation of discontinuity	As for type IV

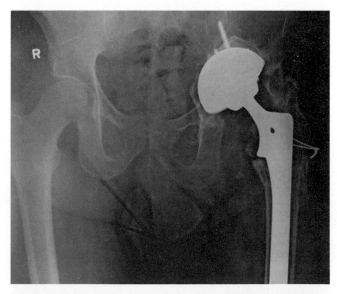

Figure 22.4 AP radiograph of both hips of the clinical case showing a trabecular metal shell in situ after a second-stage revision left total hip arthroplasty.

Quality of the evidence

- Level III: 4
- Level IV: 16
- Level V: 8

Findings

Conventional porous-coated acetabular implants have proven effective in revision THA where bone stock is sufficient for stability and ingrowth and success with these implants occurs when contact with host bone is greater that 50%.[8–10] Antiprotrusio cages are recommended for host support less than 50%, but implantation is problematic and biological bone ingrowth is not possible.[21,41] Porous tantalum acetabular cups may provide a solution.[22–36] The porosity of materials commonly used to manufacture acetabular shells approximates 30–50% of their volume. Porous tantalum exhibits almost double this porosity (80%) for bone–metal interdigitation.[42] Porous tantalum implants display high surface frictional characteristics and good osseointegration properties.[42–44] Trabecular metal revision shells are made completely of porous tantalum and have perforations for screw fixation. These shells can be positioned for maximal bone contact using a polyethylene liner locked within or cemented at the required orientation.[24,35,45] When less than 50% host bone is available to support the shell, tantalum augments are used to help fill the defect. A thin layer of cement between the shell and each augment minimizes metal fretting.[45] For pelvic discontinuity, tantalum cup and reconstruction cage constructs can be used. The cage is positioned over the cup, bridging the acetabular defect, and a polyethylene liner is cemented into the cage.[22,45,46] Trabecular metal constructs have been used effectively for severe acetabular defects. The published results to date[24–26,29–32,34–36,46–48] are presented in Table 22.5.

Table 22.5 Porous tantalum studies

Year	Author	No. of cases	Mean follow-up (years)	Survival (%)
2004	Nehme	16	2.7	87.5
2005	Unger	59	3.5	88
2006	Sporer	13	2.6	100
2007	Boscainos	14	2.5	100
2007	Weeden	43	2.8	100
2008	Flecher	23	2.9	100
2008	Kim	46	3.3	98
2009	Fernandez-Fairen	263	6.1	100
2009	Kosashvilli	26	3.7	88.5
2009	Lakstein	53	3.8	96
2009	Malkani	22	3.3	100
2009	Siegmeth	34	2.8	94
2009	Van Kleunen	97	3.8	100

Recommendation

- Porous tantalum trabecular metal shells have good survival statistics for reconstruction of severe acetabular defects in case series with short- to medium-term review [overall quality: low]

Summary of recommendations

- Classification systems for acetabular bone loss show limited reliability and should be considered a general guide to discern between simple and complex reconstructive scenarios
- There are no trials in the clinical literature to differentiate between treatment modalities for each grade of acetabular bone loss in revision hip arthroplasty. Evidence for different surgical techniques is limited to comparison of case series and expert reviews
- Porous tantalum trabecular metal shells have good survival statistics for reconstruction of severe acetabular defects in case series with short- to medium-term review

Conclusions

Revision THA where complex reconstruction of deficient acetabular bone stock is necessary provides challenges to both patients and their orthopedic surgeons.

The classification systems for acetabular bone loss vary in their description and relevance to treatment options. Most authors agree that defects where less than 50% coverage of the revision acetabular cup by remaining host bone is possible provide a much greater challenge to successful reconstruction.

There is as yet no universal agreement on which reconstructive techniques to use for each grade of periprosthetic acetabular bone deficiency. A lack of high-level evidence exists in the scientific literature to discern between different techniques.

Cavitary defects can be successfully managed with either cemented or cementless components, with or without morsellized allograft, with results approximating those of primary surgery. Segmental and mixed defects can be treated with various combinations of morsellized or structural allograft, metallic reinforcement devices and cemented or cementless components, but results for many of these constructs have been unsatisfactory.

The use of porous tantalum trabecular metal components for severe defects shows encouraging short- to medium-term results, but cannot restore bone stock for future revisions.

Clinical trials, to identify the ideal allograft, reinforcement device, and acetabular component combination may be necessary to maximize survival of revision hip arthroplasty while preserving adequate bone stock for future revision surgeries in younger patients.

Acknowledgement

The authors wish to thank Dr. David Zukor for his contribution to the clinical case.

References

1. Hall MJ, Owings MF. 2000 National Hospital Discharge Survey. Adv Data 2002;329:1–18.
2. Kurtz S, Mowat F, Ong K, Chan N, Lau E, Halpern M. Prevalence of primary and revision total hip and knee arthroplasty in the United States from 1990 through 2002. J Bone Joint Surg Am 2005;87(7):1487–97.
3. Havelin LI, Fenstad AM, Salomonsson R, Mehnert F, Furnes O, Overgaard S, et al. The Nordic Arthroplasty Register Association. Acta Orthop 2009;80:1–9.
4. D'Antonio JA. Periprosthetic bone loss of the acetabulum. Classification and management. Orthop Clin North Am 1992; 23(2):279–90.
5. Paprosky WG, Perona PG, Lawrence JM. Acetabular defect classification and surgical reconstruction in revision arthroplasty. A 6-year follow-up evaluation. J Arthroplasty 1994;9(1): 33–44.
6. Gross AE, Allan DG, Catre M, Garbuz DS, Stockley I. Bone grafts in hip replacement surgery. The pelvic side. Orthop Clin North Am 1993;24(4):679–95.
7. Campbell DG, Garbuz DS, Masri BA, Duncan CP. Reliability of acetabular bone defect classification systems in revision total hip arthroplasty. J Arthroplasty 2001;16(1):83–6.
8. Della Valle CJ, Berger RA, Rosenberg AG, Galante JO. Cementless acetabular reconstruction in revision total hip arthroplasty. Clin Orthop Relat Res 2004;420:96–100.
9. Della Valle CJ, Shuaipaj T, Berger RA, Rosenberg AG, Shott S, Jacobs JJ, et al. Revision of the acetabular component without cement after total hip arthroplasty. A concise follow-up, at fifteen to nineteen years, of a previous report. J Bone Joint Surg Am 2005;87(8):1795–800.
10. Weeden SH, Paprosky WG. Porous-ingrowth revision acetabular implants secured with peripheral screws. A minimum twelve-year follow-up. J Bone Joint Surg Am 2006;88(6):1266–71.
11. Sporer SM, O'Rourke M, Chong P, Paprosky WG. The use of structural distal femoral allografts for acetabular reconstruction. Average ten-year follow-up. J Bone Joint Surg Am 2005;87(4): 760–5.
12. Argenson JN, Paratte S, Flecher X, Aubaniac JM. Impaction grafting for acetabular revision: bringing back the bone. Orthopedics 2004;27(9):967–8.
13. Chen XD, Waddell JP, Morton J, Schemitsch EH. Isolated acetabular revision after total hip arthroplasty: results at 5–9 years of follow-up. Int Orthop 2005;29(5):277–80.
14. Somers JF, Timperley AJ, Norton M, Taylor R, Gie GA. Block allografts in revision total hip arthroplasty. J Arthroplasty 2002;17(5):562–8.
15. Reikeraas O, Folleraas G, Winge JF. Allografting in uncemented acetabular revision. Orthopedics 1998;21(11):1191–5.
16. Hooten JP, Jr., Engh CA, Jr., Engh CA. Failure of structural acetabular allografts in cementless revision hip arthroplasty. J Bone Joint Surg Br 1994;76(3):419–22.
17. Jasty M, Freiberg AA. The use of a high-hip center in revision total hip arthroplasty. Semin Arthroplasty 1995;6(2):103–8.
18. Dearborn JT, Harris WH. High placement of an acetabular component inserted without cement in a revision total hip arthroplasty. Results after a mean of ten years. J Bone Joint Surg Am 1999;81(4):469–80.
19. Garbuz D, Morsi E, Gross AE. Revision of the acetabular component of a total hip arthroplasty with a massive structural allograft. Study with a minimum five-year follow-up. J Bone Joint Surg Am 1996;78(5):693–7.
20. Schelfaut S, Cool S, Mulier M. The use of structural periacetabular allografts in acetabular revision surgery: 2.5–5 years follow-up. Arch Orthop Trauma Surg 2009;129(4):455–61.
21. Berry DJ. Antiprotrusio cages for acetabular revision. Clin Orthop Relat Res 2004;420:106–12.
22. Gross AE, Goodman SB. Rebuilding the skeleton: the intraoperative use of trabecular metal in revision total hip arthroplasty. J Arthroplasty 2005;20(4 Suppl 2):91–3.
23. Macheras GA, Papagelopoulos PJ, Kateros K, Kostakos AT, Baltas D, Karachalios TS. Radiological evaluation of the metal-bone interface of a porous tantalum monoblock acetabular component. J Bone Joint Surg Br 2006;88(3):304–9.
24. Kim WY, Greidanus NV, Duncan CP, Masri BA, Garbuz DS. Porous tantalum uncemented acetabular shells in revision total hip replacement: two to four year clinical and radiographic results. Hip Int 2008;18(1):17–22.
25. Unger AS, Lewis RJ, Gruen T. Evaluation of a porous tantalum uncemented acetabular cup in revision total hip arthroplasty: clinical and radiological results of 60 hips. J Arthroplasty 2005;20(8):1002–9.
26. Sporer SM, Paprosky WG. Acetabular revision using a trabecular metal acetabular component for severe acetabular bone loss associated with a pelvic discontinuity. J Arthroplasty 2006; 21(6 Suppl 2):87–90.
27. Rose PS, Halasy M, Trousdale RT, Hanssen AD, Sim FH, Berry DJ, et al. Preliminary results of tantalum acetabular components for THA after pelvic radiation. Clin Orthop Relat Res 2006;453:195–8.
28. Malizos KN, Bargiotas K, Papatheodorou L, Hantes M, Karachalios T. Survivorship of monoblock trabecular metal cups in primary THA : midterm results. Clin Orthop Relat Res 2008;466(1):159–66.
29. Malkani AL, Price MR, Crawford CH, 3rd, Baker DL. Acetabular component revision using a porous tantalum biomaterial: a case series. J Arthroplasty 2009;24(7):1068–73.
30. Flecher X, Sporer S, Paprosky W. Management of severe bone loss in acetabular revision using a trabecular metal shell. J Arthroplasty 2008;23(7):949–55.
31. Siegmeth A, Duncan CP, Masri BA, Kim WY, Garbuz DS. Modular tantalum augments for acetabular defects in revision hip arthroplasty. Clin Orthop Relat Res 2009;467(1):199–205.
32. Kosashvili Y, Backstein D, Safir O, Lakstein D, Gross AE. Acetabular revision using an anti-protrusion (ilio-ischial) cage and trabecular metal acetabular component for severe acetabular bone loss associated with pelvic discontinuity. J Bone Joint Surg Br 2009;91(7):870–6.

33. Xenakis TA, Macheras GA, Stafilas KS, Kostakos AT, Bargiotas K, Malizos KN. Multicentre use of a porous tantalum monoblock acetabular component. Int Orthop 2009;33(4):911–6.

34. Van Kleunen JP, Lee GC, Lementowski PW, Nelson CL, Garino JP. Acetabular revisions using trabecular metal cups and augments. J Arthroplasty 2009;24(6 Suppl):64–8.

35. Lakstein D, Backstein D, Safir O, Kosashvili Y, Gross AE. Trabecular Metal cups for acetabular defects with 50% or less host bone contact. Clin Orthop Relat Res 2009;467(9):2318–24.

36. Fernandez-Fairen M, Murcia A, Blanco A, Merono A, Murcia A, Jr., Ballester J. Revision of failed total hip arthroplasty acetabular cups to porous tantalum components: a 5-year follow-up study. J Arthroplasty 2010;25(6):865–72.

37. Brubaker SM, Brown TE, Manaswi A, Mihalko WM, Cui Q, Saleh KJ. Treatment options and allograft use in revision total hip arthroplasty the acetabulum. J Arthroplasty 2007;22(7 Suppl 3):52–6.

38. Saleh KJ, Holtzman J, Gafni A, Saleh L, Davis A, Resig S, et al. Reliability and intraoperative validity of preoperative assessment of standardized plain radiographs in predicting bone loss at revision hip surgery. J Bone Joint Surg Am 2001;83(7): 1040–6.

39. Christie MJ. Clinical applications of Trabecular Metal. Am J Orthop 2002;31(4):219–20.

40. Bobyn JD, Poggie RA, Krygier JJ, Lewallen DG, Hanssen AD, Lewis RJ, et al. Clinical validation of a structural porous tantalum biomaterial for adult reconstruction. J Bone Joint Surg Am 2004;86(Suppl 2):123–9.

41. Gross AE, Goodman S. The current role of structural grafts and cages in revision arthroplasty of the hip. Clin Orthop Relat Res 2004;429:193–200.

42. Bobyn JD, Stackpool GJ, Hacking SA, Tanzer M, Krygier JJ. Characteristics of bone ingrowth and interface mechanics of a new porous tantalum biomaterial. J Bone Joint Surg Br 1999;81(5):907–14.

43. Levine BR, Sporer S, Poggie RA, Della Valle CJ, Jacobs JJ. Experimental and clinical performance of porous tantalum in orthopedic surgery. Biomaterials 2006;27(27):4671–81.

44. Bobyn JD, Toh KK, Hacking SA, Tanzer M, Krygier JJ. Tissue response to porous tantalum acetabular cups: a canine model. J Arthroplasty 1999;14(3):347–54.

45. Patil N, Lee K, Goodman SB. Porous tantalum in hip and knee reconstructive surgery. J Biomed Mater Res B Appl Biomater 2009;89(1):242–51.

46. Boscainos PJ, Kellett CF, Maury AC, Backstein D, Gross AE. Management of periacetabular bone loss in revision hip arthroplasty. Clin Orthop Relat Res 2007;465:159–65.

47. Nehme A, Lewallen DG, Hanssen AD. Modular porous metal augments for treatment of severe acetabular bone loss during revision hip arthroplasty. Clin Orthop Relat Res 2004;429: 201–8.

48. Weeden SH, Schmidt RH. The use of tantalum porous metal implants for Paprosky 3A and 3B defects. J Arthroplasty 2007;22(6 Suppl 2):151–5.

Antibiotic Cement in Total Knee Arthroplasty

Philip A. O'Connor and Steven J. MacDonald
University of Western Ontario and University Hospital, London, ON, Canada

Case scenarios

Case 1

A 49 year old woman with tricompartmental osteoarthritis undergoes a primary total knee arthroplasty (TKA).

Case 2

A 75 year old man, with a history of of type 2 diabetes mellitus, undergoes a revision of an infected TKA.

Top six questions

Therapy

1. What are the benefits of routine use of antibiotic-loaded bone cement in primary TKA?
2. Is the routine use of antibiotic-loaded bone cement in primary TKA cost-effective?
3. What is the role of antibiotic-loaded bone cement in the treatment of established prosthetic knee infection?

Prognosis

4. Does the use of antibiotic-loaded bone cement in primary TKA lead to earlier mechanical failure rates?

Harm

5. Can the routine use of antibiotic-loaded bone cement lead to the development of resistant organisms in TKA?
6. Is there a risk of developing systemic toxicity or an allergic reaction with the use of antibiotic-loaded bone cement in TKA?

Question 1: What are the benefits of the routine use of antibiotic-loaded bone cement in primary TKA?

Case clarification

Antibiotic laden bone cement (ALBC) has two distinct roles in TKA. It can be used as a prophylactic measure or as treatment modality for established implant-related infection. Dosages of combined antibiotics can be arbitarily divided into *low* (<2g antibiotic per 40g acrylic cement) and *high* (>2g per 40g acrylic cement). It is the use of low-dose ALBC for supplemental prophylaxis in TKA that remains controversial.

Relevance

The use of systemic periopertaive prophylactic antibiotics is well-accepted practice but deep infection rates persist and on average occur in 2% of cases with osteoarthrosis and in 4% of patients with rheumatoid arthritis.[1]

Evidence-Based Orthopedics, First Edition. Edited by Mohit Bhandari.
© 2012 Blackwell Publishing Ltd. Published 2012 by Blackwell Publishing Ltd.

Current opinion

Current opinion is divided on this subject. There are significant geographic differences. In North America, the majority of primary TKAs use acrylic bone cement that does not contain antibiotics. In Europe, ALBC is commonly employed for primary TKAs.

Finding the evidence

• Cochrane Database: no reviews on this topic were identified.
• PubMed, using the following search terms: "antibiotic cement primary knee arthroplasty," "antibiotic laden bone cement"
• Manual review of cited references from identified articles

Quality of the evidence

We found 37 articles, 3 of which were review articles.[2-4]

Level I
• 3 randomized trials[5-7]

Level II
• 1 systemic review of cohort studies[8]
• 4 individual cohort studies[9-12]

Findings

The advantage of using ALBC is a reduction of perioperative infections following TKA. With an already low rate of deep periprosthetic infection, most studies are underpowered to demonstrate efficacy in the use of ALBC. It is estimated that 8,800 patients would have to be entered into a randomized controlled trial (RCT) to detect a significant effect. To date only three RCTs have been identified that have reported on the prophylactic use of ALBC in arthroplasty.[5-7].

McQueen[6] reported on a prospective randomized trial of 295 arthroplasties (both hip and knee). Patients were randomized to receive cefuroxime either in bone cement or parenterally. No statistically significant difference in the rate of superficial or deep infection between the groups was observed. Follow-up was for 3 months only and the method of randomization was not made clear. A follow-up report[13] of 401 patients confirmed their earlier results.

Josefsson performed a prospective RCT, again comparing systemic antibiotic administration with ALBC (containing gentamicin) in 1688 consecutive total hip arthroplasties (THAs). Three separate reports at follow-up intervals of 2, 5, and 10 years were published.[7,14,15] This was a multicenter trial, with different regimes of parental antibiotic administered and compared against ALBC with gentamicin. At intervals of 2 and 5 years postoperatively, a statistically significant difference was observed in favour of the use of ALBC. However, no difference was detected at follow-up

after 10 years postoperatively. Reclassification of cases had ensued at the latest follow-up.

Chiu et al.[5] performed an RCT of 340 primary TKAs on the use of ALBC against plain bone cement (PBC). There was a statistically significant reduction (p = 0.02) in the rate of deep infection in ALBC group (0 out of 162) vs. PBC (5 out of 162). In a further trial the same authors[16] examined the role of antibiotic-impregnated cement in the prevention of deep infection at primary TKA in a cohort of diabetic patients undergoing TKA. In this study 41 TKAs were randomized to receive ALBC (with cefuroxime) vs. 31 TKAs with PBC. There was a statistically significant difference between the two groups, with five cases of deep infection occuring in the PBC group (5/37) and none in the ALBC group (0/41).

The strongest evidence for the use of ALBC comes from large registries; the Scandinavian countries have the longest history of data collection. In a study from the Finnish Arthroplasty Register, Jämsen[12] reports on all primary and revision knee arthroplasties that were performed from January 1997 to June 2004. The minimum duration of follow-up was 6 months. The data of the study related to 43,149 operations, of which 40,135 were primary TKAs, 2166 were revision TKAs and 848 were partial revision arthroplasties. Antibiotic-impregnated cement was used for the fixation of at least one prosthetic component in 84% of the knees. The combination of parenteral antibiotic prophylaxis and prosthetic fixation with antibiotic-impregnated cement was found to protect against septic failure. Specifically, the risk of periprosthetic infection following a primary TKA was 0.68% when antibiotics were used both in the cement and intravenously, 0.81% when used in the cement only, and 1.05% when used intravenously only.

Epsehaung et al.[9] published data from the Norwegian arthroplasty registry on 10,905 primary THAs. The infected revision rate of patients who had combined prophylaxis with systemically adminstered antibiotics and the use of ALBC had the lowest revision rate when compared with the use of either prophylactic regimen in isolotaion (systemically adminstered antibiotics alone 4.3 times higher, ALBC alone 6.4 times higher). The authors also report that the use of ALBC resulted in reduced rate of aseptic loosening. The conclusion was that some of these cases represent subclinical infections and that the use of ALBC leads to a reduction in the incidence of these cases.

In a report on the Swedish register of 120,000 arthroplasty cases, Persson et al.[10] documents a deep wound infection rate of 0.44% (72/16,400) with the use of systemic antibiotics and a reduction to 0.23% (18/7,674) when combined with ALBC. All cases were preformed in an ultra-clean environment.

In contrast, Namba et al. analyzed a community-based total joint registry in the United States.[11] The found that ALBC was used in 8.9% of 22,889 primary TKAs. The rate of deep infection was found to be statistically higher with the use of ALBC. In their analysis, diabetes (2,449 cases) and operative time were not found to be factors associated with the development of infection.

Recommendation

• The use of ALBC decreases the rate of deep infection following TKA [overall quality: moderate]

Question 2: Is the routine use of ALBC in primary TKA cost-effective?

Case clarification

The question related to the use of low-dose ALBC as supplemental prophylaxis against infection for the patient in Case 1.

Relevance

TKA is a cost-effective and successful solution to gonoarthrosis.[17] Infection is a devastating event and associated with poorer outcomes.

Current opinion

Opinion is divided on the subject. The unavailabilty of commerically premixed ALBC in North America resulted in surgeons hand-mixing antibiotics into bone cement at the time of surgery. In May 2003 the US Food and Drug Administration (FDA) approved the use of commercially premixed ABLC but only for reimplantation as part of a staged arthroplasty for the treatment of implant-related sepsis. Off-label use in primary arthroplasty is increasing. A survey of 1,015 orthopedic surgeons in the United States revealed that 56% use ABLC for at least some cases. Surgeons specializing in joint reconstruction were more likely to use antibiotic in bone cement (88%),[18] and 13% always used ALBC in primary joint arthroplasty. Historically, the majority of THAs in North America have not involved the use of bone cement, but it is estimated that cemented components are used in 85% of all TKAs performed in the US.[19] Some advocate the use of ALBC only in high-risk patients.[4]

Finding the evidence

• PubMed, using search terms: "cost effectiveness arthroplasty bone cement antibiotic" with limits: "Humans," "All Adults: 19 + years," and "English language"

Quality of the evidence

Level II
• 2 studies[10,20]

Findings

Cummins[20] performed an economic modelling analysis of the cost-effectivness of using antibiotic-impregnated bone

cement in THA. Data from published cohorts, the National Inpatient Survey, and local purchase costs were entered into a computerized decsion tree model to tabulate costs and quality-adjusted life years (QALYs) accumulated per patient. All cost were in US dollars and based on 2002 values. The estimated cost differential per case for ALBC vs. PBC was $600 per primary THA. The cost assigned to a revision due to infection was $96,166. The model was strongly influenced by the average age of the patients and by the cost of bone cement. Older patients undergoing revision due to infection have reduced cost efficiency based on calculated QALYs. The analysis concluded that the use of ALBC is cost-effective until the average age of patients exceeds 71 years.

Proponents of the use of ALBC cite a reduction in the rate of infection as a direct result of their usuage. The higher cost (US$284–$349[21]) is accepted to offset the cost of treating an infected arthroplasty. Jiranek has proprosed that a reduction of the rates of infection from 1.5% to 0.3% would need to be achieved in order to offset the extra cost incurred by the routine use of ALBC.

Effective treatment of deep-seated infection following TKA often entails exchange arthroplasty, usually staged, and with the prolonged administration of systemically adminstered antibiotics. This represents a significant burden for the patient. The cost of treatment in the US has been estimated to exceed $55,000.[22] This fails to account for the hidden costs incurred by the patient and for the morbidity and mortality associated with treatment. Eradication is not always possible and rates of success for revision arthroplasty following infection are typically no greater than 90%.[23] Hence, prevention of infection in the performance of arthroplasty is vital.

Recommendations

• The use of ALBC is cost-effective and its use is fully justified based on potential savings from the reduction of the number of revision procedures performed for infection and the avoidance of the associated morbidity which may be unquantifiable [overall quality: poor]
• There are no proven disadvantages with the routine use of ALBC in primary TKA [overall quality: moderate]

Question 3: What is the role of ALBC in the treatment of established prosthetic knee infection?

Case clarification

Use of high-dose ALBC (at least 3.6g antibiotic per 40g bone cement) is required for the treatment of deep infection following arthroplasty and is typically used as a spacer during staged exchange arthroplasty. With high-dose ABLC the mechanical properties of the acrylic bone cement are altered, rendering it unsuitable for long-term fixation of components.[24]

Relevance

Buchholz and Engelbrech were the first to combine antibiotics with acrylic bone cement as a prophylactic measure in arthroplasty.[25] Antibiotics can be added to acrylic cement in the form of powder, either commercially mixed or mixed by hand at the time of surgery. Elution characteristics for various antibiotics have been documented.[26,27]

Current opinion

The value of high-dose ALBC in established prosthesis-related infection is well established.

Finding the evidence

See Question 1.

Quality of the evidence

Level IV
• 1 case series[28]

Findings

Antibiotics added to acrylic bone cement must be thermally stable to resist the heat of polymerization. Elution characteristics vary between antibiotics and between bone cement types. Gentamicin added to bone cement has been the most extensively studied. It elutes levels above the minimum concentration level for staphylococci and aerobic gram-negative rods for up to 5 days.[29] In North America tobramycin is more commonly employed, due to its availability in powdered form. The elution characteristics of ALBC are enhanced with the addition of more than one antibiotic.[27] The value of ALBC in established prosthesis-related infection is irrefutable.[28,30,31]

Recommendations

• High-dose ALBC is an established regime for the treatment of infection in TKA [overall quality: moderate]
• High-dose ABLC is unsuitable for long-term fixation of components in revision TKA [overall quality: moderate]

Question 4: Does the use of ALBC in primary TKA lead to earlier mechanical failure rates?

Case clarification

See Question 1.

Relevance

Mentioned as a theoretical adverse effect to the use of ALBC in primary TKA.

Current opinion

See Question 1.

Finding the evidence

See Question 1.

Quality of the evidence

• Level II[9,32,33]

Findings

There is good evidence that the addition of low-dose antibiotics to bone cement does not alter its mechanical properties to any clinically relevant extent and is suitable for long-term implant fixation.[34] In-vitro testing has shown that low-dose ALBC shows negligible reduction in fatigue strength.[35] To date, clinical studies and joint registries have not shown an increased mechanical loosening rate with the use of low-dose ALBC.

Recommendation

• No adverse affect on mechanical loosening rates has been documented with the routine use of low-dose ALBC in TKA [overall quality: moderate]

Question 5: Can the routine use of ALBC lead to the development of resistant organisms in TKA?

Case clarification

See Question 1.

Relevance

Reports of infected joint replacements with microbes resistant to gentamicin have raised concern regarding the routine use of low-dose ALBC in TKA.

Current opinion

This is a subject of controversy.

Finding the evidence

• PubMed, using the search term: "microbiology of the infected knee arthroplasty"

Quality of the evidence

Level II
• 1 systemic review of cohort studies[36]

Findings

Recently, antimicrobial resistance among bacteria found after use of ALBC in prosthesis-related infection has been ascribed to the use of ALBC. In a report on 426 surgically revised knee arthroplasties over a 14 year period, gentamicin resistance was found in 1/28 tested isolates of *Staphylococcus aureus* and 19/29 of tested coagulase-negative staphylococci.[36] In an animal model of ALBC vs. PBC, Thornes[37] noted a lower rate of infection with the addition of gentamicin to bone cement. A statisically significant increase in gentamicin-resistant *Staphylococcus epidermidis* was reported. It is unknown whether this represents eradication of gentamicin-sensitive strains of bacteria and the resultant demonstration of resistant strains.

Recommendation
• There is no evidence to support the hypothesis that the emergence of bacterial resistance is related to the use of ALBC as a prophylactic measure [overall quality: low]

Question 6: Is there a risk of developing systemic toxicity or an allergic reaction with the use of ALBC in TKA?

Case clarification
See Question 1.

Relevance
This has been mentioned as a theoretical adverse effect to the use of ALBC.

Current opinion
Low- or high-dose ABLC cement has been proven to be safe through three decades of use.

Finding the evidence
• PubMed, using the search term: "nephrotoxicity antibiotic bone cement"

Quality of the evidence
Level IV
• 3 case reports[38-40]

Findings
No reports of systemic toxcity have been reported from the routine use of low-dose ALBC despite three decades of documented usage decades in Scandanivia and other European countries. Scant reports exist of patient toxicity following use of high-dose ALBC.[38-40] Gentamicin is the the most studied antiobiotic in ALBCs. It is typically associated with a lack of allergic reactions. There have been no reports of allergic reactions associated with its use in ALBC in more than 100,000 arthroplasty cases in the literature thus far.[3]

Recommendation
• Low- or high-dose ABLC cement has been proven to be safe through three decades of documented use [overall quality: very low]

Summary of recommendations

• The use of ALBC decreases the rate of deep infection following TKA
• The use of ALBC is cost-effective and its use is fully justified based on potential savings from the reduction of the number of revision procedures performed for infection and the avoidance of the associated morbidity which may be unquantifiable

• There are no proven disadvantages with the routine use of ALBC in primary TKA
• High-dose ALBC is an established regime for the treatment of infection in TKA
• High-dose ALBC is unsuitable for long-term fixation of components in revision TKA
• No adverse affect on mechanical loosening rates have been documented with the routine use of low-dose ALBC in TKA
• There is no evidence to support the hypothesis that the emergence of bacterial resistance is related to the use of ALBC as a prophylactic measure
• Low- or high-dose ALBC cement has been proven to be safe through three decades of documented use.

Conclusions

Infection following TKA is associated with poor outcomes. The routine use of low-dose ALBC has excellent outcomes documented for over three decades. The incidence of septic loosening is reduced. Current evidence indicates that ALBC should be used routinely in all primary TKAs. The studies reviewed here are summarized in Figure 23.1 and Table 23.1.

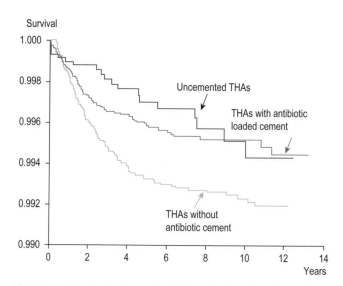

Figure 23.1 Survival analysis in total hip arthroplasty. Cox-adjusted survival curves with infection as endpoint for uncemented total hip arthroplasties (THAs), cemented THAs with antiobiotic-loaded cement, and cemented THAs without antibiotic cement. (Reprinted with permission from Engesaeter LB, Epshaug B, Lie SA, Furnes O, Havelin LI Does cement increase the risk of infection in primary total hip arthroplasty? Revision rates in 56,275 cemented and uncemented primary THAs followed for 0–16 years in the Norwegian Arthroplasty Register. Acta Orthop Scand, 2006; 77, 351–358. © Nordic Orthopaedic Federation.)

Table 23.1 Studies on ALBC in joint arthroplasty

Author	Study type	No. of joints studied	Mean age (range) (years)	Diagnosis	Mean follow-up (range)	Outcome
Chiu et al.[41]	Prospective Randomized Level I	183 Revision TKA	70	Aseptic loosening—69 Severe wear—21	5 years (3–13)	ALBC (vancomycin) vs. PBC ALBC 0/93 (0%) PBC 6/90 (6.7%) infected
Chiu et al.[5]	Prospective Randomized Level I	340 Primary TKA	70	OA—300 RA—16 2° OA—16 Gout—3 AVn—5	49 (26–81) months	ALBC (cefuroxime) Vs PBC ALBC 0/178 (0%) PBC 5/162 (3.1%) infected
Chiu et al.[16]	Prospective Randomized Level I	78 TKA	70	OA—78 DM—78	50 (26–88) months	ALBC (cefuroxime) vs. PBC ALBC 0/41 (0%) PBC 5/37 (13.5%) infected
Josefsson et al.[7]	Prospective Randomized Controlled Level I	1688 THA	69 (25–98)	OA—1434 RA—69 2° OA—128 Others—57	10.3 (8.4–12.6) years	Systemic Ab—different regimes vs. ABLC (gentamicin) only Systemic Ab alone 13/835(1.6%) ALBC alone 9/853 (1.1%) No significant difference
McQueen et al.[6]	Prospective Randomized Controlled Level I	295 269 THA 26 TKA	68 (41–93)	OA—253 RA—17 AVN—11 2° OA—4 Ank. Spond.—1 Malignancy—1 Post sepsis—1 Revision—7	3 months	Systemic Ab alone vs. ABLC alone—No difference
Parvizi et al.[8]	Meta-analysis (6 papers) Level II	21,445 THA				ALBC (gentamicin) vs. PBC ALBC (1.2%) PBC (2.3%) infected
Gandhi et al.[42]	Prospective Comparative Level II	1625 TKA	66.1	OA 2° OA RA	1 year	ALBC vs. PBC ALBC 18/814 infected PBC 25/811 infected Adjusted analysis—not significant
Lynch et al.[43]	Retrospective Comparitive Level III	1542 THA		OA—994 RA—70 Others—478	8.1 years	ALBC (gentamicin) vs. PBC ALBC 9/671 (1.34%) infected PBC 19/871 (2.18%) infected
Namba et al.[11]	Retrospective Comparative Level III	22,889 TKA	68	OA—21,139 Other—1,750		ALBC 28/2030 (1.4%) PBC 154/20,869 (0/7%)

2°OA, secondary osteoarthritis; Ab, antibiotics; ALBC, antibiotic-loaded bone cement; Ank. Spond., ankylosing spondylitis; AVN, avascular necrosis; DM, diabetes mellitus; OA, osteoarthritis; PBC, plain bone cement; RA, rheumatoid arthritis.

References

1. Bongartz T, Halligan CS, Osmon DR, et al. Incidence and risk factors of prosthetic joint infection after total hip or knee replacement in patients with rheumatoid arthritis. Arthritis Rheum 2008;59:1713–20.

2. Dunbar MJ. Antibiotic bone cements: their use in routine primary total joint arthroplasty is justified. Orthopedics 2009;32.

3. Bourne RB. Prophylactic use of antibiotic bone cement: an emerging standard—in the affirmative. J Arthroplasty 2004;19: 69–72.

4. Hanssen AD. Prophylactic use of antibiotic bone cement: an emerging standard—in opposition. J Arthroplasty 2004;19: 73–7.

5. Chiu FY, Chen CM, Lin CF, Lo WH. Cefuroxime-impregnated cement in primary total knee arthroplasty: a prospective, randomized study of three hundred and forty knees. J Bone Joint Surg Am 2002;84:759–62.

6. McQueen M, Littlejohn A, Hughes SP. A comparison of systemic cefuroxime and cefuroxime loaded bone cement in the prevention of early infection after total joint replacement. Int Orthop 1987;11:241–3.

7. Josefsson G, Kolmert L. Prophylaxis with systematic antibiotics versus gentamicin bone cement in total hip arthroplasty. A ten-year survey of 1,688 hips. Clin Orthop Relat Res 1993;210–14.

8. Parvizi J, Saleh KJ, Ragland PS, Pour AE, Mont MA. Efficacy of antibiotic-impregnated cement in total hip replacement. Acta Orthop 2008;79:335–41.

9. Espehaung B ELB, Vollset SE, Havelin LI, Langeland N. Antibiotic prophylaxis in total hip arthroplasty. J Bone Joint Surg Br 1997;79:590–5.

10. Persson U, Persson M, Malchau H. The economics of preventing revisions in total hip replacement. Acta Orthop Scand 1999;70:163–9.

11. Namba RS, Chen Y, Paxton EW, Slipchenko T, Fithian DC. Outcomes of routine use of antibiotic-loaded cement in primary total knee arthroplasty. J Arthroplasty 2009;24:44–7.

12. Jämsen E, Huhtala H, Puolakka T, Moilanen T. Risk factors for infection after knee arthroplasty. A register-based analysis of 43,149 cases. J Bone Joint Surg Am 2009;91:38–47.

13. McQueen MM, Hughes SP, May P, Verity L. Cefuroxime in total joint arthroplasty. Intravenous or in bone cement. J Arthroplasty 1990;5:169–72.

14. Josefsson G, Lindberg L, Wiklander B. Systemic antibiotics and gentamicin-containing bone cement in the prophylaxis of postoperative infections in total hip arthroplasty. Clin Orthop Relat Res 1981;194–200.

15. Josefsson G, Gudmundsson G, Kolmert L, Wijkstrom S. Prophylaxis with systemic antibiotics versus gentamicin bone cement in total hip arthroplasty. A five-year survey of 1688 hips. Clin Orthop Relat Res 1990;173–8.

16. Chiu FY, Lin CF, Chen CM, Lo WH, Chaung TY. Cefuroxime-impregnated cement at primary total knee arthroplasty in diabetes mellitus. A prospective, randomised study. J Bone Joint Surg Br 2001;83:691–5.

17. Lavernia CJ, Guzman JF, Gachupin-Garcia A. Cost effectiveness and quality of life in knee arthroplasty. Clin Orthop Relat Res 1997;134–9.

18. Heck D, Rosenberg A, Schink-Ascani M, Garbus S, Kiewitt T. Use of antibiotic-impregnated cement during hip and knee arthroplasty in the United States. J Arthroplasty 1995;10: 470–5.

19. Wood JEJ. Uncemented fixation in total knee replacement: a promising future. Curr Opin Orthop 2007;18:61–5.

20. Cummins JS, Tomek IM, Kantor SR, Furnes O, Engesaeter LB, Finlayson SR. Cost-effectiveness of antibiotic-impregnated bone cement used in primary total hip arthroplasty. J Bone Joint Surg Am 2009;91:634–41.

21. Jiranek WA, Hanssen AD, Greenwald AS. Antibiotic-loaded bone cement for infection prophylaxis in total joint replacement. J Bone Joint Surg Am 2006;88:2487.

22. Sculco TP. The economic impact of infected total joint arthroplasty. Instr Course Lect 1993;42:349–51.

23. Haleem AA, Berry DJ, Hanssen AD. Mid-term to long-term followup of two-stage reimplantation for infected total knee arthroplasty. Clin Orthop Relat Res 2004;35–9.

24. Pelletier MH, Malisano L, Smitham PJ, Okamoto K, Walsh WR. The compressive properties of bone cements containing large doses of antibiotics. J Arthroplasty 2009;24:454–60.

25. Buchholz HW, Engelbrecht H. [Depot effects of various antibiotics mixed with Palacos resins]. Chirurg 1970;41:511–15.

26. Anagnostakos K, Wilmes P, Schmitt E, Kelm J. Elution of gentamicin and vancomycin from polymethylmethacrylate beads and hip spacers in vivo. Acta Orthop 2009;80:193–7.

27. Penner MJ, Masri BA, Duncan CP. Elution characteristics of vancomycin and tobramycin combined in acrylic bone-cement. J Arthroplasty 1996;11:939–44.

28. Hanssen AD, Rand JA, Osmon DR. Treatment of the infected total knee arthroplasty with insertion of another prosthesis. The effect of antibiotic-impregnated bone cement. Clin Orthop Relat Res 1994;44–55.

29. Sorensen TS, Andersen MR, Glenthoj J, Petersen O. Pharmacokinetics of topical gentamicin in total hip arthroplasty. Acta Orthop Scand 1984;55:156–9.

30. Hanssen AD, Osmon DR. The use of prophylactic antimicrobial agents during and after hip arthroplasty. Clin Orthop Relat Res 1999;124–38.

31. Haddad FS, Masri BA, Campbell D, McGraw RW, Beauchamp CP, Duncan CP. The PROSTALAC functional spacer in two-stage revision for infected knee replacements. Prosthesis of antibiotic-loaded acrylic cement. J Bone Joint Surg Br 2000;82:807–12.

32. Malchau H, Herberts P, Ahnfelt L. Prognosis of total hip replacement in Sweden. Follow-up of 92,675 operations performed 1978–1990. Acta Orthop Scand 1993;64:497–506.

33. Engesaeter LB, Lie SA, Espehaug B, Furnes O, Vollset SE, Havelin LI. Antibiotic prophylaxis in total hip arthroplasty: effects of antibiotic prophylaxis systemically and in bone cement on the revision rate of 22,170 primary hip replacements followed 0–14 years in the Norwegian Arthroplasty Register. Acta Orthop Scand 2003;74:644–51.

34. He Y, Trotignon JP, Loty B, Tcharkhtchi A, Verdu J. Effect of antibiotics on the properties of poly(methylmethacrylate)-based bone cement. J Biomed Mater Res 2002;63:800–6.

35. Lewis G, Bhattaram A. Influence of a pre-blended antibiotic (gentamicin sulfate powder) on various mechanical, thermal, and physical properties of three acrylic bone cements. J Biomater Appl 2006;20:377–408.

36. Stefansdottir A, Johansson D, Knutson K, Lidgren L, Robertsson O. Microbiology of the infected knee arthroplasty: report from the Swedish Knee Arthroplasty Register on 426 surgically revised cases. Scand J Infect Dis 2009;41:831–40.

37. Thornes B, Murray P, Bouchier-Hayes D. Development of resistant strains of *Staphylococcus epidermidis* on gentamicin-loaded bone cement in vivo. J Bone Joint Surg Br 2002;84:758–60.

38. Curtis JM, Sternhagen V, Batts D. Acute renal failure after placement of tobramycin-impregnated bone cement in an infected total knee arthroplasty. Pharmacotherapy 2005;25:876–80.

39. Patrick BN, Rivey MP, Allington DR. Acute renal failure associated with vancomycin- and tobramycin-laden cement in total hip arthroplasty. Ann Pharmacother 2006;40:2037–42.

40. Dovas S, Liakopoulos V, Papatheodorou L, et al. Acute renal failure after antibiotic-impregnated bone cement treatment of an infected total knee arthroplasty. Clin Nephrol 2008;69:207–12.

41. Chiu FY, Lin CF. Antibiotic-impregnated cement in revision total knee arthroplasty. A prospective cohort study of one hundred and eighty-three knees. J Bone Joint Surg Am 2009;91:628–33.

42. Gandhi R, Razak F, Pathy R, Davey JR, Syed K, Mahomed NN. Antibiotic bone cement and the incidence of deep infection after total knee arthroplasty. J Arthroplasty 2009;24:1015–18.

43. Lynch M, Esser MP, Shelley P, Wroblewski BM. Deep infection in Charnley low-friction arthroplasty. Comparison of plain and gentamicin-loaded cement. J Bone Joint Surg Br 1987;69:355–60.

44. Engesaeter LB, Espehaug B, Lie SA, Furnes O, Havelin LI. Does cement increase the risk of infection in primary total hip arthroplasty? Revision rates in 56,275 cemented and uncemented primary THAs followed for 0–16 years in the Norwegian Arthroplasty Register. Acta Orthop Scand 2006;77:351–8.

24 Cemented vs. Uncemented Fixation in Total Knee Arthroplasty

Eric R. Bohm[1], Ili Slobodian[1], Thomas R. Turgeon[1], and Martin Petrak[2]

[1]University of Manitoba and Concordia Joint Replacement Group, Winnipeg, MB, Canada
[2]Concordia Hip and Knee Institute, Winnipeg, MB, Canada

Case scenario

A 58 year old nurse tells you that she has exhausted non-operative management of her bilateral knee osteoarthritis. She is tired of the resulting pain and disability, and wants to proceed with total knee arthroplasty (TKA). Physical examination reveals a body mass index (BMI) of 34, an antalgic gait, painful passive range of motion of both knees, correctable varus deformity, and a normal neurovascular examination. Radiographs confirm medial and patellofemoral osteoarthritis. She tells you that she wants the "best" type of knee replacement.

Relevant background

The three components that make up a total knee replacement (Figure 24.1) can be secured to bone using either cemented or cementless fixation. Cemented fixation relies on the polymer polymethylmethacrylate (PMMA) to secure the implants. Cementless fixation relies on either a porous metal surface or a contoured surface coated with hydroxyapatite (HA) to promote bone ingrowth and subsequent stability (Figure 24.2).[1] The articulation (and wear) occurs between the metal femoral component and the polyethylene of the tibial component. Tibial components can either be manufactured entirely from polyethylene, or from metal on to which a polyethylene insert is secured. Although cementless patellas have fallen out of favor due to high failure rates[2] (a result of thin polyethylene necessitated by the metal backing), there still remains some interest within the orthopedic world about the role of cementless fixation, particularly of the tibial component. This is because the most common noninfectious failure mechanism of TKA is loosening of the tibial component secondary to tibial bone osteolysis (resorption) caused by polyethylene debris

arising from wear of the bearing surface.[3] It is postulated that cementless fixation may ultimately result in improved TKA longevity by preventing polyethylene debris from gaining access to the bone–implant interface.

Importance of the problem

TKA is on the rise worldwide. Canadian volumes increased by 141% between 1996 and 2006,[3] volumes in the UK increased by 43% between 2003 and 2008 (Professor Paul Gregg, personal communication) and in the United States volumes are predicted to increase by 674% between 2005 and 2030.[4] TKA has a finite survivorship, with approximately 5% of implants being revised by 10 years.[5] The increasing volumes of primary TKAs will ultimately lead to increasing numbers of revision TKAs, the clinical results of which are inferior to[6] and the costs approximately 140% higher[7] than the primary surgery.

The assumption of improved outcome with cementless implants was predicated on the survival being at least equal to that of traditional cemented designs. Some early cementless designs did not meet the goals for long-term survival, with early loosening occurring more commonly with the tibial component.[2,8–9] The large majority of TKAs performed today use cemented fixation,[10–13] but cementless technology continues to evolve and develop in an attempt to achieve the original goals of improved survival and outcomes in younger, active patients.

Top five questions

1. Are there differences in survivorship between cemented and noncemented TKA?
2. Is there a difference in functional outcome between the two fixation types?

3. Are there differences in complication rates between the two fixation methods?

4. Are there differences in ease of revision or quality of outcome of revision following cemented and cementless TKA?

5. Are there differences in costs between cemented and cementless TKA?

Question 1: Are there differences in survivorship between cemented and noncemented TKAs?

Case clarification

Patients often ask how long they can expect their knee replacement to last.

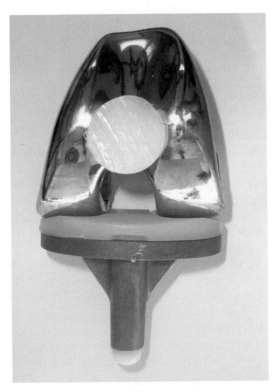

Figure 24.1 Modular total knee replacement system.

Relevance

Young patients appear to be at higher risk of revision due to loosening;[5] it is therefore worthwhile to explore other fixation options that may improve longevity.

Current opinion

Worldwide registry data demonstrates that the majority of TKAs are inserted using cement.[5,14–17]

Finding the evidence

• Cochrane Database: search terms "cemented knee," "uncemented knee," and "cementless knee"

• PubMed: search terms "cemented knee," "uncemented knee," "cementless knee," "cemented fixation," "total knee arthroplasty." Limited to humans, clinical trials, meta-analysis, practice guidelines, randomized controlled trial, review, comparative study, controlled clinical trial, English

• Google: joint replacement registries

Quality of the evidence

Level I

• 1 randomized controlled trial (RCT) specifically powered to detect clinically significant functional differences based on tibial component fixation method[18]

Level II

• 1 meta-analysis with methodological flaws (inconsistent application of trial inclusion criteria, inclusion of two RCTs reporting on the same set of patients)[19]

• 2 RCTs comparing cementless to cemented TKA (randomization method flaws)[20,21]

• 10 RCTs comparing hybrid fixation (typically a cemented femur combined with a cementless tibia) to either entirely cemented or cementless fixation (either no a-priori sample size calculation, powered to detect radiographic changes only, insufficient power to detect clinically significant differences, or unclear description of fixation method)[22–31]

• 13 cohort studies with control groups (usually matched control groups)[2,32–43]

• 4 national joint replacement registries contain information on TKA survival based on fixation method[5,14–16]

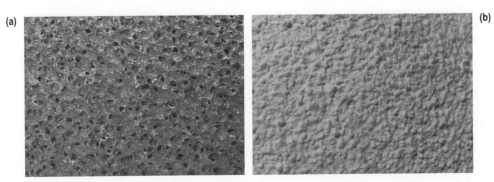

Figure 24.2 (a) Porous metal surface. (b) Hydroxyapatite coating.

Findings

A recent meta-analysis compared survival and clinical outcomes of cemented and cementless TKAs.[19] It included 5 RCTs and 10 cohort studies with control groups. Limitations in the analysis include the overall quality of studies, inconsistent application of their criteria for determining if a study should be included in the analysis, and inclusion of 2 RCTs that reported two different follow-up periods on the same cohort of patients. Nonetheless, they concluded that the combined odds ratio for failure of cementless TKA was 4.2 (95% CI 2.7–6.5) compared to cemented TKA.

Thirteen RCTs were found; however none were either adequately powered or had sufficient follow-up to detect clinically significant differences in survival. Three RCTs reported on the same cohort of patients;[20,44,45] two of these were therefore excluded from the current analysis.[44,45]

Several studies employing radiostereometric analysis (RSA) to examine differences in implant–bone micromotion between the fixation methods were found.[22–25,27–31,40,46–49] RSA is a highly accurate, noninvasive radiographic method that can predict long-term survivorship of an implant based upon micromotion occurring between the implant and surrounding bone.[46,47,50,51] It requires small numbers of subjects and a relatively short postoperative follow-up period (typically 2 years).[46,47,50,51] It appears that the femoral fixation method has little impact on component migration. However, cementless tibial components tend to migrate for the first 3–12 months before final bone ingrowth and subsequent stability occurs.[23,40,46] The addition of HA to the cementless tibial component appears to improve stability through improved bone ingrowth.[22,25,31] Cemented tibial components tend to have increasing migration with time,[28,48] but the impact of this late migration on long-term survivorship is poorly understood.

Thirteen cohort studies that had a control group were identified. Five of these studies[2,13,34,35,38] with a total of 1958 TKAs found that cemented TKAs had higher survivorship than cementless TKAs primarily due to a lower aseptic loosening rate. Basset reported on his personal series of 584 cementless TKAs and 416 cemented TKAs and found no difference in survivorship at 5 years. The decision to use cement was subjectively based upon the amount of porosity of the cut tibial surface, with the more porous tibias receiving cemented fixation.[33] Seven studies had insufficient power to detect clinically significant differences.[36,37,39–43]

Four national joint registries examine TKA survivorship in relation to fixation method: those of England and Wales,[14] New Zealand,[15] Australia,[16] and Sweden.[5] All four report that cemented fixation is most common, followed by hybrid and then cementless. The Swedish registry has the longest follow-up data (18 years), and has found a 1.5 (1.2–2.8) times higher revision rate for cementless TKAs secondary to tibial component failure; subsequently they have essen-

tially abandoned the use of cementless TKA. The Australians have data on 3713 TKAs equally divided into cementless and cemented fixation out to 7 years; they are unable to detect any differences in survival based on fixation method. The National Joint Registry of England and Wales have followed more than 111,000 TKAs out to 3 years (13% cementless). Although they found a trend towards higher revision rates in the cementless and hybrid groups, it did not reach statistical significance. New Zealand surgeons have found that uncemented TKAs have twice the revision rate of either cemented or hybrid TKA. It appears that the majority of their hybrid TKAs employ a cementless femur and a cemented tibia, a configuration that one would expect to have good survivorship, as it appears that the uncemented tibial component is usually the reason for revision in cementless TKAs.[5]

Recommendation

- Cemented fixation demonstrates improved survivorship over cementless procedures in TKA [overall quality: high]

Question 2: Is there a difference in functional outcome between the two fixation types?

Case clarification

While the patient is concerned about the longevity of her impending knee replacement, she is also concerned about any functional differences that may exist between the two fixation methods.

Relevance

Patient satisfaction following knee replacement is tied closely to relief of pain and restoration of function.[6] Any differences in functional outcome according to fixation method would therefore be of interest.

Current opinion

The vast majority of total knees are inserted using cemented fixation,[3,5,13,15–17] implying that surgeons may feel that no significant functional benefit is realized from cementless fixation.

Finding the evidence

The same search method employed to answer Question 1 above was used. Due to a general lack of functional data, joint replacement registries were excluded.

Quality of the evidence

See Question 1 above.

Findings

As noted above, a recent meta-analysis[19] with some design limitations was found. Analyzing pooled data from both RCTs and cohort studies, they could not detect any differences in joint function as measured by the Knee Society score.[52]

A review of the 13 RCTs found in our search revealed one well-designed study[18] powered to detect clinically significant differences in WOMAC knee function scores[53] between 81 patients randomized to receive either cementless or cemented tibial component fixation. They found that those patients receiving cementless fixation reported higher pain at the 6 month assessment as measured by both the SF-36 and WOMAC; however, this difference disappeared by 5 years postoperatively. They postulated that the higher pain scores were a result of early migration of the tibial component before ingrowth occurred. This clinical finding of slower pain resolution in cementless components has previously been reported in an RCT whose authors also noted that, when assessed using RSA, cementless tibial components demonstrate higher early micromotion before ingrowth and stabilization occurs.[27] The remaining 11 RCTs either did not report on functional outcomes (as they focused mainly on radiographic differences), or had an inadequate sample size to detect clinical differences, or did not do appropriate statistical testing

Thirteen cohort studies that had a control group were identified. Barrack's study of 158 knees found that cementless TKAs had poorer postoperative Knee Society scores; this was likely due to loose and painful tibial components that led to a higher rate of revision in this group.[32] Two adequately powered studies incorporating a total of 1118 knees found no differences in functional scores; both reported low rates of revision for either cementless femoral or tibial components.[13,33] However, patients in both cementless groups were younger, and in Rand's study the cementless group started with higher preoperative scores, both of which should bias scores towards the cementless groups. The remaining studies had inadequate statistical power,[36,37] did not report on functional outcomes,[34,35,38–41] or did not do appropriate statistical testing.[42,43] It would appear that functional scores are equivalent as long as bony fixation is obtained with cementless implants; if not, both revision rates and functional scores are worse.

Recommendation
• Cementless TKAs appear to provide equivalent midterm (5 year) functional outcomes compared to cemented TKAs as long as loosening does not occur [overall quality: high]

Question 3: Are there differences in complication rates between the two fixation methods?

Case clarification
After you review the risks generally associated with elective knee replacement surgery, the patient asks if complication rates are different between the two fixation methods.

Relevance
Since TKA is an elective surgical procedure, one always aims to minimize the possibility of complications.

Current opinion
The surgical technique for cemented and cementless TKA is essentially identical. Both involve bone cuts to tibia and femur, soft tissue releases as required, and then insertion of components In the case of cemented fixation, cement is applied to the bone surfaces immediately before component insertion. It is the authors' experience that most intraoperative complications (ligament rupture or bone fracture) occur before insertion of the final implants, and arise as a result of difficulties encountered undertaking the bone cuts or ligament balancing. Accordingly, we have not found any differences in intraoperative complications.

The use of cement during TKA offers two theoretical advantages: antibiotics can be added in an effort to reduce infection rates, and the application of cement to the cut bone surfaces may reduce postoperative blood loss.

Finding the evidence
The RCTs and controlled series identified for Question 1 were reviewed.

Quality of the evidence
See Question 1 above.

Findings
Intraoperative complications during TKA are quite infrequent;[54] accordingly, none of the RCTs or series identified were adequately powered to detect differences in these areas. One RCT reported more blood loss in the cementless group (783 mL vs. 519 mL, p = 0.02) but did not indicate how this was measured or if it had any effect on transfusion rates. The Australian Joint Registry is the only registry to report on the impact of cement type (with or without antibiotics) on revision rates; they noted a trend towards a lower revision rate for infection in cemented knees when antibiotics were present in the cement. However, they did not make a comparison in rates of revision for infection between cemented knees (containing cement) and cementless knees.

Recommendation
• The use of cement for TKA fixation may result in lower blood loss [overall quality: very low]

Question 4: Are there differences in ease of revision or quality of outcome of revision following cemented and cementless TKA?

Case clarification

Given the relatively young age of the patient, you consider her need for future revision TKA and consider whether cemented or uncemented implants will serve the patient in preservation of bone and other tissue for possible future revision.

Relevance

Uncemented implants tend to be used in younger patients, based on the premise that the bone adjacent to the implant may be better preserved for future surgeries.

Current opinion

The majority of TKAs performed in both young and old patients continue to be cemented.

Finding the evidence

Search terms used were:
- Uncemented knee revision
- Cementless knee revision
- (Cemented OR cementless) AND knee AND bone AND (density OR densitometry)
- Trabecular metal AND knee AND bone (density OR densitometry)

Quality of evidence

Level II
- 2 randomized trials with methodologic limitations

Level III
- 3 retrospective cohort studies

Findings

There are five published comparative studies assessing the bone mineral density adjacent to total knee implants between cemented and cementless designs. Three of the studies compared cemented to cementless versions of the same implant system, while the other two studies used cemented and cementless designs from different arthroplasty systems.[55–59] Measurement technique of bone density varied between the studies as well, with some studies using radiograph measurements and others using triple or dual energy X-ray absorption (DEXA). Additionally, the areas of bone assessed relative to the implants varied. Bone density findings were inconsistent between the studies. One study found a 50% reduction in bone density posterior to the anterior femoral flange with cemented implants vs. cementless.[59] A second study found a trend toward this finding that did not achieve statistical significance with a slightly smaller difference between the two fixation types.[56]

The remaining studies found no change in femoral bone density. Of the three studies that assessed bone density of the tibia, one found reduced bone density,[58] one a trend to reduced density,[56] and the third increased density[55] of one zone of the tibia adjacent to the implant with cementless implants. The location of the altered bone density differed, as did the design of the implants. There were no comparative assessments of the results of revision of the two fixation techniques.

Recommendations

- Some possible improvement in bone density under the anterior flange of the femoral component with the use of cementless implants vs. cemented [overall quality: very low]
- No reported evidence of improved ease of revision or beneficial effect from cementless implants beyond measurement of bone density [overall quality: very low]

Question 5: Are there differences in costs between cemented and cementless TKA?

Case clarification

Your hospital resists the use of cementless knee components and suggests that patients should be responsible for any additional implant costs.

Relevance

Cementless TKA components generally carry a 30–100% premium cost compared to cemented implants. However, there is a reduction in costs from cement, cement gun, and mixing equipment disposables. There is also the potential for reduced operating room time by avoiding the cementing steps and no longer having to wait for cement to cure.

Current opinion

Cementless TKA is viewed as a more costly option for the healthcare payer.

Finding the evidence

Search terms used were:
- PubMed: (uncemented OR cementless) AND knee and (cost OR financial) 2000–2009
  - No results
- Econlit: Knee AND replacement, Knee AND arthroplasty
  - No results
- Health Reference Centre: Knee replacement cost, Knee arthroplasty cost
  - No results
- Business Source Premier: Knee replacement cost, Knee arthroplasty cost
  - No results

Quality of the evidence
- Level V: 2

Findings

Due to the complex nature of implant pricing, little information has been published allowing for comparison of cemented vs. cementless TKA. Cementless implants are 30–100% more expensive than cemented implants of the same design.[60] The addition of cement and related disposables adds $500–1000 per case depending on contract pricing, number of units of cement used, use of premixed antibiotics in the cement, and the types of mixing disposables selected. At best, cementless TKA will break even with cemented TKA, but in most contract scenarios the cementless implants will cost more for the healthcare payer

Recommendation
- While the cost of implants must be considered in all arthroplasty cases, ultimate selection of implants should be determined by the clinical effectiveness [overall quality: very low]

Summary of recommendations

- Cemented fixation demonstrates improved survivorship over cementless procedures in total knee arthroplasty
- Cementless TKAs appear to provide equivalent mid-term (5 year) functional outcomes compared to cemented TKAs as long as loosening does not occur
- The use of cement for TKA fixation may result in lower blood loss
- Some possible improvement in bone density under the anterior flange of the femoral component may occur with the use of cementless implants
- No reported evidence of improved ease of revision or beneficial effect from cementless implants beyond measurement of bone density
- While the cost of implants must be considered in all arthroplasty cases, ultimate selection of implants should be determined by the clinical effectiveness

Conclusions

Cemented TKA appears to more reliably provide early fixation and relief of pain compared to cementless TKA; however, mid-term (5 year) functional outcomes appear equivalent if loosening does not occur. Differences in cost, complications, and ease of revision are not well studied in the available literature. Interest in cementless fixation, particularly with the use of HA coating to improve ingrowth, will likely remain high as efforts continue to improve long-term (>15 year) survivalship of implants. High-quality long-term data is required in order to make this determination.

References

1. Freeman MA, Tennant R. The scientific basis of cement versus cementless fixation. Clin Orthop Relat Res 1992(276):19–25.
2. Duffy GP, Berry DJ, Rand JA. Cement versus cementless fixation in total knee arthroplasty. Clin Orthop Relat Res 1998;356:66–72.
3. Canadian Institute for Health Information. Hip and Knee Replacements in Canada—Canadian Joint Replacement Registry (CJRR), 2008–2009 Annual Report. CIHI, Ottawa, 2009.
4. Kurtz S, Ong K, Lau E, Mowat F, Halpern M. Projections of primary and revision hip and knee arthroplasty in the United States from 2005 to 2030. J Bone Joint Surg Am 2007;89(4):780–5.
5. The Swedish Knee Arthroplasty Register, Annual Report 2008. Dept. of Orthopedics, Lund University Hospital, Lund, 2009.
6. Robertsson O, Dunbar MJ. Patient satisfaction compared with general health and disease-specific questionnaires in knee arthroplasty patients. J Arthroplasty 2001;16(4):476–82.
7. Bozic KJ, Durbhakula S, Berry DJ, Naessens JM, Rappaport K, Cisternas M, et al. Differences in patient and procedure characteristics and hospital resource use in primary and revision total joint arthroplasty: a multicenter study. J Arthroplasty 2005;20(7 Suppl 3):17–25.
8. Berger RA, Lyon JH, Jacobs JJ, Barden RM, Berkson EM, Sheinkop MB, et al. Problems with cementless total knee arthroplasty at 11 years followup. Clin Orthop Relat Res 2001;392:196–207.
9. Regner L, Carlsson L, Karrholm J, Herberts P. Clinical and radiologic survivorship of cementless tibial components fixed with finned polyethylene pegs. J Arthroplasty 1997;12(7):751–8.
10. Furnes O, Espehaug B, Lie SA, Vollset SE, Engesaeter LB, Havelin LI. Early failures among 7,174 primary total knee replacements: a follow-up study from the Norwegian Arthroplasty Register 1994–2000. Acta Orthop Scand 2002;73(2):117–29.
11. Jamsen E, Huhtala H, Puolakka T, Moilanen T. Risk factors for infection after knee arthroplasty. A register-based analysis of 43,149 cases. J Bone Joint Surg Am 2009;91(1):38–47.
12. Malik MH, Chougle A, Pradhan N, Gambhir AK, Porter ML. Primary total knee replacement: a comparison of a nationally agreed guide to best practice and current surgical technique as determined by the North West Regional Arthroplasty Register. Ann R Coll Surg Engl 2005;87(2):117–22.
13. Rand JA, Trousdale RT, Ilstrup DM, Harmsen WS. Factors affecting the durability of primary total knee prostheses. J Bone Joint Surg Am 2003;85(2):259–65.
14. National Joint Registry for England and Wales, 5th Annual Report, 2009.
15. The New Zealand Joint Registry Nine Year Report, January 1999 to December 2007. Christchurch, 2008.
16. Australian Orthopedic Association National Joint Replacement Registry Annual Report. AOA, Adelaide, 2008.
17. The Norwegian Arthroplasty Register Report 2008. Haukeland University Hospital, 2008.

18. Beaupre LA, al-Yamani M, Huckell JR, Johnston DW. Hydroxyapatite-coated tibial implants compared with cemented tibial fixation in primary total knee arthroplasty. A randomized trial of outcomes at five years. J Bone Joint Surg Am 2007;89(10): 2204–11.

19. Gandhi R, Tsvetkov D, Davey JR, Mahomed NN. Survival and clinical function of cemented and uncemented prostheses in total knee replacement: a meta-analysis. J Bone Joint Surg Br 2009;91(7):889–95.

20. Baker PN, Khaw FM, Kirk LM, Esler CN, Gregg PJ. A randomised controlled trial of cemented versus cementless press-fit condylar total knee replacement: 15-year survival analysis. J Bone Joint Surg Br 2007;89(12):1608–14.

21. Nilsson KG, Bjornebrink J, Hietala SO, Karrholm J. Scintimetry after total knee arthroplasty. Prospective 2-year study of 18 cases of arthrosis and 15 cases of rheumatoid arthritis. Acta Orthop Scand 1992;63(2):159–65.

22. Carlsson A, Bjorkman A, Besjakov J, Onsten I. Cemented tibial component fixation performs better than cementless fixation: a randomized radiostereometric study comparing porous-coated, hydroxyapatite-coated and cemented tibial components over 5 years. Acta Orthop 2005;76(3):362–9.

23. Dunbar MJ, Wilson DA, Hennigar AW, Amirault JD, Gross M, Reardon GP. Fixation of a trabecular metal knee arthroplasty component. A prospective randomized study. J Bone Joint Surg Am 2009;91(7):1578–86.

24. Gao F, Henricson A, Nilsson KG. Cemented versus uncemented fixation of the femoral component of the NexGen CR total knee replacement in patients younger than 60 years: a prospective randomised controlled RSA study. Knee 2009;16(3): 200–6.

25. Nelissen RG, Valstar ER, Rozing PM. The effect of hydroxyapatite on the micromotion of total knee prostheses. A prospective, randomized, double-blind study. J Bone Joint Surg Am 1998; 80(11):1665–72.

26. Nilsson KG, Henricson A, Norgren B, Dalen T. Uncemented HA-coated implant is the optimum fixation for TKA in the young patient. Clin Orthop Relat Res 2006;448:129–39.

27. Nilsson KG, Karrholm J. Increased varus-valgus tilting of screw-fixated knee prostheses. Stereoradiographic study of uncemented versus cemented tibial components. J Arthroplasty 1993; 8(5):529–40.

28. Nilsson KG, Karrholm J, Carlsson L, Dalen T. Hydroxyapatite coating versus cemented fixation of the tibial component in total knee arthroplasty: prospective randomized comparison of hydroxyapatite-coated and cemented tibial components with 5-year follow-up using radiostereometry. J Arthroplasty 1999; 14(1):9–20.

29. Nilsson KG, Karrholm J, Ekelund L, Magnusson P. Evaluation of micromotion in cemented vs uncemented knee arthroplasty in osteoarthrosis and rheumatoid arthritis. Randomized study using roentgen stereophotogrammetric analysis. J Arthroplasty 1991;6(3):265–78.

30. Nilsson KG, Karrholm J, Linder L. Femoral component migration in total knee arthroplasty: randomized study comparing cemented and uncemented fixation of the Miller-Galante I design. J Orthop Res 1995;13(3):347–56.

31. Onsten I, Nordqvist A, Carlsson AS, Besjakov J, Shott S. Hydroxyapatite augmentation of the porous coating improves fixation of tibial components. A randomised RSA study in 116 patients. J Bone Joint Surg Br 1998;80(3):417–25.

32. Barrack RL, Nakamura SJ, Hopkins SG, Rosenzweig S. Winner of the 2003 James A. Rand Young Investigator's Award. Early failure of cementless mobile-bearing total knee arthroplasty. J Arthroplasty 2004;19(7 Suppl 2):101–6.

33. Bassett RW. Results of 1,000 Performance knees: cementless versus cemented fixation. J Arthroplasty 1998;13(4):409–13.

34. Chockalingam S, Scott G. The outcome of cemented vs. cementless fixation of a femoral component in total knee replacement (TKA) with the identification of radiological signs for the prediction of failure. Knee 2000;7(4):233–38.

35. Cloke DJ, Khatri M, Pinder IM, McCaskie AW, Lingard EA. 284 press-fit Kinemax total knee arthroplasties followed for 10 years: poor survival of uncemented prostheses. Acta Orthop 2008;79(1): 28–33.

36. Collins DN, Heim SA, Nelson CL, Smith P, 3rd. Porous-coated anatomic total knee arthroplasty. A prospective analysis comparing cemented and cementless fixation. Clin Orthop Relat Res 1991;267:128–36.

37. Dodd CA, Hungerford DS, Krackow KA. Total knee arthroplasty fixation. Comparison of the early results of paired cemented versus uncemented porous coated anatomic knee prostheses. Clin Orthop Relat Res 1990;260:66–70.

38. Gioe TJ, Novak C, Sinner P, Ma W, Mehle S. Knee arthroplasty in the young patient: survival in a community registry. Clin Orthop Relat Res 2007;464:83–7.

39. Grewal R, Rimmer MG, Freeman MA. Early migration of prostheses related to long-term survivorship. Comparison of tibial components in knee replacement. J Bone Joint Surg Br 1992;74(2):239–42.

40. Henricson A, Linder L, Nilsson KG. A trabecular metal tibial component in total knee replacement in patients younger than 60 years: a two-year radiostereophotogrammetric analysis. J Bone Joint Surg Br 2008;90(12):1585–93.

41. Pecina M, Djapic T, Haspl M. Survival of cementless and cemented porous-coated anatomic knee replacements: retrospective cohort study. Croat Med J 2000;41(2):168–72.

42. Rorabeck CH, Bourne RB, Nott L. The cemented kinematic-II and the non-cemented porous-coated anatomic prostheses for total knee replacement. A prospective evaluation. J Bone Joint Surg Am 1988;70(4):483–90.

43. Rosenberg AG, Barden RM, Galante JO. Cemented and ingrowth fixation of the Miller-Galante prosthesis. Clinical and roentgenographic comparison after three- to six-year follow-up studies. Clin Orthop Relat Res 1990;260:71–9.

44. Khaw FM, Kirk LM, Morris RW, Gregg PJ. A randomised, controlled trial of cemented versus cementless press-fit condylar total knee replacement. Ten-year survival analysis. J Bone Joint Surg Br 2002;84(5):658–66.

45. McCaskie AW, Deehan DJ, Green TP, Lock KR, Thompson JR, Harper WM, et al. Randomised, prospective study comparing cemented and cementless total knee replacement: results of press-fit condylar total knee replacement at five years. J Bone Joint Surg Br 1998;80(6):971–5.

46. Nilsson KG, Karrholm J. RSA in the assessment of aseptic loosening. J Bone Joint Surg Br 1996;78(1):1–3.

47. Ryd L. Roentgen stereophotogrammetric analysis of prosthetic fixation in the hip and knee joint. Clin Orthop Relat Res 1992;276: 56–65.

48. Ryd L, Albrektsson BE, Carlsson L, Dansgard F, Herberts P, Lindstrand A, et al. Roentgen stereophotogrammetric analysis as a predictor of mechanical loosening of knee prostheses. J Bone Joint Surg Br 1995;77(3):377–83.

49. Uvehammer J, Karrholm J, Carlsson L. Cemented versus hydroxyapatite fixation of the femoral component of the Freeman-Samuelson total knee replacement: a radiostereometric analysis. J Bone Joint Surg Br 2007;89(1):39–44.

50. Valstar ER, Gill R, Ryd L, Flivik G, Borlin N, Karrholm J. Guidelines for standardization of radiostereometry (RSA) of implants. Acta Orthop 2005;76(4):563–72.

51. Derbyshire B, Prescott RJ, Porter ML. Notes on the use and interpretation of radiostereometric analysis. Acta Orthop 2009;80(1):124–30.

52. Insall JN, Dorr LD, Scott RD, Scott WN. Rationale of the Knee Society clinical rating system. Clin Orthop Relat Res 1989;248: 13–14.

53. Ehrich EW, Davies GM, Watson DJ, Bolognese JA, Seidenberg BC, Bellamy N. Minimal perceptible clinical improvement with the Western Ontario and McMaster Universities osteoarthritis index questionnaire and global assessments in patients with osteoarthritis. J Rheumatol 2000;27(11):2635–41.

54. Pinaroli A, Piedade SR, Servien E, Neyret P. Intraoperative fractures and ligament tears during total knee arthroplasty. A 1795 posterostabilized TKA continuous series. Orthop Traumatol Surg Res 2009;95(3):183–9.

55. Abu-Rajab RB, Watson WS, Walker B, Roberts J, Gallacher SJ, Meek RM. Peri-prosthetic bone mineral density after total knee arthroplasty. Cemented versus cementless fixation. J Bone Joint Surg Br 2006;88(5):606–13.

56. Kamath S, Chang W, Shaari E, Bridges A, Campbell A, McGill P. Comparison of peri-prosthetic bone density in cemented and uncemented total knee arthroplasty. Acta Orthop Belg 2008;74(3): 354–9.

57. Petersen MM, Lauritzen JB, Pedersen JG, Lund B. Decreased bone density of the distal femur after uncemented knee arthroplasty. A 1-year follow-up of 29 knees. Acta Orthop Scand 1996;67(4):339–44.

58. Regner LR, Carlsson LV, Karrholm JN, Hansson TH, Herberts PG, Swanpalmer J. Bone mineral and migratory patterns in uncemented total knee arthroplasties: a randomized 5-year follow-up study of 38 knees. Acta Orthop Scand 1999;70(6): 603–8.

59. Seki T, Omori G, Koga Y, Suzuki Y, Ishii Y, Takahashi HE. Is bone density in the distal femur affected by use of cement and by femoral component design in total knee arthroplasty? J Orthop Sci 1999;4(3):180–6.

60. Lasarkis J. The impact of consumables: orthopedic joint replacement. MD Buyline 2008;1(2):1–5.

25 High-Flexion Implants vs. Conventional Design Implants

Nicholas Paterson[1], Robert J. Orec[2], and Douglas D.R. Naudie[1]

[1]University of Western Ontario, London, ON, Canada
[2]Middlemore Hospital, Otahuhu, Manukau, New Zealand

Case scenarios

Case 1

A 65 year old man is referred to an orthopedic surgeon with a diagnosis of primary knee osteoarthritis. He complains of global knee pain that is insufficiently relieved by rest, anti-inflammatory medication, bracing, or injections. He has a good range of motion (ROM) and no flexion contracture. Radiographic findings indicate bicompartmental joint space narrowing and presence of osteophytes. He wishes to return to his previous recreational activities, including golf and yoga.

Case 2

A 55 year old Muslim woman presents with endstage degenerative joint disease of her knee. She has marked varus angular deformity with limited knee flexion to 100°. Radiographic evaluation demonstrates severe varus osteoarthritis. The patient has exhausted conservative treatment, experiences night pain, and wishes to pursue surgical relief. She explains how it is very important for her to position herself properly for prayer. She has read about high-flexion total knee replacement prostheses and insists this is the only solution for her.

Importance of the problem

Total knee arthroplasty (TKA) is a highly successful operation that delivers noticeable and measurable improvement in pain, function, and satisfaction. The ultimate goal of a painless knee with normal function that lasts indefinitely has yet to be reached. A prominent source of dissatisfaction among TKA patients is postoperative stiffness and an inadequate ROM to perform everyday activities. The concept of a knee replacement with a greater ROM while retaining the overall success of TKA has become a strong marketing point, both for companies to surgeons and for surgeons to their patients.

Relevant anatomy and background

The native knee achieves flexion past 120° by the lateral femoral condyle rolling back and perching on the edge of the lateral tibial plateau, while the medial femoral condyle rides up on to the posterior horn of the medial meniscus, effectively "lifting-off" and losing contact with the tibial plateau.[1] The re-creation of such kinematics has been actively avoided by arthroplasty designers for fear of excessive forces being applied to the polyethylene inserts and potential dislocation of the prosthetic components. Currently, conventional primary TKA systems are designed to achieve maximum flexion up to 130°.[2]

High-flexion (HF) implants have embraced design modifications including: changes to the posterior femoral condylar resection, femoral component, and polyethylene liner. Different companies have incorporated some or all of these changes into their HF designs in the hope of creating a stable knee that can achieve flexion up to 150° or more. The changes to the femoral component aim to make the most posterior lip of the posterior femoral condyles more rounded in order to increase the weightbearing area of this edge while the prosthesis is in deep flexion (Figure 25.1). These changes are necessary to avoid impingement or edge

Evidence-Based Orthopedics, First Edition. Edited by Mohit Bhandari.
© 2012 Blackwell Publishing Ltd. Published 2012 by Blackwell Publishing Ltd.

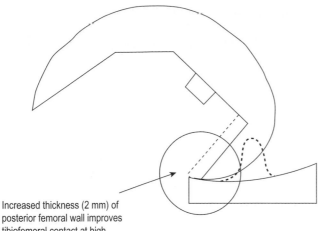

Increased thickness (2 mm) of posterior femoral wall improves tibiofemoral contact at high flexion

Figure 25.1 Schematic drawing of a high-flexion femoral component demonstrating the increased thickness of the posterior condyles required to avoid impingement of the flanges into the polyethylene at high flexion angles.

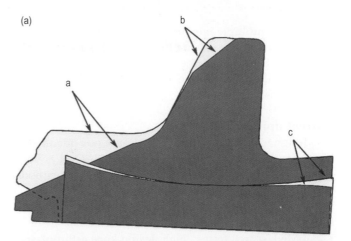

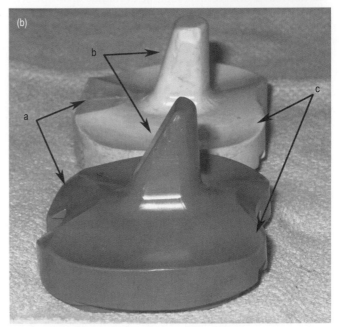

loading of the component into the polyethylene insert, thus preventing fractures and/or delamination of the insert.[3] The femoral modifications require resection of extra host bone, which is replaced by the more rounded edge of the implant. Changes to the polyethylene insert have consisted of decreasing the congruency of the posterior portion to avoid impingement on the femur and creating a recess in the polyethylene anteriorly to accept the patellar tendon as it "leans back" in deep flexion. Additionally, in posterior stabilizing (PS) models, increasing the height of the posterior cam and altering its geometry has been addressed to decrease the chance of "jumping the post" with increased flexion (Figure 25.2).

Figure 25.2 (a-b) Schematic drawings showing differences between a Genesis II (Smith and Nephew, Memphis, TN) standard posterior stabilized (white, background) and high-flexion posterior stabilized (gray, foreground). (a) The cutout of polyethylene at the anterior aspect of the inserts is shown. (b) The slope of the polyethylene at the proximal anterior portion of the post is demonstrated. (c) Changes in the radius of curvature of the posterior portion of the articulating surfaces is shown. (With kind permission from Springer Science+Business Media: McCalden RW, Macdonald SJ, Charron KD, Bourne RB, Naudie D. The role of polyethylene design on postoperative TKA flexion: an analysis of 1534 cases. Clin Orthop Relat Res 2010;468(1):108–114.)

Top four questions

Complications

1. Have the design changes associated with HF implants resulted in increased complication rates?

Outcome measures

2. What are the available clinical tools to measure ROM and what are their limitations?
3. Do HF implants achieve greater postoperative ROM and patient satisfaction scores than conventional TKA?

Indications

4. Are there specific patient population demographics or individual traits that indicate the use of HF implants?

Question 1: Have the design changes associated with HF implants resulted in increased complication rates?

Case clarification

In both Cases 1 and 2, while the patients are concerned about their ability to achieve deep flexion postoperatively, they are aware of the importance of implant longevity and ask if there are any trade-offs.

Relevance

In HF TKA, multiple implant modifications were simultaneously introduced. Teasing their effects apart can be difficult. As HF TKA data does not yet exist beyond 5 years, it is critical that we continue to monitor and appraise these new designs.

Current opinion

The design modifications in HF TKA pose no added risk to the patient during surgery. Similarly, the rates of adverse events and complications remain parallel to conventional TKA at short-term follow-up.

Finding the evidence

- PubMed: search terms "high flexion knee arthroplasty," "high flexion TKA," "high flexion knee complications" with limits: "humans" and "English language"

Quality of the evidence

Level I

- 3 randomized controlled trials powered to detect outcomes and differences in ROM[6]
- 1 meta-analysis examining only RCTs[7]

Level II

- 5 RCTs with methodological limitations: lacking a-priori sample size calculation;[8,9] insufficient power or flawed inclusion confounders[10–12]
- 2 meta-analyses including lower-level study methodologies[13,14]
- 4 prospective cohort studies with matched control groups[15–18]

Level III

- 5 retrospective case-control studies (comparison observational studies)[19–23]

Level IV

- 1 study with methodological limitations: a retrospective single-surgeon series following a small sample of HF PS knees[24]

Findings

Concerns have been expressed regarding the HF design changes and their potential long-term indications. Any knee joint that undergoes deep flexion is subject to high shear forces between the tibia and femur, estimated to be several orders of magnitude more than the one's body weight.[25,26] To reach deep flexion the amount of posterior translation required by the normal knee leads to posterior subluxation of the lateral femoral condyle and a small amount of lift-off of the medial femoral condyle as it rides up on the more tethered posterior horn of the medial meniscus. This mechanism causes significant posterior loading on the polyethylene insert and tibial tray.[1]

Although HF designs have improved the amount of articulating surface area when compared to standard designs according to dual fluoroscopy and three-dimensional modeling in vivo,[23] the contact area of all designs is known to decrease markedly in deep flexion. During deep flexion, as contact area is decreased, contact pressure stresses demonstrate corresponding increases.[25] What is not known is how much stress is problematic with contemporary polyethylene inserts.

The introduction of multiple implant modifications introduced simultaneously raised warranted initial concerns. Both the structural integrity of a thinner and taller cam–post mechanism in PS designs and the necessary extra bone resected to allow HF femoral components were anticipated to be problematic.[24,27,28] Han et al. reported a 38% incidence of aseptic loosening of the femoral component at just less than 3 years in one manufacturer's HF design.[24] That being said, all of the level I and II evidence at short- and mid-term follow-ups suggests there are no differences between complication rates in HF and conventional TKA.[5–12,29]

Recommendations

- HF TKA may result in higher rates of short-term aseptic loosening [overall quality: very low]
- HF components have better contact forces in deep flexion [overall quality: low]
- Rates of complications are comparable in conventional and HF TKA at short-term follow-up [overall quality: high]

Question 2: What are the available clinical tools to measure ROM and what are their limitations?

Case clarification

When discussing with the patient the increased ROM they may receive from a HF implant it is important to consider and explain the limitations of our measurement techniques, and whether these gains may be clinically significant in their everyday life.

Relevance

The simple act of measuring knee flexion has been debated. The clinically predictive worth of passive, active, or "drop" flexion is unclear. Comparing ROM between HF and conventional models in most of the studies reveals differences in flexion that are small enough to be clinically irrelevant. A difference of several degrees may reach significance but is often well within the accuracy limitations of any measurement tool used.

Current opinion

The measured radiographic angulations between the long axis of the tibia and the long axis of the femur under active and passive knee ROM is widely considered the gold standard.[30]

Finding the evidence
PubMed: search terms "knee kinematics," "knee ROM," "deep knee flexion," "ROM knee arthroplasty" with limits: "humans" and "English language"

Quality of the evidence
Level III
• Case-control studies and exploratory validation observational studies,[30–32] prospective[33] and retrospective observational studies[34,35]

Findings
Goniometric measurements used by a single assessor are seen as being reliable[30,31,36] but do not guarantee comparability between studies. Electrogoniometry and deep flexion radiography are also used at an increased expense and can introduce sources of error such as marker placement and stability or operator variation.[36] The justification of using such techniques under the pretense of improving accuracy is questionable given the increase in flexion required to be clinically relevant—an undefined amount that is unique to each patient's demands. Roentgenographic measurements remain the gold standard but are less used clinically compared with visual ROM estimations and goniometric measurements. Several studies have found that assessors tended to underestimate flexion,[30,36] increasingly so as the flexion angle increased, when using visual and goniometric measurements compared against radiographic standards.[36] It is important to note that while gains obtained in conventional and HF studies may appear statistically different; they may not be clinically significant given the limitations of accuracy for goniometric measurement.[30,36]

Active ROM testing has been shown to under-represent the flexion when compared to passive methods of testing.[6,30] However, proponents of the use of active ROM claim that it is a better representation of the range used functionally.[32,33,35] Others feel that preoperative and early postoperative assessments are hampered by pain and that patients would not perform an active test exercise (kneeling) in the early postoperative period for fear of damaging the implant.[34]

Clinical outcome tools are too blunt and limited in their ability to detect changes in deep-flexion specific tasks.[37] For instance, Knee Society scores lack an option to record flexion beyond 125° and Oxford knee scores have only a single question that addresses deep flexion. This creates a ceiling effect where assessment scores are inadequate in patients with higher function.[29]

Recommendations
• Goniometry provides reliable and accurate ROM results [overall quality: moderate]

• Visual assessment may underestimate flexion, especially deep flexion [overall quality: low]

Question 3: Do HF implants achieve greater postoperative ROM and patient satisfaction scores than conventional TKA?

Case clarification
When recommending (or not recommending) a particular implant to a patient, such as those in Cases 1 or 2, it is important to consider the available evidence that should guide our clinical practice.

Relevance
Patient satisfaction following TKA is closely associated with restoration of function (including ROM and the ability to perform activities of daily living)[38] and as such warrants discussions of whether the patients may benefit from a HF implant.

Current opinion
HF implants perform at least on a par to conventional TKA in increasing ROM postoperatively. Some HF designs have shown improved ROM compared to conventional TKA, but it remains unclear whether these ROM changes are clinically significant and lead to improved patient satisfaction in the long-term.

Finding the evidence
See Question 1.

Quality of the evidence
See Question 1.

Findings
Studies utilizing *in-vivo fluoroscopy* comparing flexion, contact areas and contact stresses have found either no significant differences between standard and HF designs or a small improvement in favor of the HF design.[23,39,40]

A number of *nonrandomized* studies compared flexion and clinical outcomes between a variety of standard and HF designs,[15–18,20–23] and reveal conflicting results and conclusions. Five of these studies revealed a modest improvement in flexion,[17,18,20–22] with no improvement in clinical rating scores found in any of the studies that utilized them. An early meta-analysis[13] included two RCTs[4,12] and four non-RCT studies.[19–22] The authors concluded that while there are marginal gains in knee flexion and ROM, there is no clinical advantage over traditional TKA. A more recent systematic review[29] included RCTs,[4,8,12] retrospective[15,20–22] and prospective[11] studies. The authors contend that methodological limitations and inconsistent results in HF TKA research suggests that there is currently no established benefit in postoperative ROM or physical function when

Table 25.1 Published results of RCT trials

Reference	Seon et al.[11]	McCalden et al.[5]	Kim et al.[6]	Kim et al.[12]	Nutton et al.[4]	Weeden and Schmidt[8]	Choi et al.[10]	Seng et al.[9]
Location	South Korea	Ontario	South Korea	South Korea	Scotland	Texas	South Korea	Singapore
Implant	Nexgen CR vs. CR Flex	Genesis II PS vs. HF	Nexgen CR vs. CR Flex	Nexgen LPS vs. LPSFlex	Nexgen LPS vs. LPSFlex	Nexgen LPS vs. LPSFlex	PFC Sigma RPF vs. PFC Sigma RP	DePuy PFC Modular vs. Nexgen LPSFlex
Power calculation	Y	Y	Y	Y	Y	Y	Y	N
Groups	52/52	50/50	59 knees (simultaneous bilateral)	50/50 (simultaneous bilateral)	30/30	25/25	85/85	35/41
Randomized?	Y	Y	Y	Y	Y	Y	Y	Y
Concealed?	Y	Y	Y	Y	Y	Y	Y	Y
Intention to treat?	Y	Y	Y	Y	Y	Y	Y	Y
Groups similar?	Unclear	Implied	Implied	Implied	Y	Implied	Implied	Y
Patients blinded?	Y	Y	Y	Y	Y	Y	Y	Y
Surgeons blinded?	N	N	N	N	N	N	N	N
Assessors blinded?	Y	Y	Y	Y	Y	unclear	Y	Y
Follow-up?	>2 years	>2 years	3 years	2 years	1 years	1 year	>2 years	5 years
Conclusion	No early benefit	No early benefit	No early benefit	No early benefit	No early benefit	Recommended high flexion	No early benefit	Greater post-op flexion and quality of life test scores in high-flexion group

CR, cruciate retaining; HF, high flexion; LPS, legacy PS; PFC press-fit condylar; Std, standard.

using these implants. Additionally, two recent meta-analyses with stronger inclusion criteria[7,14] suggested that no clinically relevant or statistically significant improvement was obtained in flexion with the HF prostheses.

Table 25.1 summarizes the relevant methodological details of eight randomized controlled trials.[4–6,8–12] Of these eight studies, only Weeden et al.[8] and Seng et al.[9] found a significant advantage to the HF design implants. Moreover, the study by Seng et al.[9] found that at 5 years, the increase in postoperative knee flexion correlated with a significant improvement in general health, vitality, and physical functioning scales of the SF-36.

Although they are RCTs, these studies do have several of the limitations mentioned above. The validity of performing simultaneous knee replacements (one of either design) and using the patient as their own control[6,12] is debatable. While bilateral simultaneous TKA may be ideal for comparison as it controls for patient motivation,[15] others contend that it may confound results with the patient comparing the two sides in an attempt to keep the sides equal in their flexion.[29] Moreover, performing simultaneous bilateral TKA may confound clinical scoring parameters, with scoring systems unable to detect which knee is causing an inability to perform a global function such as climbing stairs.[6]

Recommendations

• No short-term differences in ROM or patient satisfaction scores exist between conventional and HF implants [overall quality: high]
• HF TKA produces greater ROM and deep flexion [overall quality: moderate]
• HF TKA can increase patient scores on the general health, vitality, and physical functioning scales of the SF-36 [overall quality: low]

Question 4: Are there specific patient population demographics or individual traits that indicate the use of HF implants?

Case clarification
Patients may ask if they are suitable candidates for this design or directly request it as a result of their desire to achieve deep flexion for cultural, recreational, or religious reasons.

Relevance
A notable shortfall of contemporary TKA is the ROM routinely obtained after surgical intervention and its comparison to the amounts necessary to perform routine activities of daily living (ADLs) (Table 25.2). Postoperative outcome studies reveal stiffness as a leading cause of dissatisfaction amongst patients.[38,41]

Current opinion
It is important to consider patient, instrument, design, and material factors in recommending the use of an HF implant. A patient's preoperative ROM is an important predictor of their postoperative ROM. Many implant and material (such as highly cross-linked polyethylene) modifications have been introduced simultaneously, making it difficult to tease out the individual effects of a HF design.

Finding the evidence
See Question 1 above.

Quality of the evidence
See Question 1 evidence, as well as
• Several level II[3,42–44] and level III[37,45–48] observational and cohort studies

Table 25.2 Values of knee flexion used in various daily activities of living

Activity	Range of motion (°)
Level walking	≤ 90
Gentle slope	≤110
Rising from a seated position	≤120
Getting up and down stairs	≤120
Getting in and out of the bathtub	≤135
Sitting cross-legged	≤110
Squatting	≤160
Sitting on calves plantar flexed (Japanese formal floor sitting or Islamic Su'ud sitting)	≤160

Findings
Cultural, religious, and recreational considerations should be weighed into the decision to use a HF implant. Table 25.2 lists commonly quoted values of knee flexion used in various routine daily activities. Although the highest-flexion actions listed in Table 25.2 appear to be more relevant in Eastern cultures, Western cultures still regularly partake in activities using these movements, such as golf, gardening, yoga, and kneeling.[49,50] Variations between cultures in normal knees have been noted[51] and are attributed to differences in routine daily activities. Similarly, ADLs have accounted for different wear patterns in osteoarthritic knees of Arabian and North American people.[52]

Patients' expectations are also a determining factor. One study found that patients who were less mobile than they expected postoperatively were highly likely to be dissatisfied with the TKA,[37] suggesting that significant postoperative ROM gains may improve mobility and thus patient satisfaction. Moreover, while an improvement in the ability to kneel is often anticipated,[45] preoperative expectation surveys in one study revealed that, while the inability to perform HF activities was seen as the most disabling, they were not perceived as being the most important.[42] Pain relief, perioperative complications, and the ability to perform basic ADLs were all valued as being of greater significance.[42] These results mirrored previous studies of European patients[53] and Indian patients.[47] Similarly, postoperative outcome studies have shown that while a severe lack of flexion (<90°) correlates with overall physical impairment and dissatisfaction,[38,44,54] factors such as pain, inability to meet expectations, operative complications, and mental, social, and emotional scores have been shown to be stronger indicators of unsatisfied patients.[37,38,44,50,55,56] However, while poor ROM has been quoted as a leading cause of dissatisfaction,[2] there is no guarantee that higher flexion will lead to greater satisfaction.[47] This idea is supported by studies that show no increase in clinical outcome scores despite those individuals achieving high flexion.[18,20–22]

Preoperative ROM remains the greatest predictor of postoperative ROM in TKA and HF TKA alike.[43,46] Controlling for implant design, patients with good preoperative ROM, especially with very high preoperative ROM (>120°), may be more likely to gain flexion with a HF than a conventional TKA design.[48] Patients' anatomy and quality of cruciate ligaments may also be important as one study found HFPS designs to achieve greater improvements in ROM over HFCR designs.[3]

Recommendation
• Patients with high preoperative flexion may be more likely to gain flexion with a HF over a conventional TKA design [overall quality: low]

Summary of recommendations

- HF TKA may result in higher rates of short-term aseptic loosening
- HF components have better contact forces in deep flexion
- Rates of complications are comparable in conventional and HF TKA at short-term follow-up
- Goniometry provides reliable and accurate ROM results
- Visual assessment may underestimate flexion, especially deep flexion
- No short-term differences in ROM or patient satisfaction scores exist between conventional and HF implants
- HF TKA produces greater ROM and deep flexion
- HF TKA can increase patient scores on the general health, vitality, and physical functioning scales of the SF-36
- Patients with high preoperative flexion may be more likely to gain flexion with a HF over a conventional TKA design

Conclusion

Postoperative ROM after TKA is related to many factors. New HF TKA design changes have aimed to improve post-operative flexion and ameliorate patient satisfaction outcomes. There remain inconsistent results, despite the vast array of clinical evidence evaluating these designs over the past half-decade. Reported improvements in ROM have been identified in high (level I) and lesser quality (level II) RCTs. However, these improvements have not proven to be of major clinical significance with the exception of one study by Seng et al.[51] with a mid-term follow-up. One major limitation in performing these studies remains our rudimentary tools for measuring ROM changes. The concept of performing or receiving a TKA with a higher ROM remains attractive to companies, surgeons, and patients alike. However, the long-term effects of these design changes are as of yet unknown, and we as surgeons and consumers must continue to evaluate them before fully embracing this technology.

References

1. Pinskerova V, Samuelson KM, Stammers J, Maruthainar K, Sosna A, Freeman M. The knee in full flexion: an anatomical study. J Bone Joint Surg Br 2009;91(6):830–4.
2. Tarabichi S, Tarabichi Y, Hawari M. Achieving deep flexion after primary total knee arthroplasty. J Arthroplasty 2010;25(2):219–24.
3. McCalden RW, MacDonald SJ, Charron KDJ, Bourne RB, Naudie DD. The role of polyethylene design on postoperative TKA flexion: an analysis of 1534 cases. Clin Orthop Relat Res 2010;468(1):108–14.
4. Nutton R, Van Der Linden M, Rowe P, Gaston P, Wade F. A prospective randomised double-blind study of functional outcome and range of flexion following total knee replacement with the NexGen standard and high flexion components. J Bone Joint Surg Br 2008;90(1):37–42.
5. McCalden RW, MacDonald SJ, Bourne RB, Marr JT. A randomized controlled trial comparing "high-flex" vs "standard" posterior cruciate substituting polyethylene tibial inserts in total knee arthroplasty. J Arthroplasty 2009;24(6):33–8.
6. Kim Y-H, Choi Y, Kwon O-R, Kim J-S. Functional outcome and range of motion of high-flexion posterior cruciate-retaining and high-flexion posterior cruciate-substituting total knee prostheses. A prospective, randomized study. J Bone Joint Surg Am 2009;91(4):753–60.
7. Mehin R, Burnett R, Brasher P. Does the new generation of high-flex knee prostheses improve the post-operative range of movement? A meta-analysis. J Bone Joint Surg Br 2010;92(10):1429–34.
8. Weeden SH, Schmidt R. A randomized, prospective study of primary total knee components designed for increased flexion. J Arthroplasty 2007;22(3):349–52.
9. Seng C, Yeo SJ, Wee JL, Sri S, Chong HC, Lo NN. Improved clinical outcomes after high-flexion total knee arthroplasty a 5-year follow-up study. J Arthroplasty 2010;12 Nov (E-Pub ahead of print.)
10. Choi WC, Lee S, Seong SC, Jung JH, Lee MC. Comparison between standard and high-flexion posterior-stabilized rotating-platform mobile-bearing total knee arthroplasties: a randomized controlled study. J Bone Joint Surg Am 2010;92(16):2634–42.
11. Seon JK, Park SJ, Lee KB, Yoon TR, Kozanek M, Song EK. Range of motion in total knee arthroplasty: a prospective comparison of high-flexion and standard cruciate-retaining designs. J Bone Joint Surg Am 2009;91(3):672–9.
12. Kim Y-H, Sohn K-S, Kim J-S. Range of motion of standard and high-flexion posterior stabilized total knee prostheses. A prospective, randomized study. J Bone Joint Surg Am 2005;87(7):1470–5.
13. Gandhi R, Tso P, Davey JR, Mahomed NN. High-flexion implants in primary total knee arthroplasty: a meta-analysis. Knee 2009;16(1):14–7.
14. Luo S-X, Su W, Zhao J-M, Sha K, Wei Q-J, Li X-F. High-flexion vs conventional prostheses total knee arthroplasty: a meta-analysis. J Arthroplasty 2010 Nov 11;(Epub ahead of print)
15. Ng F, Wong H, Yau W, Chiu K, Tang W. Comparison of range of motion after standard and high-flexion posterior stabilised total knee replacement. Int Orthop 2008;32(6):795–798.
16. Minoda Y, Aihara M, Sakawa A, Fukuoka S, Hayakawa K, Ohzono K. Range of motion of standard and high-flexion cruciate retaining total knee prostheses. J Arthroplasty 2009;24(5):674–80.
17. Crow B, McCaluey J, Ezzet K. Can high-flexion tibial inserts improve range of motion after posterio cruciate-retaining total knee arthroplasty. Orthop 2010;33(9):667.
18. Gupta SK, Ranawat A, Shah V, Zikria B, Zikria J, Ranawat C. The P.F.C. sigma RP-F TKA designed for improved performance: a matched-pair study. Orthop 2006;29(9):S49–52.

19. Bajammal SS, Petruccelli D, Adili A, Winemaker M, De Beer J. Can a change in implant articular geometry affect postoperative range of movement in patients undergoing primary TKA or osteoarthritis? S A Orthop J 2006;34–42.

20. Bin SI, Nam TS. Early results of high-flex total knee arthroplasty: comparison study at 1 year after surgery. Knee Surg Sports Traumatol Arthrosc 2007;15(4):350–5.

21. Huang H-T, Su JY, Wang G-J. The early results of high-flex total knee arthroplasty: a minimum of 2 years of follow-up. J Arthroplasty 2005;20(5):674–9.

22. Laskin RS. The effect of a high-flex implant on postoperative flexion after primary total knee arthroplasty. Orthop 2007;30(8):86–8.

23. Suggs JF, Kwon Y-M, Durbhakula SM, Hanson GR, Li G. In vivo flexion and kinematics of the knee after TKA: comparison of a conventional and a high flexion cruciate-retaining TKA design. Knee Surg Sports Traumatol Arthrosc 2009;17(2):150–6.

24. Han HS, Kang S-B, Yoon KS. High incidence of loosening of the femoral component in legacy posterior stabilised-flex total knee replacement. J Bone Joint Surg Br 2007;89(11):1457–61.

25. Shiramizu K, Vizesi F, Bruce W, Herrmann S, Walsh WR. Tibiofemoral contact areas and pressures in six high flexion knees. Int Orthop 2009;33(2):403–6.

26. Smith SM, Cockburn RA, Hemmerich A, Li RM, Wyss UP. Tibiofemoral joint contact forces and knee kinematics during squatting. Gait Posture 2008;27(3):376–86.

27. Ranawat CS. Design may be counterproductive for optimizing flexion after TKR. Clin Orthop Relat Res 2003;416(1):174–6.

28. Ritter M. High-flexion knee designs: more hype than hope? In the affirmative. J Arthroplasty 2006;21(4):40–1.

29. Murphy M, Journeaux S, Russell T. High-flexion total knee arthroplasty: a systematic review. Int Orthop 2009;33(4):887–93.

30. Lavernia C, D'Apuzzo M, Rossi MD, Lee D. Accuracy of knee range of motion assessment after total knee arthroplasty. J Arthroplasty 2008;23(6):85–91.

31. Gogia PP, Braatz JH, Rose SJ, Norton BJ. Reliability and validity of goniometric measurements at the knee. Phys Ther 1987;67(2):192–5.

32. Rowe PJ, Myles CM, Walker C, Nutton R. Knee joint kinematics in gait and other functional activities measured using flexible electrogoniometry: how much knee motion is sufficient for normal daily life? Gait Posture 2000;12(2):143–55.

33. Myles CM, Rowe PJ, Walker CRC, Nutton RW. Knee joint functional range of movement prior to and following total knee arthroplasty measured using flexible electrogoniometry. Gait Posture 2002;16(1):46–54.

34. Schai P, Gibbon A, Scott R. Kneeling ability after total knee arthroplasty: perception and reality. Clin Orthop Relat Res 1999;367(1):195–200.

35. Rowe PJ, Myles CM, Nutton R. The effect of total knee arthroplasty on joint movement during functional activities and joint range of motion with particular regard to higher flexion users. J Orthop Surg (Hong Kong) 2005;13(2):131–8.

36. Edwards JZ, Greene KA, Davis RS, Kovacik MW, Noe DA, Askew MJ. Measuring flexion in knee arthroplasty patients. J Arthroplasty 2004;19(3):369–372.

37. Noble PC, Conditt MA, Cook KF, Mathis KB. The John Insall Award: Patient expectations affect satisfaction with total knee arthroplasty. Clin Orthop Relat Res 2006;452(1):35–43.

38. Bourne RB, Chesworth BM, Davis AM, Mahomed NN, Charron KDJ. Patient satisfaction after total knee arthroplasty: who is satisfied and who is not? Clin Orthop Relat Res 2010;468(1):57–63.

39. Sharma A, Komistek RD, Scuderi GR, Cates HE. High-flexion TKA designs: what are their in vivo contact mechanics? Clin Orthop Relat Res 2007;464(1):117–26.

40. Coughlin KM, Incavo SJ, Doohen RR, Gamada K, Banks S, Beynnon BD. Kneeling kinematics after total knee arthroplasty: anterior-posterior contact position of a standard and a high-flex tibial insert design. J Arthroplasty 2007;22(2):160–5.

41. Anderson JG, Wixson RL, Tsai D, Stulberg DS, Chang R. Functional outcome and patient satisfaction in total knee patients over the age of 75. J Arthroplasty 1996;11(7):831–840.

42. Park KK, Shin KS, Chang CB, Kim SJ, Kim TK. Functional disabilities and issues of concern in female Asian patients before TKA. Clin Orthop Relat Res 2007;461(1):143–152.

43. Ritter M, Harty L, Davis K, Meding J, Berend M. Predicting range of motion after total knee arthroplasy: clustering, log linear regression, and regression tree analysis. J Bone Joint Surg Am 2003;85(1):1278–1285.

44. Bourne RB, McCalden RW, MacDonald SJ, Mokete L, Guerin J. Influence of patient factors on TKA outcomes at 5 to 11 years followup. Clin Orthop Relat Res 2007;464(1):27–31.

45. Mancuso CA, Sculco TP, Wickiewicz TL, Jones EC, Robbins L, Warren RF, et al. Patients' expectations of knee surgery. J Bone Joint Surg Am 2001;83(7):1005–12.

46. Kawamura H, Bourne RB. Factors affecting range of flexion after total knee arthroplasty. J Orthop Sci 2001;6(3):248–52.

47. Narayan K, Thomas G, Kumar R. Is extreme flexion of the knee after total knee replacement a prerequisite for patient satisfaction? Int Orthop 2009;33(3):671–4.

48. Victor J, Reis M, Bellemans J, Robb W, Van Hellemondt G. Knee arthroplasty: who benefits the most? Orthop 2007;30(8):77–80.

49. Huddleston JI, Scarborough DM, Goldvasser D, Freiberg AA, Malchau H. 2009 Marshall Urist Young Investigator Award: how often do patients with high-flex total knee arthroplasty use high flexion? Clin Orthop Relat Res 2009;467(7):1898–906.

50. Weiss JM, Noble PC, Conditt MA, Kohl HW, Roberts S, Cook KF, et al. What functional activities are important to patients with knee replacements? Clin Orthop Relat Res 2002;404(1):172–188.

51. Ahlberg A, Moussa A, Al-Nahdi M. On geographic variations in the normal range of joint motion. Clin Orthop Relat Res 1988;234(1):229–31.

52. Hodge WA, Harman MK, Banks SA. Patterns of knee osteoarthritis in Arabian and American knees. J Arthroplasty 2009;24(3):448–53.

53. Moran M. Evaluation of patient concerns before total knee and hip arthroplasty. J Arthroplasty 2003;18(4):442–5.

54. Ritter M, Campbell E. Effect of range of motion on the success of a total knee arthroplasty. J Arthroplasty 1987;295–7.

55. Park KK, Chang CB, Kang YG, Seong SC, Kim TK. Correlation of maximum flexion with clinical outcome after total knee replacement in Asian patients. J Bone Joint Surg Br 2007;89(5):604–8.

56. Fisher D, Dierckman B, Watts M, Davis K. Looks good but feels bad: factors that contribute to poor results after total knee arthroplasty. J Arthroplasty 2007;22(6 Suppl 2):39–42.

26 The Neuropathic/Charcot Joint

Rajrishi Sharma[1] and Mitchell J. Winemaker[2]
[1]University of Western Ontario, London, ON, Canada
[2]McMaster University, Hamilton, ON, Canada

Case scenario

A 55 year old woman diagnosed with spina bifida occulta and relative insensate lower limbs presents to clinic using two canes and a lateral unloading brace. She states that over the past month she has been having increasing pain to the lateral joint line and major instability on weightbearing without her brace. She has tried anti-inflammatories, bracing, non-weightbearing, and physiotherapy with limited benefit. She has become a minimal ambulatory and has had to go on sick leave from work. On examination, weightbearing without the brace reveals a 45° valgus deformity correctable to neutral. She has some sensory deficit in the peroneal nerve distribution but has intact motor and vascular function. Radiographs show severe lateral compartment arthritis with bony fragmentation in the surrounding synovial tissue and medial subluxation of tibiofemoral joint. The patella was subluxed laterally. She was diagnosed with a Charcot joint.

Relevant anatomy

The knee joint moves in both flexion/extension and internal/external rotation and is determined by the shape of the articulating surfaces and the orientation of the four major knee ligaments. This four-bar linkage system includes the anterior and posterior cruciate ligaments and the medial and lateral collateral ligaments. The posterior cruciate ligament (PCL) also facilitates the femoral rollback, which allows for increased flexion. Due to asymmetry of the lateral and medial femoral condyles, the lateral condyle rolls a greater distance than medial at 20° flexion causing external rotation of the tibia, called the screw-home mechanism.

The primary function of the medial collateral ligament (MCL) is to restrain valgus rotation, while its secondary function controls external rotation. The lateral collateral ligament (LCL) restrains varus rotation and resists internal rotation. Numerous implants are available to accommodate for ligamentous laxity and bone loss. Cruciate retaining (CR) and posterior stabilizing (PS) knee implants are generally used for knees with a competent MCL and LCL. Total stabilizing (TS) knee implants are used for knees with incompetent collateral ligaments, while rotating hinged implants are reserved for complex instability involving bone loss and ligament incompetence.[1]

Importance of the problem

Charcot arthropathy or neuropathic arthropathy is a progressive, relatively painless degenerative condition of the musculoskeletal system, caused by an underlying neurological or neurovascular disorder.[2-5] It is a progressive arthropathy characterized by joint dislocations, pathologic fractures, pronounced new bone formation, and debilitating deformities with severe destruction and elongation of supporting structures.[6] This disorder results in progressive destruction of bone and soft tissues, mainly at weightbearing, lower extremity joints. Definitive treatment for individuals suffering from this devastating disease remains controversial.[5-9]

The actual incidence of Charcot arthropathy is perhaps greater than reported, as a result of delay or missed diag-

Evidence-Based Orthopedics, First Edition. Edited by Mohit Bhandari.
© 2012 Blackwell Publishing Ltd. Published 2012 by Blackwell Publishing Ltd.

nosis in as many as 25% of patients.[10–12] Disorders that have the potential to produce Charcot joints include amyloidosis, alcoholism, cerebral palsy, Charcot–Marie–Tooth disease, congenital insensitivity to pain, idiopathic sensorimotor neuropathy, infection, leprosy, pernicious anemia, poliomyelitis, steroids, syringomyelia, spina bifida, spinal or peripheral nerve injury, and trauma. Tabes dorsalis due to syphilis was the most predominant cause until improved antimicrobial therapy was implemented; diabetic neuropathy has now replaced it as the leading cause of Charcot joint disease.[2,3,12,13]

The overall international incidence of Charcot arthropathy seems to be the same as that found within the United States alone. The incidence ranges from 0.10% to 3% in a general population of diabetics and up to 13% in high-risk diabetic patients presenting to specialized clinics.[13] Radiographic changes have been noted in up to 29% of patients with established peripheral neuropathy.[13,14] The most common sites affected include the foot, ankle, and rarely the knee.[4]

The neuropathic joint causes immense morbidity to patients. Because of the rarity of this clinical entity, no management guidelines have been established to date. A few retrospective studies have been identified within the literature, but no prospective, case-control studies, or randomized control trials have been identified. Despite difficulty in diagnosis and treatment, patient interest remains strong. Over 250,000 hits result from a Google search using the terms "Charcot joint" and over 150,000 hits appear when searching the terms "neuropathic arthropathy."

Finding the evidence

Since the evidence in the literature is lacking, it is difficult to critically analyze and formulate knowledgeable answers to the key clinical questions. As such, we present all the available evidence within Charcot neuroarthropathy first, followed by attempts to answer the clinical questions.
- Cochrane Database, with search term "neuropathic arthropathy," "Charcot arthropathy," "neuroarthropathy"
  ◦ No articles found
- PubMed (www.ncbi.nlm.nih.gov/pubmed/) clinical queries search/ systematic reviews: "neuropathic arthropathy," "Charcot arthropathy," "neuroarthropathy"
  ◦ No articles found
- MEDLINE search identifying the population ("knee" AND "neuropathic arthropathy")
  ◦ 29 articles identified
- PubMed (www.ncbi.nlm.nih.gov/pubmed/): sensitivity search using keywords "knee neuropathic arthropathy"
  ◦ 145 hits and, after review, 25 potentially relevant articles

Quality of evidence

High-quality evidence is lacking within this field.

Level II
- 1 prognostic study

Level III
- 2 retrospective studies

Level IV
- 3 case series

Level V
- 19 case reports and expert opinion

Top four questions

Diagnosis

1. How accurate is the clinical and radiographic examination in the diagnosis of Charcot neuroarthropathy?

Therapy

2. What is the role of nonoperative treatment for the Charcot joint?
3. Is arthroplasty better than fusion for large joints affected by neuroarthropathy?

Harm

4. What are the complications of fusion and total joint arthroplasty?

Question 1: How accurate is the clinical and radiographic examination in the diagnosis of Charcot neuroarthropathy?

Case clarification

This 55 year old woman presented with a warm, effused knee in valgus alignment which was accentuated during her unstable gait. Radiographs showed complete lateral compartment joint space loss with bone fragmentation and debris within the synovium. Marked (45°) clinical valgus malalignment was noted in stance without the valgus unloading brace.

Relevance

Because of its rarity, delay in diagnosis is one of the common problems when dealing with patients with neuroarthropathy. Commonly, once presented to the orthopedic surgeon, the disease is markedly advanced, beyond nonoperative treatment. In fact, up to 25% cases of Charcot neuroarthropathy are missed.

Current opinion

It is not surprising that Charcot neuroarthropathy is commonly missed since the presentation can be confused with cellulitis, rheumatoid arthritis, and advanced osteoarthritis. Attention to a detailed history, the extent of disease progression, and radiological appearance should alert one to the diagnosis. The patient commonly presents with a hot, swollen joint (typically more than 2 °C warmer than the opposite limb), relatively little pain considering the extent of disease, and deformity. Radiography reveals an advanced degenerative joint with fragmentation and joint line collapse. Commonly there is bony debris within the synovium with associated stress fractures or joint line subluxation. Abutting articular bone may show signs of osteonecrosis.

Findings

Despite the lack of high-quality data, a retrospective descriptive study of 24 patients with tabes arthropathy was performed from 1983 to 2003.[15] Their inclusion criteria were typical radiological findings and positive syphilitic serology in blood and/or synovial fluid and/or cerebrospinal fluid. Fifteen men and nine women with mean age of 53.71±12.25 years were included, with the delay in diagnosis being 36.83±53.03 months. Overall clinical, biological, and radiological characteristics were described.

They found most patients presented with a single painless, swollen, and deformed joint with significant crepitations. Peripheral neuropathy was found in 29% patients. Loosening of periarticular soft tissues and bone destruction both lead to articular subluxation.[15] Most patients have symptoms that are much milder than would be expected on the basis of radiological findings.

Typical radiological findings include joint destruction, disorganization, and effusion with osseous debris. Additionally, subchondral sclerosis, osteophytosis, subluxation, and soft tissue swelling are also typically seen.[16]

A prognostic level II paper showed that in 44 of 547 patients with hereditary sensory and autonomic neuropathies type III, osteonecrosis is the initial lesion preceding destructive arthropathy. Osteonecrosis and osteochondral fragmentation were always isolated at the distal posterior lateral femoral condyle in the knee.[17]

The differential diagnosis of the neuropathic joint includes infection, osteonecrosis, calcium pyrophosphate dihydrate crystal deposition disease, psoriatic arthritis, osteoarthritis, and osteolysis with detritic synovitis. Advanced imaging combined with physical examination may help differentiate.[15,16,18]

Recommendations

- Clinical manifestations of this disorder classically include gross deformity, crepitus, lack of proprioception, warm joint with an effusion, and decreased awareness of pain in the affected joint [overall quality: low]
- Radiological findings include joint destruction, disorganization, effusion with osseous debris, subchondral sclerosis, osteophytosis, subluxation, and soft tissue swelling [overall quality: moderate]

Question 2: What is the role of nonoperative treatment for the Charcot joint?

Case clarification

Our 55 year old patient with spina bifida had noticed some improved stability in an unloader brace which became less effective over time as the deformity progressed. Given her relatively young age and productive lifestyle, the utility of nonoperative treatment provided relative short-term benefit.

Relevance

Generally, patients diagnosed with neuroarthropathy are younger and concern is typically raised about the longevity of operative treatment. As such, optimizing non-operative treatments, especially early in the disease is beneficial to delay operative treatment as long as possible.

Current opinion

Optimizing nonoperative treatment is beneficial primarily in early stages of the disease. Unfortunately, many of these patients present with advanced disease.

Findings

Extremely poor (level V) evidence, exists for nonoperative treatment for the neuropathic joint. This is likely due to the delayed presentation to the orthopedic surgeon.[2-6] During the early stages, conservative treatments, such as bracing and protective weightbearing, are effective. It has been stressed that early recognition and conservative treatment may alter the course of the disease.[19,20]

Recommendation

- Bracing and protective weightbearing may be effective early in the course of the disease [overall quality: very low]

Question 3: Is arthroplasty better than fusion for large joints affected by neuroarthropathy?

Case clarification

Having failed nonoperative treatment with progressive functional decline, our patient elected to proceed with a surgical alternative. Given her advanced disease and severe instability and deformity, both knee arthrodesis and total joint arthroplasty were discussed.

Relevance

The goals of surgery are to achieve patient satisfaction through relieving pain, correcting deformity, and improving function. This must be weighed against the risks and complications relating to the surgical intervention.

Operative treatments on the neuropathic joint have resulted in high complication rates. A few case series have reported complications in up to 47% of cases treated with total knee arthroplasty (TKA).[8,9] Similar high complication rates are seen in knee arthrodesis for this problem with a high incidence of nonunion.[4,5,21] Arthrodesis, if successful, can yield a long-term durable result, but patient satisfaction and function remain poor.[22] This must be weighed against the improved patient satisfaction and function from a TKA that may ultimately fail and require revision surgeries and more potential future risk.[8,9]

Current opinion

There remains limited use for arthrodesis as joint implants improve with time. The increased patient satisfaction and continued knee range of motion (ROM) and ability to maintain arthrodesis as the fallback plan strengthen the arthroplasty decision. With meticulous ligamentous balancing, bony alignment, augmentation of bony defects, selection of appropriate prosthesis, and patient compliance, TKA is the current preferred surgical intervention.

Findings

At present there are no comparative trials to solve this question definitively. Historically, arthrodesis was the surgical treatment for the neuropathic knee joint.[2,4,5] However, the results were variable and solid arthrodesis was difficult to obtain. It was emphasized that a successful arthrodesis was promoted by adequate bone resection, complete synovectomy, and rigid internal fixation.[4,5,21] This procedure had a wide spectrum of results and a relatively small number within each series, not lending itself to the conclusive treatment.

No randomized controlled trials (RCTs) or prospective studies exist to date. The best available evidence stems from a retrospective review of 40 condylar TKAs in 29 patients with 7.9 years of clinical and 6.4 years of radiographic follow-up. They found a significant improvement in the Knee Society pain and function scores and ROM after TKA.[9]

Due to increased complexity of bone loss and ligamentous attenuation or incompetence resulting in instability, it may become necessary to place a more constrained prosthesis or stems. Proper arrangements must be made prior to beginning any surgical intervention to make sure reconstruction prostheses are available.[2,5,8,9] The key to successful

TKA in the neuropathic joint is to achieve adequate postoperative stability.

Earlier reports have emphasized the importance of surgical timing in the treatment of the Charcot joint. Osteolysis and bone destruction must have ceased and bone reconstruction or coalescence must have begun prior to surgical intervention.[4] Difficulty exists, however, when attempting to categorize radiographs into distinct presentations, since fragmentation, destruction, and coalescence often exist simultaneously.[9] Controversy as to the timing of intervention therefore still remains.

Recommendation

• Total joint arthroplasty is the current preferred method of treatment for neuropathic joint arthropathy [overall quality: moderate]

Question 4: What are the complications of fusion and total joint arthroplasty?

Case clarification

Our patient was informed of the potential consequences of all treatments. She discounted nonsurgical treatment becausee of her desire for improved mobility and pain relief while she remains relatively young. She chose surgery, with the understanding that it may result in a complication and potential for loss of function later in life. The reality is that an above-knee amputation is a possible outcome with or without treatment in this individual's lifetime, and she has accepted this possibility prior to embarking on a surgical treatment.

Relevance

Medicine is a continuous balance between benefit and harm. Without a clear understanding of these complications weighed against the potential benefits, appropriate decisions cannot be made.

Current opinion

Charcot joint arthropathy of the knee is a devastating problem, with the potential for a poor outcome with or without surgery. With this in mind, both patient and surgeon accept a higher tolerance for risk in the hopes of achieving a better outcome, even if it has limitations. When given the choice between no surgery, arthrodesis, and arthroplasty, with complications and functional outcomes discussed for each, patients invariably choose arthroplasty.

Findings

No adequate studies exist that adequately document the complications after operative (TKA or arthrodesis) fixation of a neuropathic joint. Only expert opinions and case reports (level V) discuss the complications. For fixation by arthroplasty these include aseptic loosening, further collapse, infection, progressive ligamentous instability, and periprosthetic fractures.[4,5,9] Complications of knee arthrodesis include nonunion, malunion, infection, shortening, and loss of fixation.[2,5,21]

Although not commonly reported, advancing to a more highly constrained prosthesis is possible.[9] If continued instability exists despite trying to achieve a stable joint, arthrodesis, despite being much more difficult, can be considered at a later stage.[9]

Overall, patients treated with arthrodesis do not function well long term. In fact, a level III retrospective study with a small sample population of 15 patients with average follow-up of 7 years showed overall decreased functional status compared with comparable age group norms by SF-36 score. Patients treated with arthrodesis did significantly worse with regard to physical functioning, physical role, bodily pain, vitality, and social functioning. A second retrospective study observed 29 patients at an average of 48 months with arthrodesis secondary to infected TKA. They found 28% of the patients who achieved fusion complained of pain in the fused knee, 16% remained nonambulatory, and 68% required some sort of walking aid.[23]

Recommendations
- Complications of TKA include aseptic loosening, further collapse, infection, progressive ligamentous instability and periprosthetic fractures (overall quality: low)
- Complications of arthrodesis include nonunion, malunion, infection, shortening, and loss of fixation (overall quality: low)

Summary of recommendations

- Clinical manifestations of this disorder classically include gross deformity, crepitus, lack of proprioception, joint effusion, calor, and decreased awareness of pain in the affected joint
- Radiological findings include joint destruction, disorganization, effusion with osseous debris, subchondral sclerosis, osteophytosis, subluxation, and soft tissue swelling
- Bracing and protective weight bearing may be effective early in the course of the disease
- Total joint arthroplasty is the current preferred method of treatment for the neurogenic joint arthropathy
- Complications of TKA include aseptic loosening, further collapse, infection, progressive ligamentous instability and periprosthetic fractures
- Complications of arthrodesis include nonunion, malunion, infection, shortening, and loss of fixation

Conclusion

Owing to the extreme lack of high-quality literature, many questions remain unanswered or poorly answered. Due to the rarity of this condition, an RCT would likely be difficult. However, strong case-control or cohort studies may be appropriate and attainable. As such, more research within this area needs to be performed.

Our 55 year old patient with spina bifida did in fact elect to proceed with a TKA. Despite preparing for either a TS or rotating hinged prosthesis, a well-balanced knee was achieved allowing full ROM and adequate static stability using a PS knee prosthesis. The MCL and LCL were both competent and intact, and minimal constraint was chosen to reduce stress at the bone fixation interface and improve implant longevity. This will allow for more constraint if future revision is required. Our patient is currently happy with her short-term outcome.

References

1. Hannah M, Battista V, Seth S. Constraint in primary total knee arthroplasty. J Acad Orthop Surg 2005;13(8):515–24.
2. Yoshino S, Fujimori J, Uchida S. Total knee arthroplasty in Charcot's joint. J Arthroplasty 1993;8(3):335–40.
3. Lambert A, Close C. Charcot neuroarthropathy of the knee in type 1 diabetes: Treatment with total knee arthroplasty. Diabet Med 2002;19:338–41.
4. Fullerton B, Browngoehl L. Total knee arthoplasty in a patient with bilateral Charcot knees. Arch Phys Med Rehabil 1997;78:780–2.
5. Soudry M, Binazzi R, Johanson NA, Bullough PG, Insall JN. Total knee arthroplasty in Charcot and Charcot-like joints. Clin Orthop Relat Res 1986;208:199–204.
6. Vince K, Cameron HU, Hungerford DS, Laskin RS, Ranawat CS, Scuderi GR. What would you do? case challenges in knee surgery. J Arthroplasty 2005;20(4 Suppl. 2):44–50.
7. Chong A, Bruce W, Goldberg J. Treatment of the neuropathic knee by arthroplasty. Aust N Z J Surg 1995;65:370–1.
8. Kim Y, Kim J, Oh S. Total knee arthroplasty in neuropathic arthropathy. J Bone Joint Surg Br 2002;84(2):216–19.
9. Parvizi J, Marrs J, Morrey B. Total knee arthroplasty for neuropathic (Charcot) joints. Clin Orthop Relat Res 2003;416:145–50.
10. Chantelau E. The perils of procrastination: effects of early vs delayed detection and treatment of incipient Charcot fracture. Diabet Med 2005;22(12):1707–12.
11. Marks R. Complications of foot and ankle surgery in patients with diabetes. Clin Orthop Relat Res 2001;391:153–61.
12. Myerson M, Henderson M, Saxby T. Management of midfoot diabetic neuroarthropathy. Foot Ankle Int 1994;15(5):233–241.
13. Frykberg R, Belczyk R. Epidemiology of the Charcot foot. Clin Podiatr Med Surg 2008;25:17–28.
14. Cofield R, Motrisin M, Beabout J. Diabetic neuroarthropathy in the foot: patient characteristics and patterns of radiographic changes. Foot Ankle Int 1983;4:15–22.

15. Allali F, Rahmouni R, Hajjaj-Hassouni N. Tabetic arthropathy. A report of 43 cases. Clin Rheumatol 2006;25:858–60.

16. Jones E, Manaster BJ, May DA, Disler DG. Neuropathic osteoarthropathy: diagnostic dilemmas and differential diagnosis. Radiographics 2000;20(Spec No):S279–293.

17. Feldman DS, Ruchelsman DE, Spencer DB, Straight JJ, Schweitzer ME, Axelrod FB. Peripheral arthropathy in hereditary sensory and autonomic neuropathy types III and IV. J Pediatr Orthop 2009;39:91–7.

18. Troyer J, Levine B. Proximal tibia reconstruction with a porous tantalum cone in patient with Charcot arthropathy. Orthopaedics 2009;32(5).

19. Harris J, Brand P. Patterns of disintegration of the tarsus in the anesthetic foot. J Bone Joint Surg Br 1966;48:4.

20. Johnson J. Neuropathic fractures and joint injuries. J Bone Joint Surg Am 1967;49:1.

21. Drennan D, Fahey J, Maylahn D. Important factors in achieving arthrodesis of the Charcot knee. J Bone Joint Surg Am 1971;53:1180.

22. Crockarell J, Mihalko M. Knee arthrodesis using an intramedullary nail. J Arthroplasty 2005;20(6):703–8.

23. Talmo C, Bono JV, Figgie MP, Sculco TP, Laskin RS, Windsor RE. Intramedullary arthrodesis of the knee in the treatment of sepsis after TKR. HSS J, 2007;3(1):83–8.

27 Cemented vs. Uncemented Stems in Revision Knee Arthroplasty: Indications, Technique, and Outcomes

Gerard M.J. March and Paul R. Kim
University of Ottawa, Ottawa, ON, Canada

Case scenario

An 82 year old woman presents with a painful cemented primary total knee arthroplasty (TKA) done 10 years ago for osteoarthritis. Radiographs show tibial and femoral component loosening with loss of medial tibial bone stock and osteolysis (Figure 27.1).

Importance of the problem

The use of stemmed components in revision TKA surgery has been well established. Stems can aid in diaphyseal referencing which is thought to improve mechanical alignment intraoperatively in addition to offloading stress on damaged or absent metaphyseal bone.[1-9] The optimal fixation method of these stemmed components is still not established. A press-fit stem has the theoretical advantage of reduced bone loss with component insertion and provides for ease of extraction if this becomes necessary. The primary concerns with uncemented stems include a lack of long-term fixation, increased incidence of malalignment, and an increased incidence of clinically significant stem-tip pain.[10,11] Fully cemented stems have a good long-term clinical track record, but potential difficulty with future extraction is a major downside to their use.[9,12,13] Presently cemented fixation of a stemmed revision prosthesis is considered the gold standard.[9,12,13] Hybrid fixation with cemented articular components and a press-fit uncemented stem has gained increasing use recently. This chapter reviews the available literature regarding revision TKA with a focus on the use of cemented vs. uncemented stemmed components.

Top three questions

1. What are the advantages and disadvantages of uncemented revision components?
2. What are the advantages and disadvantages of hybrid revision components?
3. What are the advantages and disadvantages of cemented revision components?

Question 1: What are the advantages and disadvantages of uncemented revision components?

Relevance

Further interest in uncemented components has increased in recent years with the advancement of foam metal technology. These implants are made of elemental tantalum or titanium and are highly porous to allow for significant bio-interlock. Foam metal has a modulus of elasticity similar to cancellous bone, allowing for physiological transfer of force and stress from implant to the periprosthetic bone interface. In 2008, Meneghini et al. showed early results of

Evidence-Based Orthopedics, First Edition. Edited by Mohit Bhandari.
© 2012 Blackwell Publishing Ltd. Published 2012 by Blackwell Publishing Ltd.

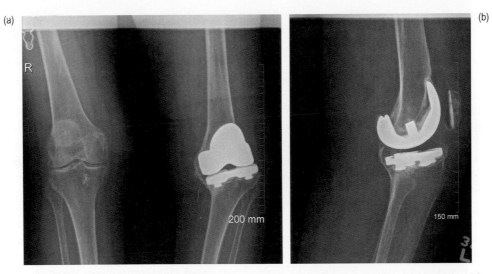

Figure 27.1 Preoperative radiographs (a, AP; b, lateral) demonstrating a loose primary TKA with significant loss of both tibial and femoral bone stock:

a porous tantalum cone used for severe metaphyseal bone stock deficit. Results were considered successful in all 15 revision TKAs, but the average follow-up was only 34 months (range 24–47).[14] These components may help to decrease bone loss during insertion, lead to stable long-term fixation, and have predictable bony ingrowth with a reduction of proximal stress shielding.[15]

Finding the evidence
• PubMed: (www.ncbi.nlm.nih.gov/pubmed): clinical queries and systematic review search using keywords: "total knee replacement revision uncemented"

Quality of the evidence
None of the evidence was higher than level III.

Findings
End-of-stem pain can occur with both cemented and uncemented stems. Methods to reduce stem stiffness with fluting or slots have been undertaken by most manufacturers to try to minimize stem-tip pain. So far there are no clinical results comparing these types of stems to nonfluted stems with respect to stem-tip pain. In 1999, Barrack et al. reported a retrospective review of 80 consecutive revision TKAs. With a minimum follow-up of 2 years they reported localized pain at the end of the stem in 11% of uncemented femurs and 14% of uncemented tibias.[6] It was also noted that end-of-stem pain does not seem to be eliminated completely by the use of a cemented prosthesis.[6]

Concerns about proximal stress shielding remain, especially if the stem is well fixed distally. Presently, highly polished titanium alloy stems are used to reduce the possibility of osteointegration.[16] The cylindrical smooth stem is used for prosthesis positioning and stability only. Axial load transfer occurs mainly proximally and not through the

stem itself.[13,17,18] There is also no definitive answer on optimal stem size relative to the endosteal canal. Canal-filling stems would seem to provide better initial stability and alignment compared to thin dangling stems, but long-term concerns with proximal stress shielding remain with canal-filling stems.[19–21]

Theoretical concern exists with greater access areas for polyethylene wear debris to enter the metaphyseal bone compared to a cemented implant.[12] It is thought that cement offers an immediate barrier to third-body debris that is absent with an uncemented prosthesis. This is especially concerning if one considers that increased levels of constraint (and hence polyethylene wear) are commonly needed in revision TKA surgery. The presence of radiolucent lines and its potential association with loosening also remains a concern with uncemented prostheses.[21]

It has been demonstrated that establishing secure initial stability is crucial when trying to encourage biological interlock. Minimal tolerances of micromotion must exist if true osteointegration is to occur.[22,23] Porous tantalum metal has the potential for greater bony ingrowth (80%) compared to fibre metal coatings (50%). However, it is postulated that the rate of fixation or time to secondary stabilization is more important to long-term clinical outcome.[24] Finally, a long uncemented stem will not be useful in all deformities. The basis of press-fit stability is reliant upon complete canal fill in cases with significant proximal bone loss. This process can be disrupted by deformities that affect the diaphysis of either the femur or tibia.[25]

An uncemented total knee revision technique offers several advantages, including endosteal referencing and subsequent stabilization of the construct without the difficulty of future extraction compared to cemented stems. Reported results with uncemented components in revision

TKA have been good in the short term.[26] However, no long-term results have been published.

Recommendations

• In the setting of severe bone loss, cement augmentation may be less than ideal. Uncemented TKA in these situations is an attractive option with published results[14,27,28] [overall quality: low]

• Application of foam metal technology to revision TKA is in its early stages. It is hoped that the use of these metals in the setting of uncemented revision knee surgery will lead to stable long-term fixation and a reduction of proximal stress shielding. This is dependent upon reliable bony ingrowth[14,15] [overall quality: low]

• It has yet to be characterized if an uncemented prosthesis is more or less susceptible to third-body-induced osteolysis. This remains a theoretical concern for the long-term clinical outcome of uncemented revision procedures[12] [overall quality: low]

• For long-term stable fixation of uncemented components, biological interlock is a necessity. In order for this to occur, initial press-fit stability must be achieved, otherwise fibrous ingrowth will occur ensue secondary to micromotion.[12,22] This is a concern with uncemented components in revision TKA[24] [overall quality: low]

Question 2: What are the advantages and disadvantages of hybrid revision components?

Finding the evidence

• PubMed: (www.ncbi.nlm.nih.gov/pubmed): clinical queries and systematic review search using keywords: "total knee replacement revision hybrid fixation"

Quality of the evidence

None of the evidence was higher than level III.

Findings

Early work by Bertin et al. introduced smooth uncemented intramedullary stems with cemented tibial components. The polymethylmethacrylate bone cement replaced small surface defects and afforded immediate stable fixation.[7,29] Bertin reviewed 53 revision TKAs with an average follow-up of 18 months. There were no radiographic failures and they found no evidence of progressive radiolucent lines near the prosthesis or the bone–cement interface.[7] Parsley et al. showed in a 2003 retrospective study that tibial AP alignment was more predictable with long canal-filling cementless stems.[30]

Gofton et al. published a review of 89 revision TKAs completed with a hybrid fixation technique. The results showed survivorship of 93.5% at 8.6 years.[4] They found the rate of aseptic loosening either clinically or radiographically in this patient group matched previously published

results. In 1995 Vince et al. reported on a series of 44 revision TKAs. Of the 13 patients who needed a constrained articulation due to intraoperative instability, 3 failed. No patients with a nonconstrained insert showed signs of failure at the time of final review (range 2–6 years).[29]

Wood et al. in 2009 reported on 135 revision TKAs using a press-fit hybrid technique. Kaplan–Meier survivorship analysis calculated a 13% revision rate at 12 years.[3] Use of antibiotic-impregnated cement is a common stated advantage to the fully cemented stem technique. In this retrospective review of hybrid press-fit stems, there was no increase in the rate of septic loosening with uncemented stems.[3] Barrack et al. published a retrospective review of 80 consecutive revision TKAs. They reported their early results showing no radiographic or clinical sign of loosening. The majority of patients received hybrid fixation but 16 (20%) had fully cemented tibial components based on surgeon discretion.[6]

Bottner et al. reported on 33 revision TKAs completed with hybrid fixation with an average follow-up of 38 months. They had a revision rate of 9.1%.[31] Concerns were raised regarding the ability to gain appropriate fixation in the face of poor bone quality, which is commonly found in revision knee arthroplasty. Loss of cortical contact by the tibial tray can increase strain across the proximal tibia by up to 60%. It has been reported that a cemented long intramedullary stem can reduce the axial load to the tibia plateau by up to 38%.[2] Despite the acceptable outcome in this series of hybrid fixation revision knees, they recommended that fully cemented stems be considered in scenarios of severe bone loss with increased strain to the periarticular region.[11]

Haas et al. reviewed 76 revision TKAs from 1980–1989 completed with a press-fit stem hybrid technique.[32] They felt that fluted or splined press-fit stems would offer an alternative to cementation in the situation of poor proximal bone stock. A failure rate of 7.9% was reported at an average of 42 months follow-up. In 2005, Peters et al. reviewed 50 revision press-fit TKAs at an average of 36 months.[33] Despite good results the authors stated that at that time there was no evidence that the press-fit method provided durable long-term fixation.

In 2003 Shannon et al. presented a retrospective review of 63 revision TKAs with a mean follow-up of 5.75 years. They reported a relatively high failure rate of their hybrid fixation components. Twelve knees (19%) failed, of which half were revised a second time for aseptic loosening.[34] Nonprogressive radiolucencies were also found in over 90% of the surviving prostheses but had no effect on clinical outcome. A further 10 knees (16%) were deemed at risk for failure based on radiographic signs.[34]

The hybrid fixation technique was developed out of a desire to avoid bone loss associated with revision of a fully cemented stem. The cemented articular prosthesis is able to accommodate minor bony defects at the revision surface.[7,29] The uncemented stem attempts to achieve press-fit stabilization within the diaphysis.[32,33] Results in the literature show that the hybrid technique is able to achieve immediate and stable fixation of the prosthesis.[34] It appears that in the properly selected patient, one with adequate bone stock and minimal diaphyseal deformity, the hybrid technique is a viable option. Long-term studies have yet to be completed, thus the question of hybrid fixation longevity remains outstanding.[33]

Recommendations

• The cemented articular prosthesis in a hybrid technique is able to achieve immediate and stable fixation. Additionally, small bony surface defects are easily dealt with by a cemented articular prosthesis[7,29] [overall quality: low]
• Short-term clinical review show the hybrid technique has a high percentage of good to excellent outcomes and universal improvement to Knee Society scores[3,4,6,7,11,32,33] [overall quality: low]
• Published reviews of hybrid technique revision TKAs included selection bias. Cases not deemed appropriate in terms of bone stock were treated with a fully cemented prosthesis. Selection criteria for full cementation include low-demand patients, large canals, diaphyseal deformity, or severe loss of bone stock[3,6,11] [overall quality: low]
• Despite good short-term outcomes of hybrid fixation, the longevity of this construct cannot be clarified at this point in time because of a lack of long-term studies[33] [overall quality: low]

Question 3: What are the advantages and disadvantages of cemented revision components?

Current practice

Proponents of fully cemented fixation are supported by the successful published long-term results of cemented tibial components in primary knee arthroplasty. The use of cement has an important advantage of offering stable and immediate fixation.[26,35,36] Additionally, cemented fixation is able to distribute load evenly across the prosthesis to the available bone stock thereby preventing point stress shielding.

Finding the evidence

• PubMed: (www.ncbi.nlm.nih.gov/pubmed): clinical queries and systematic review search using keywords: "total knee replacement revision cemented"

Quality of the evidence

None of the evidence was higher than level III.

Findings

In 1994, Murray et al. published on 40 cemented long-stemmed kinematic stabilizer revision TKAs.[5] No revisions were performed for mechanical loosening. The early incidence of radiolucent lines was high (32%) but progression was not seen.[5] In 2007 Mabry echoed the concern of stress shielding with cemented stems in revision TKA. This retrospective review of 70 fully cemented revision TKAs showed a 10-year survivorship of 92%.[26]

In an attempt to directly compare stem fixation in revision TKA, Fehring in 2003 presented a retrospective review of 475 revision TKAs completed from 1986 to 2000. They identified 113 cases with 202 metaphyseal engaging stems. Of these, 107 were fully cemented and 95 had press-fit fixation.[37] The choice of cemented vs. cementless technique was not randomized but remained at the discretion of the treating surgeon. The authors showed that implants with fully cemented fixation appeared radiographically more stable.[37] Of the cemented population, 93% were found to be stable, 7% required close follow-up, and none were found to be overtly loose. By comparison, in the uncemented population, 71% were classified as stable, 19% required close follow-up due to possible loosening, and 10% were documented as being loose. The uncemented stems had a re-revision rate for aseptic loosening of 4% while the cemented group had no such cases. They concluded that cemented metaphyseal stemmed components were more stable than their uncemented counterparts (p = 0.0001).[37]

Biomechanical data has also shown support for cemented stem fixation. In 1997, Stern et al. submitted cadaveric tibial base plates to axial and eccentric loading cycles. They compared cemented to cementless specimens documenting micromotion and evidence of subsidence. Results showed that for all configurations of stem length and loading pattern tested, the cemented components showed significantly less micromotion and migration when compared with an uncemented component.[38] In 2001, Jazrawi et al. investigated 12 cadaveric tibial base plates under central, varus, and valgus loading conditions. They were able to show a statistically significant improvement in stability with 75mm and 150mm cemented stems when compared to their uncemented press-fit counterparts.

Despite reservations about stress shielding and stress riser formation, the literature supports the use of fully cemented stemmed components as a stable and durable construct. The lack of randomized trials comparing these two fixation methods presents a challenge for selection of implant technique. It is clear that the fully cemented option has shown favourable survivorship in the long-term. Cadaveric experiments indicate reduced micromotion with cemented stemmed components compared to their uncemented counterparts.[38,39] Despite the acknowledged difficulty with component extraction if the need for re-revision arises, cemented stemmed components remain the gold standard in revision TKA.

Recommendations

- Apprehension with the use of fully cemented stems due to concerns regarding stem length stress shielding and stem-tip stress riser formation have not been confirmed with currently published retrospective reviews. The major concern with fully cemented stems is the difficulty with later extraction if necessary[5,26] [overall quality: low]
- In a retrospective comparison of cemented and uncemented metaphyseal engaging stems, the cemented group had better radiographic stability and less revisions for aseptic loosening (0 vs. 4%) compared to the uncemented stem group[37] [overall quality: low]
- A 2003 retrospective review of 38 fully cemented revision TKAs showed component survivorship of 96.7% at 10 years indicating that cemented stemmed revision TKA offers reliable long-term fixation[34] [overall quality: low]
- Biomechanical data in cadaveric studies support the stability of fully cemented stemmed tibial components[38,39] [overall quality: low]

Case scenario continued

The patient was diagnosed with aseptic loosening and underwent revision TKA. Fully cemented stemmed components with metal augmentation were used because of the significant loss of tibial and femoral bone stock (Figure 27.2).

Summary of recommendations

- In the setting of severe bone loss, cement augmentation may be less than ideal. Uncemented TKA in these situations is an attractive option with published results[14,27,28]

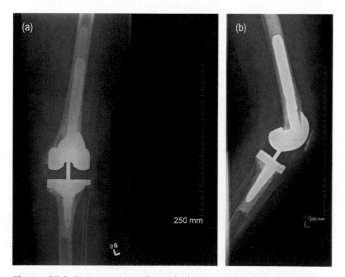

Figure 27.2 Postoperative radiographs (a, AP; b, lateral) showing a revision TKA utilizing a fully cemented stem technique on both the tibial and femoral sides.

- Application of foam metal technology to revision TKA is in its early stages. It is hoped that the use of these metals in the setting of uncemented revision knee surgery will lead to stable long-term fixation and a reduction of proximal stress shielding. This is dependent upon reliable bony ingrowth[14,15]
- It has yet to be characterized if an uncemented prosthesis is more or less susceptible to third-body-induced osteolysis. This remains a theoretical concern for the long-term clinical outcome of uncemented revision procedures[12]
- For long-term stable fixation of uncemented components, biological interlock is a necessity. In order for this to occur, initial press-fit stability must be achieved, otherwise fibrous ingrowth will occur ensue secondary to micromotion.[12,22] This is a concern with uncemented components in revision TKA[24]
- The cemented articular prosthesis in a hybrid technique is able to achieve immediate and stable fixation. Additionally, small bony surface defects are easily dealt with by a cemented articular prosthesis[7,29]
- Short-term clinical review show the hybrid technique has a high percentage of good to excellent outcomes and universal improvement to Knee Society scores[3,4,6,7,11,32,33]
- Published reviews of hybrid technique revision TKAs included selection bias. Cases not deemed appropriate in terms of bone stock were treated with a fully cemented prosthesis. Selection criteria for full cementation include low-demand patients, large canals, diaphyseal deformity, or severe loss of bone stock[3,6,11]
- Despite good short-term outcomes of hybrid fixation, the longevity of this construct cannot be clarified at this point in time because of a lack of long-term studies[33]
- Apprehension with the use of fully cemented stems due to concerns regarding stem length stress shielding and stem-tip stress riser formation have not been confirmed with currently published retrospective reviews. The major concern with fully cemented stems is the difficulty with later extraction if necessary[5,26]
- In a retrospective comparison of cemented and uncemented metaphyseal engaging stems, the cemented group had better radiographic stability and less revisions for aseptic loosening (0 vs. 4%) compared to the uncemented stem group[37]
- A 2003 retrospective review of 38 fully cemented revision TKAs showed component survivorship of 96.7% at 10 years indicating that cemented stemmed revision TKA offers reliable long-term fixation[34]
- Biomechanical data in cadaveric studies support the stability of fully cemented stemmed tibial components[38,39]

Conclusions

Stemmed components are the implant of choice in revision TKA. The type of stem fixation continues to remain controversial. Direct comparisons of fixation methods are rare, and choice of technique is left to an analysis of retrospective reviews complemented by biomechanical results from cadaveric experiments.

On the basis of available data, we recommend the use of a hybrid cement technique in the optimal patient where press-fit stemmed components are appropriate. This is contingent upon the presence of adequate periarticular bone stock (cortical/metaphyseal) allowing for successful cementation of the articular portion of the prosthesis. Overall alignment and component stability are supplemented with the use of an uncemented stem which is canal filling. Surgeon discretion should be used to identify patients better suited for a fully cemented technique. Patients with large intramedullary canals, diaphyseal deformity, or severe bone loss would be better served with a cemented component which includes a cemented stemmed component. The choice of stem length for cementation depends on available proximal bone stock and the possibility of future revision surgery. Our recommendation is to cement the shortest stem possible, as this avoids loss of bone stock and may make future revision surgery easier if component extraction becomes necessary. Use of a cement restrictor and having an adequate cement mantle around the stem are recommended technical points for this technique.

References

1. Parsley BS, Sugano N, Bertolusso R, Conditt MA Mechanical alignment of tibial stems in revision total knee arthroplasty. J Arthroplasty 2003;18(7 Suppl 1):33–6.

2. Brooks PJ, Walker PS, Scott RD, Tibial component fixation in deficient tibial bone stock. Clin Orthop Relat Res 1984;184: 302–8.

3. Wood GC, Naudie DD, MacDonald SJ, McCalden RW, Bourne RB. Results of press-fit stems in revision knee arthroplasties. Clin Orthop Relat Res 2009;467(3):810–17.

4. Gofton WT, Tsigaras H, Butler RA, Patterson JJ, Barrack RL, Rorabeck CH. Revision total knee arthroplasty: fixation with modular stems. Clin Orthop Relat Res 2002;404:158–68.

5. Murray PB, Rand JA, Hanssen AD. Cemented long-stem revision total knee arthroplasty. Clin Orthop Relat Res 1994;309: 116–23.

6. Barrack RL, Rorabeck C, Burt M, Sawhney J. Pain at the end of the stem after revision total knee arthroplasty. Clin Orthop Relat Res 1999;367:216–25.

7. Bertin, KC, Freeman MA, Samuelson KM, Ratcliffe SS, Todd RC. Stemmed revision arthroplasty for aseptic loosening of total knee replacement. J Bone Joint Surg Br 1985;67(2):242–8.

8. Bauer TW, Schils J. The pathology of total joint arthroplasty. I. Mechanisms of implant fixation. Skeletal Radiol 1999;28(8): 423–32.

9. Kim PRC. Results of cemented revision total knee arthroplasty. In: Engh GRC, ed., Revision Total Knee Arthroplasty, pp. 427–42. Williams &Wilkins, Baltimore, 1997.

10. Hanssen AD. Cemented stems are requisite in revision knee replacement. Orthopedics 2004;27(9):990, 1003.

11. Bottner F, Laskin R, Windsor RE, Haas SB. Hybrid component fixation in revision total knee arthroplasty. Clin Orthop Relat Res 2006;446:127–31.

12. Mow CS, Wiedel JD. Noncemented revision total knee arthroplasty. Clin Orthop Relat Res 1994;309:110–15.

13. Mears S. Results of revision total knee arthroplasty. Curr Opin Orthop 2004;15(1):37–40.

14. Meneghini RM, Lewallen DG, Hanssen AD. Use of porous tantalum metaphyseal cones for severe tibial bone loss during revision total knee replacement. J Bone Joint Surg Am 2008;90(1): 78–84.

15. Whittaker JP, Dharmarajan R, Toms AD. The management of bone loss in revision total knee replacement. J Bone Joint Surg Br 2008;90(8):981–7.

16. Cameron HU. Clinical and radiologic effects of diaphyseal stem extension in noncemented total knee replacement. Can J Surg 1995;38(1):45–50.

17. Whiteside LA. Cementless reconstruction of massive tibial bone loss in revision total knee arthroplasty. Clin Orthop Relat Res 1989;248:80–6.

18. Chockalingam S, Scott G. The outcome of cemented vs. cementless fixation of a femoral component in total knee replacement (TKR) with the identification of radiological signs for the prediction of failure. Knee 2000;7(4):233–8.

19. Conditt, MA, Parsley BS, Alexander JW, Doherty SD, Noble PC. The optimal strategy for stable tibial fixation in revision total knee arthroplasty. J Arthroplasty 2004;19(7 Suppl 2):113–18.

20. Nakasone, CK, Abdeen A, Khachatourians AG, Sugimori T, Vince KG. Component alignment in revision total knee arthroplasty using diaphyseal engaging modular offset press-fit stems. J Arthroplasty 2008;23(8):1178–81.

21. Bourne RB, Finlay JB. The influence of tibial component intramedullary stems and implant-cortex contact on the strain distribution of the proximal tibia following total knee arthroplasty. An in vitro study. Clin Orthop Relat Res 1986;208:95–9.

22. Bobyn JD, Toh KK, Hacking SA, Tanzer M, Krygier JJ. Tissue response to porous tantalum acetabular cups: a canine model. J Arthroplasty 1999;14(3):347–54.

23. Volz RG, Nisbet JK, Lee RW, McMurtry MG. The mechanical stability of various noncemented tibial components. Clin Orthop Relat Res 1988;226:38–42.

24. Bobyn JD, Stackpool GJ, Hacking SA, Tanzer M, Krygier JJ. Characteristics of bone ingrowth and interface mechanics of a new porous tantalum biomaterial. J Bone Joint Surg Br 1999;81(5): 907–14.

25. Dennis DA, Berry DJ, Engh G, Fehring T, MacDonald SJ, Rosenberg AG, Scuderi G. Revision total knee arthroplasty. J Am Acad Orthop Surg 2008;16(8):442–54.

26. Mabry TM, Vessely MB, Schleck CD, Harmsen WS, Berry DJ. Revision total knee arthroplasty with modular cemented stems: long-term follow-up. J Arthroplasty 2007;22(6 Suppl 2):100–5.

27. Pellicci PM, Wilson PD Jr, Sledge CB, Salvati EA, Ranawat CS, Poss R, Callaghan JJ. Long-term results of revision total hip replacement. A follow-up report. J Bone Joint Surg Am 1985;67(4): 513–16.

28. Sierra RJ, Cooney WP 4th, Pagnano MW, Trousdale RT, Rand JA. Reoperations after 3200 revision TKAs: rates, etiology, and lessons learned. Clin Orthop Relat Res 2004;425:200–6.

29. Vince KG, Long W. Revision knee arthroplasty. The limits of press fit medullary fixation. Clin Orthop Relat Res 1995;317:172–7.

30. Shannon BD, Klassen JF, Rand JA, Berry DJ, Trousdale RT. Revision total knee arthroplasty with cemented components and uncemented intramedullary stems. J Arthroplasty 2003;18(7 Suppl 1):27–32.

31. Nazarian, DG, Mehta S, Booth RE Jr., A comparison of stemmed and unstemmed components in revision knee arthroplasty. Clin Orthop Relat Res 2002;404:256–62.

32. Haas SB, Insall JN, Montgomery W 3rd, Windsor RE. Revision total knee arthroplasty with use of modular components with stems inserted without cement. J Bone Joint Surg Am 1995;77(11):1700–7.

33. Peters CL, Erickson J, Kloepper RG, Mohr RA. Revision total knee arthroplasty with modular components inserted with metaphyseal cement and stems without cement. J Arthroplasty 2005;20(3):302–8.

34. Whaley AL, Trousdale RT, Rand JA, Hanssen AD. Cemented long-stem revision total knee arthroplasty. J Arthroplasty 2003;18(5):592–9.

35. Sheng PY, Konttinen L, Lehto M, Ogino D, Jämsen E, Nevalainen J, et al. Revision total knee arthroplasty: 1990 through 2002. A review of the Finnish arthroplasty registry. J Bone Joint Surg Am 2006;88(7):1425–30.

36. Ritter MA, Berend ME, Meding JB, Keating EM, Faris PM, Crites BM. Long-term followup of anatomic graduated components posterior cruciate-retaining total knee replacement. Clin Orthop Relat Res 2001;388:51–7.

37. Fehring TK, Odum S, Olekson C, Griffin WL, Mason JB, McCoy TH. Stem fixation in revision total knee arthroplasty: a comparative analysis. Clin Orthop Relat Res 2003;416:217–24.

38. Stern SH, Wills RD, Gilbert JL. The effect of tibial stem design on component micromotion in knee arthroplasty. Clin Orthop Relat Res 1997;345:44–52.

39. Jazrawi LM, Bai B, Kummer FJ, Hiebert R, Stuchin SA. The effect of stem modularity and mode of fixation on tibial component stability in revision total knee arthroplasty. J Arthroplasty 2001;16(6):759–67.

28 Management of Structural Defects in Revision Knee Arthroplasty: Femoral Side

Sandor Gyomorey[1], Paul T.H. Lee[2], and David J. Backstein[3]

[1]William Osler Health Center, Etobicoke General Hospital, Toronto, ON, Canada
[2]The Royal Orthopaedic Hospital, Birmingham, UK
[3]Mount Sinai Hospital, Toronto, ON, Canada

Case scenario

An active 69 year old man with history of remote right total knee arthroplasty (TKA) presents with increasing right knee pain and instability. On examination, the right knee is unstable to varus and valgus forces with good range of motion (ROM). The neurovascular examination is normal.

Importance of the problem

Among the major challenge of revision TKA is assessment and restoration of bony defects. Bone loss is often classified according to the Anderson Orthopaedic Research Institute (AORI) bone defect classification (Table 28.1).[1]

Defects may be characterized as contained or uncontained. *Contained defects* may be cavitary or central, representing loss of cancellous bone with intact cortical rim. *Uncontained defects* represent cancellous bone loss in addition to significant loss of surrounding supportive cortical bone. Uncontained defects may be *segmental*, involving the medial or lateral side of the femur, or *circumferential*, involving the entire bone.[2]

For patients with endstage knee arthritis, TKA is a common and successful procedure with 90% survivorship at more than 15 years follow-up.[3–5] It is estimated that from 1996 to 2030 the number of TKAs will increase by 85%, raising the annual rate to almost 500,000 in the United States.[6] The number of revision TKAs is also on the rise.[7–9] In 1995, 19,138 revision TKAs were performed in the US.[10] Coyte et al. estimated an annual increase of 14.1% for primary TKA and 19.3% for revision TKA.[11]

In the US the yearly costs for arthroplasty procedures are estimated at $10 billion.[12] A primary TKA has been estimated to cost $11,826, whereas a revision TKA cost nearly double that at $21,888.[12,13] Revision TKA requires longer operating times, costlier implants, additional materials, longer hospital stays, and longer periods of convalescence; it also has higher complication rates.[14]

Unfortunately, outcomes and success rates of revision TKA are not comparable with those for primary TKA.[15,16] Structural bone defects commonly contribute to the complexity of revision TKA.[17,18] The major etiologies of bone loss being: aseptic loosening, infection, osteolysis, stress shielding, wear and implant loosening.[19,20]

Top five questions

Diagnosis

1. How effective are radiographs and CT scans in assessing defect size?

Therapy/prognosis

2. How can smaller defects be managed?
3. How can large uncontained defects be managed?
4. What is the role of tumor prostheses in the treatment of massive defects?

Future direction

5. What is the role of trabecular metal in the treatment of defects?

Evidence-Based Orthopedics, First Edition. Edited by Mohit Bhandari.
© 2012 Blackwell Publishing Ltd. Published 2012 by Blackwell Publishing Ltd.

Table 28.1 AORI classification of bone defects

AORI type	Characteristic	Treatment
1	Intact structural bone (contained, minor defect): good cancellous bone at or near a normal joint-line level not compromising implant stability	Cement or morselized bone graft
2	Deficient structural (noncontained) bone: bone damage with loss of cancellous bone, which requires the use of cement fills, augments, or small bone grafts to restore the joint line	<5 mm: cement >5–10 mm: augmentation and bone grafts may be required
3	Severe structural (noncontained) bone loss with ligamentous instability: deficiencies that compromise major portion of either condyle with associated ligamentous dysfunction	Femoral defects >10–20 mm: A custom or stemmed (collateral constrained) component with a structural allograft is required or allograft-prosthesis composite

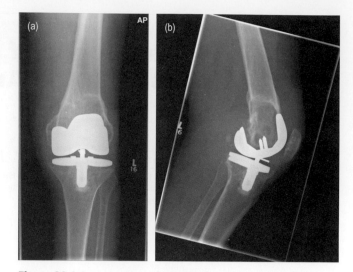

Figure 28.1 Representative radiographs of a 69 year old man with osteolysis around TKA implants. (a) AP and (b) lateral radiograph of TKA with femoral bone loss secondary to osteolysis.

Question 1: How effective are radiographs and CT scans in assessing defect size?

Case clarification
Although radiographs demonstrate the process of osteolysis, CT scans are more effective in demonstrating the extent of the defect, as seen in Figure 28.1 and Figure 28.2.

Relevance
Delineating the extent of osteolysis is essential for proper planning and management.

Current opinion
A thorough clinical assessment is essential prior to surgery to evaluate the patient's health status, with possible consultation from Internal Medicine and Anesthesia. The operative site is assessed for previous incisions and potential wound complications and work-up for infection is performed using blood work, imaging, and possibly joint aspiration.

Component loosening and position and degree and location of bone loss should be assessed with radiography and CT. The reason for failure should be established and a management plan formulated.

Finding the evidence
• PubMed: search terms "osteolysis," "radiographic," "evaluation," "total knee arthroplasty"

Quality of the evidence
Level II
• 1 prospective study[21]
• 1 cadaveric study[22]
• 2 retrospective studies[23–25]

Findings
Assessment of bone loss using routine radiographs is known to lead to underestimation and further imaging should be obtained including oblique views or CT to achieve reasonable prediction of defect size (Figures 28.1, Figure 28.2).[21–24] Agreement between plain radiographs and intraoperative assessment of bone loss has been shown to be fair, based on the AORI classification.[22] Also, in an analysis of 31 patients who had osteolytic lesions confirmed by multidetector CT, plain radiography detected only 17% of lesions.[25]

Recommendation
• Although plain radiographs can aid in the assessment of osteolysis, CT scans should be performed for more accurate delineation of defect size and location [overall quality: moderate]

Question 2: How can smaller defects be managed?

Case clarification
The defects seen in Figure 28.1 and Figure 28.2 appear to be a combination of contained and uncontained defects

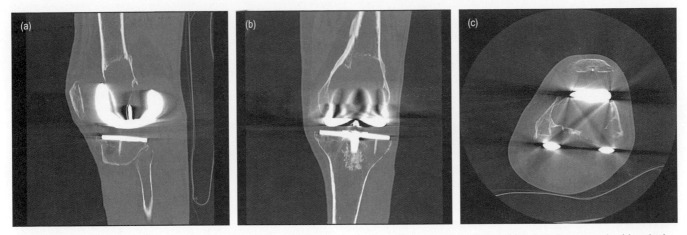

Figure 28.2 CT scan showing femoral bone loss due to osteolysis on cross-sectional imaging in the same 69 year old patient. Representative (a) sagittal, (b) coronal, and (c) axial images showing degree of bone loss.

and may require more than just cement or bone graft for stabilization.

Relevance

Defect size and character will determine the method of reconstruction for achievement of a stable joint.

Current opinion

Few studies report on treatment of femoral defects in TKA (Table 28.2). Contained defects are generally simpler to manage. Small contained defects can be addressed with impacted morselized bone graft or cement. Although the primary function of cement is to supply component fixation, small defects (<5 mm) may be filled with cement.[26,27] Cement provides inferior load transfer with poor fatigue properties,[28–30] however, and bone grafting is preferable to cement augmentation because of its biological advantage.[31,32]

Finding the evidence

- PubMed: search terms "osteolysis," "femoral," "defect," "small," "revision," "treatment," "total knee arthroplasty," "augmentation," "bone grafting"

Quality of the evidence

Level II
- 3 prospective studies[32,35,36]
- 3 retrospective studies[31,38,39]
- 1 case report[34]

Findings

The majority of studies assessing patients treated with morselized bone graft are reported in combined series for tibial/femoral reconstruction and report good outcomes.[2,32–35] Van Loon et al.[36] reported on a series of 22 patients treated for femoral defects with bone grafting and advocated the use of impacted morselized bone grafts for

contained and uncontained defects (up to 4–10 cm^3) in combination with cemented TKA.

Uncontained defects are more challenging. Small uncontained defects on the femoral side can be managed with metallic blocks or wedges. These metal inlays are fixed to the distal and posterior parts of the femoral component, providing a stable platform for support and allowing for rebuilding of condyles. Uncontained, segmental defects larger than 5 mm can be treated with metal augments; however, most systems have a limit of 20 mm for augment size. Radney et al.[37] recommended the use of cement for defects smaller than 5 mm, and metal augmentation for defects 5–10 mm. Hass et al.[38] have reported 83% survival at 8 years follow-up of distal femoral augments.

Interestingly, Hockman et al.[39] reported on a series of revision TKAs in which modular femoral augmentation was used in 35 knees. They found a trend towards increased failure rates (59%) in knees with less severe bone defects, which were revised with metal augmentation alone. They speculated that this might be a result of reduced surface area for bonding between host bone and implant and secondly due to lack of cancellous bone structure reducing the quality of the cement–bone bond.

Recommendation

- Small contained defects can be addressed with impacted morsellized bone graft or cement. Small uncontained defects on the femoral side can be managed with metallic blocks or wedges and may also require bone grafting for a successful outcome [overall quality: moderate]

Question 3: How can large uncontained defects be managed?

Case clarification

As the CT scans (Figure 28.2) indicate, bone grafting and augmentation may not be enough for reconstruction of the

Table 28.2 Treatment of femoral defects in TKA

Study	Number of femurs	Procedures	Level of evidence	Survivorship
Mow et al.[31]	7 femurs 1 segmental 4 cavitary 2 combined	Cavitary: Femoral head allograft Segmental/combination defects: size-matched allografts were used	Retrospective Level II	80% at 47 mnth
De Wall et al.[32]	14 femurs 6 contained 8 noncontained	Morselized graft vs. solid corticocancellous or solid cancellous graft and internal fixation	Prospective Level II	75% at 3 years
Ullmark et al.[34]	3 femurs contained	Impaction grafting and stem	Case report Level 4	100% at 18–28 mnth
Whiteside[35]	39 femurs	39 long-stem femoral component with morselized allograft	Prospective Level II	100% at 24 mnth
Van Loon et al.[36]	24 femurs 10 contained 14 uncontained	Morselized or trabecular or combined bone graft	Prospective Level II	92% at 38 mnth
Haas et al.[38]	23 femurs	Distal or posterior femoral augments	Retrospective Level II	83% at 8 yrs
Hockman et al.[39]	43 knees	35 modular femoral augments 17 femoral allografts with 6 also requiring augments	Retrospective Level II	79% at 8 yrs
Tsahakis et al.[40]	13 femurs	Distal femoral allograft	Retrospective Level II	100 % at 2.1 yrs
Stockley et al.[2]	16 femurs	Structural allografts and morselized bone 12 bulk allograft 3 morselized 1 strut allograft	Retrospective Level II	85% at 4.2years
Clatworthy et al.[41]	39 femurs all uncontained	Allograft-prosthesis composites and large structural allografts 31 segmental grafts 2 noncircumferential grafts 6 femoral head grafts	Prospective Level II	92% at 5yrs, 72% at 10 yrs
Ghazivi et al.[42]	12 femurs	Allograft-prosthesis composites and large structural allografts	Retrospective Level II	67% at 5 years
Backstein et al.[43]	61 knees site not specified	Allograft-prosthesis composites and large structural allografts	Retrospective Level II	79% at 5.4yrs
Mnaymneh et al.[45]	7 femurs	Allograft-prosthesis composites	Prospective" Level II	40 mnth 86% survival
Engh et al.[47]	13 femoral 8 femoral head 3 distal femoral	Femoral head and allograft-prosthesis composites	Retrospective Level II	100% at 50 months
Bauman et al.[48]	50 femurs uncontained	Allograft-prosthesis composites and large structural allografts: 33 femoral head 17 femoral head and allograft-prosthesis composites	Retrospective Level II	5 yr 80%

femoral defects in the case presented, and other methods of reconstruction may be needed to regain joint stability and function.

Relevance

Large defects are not only difficult to manage intraoperatively, but also present a great challenge with respect to functional outcomes and survival of the construct.

Current opinion

Very large segmental or circumferential uncontained defects may be beyond the capacity of augments and require structural allografts to rebuild a cortical rim to support the femoral component. These can be managed with an allograft–implant composite, which consists of a stemmed femoral component cemented to a corresponding distal femoral allograft. This allograft–implant composite is in turn fixed to host bone via a step-cut, with circlage wires and a bridging strut–allograft in some circumstances.

Finding the evidence

- PubMed: search terms "revision total knee arthroplasty," "femoral," "structural allograft," "outcomes"

Quality of the evidence

Level II
- 2 prospective studies[41,45]
- 6 retrospective studies[2,40,42,43,47,48]

Findings

In the short term, good success has been reported with 100% incorporation of structural allograft and improved functional outcomes.[40] Stockley et al.[2] showed union of the allograft to host in 16 of 16 cases at an average of 4.2 years follow-up. In the intermediate to long term, Clatworthy et al.[41] reported on treatment of large bony defects with structural allograft and showed that the rate of survival of the allografts was 92% (95% CI 89–95%) at 5 years and 72% (95% CI 69–75%) at 10 years. Similar findings were reported by Ghazavi et al.[42] on the management of uncontained defects larger than 3 cm using massive structural allograft. Their success rate was 77% at a mean of 50 months, with a Kaplan–Meier probability of graft survival at 5 years of 67%. Backstein et al.[43] reported satisfactory results after 5 years when using structural allograft in 58 patients with uncontained bone defects which were too large to be reconstructed with metal augments. Radiological allograft–host union was observed in 98%, although allograft-related complications required additional intervention in 21% with one graft nonunion and three graft resorptions. Parks and Engh have reported peripheral new bone formation at 41 months through histological assessment confirming the clinical assessment of graft incorporation.[44]

Using 14 large allografts for reconstruction of massive defects of the distal femur and proximal tibia in failed TKA, Mnaymneh et al.[45] reported 86% survival at an average of 40 month follow-up. Similar results were reported in treating 15 patients with large segmental, cavitary, or combination defects of the femur and/or tibia with an average follow-up of 47 months showing full incorporation of all allografts.[46]

Engh et al.[47] reported an 87% excellent to good clinical outcome of solid allografts for the treatment of femoral and/or tibial bone loss at an average of 50 months and suggested the use of stemmed femoral components when large structural allografts are used to protect the graft. More recently Bauman et al.[48] retrospectively reviewed outcomes of treatment of major bone defects for 74 patients treated with structural allografts and showed revision-free survival of grafts of 80.7% (95% CI 71.7–90.8) at 5 years and 75.9% (95% CI 65.6–87.8) at 10 years with good clinical outcomes.

Recommendation

- Massive bony defects can successfully be managed with structural allografts or allograft-implant composites [overall quality: moderate]

Question 4: What is the role of tumor prosthesis in the treatment of massive defects?

Case clarification

Our patient is 69 years old with an active lifestyle, so reconstructive measures have to focus on regaining his quality of life while keeping in mind the potential need for future revision.

Relevance

The patient's age, activity level, and health status play an important role in the choice of reconstructive method to optimize quality of life.

Current opinion

An alternative management option for massive distal femoral bone loss is distal femoral replacement with so-called "tumor prostheses." These devices provide immediate ligamentous and bony stability without the need for bone graft ingrowth. However, a high degree of constraint predisposes to early prosthetic loosening, particularly in active patients. It is therefore the authors' recommendation that distal femoral replacement implants be used for older, more sedentary individuals while allograft–implant composites should be the treatment of choice for younger, more active patients.

Finding the evidence

- PubMed: search terms "revision total knee arthroplasty," "tumor prosthesis," "hinged knee," "outcomes"

Quality of the evidence
Level II
- 4 retrospective studies[49–52]

Findings
Jones et al.[49] reported satisfactory results on 15 patients with a mean follow-up of 3.9 years using a mobile-bearing hinged prosthesis. The mean age at surgery was 63 years. There was no evidence of loosening, and complete bone apposition was seen in nearly all cases. Pour et al.[50] reported 79.6% survival at 1 year and 68.2% at 5 years with the use of rotating hinged knee implants in 44 cases with a mean follow-up of 4.2 years. The mean patient age at surgery was 71.8 years and the authors cautioned against the use of these prostheses in active or younger patients. Survivorships following megaprosthetic reconstruction of the distal femur are mainly available for patients post tumor surgery and reveal average implant survival of 85% at 3 years, 65% at 5 years, and 45% at 10 years.[51–52]

Recommendation
- Although proper assessment of bony defects is important when selecting the method of reconstruction, consideration must also be paid to potential future revision on an individual basis, factoring in comorbidities, functional demand, and life expectancy of the particular patient. Thus, restoration of bone stock becomes more important if future revision surgery is more likely [overall quality: moderate]

Question 5: What is the role of trabecular metal in the treatment of defects?

Case clarification
The defects in the sample case may be amenable to reconstruction using trabecular metal.

Relevance
Recently, encouraging results using new technologies have been utilized in the treatment of large distal femoral bony defects.

Current opinion
The use of trabecular metal may provide a means of structural reconstruction with a biologic advantage, allowing for faster bony ingrowth and reconstitution than structural allografts.

Finding the evidence
- PubMed: search terms "revision total knee arthroplasty," "new technology," "trabecular metal," "cones," "tantalum"

Quality of the evidence
Level II
- 1 prospective study[53]

Findings
Trabecular metal cones, constructed of highly porous tantalum with excellent ingrowth potential, are designed to fill defects. Radney and Scuderi[53] reported on the use of nine trabecular metal cones for severe defects in the intercondylar area at the metaphyseal–diaphyseal junction, with a mean follow-up of 10.2 months. The cones provided support for the femoral component and created a base onto which further femoral augmentation could be added. Radiographic evaluation revealed incorporation of the femoral cones into adjacent bone with no evidence of subsidence, change in position, or bone resorption.

Recommendation
- The use of trabecular metal in the reconstruction of femoral defects holds potential solution to the provision of structural support in combination with biologic ingrowth [overall quality: moderate]

Summary of recommendations

- Determination of the extent of femoral defects: CT scans are essential for more accurate delineation of defect size and location
- Treatment of small defects:
  - Small, contained: impacted morselized bone graft or cement.
  - Small, uncontained: metallic blocks or wedges and may also require bone grafting for a successful outcome
- Treatment of large defects: Massive bony defects can successfully be managed with structural allografts or allograft-implant composites
- Use of megaprosthesis to be considered in the low-demand patient with low likelihood of future revision surgery
- Use of trabecular metal may provide a potential solution to the provision of structural support in combination with biologic ingrowth

Conclusions

Massive bone defects are a reconstructive challenge in revision TKA. Management decisions for femoral-sided structural defects must take into account size and degree of containment. Contained defects may be treated using cement filling for very small areas or morselized allografts for larger defects. Most complex to treat are the large uncontained defects, which require structural allograft for reconstruction. Clinical outcomes are not on a level with primary TKA, although evidence suggests that allograft reconstruction has the potential to result in satisfactory outcomes. The use of megaprostheses should be reserved for patients with a low likelihood for revision surgery. The more active patients may benefit from newer technologies such as trabecular metal augmentation for large defects as an alternate to allograft reconstruction.

References

1. Engh G, Parks NL. The classification and treatment options of bone defects in revision knee surgery. Trans AAOS, 1994: 1–8.

2. Stockley M, McAuley JP, Gross AE. Allograft reconstruction in total knee arthroplasty. J Bone Joint Surg Br 1992;74:393–7.

3. Clarke HD, Scuderi GR. Revision total knee arthroplasty: planning, management, controversies, and surgical approaches. Instr Course Lect 2001;50:359–65.

4. Font-Rodriguez DE, Scuderi GR, Insall JN. Survivorship of cemented total knee arthroplasty. Clin Orthop Relat Res 1997;345: 79–86.

5. Windsor RE, Scuderi GR, Moran MC, Insall JN. Mechanisms of failure of the femoral and tibial components in total knee arthroplasty. Clin Orthop Relat Res 1989;248:15–20.

6. American Academy of Orthopaedic Surgeons. Musculoskeletal Conditions in the United States, 1999. www2.aaos.org/aaos/archives/bulletin/oct99/musculo.htm

7. Australian Orthopaedic Association. National Joint Replacement Registry, Annual Report 2008.

8. CJRR: Total Hip and Total Knee Replacements in Canada, Annual Report 2008.

9. The Swedish Knee Arthroplasty Register, Annual Report 2008.

10. Mendenhall S. Get the lowdown on orthopedic implants. Mater Manag Health Care 1996;5:30–2.

11. Coyte PC, Young W, Williams JI. Devolution on hip and knee replacement surgery? Can J Surg 1996;39:373–8.

12. Lavernia CJ, Drakeford MK, Tsao AK, Gittelsohn A, Krackow KA, Hungerford DS. Revision and primary hip and knee arthroplasty. A cost analysis. Clin Orthop 1995;311:136–41.

13. Healy WL, Finn D. The hospital cost and the cost of the implant for total knee arthroplasty. A comparison between 1983 and 1991 for one hospital. J Bone Joint Surg Am 1994;76:801–6.

14. NIH Consensus Development Panel on Total Hip Replacement. NIH consensus conference: total hip replacement. JAMA 1995; 273:1950–6.

15. Bartel DL, Burstein AH, Santavicca EA, Insall JN. Performance of the tibial component in total knee replacement. J Bone Joint Surg Am 1982;64:1026.

16. Donaldson WF, Sculco TP, Insall JN, Ranawat CS. Total condylar III knee prosthesis: long term follow-up study. Clin Orthop 1988;226:21.

17. Whiteside LA. Cementless revision total knee arthroplasty. Clin Orthop 1993;286:160.

18. Windsor RE, Insall JN, Sculco TP. Bone grafting of tibial defects in primary and revision total knee arthroplasty. Clin Orthop 1986;205:132.

19. van Loon CJ, Waal MC, Buma P, Verdonschot N, Veth RP. Femoral bone loss in total knee arthroplasty. A review. Acta Orthop Belg 1999;65:154.

20. Sharkey PF, Hozak WJ, Rothman RH, Shastri S. Jacoby Sm. Insall Award Paper. Why are total knee arthroplasties failing today? Clin Orthop Relat Res 2002;404:7–13.

21. Mulhall KJ, Ghamrawi HM, Engh GA. Radiographic prediction of intraoperative bone loss in knee arthroplasty revision. Clin Orthop 2006;446:51–8.

22. Nadaud MC, Fehring TK, Fehring K. Underestimation of osteolysis in posterior stabilized total knee arthroplasty. J Arthroplasty 2004;19:110–15.

23. Vyskocil P, Gerber C, Bamert P. Radiolucent lines and component stability in knee arthroplasty: standard versus fluoroscopically-assisted radiographs. J Bone Joint Surg Br 1999;81:24–6.

24. Miura H, Matsuda S, Okazaki K, et al. Validity of an oblique posterior condylar radiographic view for revision total knee arthroplasty. J Bone Joint Surg Br 2005;87:1643–6.

25. Reish TG, Clarke HD, Scuderi GR, Math KR, Scott WN. Use of multi-detector computed tomography for the detection of periprosthetic osteolysis in total knee arthroplasty. J Knee Surg. 2006;19(4):259–64.

26. Scuderi GR, Insall JN. Revision total knee arthroplasty with cemented fixation. Tech Orthop, 1993;7:96–105.

27. Faris PM. Autografting in total knee replacement. In: Insall JN, Scott WN, Scuderi GR, eds., Current Concepts in Primary and Revision Total Knee Arthroplasty, pp. 203–7. Lippincott-Raven, Philadelphia, 1996.

28. Dennis DA. Repairing minor bone defects: augmentation and autograft. Orthopedics 1998;21:1036–8.

29. Brooks PJ, Walker PS, Scott RD. Tibial component fixation in deficient tibial bone stock. Clin Orthop 1984;184:302–8.

30. Saha S, Pal S. Mechanical properties of bone cement: a review. J Biomed Mater Res 1984;18:435–62.

31. Mow CS, Wiedel JD. Structural allografting in revision total knee arthroplasty. J Arthroplasty 1996;11:235–41.

32. de Waal Malefijt MC, van Kampen A, Slooff TJ. Bone grafting in cemented knee replacement. 45 primary and secondary cases followed for 2–5 years. Acta Orthop Scand 1995;66(4):325–8.

33. Samuelson KM. Bone grafting and noncemented revision arthroplasty of the knee. Clin Orthop 1988;226:93–101.

34. Ullmark G, Hovelius L. Impacted morsellized allograft and cement for revision total knee arthroplasty: a preliminary report of 3 cases. Acta Orthop Scand 1996;67(1):10–12.

35. Whiteside LA. Cementless revision total knee arthroplasty. Clin Orthop Relat Res 1994;299:169–72.

36. van Loon CJ, Wijers MM, de Waal Malefijt MC, Buma P, Veth RP. Femoral bone grafting in primary and revision total knee arthroplasty. Acta Orthop Belg 1999;65(3):357–63.

37. Radnay CS, Scuderi GR. Management of bone loss: augments, cones, offset stems. Clin Orthop Relat Res 2006;446:83–92.

38. Haas SB, Insall JN, Montgomery W, Windsor RE. Revision total knee arthroplasty with use of modular components with stems inserted without cement. J Bone Joint Surg Am 1995;77:1700–1707.

39. Hockman D, Ammeen D, Engh GA. Augments and allografts in revision total knee arthroplasty: usage and outcome using one modular revision prosthesis. J Arthroplasty 2005;1:35–41.

40. Tsahakis PJ, Beaver WB, Brick GW. Technique and results of allograft reconstruction in revision total knee arthroplasty. Clin Orthop Relat Res 1994;303:86–94.

41. Clatworthy MG, Ballance J, Brick GW, Chandler HP, Gross AE. The use of structural allograft for uncontained defects in revision total knee arthroplasty: a minimum five-year review. J Bone Joint Surg Am 2001;83:404–11.

42. Ghazavi MT, Stockley I, Yee G, Davis A, Gross AE. Reconstruction of massive bone defects with allograft in revision total knee arthroplasty. J Bone Joint Surg Am 1997;79:17–25.

43. Backstein D, Safir O, Gross A. Management of bone loss: structural grafts in revision total knee arthroplasty. Clin Orthop Relat Res 2006;446:104–12.

44. Parks NL, Engh GA. Histology of nine structural bone grafts used in total knee arthroplasty. Clin Orthop Relat Res 1997;345:17–23.

45. Mnaymneh W, Emerson RH, Borja F, Head WC, Malinin TI. Massive allografts in salvage revisions of failed total knee arthroplasties. Clin. Orthop Relat Res 1990;260:144–53.

46. Mow CS, Wiedel JD. Structural allografting in revision total knee arthroplasty. J Arthroplasty 1996;11:235–41.

47. Engh GA, Herzwurm PJ, Parks NL. Treatment of major defects of bone with bulk allografts and stemmed components during total knee arthroplasty. J Bone Joint Surg Am. 1997;79:1030–9.

48. Bauman RD, Lewallen DG, Hanssen AD. Limitations of structural allograft in revision total knee arthroplasty. Clin Orthop Relat Res 2009;467(3):818–24.

49. Jones RE, Skedros JG, Chan AJ, Beauchamp DH, Harkins PC. Total knee arthroplasty using the S-ROM mobile-bearing hinge prosthesis. J Arthroplasty 2001;16:279–87.

50. Pour AE, Parvizi J, Slenker N, Purtill JJ, Sharkey PF. Rotating hinged total knee replacement: use with caution. J Bone Joint Surg 2007;89:1735–41.

51. Kawai A, Muschler GF, Lane JM, Otis JC, Healey JH. Prosthetic knee replacement after resection of a malignant tumor of the distal part of the femur. medium to long-term results. J Bone Joint Surg Am 1998;80(5):636–47.

52. Yasko AW, Rutledge J, Tolley S, Lin P, Weber KL. The Finn rotating hinge segmental knee prosthesis. Clinical results at 5–10 year follow up. Annual Meeting of the Musculoskeletal Tumor Society, Toronto, Ontario, Canada, April 26, 2002.

53. Radnay CS, Scuderi GR. Management of bone loss: augments, cones, offset stems. Clin Orthop Relat Res 2006;446:83–92.

29 Patellar Options in Revision Knee Arthroplasty

Hatem Al-Harbi and Paul Zalzal
McMaster University, Hamilton, ON, Canada

Case scenario

A 75 year old relatively active woman with a right total knee replacement 14 years ago complains of pain and instability in her right knee. She has difficulty ascending and descending stairs, requires a cane for walking, and can only walk for short distances. On examination, the right knee has an effusion and varus and valgus instability.

Relevant anatomy

Revision knee arthroplasty can consist of replacement of some or all of the existing components of a total knee replacement. It can include the revision, excision, or addition of a patellar component. These procedures can be complicated by reduced bone stock. This chapter will focus on the surgical options available for the patella during revision knee arthroplasty.

Importance of the problem

The number of total knee arthroplasties (TKAs) being performed in North America and around the world is increasing at a steady rate.[1-3] In addition, TKA is being used to treat endstage osteoarthritis in younger, more active people

compared to a decade ago. Many TKA recipients are still active members of the workforce, while others who may be retired expect to remain active throughout their later years. This combination of an increasing number of procedures and a younger, more active patient population will likely lead to an increased number of revision TKAs being performed, and some patients may require more than one revision in their lifetime. Currently, however, the functional outcome and survivorship of revision TKA are thought to be inferior to those of a primary TKA. In addition, the leading cause of failure of a primary TKA has been shown to be problems with the extensor mechanism.[4-6] Therefore treatment of the patella, which is an integral part of the knee extensor mechanism, is an important consideration during revision TKA. A better understanding of options available for the patella during revision TKA may serve to improve functional outcomes and survivorship of these procedures.

Although the patella and extensor mechanism play an important role in primary and revision TKA, there is a paucity of information available in the medical literature regarding how to treat the patella during revision TKA. A PubMed search for "patella and revision TKA" yielded only 47 results. There is little high-level evidence available, making it difficult to guide practice, and most of the review literature available reports on case series and expert opinion.[7] It is therefore necessary to develop a guide based on the best data available, butthe quality of the data must be scrutinized and highlighted.

Evidence-Based Orthopedics, First Edition. Edited by Mohit Bhandari.
© 2012 Blackwell Publishing Ltd. Published 2012 by Blackwell Publishing Ltd.

Top five questions

1. How can patellar problems in a TKA be preoperatively diagnosed?
2. Can an existing patellar implant be left in place at the time of revision TKA?
3. Should an unresurfaced patella be resurfaced during revision TKA?
4. What options are available for the patella in the presence of poor patellar bone stock?
5. Should an isolated patellar procedure be performed in a TKA with a loose patellar component and well-fixed tibial and femoral components?

Question 1: How can patellar problems in a TKA be preoperatively diagnosed?

Case clarification

The patient is complaining of anterior knee pain. Radiographs show the patella has been resurfaced and a lucency is detected at the interface between the patellar cement and the bone.

Relevance

Several options are available for the patella during revision TKA. The key to successful surgical outcome in revision TKA is identifying a clear cause for patient symptoms.[8] Therefore, it is important to have as much information as possible about the patella before the revision procedure is performed. This can help the surgeon choose which patellar option may be appropriate so that a proper preoperative plan can be achieved and the necessary equipment and components can be made available for the revision procedure.

Current opinion

A thorough history and physical examination with specific attention paid to the patella and the extensor mechanism is required for all patients undergoing a revision TKA. Infection needs to be ruled out if the surgeon is considering keeping a well-fixed patellar component. A full set of radiographs including skyline views should be obtained preoperatively to look for signs of loosening, fracture, and patellar maltracking. Bone scans can also be helpful.

Finding the evidence

• Cochrane, PubMed, and Ovid MEDLINE databases were searched with the following terms: "patella revision," "loose patella," "diagnosis of loose patella," "maltracking patella"

Quality of the evidence

• Level IV: 4

Findings

In order to perform an effective preoperative workup for a patient undergoing a revision TKA, it is important to be cognizant of the possible indications for revising a patella. These include a loose or worn patellar component, malpositioning of the patellar component, maltracking, poor implant design, periprosthetic patellar fracture, and in some cases anterior knee pain. History starts with gathering detailed information from the preoperative, perioperative, and postoperative periods around the initial TKA from the patient and any available medical records and previous operative notes. The physical examination starts with assessing gait, alignment, and extensor mechanism continuity. Palpation of the patella during active range of motion may detect the presence of patella subluxation or dislocation. Preoperative workup should include a complete blood count, C-reactive protein, erythrocyte sedimentation rate (ESR) and a joint aspirate for cell count, Gram stain, and culture which have been recommended for diagnosing prosthetic infection.[9] Imaging also plays an important role in identifying the etiology of patient symptoms. Features associated with patellar component loosening on radiograph include bone-cement radiolucency, increased bone density, trabecular collapse , fragmentation, and fracture.[10] A CT scan can add valuable information about femoral component rotation which may affect patellar tracking.[11]

Recommendation

• In order to diagnose patellar problems preoperatively, a thorough history, physical examination, blood work, and radiological workup is required [overall quality: low]

Question 2: Can an existing patellar implant be left in place at the time of revision TKA?

Case clarification

Review of the operative notes of the primary TKA indicate that the patella was resurfaced using a universal dome, all-polyethylene, onset patella. The preoperative radiographs do not suggest loosening of the patellar component.

Relevance

Surgical time, exposure, risk of fracture, and morbidity of revision TKA can be reduced by retaining an existing patellar component. In addition, patellar bone stock is preserved. However, disadvantages of retaining an existing patellar component include the fact that the component may be damaged or a geometric mismatch may occur between the patella and the femoral component, which could lead to increased polyethylene wear and pain.

Current opinion

Current opinion suggests that the majority of arthroplasty surgeons would leave a well-fixed, well-tracking, and well-articulating patella in place at the time of revision surgery.

Finding the evidence

- Cochrane, PubMed, and Ovid MEDLINE databases were searched with the following terms: "patella revision," "loose patella," "well-fixed patella," "metal-backed patella"

Quality of the evidence

- Level IV: 4
- Level V: 1

Findings

The results of patellar component revision have been reported by several authors. Barrack et al.[12] retrospectively compared the results of retention vs. revision of patellar components in 73 knees with a minimum and mean follow-up of 24 and 36 months respectively. In 34 cases a well-fixed and well-positioned patellar component with minimal to no surface damage was retained; 12 of these knees had metal-backed components. The remaining 39 cases involved patellar component revision for reasons such as loosening, wear, osteolysis, and malpositioning. For patients with metal-backed components, revision was undertaken only if the surgeon thought that the remaining bone stock would allow for implantation of another component. Both groups were assessed clinically and radiographically. The authors found no difference between the two groups. Lonner et al.[13] reviewed a series of revision TKAs that retained the all-polyethylene patella. They reported that 10% of patients had anterior knee pain at an average period of 7.3 years and concluded that retaining a well-positioned, stable all-polyethylene patellar component at the time of revision TKA can be successful, provided that the polyethylene has not oxidized. Manufacturing mismatch is acceptable with most contemporary designs, provided that the patellar component articulates appropriately with the femoral implant.

The type of patellar prosthesis (all-polyethylene vs. metal-backed) is thought to be an important variable. Most of the authors recommend revising the metal-backed prosthesis at the time of revision TKA if possible because of the high failure rates associated with metal-backed patellar components.[7,14-16]

Recommendations

- If the patella is an all-polyethylene design, well fixed, and articulates well with the revision femoral component it should be left in place [overall quality: low]
- If the patella is of a metal-backed design and there is good bone stock, it should be revised at the time of revision TKA even if it is well fixed [overall quality: low]

Question 3: Should an unresurfaced patella be resurfaced during revision TKA?

Case clarification

The patient is complaining of anterior knee pain. Radiographs and operative records indicate that the patella was not resurfaced during the initial TKA. Radiographs also suggest minimal joint space narrowing under the patella.

Relevance

There is no consensus in the orthopedic literature regarding whether or not to resurface the patella during primary TKA.[17] Therefore, it is possible to encounter a situation where a patient requires a revision TKA and the patella was not resurfaced. The decision whether or not to resurface the patella at the time of revision needs to be made.

Current opinion

Current opinion suggests that if a patient has anterior knee pain in the presence of a TKA with an unresurfaced patella, going to the operating room for the sole purpose of resurfacing the patella may be of some benefit. If the patient is undergoing revision TKA for another reason, such as loosening of the tibial or femoral components, and the patient is not complaining of anterior knee pain, the patella may be left unresurfaced.

Finding the evidence

- Cochrane, PubMed, and Ovid MEDLINE databases were searched with the following terms: "anterior knee pain," "unresurfaced patella"

Quality of the evidence

- Level IV: 4
- Level V: 1

Findings

There is very little information in the literature regarding whether or not to resurface an unresurfaced patella during a revision TKA. Deirmengian and Israelite recommend resurfacing an unresurfaced patella during revision TKA, but this appears to be expert opinion only and is not backed by clinical data.[18] However, there is some clinical data available regarding performing a revision procedure for a TKA with an unresurfaced patella and persistent anterior knee pain. Barrack reported on seven patients who underwent a secondary resurfacing of the patella: four of the seven patients continued to experience anterior knee pain.[19] Muoneke et al. reported on 20 patients who underwent a revision procedure to resurface only the patella for anterior knee pain and found that 44.4% reported some improvement.[20] Other investigators also reported poor outcome with secondary resurfacing procedures, based on retrospective reviews.[21] Karnezis et al. reported significant clinical improvement after secondary patellar resurfacing, however, the results were inferior to primary patellar resufacing.[22]

Recommendation

- If a patient has an unresurfaced patella and anterior knee pain with a TKA and no other etiology for pain, performing a secondary patellar resurfacing may be of some benefit [overall quality: low]

Question 4: What options are available for the patella in the presence of poor patellar bone stock?

Case clarification

Review of the radiographs suggest the patella is loose and the underlying bone stock is extremely poor.

Relevance

Revision of the patellar component in the presence of poor bone stock can be challenging and can lead to poor outcomes. With insufficient bone, it is difficult to achieve good fixation and the risk of patella fracture is increased.

Current opinion

If the bone stock is poor and the patellar component is loose, the component should be removed and patelloplasty should be performed to insure the remaining bone articulates as well as possible with the femoral component without catching or locking.

Finding the evidence

- Cochrane, PubMed, and Ovid MEDLINE databases were searched with the following terms: "patella revision," "loose patella," "poor bone stock," "patelloplasty," "patellectomy," "trabecular metal," "patellar bone graft"

Quality of the evidence

- Level IV: 9

Findings

Available surgical options to treat the bone-deficient patella include patelloplasty, patellectomy (partial or total), the use of a porous metal implant, and bone grafting procedures. Patellectomy has been shown to result in poor functional outcomes with persistent pain, quadriceps weakness, and extensor lag.[23,24] Patelloplasty usually results in better clinical outcomes than patallectomy. It consists of consists of removing the old implant and using a rongeur or high-speed burr to smooth out the remaining patellar bone. The results are still less than ideal, as shown by generally low knee scores and complications such as patellar maltracking, fracture, and avascular necrosis (AVN).[25–27] Bone grafting procedures have been described to address poor

patellar bone stock. Two such techniques have shown promising clinical results, possibly due to the restoration of patellofemoral biomechanics and quadriceps function.[28,29] These techniques appear to be technically demanding and are described by only a few authors. An emerging technology involves the use of a porous metal-backed implant with a polyethylene articulating surface. Early results suggest reasonable clinical results.[30,31]

Recommendations

- Patelloplasty is an option for treatment of a patella during revision TKA with poor patellar bone stock, however results are not ideal and may be associated with complications [overall quality: low]
- Patellectomy should be avoided due to poor functional outcomes, pain, and extensor lag [overall quality: low]
- Porous metal-backed implants represent a new technology with promising results [overall quality: low]

Question 5: Should an isolated patellar procedure be performed in a TKA with a loose patellar component and well-fixed tibial and femoral components?

Case clarification

The patient is complaining of anterior knee pain. Physical examination revealed an effusion and crepitus with range of motion. Radiographs and a bone scan suggest the tibial and femoral components are well fixed, but the cemented all-polyethylene patella appears to be loose.

Relevance

Extensor mechanism problems are the leading cause for revision TKA. Therefore, the situation may be encountered where the tibial and femoral components are well fixed and the patellar component is loose. Treating the patellar problem, such as revising or removing the patellar component, and leaving the femoral and tibial components in situ, is a technically easier and quicker procedure than revising all the components. However, the functional outcome and survivorship of isolated patellar revision needs to be determined.

Current opinion

Isolated patellar revision in the setting of a well-fixed tibia and femur is an attractive option due to the suspected reduced morbidity and quicker recovery compared to a revision procedure where all components are replaced. Furthermore, isolated patellar revision avoids the need for stemmed tibial and femoral components.

Finding the evidence

- Cochrane Database, PubMed, and Ovid MEDLINE were searched with the following terms "patella revision," "loose patella," "isolated patellar revision," "secondary patellar revision"

Quality of the evidence
• Level V: 5

Findings
Leopold et al.[32] investigated the success of isolated patellar component revision in 40 knees with a mean follow-up of 62 months. The authors found a 38% rate of subsequent failure of the patellar component with about half of these patients requiring further surgical intervention. Berry and Rand[33] found 83% of patients achieved good or excellent results, significant improvement in knee scores, and no definite radiographic loosening at an average of 3.5 years. However, this procedure is associated with a high rate of complications: 33% of patients had a significant complication and 19% of patients had reoperation for problems directly related to the patellar revision. Most common complications were patellar fracture and patellar instability. Parvize[25] found that individuals who had isolated patellar procedures had more pain and more reoperations compared with those who had a combined procedure with femoral revision. It is important to evaluate the rotation of the tibial and femoral components before deciding to do an isolated patellar revision.[34] Malrotation of either or both of these components can lead to patellar maltracking or anterior knee pain that would likely not be corrected with an isolated patellar procedure.

Recommendation
• Isolated patellar revision can be undertaken only after all other possible causes of patellar problems, such as femoral or tibial malrotation, have been ruled out, but a high complication rate has been reported [overall quality: low]

Summary of recommendations

• In order to diagnose patellar problems preoperatively, a thorough history, physical examination, blood work, and radiological workup is required
• If the patella is an all-polyethylene design, well fixed, and articulates well with the revision femoral component it should be left in place
• If the patella is of a metal-backed design, it should be revised at the time of revision TKA
• If a patient has an unresurfaced patella and anterior knee pain with a TKA and no other etiology for pain, performing a secondary patellar resurfacing may be of some benefit
• Patelloplasty is an option for treament of a patella during revision TKA with poor patellar bone stock, however results are not ideal and may be associated with complications

• Patellectomy should be avoided due to poor functional outcomes, pain, and extensor lag
• Porous metal-backed implants represent a new technology with promising results
• Isolated patellar revision can be undertaken only after all other possible causes of patellar problems, such as femoral or tibial malrotation, have been ruled out, but a high complication rate has been reported

---

Conclusion

Several options are available for dealing with the patella during a revision TKA. Unfortunately, there is a lack of high-level evidence in the literature to help guide the surgeon in deciding which option will result in the best functional outcome. Most of the published data available is based on retrospective case series.

References

1. Vesseley M, Harmsen WS, Schleck C, et al. James A. Rand Award Paper: a population based study of trends in use of total hip and knee arthroplasty. J Arthroplasty 2007;22:303.
2. Kurtz S, Mowat F, Ong K, et al. Prevalence of primary and revision total hip and knee arthroplasty in the United States from 1990 through 2002. J Bone Joint Surg Am 2005;87:1487.
3. Surgeons. AAOS: primary total hip and total knee arthroplasty projections to 2030. Am Acad Orthop Surg 1998;7.
4. Thornhill TS, Hood RW, Dalziel RE, Ewald FC, Insall JN, Sledge CB. Knee revision in failed non-infected total knee athroplasty—the Robert B. Brigham Hospital and Hospital for Special Surgery experience. Orthop Trans 1982;6:368–9.
5. Aglietti P, Buzzi R, De Felice R, Giron F. The Insall-Burstein total knee arthroplasty in osteoarthritis: a 10-year minimum follow-up. J Arthroplasty 1999;14:560–5.
6. Boyd Jr AD, Ewald FC, Thomas WH, Poss R, Sledge CB. Long-term complications after total knee arthroplasty with or without resurfacing of the patella. J Bone Joint Surg Am 1993;75:674–81.
7. Rorabeck CH, Mehin R, Barrack R. Patellar options in revision total knee arthroplasty. Clin Orthop Relat Res 2003;416:84–92.
8. Mont MA, Serna FK, Krockow KA, et al. Exploration of radiographically normal total knee arthroplasties for unexplained pain. Clin Orthop 1996;331:216–20.
9. Gonzalez MH, Mekhail AO. The failed total knee arthroplasty: Evaluation and etiology. J Am Acad Orthop Surg 2004;12:436–46.
10. Berend ME, Ritter MA, Keating EM, et al. The failure of all-polyethylene components in total knee arthroplasty. Clin Orthop Relat Res 2001;388:105–11.
11. Berger RA, Crossett LS, Jacobs JJ, Rubash HE. Malrotation causing patellofemoral complications after total knee arthroplasty. Clin Orthop 1998;356:144–53.
12. Barrack RL, Rorabeck C, Partington P, et al. The results of retaining a well-fixed patellar component in revision total knee arthroplasty. J Arthroplasty 2000; 15:413–17.

13. Lonner JH, Mont MA, Sharkey PF, et al. Fate of the unrevised all-polyethylene patellar component in revision total knee arthroplasty. J Bone Joint Surg Am 2003;85: 56–59.

14. Bayley JC, Scott RD, Ewald FC, Holmes GB: Failure of the metal-backed patellar component after total knee arthroplasty. J Bone Joint Surg Am 1998;70:668–74.

15. Kraay MJ, Darr OJ, Salata MJ, Goldberg VM: Outcome of metal-backed cementless patellar components: The effect of implant design. Clin Orthop 2001;392:239–44.

16. Levi N, Kofoed H. Early failure of metal-backed patellar arthroplasty. J Bone Joint Surg Br 1994;76:675.

17. Burnett RS, Bourne RB. Indications for patellar resurfacing in total knee arthroplasty. J Bone Joint Surg Am 2003;85:728–45.

18. Brown TE, Cui Q, Mihalko WM, Saleh KJ. Patellar revision/reconstruction. In: Deirmengian GK, Israelite CL, eds, Arthritis and Arthroplasty: The Knee, pp. 247–256. Saunders Elsevier, Phildelphia, 2009.

19. Barrack RL, Bertot AJ, Wolfe MW, et al. Patellar resurfacing in total knee arthroplasty: A prospective, randomized, double blind study with five to seven years of follow-up. J Bone Joint Surg Am 2001; 83A:1376–81.

20. Muoneke HE, Khan AM, Giannikas KA, Hagglund E, Dunningham TH. Secondary resurfacing of the patella for persistent anterior knee pain after primary kneearthroplasty. J Bone Jt Surg Br 2003;85:675–8.

21. Mockford BJ, Beverland DE. Secondary resurfacing of the patella in mobile-bearing total knee arthroplasty. J Arthroplasty 2005;20 :898–902.

22. Karnezis IA, Vossinakis IC, Rex C, Fragkiadakis EG, Newman JH. Secondary patellar resurfacing in total knee arthroplasty: results of multivariate analysis in two casematched groups. J Arthroplasty 2003;18:993–8.

23. Laskin RS. Management of the patella during revision total knee arthroplasty. Orthop Clin North Am 1998;29:355–60.

24. Busfield BT, Ries MD. Whole patellar allograft for total knee arthroplasty after previous patellectomy. Clin Orthop Relat Res 2006;450:145–9.

25. Parvizi J, Seel MJ, Hanssen AD, Berry D, Morrey BF: Patellar component resection arthroplasty for the severely compromised patella. Clin Orthop 2002;397:356–61.

26. Pagnano MW, Scuderi GR, Insall JN. Patellar component resection in revision and reimplantation total knee arthroplasty. Clin Orthop 1998;356:134–8.

27. Barrack RL, Matzkin E, Ingraham R, et al. Revision knee arthroplasty with patella replacement versus bony shell. Clin Orthop 1998;356:139–43.

28. Hanssen AD: Bone-grafting for severe patellar bone loss during revision knee arthroplasty. J Bone Joint Surg Am 2001;83: 171–6.

29. Buechel FF. Patellar tendon bone grafting for patellectomized patients having total knee arthroplasty. Clin Orthop 1991;271: 72–8.

30. Nelson CL, Lonner JH, Lahiji A, et al.:Use of trabecular metal patella for marked patellar bone loss during revision total knee arthroplasty. J Arthroplasty 2003;18(suppl 1):37–41.

31. Nasser S, Poggie RA. Revision and salvage patellar arthroplasty using a porous tantalum implant. J Arthroplasty 2004;19: 562–72.

32. Leopold SS, Silverton CD, Barden RM, et al. Isolated revision of the patellar component in total knee arthroplasty. J Bone Joint Surg Am 2003;85:41–7.

33. Berry DJ, Rand JA: Isolated patellar component revision of total knee arthroplasty. Clin Orthop 1993;286:110–15.

34. Barrack RL, Schrader T, Bertot A, Wolfe MW, Myers L. Component rotation and anterior knee pain after total knee arthroplasty. Clin Orthop 2001;392:46–55.

30 Total Shoulder Replacement vs. Hemiarthroplasty in the Treatment of Shoulder Osteoarthritis

Olivia Y.Y. Cheng and Michael D. McKee
St.Michael's Hospital, University of Toronto, Toronto, ON, Canada

Case scenario

A 65 year old healthy woman presents with right shoulder stiffness and pain. Physical examination shows that she is neurologically intact. She is able to externally rotate to neutral with pain at extremes of motion. Rotator cuff examination is normal (Figure 30.1).

Relevant anatomy

The glenohumeral joint is the most important joint of the shoulder. It is a spheroidal joint. The glenohumeral contact occurs between the spherical humeral head and a shallow glenoid fossa. The shallow glenoid articular surface allows for large range of motion at the expense of stability. The normal glenohumeral motion is dependent on the shape of the bony architecture and the soft tissue balances. There are static and dynamic restraints of shoulder motion. Static restraints include articular anatomy, glenoid labrum, negative pressure, capsule, and ligaments. Dynamic restraints include the rotator cuff muscles and the biceps tendon.

In primary osteoarthritis (OA) of the glenohumeral joint, the cartilage wears away and the bones begin to grind against each other, leading to pain and stiffness. It is commonly associated with osteophyte formation and eccentric posterior glenoid wear. The osteoarthritic shoulder demonstrates increased stress of the posterior glenoid which leads to increased bone remodelling and posterior subluxation.[1] The goal in the treatment of severe osteoarthritis is to eliminate pain, to restore shoulder soft tissue balance and improve function.[2]

Importance of the problem

Musculoskeletal disorders have a significant impact on the world's population. In the United States, musculoskeletal conditions account for 131 million patient visits per year, costing society about $215 billion. The incidence of primary OA of the shoulder is not as common as that involving the knee or the hip and is estimated to be less than 1% of the population.[3] Although shoulder OA is not as common as other locations, loss of function can lead to depression, anxiety, activity limitations, and job performance problems.[4]

Over 11,000,000 hits appear on Google when the search term "shoulder osteoarthritis" is entered. The vast number of websites targeted at this topic and the lack of quality control of the information provided indicates a need for a preappraised, evidence-based guide for patients and surgeons.

Top six questions

Diagnosis

1. How much do the radiological findings correlate with clinical symptoms?

Evidence-Based Orthopedics, First Edition. Edited by Mohit Bhandari.
© 2012 Blackwell Publishing Ltd. Published 2012 by Blackwell Publishing Ltd.

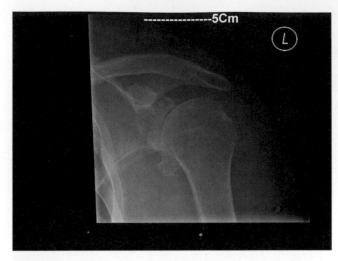

Figure 30.1 Radiograph of right shoulder with endstage osteoarthritis.

2. CT scan vs. plain radiographs as tools in estimating posterior glenoid wear and glenoid bone stock?

Treatment

3. What is the outcome of total shoulder arthroplasty (TSA) vs. humeral head replacement (HHR) for the treatment of shoulder OA?
4. What is the survivorship of TSA in young, active patients?

Complications

5. What are the results of converting a HHR to TSA after glenoid erosion?
6. How do the rates of revision in HHR compare with TSA?

Question 1: How much do the radiological findings correlate with clinical symptoms?

Case clarification
In this 65 year old woman who complains of shoulder pain and stiffness, the radiographs are consistent with severe shoulder OA. How do the radiological findings correlate with her clinical presentation?

Relevance
Surgeons use radiographs as part of the assessment in patients with shoulder OA. What degree of correlation is there between radiographic findings and patient's clinical symptoms?

Current opinion
Most surgeons would agree that TSA and HHR are the main treatments for patients with primary OA of the shoul-

der who experience pain. Radiographic findings are used as adjuncts in making this decision, but alone are not sufficient to justify surgical intervention.

Finding the evidence
• PubMed (www.ncbi.nlm.nih.gov/pubmed/): sensitivity search using keywords "radiological parameters" AND "shoulder osteoarthritis" as well as "symptoms" AND "functions"

Quality of the evidence
Level III 1 retrospective review

Findings
Kircher et al. retrospectively examined 120 standardized radiographs of patients with advanced shoulder OA using the true AP and axillary views.[5] Seventy-five of these patients had a complete record that documented pain, active and passive range of motion, and the Constant Score. The result of this study showed that the joint space width was not correlated with pain or range of motion. The size of the osteophytes were negatively correlated with range of motion. The size of the caudal humeral osteophyte was a predictive factor for function. Overall, the primary clinical feature, pain, as the main indication for surgery, is not related to radiological parameters.

Recommendation
• Radiographic parameters of osteoarthritis do not correlate with degree of pain. Therefore, isolated radiographic shoulder OA is not an indication for operative intervention in the absence of symptoms [overall quality: low]

Question 2: CT scan vs. plain radiographs as tools in estimating posterior glenoid wear and glenoid bone stock?

Case clarification
Examination of this 65 year old woman with primary shoulder OA and pain showed decreased range of motion and pain. The radiographic findings were consistent with severe OA. The axillary view shows posterior glenoid wear. Do we need a CT scan of the glenoid for preoperative planning for this patient?

Relevance
Abnormalities of glenoid version have been associated with abnormal loading of the glenoid component and poor clinical results. CT scans provide better imaging of the glenoid than plain radiographs, at higher cost and radiation exposure.

Current opinion
Pathological processes involving OA of the shoulder leads to severe geometric bony changes. Most surgeons would

obtain a CT scan of the glenoid for preoperative planning of TSA in patient with radiographic images showing medial erosion of the glenoid to the level of the coracoid, or posterior glenoid wear on the axillary view.

Finding the evidence

• PubMed (www.ncbi.nlm.nih.gov/pubmed/): sensitivity search using keywords "computed tomography" AND "radiography" as well as "shoulder arthroplasty"

Quality of the evidence

Level III

• 2 retrospective reviews

Findings

Nyffeler et al. compared conventional radiographs with CT scans for the measurement of glenoid version.[6] Three independent observers retrospectively analyzed the radiographs and CT scans of 50 patients. The results from this study indicated poor correlation between plain radiographs and CT scans in measuring glenoid version. Glenoid retroversion was overestimated on plain radiographs in 86% of the cases, with a maximum difference of 21° (mean 6.4°) compared with the values measured on CT scan. This study indicated that glenoid version cannot be determined accurately on standard axillary radiographs, either preoperatively or postoperatively.

A previous study by Friedman et al. also demonstrated the usefulness of CT images in determining glenoid morphology.[7] In that study, CT was done preoperatively on 20 shoulders with severe arthritic change. This was compared with CT scans of 63 shoulders without evidence of arthritis. In the group with severe arthritis the mean glenoid orientation was 11° of retroversion (range 2–32° of retroversion). The glenoid version in the control group was 2° of anteversion (range 14° of anteversion to 12° of retroversion). The difference between the two groups was significant (p < 0.0001). This study concluded that in severe shoulder arthritis, the glenoid is retroverted and CT scan accurately reveals the extent and pattern of erosion.

Morphologic changes such as humeral head subluxation, humeral and glenoid version, glenoid tilt, or changes in dimensions are generally assessed by measuring geometric parameters on medical images. Successful TSA is highly dependent on the quality and morphology of the glenoid bone. Therefore, accurate preoperative assessment of the bone quality can help surgeons in planning the surgery.

Recommendation

• In patients with severe osteoarthritis of the shoulder with bone loss on the glenoid side, CT scanning is useful in assessing glenoid version, glenoid tilt, and glenoid bone stock when planning a TSA procedure [overall quality: low]

Question 3: What is the outcome of HHR vs. TSA for the treatment of shoulder OA?

Case clarification

HHR (Figure 30.2) and TSA (Figure 30.3) are the two primary methods of treatment for shoulder OA. What is the outcome of HHR vs. TSA?

Relevance

There is ongoing controversy concerning the ideal management of primary glenohumeral OA[8–12]

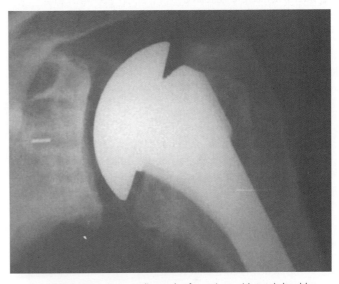

Figure 30.2 Postoperative radiograph of a patient with total shoulder replacement.

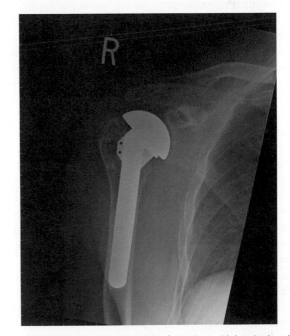

Figure 30.3 Postoperative radiograph of a patient with hemiarthroplasty of the shoulder.

Current opinion

Most surgeons would perform TSA for primary osteoarthritis of the shoulder with an intact rotator cuff and adequate glenoid bone stock.

Finding the evidence

• PubMed (www.ncbi.nlm.nih.gov/pubmed/): sensitivity search using keywords "total shoulder arthroplasty" AND "hemiarthroplasty of the shoulder" as well as "shoulder arthritis" AND "outcome"

Quality of the evidence

Level I
• 1 prospective randomized trial
• 2 systemic reviews and meta-analysis

Level II
• 1 prospective comparative study

Findings

In HHR the humeral articular surface is replaced with a stemmed humeral component coupled with a humeral head. TSA involves replacement of the humeral articular surface as well as replacement of the glenoid articular surface with a polyethylene glenoid component. HHR of the shoulder is technically easier to perform. For patients who have undergone HHR, pain and the radiographic appearance of subchondral sclerosis and joint space narrowing may develop, leading to revision surgery. TSA is associated with risk of glenoid loosening. However, multiple studies have shown that the risk of symptomatic glenoid loosening is low and overall revision surgery for TSA is significantly lower than HHR (especially when current cemented all-polyethylene glenoid components are used).[12–22]

Edwards et al. conducted a large multicenter retrospective study (n = 690) comparing HHR vs. TSA in the treatment of primary glenohumeral OA,[11] with an average follow-up of 43 months. The following parameters were significantly better for patients receiving TSA: active forward elevation (p < 0.0005), active external rotation (p < 0.015), Constant Score (p < 0.0005), incidence of radiolucent lines around the humeral component (p < 0.001), and humeral implant migration (p < 0.033). Good or excellent results were seen in 86% of HHR and 94% of TSA. Overall, this study shows that TSA is more effective than HHR in patients with primary glenohumeral osteoarthritis with no significant increase in complication rate associated with glenoid resurfacing.

In contrast, Lo et al. found no significant difference in quality of life measures between HHR and TSA in a prospective, randomized study with minimum 2 year follow-up.[19] In this study 42 patients with OA of the shoulder were randomized to receive a HHR or a TSA. All patients were evaluated preoperatively and at 6 weeks and 3, 6, 12, 18, and 24 months postoperatively with both subjective and objective parameters. The primary outcome measure in this study was the Western Ontario Osteoarthritis of the Shoulder (WOO) index. Significant improvements in disease-specific quality of life were seen at 2 years for both the TSA and HHR. There were no significant differences in the WOO score between the two groups. However, there was a trend toward superior results in the TSA group. It is possible that there was a beta error due to the study being underpowered (n = 42).

In a recent meta-analysis comparing HHR with TSA for the treatment of primary glenohumeral OA, Radnay et al. identified 23 studies published between 1966 and 2004, (total of 1952 patients), and a mean follow-up of 43.3 months.[23] The results showed significantly greater pain relief (p < 0.0001), forward elevation (p < 0.0001), gain in forward elevation (p < 0.0001), gain in external rotation (p = 0.0002), and patient satisfaction (p < 0.0001) with TSA compared with HHR. Furthermore, the TSA group had a significantly lower revision rate than the HHR group. Overall, the conclusion reached by this study was that TSA is the surgical treatment of choice for patients with end-stage primary glenohumeral OA.

Recommendation

• In recent years, multiple studies show that with proper patient selection TSA is superior to HHR for patients with endstage primary shoulder OA [overall quality: high]

Question 4: What is the survivorship of TSA in young, active patients?

Case clarification

A 50 year old man, active and healthy, has severe primary OA of the shoulder. Before he proceeds with a TSA he would like to know what the survivorship of TSA is in individuals like him.

Relevance

TSA is a reliable treatment option for patients with primary osteoarthritis. Many surgeons are reluctant to perform TSA on young and middle-aged patients because of the risk of late implant loosening.

Current opinion

• Most orthopedic surgeons would caution against doing a TSA in a young, active patient due to the risk of implant loosening and possible future revision surgeries.

Finding the evidence

• PubMed (www.ncbi.nlm.nih.gov/pubmed/): sensitivity search using keywords "total shoulder arthroplasty" AND "young patient" as well as "total shoulder arthroplasty" AND "outcome"

Quality of the evidence
Level II
- 1 prospective comparative study

Level III
- 1 retrospective review

Findings
Sperling et al. published a retrospective series of 98 patients younger than 50 years old who underwent HHR or TSA between 1976 and 1985 with a mean follow-up of 12.3 years.[10] Both TSA and HHR resulted in significant long-term pain relief and improvement in function. The estimated survival of the HHR prostheses was 92% (86–98%) at 5 years, 83% (75–93%) at 10 years, and 73% (59–88%) at 15 years. The estimated survival of the TSA was 97% (92–100%) at 5 years, 97% (91–100%) at 10 years, and 84% (70–100%) at 15 years. The data from this study indicates that TSA provides marked long-term relief of pain and improvement in motion; however, nearly half of all young patients who have a shoulder arthroplasty have an unsatisfactory result according to a strict rating system. Care should be exercised when either a HHR or a TSA is offered to patients who are 50 years old or less.

A recent prospective study done by Raiss et al., looking at TSA in young and middle-aged patients with glenohumeral OA, showed that third-generation TSA is a viable method of treatment with a low complication rate and excellent mid-term results.[24] They studied 21 patients less than 60 years old (mean age 55 years) with primary shoulder OA treated with either HHR or TSA. At a minimum of 5 years follow-up there were no revisions. Significant improvements in Constant scores, pain relief, power, activity, mobility, and range of motion were noted at a mean follow-up of 7 years. This study showed the patient satisfaction rate after TSA was 95% with significant relief from pain and improvement in range of motion. For young and middle-aged patients with OA, third-generation TSA is a viable treatment method with low rate of complications and excellent mid-term results.

Recommendations
- TSA is a safe method of treatment for middle-aged active patients with primary OA of the shoulder in patients who are more than 50 years old [overall quality: moderate]
- Caution needs to be exercised when performing TSA in active patients who are less than 50 years old [overall quality: moderate]

Question 5: What is the result of converting hemiarthroplasty into TSA after glenoid erosion?

Case clarification
A 65 year old woman with endstage OA of the shoulder would like to know if HHR converted to TSA would have the same result as a primary TSA.

Relevance
For patients who had HHR for primary glenohumeral OA, the glenoid can undergo progressive erosion over time (Figure 30.4). This often leads to conversion to TSA at a later date. What are the results of revision of HHR to TSA?

Current opinion
Most orthopedic surgeons would agree that patients undergoing revision surgery from HHR to TSA after failed HHR due to glenoid arthrosis do not do as well as patients who underwent primary TSA.

Finding the evidence
- PubMed (www.ncbi.nlm.nih.gov/pubmed/): sensitivity search using keywords "shoulder hemiarthroplasty" AND "revision surgery" as well as "total shoulder arthroplasty" AND "outcome"

Quality of the evidence
Level III
- 1 retrospective review

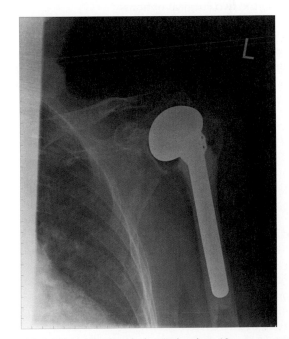

Figure 30.4 Patient with shoulder hemiarthroplasty 10 years ago now showing evidence of glenoid erosion.

Findings

The revision of HHR to TSA for glenoid arthrosis is not as successful as primary TSA for glenohumeral OA. Carroll et al. identified 16 consecutive patients who underwent revision TSA for failed HHR.[25] The mean interval from the time of HHR to revision TSA was 3.5 years. All patients had significant glenoid arthrosis on radiograph. They found that 47% of patients had an unsatisfactory clinical result at a mean of 5.5 years after the revision and one-third had incomplete pain relief after the conversion of failed HHR to TSA. Furthermore, HHR did not preserve glenoid bone stock, with posterior and superior glenoid wear evident in many patients. In addition, many of these patients had contractures of the anterior capsule and the subscapularis. The combined bony and soft tissue abnormalities made revision surgery much more challenging.

Recommendation

• After assessing the evidence, we do not recommend HHR as the first line of treatment for primary OA of the shoulder due to its high rate of revision and the inferior results of the revision surgeries when compared to primary TSA.

Question 6: How do the rates of revision in HHR compare with TSA?

Case clarification

A 65 year old woman with severe OA of the shoulder understands that both HHR and TSA are options for treating her shoulder. However, how do the revision rates differ between the two surgical options?

Relevance

For primary OA of the shoulder, both HHR and TSA are treatment options. Each has its own advantages and disadvantages. So how do the rate of revision between these two procedures compare?

Current opinion

Most surgeons feel that revision surgery involving conversion of HHR to TSA for glenoid arthrosis is higher than revision surgery involving TSA for glenoid loosening. This is especially true with modern cemented all-polyethylene pegged glenoid components.

Finding the evidence

• PubMed (www.ncbi.nlm.nih.gov/pubmed/): sensitivity search using keywords "total shoulder arthroplasty" AND "revision surgery" as well as "hemiarthroplasty of the shoulder"

Quality of the evidence

Level I

• 2 randomized control trials
• 2 systemic review and meta-analyses

Findings

Gartsman et al. performed a randomized prospective study comparing TSA with HHR in patients with shoulder OA.[26] In this study 51 patients were randomized to be treated with either TSA (27 shoulders) or HHR (24 shoulders) and were evaluated at a mean of 35 months postoperatively. The TSA group had significant improvements in pain relief and internal rotation compared to the HHR group. There were no revisions in the TSA procedures. Three shoulders that had been treated with a HHR were revised to TSA secondary to increased pain and glenoid wear.

Bryant et al. published a systemic review and meta-analysis comparing HHR and TSA in patients with shoulder OA.[15] This study included 112 patients (50 received HHR and 62 received TSA) with a minimum of 2 years of follow-up, and 10 patients from the HHR group crossed over to the TSA group because of excess pain or stiffness. There were no revisions in the TSA group.

A recent meta-analysis looking at HHR vs. TSA examined 23 studies involving 1952 patients.[23] Only 80 of 1238 TSAs (6.5%) required revision surgery for any cause. Of the TSAs that used metal-backed glenoids, 6.8% required revision. However, the revision rate for loosening in TSAs with all-polyethylene glenoids was only 1.7%. Meanwhile, 10.2% of HHRs required additional surgical procedures for any cause; 8.1% of HHRs required conversion to TSA because of pain. The difference in the rate of revision surgery was significantly in favor of TSA.

Recommendation

• TSA has a lower rate of revision surgery than HHR, especially when cemented all-polyethylene glenoid components are used [overall quality: high]

Summary of recommendations

• Isolated radiographic shoulder OA is not an indication for operative intervention in the absence of symptoms
• CT scan is useful in assessing glenoid version, glenoid tilt, and glenoid bone stock when planning a TSA procedure
• TSA outperforms HHR for the treatment of primary shoulder OA in terms of pain relief, range of motion, and patient satisfaction. In addition, the revision rate for TSA is significantly lower than for HHR
• TSA is a safe method of treatment for middle-aged active patients with primary OA of the shoulder in patients who are older than 50
• Caution needs to be exercised when performing TSA in active patients who are younger than 50 years old
• After assessing the evidence, we do not recommend HHR as the first line of treatment for primary OA of the shoulder due to its high rate of revision and the inferior

results of the revision surgeries when compared to primary TSA

• TSA has a lower rate of revision surgery than HHR, especially when cemented all-polyethylene glenoid components are used

References

1. Buchler P, Ramaniraka NA, Rakotomanana LR, et al. A finite element model of the shoulder: application to the comparison of normal and osteoarthritic joints. Clin Biomech (Bristol, Avon) 2002;17(9–10):630–9.

2. Caniggia M, Fornara P, Franci M, et al. Shoulder arthroplasty. Indications, contraindications and complications. Panminerva Med 1999;41(4):341–9.

3. Marx RG, McCarty EC, Montemurono TD, et al., Development of arthrosis following dislocation of the shoulder: a case-control study. J Shoulder Elbow Surg 2002;11(1):1–5.

4. Memel DS, Kirwan JR, Sharp DJ, et al. General practitioners miss disability and anxiety as well as depression in their patients with osteoarthritis. Br J Gen Pract 2000;50(457):645–8.

5. Kircher J, Morhard M, Magosch P, et al. How much are radiological parameters related to clinical symptoms and function in osteoarthritis of the shoulder? Int Orthop 2010;34(5):677–81.

6. Nyffeler RW, Jost B, Pfirrmann CW, et al. Measurement of glenoid version: conventional radiographs versus computed tomography scans. J Shoulder Elbow Surg 2003;12(5):493–6.

7. Friedman RJ, Hawthorne KB, Genez BM. The use of computerized tomography in the measurement of glenoid version. J Bone Joint Surg Am 1992;74(7):1032–7.

8. Rodosky MW, Bigliani LU. Indications for glenoid resurfacing in shoulder arthroplasty. J Shoulder Elbow Surg 1996; 5(3):231–48.

9. Haines JF, Trail IA, Nuttall D, et al. The results of arthroplasty in osteoarthritis of the shoulder. J Bone Joint Surg Br 2006;88(4): 496–501.

10. Sperling, JW, Cofield RH, Rowland CM, Minimum fifteen-year follow-up of Neer hemiarthroplasty and total shoulder arthroplasty in patients aged fifty years or younger. J Shoulder Elbow Surg 2004;13(6):604–13.

11. Edwards TB, Kadakia NR, Boulahia A, et al. A comparison of hemiarthroplasty and total shoulder arthroplasty in the treatment of primary glenohumeral osteoarthritis: results of a multicenter study. J Shoulder Elbow Surg 2003;12(3):207–13.

12. Adams JE, Sperling JW, Schleck CD, et al. Outcomes of shoulder arthroplasty in Olmsted County, Minnesota: a population-based study. Clin Orthop Relat Res 2007;455:176–82.

13. Angst F, Pap G, Mannion AF, et al., Comprehensive assessment of clinical outcome and quality of life after total shoulder arthroplasty: usefulness and validity of subjective outcome measures. Arthritis Rheum 2004;15;51(5):819–28.

14. Boorman RS, Kopjar B, Fehringer E, et al. The effect of total shoulder arthroplasty on self-assessed health status is comparable to that of total hip arthroplasty and coronary artery bypass grafting. J Shoulder Elbow Surg 2003;12(2):158–63.

15. Bryant D, Litchfield R, Sandow M, et al. A comparison of pain, strength, range of motion, and functional outcomes after hemiarthroplasty and total shoulder arthroplasty in patients with osteoarthritis of the shoulder. A systematic review and meta-analysis. J Bone Joint Surg Am 2005;87(9):1947–56.

16. Buchner M, Eschbach N, Loew M. Comparison of the short-term functional results after surface replacement and total shoulder arthroplasty for osteoarthritis of the shoulder: a matched-pair analysis. Arch Orthop Trauma Surg 2008;128(4):347–54.

17. Orfaly RM, Rockwood CA, Jr., Esenyel CZ, et al. A prospective functional outcome study of shoulder arthroplasty for osteoarthritis with an intact rotator cuff. J Shoulder Elbow Surg 2003;12(3):214–21.

18. Torchia ME, Cofield RH, Settergren CR. Total shoulder arthroplasty with the Neer prosthesis: long-term results. J Shoulder Elbow Surg 1997;6(6):495–505.

19. Kay SP, Amstutz HC, Shoulder hemiarthroplasty at UCLA. Clin Orthop Relat Res 1988;228:42–8.

20. Krepler P, Wanivenhaus AH, Wurnig C. Outcome assessment of hemiarthroplasty of the shoulder: a 5-year follow-up with 4 evaluation tools. Acta Orthop 2006;77(5):778–84.

21. Lo IK, Litchfield RB, Griffin S, et al. Quality-of-life outcome following hemiarthroplasty or total shoulder arthroplasty in patients with osteoarthritis. A prospective, randomized trial. J Bone Joint Surg Am 2005;87(10):2178–85.

22. Pfahler M, Jena F, Neyton L, et al. Hemiarthroplasty versus total shoulder prosthesis: results of cemented glenoid components. J Shoulder Elbow Surg 2006;15(2):154–63.

23. Radnay CS, Setter KJ, Chambers L, et al. Total shoulder replacement compared with humeral head replacement for the treatment of primary glenohumeral osteoarthritis: a systematic review. J Shoulder Elbow Surg 2007;16(4):396–402.

24. Raiss P, Aldinger PR, Kasten P, et al. Total shoulder replacement in young and middle-aged patients with glenohumeral osteoarthritis. J Bone Joint Surg Br 2008;90(6):764–9.

25. Carroll RM, Izquierdo R, Vazquez M, et al. Conversion of painful hemi-arthroplasty to total shoulder arthroplasty: long-term results. J Shoulder Elbow Surg. 2004;13(6):599–603.

26. Gartsman GM, Roddey TS, Hammerman HS, Shoulder arthroplasty with or without resurfacing of the glenoid in patients who have osteoarthritis. J Bone Joint Surg Am 2000;82(1):26–34.

31 Cemented vs. Uncemented Fixation in Shoulder Arthroplasty

Shahryar Ahmadi[1] and Christian Veillette[2]

[1]University of Arkansas for Medical Sciences, Fayetteville, AR, USA
[2]Toronto Western Hospital, University Health Network and University of Toronto, Toronto, ON, Canada

Case scenario

A 65 year old man who is right-hand dominant and a semi-retired chartered accountant presents with progressively increasing left shoulder pain and decreased range of motion. He complains of pain with any range of motion of his shoulder and has noted difficulty golfing. He has difficulty sleeping at night due to shoulder pain. On examination, his active and passive range of motion is forward elevation to 100°, abduction to 60°, and external rotation to neutral. There is abundant grinding and catching with motion. He is neurovascularly intact. Relevant radiographs are shown in Figure 31.1.

Relevant anatomy

Shoulder arthritis is a condition in which the cartilage that normally provides a smooth surface over the humeral head and glenoid is lost. The cartilage loss can result from either primary or secondary causes such as trauma, inflammatory disease, infection, rotator cuff disease, instability, or avascular necrosis of humeral head. Patients with shoulder arthritis often have coexisting synovial joint pathology, including bursitis, synovitis, loose bodies, labral tears, osteophytes, and capsular contractures. The final common clinical pathway is disabling pain, decreased range of motion, and functional limitations. Joint replacement surgery is the most reliable treatment for advanced shoulder osteoarthritis.

The angle between the humeral neck and shaft is about 130°. The humeral head is retroverted 20–40° relative to the epicondylar axis. The glenoid in the resting position has an average of 5° superior tilt and 7° retroversion (range from 10° anteversion to 10° retroversion). The glenoid fossa provides a shallow socket in which the humeral head articulates. It is composed of the bony glenoid and the glenoid labrum. The fibrocartilaginous labrum provides a 50% increase in the depth of the concavity. The glenoid has an average depth of 9 mm in the superoinferior direction and 5 mm in the anteroposterior direction with an intact labrum.

Importance of the problem

The shoulder is the third most common joint for replacement. Cofield et al. reported a rate of 10.1 per 100,000 person-years for shoulder arthroplasty from 1996 to 2000 in Olmsted County, Minnesota. In contrast, the rates for hip and knee replacement were 125 and 60.8 per 100,000 respectively.[1]

Since the first shoulder arthroplasty by Pean in 1893, there has been a significant improvement in both implant design and technique. Based on the Nationwide Inpatient Sample database, 12,758 total shoulder arthroplasties (TSAs) were performed in the US from 1990 to 2000.[2] In addition, a steady increase has been shown in the age- and sex-adjusted annual operative incidence rate of 1.4 per 100,000 person-years in 1976–1980 to 10.1 per 100,000 person-years in 1996–2000.[1] This increased use of shoulder arthroplasty was mainly due to increased use for osteoarthritis (OA).

Shoulder arthroplasty for OA is very effective in improving pain, function, and patient satisfaction.[3] Boorman et al. showed that improvement in self-assessed health status is comparable to total hip arthroplasty and coronary artery bypass grafting.[4]

Evidence-Based Orthopedics, First Edition. Edited by Mohit Bhandari.
© 2012 Blackwell Publishing Ltd. Published 2012 by Blackwell Publishing Ltd.

(a)

(b)

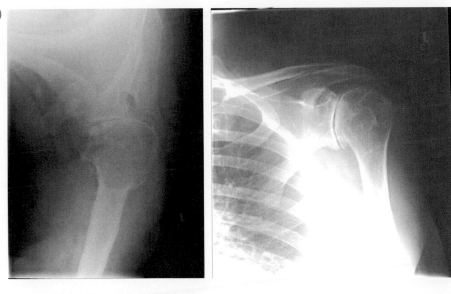

Figure 31.1 Standard AP radiograph (a) demonstrates endstage osteoarthritis with joint space narrowing, subchondral sclerosis, inferior humeral head osteophyte. Axillary radiograph (b) shows flattening of humeral head, joint space narrowing and posterior glenoid wear.

Top nine questions

Diagnosis

1. Is there a role for CT scan/MRI in preoperative planning?

Therapy

2. What is the relative effect of a cemented vs. uncemented humeral component on the functional outcome of patients with shoulder OA?
3. Is there a role for the use of antibiotic-impregnated cement?
4. What is the optimal approach to a cemented humeral component?
5. What is the optimal approach to an uncemented humeral component?
6. What is the optimal approach to cementing a glenoid component?
7. What is the relative effect of all-polyethylene vs. metal-backed glenoid component?

Prognosis

8. Is postoperative management different for cemented vs. uncemented arthroplasty?
9. Is there a significant difference in survival of cemented vs. uncemented arthroplasty?

Question 1: Is there a role for CT scan in preoperative planning?

Clarification

The patient's radiographs shows severe OA of the left shoulder. There is mild posterior glenoid erosion on the axillary view. A CT scan accurately shows the amount of glenoid bone loss and its correct version.

Relevance

Glenoid component loosening is one of the most common reasons for revision surgery after TSA.[5-7] Malposition of the glenoid component increases the risk of glenoid component loosening.[8-11]

Current opinion

Current opinion suggests that the majority of surgeons use CT scan for preoperative assessment of glenoid bone stock and more accurate assessment of version if an axillary radiograph shows any evidence of erosion in the glenoid.

Finding the evidence

- PubMed, with search terms: "glenoid loosening" AND "total shoulder arthroplasty," "glenoid version" AND "total shoulder arthroplasty," "complication of total shoulder arthroplasty," "preoperative CT scan AND total shoulder arthroplasty"

Quality of the evidence

- 3 biomechanical studies
- 3 basic science studies

Findings

Effect of glenoid component version in TSA. Three different biomechanical studies showed that:
- Every 4° change in version caused a 2° change in the force vector away from the center of glenoid[8]
- Retroversion was worse than anteversion, and superoinferior misalignment was worse than anteroposterior[9]
- Glenoid retroversion induced a posterior displacement of the glenohumeral contact point during internal and external rotation, inducing a significant increase of stress

within the cement mantle (+326%) and within the glenoid bone (+162%)[10]

Accuracy of plain radiograph compared to CT scan in assessing glenoid version
- The medial border of scapula cannot be seen in axillary view (mean visible length 4.9 cm) and thus it will be difficult to define the true scapular axis. Also glenoid version (n = 50 patients) varied from 11° of anteversion in extension to 7° of retroversion in flexion[12]
- The glenoid version angle measured from the three-dimensional (3-D) CT imaging (12 normal cadaveric scapula) was within $1.0 \pm 0.7°$ (mean ± SD) of those from the actual specimen (95% CI <2.2° for all observers)[13]
- Surgical decisions that were made on the basis of two-dimensional (2-D) data differed from those that were made on the basis of 3-D data in 37 of 96 cases (39%)[14]

Recommendation
- Pattern and extent of glenoid bone loss and glenoid version can be most accurately assessed by 3-D CT imaging [overall quality: high]

Question 2: What is the relative effect of a cemented vs. uncemented humeral component on the functional outcome of patients with shoulder OA?

Clarification
The patient wishes to proceed with a TSA. Should a cemented or uncemented humeral component be used to optimize functional outcome?

Relevance
The survivorship of the humeral component in TSA has been reported as 86.7% (95% CI 84.2–89.4) at 15 years and 82.8% (95% CI 78.5–87.5) at 20 years.[15] Revision of an uncemented humeral stem is often easier than a cemented humeral stem. Bone ingrowth into the proximal porous coating of uncemented humeral stems may provide improved survivorship and functional outcome. Based on these factors, should uncemented TSA be performed in younger patients? Is there any significant difference in functional outcome after shoulder arthroplasty between cemented and uncemented humeral components?

Current opinion
Current opinion suggests that the majority of surgeons preferentially use an uncemented humeral component in the management of shoulder OA in patients in North America. Implant manufacturers have preferentially developed and marketed uncemented implants over recent years.

Finding the evidence
- PubMed, with search terms: "cemented versus uncemented humeral component" AND "total shoulder arthroplasty," "cemented versus uncemented humeral component"

Quality of the evidence
Level I
- 1 prospective randomized study

Findings
In a prospective randomized study, Litchfield et al. compared cemented (n = 80 patients) with uncemented (n = 81) humeral components (Bigliani/Flatow, Zimmer) for TSA. They showed a significant difference in WOOS score at postoperative intervals of 12, 18, and 24 months (p = 0.009, 0.001, 0.028 respectively) in favor of the cemented humeral component. Also they noticed better strength (3 mo p = 0.038, 12 mo p = 0.036, 18 mo p = 0.051, 24 mo p = 0.053) and forward flexion (6 mo p = 0.031, 12 mo p = 0.04) in the cemented group. Operative time was significantly less for the uncemented group (C = 2.26 ± 0.63 h; U = 1.69 ± 1.9 h, p = 0.03). The authors concluded that a cemented humeral component provides better quality of life, strength, and range of motion than an uncemented humeral component.[16]

Recommendation
To best of our knowledge, this is the only level I study that has compared the functional outcome after cemented vs. uncemented humeral component fixation. The major limitation of this study is that results can only be applied to the use of the Zimmer BF implant and are not necessarily generalizable to all uncemented humeral components. In addition, this study only reports on the short term outcome and we do not know if the results can be extrapolated to long term follow-up.
- The authors recommend that all of the factors, including potential difference in functional outcome, ease of revision, survivorship, and complications, be discussed with the patient. Also the patient's age, expectations, functional level, and proximal humeral bone quality must be considered. The final decision should be individualized on the basis of these parameters [overall quality: low]

Question 3: Is there a role for the use of antibiotic-impregnated cement?

Clarification
The patient wishes to proceed with a TSA. Should antibiotics be added to the cement for the glenoid component and/ or the humeral component?

Relevance
The addition of antibiotics to cement can potentially affect the properties of the cement and subsequent fixation. In addition, antibiotics may decrease infection rates but increase the risk of developing antibiotic-resistant bacteria.

Current opinion

Current opinion suggests that the majority of North American surgeons use antibiotic-impregnated cement if cement is utilized for glenoid or humeral component fixation in TSA.

Finding the evidence

• PubMed, with search terms: "antibiotic cement" AND "total shoulder arthroplasty"

Quality of the evidence

Level I
• 1 prospective randomized study

Level II
• 1 prospective randomized study
• 1 review study

Findings

A prospective randomized study of 1688 total hip replacements in Sweden with a follow-up of 10 years did not show any significant difference between the systemic antibiotic group and the gentamicin-impregnated cement group ($p < 0.05$).[17]

A prospective randomized study of 401 total hip and knee arthroplasties in two British centers with a follow-up of 2 years, did not show any significant difference between the systemic cefuroxime group and the cefuroxime-impregnated cement group.[18]

Recommendation

To the best of our knowledge, there are no studies that evaluate the use of antibiotic-impregnated cemented for TSA. The reviewed studies are from total hip and knee arthroplasty and therefore we are uncertain whether the conclusions are applicable in TSA.
• In conclusion, there is no evidence to justify using antibiotic-impregnated cement in TSA [overall quality: low][17–19]

Question 4: What is the optimal approach to a cemented humeral component?

Relevance

Does first-, second-, or third-generation cementing technique or use of cement restrictor make any significant difference in complication, component survival or functional outcome?

Current opinion

Current opinion shows that all—first-, second-, or third-generation—cementing techniques are being used by surgeons. The use of cement restrictors for humeral component cementing is not routine. The presence of a poor cement mantle and early postoperative radiolucent lines may lead to higher loosening rates.

Finding the evidence

• PubMed, with search terms: "cement technique" AND "total shoulder arthroplasty," "cement technique" AND "humeral component"

Quality of the evidence

There are no studies comparing cementing techniques or the use of cement restrictors for shoulder arthroplasty.

Recommendation

There are a few case reports of radial nerve palsy due to cement extrusion after using a cemented humeral component.[20] However, there is no evidence whether using a cement restrictor or different cementing technique affects the risk of this complication. In addition, there is no evidence that cementing techniques affect the survivorship of the humeral component [overall quality: low].

Question 5: What is the optimal approach to an uncemented humeral component?

Relevance

Is there any evidence to support the use of hydroxyapatite (HA) coated compared with non-HA-coated implants or press-fit compared with porous ingrowth fixation for uncemented humeral components?

Current opinion

Current opinion suggests that HA-coated, non-HA-coated, press-fit, and porous ingrowth implants are all commonly used for uncemented humeral component fixation.

Finding the evidence

• PubMed, with search terms: "hydroxyapatite" AND "total shoulder arthroplasty," "hydroxyapatite coated humeral component," "ingrowth humeral component," "press fit humeral component," "humeral fixation press fit," "humeral fixation porous ingrowth"

Findings

There is no evidence to show that a specific method of uncemented humeral component fixation provides improved implant survivorship.

Recommendation

• Surgeons need to be aware of the lack of comparative studies that evaluate different methods of uncemented humeral component fixation

Question 6: What is the optimal approach to cementing a glenoid component?

Clarification

How should the glenoid be prepared for cementing? Should the cement be pressurized?

Relevance

Preparation and cementing technique have very important implication for outcome.

Current opinion

Current opinion suggests that the majority of surgeons pressurize the cement using a variety of techniques and there is a lack of consensus on glenoid preparation methods.

Finding the evidence

• PubMed, with search terms: "optimal cementing technique" AND "glenoid," "glenoid preparation," "glenoid cemented fixation"

Quality of the evidence

Level I
• 1 prospective randomized study

Nonclinical studies
• 3 biomechanical studies

Findings

In a prospective randomized study, Edwards et al. compared the immediate postoperative periglenoid radiolucencies between three glenoid-drying techniques (n = 71 patients). They prepared the glenoid with thrombin-soaked gel foam compresses, gas lavage, and saline solution lavage with sponge drying. The mean total radiolucent line score was 0.63 (p = 0.94), with no significant difference among the three groups (p = 0.89).[21]

In a biomechanical study on glenoid cement mantle, Terrier et al. demonstrated that, cement thickness less than 1 mm weakens the cement mantle and puts excessive peak stress at the bone–cement interface, around the back-keel edges. Also, thickening of the cement mantle rigidifies the cemented implant and increases the stress at the bone–cement interface and the underlying bone. They identified an ideal value of 1 mm for cement mantle to avoid both excessive cement fatigue and fatigue of the bone–cement interface.[22]

A biomechanical study by Nyffeler et al. compared two cementing techniques for glenoid component fixation. In the first group they put cement on the back of the glenoid component and into the peg-receiving holes of the glenoid and pressurized them with a syringe. In the second group, they applied cement just into the peg-receiving holes of

glenoid and pressurized them with finger pressure. They assessed all of the specimens with microCT scan. There was an intact cement mantle around all 12 pegs (100%) in first group and an incomplete cement plug in 7 of 15 pegs (47%) in second group.[23]

In a cadaver study Hassan et al. compared syringe pressurization (SP) with weephole technique (WH) and modified weephole technique (MWH). Both WH and MWH techniques increase cement mantle volume around individual pegs and decrease the amount of glenoid face cement compared to conventional SP. Whether this improves the clinical outcome and survivorship requires further study.[24]

Recommendation

• On the basis of current evidence we recommend saline solution lavage with sponge drying for glenoid preparation, and also pressurizing glenoid cement with a syringe associated with application of cement on the back of glenoid component and 1 mm cement mantle thickness [overall quality: moderate]

Question 7: What is the relative effect of all-polyethylene vs. metal-backed glenoid component?

Clarification

There are two option for glenoid component fixation—cemented all-polyethylene glenoid components and uncemented metal-backed glenoid components.

Relevance

There is a significant difference in survival of these two components.

Current opinion

Current opinion suggests that the majority of surgeons use all-polyethylene glenoid components.

Finding the evidence

• PubMed, with search terms: "metal backed glenoid," "cemented" AND "uncemented glenoid"

Quality of the evidence

Level I
• 1 prospective double-blind randomized study

Level IV
• 2 case series

Findings

In a prospective double-blind randomized study of cemented polyethylene vs. uncemented metal-backed glenoid component (n = 39) with a 3 years follow-up,

Boileau et al. showed 20% (4 cases) loosening of metal-backed implant vs. 0% of polyethylene glenoid components (p < 0.001).[25]

In a review of 83 metal-backed glenoid components with 9.5 years follow-up, Cofield et al. showed a 5 year survival of 79.9% (95% CI 71.6–89.3%), and a 10-year survival of 51.9% (95% CI 41.0–65.8%).[26]

In a review of 147 metal-backed glenoid components with 7.5 years follow-up, Martin et al. showed a 5 year survival of 95%, and a 10 year survival of 85%. These authors report a higher failure rate of metal-backed glenoid compared to a previous report of polyethylene glenoid.[27]

Recommendation
• On the basis of current evidence we recommend use of a cemented all-polyethylene glenoid component [overall quality: moderate]

Question 8: Is postoperative management different for cemented vs. uncemented arthroplasty?

Clarification
There are several rehabilitation protocols after TSA.

Relevance
There is no study suggesting different protocol for cemented vs. uncemented TSA.

Current opinion
Current opinion suggests that the majority of surgeons set the postoperative rehabilitation protocol based on the following factors:
• Underlying pathology and preoperative function of shoulder
• Surgical approach
• Quality of component fixation and soft tissue repair
• Quality of bone and soft tissue, including rotator cuff
• Presence of intra-/postoperative complication
• Patient factors: age, functional level, comorbidities, cooperation, etc.

Finding the evidence
• PubMed, with search terms: "post operative management" AND "total shoulder arthroplasty," "rehabilitation" AND "total shoulder arthroplasty," "physiotherapy" AND "total shoulder arthroplasty"

Quality of the evidence
Level V
• 1 expert opinion

Findings
Millett et al. in their article about rehabilitation after TSA emphasized the importance of underlying pathology and

tissue healing time frame as a base for rehabilitation protocol after surgery.[28]

Recommendation
There is inadequate evidence to support different rehabilitation protocols for cemented vs. uncemented TSA.
• We recommend that the surgeon consider the six factors outlined above and tailor the protocol accordingly [overall quality: low]

Question 9: Is there a significant difference in survival of cemented vs. uncemented humeral component fixation in shoulder arthroplasty?

Clarification
The two options for humeral component fixation in shoulder arthroplasty are cement fixation and uncemented tissue ingrowth or press-fitted fixation.

Relevance
Loosening of the humeral component is rarely a cause for revision in shoulder arthroplasty. There is no long-term comparative level I evidence to justify the use of cemented or uncemented (either press-fit or ingrowth) for humeral component fixation. However, each option has its own advantages and disadvantages.

Current opinion
Current opinion suggests that the majority of surgeons use uncemented humeral component fixation when possible.

Finding the evidence
• PubMed, with search terms: "survival" AND "total shoulder arthroplasty," "outcome" AND "total shoulder arthroplasty"

Quality of the evidence
Level I
• 1 prospective randomized study

Level IV
• 4 case series

Findings
In a review of 1584 shoulder arthroplasties, Cil et al. reported no significant difference in survivorship (HR 0.79; 95% CI 0.22–2.83; p = 0.72) between uncemented and cemented Neer II implants.[15] For the Cofield 1 humeral component, survivorship was significantly increased for cement fixation relative to fixation without cement (HR 0.33; 95% CI 0.13–0.81; p = 0.02). Overall, there was an increased survivorship across all implants (Neer II, Cofield I and II) for cement fixation compared to a component without cement fixation (HR 0.37; 95% CI 0.18–0.76; p = 0.007).

In a review of 37 uncemented shoulder replacements with a mean follow-up of 9.2 years (range 5.8–13.6 years), Verborgt et al. reported 0% loosening.[29]

In a review of 730 cemented shoulder arthroplasty and 570 uncemented shoulder arthroplasty from different centers, Cofield reported 6 implants with radiographic and 0 implants with clinical evidence of humeral component loosening in the cemented group compared with 63–70 implants with radiographic evidence and 2 implants with clinical evidence of humeral component loosening in the uncemented group.[30]

In a prospective randomized study of 26 total shoulder replacements in patients with rheumatoid arthritis with 2 year follow-up, Rahme et al. reported no loosening or difference in micromotion between cemented and uncemented groups.[31]

In a review of 431 shoulder arthroplasty with an average follow-up of 4.2 years, Cofield et al. reported no significant difference in complication rate between cemented and uncemented humeral stems in shoulder arthroplasty.[7]

Recommendation

Based on current evidence, the result of new designs of uncemented (tissue ingrowth) humeral component fixation is similar to cemented fixation. The choice between the use of a cemented or uncemented humeral component, should be individualized based on patient and diagnostic factors.[15]
- There is currently insufficient evidence to recommend the routine use of a single method of fixation; however, in younger patients with good bone quality uncemented humeral fixation is recommended [overall quality: moderate]

Summary of recommendations

- Pattern and extent of glenoid bone loss and glenoid version can be most accurately assessed by 3-D CT imaging
- 3-D CT imaging is not recommended for routine use
- We do not recommend routine use of antibiotic-impregnated cement in primary TSA
- There are a few case reports of radial nerve palsy due to cement extrusion after using a cemented humeral component.[20] However, there is no evidence whether using a cement restrictor or different cementing technique affects the risk of this complication. In addition, there is no evidence that cementing techniques affect the survivorship of the humeral component
- Surgeons need to be aware of the lack of comparative studies that evaluate different methods of uncemented humeral component fixation
- We recommend saline solution lavage with sponge drying for glenoid preparation and also pressurizing glenoid cement
- We recommend that cement fixation of an all-polyethylene glenoid component be used for glenoid resurfacing

- The patient's age, expectations, functional level, and proximal humeral bone quality must be considered in the selection of method of humeral component fixation
- We recommend that the surgeon consider the six factors outlined on p. 275 and tailor the protocol accordingly
- In younger patients with good bone quality, uncemented humeral fixation is recommended

Conclusion

In conclusion, advanced imaging modalities such as 2-D and 3-D CT scans are valuable in selected cases with significant and/or asymmetric glenoid erosion to improve glenoid component placement. There is sufficient evidence to recommend the use of cement fixation over tissue ingrowth fixation for the glenoid component. There are no clear-cut indications for cement fixation vs. uncemented tissue ingrowth fixation for the humeral component other than those intuitively based on bone quality and perceived ease of revision.

References

1. Adams JE, Sperling JW, Hoskin TL, Malton III LJ, Cofield RH. Shoulder arthroplasty in Olmsted County, Minnesota, 1976–2000: A population-based study. J Shoulder Elbow Surg 2006;15: 50–5.
2. Jain NB, Higgins LD, Guller U, Pietrobon R, Katz JN. Trends in the epidemiology of total shoulder arthroplasty in the United States from 1990–2000. Arthritis Rheum 2006;55: 591–7.
3. NorrisTR, Iannotti JP. Functional outcome after shoulder arthroplasty for primary osteoarthritis: a multicenter study. J Shoulder Elbow Surg 2002;11:130–5.
4. Boorman RS, Kopjar B, Fehringer E, Churchill RS, Smith K, Matsen III FA. The effect of total shoulder arthroplasty on self-assessed health status is comparable to that of total hip arthroplasty and coronary artery bypass grafting. J Shoulder Elbow Surg 2003;12:153–63.
5. Hasan SS, Leith JM, Campbell B, Kapil R, Smith KL, Matsen III FA. Characteristics of unsatisfactory shoulder arthroplasties. J Shoulder Elbow Surg 2002;11:431–41.
6. Bohsali KI, Wirth MA, Rockwood Jr CA. Complications of total shoulder arthroplasty. J Bone Joint Surg 2006;88:2279–92.
7. Chin PYK, Sperling JW, Cofield RH, Schleck C. Complications of total shoulder arthroplasty: Are they fewer or different? J Shoulder Elbow Surg 2006;15:19–22.
8. Nyffeler RW, Sheikh R, Atkinson TS, Jacob HAC, Favre P, Gerber C. Effects of glenoid component version on humeral head displacement and joint reaction forces: An experimental study. J Shoulder Elbow Surg 2006;15:625–9.
9. Hopkins AR, Hansen UN, Amis AA, Emery R. The effect of glenoid component alignment variations on cement mantle stresses in total shoulder arthroplasty. J Shoulder Elbow Surg 2004;13:668–75.

10. Farron A, Terrier A, Buchler P. Risks of loosening of a prosthetic glenoid implanted in retroversion. J Shoulder Elbow Surg 2006;15:521–6.

11. Shapiro TA, McGarry MH, Gupta R, Lee YS, Lee TQ. Biomechanical effects of glenoid retroversion in total shoulder arthroplasty. J Shoulder Elbow Surg 2007;16:90–5S.

12. Nyffeler RW, Jost B, Pfirrmann CWA, Gerber C. Measurement of glenoid version: Conventional radiographs versus computed tomograghy scans. J Shoulder Elbow Surg 2003;12:493–6.

13. Kwon YW, Powell KA, Yum JK, Brems JJ, Iannotti JP. Use of three-dimensional computed tomography for the analysis of the glenoid anatomy. J Shoulder Elbow Surg 2005;14:85–90.

14. Scalise JJ, Codsi MJ, Bryan J, Brems JJ, Iannotti JP. The influence of three-dimensional computed tomography images of the shoulder in progressive planning for total shoulder arthroplasty. J Bone Joint Surg 2008;90:2438–45.

15. Cil A, Veillette CJH, Sanchez-Sotelo J, Sperling JW, Schleck CD, Cofield RH. Survivorship of the humeral component in shoulder arthroplasty. J Shoulder Elbow Surg 2009;18:1–8.

16. Litchfield RB, McKee M, Balyk R, Mandel S, Holtby R, Hollinshead R, et al. Cemented versus uncemented fixation of humeral components in total shoulder arthroplasty for osteoarthritis of the shoulder. Presented at ASES meeting, Feb 28, 2009.

17. Josefsson G, Kolmert L. Prophylaxis with systemic antibiotics versus gentamicin bone cement in total hip arthroplasty. A ten-year survey of 1688 hips. Clin Orthop Relat Res 1993;292: 210–14.

18. McQueen MM, Hughes SPF, May P, Verity L. Cefuroxime in total joint arthroplasty. J Arthroplasty 1990;2:169–72.

19. Joseph TN, Chen AL, Di Cesare PE. Use of antibiotic-impregnated cement in total joint arthroplasty. J Am Acad Orthop Surg 2003;11:38–47.

20. Sherfey MC, Edwards TB. Cement extrusion causing radial nerve palsy after shoulder arthroplasty: a case report. J Shoulder Elbow Surg 2009;18:e21–4.

21. Edwards TB, Sabonghy EP, Elkousy H, Warnock M, Hammerman SM, O'Connor DP, Gartsman GM. Glenoid component insertion in total shoulder arthroplasty: comparison of three techniques for drying the glenoid before cementation. J Shoulder Elbow Surg 2007;16: 107S-110S.

22. Terrier A, Buchler P, Farron A. Bone-cement interface of the glenoid component: stress analysis for varying cement thickness. Clin Biomechanics 2005;20:710–17.

23. Nyffeler RW, Meyer D, Sheikh R, Koller BJ, Gerber C. The effect of cementing technique on structural fixation of pegged glenoid components in total shoulder arthroplasty. J Shoulder Elbow Surg 2006;15:106–11.

24. Hasan SA, Cox WK, Syed M, Suva LJ. Microcomputed tomography assessment of glenoid component cementation techniques in total shoulder arthroplasty. J Orthop Res 2009;27:1–6.

25. Boileau P, Avidor C, Krishnan SG, Walch G, Kempf JF, Molé D. Cemented polyethylene versus uncemented metal-backed glenoid components in total shoulder arthroplasty: a prospective, double-blind, randomized study. J Shoulder Elbow Surg 2002;11:351–9.

26. Taunton MJ, McIntosh AL, Sperling JW, Cofield RH. Total shoulder arthroplasty with a metal-backed, bone-ingrowth glenoid component. medium to long-term results. J Bone Joint Surg 2008;90:2180–8.

27. Martin SD, Zurakowski D, Thornhill TS. Uncemented glenoid component in total shoulder arthroplasty. survivorship and outcomes. J Bone Joint Surg Am 2005;87:1284–92.

28. Wilcox III RB, Arslanian LE, Millett PJ. Rehabilitation following total shoulder arthroplasty. J Orthop Sports Phys Ther 2005; 35(12):821–836.

29. Verborgt O, El-Abiad R, Gazielly DF. Long-term results of uncemented humeral components in shoulder arthroplasty. J Shoulder Elbow Surg 2007;16:13–18S.

30. Cofield RH. Uncemented total shoulder arthroplasty: a review. Clin Orthop Relat Res 1994;307:86–93.

31. Rahme H, Mattsson P, Wikblad L, Larsson S. Cement and press-fit humeral stem fixation provides similar results in rheumatoid patients. Clin Orthop Relat Res 2006;448:28–32.

32 Reverse Total Shoulder Arthroplasty

Ryan T. Bicknell

Queen's University, Kingston, ON, Canada

Case scenario

A 75 year old woman who is living independently is seen with complaints of right shoulder pain. She has no history of trauma and the pain has been progressive over the past 2–3 years. On examination, she has very limited active movement and crepitus. She is neurovascularly intact.

Relevant anatomy

A rotator cuff tear can be classified as acute (no irreversible muscular fatty atrophy and generally reparable) or chronic (with irreversible muscular fatty atrophy and generally irreparable). Instability of the glenohumeral joint due to a long-standing irreparable rotator cuff tear often occurs in an anterior and superior direction, called *anterosuperior escape*, often leading to a pseudoparalysed shoulder, generally defined as a loss of active forward elevation with maintained passive movement.

Importance of the problem

Shoulder arthritis can include osteoarthritis (OA), rheumatoid arthritis (RA), post-traumatic arthritis, and cuff tear arthropathy. Each type of arthritis is not infrequently seen in combination with a rotator cuff tear. A conventional total shoulder arthroplasty (TSA) is used to relieve pain and improve function in arthritic shoulders. The articular surfaces are unconstrained and allow the healthy rotator cuff and extrinsic shoulder muscles to restore shoulder function. In most arthritic shoulders, with or without a rotator cuff tear, this "ball-and-socket" biomechanics of the glenohumeral joint are maintained. However, each type of arthritis may present in combination with rotator cuff dysfunction and loss of the normal biomechanics, often leading to instability and pseudo-paralysis. In this situation, the outcome of a traditional shoulder arthroplasty is substantially compromised.[1–3]

The incidence of rotator cuff tear dysfunction in the population of shoulder arthritis patients is difficult to determine, but occurs in a minority of patients. Although shoulder arthritis is much less common than hip or knee arthritis, the incidence and indications for shoulder arthroplasty continue to increase.

Even though reverse total shoulder arthroplasty (RTSA) is a relatively new procedure, surgeons and patients are inundated with an everincreasing easily accessible body of information. A Google search for "reverse shoulder arthroplasty" returns over 600,000 hits.

Top five questions

Diagnosis

1. What are the indications for an RTSA?

Therapy

2. What patient factors predict function after an RTSA?
3. What technical factors may affect outcome of an RTSA?

Prognosis

4. What are the results of an RTSA?

Harm

5. What complications are associated with an RTSA?

Question 1: What are the indications for an RTSA?

Case clarification

The patient has active forward elevation to 45°, but maintained passive forward elevation to 160°. The patient's radiograph reveals humeral head elevation with a complete loss of acromiohumeral distance and complete loss of glenohumeral joint space.

Relevance

Traditionally, shoulder arthritis associated with rotator cuff dysfunction has been treated with a hemiarthroplasty. However, in patients with a pseudo-paralyzed shoulder, this may not provide an improvement in active range of motion (ROM) and requires re-establishing the ball-and-socket mechanics of the shoulder.

Current opinion

Current opinion suggests that the majority of surgeons use an RTSA for the treatment of patients with shoulder arthritis and rotator cuff dysfunction that results in a pseudo-paralyzed shoulder.

Finding the evidence

- Cochrane Database, with search term "reverse arthroplasty"
- PubMed (www.ncbi.nlm.nih.gov/pubmed/): clinical queries search/systematic reviews: "reverse shoulder arthroplasty"
- PubMed (www.ncbi.nlm.nih.gov/pubmed/): search using keywords "reverse arthroplasty" OR "reverse shoulder arthroplasty" OR "reverse total shoulder arthroplasty"

Quality of the evidence

Level IV
- 1 case series

Level V
- 2 expert opinions

Findings

Overall indication RTSA may be considered when the patient presents with a clinically symptomatic, irreparable rotator cuff tear associated with an irrecoverable pseudo-paralysis. However, deltoid function must be preserved. As well, adequate glenoid bone stock must be available to allow secure glenoid component fixation. RTSA should be reserved for elderly patients with low functional demands.[1,4]

Contraindications Contraindications include infection, neuroarthropathy, and glenoid bone erosion.[1]

Specific diagnoses The initially described, and main, indication for an RTSA is cuff tear arthropathy.[1,4,5] A massive cuff tear without glenohumeral OA can also be considered. An RTSA can be considered in RA if sufficient bone stock exists, for some three- and four-part proximal humerus fractures, and revision of failed prosthesis.[1,4]

Recommendations

- In patients greater than 70 years of age, a RTSA can be considered when rotator cuff dysfunction leads to antero-superior escape and a pseudo-paralyzed shoulder [overall quality: low]
- The most common indication is cuff tear arthropathy or a massive cuff tear with glenohumeral arthritis. However, patients with RA, proximal humerus fractures, and failed arthroplasty may also be considered, when all other options are exhausted [overall quality: moderate]

Question 2: What patient factors predict function after an RTSA?

Case clarification

The patient is offered an RTSA. Preoperatively, she has no active external rotation and a positive Hornblower's sign. A preoperative CT scan is ordered.

Relevance

The level of shoulder function preoperatively may predict function postoperatively and may suggest to the surgeon to add other procedures at the time of RTSA.

Current opinion

Current opinion suggests that an RTSA does not result in an improvement in active external rotation. As well, results after an RTSA are inferior in the absence of an intact teres minor.

Finding the evidence

- Cochrane Database, with search term "reverse arthroplasty"
- PubMed (www.ncbi.nlm.nih.gov/pubmed/): clinical queries search/systematic reviews: "reverse shoulder arthroplasty"
- PubMed (www.ncbi.nlm.nih.gov/pubmed/): search using keywords "reverse arthroplasty" OR "reverse shoulder arthroplasty" OR "reverse total shoulder arthroplasty"

Quality of the evidence

Level IV
- 5 case series

Level V
- 1 expert opinion

Findings

Loss of active external rotation cannot be treated with an RTSA. Results are inferior with a nonfunctioning teres minor.[6–8] An RTSA combined with a latissimus dorsi transfer may offer an improvement in active external rotation.[9,10]

Recommendation

- In patients undergoing an RTSA, improvement in active external rotation cannot be expected, but a latissimus dorsi tendon transfer may offer some improvement [overall quality: moderate]

Question 3: What technical factors may affect outcome of an RTSA?

Case clarification

Intraoperatively, the patient undergoes an RTSA through a deltopectoral approach.

Relevance

There is debate as to preferred surgical approach and correct positioning of both the humeral and glenoid components.

Current opinion

Use of either a superolateral or deltopectoral approach is generally based on the surgeon's comfort level with either approach. The deltopectoral approach is thought to have a higher risk of instability, while the superolateral approach is thought to have a higher risk of glenoid component malpositioning and scapular notching. Subscapularis repair is thought to help prevent instability. An inferior tilt and inferior positioning of the glenoid component may prevent loosening and notching, respectively. Generally, the humeral component is inserted in neutral rotation.

Finding the evidence

- Cochrane Database, with search term "reverse arthroplasty"
- PubMed (www.ncbi.nlm.nih.gov/pubmed/) clinical queries search/systematic reviews: "reverse shoulder arthroplasty"
- PubMed (www.ncbi.nlm.nih.gov/pubmed/): search using keywords "reverse arthroplasty" OR "reverse shoulder arthroplasty" OR "reverse total shoulder arthroplasty"

Quality of the evidence

Level II
- 1 nonblinded randomized controlled trial

Level III
- 2 retrospective comparative studies

Level IV
- 1 case series

Level V
- Expert Opinion: 2

Findings

RTSA performed through a superolateral approach has been found to have a lower incidence of postoperative instability than a deltopectoral approach (0% vs. 5.1%, $p < 0.05$), but a superolateral approach has been shown to be better for preventing fractures of the scapular spine and acromion ($p < 0.05$).[7] A deltopectoral approach has been shown to have better preservation of active external rotation, better orientation of the glenoid component, and decreased glenoid loosening and scapular notching.[7] Revision surgery is more frequently and easily performed through a deltopectoral approach, but when instability is a concern, a superolateral approach is preferable.[1,4]

Subscapularis repair may decrease the rate of instability by creating an anterior envelope.[1] However, repair has no statistical effect on outcome.[7]

Inferior tilt of the glenoid component may increase notching,[11,12] but prevent glenoid loosening.[1] Placing the glenoid baseplate as inferior as possible prevents notching and improves ROM.[11,12] A larger-diameter glenosphere is associated with less pain and better strength.[7,13]

Neutral rotation of the humeral component (compared with 20° retroversion) has better outcomes in terms of activities of daily living, strength, Constant score, radiologic loosening, and glenoid complications.[7]

Recommendations

Technical considerations when performing a RTSA include:

- Surgical approach is determined by surgeon preference; however, if instability is a concern, a superolateral approach may be preferable [overall quality: high]
- Subscapularis repair, if possible, is recommended [overall quality: low]
- Glenoid component positioning should include an inferior position and inferior tilt [overall quality: moderate]
- A larger-diameter glenosphere is recommended [overall quality: low]
- Humeral component should be in neutral rotation [overall quality: low]

Question 4: What are the results of an RTSA?

Case clarification

Three months postoperatively, the patient has good pain relief and active elevation of 115°.

Relevance

The results of RTSA are very good in some situations but are highly dependent on the indication. Long-term outcomes are uncertain.

Current opinion

Results of RTSA are very good for pain relief and improved active elevation in patients with cuff tear arthropathy and massive cuff tears. However, the results when performed for other indications are unclear. Long-term outcomes are unclear.

Finding the evidence

- Cochrane Database, with search term "reverse arthroplasty"
- PubMed (www.ncbi.nlm.nih.gov/pubmed/) clinical queries search/systematic reviews: "reverse shoulder arthroplasty"
- PubMed (www.ncbi.nlm.nih.gov/pubmed/): search using keywords "reverse arthroplasty" OR "reverse shoulder arthroplasty" OR "reverse total shoulder arthroplasty"

Quality of the evidence

Level IV

- 8 case series

Findings

At 2–10 year follow-up, RTSA is effective in treating loss of active elevation associated with massive rotator cuff tears.[5,7,13–15] For cuff disease, RTSA can reliably restore elevation.[5,7,14,15] Constant score, pain scores, and elevation improve and satisfaction is high. At 10 years, survivability is approximately 90% for implant retention and 70% for a Constant score greater than 30 points.[7,15–18] Radiographic results deteriorate after 6 years, and clinical results after 6–8 years.[7,14]

Results are dependent on the indication, with cuff disease having the best results. Results are better in primary vs. revision cases.[5,13–15]

Recommendations

- Results are dependent on the indication, with cuff disease have the best results, and revision cases having the worst [overall quality: low]
- RTSA for cuff disease allows predictable improvement in pain and active elevation [overall quality: low]

Question 5: What complications are associated with an RTSA?

Case clarification

At 9 months postoperatively, the patient presents with an acute worsening of pain and an inability to move her shoulder. Radiographs reveal an anterior dislocation.

Relevance

Early series of RTSA have had high complication rates.

Current opinion

Complication rates are high but dependent on the indication.

Finding the evidence

- Cochrane Database, with search term "reverse arthroplasty"
- PubMed (www.ncbi.nlm.nih.gov/pubmed/): clinical queries search/systematic reviews: "reverse shoulder arthroplasty"
- PubMed (www.ncbi.nlm.nih.gov/pubmed/): search using keywords "reverse arthroplasty" OR "reverse shoulder arthroplasty" OR "reverse total shoulder arthroplasty"

Quality of the evidence

Level II

- 1 nonblinded randomized controlled trial

Level III

- 4 retrospective comparative studies

Level IV

- 5 case series

Level V

- 1 expert opinion

Findings

The most common complications include dislocation, infection, hematoma, acromial fracture, humeral fracture, and transient nerve palsy.[1] The reported complication rate is from 0 to 68%, with a 5–40% revision rate.[5,17,19] Revision rates are higher for revision surgery.[15]

Instability Rate of 3.4% in primary cases,[7] usually anterior with arm in extension and internal rotation.[1] Preventive measures include using a superolateral approach, avoiding retroversion of humerus, avoiding anteversion of glenoid, establishing optimal humeral length, and repairing subscapularis when possible.[7,20,21] When instability occurs within the first 3 months, closed reduction is generally not successful. However, a later dislocation (>1 year) can usually be successfully treated with closed reduction.[7]

Infection Rate of 5.1% in primary cases,[7] higher in revision cases.[15] Most infections occur early and can be treated by lavage and antibiotics, but some occurring after 3 months do not respond to prosthesis retention.[7]

Glenoid loosening Rate of 4.1%, 55% of which occur within the first 2 years postoperatively.[7] Risk factors are younger patient age (<70 years), female gender, and a superolateral approach.[1]

Scapular notching Rate of 44–96%.[12,15,22,23] Generally observed within the first 6 months postoperatively and appears to stabilize in some studies,[12,13] but increase in incidence and severity with time in other studies.[22] A superolateral approach leads to more notching (p < 0.0001).[22] Notching has been found to be associated with poorer clinical results.[12] Placing baseplate as inferior as possible prevents notching.[11,12]

Acromion fracture An acromion stress fracture does not affect outcome and may be neglected, but a scapular spine fracture often leads to painful dysfunction and may require operative treatment.[7,24]

Recommendations

- Complication rates are high but dependent on the indication, with cuff disease having the lowest complication rate and revision cases the highest [overall quality: moderate]
- The most common complications include dislocation, infection, and hematoma [overall quality: moderate]
- Scapular notching is common, but may not affect outcome [overall quality: low]

Summary of recommendations

- In patients greater than 70 years of age, a RTSA can be considered when rotator cuff dysfunction leads to antero-superior escape and a pseudo-paralyzed shoulder
- The most common indication is cuff tear arthropathy or a massive cuff tear with glenohumeral arthritis; however, patients with RA, proximal humerus fractures, and failed arthroplasty may also be considered, when all other options are exhausted
- In patients undergoing a RTSA, improvement in active external rotation cannot be expected, but a latissimus dorsi tendon transfer may offer some improvement in active external rotation
- Technical considerations when performing a RTSA include:
  - Surgical approach is determined by surgeon preference, but if instability is a concern a superolateral approach may be preferable
  - Subscapularis repair, if possible, is recommended
  - Glenoid component positioning should include an inferior position and inferior tilt
  - A larger diameter glenosphere is recommended
  - Humeral component should be in neutral rotation
- Results are dependent on the indication, with cuff disease have the best results, and revision cases having the worst
- RTSA for cuff disease allows predictable improvement in pain and active elevation

- Complication rates are high but dependent on the indication, with cuff disease having the lowest complication rate and revision cases the highest
- The most common complications include dislocation, infection, and hematoma
- Scapular notching is common, but may not affect outcome

Conclusion

In patients greater than 70 years of age, a RTSA can be considered when rotator cuff dysfunction leads to antero-superior escape and a pseudo-paralyzed shoulder. Results are dependent on the indication. RTSA allows predictable improvement in pain and active elevation. Complication rates are high but dependent on the indication. The most common complications include dislocation, infection, and hematoma.

References

1. Gerber C, Pennington SD, Nyffeler RW. Reverse total shoulder arthroplasty. J Am Acad Orthop Surg 2009;17:284–95.
2. Edwards TB, Boulahia A, Kempf JF, Boileau P, Nemoz C, Walch G. The influence of rotator cuff disease on the results of shoulder arthroplasty for primary osteoarthritis: results of a multicenter study. J Bone Joint Surg Am 2002;84:2240–8.
3. Neer CS II, Craig EV, Fukuda H. Cuff tear arthropathy. J Bone Joint Surg Am 1983;65:1232–44.
4. Matsen FA, Boileau P, Walch G, Gerber C, Bicknell RT. The reverse total shoulder arthroplasty. J Bone Joint Surg Am 2007;89:660–7.
5. Wall B, Nove-Josserand L, O'Connor DP, Edwards TB, Walch G. Reverse total shoulder arthroplasty: a review of results according to etiology. J Bone Joint Surg Am 2007;89:1476–85.
6. Grammont PM, Baulot E. Delta shoulder prosthesis for rotator cuff rupture. Orthopedics 1993;16:33–6.
7. Molé D, Favard L. Excentered scapulohumeral osteoarthritis [French]. Rev Chir Orthop Reparatrice Appar Mot 2007;93(6 suppl):37–94.
8. Simovitch RW, Helmy N, Zumstein MA, Gerber C. Impact of fatty infiltration of the teres minor muscle on the outcome of reverse total shoulder arthroplasty. J Bone Joint Surg Am 2007;89(5):934–9.
9. Boileau P, Chuinard C, Roussanne Y, Bicknell RT, Rochet N, Trojani C. Reverse shoulder arthroplasty combined with a modified latissimus dorsi and teres major tendon transfer for shoulder pseudoparalysis associated with dropping arm. Clin Orthop Relat Res 2008;466:584–93.
10. Gerber C, Pennington SD, Lingenfelter EJ, Sukthankar A. Reverse Delta-III total shoulder replacement combined with latissimus dorsi transfer. A preliminary report. J Bone Joint Surg Am 2007;89:940–7.
11. Nyffeler RW, Werner CM, Gerber C. Biomechanical relevance of glenoid component positioning in reverse Delta III total shoulder prosthesis. J Shoulder Elbow Surg 2005;14:524–8.

12. Simovitch RW, Zumstein MA, Lohri E, Helmy N, Gerber C. Predictors of scapular notching in patients managed with the Delta III reverse total shoulder replacement. J Bone Joint Surg Am 2007;89:588–600.

13. Sirveaux F, Favard L, Oudet D, Huquet D, Walch G, Mole D. Grammont inverted total shoulder arthroplasty in the treatment of glenohumeral osteoarthritis with massive rupture of the cuff: results of a multicentre study of 80 shoulders. J Bone Joint Surg Br 2004;86:388–95.

14. Guery J, Favard L, Sirveaux F, Oudet D, Mole D, Walch G. Reverse total shoulder arthroplasty: survivorship analysis of eighty replacements followed for five to ten years. J Bone Joint Surg Am 2006;88:1742–7.

15. Werner CM, Steinmann PA, Gilbart M, Gerber C. Treatment of painful pseudoparesis due to irreparable rotator cuff dysfunction with the Delta III reverse-ball-and-socket total shoulder prosthesis. J Bone Joint Surg Am 2005;87:1476–86.

16. Boileau P, Watkinson D, Hatzidakis AM, Hovorka K. Neer Award 2005: The Grammont reverse shoulder prosthesis: results in cuff tear arthritis, fracture sequelae, and revision arthroplasty. J Shoulder Elbow Surg 2006;15:527–40.

17. Boileau P, Gonzalez JF, Chuinard C, Bicknell R, Walch G. Reverse total shoulder arthroplasty after failed rotator cuff surgery. J Shoulder Elbow Surg 2009;18:600–6.

18. Cuff D, Pupello D, Virani N, Levy J, Frankle M. Reverse shoulder arthroplasty for the treatment of rotator cuff deficiency. J Bone Joint Surg Am 2008;90:1244–51.

19. Wierks C, Skolasky RL, Ji JH, McFarland EG. Reverse total shoulder replacement: intraoperative and early postoperative complications. Clin Orthop Relat Res 2009;467:225–34.

20. Ladermann A, Williams MD, Melis B, Hoffmeyer P, Walch G. Objective evaluation of lengthening in reverse shoulder arthroplasty. J Shoulder Elbow Surg 2009;18:588–95.

21. Edwards TB, Williams MD, Labriola JE, Elkousy HA, Gartsman GM, O'Connor DP. Subscapularis insufficiency and the risk of shoulder dislocation after reverse shoulder arthroplasty. J Shoulder Elbow Surg 2009;18(6):892–6.

22. Rittmeister M, Kerschbaumer F. Grammont reverse total shoulder arthroplasty in patients with rheumatoid arthritis and non-reconstructible rotator cuff lesions. J Shoulder Elbow Surg 2001;10:17–22.

23. Levigne C, Boileau P, Favard L, Garaud P, Mole D, Sirveaux F, Walch G. Scapular notching in reverse shoulder arthroplasty. J Shoulder Elbow Surg 2008; 17:925–35.

24. Walch G, Mottier F, Wall B, Boileau P, Mole D, Favard L. Acromial insufficiency in reverse shoulder arthroplasties. J Shoulder Elbow Surg 2009;18:495–502.

33 Glenoid Fixation in Total Shoulder Arthroplasty: What Type of Glenoid Component Should We Use?

Eric C. Benson[1], Kenneth J. Faber[2], and George S. Athwal[2]

[1]University of New Mexico, Albuquerque, NM, USA
[2]St. Joseph's Health Care, University of Western Ontario, London, ON, Canada

Case scenario

A 72 year old right-hand dominant man has been experiencing 3 years of right shoulder pain. He denies previous trauma. Instead, the pain has been insidious in onset and has failed nonoperative treatment. Radiographic studies including conventional radiographs and CT scan show considerable degenerative changes with loss of joint space, marginal osteophytes, subchondral sclerosis, and significant posterior glenoid erosion (Figure 33.1a,b,c).

Relevant anatomy

Total shoulder arthroplasty (TSA) appears to be the most reliable treatment option for patients with shoulder arthritis that is unresponsive to nonoperative management. Despite improvements in our understanding of the relevant anatomy and factors that influence glenoid fixation, failure of the glenoid component remains the most common mode of failure for shoulder arthroplasty. Glenoid version, the orientation of the glenoid articular surface relative to the transverse axis of the scapula, is typically between 2° of anteversion and 9° of retroversion.[1,2] Patients with osteoarthritis (OA) typically have significantly increased retroversion of the glenoid compared to normal anatomy, with up to 30° or more of retroversion.[3] This affects glenoid fixation and shoulder mechanics, and may ultimately affect the longevity of the glenoid component.

Importance of the problem

Roughly 20,000 TSAs are performed in the United States each year for OA.[4] This is compared to 7000 annually from 1996 through 2002, indicating a 185% increase.[5] As the frequency of TSA increases, the anticipated burden of revision arthroplasty is also expected to increase. One of the most important outcome measures for any joint replacement procedure is the rate of revision-free survivorship. In TSA, the most frequent cause for revision in mid- and long-term follow-up is glenoid component failure. Bohsali et al. performed a retrospective review of the literature from 1996 to 2005 to identify complications associated with TSA. They found that glenoid loosening accounted for 32% of all complications and occurred in 5.3% of 2540 shoulders.[5]

Pain, functional limitation, and occasionally mechanical symptoms can accompany glenoid loosening leading to the need for revision. Buckingham et al. evaluated the changes in patients' functional self-assessment at an average of 7.4 years after primary TSA and just prior to revision for glenoid component loosening. Although the numbers in their study were small, the data are telling of the functional decline with a failed glenoid component: mean simple shoulder test scores prior to initial arthroplasty were 4.4, they rose to 11.3 at their peak, but fell back to 4.6 just prior to revision. In addition, at the time of revision less than 50% of patients reported comfortable sleep (17%), the ability to wash the back of the contralateral shoulder (8%), place their hand behind their head (33%), lift 8 lbs (3.6 kg) to shoulder level (35%), throw a softball 20 yards (18 m) (0%), or work at their regular job (25%).[6] Failure of glenoid fixation may contribute to dramatic changes in patients' quality of life and overall functional status, emphasizing the importance of improving techniques and technologies to maximize glenoid component longevity.

As the volume of TSA increases over time, so too does the body of information related to the procedure. The available information is not always founded in sound methodology or evidence-based principles. 106,000 hits resulted from a Google internet search of the terms "glenoid

Evidence-Based Orthopedics, First Edition. Edited by Mohit Bhandari.
© 2012 Blackwell Publishing Ltd. Published 2012 by Blackwell Publishing Ltd.

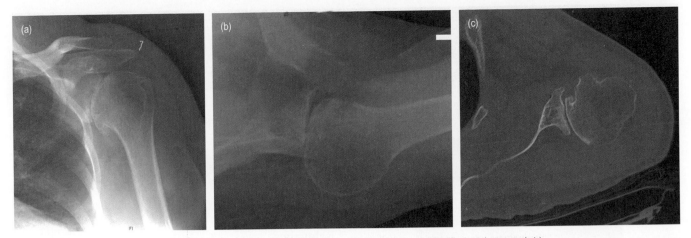

Figure 33.1 AP and axial radiographs (a,b) and axial CT scan (c) show characteristic findings in glenohumeral osteoarthritis.

fixation." The goal of this chapter is to identify and compile the best-quality information available to generate evidence-based treatment guidelines for glenoid fixation based on evidence from the last 10 years.

Top five questions

Diagnosis

1. What is the best method of determining clinically relevant glenoid loosening?

Therapy

2. What is the optimal degree of radial mismatch?
3. Which is optimal: all-polyethylene cemented or metal-backed uncemented?
4. Which is optimal: keel or pegged glenoid?

Prognosis

5. Do early radiographic lucent lines around the glenoid component predict outcomes?

Question 1: What is the best method of determining clinically relevant glenoid loosening?

Case clarification

A patient who had a previous TSA now presents with shoulder pain and popping with range of motion (ROM) of the shoulder. Their pain has returned to the level they experienced prior to their initial replacement.

Relevance

The decision to revise a loose glenoid component depends on radiographic criteria as well as clinical assessment. It is important that our imaging criteria accurately correlate to the clinical picture if they are to help guide our treatment decisions.

Current opinion

CT scan provides data that better correlates radiographic evidence of loosening and clinical symptoms when compared to conventional radiographs.

Finding the evidence

- Cochrane Database: no Cochrane reviews found
- PubMed clinical queries search/systematic reviews: "total shoulder arthroplasty" as well as "glenoid"
- PubMed sensitivity search. The following is the Query Translation:
- (glenoid[All Fields] AND total[All Fields] AND ("shoulder"[MeSH Terms] OR "shoulder"[All Fields]) AND ("arthroplasty"[MeSH Terms] OR "arthroplasty"[All Fields])) OR (total[All Fields] AND ("shoulder"[MeSH Terms] OR "shoulder"[All Fields]) AND ("replantation" [MeSH Terms] OR "replantation"[All Fields] OR "replacement"[All Fields])) NOT resurfacing[All Fields] NOT reverse[All Fields] NOT ("fractures, bone"[MeSH Terms] OR ("fractures"[All Fields] AND "bone"[All Fields]) OR "bone fractures"[All Fields] OR "fracture" [All Fields]) AND ("1999/09/30"[PDat] : "2009/09/26" [PDat])

Quality of the evidence

Level III
- 3 observational studies

Findings

Currently, the majority of clinical trials use conventional radiographs to determine glenoid loosening, but the reliability of this method remains uncertain (Figure 33.2). Mileti found that there was no correlation between pain,

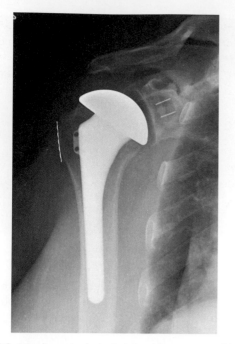

Figure 33.2 AP radiograph of a keeled glenoid component without evidence of radiolucent lines.

ROM, or satisfaction relative to conventional radiographic criteria for glenoids considered stable or those at risk for loosening.[7] In a study by Nho, conventional radiographs significantly underestimated intraoperative findings of loosening. In this retrieval study, including 73 glenoid components, the mean pre-revision radiolucency score was 7.1 (indicating they were possibly loose) whereas at revision 92% of glenoids were loose.[8] These studies, then, raise the question of whether conventional radiographic criteria accurately represent true clinical loosening.

Yian evaluated conventional radiographs and CT scans as tools to assess radiographic lucency about glenoid components. He found that conventional radiographic lucency scores did not correlate to clinical outcomes such as the Constant score, pain score, or active shoulder mobility. In contrast, he found the CT scan scores significantly, though weakly, correlated with pain scores and abduction strength. In addition, inter- and intraobserver reliability scores were both higher for CT scan evaluation (0.89 and 0.95, respectively) than for conventional radiographs (0.47 and 0.70, respectively).[9]

Recommendations

• Compared to conventional radiographic scoring criteria, CT scan radiolucency scoring criteria correlate better with clinical outcome measures [overall quality: low]
• CT scan scoring systems have better inter- and intraobserver reliability [overall quality: low]

Question 2: What is the optimal degree of radial mismatch?

Case clarification

The patient's CT scan shows 20° of glenoid retroversion preoperatively. There is no history of prior instability. You must decide whether to use a glenoid component with more or less radial mismatch.

> Radial mismatch refers to the difference in radius of curvature between the glenoid component and the humeral head.

Relevance

Glenoid component radial mismatch is broadly categorized as either more conforming (small mismatch) or less conforming (large mismatch). There remains considerable debate regarding the optimal amount of articular congruity of these implants. Theoretical advantages of a more conforming device include joint stability, concentric loading, and greater contact surface area with decreased wear rates; the disadvantages are that it does not allow coupled translation of the shoulder with resulting increased stress at the implant-bone junction as well as increased shear forces. Theoretical advantages of the less conforming device include better-coupled translation but at the risk of joint instability, decreased contact surface area with increased wear rates, and component fracture.[10,11]

Finding the evidence

• Cochrane Database: no Cochrane reviews
• PubMed clinical queries search/systematic reviews: "total shoulder arthroplasty" as well as "glenoid"
• PubMed sensitivity search: the Query Translation was the same as for Question 1

Quality of the evidence

Level III
• 1 observational study
• 2 biomechanical studies

Findings

The biomechanics of the shoulder joint demonstrate coupled translation of the humeral head during rotation.[12] Biomechanical studies demonstrate that implant designs with less conformity better recreate the normal coupled translation of the glenohumeral joint. Anglin concluded that greater radial mismatch performed better with less distraction than did the lower radial mismatch device. The authors' numbers were quite small, however, looking at only three implants of each type.[13] Harryman used seven cadaveric shoulders to compare the effect of various amounts of radial mismatch on glenohumeral translation.

Measuring radial mismatches of 0–5 mm he concluded that a radial mismatch of 5 mm best reproduces the normal joint translation. The translation was 1.5 mm for the native glenoid and 1.7 mm with a radial mismatch of 5 mm for the TSA.

In order to determine the clinical applicability of some of these results, Walch, in a retrospective multicenter trial, looked at the correlation between radial mismatch and clinical outcomes. At a mean follow-up of 53.5 months, there was a significant difference in the mean radiolucency score on AP radiographs based on the amount of joint congruity. In 319 TSAs, those with a radial mismatch of greater than 6 mm demonstrated significantly lower radiolucency scores than those with a mismatch of 4 mm or less. Patients with a mismatch of 6–7 mm had the highest Constant scores at final follow-up, but this was not statistically significant. In fact, the only significant parameter correlated with radial mismatch in this study other than mean radiolucency score was improved external rotation in patients with radial mismatch of 4.5–7 mm. There was no effect of radial mismatch on rate or type of complication (instability), forward elevation, internal rotation, the Constant score, or any component of the Constant score (pain, activity, mobility, or strength).[10]

Recommendations
• Radial mismatch of 5–7 mm best recreates normal glenohumeral joint kinematics [overall quality: low]
• Radial mismatch of 6–7 mm improves radiolucency scores at 4.5 years [overall quality: low]
• At present, no recommendation can be made regarding the effect of radial mismatch on clinical outcomes or survivorship of glenoid implants.

Question 3: Which is optimal: all-polyethylene cemented or metal-backed uncemented?

Case clarification
The patient elects to proceed with TSA and you have decided on a glenoid component with 5 mm of radial mismatch. Next, you must decide whether to use an all-polyethylene cemented component or a metal-backed uncemented component.

Relevance
Securing durable and reliable fixation of the glenoid component is critical to success in TSA. Two main categories of implant design have been widely used and studied: cemented pegged or keeled all-polyethylene components, or uncemented metal-backed components. The theoretical advantage of the uncemented designs is that the initial stability afforded by screw fixation ultimately allows for durable bone ingrowth or bone ongrowth. The theoretical disadvantage of cemented components is that temperatures generated with methylmethacrylate may rise to levels risking bone necrosis. Churchill showed that mean bone temperatures adjacent to cemented components exceeded 64 °C, well above the threshold for thermal-induced bone necrosis.[14]

Finding the evidence
• Cochrane Database: no Cochrane reviews
• PubMed clinical queries search/systematic reviews: "total shoulder arthroplasty" as well as "glenoid"
• PubMed sensitivity search. The Query Translation was the same as for Question 1

Quality of the evidence
Level II
• 1 randomized trial with limitations

Level III
• 5 observational studies
• 3 biomechanical studies

Level IV
• 1 systematic review

Findings
There is no level I study and only one level II study comparing uncemented metal-backed glenoids to cemented all-polyethylene components. In a prospective randomized study, Boileau compared 20 shoulders in each of two groups: cemented all-polyethylene keeled glenoids and uncemented metal-backed glenoids. Glenoid type was not chosen until after humeral preparation was complete and so patient and surgeon were blinded until this point. Four patients died in the study, leaving 90% follow-up of at least 3 years with a mean of 38.4 months for the metal-backed and 37 months for the polyethylene group. Clinical outcome measures included the Constant score, forward elevation, and external rotation. There was no statistical difference between the two groups at any time point, including at final follow-up for any of these outcome measures. Radiographic lucency was noted in 85% of polyethylene components vs. 25% of metal-backed components, and this was a significant difference (p < 0.001). Progression to radiographic loosening and need for revision surgery did not occur in the polyethylene group, but did occur in four shoulders (20%) of the metal-backed group. This difference in revision surgery rate (0% vs. 20%) was statistically significant. Ultimately, despite equivalent results between the two glenoid component types in this short-term follow-up study, the higher revision rate for metal-backed glenoids led the author to conclude that use of metal-backed components should be abandoned.[15] (Figure 33.3)

In addition, Boileau drew some conclusions regarding the proposed mechanisms of failure of the metal-backed

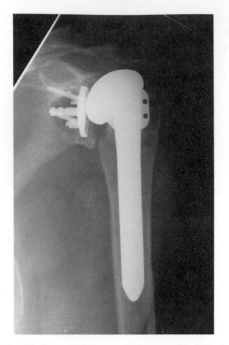

Figure 33.3 AP radiograph demonstrating severe osteolysis about an uncemented, metal-backed glenoid component.

glenoid implants. The modes of failure he described were insufficient polyethylene thickness, overtensioning of the rotator cuff due to a thicker glenoid component, stress shielding of underlying cancellous bone, increased component rigidity leading to increased polyethylene wear, and eccentric loading leading to dissociation of the polyethylene.[15]

There are several retrospective studies comparing these two groups of glenoid components. The most recent, by Fox, retrospectively assessed survival of the glenoid component in TSA. Six types of glenoid components used in 1542 TSAs are analyzed. Among these were two metal-backed designs: one cemented and one uncemented. Out of all the cases there were 121 revisions. Survival free of revision or removal for all four types of the all-polyethylene cemented glenoid designs combined were: 98% (95% CI 98–99%) at 5 years, 95% (95% CI 93–98%) at 10 years, and 92% (95% CI 88–96%) at 15 years. Revision-free survival rates for the Neer II metal-backed glenoid were 96%, 94%, and 89%; for the Cofield 1 metal-backed component they were 86%, 79%, and 67%. Metal-backed component types in this study were significantly associated with component revision (p < 0.001).[16]

There are two studies that individually analyze the results of uncemented and cemented metal-backed components. These both represent cases from the same institution and from a time period overlapping the study by Fox above, so it cannot be determined whether these are separate cases

or if they represent data points used in the calculations from Fox's analysis. The first of these, a retrospective study by Taunton, looked at the survivorship of uncemented metal-backed glenoids after 9.5 years, and it reports a calculated 10-year Kaplan–Meier survival estimate of 78.5%.[17] In an analysis of 100 metal-backed cemented glenoids, Tammachote found the following survival rates: 98% (95% CI 95–100%) at 5 years, 97% (95% CI 93–100%) at 10 years, and 93% (95% CI 87% to 99%) at 15 years.[18]

In a retrospective study of metal-backed glenoids from a different institution, Martin calculated an 85% 10-year survivorship based on 7.5 years of follow-up on 140 glenoids.[19]

Some information can be drawn from several studies comparing hemiarthroplasty to TSA. Edwards evaluated 601 TSAs in a retrospective multicenter series, of which 238 used uncemented metal-backed glenoid components. Of the 601 cases, 23 of the 25 that required revision for glenoid complications were in the metal-backed group, or 9.7%. Only 2 of the remaining cases, all of which used all-polyethylene cemented glenoids, required revision.[20]

In a systematic review investigating the results of TSA vs. hemiarthroplasty, Radnay was able to extract data specific to revision rates for all-polyethylene and metal-backed glenoid components. The mean level of evidence of the 23 studies included in this review was 3.73, and the mean follow-up was 43.4 months. Of 1238 TSAs, 6.5% required revision. Of the metal-backed glenoid components, 6.8% required revision vs. only 1.7% of all-polyethylene components. They did not report if this difference demonstrated statistical significance.[21]

In biomechanical studies, both Stone and Gupta showed that there are high stress levels at the polyethylene–metal interface, leading to the potential for backside wear.[22,23] Both Stone and Pelletier demonstrated evidence of stress shielding associated with metal-backed glenoids as compared to all-polyethylene glenoids, results that support one of Boileau's proposed mechanisms of failure of these devices.[22,24]

Recommendation

• With current designs, all-polyethylene cemented glenoid components have lower revision rates than uncemented metal-backed glenoids, and the use of metal-backed glenoids should be abandoned [overall quality: moderate]

Question 4: Which is optimal: keel or pegged glenoid?

Case clarification

In this patient with primary OA of the shoulder you have decided to use a glenoid with 5mm of radial mismatch that is an all-polyethylene, cemented component. Now you must decide whether to use a keel or a pegged design.

Relevance

Equally important in the discussion of optimal designs for secure glenoid fixation, there remains the choice between cemented keeled and pegged glenoids. There are two considerations with regard to these two designs. Keeled glenoids are typically easier to implant, requiring somewhat less exposure for instrumentation. Pegged glenoids involve less removal of glenoid bone, potentially exposing less bone to the risk of thermal necrosis. Ultimately, however, the most important question remains: which of these two designs yields improved clinical outcomes and improved longevity?

Finding the evidence

- Cochrane Database: no Cochrane reviews
- PubMed clinical queries search/systematic reviews: no results with any search terms
- PubMed sensitivity search: the Query Translation was the same as for Question 1

Quality of the evidence

Level I
- 1 randomized trial

Level II
- 1 randomized trial with limitations

Level IV
- 3 observational studies
- 5 biomechanical studies

Findings

The literature search for this question identified one level I study, one level II study, and three level III observational clinical studies. There are multiple biomechanical studies that investigate the properties of keeled and pegged glenoids.

In the only level I study pertaining to this question, Gartsman conducted a prospective randomized trial in which 23 patients were randomized to a keeled component and 20 were randomized to a pegged component. In this study, keeled components showed a higher incidence and higher overall grade of radiographic lucency as compared to pegged components. At 6 weeks, 9 of 23 (39%) of the keeled glenoids compared to 1 of 20 (5%) of the pegged glenoids showed evidence of radiographic lucency (p = 0.026). (Figure 33.4) The two main limitations to this study include the inherent limitation of radiographic interpretation and that it only addresses the acute postoperative time period. Longer follow-up is needed to see if the initial radiographic lucency correlates to increased revision rates or clinical failure. Gartsman raises the question that it is unclear how radiographic evaluation of peg and keel gle-

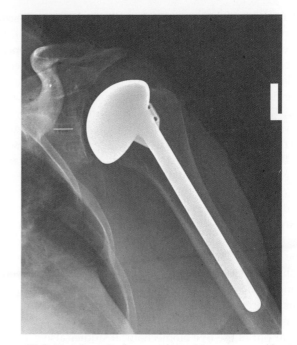

Figure 33.4 AP radiograph of a pegged glenoid component without evidence of radiolucent lines.

noids correlate. CT scan might have been a better imaging modality to determine outcomes in this study.[25]

One level II study, a prospective randomized trial with some limitations, pertains to this question. In this study, Nuttall randomized 10 patients each to pegged or keeled components. Radiostereometric analysis was used to identify movement of the glenoid implant relative to the scapula over 24-month follow-up. Keeled components showed significantly more movement than the pegged glenoids. Both types of components demonstrated positional changes over the 2 years, but the keeled components migrated to a significantly greater degree based on radiostereometric analysis. It remains unclear, however, whether there is any clinical correlation with these findings. Nuttall reports significant improvement for both types of glenoid with regard to clinical outcome measures (p < 0.001): visual analog pain score, abduction, forward flexion, American Shoulder and Elbow Surgeons (ASES) score, and Constant–Murley score. However, in interpreting the data provided, the keeled components actually showed better final ROM and ASES and Constant–Murley scores, and larger improvements for these outcomes than did the pegged components. The author does not comment on this, nor are statistical analyses provided to determine whether these differences are significant.[26]

There are three observational studies identified by this literature search that are all level IV evidence. Lazarus reviewed the initial postoperative radiographs of 328 TSAs and found a significant difference in radiolucency score favoring pegged components (1.3 vs. 1.8, p = 0.0004). He concedes that the results may be biased in that intraoperative conversion from a planned pegged implant to a keeled implant for difficulties with exposure may indicate discrepancies in the patient groups, and these cannot be accounted for in this retrospective study.[27] Klepps, in a study analyzing old vs. new cementation techniques, extrapolated significant differences favoring pegs in average radiolucency score (p < 0.05), and in a single zone showed a significantly decreased incidence of radiolucent lines greater than 1 mm. He concludes that despite these results, it is impossible to claim either design as superior to the other.[28] Trail showed a lower incidence of at least one zone with 1 mm lucency for pegs (36%) vs. keels (90%, p = 0.005) at 8-year follow-up, but none of these components were grossly loose.[29] Although all three of these studies demonstrate statistically better radiographic lucency scores for pegged vs. keeled components, at present this data cannot be correlated to improved clinical outcomes.

Four out of the five biomechanical studies also conclude that peg fixation is superior to keel fixation for the glenoid.[13,14,30,31] One biomechanical study by Roche concludes that there is no difference in glenoid fixation using keel or pegged components. This study has several limitations, including insufficient power and the use of polyurethane bone substitute rather than human bone.

Recommendations

• Based on the available outcome measures, pegged glenoid components outperform keeled components [overall quality: low]
• With the data available, and given the lack of correlation between the outcome measures and clinical results, it is impossible to recommend one component design over the other.

Question 5: Do early radiographic lucent lines around the glenoid component predict outcomes?

Case clarification

The patient underwent a right TSA and on follow-up postoperative radiographs, there is evidence of minor (<1 mm) radiolucency around part of the glenoid. How should you now counsel the patient with regard to outcomes?

Relevance

The ability to predict long-term outcomes is important in any arthroplasty setting. Many published papers that address glenoid stability and survivorship use radiographic lucency scores as one of the main outcome measures, basing this choice on the assumption that lucency may predict glenoid loosening or clinical failure. (Figure

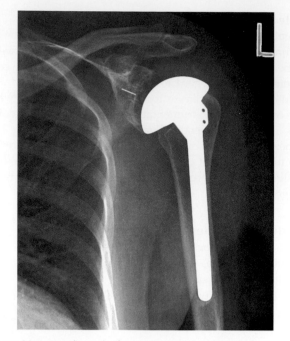

Figure 33.5 AP radiograph of a pegged component demonstrating lucent lines around the entire component.

33.5) In one paper frequently cited to support this assumption, Torchia showed that 93% of glenoids with progressive radiographic lucency had lucencies on immediate postoperative radiographs. In contrast, only 44% of glenoids without initial lucencies showed evidence of progression.[32] Despite this data, without appropriate statistical analysis and power, this observation must be interpreted with caution. The question remains, does radiographic lucency correlate with progressive loosening, clinical outcomes, or decreased survivorship? Put another way, is the use of radiographic lucency scores appropriate as a primary outcome measure for studies investigating glenoid fixation and survivorship?

Finding the evidence

• Cochrane Database: no Cochrane reviews
• PubMed clinical queries search/systematic reviews: no results with any search terms
• PubMed sensitivity search: the Query Translation was the same as for Question 1

Quality of the evidence
Level II
• 1 randomized trial with limitation

Level IV
• 4 observational studies

Findings

The literature search for this question yielded one level II study and four level IV studies. As part of his prospective randomized investigation of cemented all-polyethylene vs. uncemented metal-backed glenoids, Boileau was able to extract data regarding radiographic lucency for glenoids at 3 years follow-up. He noted that 60% of glenoids had less than 1 mm lucency on immediate postoperative radiographs, but 85% showed radiolucent lines at 3 years. He reported a 25% incidence of progression. No analysis was performed comparing progression in those with and without early radiographic lucency. Nonetheless, over 3 years, 25% showed some progression.[15]

All four level IV studies showed similar findings. Radiographic lucent lines typically progressed in short- and mid-term follow-up, but there was no correlation between initial radiographic lucent lines and progression, clinical outcome measures, or glenoid loosening.

In a study of 70 TSAs with cemented keeled glenoids, Mileti showed that in cases without initial radiolucency, 73% progressed. In those with radiolucency postoperatively, 76% progressed. There was no correlation between initial radiographic lucency and the risk of progression. There was no correlation between radiographic criteria and clinical loosening.[7]

Yian's results on 47 total shoulder replacements indicate radiolucency in 11% immediately after surgery and in 45% at 40 months. There is no comment whether there is increased risk of progression in those with early radiolucency.[9] Edwards' results were similarly inconclusive: in this study 57% of glenoids showed radiolucent lines and 50% of these progressed, but there is no description of results for those glenoids that had no radiolucencies. Progression occurs, but no predisposing factors were identified and no conclusions could be drawn with regard to clinical outcomes.[20]

Phaler's level IV series was the largest and included 705 TSAs. He used a combination of 585 keeled flat glenoids, 62 pegged flat glenoids, and 58 keeled convex glenoids. Of the entire cohort, 68% of glenoids showed some radiolucent lines at some point. In 129 shoulders where appropriate serial radiographic imaging was done, 50% were stable and 50% progressed. These scores did not correlate with functional results as determined by the Constant score. Even progression did not correlate with Constant scores.[33]

Recommendations

• With current techniques, 25–50% of cemented all-polyethylene glenoids may show progression of radiographic lucency [overall quality: moderate]
• Early radiolucent lines do not predict progression of radiolucency, clinical outcome measures, or loosening [overall quality: low]

Summary of recommendations

• Compared to conventional radiographic scoring criteria, CT scan radiolucency scoring criteria correlate better with clinical outcome measures
• CT scan scoring systems have better inter- and intraobserver reliability
• Radial mismatch of 5–7 mm best recreates normal glenohumeral joint kinematics
• Radial mismatch of 6–7 mm improves radiolucency scores at 4.5 years
• At present, no recommendation can be made regarding the effect of radial mismatch on clinical outcomes or survivorship of glenoid implants
• With current designs, all-polyethylene cemented glenoid components have lower revision rates than uncemented metal-backed glenoids, and the use of metal-backed glenoids should be abandoned
• Based on the available outcome measures, pegged glenoid components outperform keeled components
• With the data available, and given the lack of correlation between the outcome measures and clinical results, it is impossible to recommend one component design over the other
• With current techniques, 25–50% of cemented all-polyethylene glenoids may show progression of radiographic lucency
• Early radiolucent lines do not predict progression of radiolucency, clinical outcome measures, or loosening

Conclusions

Since Neer first published his report of glenohumeral joint replacement in 1975, the volume of TSAs performed worldwide has continued to increase.[4,5,34] Successful TSA requires secure and lasting fixation of the glenoid component. To date, the optimal type of glenoid design has not been determined. The current literature that addresses glenoid design and fixation lacks adequate randomization as well as statistical analysis and power to confidently report evidence-based treatment guidelines. Overall, it seems clear that existing metal-backed, uncemented glenoid components are to be abandoned due to poor survivorship relative to all-polyethylene, cemented components. Low-quality evidence suggests that glenoid implants with radial mismatch of 5–7 mm and either pegged or keeled design may represent the best choice of component. CT scans are likely useful to determine clinically significant loosening. Current evidence does not support any correlation between early radiolucent lines and clinical or functional outcomes or radiographic progression of lucency.[11,15]

Glenoid fixation is challenging as a result of the local anatomy and bone stock. Further investigation is required with better randomization, better controls, better statistical analysis and more relevant outcome measures before evidence-based guidelines of treatment can be generated.

References

1. Churchill RS, Brems JJ, Kotschi H. Glenoid size, inclination, and version: an anatomic study. J Shoulder Elbow Surg 2001;10(4): 327–32.

2. Nyffeler RW, Jost B, Pfirrmann CW, Gerber C. Measurement of glenoid version: conventional radiographs versus computed tomography scans. J Shoulder Elbow Surg 2003;12(5):493–6.

3. Scalise JJ, Codsi MJ, Bryan J, Iannotti JP. The three-dimensional glenoid vault model can estimate normal glenoid version in osteoarthritis. J Shoulder Elbow Surg 2008;17(3):487–91.

4. Strauss EJ, Roche C, Flurin PH, Wright T, Zuckerman JD. The glenoid in shoulder arthroplasty. J Shoulder Elbow Surg 2009;18(5):819–33.

5. Bohsali KI, Wirth MA, Rockwood CA,Jr. Complications of total shoulder arthroplasty. J Bone Joint Surg Am 2006;88(10): 2279–92.

6. Buckingham BP, Parsons IM, Campbell B, Titelman RM, Smith KL, Matsen FA. Patient functional self-assessment in late glenoid component failure at three to eleven years after total shoulder arthroplasty. J Shoulder Elbow Surg 2005;14(4):368–74.

7. Mileti J, Boardman ND 3rd, Sperling JW, Cofield RH, Torchia ME, O'Driscoll SW, et al. Radiographic analysis of polyethylene glenoid components using modern cementing techniques. J Shoulder Elbow Surg 2004;13(5):492–8.

8. Nho SJ, Nam D, Ala OL, Craig EV, Warren RF, Wright TM. Observations on retrieved glenoid components from total shoulder arthroplasty. J Shoulder Elbow Surg 2009;18(3):371–8.

9. Yian EH, Werner CM, Nyffeler RW, Pfirrmann CW, Ramappa A, Sukthankar A, et al. Radiographic and computed tomography analysis of cemented pegged polyethylene glenoid components in total shoulder replacement. J Bone Joint Surg.Am 2005; 87(9):1928–36.

10. Walch G, Edwards TB, Boulahia A, Boileau P, Mole D, Adeleine P. The influence of glenohumeral prosthetic mismatch on glenoid radiolucent lines: results of a multicenter study. J Bone Joint Surg Am 2002;84(12):2186–91.

11. Nho SJ, Ala OL, Dodson CC, Figgie MP, Wright TM, Craig EV, et al. Comparison of conforming and nonconforming retrieved glenoid components. J Shoulder Elbow Surg 2008;17(6):914–20.

12. Harryman DT,2nd, Sidles JA, Clark JM, McQuade KJ, Gibb TD, Matsen FA,3rd. Translation of the humeral head on the glenoid with passive glenohumeral motion. J Bone Joint Surg Am 1990;72(9):1334–43.

13. Anglin C, Wyss UP, Pichora DR. Mechanical testing of shoulder prostheses and recommendations for glenoid design. J Shoulder Elbow Surg 2000;9(4):323–31.

14. Churchill RS, Boorman RS, Fehringer EV, Matsen FA,3rd. Glenoid cementing may generate sufficient heat to endanger the surrounding bone. Clin Orthop Relat Res 2004;419:76–9.

15. Boileau P, Avidor C, Krishnan SG, Walch G, Kempf JF, Mole D. Cemented polyethylene versus uncemented metal-backed glenoid components in total shoulder arthroplasty: a prospective, double-blind, randomized study. J Shoulder Elbow Surg 2002;11(4):351–9.

16. Fox TJ, Cil A, Sperling JW, Sanchez-Sotelo J, Schleck CD, Cofield RH. Survival of the glenoid component in shoulder arthroplasty. J Shoulder Elbow Surg 2009;18(6):859–63.

17. Taunton MJ, McIntosh AL, Sperling JW, Cofield RH. Total shoulder arthroplasty with a metal-backed, bone-ingrowth glenoid component. Medium to long-term results. J Bone Joint Surg Am 2008;90(10):2180–8.

18. Tammachote N, Sperling JW, Vathana T, Cofield RH, Harmsen WS, Schleck CD. Long-term results of cemented metal-backed glenoid components for osteoarthritis of the shoulder. J Bone Joint Surg.Am 2009;91(1):160–6.

19. Martin SD, Zurakowski D, Thornhill TS. Uncemented glenoid component in total shoulder arthroplasty. Survivorship and outcomes. J Bone Joint Surg Am 2005;87(6):1284–92.

20. Edwards TB, Kadakia NR, Boulahia A, Kempf JF, Boileau P, Nemoz C, et al. A comparison of hemiarthroplasty and total shoulder arthroplasty in the treatment of primary glenohumeral osteoarthritis: results of a multicenter study. J Shoulder Elbow Surg 2003;12(3):207–13.

21. Radnay CS, Setter KJ, Chambers L, Levine WN, Bigliani LU, Ahmad CS. Total shoulder replacement compared with humeral head replacement for the treatment of primary glenohumeral osteoarthritis: a systematic review. J Shoulder Elbow Surg 2007;16(4):396–402.

22. Stone KD, Grabowski JJ, Cofield RH, Morrey BF, An KN. Stress analyses of glenoid components in total shoulder arthroplasty. J Shoulder Elbow Surg 1999;8(2):151–8.

23. Gupta S, van der Helm FC, van Keulen F. Stress analysis of cemented glenoid prostheses in total shoulder arthroplasty. J Biomech 2004;37(11):1777–86.

24. Pelletier MH, Langdown A, Gillies RM, Sonnabend DH, Walsh WR. Photoelastic comparison of strains in the underlying glenoid with metal-backed and all-polyethylene implants. J Shoulder Elbow Surg 2008;17(5):779–83.

25. Gartsman GM, Elkousy HA, Warnock KM, Edwards TB, O'Connor DP. Radiographic comparison of pegged and keeled glenoid components. J Shoulder Elbow Surg 2005;14(3):252–7.

26. Nuttall D, Haines JF, Trail II. A study of the micromovement of pegged and keeled glenoid components compared using radiostereometric analysis. J Shoulder Elbow Surg 2007;16(3 Suppl):S65–70.

27. Lazarus MD, Jensen KL, Southworth C, Matsen FA,3rd. The radiographic evaluation of keeled and pegged glenoid component insertion. J Bone Joint Surg Am 2002;84 (7):1174–82.

28. Klepps S, Chiang AS, Miller S, Jiang CY, Hazrati Y, Flatow EL. Incidence of early radiolucent glenoid lines in patients having total shoulder replacements. Clin Orthop Relat Res 2005;435: 118–25.

29. Trail IA, Nuttall D. The results of shoulder arthroplasty in patients with rheumatoid arthritis. J Bone Joint Surg Br 2002;84(8):1121–5.

30. Anglin C, Wyss UP, Nyffeler RW, Gerber C. Loosening performance of cemented glenoid prosthesis design pairs. Clin Biomech (Bristol, Avon) 2001;16(2):144–50.

31. Lacroix D, Murphy LA, Prendergast PJ. Three-dimensional finite element analysis of glenoid replacement prostheses: a comparison of keeled and pegged anchorage systems. J Biomech Eng 2000;122(4):430–6.

32. Torchia ME, Cofield RH, Settergren CR. Total shoulder arthroplasty with the Neer prosthesis: long-term results. J Shoulder Elbow Surg 1997;6(6):495–505.

33. Pfahler M, Jena F, Neyton L, Sirveaux F, Mole D. Hemiarthroplasty versus total shoulder prosthesis: results of cemented glenoid components. J Shoulder Elbow Surg 2006;15(2):154–63.

34. Hughes M, Neer CS,2nd. Glenohumeral joint replacement and postoperative rehabilitation. Phys Ther 1975;55(8):850–8.

34 Fusion vs. Arthroplasty in the Treatment of Ankle Arthritis

Timothy R. Daniels[1], Mark Glazebrook,[2] Terence Chin[2], and Roger A. Haene[1]

[1]St. Michael's Hospital, University of Toronto, Toronto, ON, Canada
[2]Queen Elizabeth II Health Sciences Centre, Halifax, NS, Canada

Case scenario

A 58 year old man in good general health but with a past history of a previous tibial pilon fracture presents with signs and symptoms of endstage ankle osteoarthritis (OA) (Figure 34.1). On examination, he has a well-aligned hindfoot with stiffness and irritability of the ankle joint. He has a supple and pain-free subtalar joint complex. He wishes to consider surgical intervention and in particular, wants to discuss the role of ankle arthrodesis vs. total ankle arthroplasty (TAA).

Top eight questions

1. What is the long-term clinical outcome of ankle arthrodesis?
2. What is the best technique for performing ankle arthrodesis?
3. Does ankle arthrodesis accelerate the development of ipsilateral subtalar complex OA?
4. What is the medium- to long-term outcome of modern TAA?
5. What are the main complications of TAA?
6. Does TAA protect the subtalar joint complex from accelerated degeneration?
7. Are there any direct comparisons of ankle arthrodesis vs. TAA in the literature?
8. Does TAA result in more normal gait compared to ankle arthrodesis?

Question 1: What is the long-term clinical outcome of ankle arthrodesis?

Case clarification

The surgical management of endstage ankle arthritis has been an area of much debate.

Relevance

For over a century now, ankle arthrodesis (Figure 34.2) has been the most commonly performed surgical procedure for the treatment of endstage ankle arthritis.[1-12] Concerns exist regarding the long-term durability of ankle arthrodesis, especially in regard to the development of ipsilateral hindfoot degeneration leading to significant pain and impaired function.[13-15]

Current opinion

Ankle arthrodesis has traditionally been seen as the most reliable surgical method of treating ankle arthritis.

Finding the evidence

• PubMed, using search terms: "ankle," together with "osteoarthritis" OR "arthrosis" OR "fusion" OR "arthrodesis". Limits included: "English language" AND "humans"
• The reference list of all eligible papers was also cross-referenced for further studies which did not come up on the original PubMed search.

Quality of the evidence

Most studies contain level III and IV evidence. The vast majority are in fact retrospective level IV case series with

Evidence-Based Orthopedics, First Edition. Edited by Mohit Bhandari.
© 2012 Blackwell Publishing Ltd. Published 2012 by Blackwell Publishing Ltd.

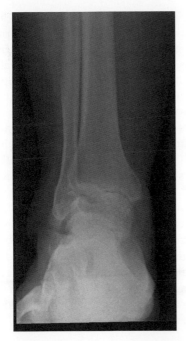

Figure 34.1 Endstage ankle arthritis.

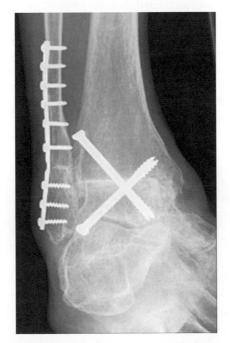

Figure 34.2 Open ankle arthrodesis with internal fixation.

heterogeneous populations, small patient numbers, and high rates of patients lost to follow-up, and do not use standardized or validated functional outcome instruments.[1–3,5–7,9,11,16–25]

Findings

The published reports on the outcomes of ankle arthrodesis have mainly been favorable, with good relief of ankle pain and high rates of patient satisfaction. Good results have

been reported in 66–90% of patients in the medium term.[1,2,5,6,10,12,16,19–23,26–29] In a meta-analysis comparing the results of ankle arthrodesis and TAA, Haddad et al. reviewed 39 studies on ankle arthrodesis from 1990 to 2005, and found between 67% and 73% good/excellent results.[30] The authors warn caution in interpreting these results as most studies reviewed are of poor scientific quality, with many studies lacking key data elements, having variable patient baseline characteristics, outcome reporting, and surgical procedures. In a recent level III study assessing functional outcomes and gait analysis, Thomas et al. reviewed 26 patients with ankle arthrodesis performed using modern screw fixation techniques with age-matched normal controls.[15] The authors utilized validated outcome scores—ankle osteoarthritis score (AOS) and the Musculoskeletal Outcomes Data Evaluation and Management Systems (MODEMS) questionnaire. Using intermediate-term follow-up of patients with ankle arthrodesis this study demonstrated acceptable pain relief, improvement in overall function, and high rates of patient satisfaction, but persistent disability with reduced foot and ankle function when compared to controls.[15]

Recommendation

- Good results may be expected in 66–90% of patients in the medium term [overall quality: very low]

Question 2: What is the best technique for performing ankle arthrodesis?

Case clarification

Arthrodesis technique in the ankle will not only influence the union process, but will also affect the long-term mechanics of the lower limb.

Relevance

Prior to the 1950s, ankle arthrodesis was performed with plaster of Paris cast immobilization.[16] Recognizing the importance of eliminating shear strain and gap formation between cut bone surfaces, Sir John Charnley described the method for compression arthrodesis of the ankle joint in his landmark paper of 1951.[6] This technique and modifications thereof was to be widely used over the next 20 years.[8,21,23,31,32] Internal fixation gained popularity in the 1970s.

Current opinion

To date, up to 35 different methods of internal fixation (screws, plates, and staples with or without inlay/onlay bone graft) have been described.[8–10,23,25,33–43]

Finding the evidence

- PubMed, using search terms: "ankle," together with "osteoarthritis" OR "arthrosis" OR "fusion" OR "arthrodesis." Limits included: "English language" AND "humans"

• The reference list of all eligible papers was also cross-referenced for further studies which did not come up on the original PubMed search

Quality of the evidence

Current recommendations on the optimum position for ankle arthrodesis are based on level III studies.

Findings

Current recommendations on the optimum position for ankle arthrodesis conclude that the ideal position is neutral dorsiflexion, 0–5° of valgus, external rotation of 5–10° or equal to the contralateral side, and with the talus positioned directly under or slightly posterior to the anatomic axis of the tibia. The latter reduces the anterior lever arm of the foot on the arthrodesis site and also improves ground clearance.[11,29,44–46] This position maximizes the compensatory potential of the subtalar and transverse tarsal joints and allows the closest approximation to normal gait patterns for the knee, foot, and ankle.[44]

Level III/IV evidence indicates lower nonunion (<10% vs. 40%) and infection rates (<5% vs. up to 40%) when ankle arthrodesis is performed with modern screw internal fixation compared to large pin external fixation.[10,12,28,29,33,36,37,47–49]

In terms of rigidity of internal fixation, biomechanical testing on cadaver models has shown the following:
• two crossed screws provide a more rigid construct than two parallel screws
• three screws provide greater compression and resistance to torque compared to two
• the addition of a fibular strut graft provides added stability compared to a two-screw construct, especially if the bone quality is poor.[50–52]

Most surgeons agree that a minimum of two screws are required for rigid fixation, and good results have been obtained with both two and three screws.[10,28,29,36,37,48]

Currently, external fixation with fine-wire or hybrid frames is recommended for complex ankle fusions in the setting of infection, poor-quality soft tissues, significant bone loss or deformity correction, and salvage of failed TAA.[53–55] Satisfactory outcomes are reported in level IV studies. The Ilizarov construct provides excellent stiffness and shear rigidity in bending and torsion while allowing for axial compression.[56] It also allows for continued adjustment to correct deformity and improve compression throughout the treatment period.

Schneider first described the technique of arthroscopic ankle arthrodesis in 1983.[57] There is level III/IV evidence suggesting lower infection rates, shorter hospital stays, shorter fusion times, and union rates at least equivalent to open ankle arthrodesis.[7,58–63] The reported advantages of arthroscopic ankle arthrodesis should, however, be interpreted with caution, as most studies report on patients with minimal ankle deformity. Level III studies comparing arthroscopic and open ankle arthrodesis are similarly biased by having patients with lesser deformities in the arthroscopic group.[61,62,64] Nevertheless, arthroscopic ankle arthrodesis is less invasive and, is theoretically beneficial in patients with poor soft tissues (previous open fractures, skin grafts, and soft tissue flaps) or those with risk factors for soft tissue complications.[61,62] Arthroscopic ankle arthrodesis requires a surgeon with experience in ankle arthroscopy.[58,61,62] Current level III/IV evidence would support its use in ankle OA with minimal deformity (<15°), although recent studies suggest its efficacy with greater degrees of deformity.[60,63]

As the outcomes of TAA improve, there is an increasing consideration to convert an arthrodesed ankle to TAA.[43,65,66] Having intact malleoli is a prerequisite for this. More recently, surgical approaches to ankle arthrodesis that preserve the malleoli have been performed. These include the fibular sparing z-osteotomy lateral approach (Figure 34.2), open anterior approach, and arthroscopic ankle arthrodesis (Figure 34.3).[7,43,61,62]

Recommendations

With regard to ankle arthrodesis, level III evidence exists to support the following:
• Use of modern internal fixation methods over older mainly external fixation techniques; three screws provide greater stability than two; any form of adjacent plate or fibular strut neutralization provides greatest stability (biomechanical cadaveric studies)
• The optimum fusion position of neutral plantar flexion, is 0–5° of valgus, external rotation of 5–10° or equal to the

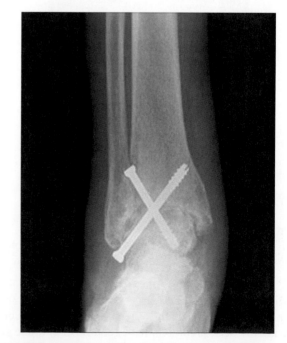

Figure 34.3 Arthroscopic ankle arthrodesis.

opposite limb, and with the talus directly under or slightly posterior to the anatomic axis of the tibia

Recommendations for ankle arthrodesis can be made for the following:
• Equivalent fusion rates, shorter time to fusion lower morbidity, and shorter hospital stays may occur with arthroscopic ankle arthrodesis (although the level III/IV evidence base for this is still debated because of potential patient selection bias in some studies) [overall quality: low to fair]

Question 3: Does ankle arthrodesis accelerate the development of ipsilateral subtalar complex OA?

Case clarification
The younger the candidate for ankle arthrodesis, the more important it becomes to consider the more distant effects of ankle arthrodesis.

Relevance
Since our patient is 58 years old and in good general health, he might reasonably expect another 10–20 years of active use from the ipsilateral lower limb. The potential to develop hindfoot degeneration may be an important factor in reaching a decision.

Current opinion
There is increasing concern regarding the detrimental effect of a fused ankle on adjacent subtalar and transverse tarsal joints, with degeneration of these joints an important contributor to pain and impaired function after ankle arthrodesis (Figure 34.4).[13–15,37,49,67,68]

Finding the evidence
• PubMed, using search terms "ankle," together with "osteoarthritis" OR "arthrosis" OR "fusion" OR "arthrodesis." Limits included "English language" AND "humans"
• The reference list of all eligible papers was also cross-referenced for further studies which did not come up on the original PubMed search.

Quality of the evidence
Most studies are of level III and IV evidence, mainly retrospective. There is one level III prospective study.

Findings
Hallock in 1945 reported poor results following ankle arthrodesis in patients who had subtalar and midtarsal OA.[16] He noted that the ipsilateral hindfoot OA is usually due to the original trauma but may develop after ankle fusion. In a recent level III prospective study Thomas et al. reported on the development of moderate to severe subtalar OA in 4 of 26 patients at an average follow-up of 4.4

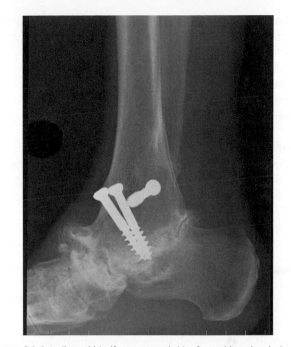

Figure 34.4 Ipsilateral hindfoot osteoarthritis after ankle arthrodesis.

years.[15] Retrospective level III/IV studies with long-term follow-up (9–23 years) report 50–90% incidence of ipsilateral hindfoot (mainly subtalar joint) degeneration following ankle arthrodesis.[13,14,49,68] Most of these studies however, describe older methods of fixation,[13,14,68] do not assess for degenerative changes in these ipsilateral joints preoperatively[14,49,68] and have a substantial proportion of patients fused in unsatisfactory positions (varus, equinus).[14,49,68] Sheridan et al. (level IV evidence) showed that a significant proportion of patients have ipsilateral hindfoot and midfoot arthritis prior to ankle arthrodesis, and therefore ipsilateral joint degeneration may not be a direct consequence of the ankle arthrodesis.[69] In a population-based level III retrospective study, SooHoo et al. noted a significantly higher rate of subtalar joint fusion following ankle arthrodesis (2.8%) compared to TAA (0.7%).[70] Evidence from level III retrospective studies suggests the presence of subtalar OA after ankle arthrodesis correlates with poorer outcomes.[13,14,68] Despite the high incidence of ipsilateral hindfoot OA after ankle arthrodesis, most patients remain satisfied.[13,14,68]

In summary, there is level III and IV evidence in the literature indicating a high incidence of ipsilateral subtalar, and to a lesser extent, talonavicular OA in the setting of an ankle arthrodesis.[1,4,13–16,67,68] A recent prospective study using modern techniques of ankle ankle arthrodesis has shown a 15% incidence of progressive subtalar OA at 4 year follow-up.[15]

Current literature suggests that the high incidence of ipsilateral hindfoot arthritis observed in long-term outcome studies is the result of abnormal hindfoot mechanics,[71] poor technique,[13,14,68] and an increased incidence of pre-existing ipsilateral hindfoot arthritis;[69] it is highly likely that with modern techniques the incidence will be lower but still substantial. Despite a high incidence of ipsilateral hindfoot OA following ankle arthrodesis, most patients derive definite benefit from the procedure, generally remain satisfied with the outcomes and many (>80–90%) would have the procedure again.[4,10,13–15,19,28,29,47,68]

Recommendation

• Improvements in pain with high rates of patient satisfaction despite a high incidence of ipsilateral (predominantly subtalar joint) OA (mainly older level IV long-term studies with one recent level III short-term study) [overall quality: low to fair]

Question 4: What is the medium to long-term outcome of modern TAA?

Case clarification

First-generation TAA designs were two-component prostheses that were fixed using bone cement. In order to accommodate the cement mantle, bone resection was substantial. Since then, much progress has been made in the biomechanics of TAA, with a change to semiconstrained, uncemented, anatomic three-component designs with mobile meniscal bearings (Figure 34.5).[72–75]

Relevance

Patients will want to know what the medium to long-term outcomes are for the newer generation designs of TAA.

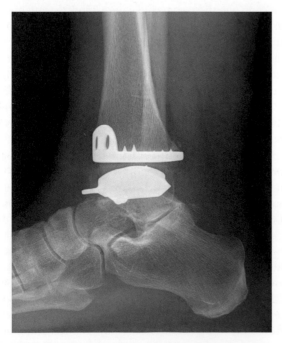

Figure 34.5 Third-generation total ankle arthroplasty

Current opinion

The first-generation versions of TAA in the 1970s and 1980s showed disappointing results, leading Kitaoka et al.[76] to recommend that surgical treatment of rheumatoid arthritis (RA) and OA using TAA should be abandoned.

A resurgence of interest in TAA for treatment of endstage ankle arthritis has emerged due to improved second- and third-generation implant results[77–80] and concurrent concerns regarding the long-term durability of ankle arthrodesis, especially in regard to the development of ipsilateral hindfoot OA leading to significant pain and impaired function.[13–15]

Finding the evidence

• PubMed, using search terms: "ankle," together with "osteoarthritis" OR "arthrosis" OR "arthroplasty" OR "replacement." Limits included "English language" AND "humans"

• The reference lists of all eligible papers were also cross-referenced for further studies which did not come up on the original PubMed search

Quality of the evidence

The majority of TAA evidence is level IV, from small numbers of patients drawn from heterogeneous populations, followed for short periods of time and assessed using inconsistent and nonvalidated measures. There are very few independent studies presenting long-term TAA outcomes. In the past decade, there has been one study with level II evidence[81] and none with level I evidence.

In spite of level III and IV studies, controversy still exists regarding the following:
• Whether patient age at time of TAA negatively influences outcome
• What the effect of preoperative coronal plane deformity has on TAA survivorship
• The significance of the relatively common finding of heterotopic ossification seen on radiographs following TAA.

Findings

Patient satisfaction Level IV evidence supports that marked pain improvement occurs after TAA in nearly all patients; however, some persistent pain is common. Postoperative range of motion following TAA will be roughly equivalent to the preoperative level.

Survival rates In papers with short- to medium-term follow-up the survival rates range from 67.7 to 98.7% with an overall mean of 87.6 % survival at 5 years (Table 34.1).[49,73–75,77–80,82–93] Similar results have been published in a recent meta-analysis by Haddad et al.[30] In 2007, results from the Norwegian, Swedish, and New Zealand registers were published. Norwegian results showed 5-year survival of 89% and 10-year survival of 76%.[84] Swedish results

Table 34.1 Short to medium-term survival rates of various total ankle arthroplasty prostheses

Study	Mean follow-up time (months)	Implant	Cases	% Survival
Spirt et al.[91]	33	Agility	306	89.2
Knecht et al.[79]	108	Agility	132	89.4
Hosman et al.[86,a]	32	Agility	117	92.3
Pyevich et al.[89]	58	Agility	86	94.2
Hurowitz et al.[87]	40	Agility	65	67.7
Schuberth et al.[73]	24	Agility	50	84.0
Ali et al.[82]	60 (3–150)	B-P	35	97.1
Kurup and Taylor[88]	34	B-P	34	88.2
San Giovanni et al.[90 was 89]	100	B-P	31	93.5
Beuchel et al.[77,a]	60	B-P (deep-sulcus)	75	98.7
Buechel et al.[77,a]	144	B-P (shallow-sulcus)	40	82.5
Su et al.[94]	77	B-P/HSS	27	92.6
Doets et al.[95]	91	B-P/LCS	93	83.9
Hintermann et al.[78]	36	HINTEGRA	271	85.6
Henricson et al.[85,a]	25	HINTEGRA	29	86.2
Henricson et al.[85 was 81,a]	54	STAR	318	77.0
Fevang et al.[84,a]	37	STAR	212	90.1
Wood and Deakin[74]	46	STAR	200	92.7
Valderrabano et al.[93]	44	STAR	68	86.8
Anderson et al.[75]	52	STAR	51	76.5
Hosman et al.[86,a]	43	STAR	45	93.3
Kofoed[80,a]	113	STAR—cemented	33	72.7
Kofoed[80,a]	113	STAR—noncemented	25	96.0
Fevang et al.[84,a]	92	TPR—cemented	32	81.3
Takakura et al.[49]	62	TNK—New ceramic	70	95.7
			Total cases	2445.0
			Overall survival rate	87.5

[a]Five of the studies included used two separate prostheses in their study; they were considered separately in the interest of more thorough interpretation. This gives a total of 25 entries for this table.

(Copyright © 2011 by the American Orthopaedic Foot and Ankle Society, Inc., originally published in Foot & Ankle International, 30(10):946 and reproduced here with permission.)

showed 5-year survival of 78%,[81] but the results for the three surgeons who performed the majority of TAAs averaged 86%. New Zealand data reflected 5-year survival rate of 86%.[86] What is clear from the outcome data is that survival rates vary among different institutions, and that increased surgeon experience is associated with better outcomes.

Predictors of outcome Level IV and III evidence supports that TAA outcomes are not significantly influenced by the underlying cause of ankle degeneration.

In a 1998 level III long-term study, Kofoed found only slight differences in outcomes between patients with OA and those with RA, with no differences in TAA survival.[72] Similar findings were reported by Anderson in 2003 from a level IV study[75] and Valderrabano in 2004 in a level IV series,[93] although Valderrabano found that the revision rate was higher in patients with post-traumatic OA.[93] Neither the Norwegian register[84] nor the Swedish register[85] found any significant influence, except for a nonsignificant tendency found in the Swedish register for TAA in the post-traumatic group to have a slightly lower survival rate.

Age at surgery is controversial. In a long-term level III study, Kofoed found that TAA outcomes were equal in patients of all ages,[96] with similar level IV evidence by Valderrabano at 4 years follow-up.[93] The Norwegian register showed no significant influence.[84] However, a level IV study by Spirt showed that at 3 years follow-up younger age negatively influenced reoperation rates,[91] and the Swedish register showed that lower age at index surgery implied increased risk of revision.[85]

Level of postoperative activity is not strictly related to age. In 2009, Naal's level IV series showed no association between increased postoperative physical activity levels and the appearance of periprosthetic radiolucencies at 3.7 years after TAA.[97]

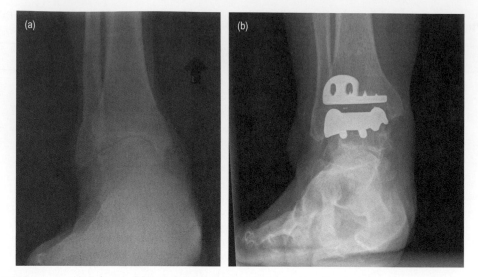

Figure 34.6 (a) Preoperative varus ankle deformity. (b) Postoperative position with total ankle arthroplasty.

Gender has no significant influence on TAA outcome, according to both Norwegian[84] and Swedish registers.[85]

Preoperative coronal plane ankle deformity (Figure 34.6) is another controversial topic. In their 2003 level IV series, Wood and Deakin[74] found that postoperative edge loading of the polyethylene bearing was more common in those with preoperative varus or valgus greater than 15°. In 2009, Wood further found that preoperative coronal plane deformity showed a significant effect on survivorship at 54 months, with the likelihood of revision being directly proportional to the size of the preoperative deformity. However, in 2009 Hobson's level III study found no significant difference in complications or outcomes between neutral ankles and those with preoperative deformity up to 30°,[98] and this has been supported by findings by Kim in a level III study.[99] Further research in this area may clarify what factors have produced the differences in outcomes, and what the safe recommendations are.

Supplementary procedures performed concurrently with TAA are common, including calcaneal osteotomy, subtalar/talonavicular fusion, ligament reconstruction, and tendon transfer. In Schuberth's level IV series,[73] concomitant procedures were not associated with an increased incidence of complications compared to TAA alone.

Radiographic findings Radiographic appearances have not yet found to be related to clinical findings.[89] However, many authors believe that it is simply a reflection of the short follow-up periods of TAA studies.

Periarticular heterotopic new bone formation is common. Two recent level IV papers from different major centers have interpreted its significance differently. Valderrabano[93] believed it to be responsible for decreased range of motion,

while Wood and Deakin[74] found that heterotopic new bone was not associated with a poor result.

Periprosthetic lucent lines are frequently found in uncemented TAA, but the fact that they are always seen within 2 years and are mostly nonprogressive suggest that they are not caused by polyethylene particle wear.[89] Progression of lucent areas, in contrast, is more indicative of prosthetic loosening.[79,89] Polyethylene wear also occurs in TAA and can eventually also produce the classical expansile osteolysis recognized in hip and knee replacements.[74,79,93]

Implant migration has been seen in some TAA series.[89,92] Knecht[79] suggested that migration of 5 mm or 5° or more places a patient at higher risk of implant failure.

Scoring systems vs. patient satisfaction The majority of scoring systems used in the literature are based on pain, general mobility, and range of motion at the ankle joint. A significant improvement in the pain scales is a near universal finding; however, some persistent pain is common (level IV).[89,93] Postoperative range of motion following TAA will be roughly equivalent to the preoperative level, even at mid- to long-term follow-up.[74,75,89] It is fairly common to find that patient satisfaction remains high with TAA, independent of whether the scoring systems produce satisfactory or unsatisfactory results.[79,89,92,93,100] This incongruence suggests that current outcome scores are not capturing the benefits of TAA as perceived by the patients.

Recommendation

• Patients can expect substantial improvement in pain following TAA, although range of motion is often the same. Survival rates range from 67.7 to 98.7% with an overall mean of 87.6 % survival at 5 years [overall quality: low to fair]

Question 5: What are the main complications of TAA?

Case clarification
Complications of TAA have the potential to consume many months and possibly require salvage surgery.

Relevance
Earlier design generations of the total ankle replacement were plagued with problems.

Current opinion
The belief that TAA is associated with high complication rates is held by many surgeons, who remain wary of the procedure because of its technical difficulty.

Finding the evidence
• PubMed, using search terms: "ankle," together with "osteoarthritis" OR "arthrosis" OR "arthroplasty" OR "replacement." Limits included: "English language" AND "humans"
• The reference lists of all eligible papers were also cross-referenced for further studies which did not come up on the original PubMed search.

Quality of the evidence
Most studies provide level IV evidence, with some level III work.

Findings
It has been well documented that a surgeon will experience an early high complication rate associated with TAA but this reduces with experience.[73,74,85,101] In 2006 Schuberth published the perioperative complication rate of the first 50 consecutive total ankle replacements performed by a single surgeon.[73] There was a 38% rate of intraoperative malleolar fractures, 24% occurrence of some degree of component malalignment, 18% incidence of minor wound healing disturbances that resolved with local wound care, and a 2% rate of major wound complications requiring flap coverage. Early component revision was required in 16%. Each of these complications, other than wound complications, decreased with surgeon experience. In 2008, Lee documented the difference in complication rates between the first 25 TAA cases and the second 25 cases performed at a single hospital.[101] In the first 25 cases, the complication rate was 60%, including a 16% incidence of intraoperative malleolar fractures. In the second 25 cases, the complication rate was 20%, and the malleolar fracture rate was 4%. Saltzman[102] has confirmed the importance of increased collective surgical experience and suggested that overall outcomes can be expected to improve in future studies.

Recently an evidence-based classification system for complications in TAA has been proposed that classifies complications according to their potential to cause failure of the prosthesis (defined as removal of implants).[103] Twenty studies identified under specific inclusion criteria revealed nine main complications of TAA. Deep infection, aseptic loosening, and implant failure were classified as "high-grade" complications since they were shown to result in failure greater than 50% of the time. Technical error, subsidence, and postoperative bone fracture were classified as "medium-grade," resulting in failure less than 50% of the time. Intraoperative bone fractures and wound healing problems were classified as "low-grade," resulting in failure less than 50% of the time.

Level IV evidence supports that supplementary extra-articular realignment procedures performed concomitantly with TAA are not associated with an increased incidence of complications.

Recommendation
• There is a well-described learning curve with TAA, and in the early stages a surgeon can experience 20–60% complication rates. However, many complications do not pose a threat to the longevity of the prosthesis itself, and a classification of complication impact has therefore been developed [overall quality: very low to low]

Question 6: Does TAA protect the subtalar joint complex from accelerated degeneration?

Case clarification
Patients hope to retain ankle and hindfoot motion following TAA.

Relevance
This is an important consideration, as it remains one of the main goals a surgeon hopes to achieve when performing TAA.

Current opinion
Interest in TAA developed as a way to treat ankle arthritis in RA while avoiding subsequent overload of adjacent hindfoot joints.

Finding the evidence
• PubMed, using search terms: "ankle," together with "osteoarthritis" OR "arthrosis" OR "arthroplasty" OR "replacement." Limits included: "English language" AND "humans"
• The reference lists of all eligible papers were also cross-referenced for further studies which did not come up on the original PubMed search

Quality of the evidence
There is level III evidence to support that patients do not go on to develop hindfoot OA following TAA.

Findings

Degeneration of ipsilateral hindfoot joints has been sought on follow-up radiographic study. Kofoed,[72] in his long-term level III study, found that none of the patients with OA went on to develop subtalar arthrosis following arthroplasty, with similar results published by Valderrabano.[93]

Recommendation

- Level III evidence supports that TAA prevents hindfoot degeneration in later years [overall quality: fair]

Question 7: Are there any direct comparisons of ankle arthrodesis vs. TAA in the literature?

Case clarification

Patients are interested in which procedure is more likely to succeed in their particular circumstance, and direct comparative studies are helpful in providing information.

Relevance

The deficiencies in historical studies looking at either ankle arthrodesis or TAA do not allow easy comparisons of results.

Current opinion

Opinions are divided on the matter, and the choice of procedure remains controversial in many cases.

Finding the evidence

- PubMed, using search terms: "ankle," together with "osteoarthritis" OR "arthrosis", AND "fusion" OR "arthrodesis," AND "arthroplasty" OR "replacement." Limits included: "English language" and "humans"
- The reference list of all eligible papers was also cross-referenced for further studies which did not come up on the original PubMed search

Quality of the evidence

The authors identified one short-term level II study, one level III meta-analysis, and one level IV paper.

Findings

Only three papers using modern surgical methods have directly compared the outcomes of ankle arthrodesis and TAA,[30,70,102] and only one of these studies compared overall clinical outcomes.

In 2009, Saltzman[102] published a prospective multicenter level II trial comparing ankle arthrodesis and TAA. By 24 months, ankles treated with TAA had better function and equivalent pain relief compared to ankles treated with fusion. Operative time, blood loss, and length of hospital stay were the same for both. Rates of secondary major surgeries were the same for both. The study

concluded that using modern implants and surgical techniques, superior overall patient success has been shown in the TAA group. The major weakness of this study, however, lies in the 2 year follow-up period, which is very short.

In 2007, SooHoo published a level III meta-analysis comparing reoperation rates between 4705 ankle arthrodesis and 480 TAA cases, based on their review of the California hospital database from 1995 to 2004.[70] Patients treated with ankle arthrodesis had a higher requirement for subtalar fusion at 5 years postoperatively than did those treated with ankle replacement. TAA had an increased risk of device-related infection and of having a major revision procedure.

The 2007 level IV publication by Haddad[30] compared the results of meta-analysis of TAA publications against meta-analysis of ankle arthrodesis publications. Patient satisfaction with their outcome in the TAA group was 78% and in the ankle arthrodesis group was 73%. The 5-year TAA survival was 78% and 10-year survival 77%. The TAA revision rate was 7%, mainly due to loosening and subsidence. The overall revision rate for ankle fusions was 9% with a non-union rate of 10%.

Recommendation

- Level II, III, and IV evidence supports that TAA and ankle arthrodesis provide equivalent results in the short term [overall quality: low to good]

Question 8: Does TAA result in more normal gait compared to ankle arthrodesis?

Case clarification

Patients undergoing arthroplasty hope to avoid a postoperative limp.

Relevance

For TAA to truly offer the patient an advantage over ankle arthrodesis, it must allow for enough motion to normalize gait.

Finding the evidence

- PubMed, using search terms "ankle," together with "osteoarthritis" OR "arthrosis", "fusion" OR "arthrodesis," "arthroplasty" OR "replacement", "gait" OR "limp." Limits included "English language" and "humans"
- The reference list of all eligible papers was also cross-referenced for further studies which did not come up on the original PubMed search

Quality of the evidence

Good-quality Level II and III studies have been performed separately for each procedure as well as combined in the same study in order to compare the effect on gait.

Findings

Gait analysis after ankle arthrodesis Level III evidence in several gait analysis reports indicates abnormal gait patterns following ankle arthrodesis. Decreased stride length, reduced walking velocity, and reduced hindfoot motion are consistent findings after ankle arthrodesis.[11,15,71,104,105] Compensatory sagittal motion in the midfoot occurs following ankle arthrodesis, giving a relatively "normal" appearance to gait.[11,46,71] Decreased anterior tibial tilt and early heel-off at the end of stance phase has also been demonstrated in patients after arthrodesis.[71] During normal gait, the tibia moves forward on the foot during midstance. This movement is due to dorsiflexion of the ankle joint. With an arthrodesed ankle, forward progression of the tibia is reduced but not eliminated, and is mediated by the compensatory midtarsal dorsi/plantarflexion. As this midtarsal compensation is incomplete, early heel-off occurs following arthrodesis. Beyaert et al.[71] were able to demonstrate that this early heel-off results in the ground reaction force normally centered close to the metatarsal heads to be shifted posteriorly to the region of the midfoot during early heel-off. The authors conclude that this provides evidence for increased pathologic stresses applied to the midfoot after arthrodesis.[71] Beyaert et al. and others also demonstrated that the abnormal gait patterns and altered foot dynamics in ankle arthrodesis are most evident when walking barefoot, are exacerbated when walking at speed, but are improved with shoe wear (especially with an elevated heel).[11,71,104]

The effect of ankle arthrodesis on the ipsilateral hip (decreased hip flexion) and knee (early knee extension in late stance) is minimal unless the ankle is fused in equinus, where upon genu recurvatum, knee external rotation with increased stress on the medial collateral ligament can occur.[11] A level II gait analysis study on patients with RA treated with ankle and hindfoot fusions demonstrated significant improvements in both kinematics and kinetics of ipsilateral hip and knee joints.[106]

Gait analysis after TAA Several gait analysis studies have been performed following patients with more recent TAA designs.[95,107,108] Dyrby's[107] and Valderrabano's[108] level II studies and Doets'[95] level III study all support improvement of muscle function during walking, with near-normal gait pattern in terms of kinematics of the knee, ankle, and foot. Ground reactive forces at midstance were improved, but patients continued to demonstrate decreased vertical peak pressures during the terminal stance phase.[95] The improved dorsiflexion during the stance phase may help decrease the abnormal shear forces to the subtalar joint complex, thereby decreasing the incidence of progressive ipsilateral hindfoot arthritis.

Direct gait analysis comparisons between ankle arthrodesis and TAA Piriou's 2008 level III paper[109] compared gait analysis after ankle arthrodesis and TAA. Neither procedure restored normal movement or walking speed. Ankle arthrodesis resulted in a faster gait with longer step length, although the timing of gait demonstrated greater asymmetry. The TAA group had greater movement at the ankle, a symmetrical timing of gait, and restored ground reaction force pattern.

Recommendation

- There is level II evidence indicating abnormal pressures through the midfoot[71] and level III evidence indicating compensatory midfoot sagittal motion following ankle arthrodesis.[11,46,71] Compared to arthrodesis, level II/III evidence demonstrates TAA improves gait analysis parameters towards normality, although normal gait kinetics or kinematics are not restored.[95,107–109]

Summary of recommendations

Analysis of the evidence presented in this chapter suggests the possibility of equivalence in the outcomes of ankle arthrodesis and TAA procedures, with both yielding satisfactory outcomes. Long-term studies of ankle arthrodesis suggest persistent alterations in gait and high incidence of ipsilateral hindfoot joint OA, with pain and poor function. The improvement in gait mechanics following TAA may help decrease this.

Conclusions

The most common cause of ankle arthritis is trauma, followed by inflammatory arthropathies and structural deformity.[110] The ankle joint is resilient to the process of aging, and primary OA is rare. Level I and II evidence shows that endstage ankle arthritis is as debilitating as endstage hip arthritis.[111,112]

Any evaluation of ankle arthrodesis needs to be done in the light of the improving results with current TAA. Prospective long-term outcome studies comparing the two are needed. Future studies on ankle arthrodesis will hopefully report on ankles fused in optimum positions and utilize validated outcome measures. Only then will valid answers be provided with regard to the effect of ankle arthrodesis on adjacent hindfoot joints, its impact on functional outcomes, and ultimately how ankle arthrodesis measures up to current TAA.

Even in the hands of well-trained and experienced surgeons, results of TAA are still likely inferior to hip arthroplasty. Further improvement in prosthesis design, surgical technique, and clarification of the indications are required.

The long-term results of most new arthroplasty designs are unknown.

At present, TAA is a valuable and equivalent alternative to ankle arthrodesis, but it is not yet known if it will in future fully replace ankle arthrodesis.

In conclusion it is clear that both ankle arthrodesis and TAA may be assigned a grade B recommendation (fair evidence, level II or III studies with consistent findings) for the surgical treatment of endstage ankle arthritis. However, clearly more well-designed level I randomized controlled trials documenting patient preoperative characteristics and postoperative outcomes are needed to assist in making recommendations on which procedure is superior.

References

1. Aaron AD. Ankle fusion: a retrospective review. Orthopedics 1990;13(11):1249–54.

2. Abdo RV, Wasilewski SA. Ankle arthrodesis: a long-term study. Foot Ankle 1992;13(6):307–12.

3. Adams JC. Arthrodesis of the ankle joint; experiences with the transfibular approach. J Bone Joint Surg Br 1948;30(3):506–11.

4. Ahlberg A, Henricson AS. Late results of ankle fusion. Acta Orthop Scand 1981;52(1):103–5.

5. Boobbyer GN. The long-term results of ankle arthrodesis. Acta Orthop Scand 1981;52(1):107–10.

6. Charnley J. Compression arthrodesis of the ankle and shoulder. J Bone Joint Surg Br 1951;33(2):180–91.

7. Ferkel RD, Hewitt M. Long-term results of arthroscopic ankle arthrodesis. Foot Ankle Int 2005;26(4):275–80.

8. Hagen RJ. Ankle arthrodesis. Problems and pitfalls. Clin Orthop Relat Res 1986;202:152–62.

9. Kopp FJ, Banks MA, Marcus RE. Clinical outcome of tibiotalar arthrodesis utilizing the chevron technique. Foot Ankle Int 2004;25(4):225–30.

10. Mann RA, Rongstad KM. Arthrodesis of the ankle: a critical analysis. Foot Ankle Int 1998;19(1):3–9.

11. Mazur JM, Schwartz E, Simon SR. Ankle arthrodesis. Long-term follow-up with gait analysis. J Bone Joint Surg Am 1979;61(7):964–75.

12. Muir DC, Amendola A, and Saltzman CL. Long-term outcome of ankle arthrodesis. Foot Ankle Clin 2002;7(4):703–8.

13. Buchner M, Sabo D. Ankle fusion attributable to posttraumatic arthrosis: a long-term followup of 48 patients. Clin Orthop Relat Res 2003;406:155–64.

14. Coester LM, Saltzman CL, Leupold J, Pontarelli W. Long-term results following ankle arthrodesis for post-traumatic arthritis. J Bone Joint Surg Am 2001;83(2):219–28.

15. Thomas R, Daniels TR, Parker K. Gait analysis and functional outcomes following ankle arthrodesis for isolated ankle arthritis. J Bone Joint Surg Am 2006;88(3):526–35.

16. Hallock H. Arthrodesis of the ankle joint for old painful fractures. J Bone Joint Surg Am 1945;27(1):49–58.

17. Jackson A, Glasgow M. Tarsal hypermobility after ankle fusion—fact or fiction? J Bone Joint Surg Br 1979;61(4):470–3.

18. Lance EM, Paval A, Fries I, Larsen I, Patterson RL Jr. Arthrodesis of the ankle joint. A follow-up study. Clin Orthop Relat Res 1979;142:146–58.

19. Lynch AF, Bourne RB, Rorabeck CH. The long-term results of ankle arthrodesis. J Bone Joint Surg Br 1988;70(1):113–16.

20. Morrey BF, Wiedeman GP Jr. Complications and long-term results of ankle arthrodeses following trauma. J Bone Joint Surg Am 1980;62(5):777–84.

21. Ratliff AH. Compression arthrodesis of the ankle. J Bone Joint Surg Br 1959;41:524–34.

22. Said E, Hunka L, Siller TN. Where ankle fusion stands today. J Bone Joint Surg Br 1978;60(2):211–14.

23. Scranton PE Jr., Fu FH, Brown TD. Ankle arthrodesis: a comparative clinical and biomechanical evaluation. Clin Orthop Relat Res 1980(151):234–43.

24. Anderson, T., Montgomery F, Besjakov J, Verdier H, Carlsson A. Arthrodesis of the ankle for non-inflammatory conditions–healing and reliability of outcome measurements. Foot Ankle Int 2002;23(5):390–3.

25. Wang GJ, Shen WJ, McLaughlin RE, Stamp WG. Transfibular compression arthrodesis of the ankle joint. Clin Orthop Relat Res 1993(289):223–7.

26. Barr JR, Record EE. Arthrodesis of the ankle joint. Indications, operative technique and clinical experience. New Engl J Med 1953;248:53–56.

27. Helm R. The results of ankle arthrodesis. J Bone Joint Surg Br 1990;72(1):141–3.

28. Monroe MT, Beals TC, Manoli A 2nd. Clinical outcome of arthrodesis of the ankle using rigid internal fixation with cancellous screws. Foot Ankle Int 1999;20(4):227–31.

29. Morgan CD, Henke JA, Bailey RW, Kaufer H. Long-term results of tibiotalar arthrodesis. J Bone Joint Surg Am 1985;67(4):546–50.

30. Haddad SL, Coetzee JC, Estok R, Fahrbach K, Banel D, Nalysnyk L. Intermediate and long-term outcomes of total ankle arthroplasty and ankle arthrodesis. A systematic review of the literature. J Bone Joint Surg Am 2007;89(9):1899–905.

31. Kenzora JE, Simmons SC, Burgess AR, Edwards CC. External fixation arthrodesis of the ankle joint following trauma. Foot Ankle 1986;7(1):49–61.

32. Stewart MJ, Beeler TC, McConnell JC. Compression arthrodesis of the ankle. Evaluation of a cosmetic modification. J Bone Joint Surg Am 1983;65(2):219–25.

33. Chen YJ, Huang TJ, Shih HN, Hsu KY, Hsu RW. Ankle arthrodesis with cross screw fixation. Good results in 36/40 cases followed 3–7 years. Acta Orthop Scand 1996;67(5):473–8.

34. Colgrove RC, Bruffey JD. Ankle arthrodesis: combined internal-external fixation. Foot Ankle Int 2001;22(2):92–7.

35. Dohm MP, Benjamin JB, Harrison J, Szivek JA. A biomechanical evaluation of three forms of internal fixation used in ankle arthrodesis. Foot Ankle Int 1994;15(6):297–300.

36. Holt ES, Hansen ST, Mayo KA, Sangeorzan BJ. Ankle arthrodesis using internal screw fixation. Clin Orthop Relat Res 1991;268:21–8.

37. Maurer RC, Cimino WR, Cox CV, Satow GK. Transarticular cross-screw fixation. A technique of ankle arthrodesis. Clin Orthop Relat Res 1991;268:56–64.

38. Morgan SJ, Thordarson DB, Shepherd LE. Salvage of tibial pilon fractures using fusion of the ankle with a 90 degrees cannulated blade-plate: a preliminary report. Foot Ankle Int 1999;20(6):375–8.

39. Plaass C, Knupp M, Barg A, Hintermann B. Anterior double plating for rigid fixation of isolated tibiotalar arthrodesis. Foot Ankle Int 2009;30(7):631–9.

40. Ross SD, Matta J. Internal compression arthrodesis of the ankle. Clin Orthop Relat Res 1985;199:54–60.

41. White AA 3rd. A precision posterior ankle fusion. Clin Orthop Relat Res 1974;98:239–50.

42. Wu CC, Shih CH, Chen WJ, Tai CL. Tension-band technique for ankle fusion. Orthopedics 2001;24(1):37–40.

43. Glazebrook M, Holden D, Mayich J, Mitchell A, Boyd G. Fibular sparing Z-osteotomy technique for ankle arthrodesis. Tech Foot Ankle Surg 2009;8(1):34–7.

44. Buck P, Morrey BF, Chao EY. The optimum position of arthrodesis of the ankle. A gait study of the knee and ankle. J Bone Joint Surg Am 1987;69(7):1052–62.

45. Hefti FL, Baumann JU, Morscher EW. Ankle joint fusion—determination of optimal position by gait analysis. Arch Orthop Trauma Surg 1980;96(3):187–95.

46. King HA, Watkins TB Jr., Samuelson KM. Analysis of foot position in ankle arthrodesis and its influence on gait. Foot Ankle 1980;1(1):44–9.

47. Colman AB Pomeroy GC. Transfibular ankle arthrodesis with rigid internal fixation: an assessment of outcome. Foot Ankle Int 2007;28(3):303–7.

48. Moeckel BH, Patterson BM, Inglis AE, Sculco TP. Ankle arthrodesis. A comparison of internal and external fixation. Clin Orthop Relat Res 1991;268:78–83.

49. Takakura Y, Tanaka Y, Sugimoto K, Akiyama K, Tamai S. Long-term results of arthrodesis for osteoarthritis of the ankle. Clin Orthop Relat Res 1999;361:178–85.

50. Friedman RL, Glisson RR, Nunley JA 2nd. A biomechanical comparative analysis of two techniques for tibiotalar arthrodesis. Foot Ankle Int 1994;15(6):301–5.

51. Ogilvie-Harris DJ, Fitsialos D, Hedman TP. Arthrodesis of the ankle. A comparison of two versus three screw fixation in a crossed configuration. Clin Orthop Relat Res 1994;304:195–9.

52. Thordarson DB, Markolf KL, Cracchiolo A 3rd. Arthrodesis of the ankle with cancellous-bone screws and fibular strut graft. Biomechanical analysis. J Bone Joint Surg Am 1990;72(9):1359–63.

53. Salem KH, Kinzl L, Schmelz A, Ankle arthrodesis using Ilizarov ring fixators: a review of 22 cases. Foot Ankle Int 2006;27(10):764–70.

54. Johnson EE, Weltmer J, Lian GJ, Cracchiolo A 3rd. Ilizarov ankle arthrodesis. Clin Orthop Relat Res 1992;280:160–9.

55. Eylon S, Porat S, Bor N, Leibner ED. Outcome of Ilizarov ankle arthrodesis. Foot Ankle Int 2007;28(8):873–9.

56. Fleming, B., Paley D, Kristiansen T, Pope M. A biomechanical analysis of the Ilizarov external fixator. Clin Orthop Relat Res 1989;241:95–105.

57. Schneider D. Arthroscopic ankle fusion. Arthroscopic Video J 1983;3.

58. Collman DR, Kaas MH, Schuberth JM. Arthroscopic ankle arthrodesis: factors influencing union in 39 consecutive patients. Foot Ankle Int 2006;27(12):1079–85.

59. Glick JM, Morgan CD, Myerson MS, Sampson TG, Mann JA. Ankle arthrodesis using an arthroscopic method: long-term follow-up of 34 cases. Arthroscopy 1996;12(4):428–34.

60. Gougoulias NE, Agathangelidis FG, Parsons SW. Arthroscopic ankle arthrodesis. Foot Ankle Int 2007;28(6):695–706.

61. Myerson MS, Quill G. Ankle arthrodesis. A comparison of an arthroscopic and an open method of treatment. Clin Orthop Relat Res 1991;268:84–95.

62. O'Brien TS, Hart TS, Shereff MJ, Stone J, Johnson J. Open versus arthroscopic ankle arthrodesis: a comparative study. Foot Ankle Int 1999;20(6):368–74.

63. Winson IG, Robinson DE, Allen PE. Arthroscopic ankle arthrodesis. J Bone Joint Surg Br 2005;87(3):343–7.

64. Nielsen KK, Linde F, Jensen NC. The outcome of arthroscopic and open surgery ankle arthrodesis: a comparative retrospective study on 107 patients. Foot Ankle Surg 2008;14(3):153–7.

65. Greisberg J., Assal M, Flueckiger G, Hansen ST Jr. Takedown of ankle fusion and conversion to total ankle replacement. Clin Orthop Relat Res 2004;424:80–8.

66. Hintermann B, Barg A, Knupp M, Valderrabano V. Conversion of painful ankle arthrodesis to total ankle arthroplasty. J Bone Joint Surg Am 2009;91(4):850–8.

67. Davis RJ, Millis MB. Ankle arthrodesis in the management of traumatic ankle arthrosis: a long-term retrospective study. J Trauma 1980;20(8):674–8.

68. Fuchs S, Sandmann C, Skwara A, Chylarecki C. Quality of life 20 years after arthrodesis of the ankle. A study of adjacent joints. J Bone Joint Surg Br 2003;85(7):994–8.

69. Sheridan BD, Robinson DE, Hubble MJ, Winson IG. Ankle arthrodesis and its relationship to ipsilateral arthritis of the hind- and mid-foot. J Bone Joint Surg Br 2006;88(2):206–7.

70. SooHoo NF, Zingmond DS, Ko CY. Comparison of reoperation rates following ankle arthrodesis and total ankle arthroplasty. J Bone Joint Surg Am 2007;89(10):2143–9.

71. Beyaert C, Sirveaux F, Paysant J, Molé D, André JM The effect of tibio-talar arthrodesis on foot kinematics and ground reaction force progression during walking. Gait Posture 2004;20(1):84–91.

72. Kofoed H, Sorensen TS. Ankle arthroplasty for rheumatoid arthritis and osteoarthritis: prospective long-term study of cemented replacements. J Bone Joint Surg Br 1998;80(2):328–32.

73. Schuberth JM, Patel S, Zarutsky E. Perioperative complications of the Agility total ankle replacement in 50 initial, consecutive cases. J Foot Ankle Surg 2006;45(3):139–46.

74. Wood PL, Deakin S. Total ankle replacement. The results in 200 ankles. J Bone Joint Surg Br 2003;85(3):334–41.

75. Anderson T, Montgomery F, Carlsson A. Uncemented STAR total ankle prostheses. Three to eight-year follow-up of fifty-one consecutive ankles. J Bone Joint Surg Am 2003;85(7):1321–9.

76. Kitaoka HB, Patzer GL. Clinical results of the Mayo total ankle arthroplasty. J Bone Joint Surg Am 1996;78(11):1658–64.

77. Buechel FF Sr., Buechel FF Jr., Pappas MJ. Twenty-year evaluation of cementless mobile-bearing total ankle replacements. Clin Orthop Relat Res 2004(424):19–26.

78. Hintermann B, Valderrabano V, Knupp M, Horisberger M. [The HINTEGRA ankle: short- and mid-term results]. Orthopade 2006;35(5):533–45.

79. Knecht SI, Estin M, Callaghan JJ, Zimmerman MB, Alliman KJ, Alvine FG, Saltzman CL. The Agility total ankle arthroplasty. Seven to sixteen-year follow-up. J Bone Joint Surg Am 2004;86(6):1161–71.

80. Kofoed H. Scandinavian Total Ankle Replacement (STAR). Clin Orthop Relat Res 2004;424:73–9.

81. Wood PL, Sutton C, Mishra V, Suneja R. A randomised, controlled trial of two mobile-bearing total ankle replacements. J Bone Joint Surg Br 2009;91(1):69–74.

82. Ali MS, Higgins GA, Mohamed M. Intermediate results of Buechel Pappas unconstrained uncemented total ankle replacement for osteoarthritis. J Foot Ankle Surg 2007;46(1):16–20.

83. Doets HC, Brand R, Nelissen RG. Total ankle arthroplasty in inflammatory joint disease with use of two mobile-bearing designs. J Bone Joint Surg Am 2006;88(6):1272–84.

84. Fevang BT, Lie SA, Havelin LI, Brun JG, Skredderstuen A, Furnes O. 257 ankle arthroplasties performed in Norway between 1994 and 2005. Acta Orthop 2007;78(5):575–83.

85. Henricson A, Skoog A, Carlsson A. The Swedish Ankle Arthroplasty Register: An analysis of 531 arthroplasties between 1993 and 2005. Acta Orthop 2007;78(5):569–74.

86. Hosman AH, Mason RB, Hobbs T, Rothwell AG. A New Zealand national joint registry review of 202 total ankle replacements followed for up to 6 years. Acta Orthop 2007;78(5):584–91.

87. Hurowitz EJ, Gould JS, Fleisig GS, Fowler R. Outcome analysis of agility total ankle replacement with prior adjunctive procedures: two to six year followup. Foot Ankle Int 2007;28(3):308–12.

88. Kurup HV, Taylor GR. Medial impingement after ankle replacement. Int Orthop 2008;32(2):243–6.

89. Pyevich MT, Saltzman CL, Callaghan JJ, Alvine FG. Total ankle arthroplasty: a unique design. Two to twelve-year follow-up. J Bone Joint Surg Am 1998;80(10):1410–20.

90. San Giovanni TP, Keblish DJ, Thomas WH, Wilson MG. Eight-year results of a minimally constrained total ankle arthroplasty. Foot Ankle Int 2006;27(6):418–26.

91. Spirt AA, Assal M, Hansen ST Jr. Complications and failure after total ankle arthroplasty. J Bone Joint Surg Am 2004;86(6):1172–8.

92. Nishikawa, M., Tomita T, Fujii M, Watanabe T, Hashimoto J, Sugamoto K, Ochi T, Yoshikawa H. Total ankle replacement in rheumatoid arthritis. Int Orthop 2004;28(2):123–6.

93. Valderrabano V, Hintermann B, Dick W. Scandinavian total ankle replacement: a 3. 7-year average followup of 65 patients. Clin Orthop Relat Res 2004;424:47–56.

94. Su EP, Kahn B, Figgie MP. Total ankle replacement in patients with rheumatoid arthritis. Clin Orthop, Relat Res 2004;424:32–8.

95. Doets H, van Middelkoop M, Houdijk H, Nelissen RG, Veeger HE. Gait analysis after successful mobile bearing total ankle replacement. Foot Ankle Int 2007;28(3):313–22.

96. Kofoed H, Lundberg-Jensen A. Ankle arthroplasty in patients younger and older than 50 years: a prospective series with long-term follow-up. Foot Ankle Int 1999;20(8):501–6.

97. Naal FD, Impellizzeri FM, Loibl M, Huber M, Rippstein PF. Habitual physical activity and sports participation after total ankle arthroplasty. Am J Sports Med 2009;37(1):95–102.

98. Hobson SA, Karantana A, Dhar S. Total ankle replacement in patients with significant pre-operative deformity of the hindfoot. J Bone Joint Surg Br 2009;91(4):481–6.

99. Kim BS, Choi WJ, Kim YS, Lee JW. Total ankle replacement in moderate to severe varus deformity of the ankle. J Bone Joint Surg Br 2009;91(9):1183–90.

100. Wood PL, Prem H, Sutton C. Total ankle replacement: medium-term results in 200 Scandinavian total ankle replacements. J Bone Joint Surg Br 2008;90(5):605–9.

101. Lee KB, Cho SG, Hur CI, Yoon TR. Perioperative complications of HINTEGRA total ankle replacement: our initial 50 cases. Foot Ankle Int 2008;29(10):978–84.

102. Saltzman CL, Mann RA, Ahrens JE, Amendola A, Anderson RB, Berlet GC, et al. Prospective controlled trial of STAR total ankle replacement versus ankle fusion: initial results. Foot Ankle Int 2009;30(7):579–96.

103. Glazebrook MA, Arsenault K, Dunbar M. Evidence-based classification of complications in total ankle arthroplasty. Foot Ankle Int 2009;30(10):945–9.

104. Trouillier H, Hänsel L, Schaff P, Rosemeyer B, Refior HJ. Long-term results after ankle arthrodesis: clinical, radiological, gait analytical aspects. Foot Ankle Int 2002;23(12):1081–90.

105. Wu WL, Su FC, Cheng YM, Huang PJ, Chou YL, Chou CK. Gait analysis after ankle arthrodesis. Gait Posture 2000;11(1):54–61.

106. Weiss RJ, Broström E, Stark A, Wick MC, Wretenberg P. Ankle/hindfoot arthrodesis in rheumatoid arthritis improves kinematics and kinetics of the knee and hip: a prospective gait analysis study. Rheumatology (Oxford) 2007;46(6):1024–8.

107. Dyrby C, Chou LB, Andriacchi TP, Mann RA. Functional evaluation of the Scandinavian Total Ankle Replacement. Foot Ankle Int 2004;25(6):377–81.

108. Valderrabano V, Nigg BM, von Tscharner V, Frank CB, Hintermann B. Total ankle replacement in ankle osteoarthritis: an analysis of muscle rehabilitation. Foot Ankle Int. 2007;28(2):281–91.

109. Piriou P, Culpan P, Mullins M, Cardon JN, Pozzi D, Judet T. Ankle replacement versus arthrodesis: a comparative gait analysis study. Foot Ankle Int 2008;29(1):3–9.

110. Thomas RH, Daniels TR. Ankle arthritis. J Bone Joint Surg Am 2003;85-A(5):923–36.

111. Agel J, Coetzee JC, Sangeorzan BJ, Roberts MM, Hansen ST Jr. Functional limitations of patients with end stage ankle arthrosis. Foot Ankle Int 2005;26(7):537–9.

112. Glazebrook M, Daniels T, Younger A, Foote CJ, Penner M, Wing K, et al. Comparison of health-related quality of life between patients with end stage ankle and hip arthrosis. J Bone Joint Surg Am 2008;90(3):499–505.

35 Fusion vs. Arthroplasty in the Treatment of 1st MTP Arthritis

Jeffrey G.M. Tan[1], Gilbert Yee,[2] and Johnny T.C. Lau[1]
[1]University of Toronto, Toronto, ON, Canada
[2]The Scarborough Hospital, Scarborough, ON, Canada

Case scenario

A 51 year old woman was seen in the clinic with pain and stiffness in her left hallux metatarsophalangeal (MTP) joint and limited walking distance. On examination, she has flexion of 0–20° and limited dorsiflexion of 0–10° in the MTP joint with pain on movement. Standing radiographs revealed dorsal osteophytes, severe decrease in joint space, and subchondral sclerosis in the MTP joint (grade III hallux rigidus). She had failed conservative therapy with podiatry-prescribed shoes, steroid injections, and analgesia.

She was keen for surgical intervention, after suffering the symptoms for several years. Being an active individual who did weekly ballroom dancing and regular jogging, she requested an outcome that would allow her to continue her current lifestyle after the surgery. Looking at the clinical picture and radiographic findings, you presented two options of surgical treatment to this particular patient: fusion (arthrodesis) vs. arthroplasty.

You started a lengthy discussion with the patient on the indications and "pros and cons" of the above options. She is especially perturbed about the idea of "fusion" of the joint, which she perceived as being functionally limited, and seemed anxious about getting back to wearing high heels, ballroom dancing, tennis, and jogging after the procedure.

She seemed to be inclined towards the option of implant replacement arthroplasty and was trying to extrapolate the excellent results of hip and knee replacements to that in the forefoot. Her initial impression is that arthroplasty seemed to "fit in" more with her lifestyle and she asked you for advice on the long-term survival results of big toe implants.

Introduction

The hallux MTP joint can be affected by a number of conditions causing arthritis, commonly degenerative arthritis (described as hallux rigidus), rheumatological conditions, crystal deposition arthropathies (such as gouty arthritis), and neuropathic arthropathy as well as post-traumatic arthritis. This chapter focuses on the management options of endstage hallux rigidus, which is the most common form of arthritis affecting the great toe MTP joint.

The grading of hallux rigidus

In 1988, Hattrup and Johnson[1] described the following radiographic classification system:

- Grade 1: mild changes with a maintained joint space and minimal spurring
- Grade 2: Moderate changes, joint space narrowing, bony proliferation of the metatarsal head, and phalanx and subchondral sclerosis or cysts
- Grade 3: Severe changes with significant joint space narrowing, extensive bony proliferation, and loose bodies or a dorsal ossicle

---

Relevant anatomy

Degenerative arthritis or hallux rigidus of the great toe is the next common affliction of the MTP joint after hallux valgus. Hallux rigidus is the *most common* arthritis in the foot, with an incidence of 1 in 40 in persons aged 50 and above.[2,3] Women are more commonly affected than men in

---

Evidence-Based Orthopedics, First Edition. Edited by Mohit Bhandari.
© 2012 Blackwell Publishing Ltd. Published 2012 by Blackwell Publishing Ltd.

all age groups. The condition is more prevalent in North America and Europe than in Asia.

Many surgical options have been described such as arthrodesis, excisional arthroplasty, osteotomy, implant arthroplasty, cheilectomy, and interpositional arthroplasty. Despite the frequency of hallux rigidus, the remains some degree of controversy about its surgical treatment.

The 1st MTP joint consists of the articulation between the metatarsal head, proximal phalanx, and metatarso-sesamoid articulation. The plantar aspect of the metatarsal head has an undulating surface with the intersesamoid ridge and respective grooves on either side for articulation with the sesamoids. The range of motion of the 1st MTP joint is greatest in the sagittal plane and consists of approximately 30° of plantar flexion to 90° of dorsiflexion.[4]

In hallux rigidus, there is a decreased total arc of motion with relatively normal plantar flexion and markedly decreased dorsiflexion secondary to mechanical block by dorsal osteophytes and scarring of plantar structures. A small degree of transverse motion in the medial and lateral direction also occurs in the sagittal range of motion, but this transverse motion has a 50% reduction in hallux rigidus, and is thought to be due to contracture of the collateral ligaments and joint capsule.[4]

Stability of the 1st MTP joint in turns leads to stability of the medial column of the foot. Approximately 40–60% of body weight passes through the 1st MTP joint and great toe during normal gait.[5] During athletic activities like jogging and running, these forces can approach two to three times body weight.

Importance of the problem

The two main surgical procedures for the more advanced arthritis of the 1st MTP joint are arthrodesis or arthroplasty. There is still much debate between surgeons on the differing opinions on methods of surgical treatment for this condition.

Over the last decade, several designs of great toe MTP implant options are becoming widely available in the market and various trials have been conducted and published, mostly in small sample studies. The long-term results of these newer metal-on-polyethylene and metal resurfacing implants remain to be seen.

Surgical decision depends on the age of the patient, functional level and demand, comorbidities, and competency of the soft tissue restraint.

Top five questions

Therapy

1. What are the optimal techniques available for the fusion of the 1st MTP joint?

2. Does 1st MTP arthrodesis or arthroplasty effect a change in gait?

3. What are the effect of Keller's arthroplasty and interpositional arthroplasty on the treatment of 1st MTP arthritis?

4. What is the relative effect of arthrodesis vs. implant arthroplasty on the patient's satisfaction and complication rate?

Prognosis

5. What is the current survival analysis on the implants used in arthroplasty?

Question 1: What are the optimal techniques available for the fusion of the 1st MTP joint?

Relevance

There are multiple techniques to achieve optimal fusion of the 1st MTP joint. Good bone preparation and a reliable and stable fixation construct with good position of the joint is crucial to achieve satisfactory result in arthrodesis of the 1st MTP joint.

Current opinion

Arthrodesis is an accepted surgical option for advanced-stage osteoarthritis of the 1st MTP joint, as it is a reliable and predictable procedure with consistently favorable long-term results.[6] The more common methods of preparation and fixation include conical reaming with a combination of lag screws and low profile dorsal plating.

Finding the evidence

• Cochrane Database, with search terms "MTP arthrodesis," "MTP fusion," "hallux arthrodesis," "MTP arthrodesis versus arthroplasty" or "hallux arthrodesis versus arthroplasty"

• PubMed (www.ncbi.nlm.nih.gov/pubmed/) clinical queries search/systematic reviews: "MTP arthrodesis," "MTP fusion," "hallux arthrodesis," "MTP arthrodesis versus arthroplasty," or "hallux arthrodesis versus arthroplasty"

Quality of the evidence
Level I
• 1 randomized trials

Level II
• 2 prospective comparative studies

Level IV
• 6 retrospective case series

Findings
Various methods of preparation of the bone ends and fixation of the fusion site have been described in the literature.

Methods of preparation includes conical reamers,[7] ball and socket reamers,[8] peg and cone preparation,[9] and flat planar cuts of the metatarsal heads and phalangeal base, denuding the joint surfaces of cartilage and inserting small drill holes into subchondral bones.

Methods of fixation include cross screws, Kirschner wires, wire loops, external compression devices, Steinman pins, staples, and compression plating as well as a lag screw and plate combination.[9–13] Fusion rates of 90–100%[7–9,11,13] have been reported (Table 35.1). Several authors noted that the majority of nonunions were asymptomatic and did not necessarily serve as a predictor of poor outcome.[7,13–15]

Complications of 1st MTP arthrodesis include shortening of the first ray, malunion, nonunion, transfer metatarsalgia, infection, and prominent implants. The average load across a fused MTP joint could reach approximately 172 N.[16]

A crucial aspect of arthrodesis of the 1st MTP joint and maintenance of the biomechanics of the first ray requires minimal shortening and correct anatomical positioning of the fused joint.

Various biomechanical and clinical studies demonstrated that a dorsal plate with an oblique compression lag screw gave the most biomechanical stability after the bone ends were prepared by machined conical reaming, followed by conical reaming with either dorsal plating or interfragmentary screws alone.[17–20] Memory staples or Kirschner wires, in turn, were weaker than the compression screw fixation or dorsal plate fixation.[21]

Effect on shortening The effect of arthrodesis of the 1st MTP joint results in shortening. Two studies investigate the effect of shortening of the first ray on the biomechanics of the foot. Jung et al.[22] showed that a decrease in the length of the first ray by 5–10 mm can cause significant plantar pressure changes which can lead to metatarsalgia of the second ray ($p < 0.016$) in 12 pairs of cadaver feet.

A study[23] with six paired cadaver feet comparing the effect of two fusion techniques between flat bone cut and machined conical reamer preparation found that there was no statistically significant difference ($p = 0.44$) in the

Table 35.1 Summary of fusion rates of 1st MTP arthrodesis using various methods of joint preparation and internal fixation

Series (year)	N	Preparation method	Fixation method	Position of fusion	Postoperative regime	Fusion rate (%)
O'Doherty[15] (1990)	50	Debridement of cartilage and subchondral bone	20 gauge cerclage wire loop and Kirschner wire	–	Weight bear in cast slipper at 2 weeks Cast removed at 6 weeks	56.0
Gibson[27] (2005)	38	Debridement of cartilage and subchondral bone	20 gauge cerclage wire loop and 2 mm crossed Kirschner wire	10 DF	Partial weightbear in fiberglass cast after surgery	100.0 (6 delayed unions with final union at 12 months)
Brodsky[29] (2005)	60	Curettage and rongeur to exposed cancelleous surface	Parallel 3.5 mm cortical screws	10–25 DF 5–10 valgus	Postop shoes for 8 weeks Non-weightbear for the first 4 weeks	100.0
Hyer[19] (2008) comparative study	14 31	Simple curettage and rongeur to remove cartilage Subchondral bone drilled and "rose petalled" As above	2 crossed 4.0 mm cannulated screws or 2.7 mm Herbert type cannulated screws 5-hole low profile titanium plate	0 valgus or varus As above	Partial weight bear with postop shoes after surgery As above	92.9 90.3
Goucher[9] (2006)	53	Dome-shaped power reamers	Dorsal titanium plate with a cross lag screw	10–15 DF 10 valgus	Postop shoe for 12 weeks Weight bear on heel and lateral border of foot	92.0
Coughlin[11] (1994)	58	Cup- or cone-shaped reamers	Vitallium low profile dorsal plate	20–30 DF 15–20 valgus	Postop shoe with weight bear on heel and lateral aspect of foot Cast used if patient is unreliable	98.0

DF, dorsiflexion with respect to metatarsal shaft; N, sample size.

postprocedure lengths of the first ray between the two techniques. The authors concluded that neither of the techniques is likely to lead to transfer metatarsalgia as the length of shortening is similar.

Recommendation

• There is no consensus on the optimal method of preparation and fixation. In most studies, a combination of a lag screw with dorsal plating, followed by lag screws or dorsal plating alone, gives better biomechanical stability. A fusion rate of 90–100% is expected.

Question 2: Does 1st MTP arthrodesis or arthroplasty effect a change in gait?

Relevance

Surgeons may have some reservation about fusing the 1st MTP joint as this takes away a functional range of movement and causes gait cycle changes. There is also concern about weakness in push-off and developing arthritis in the interphalangeal joint.

Current opinion

Arthrodesis eliminates painful motion at the MTP joint, gives stability to the medial column of the foot but effects in a decrease of push-off power at toe-off.

Quality of the evidence

Level II

• 3 prospective comparative study

Level III

• 1 retrospective case control studies

Level IV

• 2 retrospective case series

Findings

Two studies comparing the effects of arthrodesis vs. Keller's arthroplasty and demonstrated that arthrodesis re-establishes the normal weightbearing pattern of the forefoot and redistributes more weight through the medial ray when the 1st MTP joint is fused.[24,25] This results from a stabilization of the medial column when pain is eliminated although motion is lost in the MTP joint. After arthrodesis, the big toe bore weight in 80% compared with 40% after Keller's operation.[24]

Three prospective studies showed inconsistent evidence with regards to plantar pressures under the hallux and push-off power. Two of the studies[26,27] showed increased pressure under the first metatarsal (p = 0.01 and p = 0.16 respectively), while one study[28] suggested postoperative improvement in stability of the foot after arthrodesis. There is no consensus on the effect of push-off power.

Functional limitation In a functional evaluation of MTP arthrodesis (level IV study) by Brodsky et al.,[29] patients retained good function and were able to return to athletic activities such as jogging, golfing, hiking, and tennis. Good outcome and function was achieved when the fused joint is well positioned. More prospective studies would be needed to validate these observations as these data would be useful as a reference to counsel patients preoperatively regarding the functional outcome after arthrodesis.

Recommendation

• There is inconsistent evidence in prospective studies (level II) regarding plantar pressures and push-off power after arthrodesis or arthroplasty. However, a properly positioned and fused stable 1st MTP joint redistributes loads back to the first ray and medial column and provides stability during gait.

Question 3: What are the effects of Keller's resection arthroplasty and interpositional arthroplasty on the treatment of 1st MTP arthritis?

Relevance

Keller's arthroplasty has been performed since 1904 and involved a resection of the base of the proximal phalanx. Its indication has extended beyond the use in hallux valgus to hallux rigidus and has been a popular procedure for many decades. Since Keller's first description of the procedure, there has been several modification of the technique by using soft tissue interposition with an aim to improve stability and function as well as to reduce pain.

Current opinion

Keller's procedure is a resection arthroplasty that decompresses the joint at the expense of stability. Common complications include transfer metatarsalgia, claw toe, cock-up deformity, and hallux weakness. For this reason, the Keller's resection arthroplasty has been used for low-demand and elderly patients.[6,15]

Interposition arthroplasty provides an alternative for treatment of endstage 1st MTP arthritis in a low-demand patient with pain relief and preservation of motion. There are inconsistent results, techniques and lack of comparison studies, and some authors consider it a salvage procedure.

Finding the evidence

• Cochrane Database, with search terms: "MTP excision arthroplasty," "MTP resection arthroplasty," "hallux resection arthroplasty," "Keller arthroplasty," or "MTP interpositional arthroplasty"
• PubMed (www.ncbi.nlm.nih.gov/pubmed/) clinical queries and sensitivity search/ systematic reviews: "MTP

excision arthroplasty," "hallux resection arthroplasty," "Keller arthroplasty," "MTP interpositional arthroplasty," or "hallux interpositional arthroplasty"

Quality of the evidence

Level II
- 1 prospective comparative study

Level III
- 1 retrospective case control studies

Level IV
- 9 retrospective case series

Findings

Keller's arthroplasty In 1904, Keller[30] described a technique involving resection of the base of the proximal phalanx for treatment of hallux valgus with associated OA of the 1st MTP joint. This procedure has since been adapted for treatment of hallux rigidus as well. Following that, other level IV studies with Keller's procedure reported good satisfaction with pain relief.[31,32] However complications such as transfer metatarsalgia and postoperative cock-up deformity were common.

In a randomized trial, O'Doherty et al.[15] published the results comparing 50 arthrodeses and 60 Keller's arthroplasty in older patients (average age 60.5 years) with a minimum follow-up period of 2 years. Both groups gave a similar degree of patient satisfaction and symptom relief. No significant difference was noted in terms of the incidence of postoperative transfer metatarsalgia or cock-up deformity(p > 0.01).

The above study had limitations as the method of arthrodesis using cerclage wire loops and Kirschner wires contributed to the high incidence of nonunion (44%) and malrotation of the hallux. Although the authors had suggested that Keller's arthroplasty is the better operation in older and lower-demand patients, it was felt that the arthrodesis could have been optimized with more rigid fixation to improve the fusion rate.

Interpositional arthroplasty Interpositional arthroplasty combines a resection arthroplasty of the proximal phalanx and cheilectomy with the insertion of a biological tissue or spacer into the joint so as to avoid some of the problems associated with an isolated resection arthroplasty.

Various tissues including the extensor hallucis brevis (EHB), joint capsule, and plantaris and gracilis tendons have been utilized as the interpositional graft.[33,34] This procedure requires less bone resection and maintains joint stability and range of motion. Soft tissue tension plays an important aspect in this procedure.

Complications from this procedure are common; they include transfer metatarsalgia, floppy hallux, stiffness, short hallux, first toe weakness, and, less commonly, osteonecrosis of the metatarsal head.[34]

Hamilton et al.[33] treated 37 feet with advanced-stage hallux rigidus using EHB tendon interposition over a 10 year period, and yielded satisfactory results in term of American Orthopaedic Foot and Ankle Score (AOFAS), improved dorsiflexion, and patient satisfaction. No weakness, transfer metatarsalgia, or metatarsal callosities were reported.

Subsequent investigators could not reproduce the results of Hamilton et al. in terms of satisfaction and complication rates. There is also a decrease in sample size in subsequent studies, variation in techniques and nonuniformity in patient selection and outcome measures.[34–38] One study comparing EHB interpositional arthroplasty with Keller arthroplasty(level III) found no significant difference in terms of AOFAS, patient satisfaction, range of motion, and clinical and radiological outcome.[39]

Recommendations

- Given the favorable results from level II and level IV studies, there is fair evidence to support the use of Keller's resection arthroplasty for the treatment of hallux rigidus in older and low-demand patients. Patient selection is important and the possibility of cock-up deformity and transfer metatarsalgia must be considered [overall quality: moderate]
- Considering the level of evidence (level III and IV), sample sizes of study, and differences in methods of outcome analysis and patient selection, there is insufficient evidence to recommend interpositional arthroplasty for the treatment of advanced arthritis of the 1st MTP joint [overall quality: low]

Question 4: What is the relative effect of arthrodesis vs. implant arthroplasty on the patient's satisfaction and revision rate?

Relevance

Arthrodesis is an accepted surgical option for advanced-stage osteoarthritis of the 1st MTP joint. Arthroplasty maintains range of motion of the 1st MTP joint and provides pain relief but the issue of longevity remains. Silastic implants have been used widely in the past but unfortunately late complications of silicone particulate synovitis and failure were a concern.

Current opinion

Most surgeons uses arthrodesis for the surgical treatment of endstage arthritis of the 1st MTP joint as it is a reliable and predictable procedure (gold standard) with consistently favorable long-term results.[6,19]

Finding the evidence

- Cochrane Database, with search terms "MTP arthrodesis," "hallux arthrodesis," "MTP arthrodesis versus arthroplasty" or "hallux arthrodesis versus arthroplasty"

• PubMed (www.ncbi.nlm.nih.gov/pubmed/) clinical queries search/systematic reviews and sensitivity search using keywords: "MTP arthrodesis," "hallux arthrodesis," "MTP arthrodesis versus arthroplasty" or "hallux arthrodesis versus arthroplasty"

Quality of the evidence

Level II
• 1 randomized trial with methodological limitations

Level III
• 1 retrospective case control study

Level IV
• 4 retrospective case series

Findings

Arthrodesis provides pain relief and stability of the MTP joint at the expense of loss of motion. Besides hallux rigidus, it is also indicated for rheumatoid arthritis, hallux valgus or hallux varus with degenerative arthritis, and as a salvage procedure for failed implant arthroplasty or failed Keller's operation. Arthrodesis is generally preferred for young and active patients.

Two studies (level II and level III evidence) have compared arthrodesis with an implant arthroplasty of the 1st MTP joint. In these studies, arthrodesis demonstrated equivalent or superior results with fewer complications.

Gibson et al.[27] reported the results of a randomized controlled trial involving 38 cases of arthrodesis and 39 cases of arthroplasty for treatment of arthritis of the 1st MTP joint. The arthrodesis technique involves cerclage wire and a Kirschner cross wire. The replacement studied is an unconstrained joint with a polyethylene insert. However, there was a protocol deviation within 18 months of the trial: 5 of the first 30 patients were found to have radiographic signs of loosening and the protocol was then revised to cement the phalangeal component in the remaining 9 patients.

At 24 months, pain was more significantly improved in the arthrodesis group (p = 0.01). Six of the 39 implants had to be removed because of phalangeal component loosening. All the 38 arthrodeses united. The cost ratio was 2:1 in favor of arthrodesis. Arthroplasty has more complication rates in terms of revision surgery.

Raikin et al.[40] compared the long-term outcome of a metallic hemiarthroplasty of the proximal phalanx base (Biopro, Port Huron, MI) with arthrodesis for advanced arthritis of the 1st MTP joint.

The results of 21 hemiarthroplasties with a mean follow-up of 79 months were compared with 27 arthrodeses with a mean follow-up of 30 months. All arthrodeses united and 2 required hardware removal. Five (24%) of the hemiarthroplasties failed; most failures occurred within the first 2 years after surgery. The patients who underwent arthrodesis had significantly higher satisfaction rates(p < 0.01), higher AOFAS scores(p = 0.006), lower VAS scores (p = 0.021), and lower incidences of plantar callosities(p = 0.041). The authors concluded that arthrodesis was more predictable for alleviating symptoms and restoring function in patients with severe hallux rigidus. The study had limitations, as one surgeon performed the arthrodesis between 1999 and 2000, and another surgeon performed the arthroplasty after year 2000.

Incidence of interphalangeal joint arthritis after arthrodesis The reported incidence of developing osteoarthritis in the interphalangeal joint after 1st MTP joint arthrodesis varies from 10% to 15% (level IV studies), with most of the degenerative changes being usually asymptomatic.[41-43]

Recommendations

• The favorable results reported in these level II and III studies constitute fair evidence to support the use of arthrodesis over arthroplasty for the treatment of advanced-stage osteoarthritis of the 1st MTP [overall quality: moderate]

Question 5: What is the current survival analysis on the implants used in arthroplasty?

Relevance

Over the last decade, newer generation implants have been developed with clinical trials under way for surgical replacement of the MTP joint. A search of the literature revealed various options of hemiarthroplasty resurfacing prostheses and total replacement prostheses, some of which are still undergoing clinical trials.

Current opinion

The newer prostheses for the big toe MTP joint currently in use have limited short-term results, and long-term outcomes remains to be seen. MTP resurfacing or total joint replacement provides an alternative in a selected group of patients who desire preservation of joint motion, function, and symptom relief.

Finding the evidence

• Cochrane Database, with search terms "survival analysis," "survivorship," "MTP arthrodesis versus arthroplasty," "long term survival"
• PubMed (www.ncbi.nlm.nih.gov/pubmed/) clinical queries search/ systematic reviews and sensitivity search using keywords: "survival analysis," "survivorship," "MTP arthrodesis versus arthroplasty," "long term survival"

Quality of the evidence

Level II
• 1 randomized trials with methodological limitations

Table 35.2 Results of hemiarthroplasty of the 1st MTP joint

Series (year)	Implant	N	Follow-up[a] (years) (range)	Age (range)	Complications
Konkel [58] (2006)	Futura Hemi- Toe	13	8 (7.2–8.9)	59 (42–77)	11 radiographic sign of loosening 6 recurrent osteophytes 1 transfer metatarsalgia
Sorbie [59] (2008)	cobalt chrome Trihedron	19	5.7 (2.8–6.0)	53 (35–70)	1 loss of alignment due to pre-existing hallux valgus (requiring further surgery)
Raikin [40] (2007)	Biopro	21	6.6 (5.7–7.1)	59.7 (39–70)	5 failures (1 required revision and 4 required arthrodesis) . Additional 8 had radiographic cut-out of stem through plantar cortex
Giza [56] (2005)	Biopro (preliminary results)	103	(0.5–4) (preliminary results)	60.7 (55–80)	17 cases underwent MUA at 3 months for postoperative stiffness
Townley [57] (1994)	Biopro	279	(0.67–33)	54.4 (22–91)	13 failures (11 in patients with HV and RA), of which 12 required revision surgeries

HV, hallux valgus; MUA, manipulation under anesthesia; N, sample size; RA, rheumatoid arthritis.
[a] Mean follow-up.

Level III

• 2 retrospective case control studies

Level IV

• 16 retrospective case series

Findings

There is sparse data in the literature regarding survivorship analysis of the implants used in arthroplasty of the MTP joint.

Silastic implants for the great toe of the Swanson design[44] have been used since 1967, albeit with high failure rates.[45,46] Radiographic loosening and fragmentation coupled with silicone granulomatous disease, synovitis, and lymphadenitis were common complications on long-term outcomes.[47–51] Salvage of failed silastic implants with poor bone stock was a challenging surgical problem.[45,52]

It is beyond the scope of this chapter to assess the different types of big toe MTP implants used today. In brief, they can be divided into hemiarthroplasty resurfacing, and total joint replacement metal-on-polyethylene implants (usually nonconstrained). The majority of hemiarthroplasty implants involve resurfacing the proximal phalanx, which does not address the cartilage damage or degeneration on the metatarsal head. Some form of debridement, cheilectomy of the dorsal osteophytes on the metatarsals, and soft tissue release is required.[53,54] A minority of the hemiarthropalsty implants involve resurfacing of the metatarsal head.[55] The Biopro implant (Biopro Inc, Port Huron, MI) has the most extensively published data and long-term results for its clinical use.[40,53,56,57] A Kaplan–Meier analysis of a hemiarthroplasty population using Biopro has an implant failure rate of 23.8% at 18 months postoperatively.[40]

Results of the hemiarthroplasty and total replacement trials are summarized in Table 35.2 and 35.3 respectively. There is no published trial comparing the outcome between hemiarthroplasty and total joint replacement.

Implant cut-out, loosening, recurrent osteophytes with impingement, and metatarsalgia are reported complications with the hemiarthroplasties.[39,52,54–56,58,59] Many of the total toe implants suffer from loosening and early failure requiring revision in short to medium-term results,[27,60–63] with complications such as implant subluxation, subsidence, periprosthetic fracture, postoperative stiffness, infection, and transfer metatarsalgia.

Most of the published studies are mid-term (3–5 years) results with small sample sizes. There is a lack of large randomized multicenter trials, survivorship analysis, and long-term results. In addition, it is difficult to standardize the studies (level III and IV evidence) because of the many available implant types with different design rationale and surgical techniques. The study groups consisted of a vast distribution of patients with hallux valgus, hallux rigidus, inflammatory arthritis, and those undergoing revision surgery, all with different types of outcome measures. More data is needed for the salvage options for failure of the newer implants.

Recommendations

• Taking into consideration the above known common complications and long-term durability of silicone implants, there is insufficient evidence to recommend silastic/silicone implants for the treatment of 1st MTP arthritis [overall quality: high]

Table 35.3 Results of the 1st MTP total joint arthroplasty trials

Series (year)	Implant	N	Follow-up (years) (range)	Age (range)	Complications
Kundert[62] (2005)	Toefit-Plus (hemi- & total- modularity)	14	4 (3.0–5.3)	–	3 cases require revision before 3 years
Pulavarti[63] (2005)	Bio-Action Great Toe	36	3.9 (3.0–5.8)	57 (38–72)	3 persistent pain (2 cases required revision at 2.5 years to arthrodesis or excision arthroplasty) 12 implant subsidence at 3 years
Gibson[27] (2005)	Biomet Total Toe System	39	2.0 (2.0)	55.5 (34–69)	6 implants with phalangeal component loosening were revised before 2 years
Fuhrmann[61] (2005)	ReFlexion	43	3.3 (2.1–4.8)	-	4 cases with persistent pain were revised to arthrodesis at average 2.2 years Radiographic signs of loosening in 14 implants

N, sample size.

ª Mean follow-up.

- Except for the study by Townley, the use of hemiarthroplasty in the management of 1st MTP arthritis is supported by poor quality evidence [overall quality: low]
- Given these conflicting results in multiple studies with different implants, there is weak and inconsistent evidence to support total joint arthroplasty as a standard procedure for advanced arthritis of the 1st MTP joint [overall quality: low]

Summary of recommendations

- There is no consensus on the optimal method of preparation and fixation. In most studies, a combination of a lag screw with dorsal plating, followed by lag screws or dorsal plating alone, gives better biomechanical stability. A fusion rate of 90–100% is expected.
- The consistently favorable results in many level II and IV studies constitute fair evidence to support the use of arthrodesis for the surgical treatment of advanced-stage arthritis of the 1st MTP joint
- Keller resection arthroplasty can be considered for advanced-stage of arthritis in elderly patients with low physical demand. However, complications such as cock-up deformity, weakness, and lateral metatarsalgia may develop for this procedure
- There is insufficient evidence to recommend interpositional arthroplasty as a standard treatment for end stage arthritis of the 1st MTP joint
- Though the evidence comparing arthrodesis with arthroplasty is rather weak with certain limitations, arthrodesis provides a predictable and reliable treatment for pain relief

- Given the inconsistent results, small sample size and quality of evidence, there is insufficient evidence to support total joint arthroplasty in the treatment of 1st MTP arthritis
- The use of hemiarthroplasty for resurfacing of the proximal phalanx in the management of 1st MTP arthritis is supported by poor quality evidence
- There is paucity of survivor analysis on the longevity of various implants including total prosthetic arthroplasty and hemiarthroplasty. Further long-term prospective trials are needed to investigate the long-term effects of these implants
- Taking into consideration the above known common complications and long-term durability of silicone implants, there is insufficient evidence to recommend silastic/silicone implants for the treatment of 1st MTP arthritis

Conclusions

- The evidence in the literature supports arthrodesis as a standard treatment for 1st MTP arthritis with successful fusion rates of 90–100%. In comparative trials with implant arthroplasty, arthrodesis provides superior and durable results as well as more reliable and predictable treatment for symptom relief
- There is also fair evidence to support Keller's resection arthroplasty for a selected group of elderly patients with low functional demand
- At present, there is insufficient evidence to support the use of total joint arthroplasty and interpositional arthro-

plasty. The use of hemiarthroplasty for the proximal phalanx is weakly supported.

Acknowledgements and disclosures

The authors did not receive any supporting research grants or sponsorships in the preparation and writing of this manuscript.

References

1. Hattrup SJ, Johnson KA. Subjective results of hallux rigidus following treatment with cheilectomy. Clin Orthop Relat Res 1988;226:182–91.
2. Thordarson DB. Hallux valgus, hallux varus and sesamoid disorders. Normal anatomy of the 1st metatarsophalangeal joint. Chapter 6 in: Foot and Ankle. Lippincott Williams & Wilkins, Philadelphia, 2004.
3. Coughlin MJ. Hallux rigidus: demographics, etiology, and radiographic. Foot Ankle Int 2003;24:731–43.
4. Shereff MJ, Bejjani FJ, Kummer FJ. Kinematics of the first metatarso-phalangeal joint. J Bone Joint Surg Am 1986;68:392–8.
5. Stokes IA, Hutton WC, Stott JRR, et al. Forces under the hallux valgus foot before and after surgery. Clin Orthop Relat Res 1979;142:64–72.
6. Yee G, Lau J. Current concepts review: hallux rigidus. Foot Ankle Int 2008;29:637–46.
7. Johansson JE, Barrington TW. Cone arthrodesis of the first metatarsophalangeal joint. Foot Ankle 1984;4:244 –48.
8. Flavin R, Stephens NM. Arthrodesis of the first metatarsophalangeal joint using a dorsal titanium contoured plate. Foot Ankle Int 2004;25:783–7.
9. Goucher NR, Couglin MJ. Hallux metatarsophlangeal joint arthrodesis using dome-shaped reamers and dorsal plate fixation: a prospective study. Foot Ankle Int 2006;27:869–76.
10. Bennett GL, Sabetta J. First metatarsophalangeal joint arthrodesis: evaluation of plate and screw fixation. Foot Ankle Int 2009;30:752–7.
11. Coughlin MJ, Abdo RV. Arthrodesis of the first metatarsophalangeal joint with vitallium plate fixation. Foot Ankle Int 1994;15:18 –28.
12. Rongstad, KM, Miller GJ, VanderGriend RA, et al. A biomechanical comparison of four fixation methods of the first metatarsal phalangeal joint arthrodesis. Foot Ankle Int 1994;15:415 –19.
13. Lombardi CM, Silhanek AD, Connolly FG et al. First metatarsophalangeal arthrodesis for treatment of hallux rigidus: a retrospective study. J Foot Ankle Surg 2001;40:137–43.
14. Riggs SA Jr, Johnson EW Jr. McKeever arthrodesis for the painful hallux. Foot Ankle 1983;3:248–53.
15. O'Doherty DP, Lowrie IG, Magnussen PA et al. The management of the painful first metatarsophalangeal joint in the older patient: Arthrodesis or Keller's arthroplasty. J Bone Joint Surg 1990;72B, 839–42.
16. Samnegard E, Turan I, Lanshammar H. Postoperative evaluation of Keller's arthroplasty and arthrodesis of the first metatarsophalangeal joint using the EMED gait analysis system. J Foot Surg 1991;30:373–4.
17. Politi J, Hayes J, Njus G et al. First metatarsal-phalangeal joint arthrodesis. a biomechanical assessment of stability. Foot Ankle Int 2003;24:332–37.
18. Curtis MJ, Myerson M, Jinnah RH. Arthrodesis of the first metatarsophalangeal joint: a biomechanical study of internal fixation techniques. Foot Ankle 1993;14:395–9.
19. Hyer CF, Glover JP, Berlet GC et al. Cost comparison of crossed screws versus dorsal plate construct for first metatarsophalangeal joint arthrodesis. J Foot Ankle Surg 2008; 47:13–8.
20. Buranosky DJ, Taylor DT, Sage RA, et al. First metatarsophalangeal joint arthrodesis: quantitative mechanical testing of six-hole dorsal plate versus crossed screw fixation in cadaveric specimens. J Foot Ankle Surg 2001;40:208–13.
21. Neufeld SK, Parks BG, Naseef GS et al. Arthrodesis of the first metatarso-phalangeal joint: a biomechanical study comparing memory compression staples, cannulated screws and a dorsal plate. Foot Ankle Int 2002;23:97–101.
22. Jung HG, Zaret DI, Park BG et al. Effect of first metatarsal shortening and dorsiflexion osteotomies on forefoot plantar pressure in a cadaver model. Foot Ankle Int 2005;26:748–53.
23. Singh B, Draeger R, Del Gaizo DJ et al. Changes in length of the first ray with two different first MTP fusion techniques: a cadaveric study. Foot Ankle Int 2008;29:722–5.
24. Henry APT, Waugh W. The use of footprints in assessing the results of hallux valgus. A comparison of Keller's operation and arthrodesis. J Bone Joint Surg Br 1975;57:478–81.
25. Beauchamp CG, Kirby T, Rudge SR et al. Fusion of the first metatarso-phalangeal joint in forefoot arthroplasty. Clin Orthop Relat Res 1984;190:249–53.
26. DeFrino PF, Brodsky JW, Pollo FE, et al. First metatarsophalangeal arthrodesis: a clinical, pedobarographic, and gait analysis study. Foot Ankle Int 2002;23:496–502.
27. Gibson JN, Thomson CE. Arthrodesis or total replacement arthroplasty for hallux rigidus: a randomized controlled trial. Foot Ankle Int 2005;26:680–90.
28. Brodsky JW, Baum BS, Pollo FE et al. Prospective gait analysis in patients with first metatarsophalangeal joint arthrodesis for hallux rigidus. Foot Ankle Int 2007;28,162–5.
29. Brodsky JW, Passmore RN, Pollo FE et al. Functional outcome of arthrodesis of the first metatarsophalangeal joint using parallel screw fixation. Foot Ankle Int 2005;26,140–6.
30. Keller WL. The surgical treatment of bunions and hallux valgus. New York Med J 1904;80:741–2.
31. Wrighton JD. A ten-year review of Keller's operation. Review of Keller's operation at the Princess Elizabeth Hospital, Exeter. Clin Orthop Relat Res 1972;89:207–14.
32. Love TR, Whynot AS, Farine I et al. Keller's arthroplasty: a prospective review. Foot Ankle 1987;8:46–54.
33. Hamilton, WG O'Malley MJ, Thompson FM et al. Capsular interposition arthroplasty for severe hallux rigidus. Foot Ankle Int 1997;18:68–70.
34. Can Akgun R, Sahin O, Demirors H et al. Analysis of modified oblique Keller procedure for severe hallux rigidus. Foot Ankle Int 2008;29:1203–8.
35. Kennedy JG, Chow FY, Dines J et al. Outcomes after interposition arthroplasty for treatment of hallux rigidus. Clin Orthop Relat Res 2006;445:210–5.

36. Lau JT, Daniels TR. Outcomes following cheilectomy and inter-positional arthroplasty in hallux rigidus foot. Foot Ankle Int 2001;22:462–70.

37. Barca F. Tendon arthroplasty of the first metatarsophalangeal joint in hallux rigidus:preliminary communication. Foot Ankle Int 1997;18:222–8.

38. Mroczek KJ, Miller SD. The modified oblique Keller procedure: a technique for dorsal approach interposition arthroplasty sparing the flexor tendons. Foot Ankle Int 2003;24:521–2.

39. Schenk S, Meizer R, Kramer R et al. Resection arthroplasty with and without capsular interposition for treatment of severe hallux rigidus. Int Orthop 2009;33:145–50.

40. Raikin SM, Ahmad J, Pour AR et al. Comparison of arthrodesis and metallic arthroplasty of the hallux metatarsophalangeal joint. J Bone Joint Surg Am 8 2007;9:1979–85.

41. Moynihan FJ. Arthrodesis of the metatarso-phalangeal joint of the great toe. J Bone Joint Surg Br 1967;49:544–51.

42. Fitzgerald JA. A review of long-term results of arthrodesis of the first metatarso-phalangeal joint. J Bone Joint Surg Br 1969; 51:488–93.

43. Suckel A, Wulker N. Arthrodesis of the first metatarsophalangeal joint. Orthopade 2006;35:443–9.

44. Swanson AB, Lumsden RM II, Swanson GD. Silicone implant arthroplasty of the great toe. A review of single stem and flexible hinge implants. Clin Orthop Relat Res 1979;142:30–43.

45. Shereff MJ, Jahss MH. Complications of silastic implant arthroplasty in the hallux. Foot Ankle 1980;1:95–101.

46. Sebold EJ, Cracchiolo A. Use of titanium grommets in silicone implant arthroplasty of the hallux metatarsophalangeal joint. Foot Ankle Int 1996;17:145–51.

47. Cracchiolo A 3rd, Weltmer JB Jr, Lian G et al. Arthroplasty of the first metatarso-hlangeal joint with a double stem silicone implant. Results in patients who have degenerative joint disease, failure of previous operations or rheumatoid arthritis. J Bone Joint Surg Am 1992;92:552–63.

48. Smetana M, Vencálková S. Use of a silicone metatarsophalangeal joint endoprosthesis in hallux rigidus over a 15-year period. Acta Chir Orthop Traumatol Cech 2003;70:177–81.

49. Granberry WM, Noble PC, Bishop JO, et al. Use of a hinged silicone prosthesis for replacement arthroplasty of the first metatarsophalangeal joint. J Bone Joint Surg Am 1991;10:1453–9.

50. Shankar NS, Asaad SS, Craxford AD. Hinged silastic implants of the great toe. Clin Orthop Relat Res 1991;272:227–34.

51. Papagelopoulos PJ, Kitaoka HB, Ilstrup DM. Survivorship analysis of implant arthroplasty for the first metatarsophalangeal joint. Clin Orthop Relat Res 1994;302:164–172.

52. Hecht, PJ, Gibbons MJ, Wapner KL, et al. Arthrodesis of the first metatarsophalangeal joint to salvage failed silicone implant arthroplasty. Foot Ankle Int 1997;18:383–90.

53. Leavitt KM, Nirenberg MS, Wood B, et al. Titanium hemi-great toe implant: A preliminary study of its efficacy. J Foot Ankle Surg 1991;30:289–93.

54. Koenig RD, Horwitz LR. The Biomet Total Toe System utilizing the Koenig score: a five-year review. J Foot Ankle Surg 1996;35:23–6.

55. Hasselman CT, Shields N. Resurfacing of the first metatarsal head in the treatment of hallux rigidus. Tech Foot Ankle Surg 2008;7:31–40.

56. Giza E, Sullivan MR. First metatarsophalangeal hemiarthroplasty for grade III and IV hallux rigidus. Tech Foot Ankle Surg 2005;4:10–17.

57. Townley CO, Taranow, WS. A Metallic hemiarthroplasty resurfacing prosthesis for the hallux metatarsophalangeal joint. Foot Ankle Int 1994;15:575–80.

58. Konkel KF, Menger AG, Retzlaff SA. Mid-term results of Futura Hemi-Great Toe implants. Foot Ankle Int 2008;29:831–7.

59. Sorbie C. Hemiarthroplasty in the treatment of hallux rigidus. Foot Ankle Int 2008;29:273–81.

60. Esway JE, Conti SF. Joint replacement in the hallux metatarsophalangeal joint. Foot Ankle Clin 2005;10:97–115.

61. Fuhrmann, RA. MTP prosthesis (ReFlexion) for hallux rigidus. Tech Foot Ankle Surg 2005;4:2–9.

62. Kundert HP, Knessl J, Zollinger-Kies H. Replacement of the first metatarso-phalangeal joint. Tech Foot Ankle Surg 2005;4:190–5.

63. Pulavarti RS, McVie JL, Tulloch CJ. First metatarsophalangeal joint replacement using the bio-action great toe implant: intermediate results. Foot Ankle Int 2005;26:1033–7.

36 Charcot–Marie–Tooth Disease and the Treatment of the Cavo-Varus Foot

David N. Townshend and Alastair S.E. Younger
University of British Columbia, Vancouver, BC, Canada

Case scenario

A 35 year old man presents with recurrent ankle instability and overload of the lateral border of his foot. This has worsened over the last few years. He is otherwise fit and well. His father had a similar problem, with a similar foot shape. On examination he has a bilateral high arches and varus heels with callosities under the lateral borders of his feet. He has some clawing of the toes.

Charcot–Marie–Tooth disease and cavo-varus foot deformity

Cavo-varus foot deformity results from an imbalance of muscle forces. Charcot–Marie–Tooth disease (CMT) is a hereditary motor sensory neuropathy (HSMN) and is a common cause of cavo-varus deformity. Cavo-varus foot may also be caused by cerebral palsy, cerebral injury (stroke), anterior horn cell disease (polio, spinal root injury), talar neck injury, and residual clubfoot.[1] CMT as a clinical entity was described in 1886 by Jean-Martin Charcot and Pierre Marie in France, and Howard Henry Tooth in England. It has since become apparent that the condition is a result of many different genetic mutations which result in phenotypically similar deformities. More than 30 different gene defects have been identified in relation to CMT. More recently it has been recognized that the heterogeneity of this disease precludes a standard treatment "recipe" approach to managing individual patients.[2]

Limitations of outcome studies

The variation in phenotypic expression of this disease group makes evaluation of prior studies difficult, as the preoperative deformities are often not outlined. The major-ity of the literature represents level V or expert opinion only and there are no more than level IV studies to guide operative management. Many series do not differentiate progressive from nonprogressive etiologies of the cavo-varus foot, further complicating interpretation of outcome data. Description of the anatomic deformity and the procedures required to correct this will be required in future studies.

Relevant anatomy

CMT is a progressive disease characterized by muscle imbalance. The tibialis anterior and peroneus brevis are often weak, with relative preservation of tibialis posterior, peroneus longus, and extensor hallucis longus. The posterior compartment is usually spared until late in the disease. Foot intrinsics are often weak, resulting in claw toes.

Importance of the problem

The true incidence of CMT and its impact on society is unknown. Many patients will live with milder forms of the disease without ever presenting to a physician. Cavo-varus deformity may present with ankle instability, metatarsalgia, stress fracture, degenerative joint pain, and/or difficulties with shoe wear. A Google search for "Charcot Marie Tooth" gives 297,000 hits, which compares with 731,000 for hip fracture.

Top four questions

1. Is there any evidence for orthotics in the management of the foot deformity in CMT?
2. Should the patient be referred for physiotherapy?

Evidence-Based Orthopedics, First Edition. Edited by Mohit Bhandari.
© 2012 Blackwell Publishing Ltd. Published 2012 by Blackwell Publishing Ltd.

Table 36.1 Outcomes of orthotic interventions

Author	Year	Patients (n)	CMT	Intervention	Outcome	Level
Bean et al.[4]	2001	1	1	AFO		IV
Refshauge et al.[3]	2006	14	14	Night splints	No improvement with night splints	IV
Vinci and Gargiulo[5]	2008	25	25	AFOs	Poor compliance with AFO	IV
Burns et al.[6]	2006	154	Unknown	Custom orthoses	Custom orthoses improved pain and function	I

AFO, ankle–foot orthosis.

3. When is the best time to recommend reconstructive surgery?
4. What are the outcomes from surgical reconstruction of the cavo-varus foot in a patient with CMT?

Question 1: Is there any evidence for orthotics in the management of the foot deformity in CMT?

Relevance

Abnormal distribution of pressure leading to pain, foot drop, and ankle instability can all be managed with an orthotic shoe insert or brace. Orthoses are the first line of management for many foot and ankle disorders, but custom orthoses can be expensive.

Current opinion

Patients should try orthoses before proceeding to surgery. CMT is a neurogenic, progressive disorder and as such early surgery may prevent or slow secondary joint degeneration.

Finding the evidence

- Cochrane Database with search term "(Charcot Marie Tooth OR Pes Cavus OR Cavo-varus)"
- PubMed (www.ncbi.nlm.nih.gov/pubmed/) clinical queries search/systematic reviews: ("Charcot Marie Tooth" OR "Pes Cavus" OR cavo-varus) AND orthotics
- PubMed (www.ncbi.nlm.nih.gov/pubmed/): sensitivity search using keywords ("Charcot Marie Tooth" OR "Pes Cavus" OR "Cavo-varus") AND orthotics

Quality of the evidence

Level I
- 1 randomized trial

Level II
- 1 randomized trial with methodological limitations
- 3 systematic reviews/meta-analyses (of no more than level II studies)

Findings

The most comprehensive study looking solely at patients with CMT was a (level II) randomized controlled trial (RCT) of night splints but with only 14 patients.[3] Wearing night splints was not found to improve dorsiflexion strength or range of motion. Two further (level IV) studies found that optimizing CMT patients' ankle–foot orthosis (AFO) prescription improved physiological performance and perceived exertion,[4] but compliance with AFOs in CMT patients is poor.[5]

In a good-quality (Level I) RCT of 154 symptomatic cavus feet (9 with CMT) Burns et al. found significant improvement in pain, function, and distribution of plantar pressure with custom orthotics vs. sham insoles.[6] Nine of these patients had CMT. The results of orthotic interventions are summarized in Table 36.1.

Recommendations

- There is insufficient evidence to support the use of orthotics specifically in CMT [overall quality: low]
- There is, however, strong evidence to support the use of custom-made orthotics in the symptomatic cavus foot [overall quality: high]

Question 2: Should the patient be referred for physiotherapy?

Relevance

Lateral ligament instability and/or foot drop, disorders which conventionally are referred for physiotherapy, can be manifestations of CMT.

Current opinion

Depending on the degree of symptoms a course of physiotherapy may be beneficial, In the presence of progressive motor and sensory deficits, strengthening and proprioceptive training are less likely to be of benefit.[2]

Finding the evidence

- Cochrane Database with search term "(Charcot Marie Tooth OR Pes Cavus OR Cavo-varus)"

Table 36.2 Outcomes of physiotherapy interventions

Author	Year	Patients (n)	CMT	Intervention	Outcome	Level
Lindeman [7]	1995	62	29	Strength training	Moderate benefit	II
Chetlin et al.[8]	2004	40	40	Resistance training ± creatine	No benefit from creatine	II
Chetlin et al.[9]	2004	20	20	Resistance training	Moderate benefit	IV
El Mhandi et al.[10]	2008	8	8	Interval training	Moderate benefit	IV

- PubMed (www.ncbi.nlm.nih.gov/pubmed/) clinical queries search/systematic reviews: ("Charcot Marie Tooth" OR "Pes Cavus" OR cavo-varus) AND physiotherapy
- PubMed sensitivity search using keywords: ("Charcot Marie Tooth" OR "Pes Cavus" OR cavo-varus) AND physiotherapy

Quality of the evidence

Level II
- 1 randomized trial with methodological limitations
- 1 prospective comparative study
- 3 systematic reviews/meta-analyses (of no more than level II studies)

Findings

In one RCT of poor quality with small numbers (level II), a moderate increase in strength and leg-related functional performance was demonstrated with strength training in patients with HSMN.[7] A prospective comparative study (level II) of resistance training with and without creatine supplementation showed no additional benefit.[8] Two small case series (level IV) also showed that resistance training[9] and interval training exercise[10] could improve functional performance and subjective perception of pain and fatigue. Outcomes of physiotherapy interventions are summarized in Table 36.2.

Recommendation

- In light of the poor quality of the level II studies, only a limited recommendation can be given for physiotherapy-directed exercise in CMT [overall quality: moderate]

Question 3: When is the best time to recommend reconstructive surgery?

Relevance

CMT is a progressive disorder. Benefits of surgery must be weighed against risks; in general, flexible deformities are more easily corrected than late, fixed deformity.

Current opinion

Some surgeons believe that tendon surgery should be performed early to prevent progression of deformity.[1]

Finding the evidence

- Cochrane Database with search term "(Charcot Marie Tooth OR Pes Cavus OR Cavo-varus)"
- PubMed (www.ncbi.nlm.nih.gov/pubmed/) clinical queries search/systematic reviews: ("Charcot Marie Tooth" OR "Pes Cavus" OR cavo-varus) AND physiotherapy
- PubMed sensitivity search using keywords : ("Charcot Marie Tooth" OR "Pes Cavus" OR cavo-varus) AND physiotherapy

Quality of evidence

Level IV
- 1 observational study
- 1 case-control study

Findings

There is no evidence to guide timing of surgical intervention. One observational study demonstrated a reduction in muscle strength and sensory function over a 2 year period in patients with CMT type 1A.[11] Another case-control study demonstrated an increase in physical disability over 5 years but, interestingly, a similar deterioration in muscle strength compared to a control group.[12]

Recommendation

- No recommendation can be made for early surgical intervention due to insufficient evidence [overall quality; low]

Question 4: What are the outcomes from surgical reconstruction of the cavo-varus foot in a patient with CMT?

Case clarification

The patient may have failed the nonoperative interventions described above and/or you believe that early surgical intervention is warranted.

Relevance

CMT is a progressive disorder characterized by muscle imbalance. The goals of surgical reconstruction are to rebalance the foot, to reduce pain, and to maintain a plantigrade, shoeable foot. Traditionally this was performed with a triple arthrodesis but the poor long-term results, particularly in the adolescent population, have directed attention towards more joint-sparing procedures.

Finding the evidence

• Cochrane Database with search term "(Charcot Marie Tooth OR Pes Cavus OR Cavo-varus)"
• PubMed (www.ncbi.nlm.nih.gov/pubmed/) clinical queries search/systematic reviews: ("Charcot Marie Tooth" OR "Pes Cavus" OR cavo-varus) AND surgery
• PubMed sensitivity search using keywords : ("Charcot Marie Tooth" OR "Pes Cavus" OR cavo-varus) AND surgery

Quality of the evidence

A number of scientific articles have been written on the surgical management of CMT but no more than level IV evidence is available and most of the literature is expert opinion. This reflects the complex nature and heterogeneity of the disease.

Findings

Surgeries can be broadly classified into soft tissue procedures, osteotomies, and fusions. These procedures will, however, usually be combined.

In one of the longest case series (level IV), Ward et al.[13] reviewed 41 feet in 25 consecutive patients with CMT who underwent an "algorithmic" approach to reconstruction of their cavo-varus feet at an average of 26.1 years of age. This included a dorsiflexion osteotomy of the 1st metatarsal, transfer of the peroneus longus to the peroneus brevis, plantar fascia release, transfer of the extensor hallucis longus to the neck of the 1st metatarsal, and in selected cases transfer of the tibialis anterior tendon to the lateral cuneiform. Although 11 patients required subsequent procedures, no patients required a triple arthrodesis and reoperation rates and rates of degenerative changes were lower than reports following triple arthrodesis.

Soft tissue surgery Frequently described soft tissue procedures include gastrosoleus lengthening, plantar fascia release, and tendon transfers. One of the few series (level IV) of soft tissue procedure only was described by Roper and Tibrewal.[14] Surgery included tendo achilles (TA) lengthening, tibialis anterior transfer, Jones transfer, plantar fascia release, and Girdlestone Taylor transfer for claw toes. Follow-up was to an average of 14 years with a "good" outcome reported in all 10 patients. No patients had required a triple fusion. Tynan and Klenerman[15] described a case series (level IV) of isolated Jones transfers in 28 feet with pes cavus of varying etiology. The procedures were successful for clawing but not first ray overload and the authors recommended adjunctive procedures.

Osteotomies Where a CMT foot demonstrates a combination of fixed and flexible deformity, osteotomies may be employed to supplement soft tissue correction.

Kucukkaya et al.[16] reported a case series (level IV) of pes cavus including two feet with CMT treated with V-osteotomy and Ilizarov method. Of nine feet treated, eight achieved a painless, plantigrade foot but follow-up was only to average 9 months. Sammarco and Taylor[17] reported on 21 feet in 15 patients treated with calcaneal osteotomy and one or more metatarsal osteotomies; 15 patients had CMT. These authors advocated an adjunctive plantar fascia release.

Fusions More literature is available documenting triple arthrodesis than any other single intervention for CMT, although there are still no more than level IV studies to guide practice and outcome measures are also inconsistent between the studies.

Wetmore and Drennan[18] reported a series of 16 patients with CMT, average age 15 years, with a total of 30 triple arthrodesis. Average length of follow-up was 21 years. Of 30 feet, 2 were excellent, 5 good, 9 fair, and 14 poor; 23 feet had evidence of ankle and/or midfoot arthritis and 6 had required ankle arthrodesis. Wukich and Bowen[19] reported a series of 22 patients reviewed at average of 12.4 years with 88% good or excellent results and 86% satisfied; 24% had ankle arthritis and 62% rest of foot arthritis on radiographs, and 15% had talo-navicular pseudarthroses. Mann and Hsu[20] reported on 12 feet in 10 adolescent patients with CMT with an average follow-up 7.7 years. Only 5 feet were plantigrade and asymptomatic and radiographically fused; 3 had asymptomatic pseudarthroses. The authors comment that achieving plantigrade foot is most important.

In the single largest and longest review of triple fusions, Saltzman et al.[21] reported on 67 feet in 57 patients of whom 6 had CMT. With an average follow-up 44 years, 78% had residual deformity, 28% were good, 69% fair and 3% poor at final follow-up. All had radiographic arthritis at ankle and midfoot. Note that in this series, soft tissue procedures were performed as necessary. Outcomes of surgical interventions are summarized in Table 36.3.

Recommendations

• No more than level IV evidence exists for any surgical intervention;only a limited recommendation can therefore be given for an appropriate combination of soft tissue and bony procedures [overall quality: low]
• More evidence is available for triple arthrodesis, but the relatively poor long-term outcomes of surgery performed in adolescents should be noted [overall quality: low]

Table 36.3 Outcomes of surgical interventions

Author	Year	Patients (n)	CMT	Intervention	Outcome	Level
Wetmore and Drennan[18]	1989	16 (30 feet)	16	Triple arthrodesis	At mean 21 yrs, 2 excellent, 5 good, 9 fair, 14 poor	IV
Roper and Tibrewal[14]	1989	10	10	Soft tissue procedures	Mean 14 yrs, no triples, all "satisfactory"	IV
Wukich and Bowen[19]	1989	22	22	Triple arthrodesis	Mean 12 yrs, 88% good/ excellent	IV
Mann and Hsu[20]	1992	10 (12 feet)	10	Triple arthrodesis	Non-plantigrade foot poorer outcome	IV
Santavirta et al.[22]	1993	15 (26 feet)	15	Various fusions	Mean 14 yrs, 4 excellent, 15 good, 4 fair, 3 poor	IV
Saltzman et al.[21]	1999	57 (67 feet)	6	Triple arthrodesis	Mean 44 yrs, 19 good, 46 fair, 17 poor	IV
Kucukkaya et al.[16]	2002	9	2	Ilizarov frame	Mean 9 months, 8 satisfactory	IV
Ward et al.[13]	2008	21 (45 feet)	21	Combined approach	Mean 26 yrs, 31 feet no further surgery	IV

Summary of recommendations

- There is insufficient evidence to support the use of orthotics specifically in CMT, but strong evidence to support the use of custom-made orthotics in the symptomatic cavus foot.
- There is fair evidence for physiotherapy-directed exercise in CMT.
- There is insufficient evidence to guide timing of surgical intervention.
- No more than Level IV evidence exists for any surgical intervention.
- There is poor evidence to guide selection of appropriate combination of soft tissue and bony procedures.
- There is poor evidence for triple arthrodesis. The relatively poor long-term outcomes of surgery performed in adolescents should be noted.

Conclusion

The cavo-varus foot deformity resulting from CMT represents a challenging problem. The relative heterogeneity of the problem makes evaluation of the literature difficult. A thorough knowledge of the disease process and resulting deformities is essential to guide the surgeon in selecting appropriate soft tissue and bony procedures. Future outcome studies should include details of the specific deformities and the procedures used to address them.

References

1. Younger AS, Hansen ST. Adult cavovarus foot. J Am Acad Orthop Surg 2005;13(5):302–15.
2. Beals TC, Nickisch F. Charcot–Marie–Tooth disease and the cavovarus foot. Foot Ankle Clin 2008;13(2):259–74, vi–vii.
3. Refshauge KM, Raymond J, Nicholson G, van den Dolder PA. Night splinting does not increase ankle range of motion in people with Charcot–Marie–Tooth disease: A randomised, crossover trial. Aust J Physiother 2006;52(3):193–9.
4. Bean J, Walsh A, Frontera W. Brace modification improves aerobic performance in Charcot–Marie–Tooth disease: A single-subject design. Am J Phys Med Rehabil 2001;80(8):578–82.
5. Vinci P, Gargiulo P. Poor compliance with ankle-foot-orthoses in Charcot–Marie–Tooth disease. Eur J Phys Rehabil Med 2008;44(1):27–31.
6. Burns J, Crosbie J, Ouvrier R, Hunt A. Effective orthotic therapy for the painful cavus foot: A randomized controlled trial. J Am Podiatr Med Assoc 2006;96(3):205–11.
7. Lindeman E, Leffers P, Spaans F, Drukker J, Reulen J, Kerckhoffs M, et al.. Strength training in patients with myotonic dystrophy and hereditary motor and sensory neuropathy: A randomized clinical trial. Arch Phys Med Rehabil 1995;76(7):612–20.
8. Chetlin RD, Gutmann L, Tarnopolsky MA, Ullrich IH, Yeater RA. Resistance training exercise and creatine in patients with Charcot–Marie–Tooth disease. Muscle Nerve 2004;30(1):69–76.
9. Chetlin RD, Gutmann L, Tarnopolsky M, Ullrich IH, Yeater RA. Resistance training effectiveness in patients with Charcot–Marie–Tooth disease: Recommendations for exercise prescription. Arch Phys Med Rehabil 2004;85(8):1217–23.
10. El Mhandi L, Millet GY, Calmels P, Richard A, Oullion R, Gautheron V, et al.. Benefits of interval-training on fatigue and functional capacities in Charcot–Marie–Tooth disease. Muscle Nerve 2008;37(5):601–10.
11. Padua L, Pareyson D, Aprile I, Cavallaro T, Quattrone A, Rizzuto N, et al. Natural history of CMT1A including QoL: A 2-year prospective study. Neuromuscul Disord 2008; 18(3):199–203.
12. Verhamme C, van Schaik IN, Koelman JH, de Haan RJ, de Visser M. The natural history of Charcot–Marie–Tooth type 1A in adults: A 5-year follow-up study. Brain 2009;132(Pt 12):3252–62.
13. Ward CM, Dolan LA, Bennett DL, Morcuende JA, Cooper RR. Long-term results of reconstruction for treatment of a flexible cavovarus foot in Charcot–Marie–Tooth disease. J Bone Joint Surg Am 2008;90(12):2631–42.
14. Roper BA, Tibrewal SB. Soft tissue surgery in Charcot–Marie–Tooth disease. J Bone Joint Surg Br 1989;71(1):17–20.
15. Tynan MC, Klenerman L. The modified Robert Jones tendon transfer in cases of pes cavus and clawed hallux. Foot Ankle 1994; 15:68–71.

16. Kucukkaya M, Kabukcuoglu Y, Kuzgun U. Management of the neuromuscular foot deformities with the ilizarov method. Foot Ankle Int 2002;23(2):135–41.

17. Sammarco GJ, Taylor, R. Cavovarus foot treated with combined calcaneus and metatarsal osteotomies. Foot Ankle Int 2001; 22(1):19–30.

18. Wetmore RS, Drennan JC. Long-term results of triple arthrodesis in Charcot–Marie–Tooth disease. J Bone Joint Surg Am 1989;71(3): 417–22.

19. Wukich DK, Bowen JR. A long-term study of triple arthrodesis for correction of pes cavovarus in Charcot–Marie–Tooth disease. J Pediatr Orthop 1989;9(4):433–7.

20. Mann DC, Hsu JD. Triple arthrodesis in the treatment of fixed cavovarus deformity in adolescent patients with Charcot–Marie–Tooth disease. Foot Ankle 1992;13(1):1–6.

21. Saltzman CL, Fehrle MJ, Cooper RR, Spencer EC, Ponseti IV. Triple arthrodesis: twenty-five and forty-four-year average follow-up of the same patients. J Bone Joint Surg Am 1999;81(10): 1391–402.

22. Santavirta S, Turunen V, Ylinen P, Konttinen YT, Tallroth K. Foot and ankle fusions in Charcot–Marie–Tooth disease. Arch Orthop Trauma Surg 1993;112(4):175–9.

IV Trauma

37 Acromioclavicular Joint

Bill Ristevski and Michael D. McKee

St. Michael's Hospital and University of Toronto, Toronto, ON, Canada

Case scenario

A 23 year old man comes to the Emergency Department after being tackled during a football game and injuring his left shoulder. He has swelling and deformity at the distal end of his clavicle. His upper extremity is neurovascularly intact. It is an isolated injury.

Relevant anatomy

The lateral end of the clavicle and the acromion meet to form the acromioclavicular (AC) joint. The capsule resists mainly anterior and posterior motion while the vertical checkrein is the coracoclavicular (CC) ligament complex. Increasing disruption of these anatomic structures usually results in higher-grade injuries.

> AC joint injuries are typically classified into six grades:
> I   AC joint strain
> II AC joint subluxated and the CC ligaments are intact
> III AC joint dislocated and the CC ligaments are disrupted
> IV AC joint superiorly and posteriorly dislocated
> V   AC joint dislocated with 100–300% separation
> VI AC joint dislocated and Inferiorly displaced under the coracoid

Importance of the problem

A Google search for "AC joint separation" returns over 7,000,000 hits. This high hit rate correlates with how common AC joint injuries are, and the various treatments that have been put forward for such injuries. The AC joint remains one of few major joints in the body where dislocation is often accepted without intervention.

Top five questions

Diagnosis

1. Is there a role for MRI rather than standard radiographs in the diagnosis of AC joint injuries?

Therapy

2. What is the optimal nonoperative treatment of an AC joint injury?
3. What type of AC joint injuries should be considered for operative intervention?
4. What is the best operative repair for an AC joint injury?

Prognosis

5. What is the outcome of acute repair vs. delayed reconstruction of an AC joint injury?

Question 1: Is there a role for MRI rather than standard radiographs in the diagnosis of AC joint injuries?

Case clarification

Most AC injuries can be accurately graded using plain radiographs (Figure 37.1). However, this is not always the case and some injuries may be graded incorrectly due to their benign appearance on radiographs secondary to changes in the positioning of the upper extremity, angle of the radiograph beam, or position of the patient. The role of MRI in assessing the extent of injury is brought up by the patient.

Relevance

The classification of AC joint injuries is important as it aids decision-making for potential treatments. Most surgeons

Evidence-Based Orthopedics, First Edition. Edited by Mohit Bhandari.
© 2012 Blackwell Publishing Ltd. Published 2012 by Blackwell Publishing Ltd.

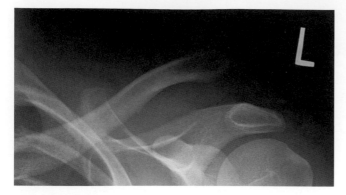

Figure 37.1 Radiograph demonstrating a left grade V AC joint dislocation from the patient in our case scenario.

treat types I and II AC joint injuries nonoperatively. Types IV–VI usually require operative stabilization secondary to their displacement, instability, and associated soft tissue damage. The current debate centers on the optimal management of type III AC joint injuries. Typically, type III injuries have AC joint capsule disruption as well as tearing of the CC ligaments or, rarely, fracture of the coracoid process. Hence the role of MRI is being investigated to define injury severity and perhaps aid in accuracy of classification and improve treatment.

Current opinion

Most orthopedic surgeons would treat type III AC joint injuries nonoperatively.

Finding the evidence

- Cochrane Database, with search term "acromioclavicular"
- PubMed (www.ncbi.nlm.nih.gov/pubmed/) clinical queries search: "acromioclavicular joint"
- PubMed (www.ncbi.nlm.nih.gov/pubmed/) randomized controlled trials: "acromioclavicular"
- PubMed (www.ncbi.nlm.nih.gov/pubmed/) comparative study: "acromioclavicular"
- PubMed (www.ncbi.nlm.nih.gov/pubmed/) Meta-analysis: "acromioclavicular"
- Repeat searches with "acromioclavicular dislocation" and "acromioclavicular injury"
- Repeat searches with "acromioclavicular AND nonoperative"
- Repeat searches with "acromioclavicular AND chronic OR delay"

Quality of the evidence

- Level IV

Findings

The most commonly accepted classification of AC joint injuries by Rockwood is based on the radiographic appearance of the distal clavicle relative to the acromion and coracoid process. The grades essentially escalate with increasing soft tissue disruption about the AC joint. With little disruption of soft tissues (grades I and II) nonoperative treatment is preferred. With significant soft tissue damage (grades IV–VI) most surgeons favor operative treatment in order to reduce and restore stability to the AC joint. Grade III injuries have intermediate soft tissue disruption, with tearing of the AC joint capsule along with the coracoclavicular ligaments. Unfortunately, as in many classification systems, inter- and intraobserver reliability is such that absolute concordance of classification is not possible. In addition, occasionally, patient positioning, support of the extremity, or X-ray beam angle can cause more serious separations of the AC joint to be misdiagnosed. To avoid this, many authors have suggested stress or weighted radiographs of the AC joint, which would in theory separate the acromion from the clavicle allowing the full extent of the AC joint injury to be documented. Bossart et al. evaluated the efficacy of weighted films and found that only 4% of weighted films unmasked a more severe injury (level III).[1] In some instances weighted films made the injury less severe secondary to the uninjured contralateral side, increasing its coracoclavicular distance under stress or muscular contraction secondary to weighted limbs reducing the clavicle separation on the injured side. Their conclusion was that weighted films were not necessary for AC joint injuries. This, combined with the pain the patient endures to obtain these radiographs, as well as the greater radiation exposure, has made stress films less popular in recent times.

With stress films losing popularity, attention has turned to other imaging modalities such as MRI. However, no comparative data exists in sufficient quantity to judge radiographic appearances of AC joint injuries with MRI and correlate this with classifications of the injuries. It is evident that MRI has the ability to demonstrate injury to the AC joint and evaluate the integrity of the coracoclavicular ligaments (level IV).[2,3] This has allowed some authors to use MRI results to classify AC joint injuries on the basis of Rockwood's classification. However, the sensitivity and specificity of injury detection and accuracy of classification via MRI compared to radiograph remains to be determined, and indications for MRI in this setting remain controversial.

Recommendation

Most patients can be reliably diagnosed and classification of their AC joint injury can be determined by an accurate focused history and physical examination along with standardized radiographs including AP, axillary, and upshot (Zanca) view where the arm is resting at the side, without use of a sling. Typically grade I, as well as grades IV–VI, can be reliably distinguished on radiographs. In the rare circumstances where a patient's treatment might be altered because clinical and radiographic findings are equivocal,

MRI will give the physician and patient more information on the integrity of the AC joint soft tissues restraints. How this additional information factors into the ultimate outcome following such injuries has yet to be determined.

- There is insufficient evidence to recommend use of MRI imaging for AC joint injuries. [overall quality: low]

Question 2: What is the optimal nonoperative treatment of an AC separation?

Case clarification
Once an AC joint separation is diagnosed and classified the clinician and patient must decide on operative vs. nonoperative treatment. If nonoperative treatment is decided upon, what form of nonoperative treatment leads to the best outcome?

Relevance
The majority of patients with an AC joint injury will benefit from nonoperative treatment. Taping, bracing/splinting, simple sling, and casting have all had proponents and opponents over time. The issue remains if one method has been able to show benefits when compared to alternate treatments.

Current opinion
Most orthopedic surgeons use a simple sling as their preferred nonoperative management of AC joint injuries.

Finding the evidence
- See Question 1

Quality of the evidence
- Level III

Findings
AC joint separations have been recognized at least since the time of Hippocrates. Many nonoperative treatments have been proposed, with variable success. Lazcano et al. divided nonoperative treatments into three groups: (1) adhesive dressings, (2) various harnesses and braces, or (3) hanging-type casts (suspension casts).[4] Some authors have reported success with various devices, achieving healing in the reduced position (level IV).[5] However, there has been little in the way of direct comparative studies looking at simple sling vs. other more elaborate splints/braces that effectively elevate the arm and acromion and/or depress the clavicle dynamically. In one study operative vs. nonoperative treatment was studied. The nonoperative treatment arm consisted of simple sling, a Kenny–Howard splint (a combination of straps that are designed to elevate the acromion while depressing the clavicle) and casting/taping. Overall the authors felt that the Kenny–Howard splint was superior in reducing the AC joint separation radiographically. However, only 1 in 10 patients ended

with an anatomic reduction of the joint vs. 0 out of 43 patients with simple sling treatment (level III).[6]

Overall, there appears to be evidence that it is possible to reduce an AC joint and maintain this position with various splinting techniques. However, these devices are often elaborate, must be positioned correctly, can be painful to wear, and have questionable patient compliance. The combination of these factors has likely negated the potential benefits that can be demonstrated by such splints.

Recommendation
- Although there are reports that can demonstrate reduction of displaced AC joint with splints, there is insufficient evidence to support the use of a reduction splint vs. simple sling for the nonoperative treatment of AC joint injuries [overall quality: low]

Question 3: What type of AC joint injuries should be considered for operative intervention?

Case clarification
Our patient presents after an isolated, closed injury to the AC joint. He is neurovascularly intact and otherwise healthy with no comorbidities. The patient inquires about surgical treatment vs. nonoperative treatment of this injury.

Relevance
The patient's understanding of the result of nonoperative treatment of their injury vs. the expected risks and benefits of operative intervention forms the basis of treatment decisions. With AC joint injuries the goals of operative intervention are restoration of preinjury anatomy, restoration of preinjury strength and function. and restoration of shoulder appearance.

Current opinion
Most orthopedic surgeons would treat grade I and II AC joint injuries nonoperatively and grade IV–VI AC joint injuries operatively with their preferred technique. Grade III injuries receive variable treatment, with mixed opinion on whether operative treatment is warranted or not.

Finding the evidence
- See Question 1

Quality of the evidence
Level II
- 2 meta-analyses
- 3 randomized controlled trials (RCTs)

Findings
Most of the literature detailing the treatment of severe AC joint injuries (grade IV–VI) is based on expert opinion.

Most authors recommend operative treatment based on their experience of patient outcome following such injuries. Authors have noted deformity, shoulder weakness, loss of shoulder motion, and pain. Unfortunately, there is a paucity of objective data on these injuries. Intuitively, increasing soft tissue damage with increasing grades of AC joint injury would lead to greater functional deficits and pain. Particularly poor outcome has been noted when the clavicle tears through the deltotrapezial fascia and remains directly subcutaneous. Lying subcutaneous makes the clavicle deformity more prominent, and lack of muscular attachments contributes to ongoing shoulder dysfunction.

Three RCTs focusing on AC dislocations were identified. Bannister et al. completed two of these trials (level II).[7,8] Patients were randomized to nonoperative treatment vs. surgical treatment, which consisted of removal of the AC joint meniscus and screw fixation of the clavicle to the coracoid, as well as repair of the anterior deltoid if torn. Hardware was removed 6 weeks after surgery. Patients were ranked as excellent or not excellent in one study or perfect, excellent, good, or fair in another study. Overall, in both studies the authors felt that nonoperative treatment was favorable as patients returned to full activity sooner with avoidance of surgical complications. However, in severely displaced AC joints (defined as >2 cm above the acromion), operative fixation was deemed to give more favorable results.

Larsen et al. completed a randomized study on dislocated AC joints comparing nonoperative treatment to operative treatment which consisted of removal of the AC joint meniscus, reduction and transarticular pinning of the AC joint with Kirschner wires (K-wires), and repair of the CC ligaments and any associated muscle damage (level II).[9] Wires were removed 5–12 weeks after surgery. Points were assigned to patients based on their strength (gauged by spring weights), motion, and subjective pain. Their conclusion was that nonoperative treatment was superior because of the lack of complications seen in the operative group including pin breakage/migration, infection, loss of reduction, and prolonged rehabilitation vs. nonoperative treatment. Outcomes were not significantly different.

Systematic reviews on grade III AC joint injuries have come to the conclusion that operative treatment is not warranted as it shows no difference compared to nonoperative treatment (typically with a sling) and exposes patients to increased risk of complications (level II).[10,11] From the data that is available no appreciable difference in range of motion, pain control, or ultimate shoulder strength was found.

These studies and meta-analyses unfortunately contain flaws that render the conclusions questionable. Many of the authors subjectively felt that their studies were underpowered and that younger patients with greater demands on

their shoulder (athletes, laborers who perform overhead activities, etc.) actually did better with surgery.[7,9] In addition, these studies employed fixation techniques/procedures that are inferior to modern techniques. Fixation devices including hook plates, autograft/allograft fixation, or combinations of fixation techniques are felt to be superior (level IV).[12–17] A recent retrospective comparative study by Gsettetner et al. showed a statistically significant higher Constant score achieved by patients in the operative fixation group via hook plate compared to the nonoperative group in patients with a Rockwood grade III AC joint injury (level III).[18] Such studies and author inferences combined with presumed better operative techniques have added to the debate on the optimal treatment of grade III AC joint injuries.

Recommendation

There is mounting level III/IV evidence that modern operative techniques can result in improved outcomes compared to Bosworth screw or K-wire fixation of grade III AC joint injuries. Higher-quality randomized clinical trials with validated outcome measures and objective testing will be required to elucidate whether the benefits of improved surgical intervention outweigh the potential risks of surgery for such injuries.

• There is insufficient evidence to recommend surgical intervention for grade III AC joint injuries. [overall quality: low]

Question 4: What is the best operative repair for an AC joint injury?

Case clarification

This patient has a widely displaced grade V AC joint injury. He is a young active man with no other comorbidities. The injury is closed and isolated and his upper extremity is neurovascularly intact. The recommendation for operative intervention is made.

Relevance

In high-grade (IV–VI) AC joint injuries most surgeons agree that operative intervention is warranted. Many techniques have been reported with variable success. The ideal repair would achieve and maintain an anatomic reduction, and promote healing in such a way as to preserve the physiological motion demonstrated by the AC joint.

Current opinion

Opinion is divergent on the best operative intervention for AC joint injuries

Finding the evidence

• See Question 1

Findings

No RCTs or meta-analyses exist in the literature comparing fixation techniques for AC joint dislocations. Previous RCTs looking at nonoperative vs. operative treatment for grade III AC joint injuries have demonstrated that clavicular-coracoid screw fixation alone or transfixation of the AC joint via K-wires is not superior to nonoperative treatment (level II).[7–9,19,20] Bannister et al. felt that widely displaced AC joint injuries did have superior results with clavicular-coracoid screw fixation alone.

Many other procedures have been described, including both intra-articular and extra-articular procedures. Authors have reported using various fixation devices, coracoclavicular slings (either biologic or synthetic), coracoacromial ligament transfer to the distal end of the clavicle, or dynamic transfers of the conjoint tendon/coracoid process (level IV).[12,14–18,21–25] Comparison is extremely difficult, with multiple different techniques and implants being employed on various grades of injuries. In addition, these case series are typically small and combine acute and chronic injuries.

Recommendation

Our preferred method of treatment involves the use of a hook plate (Figure 37.2), which we have found to provide stable fixation and adequate reduction for these types of injuries. A disadvantage of this technique is the need for subsequent reoperation for removal in most cases. Although many authors have been able to show good results with K-wire fixation, we would not employ this technique secondary to the rare but potentially devastating complications of K-wire migration to vital organs, especially when other alternative modes of fixation are available that avoid such major complications (level IV).[26–30] The patient in our case scenario elected to undergo operative fixation of his AC joint injury via open reduction and internal fixation with a hook plate.

- There is insufficient data to recommend one type of operative repair over another for dislocated AC joints.

Question 5: What is the outcome of acute repair vs. delayed reconstruction of an AC joint injury?

Case clarification

The patient's radiograph reveals a grade V separation of the AC joint. Surgery is offered to the patient. The patient inquires about waiting to see if the injury is symptomatic and if so can surgery be completed then.

Relevance

Prediction of which patients will be symptomatic following a particular grade of injury is extremely difficult. A patient's ultimate outcome is influenced by their injury, age, handedness, functional demand, expectations, etc. A reasonable question is whether delayed reconstruction is as effective as acute operative intervention.

Current opinion

Most orthopedic surgeons feel that delayed reconstruction of AC joint injuries has inferior results compared to acute repair in comparable injuries.

Finding the evidence

- See Question 1

Quality of the evidence

- Level III

Findings

No RCTs or meta-analyses exist on this topic. Many authors have been able to show improved outcomes following reconstruction of chronic AC joint dislocations in case series but have not compared their results to acute reconstruction (level IV).[16,21,24,31,32] Rolf et al. looked retrospectively at a total of 49 patients, 20 with delayed repair of their AC joint injury and 29 with acute repair. Acute repair consisted of reduction of the AC joint with PDS coracoclavicular sling and repair of the AC joint ligaments with

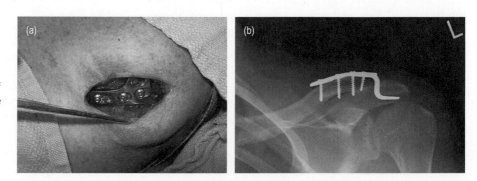

Figure 37.2 (a) Intraoperative photograph of a clavicular hook plate in situ. (b) Postoperative radiograph demonstrating a reduced AC joint held by a hook plate. Note the hook portion of the plate resting in the subacromial space, resisting the superior displacement of the clavicle.

temporary K-wire transfixation. Delayed reconstruction consisted of distal clavicular excision with transfer of the coracoacromial ligament to the distal clavicle and augmentation with PDS coracoclavicular sling. Overall, a significant nine point difference in Constant scores was demonstrated, favoring acute repair (level III).[13]

Recommendation

- Early level III evidence supports that patients with acute reconstruction ultimately have marginally better outcomes [overall quality: low]

Summary of recommendations

- There is insufficient evidence to recommend use of MRI imaging for AC joint injuries. Most patients can be reliably diagnosed and classification of their AC joint injury can be determined by an accurate focused history and physical examination along with standardized radiographs including AP, axillary, and 20° upshot (Zanca) view.
- Although there are reports that demonstrate reduction of displaced AC joint with specialized splints, there is insufficient evidence to support the use of a reduction splint vs. simple sling for the nonoperative treatment of AC joint separation.
- There is insufficient high quality evidence to recommend surgical intervention for grade III AC joint injuries in general.
- There is insufficient data to recommend one type of operative repair over another for dislocated AC joints.
- Early level III evidence supports that patients with acute repair ultimately have marginally better outcomes, compared with delayed reconstruction of AC joint injuries.

Conclusion

The literature on the treatment of AC joint injuries has been extremely varied. Conventional opinion dictates primary repair is indicated for higher-grade (IV–VI) injuries. Careful injury classification and patient selection is critical to successful operative treatment. RCTs are in progress to better delineate which patients would benefit with operative treatment and which techniques can optimize the ultimate function and satisfaction of patients.

References

1. Bossart PJ, Joyce SM, Manaster BJ, Packer SM. Lack of efficacy of "weighted" radiographs in diagnosing acute acromioclavicular separation. Ann Emerg Med 1988;17(1):20–4.

2. Alyas F, Curtis M, Speed C, Saifuddin A, Connell D. MR imaging appearances of acromioclavicular joint dislocation. Radiographics 2008;28(2):463–79; quiz 619.

3. Antonio GE, Cho JH, Chung CB, Trudell DJ, Resnick D. Pictorial essay. MR imaging appearance and classification of acromioclavicular joint injury. AJR Am J Roentgenol 2003 Apr;180(4): 1103–10.

4. Lazcano MA, Anzel SH, Patrick JK. Complete dislocation and subluxation of the acromioclavicular joint: end results in seventy-three cases. J Bone Joint Surg Am 1961;43:379–91.

5. Giannestras NJ. A method of immobilization of acute acromioclavicular separation. J Bone Joint Surg Am 1944;26:597–9.

6. Taft TN, Wilson FC, Oglesby JW. Dislocation of the acromioclavicular joint. An end-result study. J Bone Joint Surg Am 1987;69(7):1045–51.

7. Bannister GC, Wallace WA, Stableforth PG, Hutson MA. The management of acute acromioclavicular dislocation. A randomised prospective controlled trial. J Bone Joint Surg Br 1989;71(5):848–50.

8. Bannister GC, Wallace WA, Stableforth PG, Hutson MA. A classification of acute acromioclavicular dislocation: a clinical, radiological and anatomical study. Injury 1992;23(3):194–6.

9. Larsen E, Bjerg-Nielsen A, Christensen P. Conservative or surgical treatment of acromioclavicular dislocation. A prospective, controlled, randomized study. J Bone Joint Surg Am 1986;68(4):552–5.

10. Bathis H, Tingart M, Bouillon B, Tiling T. [Conservative or surgical therapy of acromioclavicular joint injury—what is reliable? A systematic analysis of the literature using "evidence-based medicine" criteria]. Chirurg 2000;71(9):1082–9.

11. Phillips AM, Smart C, Groom AF. Acromioclavicular dislocation. Conservative or surgical therapy. Clin Orthop Relat Res 1998;353: 10–7.

12. Hosseini H, Friedmann S, Troger M, Lobenhoffer P, Agneskirchner JD. Arthroscopic reconstruction of chronic AC joint dislocations by transposition of the coracoacromial ligament augmented by the Tight Rope device: a technical note. Knee Surg Sports Traumatol Arthrosc 2009;17(1):92–7.

13. Rolf O, Hann von Weyhern A, Ewers A, Boehm TD, Gohlke F. Acromioclavicular dislocation Rockwood III-V: results of early versus delayed surgical treatment. Arch Orthop Trauma Surg 2008;128(10):1153–7.

14. Lim YW. Triple endobutton technique in acromioclavicular joint reduction and reconstruction. Ann Acad Med Singapore 2008; 37(4):294–9.

15. Ejam S, Lind T, Falkenberg B. Surgical treatment of acute and chronic acromioclavicular dislocation Tossy type III and V using the Hook plate. Acta Orthop Belg 2008;74(4):441–5.

16. Tauber M, Eppel M, Resch H. Acromioclavicular reconstruction using autogenous semitendinosus tendon graft: results of revision surgery in chronic cases. J Shoulder Elbow Surg 2007;16(4): 429–33.

17. Tienen TG, Oyen JF, Eggen PJ. A modified technique of reconstruction for complete acromioclavicular dislocation: a prospective study. Am J Sports Med 2003;31(5):655–9.

18. Gstettner C, Tauber M, Hitzl W, Resch H. Rockwood type III acromioclavicular dislocation: surgical versus conservative treatment. J Shoulder Elbow Surg 2008;17(2):220–5.

19. Eskola A, Vainionpaa S, Korkala O, Rokkanen P. Acute complete acromioclavicular dislocation. A prospective randomized trial of

fixation with smooth or threaded Kirschner wires or cortical screw. Ann Chirurg Gynaecol 1987;76(6):323–6.

20. Eskola A, Vainionpaa S, Korkala S, Santavirta S, Gronblad M, Rokkanen P. Four-year outcome of operative treatment of acute acromioclavicular dislocation. J Ortho Trauma 1991;5(1):9–13.

21. Bircher HP, Julke M, Thur C. [Reconstruction of chronic symptomatic acromioclavicular joint dislocation (Rockwood III-V) using the modified Weaver-Dunn method. 24 operated patients (1988–95), surgical technique, results]. Swiss Surg 1996;2:46–50.

22. Clayer M, Slavotinek J, Krishnan J. The results of coracoclavicular slings for acromio-clavicular dislocation. Austral N Z J Surg 1997;67(6):343–6.

23. De Baets T, Truijen J, Driesen R, Pittevils T. The treatment of acromioclavicular joint dislocation Tossy grade III with a clavicle hook plate. Acta Orthop Belg 2004;70(6):515–19.

24. Ferris BD, Bhamra M, Paton DF. Coracoid process transfer for acromioclavicular dislocations. A report of 20 cases. Clin Orthop Relat Res 1989;242:184–94.

25. Jiang C, Wang M, Rong G. Proximally based conjoined tendon transfer for coracoclavicular reconstruction in the treatment of acromioclavicular dislocation. surgical technique. J Bone Joint Surg Am 2008;90(Suppl 2 Part 2):299–308.

26. Tsai C-H, Hsu H-C, Huan C-Y, Chen H-T, Fong Y-C. Late migration of threaded wire (schanz screw) from right distal clavicle to the cervical spine. J Chinese Med Assoc JCMA 2009;72(1): 48–51.

27. Nakayama M, Gika M, Fukuda H, Yamahata T, Aoki K, Shiba S, et al. Migration of a Kirschner wire from the clavicle into the intrathoracic trachea. Ann Thorac Surg 2009;88(2):653–4.

28. Marchi E, Reis MP, Carvalho MV. Transmediastinal migration of Kirschner wire. Interact Cardiovasc Thorac Surg 2008;7(5): 869–70.

29. Nishizaki K, Seki T. Intracardiac migration of a Kirschner wire from the right clavicle. Asian Cardiovasc Thorac Ann 2007; 15(3):272–3.

30. Fransen P, Bourgeois S, Rommens J. Kirschner wire migration causing spinal cord injury one year after internal fixation of a clavicle fracture. Acta Orthop Belg 2007;73(3):390–2.

31. Jeon IH, Dewnany G, Hartley R, Neumann L, Wallace WA. Chronic acromioclavicular separation: the medium term results of coracoclavicular ligament reconstruction using braided polyester prosthetic ligament. Injury 2007;38(11):1247–53.

32. Larsen E, Petersen V. Operative treatment of chronic acromioclavicular dislocation. Injury 1987;18(1):55–6.

38 Clavicle

Bill Ristevski and Michael D. McKee
University of Toronto and St. Michael's Hospital, Toronto, ON, Canada

Case scenario

A 30 year old man who is left-hand dominant and currently employed as a carpenter presents with intense pain in his shoulder after falling off of his mountain bike. On examination his left shoulder is deformed, appearing shortened and "ptotic." It is a closed injury and his left upper extremity is neurovascularly intact (Figure 38.1).

Relevant anatomy

The etymology of clavicle is from the Latin clavicula meaning "tendril, small key, rod, or bolt." Appropriately this relatively thin, double-curved bony "rod" struts the shoulder from the axial skeleton and was deemed to demonstrate "key-like" motion with shoulder movement.

According to the Arbeitsgemeinschaft für Osteosythesefragen/Orthopaedic Trauma Association (AO/OTA) classification (Figure 38.2), clavicular injuries are typically divided into medial, shaft, and distal fractures. Shaft fractures may be simple, wedge, or complex.

Importance of the problem

Clavicle fractures represent approximately 2.6% of all fractures.[1] The majority can be treated successfully by nonoperative techniques. Historically, orthopedic dogma based on large studies using clavicular union as the ultimate successful endpoint, molded surgical belief in such a way that operative intervention was deemed unnecessary and dangerous.

Recently, other outcomes such as patient satisfaction, shoulder strength/endurance, time to recovery, and shoulder appearance have come to the fore. Modern studies have demonstrated functional deficiencies and higher nonunion rates with displaced clavicle fractures compared to previous reports. In some patients there is evidence many of these issues, and resultant disabilities, can be improved by acute operative intervention.

Many patients attempt to weigh fact and opinion from an increasingly massive amount of information that is directed toward them. A Google search for "collarbone fracture" yields 970,000 hits. With expanding treatment options for clavicle fractures, orthopedic surgeons together with their patients must decide on appropriate treatment.

Top five questions

Therapy

1. What is the optimal nonoperative treatment of a closed midshaft clavicle fracture?
2. What factors are associated with poor outcomes following nonoperative treatment of displaced clavicle fractures?
3. What is the optimal treatment of a displaced midshaft clavicle fracture?
4. What is the best operative technique for a clavicle fracture: intramedullary pin or plate?

Prognosis

5. What are the results of acute repair vs. delayed reconstruction secondary to nonunion or malunion for clavicle fractures?

Evidence-Based Orthopedics, First Edition. Edited by Mohit Bhandari.
© 2012 Blackwell Publishing Ltd. Published 2012 by Blackwell Publishing Ltd.

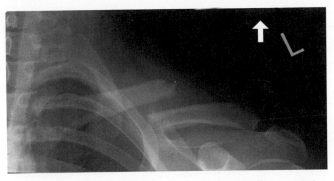

Figure 38.1 Radiograph of a 30 year old man who fell off his mountain bike and sustained a midshaft clavicle fracture. Displacement and shortening is evident.

Question 1: What is the optimal nonoperative treatment of a closed midshaft clavicle fracture?

Case clarification

The patient's radiograph reveals a displaced midshaft clavicle fracture. Many surgeons would now offer operative treatment for such an injury. However, this patient is strongly against surgery. Two nonoperative options are offered: a figure-of-eight bandage or a simple sling.

Relevance

Obtaining and maintaining reduction for clavicle fractures via closed reduction techniques has eluded practitioners of medicine, despite literally hundreds of immobilization devices since the advent of bandaging fractures. The two nonoperative treatment methods that are most popular are figure-of-eight immobilization (believed to help control shoulder position to aid in the reduction of the fracture) or a simple sling.

Current opinion

Current opinion suggests that the majority of surgeons use a simple sling for the nonoperative treatment of a midshaft clavicle fracture.

Finding the evidence

- Cochrane Database, with search term "clavicle fracture"
- PubMed (www.ncbi.nlm.nih.gov/pubmed/) systematic reviews: "clavicle"
- PubMed (www.ncbi.nlm.nih.gov/pubmed/) randomized controlled trials: "clavicle"
- PubMed (www.ncbi.nlm.nih.gov/pubmed/) clinical trial: "clavicle AND fracture, clavicle AND malunion, clavicle AND nonunion"
- American Academy of Orthopedic Surgeons, proceedings of the 2003–2008 annual meetings.
- MEDLINE OVID clavicle and fracture and plate limited to comparative study

Quality of the evidence
Level II
- 1 meta-analysis
- 2 randomized trials with methodologic limitation

Findings

Meta-analysis of the current evidence does not allow definitive conclusions on which intervention is better (level II).[2] Two trials were included in the meta-analysis, one by Andersen et al. in 1987 and the other by Hoofwick et al. in 1988 (level II).[3,4] Both trials were underpowered, with the total number of participants being 234. Data pooling was not possible because of the different and/or unvalidated outcome measures used by the authors.

Pain, union, and function Between the two treatment groups both authors reported no difference in union, malunion, or shoulder function with the use of a sling or figure-of-eight bandage. Andersen reported 9/34 patients were dissatisfied with figure-of-eight treatment vs. 2/27 for sling treatment.[3] Some of the reasons for this were secondary to the figure-of-eight bandage causing pain, difficulty sleeping, edema, and parasthesias of the arm.

Pain as measured by a visual analogue scale in the Hoofwijk study was better at 15 days in the group treated by sling vs. figure-of-eight bandage, (mean difference 0.80, 95% CI 0.34–1.26; visual analogue scale, 0 (no pain) to 10 (worst pain)).[2]

Recommendation

In adult patients with closed midshaft clavicle fractures:
- Sling immobilization is as effective as figure-of-eight bandage, with superior patient tolerance [overall quality: moderate]

Question 2: What factors are associated with poor outcomes following nonoperative treatment of displaced clavicle fractures?

Case clarification

This young man has a displaced, shortened, midshaft clavicle fracture with minimal comminution. Clinically his scapula is malpositioned with prominence of the medial border and inferior tip. The natural history of this particular injury vs. an undisplaced clavicle fracture is discussed with the patient.

Relevance

Neer and Rowe independently reported on 2236 and 566 clavicle fractures and observed nonunion rates of 0.13% and 0.8% respectively.[5,6] This helped support the overwhelming notion that these injuries were best treated nonoperatively.

BONE: CLAVICLE (15)

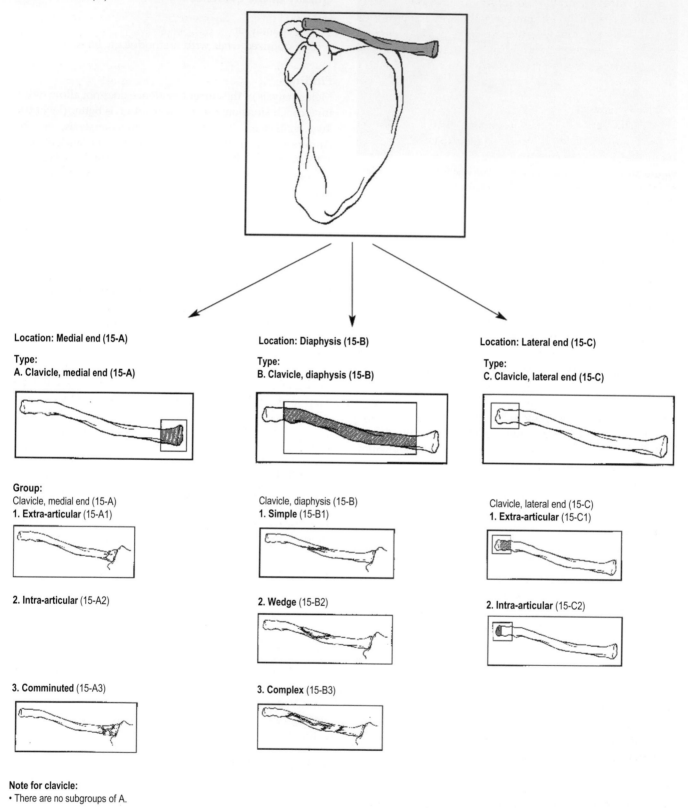

Location: Medial end (15-A)

Type:
A. Clavicle, medial end (15-A)

Location: Diaphysis (15-B)

Type:
B. Clavicle, diaphysis (15-B)

Location: Lateral end (15-C)

Type:
C. Clavicle, lateral end (15-C)

Group:
Clavicle, medial end (15-A)
1. Extra-articular (15-A1)

Clavicle, diaphysis (15-B)
1. Simple (15-B1)

Clavicle, lateral end (15-C)
1. Extra-articular (15-C1)

2. Intra-articular (15-A2)

2. Wedge (15-B2)

2. Intra-articular (15-C2)

3. Comminuted (15-A3)

3. Complex (15-B3)

Note for clavicle:
• There are no subgroups of A.

Figure 38.2 The OTA classification of clavicle fractures.

More recent literature, contrary to previous reports, demonstrated a subset of patients with permanent disability following the non-operative treatment of a clavicle fracture. This prompted further investigations to elucidate the potential negative sequelae of clavicle fractures and how to avoid them.

Current opinion

Most orthopedic surgeons recognize that a subset of patients with clavicle fractures will go on to have sustained pain and/or functional impairment.

Finding the evidence

- See Question 1

Quality of the evidence

Level I

- 1 systematic review
- 2 prospective prognostic studies

Findings

Most patients with a clavicle fracture will heal uneventfully via nonoperative treatment and most will have a satisfactory functional outcome with subjectively acceptable shoulder appearance. A minority of patients will have ongoing sequelae from a clavicle fracture.

In their 1997 study Hill et al. identified a subset of patients who had persistent symptoms and shoulder complaints following clavicle fracture. Patients with a completely displaced middle third clavicle fracture had a 15% nonunion rate and 31% expressed dissatisfaction with their ultimate outcome (level II).[7]

In 2005 Zlowodzki et al. performed a systematic review of the literature focusing on papers on clavicle fractures published from 1975 to 2005. A total of 22 studies were deemed acceptable, reporting on a total of 2144 fractures. Of these 1145 were treated nonoperatively with a resultant nonunion rate of 5.9%. Subset analysis identified 159 displaced fractures, whose nonunion rate was 15.1%, consistent with Hill's earlier findings (level I).[8]

Encompassed within this systematic review were important prospective observational cohort studies that provided insight into factors that are associated with negative outcomes after clavicle fracture. Robinson's study employing multivariate analysis found increasing fracture displacement, comminution, advancing age, and female gender all to be independent predictors of nonunion in shaft fractures (level I).[9] Nowak et al. also found that displacement, comminution, and older age were predictors for sequelae (pain and deformity) following clavicle fracture (level I).[10] Other authors have found association of long-term symptoms to be related to the degree of shortening. Patients with overall shortening of the clavicle by more than 15–20 mm had increasingly prominent symptoms.[7,8,11–15]

Recommendation

Increased risks for having ongoing symptoms or nonunion after clavicle fracture include no cortical contact at fracture site (amount of displacement), comminution, excessive shortening (>20 mm), advancing age, and female gender.

- If risk factors are present, a more objective prognostication of potential negative outcomes can be offered to the patient and treatment alternatives considered [overall quality: high]

Question 3: What is the optimal treatment of a displaced midshaft clavicle fracture?

Case clarification

This patient is a healthy, active young man whose job entails heavy lifting, repetitive motions, and overhead activity. His radiograph shows a widely displaced and shortened clavicle. On physical exam he has shoulder "ptosis" and a prominent medial border of his scapula (a form of scapular winging). The risks and benefits of two options are discussed with the patient: reduction with internal fixation vs. nonoperative management.

Relevance

A logical sequence of investigational questions can be temporally mapped in the literature, leading to a renewed interest in operative treatments for clavicle fractures. First, compelling evidence from patient-based studies showed some patients have poor outcomes following specific types of clavicle fractures. Second, investigations directed at categorizing patient or fracture types identified an at-risk population for poor outcome. Third, studies objectively demonstrated functional deficits following nonoperative treatment of displaced clavicle fractures. Fourth, studies investigating the use of acute operative fixation to potentially improve outcomes for patients at risk of long-term sequelae were performed. Debate continues with regard to which patients would benefit from acute fixation of clavicle fractures. Mitigation of overtreatment secondary to poor patient selection for operative stabilization is critical to avoid unnecessary risk exposure for patients.

Current opinion

Most surgeons acknowledge a benefit from acute operative fixation of widely displaced midshaft clavicle fractures in young healthy adults.

Finding the evidence

- See Question 1

Quality of the evidence

Level I

- 1 randomized trial

Level II

- 1 systematic review
- 3 randomized trials

Findings

In a systematic review, Zlowodzki et al. on behalf of the Evidence-Based Orthopaedic Trauma Working Group reported on 2144 clavicle fractures. Plated fractures (N = 635) had a nonunion rate of 2.5% vs. 5.9% for nonoperative treatment (relative nonunion risk for nonoperative treatment, 2.4 (95% CI 1.4–4), and a relative risk reduction for plating of 57% (95% CI 27–75%; p = 0.001). (level II).[8]

When subset analysis of displaced fractures was reviewed, 460 plated fractures had an ultimate nonunion rate of 2.2% vs. 15.1% for nonoperatively treated displaced fractures. Therefore, the relative nonunion risk for nonoperative treatment was 6.9 (95% CI 3.4–14.2), with a relative risk reduction for plating of 86% (95% CI 71–93%); p < 0.001). Intramedullary pin fixation of the clavicle showed a similar improvement in nonunion rates vs. nonoperative treatment (level II).[8]

In 2007 The Canadian Orthopaedic Trauma Society (COTS) published their results from a multicenter prospective randomized controlled trial (RCT) of plate fixation vs. nonoperative treatment for displaced midshaft clavicle fractures. Outcomes included analysis of the Constant shoulder score, Disability of the Arm, Shoulder and Hand (DASH) score, radiographs, and standard clinical follow-up for duration of 1 year. The operative arm of the study had patients that demonstrated statistically significant differences including a shorter time to union (16.4 vs. 28.4 weeks), improved Constant and DASH scores, as well as being more satisfied with their outcomes and appearance (level I).[16] The operative group had Constant and DASH scores that were improved by approximately 10 points, a difference that has been shown to be clinically relevant.[17,18]

Complications for the operative group were 37% vs. 63% for nonoperative treatment. The operative group's complications included hardware irritation (with some patient requests for removal), transient brachial plexus irritations, and wound complications (4.8%). The nonoperative group had complications predominated by nonunion, malunion (requiring corrective surgery), and transient brachial plexus irritation. The only statistically significant difference in complications was a lower incidence of symptomatic malunion and nonunion in the operative group (level I).[16]

RCTs by both Smith and Smekal noted excellent results following operative fixation of displaced midshaft clavicle fractures (level II).[19,20] Smekal et al., looked at operative fixation via elastic stable intramedullary nailing of fully displaced clavicle fractures vs. nonoperative treatment. A total of 60 patients were enrolled in the study. A significant difference was found in favor of the operative group in terms of the DASH score (first 18 weeks postoperatively) and the Constant score up until 2 years (Figure 38.3). In the nonoperative group 3 patients (10%) had a nonunion vs. 0 in the operative group, with 7 patients in the operative group having medial nail protrusion and 2 implant failures

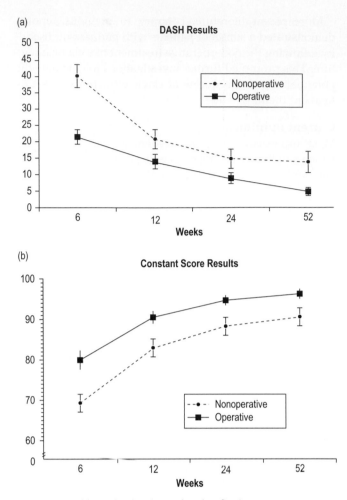

Figure 38.3 (a) Graphical DASH results, plate fixation group vs. nonoperative group for acutely displaced clavicle fractures. The DASH is a disability score with a "perfect" upper extremity achieving a score of 0. The operative group scores are significantly improved (lower DASH score) at every follow-up time point. (b) Graphical Constant score results, plate fixation group vs. nonoperative group for acutely displaced clavicle fractures. The operative group scores are significantly improved at every follow-up time point (p = 0.01). (Adapted from Canadian Orthopaedic Trauma Society. Nonoperative Treatment compared with plate fixation of displaced midshaft clavicle fractures. A multicenter, randomized clinical trial. J Bone Joint Surg(A) 89:1–10, 2007. Reprinted with permission of the Journal of Bone and Joint Surgery. www.jbjs.org)

requiring revision surgery after repeat trauma. Overall, Smekal noted operatively treated patients returned to daily activities quicker, and had a higher degree of satisfaction. Smith et al. found similar results in their prospective randomized study,[20] where 12 out of 35 patients in the nonoperative group developed a nonunion, whereas all 30 patients treated with plate fixation went on to unite (p = 0.001). There was a 30% rate of hardware removal in their study.

Recently, Judd et al. published a prospective randomized trial looking at nonoperative treatment vs. operative treatment employing a modified Hagie pin for displaced mid-shaft clavicle fractures (level II).[21] No significant difference in outcome was identified at 1 year after the interventions, except the operative group had a higher amount of complications particularly related to hardware prominence.

Recommendation

• Young active individuals who are low risk for general anesthetic and have a completely displaced clavicle fracture demonstrate a functional benefit and overall higher satisfaction level with operative vs. nonoperative treatment. A discussion with such patients should be had outlining the relative risks of operative fixation vs. nonoperative treatment [overall quality: moderate]

Question 4: What is the best operative technique for a clavicle fracture: intramedullary pin or plate?

Case clarification

This young adult man has a displaced, shortened clavicle fracture with minimal comminution and clinically malaligned scapula. After patient counseling a decision to proceed with operative treatment is made (Figure 38.4). Two options are offered: intramedullary pinning vs. plate fixation.

Relevance

Early studies of clavicle fixation demonstrated that small plates and/or cerclage wires for clavicle fractures were inadequate and would commonly lead to catastrophic failure or nonunion.[5,6] This certainly added to the impetus to avoid operating on clavicle injuries. In addition, the clavicle poses other difficulties in terms of operative treatment. It is a superficially located, irregularly shaped bone

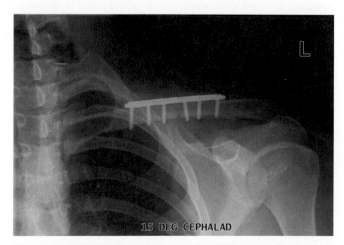

Figure 38.4 The patient in the above case scenario elected to have operative treatment. This radiograph was obtained during follow-up and demonstrates fixation with a precontoured clavicle plate.

in close proximity to neurovascular structures. Depending on the position of the arm the clavicle undergoes motion, which alternates the topography of compressive, tensile, and rotation forces on the bone. This provides an extremely challenging stress on implants used for fixation. Although many methods of internal fixation exist, two general categories have been popular: intramedullary fixation and plate fixation.

Current opinion

Plate fixation for clavicle fractures provides increased stability and more reliable results for maintenance of reduction vs. intramedullary devices.

Finding the evidence

• See Question 1

Quality of the evidence

Level I

• 1 randomized trial

Level II

• 1 systematic reviews/meta-analyses
• 4 randomized trials

Findings

RCTs have shown benefits in terms of union rates, avoidance of malunion, and quicker return to baseline function with internal fixation vs. nonoperative treatment for displaced midshaft clavicle fractures (level I/II).[16,20] Other studies employing intramedullary fixation have demonstrated mixed results, some comparable to plate fixation (level II)[19] with other studies showing no benefit of intramedullary fixation (level II/III).[21,22] Some authors have suggested that the benefit of intramedullary stabilization of clavicle fractures is negated by the complications—mainly hardware migration, infections, and loss of reduction associated with this type of hardware (level II/III).[21,22]

There has been only one RCT directly comparing intramedullary pinning vs. plate fixation, by Lee et al. (level II).[23] The difference between Knowles pins and plate fixation was investigated in elderly patients. Overall, the authors felt Knowles pins were superior, secondary to a smaller incision and decreased pain rate. No difference in healing time, shoulder scores, or union was observed. However, interpretation of this data is difficult as this study focused on elderly patients with lower functional demands. In addition, some patients had cerclage wire in addition to implantation of the Knowles pin or plate fixation, which included the use of reconstruction plates, tubular plates (which are suboptimal in higher-demand patients), or dynamic compression plates.

Recommendation

Most of the complications with intramedullary devices are centered on hardware migration (skin protrusion/hardware irritation), loss of reduction, and infection vs. hardware prominence and potential for more wound complications/ infections with the larger incision needed for plating. More studies are necessary to determine if the potential advantage of smaller incisions with intramedullary fixation can outweigh the risks of losing fracture reduction via shortening or rotation, problems associated with any unlocked intramedullary device.

• There is insufficient evidence to determine if plating or intramedullary fixation provides a superior outcome for displaced midshaft clavicle fractures [overall quality: insufficient]

Question 5: What are the results of acute repair vs. delayed reconstruction secondary to nonunion or malunion for clavicle fractures?

Case clarification
This young adult has a completely displaced midshaft clavicle fracture, with a clinically obvious shoulder deformity. The expected benefits of acute fixation are discussed vs. the potential benefits of delayed reconstruction of a nonunion or malunion.

Relevance
Improper healing of a clavicle fracture can be problematic. However, a proportion of patients with significant malunions and to lesser degree nonunions of their clavicle may be asymptomatic. This suggests that a possible treatment approach would be delayed reconstruction of a symptomatic malunion or nonunion vs. acute fixation.

Current opinion
Most orthopedic surgeons recognize that acute fixation of displaced clavicle fractures provides a better functional outcome than reconstructive procedures.

Finding the evidence
• See Question 1

Quality of the evidence
• Level III

Findings
There is limited information available comparing delayed reconstruction of clavicle fracture malunion and nonunions to acute fixation. Potter et al. found that patients with delayed reconstruction had a significant difference in their Constant scores, with the acute fixation group scoring on average 6 points higher than the group who underwent delayed reconstruction (level III).[14,24] Patients with delayed reconstruction also had significantly poorer endurance strength of their shoulders.

Other studies have demonstrated improved Constant and/or DASH scores with delayed reconstructions but unfortunately did not have an acute clavicle fixation group to compare with (level IV).[14,15,25–27]

Answering such questions by the scientific method is difficult, as a delayed reconstruction implies bias; patients who underwent nonoperative treatment and are displeased with their outcome. This may select a subgroup of patients with intrinsically poor results.

Recommendation
Debate continues as to how significant the differences of acute fixation are relative to delayed reconstruction. This should be discussed with the patient and overall suitability ascertained by the patients' age, expectations, timeline to return to activities, occupation/recreational activities, comorbidities, operative suitability, level of risk aversion, and possible need for reoperation secondary to complication or for hardware removal.

• There is no level I evidence to suggest that acute fixation of a displaced midshaft clavicle fracture provides superior outcome compared with delayed reconstruction. What evidence is available supports a marginally improved Constant shoulder score and improved endurance strength with acute fixation. In isolation this information should not be used to make a decision between nonoperative vs. operative treatment, but can be relayed to patients to allow a complete discussion of such injuries [overall quality: low]

Summary of recommendations

• In adult patients with a closed midshaft clavicle fracture, sling immobilization is as effective as a figure-of-eight bandage with superior patient satisfaction. Our recommendation is nonoperative treatment with a sling

• Prognostic factors for poor outcome following a clavicle fracture include:
  ○ No cortical contact at fracture site (amount of displacement)
  ○ Comminution
  ○ Excessive shortening (>20 mm)
  ○ Advancing age
  ○ Female gender

• Young active individuals who are low risk for anesthetic and have a completely displaced midshaft clavicle fracture demonstrate a functional benefit and overall higher satisfaction level with operative vs. nonoperative treatment

• There is insufficient evidence to determine if plates or intramedullary fixation provides a superior outcome for displaced midshaft clavicle fractures treated operatively. Complications of intramedullary nailing include hardware migration with subsequent loss of reduction, and hardware irritation. Hardware prominence and wound complications are more common with plating. In general, results appear to be more consistent with plating

- There is no level I evidence to suggest that acute fixation of a displaced midshaft clavicle fracture provides superior outcome compared with delayed reconstruction. What evidence is available supports an improved Constant shoulder score and activity endurance with acute fixation

Conclusion

The treatment of clavicle fractures has changed dramatically over the last two decades, with high-quality prospective and randomized trials supporting primary operative fixation of completely displaced clavicle fractures in select patients.

References

1. Postacchini F, Gumina S, De Santis P, Albo F. Epidemiology of clavicle fractures. J Shoulder Elbow Surg 2002;11(5):452–6.
2. Lenza M, Belloti JC, Andriolo RB, Gomes Dos Santos JB, Faloppa F. Conservative interventions for treating middle third clavicle fractures in adolescents and adults. Cochrane Database Syst Rev 2009;2:CD007121.
3. Andersen K, Jensen PO, Lauritzen J. Treatment of clavicular fractures. Figure-of-eight bandage versus a simple sling. Acta Orthop Scand 1987;58(1):71–4.
4. Hoofwijk AG, van der Werken C. [Conservative treatment of clavicular fractures]. Z Unfallchir Versicherungsmed Berufskr 1988;81(3):151–6.
5. Neer CS, 2nd. Nonunion of the clavicle. J Am Med Assoc 1960;172:1006–11.
6. Rowe CR. An atlas of anatomy and treatment of midclavicular fractures. Clin Orthop Relat Res 1968;58:29–42.
7. Hill JM, McGuire MH, Crosby LA. Closed treatment of displaced middle-third fractures of the clavicle gives poor results.[see comment]. J Bone Joint Surgery Br 1997;79(4): 537–9.
8. Zlowodzki M, Zelle BA, Cole PA, Jeray K, McKee MD, et al. Treatment of acute midshaft clavicle fractures: systematic review of 2144 fractures: on behalf of the Evidence-Based Orthopaedic Trauma Working Group. J Orthop Trauma 2005;19(7):504–7.
9. Robinson CM, Court-Brown CM, McQueen MM, Wakefield AE. Estimating the risk of nonunion following nonoperative treatment of a clavicular fracture.[see comment]. J Bone Joint Surg Am 2004;86(7):1359–65.
10. Nowak J, Holgersson M, Larsson S. Can we predict long-term sequelae after fractures of the clavicle based on initial findings? A prospective study with nine to ten years of follow-up. J Shoulder Elbow Surg 2004;13(5):479–86.
11. Eskola A, Vainionpaa S, Myllynen P, Patiala H, Rokkanen P. Outcome of clavicular fracture in 89 patients. Arch Orthop Trauma Surg 1986;105(6):337–8.
12. Lazarides S, Zafiropoulos G. Conservative treatment of fractures at the middle third of the clavicle: the relevance of shortening and clinical outcome. J Shoulder Elbow Surg 2006;15(2): 191–4.
13. McKee MD, Pedersen EM, Jones C, Stephen DJG, Kreder HJ, Schemitsch EH, et al. Deficits following nonoperative treatment of displaced midshaft clavicular fractures. J Bone Joint Surg Am 2006;88(1):35–40.
14. Rosenberg N, Neumann L, Wallace AW. Functional outcome of surgical treatment of symptomatic nonunion and malunion of midshaft clavicle fractures. J Shoulder Elbow Surg 2007; 16(5):510–13.
15. Wick M, Muller EJ, Kollig E, Muhr G. Midshaft fractures of the clavicle with a shortening of more than 2 cm predispose to nonunion. Arch Orthop Trauma Surg 2001;121(4): 207–11.
16. Canadian Orthopaedic Trauma Society. Nonoperative treatment compared with plate fixation of displaced midshaft clavicular fractures. A multicenter, randomized clinical trial.[see comment]. J Bone Joint Surgery Am 2007;89(1):1–10.
17. Hudak PL, Amadio PC, Bombardier C. Development of an upper extremity outcome measure: the DASH (disabilities of the arm, shoulder and hand) [corrected]. The Upper Extremity Collaborative Group (UECG)[erratum appears in Am J Ind Med 1996;30(3):372]. Am J Ind Med 1996;29(6): 602–8.
18. Yian EH, Ramappa AJ, Arneberg O, Gerber C. The Constant score in normal shoulders. J Shoulder Elbow Surg 2005;14(2): 128–33.
19. Smekal V, Irenberger A, Struve P, Wambacher M, Krappinger D, Kralinger FS. Elastic stable intramedullary nailing versus nonoperative treatment of displaced midshaft clavicular fractures—a randomized, controlled, clinical trial. J Orthop Trauma 2009;23(2):106–12.
20. Smith CA, Rudd J, Crosby LA, eds. Results of Operative versus Nonoperative Treatment for 100% Displaced Midshaft Clavicle Fractures: A Prospective Randomized Clinical Trial. 16th Annual Open Meeting of the American Shoulder and Elbow Surgeons, March 18, 2000.
21. Judd DB, Pallis MP, Smith E, Bottoni CR. Acute operative stabilization versus nonoperative management of clavicle fractures. Am J Orthop 2009;38(7):341–5.
22. Grassi FA, Tajana MS, D'Angelo F. Management of midclavicular fractures: comparison between nonoperative treatment and open intramedullary fixation in 80 patients. J Trauma 2001;50(6):1096–100.
23. Lee Y-S, Lin C-C, Huang C-R, Chen C-N, Liao W-Y. Operative treatment of midclavicular fractures in 62 elderly patients: Knowles pin versus plate. Orthopedics. 2007;30(11): 959–64.
24. Potter JM, Jones C, Wild LM, Schemitsch EH, McKee MD. Does delay matter? The restoration of objectively measured shoulder strength and patient-oriented outcome after immediate

fixation versus delayed reconstruction of displaced midshaft fractures of the clavicle. J Shoulder Elbow Surg 2007;16(5):514–18.

25. Ledger M, Leeks N, Ackland T, Wang A. Short malunions of the clavicle: an anatomic and functional study. J Shoulder Elbow Surg 2005;14(4):349–54.

26. Kitsis CK, Marino AJ, Krikler SJ, Birch R. Late complications following clavicular fractures and their operative management. [see comment]. Injury 2003;34(1):69–74.

27. Hillen RJ, Eygendaal D. Corrective osteotomy after malunion of mid shaft fractures of the clavicle. Strategies Trauma Limb Reconstr 2007;2(2–3):59–61.

39 Scapula

Peter A. Cole and Lisa K. Schroder
University of Minnesota–Regions Hospital, Saint Paul, MN, USA

Case scenario

History and physical examination

A 28 year old snowboarder crashed into a tree. He was dazed at the scene, had labored respirations, and was carried off via stretcher and airlifted to a level I trauma center.

A trauma workup revealed a Glasgow Coma Score of 13 in a mildly disoriented man who complained of severe shoulder, chest, and back pain.

History revealed that he was a right-handed warehouse stockman who was otherwise healthy. Physical examination revealed left-sided facial lacerations and an abrasion over a tender mass at the acromion. He had a strong grip and intact sensation of C5–T1, but an inability to forward elevate or externally rotate the shoulder.

Radiography

A chest radiograph revealed four consecutive left-sided rib fractures and a pneumothorax, prompting dedicated shoulder radiographs. A fracture of the scapula in the region of the glenoid neck in addition to a displaced acromioclavicular (AC) joint was diagnosed (Figure 39.1). Moderate displacement at the lateral scapula border, and a glenopolar angle (GPA) of 63° as seen on the anteroposterior (AP) view, with an angular deformity of 21° measured on the scapula Y radiograph, prompted a CT scan (Figure 39.2).

On 3-D CT, the patient had 20° of angulation, 150% translation and 0.5 cm of displacement of the lateral border. Fracture lines propagated into the spinoglenoid notch, and out the scapular spine, and vertebral border. A 2-D CT revealed no intra-articular involvement, but significant displacement at the base of the coracoid, and a retroverted glenoid neck of 11° (Figure 39.2C).

Relevant anatomy

Often, the "neck" of the scapula is referred to as the anatomy just proximal to the glenoid extending up to the coracoid, though some refer to a fracture of the neck as one which remains lateral to the acromion base. Others refer to the neck as simply involving the high lateral border. The coracoid and acromion processes are vulnerable to fracture because of their narrow stalks, though variation in fracture patterns of these scapular extensions is wide, as evidenced by the mapping of these injuries (level IV).[1] On the other hand, fracture patterns involving the scapula neck and body are quite consistent, as reported by Armitage et al. (level IV),[2] and emanate from just inferior to the glenoid and out the vertebral border at the base of the spine in over two thirds of cases. The spinoglenoid notch is involved in about 20% of cases (Figure 39.3). The best opportunities for fixation are at the glenoid neck and lateral border, though the spine of the scapula and the vertebral border are also used, but provide lesser purchase.

Neurovascular structures at risk during typical posterior surgical approaches include the suprascapular neurovascular bundle, which must be protected from iatrogenic harm. The circumflex scapular artery, a mean 5.6 cm (range 4.5–7.0) from the spinoglenoid notch must also be protected or coagulated (Figure 39.4A,B).[3]

Importance of the problem

Scapula fractures account for approximately 1% of all fractures, about the same percentage as calcaneus fractures and exceeding that of talus fractures. Therefore, this injury is quite relevant, particularly for trauma centers, where such injuries are filtered with regularity.

Evidence-Based Orthopedics, First Edition. Edited by Mohit Bhandari.
© 2012 Blackwell Publishing Ltd. Published 2012 by Blackwell Publishing Ltd.

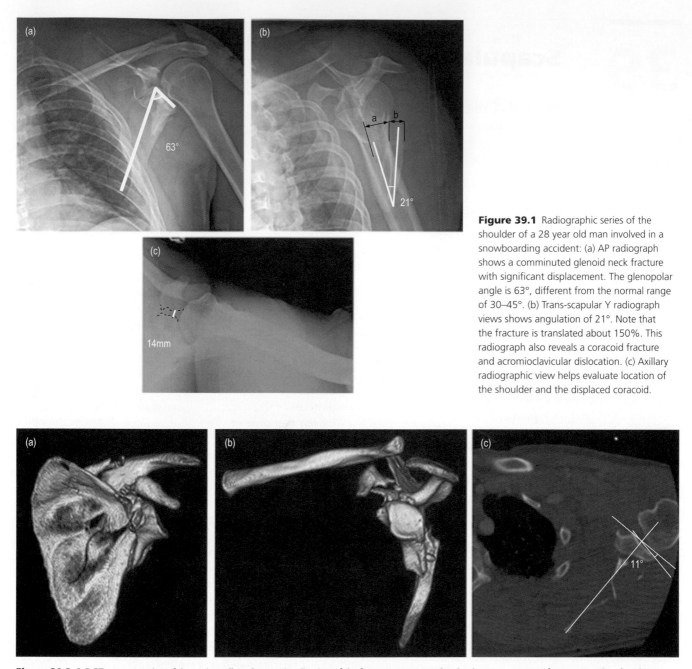

Figure 39.1 Radiographic series of the shoulder of a 28 year old man involved in a snowboarding accident: (a) AP radiograph shows a comminuted glenoid neck fracture with significant displacement. The glenopolar angle is 63°, different from the normal range of 30–45°. (b) Trans-scapular Y radiograph views shows angulation of 21°. Note that the fracture is translated about 150%. This radiograph also reveals a coracoid fracture and acromioclavicular dislocation. (c) Axillary radiographic view helps evaluate location of the shoulder and the displaced coracoid.

Figure 39.2 3-DCT reconstruction of the patient allows better visualization of the fracture pattern and assists in measurements for preoperative planning: (a) The AP radiographic view shows a comminuted glenoid neck fracture with an associated displaced coracoid. (b) Scapula Y reveals dislocation of the acromioclavicular joint. This patient has a triple disruption of the superior shoulder suspensory complex. (c) The 2-D CT demonstrates glenoid retroversion of 11°.

Eighteen muscles insert on, originate from, or traverse the scapula. This bone provides interplay between the clavicle, humerus, and thoracic cage, as well as providing the conduit for the suprascapular nerve and protection of the brachial plexus. A displaced scapula fracture therefore has a number of clinical implications.

Displacement of the glenoid relative to the lateral border, anteversion of the glenohumeral joint with the proximal scapular fragment, and the tendency for gravity to rotate the glenoid caudad, all manifest in displacements that adversely affect shoulder biomechanics.[4] If the scapula heals in the typical malunited position, multiple muscles are shortened, the rotator cuff and deltoid yield a shearing rather than compressive force on the glenohumeral joint, and the arc of motion of the glenohumeral joint is shifted, compromising forward elevation, abduction, and external rotation.

Concomitant injuries to the shoulder girdle also need to be taken into consideration during treatment, particularly in the context of the superior shoulder suspensory complex (SSSC) described by Goss (level V).[5] Massive thoracic injury

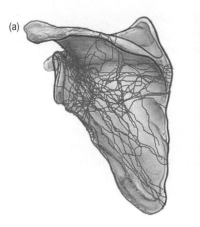

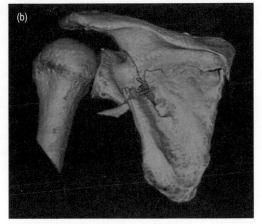

Figure 39.3 (a) A study of 90 3-D CT scans of surgically treated scapula fractures demonstrated that 20 (22%) involved the spinoglenoid notch. (b) 3-D CT scan showing a typical fracture pattern involving the spinoglenoid notch.

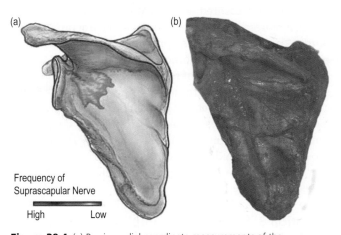

Frequency of
Suprascapular Nerve

High   Low

Figure 39.4 (a) Precise radial coordinate measurements of the suprascapular nerve were made on 24 cadaveric scapulae to create a frequency distribution of the suprascapular nerve. (b) Posterior view of a cadaveric scapula after removal of infraspinatus showing the suprascapular nerve at the base of the acromion before it branches to innervate infraspinatus and teres minor muscles.

from the force vector hitting the superior or lateral shoulder may also result in many consecutive segmental rib fractures. Ultimately, treatment decisions will be influenced by these factors as well as patient functional demands, age, activity level, handedness, and occupation. Not unlike other fractures, the well-stabilized shoulder girdle will yield more immediate patient comfort and effective rehabilitation.

Top seven questions

Diagnosis

1. What should the appropriate preoperative workup include?
2. What displacements are important to measure in deciding which cases should be considered for surgery?

Therapy

3. What are the implications for treating patients nonoperatively?
4. What are the indications for open reduction and internal fixation (ORIF)?
5. What approach should be utilized for ORIF?
6. How should an operative or nonoperative patient be rehabilitated?

Prognosis and harm

7. What is known about outcomes and complications of ORIF?

Finding the evidence

Study identification followed the following steps (April 2010 search date):
- Cochrane Database, with search term "scapula OR glenoid AND fracture" in Title, Abstract or Keywords in Cochrane Database of Systematic Reviews
  - 1 hit, not relevant
- PubMed (www.ncbi.nlm.nih.gov/PubMed/) clinical queries search/ systematic reviews: ((scapula* [ti] OR glenoid* [ti] AND fracture* [ti] NOT rim* [ti])) AND systematic[sb]
  - 2 hits, both relevant
- PubMed-MEDLINE (www.ncbi.nlm.nih.gov/PubMed/) -sensitivity search using keywords "scapula* [ti] OR glenoid* [ti] AND fracture* [ti]"
  - 295 hits

Question 1: What should the appropriate preoperative workup include?

Case clarification

Our patient had injuries which required prioritization over the scapula (massive facial lacerations, a painful neck, and a pneumothorax). The obvious recognition of a scapula fracture on the chest radiograph led to shoulder films, and then, on the basis of the displacement, to a dedicated CT scan.

The scapula fracture was complex and displaced at the spinoglenoid notch, a pattern which is associated with suprascapular nerve lesions. The pattern of displacement was atypical because the glenoid was actually tilted superior (glenopolar angle (GPA) 63°) and it was retroverted (11°) rather than anteverted. Postoperative electromyography (EMG) and nerve conduction study revealed that he had a complete lesion of the suprascapular nerve, also witnessed at the time of surgery.

Relevance and current opinion

A history should include the patient's job description and recreational activities. The shoulder can compensate adequately in lower-functioning individuals; therefore, not every displaced scapula fracture requires surgery. A physical examination should include whether or not abrasions exist over the shoulder, palpation of the acromioclavicular and sternoclavicular joints, and a neurovascular examination of the extremity. When the patient can be upright, they must be examined disrobed to appreciate shoulder drooping, which is bothersome in severe cases.

Shoulder radiographs yield the detail necessary to determine whether or not there is displacement of a fracture. If on the radiographs, there is displacement of a fracture greater than 1 cm, a 3-D CT should be obtained to specifically measure displacement and angulation. In nondisplaced fractures in which nonoperative treatment has been selected, weekly follow-up films over 2 weeks should be obtained due to the risk of displacement (level IV).[6]

Often, scapula fractures are delayed in referral or workup, either because of missed injury, or treatment of other bodily injuries, or the time it takes to refer to an appropriate medical center (level IV).[7] In cases when such delay is greater than 2 weeks, an EMG and nerve conduction study should be performed because this injury has a high association with nerve injuries (level V).[8] This information is helpful for preoperative planning and prognostication. A 2-D CT scan is useful when there is intra-articular involvement to determine step, gap, and number of fragments.

Recommendations

• If radiographs show displacement of a fracture greater than 1 cm, a 3-D CT should be obtained to specifically measure displacement and angulation
• In nondisplaced fractures in which nonoperative treatment has been selected, weekly follow-up films over 2 weeks should be obtained due to the risk of displacement
• When referral is delayed longer than 2 weeks, an EMG and nerve conduction study should be performed because scapula fracture has a high association with nerve injuries

Question 2: What displacements are important to measure in deciding which cases should be considered for surgery?

Case clarification

Our patient had multiple indications for surgery, as is commonly the case: a displaced "triple lesion", (acromioclavicular joint, coracoid, and neck) and an excessive GPA. The patient also had dramatic translational deformity of the lateral border (150%) indicating a very unstable injury. He was a young manual laborer who would depend on maximum upper extremity function for his livelihood.

Relevance and current opinion

Medialization, angulation, GPA, and intra-articular step-off should be measured. Medialization is often misunderstood: it represents the displacement at the fractured lateral border, or the position of the proximal relative to the distal main fragments. This definition is most relevant because it defines the relationships of muscles acting on or across the scapula and glenohumeral joint. Angulation refers to the angle measured between the lateral borders on the scapula Y view. GPA measures the inferior rotation of the glenoid (on its proximal fragment) relative to the body as measured off an AP image. A 3-D CT scan is vital for accuracy since this modality allows for the perfect rotation of the images to get an accurate "AP and Y view."

Question 3: What are the implications for treating patients nonoperatively?

Case clarification

With this constellation of fractures and displacement, our patient would have fared very poorly, particularly in the first months after injury. With a floating shoulder and all the displacement and rib fractures, he would have required immobilization for at least 3 weeks, coming out very stiff and requiring months of therapy just to get to a plateau in function. He would have lost the internal rotation that his retroverted neck would have measured and the extension that his GPA side-to-side difference was, and he would have been weakened as a result of changing the Blick's curve of all the shoulder muscles. He would have had a high risk for a painful coracoid nonunion, and impingement from an acromion which was tilted into the subacromial space from downward rotation.

Relevance and current opinion

Though nonoperative treatment of double lesions of the SSSC have been shown to result in good or excellent outcomes, it is likely that such series reflected minimally displaced injuries since almost no malunions were reported (all level IV; Table 39.1).[9–12] Nonoperative series to date have not stratified data based on measured displacement, and rigorous outcome assessment of strength, motion, and function are lacking in

Table 39.1 Current evidence in floating shoulder fractures

Author	Level of evidence No. of patients No. followed/total (% follow-up)	Summary
Therapy		
Herscovici et al. (1992)	IV 2 Nonop/7 Op/2 LTF 9/11 (82%)	The authors reviewed 9 patients having double lesion injuries and recommended the use of anteroposterior radiographs of the clavicle and scapula, and trans-scapular Y views. Internal fixation of the clavicle should be performed as soon as possible to prevent malunion of the scapular neck fracture
Leung and Lam (1993)	IV 15 Operative 15/15 (100%)	The authors found that operative treatment for ipsilateral fractures of the scapular neck and the clavicle is safe and that functional recovery is predictably good with most patients regaining normal function of the shoulder soon after injury. With fixation of both fractures, postoperative rehabilitation is greatly facilitated
Rikli et al. (1995)	IV 12 Operative 12/12 (100%)	The authors found that in an unstable shoulder girdle, the therapeutic goal can be reached with ORIF of the clavicle alone. The fracture of the scapular neck is usually reduced indirectly and sufficiently stable for functional after treatment. ORIF of the scapula is therefore, only necessary in displaced intra-articular fractures
Oh et al. (2002)	IV 3 Nonop/10 Op 13/13 (100%)	The authors found that surgical treatment for double disruption of the SSSC is a good option, allowing for early rehabilitation and giving good functional results
Prognosis		
Ramos et al. (1997)	IV 16 Nonoperative 13/16 (81%)	The authors found that after a mean follow-up of 7.5 years, the functional results were good or excellent in 92% of the cases and propose that successful nonoperative treatment was due to intense physical therapy, and to the fact that most clavicular and scapular fractures do not require formal reduction for healing, and even vicious callus is well tolerated by most patients
Edwards et al. (2000)	IV 36 Nonoperative 20/36 (56%)	The authors concluded that many floating shoulder injuries are not as unstable as was previously thought and do not require operative fixation. None of the functional assessments utilized identified poor outcomes and thus, it is difficult to identify factors that might predict which fractures will do well with non operative treatment and which will have a better result with surgery
Egol et al. (2001)	IV 12 Nonop/7 Op/4 LTF 19/23 (83%)	The authors concluded that good results may be seen both with and without operative treatment, and therefore do not universally recommend operative treatment for double disruption of the superior shoulder suspensory complex. Treatment must be individualized for each patient
Van Noort et al. (2001)	IV 31 Nonop/4 Op/11 LTF 35/46 (76%)	The authors conclude that ipsilateral fractures of the neck of the scapula and of the clavicle is not inherently unstable and, in the absence of caudal dislocation of the glenoid, conservative treatment gives a good functional outcome
Hashiguchi and Ito (2003)	IV 5 Operative 5/5 (100%)	The authors conclude that for a patient with a floating shoulder, it is important to determine the severity of fracture displacement accurately and the presence or absence of coracoclavicular ligament rupture radiographically. On the basis of those factors, an appropriate treatment for both fractures that may lead to a satisfactory clinical outcome can be determined
Labler et al. (2004)	IV 8 Nonop/9 Op 17/17 (100%)	The authors concluded that nondisplaced or less displaced floating shoulders are expected to give good results after nonoperative treatment and recommend operative treatment in cases of displacement of scapular neck fracture of more than 25 mm and/or reduction of the glenopolar angle less than 30° as an indirect sign for ruptured associated ligaments

those series (all level IV; Table 39.1).[9–13] Furthermore, other authors have reported patients with malunion which eventuated in poor outcomes, indicating that not all malunions are benign (all level IV).[14–16] One study demonstrated increased pain and dysfunction and/or decreased motion in almost half of patients who were malunited.[12]

Question 4: What are the indications for ORIF?

Case clarification
By almost anyone's criteria, our patient warranted surgical intervention on the basis of a highly displaced double (triple) lesion, a displaced coracoid and acromion, and an angulated glenoid neck.

Relevance and current opinion
There are multiple opinions on the degree of displacement or angular deformity which warrant ORIF. These have included articular injuries displaced by 4–10 mm (all level IV),[7,17–19] fractures with lateral border displacement ("medialization") of 10–20 mm (all level IV),[7,16,17,20] angular deformity of 25–45°,[7,16,17,20] and a GPA of less than 20° (all level IV).[14,15] Some authors feel that excessive translation and version of the proximal relative to the distal fragment should be considered a relative indication for surgery (level IV, V respectively).[6,21] Though there is no "high-level" evidence to date, deductive reasoning would lead us to believe that some degree of displacement and angular deformity will yield an adverse clinical result. If the clinician believes that function and form are interdependent, then malunion results in compensation, and by definition, compensation costs something. Experts differ as to what amount and type of displacement warrants intervention, but there is growing consensus, given the positive surgical results on record, that operative correction of displaced scapula fractures is beneficial for a subset of patients.

Recommendation
• There is growing consensus that operative correction of displaced scapula fractures is beneficial for a subset of patients

Question 5: What approach should be utilized for ORIF?

Case clarification
Our patient had a staged posterior and anterior approach to his shoulder. The surgeon began with the posterior approach to reduce and fix the neck and body of the scapula. During this approach, the suprascapular nerve was found trapped in the fracture and partially lacerated. Decompression from the callus was required, with reattachment of a torn branch. The patient was in a lateral slightly forward position for this part of the procedure. Now there was a stable base on to which the coracoid could be fixed from anterior.

An anterior approach from a beach chair position was used to address both the coracoid and the acromioclavicular (AC) dislocation. A single incision was drafted from medial to lateral along the distal clavicle to within a centimeter of the AC joint, and then caudad over the coracoid down along the superior limb of the deltopectoral approach. The AC joint relocation and fixation was necessary to effect the reduction of the coracoid, since the coracoid was attached to the displaced clavicle via the coracoclavicular ligaments.

Relevance and current opinion
Fractures of the scapula neck and body should be addressed through a posterior approach. There have been a number of modifications to the posterior Judet approach,[22] which are variations on the theme of more or less invasiveness (level IV and V).[17,23,24] Either the entire rotator cuff (and deltoid) can be mobilized from the vertebral border to the lateral border on the neurovascular pedicle, or muscular intervals between the infraspinatus and teres minor can be utilized to spare the muscles of detachment from their origins. Such an interval allows good access to the articular surface (level IV).[24] A straight posterior approach to the glenoid neck can be used for fractures isolated to the posterior glenoid or those lateral to the acromial base. The only glenoid fractures associated with the scapula body which should be addressed from anterior rather than posterior are those involving the superior coronal half extending into the superior fossa, usually inferior to the coracoid. Sometimes the coracoid itself is detached at the base in these variants.

Most articular fractures, however, are best accessed through a deltopectoral approach, as the version of the glenoid allows for better visualization from anterior, either through an arthrotomy or through a fracture interval. A transaxillary approach has also been described for inferior glenoid fractures in the frontal plane (level V).[25]

Recommendation
• Fractures of the scapula neck and body should be addressed through a posterior approach. Most articular fractures, however, are best accessed through a deltopectoral approach, and a transaxillary approach has also been described for inferior glenoid fractures in the frontal plane

Question 6: How should an operative or nonoperative patient be rehabilitated?

Case clarification
Our patient began full passive range of motion as his symptoms allowed the day after surgery. He was taught how to use pulleys, the help of his spouse, and the use of his opposite hand, pushing himself to discomfort. The second month consisted of full active range of motion. The third month consisted of a strength program beginning with 3–5 lb (1.5–2.5 kg) weights and working up to no

restrictions after 3 months. In the fourth month, endurance activities were promoted, swimming when possible, with an attempt to return to normality.

Relevance and current opinion

One of the goals of surgery is to achieve stability, which means that the fixation can withstand physiologic motion. Intraoperatively, the patient should be taken through a range of motion to prove such stability has been accomplished. Often, the patient is well ahead of the schedule detailed for our patient, as the resolution of pain after ORIF is rather rapid. To our knowledge, different rehabilitation regimens have not been studied or compared after scapula fractures.

The only caveat for physical therapy and rehabilitation in nonoperated scapula fractures is that the patient requires a period of immobilization due to the instability of the fragments. Not only are they too painful for a few weeks to begin motion, but there is a risk of further displacement if motion ensues too early.[6] This period of immobilization is not benign, as extrinsic adhesions establish, and must be overcome.

Question 7: What is known about outcomes and complications of ORIF?

Case clarification

At seven months after surgery, the patient's Disability of Arm Shoulder and Hand Index (DASH score) was 4.2, indicating a good outcome, based on normative data from uninjured populations.[26] The patient's active forward flexion was 135° and external rotation with the arm at his side was 18° (normal side 145°, 55° respectively). His strength measured with a handheld dynamometer, was 9 lb (4 kg) of force relative to the opposite side of 35 lb (16 kg) for forward flexion, and 13 lb (6 kg) of force relative to the opposite side of 36 lb (16 kg) for external rotation. The patient claimed to have no pain, and was eager to get back on his snowboard for the upcoming season. These results, though not perfect, represent a significant improvement over his 3 months measures, which still reflected the incomplete but significant injury to the suprascapular and axillary nerve.

Relevance and current opinion

The literature is replete with many retrospective series of operative intra-articular (Table 39.2) and extra-articular

Table 39.2 Current evidence in exclusive articular glenoid fractures

Author	Level of evidence No. of patients No. followed/total (% follow-up)	Summary
Therapy		
Kavanagh et al. (1993)	IV 10 Operative 9/10 (90%)	The authors concluded the posterior operative approach described allowed excellent visualization of both intra-articular and extra-articular components of the fractures and that open reduction and internal fixation should be seriously considered for patients who have this type of injury and wish to remain active
Leung et al. (1993)	IV 14 Operative 14/14 (100%)	The authors concluded that operative treatment is indicated in displaced intra-articular fractures of the glenoid. This report shows that the operation is safe and the result is good. Special attention must be paid to prevent and treat the complications resulting from the common association of chest injuries in these patients
Mayo et al. (1998)	IV 31 Operative 27/31 (87%)	The authors reported that this series documents the assertion that these difficult and unusual injuries can be successfully treated surgically in most cases. Perfect joint reduction is the goal and can be achieved in a high percentage of cases. Complications are uncommon and the poor outcomes usually are not related to glenohumeral arthritis. Rather, they are most often the result of associated injuries or poor rehabilitative effort
Adam (2002)	IV 10 Operative 10/10 (100%)	The authors found that displaced intra-articular fractures are managed better by operative than by nonoperative treatment. Functional end result and avoidance of post traumatic instability or degenerative joint changes after surgery for these markedly displaced intra-articular fractures demand experience and a thorough knowledge of anatomical approaches, and a strict postoperative rehabilitation program
Schandelmaier et al. (2002)	IV 22 Operative 22/22 (100%)	The authors conclude that open reduction and fixation can give good results for patients with displacement of the glenoid fossa.. Additional factors such as polytrauma, brachial plexus injury, and the general condition of the patient should be taken into consideration. The Ideberg classification is useful when planning surgical approach
Nork et al. (2008)	IV 17 Operative 17/17 (100%)	The authors conclude that in the surgical treatment of displaced type IV, V, and VI intra-articular fractures of the glenoid, the ease and accuracy of anatomic articular reduction is improved by initially addressing the medial fracture displacement. Use of the modified surgical approach allows for medial fracture reduction, reconstitution of the overall scapular morphology, and subsequent articular reduction using the infraspinatus-teres minor interval

(Table 39.3) fractures, demonstrating good and excellent outcomes with very low complication rates, including almost no reports of a nonunion, and less than 2% infection rate in over 300 operated patients in the literature (level IV).[27,28] Several authors note that the rare poor results were associated with brachial plexus or neurological lesions,[19] much like the patient described in this chapter.

Recommendation

• A 2-D CT scan is useful when there is intra-articular involvement to determine step, gap, and number of fragments

Summary of recommendations

• If radiographs show displacement of a fracture greater than 1 cm, a 3-D CT should be obtained to specifically measure displacement and angulation

• In nondisplaced fractures in which nonoperative treatment has been selected, weekly follow-up films over 2 weeks should be obtained due to the risk of displacement

• When referral is delayed longer than 2 weeks, an EMG and nerve conduction study should be performed because scapula fracture has a high association with nerve injuries

• A 2-D CT scan is useful when there is intra-articular involvement to determine step, gap, and number of fragments

• There is growing consensus that operative correction of displaced scapula fractures is beneficial for patients having displaced articular injuries, fractures with substantial lateral border displacement, angular deformity or a GPA of less than 20°

• Fractures of the scapula neck and body should be addressed through a posterior approach. Most articular fractures, however, are best accessed through a deltopectoral approach, and a transaxillary approach has also been described for inferior glenoid fractures in the frontal plane

Table 39.3 Current evidence in scapular neck and body fractures (± articular involvement)

Author	Level of evidence No. of patients No. followed/total (% follow-up)	Summary
Therapy		
Wilber and Evans (1977)	IV 38 Nonop/2 Op 6/40 (15%)	The authors concluded that fractures of the scapular body, neck or spine can be treated conservatively and good clinical results can be anticipated. Fractures involving the acromion, glenoid, or coracoid processes should be treated by immobilization in abduction for 6 weeks, with early active abduction exercises to prevent the contractures that commonly result after these fractures. Open reduction is rarely necessary
Armstrong and Van der Spuy (1984)	IV 62 Nonoperative 52/62 (84%)	The authors concluded that the combination of a fracture of the scapula and the underlying 1st rib appear to be a particularly severe injury. Good results can be obtained with conservative therapy in fractures of the body, spine, coracoid and acromion. Less favorable results follow fractures of the neck and glenoid. In young and fit patients open reduction may be indicated in fractures of the neck and glenoid
Bauer et al. (1995)	IV 25 Operative 20/25 (80%)	Depending on age, activity, and general condition of the patient, ORIF is recommended in: grossly displaced fractures of the acromion and coracoid process; displaced fractures of the anatomical neck; unstable fractures of the surgical neck; displaced fractures of the glenoid fossa. The authors recommend early operative treatment for these types of fractures in order to achieve good results
Khallaf et al. (2006)	IV 5 Nonop/14 Op	The authors found that ORIF of grossly displaced scapular neck fractures can restore the normal biomechanics of both glenohumeral and scapulothoracic joints and allow favorable clinical outcome
Herrera et al. (2009)	IV 22 Operative 16/22 (73%)	The purpose of this retrospective study was to examine the safety and efficacy of delayed operative management of displaced fractures of the scapula and to describe early functional outcomes. The authors found that their results suggest that safe surgery can be accomplished and good outcomes achieved even with late presentation and surgery
Jones et al. (2009)	IV 37 Operative 37/37 (100%)	The authors found that the modified Judet approach allows for excellent scapular and glenoid fracture visualization and reduction while preserving rotator cuff function. Minifragment fixation along the lateral scapular border provides excellent plate position and fracture stability

Table 39.3 (*Continued*)

Author	Level of evidence No. of patients No. followed/total (% follow-up)	Summary
Prognosis		
Hardegger et al. (1984)	IV 37 Operative 33/37 (89%)	Two groups of scapular fractures can be distinguished: those which will probably heal without long-term complications, and those liable to cause significant disability. The first group inlcudes most fractures of the scapular body, and also those fractures of the scapular neck and apophyses (coracoid, acromion, scapular spine) which have minimal displacement. The second group is composed of glenoid fracture-dislocations, unstable fractures of the scapular neck and significantly displaced apophyseal fractures
Ada and Miller (1991)	IV 113 Nonop/8 Op 32/121** (26%)	There is a high incidence of significant associated injuries with scapular fractures. Displaced scapular neck and comminuted spine fractures present major long-term and immediate problems, such as dysfunction of the rotator cuff and pain. The majority can be treated non operatively, but indications for surgical management should be extended to include some types of displaced scapular neck and spine fractures, as well as intra-articular injuries
Nordqvist and Petersson (1992)	IV 129 Nonoperative 84/129 (65%)	The authors' results indicate that patients with persisting shoulder deformity and persisting symptoms often sustained a more serious trauma. The treatment of concomitant injuries was sometimes given a higher priority. In some cases with displaced fractures of the scapula, initial open surgical procedures could perhaps have improved the long-term result
Romero et al. (2001)	IV 16 Nonop/ 3 Op	Pain, reduced activities of daily living, and abduction weakness at follow-up were significantly more common among patients with severe rotational malalignment of the glenoid neck (GPA < 20°) than among patients with no or mild glenoid malunion. The simple measurement of GPA may yield useful prognostic information
Bozkurt et al. (2005)	IV 18 Nonoperative	The authors report that in the determination of the degree of dysfunction, decreased GPA has proven more reliable evidence than the fracture type. Patient age and associated injuries were also found as effective determinants of the functional outcome
Pace et al. (2005)	IV 12 Nonoperative 9/12 (75%)	The authors found that the majority of glenoid neck fractures treated nonoperatively have some activity-related pain, which in turn seems to be associated with glenoid neck malunion
van Noort and van Kampen (2005)	IV 23 Nonop/1 Op 13/24 (54%)	The authors found that nonoperative treatment of a surgical neck fracture of the scapula in the absence of an ipsilateral shoulder injury and associated permanent neurological impairment leads to a good to excellent functional outcome, with or without significant translational displacement
Schofer et al. (2009)	IV 137 Nonop/7 Op 50/137 pts (37%)	The purpose of this study was to determine the long-term prognoses for nonoperatively treated fractures of the scapula. The authors found that after conservative treatment, scapular fractures heal with a good functional result despite measureable restrictions
Diagnosis		
McGinnis and Denton (1989)	IV 39 Nonoperative	Patients with a fractured scapula should be thoroughly examined for associated injuries. The scapula fracture should not be neglected due to the associated injuries. Even if the scapula fracture is an isolated injury, the patient should be admitted to a hospital with a follow-up chest radiograph to rule out the late development of pneumothorax, hemothorax, or pulmonary contusion. 73% of the patients in this series had excellent or good results
McAdams et al. (2002)	IV 20	The authors found that scapular neck fracture displacement, angulation, and anatomic classification showed moderate interobserver reliability by plain films but were not enhanced by 2-D CT. 2-D CT may be useful in selected cases in which intra-articular extension is noted on plain films

Acknowledgments

The authors would like to acknowledge Dr. Erich Gauger for his support in preparing this manuscript. In addition, we wish to thank Synthes, Inc. for the research grant funding which supports the research of the Scapula Institute at the University of Minnesota Regions Hospital.

References

1. Anavian J, Wijdicks CA, Schroder LK, Vang S, Cole PA. Surgery for scapula process fractures. Acta Orthop 2009;80(3):344–50.
2. Armitage BM, Wijdicks CA, Tarkin IS, Schroder LK, Marek DJ, Zlowodzki M, et al. Mapping of scapular fractures with three-dimensional computed tomography. J Bone Joint Surg Am 2009; 91(9):2222–8.
3. Wijdicks CA, Armitage BM, Anavian J, Schroder LK, Cole PA. Vulnerable neurovasculature with a posterior approach to the scapula. Clin Orthop Relat Res 2009;467(8):2011–17.
4. Chadwick EK, van Noort A, van der Helm FC. Biomechanical analysis of scapular neck malunion–a simulation study. Clin Biomech (Bristol, Avon) 2004;19(9):906–12.
5. Goss TP. Double disruptions of the superior shoulder suspensory complex. J Orthop Trauma 1993;7(2):99–106.
6. Anavian J, Khanna G, Plocher EK, Wijdicks CA, Cole PA. Progressive displacement of scapula fractures. J Trauma 2010; 69(1):156–61.
7. Herrera DA, Anavian J, Tarkin IS, Armitage BA, Schroder LK, Cole PA. Delayed operative management of fractures of the scapula. J Bone Joint Surg Br 2009;91(5):619–26.
8. Robinson LR. Role of neurophysiologic evaluation in diagnosis. J Am Acad Orthop Surg 2000;8(3):190–9.
9. Ramos L, Mencia R, Alonso A, Ferrandez L. Conservative treatment of ipsilateral fractures of the scapula and clavicle. J Trauma 1997;42(2):239–42.
10. Edwards SG, Whittle AP, Wood GW, 2nd. Nonoperative treatment of ipsilateral fractures of the scapula and clavicle. J Bone Joint Surg Am 2000;82(6):774–80.
11. Egol KA, Connor PM, Karunakar MA, Sims SH, Bosse MJ, Kellam JF. The floating shoulder: clinical and functional results. J Bone Joint Surg Am 2001;83(8):1188–94.
12. van Noort A, te Slaa RL, Marti RK, van der Werken C. The floating shoulder. A multicentre study. J Bone Joint Surg Br 2001;83(6): 795–8.
13. Labler L, Platz A, Weishaupt D, Trentz O. Clinical and functional results after floating shoulder injuries. J Trauma 2004;57(3): 595–602.
14. Bozkurt M, Can F, Kirdemir V, Erden Z, Demirkale I, Basbozkurt M. Conservative treatment of scapular neck fracture: the effect of stability and glenopolar angle on clinical outcome. Injury 2005;36(10):1176–81.
15. Pace AM, Stuart R, Brownlow H. Outcome of glenoid neck fractures. J Shoulder Elbow Surg 2005;14(6):585–90.
16. Ada JR, Miller ME. Scapular fractures. Analysis of 113 cases. Clin Orthop Relat Res 1991;269:174–80.
17. Jones CB, Cornelius JP, Sietsema DL, Ringler JR, Endres TJ. Modified Judet approach and minifragment fixation of scapular body and glenoid neck fractures. J Orthop Trauma 2009;23(8): 558–64.
18. Kavanagh BF, Bradway JK, Cofield RH. Open reduction and internal fixation of displaced intra-articular fractures of the glenoid fossa. J Bone Joint Surg Am 1993;75(4):479–84.
19. Mayo KA, Benirschke SK, Mast JW. Displaced fractures of the glenoid fossa. Results of open reduction and internal fixation. Clin Orthop Relat Res 1998;347:122–30.
20. Khallaf F, Mikami A, Al-Akkad M. The use of surgery in displaced scapular neck fractures. Med Princ Pract 2006;15(6): 443–8.
21. Cole PA, Marek DA. Shoulder girdle injuries. In: Stannard JP, Schmidt AH, Kregor PJ, eds, Surgical Treatment of Orthopaedic Trauma, pp. 207–36. Thieme, Boston, 2007.
22. Judet R. Surgical treatment of scapular fractures. Acta Orthop Belg 1964;30:673–8.
23. Obremskey WT, Lyman JR. A modified Judet approach to the scapula. J Orthop Trauma 2004;18(10):696–9.
24. Nork SE, Barei DP, Gardner MJ, Schildhauer TA, Mayo KA, Benirschke SK. Surgical exposure and fixation of displaced type IV, V, and VI glenoid fractures. J Orthop Trauma 2008;22(7):487–93.
25. Wiedemann E. Fractures of the scapula. Unfallchirurg 2004; 107(12):1124–33.
26. Hunsaker FG, Cioffi DA, Amadio PC, Wright JG, Caughlin B. The American Academy of Orthopaedic Surgeons outcomes instruments: normative values from the general population. J Bone Joint Surg Am 2002;84:208–215.
27. Zlowodzki M, Bhandari M, Zelle BA, Kregor PJ, Cole PA. Treatment of scapula fractures: systematic review of 520 fractures in 22 case series. J Orthop Trauma 2006;20(3):230–3.
28. Lantry JM, Roberts CS, Giannoudis PV. Operative treatment of scapular fractures: a systematic review. Injury 2008;39(3):271–83.

40 Post-Traumatic Avascular Necrosis of the Proximal Humerus

Ilia Elkinson and Darren S. Drosdowech

St Joseph's Health Care, London, ON, Canada

Case scenario

A 60 year old woman presented to clinic complaining of activity-related pain and stiffness of the shoulder joint. Two years ago she fell over and sustained a fracture of the proximal humerus. She was treated at a different institution with a locking proximal humeral plate and screw fixation. The metalware was removed 9 months ago. Clinical examination revealed a healed scar from the previous anterior deltopectoral approach to the shoulder. She has 100° of active forward elevation, 60° of scapular abduction, 25° of external rotation, and limited internal rotation to her buttocks.

Relevant anatomy

Gerber et al. performed an anatomical perfusion study of the arterial vascularization of the humeral head.[1] They found that the humeral head was consistently perfused by the anterolateral ascending branch of the anterior circumflex humeral artery, known as the arcuate artery.

In 1993 Brooks performed an experimental cadaver perfusion study looking at the effects of simulated four-part fracture on the vascularity of the proximal humerus.[2] A simulated four-part fracture interrupted the perfusion of the humeral head in all specimens.

Importance of the problem

Codman in 1934 discussed the importance of the soft tissue attachments in fractures of the proximal end of the humerus.[3] Neer in 1963 and Baux in 1969 reported on cases of aseptic osteonecrosis after displaced fractures of the humeral neck.[4,5]

In 1970, Neer introduced the "four-part" classification system of proximal humerus fractures.[6,7] Fracture pattern was linked to prognosis and the development of osteonecrosis of the humeral head.

Reported incidence of avascular necrosis (AVN) following a three-part fracture was found to be between 3% and 21%. Four-part fractures have been associated with much higher rates of AVN, with reported incidence between 21% and 75%. Table 40.1 summarizes reported incidence of AVN following a four-part fracture of the proximal humerus.[7-16]

The most commonly used classification of AVN in the humeral head is that of Cruess, who modified the Ficat and Arlet classification system of AVN in the femoral head.[17-20] There are five stages of AVN, according to radiographic appearance ranging from stage I to stage V. (Figure 40.1)

Top four questions

Diagnosis

1. What is the natural history of post-traumatic AVN in the humeral head, and the relationship between extent of the disease at presentation and prognosis?

Management and prognosis

2. What are the nonarthroplasty treatment options in managing post-traumatic AVN of the humeral head?
3. What are the indications for arthroplasty in post-traumatic AVN, and what type of arthroplasty should we recommend?
4. What are the rates of revision in arthroplasty for post-traumatic AVN?

Evidence-Based Orthopedics, First Edition. Edited by Mohit Bhandari.
© 2012 Blackwell Publishing Ltd. Published 2012 by Blackwell Publishing Ltd.

Question 1: What is the natural history of post-traumatic AVN of the humeral head, and the relationship between extent of the disease at presentation and prognosis?

Case clarification

The patient's plain radiographs revealed a partially collapsed humeral head with no evidence of glenoid involvement. We diagnosed this patient with stage IV AVN of the humeral head.

> Cruess stage IV denotes progression to subchondral humeral head collapse and fragmentation, without glenoid involvement.

Relevance

Knowledge of the natural history will determine the most appropriate type of treatment and will have important implications for outcome and function.

Table 40.1 Incidence of avascular necrosis following four-part fractures

Author (year)	Number	%
Neer (1970)	6/13	46
Lee and Hansen (1981)	4/19	21
Sturzenegger, Fornaro and Jacob (1982)	5/14	36
Leysbon (1984)	6/8	75
Marti, Lim and Jolles (1987)	6/13	46
Jacob et al. (1991)	5/19	26
Schai (1995)	10/13	77
Wijgman et al. (2002)	8/9	88
Gerber, Werner and Vienne (2004)	7/18	39
Solberg et al. (2009)	6/15	40

Current opinion

Post-traumatic AVN is associated with significant patient morbidity.

Finding the evidence

• Cochrane Database, with search term "osteonecrosis humeral head," "avascular necrosis humeral head"
• PubMed: search using keywords: "avascular necrosis humeral head" OR "osteonecrosis humeral head" AND "post-traumatic"

Quality of the evidence

Level IV

• 4 retrospective case series

Findings

There is a small number of retrospective case series on the natural history of post-traumatic AVN. Basamania et al. reported on the long-term outcome of post-traumatic vs. atraumatic AVN in 55 shoulders.[21] They found 41% of patients with atraumatic AVN responded well to nonoperative treatment but 100 % of patients with post-traumatic AVN required surgical intervention.

Bigliani in 1991 reported that AVN in this subgroup of patients invariably leads to a stiff and painful shoulder.[22] Gerber in 1998 reported on the clinical outcomes of post-traumatic AVN of the shoulder in 25 patients with partial or complete head collapse over a 15 year period.[8] The global shoulder function was poor, with a Constant score of 46, which corresponded to a functional shoulder value of 51% of a matched normal control group.

Hattrup and Cofield in 1999 reported their results in a large cohort of 200 shoulders in 151 patients with AVN.[23] The need for arthroplasty was examined in the context of disease extent, staging at presentation and diagnosis. In

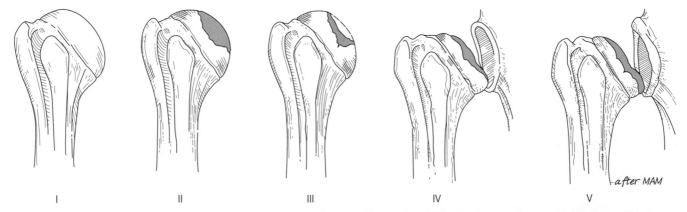

| I | II | III | IV | V |

after MAM

Figure 40.1 Stages of progression from pre-collapse lesion to late stage disease and humeral head collapse in the avascular necrosis of the humeral head: Stage I: No radiographic evidence of osteonecrosis. The humeral head appears normal, with no sclerosis, and sphericity is maintained. Stage II: Signs of mottled sclerosis appear, but the curvature of the humeral head remains intact. Stage III: A crescent sign is indicative of subchondral fracturing; humeral head loses its sphericity. Stage IV: progression to collapse of the subchondral bone. Stage V: there are degenerative changes in the glenoid fossa. (©1997 American Academy of Orthopaedic Surgeons. Reprinted from the Journal of the American Academy of Orthopaedic Surgeons, Volume 5(6), pp. 339–346 with permission.)

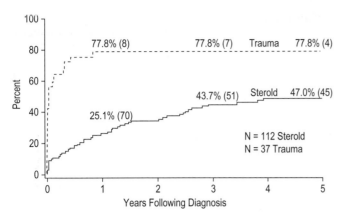

Figure 40.2 Diagnosis of avascular necrosis and shoulder arthroplasty over time. Kaplan–Meier survivorship analysis. Percentage is cumulative incidence of replacement. Number in parenthesis is number of patients remaining at risk at each time point. (Reprinted from Journal of Shoulder and Elbow Surgery, 8,Hattrup SJ, Cofield RH, Osteonecrosis of the humeral head: Relationship of disease stage, extent, and cause to natural history, 559–564, 1999, with permission from Elsevier.)

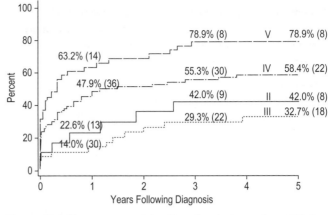

Figure 40.3 Disease stage and shoulder arthroplasty over time. With the Kaplan–Meier survivorship analysis method, need for shoulder arthroplasty is shown for stage of disease at presentation. Percentage is cumulative incidence. Number in parenthesis is number of patients remaining are risk at each time point. (Reprinted from Journal of Shoulder and Elbow Surgery, 8,Hattrup SJ, Cofield RH, Osteonecrosis of the humeral head: Relationship of disease stage, extent, and cause to natural history, 559–564, 1999, with permission from Elsevier.)

this study 112 (56%) had a previous history of corticosteroid use, followed by 37 patients (18.5%) who had post-traumatic AVN. Among the 97 shoulders that had undergone arthroplasty, the average time to surgery was 0.9 years. The range was between 1 day and 11.9 years.

Shoulders in the post-traumatic group did considerably worse. By 3 years after initial diagnosis, 77.8% with post-traumatic AVN required surgery vs. 43.7% with a history of corticosteroid use (p < 0.001) (Figure 40.2).

Extent of involvement and the stage at presentation were directly related to the need for further surgery. With the Kaplan–Meier survivorship analysis at 3 years from diagnosis, the authors reported that 42% of shoulders with stage II disease and 29.3% with stage III disease required surgery. The difference was not statistically significant (p < 0.465). However, 55% with stage IV and 79% with stage V disease had required shoulder arthroplasty within 3 years from presentation (Figure 40.3). The overall difference in the need for arthroplasty was statistically significant (p < 0.001) between stages II vs. III vs. IV vs. V.

Recommendations

- Patients with post-traumatic AVN tend to require surgery more often than patients with atraumatic AVN [overall quality: very low]
- At 3 years after initial diagnosis, up to 78% of patients with post-traumatic AVN need shoulder arthroplasty [overall quality: very low]
- Up to 30% of patients in stage III disease and up to 80% in stage IV disease at presentation required arthroplasty [overall quality: very low]
- Similarly, at 3 years, more patients with greater extent of humeral head involvement required arthroplasty [overall quality: very low]

Question 2: What are the nonarthroplasty treatment options in managing post-traumatic AVN of the humeral head?

Case clarification

This patient has stage IV disease and has painful restriction of shoulder motion. She has difficulty with most activities of daily living. We propose that this patient should be treated with prosthetic replacement. The patient would like to know if there are any other alternatives to prosthetic replacement of the shoulder.

Relevance

The treating surgeon has to be familiar with all treatment modalities, which also include nonarthroplasty options.

Current opinion

Nonarthroplasty treatments can be considered in the management of early stage disease.

Finding evidence

- Cochrane Database, with search terms "osteonecrosis humeral head," "avascular necrosis humeral head"
- PubMed: search using keywords: "avascular necrosis humeral head" OR "osteonecrosis humeral head" AND "post-traumatic" AND "core decompression" AND "bisphosphonates"

Quality of the evidence

Level IV

- 3 case series

Level V

- 2 expert opinions

Table 40.2 Results of core decompression in avascular necrosis

Author (year)	Mean follow-up (months)	No. of shoulders with AVN post trauma	No. of shoulders with atraumatic AVN	Successful outcomes			
				Stage I	Stage II	Stage III	Stage IV
Dines (2007)	7	0	3	—	1 (100%)	—	—
Chapman (2004)	—	0	1	1 (100%)	—	—	—
LaPorte (1998)	120	3	60	15/16 (94%)	15/17 (88%)	16/23 (70%)	1/7(14%)
Mont (1993)	67.2	5	25	6/6 (100%)	8/8 (100%)	7/10 (70%)	1/6 (16%)

Findings

Nonsurgical management of post-traumatic AVN must include range of motion and muscle strengthening exercises to maintain glenohumeral joint function and prevent disuse-related stiffness. These measures are thought to be more successful in the shoulder joint than in the hip.

Bisphosphonates represent the most clinically relevant class of antiresorptive drugs available. There are no published reports on the use of bisphosphonates in post-traumatic AVN of the humeral head.

Arthroscopic debridement as a minimally invasive treatment modality of AVN was first described by Johnson in 1986.[24] Arthroscopy allows direct visualization of the entire humeral head, hence it may aid diagnosis and staging of AVN. Surgical debridement of osteochondral flaps and removal of loose intra-articular bodies has been shown to alleviate mechanical symptoms.[25,26]

Hungerford (1979), followed by Ficat (1985), first reported on the use of core decompression in the shoulder.[27,28] Mont (1993) reported his results in a retrospective review of 20 patients (30 shoulders) at a mean follow-up of 5.6 years (range 2–14 years).[29] Their technique involved using a 6–10-mm trephine to perform an open core decompression. Of the 30 shoulders, 22 (73%) had good or excellent results and did not require shoulder arthroplasty. All 14 patients (100%) with stage I and II disease avoided further surgery and 7 of 10 (70%) with radiographic stage III disease also had good and excellent results. The remaining 6 patients in stage IV disease progressed to require shoulder arthroplasty, although progression was delayed in 4 of those 6 patients by up to 5 years.

LaPorte and Mont (1998) expanded their earlier study to include 63 shoulders in 43 patients with 2–20 year follow-up (mean 10 years).[30] Successful outcome was observed in 15 of 16 (94%) patients with stage I disease and 15 of 17 (88%) with stage II disease. Of the patients in stage III, 16 of 23 (70%) had good and excellent results and only 1 of 7 (14%) patients with stage IV disease did not require arthroplasty.

Harreld et al. reported on the use of the percutaneous small diameter technique with a 3.2 mm Steinmann pin in 15 patients (26 shoulders).[31] At a mean follow-up of 32 months no patient had progressed to shoulder arthroplasty.

A new arthroscopic-assisted technique of core decompression was described by Chapman et al. (2004). A similar technique was also reported by Dines et al. (2007).[32,33] Table 40.2 summarizes current studies on core decompression for AVN.[29,30,32,33]

Recommendations

• Currently there is no data concerning safety or efficacy of bisphosphonates for cases specific to the shoulder [overall quality: very low]
• Core decompression should be considered for stages i, ii and iii [overall quality: very low]

Question 3: What are the indications for arthroplasty in post-traumatic AVN, and what type of arthroplasty should we recommend?

Case clarification

We would recommend prosthetic replacement for this patient. The arthroplasty options include resurfacing arthroplasty, humeral head replacement (hemiarthroplasty), and total shoulder arthroplasty.

Relevance

Arthroplasty in the setting of post-traumatic AVN presents multiple challenges which include dealing with deformity, contracted soft tissues and cuff pathology.

Current opinion

Patients with stage IV disease should be considered for hemiarthroplasty while those with stage V disease will be candidates for a total shoulder arthroplasty.

Finding evidence

• Cochrane Database, with search term "osteonecrosis humeral head," "avascular necrosis humeral head"
• PubMed: sensitivity search using keywords: "avascular necrosis humeral head" OR "osteonecrosis humeral head" AND "post-traumatic," "shoulder arthroplasty," "shoulder resurfacing," "surface replacement arthroplasty"

Quality of the evidence
Level II
- 2 prospective cohort studies

Level IV
- 14 case series

Findings
Hemiarthroplasty and total shoulder arthroplasty data
Arthroplasty was reserved for management of advanced AVN of the humeral head. Indications for arthroplasty included failure of nonoperative treatment, progression of AVN to head collapse with advanced arthritis (Cruess stages IV and V) despite core decompression, or arthroscopy. Neer as early as 1955 reported his results of arthroplasty in 3 patients with AVN.[34]

- Cruess stage IV: humeral head collapse, glenoid not involved
- Cruess stage V: head collapse with glenoid degenerative changes[2]

Information on outcomes of shoulder arthroplasty in post-traumatic AVN was provided in 11 published studies (N = 325). There were 10 retrospective case series and 1 prospective cohort treatment study by Orfaly et al.[35–43] Studies of arthroplasty for atraumatic AVN were not included in this review. Table 40.3 summarizes results of arthroplasty for post-traumatic AVN of the humeral head.

Our review found that there was a high degree of variability in data reporting in the literature. Reported sample sizes tended to vary greatly (N = 3 patients in a study by Dines[43] and N = 137 in the largest retrospective case series

Table 40.3 Published results of arthroplasty for post-traumatic avascular necrosis of the humeral head

Study	No. of shoulders	HHR vs. TSA vs. reverse	Follow-up (mo)	Improved or satisfactory Result (%)	No or slight pain (%)	Normalized Constant score	Mean ASES score	Mean active elevation and external rotation (°)	Complications (%)	Revisions
Feeley 2008[35] Retrospective	17	9/8	58	—	—	—	64	119/39	—	—
Tauber 2007[36] Retrospective	38	31/3/4	96	95	95	57	—	120/39	5%	2
Orfaly 2007[37] Prospective	9	7/2	56	—	83	—	81	114/34	0	0
Boileau 2006[38] Retrospective Mjlti Centre	137	—	42	—	80	62	—	125/32	21 (16%)	15 (11%)
Mansat 2004[39] Retrospective	7	—	47	64	73	69	—	108/29	—	—
Hettrich 2004[40] Retrospective	11	11/0	51	83	—	—	—	—	—	—
Boileau 2001[41] Retrospective	40	—	19	81	80	75	—	133/40	—	0
Hattrup 2000[42] Retrospective	46	—	107	80	77	—	55	107/49	28%	—
Norris 1995[54] Retrospective	9	2/7	24	—	90	—	—	—	—	—
Dines 1993[43] Retrospective	3	—	—	90	70	—	—	110/31	0	0
Tonner 1983[52] Retrospective	8	—	40	89	89	—	—	112/42	—	—

by Boileau[38]). The mean follow-up was 54 months (range 19–107 months).

All reviewed literature demonstrated the ability of arthroplasty to improve shoulder function, pain, and range of motion. Satisfactory or improved results were reported to occur in between 64% of cases (study by Mansat et al.,[39] N = 7 shoulders) and more recently 95% (study by Tauber et al.,[36] N = 38 shoulders).

Between 70% and 95% reported no or slight pain postoperatively. Constant scores and ASES (American Shoulder and Elbow Surgeons score) improved, but four earlier studies did not use these outcome measures in their results.

- Constant score (Constant–Murley Shoulder Outcome Score): This 100 point scoring system consists of four variables: pain, daily activities, motion, and strength. Subjective assessment includes pain (15 points), activities of daily living (20 points); objective assessment includes range of motion (40 points) and strength (25 points). Higher score indicates better-functioning shoulder.[44]
- ASES (American Shoulder and Elbow Surgeons score): A 100 point system based on pain and function. 50 points are assigned based on the pain indicated on a visual analog scale (VAS), and 50 points are given based on the ability to perform 10 activities of daily living.[45]

The longest published follow-up was reported recently by Tauber et al. (mean 96 months, range 60–156 months).[36] Constant scores improved overall form 27 points preoperativley (range 11–59 points) to 57 points at follow-up (range 6–95 points). The overall range of motion improved substantially in all planes. Active forward elevation increased from mean 66° preoperatively (range 10–120°) to mean 120° at follow-up (range, 10–180°), p < 0.01. External rotation improved significantly from 15° preoperativley (range 5–50°) to 39° at follow-up (range 0–80°), p < 0.01.

The only prospective cohort treatment study was by Orfaly et al. (N = 9/21 shoulders with post-traumatic AVN). Significant overall improvement was observed. The mean pain level measured by VAS was 45 points preoperatively to 17 points at follow-up (p < 0.01). Active forward elevation increased from 87° to 114° (statistically not significant, p-value not provided). External rotation improved from a mean of –7° (range –45° to –35°) to a mean of 34° (range –10° to 60°), p < 0.001.

Visual analog scale (VAS): A 100-point score was used for pain and function. A score of 0 indicated no pain, and 100 meant a constant, severe pain. For the functional assessment, a score of 0 indicated comfortable use of shoulder for all activities, and 100 indicated an inability to perform any of the normal tasks.

Functional scores at follow-up improved from a mean score of 57 points to 14 points at follow-up, p < 0.001. When comparing outcomes between the atraumatic and post-traumatic groups, there was no statistically significant difference at follow-up.[37]

Hattrup and Cofield in 2000 retrospectively reviewed a large cohort of 88 arthroplasties which included 42 shoulders with atraumatic AVN and 46 shoulders with post-traumatic AVN.[42] In contrast to the previous report, they found statistically significant difference in ASES scores between the two groups. The mean ASES score was 69 in the atraumatic group, compared to 55 in the post-traumatic group (p < 0.017). Shoulder motion in every direction at follow-up also showed significantly better results in the atraumatic group (p > 0.003).

Resurfacing arthroplasty data Surface replacement was considered when nonarthroplasty treatments failed and there was sufficient bone stock for implant fixation (up to 70% of the head).

The literature on the use of surface replacement for post-traumatic AVN was limited to four reports: one prospective cohort study (N = 6/12 shoulders) and three retrospective series (N = 23).

In 2001, Levy and Copeland reported results from 94 patients with a mean follow-up 81.6 months (range 60–120 months).[46] There were 4 patients with AVN (etiology was not specified). For the AVN group, Constant scores improved from 11 to 74 points, active forward elevation improved from 63° to 133°, and external rotation improved from –3° to 81° (p < 0.001) There was 1 revision to a TSA at 21 months due to an acute fracture.

In 2009, Raiss et al. reported on 17 shoulders with atraumatic (n = 9) and post-traumatic (n = 8) AVN.[47] On average, the necrotic area occupied 18.6% of the humeral head (range 8.9–30.9%). All of the final outcome measures were significantly better in the atraumatic group. The mean final Constant score was 69.8 in the atraumatic group (SD 12.6, range 52–81) vs. 52.4 in the post-traumatic group (SD 18.1, range 27–83), p < 0.05. Significant postoperative differences were also found for shoulder abduction and power (p < 0.05), with higher scores in the atraumatic group.

There were 2 published studies of partial resurfacing for AVN. Scalise et al. (2007) reported short-term multicenter results in 62 patients, which included 8 patients with AVN (etiology was not specified).[48] Uribe et al. (2009) published a prospective cohort treatment study of partial resurfacing in 12 shoulders, including 6 patients with post-traumatic AVN.[49] At an average follow-up of 30 months (range 21–57 months), there was no statistically significant difference between the atraumatic and post-traumatic groups.

Recommendation

• Shoulder hemiarthroplasty is indicated in humeral head collapse in stage IV disease [overall quality: very low]
• Total shoulder arthroplasty is reserved for patients with glenoid involvement as seen in stage V [overall quality: very low]
• There are no long-term evidence for resurfacing arthroplasty for post-traumatic AVN [overall quality: very low]

Question 4: What are the rates of revision in arthroplasty for post-traumatic AVN?

Case clarification

The patient has consented to undergo shoulder hemiarthroplasty. She would like to know more about the possibility of requiring further revision surgery.

Relevance

Revision arthroplasty in the post-traumatic AVN setting poses great challenges. Failure of hemiarthroplasty due to glenoid wear is a major reason for revision to a total arthroplasty.

Current opinion

Outcomes of arthroplasty in the post-traumatic and atraumatic groups are similar.

Finding the evidence

• Cochrane Database, with search terms "osteonecrosis humeral head," "avascular necrosis humeral head"
• PubMed: sensitivity search using the following keywords: "avascular necrosis humeral head" OR "osteonecrosis humeral head" AND "post-traumatic," "shoulder arthroplasty," "shoulder resurfacing," "surface replacement arthroplasty"

Quality of the evidence

Level II
• 2 prospective cohort studies

Level IV
• 14 case series

Findings

As there were a limited number of studies and data reporting was variable, it was difficult to evaluate revision rates for post-traumatic AVN. We found that most studies did not expand on the etiology of their revision cases. The largest retrospective case series was reported by Boileau and colleagues in 2006.[38] Their revision rate for post-traumatic AVN was 11% (15/137). Tauber et al. reported a revision rate of 5% (2/38 shoulders).[36] No hemiarthroplasties had to be revised to a total shoulder replacement.

Most available revision data comes from the studies of atraumatic AVN. Five studies with longer follow-up of up to 12 years showed glenoid involvement as a major reason for conversion of humeral head replacement to a total shoulder arthroplasty.[20,37,42,50,51] Revision rates ranged from 6% in two reports with mean follow-up to 12 years, to 20% in an earlier study of 5 patients by Cruess.

Recommendation

• Current evidence lacks specific information of the rate of revision of arthroplasty in the setting of post-traumatic AVN [overall quality: very low]

Summary of recommendations

• Patients with post-traumatic AVN tend to require surgery more often than patients with atraumatic AVN
• At 3 years after initial diagnosis, up to 78% of patients with post-traumatic AVN need shoulder arthroplasty
• Up to 30% of patients in stage III disease and up to 80% in stage IV disease at presentation required arthroplasty
• Similarly, at 3 years, more patients with greater extent of humeral head involvement required arthroplasty
• Currently there is no data concerning safety or efficacy of bisphosphonates for cases specific to the shoulder
• Core decompression should be considered for stages I, II and III
• Shoulder hemiarthroplasty is indicated in humeral head collapse in stage IV disease
• Total shoulder arthroplasty is reserved for patients with glenoid involvement as seen in stage V
• There is no long-term evidence for resurfacing arthroplasty for post-traumatic AVN
• Current evidence lacks specific information of the rate of revision of arthroplasty in the setting of post-traumatic AVN

Conclusion

Post-traumatic AVN of the humeral head is associated with displaced fractures of the proximal humerus. Three- and four-part fractures have been shown to result in AVN in 21–75% of patients. Studies of the natural history of this disease demonstrated rapid progression to surgical treatment, which included core decompression and arthroplasty. The stage at presentation and extent of the lesion were directly associated with disease progression and need for arthroplasty. Currently there is no evidence on safety and efficacy of bisphosphonate treatment in post-traumatic AVN of the shoulder. Core decompression and arthroscopic debridement may be considered for stages I–III disease.

Hemiarthroplasty should be reserved for stage IV disease and total shoulder replacement for stage V disease. There is no long-term data on the resurfacing arthroplasty for post-traumatic AVN.

References

1. Gerber C, Schneeberger AG, Vinh iS. The arterial vascularization of the humeral head: an anatomical study. J Bone Joint Surg Am 1990;72:1486–94.

2. Brooks CH, Revell WJ, Heatley FW. Vascularity of the humeral head after proximal humeral fractures. J Bone Joint Surg Br 1993;75:132–6.

3. Codman EA. The shoulder, 2nd edn. Thomas Todd, Boston, 1934.

4. Neer, CS II. Prosthetic replacement of the humeral head. Indication hand operative technique. Surg Clin North Am 1963;43:1581–97.

5. Baux, S., Razemon, J. P. Les fractures et fractures-luxations de l'extrémité supérieure de l'humérus. Rev Chirurg Orth 1969;55:388–96.

6. Neer CS II. Displaced proximal humeral fractures: Classification and evaluation. *J Bone Joint Surg* Am 1970;52:1077–89.

7. Neer CS II. Displaced proximal humeral fractures: Treatment of 3-part and 4-part displacement. J Bone Joint Surg Am 1970;52:1090–103.

8. Gerber C, Hersche O, Berberat C. The clinical relevance of post-traumatic avascular necrosis of the humeral head. J Shoulder Elbow Surg 1998;7:586–90.

9. Gerber C, Werner CM, Vienne P. Internal fixation of complex fractures of the proximal humerus. J Bone Joint Surg Br 2004;86:848–55.

10. Lee CK, Hansen HR. Post-traumatic avascular necrosis of the humeral head in displaced proximal humeral fractures. J Trauma 1981;21:788–91.

11. Leysbon RL. Closed treatment of fractures of the proximal humerus. Acta Orthop Scand 1984;55:48–51.

12. Marti R, Lim TE, Jolles CW. On the treatment of comminuted fracture-dislocations of the proximal humerus: internal fixation or prosthetic replacement. In: Kölbel R, Helbig B, Blauth W, eds., Shoulder Replacement, pp. 135–48. Springer-Verlag, Berlin, 1987.

13. Jakob RJ, Miniaci A, Anson PS, et al. Four-part valgus impacted fractures of the proximal humerus. J Bone Joint Surg Br 1991;73:295–8.

14. Wijgman AJ, Roolker W, Patt TW, et al. Open reduction and internal fixation of three and four-part fractures of the proximal part of the humerus. J Bone Joint Surg Am 2002;84:1919–25.

15. Solberg BD, Moon CN, Franco DP, et al. Surgical treatment of 3 and 4-part proximal humeral fractures. J Bone Joint Surg 2009;91:1689–97.

16. Schai P, Imhoff A, Peiss S. Comminuted humeral head fractures: A multicenter analysis. J Shoulder Elbow Surg 1995;4:319–30.

17. Ficat RP. Idiopathic bone necrosis of the femoral head: Early diagnosis and treatment. J Bone Joint Surg 1985;67:3–9.

18. Ficat RP, Arlet TJ. Necrosis of the femoral head. In: Hungerford DS, ed., Ischemia and Necrosis of Bone, pp.171–82. Williams & Wilkins, Baltimore,MD, 1980.

19. Cruess RL. Steroid-induced avascular necrosis of the head of the humerus. J Bone Joint Surg 1976;58:313–17.

20. Cruess RL. Experience with steroid induced avascular necrosis of the shoulder and etiologic considerations regarding osteonecrosis of the hip. Clin Orthop 1978;130:86–93.

21. Basamania CJ, et al. Treatment of post-traumatic vs. atraumatic avascular necrosis of the shoulder. Abstracts from the AAOS 64th Annual Open Meeting, 51. San Francisco, 1997.

22. Bigliani L. In: Rockwood and Green's Fractures in Adults, Vol. 1,3rd edn. JB Lippincott, Philadelphia, 1991.

23. Hattrup SJ, Cofield RH. Osteonecrosis of the humeral head: Relationship of disease stage, extent, and cause to natural history. J Shoulder Elbow Surg 1999; 8:559–564.

24. Johnson LL. Arthroscopic abrasion arthroplasty historical and pathologic perspective. Arthroscopy 1986;2:54–69.

25. Hardy P, Decrette E, Jeanrot C et al. Arthroscopic treatment of bilateral humeral head osteonecrosis. Arthroscopy 2000;16:332–35.

26. Hayes JM. Arthroscopic treatment of steroid-induced osteonecrosis of the humeral head. Arthroscopy 1989;5:218–21.

27. Hungerford DS. Bone marrow pressure, venography, and core decompression in ischemic necrosis of the femoral head. In: The Hip: Proceedings of the Seventh Open Scientific Meeting of the Hip Society, p.1. CV Mosby, St. Louis, 1979.

28. Ficat RP. Idiopathic bone necrosis of the femoral head: Early diagnosis and treatment. J Bone Joint Surg Br 1985;67:3–9.

29. Mont MA, Maar DC, Urquhart MW et al. Avascular necrosis of the humeral head treated by core decompression. J Bone *Joint Surg* 1993;75:785–88.

30. LaPorte DM, Mont MA, Mohan V, et al. Osteonecrosis of the humeral head treated by core decompression. Clin Orthop Relat Res 1988;355:254–60.

31. Harreld KL, Marulanda GA, Ulrich SD, et al. Small-diameter percutaneous decompression for osteonecrosis of the shoulder. Am J Orthop 2009;38:348–54.

32. Dines JS, Strauss EJ, Fealy S, et al. Arthroscopic-assisted core decompression of the humeral head. Arthroscopy 2007;23:103.

33. Chapman C, Mattern C, Levine WN. Arthroscopically assisted core decompression of the proximal humerus for avascular necrosis. Arthroscopy 2004;20:1003–6.

34. Neer CS II. Articular replacement for the humeral head. J Bone Joint Surg Am 1955;37:215–28.

35. Feeley BT, Fealy S, Dines DM et al.. Hemiartroplasty and total shoulder arthroplasty for avascular necrosis of the humeral head. J Shoulder Elbow Surg 2008;17:689–94.

36. Tauber M, Karpik S, Matis N, et al. Shoulder arthroplasty for traumatic avascular necrosis. Clin Orthop 2007;465:208–14.

37. Orfaly RM, Rockwood CA Jr, Esenyel CZ, Wirth MA. Shoulder arthroplasty in cases with avascular necrosis of the humeral head. J Shoulder Elbow Surg 2007;16:S27–32.

38. Boileau P, Chuinard C, Le Huec JC, Walch G, Trojani C. Proximal humerus fracture sequelae: impact of a new radiographic classification on arthroplasty. Clin Orthop Relat Res 2006;442:121–30.

39. Mansat P, Guity MR, Bellumore Y, Mansat M. Shoulder arthroplasty for late sequelae of proximal humeral fractures. J Shoulder Elbow Surg 2004;13:305–12.

40. Hettrich CM, Weldon E III, Boorman RS, et al. Preoperative factors associated with improvements in shoulder function after

humeral hemiarthroplasty. J Bone Joint Surg Am 2004;86: 1446–51.

41. Boileau P, Trojani C, Walch G et al. Shoulder arthroplasty for the treatment of the sequelae of fractures of the proximal humerus. J Shoulder Elbow Surg 2001;10:299–30.

42. Hattrup SJ, Cofield RH. Osteonecrosis of the humeral head: Results of replacement. J Shoulder Elbow Surg 2000;9:177–82.

43. Dines DM, Warren RF, Altchek DW, et al. Posttraumatic changes of the proximal humerus: malunion, nonunion, and osteonecrosis: treatment with modular hemiarthroplasty or total shoulder arthroplasty. J Shoulder Elbow Surg 1993;2:11–21.

44. Constant CR, Murley AH. A clinical method of functional assessment of the shoulder. Clin Orthop Relat Res 1987;214:160–4.

45. Research Committee ASES. A standardised method for the assessment of shoulder function. J Shoulder Elbow Surg 1994; 3:347–52.

46. Levy O, Copeland SA. Cementless surface replacement arthroplasty of the shoulder: 5- to 10-year results with the Copeland mark-2 prosthesis. J Bone Joint Surg Br 2001;83:213–21.

47. Raiss P, Kasten P, Baumann F, et al. Treatment of osteonecrosis of the humeral head with cementless surface replacement arthroplasty. J Bone Joint Surg Am 2009;91:340–49.

48. Scalise JJ, Miniaci A, Iannotti JP. Resurfacing arthroplasty of the humerus: Indications, surgical technique, and clinical results. Tech Shoulder and Elbow Surg 2007; 8:152–60.

49. Uribe JW, Botto-van Bemden A. Partial humeral head resurfacing for osteonecrosis. J Shoulder Elbow Surg 2009;18:711–16.

50. Lau MW, Blinder MA, Williams K, et al. Shoulder arthroplasty in sickle cell patients with humeral head avascular necrosis. J Shoulder Elbow Surg 2007;16:129–34.

51. Smith RG, Sperling JW, Cofield RH, et al. Hattrup SJ, Schleck CD: Shoulder hemiarthroplasty for steroid-associated osteonecrosis. J Shoulder Elbow Surg 2008;17:685–88.

52. Tonner MW, Cofield RH. Prosthetic arthroplasty for fracture ad fracture-dislocations of the proximal humerus. Clin Orthop 1983;179:116–128.

53. Cushner MA, Friedman RJ. Osteonecrosis of the humeral head. J Am Acad Orthop Surg 1997;5(6):339–46.

54. Norris TR, Green A, McGuigan FX. Late prosthetic shoulder arthroplasty for displaced proximal humerus fractures. J Shoulder Elbow Surg 1995;4:271–80.

41 Proximal Humerus Fractures

Job N. Doornberg[1] and David Ring[2]

[1]Orthotrauma Research Center Amsterdam, Academic Medical Center Amsterdam, and St. Lucas Andreas Hospital, Amsterdam, The Netherlands
[2]Harvard Medical School and Massachusetts General Hospital, Boston, MA, USA

Case scenario

A 69 year old woman presents to the emergency department after a slip and fall at home. She is an avid golfer and does not take any medication. On examination, she has pain, swelling, and ecchymosis of her right dominant shoulder and arm and a normal neurovascular examination. Radiographs reveal a fracture of the proximal humerus.

Relevant anatomy

Fractures of the proximal humerus may be (1) avulsion fractures of the tuberosities; (2) stable impacted fractures of the surgical or anatomical neck; (3) displaced fractures; or (4) fractures associated with dislocation of the glenohumeral joint. Neer[1] suggested classification according to four parts as follows: (1) the articular segment or anatomical neck, (2) the greater tuberosity, (3) the lesser tuberosity, and (4) the shaft or surgical neck. To be considered a separate part, a fragment has to be at least 1 cm displaced or 45° angulated.

Importance of the problem

Proximal humeral fractures occur largely in older men and women in a 30:70 ratio,[2] usually after a simple fall.[3] Proximal humerus fractures are among the most common fractures associated with osteoporosis, accounting for 18% of osteoporotic fractures in postmenopausal women and 43% of osteoporotic fractures in patients older than 75 years.[4] Most fractures of the proximal humerus are minimally displaced, stable, and associated with limited functional impairment after nonoperative treatment.[3,5] Displaced fractures that heal with malunion or are treated with arthroplasty can be associated with severe shoulder impairment.[6]

Top five questions

Diagnosis

1. Is there a role for CT scan in the classification and management of fractures of the proximal humerus?

Therapy

2. When should patients with minimally displaced fractures of the proximal humerus start exercises to regain motion?
3. What are the indications for operative vs. nonoperative treatment of displaced proximal humerus fractures?
4. When treated operatively, what is the best treatment for displaced three- and four-part fractures and fracture-dislocations of the proximal humerus: arthroplasty or open reduction and internal fixation (ORIF)?

Prognosis

5. Which factors predict outcome after a proximal humeral fracture in an elderly patient?

Question 1: Is there a role for CT scan in the classification and management of fractures of the proximal humerus?

Case clarification

The patient's radiographs are reviewed at a morning fracture conference. The surgeons present at the conference

Evidence-Based Orthopedics, First Edition. Edited by Mohit Bhandari.
© 2012 Blackwell Publishing Ltd. Published 2012 by Blackwell Publishing Ltd.

disagree whether the amount of displacement merits consideration of operative treatment. They also debate whether CT will help guide management and lead to an improved outcome.

Relevance

Surgeons and patients hope that more detailed imaging will help improve management and outcome.

Current opinion

Surgeons debate whether CT helps to characterize complex fractures or facilitates preoperative planning.

Finding the evidence

- PubMed (www.ncbi.nlm.nih.gov/pubmed/): sensitivity search using keywords "proximal humerus fracture" AND "imaging"
- Bibliography of eligible articles
- It is recommended to include only the most recent studies in decision-making, as CT imaging protocols have become significantly more advanced over the last few years.

Quality of the evidence

Level II
- 2 diagnostic test accuracy/observer reliability studies with methodological limitations[7,8]

Findings

Conventional radiographs vs. 2-D and 3-D CT imaging One prospective diagnostic study[7] (44 consecutive cases, all fracture types included, 3 independent observers) with methodological limitations (no gold standard, no power calculation) showed a significantly better assessment (p < 0.05) of relevant structures (tuberosities, the glenoid and humeral head) using a four-grade scoring system (1, excellent; 2, good; 3, fair; 4, inadequate) based on CT diagnostics than conventional radiographs (AP view, scapular Y views and axillary views) independently of fracture severity (i.e. two-, three-, or four-part fractures) (level II).

An intra- and interobserver study[8] using kappa statistics (40 consecutive patients, 4 independent observers) with methodological limitations (no gold standard, no power calculation, retrospective design) showed a significantly (p < 0.001) improved interobserver reliability from 'moderate' for radiographs ($\kappa = 0.42$) and 2-D CT ($\kappa = 0.56$), to 'good' for the Neer classification system ($\kappa = 0.76$). Intraobserver reliability improved (p < 0.001) from 'moderate' for conventional radiographs ($\kappa = 0.48$) and 2-D CT ($\kappa = 0.63$), to 'excellent' for the Neer classification ($\kappa = 0.84$) (level II).

Recommendations

- CT imaging improves the reliability of classification of proximal humerus fractures [overall quality: moderate]

- 3-D CT improves the reliability of classification over 2-D CT [overall quality: low]
- It is not known whether more reliable classification leads to more accurate classification or improved outcomes

Question 2: When should patients with minimally displaced fractures of the proximal humerus start exercises to regain motion?

Case clarification

The fracture is stable with limited displacement and the patient and surgeon elect nonoperative treatment. The patients wants to know she should begin exercises to regain motion.

Relevance

Immediate initiation of exercises might result in better final shoulder motion and function but could also interfere with healing.

Current opinion

There is debate between early (within 1 week) or late (3 weeks or more, once healing is established) initiation of exercises after a proximal humerus fracture.

Finding the evidence

- Cochrane Database, with search term "humerus fracture".
- PubMed (www.ncbi.nlm.nih.gov/pubmed/) clinical queries search/systematic reviews: "humerus fracture"
- PubMed (www.ncbi.nlm.nih.gov/pubmed/): sensitivity search using keywords "proximal humeral fracture," as well as "proximal humerus fracture" AND "treatment"
- Bibliography of eligible articles

Quality of the evidence

Level I
- 1 multicenter randomized controlled trial (RCT)[9]

Level II
- 2 systematic reviews/meta-analyses (of level II RCTs)[10,11]
- 4 randomized trials with methodological limitations[12–15]

Findings

Shoulder function (Constant score) Two prospective RCTs[12,13] (160 patients) with methodological limitations (possible bias; allocation concealment unclear, some blinding outcome assessors, blinding patients impossible, inclusion/exclusion criteria not (clearly) defined) showed that early mobilization within one week resulted in significantly better Constant shoulder scores at 12 weeks[12] for impacted (stable) proximal humeral fractures (weighted mean difference 9.9, 95% CI 2.1–17.7, p < 0.05) and 16 weeks[13] for non- and minimally displaced two-part fractures (mean difference 16.0, 95% CI 7.1–24.9, p < 0.001). There were no significant differences 6 months[12] (mean difference 6.1, 95%

CI −0.2–12.4, p = 0.06) and 1 year[13] (mean difference 7.0, 95% CI −3.4–17.4, p = 0.19) after fracture (level II).

General health status (Short Form-36) One prospective RCT[13] (86 patients) showed that early mobilization within 1 week for patients with non- and minimally displaced proximal humerus fractures resulted in significantly better health-related quality of life scores at 16 weeks in two dimensions of the SF-36 (role limitation physical: mean difference 22.2, 95% CI 3.8–40.6; pain: mean difference 12.1, 95% CI 3.2–20.9). There were no statistically significant differences between the two treatment groups in the other six dimensions (e.g., physical functioning) of SF-36, nor in any of the eight dimensions at 1 year (level II).

Pain One prospective controlled trial of patients with impacted proximal humeral fractures[12] (64 patients) reported significantly less pain in patients that started pendulum exercises immediately compared to those who were immobilized for 1 month as measured on a 100 mm visual analog scale (VAS) pain score at 3 months (mean difference 15.7, 95% CI 0.52–30.9, p < 0.05), but not at 6 weeks (mean difference 3.6, 95% CI −13.6–20.8, p = 0.68) or 6 months (mean difference −0.20, 95% CI −14.4 to 14.0, p = 0.98) (level II).

Recommendation

Limited evidence suggests that for patients with non- and minimally displaced two-part fractures and impacted fractures of the proximal humerus:

• Early initiation of exercises does not affect impairment or disability 6 months or more after fracture of the proximal humerus [overall quality: moderate]
• No risk of nonunion was seen with early initiation of exercises [overall quality: moderate]
• The decision regarding when to start exercises can be left to the preferences of patient and surgeon

Question 3: What are the indications for operative *vs.* nonoperative treatment of displaced proximal humerus fractures?

Case clarification

The fracture is unstable with displacement and the patient and surgeon have to decide between operative and nonoperative treatment.

Relevance

The indications for operative treatment are incompletely defined.

Current opinion

The decision regarding optimal treatment is based on the preferences of patient and surgeon.

Finding the evidence

• Cochrane Database, with search term "humerus fracture"
• PubMed (www.ncbi.nlm.nih.gov/pubmed/) clinical queries search/systematic reviews: "humerus fracture"
• PubMed (www.ncbi.nlm.nih.gov/pubmed/): sensitivity search using keywords "proximal humeral fracture," as well as "proximal humerus fracture" AND "treatment"
• Bibliography of eligible articles

Quality of the evidence
Level I
• 1 multicenter randomized controlled trial[9,16]

Level II
• 3 systematic reviews/meta-analyses (of level II studies)[10,17]
• 3 randomized trials[18–20]

Findings
Shoulder function Three prospective controlled trials[18–20] (103 patients) with serious methodological limitations (possible bias; unclear allocation concealment, unable to blind patients and caregivers, outcome assessors not blinded, >25% loss to follow-up) randomized patients to nonoperative treatment; vs. arthroplasty with a Neer prosthesis for displaced fractures (32 patients);[20] vs. transcutaneous reduction and external fixation for displaced two-, three-, and four-part fractures (31 patients);[18] and vs. tension-band osteosynthesis for three- or four-part proximal humerus fractures (40 elderly patients, mean age 74 years).[19] Two studies[18,19] using standardized outcome instruments found no statistically significant differences in Constant[21] (mean difference 5.0, 95% CI −7.5 to 17.5, p = 0.43)[19] or Neer[1] scores (RR = 2.2, 95% CI 0.74–6.54, p = 0.16) (level II).[18] One study[20] did not use standardized outcome instruments, but reported significantly more patients who were dependent in activities of daily living (RR = 4.5, 95% CI 1.2–17.4, p = 0.03) and significantly more patients with constant pain (RR = 4.8, 95% CI 1.2–18.47, p = 0.02) in the nonoperative treatment group as compared with the group treated with a Neer prosthesis (level II).

Complications There were no differences in major complications;[18–20] deep infections (RR = 0.27, 95% CI 0.1–1.6, p = 0.15) nonunion (RR = 4.0, 95% CI 0.5–30.3, p = 0.18) osteonecrosis (RR = 1.06, 95% CI 0.2–5.5, p = 0.95) or refractures (RR = 1.06, 95% CI 0.7–14.1, p = 1.00) (level II).

Recommendations

There is insufficient evidence to determine if operative treatment will produce consistently better outcomes for displaced proximal humerus fractures than nonoperative treatment.

• Although fewer patients in the operative treatment groups had unsatisfactory ratings of function, with current

small sample sizes there is no significant difference in shoulder scores [overall quality: very low]
- Operative treatment is associated with nonsignificantly more complications [overall quality: very low]

Question 4: What is the best operative treatment for displaced three- and four-part fractures and fracture-dislocations of the proximal humerus: arthroplasty or ORIF?

Case clarification
Radiographs and 2-D and 3-D CT show a complex four-part fracture of the proximal humerus. Patient and surgeon elect operative treatment. Which type of operative intervention is preferred?

Relevance
Difficulties associated with loss of fixation, nonunion, malunion, and osteonecrosis make prosthetic arthroplasty an appealing treatment option, but function after arthroplasty has been poor and prostheses gradually loosen, particularly in active patients.

Current opinion
There is a lack of consensus regarding the optimal operative treatment strategy.

Finding the evidence
- Cochrane Database, with search term "humerus fracture"
- PubMed (www.ncbi.nlm.nih.gov/pubmed/): clinical queries search/systematic reviews: "humerus fracture"
- PubMed (www.ncbi.nlm.nih.gov/pubmed/): sensitivity search using keywords "proximal humeral fracture," as well as "proximal humerus fracture" AND "arthroplasty"
- Bibliography of eligible articles

Quality of the evidence
Level I
- 1 multicenter randomized controlled trial[9]

Level II
- 3 systematic reviews/meta-analyses (of level II RCTs)[10,17,22]
- 1 randomized trial with methodologic limitations[23]

Findings
Tension-band wiring vs. arthroplasty One RCT[23] (30 patients) with methodological limitations (unclear allocation concealment, unable to blind caregivers, patients not blinded, outcome assessors not blinded, >25% loss to follow-up) showed no difference in shoulder function as measured with the Constant score (minus power component) between patients with four-part proximal humerus fractures treated with tension-band wiring vs. arthroplasty (49 vs. 48 points).

Patients in the arthroplasty group had significantly fewer subsequent surgeries within 1 year (RR = 0.09, 95% CI 0.01–1.5, p < 0.05), but no difference in implant removal (RR = 0.1, 95% CI, 0.01–1.9, p = 0.13) or pain (RR = 0.5, 95% CI 0.05–4.6, p = 0.54) (level II).

Recommendation
- There is insufficient evidence from randomized trials to determine the preferred (operative) intervention in patients with displaced four-part fractures of the proximal humerus.

Question 5: Which factors predict outcome after a proximal humeral fracture in an elderly patient?

Case clarification
The patient loves to swim and wonders whether this will be possible.

Relevance
Patients and surgeons often make decisions based on prognosis.

Current opinion
A growing body of evidence suggests that pain is a stronger correlate with disability than impairment at many anatomical sites. Even pathophysiological changes such as osteonecrosis do not seem to affect outcome as much as one might imagine.

Finding the evidence
- PubMed (www.ncbi.nlm.nih.gov/pubmed/): sensitivity search using keywords "proximal humeral fracture," "proximal humerus fracture" AND "prognostic factors" as well as "proximal humerus fracture" AND "outcome"
- Bibliography of eligible articles

Quality of the evidence
Level II
- 1 prospective case series[24]

Level III
- 1 systematic review (of level III) studies[25]
- 2 retrospective case series[26]

Findings
Predictors of humeral head ischemia One prospective study[24] evaluated predictors of fracture-induced ischemia in a consecutive series of 100 proximal humerus fractures in 98 patients (mean age 60 years). Fifty-five heads were considered ischemic and 45 perfused according to a definition of borehole bleeding and pulsatile Doppler signal. Less than 8 mm of metaphyseal extension remaining attached to the

head (p < 0.0001; PPV = 0.77, NPV = 1), disruption of the medial hinge (displacement of the shaft) greater than 2 mm (p < 0.0001; PPV = 0.83, NPV = 0.75) and anatomical neck fractures (p < 0.0001; PPV = 0.71, NPV = 0.68) were good predictors of ischemia. Four-part fractures (PPV = 0.74, NPV = 0.61), more than 45° of angular displacement of the head (PPV = 0.79, NPV = 0.55), more than 10 mm displacement of the tuberosities (PPV = 0.63, NPV = 0.58), glenohumeral dislocation (PPV = 0.6, NPV = 0.46), head-split components (PPV = 0.61, NPV = 0.46) and three-part fractures (PPV = 0.43, NPV = 0.34) were moderate and poor predictors of ischemia (level II).

Internal fixation and avascular necrosis A systematic review[25] of 12 studies with 791 patients treated with locking plates of two-, three-, and four-part fractures reported an incidence of avascular necrosis of 7.9%.

One retrospective study[26] of a consecutive series of 34 two-, three-, and four-part fractures found a significant difference in function as measured with the Constant shoulder score between patients with and without complete or partial avascular necrosis (66 point vs. 81 points; p < 0.0005) (level III).

Prognostic factors after arthroplasty One retrospective study[27] investigated prognostic factors on the outcome of arthroplasty in a consecutive series of 38 patients (mean age 58 years) with 2 Neer type III, 15 type IV, and 15 fracture-dislocations of the proximal humerus. Ninety-seven percent had no or mild pain. Patients treated within 14 days (r = 0.60; p = 0.005) and patients with superior radiological parameters describing the position of the greater tuberosity relative to the humeral head (humeral offset; p = 0.002) and humeral head height (r = −0.57; p = 0.002) had significantly better outcome according to the Constant shoulder score (level III).

Recommendation

There is insufficient evidence from prospective case studies to identify predictors of outcome in patients with complex fractures of the proximal humerus. The following trends were noted:
• Patients with proximal humeral fractures with the following radiographic characteristics are more likely to develop avascular necrosis: less than 8 mm of metaphyseal extension remaining attached to the head, disruption of the medial hinge (displacement of the shaft) greater than 2 mm and anatomical neck fractures [overall quality: moderate]
• 7.9% of patients with complex two-, three-, and four-part fractures develop avascular necrosis [overall quality: very low]
• Patients with avascular necrosis have significantly impaired shoulder function [overall quality: very low]

Summary of recommendations

• CT imaging improves the reliability of fracture classification over radiographs alone, but there is no evidence that CT improves outcome
• 3-D CT improves the reliability of classification over 2-D CT
• Although fewer patients in the operative treatment groups had unsatisfactory ratings of function, with current small sample sizes there is no significant difference in shoulder scores
• Operative treatment is associated with nonsignificantly more complications
• For patients with non- and minimally displaced two-part fractures and impacted fractures of the proximal humerus, early mobilization and physical therapy results in less pain and faster and better recovery without compromising long-term outcome
• In patients with displaced four-part fractures of the proximal humerus, there is no difference in shoulder function between arthroplasty and tension-band wiring, but patients treated with arthroplasty had significantly fewer subsequent procedures and arthroplasty nonsignificantly reduces pain compared to tension-band wiring
• Patients with proximal humeral fractures with the following radiographic characteristics are more likely to develop avascular necrosis: less than 8 mm of metaphyseal extension remaining attached to the head, disruption of the medial hinge (displacement of the shaft) greater than 2 mm and anatomical neck fractures
• 7.9% of patients with complex two-, three-, and four-part fractures develop avascular necrosis
• Patients with avascular necrosis have significantly impaired shoulder function

Conclusion

There is insufficient evidence from randomized trials to determine the optimal intervention in patients with proximal humeral fractures.

References

1. Neer CS, 2nd. Displaced proximal humeral fractures. I. Classification and evaluation. J Bone Joint Surg Am 1970;52(6): 1077–89.
2. Court-Brown CM, Caesar B. Epidemiology of adult fractures: A review. Injury 2006;37(8):691–7.
3. Court-Brown CM, Garg A, McQueen MM. The epidemiology of proximal humeral fractures. Acta Orthop Scand 2001;72(4): 365–71.
4. Calvo E, Osorio-Picone F, Redondo-Santamaria E, Avila F, Herrara A. Non-displaced proximal humeral fractures limit

shoulder function and patient's perception of health. In: Jones CB, Lee Ramsey M, eds. 73rd Annual Meeting of the American Academy of Orthopaedic Surgeons, 25 Feb2009, Las Vegas, NV.

5. Koval KJ, Gallagher MA, Marsicano JG, Cuomo F, McShinawy A, Zuckerman JD. Functional outcome after minimally displaced fractures of the proximal part of the humerus. J Bone Joint Surg Am 1997;79(2):203–7.

6. Beredjiklian PK, Iannotti JP, Norris TR, Williams GR. Operative treatment of malunion of a fracture of the proximal aspect of the humerus. J Bone Joint Surg Am 1998;80(10):1484–97.

7. Bahrs C, Rolauffs B, Sudkamp NP, et al. Indications for computed tomography (CT-) diagnostics in proximal humeral fractures: a comparative study of plain radiography and computed tomography. BMC Musculoskelet Disord. 2009;10:33.

8. Brunner A, Horisberger M, Ulmar B, Hoffmann A, Babst R. Classification systems for tibial plateau fractures; Does computed tomography scanning improve their reliability? Injury 2010;41(2):173–8.

9. Brorson S, Olsen BS, Frich LH, et al. Effect of osteosynthesis, primary hemiarthroplasty, and non-surgical management for displaced four-part fractures of the proximal humerus in elderly: a multi-centre, randomised clinical trial. Trials 2009;10:51.

10. Handoll HH, Gibson JN, Madhok R. Interventions for treating proximal humeral fractures in adults. Cochrane Database Syst Rev 2003;4:CD000434.

11. Hodgson S. Proximal humerus fracture rehabilitation. Clin Orthop Relat Res 2006;442:131–8.

12. Lefevre-Colau MM, Babinet A, Fayad F, et al. Immediate mobilization compared with conventional immobilization for the impacted nonoperatively treated proximal humeral fracture. A randomized controlled trial. J Bone Joint Surg Am 2007;89(12):2582–90.

13. Hodgson SA, Mawson SJ, Stanley D. Rehabilitation after two-part fractures of the neck of the humerus. J Bone Joint Surg Br 2003;85(3):419–22.

14. Kristiansen B, Angermann P, Larsen TK. Functional results following fractures of the proximal humerus. A controlled clinical study comparing two periods of immobilization. Arch Orthop Trauma Surg 1989;108(6):339–41.

15. Hodgson SA, Mawson SJ, Saxton JM, Stanley D. Rehabilitation of two-part fractures of the neck of the humerus (two-year follow-up). J Shoulder Elbow Surg 2007;16(2):143–5.

16. Handoll H, Brealey S, Rangan A, et al. Protocol for the ProFHER (PROximal Fracture of the Humerus: Evaluation by Randomisation) trial: a pragmatic multi-centre randomised controlled trial of surgical versus non-surgical treatment for proximal fracture of the humerus in adults. BMC Musculoskelet Disord 2009;10:140.

17. Misra A, Kapur R, Maffulli N. Complex proximal humeral fractures in adults–a systematic review of management. Injury 2001;32(5):363–72.

18. Kristiansen B, Kofoed H. Transcutaneous reduction and external fixation of displaced fractures of the proximal humerus. A controlled clinical trial. J Bone Joint Surg Br 1988;70(5):821–4.

19. Zyto K, Ahrengart L, Sperber A, Tornkvist H. Treatment of displaced proximal humeral fractures in elderly patients. J Bone Joint Surg Br 1997;79(3):412–17.

20. Stableforth PG. Four-part fractures of the neck of the humerus. J Bone Joint Surg Br 1984;66(1):104–8.

21. Constant CR, Murley AH. A clinical method of functional assessment of the shoulder. Clin Orthop 1987;214:160–4.

22. Bhandari M, Matthys G, McKee MD. Four part fractures of the proximal humerus. J Orthop Trauma 2004;18(2):126–7.

23. Hoellen IP, Bauer G, Holbein O. [Prosthetic humeral head replacement in dislocated humerus multi-fragment fracture in the elderly—an alternative to minimal osteosynthesis?] Zentralbl Chir 1997;122(11):994–1001.

24. Hertel R, Hempfing A, Stiehler M, Leunig M. Predictors of humeral head ischemia after intracapsular fracture of the proximal humerus. J Shoulder Elbow Surg 2004;13(4):427–33.

25. Thanasas C, Kontakis G, Angoules A, Limb D, Giannoudis P. Treatment of proximal humerus fractures with locking plates: a systematic review. J Shoulder Elbow Surg 2009;18(6):837–44.

26. Gerber C, Werner CM, Vienne P. Internal fixation of complex fractures of the proximal humerus. J Bone Joint Surg Br 2004;86(6):848–55.

27. Demirhan M, Kilicoglu O, Altinel L, Eralp L, Akalin Y. Prognostic factors in prosthetic replacement for acute proximal humerus fractures. J Orthop Trauma. 2003;17(3):181–8; discussion 8–9.

42 Humeral Shaft Fractures

Amy Hoang-Kim[1], Jörg Goldhahn[2], and David J. Hak[3]

[1]St. Michael's Hospital, University of Toronto, Toronto, ON, Canada
[2]Schulthess Clinic, Zurich, Switzerland
[3]Denver Health, University of Colorado, Denver, CO, USA

Case scenario

A 35 year old man is brought to the Emergency Department following a motor vehicle accident. He is complaining of right arm pain. He has an obvious deformity of his right upper arm, which appears to be his only orthopedic injury.

Relevant anatomy

Surgical approaches to the humerus must take into account the neurovascular anatomy of the brachium (Figure 42.1). Proximally, the circumflex humeral vessels and the axillary nerve divide the humerus at the surgical neck. Distally, the radial and ulnar nerves cross the intermuscular septae to leave the posterior compartment between the brachioradialis and brachialis muscles. Innervation is provided by branches of the radial nerve which passes through the lateral intermuscular septum to innervate the lateral third of the brachialis. The medial two thirds of the brachialis muscle and the remainder of the anterior compartment are innervated by the musculocutaneous nerve.

Importance of the problem

Fractures of the humeral shaft account for 1–5% of all fractures.[1,2] Over 66,000 humeral shaft fractures occur annually in the United States and account for over 363,000 days in the hospital.[3] Google Scholar returns 17,100 hits for "humeral shaft fractures" proving the topic to be much discussed, and the body of unfiltered literature contains conflicting opinions.

Top five questions

Therapy

1. What is the optimal nonoperative approach in patients with humeral shaft fractures?
2. What is the relative effect of plate fixation vs. intramedullary nailing in the management of displaced or comminuted humeral shaft fractures?
3. What is the approach for radial nerve injury when the nerve is out vs. when the nerve is initially in, but goes out following closed reduction or fracture manipulation?
4. What predictors of plate fixation failure indicate use of a locking plate vs. a nonlocking plate?

Harm

5. What are the complications associated with plate/screw fixation of humeral shaft fractures?

Finding the evidence

A search was conducted of the literature published from 1950 to June 2009 using the following computer databases: Cochrane Database of Systematic Reviews, CINAHL, Embase, OVID MEDLINE and experts in the field.
1. Exp humeral fractures/ or (exp fractures, bone/ and ((exp humerus/ or humeral.mp.))
2. (humer$ adj1 fracture$).mp.
3. 1 or 2
4. Exp diaphysis/ or diaphys$s.mp.
5. Shaft$.mp. or shaft$.tw.
6. 3 and (4 or 5)

Evidence-Based Orthopedics, First Edition. Edited by Mohit Bhandari.
© 2012 Blackwell Publishing Ltd. Published 2012 by Blackwell Publishing Ltd.

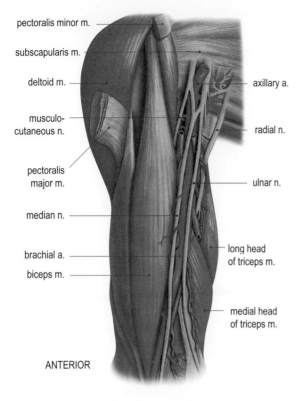

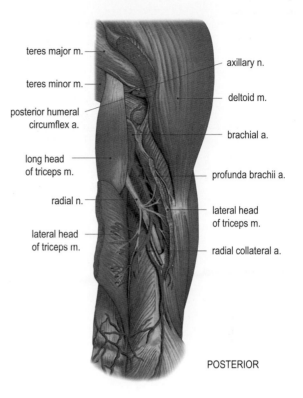

Figure 42.1 Anatomy and innervation of the humerus.

- Cochrane Database of systematic reviews, with text words "humeral fracture$" (fracture or fractures) or ('humerus' and 'fracture') + diaphys$s or shaft.
- PubMed: "humerus' + 'fracture' or 'humeral fracture' + ('shaft' or diaphysis')
- CINAHL, exp humeral fractures + ('shaft' or 'diaphys$s' or 'long')
- EMBASE exp Humeral fractures or (exp humerus + exp fracture) + diaphysis

Question 1: What is the optimal nonoperative approach in patients with humeral shaft fractures?

Case clarification

The patient's neurological examination is normal. His arm is splinted in the Emergency Department. He follows up a week later with an orthopedic surgeon who places him in a humeral fracture brace. The patient returns to his orthopedic surgeon 2 weeks after placement of the humeral fracture brace. Radiographs are obtained, and to the patient they appear to show that his bone is quite crooked. He expresses concerns to his orthopedic surgeon that the fracture is not properly aligned.

Relevance of the question

Nonoperative modalities include hanging cast, functional bracing, and plaster U splint. Residual deformity may influence active and passive range of motion as well as the function of the adjacent joints. However, the high degree of freedom provided by the shoulder joint may overcompensate deformities of the humeral shaft resulting from a misaligned humeral fracture.

Current opinion

Humeral shaft fractures can be effectively treated by functional fracture-bracing as developed by Sarmiento.

Quality of the evidence

Level I

- 1 systematic review

Findings

Union rates Following an initial 2 week period of immobilization in a plaster cast, functional bracing is indicated provided that the patient is compliant. Nonunion rates, associated with fracture pattern, are 12.8% for spiral, 4.9% for oblique, 8.9% for transverse, and 2.2% for comminuted and segmental fractures.[4]

Angulation and shortening Angulation of less than 10° is reported with an acceptable 2 cm shortening of the fracture.[4] Even slight residual angulation when managing a spiral or comminuted fracture does not produce a clinically significant deformity at this level.

Table 42.1 Summary of evidence of trials reporting health status and region-specific scores for functional bracing in patients following humeral fracture

Author (year)	Intervention	No. of patients for functional outcome (%), loss to follow-up	Level of evidence, patient characteristics	Final follow-up (months)	Health status	Region-specific scores	No. of patients recovered (%)
Ekholm et al. (2006)	Functional brace	49 (78), 1	Level III	N = 43 patients healed fracture after nonoperative treatment N = 6 patients healed fracture after operative treatment	26.4	SF-36 lower results compared to Swedish reference population. Bodily pain was the exception	Better SMFA scores for nonoperative treatment than surgical intervention	21 (49) nonoperative vs. 0 (0) surgically treated (p < 0.05)
Rosenberg et al. (2006)	Functional brace	15 (100), 0	Level V	n = 9 midshaft fractures n = 3 proximal third fractures n = 3 distal third fractures	30	NR	Constant score significantly lower in injured limb vs. normal contralateral side (p < 0.001) Oxford shoulder score of 34 (range 17–54) in injured extremities vs. contralateral side	6 (40)

NR, not reported.

Functional outcome Two studies (N = 64 patients) reported worse region-specific scores; one of them reported lower health status (Table 42.1).

Recommendations
• Functional bracing follows an initial 2 week period of immobilization in a plaster splint [overall quality: moderate]
• Angulation up to 10° can be tolerated and shortening should not exceed 2 cm [overall quality: moderate]

Question 2: What is the relative effect of plate fixation vs. intramedullary nailing in the management of displaced or comminuted humeral shaft fractures?

Case clarification
Follow-up radiographs show persistent distraction at the fracture site, suggesting the possibility of soft tissue interposition, an indication for operative treatment. The surgeon discusses two surgical fixation options with the patient: plate fixation or intramedullary nail (IMN) fixation.

Relevance of the question
Surgical intervention using both open reduction and internal fixation (ORIF) with plate and screws, or IMN and external fixation has specific indications (Table 42.2). Two

Table 42.2 Some indications for operative treatment of humeral shaft fractures

Inability to obtain and maintain an acceptable closed reduction: common examples include: obesity, segmental fractures, patients requiring prolonged recumbency

Floating elbow (ipsilateral forearm fracture)

Multiply injured patients

Open fractures

Vascular injury

Pathologic fractures

Spinal cord injury

Brachial plexus injury

Bilateral humeral shaft fractures

Progressive or new onset nerve palsy

Patients noncompliant for bracing

Table 42.3 Characteristics of randomized controlled trials comparing intramedullary nailing to plate fixation

Author (year)	Study design	Sample	Fracture type	IMN intervention	DCP intervention	Outcomes	Follow-up months (%)	Level of evidence
Changulani (2007) [14]	RCT	N = 47 patients Male: 87% Female: 13% Age: 37 years (24–51)	Comprehensive classification type A, B, and C	Antegrade nail: n = 23	n = 24	Infection, nonunion, implant failure, iatrogenic nerve injury	6–33 (96)	II
Chapman (2000) [6]	RCT	N = 84 Male: 62% Female: 38% Age: 34 years (18–83)	Closed and open type I, II, IIIA, IIIB, and IIIC	Antegrade nail: n = 38	n = 46	Infection, malunion, nonunion, iatrogenic nerve injury, elbow and shoulder pain, elbow and shoulder ROM, hardware removal	13 (4–48) NR	II
McCormack (2000) [7]	RCT	N = 44 Male: 64% Female: 36% Age: 45 years (19–82)	Comprehensive classification type A, B, and C	Antegrade nail: n = 23	n = 24	Infection, nonunion, implant failure, iatrogenic nerve injury, impingement	6–33 (96)	II
Rodriguez-Merchan (1995) [15]	RCT	N = 40 Male: 78% Female: 22% Age: 46 years (20–65)	Closed transverse fractures	Flexible nail : n = 20	n = 20	Infection, nonunion, implant failure, elbow and shoulder ROM, pain, disability	18.5 (12–50) NR	II

IMN, intramedullary nail; RCT, randomized controlled trial; ROM, range of motion.

indications for ORIF are a coexisting injury to the brachial artery that requires arterial repair and a progressive loss of radial nerve function.

Current opinion

ORIF with compression plate fixation has the advantage of accurate fracture reduction, but has disadvantages of additional soft tissue and periosteal stripping, infection, and potential risk of radial nerve injury. Biomechanical studies show increased initial stability when an IMN is inserted antegrade for proximal fractures and retrograde for distal fractures.[5]

Quality of the evidence

Level I
- 1 systematic review/meta-analysis

Level II
- 4 studies

Findings

Impairment Three studies demonstrated overall more shoulder pain and reduced shoulder range of motion with IMN (Table 42.3). Chapman et al. reported 93% healing in those patients treated with plate fixation and 87% with IMN at 16 weeks.[6] In the plate fixation group, a significant decrease in elbow range of motion was seen especially for distal third diaphyseal fractures (p = 0.003).

Shoulder pain following antegrade vs. retrograde nail insertion ranges from 16% to 37%, and can be reduced by carefully splitting, retracting and repairing the rotator cuff.[7,8] Cheng et al. (RCT: level II) reported similar fracture healing rate and time to healing did not differ significantly between retrograde and antegrade IMN.[9] Active range of motion exercises should be started in the early postoperative period, 4–7 days after surgery. Crutch ambulation is possible if the fixation is stable and will axially load the fracture site, aiding union.[5]

Disability McCormack (RCT; level II) and Gregory et al. (meta-analysis; level II), found no significant differences in the function of the shoulder and elbow between groups.[7,10] McCormack used the American Shoulder and Elbow Surgeons score (ASES) for 16 activities involving the shoulder and elbow movement (p = 0.713). In the randomized trial by Cheng, the authors sustain a better average Neer shoulder score for the antegrade group than the retrograde

IMN (90.8 ± 6.5 vs. 93.5 ± 4.6, respectively. p = 0.03, 95% CI −3.53 to 0.33). There were no significant differences in the Mayo elbow performance score between the two nail insertion groups (p = 0.16, 95% CI −0.62 to 3.62).

The American Shoulder and Elbow Surgeons (ASES) shoulder scale contains both a patient-derived subjective assessment and a physician-derived objective assessment. It was published in 1994 by the Research Committee of the American Shoulder and Elbow Surgeons. The subjective patient self-report section consists of two equally weighted domains, pain and function, and has been widely used for outcomes assessment in patients with shoulder instability, rotator cuff disease, and glenohumeral arthritis. Pain is recorded on an ordinal scale, ranging from 0 to 10, and accounts for 50% of the overall ASES score. Function accounts for the other 50% of the overall score and is divided into ten questions.

Recommendations
- Plate fixation and IMN can result in similar healing patterns at 16 weeks [overall quality: moderate]
- Antegrade and retrograde IMN can be inserted using either an antegrade or a retrograde approach [overall quality: low]
- IMN is associated with more shoulder pain and reduced range of motion. Both IMN and compression plating can achieve similar functional results [overall quality: low]

Question 3: What is the recovery rate of radial nerve injury when the nerve is out vs. the nerve is initially in, but goes out following closed reduction or fracture manipulation?

Case clarification
Scenario 1: When the patient initially presents to the Emergency Department, physical examination reveals that he is unable to actively extend his wrist or fingers. This deficit persists following closed reduction and splint placement. Scenario 2: On initial presentation to the Emergency Department, the patient's physical examination shows intact motor function. He undergoes closed reduction and application of a splint. Following the reduction physical examination, indicates an inability to actively extend his wrist or fingers.

Relevance of the question
When radial nerve palsy develops following fracture manipulation, many surgeons have advocated radial nerve exploration because this scenario suggests that the radial nerve might be trapped within the fracture.

Current opinion
A survey of current practice among trauma surgeons in England showed that surgeons still differ in the ways of managing radial nerve palsy associated with humeral fractures, with a slightly higher percentage of surgeons preferring conservative treatment.[11]

Quality of the evidence
Level II
- 2 studies

Findings
Recovery rate Shao et al. reported that a spiral fracture pattern of the distal humerus with associated nerve palsy is not an absolute indication for radial nerve exploration and showed no significant difference in the rate of recovery between primary (88.6%) and secondary nerve palsies (93.1%).[12] A limited period of waiting also had no effect on the final recovery. Eleven studies (n = 98 patients) showed that the mean delay to first exploration was 4.3 months (range 1–15). In 101 cases treated expectantly at first, the mean spontaneous recovery onset time was 7.3 weeks, which may indicate the minimum waiting time before exploration.

The rationale for this type of injury is not to be indicated for open reduction unless it constitutes an increase in radial nerve deficit. It is reported that nerve fibers will regenerate in 3 months' time. When recovery in this time period has failed, appropriate tendon transfers can improve irreparable nerve damage. Because irrigation and debridement is required for open fractures, it is reasonable to explore the nerve at this same operation. Shao et al. did not identify a significant difference in the spontaneous recovery of radial nerve palsies in open vs. closed fractures.[12]

Recommendation
- Exploration is at 4–6 months if there is no resolution following a primary radial nerve palsy [overall quality: low]
- In patients with indications for earlier operative fixation, exploration of the nerve should be at the time of internal fixation [overall quality: low]
- Primary and secondary nerve palsies show no difference in recovery rate [overall quality: moderate]

Question 4: What predictors of plate fixation failure indicate use of a locking plate vs. a nonlocking plate?

Case clarification
Following discussion with his surgeon regarding surgical treatment options, the patient elects to undergo open reduction and plate fixation. In planning for the surgical procedure, the surgeon wonders whether he should request a traditional nonlocking plate or a more expensive locking plate.

Table 42.4 Summary of the biomechanical evidence for locking screw/plate fixation in cadaveric humeral shaft fractures

Author (year)	Study design	Intervention	Outcomes	Results
Simon (1999)	Biomechanical cadaver study	6 pairs of cadaveric humeri from elderly individuals with 10-hole broad DCP plate on one side and a DCP plate augmented with Schuhlis at each screw hole on contralateral side placed in cortical bone	Axial loading, torsion, and four-point bending, (AP, LM)	Locked construct showed a consistent ability to sustain larger rotational displacements and loads prior to failure by spiral fracture No significant differences for the stiffness values in the testing modalities prior to or after cycling
Jazrawi (2000)	Biomechanical cadaver study	6 pairs of Schuhli locking nuts with standard screws and cement augmented screws for fixation in humeral shaft fractures with osteoporosis	Axial compression, 4-point bending, torsion	Cement augmented screws showed no significant difference in fixation stability in all loading modes before and after cycling The Schuhli locking nuts and cement augmented screws had significantly greater fixation stability than the standard screws before and after cycling in torsional loading
Korner (2004)	Biomechanical cadaver study	10 matched pairs of humeri with two standard configurations of double-plate osteosynthesis with either conventional reconstruction plates or locking compression plates. Each plate was fixed with 3 bicortical screws in the proximal fragment and 3 monocortical screws in the distal fragment.	Stiffness testing (AP bending) torsion and axial compression loading. Failure patterns under cyclic loading and strength testing	Primary stiffness in AP bending and torsional loading is significantly increased using LCP in a 90° configuration (P<0.05) as compared with dorsally applied plates
O'Toole (2008)	Biomechanical cadaver and synthetic humeri study	10-hole 3.5mm LCP with either locking or nonlocking bicortical screws in cadaveric elderly matched pairs (n = 12) and synthetic bones (n = 6).	Stiffness testing and failure testing	No difference between axial stiffness before and after cyclic loading for the plates (p = 0.94) No difference in ultimate failure force (p = 0.87)

AP, anteroposterior; DCP, dynamic compression plate; LCP, locking compression plate; LM, lateral medial.

Relevance of the question

Locking plates provide a new mechanical paradigm for the fixation of fractures; they do not rely on compression of the plate to the bone to maintain their rigidity.

Current opinion

The use of the locking plate, which has a higher energy to failure, may compensate for loss of screw purchase typical in osteoporotic bone.

Quality of the evidence

Level V
• 3 studies

Findings

Union rates Ring and coinvestigators suggest that a better alternative, if it is anticipated that standard screws will not function adequately, is to use Schuhli nuts to transform each screw into a fixed-angle device.[13]

Biomechanical results Most biomechanical data support the use of locked screws (Table 42.4).

Recommendation

• Biomechanical data shows potential benefits in using locked screw configurations in the plating of osteoporosis humeral fractures [overall quality: moderate]

Question 5: What are the complications associated with plate/screw fixation of humeral shaft fractures?

Case clarification

In completing the informed consent the surgeon reviews the potential risks involved in the planned surgical fixation.

Relevance of the question
Potential complications will influence decision-making either for or against surgical management. It will also affect patient compliance and expectation.

Current opinion
Although all studies of humeral shaft fractures report specific complications, there is no general consensus on how to report them. This further challenges the comparison or pooling of different studies.

Quality of the evidence
Level I
• 2 systematic reviews/meta-analyses

Level II
• 4 studies

Findings
Reoperation McCormack's results (RCT, level II) demonstrate that for every three patients treated with plating as opposed to treatment with an IMN, one reoperation could be avoided.[7] Chapman (RCT, level II) reported no difference, with 13% of patients having reoperations for IMN compared with 9% in the plating group.[6] Changulani (RCT, level II) favors IMN over plating (RR 1.44, 95% CI 0.47, 4.44).[14] A recent updated review by Heineman et al. (2010) indicates potential confounding in the analysis conducted in 2006, since Rodriguez-Merchan included 19 patients treated with retrograde flexible nails.[15-17] However, there was a strong trend in favoring plates over IMN for risk of reoperation.[16,17]

Nonunion Nonunion ranges from 5% to 13% for IMN compared with 4–13% for plating.[6,7,14] In the three studies by Chapman, McCormack, and Changulani et al., when pooled, IMN and plating result in similar percentages of patients with nonunion (RR 1.1, 95% CI 0.4, 3.1).

Mean time to union Mean time to union was 6.3–9.8 weeks in the IMN group compared with 8.9–10.4 weeks in the plating group. McCormack reported no difference in time to union between IMN (9.8 weeks) and plating (10.4 weeks), p = 0.664,[6] while Changulani showed a significant difference in mean time to union, 6.3 weeks in the IMN group compared with 8.9 weeks in the plating group (p < 0.001).[14] The union rate was similar in both groups as reported in the meta-analyses.[16,17]

Infection Infection rates range from 0% to 5% for IMN compared to 0–21% for plating. Chapman and McCormack show a decreased infection risk for IMN compared with plating;[6,7] however, the difference was not significant in the Changulani study, although infectious complications were higher in the plate fixation group (20.8% vs. 4.7%; RR 0.21, 95% CI 0.03, 1.7) where RR was calculable.[14] While individual studies have shown a higher infection rate with plate fixation, meta-analyses results indicates that there are no significant differences between the two treatments.[16,17]

Iatrogenic nerve injury Rates for nerve injury range from 4% to 15% for IMN compared with 0–4% for plating.[6,7,14] Chapman and McCormack report a higher rate of nerve injury with IMN,[6,7] although, when the data are pooled, the difference between IMN and plating is not significant (RR 3.4, 95% CI 0.7, 16).

Recommendations
• There was an increase in risk of reoperation with IMN, which was significant when data were pooled across studies [overall quality: moderate]
• Evidence from three RCTs with rigid nails suggests that treatment of acute humeral shaft fractures with IMN compared with dynamic compression plating leads to comparable results with respect to rates of nonunion, infection, and iatrogenic nerve injury [overall quality: moderate]
• A more recent meta-analysis performed which also included a subsequently published RCT[18] suggests that the risk of a complication is lower with plate fixation compared to IMN

Summary of recommendations

• Functional fracture-bracing can be used following an initial 2 week period of immobilization in a plaster splint
• Angulation up to 10° can be tolerated and shortening should not exceed 2 cm
• Plate fixation and IMN can result in similar healing patterns at 16 weeks
• Antegrade and retrograde IMN can be inserted using either an antegrade or a retrograde approach
• IMN is associated with more shoulder pain and reduced range of motion. Both IMN and compression plating can achieve similar functional results
• IMN result in higher rates of reoperation and no differences between rates of nonunion, infection, or iatrogenic nerve injury when compared to compression plating
• Antegrade IMN has lower rate of nonunion and intraoperative complications
• Exploration is at 4–6 months if there is no resolution following a primary radial nerve palsy
• In patients with indications for earlier operative fixation, exploration of the nerve should be at the time of internal fixation

- Primary and secondary nerve palsies show no difference in recovery rate
- Biomechanical data shows potential benefits in using locked screw configurations in the plating of osteoporosis humeral fractures
- There was an increase in risk of reoperation with IMN, which was significant when data were pooled across studies
- Evidence from three RCTs with rigid nails suggests that treatment of acute humeral shaft fractures with IMN compared with dynamic compression plating leads to comparable results with respect to rates of nonunion, infection, and iatrogenic nerve injury
- A more recent meta-analysis performed which also included a subsequently published RCT suggests that the risk of a complication is lower with plate fixation compared to IMN

Conclusion

Evidence suggests comparable results between IMN and compression plating with respect to rates of nonunion, infection, and iatrogenic nerve injury. IMN patients have an increased risk of reoperation, with conflicting evidence concerning the mean time to union.

Acknowledgements
Special thanks to Ms. Mariapia Cumani for her artwork. AHK is supported by the David E. Hastings Scholarship.

References

1. Ward EF, Savoie FH, Balfour GW. Fractures of the Diaphyseal Humerus. WB Saunders, Philadelphia, 1998.
2. Crolla RM, de Vries LS, Clevers YE Locked intramedullary nailing systems of humeral fractures. Injury 1993;24:403.
3. Praemer MA, Furner S, Price DP. Musculoskeletal Conditions in the United States, p. 116. American Academy of Orthopaedic Surgeons, Park Ridge, IL, 1992.
4. Papasoulis E, Drosos GI, Ververidis AN, et al. Functional bracing of humeral shaft fractures. A reviw of clinical studies. Injury 2010;41(7):e21–27.
5. Pickering RM, Crenshaw AH, Zinar D. Intramedullary nailing of humeral shaft fractures. AAOS Instruct Course Lect 2002;51:271–8.
6. Chapman JR, Henley MB, Agel J, et al. Randomized prospective study of humeral shaft fracture fixation: intramedullary nails versus plates. J Orthop Trauma 2000;14:162–6.
7. McCormack RG, Brien D, Buckley RE, et al. Fixation of fractures of the shaft of the humerus by dynamic compression plate or intramedullary nail. A prospective, randomized trial. J Bone Joint Surg Br 2000;82:337–9.
8. Cox MA, Dolan M, Synnott K, et al. Closed interlocking nailing humeral shaft fractures with the Russell-Taylor nail. J Orthop Trauma 2000;14:349–53.
9. Cheng H, Lin J. Prospective randomized comparative study of antegrade and retrograde locked nailing for middle humeral shaft fracture. J Trauma 2008;65:94–102.
10. Gregory PR,Sanders RW. Compression plating versus intramedullary fixation of humeral shaft fractures. J Am Acad Orthop Surg 1997;5:215–223.
11. Shivarathre DG, Dheerendra S K, Bari A, et al. Management of clinical radial nerve palsy with closed fracture shaft of humerus—a postal questionnaire survey. Surgeon 2008;6:76–8.
12. Shao YC, Harwood P, Grotz MRW, et al. Radial nerve palsy associated with fractures of the shaft of the humerus: A systematic review. J Bone Joint Surg Br 2005; 87:1647–52.
13. Ring D, Perey B, Jupiter J. The functional outcome of operative treatment of ununited fractures of the humeral diaphysis in older patients. J Bone Joint Surg Am 1999;81:177–190.
14. Changulani M, Jain UK, Keswani T. Comparison of the use of the humerus intramedullary nail and dynamic compression plate for the management of diaphyseal fractures of the humerus. A randomised controlled study. Int Orthop 2007;31:391–5.
15. Rodriguez-Merchan EC. Compression plating versus hackethal nailing in closed humeral shaft fractures failing nonoperative reduction. J Orthop Trauma 1995;9:194–7.
16. Bhandari M, Devereaux PJ, McKee MD, et al. Compression plating versus intramedullary nailing of humeral shaft fractures—A meta-analysis. Acta Orthop 2006;77:279–284.
17. Heineman DJ, Poolman RW, Nork SE, et al. Treatment of humeral shaft fractures: meta-analysis reupdated. Acta Orthop 2010;81(4):517.
18. Putti AB, Uppin RB, Putti BB. Locked intramedullary nailing versus dynamic compression plating for humeral shaft fractures. Orthop Surg (Hong Kong) 2009;17:139–141.

43 Distal Humerus Fractures

Aaron Nauth and Emil H. Schemitsch
St. Michael's Hospital, University of Toronto, Toronto, ON, Canada

Case scenario

An 86 year old female patient, who lives independently, presents to the Emergency Department after a fall from standing height on her right arm. She is complaining of pain in her right elbow. There are no open wounds and her limb is neurovascularly intact.

Relevant anatomy

Distal humerus fractures involve the supracondylar region of the humerus with or without extension to the articular surface. They are most commonly classified according to the OTA/AO classification system (Figure 43.1). In this classification system "A" designates an extra-articular fracture, "B" designates a partial articular fracture, and "C" indicates an intra-articular fracture in which the articular surface is completely dissociated from the shaft of the humerus. These three types are further subdivided using the numbers 1–3 to indicate increasing degrees of comminution.

Importance of the problem

Distal humerus fractures occur in adults with an estimated incidence of 5.7 per 100,000 per year, based on a United Kingdom study in 2003.[1] The authors reported a distribution of 38.7% type A fractures, 24.1% type B fractures, and 37.2% type C fractures based on the OTA/AO classification. These injuries occur in a bimodal distribution with an early peak in males aged 12–19 years who sustain a sport-ing or motor vehicle accident, and a second peak in elderly women with osteoporotic bone who sustain a simple fall from standing height.

In a Finnish study based on the National Health Registry, the authors reported a threefold increase in the incidence of distal humerus fractures in women aged 60 years and older over their study period (11 per 100,000 in 1975 to 30 per 100,000 in 1995).[2] The authors concluded that the incidence of distal humerus fractures in elderly women is increasing rapidly and predicted an annual incidence of 52 per 100,000 in 2030.

These data indicate that although fractures of the distal humerus are rare, their incidence is increasing significantly. The dramatic increases reported in elderly female patients with potentially osteoporotic bone is of particular note, suggesting that fixation strategies for osteoporotic bone and possible joint replacement techniques, as well the management of osteoporotic disease itself, will play important roles in the future management of these injuries.

Top six questions

Diagnosis

1. What is the value of preoperative CT scanning in the assessment of distal humerus fractures?

Therapy

2. What is the optimal surgical approach for the fixation of distal humerus fractures?
3. What is the optimal fixation strategy for distal humerus fractures?

Evidence-Based Orthopedics, First Edition. Edited by Mohit Bhandari.
© 2012 Blackwell Publishing Ltd. Published 2012 by Blackwell Publishing Ltd.

OTA/AO Classification

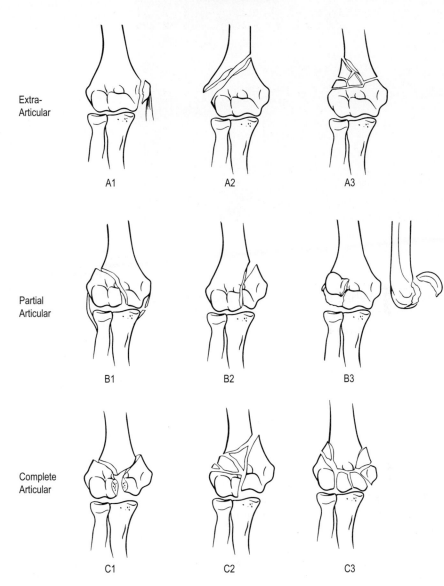

Extra-Articular

A1   A2   A3

Partial Articular

B1   B2   B3

Complete Articular

C1   C2   C3

Figure 43.1 OTA/AO Classification of distal humerus fractures.

4. What is the evidence for transposition of the ulnar nerve?

5. Should heterotopic ossification prophylaxis be used following surgical fixation of distal humerus fractures?

6. What is the evidence for open reduction and internal fixation (ORIF) vs. total elbow arthroplasty (TEA) in elderly patients?

Finding the evidence

• Cochrane Database with search term "distal humerus fracture"

• PubMed (www.ncbi.nlm.nih.gov/pubmed/) clinical queries search/ systematic reviews: "distal humerus fracture"

• PubMed (www.ncbi.nlm.nih.gov/pubmed/): sensitivity search using keywords "distal humerus" AND "fractures" as well as "distal humerus" AND "imaging," "internal fixation," "non-operative," "surgical approach," "locking plates," "ulnar nerve," "heterotopic ossification," "elbow arthroplasty"

• Manual search of AO Traumaline Database (http://www.aofoundation.org)

This search strategy was used for all of the questions discussed in this chapter.

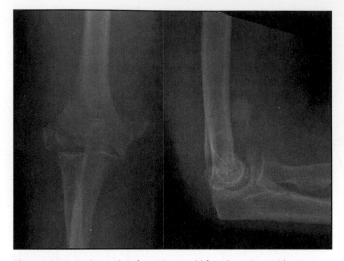

Figure 43.2 Radiographs of an 86 year old female patient with a displaced intra-articular distal humerus fracture (OTA/AO Type C3).

Question 1: What is the value of preoperative CT scanning in the assessment of distal humerus fractures?

Case clarification

Radiographs are obtained of the patient's right elbow (Figure 43.2). They show a displaced C3 type distal humerus fracture with significant comminution. You consider the value of obtaining a CT scan for preoperative planning.

Relevance

Distal humerus fractures can be difficult to characterize and classify on the basis of plain radiographs. CT scanning is a readily available modality that has been shown to influence treatment decisions in multiple other articular fractures.[3,4]

Current opinion

Most surgeons feel that CT scanning is useful for preoperative planning in distal humerus fractures that involve the articular surface, especially if articular comminution is evident on plain films.

Quality of the evidence

Level III
• 1 study[5]

Level IV
• 4 studies[6–9]

Findings

A single level III study compared the use of 3-D CT reconstructions to the use of 2-D CT and radiographs for the classification of distal humerus fractures and treatment decision-making.[5] The authors reported increased interob-

server and intraobserver reliability for fracture classification with the use of 3-D CT, as well as increased intraobserver reliability for treatment decisions. The remainder of the literature consists of level IV case series that incorporated the use of CT, primarily for the evaluation of coronal shear type fractures of the distal humerus.

Recommendation

• CT scanning can be useful for improved reliability of fracture classification and guiding treatment decisions in the management of distal humerus fractures, particularly in the setting of articular comminution [overall quality: low]

Question 2: What is the optimal surgical approach for the fixation of distal humerus fractures?

Relevance

Numerous surgical approaches have been described for the fixation of distal humerus fractures. With the exception of approach strategies for coronal shear fractures, all of these involve a posterior skin incision with various strategies of working through, or around, the triceps. Described approaches include the triceps-splitting, olecranon osteotomy, triceps-reflecting (Bryan–Morrey), triceps-reflecting anconeus pedicle (TRAP), and paratricipital approaches.

Current opinion

Surgeon opinion regarding the optimal surgical approach to distal humerus fractures is widely divergent.

Quality of the evidence

Level III
• 4 studies[10–13]

Level IV
• 10 studies[14–23]

Findings

Four level III studies retrospectively compared the triceps split approach and the olecranon osteotomy approach for the fixation of distal humerus fractures. Three of these studies showed no statistically significant differences between the approaches with regards to either objective elbow strength, range of motion, or functional outcome (n = 62 patients).[10,11,13] One of these studies found an increased rate of reoperation with the olecranon osteotomy approach due to the need for olecranon hardware removal in 27% of patients.[11] Other level IV series of patients treated with olecranon osteotomy have reported rates of hardware removal ranging from 6% to 30% and nonunion of the olecranon osteotomy in 0–9% of patients.[14–18] One level III study compared the two approaches for the fixation of open distal humerus fractures and found better functional outcomes and a trend towards improved range of motion in the triceps split group (n = 26 patients).[12] The authors hypothesized that this effect was due to the fact that open fractures had a large tear in the triceps that was easily incorporated into the triceps-splitting approach. Multiple level IV studies have reported satisfactory results using the olecranon osteotomy,[14–18] triceps-splitting,[19] triceps-reflecting,[20,21] and paratricipital[22,23] approaches.

Recommendations

• The use of a triceps-splitting approach may lead to equivalent functional outcomes and a decreased need for reoperation when compared to an olecranon osteotomy [overall quality: low]

• A triceps-splitting approach is preferred over olecranon osteotomy for the treatment of open fractures of the distal humerus [overall quality: moderate]

Question 3: What is the optimal fixation strategy for distal humerus fractures?

Relevance

Since the introduction of Arbeitsgemeinschaft für Osteosynthesefragen (AO) techniques involving dual column plating for the fixation of distal humerus fractures in the 1970s, significant improvements in surgical outcomes have been observed. However, controversy remains regarding the position/orientation of plate fixation.

Locking plates have been shown to provide improved fixation in osteoporotic bone and improved outcomes when used in other periarticular fractures.[24–26] The use of locking plates in distal humerus fractures remains controversial at present and the indications for their use in this setting are unclear.

Current opinion

Most surgeons agree that dual plate fixation is indicated for most distal humerus fractures; however, controversy exists with regard to plate configuration, with some authors recommending perpendicular plating and others recommending parallel plate fixation. Opinion among surgeons regarding the use of locking plates in the management of distal humerus fractures is highly divergent.

Quality of the evidence

Level II
• 1 study[27]

Level III
• 2 studies[28,29]

Level IV
• 20 studies[30–49]

Findings

Two level III studies retrospectively compared operative fixation with dual plates vs. minimal fixation with Kirschner (K)-wires or screws (n = 97 patients).[28,29] Both studies reported significantly improved functional outcomes following plate fixation. One study showed an almost three times higher risk of a poor outcome with the use of K-wires/screws vs. plate fixation (RR = 2.8, 95% CI 1.5–5.1).[29]

One level II study compared parallel plating to perpendicular plating in a prospective randomized fashion (n = 35 patients).[27] Although no statistically significant differences were found between the two treatment groups, there were two nonunions in the perpendicular plating group vs. no nonunions in the parallel plating group. This study may not have been sufficiently powered to detect a clinically significant difference in union rates. Multiple level IV series have reported satisfactory results with perpendicular plating techniques[30–34] and parallel plating techniques.[35–40]

Several biomechanical studies have demonstrated that parallel plate configurations at 180° to each other are biomechanically superior to perpendicular plates when a gap model is used to simulate fracture comminution.[43–45]

Two clinical level IV studies have reported on the results of locked plating of distal humerus fractures (n = 52 patients).[46,47] Pooled analysis showed good/excellent results in 79% of patients, with only a single case of implant failure.

Biomechanical studies have shown somewhat improved fixation of locking plates in models of osteoporotic or comminuted distal humerus fractures.[43,48,49]

Recommendations

• Plate fixation is favored over screw/K-wire fixation for distal humerus fractures in adults [overall quality: moderate]

• All distal humerus fractures involving both columns should be treated with dual plate fixation in either a perpendicular or parallel configuration [overall quality: moderate]

• In severely comminuted or osteoporotic fractures, a parallel plate configuration, with plates on both columns at 180° to each other, should be considered [overall quality: low]

• There is currently insufficient evidence to recommend for or against the use of locking plates in distal humerus fractures [overall quality: very low]

Question 4: What is the evidence for transposition of the ulnar nerve?

Relevance

Distal humerus fractures are often complicated by injury to the ulnar nerve either due to the original injury or as a result of surgical intervention. Controversy exists regarding the management of the ulnar nerve during surgical intervention, with some authors recommending routine anterior transposition and others recommending in-situ decompression alone.

Current opinion
Management of the ulnar nerve during the fixation of distal humerus fractures is controversial, with advocates both for and against routine anterior transposition of the ulnar nerve.

Quality of the evidence
Level II
- 1 study[50]

Level IV
- 7 studies[17,27,37,40,50–52]

Findings
A single level II study randomized patients with a distal humerus fracture and preoperative ulnar nerve symptoms to either anterior subcutaneous transposition or in situ decompression (n = 29 patients).[50] The results showed significantly improved outcomes in the transposed group, with complete nerve recovery in 12/15 transposed patients vs. 8/14 patients treated with decompression alone (p < 0.05).

Several level IV studies have reported rates of ulnar neuropathy from 0% to 12.5% with routine anterior subcutaneous transposition in patients whose ulnar nerves were normal preoperatively.[17,27,37,40,50,51] Another level IV study reported on the 12–30 year follow-up of patients who had surgical treatment of a distal humerus fracture with no transposition of the ulnar nerve.[52] Of the 30 patients evaluated, only one had symptoms of ulnar nerve dysfunction at the time of final follow-up.

Recommendations
- Anterior transposition of the ulnar nerve should be performed during the fixation of distal humerus fractures in all patients who exhibit preoperative ulnar nerve symptoms [overall quality: low]
- There is insufficient evidence to recommend for or against transposition of the ulnar nerve in patients with a distal humerus fracture who present with a normal neurological exam preoperatively [overall quality: very low]

Question 5: Should heterotopic ossification prophylaxis be used following surgical fixation of distal humerus fractures?

Relevance
Heterotopic ossification (HO) can cause significant limitations in range of motion and functional outcome when it occurs following operative intervention for distal humerus fractures.

Current opinion
Opinion among surgeons regarding the indications for HO prophylaxis following operative fixation of a distal humerus fracture is mixed, with some surgeons favoring routine prophylaxis and others recommending the selective use of prophylaxis in high risk patients.

Quality of the evidence
Level III
- 1 study[17]

Level IV
- 8 studies[27,36,37,40,53–56]

Findings
One level III study retrospectively reviewed the incidence of HO in two groups of operatively treated distal humerus fractures: one in which prophylaxis was not used, and another group which received routine prophylaxis in the form of 6 weeks of indomethacin (n = 23 patients).[17] Forty-two percent of the patients without prophylaxis developed HO, whereas only 18% of the patients who received indomethacin developed HO. The difference between the groups was not significant, although the study was likely underpowered to detect a clinically significant difference in the occurrence of HO based on the number of patients evaluated.

Results of modern series of operative fixation of distal humerus fractures which have not used routine HO prophylaxis have reported rates of clinically significant HO from 0% to 21%.[36,37,40,53–55] Pooled analysis of the data from these studies demonstrates an overall 8.6% rate of clinically symptomatic HO when routine prophylaxis is not used (n = 239 patients). Two recent level IV studies have reported on routine prophylaxis against HO in a series of distal humerus fractures treated operatively. One study used an initial dose of radiation therapy on postoperative day 1, followed by 2 weeks of indomethacin.[27] The authors reported a rate of clinically symptomatic HO of 2.9%, with a nonunion rate of 5.7% (n = 35 patients). The other study used 6 weeks of celecoxib (Celebrex) for routine prophylaxis and reported a 3.1% rate of clinically symptomatic HO (n = 32 patients).[56] No nonunions occurred in that study.

Risk factors that have been reported in the literature to significantly increase the risk of development of HO in association with a distal humerus fracture include central nervous system injury,[57] delay in surgical intervention,[55] surgery prior to definitive fixation,[40] and open fractures.[40]

Recommendations
- There is insufficient evidence to recommend for or against routine prophylaxis against HO following opera-

tive fixation of distal humerus fractures [overall quality: very low]

• Prophylaxis should be considered in patients at particularly high risk for the development of HO, such as patients with associated injuries to the central nervous system, delays in surgical intervention, surgical procedures prior to definitive fixation, and open fractures [overall quality: low]

• There is insufficient evidence to recommend a specific regimen for HO prophylaxis in distal humerus fractures (3–6 weeks of an nonsteroidal anti-inflammatory (NSAID) medication, such as indomethacin or celecoxib, is a reasonable option) [overall quality: very low]

Question 6: What is the evidence for ORIF vs. TEA in elderly patients?

Case clarification

Given your patient's advanced age, low demand, the osteopenic appearance of her bones on radiographs, and the significant articular comminution of her fracture, you elect to perform a primary TEA (Figure 43.3).

Relevance

Distal humerus fractures with comminution of the articular surface can be difficult to manage, even in young patients with excellent bone quality. In elderly patients with poor bone quality and significant articular comminution this challenge increases exponentially, and surgical outcomes have historically been poor in these patients. This has prompted many authors to investigate, and more recently advocate, the use of acute TEA in the management of distal humerus fractures in elderly patients.

Current opinion

Many surgeons feel that elderly patients with a distal humerus fracture that involves significant comminution of

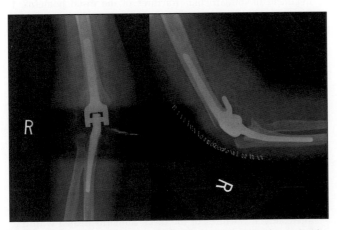

Figure 43.3 Postoperative radiographs of the same patient treated with an acute total elbow arthroplasty.

the articular surface can be treated effectively with a constrained TEA.

Quality of the evidence

Level II
• 1 study[58]

Level III
• 5 studies[59–62]

Findings

A prospective, randomized, multicenter study (level II evidence) compared ORIF vs. TEA for displaced, intra-articular fractures of the distal humerus (OTA/AO type C) in patients over the age of 65 years (n = 40 patients).[58] The authors reported better functional outcomes in the TEA group vs. the ORIF group at 2 year follow-up. In addition there was a 25% rate of intraoperative conversion to TEA in the ORIF group due to extensive comminution and inability to achieve stable fixation.

Three level III studies compared ORIF vs. TEA, in a retrospective manner, in elderly patients with intra-articular distal humerus fractures (n = 256).[59,60,63] Pooled analysis of the results suggests that TEA results in a higher proportion of patients experiencing a good/excellent functional outcome (89% in TEA vs. 76% in ORIF, p = 0.036). Complication rates did not differ significantly between the two groups.

One level III study retrospectively compared the outcome of acute TEA for distal humerus fractures vs. delayed TEA following failed ORIF or conservative treatment (n = 32 patients).[61] The authors reported a high rate of good/excellent functional outcomes (82%) with no significant differences between the two treatment groups. However, the results showed trends towards increased rates of infection, nerve injury, and implant failure in the delayed treatment group, and the study was likely underpowered to detect clinically significant differences in the rates of these complications between groups.

A final level III study performed a systematic review of level IV studies assessing ORIF or TEA for distal humerus fractures in elderly patients published prior to 2003.[62] Based on the eight studies identified, the authors reported equivalent outcomes between the two groups at less than 4 years follow-up (n = 134 patients).

Recommendation

• In elderly patients (>65 years) with displaced, intra-articular distal humerus fractures not amenable to stable internal fixation, acute TEA is preferred [overall quality: moderate]

Summary of recommendations

• CT scanning can be useful for improved reliability of fracture classification and guiding treatment decisions in the management of distal humerus fractures, particularly in the setting of articular comminution

• The use of a triceps-splitting approach may lead to equivalent functional outcomes and a decreased need for reoperation when compared to an olecranon osteotomy

• A triceps-splitting approach is preferred over olecranon osteotomy for the treatment of open fractures of the distal humerus

• Plate fixation is favored over screw/K-wire fixation for distal humerus fractures in adults

• All distal humerus fractures involving both columns should be treated with dual plate fixation in either a perpendicular or parallel configuration

• In severely comminuted or osteoporotic fractures, a parallel plate configuration with plates on both columns at 180° to each other should be considered

• There is currently insufficient evidence to recommend for or against the use of locking plates in distal humerus fractures

• Anterior transposition of the ulnar nerve should be performed during the fixation of distal humerus fractures in all patients who exhibit preoperative ulnar nerve symptoms

• There is insufficient evidence to recommend for or against transposition of the ulnar nerve in patients with a distal humerus fracture who present with a normal neurological examination preoperatively

• There is insufficient evidence to recommend for or against routine prophylaxis against HO following operative fixation of distal humerus fractures

• Prophylaxis should be considered in patients at particularly high risk for the development of HO, such as patients with associated injuries to the central nervous system, delays in surgical intervention, surgical procedures prior to definitive fixation, and open fractures

• There is insufficient evidence to recommend a specific regimen for HO prophylaxis in distal humerus fractures (3–6 weeks of an NSAID medication, such as indomethacin or celecoxib, is a reasonable option)

• In elderly patients (>65 years) with displaced, intra-articular distal humerus fractures not amenable to stable internal fixation, acute TEA is preferred

References

1. Robinson CM, Hill RM, Jacobs N, Dall G, Court-Brown CM. Adult distal humeral metaphyseal fractures: epidemiology and results of treatment. J Orthop Trauma 2003;17(1):38–47.

2. Palvanen M, Kannus P, Niemi S, Parkkari J. Secular trends in the osteoporotic fractures of the distal humerus in elderly women. Eur J Epidemiol 1998;14(2):159–64.

3. Chan PS, Klimkiewicz JJ, Luchetti WT, et al. Impact of CT scan on treatment plan and fracture classification of tibial plateau fractures. J Orthop Trauma 1997;11(7):484–9.

4. Katz MA, Beredjiklian PK, Bozentka DJ, Steinberg DR. Computed tomography scanning of intra-articular distal radius fractures: does it influence treatment? J Hand Surg Am 2001;26(3):415–21.

5. Doornberg J, Lindenhovius A, Kloen P, van Dijk CN, Zurakowski D, Ring D. Two and three-dimensional computed tomography for the classification and management of distal humeral fractures. Evaluation of reliability and diagnostic accuracy. J Bone Joint Surg Am 2006;88(8):1795–801.

6. Ashwood N, Verma M, Hamlet M, Garlapati A, Fogg Q. Transarticular shear fractures of the distal humerus. J Shoulder Elbow Surg 2010;19(1):46–52.

7. Chamseddine A, Hamdan H, Obeid B, Zein H. [Articular coronal fractures of the distal humerus]. Chir Main 2009;28(6):352–62.

8. Ruchelsman DE, Tejwani NC, Kwon YW, Egol KA. Open reduction and internal fixation of capitellar fractures with headless screws. J Bone Joint Surg Am 2008;90(6):1321–9.

9. Watts AC, Morris A, Robinson CM. Fractures of the distal humeral articular surface. J Bone Joint Surg Br 2007;89(4):510–15.

10. Mejia Silva D, Morales de los Santos R, Cienega Ramos MA, Gonzalez Perez C. [Functional results of two different surgical approaches in patients with distal humerus fractures type C (AO)]. Acta Ortop Mex 2008;22(1):26–30.

11. McKee MD, Wilson TL, Winston L, Schemitsch EH, Richards RR. Functional outcome following surgical treatment of intra-articular distal humeral fractures through a posterior approach. J Bone Joint Surg Am 2000;82(12):1701–7.

12. McKee MD, Kim J, Kebaish K, Stephen DJ, Kreder HJ, Schemitsch EH. Functional outcome after open supracondylar fractures of the humerus. The effect of the surgical approach. J Bone Joint Surg Br 2000;82(5):646–51.

13. Pajarinen J, Bjorkenheim JM. Operative treatment of type C intercondylar fractures of the distal humerus: results after a mean follow-up of 2 years in a series of 18 patients. J Shoulder Elbow Surg 2002;11(1):48–52.

14. Hewins EA, Gofton WT, Dubberly J, MacDermid JC, Faber KJ, King GJ. Plate fixation of olecranon osteotomies. J Orthop Trauma 2007;21(1):58–62.

15. Coles CP, Barei DP, Nork SE, Taitsman LA, Hanel DP, Bradford Henley M. The olecranon osteotomy: a six-year experience in the treatment of intraarticular fractures of the distal humerus. J Orthop Trauma 2006;20(3):164–71.

16. Ring D, Gulotta L, Chin K, Jupiter JB. Olecranon osteotomy for exposure of fractures and nonunions of the distal humerus. J Orthop Trauma 2004;18(7):446–9.

17. Gofton WT, Macdermid JC, Patterson SD, Faber KJ, King GJ. Functional outcome of AO type C distal humeral fractures. J Hand Surg Am 2003;28(2):294–308.

18. Henley MB, Bone LB, Parker B. Operative management of intra-articular fractures of the distal humerus. J Orthop Trauma 1987;1(1):24–35.

19. Ziran BH. A true triceps-splitting approach for treatment of distal humerus fractures: a preliminary report. J Trauma 2005;58(6):1306.

20. Ozer H, Solak S, Turanli S, Baltaci G, Colakoglu T, Bolukbasi S. Intercondylar fractures of the distal humerus treated with the triceps-reflecting anconeus pedicle approach. Arch Orthop Trauma Surg 2005;125(7):469–74.

21. Ek ET, Goldwasser M, Bonomo AL. Functional outcome of complex intercondylar fractures of the distal humerus treated through a triceps-sparing approach. J Shoulder Elbow Surg 2008;17(3):441–6.

22. Ali AM, Hassanin EY, El-Ganainy AE, Abd-Elmola T. Management of intercondylar fractures of the humerus using the extensor mechanism-sparing paratricipital posterior approach. Acta Orthop Belg 2008;74(6):747–52.

23. Schildhauer TA, Nork SE, Mills WJ, Henley MB. Extensor mechanism-sparing paratricipital posterior approach to the distal humerus. J Orthop Trauma 2003;17(5):374–8.

24. Wei DH, Raizman NM, Bottino CJ, Jobin CM, Strauch RJ, Rosenwasser MP. Unstable distal radial fractures treated with external fixation, a radial column plate, or a volar plate. A prospective randomized trial. J Bone Joint Surg Am 2009;91(7): 1568–77.

25. Rozental TD, Blazar PE, Franko OI, Chacko AT, Earp BE, Day CS. Functional outcomes for unstable distal radial fractures treated with open reduction and internal fixation or closed reduction and percutaneous fixation. A prospective randomized trial. J Bone Joint Surg Am 2009;91(8):1837–46.

26. Markmiller M, Konrad G, Sudkamp N. Femur-LISS and distal femoral nail for fixation of distal femoral fractures: are there differences in outcome and complications? Clin Orthop Relat Res 2004;426:252–7.

27. Sang-Jin S, Hoon-Sang S, Nam-Hoon D. A clinical comparison of two different double plating methods for intraarticular distal humerus fractures. J Shoulder Elbow Surg 2010;19(1): 2–9.

28. Ulusal AE, Boz U, Sertoz Z, Ustaoglu RG. [Approaches to distal humeral fractures in adults and comparison of treatment results]. Acta Orthop Traumatol Turc 2006;40(1):22–8.

29. Papaioannou N, Babis GC, Kalavritinos J, Pantazopoulos T. Operative treatment of type C intra-articular fractures of the distal humerus: the role of stability achieved at surgery on final outcome. Injury 1995;26(3):169–73.

30. Huang TL, Chiu FY, Chuang TY, Chen TH. The results of open reduction and internal fixation in elderly patients with severe fractures of the distal humerus: a critical analysis of the results. J Trauma 2005;58(1):62–9.

31. Huang TL, Chiu FY, Chuang TY, Chen TH. Surgical treatment of acute displaced fractures of adult distal humerus with reconstruction plate. Injury 2004;35(11):1143–8.

32. Aslam N, Willett K. Functional outcome following internal fixation of intraarticular fractures of the distal humerus (AO type C). Acta Orthop Belg 2004;70(2):118–22.

33. Helfet DL, Schmeling GJ. Bicondylar intraarticular fractures of the distal humerus in adults. Clin Orthop Relat Res 1993 ;292:26–36.

34. Sanders RA, Raney EM, Pipkin S. Operative treatment of bicondylar intraarticular fractures of the distal humerus. Orthopedics 1992;15(2):159–63.

35. Rebuzzi E, Vascellari A, Schiavetti S. The use of parallel pre-contoured plates in the treatment of A and C fractures of the distal humerus. Musculoskelet Surg. 2010;94(1):9–16.

36. Theivendran K, Duggan PJ, Deshmukh SC. Surgical treatment of complex distal humeral fractures: Functional outcome after internal fixation using precontoured anatomic plates. J Shoulder Elbow Surg 2010;19(4):524–32.

37. Athwal GS, Hoxie SC, Rispoli DM, Steinmann SP. Precontoured parallel plate fixation of AO/OTA type C distal humerus fractures. J Orthop Trauma 2009;23(8):575–80.

38. Atalar AC, Demirhan M, Salduz A, Kilicoglu O, Seyahi A. [Functional results of the parallel-plate technique for complex distal humerus fractures]. Acta Orthop Traumatol Turc 2009; 43(1):21–7.

39. Celli A, Donini MT, Minervini C. The use of pre-contoured plates in the treatment of C2-C3 fractures of the distal humerus: clinical experience. Chir Organi Mov 2008;91(2):57–64.

40. Sanchez-Sotelo J, Torchia ME, O'Driscoll SW. Complex distal humeral fractures: internal fixation with a principle-based parallel-plate technique. J Bone Joint Surg Am 2007;89(5): 961–9.

41. Luegmair M, Timofiev E, Chirpaz-Cerbat JM. Surgical treatment of AO type C distal humeral fractures: internal fixation with a Y-shaped reconstruction (Lambda) plate. J Shoulder Elbow Surg 2008;17(1):113–20.

42. Gupta R, Khanchandani P. Intercondylar fractures of the distal humerus in adults: a critical analysis of 55 cases. Injury 2002;33(6):511–15.

43. Stoffel K, Cunneen S, Morgan R, Nicholls R, Stachowiak G. Comparative stability of perpendicular versus parallel double-locking plating systems in osteoporotic comminuted distal humerus fractures. J Orthop Res 2008;26(6):778–84.

44. Arnander MW, Reeves A, MacLeod IA, Pinto TM, Khaleel A. A biomechanical comparison of plate configuration in distal humerus fractures. J Orthop Trauma 2008;22(5):332–6.

45. Schemitsch EH, Tencer AF, Henley MB. Biomechanical evaluation of methods of internal fixation of the distal humerus. J Orthop Trauma 1994;8(6):468–75.

46. Reising K, Hauschild O, Strohm PC, Suedkamp NP. Stabilisation of articular fractures of the distal humerus: early experience with a novel perpendicular plate system. Injury 2009;40(6):611–17.

47. Greiner S, Haas NP, Bail HJ. Outcome after open reduction and angular stable internal fixation for supra-intercondylar fractures of the distal humerus: preliminary results with the LCP distal humerus system. Arch Orthop Trauma Surg 2008;128(7): 723–9.

48. Korner J, Diederichs G, Arzdorf M, et al. A biomechanical evaluation of methods of distal humerus fracture fixation using locking compression plates versus conventional reconstruction plates. J Orthop Trauma 2004;18(5):286–93.

49. Schuster I, Korner J, Arzdorf M, Schwieger K, Diederichs G, Linke B. Mechanical comparison in cadaver specimens of three different 90-degree double-plate osteosyntheses for simulated C2-type distal humerus fractures with varying bone densities. J Orthop Trauma 2008;22(2):113–20.

50. Ruan HJ, Liu JJ, Fan CY, Jiang J, Zeng BF. Incidence, management, and prognosis of early ulnar nerve dysfunction in type C fractures of distal humerus. J Trauma 2009;67(6):1397–401.

51. Wang KC, Shih HN, Hsu KY, Shih CH. Intercondylar fractures of the distal humerus: routine anterior subcutaneous transposition of the ulnar nerve in a posterior operative approach. J Trauma 1994;36(6):770–3.

52. Doornberg JN, van Duijn PJ, Linzel D, et al. Surgical treatment of intra-articular fractures of the distal part of the humerus. Functional outcome after twelve to thirty years. J Bone Joint Surg Am 2007;89(7):1524–32.

53. Srinivasan K, Agarwal M, Matthews SJ, Giannoudis PV. Fractures of the distal humerus in the elderly: is internal fixation the treatment of choice? Clin Orthop Relat Res 2005;434:222–30.

54. Zagorski JB, Jennings JJ, Burkhalter WE, Uribe JW. Comminuted intraarticular fractures of the distal humeral condyles. Surgical vs. nonsurgical treatment. Clin Orthop Relat Res 1986;202: 197–204.

55. Kundel K, Braun W, Wieberneit J, Ruter A. Intraarticular distal humerus fractures. Factors affecting functional outcome. Clin Orthop Relat Res 1996;332:200–8.

56. Liu JJ, Ruan HJ, Wang JG, Fan CY, Zeng BF. Double-column fixation for type C fractures of the distal humerus in the elderly. J Shoulder Elbow Surg 2009;18(4):646–51.

57. Garland DE, O'Hollaren RM. Fractures and dislocations about the elbow in the head-injured adult. Clin Orthop Relat Res 1982;168:38–41.

58. McKee MD, Veillette CJ, Hall JA, et al. A multicenter, prospective, randomized, controlled trial of open reduction—internal fixation versus total elbow arthroplasty for displaced intra-articular distal humeral fractures in elderly patients. J Shoulder Elbow Surg 2009;18(1):3–12.

59. Charissoux JL, Mabit C, Fourastier J, et al. [Comminuted intra-articular fractures of the distal humerus in elderly patients]. Rev Chir Orthop Reparatrice Appar Mot 2008;94(4 Suppl):S36–62.

60. Jost B, Adams RA, Morrey BF. Management of acute distal humeral fractures in patients with rheumatoid arthritis. A case series. J Bone Joint Surg Am 2008;90(10):2197–205.

61. Prasad N, Dent C. Outcome of total elbow replacement for distal humeral fractures in the elderly: a comparison of primary surgery and surgery after failed internal fixation or conservative treatment. J Bone Joint Surg Br 2008;90(3):343–8.

62. Obremskey WT, Bhandari M, Dirschl DR, Shemitsch E. Internal fixation versus arthroplasty of comminuted fractures of the distal humerus. J Orthop Trauma 2003;17(6):463–5.

63. Frankle MA, Herscovici D, Jr., DiPasquale TG, Vasey MB, Sanders RW. A comparison of open reduction and internal fixation and primary total elbow arthroplasty in the treatment of intraarticular distal humerus fractures in women older than age 65. J Orthop Trauma 2003;17(7):473–80.

44 Fracture-Dislocations of the Elbow

Reyhan A. Chaudhary, Maurice Tompack, and J. Whitcomb Pollock
University of Ottawa, Ottawa, ON, Canada

Case scenarios

Case 1

A 35 year old man presents to the Emergency Department after a downhill skiing injury. He is an otherwise healthy, right hand dominant, high school physical education teacher. On examination he has medial and lateral tenderness, swelling, and ecchymosis of his left elbow. Neurovascular examination is normal. Radiographs demonstrate a fracture-dislocation of the elbow (Figure 44.1).

Case 2

A 20 year old man presents to the Emergency Department after falling while climbing a 10 foot (3 m) fence. He is an otherwise healthy active construction worker. On examination, he has tenderness, swelling and ecchymosis of his left elbow and a normal neurovascular examination. Radiographs reveal a fracture-dislocation of the elbow (Figure 44.2).

Importance of the problem

The incidence of elbow dislocations is approximately 6 in every 100,000 persons during their lifetime[1] and it is the second most commonly dislocated joint in the adult upper limb.[2] Dislocations constitute 10–25% of all injuries to the elbow[3] and occur at a median age of 30 years.[4] These injuries range from simple dislocation with ligamentous and musculotendinous damage to complex fracture-dislocations.

Relevant anatomy

The primary role of the elbow is to position and support the hand in space.[5,6] Stability is derived from highly congruent joint surfaces and capsuloligamentous and musculotendinous soft tissue restraints.[7] The elbow joint consists of three bony articulations: the ulnohumeral, radiocapitellar, and proximal radioulnar (PRUJ) joints.

Stability has both dynamic and static contributions. All muscles crossing the elbow joint contribute to dynamic stability. Static constraints consist of the ulnohumeral and radiocapitellar bony articulations, the medial collateral ligament (MCL), lateral collateral ligament (LCL), and the capsule. The primary stabilizers of the elbow joint are the coronoid, MCL, and LCL.[2,8,9] The secondary constraints consist of the capsule, the radiocapitellar articulation, and the common extensor and flexor origins.[2,8–10] The radial head is also a secondary valgus stabilizer[8] while the coronoid is the primary stabilizer to varus stress[11,12] and an important stabilizer to axial, posteromedial, and posterolateral rotatory forces.[9,10,13]

The MCL originates from the anterior inferior base of the medial epicondyle[13,14] and consists of three distinct bundles: anterior, posterior, and transverse.[2,14] The anterior bundle, which inserts on to the sublime tubercle of the coronoid, is considered the most important ligamentous stabilizer to valgus stress, posteromedial instability, and internal rotation of the ulna.[2,15–17]

The LCL consists of the lateral ulnar collateral ligament (LUCL), the radial collateral ligament (RCL), the annular ligament (AL), and the variably present accessory lateral collateral ligament.[2] The AL wraps around the radial head and neck and inserts on to the anterior and posterior

Evidence-Based Orthopedics, First Edition. Edited by Mohit Bhandari.
© 2012 Blackwell Publishing Ltd. Published 2012 by Blackwell Publishing Ltd.

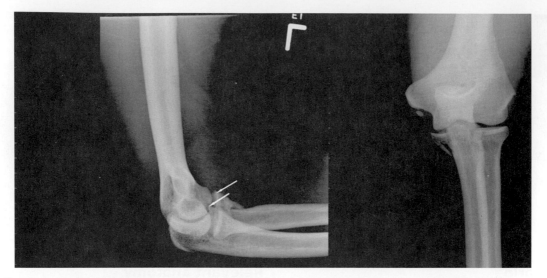

Figure 44.1 Case 1, preoperative AP and lateral radiograph of left elbow.

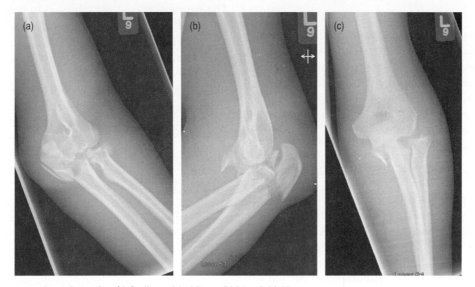

Figure 44.2 Case 2, preoperative radiographs of left elbow: (a) oblique, (b) lateral, (c) AP.

margins of the lesser sigmoid notch of the ulna.[2,15] The RCL and LUCL both originate from the lateral epicondyle.[2,15] The RCL blends with AL and LUCL inserts on to the crista supinatoris of the proximal ulna.[2,18] The LCL is the primary soft tissue stabilizer to varus or posterolateral stress at the elbow.[2,11,12,15–20]

Classification and mechanism of injury

Elbow dislocations have traditionally been classified based on the final resting position of the radius and ulna relative to the distal humerus.[12,21] Dislocations are reported as anterior, divergent, posterior, posterolateral, posteromedial, and pure lateral. This classification provides very little information as to the treatment or prognosis.

O'Driscoll has described the "ring of instability" or the progressive disruption of the LUCL, the capsule, and finally the medial ulnar collateral ligament.[21] O'Driscoll's classification consists of three stages (see box).

O'DriscFoll's classification of elbow subluxation and dislocation

- *Stage 1* involves the disruption of the LUCL
- In *stage 2* the continued force disrupts the remaining lateral ligaments, and the anterior and posterior capsule
- *Stage 3* can involve partial disruption of the MCL (3a) or complete disruption of the MCL (3b).
- *Complete dislocation* is the last of three sequential stages of elbow instability

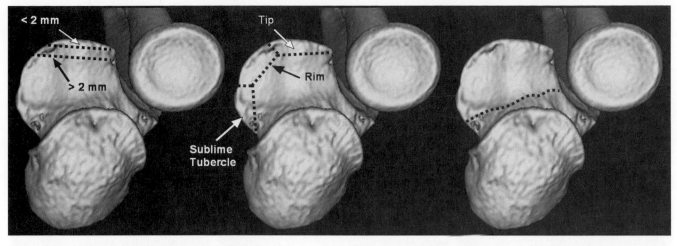

Figure 44.3 O'Driscoll's classification of coronoid fractures.

This chapter focuses on complex elbow dislocations, which by definition have associated fractures. Approximately 2–15% of patients with elbow dislocation have associated coronoid fractures.[2,22] Traditionally coronoid fractures were classified according to the height of the coronoid involved.[23] O'Driscoll has recently classified coronoid fractures to include fractures in the sagittal plane (fractures of the anteromedial facet).[24] Type 1 is a tip fracture, type 2 is an anteromedial facet fracture and type 3 is a fracture through the base. Type 2 fractures are further subdivided based on anatomical location: subtype I involves the rim of the anteromedial facet; subtype II includes the rim and tip; and subtype III involves the rim and the sublime tubercle which provides attachment for the anterior bundle of the MCL[24] (Figure 44.3). Disruption of the LCL and posterior bundle of the MCL are often associated with these injuries.[24]

Top seven questions

Diagnosis

1. What methods can be used to avoid missing the diagnosis of an anteromedial coronoid (AMC) fracture?

Therapy

2. What is the role for nonoperative vs. operative treatment of complex fracture-dislocations of the elbow?
3. When is operative fixation necessary and what the fixation methods are available for AMC fracture management?
4. In the surgical treatment of terrible triad injuries, is it necessary to address and repair the MCL?
5. When faced with a fractured radial head in the setting of a terrible triad elbow injury, is it better to perform open reduction and internal fixation (ORIF) of the fractured radial head or radial head arthroplasty?

Prognosis

6. What complications are associated with operative and nonoperative treatment of AMC fractures?
7. What functional outcomes are reported for the operative treatment of terrible triad elbow injuries?

Question 1: What methods can be used to avoid missing the diagnosis of an AMC fracture?

Case 1 clarification
An orthopedic surgeon reviews the preoperative orthogonal elbow radiographs provided (see Figure 44.1) and diagnoses a coronoid fracture. The surgeon classifies this as being a type 2 coronoid fracture according to O'Driscoll's classification system[24] (see Figure 44.3) and wonders if it represents a subtype III involving the rim and sublime tubercle. Will a CT scan aid in the proper classification and affect treatment of this fracture?

Case 2 clarification
An orthopedic surgeon reviews the preoperative orthogonal elbow radiographs provided (see Figure 44.2) and diagnoses a terrible triad variant injury. The coronoid fracture is complex and is thought to include a large coronal fracture with extension into the anteromedial facet and possibly the sublime tubercle. The radial head fracture is thought to include at least three main fracture fragments. Will a CT scan aid in the proper classification and subsequent treatment choice for this injury?

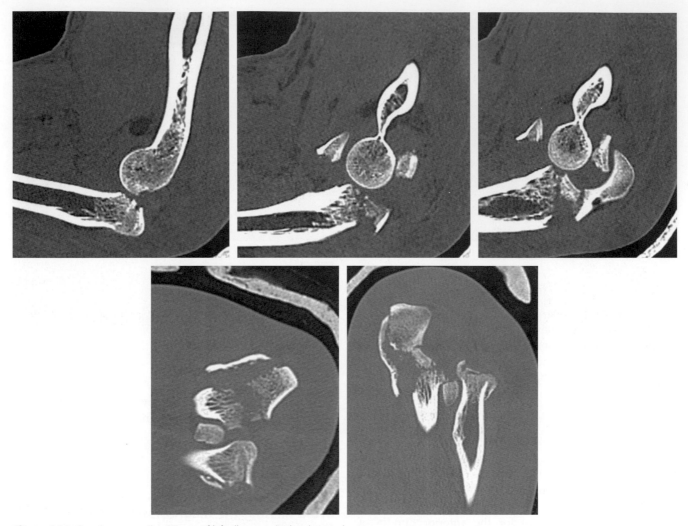

Figure 44.4 Case 2, preoperative CT scan of left elbow: sagittal and coronal cuts.

Relevance

Will more detailed cross-sectional elbow imaging improve treatment and prognosis of this injury? (See Figures 44.4 and 44.5 for for CT scan images of case 2.)

Current opinion

Surgeons use CT to better characterize complex elbow fractures to facilitate preoperative planning.

Finding the evidence

- PubMed (www.ncbi.nlm.nih.gov/pubmed/) sensitivity search using keywords "terrible triad" AND "imaging," "coronoid fracture" AND "imaging," and "radial head fracture" AND "imaging"
- Bibliography of eligible articles

It is recommended to include only the most recent studies in decision-making, as CT imaging protocols have become significantly more advanced over the last few years.

Quality of the evidence

Level III There are limited studies investigating the interobserver/intraobserver agreement between elbow radiographs vs. elbow CT scan on the classification, diagnosis, and treatment of coronoid fractures. However, most experts would agree that a CT scan better evaluates the osseous pattern of complex elbow fractures.

A prospective diagnostic study[25] tested the hypothesis that three-dimensional (3-D) CT reconstructions improve interobserver agreement on the classification and treatment of coronoid fractures when compared to 2-D CT using kappa multirater measure statistics. Twenty-nine orthopedic surgeons evaluated 10 coronoid fractures on 2 occasions, first with radiographs and 2-dimensional CT and then with radiographs and 3-D CT, separated by a minimum of 2 weeks.[25] Three-dimensional CT improved interobserver agreement in Regan and Morrey's classification[23] ($\kappa_{3\text{-}D} = 0.51$ vs. $\kappa_{2\text{-}D} = 0.40$; p < 0.001) and O'Driscoll et al.'s classifications[24] ($\kappa_{3\text{-}D} = 0.48$ vs. $\kappa_{2\text{-}D} = 0.42$; p = 0.009).[25]

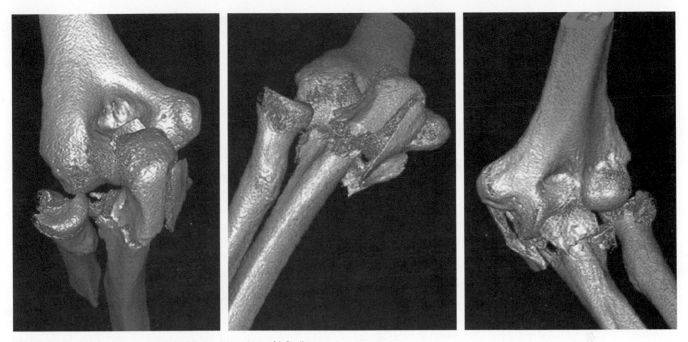

Figure 44.5 Case 2, preoperative 3-D CT reconstructions of left elbow.

There were trends toward better reliability for 3-D reconstruction in recognition of coronoid tip fractures ($\kappa_{3\text{-}D}$ = 0.19, $\kappa_{2\text{-}D}$ = 0.03; p = 0.268), comminution ($\kappa_{3\text{-}D}$ = 0.41 vs. $\kappa_{2\text{-}D}$ = 0.29; p = 0.133), and impacted fragments ($\kappa_{3\text{-}D}$ = 0.39 vs. $\kappa_{2\text{-}D}$ = 0.27; p = 0.094), and in surgeons' opinions on the need for something other than screw and/or plate fixation ($\kappa_{3\text{-}D}$ = 0.31 vs. $\kappa_{2\text{-}D}$ = 0.15; p = 0.138).[25] Interobserver agreement on treatment approach was better with 2-D CT ($\kappa_{3\text{-}D}$ = 0.27, $\kappa_{2\text{-}D}$ = 0.32; p = 0.015).[25]

Level IV: expert opinion radiology Doornberg et al.[18] investigated the interobserver/intraobserver agreement of the coronoid fracture fragment height using elbow CT scan on the classification of coronoid fractures in terrible triad injuries. They examined 3-D CT scans in 13 patients with a terrible triad injury. There were 10 men and 3 women with an average age of 50 years (range 25–73 years). Power analysis indicated that a total sample size of 13 elbows would provide 80% power to detect differences of 1.0 mm with respect to intraobserver and interobserver reliability.[18] Pearson correlations for intraobserver agreement were r = 0.95 and r = 0.97 for coronoid height and r = 0.94 and r = 0.99 for fracture fragment height. For interobserver reliability the correlation was r = 0.94 for coronoid height and r = 0.94 for coronoid fragment height (all p < 0.001).[18] The total height of the coronoid process of the ulna averaged 19 mm (range 12–25 mm). The average height of the coronoid fracture fragment was 7 mm (range 3–12 mm). This corresponds to an average of 35% of the total height of the coronoid process (range 19%–59%).[18]

In terms of the coronoid fracture component of a terrible triad injury, the prospective diagnostic study highlighted in Question 1 on AMC fractures is relevant.[25]

Guitton et al.[26] quantitatively measured the surface 3-D topography of radial head fractures with CT combined with computer analysis software. They analyzed 46 patients with radial head fractures and found that their technique could better qualify the extent of radial head fractures. No interobserver/intraobserver agreement was conducted in this study, nor was the technique compared to traditional elbow radiograph or CT interpretation.

Haapamaki et al.[27] hypothesized that CT of elbow fractures would improve fracture identification and fracture site of origin compared to plain radiographs. A total of 65 fractures and 3 main fracture types were established: 16 (25%) ulnar coronoid process fractures, 13 (20%) radial head fractures, and 12 (18%) humeral supracondylar fractures.[27] CT of the elbow revealed 13 occult fractures in the elbow joint compared to primary radiography.[27] In four patients (7%) a displaced fracture fragment was detected in primary radiography, but the origin of the fragment was unclear.[27] In all four cases, CT revealed the origin of the fragment.[27]

Recommendations
• CT imaging improves the reliability of classification of coronoid fractures [overall quality: moderate]
• 3-D CT improves the reliability of classification over 2-D CT [overall quality: moderate]
• 3-D CT may improve the reliability of classifying radial head fractures [overall quality: low]

• Radiography remains the primary imaging modality in elbow trauma, but in complex fracture patterns CT is a recommended complementary radiographic examination [overall quality: moderate]

• It is not yet known whether more reliable classification leads to more accurate classification, affects surgical management, or improves outcomes.

Question 2: What is the role for nonoperative vs. operative treatment of complex fracture-dislocations of the elbow?

Cases 1 and 2 clarification
In both cases the AMC fracture is displaced. What factures influences the decision between operative vs. nonoperative treatment.

Relevance
The indications for operative treatment for AMC and terrible triad injuries are incompletely defined.

Current opinion
The decision regarding optimal treatment, indications, and type of surgical fixation is unknown and based on expert opinion.

Finding the evidence
• PubMed (www.ncbi.nlm.nih.gov/pubmed/) clinical queries search/systematic reviews, using search term: "coronoid fracture"

• PubMed (www.ncbi.nlm.nih.gov/pubmed/) sensitivity search using keywords "coronoid fracture," as well as "coronoid fracture" AND "treatment"

• PubMed (www.ncbi.nlm.nih.gov/pubmed/) sensitivity search using keywords "terrible triad," "terrible triad" AND "treatment," "terrible triad" AND "nonoperative," "elbow fracture-dislocation" AND "treatment," as well as "elbow fracture-dislocation" AND "nonoperative"

• Bibliography of eligible articles

Quality of the evidence
Level III and IV Dornberg and Ring reported a retrospective case series of 18 consecutive patients with AMC fractures;[28] 15 patients were treated operatively and 3 were treated nonoperatively. At 26 months mean follow-up, all patients (11) with anatomical secure fixation of the AMC achieved good to excellent elbow function. In contrast, all six patients with malalignment of their AMC facets developed early post-traumatic arthrosis and had only a fair or poor result according to the system of Broberg and Morrey.[28] Finally, seven of nine patients with limited treatment of the coronoid fracture had problems with elbow stability.[28]

Pollock et al. biomechanically tested the stability of 10 cadaver elbows under varus and valgus gravitational loading with simulated AMC fractures (subtypes I, II, and III).[10] They demonstrated that the size of the anteromedial facet fracture and the presence of a concomitant LCL injury appear to be important determinants of the need for ORIF. In the varus position, the kinematics of 2.5 mm subtype I fractures with the LCL repaired were similar to those of the intact elbow. However, 5 mm fractures demonstrated a mean of $6.2 \pm 4.5°$ of internal rotation compared with a mean of $3.3 \pm 3.1°$ of external rotation in the intact elbow ($p < 0.05$). In the varus position, subtype II 2.5 mm fractures with the LCL repaired demonstrated increased internal rotation (mean $7.0 \pm 4.5°$; $p < 0.005$). Subtype II 5 mm fractures demonstrated instability in both the varus and valgus positions ($p < 0.05$). Subtype III fractures with the LCL repaired were unstable in all three testing positions ($p < 0.05$). This study suggests that the size of the coronoid fracture fragment affects elbow kinematics, particularly with varus stress. The study demonstrated that even small AMC fractures affect elbow kinematics. The authors suggested that internal fixation of AMC facet fractures larger than 2.5 mm should be considered and that LCL repair alone should not be expected to restore kinematics in the majority of patients with this injury. Only small O'Driscoll yype 2 (subtype I) fractures, with an intact MCL, can be treated with isolated LCL repair with a strict rehabilitation protocol.

A retrospective cohort study investigated the effect of delayed operative treatment (initial period of nonoperative treatment) on elbow function of patients with a terrible triad injuries.[29] Acute terrible triad patients (18) who had surgery an average of 6 days after injury were compared with patients who had delayed operative treatment (14) an average of 7 weeks after injury. The authors concluded that stability and strength were restored with both acute and subacute treatment, but earlier treatment is more straightforward and is associated with a better flexion arc (116° in the acute cohort and 93° in the subacute cohort).[29] Broberg and Morrey scores were comparable between cohorts (90 vs. 87 points).[29]

Finally, a study by Ring et al.[30] looked at 11 patients with a terrible triad injury who were evaluated after a minimum of 2 years. None of these patients had surgery on their coronoid fractures. The radial head fracture component of this injury was repaired in five patients, the radial head was resected in four, and the LCL was repaired in only three patients. All 11 patients returned for clinical examination, functional evaluation, and radiographs. Seven elbows redislocated in a splint after manipulative reduction.[30] Five, including all four treated with resection of the radial head, redislocated after operative treatment. At the time of final follow-up, three patients were considered to have a failure of the initial treatment. One of them had recurrent instability, which was treated with a total elbow arthroplasty after multiple unsuccessful operations; one had severe arthrosis and instability resembling neuropathic arthropathy; and one had an elbow flexion contracture and proximal radioulnar synostosis requiring reconstructive surgery.[30] The remaining eight patients, who were evaluated at an average of 7 years after injury, had an average of 92° (range 40–130°) of ulnohumeral motion and 126° (range 40–170°) of forearm rotation. The average Broberg and Morrey functional score was 76 points (range 34–98 points), with two results rated as excellent, two as good, three as fair, and one as poor.[30] Overall, the result of treatment was rated as unsatisfactory for 7 of the 11 patients. All four patients with a satisfactory result had retained the radial head, and two had undergone repair of the LCL. Of the 10 patients who did not go on to have a total elbow arthroplasty, 7 had radiographic signs of advanced ulnohumeral arthrosis.[30] Ulnohumeral arthrosis was less severe in those patients who had internal fixation of their radial head rather than surgical excision.[30]

Recommendations

There is evidence to suggest that operative treatment will produce consistently better outcomes for displaced AMC fractures than nonoperative treatment. Further clinical studies are needed to determine patient outcomes following operative treatment and the effectiveness of internal fixation of these fractures.

There is a general lack of evidence with regards to nonoperative treatment of terrible triad injuries. This lack of literature partially reflects the fact that these elbow injuries have significant instability requiring surgical management.

• A biomechanical study suggests that nonoperative treatment of a displaced coronoid fracture fragment larger than 2.5 mm will affect elbow kinematics [overall quality: moderate]

• Nonoperative treatment of terrible triad elbow fracture-dislocations can be attempted in minimally displaced, well-aligned fractures; however, parameters for this choice of treatment need to be further ironed out [overall quality: low]

• The results of early surgical treatment of terrible triad elbow injuries are superior to delayed. However, delayed fixation can still achieve good results [overall quality: moderate]

• Failure to repair the coronoid and/or the LCL may result in unsatisfactory patient outcomes following operative treatment for this injury [overall quality: low]

Question 3: When is operative fixation necessary and what fixation methods are available for AMC fracture management?

Case clarification

Radiographs and 2-D and 3D-CT show a type 2 subtype III AMC fracture in case 1 (see Figure 44.1) and a complex transolecranon type 2 subtype III coronoid fracture involv-

ing the rim, tip, and sublime tubercle in case 2 (see Figures 44.4 and 44.5). Should these patients undergo surgical management? Furthermore, if surgery is performed, what type of internal fixation is optimal for these fractures?

Relevance

Difficulties associated with loss of fixation, nonunion, malunion can potentially lead to poor functional outcomes such as elbow arthrosis.

Current opinion

There is a lack of consensus regarding the optimal internal fixation: sutures, Kirschner wires, screws, or buttress plate fixation have all been suggested.

Finding the evidence

• PubMed (www.ncbi.nlm.nih.gov/pubmed/) clinical queries search/ systematic reviews, using search term: "coronoid fracture"

• PubMed (www.ncbi.nlm.nih.gov/pubmed/) sensitivity search using keywords "coronoid fracture," as well as "coronoid fracture" AND "internal fixation" or "operative treatment"

• Bibliography of eligible articles

Quality of the evidence

Level IV—biomechanical study Although not specific to AMC fractures, a biomechanical study by Moon et al. compared the stability of coronoid fractures internally fixated with a 2.7 mm cortical screw inserted in the anteroposterior (AP) direction with the stability of a screw inserted in the posteroanterior (PA) direction.[31] They examined 11 pairs of fresh-frozen cadaveric ulnas and simulated a type II coronal coronoid fracture in these elbows via an osteotomy. This study found that PA screw placement yielded greater strength and stiffness of fixation than AP placement. The mean load to failure was 184 N in the PA screw group and 131 N in the AP screw group (p < 0.05).[31] The mean stiffness was 106 N/mm with PA screws and 76 N/mm with AP screws (p < 0.05).[31] These differences were statistically significant despite the fact that the screw insertion torque was similar in the PA screw (0.27 Nm) and the AP screw (0.25 Nm) (p = 0.2).[31]

Recommendation

There is insufficient clinical evidence from the literature to determine the preferred (operative) intervention in patients with AMC fractures. Biomechanical studies suggest that a PA screw is preferred to an AP screw when screw fixation is used for coronal fractures of the coronoid. There are no studies comparing the fixation options for AMC fracture subtypes which could include sutures, screws, Kirschner wires, plate, or combinations depending on the size and fracture pattern.

• Regardless of fixation used, biomechanical studies suggest that repair of the LCL is critical with this type of injury and ORIF should be performed when the size of the anteromedial facet fracture is greater than 2.5 mm.[10]

Question 4: In the surgical treatment of terrible triad injuries, is it necessary to address and repair the MCL?

Case 2 clarification

Radiographs and 2-D and 3D-CT demonstrate a variant terrible triad fracture-dislocation injury to the elbow. Both the patient and surgeon elect operative treatment. When should the MCL ligament be repaired?

Relevance

Surgeons must decide when MCL repair is necessary to provide adequate stability to allow early postoperative mobilization

Current opinion

There is a lack of consensus regarding when a torn MCL should be repaired in the setting of a terrible triad injury. Some surgeons believe that the MCL should be addressed if the elbow still demonstrates instability following surgery to the radial head, coronoid, and LCL.[32]

Finding the evidence

• PubMed (www.ncbi.nlm.nih.gov/pubmed/) clinical queries search/ systematic reviews, using search term: "terrible triad"
• PubMed (www.ncbi.nlm.nih.gov/pubmed/) sensitivity search using keywords "terrible triad," "terrible triad" AND "medial collateral ligament," "terrible triad" AND "MCL," "elbow fracture-dislocation" AND "medial collateral ligament," as well as "elbow fracture-dislocation" AND "MCL"
• Bibliography of eligible articles

Quality of the evidence

Level III Forthman et al.[33] reviewed the functional outcomes obtained after not repairing the MCL of 34 patients who had suffered an elbow dislocation with an intra-articular fracture. They hypothesized that it was unnecessary to repair the MCL if a patient's fracture and LCL were properly repaired. Of the 34 patients included in this study, 22 had a terrible triad injury. After a mean follow-up of 32 months, the authors noted that one patient with a terrible triad injury had postoperative instability related to non-compliance. Patients with terrible triad injuries had an average of 117° of ulnohumeral motion and 137° forearm rotation.[33] Seventeen of 22 patients (77%) had good or excellent results.[33]

A second study, by Jeong et al.,[34] retrospectively evaluated the functional outcomes following surgical treatment of terrible triad injuries, where all damaged medial structures were repaired. They found that concentric elbow stability was restored in all 13 patients with a mean follow-up of 25 months.[34] The flexion-extension arc of the elbow averaged 128° and forearm rotation averaged 134.6°.[34] The mean Mayo Elbow Performance Score was 95 points (range 85–100), which corresponded to 10 excellent results and 3 good results.[34]

Finally, a biomechanical study by Pollock et al.[35] evaluated the role of type II coronoid fracture fixation and collateral ligament repair in complex elbow fracture/dislocations. They submitted six fresh-frozen cadaver arms to passive varus and valgus and simulated active vertical motion. Varus/valgus angle and internal/external rotation were measured with the coronoid intact, with 50% removed, and after ORIF. Testing was performed with the collateral ligaments detached and repaired.[35] The results of this study showed that the vertical stability of the elbows were normal when both the collateral ligaments were repaired, regardless of the state of the coronoid. Elbow kinematics were altered with a repaired LCL, incompetent MCL, and type II coronoid fractures (p < 0.05).[35] On the basis of these results, the authors suggested that repair of type II coronoid fractures and injured collateral ligaments should be performed whenever possible.[35]

Recommendations

For the terrible triad injury:
• It appears that MCL repair is not always necessary to obtain elbow stability in this injury pattern. Clinical studies with longer follow-up are required [overall quality: low–moderate]
• Good elbow functional outcomes can be obtained whether or not the MCL is repaired in the surgical management of this injury. Specific rehabilitation protocols should be followed and further clinical studies with longer follow-up are required [overall quality: moderate]
• If instability persists, after repair of the radial head, coronoid and LCL, repair of the MCL should be considered.

Question 5: When faced with a fractured radial head in the setting of a terrible triad elbow injury, is it better to perform ORIF of the fractured radial head or radial head arthroplasty?

Case 2 clarification

Radiographs and 2-D and 3-D CT show a three-fragment radial head fracture associated with this terrible triad variant elbow injury. The patient and surgeon elect operative treatment. Should the surgeon perform ORIF or radial head arthroplasty?

Relevance

Difficulties associated with loss of fixation, nonunion, and malunion following ORIF of radial head fractures associated with terrible triad elbow injuries can potentially lead to poor functional outcomes. Similarly, radial head arthroplasty is not without its own set of postoperative problems and complications.

Current opinion

There is a lack of consensus regarding the optimal treatment of radial head fractures in the setting of a terrible triad elbow injury. Most authors would agree that a stable radial head (native or arthroplasty) is required to obtain stability.

Finding the evidence

- PubMed (www.ncbi.nlm.nih.gov/pubmed/) clinical queries search/ systematic reviews, using searchterm: "terrible triad"
- PubMed (www.ncbi.nlm.nih.gov/pubmed/) sensitivity search using keywords "terrible triad," "terrible triad" AND "radial head fractures," "terrible triad" AND "Mason fractures," "elbow fracture-dislocation" AND "radial head fractures," as well as "elbow fracture-dislocation" AND "Mason fractures"
- Bibliography of eligible articles

Quality of the evidence

Level III Winter et al.[36] followed 13 consecutive terrible triad patients treated with radial head arthroplasty. At 25 months, all elbows were stable and 84% of the patients were satisfied with an average elbow flexion of 131° (range 110–140°),

average elbow extension of −11° (range −30 to 0°), average pronation of 72° (range 40–80°), and average supination of 70° (range 50–80°).[36] The grip strength averaged 75% of that of the noninjured side (range 50–105%).[36]

Recommendation

There is insufficient clinical evidence to determine the preferred (operative) intervention in patients with radial head fractures in the setting of terrible triad elbow injuries. Patients with this injury pattern can do well functionally with ORIF or arthroplasty of their radial head. Isolated Mason type II radial head fractures can do well with conservative management when there is 2–5 mm of fracture displacement.[37] There is also evidence suggesting that Mason Type-III fractures with four or more fragments function poorly following ORIF and may benefit from radial head arthroplasty at the initial surgical sitting.[38]

Question 6: What complications are associated with operative and nonoperative treatment of AMC fractures?

Cases 1 and 2 clarification

The patient and surgeon elect operative treatment. ORIF is performed through a posterior incision and deep Taylor approach. The LCL was repaired in both patients. Radiographs illustrate the internal fixation used (see Figures 44.6 for postoperative radiographs of case 1, and Figures 44.7 and 44.8 for postoperative radiographs of case 2). What are the potential complications?

The patient in case 2 goes on to complain of hardware prominence and elbow stiffness at 6 months postoperatively. He undergoes hardware removal and open release

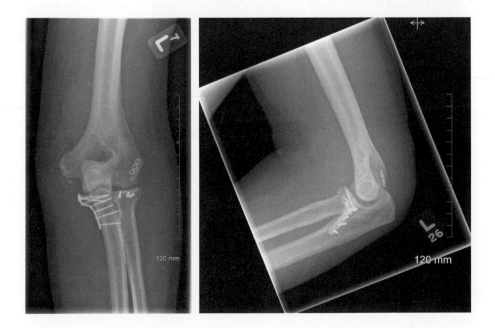

Figure 44.6 Case 1, postoperative radiographs of left elbow following ORIF of the AMC and the radial head and LCL repair.

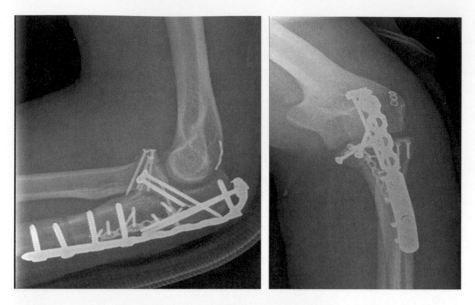

Figure 44.7 Case 2, immediate postoperative radiographs of the left elbow (following ORIF of the left elbow).

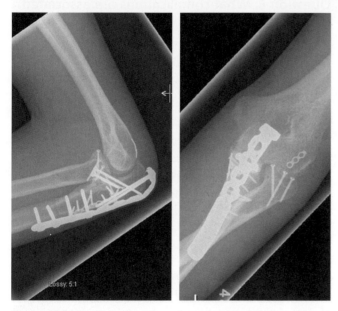

Figure 44.8 Case 2, postoperative radiographs of the left elbow taken at the 3 month postoperative follow-up patient visit.

of their elbow contracture (see Figure 44.9 for 9 month postoperative radiographs).

Relevance

Complications can impair a patient's postoperative recovery and can potentially worsen functional outcome following surgery.

Current opinion

Postoperative complications following AMC fracture fixation can include, but are not limited to, infection, bleeding, malunion, nonunion, symptomatic hardware, failure of fixation, nerve injury, arthrosis, elbow contracture, and heterotopic ossification.

Finding the evidence

- PubMed (www.ncbi.nlm.nih.gov/pubmed/) clinical queries search/systematic reviews, using search term: "coronoid fracture"
- PubMed (www.ncbi.nlm.nih.gov/pubmed/) sensitivity search using keywords "coronoid fracture," "coronoid fracture" AND "complication," and "anteromedial coronoid" AND "complication"
- Bibliography of eligible articles

Quality of the evidence

Level III: therapeutic Many studies in the literature can be found highlighting the long-term complications from both operative and nonoperative treatment of elbow dislocations with and without coronoid fractures. Despite this abundant literature, there is a lack of data on complications relating specifically to AMC fractures.

The study highlighted in Question 3 includes some data on complications related to AMC fractures. This case series examined 18 consecutive patients with AMC fractures,[28] 15 of whom were treated operatively and 3 were treated nonoperatively. At 26 months mean follow-up, Dornberg and Ring reported good to excellent elbow function in all patients (11) when anatomic secure fixation of AMC was achieved. These authors also reported on six patients who had malalignment of their AMC facets, because either their anteromedial facet fracture was not specifically treated (four patients) or because there was loss of anatomic fracture fixation (two patients). All six of these patients had development of arthrosis due to varus posteromedial subluxation of their elbow and had a fair or poor result according to the system of Broberg and Morrey.[28]

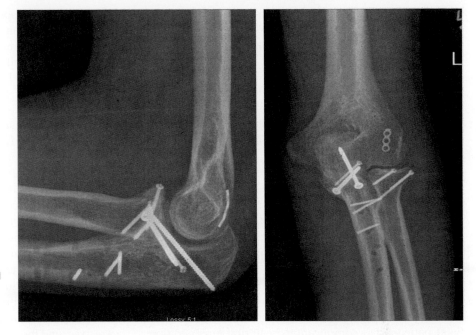

Figure 44.9 Case 2, postoperative radiographs of the left elbow taken 9 months after the initial surgery. These radiographs were taken postoperatively following a second surgery where a partial hardware removal was performed as well as an open soft tissue contracture release.

Recommendation

There is insufficient clinical evidence from the literature on AMC fractures to highlight the complications associated with the treatment of this injury. Complications can be extrapolated from the literature on other complex elbow fracture-dislocations. Common complications following treatment for terrible triad injuries include infection, malunion, nonunion, elbow instability, elbow stiffness, heterotopic ossification, hardware-related problems, and ulnar neuropathy.[21,32,33,39,40] Pugh et al. quoted a 24% complication rate using a standardized surgical protocol to treat 34 terrible triad elbow injuries with a mean follow-up of 34 months.[41]

Question 7: What functional outcomes are reported for the operative treatment of terrible triad elbow injuries?

Case 2 clarification

The patient and surgeon elect operative treatment. Radiographs illustrate the internal fixation used (see Figures 44.7 and 44.8). What functional outcomes can we expect following operative treatment of terrible triad elbow fracture-dislocations?

Relevance

The type of operative treatment for terrible triad injuries is influenced by patient outcomes.

Current opinion

Many surgeons advocate specific surgical protocols or algorithms to treat these complex elbow fracture-dislocations.

Finding the evidence

- PubMed (www.ncbi.nlm.nih.gov/pubmed/) clinical queries search/systematic reviews, using search term: "terrible triad"
- PubMed (www.ncbi.nlm.nih.gov/pubmed/) sensitivity search using keywords "terrible triad," "terrible triad" AND "functional outcome," and "elbow fracture-dislocation" AND " functional outcome"
- Bibliography of eligible articles

Quality of the evidence

Level III and level IV Ring et al.[30] evaluated 11 patients with a terrible triad injuries after a minimum of 2 years. None of these patients underwent fixation of their coronoid fractures. The radial head fracture was repaired in five patients, and the radial head was resected in four; the LCL was repaired in only three patients. All 11 patients returned for follow-up clinical examination, functional evaluation, and radiographs. Of the 11 patients with follow-up, 7 elbows redislocated.[30] Five, including all four treated with resection of the radial head, redislocated after operative treatment. At final follow-up, three patients were considered to have a failure of the initial treatment. One of them had recurrent instability, which was treated with a total elbow arthroplasty after multiple unsuccessful operations; one had severe arthrosis and instability resembling neuropathic arthropathy; and one had an elbow flexion contracture and proximal radioulnar synostosis requiring reconstructive surgery.[30] The remaining eight patients, who were evaluated at an average of 7 years after injury, had an average of 92° (range 40–130°) of ulnohumeral motion and 126° (range 40–170°) of forearm rotation.[30] The average Broberg and Morrey functional score was 76 points (range 34–98 points), with two results rated as excellent, two as good, three as fair, and one as poor.[30] Overall, the result of treatment was rated as unsatisfactory for 7 of the 11 patients.[30] All four patients with a satisfactory result had retained the radial head, and two had undergone repair of the LCL. Seven patients had radiographic signs of advanced ulnohumeral arthrosis.[30] Ulnohumeral arthrosis was less severe in those patients who had internal fixation of their radial head rather than surgical excision.[30]

Pugh et al.[41] reviewed the results of an operative treatment algorithm performed in 36 consecutive patients with a terrible triad elbow injury. Mean follow-up was 34 months. They found a flexion-extension arc of 112 ± 11° and forearm rotation averaging 136 ± 16°. The mean Mayo Elbow Performance Score was 88 points (range 45–100 points), which corresponded to 15 excellent results, 13 good results, 7 fair results, and 1 poor result.[41] Concentric stability was restored to 34 elbows.[41] Approximately 25% of patients had a complication following surgery. Eight patients had complications requiring a reoperation: two had a synostosis; one, recurrent instability; four, hardware removal and elbow release; and one, a wound infection.[41]

Zeiders et al.[42] reported on 32 patients who underwent operative treatment for their terrible triad injury. All patients had repair of the coronoid–brachialis complex.[42] The radial head was noted to be intact in six elbows. The radial head was successfully reconstructed in 7 of 13 cases in which reconstruction was attempted, and it was replaced in 19 cases.[42] A lateral repair alone was performed in 18 cases, a medial repair was performed in 2 cases, and a combined medial and lateral repair was performed in 12 cases.[42] Twenty-one elbows required protection in a hinged external fixator. After a mean follow-up of 3 years, all 32 elbows had a functional arc of motion from 30° to 130°.[42] The mean extension loss was 12° (range 0–20°), the mean flexion loss was 14° (range 0–20°), and a full range of motion was exhibited by three patients.[42] The average DASH score was 23 (range 19–28).[42] Three patients developed heterotopic ossification as a complication.

Another study by Chemama et al.[43] reported on 23 terrible triad injuries in 22 patients. ORIF of the radial head was performed in 13 cases and arthroplasty in 4 cases. The coronoid fracture was treated with ORIF in 10 cases. All torn ligaments were repaired which included 19 LCL repairs and 6 MCL repairs.[43] Of these 22 patients, 13 patients (14 elbows) had a mean follow-up of 63 months.[43] All patients had a stable elbow joint and 90% of patients reported mild or no elbow pain. The arc of extension–flexion ranged from 18° to 127°, while the average pronation-supination arc was 134°.[43] The mean Mayo Elbow Performance Score was 87. Only one patient developed symptomatic osteoarthritis at 8 years.[43]

Chen et al.[44] retrospectively evaluated the functional outcomes of operative management of terrible triad injuries in 10 patients with a mean follow-up of 24.9 months. These authors used a similar surgical approach. They fixed the coronoid and radial head and repaired the anterior capsule and LCL. Repair of the MCL along with a mobile-hinged external fixation was used in three patients. Elbow range of motion was measured at 6 months. The mean flexion–extension arc was 106.5° (range 85–130°), and the mean pronation–supination arc was 138° (range 100–160°).[44] The Hospital for Special Surgery Total Elbow Scoring System was excellent in four cases, good in four cases, and fair in two cases.[44] Complications included one radial nerve injury, six patients who developed heterotopic ossification, and one patient who developed radiographic signs of subluxation.[44]

Finally, Xun et al. retrospectively evaluated the functional outcomes after operative management of terrible triad injuries in 9 patients with a mean follow-up of 31 ± 6 months.[45] These authors used a similar surgical approach to that of previous authors. The coronoid and radial head were fixed, and the LCL and anterior capsule were repaired. If there was residual valgus instability the MCL was repaired. At 3 months follow-up, the mean flexion and extension arch was (102 ± 3)° (range 80–110°), and the mean pronation and supination arch of the forearm was (135 ± 6)° (range 100–150°).[45] According to the Mayo Elbow Scoring System, the results were excellent in five cases, good in three cases, and fair in one case. Complications included heterotopic ossification in three patients.[45]

Recommendation

- There is insufficient clinical evidence from the literature to state that a specific surgical protocol is better than another. However, there is sufficient evidence to suggest that a systematic approach to the operative treatment of terrible triad injuries is important and obtains good functional results [overall quality: moderate]

Summary of recommendations

- It is not yet known whether more reliable classification leads to more accurate classification, affects surgical management, or improves outcomes
- CT imaging improves the reliability of classification of coronoid fractures
- 3-D CT improves the reliability of classification over 2-D CT and may improve the reliability of classifying radial head fractures
- Radiography remains the primary imaging modality in elbow trauma, but in complex fracture patterns CT is a recommended complementary radiographic examination
- Biomechanical studies suggest that nonoperative treatment of a displaced coronoid fracture fragment larger than 2.5 mm will affect elbow kinematics

- Nonoperative treatment of terrible triad elbow fracture-dislocations can be attempted in minimally displaced, well-aligned fractures; however, parameters for this choice of treatment need to be further ironed out
- The results of early surgical treatment of terrible triad elbow injuries are superior to delayed. However, delayed fixation can still achieve good results
- Failure to repair the coronoid and/or the LCL may result in unsatisfactory patient outcomes following operative treatment for this injury
- Repair of the LCL is critical with this type of injury and ORIF should be performed when the size of the anteromedial facet fracture is greater than 2.5 mm
- It appears that MCL repair is not always necessary to obtain elbow stability in terrible triad injury. Clinical studies with longer follow-up are required
- Good elbow functional outcomes can be obtained whether or not the MCL is repaired in the surgical management of terrible triad injury. Specific rehabilitation protocols should be followed and further clinical studies with longer follow-up are required
- If instability persists, after repair of the radial head, coronoid and LCL, repair of the MCL should be considered
- Common complications following treatment for terrible triad injuries include infection, malunion, nonunion, elbow instability, elbow stiffness, heterotopic ossification, hardware-related problems, and ulnar neuropathy
- A systematic approach to the operative treatment of terrible triad injuries is important and obtains good functional results

References

1. Bucholz RW, Heckman JD, eds. Rockwood and Green's Fractures in Adults, 5th edn. Lippincott Williams & Wilkins, Philadelphia, 2001.
2. Morrey BF. The Elbow and its Disorders, 3rd edn. Saunders, Philadelphia, 2001.
3. Mehlhoff TL, Noble PC, Bennett JB, Tullos HS. Simple dislocation of the elbow in the adult. Results after closed treatment. J Bone Joint Surg Am 1988;70(2):244–9.
4. Josefsson PO, Nilsson BE. Incidence of elbow dislocation. Acta Orthop Scand 1986;57(6):537–8.
5. Magee DJ. Orthopedic Physical Assessment, 4th enhanced edn. Elsevier Saunders, Philadelphia, 2006.
6. Miyasaka KC. Anatomy of the elbow. Orthop Clin North Am 1999;30(1):1–13.
7. Morrey BF, An KN. Articular and ligamentous contributions to the stability of the elbow joint. Am J Sports Med 1983;11(5):315–19.
8. Morrey BF, Tanaka S, An KN. Valgus stability of the elbow. A definition of primary and secondary constraints. Clin Orthop Relat Res 1991;265:187–95.
9. Beingessner DM, Stacpoole RA, Dunning CE, Johnson JA, King GJ. The effect of suture fixation of type I coronoid fractures on the kinematics and stability of the elbow with and without medial collateral ligament repair. J Shoulder Elbow Surg 2007; 16(2):213–17.
10. Pollock JW, Brownhill J, Ferreira L, McDonald CP, Johnson J, King G. The effect of anteromedial facet fractures of the coronoid and lateral collateral ligament injury on elbow stability and kinematics. J Bone Joint Surg Am 2009;91(6):1448–58.
11. Cohen MS, Hastings H. Rotatory instability of the elbow. The anatomy and role of the lateral stabilizers. J Bone Joint Surg Am 1997;79(2):225–33.
12. Cohen MS, Hastings H. Acute elbow dislocation: evaluation and management. J Am Acad Orthop Surg 1998;6(1):15–23.
13. Schneeberger AG, Sadowski MM, Jacob HA. Coronoid process and radial head as posterolateral rotatory stabilizers of the elbow. J Bone Joint Surg Am 2004;86(5):975–82.
14. Fuss FK. The ulnar collateral ligament of the human elbow joint. Anatomy, function and biomechanics. J Anat 1991;175:203–12.
15. Seki A, Olsen BS, Jensen SL, Eygendaal D, Sojbjerg JO. Functional anatomy of the lateral collateral ligament complex of the elbow: configuration of Y and its role. J Shoulder Elbow Surg 2002; 11(1):53–9.
16. Regan WD, Korinek SL, Morrey BF, An KN. Biomechanical study of ligaments around the elbow joint. Clin Orthop Relat Res 1991;271:170–9.
17. Olsen BS, Sojbjerg JO, Nielsen KK, Vaesel MT, Dalstra M, Sneppen O. Posterolateral elbow joint instability: the basic kinematics. J Shoulder Elbow Surg 1998;7(1):19–29.
18. Doornberg JN, van DJ, Ring D. Coronoid fracture height in terrible-triad injuries. J Hand Surg Am 2006;31(5):794–7.
19. O'Driscoll SW, Bell DF, Morrey BF. Posterolateral rotatory instability of the elbow. J Bone Joint Surg Am 1991;73(3):440–6.
20. Dunning CE, Zarzour ZD, Patterson SD, Johnson JA, King GJ. Ligamentous stabilizers against posterolateral rotatory instability of the elbow. J Bone Joint Surg Am 2001;83(12):1823–8.
21. O'Driscoll SW, Morrey BF, Korinek S, An KN. Elbow subluxation and dislocation. A spectrum of instability. Clin Orthop Relat Res 1992;280:186–97.
22. Selesnick FH, Dolitsky B, Haskell SS. Fracture of the coronoid process requiring open reduction with internal fixation. A case report. J Bone Joint Surg Am 1984;66(8):1304–6.
23. Regan W, Morrey BF. Classification and treatment of coronoid process fractures. Orthopedics 1992;15(7):845–8.
24. O'Driscoll SW, Jupiter JB, Cohen MS, Ring D, McKee MD. Difficult elbow fractures: pearls and pitfalls. Instr Course Lect 2003;52:113–34.
25. Lindenhovius A, Karanicolas PJ, Bhandari M, van DN, Ring D. Interobserver reliability of coronoid fracture classification: two-dimensional versus three-dimensional computed tomography. J Hand Surg Am 2009;34(9):1640–6.
26. Guitton TG, van der Werf HJ, Ring D. Quantitative three-dimensional computed tomography measurement of radial head fractures. J Shoulder Elbow Surg 2010;19(7):973–7.
27. Haapamaki VV, Kiuru MJ, Koskinen SK. Multidetector computed tomography diagnosis of adult elbow fractures. Acta Radiol 2004;45(1):65–70.
28. Doornberg JN, Ring DC. Fracture of the anteromedial facet of the coronoid process. J Bone Joint Surg Am 2006;88(10):2216–24.
29. Lindenhovius AL, Jupiter JB, Ring D. Comparison of acute versus subacute treatment of terrible triad injuries of the elbow. J Hand Surg Am 2008;33(6):920–6.

30. Ring D, Jupiter JB, Zilberfarb J. Posterior dislocation of the elbow with fractures of the radial head and coronoid. J Bone Joint Surg Am 2002;84(4):547–51.

31. Moon JG, Zobitz ME, An KN, O'Driscoll SW. Optimal screw orientation for fixation of coronoid fractures. J Orthop Trauma 2009;23(4):277–80.

32. McKee MD, Pugh DM, Wild LM, Schemitsch EH, King GJ. Standard surgical protocol to treat elbow dislocations with radial head and coronoid fractures. Surgical technique. J Bone Joint Surg Am 2005;87(Suppl 1 Pt 1):22–32.

33. Forthman C, Henket M, Ring DC. Elbow dislocation with intra-articular fracture: the results of operative treatment without repair of the medial collateral ligament. J Hand Surg Am 2007;32(8):1200–9.

34. Jeong WK, Oh JK, Hwang JH, Hwang SM, Lee WS. Results of terrible triads in the elbow: the advantage of primary restoration of medial structure. J Orthop Sci 2010;15(5):612–9.

35. Pollock JW, Pichora J, Brownhill J, Ferreira LM, McDonald CP, Johnson JA, et al. The influence of type II coronoid fractures, collateral ligament injuries, and surgical repair on the kinematics and stability of the elbow: an in vitro biomechanical study. J Shoulder Elbow Surg 2009;18(3):408–17.

36. Winter M, Chuinard C, Cikes A, Pelegri C, Bronsard N, de Peretti F. Surgical management of elbow dislocation associated with non-reparable fractures of the radial head. Chir Main 2009;28(3):158–67.

37. Akesson T, Herbertsson P, Josefsson PO, Hasserius R, Besjakov J, Karlsson MK. Primary nonoperative treatment of moderately displaced two-part fractures of the radial head. J Bone Joint Surg Am 2006;88(9):1909–14.

38. Ring D, Quintero J, Jupiter JB. Open reduction and internal fixation of fractures of the radial head. J Bone Joint Surg Am 2002;84-A(10):1811–5.

39. Pugh DM, McKee MD. The "terrible triad" of the elbow. Tech Hand Up Extrem Surg 2002;6(1):21–9.

40. Ring D. Fractures of the coronoid process of the ulna. J Hand Surg Am 2006 Dec;31(10):1679–89.

41. Pugh DM, Wild LM, Schemitsch EH, King GJ, McKee MD. Standard surgical protocol to treat elbow dislocations with radial head and coronoid fractures. J Bone Joint Surg Am 2004;86(6):1122–30.

42. Zeiders GJ, Patel MK. Management of unstable elbows following complex fracture-dislocations—the "terrible triad" injury. J Bone Joint Surg Am 2008;90(Suppl 4):75–84.

43. Chemama B, Bonnevialle N, Peter O, Mansat P, Bonnevialle P. Terrible triad injury of the elbow: how to improve outcomes? Orthop Traumatol Surg Res 2010;96(2):147–54.

44. Chen S, Huang F, Hu X, Cen S, Xiang Z. [Operative treatment of terrible triad of the elbow]. Zhongguo Xiu Fu Chong Jian Wai Ke Za Zhi 2009;23(1):45–8.

45. Xun BT, Zhi RL, Lin Y, Qu TB. [Clinical outcome of surgical treatment of terrible triad of elbow]. Zhongguo Gu Shang 2010;23(9):650–3.

45 Radial Head Fractures

Andrea S. Bauer and David Ring

Massachusetts General Hospital, Boston, MA, USA

Case scenario

A 36-year-old woman is brought to the Emergency Department with elbow pain after a fall onto her outstretched left hand while skating. On examination, her range of elbow motion is limited due to pain, and she has tenderness over the radial head.

Relevant anatomy

Radial head fractures were classified as types I–III by Mason (se box).[1] Broberg and Morrey made the following modifications: (1) they added fractures of the radial neck; (2) defined "marginal" as less than 30% of the articular surface area; and (3) defined displacement as 2 mm step or gap of the articular surface.[2]

Mason's classification of radial head fractures
- Type I: nondisplaced or small marginal fractures
- Type II: displaced articular fractures involving part of the radial head
- Type III: displaced articular fractures of the entire radial head

Top five questions

Diagnosis

1. What is the role of aspiration/injection of the elbow joint in the initial evaluation of radial head fractures?

Therapy

2. What is the role of operative vs. nonoperative treatment of displaced isolated partial radial head fractures (modified Mason II)?
3. For unstable or displaced fractures of the radial head that are part of a complex injury, what is the evidence for open reduction and internal fixation (ORIF) vs. prosthestic replacement vs. excision?
4. Is there any role for arthroscopy in radial head fractures?

Prognosis

5. What can a patient with an isolated radial head fracture expect in the long term?

Finding the evidence

- Cochrane Database, with search term "radius fracture"
- PubMed, with search term "radial head fracture"
- Above, limited to systematic reviews
- OVID, with search term "radial head fracture" and "aspiration" or "injection"

Question 1: What is the role of aspiration/injection of the elbow joint in the initial evaluation of radial head fractures?

Case clarification

The patient's radiographs reveal a nondisplaced radial head fracture (Mason type I). She is unwilling to flex and

Evidence-Based Orthopedics, First Edition. Edited by Mohit Bhandari.
© 2012 Blackwell Publishing Ltd. Published 2012 by Blackwell Publishing Ltd.

extend her elbow more than a few degrees because of pain, and she cannot fully supinate her arm.

Relevance

The bleeding associated with fractures of the radial head can be quite painful. The inhibition of elbow motion associated with this pain might delay recovery or lead to greater loss of motion. With displaced fractures, one needs to know if the fracture blocks forearm rotation. Aspiration of the hemarthrosis, with or without local anesthesia, can help distinguish such a block from inability to rotate due to pain.

Quality of the evidence

Level I
- 1 meta-analysis
- 3 randomized trials

Findings

A meta-analysis was published in 1999 based on two randomized trials examining the role of aspiration in radial head fractures (level I).[3] In one study, 80 patients with radial head fractures were randomized to aspiration and injection of bupivacaine with initiation of exercises or exercises alone (level I).[4] There was improved comfort with immediate range of motion (ROM) in 92% of patients who underwent the aspiration and injection, but no difference in ROM. In the second study, 28 patients with modified Mason type I and II fractures were randomized to aspiration of the hemarthrosis vs. no aspiration. (level I).[5] The authors noted better pain relief and ROM in the aspiration group immediately and at 3 and 6 month evaluation. The meta-analysis concluded that the evidence for aspiration of a traumatic elbow effusion is insufficient to recommend it as a routine procedure.

A third randomized trial, not included in the above meta-analysis, randomized 40 patients with Mason I radial head fractures to aspiration alone vs. aspiration with intra-articular injection of bupivacaine (level I).[6] The authors found no difference in ROM or pain relief between the two groups at all time points examined from 1 day to 1 year.

Recommendations

For Mason I fractures of the radial head:
- Aspiration of the hematoma of the elbow joint might aid in pain relief in the acute setting [overall quality: moderate]
- There is insufficient evidence to determine whether joint aspiration and/or injection can improve the final elbow motion
- It is unclear whether injection of local anesthetic provides any benefit over joint aspiration alone

We did not identify any studies that examined the role of injection of local anesthetic to facilitate diagnosis of a block to motion by a fracture fragment in the acute setting. Given the documented pain relief with aspiration of the hemarthrosis in the acute setting, it is likely this will aid in a more comfortable examination of forearm motion. Whether this is superior to simply waiting a few days and reexamining the patient when they are more comfortable and whether assessment of a "block to forearm rotation" in any form leads to more accurate diagnosis or decision-making regarding treatment requires further study.

Question 2: What is the role of operative vs. nonoperative treatment of displaced isolated partial radial head fractures (modified Mason II)?

Case clarification

The patient's radiographs reveal an isolated, displaced (2 mm step in the articular surface) partial articular radial head fracture. What evidence exists to inform the decision between operative and nonoperative treatment?

Relevance

There is substantial debate about the best method for treating these fractures. Operative treatment is straightforward and associated with good results, but also has complications. Nonoperative treatment of isolated displaced partial articular fractures of the radial head has been associated with very good recovery in most series.

Quality of the evidence

Level II
- 1 systematic review

Findings

There is one systematic review to date examining conservative treatment vs. surgical intervention for radial head fractures (level II).[7] In this review, the authors found a maximum of level II evidence. A total of 28 studies were included; 14 studies involving 519 patients examined either pain or Broberg–Morrey outcomes in patients who underwent various surgical treatments for Mason II fractures. These same outcomes were also measured in 7 studies involving 430 patients who were treated nonoperatively for Mason II fractures. In these studies 52% of patients treated nonoperatively demonstrated good to excellent Broberg scores compared with 88% of patients who underwent surgery. Additionally, residual pain was reported in 42% of the patients treated without surgery vs. 32% of the patients who underwent operative treatment. However, the study designs and outcome measures were quite heterogeneous, preventing meaningful pooling of the results. The authors state that no conclusions can be drawn regarding the optimal management of Mason II fractures.

Recommendations

No level I studies have been completed concerning operative vs. nonoperative management of Mason II radial head fractures. The heterogeneity of existing evidence prevents meaningful conclusions regarding treatment decisions

- It may be that operative treatment of Mason II fractures is more likely to yield improved Broberg scores and less residual pain, but further study is warranted [overall quality: low]

Question 3: For unstable or displaced fractures of the radial head that are part of a complex injury, what is the evidence for ORIF vs. excision with or without prosthetic replacement?

Case clarification

The patient had a concomitant elbow dislocation that was reduced. Her radiographs reveal a displaced articular fracture involving the entire radial head (modified Mason III). You plan to treat her operatively.

Relevance

Treatment of complex radial head fractures remains controversial. Fractures that were once treated with excision are now often treated with ORIF or prosthetic replacement.

Quality of the evidence

Level II
- 1 randomized controlled trial

Level III
- 3 retrospective comparative studies

Findings

Our review of the literature identified one randomized controlled trial evaluating ORIF vs. prosthetic replacement of the radial head for modified Mason type III fractures (level II).[8] Fourteen patients were randomized to radial head replacement, while 8 patients received ORIF, and patients were followed for an average of 16 and 14 months, respectively. The authors found good to excellent results in 92% of the patients treated with radial head replacement, compared to 12.5% of patients treated with ORIF. Despite the small numbers, the magnitude of this difference was enough to achieve statistical significance (p = 0.0004). The authors conclude that type III fractures are better treated with radial head replacement.

Three nonrandomized comparative studies have examined ORIF vs. excision of the radial head in the treatment of modified Mason III fractures. The first evaluated 28 patients who were treated surgically for comminuted fractures of the radial head (a combination of modified Mason III and IV—meaning associated with a dislocation—fractures) (level III).[9] The 15 patients treated prior to 1996 received radial head excisions, while the 13 patients treated in 1996 and after underwent ORIF of the radial head. Nine of the patients who underwent ORIF later underwent plate removal. At final evaluation between 2 and 4 years after surgery, the authors noted significant improvements in visual analog scale (VAS) pain score, elbow extension, and strength in extension and supination in the group treated with ORIF vs. those treated with radial head excision. They also noted significantly improved functional scores (Broberg–Morrey and ASES) for those patients treated with ORIF.

The second study examined 20 patients at an average of 44 months following either radial head excision or ORIF for Mason II and III fractures of the radial head (level III).[10] On follow-up radiographs, signs of arthrosis were present in 90% of patients who had undergone capitellectomy and 20% of those who had undergone ORIF.

Lastly, Lindenhovius and colleagues examined 28 patients with modified Mason III fractures, 15 of whom were treated with radial head excision and 13 of whom who underwent ORIF of the radial head (level III).[11] At an average of 17 years follow-up, the authors noted that 8 patients in the excision cohort had developed arthrosis, compared with only 2 patients in the osteosynthesis group.

Recommendation

- Limited retrospective data suggest that among patients with Mason III fractures, those with associated dislocations in particular, excision of the radial head leads to greater arthrosis and worse function when compared to ORIF [overall quality: low]
- Limited retrospective and prospective data also support prosthetic replacement over ORIF for complex, displaced fractures of the entire head of the radius (Mason III). [overall quality: moderate]

Question 4: Is there any role for arthroscopy in the treatment of radial head fractures?

Case clarification

The patient has an isolated minimally displaced fracture of the radial head (Mason II), and has decided on operative treatment. She asks about a minimally invasive approach with arthroscopy that she read about on the internet.

Relevance

The indications for elbow arthroscopy are expanding to include elbow trauma.

Quality of the evidence

Level IV
- 3 retrospective case series

Findings

Only three case series exist examining the role of elbow arthroscopy in the acute treatment of radial head fractures. A total of 23 patients are reviewed in these studies. The first study examined 3 patients with radial head fractures but does not describe specific outcomes (level IV).[12]

The second study described percutaneous fixation of 6 radial head fractures: 3 Mason type II, 2 Mason type III, and 1 Mason type IV (level IV).[13] The authors cite a satisfactory functional outcome in the short term (6–18 month follow-up).

Lastly, Michels and colleagues reviewed 14 Mason II radial head fractures treated with arthroscopic percutaneous reduction and fixation (level IV).[14] At an average 5 year follow-up, the authors reported 3 good and 11 excellent Mayo elbow scores.

Recommendations

• In our opinion, only the Broberg–Morrey Mason type II fracture is suitable for arthroscopic-assisted fixation [overall quality: very low]

Given that these fractures can do very well with nonoperative treatment, as well as the fact that an open procedure is done through a 3–4 cm incision in most patients, the value of arthroscopy will need to be demonstrated in high-quality level I trials before we will change our practice.

Question 5: What can a patient with an isolated radial head fracture expect in the long term?

Case clarification

One patient has a simple Mason II fracture of the radial head, while another has an unstable modified Mason III fracture. These are young, active patients who question how these fractures will affect them in the future.

Relevance

In the acute setting, patients often question what limitations, if any, they will have in the future due to their injury, and how this may relate to treatment options. While patients can often recover quite well after simple fractures of the radial head, modified Mason III fractures can be complex, "elbow-changing" injuries.

Quality of the evidence

Level IV

• 8 retrospective case series

Findings

In 2005, Herbertsson and colleagues examined 32 patients treated nonoperatively for displaced Mason I fractures at an average 21 years of follow-up (level IV).[15] Twenty-nine

of the patients had no complaints at final follow-up, while 3 of them had occasional elbow pain. The authors found an increased prevalence of degenerative changes on radiographs in the formerly injured elbow, but found that in general displaced Mason I fractures can be successfully managed nonoperatively.

In 2006, the same group published a 19-year follow-up of 49 patients with modified Mason II fractures treated nonoperatively (level IV).[16] All patients had sustained two-fragment fractures with between 2 mm and 5 mm of articular displacement. Six patients underwent delayed radial head excision. At final follow-up, 40 of the patients had no complaints, 8 had occasional elbow pain, and 1 had daily pain. On average, there was a slight decrease in flexion, extension, and supination noted compared with the contralateral side, as well as a slightly higher prevalence of radiographic evidence of arthrosis. The authors concluded that the long-term outcome of type II fractures treated nonoperatively is favorable.

More recently, a long-term evaluation of Mason II fractures treated operatively has been published (level IV).[17] Sixteen patients were evaluated at an average of 22 years after ORIF using either screws alone or a plate and screws. Complications after surgery included 2 infections, 1 transient posterior interosseous nerve palsy, and 2 screws of excessive length that restricted elbow motion. Fourteen of the 16 patients underwent surgery for hardware removal. The authors noted a decreased ROM at final follow-up, with an average flexion arc of 129° and an average forearm rotation of 166°. They conclude that there is no appreciable advantage of operative intervention in the treatment of Mason II fractures of the radial head.

Five studies were found examining long-term results of Mason III fractures. One of these, by Herbertsson and colleagues, involves 100 patients with Mason II and III fractures followed for an average of 19 years (level IV).[18] Seventy-eight patients were treated nonoperatively and 22 operatively. Ten of the 100 patients underwent a secondary procedure—delayed radial head resection in 9 patients and an ulnar neurolysis in one patient. At final follow-up, most patients had no complaints, 21 had occasional pain, and 2 had daily pain. ROM testing demonstrated only slight deficits in flexion and extension. There was a higher incidence of radiographic arthrosis on the injured side vs. the uninjured side.

A long-term review of acute excision for Mason III fractures was published in 1998 (level IV).[19] This study reviewed 18 patients treated with radial head excision for Mason III fractures at a minimum of 16-year follow-up, and another 3 patients at 6–12 year follow-up. One patient had a poor outcome on the Broberg–Morrey scale, with pain with daily activities and a 25° loss of supination. On radiographic review, there were 12 patients with proximal migration of the radius from 1–3 mm, 11 patients with degenerative changes at the elbow, and 7 patients with periarticular ossification. The authors conclude that radial head resection is a good option for Mason III fractures, provided the medial collateral ligament is intact.

A long-term review of radial head replacement for radial head fractures was published in 2001 (level IV).[20] The authors reviewed 20 patients who had undergone acute radial head replacement for radial head fractures with associated instability (Mason IV). Using the Mayo elbow performance score, they found 12 patients had excellent results, 4 good, 2 fair, and 2 poor. No patients had recurrent instability. The authors conclude that radial head replacement should be considered for the unreconstructable radial head fracture with associated instability.

Lastly, Esser and colleagues examined 26 patients at an average follow-up of 7 years after radial head ORIF (level IV).[21] There were 11 patients with Mason II fractures, 9 with Mason III fractures, and 6 with Mason IV fractures. Using the Broberg–Morrey score, the authors found that all patients with type II and III fractures had good to excellent results, whereas 2 patients with type IV fractures had poor results. These 2 patients underwent delayed radial head excision with improved pain and ROM.

Recommendations

• In the long term, patients with a Mason I fracture of the radial head can expect minimal functional difficulties with possible radiographic evidence of arthrosis. [Overall Quality: Low]
• Patients with a modified Mason II fracture can expect some limitation of ROM with the possibility of persistent pain and dysfunction whether treated operatively or nonoperatively [overall quality: low]
• Operative intervention brings with it the risk of complications, along with the possibility of a second operation for hardware removal [overall quality: low]
• There is insufficient data to recommend any one method of treatment for unstable fractures of the radial head
• Radiographic evidence of arthrosis does not seem to correlate with patients' pain or loss of motion [overall quality: very low]

Summary of recommendations

• Aspiration of the hematoma of the elbow joint might aid in pain relief in the acute setting
• There is insufficient evidence to determine whether joint aspiration and/or injection can improve the final elbow motion
• It is unclear whether injection of local anesthetic provides any benefit over joint aspiration alone
• It may be that operative treatment of Mason II fractures is more likely to yield improved Broberg scores and less residual pain, but further study is warranted

• Limited retrospective data suggest that among patients with Mason III fractures, those with associated dislocations in particular, excision of the radial head leads to greater arthrosis and worse function when compared to ORIF
• Limited retrospective and prospective data also support prosthetic replacement over ORIF for complex, displaced fractures of the entire head of the radius (Mason III)
• In our opinion, only the Broberg–Morrey Mason type II fracture is suitable for arthroscopic-assisted fixation
• In the long term, patients with a Mason I fracture of the radial head can expect minimal functional difficulties with possible radiographic evidence of arthrosis
• Patients with a Mason II fracture can expect some limitation of ROM with the possibility of persistent pain and dysfunction whether treated operatively or nonoperatively
• Operative intervention brings with it the risk of complications, along with the possibility of a second operation for hardware removal
• There is insufficient data to recommend any one method of treatment for unstable fractures of the radial head
• Radiographic evidence of arthrosis does not seem to correlate with patients' pain or loss of motion

Conclusion

Most of the data available regarding the management of radial head fractures consists of retrospective case series, making meaningful conclusions difficult. With regards to stable fractures of the radial head, including Broberg and Morrey modified Mason I and II fractures, it is certainly not clear that operative intervention provides any benefit over nonoperative treatment. With regard to modified Mason III fractures, operative intervention does offer some advantages, but the value of ORIF vs. radial head exicision or replacement is still uncertain. For fractures associated with instability of the elbow, radial head replacement does seem to offer improved stability. Certainly, further investigation and high-quality comparative studies are needed to further elucidate the answers to these questions.

References

1. Mason ML. Some observations on fractures of the head of the radius with a review of one hundred cases. Br J Surg 1954;42:123–32.
2. Broberg MA, Morrey BF. Results of treatment of fracture-dislocations of the elbow. Clin Orthop 1987;216:109–19.
3. Carley S. The role of therapeutic needle aspiration in radial head fractures. J Accid Emerg Med 1999;16(4):282.
4. Holdsworth BJ, Clement DA, Rothwell PN. Fractures of the radial head—the benefit of aspiration: a prospective controlled trial. Injury 1987;18(1):44–7.

5. Dooley JF, Angus PD. The importance of elbow aspiration when treating radial head fractures. Arch Emerg Med. 1991;8(2): 117–21.

6. Chalidis BE, Papadopoulos PP, Sachinis NC, Dimitriou CG. Aspiration alone versus aspiration and bupivacaine injection in the treatment of undisplaced radial head fractures: a prospective randomized study. J Shoulder Elbow Surg 2009;18(5):676–9.

7. Struijs PA, Smit G, Steller EP. Radial head fractures: effectiveness of conservative treatment versus surgical intervention. A systematic review. Arch Orthop Trauma Surg 2007;127(2):125–30.

8. Ruan HJ, Fan CY, Liu JJ, Zeng BF. A comparative study of internal fixation and prosthesis replacement for radial head fractures of Mason type III. Int Orthop. 2009;33(1):249–53.

9. Ikeda M, Sugiyama K, Kang C, Takagaki T, Oka Y. Comminuted fractures of the radial head. Comparison of resection and internal fixation. J Bone Joint Surg Am 2005;87(1):76–84.

10. Pilato G, De Pietri M, Vernieri W, Bini A. The surgical treatment of fractures of the radial head: a comparison between osteosynthesis and capitellectomy. Chir Organi Mov 2004;89(3): 213–22.

11. Lindenhovius AL, Felsch Q, Doornberg JN, Ring D, Kloen P. Open reduction and internal fixation compared with excision for unstable displaced fractures of the radial head. J Hand Surg Am 2007;32(5):630–6.

12. Haddad N, Chebil M, Mili W, et al. Technique and indications of elbow arthroscopy. A twelve-cases report. Tunis Med 2009; 87(2):120–2.

13. Rolla PR, Surace MF, Bini A, Pilato G. Arthroscopic treatment of fractures of the radial head. Arthroscopy 2006;22(2):233.e1–e6.

14. Michels F, Pouliart N, Handelberg F. Arthroscopic management of Mason type 2 radial head fractures. Knee Surg Sports Traumatol Arthrosc 2007;15(10):1244–50.

15. Herbertsson P, Josefsson PO, Hasserius R, Karlsson C, Besjakov J, Karlsson MK. Displaced Mason type I fractures of the radial head and neck in adults: a fifteen- to thirty-three-year follow-up study. J Shoulder Elbow Surg 2005;14(1):73–7.

16. Akesson T, Herbertsson P, Josefsson PO, Hasserius R, Besjakov J, Karlsson MK. Primary nonoperative treatment of moderately displaced two-part fractures of the radial head. J Bone Joint Surg Am 2006;88(9):1909–14.

17. Lindenhovius AL, Felsch Q, Ring D, Kloen P. The long-term outcome of open reduction and internal fixation of stable displaced isolated partial articular fractures of the radial head. J Trauma 2009;67(1): 143–6.

18. Herbertsson P, Josefsson PO, Hasserius R, Karlsson C, Besjakov J, Karlsson M. Uncomplicated Mason type-II and III fractures of the radial head and neck in adults. A long-term follow-up study. J Bone Joint Surg Am 2004;86(3):569–74.

19. Janssen RPA, Vegter J. Resection of the radial head after Mason type-III fractures of the elbow: Follow-up at 16 to 30 years. J Bone Joint Surg Br 1998;80:231–3.

20. Harrington IJ, Sekyi-Otu A, Barrington TW, Evans DC, Tuli V. The functional outcome with metallic radial head implants in the treatment of unstable elbow fractures: a long-term review. J Trauma. 2001;50(1):46–52.

21. Esser RD, Davis S, Taavao T. Fractures of the radial head treated by internal fixation: late results in 26 cases. J Orthop Trauma 1995;9(4):318–23.

46 Monteggia Fracture-Dislocations

Bryce T. Gillespie and Jesse B. Jupiter

Massachusetts General Hospital, Boston, MA, USA

Case scenarios

Case 1

A 35 year old male carpenter comes to the Emergency Department after falling 6 feet (1.8 m) off of a ladder and landing on his outstretched right arm. He complains of right elbow and forearm pain. Examination demonstrates elbow tenderness and point tenderness with angular deformity at the proximal-third ulna border. Radiographs demonstrate an anteriorly angulated proximal-third ulnar shaft fracture and an anterior dislocation of the radial head (Figure 46.1).

Case 2

A 70 year old woman comes to the Emergency Department after tripping inside her home and landing on here outstretched left arm. She notes left elbow and forearm pain and deformity. Examination demonstrates a bony prominence at the posterolateral aspect of the elbow and deformity along the proximal ulna. Radiographs demonstrate a posteriorly angulated metaphyseal ulna fracture and a posteriorly dislocated radial head that is fractured (Figure 46.2).

Top four questions

Diagnosis

1. What methods can be used to avoid missing the diagnosis of Monteggia fracture-dislocation?

Therapy

2. Is there a role for nonplate fixation (i.e., intramedullary fixation or tension band wire fixation) of ulnar shaft fractures in Monteggia fracture-dislocations?

3. What should be done for a radial head/neck fracture in a Monteggia fracture-dislocation?

Prognosis

4. What are the complications associated with operative treatment of Monteggia fracture-dislocations?

Question 1: What methods can be used to avoid missing the diagnosis of Monteggia fracture-dislocation?

Case clarification

Radiographs in Case 1 clearly show the ulna fracture, but the radial head dislocation may be a subtle finding.

Relevance

Missing the diagnosis of an acute Monteggia fracture-dislocation can cause inappropriate and incomplete treatment leading to long-term functional deficits, including arthrosis and restricted range of motion (ROM). Chronic Monteggia fracture-dislocations may require more extensive surgical intervention. If dislocated more than 4 weeks, the radial head would likely need to be resected at the time of realignment of the ulna.

Current opinion

The correct diagnosis can usually be made by close review of elbow, forearm, and wrist radiographs, paying close attention to the congruency of the radiocapitellar joint.

Finding the evidence

- PubMed Clinical Study Category: search terms "diagnosis" AND "broad, sensitive search" AND "Monteggia" AND "fracture" with limits: "Humans" AND "All Adults: 19+ years" AND "English language"

Evidence-Based Orthopedics, First Edition. Edited by Mohit Bhandari.
© 2012 Blackwell Publishing Ltd. Published 2012 by Blackwell Publishing Ltd.

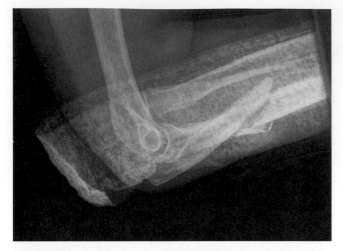

Figure 46.1 Lateral elbow radiograph for Case 1.

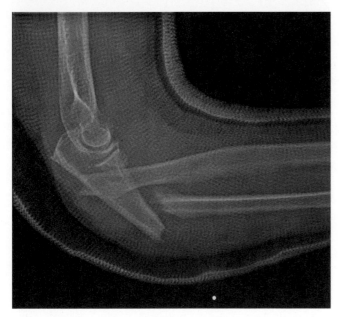

Figure 46.2 Lateral elbow radiograph for Case 2.

Quality of the evidence

Level IV
- 4 retrospective case-series[1-4]
- 1 case report[5]

Findings

Speed and Boyd recognized the importance of a high index of suspicion and complete radiographs to diagnose this injury. A radial head dislocation should be suspected with any ulna fracture not accompanied by a radius fracture. They state that elbow radiographs should always be done for ulna fractures, and that "failure to do so may lead to a grave error in diagnosis and to permanent disability."[1]

All proximal-third ulna shaft fractures should be presumed to be associated with a radial head dislocation until

proven that the radiocapitellar joint is stable. A single radiograph showing a congruent radiocapitellar joint may be deceiving. Kadakia et al. reported a missed Monteggia fracture in which static films showed a located radiocapitellar joint with a proximal ulna fracture. The patient continued to have pain and subsequent radiographic examination under anesthesia showed easily dislocatable radiocapitellar and proximal radioulnar joints. Maintaining a high index of suspicion led to the correct diagnosis.[5]

Giustra et al. found that three of five Monteggia fracture-dislocations (one adult and two pediatric) were initially misdiagnosed. Reasons for misdiagnosis included the rarity of the injury, difficult physical examination, no dedicated elbow radiographs, and midshaft, rather than proximal, ulna fractures.[2]

A line drawn along the axis of the radial shaft at the elbow should intersect the capitellum on all views with any amount of elbow flexion or extension.[3] Imaging of the contralateral, uninjured elbow in pediatric elbow trauma has not been shown to improve diagnostic accuracy,[4] which may also be true in adult cases.

Recommendations

- Maintain high index of suspicion for Monteggia fracture-dislocation with any fracture of the ulna [overall quality: very low]
- Include elbow radiographs of ulna fractures to evaluate for radiocapitellar joint dislocation [overall quality: very low]

Question 2: Is there a role for nonplate fixation (i.e., intramedullary fixation or tension band wire fixation) of ulnar shaft fractures in Monteggia fracture-dislocations?

Case clarification

The ulna fracture in Cases 1 and 2 could theoretically be addressed with intramedullary (IM) fixation instead of plate fixation.

Relevance

IM fixation has been used elsewhere in the body to provide fracture stabilization, but less commonly with adult Monteggia fracture-dislocations. An IM pin is often used to maintain reduction of the ulna fracture in pediatric Monteggia fracture-dislocations. A tension band wire (TBW) or IM screw fixation is commonly used to fix simple olecranon fractures in adults, but this method of fixation is not thought to be stable enough for adult Monteggia fracture-dislocations.

Current opinion

IM or TBW fixation of the ulna fracture in adult Monteggia fracture-dislocations does not provide sufficient stability to ensure maintained reduction of the fracture and radio-capitellar joint during healing, therefore plate fixation is the predominant treatment choice.

Finding the evidence

• PubMed and OVID, search terms "Monteggia" AND "fracture" with limits: "Humans" AND "All Adults: 19+ years" AND "English language"
• Cochrane Database, search term "fracture" AND "Monteggia" OR "ulna." One result that addressed ulna shaft fractures, but excluded Monteggia fracture-dislocations and only compared plate fixation vs. nonoperative treatment.[6]
• Manual review of cited references from identified articles.

Quality of the evidence

Level IV
• 8 retrospective case series[7–14]

Findings

TBW and IM screw fixation has been used for olecranon fractures, but these methods do not provide enough stability for ulna fractures when there are additional injuries, as seen in Monteggia fracture-dislocations.[11]

In their review of posterior (Bado type II) Monteggia fracture-dislocations, Jupiter et al. conclude that this fracture pattern is not amenable to nonplate fixation. Due to the direction of the injury, the ulnar shaft fracture is predisposed to further flexion deformity leading to redislocation of the radiocapitellar joint. They recommend fixation only with a contoured plate applied to the dorsal cortex of the proximal ulna to act as a tension band plate and assure anatomic reduction.[8]

Four of 16 adult Monteggia fracture-dislocations in one series were treated with Rush pin fixation; two required reoperation for nonunion. More recent cases were treated with plate fixation, and this is their recommended method.[7]

Only four of 38 adult Bado type II injuries in a series of 48 Monteggia fracture-dislocations were treated with nonplate fixation (3 TBW and 1 IM pin); 1 of the 3 TBW constructs required revision to a contoured dorsal plate to obtain fracture union. The fourth patient had the IM pin removed at 6 months, but the fracture healed with recurrent flexion deformity.[9]

Six patients in a series of 10 proximal ulna atrophic nonunions had initial operative treatment of Bado type II Monteggia fracture-dislocations. Three had initial plate fixation, 2 had TBW, and 1 had IM screw fixation; all required revision fixation with a contoured dorsal plate.[10]

In another series of 12 patients with proximal ulna nonunions, 7 had operative treatment of Bado types I and II Monteggia fracture-dislocations; 4 had initial plate fixation,

2 had Rush nail fixation, and 1 had TBW. All fractures healed after plate and cortical strut fixation.[14]

Eleven of 37 adult patients with Bado type II Monteggia fracture-dislocations were treated with TBW fixation in one series. The remaining 26 with Bado type II and the 7 with Bado types I, III, and IV injuries had plate fixation. Due to the selection bias of less comminuted fractures being fixed with TBW, the authors could not correlate fixation method and functional outcome. They suggest that a contoured plate along the dorsal cortex should be used to stabilize the ulna fracture.[13]

Muckley et al. have reported the use of IM nailing in 2 patients with ulnar shaft nonunion following plate fixation. Both fractures healed with near normal elbow ROM. They suggest this technique when concerned about the soft tissue envelope causing further complications with revision plating.[12]

Recommendations

• TBW fixation may be effective for certain isolated proximal ulna fractures, but the construct may not be strong enough to resist the additional instability seen with Monteggia fracture-dislocations [overall quality: low]
• IM pins are commonly used for pediatric Monteggia fracture-dislocations, but likely do not provide sufficient stability in adults. IM nails could be an option for revision fixation of nonunions [overall quality: very low]

Question 3: What should be done for a radial head/neck fracture in a Monteggia fracture-dislocation?

Case clarification

Case 2 represents a posterior Monteggia fracture-dislocation with an associated radial head fracture. In addition to fixation of the ulna fracture and reduction of the radiocapitellar joint, what should be done for the radial head fracture?

Relevance

Debate continues about the appropriate treatment of radial head fractures, especially when associated with another injury. The modified Mason classification system of radial head fractures is often utilized to help guide treatment.[15]

Treatment decisions can affect outcomes by impacting elbow stability, ROM, or arthrosis.

Current opinion

The radial head fracture in a Monteggia fracture-dislocation often requires intervention. The goal is elbow stability and functional ROM, often necessitating internal fixation or prosthetic replacement.

Finding the evidence

See Question 2.

Quality of the evidence
Level IV
• 4 retrospective case series[9,13,16,17]

Findings
In one case series, 10 of 14 adults with Bado type II Monteggia fracture-dislocations sustained radial head fractures. Two were Mason type I (treated nonoperatively), 5 were Mason type II, and 3 were Mason type III (treated with primary excision). The type II radial head fractures either had partial excision or open reduction and internal fixation (ORIF). These five patients had similar elbow flexion/extension (120/20° vs. 117/25°), but those who had ORIF had less forearm pronation/supination (60/53° vs. 35/30°). The Mason type III radial head fractures were all excised and had even more limited elbow ROM (flexion/extension of 95/12° and pronation/supination of 42/10°). No patients had prosthetic replacement. Overall, radial head fractures were more common in Bado type II than type I injuries (71% vs. 30%), and those patients with radial head fractures had poorer motion and functional results.[16]

Twenty-six of 38 adult Bado type II Monteggia fracture-dislocations had associated radial head fractures in another series. Of the 7 Mason type II fractures, 3 were treated nonoperatively, 2 had partial excision, and 2 had ORIF. Only 1 of the 19 Mason type III fractures was treated nonoperatively, 8 had ORIF and 10 had excision with 2 being replaced with silicone prostheses. Six of the 8 Mason type III fractures that had ORIF went on to have complications, including restricted ROM, secondary head excision, or migrated hardware. All patients with Bado type II injuries that had unsatisfactory results had associated radial head fractures. Ten of the 12 patients who had radial head excision without prosthetic replacement had satisfactory results.[9]

Egol et al. reviewed 20 Monteggia fracture-dislocations with radial head/neck fractures. Twelve were treated nonoperatively, 3 had ORIF, 1 was excised, and 4 had titanium prosthetic replacements. Two more patients later underwent radial head replacement for persistent instability. The Broberg–Morrey scores trended towards better functional outcome if no surgery was done for the radial head fracture. Compared to other studies, these authors concluded that radial head fractures caused restricted ROM and resulted in poorer functional outcome.[17]

In a case series of 47 adult Monteggia fracture-dislocations, 16 had concurrent radial head fractures (13 of which were Bado type II injuries). All 7 Mason type II and 5 of 9 Mason type III radial head fractures were treated with ORIF. The other 4 Mason type III fractures were treated with primary excision and no prosthetic replacement. Two patients required revision ORIF for loss of initial fracture reduction. Radial head fractures were correlated

with a "poor" Broberg–Morrey score, but no difference in scores could be determined between the ORIF and excision groups.[13]

Recommendations
• If the radial head fracture can be managed nonoperatively, this treatment method may improve long-term outcome [overall quality: very low]
• No recommendations were made regarding radial head excision alone vs. prosthetic replacement, but the goal of overall forearm stability should be considered when making this decision [overall quality: very low]

Question 4: What are the complications associated with operative treatment of Monteggia fracture-dislocations?

Case clarification
The injuries in Cases 1 and 2 and the subsequent operative intervention can be associated with complications and long-term sequelae affecting functional outcome.

Relevance
Some complications of Monteggia fracture-dislocations may be unavoidable sequelae of the injury, but careful surgical technique can help reduce their morbidity.

Current opinion
Early identification and appropriate surgical reduction and fixation of Monteggia fracture-dislocations can enhance outcomes.

Finding the evidence
See Question 2.

Quality of the evidence
Level IV
• 9 retrospective case series[7,9,13,16–21]

Findings
Two studies reported overall complication rates of 43% and 39% for adult Monteggia fracture-dislocations.[18,20] Table 46.1 highlights the difficulties associated with treating these complex injuries.

Ring et al. had 3 malunions in 48 patients and Reynders et al. noted 4 in 67 patients.[9,18] The nonunion rates in other studies (7.4–18.8% with average of 12%) included longstanding nonunions and early fixation failures that necessitated intervention.[7,13,16–21]

Incomplete reduction of the radiocapitellar joint or unstable fixation of the ulnar shaft fracture can result in persistent subluxation or dislocation. Four of 7 instances of dislocation in one series were due to non-anatomic ulna fracture fixation.[18] Overall rates were 5.6–10.4% (average 8%).[18–20]

Table 46.1 Rates of complications for operative treatment of Monteggia fracture-dislocations

Complication	Average rate (%)	No. of patients	No. of studies	References
Overall rate	41	51/121	2	Reynders 1996, Llusa 2002
Malunion	6	7/115	2	Reynders 1996, Ring 1998
Nonunion/failure of fixation	12	32/278	8	Ovesen 1990, Reynders 1996, Simpson 1996, Givon 1997, Llusa 2002, Egol 2005, Strauss 2006, Konrad 2007
Radiocapitellar joint instability	8	12/148	3	Givon 1996, Reynders 1996, Llusa 2002
HO	14	19/134	4	Reynders 1996, Simpson 1996, Egol 2005, Strauss 2006
PRUJ synostosis	7	15/216	4	Reynders 1996, Ring 1998, Llusa 2002, Konrad 2007
Radiographic osteoarthritic changes	38	58/154	5	Ovesen 1996, Ring 1998, Egol 2005, Strauss 2006, Konrad 2007
Postoperative infection	3	5/195	4	Ovesen 1996, Ring 1998, Egol 2005, Strauss 2006, Konrad 2007

HO, heterotopic ossification; PRUJ, proximal radioulnar joint.

Heterotopic ossification (HO) and synostosis of the proximal radioulnar joint (PRUJ) can have significant adverse effect on functional results. High-energy injuries and patients with head trauma appear more likely to develop HO.[20] Four case series reported their rates of HO ranging from 8.7% to 35% (average 14%).[16–18,21] The highest rate was seen in a review of 20 patients with Monteggia fracture-dislocations who had concurrent radial head fractures.[17] The average rate of PRUJ synostosis was 7% (range 4.3–8.9%).[9,13,18,20] Reynders et al. reported that 6 of their 67 patients had PRUJ synostosis and that 4 of these 6 patients had undergone open annular ligament reconstruction. Therefore they recommended against doing this procedure.[18]

Five studies reported long-term radiographic osteoarthritic changes.[7,9,13,17,21] Rates ranged from 6.3% to 70% (average 38%). Most were mild changes, but at least five patients had severe arthrosis.

Postoperative infection rates were reported in four studies.[13,18–20] Overall 5 of 195 patients had infections. The average rate was 3% (range 1.5–4.3%).

Only two studies present follow-up ROM values based upon Bado type of Monteggia fracture-dislocation. Ring et al.'s study of 48 patients included Bado types I–IV and the other study only had 24 patients with types I and II.[9,16] With these limited numbers, it is difficult to draw conclusions, but Bado types II and IV appear to have the most loss of motion (Table 46.2).

Table 46.2 Postoperative range of motion by Bado type of Monteggia fracture-dislocation

Bado type	No. of patients	Average flexion/ extension arc (°)	Average pronation/ supination arc (°)
I	17	117	142
II	52	110	122
III	1	120	120
IV	2	108	110

References: Simpson 1996, Ring 1998.

Recommendation

- These results can help an orthopedic surgeon educate a patient about the potentially poor outcomes associated with Monteggia fracture-dislocations and the risks of operative treatment of these injuries [overall quality: low]

Summary of recommendations

- Maintain high index of suspicion for Monteggia fracture-dislocation with any fracture of the ulna
- Include elbow radiographs of ulna fractures to evaluate for radiocapitellar joint dislocation
- TBW fixation may be effective for certain isolated proximal ulna fractures, but the construct may not be strong

enough to resist the additional instability seen with Monteggia fracture-dislocations

• IM pins are commonly used for pediatric Monteggia fracture-dislocations, but likely do not provide sufficient stability in adults. IM nails could be an option for revision fixation of nonunions

• If the radial head fracture can be managed nonoperatively, this treatment method may improve long-term outcome

• No recommendations were made regarding radial head excision alone vs. prosthetic replacement, but the goal of overall forearm stability should be considered when making this decision

• These results can help an orthopedic surgeon educate a patient about the potentially poor outcomes associated with Monteggia fracture-dislocations and the risks of operative treatment of these injuries

Conclusions

Monteggia fracture-dislocations represent significant injuries to the upper extremity with potentially serious functional loss. Prompt recognition and appropriate treatment can help restore function.

Ulnar fractures in Monteggia fracture-dislocations require rigid fixation to allow bone and soft tissue healing while maintaining alignment of the fracture(s) and reduction of the radiocapitellar joint. This is best accomplished with application of a contoured, stout plate along the dorsal border of the proximal ulna. This position allows for orthogonal screw fixation proximally and displaces very little muscle. Alignment of the ulna fracture usually results in reduction of the radial head dislocation, so open reduction of the radiocapitellar joint can, and should, be avoided. Dorsal plate application also has a biomechanical advantage of resisting elbow flexion forces. Newer plate technology, such as precontoured olecranon plates, has yet to be compared to other plates with regard to Monteggia fracture-dislocations.

References

1. Speed JS, Boyd HB. Treatment of fractures of ulna with dislocation of head of radius. J Am Med Assoc 1940;115:1699–705.

2. Giustra PE, Killoran PJ, Furman RS, et al. The missed Monteggia fracture. Radiology 1974;110:45–7.

3. Perron AD, Hersh RE, Brady WJ, et al. Orthopedic pitfalls in the ED: Galeazzi and Monteggia fracture-dislocation. Am J Emerg Med 2001;19:225–8.

4. Kissoon N, Galpin R, Gayle M, et al. Evaluation of the role of comparison radiographs in the diagnosis of traumatic elbow injuries. J Pediatr Orthop 1995;15:449–53.

5. Kadakia AP, Candal-Couto J. Occult Monteggia fracture in an adult: A case report. Acta Orthop Belg 2007;73:393–5.

6. Handoll HHG, Pearce P. Interventions for isolated diaphyseal fractures of the ulna in adults. Cochrane Database Syst Rev 2009;3.

7. Ovesen O, Brok KE, Arreskov J, et al. Monteggia lesions in children and adults: an analysis of etiology and long-term results of treatment. Orthopedics 1990;13:529–34.

8. Jupiter JB, Leibovic SJ, Ribbans W, et al. The posterior Monteggia lesion. J Orthop Trauma 1991;5:395–402.

9. Ring D, Jupiter JB, Simpson NS. Monteggia fractures in adults. J Bone Joint Surg Am 1998;80:1733–44.

10. Ring D, Jupiter JB, Gulotta L. Atrophic nonunions of the proximal ulna. Clin Orthop 2003;409:268–74.

11. Ring D, Tavakolian J, Kloen P, et al. Loss of alignment after surgical treatment of posterior Monteggia fractures: salvage with dorsal contoured plating. J Hand Surg Am 2004;29:694–702.

12. Muckley T, Hierholz C, Berger A, et al. Compression nailing of ulnar nonunion after Monteggia lesion. J Trauma 2005;59:249–53.

13. Konrad GG, Kundel K, Kreuz PC, et al. Monteggia fractures in adults: Long-term results and prognostic factors. J Bone Joint Surg Br 2007;89:354–60.

14. Rotini R, Antonioli D, Marinelli A, et al. Surgical treatment of proximal ulna nonunion. Chir Organi Mov 2008;91:65–70.

15. Hotchkiss RN. Displaced fractures of the radial head: internal fixation or excision? J Am Acad Orthop Surg 1997;5:1–10.

16. Simpson NS, Goodman LA, Jupiter JB. Contoured LCDC plating of the proximal ulna. Injury 1996;27:411–17.

17. Egol KA, Tejwani NC, Bazzi J. Does a Monteggia variant lesion result in a poor functional outcome? A retrospective study. Clin Orthop 2005;438:233–8.

18. Reynders P, De Groote W, Rondia J. Monteggia lesions in adults: a multicenter Bota study. Acta Orthop Belg 1996;62 (Supp 1):78–83.

19. Givon U, Pritsch M, Levy O. Monteggia and equivalent lesions: A study of 41 cases. Clin Orthop 1997;337:208–15.

20. Llusa Perez M, Lamas C, Martinez I, et al. Monteggia fractures in adults. Review of 54 cases. Chir Main 2002;21:293–7.

21. Strauss EJ, Tejwani NC, Preston CF, et al. The posterior Monteggia lesion with associated ulnohumeral instability. J Bone Joint Surg Br 2006;88:84–9.

47 Olecranon Fractures

Bryce T. Gillespie and Jesse B. Jupiter

Massachusetts General Hospital, Boston, MA, USA

Case scenarios

Case 1

A 28 year old male motorcyclist comes to the Emergency Department complaining of right elbow pain following a collision. Examination demonstrates tenderness with a palpable defect over the proximal ulna. He has no active elbow extension. Imaging studies demonstrate a displaced, comminuted olecranon fracture (Figure 47.1).

Case 2

A 75 year old woman comes to the Emergency Department complaining of left elbow pain after slipping on the ice and landing on her outstretched left arm. Examination demonstrates tenderness at the posterior elbow. She cannot actively extend her elbow. Imaging studies demonstrate a displaced, transverse, proximal olecranon fracture (Figure 47.2).

Top five questions

Diagnosis

1. What is the role of cross-sectional imaging in determining treatment method of olecranon fractures?

Treatment

2. When can fragment excision and triceps advancement be used to treat olecranon fractures?
3. Can either K-wire tension band fixation (TBF) or dorsal plating be used to treat simple or minimally comminuted olecranon fractures?

Prognosis

4. Does treatment method affect the functional outcomes of operatively treated olecranon fractures?
5. What are the complications associated with operative treatment of olecranon fractures?

Question 1: What is the role of cross-sectional imaging in determining treatment method of olecranon fractures?

Case clarification

The fractures in Cases 1 and 2 can be identified with radiographs, but would cross-sectional imaging affect treatment decisions?

Relevance

Cross-sectional imaging of the olecranon fracture in Case 1 may give further information regarding the comminution and injury to the articular surface. This may affect the planned techniques of surgical fixation. Additional imaging of the fracture in Case 2 may reveal what portion of the articular surface is involved and the overall quality of this elderly patient's bone. This may guide treatment to internal fixation or fragment excision and triceps advancement.

Current opinion

Complex intra-articular fractures benefit from cross-sectional imaging for preoperative planning. Olecranon fractures with comminution or associated injuries, vs. simple fracture patterns, are more likely to undergo this additional imaging.

Finding the evidence

- PubMed and OVID, search terms "olecranon" AND "fracture" with limits: "Humans" AND "All Adults: 19+ years" AND "English language"

Evidence-Based Orthopedics, First Edition. Edited by Mohit Bhandari.
© 2012 Blackwell Publishing Ltd. Published 2012 by Blackwell Publishing Ltd.

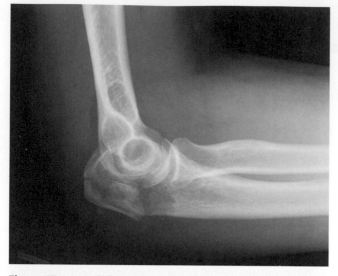

Figure 47.1 Lateral elbow radiograph for Case 1.

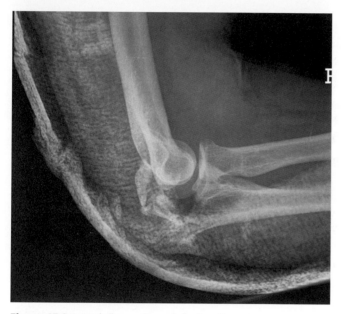

Figure 47.2 Lateral elbow radiograph for Case 2.

• Cochrane Database, search term "fracture" AND "olecranon" OR "ulna"
  ○ One result that addressed ulna shaft fractures, but not olecranon fractures[1]
• Manual review of cited references from identified articles

Quality of the evidence
Level IV
• 1 retrospective case-series[2]

Findings
No studies have systematically evaluated the role of cross-sectional imaging for evaluation and treatment planning of olecranon fractures. Several studies have demonstrated that 2-D and 3-D CT scans can improve reliability and/or accuracy of fracture characterization and influence treatment decisions for other intra-articular upper extremity fractures.[3-6]

One case series of 20 adult patients evaluated the role of MRI in detecting occult fractures in patients with acute elbow trauma and an elbow effusion seen on radiographs, but no visible fracture. Fifteen of the patients were found to have an occult fracture, but only one of these was an olecranon fracture: the remainder had radial head (13) or lateral epicondyle (1) fractures. There was no change in treatment plan based upon the MRI results.[2]

Recommendation
• Consider cross-sectional imaging (CT scan) for complex olecranon fractures to assist with selecting appropriate treatment modality, however, this recommendation requires investigation [overall quality: very low]

Question 2: When can fragment excision and triceps advancement be used to treat olecranon fractures?

Case clarification
The fracture in Case 2 may be amenable to fragment excision and triceps advancement, but it could also be addressed with internal fixation.

Relevance
As internal fixation methods and hardware technology have improved, more fractures are being addressed with surgical reduction and stabilization. This includes olecranon fractures that may previously have been addressed with fragment excision.

Current opinion
Fragment excision and triceps advancement is usually now reserved for elderly patients with low functional demands and olecranon fractures with small proximal fragments. Otherwise, internal fracture fixation is the predominant treatment method.

Finding the evidence
See Question 1.

Quality of the evidence
Level IV
• 6 retrospective case series[7-12]

Findings
Since the 1940s, fragment excision and triceps advancement has been considered a viable treatment option for olecranon fractures, especially for comminuted fractures that cannot be easily repaired.[7-9]

Instability is a valid concern when removing a portion of the olecranon, but excision is thought to produce a durable result when less than 75% of the joint surface is removed and there are no concurrent injuries to the coronoid, radial head, or collateral ligaments.

Despite range of motion results that did not differ between 4 patients treated with excision and 34 patients treated with internal fixation, Rettig et al. still recommended excision only when internal fixation is not possible.[10]

Gartsman et al. reported the largest series (53 patients) treated with primary excision.[11] Excision was used for all severely comminuted and small avulsion fractures and half of the two-part fractures. Fifteen patients who had fractures excised that were less than 50% of the joint surface were evaluated with long-term follow-up (average 3.6 years). They achieved approximately 70% of the isometric and isokinetic elbow extensor strength as compared to the uninjured side and these results were similar to the patients treated with fracture fixation.

Nonoperative treatment has also been suggested for elderly patients. One series of 12 patients aged 73–90 were treated with cast immobilization. Despite 9 patients having pseudarthrosis, 11 patients reported excellent satisfaction with their treatment result.[12]

Recommendation

- Fragment excision and triceps advancement can be considered for fractures involving up to 50% (and possibly up to 75%) of the articular surface with the expectation of similar postoperative elbow strength compared to fracture fixation [overall quality: low]
- Associated injuries may lead to instability with fragment excision, therefore this method may be best reserved for those isolated, severely comminuted fractures that are not amenable to fixation [overall quality: very low]

Question 3: Can either K-wire TBF or dorsal plating be used to treat simple or minimally comminuted olecranon fractures?

Case clarification

The fracture in Case 1 may be too comminuted for K-wire TBF, but fractures with minimal comminution or those where the fragments can be lagged together prior to K-wire fixation may be amenable to either treatment method.

Relevance

K-wire TBF was originally used for almost all olecranon fractures, but this method may fail with excessive fracture comminution. New technology has made dorsal plating a more common treatment method.

Current opinion

TBF remains an acceptable and predictable treatment for simple or minimally comminuted olecranon fractures.

Plate fixation is required for more complex multifragmented fractures.

Finding the evidence

See Question 1.

Quality of the evidence

Level II
- 1 randomized trial with methodological limitations[13]

Findings

Forty-one isolated olecranon fractures, 19 treated with K-wire TBF and 22 treated with one-third tubular plate fixation, were followed for an average of 7 months in the only prospective, randomized trial comparing these treatment options.[13] These results were evaluated in aggregate, so the results of minimally comminuted fractures could not be independently assessed (Table 47.1).

Forty-two percent of the tension band group had painful hardware vs. only 5% in the plate fixation group. There was no difference in range of motion; loss of extension averaged 7–10°.

Ten fractures treated with TBF lost reduction, including 5 that initially had perfect reduction, while only 1 fracture treated with plate fixation lost reduction. Eighty-six percent of the plate fixation group had initial reduction with less than 1mm step-off, while only 63% of the TBF group

Table 47.1 K-wire tension band fixation vs plate fixation for olecranon fractures

	K-wire tension band fixation (19 patients)	One-third tubular plate fixation (22 patients)
Postoperative infection	16% (3 pts)	5% (1 pt)
Nonunion	5% (1 pt)	0% (0 pt)
Heterotopic ossification	5% (1 pt)	0% (0 pt)
Painful hardware	42% (8 pts)	5% (1 pt)
Average loss of extension	10°	7°
Initial reduction <1 mm step-off or gap	63% (12 pts)	86% (19 pts)
Healed reduction >2 mm step-off or gap	84% (16 pts)	9% (2)
Lost reduction	53% (10 pts)	5% (1 pt)
Operative time	94.5 min (75–120 min)	120 min (85–150 min)

Reference: Hume 1992.

Table 47.2 Functional outcomes for K-wire tension band fixation and plate fixation of olecranon fractures

Study/fixation	No. of patients	Average follow-up	Flexion-extension ROM or arc	Pronation-supination ROM or arc	Avg. MEPI score	Good or excellent MEPI score[a]	Avg. DASH score	Radiographic osteoarthritic changes
K-wire tension band wire fixation								
Rommens 2004	95 total 58 at follow-up	36 months	Extension Loss >20°: 10% (6 pts)	Flexion Loss >20°: 9% (5 pts)				32% (19 pts)
Villanueva 2006	37	48 months	7–131°		88	86% (32 pts)	18	27% (10 pts)
Chalidis 2008	62	8.2 years				86% (53 pts)		48% (30 pts)
Plate fixation								
Bailey 2001	25	34 months	8.5–128.5°	76.7–67.2°	89	92% (23 pts)	10	8% (2 pts)
Anderson 2007	32 total 24 at follow-up	2.2 years	120°	158°	89	92% (22 pts)	25	
Buijze 2009	16	24 months	13–136°	74–71°	93	94% (15 pts)	13	44% (7 pts)

[a] MEPI Score greater than 74.

achieved this level of initial reduction. Sixteen patients had step-off or gapping of greater than 2 mm following TBF, while only 2 had this following plate fixation.

The authors suggest that plate fixation offers better initial reduction and better maintenance of reduction with fewer complications than TBF.

Recommendation
- For all fracture types, plate fixation was shown to provide equal or better initial reduction with less loss of reduction than did K-wire TBF [overall quality: low]

Question 4: Does treatment method affect the functional outcomes of operatively treated olecranon fractures?

Case clarification
The patient characteristics and functional demands are different in Cases 1 and 2. This may alter choice of treatment method and give varying functional outcomes.

Relevance
Most olecranon fractures require surgical treatment to restore elbow function. A consensus on appropriate treatment for the varying injury patterns could yield improved outcomes.

Current opinion
Stable fracture fixation with restoration of anatomy is the goal of operative treatment of olecranon fractures. Distinct

from treatment method, this is the most important determinant of functional outcomes.

Finding the evidence
See Question 1.

Quality of the evidence
Level IV
- 6 retrospective case series[14–19]

Findings
Villanueva et al. reported on 37 patients who underwent fixation of olecranon fractures with a K-wire tension band and had average follow-up of 4 years.[14] The worst extension loss was 25°. The average Mayo Elbow Performance Index (MEPI) score was 88.[20] The average Disabilities of the Arm, Shoulder, and Hand (DASH) score was 18. Seventy-eight percent had scores of less than 30, indicating that most patients had mild disability (Table 47.2).

Sixty-two patients who had TBF of isolated olecranon fractures were evaluated at a minimum of 6 years after surgery.[15] Eighty-six percent had good or excellent MEPI scores, although 48% had some evidence of degenerative changes on radiographs.

A majority of the 95 patients (81%) included in Rommens et al.'s study had TBF of olecranon fractures, but only 58 were available for follow-up at an average of 36 months after surgery.[16] Twenty-one percent had no loss of extension, while 53% had no loss of flexion. Arthrosis was 3.4

times more common in those fractures that had suboptimal initial osteosynthesis.

Bailey et al. reported on 25 patients who underwent fixation of olecranon fractures with various plates.[17] They reported no difference in elbow motion as compared to the uninjured elbow except for supination being limited to 67° on average, as compared to 76°. The average DASH score was 10, equivalent to almost normal function.

Twenty-four of 32 patients who had fracture fixation with congruent plates underwent follow-up on average 2.2 years after surgery.[18] The average flexion contracture was 13.5°, but four patients had contractures of more than 30°.

Buijze and Kloen reported on 16 patients who had fixation of comminuted olecranon fractures with a 3.5 mm locking compression plate.[19] Seven patients had radiographic osteoarthritis by at least 12 months postoperative follow-up.

Recommendations

• Both treatment methods seem to provide functional elbow range of motion [overall quality: very low]
• On average, 92% (58/65) of the patients who had plate fixation had good or excellent MEPI scores, while 86% (85/99) of those with TBF had similar results.[14,15,17–19] This suggests some improved function following plate fixation of olecranon fractures [overall quality: low]

Question 5: What are the complications associated with operative treatment of olecranon fractures?

Case clarification

The injuries in Cases 1 and 2 and the subsequent operative intervention can be associated with complications and long-term sequelae affecting functional outcome.

Relevance

Some complications of olecranon fracture fixation may be unavoidable sequelae of the injury, but careful surgical technique can help reduce their morbidity.

Current opinion

Appropriate surgical reduction and fixation of olecranon fractures can enhance outcomes and limit the morbidities associated with this injury.

Finding the evidence

See Question 1.

Quality of the evidence

Level II
• 1 randomized trial with methodological limitations[13]

Level IV
• 19 retrospective case series[13–19,21–32]

Findings

Overall complication rates of up to 85% have been reported for surgical treatment of olecranon fractures.[21] Higher rates are more commonly associated with K-wire TBF and usually related to prominent hardware (Table 47.3).

Rates of hardware removal are quite variable but indicate that both constructs are susceptible to becoming symptomatic. The average rate of hardware removal for tension band constructs is 57% (range 27–85%), while for plate fixation it is 20% (range 0–56%).[15,17–19,21–29]

Painful hardware, that may or may not have required removal, was separately reported in seven case series. In their randomized study, Hume and Wiss reported painful hardware for 42% of patients who had TBF and only 5% who had plate fixation.[13] Three other tension band case series had painful hardware rates of 28–75%.[21,25,28] Three case series of plate fixation had rates of 0–56% (average 19%).[18,19,29] All of the symptomatic plates were subsequently removed.

Mullett et al. compared two configurations of K-wires in TBF constructs. Forty-five patients had K-wires placed longitudinally into the ulnar intramedullary canal and 35 had transcortical K-wires that pierced the anterior cortex of the ulna distal to the coronoid. Three of the intramedullary wires and only one of the transcortical wires backed out. Therefore they recommended placing transcortical K-wires to improve construct stability and decrease backout rates.[27]

Postoperative infection rates were comparable for TBF and plate fixation at 4% (range 0–11%) and 5% (0–15%), respectively.[13,15,18,19,21–23,25–27,32]

Nonunion rates, on average, were equal for both TBF and plate fixation at 2%, ranges were 0–5% and 0–6%, respectively.[13–19,21,23,26,27,29]

Velkes et al. presented two patients with proximal radioulnar joint (PRUJ) synostosis following K-wire TBF of olecranon fractures.[30] Matthews et al. highlighted the risk of transcortical K-wires or screws approaching or engaging the radius after passing through the anterior ulna. They indicated that starting the K-wires more lateral on the tip of the olecranon and aiming them more ulnar (down the shaft of the ulna) can help prevent this complication.[31] Two case series of TBF noted heterotopic ossification (HO) in 9 of 78 patients.[14,17] Two of 25 patients who had plate fixation developed HO but did not have any block to motion.[17]

Irregularities at the articular surface can be secondary to initial malreduction or loss of initial reduction. One series of 34 patients treated with TBF reported 10 malreduced fractures and they found malreduced fractures were more likely to further displace later than those that were initially well reduced.[22] Nine of 54 patients (17%) treated with TBF in two other case series had some loss of reduction.[21,22] This rate was far lower than that reported by Hume and Wiss,

Table 47.3 Rates of complications for operative treatment of olecranon fractures

Complication	Average rate	No. of patients	No. of studies	References
K-wire tension band fixation				
Overall rate	66%	106/160	4	Macko 1985, Jensen 1986, Wolfgang 1987, Romero 2000
Hardware removal	57%	262/456	10	Holdsworth 1984, Macko 1985, Jensen 1986, Helm 1987, Wolfgang 1987, Finsen 2000, Mullett 2000, Romero 2000, Villanueva 2006, Chalidis 2008
Painful hardware	41%	50/122	4	Holdsworth 1984, Macko 1985, Hume 1992, Finsen 2000
Postoperative infection	4%	16/368	8	Holdsworth 1984, Macko 1985, Helm 1987, Wolfgang 1987, Hume 1992, Mullett 2000, Romero 2000, Chalidis 2008
Malunion	2%	2/108	2	Romero 2000, Chalidis 2008
Nonunion	2%	6/362	8	Macko 1985, Wolfgang 1987, Hume 1992, Mullett 2000, Romero 2000, Rommens 2004, Villanueva 2006, Chalidis 2008
Heterotopic ossification	12%	9/78	2	Bailey 2001, Villanueva 2006
Plate fixation				
Overall rate	0%	0/14	1	Tejwani 2002
Hardwware removal	20%	17/86	4	Bailey 2001, Tejwani 2002, Anderson 2007, Buijze 2009
Painful hardware	15%	13/84	4	Hume 1992, Tejwani 2002, Anderson 2007, Buijze 2009
Postoperative infection	5%	4/83	4	Hume 1992, Simpson 1996, Anderson 2007, Buijze 2009
Nonunion	2%	2/109	5	Hume 1992, Bailey 2001, Tejwani 2002, Anderson 2007, Buijze 2009
Heterotopic ossification	8%	2/25	1	Bailey 2001

who found 10 of 19 patients with TBF lost reduction, including five patients who had initially perfect reduction. Comparatively, only 1 of 22 patients in their study treated with plate fixation lost reduction and 19 of the 22 had initially anatomic reductions.[13]

Recommendationw

• Placing K-wire tension band hardware deep to the triceps tendon and having the K-wires engage the anterior ulnar cortex may reduce symptomatic hardware, hardware removal, and fracture displacement rates [overall quality: very low]
• Plate fixation may overall have fewer complications, but the plate can still be prominent and require subsequent removal [overall quality: very low]

Summary of recommendations

• Consider cross-sectional imaging (CT scan) for complex olecranon fractures to assist with selecting appropriate

treatment modality, however, this recommendation requires investigation
• Fragment excision and triceps advancement can be considered for fractures involving up to 50% (and possibly up to 75%) of the articular surface with the expectation of similar postoperative elbow strength compared to fracture fixation
• Associated injuries may lead to instability with fragment excision, therefore this method may be best reserved for those severely comminuted fractures that are not amenable to fixation
• For all fracture types, plate fixation was shown to provide equal or better initial reduction with less loss of reduction than did K-wire TBF
• Both K-wire TBF and plate fixation seem to provide functional elbow range of motion
• On average, 92% (58/65) of the patients who had plate fixation had good or excellent MEPI scores, while 86% (85/99) of those with TBF had similar results.[14,15,17–19] This suggests some improved function following plate fixation of olecranon fractures

- Placing K-wire tension band hardware deep to the triceps tendon and having the K-wires engage the anterior ulnar cortex may reduce symptomatic hardware, hardware removal, and fracture displacement rates
- Plate fixation may overall have fewer complications, but the plate can still be prominent and require subsequent removal

Conclusions

Displaced olecranon fractures require operative intervention. Patient and fracture characteristics can influence treatment choices that include fragment excision and triceps advancement, K-wire TBF, and plate fixation.

K-wire TBF has long been the treatment for most fractures. Done well, this construct can still be used for many fractures, but newer plate technology may continue to expand the use of plates to stabilize olecranon fractures. Plate fixation may slightly improve functional outcome and decrease the overall number of complications.

References

1. Handoll HHG, Pearce P. Interventions for isolated diaphyseal fractures of the ulna in adults. Cochrane Database Syst Rev 2009;3.
2. O'Dwyer H, O'Sullivan P, Fitzgerald D, et al. The fat pad sign following elbow trauma in adults: its usefulness and reliability in suspecting occult fracture. J Comput Assist Tomogr 2004;28:562–5.
3. Katz MA, Beredjiklian PK, Bozentka DJ, et al. Computed tomography scanning of intra-articular distal radius fractures: does it influence treatment? J Hand Surg Am 2001;26:415–21.
4. Harness NG, Ring D, Zurakowski D, et al. The influence of three-dimensional computed tomography reconstructions on the characterization and treatment of distal radius fractures. J Bone Joint Surg Am 2006;88:1315–23.
5. Doornberg J, Lindenhovius A, Kloen P, et al. Two and three-dimensional computed tomography for the classification and management of distal humeral fractures. J Bone Joint Surg Am 2006;88:1795–801.
6. Lindenhovius A, Karanicolas PJ, Bhandari M, et al. Interobserver reliability of coronoid fracture classification: two-dimensional versus three-dimensional computed tomography. J Hand Surg Am 2009; 34:1640–6.
7. McKeever FM, Buck RM. Fracture of the olecranon process of the ulna. J Am Med Assoc 1947; 135:1–5.
8. Wainwright D. Fractures of the olecranon process. Br J Surg 1942;29:403–6.
9. Adler S, Fay GF, MacAusland WR. Treatment of olecranon fractures: indications for excision of the olecranon fragment and repair of the triceps tendon. J Trauma 1962;2:597–602.
10. Rettig AC, Waugh TR, Evanski PM. Fracture of the olecranon: a problem of management. J Trauma 1979;19:23–8.
11. Gartsman GM, Sculco TP, Otis JC. Operative treatment of olecranon fractures: excision or open reduction with internal fixation. J Bone Joint Surg Am 1981;63:718–21.
12. Del Monte LV, Vercher MS, Net RB, et al. Conservative treatment of displaced fractures of the olecranon in the elderly. Injury 1999;30:105–10.
13. Hume MC, Wiss DA. Olecranon fractures: A clinical and radiographic comparison of tension band wiring and plate fixation. Clin Orthop 1992;285:229–35.
14. Villanueva P, Osorio F, Commessatti M, et al. Tension-band wiring for olecranon fractures: Analysis of risk factors for failure. J Shoulder Elbow Surg 2006;15:351–6.
15. Chalidis BE, Sachinis NC, Samoladas EP, et al. Is tension band wiring technique the "gold standard" for the treatment of olecranon fractures? A long term functional outcome study. J Orthop Surg 2008;3:9–14.
16. Rommens PM, Kuchle R, Schneider RU, et al. Olecranon fractures in adults: Factors influencing outcome. Injury 2004;35:1149–57.
17. Bailey CS, MacDermid J, Patterson SD, et al. Outcome of plate fixation of olecranon fractures. J Orthop Trauma 2001;15:542–8.
18. Anderson ML, Larson AN, Merten SM, et al. Congruent elbow plate fixation of olecranon fractures. J Orthop Trauma 2007;21:386–93.
19. Buijze G, Kloen P. Clinical evaluation of locking compression plate fixation of comminuted olecranon fractures. J Bone Joint Surg Am 2009;91(10):2416–20.
20. Morrey BF, Adams RA. Semiconstrained arthroplasty for the treatment of rheumatoid arthritis of the elbow. J Bone Joint Surg 1992;74:479–90.
21. Macko D, Szabo RM. Complications of tension-band wiring of olecranon fractures. J Bone Joint Surg Am 1985;67:1396–401.
22. Helm RH, Hornby R, Miller SWM. The complications of surgical treatment of displaced fractures of the olecranon. Injury 1987;18:48–50.
23. Romero JM, Miran A, Jensen CH. Complications and re-operation rate after tension-band wiring of olecranon fractures. J Orthop Sci 2000;5:318–20.
24. Jensen CM, Olsen BB. Drawbacks of traction-absorbing wiring (TAW) in displaced fractures of the olecranon. Injury 1986;17:174–5.
25. Holdsworth BJ, Mossad MM. Elbow function following tension band fixation of displaced fractures of the olecranon. Injury 1984;16:182–7.
26. Wolfgang G, Burke F, Bush D, et al. Surgical treatment of displaced olecranon fractures by tension band wiring technique. Clin Orthop 1987;224:192–204.
27. Mullett JH, Shannon F, Noel J, et al. K-wire position in tension band wiring of the olecranon: A comparison of two techniques. Injury 2000;31:427–31.
28. Finsen V, Lingaas PS, Storro S. AO tension-band osteosynthesis of displaced olecranon fractures. Orthopedics 2000;23:1069–72.
29. Tejwani NC, Garnham IR, Wolinsky PR, et al. Posterior olecranon plating: Biomechanical and clinical evaluation of a new operative technique. Bull Hosp Jt Dis 2002–2003;61:27–31.
30. Velkes S, Tytiun Y, Salai M. Proximal radio-ulnar synostosis complicating tension band wiring of the fractured olecranon. Injury 2005;36:1254–6.
31. Matthews F, Trentz O, Jacob AL, et al. Protrusion of hardware impairs forearm rotation after olecranon fixation. J Bone Joint Surg Am 2007;89:638–42.
32. Simpson NS, Goodman LA, Jupiter JB. Contoured LCDC plating of the proximal ulna. Injury 1996;27:411–17.

48 Forearm Fractures, Including Galeazzi Fractures

S. John Ham, Matthijs R. Krijnen, and Rudolf W. Poolman
Onze Lieve Vrouwe Gasthuis, Amsterdam, The Netherlands

Case scenarios

Case 1

A 40 year old plumber was cycling and fell on his right dominant forearm. He was taken to the local Emergency Department by his wife. Physical examination revealed an abnormal position of the forearm without neurologic deficit and normal arterial pulsations. Radiographs showed a comminuted, dislocated fracture of the distal diaphyseal part of the radius. An isolated radius fracture was diagnosed. The fracture of the radius was treated with open reduction and plate fixation. The patient was allowed to move the arm functionally without weightbearing.

Case 2

A 25 year old man presented at the Emergency Department after being involved in a fight in a local bar. Besides several bruises, he complained of pain at the midulnar region of the left, nondominant forearm. Radiographs revealed an isolated ulnar shaft fracture, with only slight (10%) dislocation. Treatment advise was cast immobilization, starting with 3 weeks long-arm cast, followed by short-arm cast.

Relevant anatomy

The ulna is a relatively straight bone. The radius, however, has a gentle lateral bowing that influences the rotational capacity of the forearm. Distally, the radius and ulna articulate in a complex relationship, held together by the dorsal and volar ligaments and the triangular fibrocartilage complex (TFCC). The interosseous membrane plays an important role in normal forearm function and in providing stability to ulnar shaft fractures. The unique anatomy provides the possibility of supination and pronation of the forearm, which are important movements in the usual activities of daily living.

Importance of the problem

The reconstruction of the anatomy of the bones and soft tissue of the forearm, including the distal radioulnar joint (DRUJ) and TFCC is important in achieving maximum functional outcome.

Four types of fractures can be considered: isolated fractures of the radius, isolated fractures of the ulna, diaphyseal fractures of both bones of the forearm, and Galeazzi fracture-dislocation.

Isolated fractures of the radial diaphysis without an ulna fracture are relatively rare. The majority of these fractures is unstable and require open reduction and internal fixation (ORIF).[1] Restoring the radial bowing is of importance to achieve restoration of rotational capacity of the forearm. A Galeazzi injury must be ruled out by thorough evaluation of the DRUJ.

Diaphyseal fractures of the ulna, also called *nightstick fractures*, are usually the result of a direct blow. The central diaphyseal fractures can often be managed with a cast or functional brace.[2] More than 50% displacement and/or 10° of angulation are considered unstable, necessitating ORIF.[2–4] Fractures of the proximal and distal third are more likely to require ORIF because of displacement.[4,5] The advantage of anatomic reduction and accelerated rehabilitation may be an argument to consider ORIF as the treatment of choice.

Evidence-Based Orthopedics, First Edition. Edited by Mohit Bhandari.
© 2012 Blackwell Publishing Ltd. Published 2012 by Blackwell Publishing Ltd.

Displacement is standard following diaphyseal fractures of both forearms. Anatomic reduction and internal fixation of the forearm fractures are mandatory for restoration of function and now form the standard treatment regimen.[1,6] This is supported by the good results of rigid plate fixation in many studies. Bone grafting of the fractures is considered in selected cases, especially in complex forearm fractures.[1,6–8] Plate removal is often advised, but the complication rate might be considerable.

Galeazzi fractures account for 6–7% of all adult forearm diaphyseal fractures.[9,10] The fracture is located at the middle to distal third of the radius and associated with dislocation and/or instability of the DRUJ. It is also called the *fracture of necessity*, which refers to its unstable nature and the need for ORIF of the radial fracture to achieve a satisfactory functional outcome in adults.[11–13] Persistent instability of the DRUJ leads to an unfavorable result, therefore a thorough examination of the DRUJ should always be conducted. Treatment of DRUJ lesions depends on the amount of instability.

Top six questions

Diagnosis

1. How accurate is radiological examination in the diagnosis of DRUJ involvement in radial shaft fractures/Galeazzi type fracture-dislocation? Is the location of the radial fracture a prognostic factor for DRUJ instability?

Therapy

2. What is the relative effect of ORIF vs. nonsurgical treatment, ORIF vs. ORIF, and nonsurgical vs. nonsurgical treatment in isolated ulnar shaft fractures?
3. Does bone grafting influence the union rate in comminuted diaphyseal fractures of the radius and/or ulna?

Prognosis

4. What is the influence of the timing of surgery due to delayed diagnosis in relation to the time of injury on functional outcome and complications in patients with Galeazzi type fractures?
5. Is there evidence that surgical reconstruction or temporary transfixion of the DRUJ prevents decrease in range of motion of the forearm and degenerative disease of the DRUJ in Galeazzi type fractures?

Harm

6. How long after surgery for forearm fracture is plate removal a safe procedure in terms of postoperative refractures or other complications?

Question 1: How accurate is radiological examination in the diagnosis of DRUJ involvement in radial shaft fractures/Galeazzi type fracture-dislocation? Is the location of the radial fracture a prognostic factor for DRUJ instability?

Case clarification

Case 1 During the rehabilitation period, the patient noticed a plopping sensation in his wrist during pro- and supination leading to a reduction in strength when using a screwdriver or pliers. A second opinion confirmed an unstable DRUJ at physical examination. In a secondary procedure, the DRUJ was stabilized and the patient recovered uneventfully, with only slightly limited pro- and supination at the final follow-up. Nevertheless, working with a screwdriver had improved after the second procedure.

Although the radiographs revealed a fracture of the distal part of the radial diaphysis, the surgeon overlooked an injury to the DRUJ.

Relevance

Distal radioulnar instability may not be obvious on radiographs and therefore missed. It is important that radiographic features suggestive of disruption of the DRUJ are recognized. This would also facilitate planning of surgery. Furthermore, DRUJ instability has to be addressed appropriately, whereas in the absence of this injury, immediate postoperative mobilization might be possible.

Current opinion

The correct diagnosis can usually be made by meticulous review of forearm and wrist radiographs paying close attention to the congruency of the DRUJ.[9]

Finding the evidence

- Cochrane Database: No reviews available
- PubMed, using search terms: "Galeazzi fracture AND distal radioulnar joint and radiograph and prognosis" as well as "Galeazzi fracture AND distal radioulnar joint AND radiograph*"

Quality of the evidence

Level IV
- 2 case series

Findings

Rettig and Raskin suggested distinguishing isolated radius fractures with and without DRUJ involvement on the basis of fracture location.[14] Fractures more than 7.5 cm from the midarticular surface of the distal radius were likely to be stable. Only 1 of 18 fractures in this location had intraoperative DRUJ instability after ORIF of the radial shaft fracture. In contrast, 12 of 22 fractures within 7.5 cm were associated with intraoperative DRUJ instability.

Ring et al. stated that the location of the fracture alone may not be sufficient to be certain that the DRUJ is stable.[15] In their series fractures of the distal third of the radius were associated with DRUJ injury in 5 of 8 patients, whereas more proximal fractures of the radius were associated with DRUJ injury in only 4 of 28 patients. Injury of the DRUJ was defined in this latter study as more than 5 mm of ulnar-positive variance on radiographs taken before any manipulative or surgical reduction. This was based on biomechanical studies that have suggested that this amount of displacement indicates injury to all of the soft tissue stabilizers of the DRUJ.

Both studies relied on retrospective data, and no formal evaluation of the DRUJ was performed. Furthermore, in the studies of Ring et al. the method of quantitatively measuring dislocation might have over- or underestimated the rate of true dislocation.

Recommendations
- Fractures of the distal third of the radius are often associated with DRUJ instability [overall quality: very low]
- DRUJ instability is best evaluated, both radiographically and physically by manipulation during surgery after stabilization of the radial fracture [overall quality: very low]
- A proximally located isolated radial fracture does not rule out traumatic DRUJ instability [overall quality: very low]

Question 2: What is the relative effect of ORIF vs. nonsurgical treatment, ORIF vs. ORIF, and nonsurgical vs. nonsurgical treatment in isolated ulnar shaft fractures?

Case clarification
Case 2 Treatment advice was cast immobilization, starting with 3 weeks long-arm cast, followed by short-arm cast. However, the patient decided that he wanted surgical stabilization so he could resume his work as a self-employed carpenter much earlier.

Relevance
Although isolated ulnar shaft fractures are relatively rare, the choice of treatment is the basis for patient satisfaction, functional results, and return to work.

Current opinion
If the displacement is less than 50% of the width of the bone and the angulation less than 10°, no closed reduction or manipulation is needed and the fracture can be treated by cast immobilization or functional bracing. Unstable fractures are treated with ORIF using compression plating.

Finding the evidence
- Cochrane Database: one Cochrane study reviewed in 2009.
- PubMed, using the search term: "isolated fractures AND ulnar shaft"

Quality of the evidence
Level II
- 3 randomized trials with methodologic limitations

Level III
- 1 case control study/retrospective comparative study

Level IV
- 3 case series

Findings
The Cochrane review included three level II trials.[16–19] A fourth trial in the Cochrane review was not found in PubMed using the above search term.[20] The objective of the Cochrane study was to assess the effects of various forms of treatment for isolated fractures of the ulnar shaft in adults. Randomized or quasi-randomized trials of conservative and surgical treatment in adults were selected. The 4 selected trials involved a total of 237 participants. All trials were methodologically flawed and potentially biased. Three trials tested conservative treatment interventions. One trial compared short-arm functional braces with long-arm plaster casts; there was no significant difference in the time it took for fracture union.[17] Patient satisfaction and return to work during treatment were significantly better in the bracing group. The other two trials, both quasi-randomized, had three treatment groups. One trial compared Ace Wrap elastic bandage vs. short-arm plaster cast vs. long-arm plaster cast.[18] The large loss to follow-up in this trial made any data analysis tentative. The need for replacement of the Ace Wrap by other methods due to pain indicated a serious problem with this intervention. The other trial which compared immediate mobilization vs. short-arm plaster cast vs. long-arm plaster cast for minimally displaced fractures, found no significant difference in outcome between these three interventions.[19] The fourth trial, which compared two types of plates for surgical fixation, found no significant differences in functional or anatomical outcomes nor complications between the two groups.[20]

The study of Goel et al. was excluded from the Cochrane review.[21] In this prospective trial, 89 people with 90 isolated ulna fractures were treated with either a cast (45) or an elastic crepe bandage support with early mobilization (45). It was not clear how the groups were derived and only 60 people were followed up. Average time to union was 10.8 weeks in the first group (28 fractures) and 7.8 weeks in the second (32 fractures). Nonunion was only reported after 2 fractures in the first group.

Finally, in three papers the results of two different treatment regimens were reported without randomization or the initial intention of comparison. Pollock et al. evaluated 71 isolated ulnar fractures: the first 12 were treated with long-arm plaster cast, and the remaining 59 without a cast or with a cast or splint for no longer than 2 weeks followed by mobilization as tolerated.[22] The average healing time in the first group was 10.5 weeks, with a nonunion rate of 8%, and in the second group 6.7 weeks with no nonunions. Szabo and Skinner treated 18 patients by immediate ORIF, and 28 closed.[5] One open fracture in the first group became infected and resulted in nonunion, whereas in the second group 7 failed to unite. Boussouga et al. treated patients with either open reduction and plate fixation or closed intramedullary pinning.[23] The results were comparable, although more nonunions and complications occurred after open intervention.

Recommendation

- Based on the present literature no conclusive recommendation is possible. [overall quality: very low]

Question 3: Does bone grafting influence the union rate in comminuted diaphyseal fractures of the radius and ulna?

Case clarification
Case 1 Did the fracture require acute bone grafting in addition to ORIF?

Relevance
Does acute bone grafting of diaphyseal forearm fractures decrease the incidence of nonunion and reduce the time to union?

Current opinion
In the past, there have been controversies over the use of bone graft in comminuted fractures of the forearm. Currently, most authors agree that acute bone grafting is not necessary, with the exception of severe comminution.

Finding the evidence
- Cochrane Database: no reviews available
- PubMed, using the search terms: "diaphyseal forearm fractures AND acute bone grafting" and "diaphyseal forearm fractures AND bone grafting"

Quality of the evidence
Level IV
- 6 case series

Findings
Anderson et al. reviewed 330 diaphyseal forearm fractures treated with ORIF.[6] Autogenic iliac crest bone was used in 90 fractures in which one third of the shaft circumference was comminuted. The union rate for the severely comminuted fractures treated with bone graft was 98%, which was comparable to the union rate for fractures with less or no comminution treated without bone grafts. Chapman et al. reviewed 129 forearm fractures of the shaft treated with compression plating, of which 68 cases involved bone grafting.[8] They routinely bone grafted open and comminuted fractures. The union rate for the comminuted and/or open fractures treated with bone graft was 99%, which was not significantly different from the union rate for the closed, noncomminuted fractures treated without bone graft. Both series did not specially evaluate the results of the comminuted fractures treated without bone graft.

The recommendation to bone graft fractures with comminution involving more than one third the diameter of the bone has been widely quoted, but also questioned. No data have been presented in support of this recommendation.

Wright et al. retrospectively reviewed 198 diaphyseal forearm fractures.[24] Although no strict criteria were used for bone grafting, the attending surgeon was more likely to use bone graft for comminuted fractures that were open. The union rate for comminuted fractures treated without bone graft was 98%, whereas the rate for comminuted fractures treated with bone graft was only 83%. They found no significant difference between the union rate for comminuted fractures that they treated without bone graft and the union rates for comminuted fractures that Anderson's and Chapman's groups treated with bone graft. They concluded that routine bone grafting of comminuted forearm shaft fractures was not indicated.

Wei et al. compared the results of the comminuted diaphyseal forearm fractures treated with and without bone grafting in a contemporaneous set of subjects derived from the same patient population.[25] Fifty-six fractures were followed for at least 1 year beyond clinical and radiological union. ORIF was done in all cases. All noncomminuted fractures were treated without bone graft. For the comminuted fractures, the decision to use bone graft was left to the discretion of the operating surgeon. Acute bone grafting of the diaphyseal forearm fractures did not affect the union rate or the time to union. Shortcomings of these studies included the mixture of various types and the inclusion of skeletally immature patients.

Ring et al. examined factors associated with nonunion in skeletally mature patients with diaphyseal fractures of both the radius and the ulna and comminution of at least one fracture treated with plates of adequate size and at least three screws on each side of the fracture.[26] Forty-one patients were followed at a minimum of 12 months follow-up. Nonunion occurred in five patients (12%). The use of bone graft was not associated with a higher rate of union.

Mikek et al. compared the union rate and time to union in fractures with different extents of comminution.[27] All fractures (319 diaphyseal fractures of forearm bones in 214 consecutive patients) were treated with ORIF without the use of bone grafting. Fractures with bone loss greater than two thirds of the diameter of the diaphysis (5% of all fractures) had a significantly prolonged time to union; there was, however, no significant difference in the union rate between groups. They concluded that primary bone grafting of comminuted diaphyseal forearm fractures was not necessary in most cases.

Recommendations
• Standard bone grafting is not required in comminuted diaphyseal fractures during initial treatment [overall quality: very low]
• If bone grafting is used, its application should possible be reserved only for fractures with bone loss greater than two thirds of the diameter of the diaphysis [overall quality: very low]

Question 4: What is the influence of the timing of surgery due to delayed diagnosis in relation to the time of injury on functional outcome and complications in patients with Galeazzi type fractures? Is there a role for nonoperative management?

Case clarification
Case 1 A delay in DRUJ reconstruction may have contributed to suboptimal outcome.

Relevance
Galeazzi fractures are known to be underdiagnosed.[11] They may be mistaken for a simple radius fracture. What is the effect of an untreated or delayed treated DRUJ injury? Has there ever been a study published comparing ORIF with conservative treatment in adults?

Current opinion
In seemingly isolated radial fractures, DRUJ may be missed. Close attention to the DRUJ is warranted. The goal of surgical intervention should be relocation of the DRUJ with anatomic reduction of the radial fracture which is rigidly fixed.

Finding the evidence
• Cochrane Database: no reviews available
• PubMed, using the search terms: "Galeazzi fracture* AND treatment," "Galeazzi fracture* AND conservative treatment," and "Galeazzi fracture* AND delay in treatment"

Quality of the evidence
Level IV
• 3 case series

Findings
One level IV study addressed the issue of delay in surgery. Moore et al. retrospectively reviewed 34 patients with 36 closed Galeazzi fractures, who were treated using standard AO compression plates with 4–7 holes.[9] Follow-up was 1.5–7 years (average 2.5 years). Loss of strength was not related to a delay in surgery for more than 10 days after injury; however, the delay had a significant influence on the final range of motion. Only 3 of 24 forearms that were operated on within 10 days had less than an excellent final range of motion, while 6 (50%) of the 12 forearms for which the operation was delayed beyond 10 days were rated good or fair. Delay in treatment was caused by various reasons, including abrasions near the fracture site and craniofacial and thoracoabdominal injuries. Of note, no statistical evaluation was performed in this paper.

Data on nonoperative management are sparse. Based on one retrospective case series, nonoperative treatment resulted in poor results in 16 out of 20 patients (80%).[12] Poor results after closed reduction were also reported by Reckling in contrast to the results of ORIF and immobilization of the forearm in full supination.[13]

Recommendations
• Anatomical fixation of the radius in Galeazzi fractures is a necessary condition to obtain DRUJ congruency [overall quality: very low]
• Surgical treatment of Galeazzi fractures should take place within 10 days after injury [overall quality: very low]

Question 5: Is there evidence that surgical reconstruction or temporary transfixion of the DRUJ prevents decrease in range of motion of the forearm and degenerative disease of the DRUJ in Galeazzi type fractures?

Case clarification
Case 1 Our patient had residual complaints located at the DRUJ even after surgical correction.

Relevance
DRUJ instability may lead to limitation in pro- and supination incapacitating forearm function. Restoring the congruency of the joint and the stability of the DRUJ could thus prevent a loss of forearm rotation.

Current opinion

If the DRUJ is reduced after ORIF of the radial fracture, cast immobilization with or without transfixion of the distal ulna to the distal radius can be performed. If the DRUJ is irreducible, open reduction should be performed with removal of interposed soft tissue and repair if necessary.

Finding the evidence

• Cochrane Database: no reviews available
• PubMed, using the search terms: "Galeazzi fracture* AND treatment" and "Galeazzi fracture* AND distal radioulnar joint repair"

Quality of the evidence

Level IV
• 3 case series

Findings

In a retrospective case series including 24 patients (adults and children) with Galeazzi fractures, 15 (62.5%) were available for follow-up.[28] In 13 cases, the DRUJ had been immobilized by pinning with Kirschner (K) wires: at follow-up, 8 of these patients revealed limited pro- or supination. In the other 5 patients, as well as in 10 cases with stable DRUJ, no decrease in range of motion was found. The authors concluded that ORIF is a requisite for healing of the radius fracture. Open reduction of the DRUJ is only indicated when soft tissue interposition prevents exact reposition. To prevent K-wire failure, postoperative cast immobilization was indicated after this procedure. Because of the retrospective nature of the study it was not definitely clear if K-wire fixation was superior to immobilization.

Two papers reported of DRUJ function after ORIF. Strehle and Gerber reviewed 19 patients after an average of 83 months.[29] They found that anatomic fracture reduction was mandatory for functional results. Open revisions, repair of the TFCC, and immobilization of the wrist were not necessary if anatomic reduction of the joint was obtained by indirect means such as ORIF of the radius.

Mestdagh et al. also reported that additional percutaneous Kirschner pinning across the ulna and the radius in order to avoid redislocation did not seem to be necessary.[30] They stressed the importance of maintaining the reduction of the DRUJ in a plaster cast for 4–6 weeks, since persistent ulnar head displacements always resulted in a lack of prosupination of more than 25°.

No comparative study surgical fixation of the DRUJ after reduction vs. plaster immobilization after reduction addressed the issue of degenerative disease of the DRUJ after Galeazzi fracture-dislocation.

Recommendations

• The DRUJ must be radiographically visualized and manually tested during surgery after ORIF of the radial fracture

to assess joint congruency and residual instability [overall quality: very low]
• If ORIF of the radial fracture leads to anatomic reduction of the DRUJ cast immobilization is sufficient and additional Kirschner wire fixation is not necessary [overall quality: very low]

Question 6: How long after surgery for forearm fracture is plate removal a safe procedure in terms of postoperative complications, especially refracture?

Case clarification

Case 1 The treating surgeon recommended plate removal after 18 months. The patient, however, is not fully convinced about the necessity for this procedure.

Relevance

Plates used for stabilization of forearm fractures can give rise to complaints, which might be a reason for removal. However, asymptomatic plates are also often removed despite the risk of complications, including refracture and injury of the superficial branch of the radial nerve.[8,31,32]

Current opinion

Because the substantial risk of refracture and injury, especially to the superficial branch of the radial nerve, elective plate removal is not indicated in asymptomatic patients.

Finding the evidence

• Cochrane Database: no reviews available
• PubMed, using the search terms "diaphyseal forearm fracture AND plate removal and complications," "forearm fracture AND plate removal AND complications," "forearm fracture AND plate removal," "forearm fracture AND plate removal AND refracture"

Quality of the evidence

Level IV
• 8 case series

Findings

Hidaka and Gustilo reported 7 refractures 2–42 weeks after removal of 32 plates in 23 patients (radius 14, ulna 18).[33] Six of these fractures were located in the radius. The interval between plate application and removal had ranged from 8 to 62 months. Average cast immobilization had been 6 weeks. The authors concluded that plates should not be removed before 12 months. Chapman suggested that use of the 4.5mm system contributed to the high incidence of refracture in this series.[8]

Deluca et al. found refracture in 7 of the 37 patients who had a total of 62 diaphyseal plates removed from the forearm.[34] Six of the 7 refractures were after an original fracture of both bones. The interval between removal of plates and refracture ranged from 42 to 121 days. Only one patient had had adequate compression of the original fracture, the other six did not. In retrospect, radiolucency at the site of the original fracture was seen in most patients when the plate was removed.

Rosson and Shearer reported refracture after plate and screw removal in 4 of 51 adults after minimal trauma.[35] According to the authors, refracture was significantly more common among those patients having plates removed within 12 months compared with those in whom plates stayed in longer. The authors stated that the incidence of refracture should be minimal using the 3.5 mm plating system.

Langkamer and Ackroyd studied 55 patients who had undergone elective removal of 44 radius and 37 ulna plates.[36] Plate removal took place at 5–84 months (average 23.7 months) after insertion. Refracture occurred in 2 patients through the previous fracture site; plate removal had taken place in those patients 9 months (4.5 mm rigid plates had been used) and 24 months after initial repair, respectively. In both, no protection or restricted activities had been prescribed. The total complication rate was 40%, with more complications occurring when junior surgeons performed the surgery. It was recommended by the authors that forearm plates should be removed only if there were significant symptoms.

Rumball and Finnegan retrospectively reviewed all patients undergoing forearm plate removal during a 5.5 year period.[37] There were 4 refractures in 63 patients, an incidence of 6%. Factors that appeared to influence the refracture rate were degree of initial displacement and comminution, physical characteristics of the plate, early removal, and lack of postremoval protection.

Labosky et al. reported 80 plates removed from the radius and/or ulna in 51 patients.[38] Removal of plates was elective in 37 patients and for clinical reasons in 14. The average time from insertion to removal was 13.6 months (range 4.4–36 months). Only one refracture occurred in one patient whose plate was taken out 6 months after surgery. According to the authors, leaving a plate in cannot be considered a benign decision considering the persistent chance for refracture and the potential complications from prolonged exposure to metal corrosion complexes and metal irons.

Beaupré and Csongradi reported a retrospective examination of 401 patients with 459 plates removed after forearm fracture.[39] These data were collected from seven studies in the literature. Various types of plates had been used, and 37 refractures had occurred in 29 patients. The refracture risk was significantly greater for the narrow large-fragment DCP system than with either the small-fragment DCP system or the one third tubular system.

Chia et al. (1996) found in a retrospective review of 82 patients with 128 diaphyseal fractures operated at a single institution that 97.5% had no complications after implant removal.[40] Two patients sustained a refracture at the site of the original fracture within 6 months after plate removal, which could be treated successfully by cast immobilization. Twenty patients experienced minor complications ranging from mild superficial wound infection to nerve injury.

Recommendations

- Elective removal of forearm plate is contraindicated and should only be considered if there is pain or another symptom resulting from hardware irritation to the soft tissues [overall quality: very low]
- If plate removal is considered, It should be delayed for at least 12–18 months after the initial fixation [overall quality: very low]
- The use of large screws (>3.5 mm) in forearm fractures should be avoided [overall quality: very low]

Summary of recommendations

- Fractures of the distal third of the radius are often associated with DRUJ instability
- DRUJ instability is best evaluated, both radiographically and physically by manipulation during surgery after stabilization of the radial fracture
- A proximal located isolated radial fracture does not rule out traumatic DRUJ instability
- Based on the present literature there is no conclusive recommendation possible for the most optimal treatment method in isolated ulnar fractures
- Standard bone grafting is not required in comminuted diaphyseal fractures during initial treatment
- If bone grafting is used, its application should possible be reserved only for fractures with bone loss greater than two thirds of the diameter of the diaphysis
- Anatomical fixation of the radius in Galeazzi fractures is a necessary condition to obtain DRUJ congruency
- Surgical treatment of Galeazzi fractures should take place within 10 days after injury
- The DRUJ must be radiographically visualized and manually tested during surgery after ORIF of the radial fracture to assess joint congruency and residual instability
- If ORIF of the radial fracture leads to anatomic reduction of the DRUJ cast immobilization is sufficient and additional K-wire fixation is not necessary
- Elective removal of forearm plate is contraindicated and should only be considered if there is pain or another symptom resulting from hardware irritation to the soft tissues
- If plate removal is considered, It should be delayed for at least 12–18 months after the initial fixation
- The use of large screws (>3.5 mm) in forearm fractures should be avoided

Conclusions

Fractures of the forearm can be divided into four groups. Isolated radial fractures (1) and fractures of both bones of the forearm (2) are routinely treated by ORIF. Acute bone grafting in comminuted fractures is not necessary in most cases. Most isolated fractures of the ulnar diaphysis (3) can be treated with immobilization in a cast or functional brace. Galeazzi fracture-dislocations (4) must be recognized and treated with stable internal fixation of the radial fracture to ensure DRUJ congruency and anatomic alignment. Thorough evaluation of the DRUJ should be performed in every isolated radial fracture, regardless of the fracture location. Temporary fixation of the DRUJ with K-wires can be of use to maintain the reduction, but there is no evidence that this should be performed in all cases. Open reduction of the DRUJ is indicated only in irreducible dislocations.

References

1. Reilly TJ. Isolated and combined fractures of the diaphysis of the radius and ulna. Hand Clin 2002;18:179–94.
2. Ostermann PA, Ekkernkamp A, Henry SL et al. Bracing of stable shaft fractures of the ulna. J Orthop Trauma 1994;8:245–8.
3. Dymond JW. The treatment of isolated fractures of the distal ulna. J Bone Joint Surg Br 1984;66:408–10.
4. Saunder DJ, Arthwal GS. Management of isolated ulnar shaft fractures. Hand Clin 2007;23:179–84.
5. Szabo RM, Skinner M. Isolated ulnar shaft fractures. Retrospective study of 46 cases. Acta Orthop Scand 1990; 61:350–2.
6. Morgan WJ, Breen TF. Complex fractures of the forearm. Hand Clin 1994;10:375–90.
7. Anderson LD, Sisk D, Tooms RE, Park WI. Compression-plate fixation in acute diaphyseal fractures of the radius and ulna. J Bone Joint Surg Am 1975;57:287–97.
8. Chapman MW, Gordon JE, Zissimos AG. Compression-plate fixation of acute fractures of the diaphyses of the radius and ulna. J Bone Joint Surg 1989;71:159–69.
9. Moore TM, Klein JP, Patzakis MJ, Harvey JP. Results of compression-plating of closed Galeazzi fractures. J Bone Joint Surg 1985;67:1015–21.
10. Faierman E, Jupiter JB. The management of acute fractures involving the distal radio-ulnar joint and distal ulna. Hand Clin 1998;14:213–29.
11. Giannoulis FS, Sotereanos DG. Galeazzi fractures and dislocations. Hand Clin 2007;23:153–63.
12. Mikić ZD. Galeazzi fracture-dislocations. J Bone Joint Surg Am 1975;57:1071–80.
13. Reckling FW. Unstable fracture-dislocations of the forearm (Monteggia and Galeazzi lesions). J Bone Joint Surg 1982;64:857–63.
14. Rettig ME, Raskin KB. Galeazzi fracture-dislocation: a new treatment-oriented classification. J Hand Surg Am 2001;26:228–235.
15. Ring D, Rhim R, Carpenter G, Jupiter JB. Isolated radial shaft fractures are more common than Galeazzi fractures. J Hand Surg Am 2006;31:17–21.
16. Handoll HHG, Pearce P. Interventions for isolated diaphyseal fractures of the ulna in adults. Cochrane Database Syst Rev 2009;3:CD000523.
17. Gebuhr P, Holmich P, Orsnes T, et al. Isolated ulnar shaft fractures: comparison of treatment by a functional brace and long-arm cast. J Bone Joint Surg Br 1992;74:757–9.
18. Atkin DM, Bohay DR, Slabaugh P, Smith BW. Treatment of ulnar shaft fractures: a prospective, randomised study. Orthopedics 1995;18:543–7.
19. Van Leemput T, Mahieu G. Conservative management of minimally displaced isolated fractures of the ulnar shaft. Acta Orthop Belg 2007;73:710–13.
20. Leung F, Chow S-P. A prospective, randomised trial comparing the limited contact dynamic compression plate with the point contact fixator for forearm fractures. J Bone Joint Surg Am 2003;85:2343–8.
21. Goel SC, Raj KB, Srivastava TP. Isolated fractures of the ulnar shaft. Injury 1991;22:212–14.
22. Pollock FH, Pankovich AM, Prieto JJ, Lorenz M. The isolated fracture of the ulnar shaft. Treatment without immobilization. J Bone Joint Surg Am 1983;65:339–42.
23. Boussouga M, Bousselmame N, Lazrek K, Taobane H. Surgical management of isolated fractures of the ulnar shaft. Acta Orthop Belg 2002;68:343–7.
24. Wright RR, Schmeling GJ, Schwab JP. The necessity of acute bone grafting in diaphyseal forearm fractures: a retrospective review. J Orthop Trauma 1997;11:288–94.
25. Wei SY, Born CT, Abene A, et al. Diaphyseal forearm fractures treated with and without bone graft. J Trauma 1999;46:1045–8.
26. Ring D, Rhim R, Carpenter G, Jupiter JB. Comminuted diaphyseal fractures of the radius and ulna: does bone grafting affect nonunion rate? J Trauma 2005;59:438–41.
27. Mikek M, Vidmar G, Tonin M, Pavlovcic V. Fracture-related and implant-specific factors influencing treatment results of comminuted diaphyseal forearm fractures without bone grafting. Arch Orthop Trauma Surg 2004;124:393–400.
28. Rothe M, Rudy T, Stankovic P, Stürmer KM. Treatment of Galeazzi's fracture: is surgical revision of the distal radioulnar joint necessary? Handchir Mikrochir Plast Chir 2001;33:252–7.
29. Strehle J, Gerber C. Distal radioulnar joint function after Galeazzi fracture-dislocations treated by open reduction and internal plate fixation. Clin Orthop 1993; 293:240–5.
30. Mestdagh H, Duquennoy A, Letendart J, et al. Long-term results in the treatment of fracture-dislocations of Galeazzi in adults. Report on twenty-nine cases. Ann Chir Main 1983;2:125–33.
31. Lindsey RW, Fenison AT, Doherty BJ, et al. Effects of retained diaphyseal plates on forearm bone density and grip strength. J Orthop Trauma 1994;8:462–7.
32. Bednar DA, Grandwilewski W. Complications of forearm-plate removal. Can J Surg 1992;35:428–31.
33. Hidaka S, Gustilo RB. Refracture of bones of the forearm after plate removal. J Bone Joint Surg Am 1984;66:1241–3.
34. DeLuca PA, Lindsey RW, Ruwe PA. Refracture of bones of the forearm after the removal of compression plates. J Bone Joint Surg Am 1988;70:1372–6.

35. Rosson JW, Shearer JR. Refracture after the removal of plates from the forearm. An avoidable complication. J Bone Joint Surg Br 1991; 73B:415–17.

36. Langkamer VG, Ackroyd CE. Removal of forearm plates. A review of the complications. J Bone Joint Surg Br 1990;72: 601–4.

37. Rumball K, Finnegan M. Refractures after forearm plate removal. J Orthop Trauma 1990;4:124–9.

38. Labosky DA, Cermak MB, Waggy CA. Forearm fracture plates: to remove or not to remove. J Hand Surg Am 1990;15:294–301.

39. Beaupre GS, Csongradi JJ. Refracture risk after plate removal in the forearm. J Orthop Trauma 1996;10:87–92.

40. Chia J, Soh CR, Wong HP, Low YP. Complications following metal removal: a follow-up of surgically treated forearm fractures. Singapore Med J 1996;37:268–9.

Distal Radius Fractures

Boris A. Zelle[1] and Michael Zlowodzki[2]

[1]University of Texas Health Science Center at San Antonio, San Antonio, TX, USA
[2]University of Minnesota, Minneapolis, MN, USA

Case scenario

A 65 year old woman presents to the Emergency Department after a fall on to her outstretched right hand. She noticed immediate onset of wrist pain and swelling.

Relevant anatomy

In the radiographic evaluation of distal radius fractures, different anatomic parameters serve as guidelines for quantifying the amount of displacement (Table 49.1).[1]

Importance of the problem

Distal radius fractures usually result from low-energy trauma and occur more frequently in women than in men.[2,3] Along with spine and hip fractures, distal radius fractures are the most common osteoporosis-related fractures in the elderly patient.[4] The lifetime risk of sustaining a distal radius fracture at the age of 50 years has been estimated to be 2% for white men and 15% for white women.[5] It has been suggested that fractures that heal with a significant intra-articular step-off appear are at risk for developing post-traumatic osteoarthritis.[6]

Top eight questions

1. Initial splinting: long-arm vs. short-arm?
2. External fixation vs. cast?
3. Bridging vs. nonbridging external fixation?
4. Kapandji vs. across-fracture pinning?
5. Injectable calcium phosphate bone cement?
6. Volar plating vs. external fixation?
7. Volar plating vs. dorsal plating?
8. Arthroscopic vs. fluoroscopic reduction?

Question 1: Initial splinting: long-arm vs. short-arm?

Case clarification

Closed reduction and splinting is performed in the Emergency Department. The healthcare staff ask if immobilization should be done with a short-arm or long-arm splint.

Relevance

Long-arm splints limit supination/pronation of the forearm and limit flexion/extension of the elbow. However, they are more uncomfortable than short-arm splints, and may result in soft tissue compromise at the elbow.

Current opinion

Sugar-tong splints should be used in the acute setting to protect against pronation/supination and flexion/extension.

Finding the evidence

• Cochrane Database: search term "(distal radi*) AND (fracture*)"
• PubMed (www.ncbi.nlm.nih.gov/pubmed/) with clinical queries search systematic reviews: search terms "(distal radi*) AND (fracture*)"
• PubMed (www.ncbi.nlm.nih.gov/pubmed/) advanced search with meta-analysis, randomized clinical trial, and review: search terms search term "(distal radi*) AND (fracture*)"

Evidence-Based Orthopedics, First Edition. Edited by Mohit Bhandari.
© 2012 Blackwell Publishing Ltd. Published 2012 by Blackwell Publishing Ltd.

Table 49.1 Radiologic parameters for the assessment of radial fracture displacement[1]

Parameter	Definition	Normal value
Radial inclination	AP radiograph, angle between (a) line drawn from tip of radial styloid to ulnar corner of articular surface of distal radius and (b) line drawn perpendicular to longitudinal radial axis	22–23°
Radial length	AP radiograph, distance between (a) line at tip of radial styloid perpendicular to the longitudinal axis of the radius and (b) second perpendicular line at level of distal ulnar articular surface	11–12 mm
Ulnar variance	AP radiograph, distance between (a) line drawn parallel to proximal surface of lunate facet and (b) line drawn parallel to distal ulnar articular surface	Neutral to ulnar 2 mm negative
Radial tilt	Lateral radiograph, angle between (a) line connecting most distal points of dorsal and volar cortical rims of distal radius and (b) line drawn perpendicular to longitudinal axis of radius	11–12° volar tilt

- PubMed (www.ncbi.nlm.nih.gov/pubmed/): search terms "(distal radi*) AND (fracture*) AND (splint* OR cast)"

Articles that were not in the English language were excluded. Data from abstracts and book chapters were not included.

Quality of the evidence
Level II
- 3 randomized clinical trials (RCT) with limitations

Level II
- 1 systematic review of cohort studies with worrisome heterogeneity

Findings
A Cochrane review included eight trials comparing above-elbow vs. below-elbow splinting of distal radius fractures.[5] Most data was retrieved from meeting abstracts and articles from the non-English literature. The authors did not identify any evidence to support recommendations for above-elbow vs. below-elbow splinting of distal radius fractures.

We identified three clinical trials comparing above-elbow vs. below-elbow splinting (Table 49.2).[7–9] These trials were heterogeneous with regard to splinting methods used and

Table 49.2 Long-arm splint vs. short-arm splint

	Bong et al.[7]	Stewart et al.[8]	Wilson et al.[9]
N	88	235	41
Level of evidence	2	2	2
Treatment	1. 38 radial gutter splints 2. 47 sugar-tong splints	1. 93 below-elbow plaster 2. 70 above-elbow brace supinated 3. 72 below-elbow brace	1. 20 below-elbow in pronation 2. 21 above-elbow in supination
Outcome anatomical Short-arm vs. long-arm	Secondary displacement: 42% vs. 36% (NS)	Mean loss of reduction dorsal tilt 1. 9.9° 2. 7.2° 3. 6.7° (NS) Mean loss of radial inclination 1. 1.7 2. 2.3 3. 2.2 (NS)	Dorsal tilt pre-/post-reduction 1. 1.2 ± 8.5/11 ± 11 2. 0.7 ± 7/7 ± 11 (NS) Radial inclination pre-/post-reduction 1. 19 ± 5/15 ± 8 2. 18 ± 3/17 ± 7 (NS)
Outcome function Short-arm vs. long-arm	DASH: 62 ± 19 vs. 70 ± 15 (significant)[a]	Modified Gartland score 1. 3.58 2. 3.22 3. 3.19 (NS)	Excellent/good/fair/poor 1. 6/11/3/0 2. 11/5/4/1 (NS)

NS, not significant.
[a] Lower scores indicate better function.

Table 49.3 Functional, clinical, and anatomical outcomes of external fixation vs. casting

	N	Events		Relative risk (95% CI)
		Ex fix	Cast	
Nonexcellent functional outcome	321	134/256	166/265	0.82 (0.71–0.95)
Pin-track infections	846	69/444	1/402	12.02 (5.07–28.49)
Osteomyelitis	332	1/182	0/150	2.47 (0.10–59.70)
Reflex sympathetic dystrophy	731	25/384	17/347	1.31 (0.74–2.32)
Redisplacement resulting in secondary treatment	694	7/356	51/338	0.17 (0.09–0.32)

CI, confidence interval; Ex fix, external fixator.

reporting of outcomes. There was no pooling of data. Significant differences in loss of reduction between long-arm and short-arm constructs were not recorded in any of these studies. Bong et al. reported improved comfort in the short-arm group at the 1 week follow-up as measured by the DASH score.[7]

Recommendations
• Short-arm splints do not increase the risk of secondary displacement in distal radius fractures [overall quality: low]
• Short-arm splints seem better tolerated by patients [overall quality: low]

Question 2: External fixation vs. cast?

Case clarification
Three days later, the patient returns to the office for follow-up. The fracture is well splinted and reduced, but she remains at risk for secondary displacement. The option of external fixation is discussed.

Relevance
Maintaining a good reduction is important in the treatment of displaced distal radius fractures.

Current opinion
External fixation may provide improved stabilization and may be associated with a decreased risk of secondary displacement.

Finding the evidence
See Question 1.

Quality of the evidence
Level I
• 1 systematic review of 15 randomized and pseudo-RCTs

Findings
In a Cochrane review[1] of 15 trials with 1022 patients, external fixation and casting of dorsally displaced distal radius fractures were compared (Table 49.3). External fixation resulted in a significantly reduced risk of fracture displacement. A significantly higher portion of patients undergoing external fixation achieved excellent functional grading. However, a sensitivity analysis showed that this finding was not robust. External fixation was associated with a significantly higher risk of minor complications, such as pin-site infections. The risk of serious complications, such as reflex sympathetic dystrophy (RSD), was not significantly different.

Recommendations
• External fixation reduces the risk of redisplacement of dorsally displaced radius fractures compared with casting [overall quality: high]
• External fixation may result in a better functional outcome [overall quality: low]
• External fixation is associated with an increased risk of pin-track complications [overall quality: high]

Question 3: Bridging vs. nonbridging external fixation?

Case clarification
Different external fixation techniques are discussed with the patient.

Relevance
Both bridging and nonbridging external fixation have been described.

Current opinion
Bridging external fixation is widely used in the treatment of distal radius fractures.

Finding the evidence
See Question 1.

Quality of the evidence
Level I
- 4 RCTs (Table 49.4)[10-13]

Findings
Only 1 study found significantly better final outcomes in the nonbridging group for volar tilt, grip strength, and wrist flexion.[13] Krishnan et al.[11] recorded significantly better wrist flexion at 6 and 52 weeks in the bridging group. Krukhaug et al.[12] reported significantly better wrist flexion in the bridging group at 6 weeks with no difference at 52 weeks.

Recommendations
- Nonbridging external fixation of distal radius fractures does not result in improved outcomes as compared with bridging external fixation [overall quality: moderate]

Question 4: Kapandji vs. across-fracture pinning?

Case clarification
The option of percutaneous pinning is discussed with the patient.

Relevance
In most percutaneous pinning techniques, the wires are placed across the fracture site. In Kapandji pinning, the wires are inserted intrafocally into the fracture gap to buttress the distal fragment.

Current opinion
Both techniques are similarly effective.

Finding the evidence
See Question 1. Trials reporting on percutaneous pinning in conjunction with other fixation methods, such as external fixation, were not included.

Quality of the evidence
Level I
- 1 RCT

Level II
- 1 RCT with methodological limitations

Findings
Two trials were identified (Table 49.5).[14,15] Lenoble et al.[14] reported a higher incidence of local nerve injury and RSD in the Kapandji group. Strohm et al.[15] reported significantly better functional outcomes in the Kapandji group as measured by a nonvalidated scoring system. Pooling of data was not feasible. The outcomes of these studies are potentially biased by the different postoperative protocols (earlier mobilization in the Kapandji groups).

Recommendations
- Kapandji and across-fracture pinning result in similar functional, anatomical, and clinical outcomes [overall quality: low]

Question 5: Injectable calcium phosphate bone cement?

Case clarification
The radiographs show overall poor bone stock and significant metaphyseal comminution. The use of injectable synthetic bone cement is discussed with the patient.

Relevance
Injectable synthetic bone cements appear to be an attractive option in the treatment of metaphyseal fractures.

Current opinion
The use of injectable calcium phosphate cements improves outcomes.

Finding the evidence
See Question 1.

Quality of the evidence
Level I
- 1 systematic review of 6 RCTs (subgroup analysis on distal radius fractures)

Findings
A recently published meta-analysis included six RCTs on the use of injectable calcium phosphate bone cement in the treatment of distal radius fractures (Table 49.6).[16] No significant difference between patients treated with and without injectable calcium phosphate bone cement was identified for functional and anatomical outcomes. Given the significant study heterogeneity, the results from this pooled analysis must be considered with caution. The use of injectable calcium phosphate bone cement was associated with a decreased risk of infection with a relative risk reduction of 85% (95% CI 58–85%, $p < 0.0001$). All infections were related to external fixator pins or Kirschner (K)-wires.

Recommendations
- The use of injectable calcium phosphate bone cement in the treatment of distal radius fractures decreases the risk of infection [overall quality: moderate]

Table 49.4 Final outcomes: bridging vs. nonbridging external fixation

	Atroshi et al.[10]	Krishnan et al.[11]	Krukhaug et al.[12]	McQueen et al.[13]
N	38	60	75	60
Level of evidence	1	1	1	1
Type of fracture	Dorsally displaced, extra- and intra-articular	Mostly intra-articular	Dorsally displaced, extra-articular	Dorsally displaced, extra- and intra-articular
Technique bridging external fixation	Hoffman, 2 pins in radius, 2 pins in 2nd MC	Hoffman, 2 pins in radius, 2 pins in 2nd MC	Dynawrist, 2 pins in radius, 2 pins in 2nd MC	2 pins in radius, 2 pins in 2nd MC
Technique nonbridging external fixation	Hoffman, 2 pins in radius, 2 pins in distal fragment	Delta frame, 1 pin in radius, 4 pins in distal fragment	Hoffman, 2 pins in radius, 2 pins in fragment	2 pins in radius, 2 pins in distal fragment
Length of FUP	52 weeks	52 weeks	52 weeks	52 weeks
DASH[b] Bridging vs. on-bridging	7 ± 8 vs. 11 ± 12 (NS)	Not recorded	13 (95%CI 8–20) vs. 9(95%CI 3–14) (NS)	Not recorded
Flexion at 6 weeks Bridging vs. nonbridging	(10 weeks) 53° ± 8 vs53° ± 12 (NS)	Median 35° vs. 28° (significant)	Loss of ROM[a] 24° (95%CI 20–28) vs. 35° (95%CI 28–40) (significant)	35 ± 22 vs. 38 ± 20 (NS)
Extension at 6 weeks Bridging vs. nonbridging	50° ± 14 vs. 49° ± 13 (NS)	Median 13° vs. 20° (NS)	Loss of ROM[a] 42° (95%CI 37–47) vs. 43° (95%CI 35–49) (NS)	14° ± 21 vs. 26° ± 22 (significant)
Flexion at 52 weeks Bridging vs. nonbridging	63° ± 9 vs. 64° ± 9 (NS)	Median 60° vs. 50° (significant)	Loss of ROM[a] 8° (95%CI 5–10) vs. 3° (95%CI −1–8) (NS)	78° ± 20 vs. 88° ± 15 (significant)
Extension at 52 weeks Bridging vs. nonbridging	62° ± 12 vs. 60° ± 12 (NS)	Median 60° vs. 50° (NS)	Loss of ROM[a] 4° (95%CI 1–6) vs. 9° (95%CI 6–12) (NS)	87° ± 15 vs. 86° ± 13 (NS)
Grip strength Bridging vs. nonbridging	22 ± 8 kg vs. 27 ± 13 kg (NS)	Median 43% vs. 45% of uninjured side (NS)	Not recorded	69% vs. 87% of uninjured side (significant)
Pin-track infections Bridging vs. nonbridging	6/19 vs. 9/19 (NS)	10/30 vs. 9/30 (NS)	9/38 vs. 9/37 (NS)	2/30 vs. 7/30
Tendon rupture Bridging vs. nonbridging	0/19 vs. 0/19 (NS)	0/30 vs. 0/30 (NS)	Not recorded	0/30 vs. 2/30
RSD Bridging vs. nonbridging	0/19 vs. 0/19 (NS)	1/30 vs. 2/30 (NS)	0/38 vs. 0/37 (NS)	2/30 vs. 0/30
Volar tilt at final FUP Bridging vs. nonbridging	4° vs. 5° (NS)	Median 7° vs. 6.5° (NS)	4°(95%CI 2–6) vs. 8° (95%CI 6–8) (NS)	−12.2° ± 13.2 vs. 5.6° ± 6.4 (significant)
Radial inclination at final FUP Bridging vs. nonbridging	19° vs. 17° (NS)	Median 22° vs. 18.5° (NS)	23(95%CI 21–24) vs. 23 (95%CI 21–24) (NS)	Not recorded

FUP, follow-up; NS, not significant; ROM, range of motion; RSD, reflex sympathetic dystrophy.

[a]Compared to uninjured side.

[b]Lower scores indicate better function.

Table 49.5 Outcomes of Kapandjii vs. across-fracture pinning

	Lenoble et al.[14]	Strohm et al.[15]
N Total	96	81
N Kapandji vs. across-fracture pinning	54 vs. 42	40 vs. 41
Level of evidence	II	I
Treatment Kapandji pinning	2 intrafocal k-wires, immediate mobilization, pin removal after 45 days	2 intrafocal k-wires plus one trans-styloid wire, 6 weeks of volar splint, PT started at 3 weeks, pin removal at 6 weeks
Treatment across-fracture pinning	2 trans-styloid k-wires, 45 days of short-arm cast, pin removal after 45 days	2 trans-styloid k-wires, 6 weeks of forearm cast, pin removal at 6 weeks
Follow-up	24 months	Median 10 months (range 6–20 months)
Pain at final FUP Kapandji vs. across-fracture pinning	7.6 vs. 6.9 (VAS 0–100) (NS)	Not recorded
Grip strength Kapandji vs. across-fracture pinning	84% vs. 83% of uninjured side at 12 months (NS)	Not recorded
Pinch strength Kapandji vs. across-fracture pinning	89% vs. 87% of uninjured side at 12 months (NS)	Not recorded
Functional outcome at final FUP Kapandji vs. across-fracture pinning	No functional outcome score recorded	Modified Martini score (0–38) Median: 34 vs. 28 (significant)
Final anatomical outcome Kapandji vs. across-fracture pinning	Similar anatomical long-term outcomes illustrated on graphs, no raw data provided	Not recorded
SBRN injuries Kapandji vs. across-fracture pinning	8/54 vs. 3/42	Not recorded
Nerve irritation Kapandji vs. across-fracture pinning	Not recorded	5/40 vs. 7/41
RSD Kapandji vs. across-fracture pinning	8/54 vs. 3/42	1/40 vs. 1/41
Superficial pin-site infection Kapandji vs. across-fracture pinning	1/54 vs. 3/42	0/40 vs. 0/41
Wire migration Kapandji vs. across-fracture pinning	0/54 vs. 0/42	3/40 vs. 5/41

NS, not significant; PT, physical therapy; RSD, reflex sympathetic dystrophy; SBRN, superficial branch radial nerve; VAS, visual analog scale.

Table 49.6 Outcomes in patients treated with and without injectable calcium phosphate bone cement

Outcome	N	No. of events calcium phosphate cement vs. control group	Point estimate (95% CI) (P value)	Tests for heterogeneity (P value, I^2)
Grip strength (mean % of uninjured side) at 1 year	494	N/A	WMD = 5.95 (−6.39 to 18.29) (p = 0.34)	<0.01, 94%
ROM flexion (mean % of uninjured side) at 1 year	456	N/A	WMD = 2.11 (−10.9 to 15.13) (p = 0.75)	<0.01, 94%
ROM supination (mean % of uninjured side) at 1 year	456	N/A	WMD = 3.18 (−7.8 to 14.16) (p = 0.57)	<0.01, 96%
Mean loss of radial inclination at 1 year	456	N/A	WMD = −4.04 (−11.78 to 3.7) (p = 0.31)	<0.01, 98%
Mean loss of dorsal angulation at 1 year	492	N/A	WMD = −2.75 (−7.45 to 1.9) (p = 0.25)	0.03, 79%
Infections	375	4/187 vs. 27/188	RR = 0.15 (0.15–0.42) (p < 0.0001)	N/A (only 2 trials)

N/A, not applicable; ROM, range of motion; WMD, weighted mean difference.

• The use of calcium phosphate bone cement does not result in improved functional or anatomical outcomes [overall quality: moderate]

Question 6: Plating vs. external fixation?

Case clarification
Articular involvement is noticed on the radiographs. More invasive options are discussed with the patient.

Relevance
Intra-articular step-off appears to be a significant predictor for the development of post-traumatic osteoarthritis.[6]

Current opinion
Multiple plating systems for distal radius fractures have become available and have reduced the use of external fixation constructs in many centers.

Finding the evidence
See Question 1. Studies comparing external fixation vs. open reduction and internal fixation (ORIF) were identified.

Quality of the evidence
Level I
• 4 RCTs

Level II
• 2 RCTs with methodological limitations

Findings
Six RCTs compared external fixation vs. ORIF (Table 49.7).[17–22] Various external fixation and ORIF techniques were used. Given the heterogeneity of these studies, pooling of data was not possible. Leung et al.[20] recorded significantly better functional outcomes in the plating group. Kreder et al.[19] recorded a faster functional recovery in the external fixation group, but no difference at final follow-up. Wei et al.[21] recorded a better restoration of radial inclination and radial length with the use of radial column plates. One trial comparing external fixation vs. dorsal plating was terminated because of the high complication rate in the dorsal plating group.[18]

Recommendations
• ORIF does not result in better functional and anatomic outcomes than external fixation [overall quality: moderate]

Question 7: Volar plating vs. dorsal plating?

Case clarification
The option of volar vs. dorsal plating is discussed with the patient.

Relevance
Most dorsally displaced fractures are amenable to volar or dorsal plating.

Table 49.7 External fixation vs. plating

	Egol et al.[17]	Grewal et al.[18]	Kreder et al.[19]	Leung et al.[20]	Wei et al.[21]	Xu et al.[22]
N	77	62	179	144	46	30
N external fixation vs. plate	38 vs. 39	33 vs. 29	88 vs. 91	74 vs. 70	22 external fixation, 12 volar plates, 12 radial column plates	14 vs. 16
Type of fracture	Intra- and extra-articular fractures	Intra-articular, >2 mm step-off	Intra-articular, dorsally displaced, >2 mm step-off	Intra-articular	Intra- and extra-articular	Intra-articular
Technique external fixation	External fixation, k-wire ± mini-open reduction	External fixation, k-wire, mini-open reduction	External fixation ± k-wire, mini-open reduction, BG, small fragment screws	External fixation, k-wire ± mini-open reduction and BG	External fixation, k-wire ± mini-open reduction and BG	External fixation ± k-wire, mini-open reduction, BG
Technique plate	Volar locked plate	Dorsal plate	Volar or dorsal plate	Volar, dorsal, or combined volar/dorsal	12 radial column plates, 12 volar plates	Volar, dorsal, or combined volar/dorsal
Level of evidence	I	I	II	II	I	I
Length of follow-up	12 months	18 months (range 6–24)	24 months	24 months	12 months	24 months
Functional outcome score external fixation vs. plate	DASH[a]: 17.2 ± 33.7 vs. 13.0 ± 30.9 (p = 0.15)	DASH and SF-36, no significant difference, no raw data provided	MFA upper limb[a]: 14.8 vs. 21 (NS)	Gartland–Werley system External fixation: 39% excellent, 55% good, 6% fair, 0% poor Plate: 67% excellent, 30% good, 3% fair, 0% poor (p = 0.04)	DASH external fixation 18 ± 14 radial plate 18 ± 12 volar plate 4 ± 5 p = 0.056 for external fixation vs. volar plate	Gartland–Werley score, no significant difference, raw data not provided
Grip strength External fixation vs. plate	% of uninjured side: 100 ± 57 vs. 85 ± 27.5 (p = 0.26)	% of uninjured side: 97% vs. 86% (p = 0.19)	lb compared to uninjured side: −8.2 vs. −11.9 (NS)	—	% of uninjured side External fixation: 69 ± 34 Radial plate: 57 ± 4 Volar plate: 75 ± 25 (NS)	% of uninjured side 95.7% (range 70.2 to 161.5) vs. 89.3 (range 64.5 to 118.7), p = 0.78
Articular step-off External fixation vs. plate	—	—	Step-off >2 mm: 3% vs. 2% (p = 0.68)	—	Step-off >2 mm External fixation: 1/12 Radial plate: 0/10 Volar plate: 0/9 (NS)	Step-off >2 mm: 3/14 vs. 4/16 (NS)

Table 49.7 (Continued)

	Egol et al.[17]	Grewal et al.[18]	Kreder et al.[19]	Leung et al.[20]	Wei et al.[21]	Xu et al.[22]
Articular gap External fixation vs. plate	—	—	Gap > 2 mm: 3% vs. 1% (p = 0.36)	—	Gap > 2 mm External fixation: 1/12 Radial plate: 0/10 Volar plate: 1/9 (NS)	—
Complications external fixation	3 nerve deficits[b], 2 pin-site infections, 1 tendon rupture	2 RSD, 1 DRUJ instability, 1 sensory loss[b], 1 stiffness, 2 pin-site infections, 1 ulnar shortening osteotomy	5 pin-site infection, 2 superficial wound infections, 1 RSD	5 loss of reduction, 5 pin-site infections, 3 wound infections, 3 SBRN injuries, 3 CTS	3 transient median nerve neuropathies, 1 pin-site infections	1 median neuropathy
Complications plate	2 nerve deficits[b], 1 wound infection, 2 tendon ruptures, 1 nonunion	3 RSD, 3 sensory loss[b], 1 ulnar shortening osteotomy, 1 compartment syndrome, 5 tendinitis, 8 HWR (symptomatic)	2 pin-site infections, 1 superficial wound infection, 3 RSD, 2 extensor tendon ruptures	5 loss of reduction, 3 wound infections, 2 CTS	3 and 2 transient median nerve neuropathies in radial plate group and volar plate group, respectively	1 median neuropathy
Remarks	—	Study terminated because of high complication rate in dorsal plating group	1. 8 patients crossed over from external to fixation to plate group to achieve reduction 2. Authors observed faster recovery in external fixation group		Radial plate group achieved significantly higher radial length and radial inclination than external fixation and volar plate group	

BG, bone graft; CTS, carpal tunnel syndrome; DRUJ, distal radioulnar joint; HWR, hardware removal; NS, not significant; RSD, reflex sympathetic dystrophy; SBRN, superficial branch of radial nerve.
[a]Lower score means better outcome.
[b]Not specified.

Current opinion

Dorsal plating allows for a better reduction of displaced dorsal fragments, but is associated with a high risk of tendinitis.

Finding the evidence

See Question 1.

Quality of the evidence

Level I
• 1 RCT

Findings

One RCT evaluated the outcomes of 30 patients with intra-articular distal radius fracture undergoing volar vs. dorsal plating.[23] The volar plating group achieved significantly better outcomes for grip strength, range of motion, and the Gartland–Werley score at 6 months follow-up (Table 49.8). Radiographic outcomes were similar in both groups.

Recommendations

• Volar plating of distal radius fractures results in superior functional short-term outcomes [overall quality: moderate]

Question 8: Arthroscopic vs. fluoroscopic reduction?

Case clarification

The plan is to proceed with external fixation and percutaneous pinning. The option of arthroscopic vs. fluoroscopic reduction is discussed.

Table 49.8 Outcomes of volar vs. dorsal plating

N	Volar plate		Dorsal plate		P
	15		15		
Gartland–Werley score[a]	1.73 ± 1.1		4.9 ± 2.1		<0.01
Grip strength % of uninjured side	95 ± 11		65 ± 15		<0.01
Pain VAS 0–10	1.2 ± 0.8		3.1 ± 1.5		>0.05
ROM					
Total arc flexion/extension (°)	115 ± 23		68 ± 17		<0.01
Total arc supination/pronation (°)	151 ± 16		130 ± 18		0.002
Radiographic outcomes					
Radial inclination (°)	21		24		0.061
Volar tilt (°)	6		10		0.145
Complications	1 RSD		2 RSD		
	0 secondary displacements		2 secondary displacements		
	1 painful scar		3 painful scars		

ROM, range of motion; RSD, reflex sympathetic dystrophy; VAS, visual analog scale.
a Lower score means better outcome.

Relevance

Wrist arthroscopy offers the potential benefit of direct visualization of intra-articular step-offs and allows for treatment of associated intra-articular soft tissue injuries.

Current opinion

Despite its potential benefits, wrist arthroscopy is rarely used in the treatment of distal radius fractures.

Finding the evidence

See Question 1. Studies comparing arthroscopic vs. fluoroscopic reduction in patients undergoing external fixation and percutaneous pinning were identified.

Quality of the evidence

Level I
- 1 RCT

Level II
- 1 prospective cohort study:

Findings

Two trials were identified.[24,25] Arthroscopically assisted reduction appeared to be associated with significantly better functional outcomes, range of motion, and articular reduction (Table 49.9). Both studies recorded that wrist arthroscopy detected a relatively high incidence of intra-articular soft tissue injuries that were addressed during the index procedure.

Recommendations

- In patients undergoing external fixation and percutaneous pinning, arthroscopically assisted reduction results in better functional and anatomic outcomes than fluoroscopic reduction alone [overall quality: moderate]

Summary of recommendations

- Short-arm splints do not increase the risk of secondary displacement in distal radius fractures
- Short-arm splints seem better tolerated by patients
- External fixation reduces the risk of redisplacement compared with casting, but is associated with increased risk of pin-site infection
- Nonbridging external fixation does not result in better outcomes than bridging external fixation
- Kapandji and across-fracture pinning result in similar functional, anatomical, and clinical outcomes
- The use of injectable calcium phosphate bone cement in the treatment of distal radius fractures decreases the risk of infection
- The use of calcium phosphate bone cement does not result in improved functional or anatomical outcomes
- ORIF does not result in better outcomes than external fixation
- Volar plating fractures results in better functional short-term outcomes than dorsal plating
- In patients undergoing external fixation and percutaneous pinning, arthroscopically assisted reduction results in

Table 49.9 Arthroscopic vs. fluoroscopic reduction

	Ruch et al.[24]	Varitimidis et al.[25]
N	30	40
N arthroscopic vs. fluoroscopic	15 vs. 15	20 vs. 20
Technique arthroscopic	External fixation, K-wires, preliminary reduction by fluoroscopyc	External fixation, k-wires, fluoroscopic and arthroscopic reduction ± mini-open reduction + BG
Technique fluoroscopic	External fixation, k-wires ± mini-open reduction	External fixation, k-wires, fluoroscopic reduction ± mini-open reduction and BG
Level of evidence	2	1
Type of fracture	Intra-articular	Intra-articular
Length of follow-up	12 months	24 months
Functional outcome score arthroscopic vs. fluoroscopic	DASH[a]: 11 vs. 19 (NS)	DASH[a]: 4.8 ± 4.2 vs. 8.3 ± 7.4 $p = 0.12$
Functional outcome score arthroscopic vs. fluoroscopic		Modified Mayo wrist score: 91.2 ± 2.2 vs. 86.7 ± 3 $p < 0.01$
Grip strength arthroscopic vs. fluoroscopic	% of uninjured side: 73% vs. 77% (NS)	% of uninjured side: 95% vs. 90%
Flexion° arthroscopic vs. fluoroscopic	78 vs. 59 $p = 0.02$	76 ± 5.2 vs. 63 ± 5.1 $p < 0.01$
Extension° arthroscopic vs. fluoroscopic	77 vs. 69 $p = 0.01$	76 ± 5 vs. 65 ± 2.6 $p < 0.01$
Supination° arthroscopic vs. fluoroscopic	88 vs. 73 $p = 0.02$	80 ± 5.8 vs 73 ± 2.3 $p < 0.01$
Pronation° arthroscopic vs. fluoroscopic	83 vs. 84 $p = 0.90$	83 ± 2.6 vs. 82 ± 2.7 $p = 0.24$
Volar tilt° at final FUP arthroscopic vs. fluoroscopic	−0.87 vs. 1.3 $p = 0.50$	7 vs. 7 $p = 0.50$
Radial inclination° at final FUP arthroscopic vs. fluoroscopic	21 vs. 25 $p = 0.10$	21 ± 1.96 vs. 24 ± 2 $p < 0.01$
Intra-articular gap at final FUP arthroscopic vs. fluoroscopic	0.29 mm vs. 0.05 mm $p = 0.09$	–
Intra-articular step-off at final FUP arthroscopic vs. fluoroscopic	0.31 mm vs. 0.18 mm $p = 0.57$	0.3 ± 0.28 vs. 0.8 ± 0.3 $p < 0.01$
Complications arthroscopic vs. fluoroscopic	Not recorded	2 RSD vs. 4 RSD, 1 superficial wound infection
Arthroscopic findings	5 SL ligament tears, 4 LT ligament tears, 10 TFCC tears	9 SL ligament tears, 4 LT ligament tears, 12 TFCC tears, 9 cartilage injuries, 8 free cartilage bodies

BG, bone graft; FUP, follow-up; LT, luno-triquetral; NS, not significant; RSD, reflex sympathetic dystrophy; SL, scapholunate; TFCC, triangular fibrocartilage complex.
[a] Lower score means better outcome.

better functional and anatomic outcomes than fluoroscopic reduction alone

Conclusions

Numerous reports on the treatment of distal radius fractures have been published. However, only few recommendations for the management of distal radius fractures are supported by high-level evidence.

References

1. Handoll HH, Huntley JS, Madhok R. External fixation vs. conservative treatment for distal radial fractures in adults. Cochrane Database Syst Rev 2007;3:CD006194.
2. Cohen MS, McMurtry RY, Jupiter JP. Fractures of the distal radius. In Browner BD, Jupiter JB, Levine AM, Trafton PG, eds. Skeletal Trauma, 3rd edn, pp. 1315–61. WB Saunders, Philadelphia, PA, 2003.
3. Sanders WE. Distal radius fractures, in Manske PR, ed., Hand Surgery Update, pp. 117–23. American Academy of Orthopaedic Surgeons, Rosemont, IL, 1996.
4. National Osteoporosis Foundation. http://www.nof.org/osteoporosis/diseasefacts.htm. Accessed October 18,2009.
5. Handoll HH, Madhok R. Conservative interventions for treating distal radial fractures in adults. Cochrane Database Syst Rev 2003;2:CD000314.
6. Knirk JL, Jupiter JB. Intra-articular fractures of the distal end of the radius in young adults. J Bone Joint Surg Am 1986;68: 647–59.
7. Bong MR, Egol KA, Leibman M, et al. A comparison of immediate postreduction splinting constructs for controlling initial displacement of fractures of the distal radius: a prospective randomized study of long-arm vs. short-arm splinting. J Hand Surg Am 2006;31:766–70.
8. Stewart HD, Innes AR, Burke FD. Functional cast-bracing for colles fractures: a comparison between cast bracing and conventional plaster casts. J Bone Joint Surg Br 1984;66:749–53.
9. Wilson C, Venner RM. Colles' fracture. Immobilisation in pronation or supination? J R Coll Surg Edinb 1984;29:109–11.
10. Atroshi I, Brogren E, Larsson GU, et al. Wrist-bridging vs. non-bridging external fixation for displaced distal radius fractures: a randomized assessor-blind clinical trial of 38 patients followed for 1 year. Acta Orthop 2006; 77:445–53.
11. Krishnan J, Wigg AE, Walker RW, et al. Intra-articular fractures of the distal radius: a prospective randomised controlled trial comparing static bridging and dynamic non-bridging external fixation. J Hand Surg Br 2003;28:417–421.
12. Krukhaug Y, Ugland S, Lie SA, et al. External fixation of fractures of the distal radius: a randomized comparison of the Hoffman compact II non-bridging fixator and the Dynawrist fixator in 75 patients followed for 1 year. Acta Orthop 2009;80:104–8.
13. McQueen MM. Redisplaced unstable fractures of the distal radius. A randomised, prospective study of bridging vs. non-bridging external fixation. J Bone Joint Surg Br 1998;80: 665–669.
14. Lenoble E, Dumontier C, Goutallier D, et al. Fracture of the distal radius. J Bone Joint Surg Br 1995;77:562–7.
15. Strohm PC, Müller CA, Boll T, et al. Two procedures for Kirschner wire osteosynthesis of distal radius fractures. J Bone Joint Surg Am 2004;86:2621–8.
16. Bajammal SS, Zlowodzki M, Lelwica A, et al. The use of calcium phosphate bone cement in fracture treatment. A meta-analysis of randomized trials. J Bone Joint Surg Am 2008;90:1186–96.
17. Egol K, Walsh M, Tejwani N, et al. Bridging external fixation and supplementary Kirschner-wire fixation vs. volar locked plating for unstable fractures of the distal radius: a randomised, prospective trial. J Bone Joint Surg Br 2008;90:1214–21.
18. Grewal R, Perey B, Wilmink M, et al. A randomized prospective study on the treatment of intra-articular distal radius fractures: open reduction and internal fixation with dorsal plating vs. mini open reduction, percutaneous fixation, and external fixation. J Hand Surg Am 2005;30:764–72.
19. Kreder HJ, Hanel DP, Agel J, et al. Indirect reduction and percutaneous fixation vs. open reduction and internal fixation for displaced intra-articular fractures of the distal radius: a randomised, controlled trial. J Bone Joint Surg Br 2005;87:829–36.
20. Leung F, Tu YK, Chew WY, et al. Comparison of external and percutaneous pin fixation with plate fixation for intra-articular distal radial fractures. A randomized study. J Bone Joint Surg Am 2008;90:16–22.
21. Wei DH, Raizman NM, Bottino CJ, et al. Unstable distal radial fractures treated with external fixation, a radial column plate, or a volar plate. A prospective randomized trial. J Bone Joint Surg Am 2009;91:1568–77.
22. Xu GG, Chan SP, Puhaindran ME, et al. Prospective randomised study of intra-articular fractures of the distal radius: comparison between external fixation and plate fixation. Ann Acad Med Singapore 2009;38:600–6.
23. Jakubietz RG, Gruenert JG, Kloss DF, et al. A randomised clinical study comparing palmar and dorsal fixed-angle plates for the internal fixation of AO C-type fractures of the distal radius in the elderly. J Hand Surg Eur 2008;33:600–4.
24. Ruch DS, Vallee J, Poehling GG, et al. Arthroscopic reduction vs. fluoroscopic reduction in the management of intra-articular distal radius fractures. Arthroscopy 2004;20:225–30.
25. Varitimidis SE, Basdekis GK, Dailiana ZH, et al. Treatment of intra-articular fractures of the distal radius: fluoroscopic or arthroscopic reduction? J Bone Joint Surg Br 2008;90:778–85.

50 Perilunate Dislocations

Geert A. Buijze[1], Job N. Doornberg[1], and David Ring[2]
[1]Orthopaedic Research Center Amsterdam, Academic Medical Center, Amsterdam, The Netherlands
[2]Harvard Medical School, Boston, MA, USA

Case scenario

A 30 year old man presents to the Emergency Department after a high-energy motorcycle collision. His only injury is to his right (dominant) wrist, which is painful, swollen, and deformed. Radiographs reveal a dorsal perilunate dislocation of the wrist. The neurovascular examination is unremarkable.

Relevant anatomy

The wrist tends to dislocate around the lunate, leaving the radiolunate relationship relatively spared. The ligaments and bones around the lunate are injured, hence the term perilunate injury. There are two types of injuries: so-called *lesser arc injuries* in which the ligament attachment of the lunate are injured and *greater arc injuries* which involve one or more fractures of surrounding carpal bones instead of a ligament injury (Figure 50.1). According to the system of Mayfield et al.,[1] perilunate injuries follow a four-stage mechanism of progressive instability from radial to ulnar (Figure 50.2; see box). In reverse perilunate injuries the mechanism is opposite, from ulnar to radial.

Four-stage mechanism of perilunate injuries
- Stage 1: scapholunate dissociation
- Stage 2: capitolunate dissociation
- Stage 3: lunotriquetral dissociation
- Stage 4: lunate dislocation

Importance of the problem

Perilunate injuries cause permanent wrist impairment and midcarpal arthrosis with effective treatment and global wrist arthrosis necessitating wrist arthrodesis with ineffective treatment.

Top seven questions

Diagnosis

1. Is there a role for CT, MRI, or arthroscopy in the diagnosis of perilunate wrist dislocations?
2. What is the relative prevalence of greater and lesser arc injuries and reverse perilunate injuries?

Therapy

3. How often is manipulative reduction successful?
4. What is the optimal timing of definitive surgery?
5. What is the preferred operative exposure in perilunate injuries?
6. What is the preferred type of temporary fixation of the carpus: screws or Kirschner (K-) wires?

Prognosis

7. What are the most important factors to predict impairment and disability after perilunate dislocations?

Evidence-Based Orthopedics, First Edition. Edited by Mohit Bhandari.
© 2012 Blackwell Publishing Ltd. Published 2012 by Blackwell Publishing Ltd.

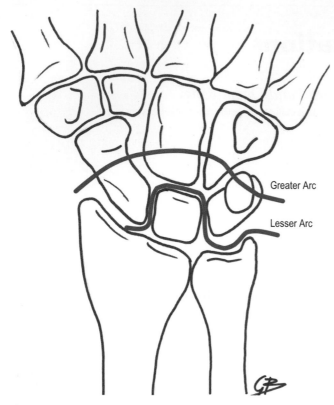

Figure 50.1 Patterns of greater arc and lesser arc injuries.

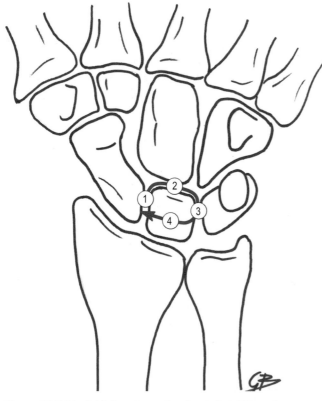

Figure 50.2 Mayfield's four stages of perilunate instability and dislocation.

Question 1: Is there a role for CT, MRI, or arthroscopy in the diagnosis of perilunate wrist dislocations?

Case clarification

Lateral and posteroanterior radiographs suggest a lesser arc perilunate injury without major fracture, but the anatomy is distorted and there are some bone fragments of unclear source.

Relevance

Perilunate dislocations are usually treated with open reduction and it is not clear that CT scanning or MRI helps with preparation or understanding of the injury beyond that gained with open visualization of the injury.

Current opinion

The role of more sophisticated imaging is debated.

Finding the evidence

• PubMed (www.ncbi.nlm.nih.gov/pubmed/): sensitivity search using keywords "perilunate injur* OR carpal dislocation" AND "imaging"
• Bibliography of eligible articles
• Articles that were not in the English language were excluded.

It is recommended to include only the most recent studies in decision-making, as CT and MRI imaging protocols have become significantly more advanced over the last few years.

Quality of the evidence

Level IV
• 1 case series[2]

Level V
• 1 expert opinion[3]

Findings

Despite the fact that posteroanterior and lateral radiographs are almost always sufficient to diagnose carpal dislocations, up to 25% of these injuries are missed at presentation, as shown by Herzberg et al. (level IV).[2] Advanced imaging is not required, but according to Kaewlai et al. (level V) CT with multiplanar and volumetric reformation can be a useful technique to demonstrate the complexity and extent of fractures and dislocations.[3] There are no methodological studies comparing plain radiographs to CT imaging, MRI, or diagnostic arthroscopy for carpal dislocations.

Recommendation

• Advanced imaging is not necessary for diagnosis of perilunate dislocations among experts, but 2-D and 3-D CT might be helpful to nonspecialists and can occasionally assist in evaluating complexity [overall quality: very low]

Question 2: What is the relative prevalence of greater and lesser arc injuries and reverse perilunate injuries?

Relevance
Greater and lesser arc injuries are managed differently and may have different prognoses.

Current opinion
Greater arc injuries are commonly believed to be less frequent than lesser arc injuries.

Finding the evidence
• PubMed (www.ncbi.nlm.nih.gov/pubmed/): sensitivity search using keywords "carpal" AND "fracture* OR injur*" AND "epidemiology OR prevalence"
• Bibliography of eligible articles

Quality of the evidence
Level III
• 1 epidemiologic study[4]

Level IV
• 2 case series[2,5]

Findings
A study by van der Molen et al. (level III), which assessed the epidemiology of functionally disabling carpal injuries (resulting in at least 6 weeks of time off work) in a 4 year period in the Netherlands, found that carpal fracture-dislocation represented 5.4% of all carpal injuries.[4] The fracture-dislocations consisted of lesser arc injuries (2.1%), greater arc injuries (3%), and radiocarpal dislocations (0.4%). In Dunn's (level IV) series of 40 carpal fracture-dislocations over a 16-year period in one center in the United States, there were 12 lesser arc injuries (30%), 13 greater arc injuries (33%), 6 (15%) radiocarpal dislocations, 5 carpometacarpal dislocations (13%), and 4 dislocations of carpals other than the lunate (10%).[5] In the largest multi-center study reported by Herzberg et al. (level IV), greater arc injuries were twice as frequent as lesser arc injuries.[2]

Recommendation
• Greater arc injuries are more common than lesser arc injuries.

Question 3: How often is manipulative reduction successful?

Relevance
Immediate successful reduction can limit the potential for median nerve dysfunction and allow for delay of definitive repair.

Current opinion
Closed reduction is often possible within a day of injury, but becomes more difficult with progressive delay.

Finding the evidence
• PubMed (www.ncbi.nlm.nih.gov/pubmed/): sensitivity search using keywords "perilunate injur* OR carpal dislocation" AND "treatment"
• Bibliography of eligible articles

Quality of the evidence
Level IV
• 1 case series[6]

Level V
• 1 case report[7]
• 1 expert opinion[8]

Findings
In the study reported by Adkison et al. (level IV) manipulative reduction was successful in 37 of 55 (67%) patients.[6] Fifty-nine percent of the wrists lost alignment during the first 6 weeks of treatment despite cast immobilization. Closed treatment alone was only successful 27% of the time. The likelihood of success decreases rapidly within a few days after injury.[7,8]

Recommendations
• Manipulative reduction is mostly successful in the acute setting and mostly unsuccessful if not performed within the first few days [overall quality: low]
• Closed reduction can only be maintained for a short period with cast immobilization [overall quality: low]

Question 4: What is the optimal timing of definitive surgery?

Relevance
Some consider these injuries emergencies.

Current opinion
If closed reduction can be achieved, surgery can be delayed for up to a week after injury.

Finding the evidence
• PubMed (www.ncbi.nlm.nih.gov/pubmed/): sensitivity search using keywords "perilunate injur* OR carpal dislocation" AND "treatment"
• Bibliography of eligible articles

Quality of the evidence
Level III
• 1 case-control studies[10]

Level IV
- 2 case series[2,9]

Level V
- 3 expert opinions[11–13]

Findings

Weir (level IV) showed that if treatment is delayed by more than 2 weeks, functional outcome is expected to be worse.[9] In the largest retrospective series reported by Herzberg et al. (level IV), delay in treatment of more than 7 days showed near-significantly worse results ($p = 0.07$) compared to treatment within 7 days.[2] Delay in treatment of more than 45 days showed significantly worse results ($p < 0.05$). However, not all patients in that series underwent surgery.

In a study by Komurcu et al. (level III) comparing the outcome of early vs. delayed treatment in 12 patients with greater arc injuries, there was a significant difference in clinical and radiological outcome in favor of early treatment[10].

Most surgeons suggest surgery between 3 and 5 days after injury for dislocations that can be manipulatively reduced.[11–13]

Recommendation

- The optimal timing of definitive surgery for a manipulatively reducible dislocation is within a week after injury [overall quality: moderate].

Question 5: What is the preferred operative exposure in perilunate injuries?

Relevance

There is controversy regarding the optimal surgical approach.

Current opinion

Approaches may be either arthroscopic-assisted percutaneous or open using a dorsal, volar, or combined exposure.

Finding the evidence

- PubMed (www.ncbi.nlm.nih.gov/pubmed/): sensitivity search using keywords "perilunate injur* OR carpal dislocation" AND "treatment"
- Bibliography of eligible articles

Quality of the evidence

Level IV
- 8 case series[2,14–20]

Level V
- 3 expert opinions[13,18,21]

Findings

There are no direct comparative studies between the different operative approaches for perilunate injuries. All three open exposures (dorsal, volar, and combined) can lead to satisfactory outcome.[2,15–20] A long-term outcome study reported by Forli et al. (level IV) of 18 greater and lesser arc injuries including all three open exposures did not show a correlation between outcome and approach.[17] Volar and dorsal approaches each have advantages and drawbacks. Herzberg (level V) reports that a combined volar and dorsal approach improves exposure, but increases the possibility of postoperative fibrosis and stiffness.[13] An arthroscopically assisted percutaneous approach can be a promising alternative in less severe cases, but to date only three patients with good outcomes have been reported by Park and Ahn (level V).[21] Moreover, one series from Wong and Ip (level IV) using a minimally invasive percutaneous approach showed good results in 21 greater arc injuries.[14] There is no evidence to determine the best methods for reduction (open or closed), ligament repair or reattachment, or immobilization. Percutaneous reduction and fixation without direct ligament repair is appealing, but the little data published on this technique suggest that it is inferior to open techniques.

Recommendation

- The surgical approach should be based on the surgeon's preference and individualized for the patient [overall quality: low].

Question 6: What is the preferred type of temporary fixation of the carpus: screws or K-wires?

Relevance

Temporary screws may reduce the likelihood of skin problems or infection and may allow earlier mobilization.

Current opinion

Most surgeons use K-wires to hold the carpus reduced while the ligaments heal.

Finding the evidence

- PubMed (www.ncbi.nlm.nih.gov/pubmed/): sensitivity search using keywords "perilunate injur* OR carpal dislocation" AND "treatment"
- Bibliography of eligible articles

Quality of the evidence

Level III
- 1 case-control study[22]

Level V
- 1 expert opinion[23]

Findings

Herbert (level V) suggested using temporary screws between the scaphoid and lunate and between the lunate and the triquetrum as an alternative to K-wire fixation.[23] In the study by Souer and colleagues (level III) comparing the two treatment methods in 18 patients there were no significant differences in radiographic and functional outcomes.[22] Although none of the outcomes were significant, there was a trend favoring screw fixation in some of the outcomes. The average flexion–extension arc was slightly higher (87° vs. 73°) and the prevalence of midcarpal arthritis was lower (29% vs. 71%) in the screw fixation group. There were 2 pin infections in the K-wire cohort and the only pin in the screw fixation cohort (used to address ulnocarpal translocation) also became infected, with 2 patients having wrist sepsis.

Recommendation

• There results of treatment with temporary screws and temporary K-wires are comparable [overall quality: moderate]

Question 7: What are the most important factors to predict impairment and disability after perilunate dislocations?

Relevance

Despite optimal management most patients with perilunate injuries experience persistent impairment and disability.

Current opinion

The most important factors predicting impairment and disability are delay in treatment, open injuries, and persistent carpal malalignment.

Finding the evidence

• PubMed (www.ncbi.nlm.nih.gov/pubmed/): sensitivity search using keywords "perilunate injur* OR carpal dislocation" AND "outcome OR prognosis"
• Bibliography of eligible articles

Quality of the evidence

Level IV
• 6 case series[2,9,16,17,19,24]

Findings

In the series of 166 perilunate injuries by Herzberg et al. (level IV), the factors significantly influencing the clinical results consisted of open injury and delay in treatment of more than 45 days, whereas the anatomical type of injury (greater vs. lesser arc) had no significant influence.[2] Delay in treatment of more than 2 weeks was associated with

poor results in a series of five late reductions, reported by Weir (level IV).[9] In two case series, additional osteochondral fractures of the head of the capitate were associated with poorer results.[19,24] In the series of 18 perilunate injuries with the longest follow-up (minimum of 10 years) reported by Forli (level IV), the presence of radiological arthritis and static carpal instability did not cause reduced function.[17] These findings are consistent with the findings of Weir et al.[9] and Hildebrand et al. (level IV).[16] The latter series of 23 perilunate injuries also investigated differences in outcome between lesser and greater arc injuries and found no significant differences in any of the clinical outcome measurements. The only significant difference was that lesser arc injuries had a significantly larger revised carpal height ratio.

Recommendations

• The most important factors predicting impairment and disability are delay in treatment, open injury, and osteochondral fracture of the capitate head [overall quality: low]
• Clinical outcomes are often substantially better than radiographic outcomes [overall quality: low]

Summary of recommendations

• Advanced imaging is not necessary for diagnosis of perilunate dislocations among experts, but 2-D and 3-D CT might be helpful to nonspecialists and can occasionally assist in evaluating of complexity
• Greater arc injuries are more common than lesser arc injuries
• Manipulative reduction is mostly successful in the acute setting and mostly unsuccessful if not performed within the first few days
• Closed reduction can only be maintained for a short period with cast immobilization
• The optimal timing of definitive surgery for a manipulatively reducible dislocation is within a week after injury
• The surgical approach should be based on the surgeon's preference and individualized for the patient
• There results of treatment with temporary screws and temporary K-wires are comparable
• The most important factors predicting impairment and disability are delay in treatment, open injury, and osteochondral fracture of the capitate head
• Clinical outcomes are often substantially better than radiographic outcomes

Conclusions

Because of the low prevalence of perilunate dislocations, there is a paucity of high-quality evidence regarding its diagnosis, treatment, and prognosis. The best available evidence on these injuries consists of retrospective comparative studies. Therefore, all recommendations in this chapter are of moderate to very low quality and thus need to be interpreted with caution.

References

1. Mayfield JK, Johnson RP, Kilcoyne RK. Carpal dislocations: pathomechanics and progressive perilunar instability. J Hand Surg Am 1980;5(3):226–41.

2. Herzberg G, Comtet JJ, Linscheid RL, Amadio PC, Cooney WP, Stalder J. Perilunate dislocations and fracture-dislocations: a multicenter study. J Hand Surg Am 1993;18(5):768–79.

3. Kaewlai R, Avery LL, Asrani AV, Abujudeh HH, Sacknoff R, Novelline RA. Multidetector CT of carpal injuries: anatomy, fractures, and fracture-dislocations. Radiographics 2008;28(6):1771–84.

4. van der Molen AB, Groothoff JW, Visser GJ, Robinson PH, Eisma WH. Time off work due to scaphoid fractures and other carpal injuries in The Netherlands in the period 1990 to 1993. J Hand Surg Br 1999;24(2):193–8.

5. Dunn AW. Fractures and dislocations of the carpus. Surg Clin North Am 1972;52(6):1513–38.

6. Adkison JW, Chapman MW. Treatment of acute lunate and perilunate dislocations. Clin Orthop Relat Res 1982;164:199–207.

7. Jasmine MS, Packer JW, Edwards GS, Jr. Irreducible transscaphoid perilunate dislocation. J Hand Surg Am 1988;13(2):212–15.

8. Blazar PE, Murray P. Treatment of perilunate dislocations by combined dorsal and palmar approaches. Tech Hand Up Extrem Surg 2001;5(1):2–7.

9. Weir IG. The late reduction of carpal dislocations. J Hand Surg Br 1992;17(2):137–9.

10. Komurcu M, Kurklu M, Ozturan KE, Mahirogullari M, Basbozkurt M. Early and delayed treatment of dorsal transscaphoid perilunate fracture-dislocations. J Orthop Trauma 2008;22(8):535–40.

11. Sauder DJ, Athwal GS, Faber KJ, Roth JH. Perilunate injuries. Orthop Clin North Am 2007;38(2):279–88, vii.

12. Budoff JE. Treatment of acute lunate and perilunate dislocations. J Hand Surg Am 2008;33(8):1424–32.

13. Herzberg G. Perilunate and axial carpal dislocations and fracture-dislocations. J Hand Surg Am. 2008 Nov;33(9):1659–68.

14. Wong TC, Ip FK. Minimally invasive management of transscaphoid perilunate fracture-dislocations. Hand Surg 2008;13(3):159–65.

15. Campbell RD, Jr., Thompson TC, Lance EM, Adler JB. Indications for open reduction of lunate and perilunate dislocations of the carpal bones. J Bone Joint Surg Am 1965;47:915–37.

16. Hildebrand KA, Ross DC, Patterson SD, Roth JH, MacDermid JC, King GJ. Dorsal perilunate dislocations and fracture-dislocations: questionnaire, clinical, and radiographic evaluation. J Hand Surg Am 2000;25(6):1069–79.

17. Forli A, Courvoisier A, Wimsey S, Corcella D, Moutet F. Perilunate dislocations and transscaphoid perilunate fracture-dislocations: a retrospective study with minimum ten-year follow-up. J Hand Surg Am;35(1):62–8.

18. Weil WM, Slade JF, 3rd, Trumble TE. Open and arthroscopic treatment of perilunate injuries. Clin Orthop Relat Res 2006;445:120–32.

19. Herzberg G, Forissier D. Acute dorsal trans-scaphoid perilunate fracture-dislocations: medium-term results. J Hand Surg Br 2002;27(6):498–502.

20. Knoll VD, Allan C, Trumble TE. Trans-scaphoid perilunate fracture dislocations: results of screw fixation of the scaphoid and lunotriquetral repair with a dorsal approach. J Hand Surg Am 2005;30(6):1145–52.

21. Park MJ, Ahn JH. Arthroscopically assisted reduction and percutaneous fixation of dorsal perilunate dislocations and fracture-dislocations. Arthroscopy 2005;21(9):1153.

22. Souer JS, Rutgers M, Andermahr J, Jupiter JB, Ring D. Perilunate fracture-dislocations of the wrist: comparison of temporary screw versus K-wire fixation. J Hand Surg Am 2007;32(3):318–25.

23. Herbert TJ. Internal fixation of the carpus with the Herbert bone screw system. J Hand Surg Am 1989;14(2 Pt 2):397–400.

24. Melone CP, Jr., Murphy MS, Raskin KB. Perilunate injuries. Repair by dual dorsal and volar approaches. Hand Clin 2000;16(3):439–48.

51 Carpal Fractures

Bertrand H. Perey[1], Anne-Marie Bedard[2], and Fay Leung[3]

[1]University of British Columbia, Port Moody, BC, Canada
[2]Laval University, Centre Hospitalier Universitaire de Quebec, Quebec, QC, Canada
[3]University of British Columbia, Vancouver, BC, Canada

Case scenario

A 30 year old laborer fell from his truck and landed on his right arm with the wrist in dorsiflexion. He presented to the Emergency Department with pain and swelling of the right wrist, at the anatomical snuffbox. Range of motion of the wrist is limited by pain. Radiographs were taken (Figure 51.1).

Relevant anatomy

The scaphoid is anatomically divided into three sections: proximal pole, waist, and distal pole. The scaphoid is largely covered with articular cartilage, and receives its blood supply primarily from the artery to the dorsal ridge of the scaphoid, a branch of the radial artery. Approximately 75% of the scaphoid, including the proximal pole, is supplied by retrograde flow from this artery. The vascularity of the proximal pole is tenuous as it depends entirely on this intraosseous blood supply. The distal pole receives abundant blood supply directly from the palmar superficial branch of the radial artery.

Scaphoid fractures are described by location (proximal, waist, or distal) and by stability (stable and unstable). An unstable scaphoid fracture is defined as greater than 1 mm of displacement on any radiological views, or greater than 15° of lunocapitate angulation, or greater than 45° scapholunate angulation on the lateral view.

The intrascaphoid angle, evaluated on a sagittal CT scan cut (Figure 51.2) is formed by the junction of two lines perpendicular to the diameter of the proximal and distal pole. The normal intrascaphoid angle is 24°.

Importance of the problem

The scaphoid is the most commonly fractured carpal bone, and accounts for approximately 60% of carpal fractures and 11% of all hand fractures. Most fractures occur in young men, many of whom are manual workers. These patients are particularly disabled when prolonged immobilization is required to achieve union.

Untreated scaphoid fractures may go on to mal- or nonunite, leading to abnormal carpal kinematics and subsequent wrist osteoarthritis (Figure 51.3), underlining the need for early diagnosis and vigilant care of an acute scaphoid injury.

Top seven questions

Diagnosis

1. What diagnostic modality should be used in the process of diagnosing, evaluating, and following a scaphoid fracture?

Treatment

2. What is the recommended treatment for an acute undisplaced fracture of the waist of the scaphoid?
3. When treating an undisplaced fracture of the scaphoid conservatively, what is the ideal method of casting?

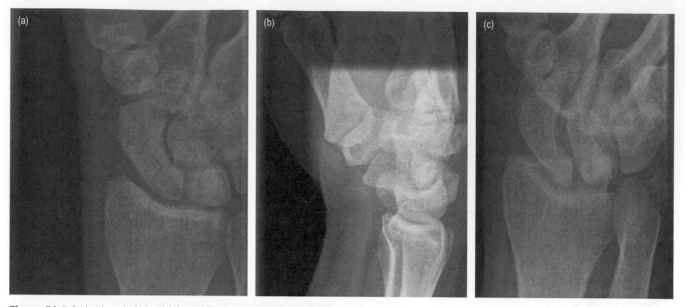

Figure 51.1 PA in ulnar deviation (a), lateral (b) and scaphoid (c) view of the right scaphoid.

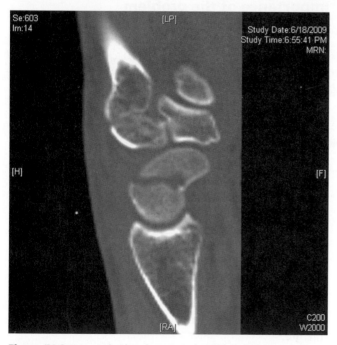

Figure 51.2 Intrascaphoid angle measured at 62° on CT scan. It is formed by the junction of two lines perpendicular to the diameter of the proximal and distal pole. Normal is 24°.

4. When treating an undisplaced scaphoid fracture with internal fixation, what is the ideal surgical technique?

5. What is the ideal treatment when faced with a delayed diagnosis of an undisplaced fracture of the scaphoid?

6. What is the ideal treatment for displaced fracture of the waist of the scaphoid?

7. What is the ideal treatment for an undisplaced proximal pole fracture?

Question 1: What diagnostic modality should be used in the process of diagnosing, evaluating and following a scaphoid fracture?

Case clarification

The patient's radiographs are initially negative. You are planning to immobilize the patient in a cast and reassess him in 2 weeks with repeat radiographs (Figure 51.4), but you wonder if an immediate bone scan, CT scan, or MRI would be more appropriate.

Relevance

A missed scaphoid fracture can have adverse outcomes. It is generally accepted that a delay in diagnosis and treatment of scaphoid fractures can lead to nonunion or malunion resulting in symptomatic osteonecrosis, carpal collapse, or secondary osteoarthritis.

Current opinion

Patients presenting with a clinically suspected scaphoid fracture, but negative initial radiographs, are treated with temporary cast immobilization for 10–14 days before a second set of radiographs is performed.

Finding the evidence

• Cochrane Database, with search term "scaphoid fracture", 1985 to present.

Quality of the evidence

Level I

• 28 diagnostic studies

• 1 therapeutic randomized controlled trial (RCT)

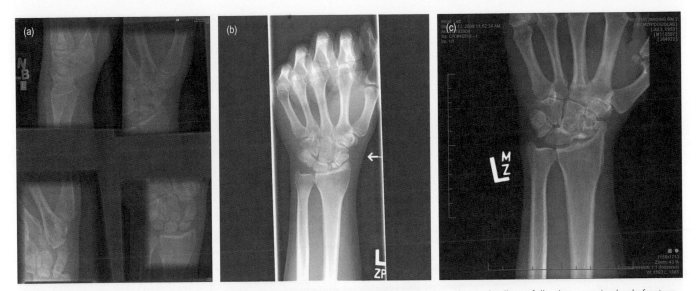

Figure 51.3 (a) Nonunion at the junction of the waist/proximal pole (b) Stage 1 scaphoid nonunion advanced collapse following a proximal pole fracture (c) Stage 3 scaphoid nonunion advanced collapse.

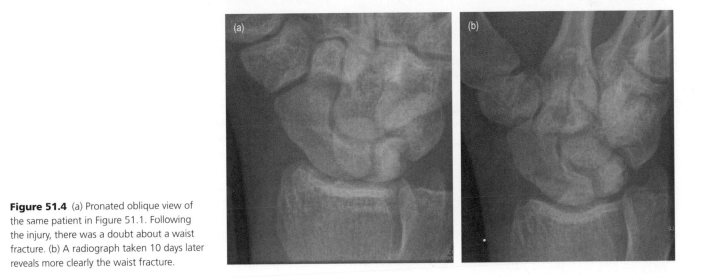

Figure 51.4 (a) Pronated oblique view of the same patient in Figure 51.1. Following the injury, there was a doubt about a waist fracture. (b) A radiograph taken 10 days later reveals more clearly the waist fracture.

Level IV
- 1 case series

Findings

Sensitivity and negative predictive value of initial radiographs
The negative predictive value (NPV) of initial radiographs varies greatly between studies. While a randomized control trial showed a sensitivity and NPV of 93% and 98.9% respectively (Table 51.1 and Table 51.2),[1] Table 51.3 shows a range between 63% and 93%. To compensate for this variation, patients with clinically suspected acute scaphoid fractures but negative initial radiographs are typically treated with 2 weeks of cast immobilization followed by repeated examination and radiographic studies. This leads

Table 51.1 Results of a prospective multicenter study on clinically suspected fractures of the scaphoid

Clinically suspected fractures	1052
True scaphoid fractures	160
Scaphoid fractures detected on initial radiographs	150
Scaphoid fractures detected on the second set of radiographs	9
Scaphoid fracture detected on the third set of radiographs	1

Table 51.2 Two-way contingency table analysis

	Positive initial radiograph	Negative initial radiograph	Total
Scaphoid fracture	150	10	160
No scaphoid fracture	0	892	892
Total	150	902	1052

Table 51.3 Negative predictive value of radiographs; frequency of scaphoid fractures in patients initially presenting with a clinical suspicion of fracture and negative radiograph

Studies	No. of clinically suspicious cases with negative radiograph	No. of scaphoid fractures	
		N	% (1-NPP)
Brismar[2]	187	21	11
Murphy[3]	54	8	15
Waizenegger[4]	84	7	8
Tiel-van Buul[5]	125	35	28
Tiel-van Buul[6]	16	5	31
Thorpe[7]	59	4	7
Hunter[8]	36	13	36
Cook[9]	8	4	50
Breitenseher[10]	42	14	33
Fowler[11]	43	6	14
Bretlau[12]	52	9	17
Roolker[13]	71	20	28
Bayer[14]	40	8	20
Raby[15]	56	7	12,5
Hauger[16]	54	5	9
Brydie[17]	195	37	19
Moller[18]	224	36	16
Brooks[19]	11	3	27
Beeres[20]	56	15	27
Memarsadeghi[21]	29	11	38
Total	1442	268	22

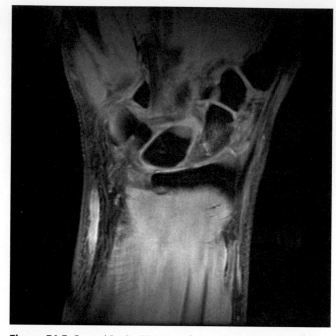

Figure 51.5 Coronal Fat Sat T2 MRI confirming a suspected proximal pole fracture of the scaphoid.

to unnecessary immobilization of probably over 75% of these patients, with the socioeconomic impact of loss of productivity, time off work, and the inappropriate use of healthcare resources.

Is immobilization necessary while waiting for the second series of radiographs? The absence of immobilization would improve the function of the patient and decrease the associated costs while waiting for the final diagnosis. However, this alternative must not compromise the outcome of being safe for fractures missed initially.

An RCT conducted by Sjolin et al.[1] studied 108 patients with a clinical suspicion of scaphoid fracture but negative initial radiographs and randomized them to treatment with either a supportive bandage or a dorsal plaster cast. Four patients proved to have incomplete waist fractures and three to have avulsions from the tuberosity. No complete fractures were seen. The average sick leave was 14 days for those in a cast and 4 days for those in a bandage, a difference that represented a significant loss of productivity. The authors concluded that occult fractures on initial radiographs are likely to be very stable, and they may be treated with a supportive bandage while awaiting definitive diagnosis.

Another argument against immediate immobilization comes from a level IV case series[22] that studied the consequences of a delay in cast treatment and the development of nonunion in 285 fractures of the scaphoid. No increase in the time to union or in the incidence of nonunion was found following a delay of immobilization of less than 4 weeks. However, when the delay exceeded 4 weeks, some fractures had healing complications.

Other diagnostic modalities and their utility in avoiding significant, unnecessary immobilization time Bone scan is sensitive but not specific for diagnosing scaphoid fractures. Sensitivity has been evaluated at approximately 95%, while specificity is around 70%. Moreover, it usually requires a delay of 72 hours following the injury before the test can be performed. Currently, MRI is thought to have sensitivity and a specificity approaching 100% (Figure 51.5).

Five level I diagnostic studies compare MRI to bone scan.[6,7,11,23] In 2005, the pooled results of four of these studies[24] showed that MRI is at least as sensitive as bone scan for diagnosing scaphoid fractures, but it has superior specificity. MRI also allows for earlier diagnosis, and the ability to detect associated soft tissue injuries. According to Thorpe et al.,[7] costs would be similar between the two options.

More recently, a new comparative diagnostic study evaluated 100 consecutive patients with suspected scaphoid fractures and negative radiographs.[25] Among the 20 cases with a proven scaphoid fracture, there were 4 false-negative cases with MRI, and 8 false-positive cases with bone scan. The authors could not confirm the superiority of MRI over bone scintigraphy and criticized the previous 4 studies for using different imaging sequences and protocols, variable timing to MRI, and small sample sizes.

Brooks[19] investigated the cost-effectiveness of MRI by randomizing 28 patients with a suspected scaphoid fracture to either MRI or immobilization with radiographs at 10–14 days. MRI reduced the days unnecessarily spent in a cast (3 days vs. 10 days, $p < 0.006$) and the use of healthcare resources. The total expenditure in the two groups was similar (MRI group = \$594 (Australian), control group = \$428, $p = 0.19$), owing to the direct cost of MRI. Costs from productivity loss and income loss secondary to immobilization were not included in the calculation; however, if considered, this may have swayed the conclusion in favor of MRI.

Dorsay[26] constructed a cost-effectiveness model based on a review of the literature pooling data on the NPV of initial radiographs (similar to Table 51.3). They found that 75% patients will be needlessly immobilized, as the diagnostic process will conclude the absence of scaphoid fracture. Their cost analysis, which did not include productivity losses, suggested that initial MRI is nearly equivalent to repeated radiographs.

CT scan can also identify occult fractures (Figure 51.6) but is more useful in defining the fracture pattern and the angular deformity.[27] It is not as sensitive, specific, or accurate as MRI for identifying acute occult fractures.[28]

Two level I diagnostic studies have looked at the results of ultrasound[29,30] and found a sensitivity of 78%, a specificity of 89%, a PPV of 88% and a NPV of 80%. This is inferior to MRI or bone scan, and only slightly better than radiographs.

Recommendations

• An initial normal radiograph cannot accurately guarantee absence of a scaphoid fracture: it is therefore recommended to proceed with further imaging, either acutely or 2 weeks later [overall quality: high]

• MRI is the study of choice to diagnose occult scaphoid fracture in the acute setting and has the advantage of avoiding unnecessary immobilization. There is good evidence to support its cost-effectiveness. The availability of

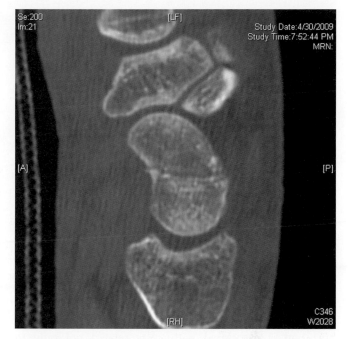

Figure 51.6 CT scan of the same patient as in Figure 51.1. CT can identify occult fracture but is more useful in assessing fracture displacement and angulation.

this modality may limit its application [overall quality: high]

• A second set of radiograph at 2 weeks is an appropriate diagnostic tool but leads to unnecessary immobilization of the majority of patients. However, there is good evidence to support that immobilization of the wrist in a cast is not necessary in the interval before the new images [overall quality: high]

Question 2: What is the recommended treatment for an acute undisplaced fracture of the waist of the scaphoid?

Case clarification

The patient's radiographs were repeated 2 weeks after the injury and now reveal an undisplaced fracture of the waist of the scaphoid (Figure 51.7). He works as a laborer and will not be able to work with a cast. He asks you about alternative options.

Relevance

Conservative treatment of undisplaced fractures by plaster cast immobilization has been reported in case series to be successful in approximately 95% of patients.[30–32] However, some have questioned the reliability of plain radiographs in diagnosing union, suggesting that reported union rates may be falsely elevated.[33] Meanwhile, many case series have shown the union rate with percutaneous technique to be close to 100%. Moreover, acute scaphoid fractures

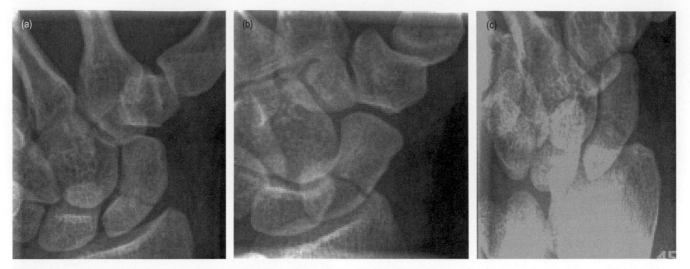

Figure 51.7 (a) AP, (b) pronated oblique and (c) scaphoid view of an undisplaced scaphoid fracture.

mainly affect young working individuals for whom immobilization is associated with costs related not only to medical treatment but also to work disability. The superiority of percutaneous treatment over cast treatment for undisplaced fractures of the scaphoid is as yet unproven.

Current opinion
Currently, the majority of acute undisplaced scaphoid fractures are treated conservatively with a cast.

Finding the evidence
• Cochrane Database, with search term "scaphoid fracture", 1985 to present.

Quality of the evidence
Level I
• 8 RCTs
• 1 meta-analysis
• 1 economic and decision analysis

Level II
• 1 RCT with methodologic limitations

Level III
• 1 retrospective comparative study

Level IV
• 2 case series

Findings
Nine RCTs have evaluated cast treatment vs. surgical fixation for undisplaced acute scaphoid fractures.[34–42] Table 51.4 summarizes the findings in each study. Derived from these randomized studies, the following observations can be drawn.

Range of motion and grip strength No negative long-term effect of cast immobilization with respect to joint stiffness and decreased grip strength was observed.

Functional scores At final follow-up, no study showed a significant difference in subjective functional scoring

Rate of union Only one study used CT scan to assess union.[42] In the remaining studies, the determination of healing was made using radiographs only, which may give an inaccurate diagnosis of union.[33] With the information available, the rate of union between conservative and surgical treatment is not different. Only Dias et al. found a difference between the two groups, but their definition of nonunion may have been too inclusive, as 5/10 nonunions diagnosed at 12 weeks eventually healed without further intervention.

Time to union For the same reason, assessment of time to union was suboptimal, and the time to union was not reported in every study. In the study by Aurora et al., the only study to include the use of CT scan, a significant difference was found in the time to union in favor of the percutaneous technique. However, the data is insufficient to conclude any advantage of the percutaneous technique over conservative treatment.

Time off work Vinnars et al. evaluated the subgroup of occupationally active individuals in an RCT[34] and published their observations in a cost-effectiveness trial.[35] The median time of absence from work was 74 days in the cast group and 39 days in the surgery group, but this difference was not significant (p = 0.32). In the subgroup of manual workers, there was a significantly longer period of absence from work in those undergoing closed treatment than those treated surgically (100 vs. 61 days, p = 0.03). Saeden et al. similarly reported that manual laborers remained on sick

Table 51.4 Conservative vs. surgical treatment of nondisplaced scaphoid fractures

Study	Fracture type	Sample size N	F/U Length (N)	Treatment	Nonunion	Time to union (weeks)	Immobilization Time (weeks)	ROM (% loss)	Grip strength	TOW (weeks)
Vinnars[34,35]	Undisplaced <28 days A_1, B_{1-2-3}	85	10 yrs (75)	BETSC Herbert Open	1/35 0/40	— —	10 3 p value unavailable	No SSD	No SSD	10.6 5.6[a]
McQueen[36]	53 undisplaced 7 displaced[b] B_{1-2}	60	1 yr (48)	Colles Acutrak Percut	4/30 1/30	13.9 9.2[c]	— —	No SSD	No SSD	11.4 3.8[c]
Dias[37,38]	Undisplaced <7 days Waist[d]	88	1 yr (81) 8 yrs (71)	Colles Herbert Open	10/44 0/44[e]	— —	— —	No SSD	No SSD	6 5
Saeden[39]	Acute, NOS	62	12 yrs (42)	BETSC Herbert Open	2/30 1/32	— —	12 2[f]	No SSD	No SSD	15 6[g]
Bond[40]	Undisplaced <2 wks Waist	25	2 yrs (25)	AETSC Acutrak Percut	0/14 0/11	12 7[h]	— —	No SSD	No SSD	15 8[i]
Adolfsson[41]	Undisplaced <2 wks B_{1-2}	53	16 wks	BETSC Acutrak Percut	0/28 1/25	No SSD	— —	13% 6%[j]	No SSD	— —
Arora[42]	Undisplaced <3 wks B_2	47	24 wks (44)	BETSC Acutrak Percut	0/23 1/21	10.6 6.1[k]	10.9 1.6[k]	No SSD	No SSD	7.9 1.1[k]

AETSC, above-elbow thumb spica cast; BETSC, below-elbow thumb spica cast; F/U, follow-up; NOS, not otherwise specified; ROM, range of motion; SSD, statistically significant difference; TOW, time off work.

[a] $p = 0.32$. But when assessed separately, patients with manual work had significantly longer time off work than the nonmanual employees/self-employed: 84 days vs. 16, statistically significant, $p < 0.001$.

[b] 2 in the nonsurgical group.

[c] Statistically significant, $p < 0.001$

[d] The original article describes 5 distal fractures, 2 proximal fractures, 10 fractures with mild displacement (amount not specified), 7 fractures with DISI and 22 fractures with comminution.

[e] Statistically significant, $p < 0.001$. Nonunion was assessed at 12 weeks. One fracture healed with continued cast treatment, whereas 4 fractures were considered healed at the time of surgery for nonunion. This leaves 5 real nonunions. Moreover, of these 10 apparent nonunions in the cast group, 5 occurred among the 11 patients with comminution.

[f] Statistically significant, $p < 0.01$

[g] Statistically significant, $p = 0.002$. The difference was significant for patients with blue-collar occupation, but not for patients with a white-collar occupation.

[h] Statistically significant, $p = 0.0003$.

[i] Statistically significant, $p = 0.0001$, but the trial was performed on U.S. Navy personnel who are not allowed to return to work with a cast.

[j] Statistically significant, $p < 0.02$, but ROM recorded at 16 weeks, just after cast removal.

[k] Statistically significant, $p < 0.05$. Only study using CT scan to assess union.

leave for a mean period of 7 weeks in the operated group and for 18 weeks in the conservative group ($p < 0.001$), whereas no significant difference was found in patients with sedentary occupations. McQueen et al. and Aurora et al. both found significantly longer periods off work in the conservative group. They did not evaluate for a difference between manual and sedentary workers. The difference found by Bond et al. can be questioned, as the trial was performed on U.S. Navy staff, who were not permitted to return to work with a cast.

Time spent off work with surgery is significantly shorter for manual workers, with lack of a clear advantage for sedentary workers. The definition of manual worker should probably be revised to encompass any individual for whom the unencumbered hand is necessary to accomplish his/her work (e.g., a surgeon or a pianist).

Cost-effectiveness There are three cost-effectiveness comparisons between the conservative and the surgical treatment of undisplaced scaphoid fractures. Two are included in the therapeutic RCTs mentioned earlier,[35] and one is a decision analytic model.[43] Aurora et al. found significant differences in the immobilization time and the time absent from work between the conservative and the surgical groups. The hospital costs were significantly higher in operated patients because of the direct cost of the surgery. The work disability costs were significantly less in operated patients (€200 vs. €1453, p < 0.01). When all costs were calculated, operative treatment (€2097) was less expensive than conservative treatment (€2363 Euros) but this was not statistically significant (p > 0.05).

As mentioned earlier, Vinnars et al. found a significant difference in time off work in manual workers treated surgically, with no such difference found in sedentary workers/self-employed group. Hospital-related costs were always higher in the operated group than in the cast group (p < 0.01) due to the direct cost of surgery. In the sedentary and self-employed workers, work disability costs were minimal, making the surgical option clearly not cost-effective for these patients. In the manual workers group, the work disability costs were numerically higher in the cast group than in the surgical group, but this did not reach statistical significance. The costs related to surgery were offset by lower work disability costs, with the final total costs being not significantly different to the cast treatment.

Davis et al.[43] designed a decision analytic model based on quality of life measures and cost differences between surgery and casting. They concluded that open reduction and internal fixation (ORIF) offers greater quality-adjusted life years and is more cost-effective than casting because less productivity is lost.

Complications Complications are variably reported, accounting for the difference in rate of complications between studies. Table 51.5 reports the complications encountered among the RCTs cited earlier. These studies all used a volar approach, either open or percutaneous.

Scaphotrapezial osteoarthritis Vinnars et al. found a significant increase in the prevalence of osteoarthritis in the scaphotrapezial joint of their surgical group (p = 0,005). No difference in the rate of osteoarthritis was found between those treated with a volar mini-incision (3/11), compared to an open approach (8/28). Subjective outcomes of patients diagnosed with scaphotrapezial osteoarthritis (STT OA) did not differ from the remaining patients.

Saeden et al. similarly reported 14/23 cases of STT OA in the surgical group, compared to 4/16 in the conservative group, as diagnosed by CT 12 years after internal fixation of scaphoid fractures. Again, these findings did not affect clinical outcome.

Recommendations
- The surgical treatment of an undisplaced scaphoid fracture does not lead to improved range of motion, grip strength, or functional outcome at final follow-up [overall quality: high]
- The rate of union and the time to union are not improved by surgical treatment of an undisplaced fracture, as assessed by radiographs. Studies with CT scan assessment of union are mandatory in the future [overall quality: moderate]
- The time off work is significantly shorter when treating a manual worker surgically, but this does not appear to be true for sedentary workers. Consequently, surgery is more cost-effective in patients who are involved in work, sports, or lifestyles incompatible with long-term immobilization [overall quality: high]
- In those where immobilization does not alter daily function, cast immobilization remains the standard treatment since patients are not subject to the attendant risks associated with surgery [overall quality: high]

Question 3: When treating an undisplaced fracture of the scaphoid conservatively, what is the ideal method of casting?

Case clarification
The patient radiographs reveal an undisplaced fracture of the waist of scaphoid (see Figure 51.7). After discussing the nonsurgical and surgical options with the patient, you decide to treat him conservatively.

Relevance
Many casting options are suggested in the literature. The ideal casting method should be one that protects the fracture fragments from moving while providing maximum function to the patient.

Current opinion
Short-arm thumb spica cast remains the most widely accepted treatment of undisplaced scaphoid fracture.

Finding the evidence
- Cochrane Database, with search term "scaphoid fracture", 1985 to present.

Quality of the evidence
Level I
- 5 RCTs

Table 51.5 Complications relating to surgical and conservative treatments of nondisplaced scaphoid fractures

Study	Percutaneous volar		Open volar		Cast treatment
	Peri-op	Post-op	Peri-op	Post-op	
Vinnars			2 screw malpositioning 1 SL ligament injury 1 FCR injury	1 CRPS 3 screw protusion 1 screw loosening[a] 2 large cysts[a] 5 screw removal for pain 1 fracture proximal to the screw	Not reported
McQueen	2 screwdriver breakage	1 screw protrusion			2 AVN 1 CRPS 3 DISI
Dias			4 screw or drill malpositioning 1 tuberosity split during insertion 2 persistant fracture mobility	1 CRPS 1 scar related problems 1 hypoesthesia PCBMN 1 wound infection 10 non-central placement[a] 3 screw loosening[a]	1 VISI
Saeden				1 screw malpositioning 1 screw loosening	Not reported
Bond		1 screw protusion			Not reported
Adolfsson	1 reaming difficulty	1 CRPS			Not reported
Arora		1 infection 2 CRPS			Not reported

PCBMN, palmar cutaneous branch of median nerve.
[a] Patients asymptomatic.

Level II
- 1 prospective comparative study

Level III
- 2 retrospective comparative study

Level IV
- 1 case series

Findings

Long-arm vs. short-arm cast One RCT[44] studied the results of a long-arm vs. a short-arm cast immobilization for acute undisplaced fracture of the scaphoid. Proximal, middle, distal third, and tuberosity fractures were included. This study showed significantly shorter time to union in the long-arm group (9.5 vs. 12.5 weeks, $p < 0.05$), and higher rate of nonunions and delayed unions (p value not mentioned). Union was assessed using plain radiographs only, which brings into question the validity of the results.[33] Nevertheless, this study remains the only level I paper addressing the long-arm vs. short-arm cast issue.

One level II prospective comparative study[45] failed to show any difference in the time to union between the two methods of casting. Level III[46,47] and level IV[30] studies show conflicting results, and no conclusion can be drawn in favor of either of the two methods.

Many biomechanical comparative studies have been conducted, again showing conflicting results.[48–51] A cadaveric study[52] used CT scan to evaluate amount of fracture displacement during prosupination between unprotected scaphoids and scaphoids immobilized in below-elbow thumb spica cast. Long-arm casting was not tested. Less than 1 mm of displacement was judged to be acceptable. The total magnitude of motion from pronation to supination averaged 0.2 mm in the specimens immobilized with a below-elbow thumb spica cast, suggesting that a short-arm cast would be appropriate in preventing motion at the fracture site.

Table 51.6 Union rate according to type of casting, at 6 months postinjury

Cast	Definitely united		Probably united		Nonunion	
	N	%	N	%	N	%
Thumb spica	111	78	18	12	14	10
Colles	114	77	19	13	15	10

NB: no p value provided in the article.

Lawton et al.[53] compared the forearm rotation allowed by a long-arm thumb spica cast vs. an epicondylar bearing (Munster) thumb spica cast on healthy individuals with no fracture. The authors suggested that the Munster cast could still limit enough forearm rotation to avoid healing complications while allowing more elbow flexion/extension than a long-arm cast; however, the clinical advantages of this type of casting have not been demonstrated.

Inclusion of the thumb One RCT[54] showed that immobilization with a thumb spica cast is no more likely to achieve union than immobilization of the wrist alone with a Colles type of cast (Table 51.6).

Furthermore, Karantana et al.,[55] in another level I trial, compared the effect of the two types of casts on hand function in 20 healthy volunteers. Both casts prolonged the time taken to complete the hand function test compared to controls, but the thumb spica cast group took significantly longer than the group in the Colles cast (thumb spica cast = 48.2 seconds, Colles cast = 58.5 seconds, no p value provided) to complete the test.

Position of immobilization of the wrist In the 1950s and 1960s, authors advocated numerous wrist positions, with the goal of reducing displaced fractures and maintaining the reduction in a cast. In the only level I RCT addressing this issue, Hambridge et al.[56] showed that wrist position does not influence rate of union (union rate 89%, p = 0.46) but does influence function. At 6 months, the patients with a Colles cast in 20° of flexion had significantly greater restriction in extension than those immobilized with 20° of extension (61° vs. 73° of dorsiflexion, p < 0.01). Flexion, radial deviation, and ulnar deviation were not impaired by any type of immobilization.

Recommendations

• The evidence is not strong enough to support the use of a long-arm cast in the treatment of an undisplaced scaphoid fracture [overall quality: moderate]
• Inclusion of the thumb in the cast is not critical for scaphoid fracture healing [overall quality: high]

Table 51.7 Advantages and disadvantages of the volar and dorsal open approaches

Advantages	Disadvantages
Volar	
Preservation of main blood supply	Violation of radiocarpal ligaments
Better access to middle and distal third fractures	Poor access to proximal pole
Easier correction of humpback deformity	Central placement of screw more difficult[a]
Dorsal	
Preservation of radiocarpal ligaments	Risk for dorsal branch of radial artery
Better access to proximal pole	Poor access to distal third
Central placement of screw easier	Difficult correction of humpback deformity
Less tourniquet time	

[a] See discussion in the section on percutaneous technique.

Question 4: When treating an undisplaced scaphoid fracture with internal fixation, what is the ideal surgical technique?

Case clarification

The patient's radiograph reveals an undisplaced fracture of the waist of scaphoid (Figure 51.7). After discussing the nonsurgical and surgical options with the patient, you decide to treat him surgically.

Relevance

When planning the surgery, the specialist must decide between an open or percutaneous technique. Each technique can further be accomplished with a volar or a dorsal approach. The surgeon must know the advantages and possible concerns/complications of each strategy.

Current opinion

The majority of surgeons prefer to use the percutaneous volar retrograde technique when treating an undisplaced fracture of the scaphoid.

Finding the evidence

• Cochrane Database, with search term "scaphoid fracture", 1985 to present.

Quality of the evidence
Level I
• 5 RCTs

Level III
- 4 retrospective comparative studies

Level IV
- 5 case series

Findings

Open approach The majority of case series discussing ORIF of scaphoid fractures have used a volar approach, which avoids disruption of the dorsal branch of the radial artery. However, violating the volar radiocarpal ligaments may subsequently create carpal instability. The dorsal approach for scaphoid fracture fixation has also been described.[57,58] Table 51.7 summarizes the advantages and disadvantages of the volar and dorsal open approaches.

There are two retrospective level III studies comparing the open volar and dorsal approaches. Polsky et al.[59] studied 26 patients with scaphoid fractures treated with a cannulated screw. Sixteen patients underwent a dorsal approach and 10 patients a volar approach. There was no difference in the rate of union between the two approaches (dorsal 81%, volar 80%, p value not reported). No significant differences were noted between the groups for range of motion, grip strength or pain level ($p > 0.08$). There was a significantly shorter tourniquet time with the dorsal approach ($p = 0.047$), explained by easier exposure with dorsal approach, with no risk of violating the radiocarpal ligaments and easier targeting of the central axis of the scaphoid (see later discussion on percutaneous approaches).

Garcia-Elias et al.[60] compared the volar approach to the dorsal approach in cases of scaphoid nonunions treated with inlay bone grafting and found a similar union rate (around 80%). The volar approach resulted in a significant increase in the scapholunate angle ($p < 0.001$) and in the lunocapitate angle ($p < 0.05$). Surgical division of the palmar radiocarpal ligaments was thought to be responsible for these findings.

To our knowledge, there is no randomized study comparing the open volar and dorsal approaches in cases involving only acute scaphoid fractures.

Percutaneous vs. open approaches There is no study directly comparing percutaneous and open approaches. It is generally accepted that the percutaneous approach reduces the surgical morbidity associated with an open procedure.

Indications for percutaneous technique are listed in Table 51.8.

Positioning of the screw Trumble et al.[61] showed decreased time to fracture union ($p < 0.05$) in open scaphoid fixation with screws located more centrally in the proximal fragment. This was true with the use of either a cannulated or noncannulated screw, but significantly more cannulated

Table 51.8 Indications for the use of a percutaneous technique

Indications	Contrindications
Nondisplaced fracture[a]	Irreducible fracture
Displaced reducible fracture	Nonunion with severe sclerosis
Proximal pole fracture	Nonunion with bone loss >1 mm
Fracture with delayed presentation	Presence of humpback deformity
Fracture with fibrous union	Pseudarthrosis
Nonunion with minimal sclerosis, bone loss <1 mm[b]	AVN of proximal pole
Presence of associated fractures, if scaphoid fracture meet the above criteria	

[a] If surgical treatment chosen.
[b] No angulation present. Consider percutaneous curettage and bone grafting.

screws were placed centrally (17/18 in the cannulated group, 7/16 in the noncannulated group, $p < 0.01$).

Trumble further stressed the importance of central screw placement after conducting a comparative biomechanical study between centrally and eccentrically placed screws.[62] This study confirmed that screws placed centrally in the proximal fragment are stronger, with greater stiffness (43%, $p < 0.01$) and increased load to displacement (113%, $p < 0.01$) and provide more secure fixation and lower risk of screw migration or fracture at the screw–bone interface.

Choice of screw Trumble's work suggests that the type of screw is not as important as its central positioning. The use of cannulated systems greatly facilitates central placement of the screw. Surgeons also favor the use of headless designs, which allow the screw to be fully buried in the bone and prevent erosion on adjacent structures. In a biomechanical comparative study, the Herbert–Whipple and the standard Acutrak were not different in their ability to resist cyclical bending load.[63]

Volar vs. dorsal percutaneous approach The volar percutaneous technique is the most commonly used (Figure 51.8). Extension and ulnar deviation of the wrist during the procedure facilitates maintenance of fracture reduction and introduction of the screw. It is more difficult to place the screw centrally with this approach, first because the surgeon cannot rely on the ring sign under fluoroscopy to target the central scaphoid axis, and, secondly, the volar lip of the trapezium limits the ability to enter the scaphoid in a

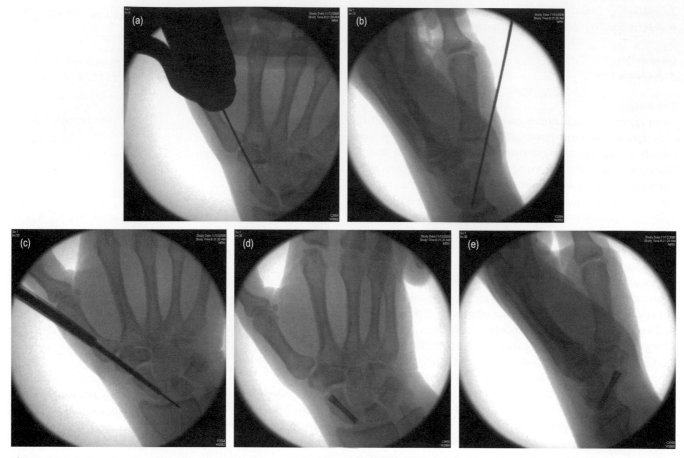

Figure 51.8 Retrograde volar percutaneous technique. (a) and (b): insertion of the KW in a retrograde fashion, through the trapezium in order to achieve central placement of the screw. (c) insertion of the screw. (d) and (e): final result.

central position unless a transtrapezial technique is used.[64] Finally, with the volar approach, there is concern about injury to the superficial branch of the radial artery or to the scaphotrapezial joint.

With the dorsal approach, the position of flexion and pronation of the wrist under fluoroscopy makes the proximal pole of the scaphoid look like a circle (ring sign). This facilitates placement of the Kirschner (K)-wire into the center of the circle. It is imperative, but technically challenging, to maintain this position throughout the surgery to prevent the K-wire from bending or breaking. There is also a risk of fracture displacement with this position. While avoiding the scaphotrapezial joint, the dorsal approach raises concerns about violating the radiocarpal joint, as well as injuring the extensor tendons.

The only situation where there is a clear advantage of a given approach is in the case of a proximal pole fracture, where the dorsal/proximal approach is more effective in securely fixing and compressing the small proximal fragment.[65] Proximal pole fractures are discussed under Question 7.

The two approaches have been directly compared in only one level III retrospective study published in 2009.[66] The two approaches were similar for all outcomes measures, namely pain, range of motion, grip strength, and Mayo wrist score. No statistically significant difference regarding union rate could be detected between the two groups (p = 0.683). The same authors also evaluated the effect of dorsal vs. volar approach on screw placement. While the dorsal approach appeared to allow for a more perpendicular placement of the screw relative to the fracture line (p < 0.05), and screw placement more parallel to the long axis of the scaphoid in the semipronated oblique view only (p = 0.019), there was no difference in union rate between the dorsal and volar groups. A cadaveric comparison of the two approaches also observed that the dorsal approach allows for a more central placement of the screw, but in the distal third only (p = 0.045).[67] While previous studies have insisted on central placement of the screw in the proximal fragment,[61,62] it remains unclear whether a more central placement in the distal pole only translates into improved clinical outcome.

As mentioned earlier in Question 2, a lack of standardization in complication reporting makes comparison of complication rates across studies difficult. Complication rates ranging from 0% to 30% have been reported in series using a volar percutaneous approach. The majority are case series but among them figure also the controlled trials of Dias et al.,[37,38] Bond et al.,[40] Adolfsson et al.,[41] and Arora et al.[42] (see Question 2, section on complications). Complications reported for the dorsal percutaneous techniques are derived from five case series[67-71] and range from 0% to 29%. Each approach brings different concerns, but generally, no approach is superior in terms of rate of complications.

The special concern about scaphotrapezial osteoarthritis with the volar percutaneous approach was discussed in Question 2.

Recommendations

- For an undisplaced fracture of the scaphoid, a percutaneous technique reduces the surgical risks compared to an open approach and is therefore the technique of choice [overall quality: moderate]
- Both the antegrade and retrograde percutaneous techniques can be used: the surgeon has to learn the technical aspects and inherent risks associated with each approach [overall quality: moderate]
- Central placement of the screw in the scaphoid is critical, as it tends to increase the rate of union and decrease the time to union [overall quality: high]
- Scaphotrapezial changes are common in patients treated with the retrograde technique, but long-term outcomes are the same in these patients [overall quality: high]

Question 5: What is the ideal treatment when faced with a delayed diagnosis of an undisplaced fracture of the scaphoid?

Case clarification

The patient presents 5 weeks after injury to his wrist. Radiographs show an undisplaced scaphoid waist fracture.

Relevance

Scaphoid fractures can escape early detection because the initial symptoms can be minimal, and the clinical and radiographic signs can be subtle. Many authors suggest that any fracture that presents more than 4 weeks from injury is at high risk of nonunion.

Current opinion

When there is a delay in diagnosis, most scaphoid fractures should be treated operatively.

Finding the evidence

- Cochrane Database from 1980 to 2009, with search terms "scaphoid," "carpal," and "delay"

- MEDLINE (OVIDSp) search from 1980 to 2009 identifying population (adult), with keywords "scaphoid," "fracture," and "delay"
- The above searches were supported by additional cross-referencing of the bibliographies of eligible published reports

Quality of the evidence

Level IV
- 3 case series

Findings

Russe[72] reported 27 cases of delayed presentation of scaphoid fractures (range 3 weeks to 3 years). All fractures eventually achieved union with cast treatment, but the duration of immobilization was considerable.

Eddleland et al.[32] reported that the rate of nonunion was 73.3% (11/15) when immobilization was initiated between 4 weeks and 1 year, and 96.3% (26/27) when it was initiated at more than 1 year. They concluded that a delay in treatment of more than 4 weeks from injury is highly predictive for the development of scaphoid nonunion.

Finally, another retrospective review of 285 scaphoid fractures demonstrated that, while the incidence of nonunion was negligible if treatment was initiated within 0–28 days of injury, the frequency of nonunion significantly increased with a delay in treatment of greater than 4 weeks ($p < 0.01$).[22] The frequency of nonunion increased incrementally with length of treatment delay ($p < 0.02$). Of the fractures that eventually healed, a treatment delay of more than 4 weeks was associated with a significantly increased time to union ($p < 0.001$).

Recommendation

- Delay in treatment exceeding 4 weeks from time of injury is associated with high risk of nonunion or delayed union, and therefore surgical intervention is warranted [overall quality: low]

Question 6: What is the ideal treatment for a displaced fracture of the waist of the scaphoid?

Case clarification

The patient elected to be treated with a cast, and returns 1 week after his original injury. He has been noncompliant with the cast, and has removed it. While mountain biking, he sustained a fall on to the affected hand. The new radiographs are as shown in Figure 51.9.

Relevance

It is assumed that a displaced fracture has greater disruption of the blood supply, as well as more fracture instability, leading to a higher risk of nonunion. The generally accepted criteria for displacement in scaphoid fractures are provided

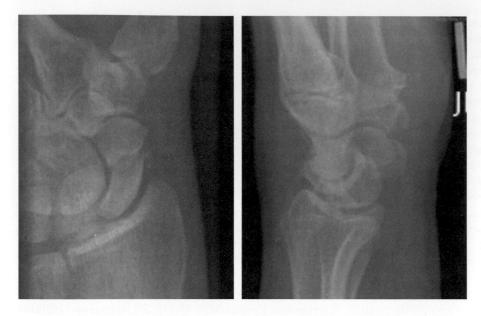

Figure 51.9 AP and lateral radiographs of a displaced scaphoid fracture. Note the increased lunocapitate and scapholunate angles, implying scaphoid shortening and angulation.

by Cooney et al.,[30] who defined a displaced or unstable fracture as greater than 1 mm offset on the AP radiograph or oblique views, or a lunocapitate angle greater than 15° or scapholunate angle greater than 45° on lateral radiograph.

Current opinion

Displaced scaphoid fractures treated conservatively are associated with an unacceptable risk of nonunion or malunion, and thus surgical treatment, by either an open or percutaneous technique, is generally preferred.

Finding the evidence

• Cochrane Database of systematic reviews, from 1980 to 2009, with search terms "scaphoid," "carpal," "displaced"
• MEDLINE (OVIDSp) search, from 1980 to 2009, identifying population (adult), with keywords "scaphoid," "fracture," and "displaced"
• The above searches were supported by additional cross-referencing of the bibliographies of eligible published reports.

Quality of evidence

Level IV
• Natural history of displaced scaphoid fractures treated nonoperatively: 4 case series
• Surgical treatment of displaced scaphoid fractures: 11 case series
• Postoperative immobilization: 1 meta-analysis of level IV evidence
• Bone graft: 8 case series

Findings

Cast immobilization Several studies have described delayed union or nonunion associated with cast treatment for dis-

placed scaphoid fractures.[30,32,73,74] However these studies are case series that often consist of heterogenous groups of acute and chronic fractures of varying morphology, and they assess the outcome of different types of treatments, either conservative or surgical. Despite the limitations of these studies, the available literature uniformly suggests that cast immobilization is associated with increased healing time, and a higher risk of nonunion. The reported success rates following surgical treatment of displaced scaphoid fractures are high, precluding further studies comparing nonsurgical and surgical treatment strategies.

Surgical treatment Many surgical techniques have been described for the treatment of displaced scaphoid fractures, demonstrating union rates of 88–100%.[58,67–69,75–84] The choice of approach has been discussed in Question 4. Most case series describe treatment with the volar approach, using a variety of fixation techniques.[75–79] Two prospective case series reported on the outcome of an open dorsal approach for displaced fractures.[58,80] The authors both reported a 100% union rate, with low complication rate.

The use of percutaneous fixation techniques is becoming increasingly favorable, even for displaced fracture. Union rates have varied from 89% to 100% union with arthroscopically assisted techniques.[67–69,81–84]

Arthroscopy has been used both to evaluate fracture reduction and to identify associated injuries not apparent on imaging.[67–69,82–84] One study of 15 patients treated with arthroscopically assisted reduction and percutaneous fixation found that 73% of displaced fractures were associated with injury to adjacent structures.[83] Thirteen percent had scapholunate ligament injury, 26.7% lunotriquetral ligament injury, 40% chondral injury to the capitate or lunate,

33% radiolunate or radioscapholuate ligament injury, and 33% triangular fibrocartilage complex (TFCC) tear.

While the available literature of varying fixation techniques consistently demonstrates high rates of union for displaced scaphoid fractures, these studies are limited to retrospective case series. There are no clinical trials comparing open and percutaneous fixation techniques, and the addition of arthroscopy has not been shown to yield better functional outcome.

Postoperative immobilization There are no studies directly evaluating the postoperative protocol following surgical treatment of acute scaphoid fractures. Most authors use a thumb spica splint for approximately 1–2 weeks. The splint is then removed, range of motion is initiated, and a removable splint is worn for 3 months. When fixation of the fracture is deemed to be tenuous or for fractures of the proximal pole, authors advocate a 4–6 week course of cast immobilization.[81,82,85]

A recent meta-analysis on scaphoid nonunions reviewed data from 36 case series, and found a union rate of 74% regardless of immobilization in a pooled sample of 500 patients.[86] The authors concluded that there is no compelling necessity for postoperative cast immobilization when fixation with a screw is stable.

Bone graft The need for bone graft in the setting of acute scaphoid fracture is not well addressed in the literature. A biomechanical study comparing various screw types showed that loss of volar cortex of the scaphoid greatly decreased the quality of fixation provided by screws.[63] In clinical studies describing an open approach to scaphoid fractures, cancellous or corticocancellous graft has been used in the presence of fracture comminution and bone loss.[76,77,79] With the advent of percutaneous reduction and fixation techniques, most studies have not described the use of bone graft.[67,81,83,84] Most recently, Slade et al.[82] suggested that scaphoid fractures and nonunions with significant gaps require bone grafting. However, in his retrospective review of 126 acute fractures treated with arthroscopically assisted dorsal percutaneous fixation, no bone graft was required acutely.

Recommendations

In patients with a displaced scaphoid fracture, evidence suggests:
• Nonoperative treatment is associated with a high risk of nonunion or malunion [overall quality: low]
• Operative management, using open dorsal or volar approach for fracture reduction and fixation or reduction and percutaneous fixation, is associated with high rate of fracture union [overall quality: low]
• When stable fixation is achieved, postoperative immobilization is unnecessary [overall quality: very low]

• There is no evidence to support use of bone graft for the treatment of acute scaphoid fractures [overall quality: low]

Question 7: What is the ideal treatment for an undisplaced proximal pole fracture?

Case clarification
The patient presents with an undisplaced proximal pole fracture (see Figure 51.10). He would like to know his treatment options.

Relevance
Cadaveric studies have indicated a tenuous blood supply to the proximal pole of the scaphoid. Fractures to this area therefore require longer fracture healing time, and present higher risk of nonunion.[87,88]

Current opinion
Because of the presumed risk of delayed union and nonunion of fractures of the proximal pole, many surgeons favor early operative intervention for acute proximal pole fractures, using a dorsal approach (Figure 51.11).

Finding the evidence
• Cochrane Database of systematic reviews from 1980 to 2009, with search terms "scaphoid," "carpal," and "proximal pole"
• MEDLINE (OVIDSp) search from 1980 to 2009, identifying population (adult), with keywords "scaphoid," "fracture," and "proximal pole"
• The above searches were supported by additional cross-referencing of the bibliographies of eligible published reports

Quality of the evidence

Level IV
• Nonoperative management of proximal pole fractures: 5 case series
• Surgical management of proximal pole fractures: 4 case series

Findings
Nonoperative management The available data is derived from level IV cases series only.[22,54,72,89] They suggest that nonoperatively treated proximal pole fractures are at risk for developing non- or delayed union. All these studies involve small numbers and do not include statistical analysis comparing healing time of proximal pole fractures to waist fractures. Furthermore, evaluation of healing was performed using radiographs, which may not represent a reliable measure of fracture union.

Surgical treatment Although there have not been any studies comparing volar vs. dorsal approach for proximal

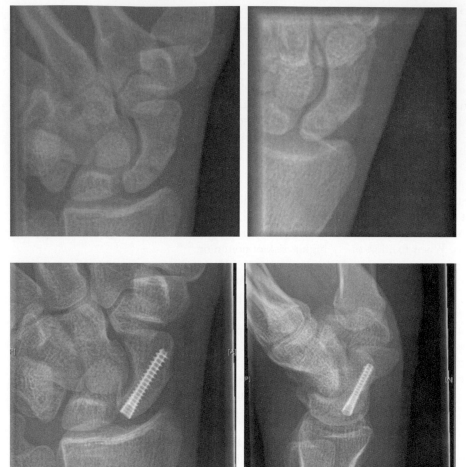

Figure 51.10 AP and pronated oblique view of proximal pole scaphoid fracture

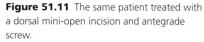

Figure 51.11 The same patient treated with a dorsal mini-open incision and antegrade screw.

scaphoid fractures, the dorsal approach is favored as it allows for easier exposure of the fracture site and maximizes fracture stability.[67,90]

There are no RCTs or comparative trials evaluating surgical treatment of proximal pole fractures. The only focused series of acute proximal pole fractures treated surgically is reported by Rettig et al.[91] Seventeen proximal pole fractures were treated within 15 days using a dorsal approach with a Herbert screw inserted in a retrograde fashion. Thirteen of these fractures were comminuted and were bone grafted. At an average follow-up of 37 weeks, the authors reported 100% of fractures achieved union as evaluated by CT, and no complications were encountered.

The literature on surgical treatment of proximal pole fracture is thus mainly derived from series where waist fractures, proximal pole fractures, and distal pole fractures are pooled together.[67,77,82,83] The high variability among those studies precludes any conclusion specific to proximal pole fracture.

Recommendations

• Nonoperative management of proximal pole scaphoid fractures is associated with a high risk of delayed union or nonunion. Surgical management is preferred [overall quality: low]
• The dorsal approach is preferred for surgical stabilization of proximal pole fractures [overall quality: very low]

Summary of recommendations

• An initial normal radiograph cannot accurately predict the absence of a scaphoid fracture: it is therefore recommended to proceed with further imaging, either acutely or 2 weeks later
• MRI is the study of choice to diagnose occult scaphoid fracture in the acute setting and has the advantage of avoiding unnecessary immobilization. There is good evidence to support its cost-effectiveness. The availability of this modality may limit its application
• A second set of radiographs at 2 weeks is an appropriate diagnostic tool but leads to unnecessary immobilization of the majority of patients. However, there is good evidence to support that immobilization of the wrist in a cast is not necessary in the interval before the new images

- The surgical treatment of an undisplaced scaphoid fracture does not lead to improved range of motion, grip strength or functional outcome at final follow-up
- The rate of union and the time to union are not improved by surgical treatment of an undisplaced fracture, but studies with CT scan assessment of union are mandatory in future
- The time off work is significantly shorter when treating a manual worker surgically, but this does not appear to be true for sedentary workers. Consequently, surgery is cost-effective and more beneficial to patients who are involved in work, sports or lifestyles incompatible with long-term immobilization
- In those where immobilization does not alter daily function, cast immobilization remains the standard treatment since patients are not subject to the attendant risks associated with surgery
- The evidence is not strong enough to support the use of a long-arm cast in the treatment of an undisplaced scaphoid fracture
- Inclusion of the thumb in the cast is not critical for scaphoid fracture healing
- For an undisplaced fracture of the scaphoid, a percutaneous technique reduces the surgical risks compared to an open approach and is therefore the technique of choice
- Both the antegrade and retrograde percutaneous technique can be used: there are technical aspects and inherent risks associated with each approach
- Central placement of the screw in the scaphoid is critical, as it tends to increase the rate of union and decrease the time to union
- Scaphotrapezial arthritic changes are common in patients treated with the retrograde technique, but long-term outcomes are the same as in patients without scaphotrapezial changes
- Delay in treatment exceeding 4 weeks from time of injury is associated with high risk of nonunion or delayed union, and therefore surgical intervention is warranted
- Nonoperative treatment of displaced scaphoid fractures is associated with a high risk of nonunion or malunion
- Operative management of displaced scaphoid fractures, using open dorsal or volar approach for fracture reduction and fixation or reduction and percutaneous fixation, is associated with high rate of fracture union
- When stable fixation is achieved, postoperative immobilization is unnecessary
- There is no evidence to support use of bone graft for the treatment of acute scaphoid fractures
- Nonoperative management of proximal pole scaphoid fractures is associated with a high risk of delayed union or nonunion. Surgical management is preferred
- The dorsal approach is preferred for surgical stabilization of proximal pole fractures

References

1. Sjolin SU, Anderson JC. Clinical fracture of the carpal scaphoid; supportive bandage or plaster cast immobilization? J Hand Surg Br 1988;13(1):75–6.
2. Brisnmar J. Skeletal scintigraphy of the wrist in suggested scaphoid fracture. Acta Radiol 1988;29:101–7.
3. Murphy D, Eisenhauer M. The utility of a bone scan in the diagnosis of clinical scaphoid fracture. J Emerg Med 1994;12:709–12.
4. Waizenegger M, Wastie ML, Barton NJ, Davis TR. Scintigraphy in the evaluation of the "clinical" scaphoid fracture. J Hand Surg Br 1994;19:750–3.
5. Tiel-van Buul MM, Broekhuizen TH, van Beek EJ, Bossuyt PM. Choosing a strategy for the diagnostic management of suspected scaphoid fracture: a cost-effectiveness analysis. J Nucl Med 1995;36:45–8.
6. Tiel-van Buul MM, Roolker W, Verbeeten BW, Broekhuizen AH. Magnetic resonance imaging versus bone scintigraphy in suspected scaphoid fracture. Eur J Nucl Med 1996;23:971–5.
7. Thorpe AP, Murray AD, Smith FW, Ferguson J. Clinically suspected scaphoid fracture: a comparison of magnetic resonance imaging and bone scintigraphy. Br J Radiol 1996;69:109–13.
8. Hunter JC, Escobedo EM, Wilson AJ, Hanel DP, Zink-Brody GC, Mann FA. MR imaging of clinically suspected scaphoid fractures. AJR 1997;168:1287–93.
9. Cook PA, Yu JS, Wiand W, Cook AJ 2nd, Coleman CR, Cook AJ. Suspected scaphoid fractures in skeletally immature patients: application of MRI. J Comput Assist Tomogr 1997;21:511–15.
10. Breitenseher MJ, Metz VM, Gilula LA, et al. Radiographically occult scaphoid fractures: value of MR imaging in detection. Radiology 1997;203:245–50.
11. Fowler C, Sullivan B, Williams LA, McCarthy G, Savage R, Palmer A. A comparison of bone scintigraphy and MRI in the early diagnosis of the occult scaphoid wrist fracture. Skeletal Radiol 1998;27:683–7.
12. Bretlau T, Christensen OM, Edstrom P, Thomsen HS, Lausten GS. Diagnosis of scaphoid fracture and dedicated extremity MRI. Acta Orthop Scand 1999;70:504–8.
13. Roolker W, Maas M, Broekhuizen AH. Diagnosis and treatment of scaphoid fractures, can non-union be prevented? Arch Orthop Trauma Surg 1999;119:428–31.
14. Bayer LR, Widding A, Diemer H. Fifteen minutes bone scintigraphy in patients with clinically suspected scaphoid fracture and normal x-rays. Injury 2000;31:243–8.
15. Raby N. Magnetic resonance imaging of suspected scaphoid fractures using a low field dedicated extremity MR system. Clin Radiol 2001;56:316–20.
16. Hauger O, Bonnefoy O, Moinard M, Bersani D, Diard F. Occult fractures of the wrist of the scaphoid: early diagnosis by high-spatial resolution sonography. AJR 2002;178:1239–45.
17. Brydie A, Raby N. Early MRI in the management of clinical scaphoid fracture. Br J Radiol 2003;76:296–300.
18. Moller JM, Larsen L, Bovin J, et al. MRI diagnosis of fracture of the scaphoid bone: impact of a new practice where the images are read by radiographers. Acad Radiol 2004;11:724–8.
19. Brooks S, Cicuttini FM, Lim S, Taylor D, Stuckey SL, Wluka AE. Cost effectiveness of adding magnetic resonance imaging to the

usual management of suspected scaphoid fractures. Br J Sports Med 2005;39:75–9.

20. Beeres FJ, Hogervorst M, Hollander P, Rhemrev S. Outcome of routine bone scintigraphy in suspected scaphoid fractures. Injury 2005;36:1233–6.

21. Memarsadeghi M, Breitenseher MJ, Schaefer-Prokop C, et al. Occult scaphoid fractures: comparison of multidetector CT and MR imaging—initial experience. Radiology 2006;240:169–76.

22. Langhoff O, Andersen JL, Consequences of late immobilization of scaphoid fractures. J Hand Surg 1988;13:77–9.

23. Kitsis C, Taylor M, Chandey J, Smith R, Latham J, Turner S, Wade P. Imaging the problem scaphoid. Injury 1998;29:515–20.

24. Foex B, Speake P, Body R. Best evidence topic report. Magnetic resonance imaging or bone scintigraphy in the diagnosis of plain x ray occult scaphoid fractures. Emerg Med J 2005;22(6): 434–5.

25. Beeres FJP, Rhemrev SJ, den Hollander PD, et al. Early magnetic resonance imaging compared with bone scintigraphy in suspected scaphoid fractures. J Bone Joint Surg Br 2008;90:1205–9.

26. Dorsay TA, Major NM, Helms CA. Cost-effectiveness of immediate MR imaging versus traditional follow-up for revealing radiographically occult scaphoid fractures. Am J Roentgenol 2001;177(6):1257–63.

27. Temple CLF, Ross DC, Bennett JD, Garvin GJ, King GJW, Faber KJ. Comparison of sagittal computed tomography and plain film radiography in a scaphoid fracture model. J Hand Surg Am 2005;30:534–42.

28. Adey L, Souer S, Lozano-Calderon S, Palmer W, Lee SG, Ring D. Computed tomography of suspected scaphoid fractures. J Hand Surg Am 2007;32:61–6.

29. Senall JA, Failla JM, Bouffard JA, Holsbeeck M, Ultrasound for the early diagnosis of clinically suspected scahpoid fracture. J Hand Surg Am 2004;29(3):400–5.

30. Cooney WP, Dobyns JH, Linscheid RL. Fractures of the scaphoid: A rational approach to management. Clin Orthop 1980;149: 90–7.

31. Leslie IJ, Dickson RA. The fractured carpal scaphoid: Natural history and factors influencing outcome. J Bone Joint Surg Br 1981;63:225–30.

32. Eddeland A, Eiken O, Hellgren E, Ohlsson NM. Fractures of the scaphoid. Scand J Plast Reconstr Surg 1975;9: 234–9.

33. Dias JJ, Taylor M, Thompson J et al., Radiographic signs of union of scaphoid fractures. An analysis of inter-observer agreement and reproducibility. J Bone Joint Surg Br 1988;70:299–301.

34. Vinnars B, Pietreanu M, Bodestedt A, Ekenstam F, Gerdin B. Nonoperative compared with operative treatment of acute scaphoid fractures: a randomized clinical trial. J Bone Joint Surg Am 2008;90:1175–85.

35. Vinnars B, Ekenstam F, Gerdin B. Comparison of direct and indirect costs of internal fixation and cast treatment in acute scaphoid fractures: a randomized trial involving 52 patients. Acta Orthop 2007;78(5):672–9.

36. McQueen MM, Gelbke MK, Wakefield A, Will EM, Gaebler C. Percutaneous screw fixation versus conservative treatment for fractures of the waist of the scaphoid: a prospective randomised study. J Bone Joint Surg Br 2008;90:66–71.

37. Dias JJ, Wildin CJ, Bhowal B, Thompson JR. Should acute scaphoid fractures be fixed? A randomized controlled trial. J Bone Joint Surg Am 2005;87(10):2160–8.

38. Dias JJ, Dhukaram V, Abhinav A, Bhowal B, Wildin CJ. Clinical and radiological outcome of cast immobilisation versus surgical treatment of acute scaphoid fractures at a mean follow-up of 93 months. J Bone Joint Surg Br 2008;90:899–905.

39. Saeden B, Tornkvist H, Ponzer S, Hoglund M. Fracture of the carpal scaphoid: a prospective, randomised 12-year follow-up comparing operative and conservative treatment. J Bone Joint Surg Br 2001;83:230–4.

40. Bond CD, Shin AY, McBride MT, Dao KD. Percutaneous screw fixation of cast immobilization for nondisplace scaphoid fractures. J Bone Joint Surg Am 2001;83(4):483–8.

41. Adolfsson L, Lindau T, Arner M. Acutrak screw fixation versus cast immobilisation for undisplaced scaphoid waist fractures. J Hand Surg Br 2001;26(3):192–5.

42. Arora R, Gschwentner M, Krappinger D, Lutz M, Blauth M, Gabl M. Fixation of non-displaced scaphoid fractures: making treatment cost effective: prospective controlled trial. Arch Orthop Trauma Surg 2007;127:39–46.

43. Davis EN, Chung KC, Kotsis SV, Lau SH, Vijan S. A cost/utility analysis of open reduction and internal fixation versus cast immobilization for acute non-displaced mid-waist scaphoid fractures. Plast Reconstr Surg 2006;117:1223–35.

44. Gellman H, Caputo RJ, Carter V, Aboulafia A, McKay M. Comparison of short and long thumb-spica casts for non-displaced fractures of the carpal scaphoid. J Bone Joint Surg Am 1989;71(3):354–7.

45. Alho A, Kankaanpää U. Management of fractured scaphoid bone. A prospective study of 100 fractures. Acta Orthop Scand 1975;46(5):737–43.

46. Broome A, Cedell CA, Colleen S. High plaster immobilisation for fracture of the carpal scaphoid bone. Acta Chir Scand 1964; 128:42–4.

47. Goldman S, Lipscomb PR, Taylor WF. Immobilization for acute carpal scaphoid fractures. Surg Gynecol Obstet 1969;129(2): 281–4.

48. Verdan C, Narakas A. Fractures and pseudarthrosis of the scaphoid. Surg Clin North Am 1968;48:1083–95.

49. Kaneshiro SA, Failla JM, Tashman S. Scaphoid fracture displacement with forearm rotation in a short arm thumb spica cast. J Hand Surg Am 1999;24:984–91.

50. Romdhane L, Chidgey L, Miller G, Dell P. Experimental investigation of the scaphoid strain during wrist motion. J Biomech 1990;23:1277–84.

51. Falkenberg P. An experimental study of instability during supination and pronation of the fractured scaphoid. J Hand Surg Br 1985;10:211–13.

52. McAdams TR, Spisak S, Beaulieu CF, Ladd AL. The effect of pronation and supination on the minimally displaced scaphoid fracture. Clin Orthop 2003:411;255–9.

53. Lawton JN, Nicholls MA, Charogul CP. Immobilization for scaphoid fracture: forearm rotation in long arm thumb-spica versus Munster thumb-spica casts. Orthopedics 2007;30(8): 612–14.

54. Clay NR, Dias JJ, Costigan PS, Gregg PJ, Barton NJ. Need the thumb be immobilised in scaphoid fractures? A randomized prospective trial. J Bone Joint Surg Br 1991;73: 828–32.

55. Karantana A, Downs-Wheeler MJ, Webb K, Pearce CA, Johnson A, Bannister GC. The effects of scaphoid and Colles casts on hand function. J Hand Surg Br 2006;31:436–8.

56. Hambidge JE, Desai VV, Schranz PJ, Compson JP, Davis TR, Barton NJ. Acute fractures of the scaphoid. Treatment by cast immobilisation with the wrist in flexion or extension? J Bone Joint Surg Br 1999;81:91–2.

57. Watson HK, Pitts EC, Ashmead D, Makhlouf MV, Kauer J. Dorsal approach to scaphoid nonunion. J Hand Surg Am 1993; 18:359–65.

58. Dos Reis FB, Koeberle G, Leite NM, Katchburian MV. Internal fixation of scaphoid injuries using the Herbert screw through a dorsal approach. J Hand Surg Am 1993;18:792–7.

59. Polsky MB, Kozin SH, Porter ST, Thoder JJ. Scaphoid fractures: dorsal vs. volar approach. Orthopedics 2002;25(8):817–19.

60. Garcia-Elias M, Vall A, Salo JM, Lluch AL. Carpal alignment after different surgical approaches to the scaphoid: a comparative study. J Hand Surg Am 1988;13(4):604–12.

61. Trumble TE, Clarke T, Kreder HJ. Non-union of the scaphoid. Treatment with cannulated screws compared with treatment with Herbert screws. J Bone Joint Surg Am 1996;78:1829–37.

62. McCallister WV, Knight J, Kaliappan R, Trumble TE. Central placement of the screw in simulated fractures of the scaphoid waist: a biomechanical study. J Bone Joint Surg Am 2003;85: 72–7.

63. Toby ER, Butler TE, McCormack TJ, Jayaraman G. A comparison of fixation screws for the scaphoid during application of cyclical bending loads. J Bone Joint Surg Am 1997;79(8):1190–7.

64. Meermans G, Verstreken F. Percutaneous transtrapezial fixation of acute scaphoid fractures. J Hand Surg Eur Vol 2008;33(6): 791–6.

65. Faran KJ, Ichioka N, Trzeciak MA, Han S, Medige J, Moy OJ. Effect of bone quality on the forces generated by compression screws. J Biomech 1999;32:861–4.

66. Jeon IH, Micic ID, Oh CW, Park BC, Kim PT. Percutaneous screw fixation for scaphoid fractures: a comparison between the dorsal and the volar approaches. J Hand Surg Am 2009;34:228–36.

67. Slade JF III, Grauer JN, Mahoney JD. Arthroscopic reduction and percutaneous fixation of scaphoid fractures with a novel dorsal technique. Orthop Clin North Am 2001;32:247–61.

68. Slade JF III, Gutow AP, Geissler WB. Percutaneous internal fixation of scaphoid fractures via an arthroscopically assisted dorsal approach. J Bone Joint Surg 2002;84:21–36.

69. Slade JF III, Taksali S, Safanda J. Combined fractures of the scaphoid and distal radius: a revised treatment rationale using percutaneous and arthroscopic techniques. Hand Clin 2005;31: 427–41.

70. Bedi A, Jebson PJL, Hayden RJ, Jacobson JA, Martus JE. Internal fixation of acute, non-displaced scaphoid fractures via a limited dorsal approach: an assessment of radiographic and functional outcomes. J Hand Surg Am 2007;32:326–33.

71. Brushness BD, McWilliams AD, Messer TM. Complications in dorsal percutaneous cannulated screw fixation of non-displaced scaphoid waist fractures. J Hand Surg Am 2007;32:827–33.

72. Russe O. Fracture of the carpal navicular: diagnosis, non-operative treatment and operative treatment. J Bone Joint Surg Am 1960;42:759–68.

73. Stewart MJ. Fractures of the carpal navicular (scaphoid): A report of 436 cases. J Bone Joint Surg Am 1954;36:998–1006.

74. Weber ER. Biomechanical implications of scaphoid waist fractures. Clin Orthop Rel Res 1980;149:83–9.

75. Rettig ME, Kozin SH, Cooney WP. Open reduction and internal fixation of acute displaced scaphoid waist fractures. J Hand Surg Am 2001;26:271–6.

76. Filan LS, Herbert TJ. Herbert screw fixation of scaphoid fractures. J Bone Joint Surg Br 1996;78:519–29.

77. Herbert TJ, Fisher WE. Management of the fractured scaphoid using a new bone screw. J Bone Joint Surg Br 1984:66:114–23.

78. Bunker TD, McNamee PB, Scott TD. The Herbert screw for scaphoid fractures; a multicentre study. J Bone Joint Surg Br 1987;69:631–4.

79. Trumble TE, Gilbert M, Murray LW, Smith J, McCallister WV. Displaced scaphoid fractures treated with open reduction internal fixation with a cannulated screw. J Bone Joint Surg Am 2000:82:633–41.

80. Chung KC. A simplified approach for unstable scaphoid fracture fixation using the Acutrak screw. Plast Recon Surg 2002;110(7); 1697–703.

81. Wozasek GE, Moser KD. Percutaneous screw fixation for fractures of the scaphoid. J Bone Joint Surg Br 1991;73:138–42.

82. Slade JF, Gillon T. Retrospective review of 234 scaphoid fractures and nonunions treated with arthroscopy for union and complications. Scand J Surg 2008:97:280–9.

83. Shih JT, Lee HM, Hou YT, Tan CM. Results of arthroscopic reduction and percutaneous fixation for acute displaced scaphoid fractures. J Arthroscop Rel Surg 2005;21(5):620–626.

84. Muller M, Germann G. Minimal invasive screw fixation and early mobilization of acute scaphoid fractures in the middle third: operative technique and early functional outcome. Tech Hand Upper Extrem Surg 2008;12(2):107–13.

85. Merrell GA, Slade JF. Technique for percutaneous fixation of displaced and nondisplaced acute scaphoid fractures and select nonunions. J Hand Surg Am 2008;33:966–73.

86. Merrell GA, Wolf SW, Slade JF. Treatment of scaphoid nonunions; quantitative meta-analysis of the literature. J Hand Surg Am 2002;27:685–91.

87. Obletz BE, Halbstein BM. Non-union of fractures of the carpal navicular. J Bone Joint Surg Am 1930;20:424–8.

88. Taleisnik J, Kelly PJ. The extraosseous and intraosseous blood supply of the scaphoid bone. J Bone Joint Surg Am 1966;48: 1125–37.

89. Bohler L, Trojan E, Jahna H. The results of treatment of 734 fresh, simple fractures of the scaphoid. J Hand Surg Br 1954;28: 319–31.

90. Segalman KA, Graham TJ. Scaphoid proximal pole fractures and nonunions. J Am Soc Surg Hand 2004;4(4):233–47.

91. Rettig ME, Raskin KB. Retrograde compression screw fixation of acute proximal pole scaphoid fractures. J Hand Surg Am 1999;24:1206–10.

52 Metacarpal Fractures

Brent Graham

Toronto Western Hospital, Toronto, ON, Canada

Case scenario

A 22 year old man is referred to the hand a clinic 3 days after having sustained an injury to the right hand as a result of an altercation. The patient came to the Emergency Department a few hours after the injury where radiographs were obtained showing the presence of a fracture involving the 5th metacarpal. The patient was immobilized in an ulnar gutter cast from the fingertips of the ring and small fingers to the proximal forearm without a prior reduction. This individual's health is entirely satisfactory. He is normally employed as a carpenter. The injured hand is the dominant limb.

The physical examination showed the presence of extensive edema and ecchymosis around the ulnar border of the hand and in the palm. The contour of the hand in this area was obscured by edema but it appeared that the prominence of the metacarpal head at the metacarpophalangeal joint of the small finger was decreased. There was an angular deformity of the distal diaphyseal area of the 5th metacarpal and this corresponded to the area of maximal tenderness to palpation. Movements of the digits were limited by voluntary guarding because of pain but the patient was capable of nearly full composite flexion with no indication of rotational deformity involving the small finger. The sensory and vascular condition of the hand was normal.

The radiographs obtained in the Emergency Department showed a fracture through the distal diaphyseal/metaphyseal junction of the 5th metacarpal with angulation of the distal fragment volarly by 50°. There was no displacement of the distal fragment, which appeared to be impacted onto the proximal fragment. No judgment could be made of rotation of the distal fragment.

Relevant anatomy

Fractures of the metacarpal bones are among the most common of all fractures incurred by the hand and the 5th metacarpal is by far the most common metacarpal fractured. The bone is slightly curved volarly when viewed from the side. As a result, angular forces applied to the dorsal surface of the distal end of the bone result in a palmarly angulated fracture when the bending tolerance of the bone is exceeded. This is a frequent occurrence when the closed fist of an individual strikes a hard object.

Painless movement of the 5th ray at the metacarpophalangeal and interphalangeal joints is critical to the ability to generate a composite grasp of adequate strength. Restoration of this ability is the principle goal of treatment for fractures of the 5th metacarpal

Importance of the problem

The most common mechanism of injury is an altercation, and the typical patient is a man between the ages of 18 and 40. The demographic group most frequently affected by this injury is an important component of the workforce and because the injury is infrequently related to work, time away from activities—both work-related and recreational—is an important consideration.

Evidence-Based Orthopedics, First Edition. Edited by Mohit Bhandari.
© 2012 Blackwell Publishing Ltd. Published 2012 by Blackwell Publishing Ltd.

Top five questions

1. What is optimal treatment for an angulated fracture of the 5th metacarpal that is not affected by rotation of the distal fragment?
2. How is rotational deformity at the fracture site most effectively established?
3. What is the long-term outcome of fractures of the 5th metacarpal? Is there a difference in long-term prognosis between cases treated surgically and those treated nonoperatively?
4. Is a supervised course of physical or occupational therapy usually required for the optimal treatment of fractures of the 5th metacarpal?
5. What is the optimal treatment for fractures at the base of the 1st metacarpal?

Question 1: What is optimal treatment for an angulated fracture of the 5th metacarpal that is not affected by rotation of the distal fragment?

Case clarification

The patient is a young man employed in a manual occupation. The injured hand is his dominant limb. There is moderate, clinically visible deformity at the fracture site but the fragments themselves are stable.

Relevance

The patient should be treated with strategy that optimizes the functional outcome with as short a period of treatment as possible.

Current opinion

Nonoperative treatment, consisting of about 3 weeks of immobilization in a plaster cast, is associated with a rapid restoration of movement and strength despite substantial angulation at the fracture site. Treating the patient nonoperatively implicitly accepts the fracture deformity but obviates any of the risks associated with surgery, even though those are probably small. Later reconstruction, if required, is entirely feasible if nonoperative treatment fails to lead to a satisfactory outcome, but this is very rarely required.

Finding the evidence

• Cochrane Database, with search term "metacarpal fracture"
• PubMed (www.ncbi.nlm.nih.gov/pubmed/), with search terms: "metacarpal fractures" AND "treatment," "metacarpal fractures" AND "surgical treatment," and "metacarpal fractures" AND "outcome"

Quality of the evidence

There have been no level I studies evaluating treatment for metacarpal fractures. There has been a Cochrane review of the topic.

Findings

Despite the frequency with which this injury is encountered, little evidence exists in the literature supporting one method of treatment over another. In some measure this may be related to the fact that the condition is so common that anecdotal experience has been substantial and so the effort to accumulate actual evidence has not been made. An additional important factor is likely the difficulty in completing prospective studies, even those with a relatively short ascertainment period, in this young, mobile patient population. Added to this obstacle is the near universal experience that outcomes with this injury are generally excellent, hence the low priority given to studying the injury in detail.

One of the main controversies related to the treatment of fractures of the 5th metacarpal has been the indication for surgical intervention. The principle that has been promulgated in the literature by the advocates of surgical treatment has related to the extent of angulation of the distal fragment beyond which operative management should be considered. The concern is that, if left untreated, excessive angulation will subsequently lead to problems with hand function, although this conclusion has been based mostly on biomechanical rather than clinical observations. However, there has been wide variation in the threshold amount of angulation that should be considered excessive. In addition, the reliability of radiographic evaluation for fracture angulation has been found to be poor.[1] The relative roles of operative and nonoperative treatment for this injury therefore remain unclear.

A Cochrane review on the topic of nonoperative treatment for closed treatment of fractures in the 5th metacarpal found the quality of existing literature on the subject to be poor.[2] There were no studies that used a validated hand function measure as a primary outcome measure and the conclusions were based on a variety of secondary measures of outcome including pain after treatment, return to activities, cosmesis, and patient satisfaction.

The treatments that were compared were cast immobilization of the hand and wrist and a variety of "functional" treatments including bracing in the hand only, immobilization with taping or an elastic bandage in the hand, and complete freedom to move without any kind of immobilization. Most of the patients had an initial angulation at the fracture site of about 40°, and where this was measured in follow-up there was little or no change. In the early weeks after treatment, patients who were immobilized in a cast were less likely to report pain than were patients who were treated in a functional brace and, in turn, these patients were less likely to report moderate pain than were those treated with bandaging alone. At 12 weeks of follow-up more than 90% of patients did not report pain regardless of the method of treatment. The prevalence of reporting severe pain was approximately the same in all groups for whom this symptom was evaluated: 5–7%. Mobility was greater in the early weeks after treatment in patients who were treated with the various forms of mobilization. At 3 months follow-up a small percentage of patients treated with cast immobilization had incomplete movement. Strength was also reduced in the first 6 weeks among patients treated with cast immobilization in comparison to those allowed mobility. No long-term data on this outcome was available. One study[3] showed that a larger proportion of patients treated with functional bracing experienced an early return to work activities than did patients treated with "neighbor strapping." Very small percentages of patients reported concerns about cosmesis, regardless of the treatment.

Where management of fractures of the 5th metacarpal is surgical, there is limited evidence in the literature to guide the selection of treatment. Winter et al.[4] compared intramedullary fixation to transverse pin fixation in a small group of patients randomized to receive one or the other of the treatments. The indication for surgery in two thirds of the patients was a rotary deformity. Patients who underwent intramedullary pinning had a slightly larger range of motion and grip strength at 3 months, although it was not clear whether the differences observed were clinically relevant. The study did not give any details about many of the important methodologic aspects of a randomized trial, including the process of randomization and blinding/masking of the evaluators.

A parallel case series comparing the same two procedures by Wong et al.[5] did not find statistically significant differences on any of the radiologic parameters or measures of impairment between the two groups. The indication for surgery in these patients was rotation or angulation of more than 30°, but the proportion meeting each of these indications was not specified.

Recommendation

• There is no clear difference in the outcome of metacarpal fractures that have been treated operatively vs. those that have been treated nonoperatively [overall quality: very low]

Question 2: How is rotational deformity at the fracture site most effectively established?

Case clarification

Most clinical experts accept the idea that a rotary malunion leads to a substantial decrease in hand function because of scissoring of the fingers. As a result, the conventional wisdom has been for fractures with rotary instability to be treated with some kind of operative stabilization although

this idea has not been tested in a randomized trial, nor is it likely to be so evaluated in the future because of the degree to which this concept has become entrenched in clinical practice.

Relevance

Identifying the need for surgical intervention depends on the recognition of this kind of fracture deformity.

Current opinion

A carefully conducted physical examination should allow even small degrees of rotary malalignment to be identified. This requires the patients to make a full, or nearly full, composite fist, which may not be practical for some patients because of pain.

Finding the evidence

• Cochrane Database, with search term: "metacarpal fracture"
• PubMed (www.ncbi.nlm.nih.gov/pubmed/), with search terms: "metacarpal fractures" AND "clinical evaluation" and "metacarpal fractures" AND "imaging"

Quality of the evidence

There have been no studies that compare various methods of establishing the presence of absence of rotary malalignment after a metacarpal fracture.

Findings

One clear indication for the operative treatment of metacarpal fractures in general is the presence of rotational deformity at the fracture site. The reasons operative management for these injuries is favored are the inability to control the fragments and maintain a satisfactory reduction with nonoperative measures and the important functional problems that occur with a rotational malunion, mainly scissoring of the digits. This may impair both strength and dexterity.

The evaluation of metacarpal fractures for rotational deformity is primarily clinical. The reliability of imaging, including plain radiographs and more advanced axial imaging such as CT scanning, is insufficient. The observation of the digits in a position of extension at the metacarpophalangeal joints may not allow identification of important rotational displacement. This is more easily and reliably identified by the observation of the digits during active composite flexion. Although there may be pain at the fracture site during this maneuver, most patients can accomplish this sufficiently that a judgment of rotational deformity can be made.

Recommendation

• Rotatory malalignment of fractures in the 5th metacarpal can be established clinically. There is no evidence to support the use of advanced imaging studies to assist in this evaluation. The topic has not been studied [overall quality: cannot assess]

Question 3: What is the long-term outcome of fractures of the 5th metacarpal? Is there a difference in long-term prognosis between cases treated surgically and those treated nonoperatively?

Case clarification

The patient is a 22 year old manual worker.

Relevance

Most of the patients who sustain fractures of the metacarpal are young men. In general this demographic group encompasses individuals who are active and who are frequently employed in manual occupations.

Current opinion

The long-term outcome of these injuries appears to be satisfactory. Even where there is substantial angulation at the fracture site, the impact on hand function seems to be very limited. While there may be measureable differences in some hand functions, in comparison to individuals matched for age, gender, and hand dominance, these do not appear to be clinically relevant. It is rare for patients to present for some kind of reconstruction after a malunion of a fracture of a single metacarpal.

Finding the evidence

- Cochrane Database, with search term "metacarpal fracture"
- PubMed (www.ncbi.nlm.nih.gov/pubmed/) with search terms: "metacarpal fractures" AND "treatment," "metacarpal fractures" AND "surgical treatment," and "metacarpal fractures" AND "outcome"

Quality of the evidence

There have been no level I studies evaluating treatment for metacarpal fractures. There has been a Cochrane review of the topic.

Findings

The Cochrane review on methods of nonoperative treatment[2] showed that pain control was satisfactory for a larger proportion of patients who were treated with cast immobilization than with all other forms of treatment. The long-term results with respect to what was termed "severe pain" were the same in all groups. Normal movement was reported to be restored at an earlier point after treatment with the methods that allowed mobilization as opposed to cast immobilization, although after pooling the data no statistically significant difference was identified for range of motion between any of the treatment groups.

There have been no prospective trials comparing nonoperative treatment to surgical management with any of the many available techniques. There has been one comparative case series[6] that evaluated 258 patients with metacarpal fractures. Approximately 80% of these patients had been treated with brief cast immobilization without any attempt at reduction, while the remaining patients were treated with a variety of percutaneous and open fixation techniques. The follow-up time was not specified in the study but the authors demonstrated that on average there was no difference between the patients treated operatively and those treated nonoperatively for outcome measured with the DASH score, grip strength, or cosmetic appearance of the hand. This result was observed for fractures of the neck of the 5th metacarpal with angulation up to 50° and fractures of the metacarpal diaphysis with angulation up to 40°. This would represent the large majority of patients with this injury. In all cases the DASH score was very low (range 3–5), indicating that the overall disability regardless of fracture location, unresolved angulation, and method of treatment was extremely limited.

In addition to its retrospective nature and lack of random assignment of treatment, the main deficiency of this study was the small proportion of patients that were successfully located for follow-up, approximately 17% of a possible sample of over 1200 individuals. However, despite this shortcoming the findings are consistent with contemporary anecdotal experience and seem likely to be reliable.

Recommendation

- Either operative or nonoperative treatment for angulated fractures of the 5th metacarpal is acceptable management [overall quality: very low]

Question 4: Is a supervised course of physical or occupational therapy usually required for the optimal treatment of fractures of the 5th metacarpal?

Case clarification

The patient is a 22 year old manual worker.

Relevance

The focus for most young, active individuals will be on a rapid return to those normal activities that may be temporarily interrupted by treatment for a fracture of a metacarpal.

Current opinion

Most patients will not require a formal course of rehabilitation, especially if management has consisted of nonoperative treatment. A spontaneous restoration of mobility and strength is the usual expectation. If this fails to occur within 2–3 weeks after immobilization is discontinued, introduction of a formal therapy program at that point will be as effective in maximizing the quality of the result as if this were immediately instituted.

Finding the evidence
• Cochrane Database, with search term: "metacarpal fracture"
• PubMed (www.ncbi.nlm.nih.gov/pubmed/), with search terms: "metacarpal fractures" AND "treatment," "metacarpal fractures" AND "therapy," metacarpal fractures" AND "rehabilitation," and "metacarpal fractures" AND "outcome"

Quality of the evidence
No level I studies have been reported, but a single well-performed systematic review has been published.

Findings
Feehan and Bassett[7] reported a carefully conducted systematic review of the literature on the topic of early mobilization following extra-articular fractures in the hand. Their conclusions were based on a total of six quasi-randomized studies, all of which concerned treatment of metacarpal fractures. No level I studies were identified. The outcomes of interest concerned the two main contrasting issues around early mobilization, concern about fracture stability and loss of position vs. an advantage to early mobilization with respect to functional outcome. No adverse effects on fracture healing were identified. One study reported complications relating to adverse skin reactions in approximately 25% of patients treated with a removable brace, but the authors of this systematic review attributed this to the use of a commercial splint because two other studies, which utilized custom orthoses, did not report similar observations. All of the studies reported transient advantages to early mobilization with respect to restoration of motion and grip strength and in return to activities, but at final follow-up there were no differences, suggesting that there are no fundamental benefits or disadvantages to early mobilization beyond what might be considered convenience.

Recommendation
• Early mobilization of fractures of the 5th metacarpal is associated with more movement, greater strength, and an earlier return to activity at early follow-up. There is no clearly deleterious effect of early motion of fracture healing [overall quality: moderate]

Question 5: What is the optimal treatment for fractures at the base of the 1st metacarpal?

Case clarification
This patient suffered a fracture of the 5th metacarpal, which may be fundamentally distinct from a fracture of the 1st

(thumb) metacarpal because of the basic differences in overall hand function that are served by the small finger and by the thumb.

Relevance
In contrast to fractures involving the other metacarpals, fractures of the thumb metacarpal frequently involve the proximal articular surface and may be associated with subluxation of the trapeziometacarpal joint.

Current opinion
Even in cases where there is substantial deformity of the proximal articular surface of the 1st metacarpal, operative treatment is rarely required. This appears to be due to the fact the tolerance of the joint surface for moderate incongruity is high. Although there may be radiographic evidence of post-traumatic degenerative changes in the trapeziometacarpal joint, these seem to be only rarely associated with clinical complaints that require treatment.

Finding the evidence
• Cochrane Database, with search term: "metacarpal fracture"
• PubMed (www.ncbi.nlm.nih.gov/pubmed/), with search terms: "metacarpal fractures" AND "treatment," "metacarpal fractures" AND "surgical treatment," "metacarpal fractures" AND "outcome," "Bennett's fractures" AND "treatment," "Bennett's fracture" AND "surgical treatment," and "Bennett's fracture" AND "outcome"

Quality of the evidence
The only literature on the topic of treatment for intra-articular fractures of the first metacarpal consists of level IV and V studies that report small comparative case series.

Findings
Fractures of the thumb metacarpal most typically occur at the base of the bone and frequently involve the proximal articular surface of the bone and the trapeziometacarpal joint. Displacement is often considerable because the medial fragment is held in place by the volar beak ligament, the main stabilizer of the trapeziometacarpal joint, while the larger lateral fragment, which usually consists of the remainder of the metacarpal, is displaced by the abductor pollicis longus. Without a reduction there will be substantial articular incongruity and the concern is that this will lead to changes of osteoarthritis. This expectation is based on the usual outcome in other joints which are affected by intra-articular deformity after fractures; however, whether or not this principle applies to injuries to the base of the 1st metacarpal remains unclear. Osteoarthritis of the trapeziometacarpal joint is an extremely prevalent condition in most industrialized socie-

ties and yet evidence of a previous, unreduced fracture of the base of the 1st metacarpal is rarely observed in these cases. Conversely, patients in whom articular incongruity persists after a fracture of the base of the 1st metacarpal very infrequently present with arthritis-related pain in this area. As a result, the need for an anatomic reduction of these fractures is unknown but this is an important question because this goal usually cannot be met without operative treatment.

There have been no randomized trials comparing treatments for fractures of the base of the 1st metacarpal. All of the literature on this topic reports level IV and V evidence, and these studies report conflicting results following operative and nonoperative treatment. Cannon et al.[8] followed a small series of patients at least 5 years after an intra-articular fracture of the 1st metacarpal. Almost 90% of the patients had been treated nonoperatively, and most of them did not report significant symptoms related to the thumb despite the presence of clinical and radiographic deformity.

Timmenga et al.[9] evaluated a small series of patients treated with either open reduction and internal fixation (ORIF) or closed reduction and percutaneous pinning. Although radiographic changes of post-traumatic arthritis appeared to be related to the quality of the reduction, the results appeared to be satisfactory regardless of the method of stabilization or the quality of reduction.

The literature is bereft of any reliable evidence with which to guide treatment recommendations and so there is no consensus on the indications for operative treatment, especially with respect to the extent of articular displacement that should be considered as acceptable. The conflicting results reported in the literature suggest that any differences in outcome that might be associated with various treatments may be small.

Recommendation

• Fractures of the base of the first metacarpal may be treated either operatively or nonoperatively [overall quality: very low]

Summary of recommendations

• There is no clear difference in the outcome of metacarpal fractures that have been treated operatively vs. those that have been treated nonoperatively
• Either operative or nonoperative treatment for angulated fractures of the 5th metacarpal is acceptable management
• Rotatory malalignment of fractures in the 5th metacarpal can be established clinically. There is no evidence to support

the use of advanced imaging studies to assist in this evaluation. The topic has not been studied
• Early mobilization of fractures of the 5th metacarpal is associated with more movement, greater strength, and an earlier return to activity at early follow-up. There is no clearly deleterious effect of early motion of fracture healing
• Fractures of the base of the first metacarpal may be treated either operatively or nonoperatively

Conclusions

There are no clear guidelines for the treatment of most fractures of the metacarpals because there is a dearth of evidence on the subject. Satisfactory results appear to be associated with either operative or nonoperative treatment. Early mobilization either after operative or nonoperative treatment may lead to a restoration of function more quickly than a period of immobilization, but these early advantages do not necessarily result in better outcomes in the long-term.

References

1. Leung YL, Beredjiklian PK, Monaghan BA, Bozentka DJ. Radiographic assessment of small finger metacarpal neck fractures. J Hand Surg Am 2002;27(3):443–8.
2. Poolman RW, Goslings JC, Lee JB, Statius Muller M, Steller EP, Struijs PA. Conservative treatment for closed 5th (small finger) metacarpal neck fractures. Cochrane Database Syst Rev 2005;3:CD003210.
3. Harding IJ, Parry D, Barrington RL. The use of a moulded metacarpal brace versus neighbour strapping for fractures of the little finger metacarpal neck. J Hand Surg Br 2001;26(3):261–3.
4. Winter M, Balaguer T, Bessiere C, Carles M, Lebreton E. Surgical treatment of the boxer's fracture: transverse pinning versus intramedullary pinning. J Hand Surg Br 2007;32(6):709–13.
5. Wong TC, Ip FK, Yeung SH. Comparison between percutaneous transverse fixation and intramedullary K-wires in treating closed fractures of the metacarpal neck of the little finger. J Hand Surg Br 2006;31(1):61–5.
6. Westbrook AP, Davis TR, Armstrong D, Burke FD. The clinical significance of malunion of fractures of the neck and shaft of the little finger metacarpal. J Hand Surg Br 2008;33(6):732–9.
7. Feehan LM, Bassett K. Is there evidence for early mobilization following an extraarticular hand fracture? J Hand Ther 2004;17(2):300–8.
8. Cannon SR, Dowd GS, Williams DH, Scott JM. A long-term study following Bennett's fracture. J Hand Surg Br 1986;11(3):426–31.
9. Timmenga EJ, Blokhuis TJ, Maas, M., Raaijmakers EL. Long-term evaluation of Bennett's fracture. A comparison between open and closed reduction. J Hand Surg Br 1994;19(3):373–7.

53 Hip Dislocations

Gregory J. Della Rocca, Brett D. Crist, and Yvonne M. Murtha

University of Missouri, Columbia, MO, USA

Case scenario

A 47 year-old otherwise healthy man is the restrained driver involved in a high-speed motor vehicle crash. He complains of left hip pain and is unable to bear weight. He is brought to the local Emergency Department for evaluation, which reveals an externally rotated, abducted, and extended left lower extremity. Neurovascular examination is normal, and no other injuries are noted.

Relevant anatomy

The hip joint represents the junction between the acetabulum and the femoral head. Stability is based upon bony architecture and soft tissue attachments. The acetabulum is recessed into the pelvis and surrounds the femoral head in a nearly hemispherical fashion, providing good inherent stability. Further stability is provided by the ligamentum teres, which takes its origin in the fossa acetabuli and inserts in the fovea centralis of the femoral head, as well as the acetabular labrum and the hip capsule.

Dislocation of the femoral head from the acetabulum can occur in isolation, or it can occur with associated fractures. Isolated dislocations of the native hip without fracture are unusual because of the high degree of constraint provided by the deep acetabular socket. Associated fractures can include acetabular fractures, femoral head fractures, or both. Soft tissues surrounding the hip, such as the acetabular labrum and the hip capsule, are almost invariably damaged during traumatic hip dislocation. Posterior dislocations are the most common dislocation type, although anterior dislocations also occur (Figure 53.1).

The blood supply to the femoral head is derived primarily from the medial femoral circumflex artery, which sends retinacular vessels into the posterior hip capsule. Further minor contributions to femoral head blood supply are provided by the lateral femoral circumflex artery and the artery of the ligamentum teres.

Importance of the problem

Traumatic hip dislocation in the young patient requires high amounts of energy, which often causes multiple injuries (level IV).[1,2] Motor vehicle crashes are a prime example of injury mechanism causing hip dislocation (level IV).[3] All of this can contribute to prolonged rehabilitation requirements. Complications of hip dislocation include osteoarthrosis (OA) and osteonecrosis (ON). OA has been described in up to 25% of patients who sustained isolated traumatic hip dislocations without fracture (level IV).[4] Acetabular fracture associated with hip dislocation increases the rate of OA substantially. ON has been described in up to 19% of patients following hip dislocation (level IV).[5,6]

Costs associated with isolated traumatic hip dislocation have not been extensively analyzed. Short-term costs include those associated with hospitalization and rehabilitation, plus opportunity cost related to lost wages. Long-term costs include those associated with adverse long-term sequelae of hip dislocation, such as recurrent instability requiring repeat hospitalization or OA/ON which leads to further surgical procedures, rehabilitation, and lost wages.

A Google search for the term "hip dislocation" (without quotation marks) yields approximately 350,000 results. Much of this information is not peer-reviewed or based on scientific evidence.

Evidence-Based Orthopedics, First Edition. Edited by Mohit Bhandari.
© 2012 Blackwell Publishing Ltd. Published 2012 by Blackwell Publishing Ltd.

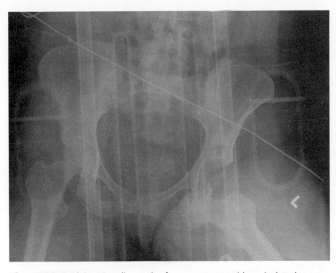

Figure 53.1 Plain AP radiograph of a young man with an isolated anterior dislocation of the left hip.

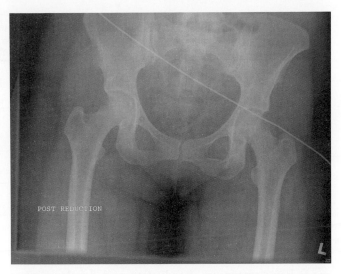

POST REDUCTION

Figure 53.2 Plain AP radiograph of a young man taken after closed reduction of an isolated traumatic anterior left hip dislocation. Note concentric reduction of the hip joint.

Finding the evidence

- Cochrane Database, with search term "hip dislocation"
- PubMed queries, with search terms "'hip dislocation" AND XXX, with XXX representing "osteonecrosis AND reduction" or "osteonecrosis AND trauma," "arthrosis AND reduction" or "arthrosis AND trauma," "CT" or "MRI", or "arthroscopy"

Top four questions

1. What is the urgency of hip reduction after traumatic dislocation, as it relates to osteonecrosis of the femoral head?
2. What is the risk of arthrosis after traumatic hip dislocation?
3. Is CT or MRI indicated after reduction of a traumatic hip dislocation?
4. Is hip arthroscopy indicated after traumatic hip dislocation?

Question 1: What is the urgency of hip reduction after traumatic dislocation, as it relates to osteonecrosis of the femoral head?

Case clarification

The patient undergoes radiographic examination of the pelvis and left femur. An anterior dislocation of the left hip is noted, without apparent bony injury (Figure 53.1). Orthopedic consultation is requested, but is delayed due to arrival of other multiply injured patients in the Emergency Department at the same time. Once the orthopedic consult-

ant is prepared to perform reduction of the patient's left hip, a further delay occurs while sedation is being prepared. Reduction of the patient's left hip is accomplished without difficulty (Figure 53.2), approximately 6 hours after the motor vehicle crash.

Relevance

Delay in reduction is associated with prolonged patient discomfort and may be associated with increased risk of ON of the femoral head.

Current opinion

Rapid reduction of the dislocated hip is associated with improvements in patient comfort and therefore should be expedited. Early reduction of the dislocated hip may be associated with lower rates of ON.

Quality of the evidence

Studies were only included if definitive patient numbers and times of reduction of hip dislocation were available from the body of the manuscripts.

Level III
- 1 prospective cohort with methodologic limitations

Level IV
- 5 retrospective case series

Findings

Six studies were identified (a total of 554 hip dislocations and fracture-dislocations) in which correlations could be

Table 53.1 Percentages of patients developing osteonecrosis after isolated traumatic hip dislocation (without fracture of the ipsilateral acetabulum or femoral head), as it correlates with speed of reduction of hip (<6 hours from injury vs. >6 hours from injury)

Study	Total patients	Early reduction (<6 h)	Osteonecrosis	Late reduction (>6 h)	Osteonecrosis
Brav 1962[9]	262	204	36	58	33
Reigstad 1980[7]	56	43	2.0	13	1.0
Hougaard 1987[4]	100	83	4.0	17	9
Dreinhofer 1994[6]	35	35	3	0	0
Sahin 2003[2]	62	35	2.0	27	3.0
Onche 2008[8]	39	22	0	17	8
Totals		422	47	132	54
Percentage			11%		41%

made between timing of reduction and development of osteonecrosis, out of a total of 11 that suggested a positive correlation between delay in reduction and development of osteonecrosis (Table 53.1) (levels III and IV).[2,4,6–9] The remaining studies did not provide direct data evidence for their suggestion that delayed reduction of hip dislocations is associated with development of ON. Early reduction was defined in some studies as less than 6 hours from injury, and in others as less than 12 hours from injury, creating heterogeneity of results which demands cautious interpretation. Early reduction was associated with an ON rate of 11%, while late reduction was associated with an ON rate of 41%. Early reduction was associated with a decreased risk of ON relative to delayed reduction (relative risk: 0.27).

Recommendation

- In adult patients with traumatic hip dislocations, rapid reduction of the dislocation is associated with a decreased rate of ON of the femoral head [overall quality: very low]

Question 2: What is the risk of arthrosis after traumatic hip dislocation?

Case clarification

The patient underwent uncomplicated closed reduction under conscious sedation approximately 6 hours after the motor vehicle crash. What is the likelihood that he will develop arthrosis of the hip, and is there a relationship to the time delay to reduction?

Relevance

Hip arthrosis may be a common sequela of hip dislocation.

Current opinion

Likelihood of future arthrosis is increased after hip dislocation, and may not be related to speed of reduction in the absence of ON.

Quality of the evidence

Studies were only included if the following could be elucidated: total number of patients with isolated dislocation (fracture-dislocations were excluded) and total number of patients developing arthrosis. Total follow-up times for studies were extremely variable.

Level IV

- 12 retrospective case series

Findings

Twelve studies were identified in which the number of patients sustaining an isolated hip dislocation (i.e., no fracture of the ipsilateral femoral head or acetabulum) was able to be discerned (584 patients) and the number of patients developing ipsilateral hip arthrosis was also able to be discerned (level IV).[2–7,9–14] Other studies did not differentiate between isolated dislocations and fracture-dislocations in such a manner that patients with post-traumatic arthrosis could be delineated based upon type of initial injury. Arthrosis was noted in 109 of 584 hips, correlating with a rate of 18.7% (Table 53.2).

Recommendation

- Patients sustaining an isolated, traumatic dislocation of the hip may be advised that their risk of developing post-traumatic ipsilateral hip arthrosis is approximately 18.7%. Prevalence of hip arthrosis in the general population approximates 3.5% (level IV).[15] This correlates with an increased risk of arthrosis related to isolated hip dislocation (relative risk: 5.33) [overall quality: very low]

Question 3: Is CT or MRI indicated after reduction of a traumatic hip dislocation?

Case clarification

The patient has undergone uncomplicated reduction of his hip dislocation under sedation in the Emergency

Table 53.2 Percentages of patients developing coxarthrosis after sustaining an isolated, traumatic hip dislocation (without fracture of the ipsilateral acetabulum or femoral head).

Study	Total patients	Arthrosis	Percentage
Armstrong 1948[10a]	19	4	21.05
Thompson 1951[3]	30	2	6.67
Paus 1951[11]	76	15	19.74
Stewart 1954[5]	28	7	25.00
Brav 1962[9]	144	32	22.22
Reigstad 1980[7]	28	0	0.00
Upadhyay 1983[12]	74	18	24.32
Hougaard 1987[4]	48	12	25.00
Yang 1991[13]	31	5	16.13
Schlickewei 1993[14]	41	4	9.76
Dreinhofer 1994[6]	43	9	20.93
Sahin 2003[2]	22	1	4.55
Totals	584	109	18.66

[a]Two different sets of values were given by the authors, one with early follow-up and one with late follow-up. There was significant loss to follow-up at the late time points. Only the late time points are included in this table.

Department. Postreduction plain radiographs reveal a concentric reduction of the hip joint. Is a CT scan or MRI necessary for full evaluation of the hip joint, in order to rule out interposed soft tissues or free chondral or osteochondral fragments?

Relevance

Reduction of an apparently isolated hip dislocation may entrap soft tissues, chondral fragments, or osseous fragments within the joint. Large fragments prevent a concentric reduction, which may be apparent on plain radiographs. Smaller fragments may not be seen on plain radiographs, and reduction may still appear concentric on plain radiographs.

Current opinion

Plain radiographs, after reduction of an apparently isolated hip dislocation (without associated acetabular or femoral head fracture), which reveal a concentric reduction of the hip joint are sufficient to guide further treatment of the hip dislocation patient.

Quality of the evidence

Studies were only included if the following could be elucidated: total number of patients with isolated dislocation (fracture-dislocations were excluded) and total number of patients undergoing CT or MR scanning.

Level IV
- 4 retrospective case series (CT)
- 3 retrospective case series (MRI)

Findings

Four studies were identified in which patients with isolated hip dislocations (without fracture and nonrecurrent) had undergone CT scans for further evaluation of a concentrically reduced joint (level IV).[16–19] Other identified studies either were nonclinical, dealt purely with the pediatric population, described treatment of known fracture-dislocations, or did not describe findings quantitatively. A total of 226 hip dislocations with concentric reductions underwent CT imaging. No loose bodies were noted in any of these hip joints. Out of 199 hip dislocations imaged by CT scanning, femoral head impaction injuries were noted in 41. One study,[18] describing 20 impaction injuries, reported surgical repair in 12 without reporting indications for such repair. The other study,[17] describing 21 impaction injuries, reported an incidental finding of 18 posterior wall acetabular fractures not apparently noted on plain radiographs.

Only 3 studies were identified which detailed use of early MRI after isolated hip dislocation in the adult patient (40 hip dislocations) (level IV).[20–22] One study, with MRI occurring within 5 weeks of injury, demonstrated intra-articular loose bodies in 4 and an entrapped ligamentum teres in 1 of 18 reduced dislocations without reference to concentricity of reduction on plain radiographs.[20] The other two studies demonstrated no loose bodies within the hip joints of 22 reduced dislocations. In one of these studies, a series of 8 football-associated dislocations demonstrated a triad of posterior lip fractures of the acetabulum, disruption of the ligamentum teres, and hemarthrosis in all patients.[22] Of 14 patients undergoing serial MRI of reduced hip dislocations in the other study, 8 patients were noted to have abnormal marrow signals in the femoral head. Five of these were noted to resolve and 3 progressed to frank ON, questioning the significance of abnormal marrow signals and MRI acutely after reduction of hip dislocation.[21]

Recommendations

- CT scanning of patients with a concentric reduction after isolated hip dislocation is likely of little value in identifying potentially problematic loose intra-articular bodies [overall quality: very low]
- MRI of patients with a concentric reduction after isolated hip dislocation is unlikely to yield valuable early information, although it can delineate the spectrum of soft tissue injury. It is of uncertain prognostic significance [overall quality: very low]

Question 4: Is hip arthroscopy indicated after traumatic hip dislocation?

Case clarification

After uncomplicated reduction of the hip dislocation under sedation in the Emergency Department, a concentric hip joint reduction is noted on plain radiographs. However, a small fragment of bone is noted within the fossa acetabuli. CT scan reveals the presence of a concentric hip reduction and a small osseous fragment within the fossa acetabuli that does not appear to be in contact with the femoral head. Should the patient be taken to the operating room for removal of the loose body and joint exploration for other loose bodies, utilizing an arthroscopic technique?

Relevance

Loose bodies that require removal may be present within the hip joint and not detectable after reduction of a traumatic hip dislocation, whether by plain radiographs, CT scans, or MRI.

Current opinion

Small osseous fragments within the fossa acetabuli do not mandate operative removal. Fragments noted to be incarcerated between the articular surfaces of the acetabulum and femoral head, or the presence of nonconcentric joint reduction, mandate operative exploration with removal and/or fixation.

Quality of the evidence

Studies were only included if the following could be elucidated: total number of patients with isolated dislocation (fracture-dislocations were excluded) and total number of patients undergoing arthroscopy. Other studies were included in the analysis if arthroscopy was utilized for known intra-articular pathology.

Level IV
- Arthroscopy without known loose bodies: 4 retrospective case series
- Arthroscopy for treatment of known loose bodies: 2 retrospective case series and 2 case reports

Findings

Four studies were identified in which the number of patients sustaining an isolated hip dislocation or fracture-dislocation underwent arthroscopy in the setting of normal postreduction imaging studies could be elucidated (44 patients) (level IV).[23–26] and four further publications (two series, two case reports) reported on arthroscopy for retrieval of known intra-articular loose bodies after reduction of an isolated hip dislocation (20 patients) (level IV).[27–30] Out of 44 cases of isolated hip dislocations and fracture-dislocations (Byrd and Jones[24] did not subdivide between these groups), 40 were found to have previously unrecognized articular pathology, including intra-articular loose bodies, labral tears, or chondral damage. In the 20 patients undergoing arthroscopy for removal of known intra-articular loose bodies, arthroscopic removal was successful.

Recommendation
- Patients sustaining an isolated, traumatic dislocation of the hip may have intra-articular pathology, such as loose bodies, labral tears, or articular chondral damage, which may not be evident on postreduction imaging, and which may be treated successfully with hip arthroscopy [overall quality: very low]

Summary of recommendations

- In adult patients with traumatic hip dislocations, rapid reduction of the dislocation is associated with a decreased rate of ON of the femoral head
- Patients sustaining an isolated, traumatic dislocation of the hip may be advised that the have an increased risk of developing post-traumatic ipsilateral hip arthrosis
- CT scanning of patients with a concentric reduction after isolated hip dislocation is likely of little value in identifying potentially problematic loose intra-articular bodies
- MRI of patients with a concentric reduction after isolated hip dislocation is unlikely to yield valuable early information, although it can delineate the spectrum of soft tissue injury. It is of uncertain prognostic significance
- Patients sustaining an isolated, traumatic dislocation of the hip may have intra-articular pathology, such as loose bodies, labral tears, or articular chondral damage, which may not be evident on postreduction imaging, and which may be treated successfully with hip arthroscopy

Conclusion

Patients sustaining a traumatic hip dislocation appear to have an increased risk of coxarthrosis as compared to the general population (18.7%, as compared to 3.5%). Patients also have a risk of ON, and this risk appears to be increased with delays in reduction (11% risk with early reduction, 41% risk with late reduction). Evidence supporting both of these statements is of low quality and primarily consists of retrospective case series. Only one study offering level III evidence was available which demonstrated a reduced risk of ON when reduction of the hip dislocation was undertaken expeditiously.

References

1. Epstein HC. Traumatic dislocations of the hip. Clin Orthop 1973;92:116–42.
2. Sahin V, Karakas ES, Aksu S, Atlihan D, Turk CY, Halici M. Traumatic dislocation and fracture-dislocation of the hip: a long-term follow-up study. J Trauma 2003;54:520–9.

3. Thompson VP, Epstein HC. Traumatic dislocation of the hip: a survey of two hundred and four cases covering a period of twenty-one years. J Bone Joint Surg Am 1951;33:746–78.

4. Hougaard K, Thomsen PB. Coxarthrosis following traumatic posterior dislocation of the hip. J Bone Joint Surg Am 1987;69:679–83.

5. Stewart MJ, Milford LW. Fracture-dislocation of the hip: an end-result study. J Bone Joint Surg Am 1954;36:315–42.

6. Dreinhofer KE, Schwarzkopf SR, Haas NP, Tscherne H. Isolated traumatic dislocation of the hip: long-term results in 50 patients. J Bone Joint Surg Br 1994;76:6–12.

7. Reigstad A. Traumatic dislocation of the hip. J Trauma 1980;20:603–6.

8. Onche II, Obiano SK, Udoh MK. A prospective evaluation of the management and outcome of traumatic posterior dislocation of the hip—a preliminary report. Niger J Med 2008;17:163–7.

9. Brav EA. Traumatic dislocation of the hip: army experience and results over a twelve-year period. J Bone Joint Surg Am 1962;44:1115–34.

10. Armstrong JR. Traumatic dislocation of the hip joint: review of one hundred and one dislocations. J Bone Joint Surg Br 1948;30:430–45.

11. Paus B. Traumatic dislocations of the hip: late results in 76 cases. Acta Orthop Scand 1951;21:99–112.

12. Upadhyay SS, Moulton A, Srikrishnamurthy K. An analysis of the late effects of traumatic posterior dislocation of the hip without fractures. J Bone Joint Surg Br 1983;65:150–2.

13. Yang RS, Tsuang YH, Hang YS, Liu TK. Traumatic dislocation of the hip. Clin Orthop 1991;265:218–27.

14. Schlickewei W, Elsasser B, Mullaji AB, Kuner EH. Hip dislocation without fracture: traction or mobilization after reduction? Injury 1993;24:27–31.

15. Hoaglund FT, Steinbach LS. Primary osteoarthritis of the hip: etiology and epidemiology. J Am Acad Orthop Surg 2001;9:320–7.

16. Hougaard K, Lindequist S, Nielsen LB. Computerised tomography after posterior dislocation of the hip. J Bone Joint Surg Br 1987;69:556–7.

17. Richardson P, Young JW, Porter D. CT detection of cortical fracture of the femoral head associated with posterior hip dislocation. Am J Roentgenol 1990;155:93–4.

18. Tehranzadeh J, Vanarthos W, Pais MJ. Osteochondral impaction of the femoral head associated with hip dislocation: CT study in 35 patients. Am J Roentgenol 1990;155:1049–52.

19. Frick SL, Sims SH. Is computed tomography useful after simple posterior hip dislocation? J Orthop Trauma 1995;9:388–91.

20. Laorr A, Greenspan A, Anderson MW, Moehring HD, McKinley T. Traumatic hip dislocation: early MRI findings. Skeletal Radiol 1995;24:239–45.

21. Poggi JJ, Callaghan JJ, Spritzer CE, Roark T, Goldner RD. Changes on magnetic resonance images after traumatic hip dislocation. Clin Orthop 1995;319:249–59.

22. Moorman CTr, Warren RF, Hershman EB, Crowe JF, Potter HG, Barnes R, et al. Traumatic posterior hip subluxation in American football. J Bone Joint Surg Am 2003;85:1190–6.

23. Yamamoto Y, Ide T, Ono T, Hamada Y. Usefulness of arthroscopic surgery in hip trauma cases. Arthroscopy 2003;19:269–73.

24. Byrd JW, Jones KS. Traumatic rupture of the ligamentum teres as a source of hip pain. Arthroscopy 2004;20:385–91.

25. Mullis BH, Dahners LE. Hip arthroscopy to remove loose bodies after traumatic dislocation. J Orthop Trauma 2006;20:22–6.

26. Philippon MJ, Kuppersmith DA, Wolff AB, Briggs KK. Arthroscopic findings following traumatic hip dislocation in 14 professional athletes. Arthroscopy 2009;25:169–74.

27. Kashiwagi N, Suzuki S, Seto Y. Arthroscopic treatment for traumatic hip dislocation with avulsion fracture of the ligamentum teres. Arthroscopy 2001;17:67–9.

28. Svoboda SJ, Williams DM, Murphy KP. Hip arthroscopy for osteochondral loose body removal after a posterior hip dislocation. Arthroscopy 2003;19:777–81.

29. Owens BD, Busconi BD. Arthroscopy for hip dislocation and fracture-dislocation. Am J Orthop 2006;35:584–7.

30. Chernchujit B, Sanguanjit P, Arunakul M, Jitapankul C, Waitayawinyu T. Arthroscopic loose body removal after hip fracture dislocation: experiences in 7 cases. J Med Assoc Thai 2009;92(Suppl 6):S161–4.

54 Femoral Head Fractures

Chad P. Coles

Dalhousie University, Halifax, NS, Canada

Case scenario

A 22 year old man is involved in a head-on motor vehicle collision. He presents complaining of left hip pain. On examination, the hip is held in a flexed, adducted, and internally rotated position.

Relevant anatomy

Originally described by Birkett in 1869,[1] femoral head fractures are relatively uncommon injuries. They typically occur as a result of a posterior dislocation of the hip, and may be associated with fractures of the acetabulum or femoral neck. Femoral head fractures were further classified by Pipkin in 1957 into four types (see box).[2]

Classification of femoral head fractures
- *Type I:* Dislocation with fracture of the femoral head caudad to the fovea
- *Type II:* Dislocation with fracture of the femoral head cephalad to the fovea
- *Type III:* Type I or type II injury associated with fracture of the femoral neck
- *Type IV:* Type I or type II injury associated with fracture of the acetabular rim

Fractures above the fovea (type II) involve the weight-bearing surface of the femoral head, whereas those below the fovea (type I) have less impact on force distribution. Only approximately 10% of hip dislocations are anterior,[3] and these can be associated with impaction fractures of the femoral head, often with a poor outcome.[4]

The blood supply to the femoral head is quite precarious, and may be disrupted either by the traumatic dislocation itself, or the surgical approach to address the fracture.[5] This may result in avascular necrosis (AVN) of the femoral head, leading to head collapse and early hip arthrosis.

Importance of the problem

Femoral head fractures are high-energy injuries, and often occur in a young, active population. They have been documented to occur in up to 7% of posterior hip dislocations.[6] These articular injuries can lead to early post-traumatic arthrosis in many patients.[7] Similarly, there is a significant risk of AVN of the femoral head as a result of the injury and its treatment. Both situations can lead to significant pain, disability, and an eventual need for total hip arthroplasty. These complications can have a significant impact on employment status and quality of life for the patient.

Despite the importance of these injuries, their relative rarity has resulted in little high-quality evidence in the published literature. Much of our treatment of femoral head fractures is based on level IV and level V evidence, which emphasizes the need for an evidence-based approach to this problem.

Top six questions

Therapy

1. Should I attempt a closed reduction?
2. Is there a role for nonoperative treatment?
3. Which surgical approach should I use?
4. Should the fragment be excised or repaired?

Evidence-Based Orthopedics, First Edition. Edited by Mohit Bhandari.
© 2012 Blackwell Publishing Ltd. Published 2012 by Blackwell Publishing Ltd.

Prognosis

5. What complications should be anticipated?
6. What is the expected outcome?

Question 1: Should I attempt a closed reduction?

Case clarification
You begin to prepare for a conscious sedation and attempt at closed reduction in the Emergency Department. The nurse asks if this is safe, or if you should be proceeding directly to the operating room?

Current opinion
Emergent reduction of hip fracture-dislocations is routinely performed in the Emergency Department.

Relevance
While delay to reduction has been implicated in the development of AVN following hip dislocation, there are also risks associated with attempts at closed reduction.

Finding the evidence
• Cochrane Database, with search term: "femoral head"
• PUBMED (www.ncbi.nlm.nih.gov/pubmed/) search using keywords: "femoral head fracture"
• Manual search of references cited in identified articles

Quality of the evidence
Level III
• 1 retrospective case-control study[18]

Level IV
• 20 retrospective case series [2,8–17,19–27]

Findings
Of the 410 femoral head fractures for which reduction method was described,[2,8–27] closed reduction was attempted in 366 (89.3%) (Table 54.1). Primary open reduction was performed in the remaining cases, based on surgeon preference or presence of an associated femoral neck fracture. Of those 366 attempted reductions, successful reduction was accomplished in 312 (85.2%). Nine patients (2.5%) had an associated unrecognized femoral neck fracture that dis-

placed,[13] or sustained an iatrogenic femoral neck fracture during the reduction attempt.[2,13,15,16,26] The remaining 45 (12.3%) were irreducible, and required open reduction. While some authors showed better outcomes with early reduction,[15,28] others showed no difference with delay to reduction.[19] There was inadequate data to draw a conclusion regarding timing of reduction.

Recommendations
• In the absence of a femoral neck fracture, a timely attempt at a closed reduction in the Emergency Department or operating room is recommended [overall quality: moderate]

Question 2: Is there a role for nonoperative treatment?

Case clarification
After successful closed reduction, CT scan reveals concentric reduction of the hip joint, but persistent displacement of the femoral head fragment. The patient wants to know if he really needs surgery.

Current opinion
Displaced femoral head fractures are typically treated with open reduction and internal fixation (ORIF).

Relevance
Historically, many fractures were managed nonoperatively. With advances in surgical techniques and implants, more fractures are now treated surgically. Has this improved the outcome of femoral head fractures?

Finding the evidence
See Question 1.

Quality of the evidence
Level IV
• 11 retrospective case series[2,12–16,19,20,22,29,30]

Findings
Eleven articles[2,12–16,19,20,22,29,30] gave details of the outcomes, according to the classification of Thompson and Epstein,[30] of nonoperatively treated femoral head fractures, in addition to the results of those treated operatively (Table 54.2). Of the 57 cases managed nonoperatively, there were 8 (14.0%) excellent, 16 (28.1%) good, 16 (28.1%) fair, and 17 (29.8%) poor results. In comparison, the 139 operatively treated fractures yielded 5 (3.6%) excellent, 66 (47.5%) good, 30 (21.6%) fair, and 38 (27.3%) poor results. Very little information was provided as to the criteria used to select these cases for nonoperative treatment. There may also be some selection bias, as less severe cases may have been those chosen for nonoperative treatment.

Table 54.1 Results of attempted closed reduction (n = 366)

Successful closed reduction	Iatrogenic femoral neck fracture	Required open reduction
312 (85.2%)	9 (2.5%)	45 (12.3%)

Table 54.2 Results of nonoperative vs. operative treatment of femoral head fractures

Results	Nonoperative(n = 57)	Operative(n = 139)
Excellent	8 (14.0%)	5 (3.6%)
Good	16 (28.1%)	66 (47.5%)
Fair	16 (28.1%)	30 (21.6%)
Poor	17 (29.8%)	38 (27.3%)

Table 54.3 Complications related to surgical approach (n = 151)

Approach	Anterior (n = 45)	Posterior (n = 62)	Trochanteric flip (n = 44)
Avascular necrosis	4 (8.9%)	10 (16.1%)	4 (9.1%)
Heterotopic ossification	17 (37.8%)	22 (35.5)	19 (43.2%)

Table 54.4 Outcomes related to surgical approach used (n = 137)

Result	Anterior (n = 38)	Posterior (n = 62)	Trochanteric flip (n = 37)
Good/excellent	25 (65.8%)	33 (53.2%)	31 (83.8%)
Fair/poor	13 (34.2%)	29 (46.8%)	6 (16.2%)

Recommendations

- In a stable hip with minimal fracture displacement, nonoperative management may be a reasonable treatment option [overall quality: very low]

Question 3: Which surgical approach should I use?

Case clarification

You determine there is sufficient displacement of the head fragment to warrant surgical intervention. But how are you going to get there?

Current opinion

Femoral head fractures are currently addressed through a variety of surgical exposures, based on surgeon preference and associated fractures.

Relevance

Multiple surgical approaches are available, and each has potential advantages and disadvantages that must be considered.

Finding the evidence

See Question 1.

Quality of the evidence

Level III

- 1 retrospective case-control study[18]

Level IV

- 10 retrospective case series[14,19,22–27,31,32]

Findings

While medial (Ludloff)[8] and anterolateral (Watson–Jones)[22] approaches have been described for the fixation of femoral head fractures, the most commonly utilized approaches are the anterior (Smith–Peterson), posterolateral (Kocher–Langenbeck), and the trochanteric flip osteotomy. Eleven articles provided adequate description of the surgical approach and complications in 151 cases to permit further analysis (Table 54.3).[14,18,19,22–27,31,32] The anterior approach was used in 45 (29.8%), a posterolateral approach in 62 (41.1%), and a trochanteric flip in 44 (29.1%) of cases.

Poor visualization of the head fragment was noted by two authors via the posterolateral approach[18,22] and in three of the case series[18,22,31] excision of the fragment was performed in 18/33 (54.5%) of cases via a posterolateral approach, compared with only 4/28 (14.3%) via an anterior approach, at least in part due to impaired visualization. AVN occurred with 4/45 (8.9%) anterior, 10/62 (16.1%) posterolateral, and 4/44 (9.1%) trochanteric flip approaches. Heterotopic ossification (HO) was noted in 17/45 (37.8%) anterior, 22/62 (35.5%) posterolateral, and 19/44 (43.2%) of the trochanteric flip approaches. This occurred despite HO prophylaxis with either indomethacin or radiation therapy in 11/34 (32.4%) of cases.[23–27]

Nine articles provided functional outcomes according to Thompson and Epstein[30] for the various approaches in 137 cases (Table 54.4).[14,18,19,22–25,31,32] A posterior approach was used more commonly when there was an associated fracture of the posterior acetabulum, which may have influenced these results.

Recommendations

- Isolated femoral head fractures are best approached using an anterior approach or trochanteric flip to improve visualization and minimize the risk of AVN [overall quality: low]
- Femoral head fractures with associated acetabular fractures (Pipkin IV) are best approached with a trochanteric flip osteotomy [overall quality: low]

Question 4: Should the fragment be excised or repaired?

Case clarification

Once you reach the femoral head fragment, should you attempt to fix the fragment, or simply excise it?

Current opinion

Most surgeons recommend fixation of displaced femoral head fractures.

Relevance

The size and extent of comminution of the femoral head fragment can vary. When should the fragment be preserved, and should it ever be excised?

Finding the evidence

See Question 1.

Quality of the evidence

Level IV
- 8 retrospective case series[13,14,16,19,21–23,31]

Findings

Eight papers described the outcomes of 123 patients treated by either fragment excision or fixation.[13,14,16,19,21–23,31] Insufficient data was provided to clearly determine the indication for excision. In 53 cases where excision was performed, there were 5 (9.4%) excellent, 30 (56.6%) good, 8 (15.1%) fair, and 10 (18.9%) poor results. Better results were obtained with open reduction and internal fixation, with 16 (22.9%) excellent, 30 (42.9%) good, 9 (12.9%) fair, and 15 (21.4%) poor results (Table 54.5).

Earlier authors suggested excision of fragments up to 1/3 of the weightbearing surface of the femoral head,[6] but most authors now advocate fixation of any fragment large enough to salvage, excising only smaller, comminuted fragments not amenable to fixation.[18,22,31]

Recommendations

- Excision of small, comminuted fragments can yield reasonable results, but fixation of larger head fragments is recommended [overall quality: low]

Question 5: What complications should be anticipated?

Case clarification

As you discuss the results of surgery with the patient's family, they ask if there are any complications to worry about.

Current opinion

Femoral head fractures are associated with complications including sciatic nerve palsy, heterotopic bone formation, AVN, arthritis, and infection.

Relevance

These potentially significant complications can lead to inferior outcomes, impaired function, and result in the need for further surgery.

Finding the evidence

See Question 1.

Quality of the evidence

Level III
- 1 retrospective case-control study[18]

Level IV
- 19 retrospective case series[7–9,13–17,19,22–30,32]

Findings

Twenty papers provided data on complications in 329 femoral head fractures (Table 54.6).[7–9,13–19,22–30,32] Traumatic sciatic nerve palsy occurred in 19 (5.8%) of cases. HO developed in 59 (17.9%) cases, 38 (11.6%) of patients went on to develop AVN, and 67 (20.4%) showed radiographic signs of arthritis. Deep infection occurred in 8 (2.4%) of cases. Length of follow-up varied significantly among studies.

Recommendations

- Long-term follow-up is recommended to monitor for the development of complications frequently observed following femoral head fractures [overall quality: low]

Table 54.5 Outcomes observed with fragment excision or fixation (n = 123)

Result	Excision (n = 57)	Fixation (n = 70)
Excellent	5 (9.4%)	16 (22.9%)
Good	30 (56.6%)	30 (42.9%)
Fair	8 (15.1%)	9 (12.9%)
Poor	10 (18.9%)	15 (21.4%)

Table 54.6 Complications observed with femoral head fractures (n = 329)

Complication	Incidence
Sciatic nerve palsy	19 (5.8%)
Heterotopic ossification	59 (17.9%)
Avascular necrosis	38 (11.6%)
Arthritis	67 (20.4%)
Deep infection	8 (2.4%)

Question 6: What is the expected outcome?

Case clarification

Your patient asks what kind of outcome he can expect.

Current opinion

Femoral head fractures have a significant complication rate, and often have a poor clinical outcome.

Relevance

As these injuries typically occur in young, active individuals, the potential impact of these injuries on their long-term function and productivity is significant.

Finding the evidence

See Question 1.

Quality of the evidence

Level IV
• 19 retrospective case series[7,12–17,19–25,28–32]

Findings

Nineteen studies described the outcome according to Thompson and Epstein[30] of 294 patients.[7,12–17,19–25,28–32] Overall there were 43 (14.6%) excellent, 120 (40.8%) good, 53 (18.0%) fair, and 78 (26.5%) poor results (Table 54.7).

Fourteen of these studies further described the results by fracture type in 202 of these patients (Table 54.7).[12–14,16,17,19,20–25,31,32] While quite similar results were reported for isolated femoral head fractures, the addition of an acetabular fracture resulted in slightly inferior outcomes, and an associated femoral neck fracture (although small numbers) resulted in significantly worse outcomes.

Recommendations

• Patients should be counseled regarding expectations following these significant articular injuries, with only slightly more than half of patients obtaining good or excellent results [overall quality: moderate]

Summary of recommendations

• In the absence of a femoral neck fracture, a timely attempt at a closed reduction in the Emergency Department or operating room is recommended
• In a stable hip with minimal fracture displacement, non-operative management may be a reasonable treatment option
• Isolated femoral head fractures are best approached using an anterior approach or trochanteric flip to improve visualization and minimize the risk of AVN
• Femoral head fractures with associated acetabular fractures (Pipkin IV) are best approached with a trochanteric flip osteotomy
• Excision of small, comminuted fragments can yield reasonable results, but fixation of larger head fragments is recommended
• Long-term follow-up is recommended to monitor for the development of complications frequently observed following femoral head fractures
• Patients should be counseled regarding expectations following these significant articular injuries, with only slightly more than half of patients obtaining good or excellent results

Conclusions

Although no high-quality studies have been published on these relatively rare injuries, an organized review of the available literature provides some useful guidance in the management of these challenging injuries. Advances in surgical technique may provide enhanced visualization, while minimizing postoperative complications. Despite our best efforts in the treatment of these high-energy injuries, the results remain unsatisfactory in many cases, and patients should be counseled with regard to potential complications and expected functional outcomes from the outset of treatment.

Table 54.7 Outcomes (Thompson and Epstein) reported for femoral head fractures

Result	Total Pipkin (n = 294)	Pipkin I (n = 68)	Pipkin II (n = 59)	Pipkin III (n = 8)	Pipkin IV (n = 65)
Excellent	43 (14.6%)	12 (17.6%)	14 (23.7%)	0 (0%)	11 (16.9%)
Good	120 (40.8%)	39 (57.4%)	30 (50.8%)	3 (37.5%)	27 (41.5%)
Fair	53 (18.0%)	11 (16.2%)	6 (10.2%)	2 (25%)	9 (13.8%)
Poor	78 (26.5%)	6 (8.8%)	9 (15.3%)	3 (37.5%)	18 (27.7%)

References

1. Birkett J. Description of a dislocation of the head of the femur, complicated with its fracture; with remarks. Med Circ Trans 1869;52:133–8.
2. Pipkin G. Treatment of Grade IV fracture-dislocation of the hip. J Bone Joint Surg Am 1957;39:1027–42.
3. Brumback RJ, Kenzora JE, Levitt LE, et al. Fractures of the femoral head. Hip 1987;181–206.
4. DeLee JC, Evans JA, Thomas J. Anterior dislocation of the hip and associated femoral head fractures. J Bone Joint Surg Am 1980;62:960–4.
5. Gautier E, Ganz K, Krügel N, et al. Anatomy of the medial femoral circumflex artery and its surgical implications. J Bone Joint Surg Br 2000;82:679–83.
6. Epstein HC. Posterior fracture-dislocations of the hip. Long-term follow-up. J Bone Joint Surg Am 1974;56:1103–27.
7. Hougaard K, Thomsen PB. Coxarthrosis following traumatic posterior dislocation of the hip. J Bone Joint Surg Am 1987;69:679–83.
8. Kelly RP, Yarbrough 3rd SH. Posterior fracture-dislocation of the femoral head with retained medial head fragment. J Trauma 1971;11(2):97–108.
9. Sarmiento A, Laird CA. Posterior fracture-dislocation of the femoral head. Report of a case. Clin Orthop Relat Res 1973;92:143–6.
10. Larson CB. Fracture dislocations of the hip. Clin Orthop Relat Res 1973;92:147–54.
11. Kristensen O, Stougaard J. Traumatic dislocation of the hip. Results of conservative treatment. Acta Orthop Scand 1974;45(2):206–12.
12. Chakraborti S, Miller IM. Dislocation of the hip associated with fracture of the femoral head. Injury 1975;7(2):134–42.
13. Roeder Jr LF, DeLee JC. Femoral head fractures associated with posterior hip dislocation. Clin Orthop Relat Res 1980;147:121–30.
14. Butler JE. Pipkin type-II fractures of the femoral head. J Bone Joint Surg Am 1981;63(8):1292–6.
15. Epstein HC, Wiss DA, Cozen L. Posterior fracture dislocation of the hip with fractures of the femoral head. Clin Orthop Relat Res 1985;201:9–17.
16. Lang-Stevenson A, Getty CJ. The Pipkin fracture-dislocation of the hip. Injury 1987;18(4):264–9.
17. Hougaard K, Thomsen PB. Traumatic posterior fracture-dislocation of the hip with fracture of the femoral head or neck, or both. J Bone Joint Surg Am 1988;70(2):233–9.
18. Swiontkowski MF, Thorpe M, Seiler JG, et al. Operative management of displaced femoral head fractures: case-matched comparison of anterior versus posterior approaches for Pipkin I and Pipkin II fractures. J Orthop Trauma 1992;6(4):437–42.
19. Marchetti ME, Steinberg GG, Coumas JM. Intermediate-term experience of Pipkin fracture-dislocations of the hip. J Orthop Trauma 1996;10(7):455–61.
20. Mostafa MM. Femoral head fractures. Int Orthop 2001;25(1):51–4.
21. Yoon TR, Rowe SM, Chung JY, et al. Clinical and radiographic outcome of femoral head fractures: 30 patients followed for 3–10 years. Acta Orthop Scan 2001;72(4):348–53.
22. Kloen P, Siebenrock KA, Raaymakers E, et al. Femoral head fractures revisited. Eur J Trauma 2002;4:221–33.
23. Keel M, Eid K, Isler B, et al. The role of surgical hip dislocation in the treatment of acetabular and femoral head fractures. Eur J Trauma 2005;2:138–47.
24. Prokop A, Helling HJ, Hahn U, et al. Biodegradable implants for Pipkin fractures. Clin Orthop Relat Res 2005;432:226–33.
25. Gardner MJ, Suk M, Pearle A, et al. Surgical dislocation of the hip for fractures of the femoral head. J Orthop Trauma 2005;19(5):334–42.
26. Mehta S, Routt ML Jr. Irreducible fracture-dislocations of the femoral head without posterior wall acetabular fractures. J Orthop Trauma 2008;22(10):686–92.
27. Solberg BD, Moon CN, Franco DP. Use of a trochanteric flip osteotomy improves outcomes in Pipkin IV fractures. Clin Orthop Relat Res 2009;467(4):929–33.
28. Yang RS, Tsuang YH, Hang YS, et al. Traumatic dislocation of the hip. Clin Orthop Relat Res 1991;265:218–27.
29. Jacob JR, Rao JP, Ciccarelli C. Traumatic dislocation and fracture dislocation of the hip. A long-term follow-up study. Clin Orthop Relat Res 1987;214:249–63.
30. Thompson VP, Epstein HC. Traumatic dislocation of the hip; a survey of two hundred and four cases covering a period of twenty-one years. J Bone Joint Surg Am 1951;33(3):746–78.
31. Stannard JP, Harris HW, Volgas DA, Alonso JE. Functional outcome of patients with femoral head fractures associated with hip dislocations. Clin Orthop Relat Res 2000;377:44–56.
32. Henle P, Kloen P, Siebenrock KA. Femoral head injuries: Which treatment strategy can be recommended? Injury 2007;38(4):478–88.

55 Intracapsular Fractures

Jennifer A. Klok[1], Marc Swiontkowski[2], and Mohit Bhandari[3]

[1]University of Ottawa, Ottawa, ON, Canada
[2]University of Minnesota, Minneapolis, MN, USA
[3]McMaster University, Hamilton, ON, Canada

Case scenario

A 75 year old woman who is currently ambulatory and living independently is brought to the Emergency Department with complaints of left hip pain after a slip in her kitchen. She is currently unable to bear weight. On examination, her left leg is shortened and externally rotated. She is neurovascularly intact.

Relevant anatomy

Hip fractures are anatomically classified in relation to the hip capsule as intracapsular fractures (i.e., femoral neck) or extracapsular fractures (intertrochanteric and subtrochanteric). This chapter focuses on management options for fractures of the femoral neck.

Importance of the problem

The disability adjusted life-years (DALYs) lost as a result of hip fractures ranks in the top 10 of all-cause disability globally. Over 4.5 million persons sustain hip fractures around the world each year. In North America, hip fractures occur in 280,000 Americans (over 5000 per week) and 36,000 (over 690 per week) Canadians annually. By the year 2040, the number of people aged 65 or older will increase from 34.8 million to 77.2 million. The number of hip fractures is likely to exceed 500,000 annually in the United States and 88,000 in Canada over the next 40 years.[1-3]

Hip fractures are associated with a 30% mortality rate at 1 year and profound temporary, and sometimes perma-nent, impairment of independence and quality of life. Furthermore, approximately 30% of surgically treated hip fractures require revision surgery.[4] These revisions are associated with a large burden of morbidity and mortality. By the year 2040, the estimated annual healthcare costs will reach $9.8 billion in the United States and $650 million in Canada.[5]

Surgeons and patients are inundated with an ever-increasing and easily accessible body of information about hip fractures. A Google search for "hip fractures" returns over 2,000,000 hits. The variable quality and lack of filtering mandates need for preappraised evidence-based guides.

Top six questions

Treatment

1. What is the relative effect of internal fixation vs. arthroplasty in the management of displaced femoral neck fractures?
2. What is the optimal implant for fixing femoral neck fractures?
3. What is the optimal approach to fixing femoral neck fractures?
4. What is the optimal approach to replacing femoral neck fractures?
5. What is the optimal perioperative care in patients with femoral neck fractures?

Prognosis

6. What is the effect of surgical delay on morbidity and mortality after a femoral neck fracture?

Evidence-Based Orthopedics, First Edition. Edited by Mohit Bhandari.
© 2012 Blackwell Publishing Ltd. Published 2012 by Blackwell Publishing Ltd.

Finding the evidence

The following general searches were undertaken to identify the best evidence (meta-analyses, systematic reviews, and clinical trials) on intracapsular hip fractures. In addition to this, more detailed search steps are outlined under each respective question.

• Cochrane Database, using the search term: "hip fractures"
• PubMed: (www.ncbi.nlm.nih.gov/pubmed/) clinical queries search/systematic reviews: "hip fracture" OR "femoral neck fracture"
• PubMed: Advanced search/type of article/randomized control trials: "femoral neck fractures"
• MEDLINE search: population ("femoral neck fracture") and methodology (clinical trial)

Question 1: What is the relative effect of internal fixation vs. arthroplasty in the management of displaced femoral neck fractures?

Case clarification

The patient's radiograph reveals a displaced femoral neck fracture (Garden type IV). You present two options for treatment to your patient: arthroplasty or internal fixation.

Garden type IV denotes a displaced femoral neck fracture; Garden types I and II are typically nondisplaced whereas types III/IV are displaced.

Relevance

Maintaining the patient's original hip with a fixation device vs. removing the femoral head and replacing the hip with

a prosthesis has important implications for outcome and function. Current opinion is highly divergent among orthopedic surgeons on whether to fix or replace the hip.

Current opinion

Current opinion suggests that the majority of surgeons use arthroplasty for the treatment of displaced femoral neck fractures.

Finding the evidence

• Search terms: "femoral neck fracture" AND "arthroplasty" OR "internal fixation"

Quality of the evidence

Level I

• 4 systematic reviews/meta-analyses[6,7]
• 10 randomized trials

Level II

• 5 randomized trials with methodological limitations

Findings

A meta-analysis by Bhandari et al. is summarized below.[8]

Mortality Nine trials (n = 1162 patients) provided postoperative mortality data at 4 months or less and 12 trials (n = 1767 patients) provided 1 year mortality data (Table 55.1).

Revision surgery All fourteen studies (n = 1901) provided information on revision surgery (Table 55.1). Arthroplasty substantially reduced the risk of revision, and the results were consistent from study to study.

Pain, function, and infection rates Information on secondary outcomes was available for 6 studies (N = 1153 patients)

Table 55.1 Mortality and revision surgery

	Events			RR[a]	95% CI	p value
	N	A	IF			
Mortality (<4 months)						
All arthroplasty vs. IF	1162	55/615	34/547	1.27	0.84–1.92	0.25
Mortality (1 year)						
All arthroplasty vs. IF	1767	226/984	160/783	1.04	0.84–1.29	0.68
Mortality (>1 year)						
All arthroplasty vs. IF	1596	412/895	251/701	1.12	0.90–1.43	0.30
Revision surgery						
All arthroplasty vs. IF	1901	111/1051	299/850	0.23	0.13–0.42	0.0003

A, all arthroplasty; CI, confidence interval; IF, internal fixation; N, total sample size pooled; RR, relative risk.
[a]The relative risk of outcome (i.e., mortality or revision surgery) with arthroplasty compared to internal fixation. Values>1.0 favor internal fixation, values <1.0 favor arthroplasty).

reporting on pain relief and 12 on function (N = 1179 patients). Pain relief and function were similar in patients treated with arthroplasty or internal fixation (RR of no/little pain 1.12, 95% CI 0.88–1.35 and good function 0.99, 95% CI 0.90–1.10). Arthroplasty significantly increased the risk of infection (12 studies, n = 1822) compared to internal fixation (RR 1.81, 95% CI 1.16–2.85, p = 0.009, homogeneity p = 0.16). The risk difference between the two treatments was 3.4%. This meant that for every 29 patients treated with internal fixation, 1 infection could be prevented (NNT = 1/0.034 = 29.4).

Blood loss and surgical time Four studies (N = 343 patients) reported on estimated blood loss, and 5 (N = 447 patients) and surgical time. Patients who underwent arthroplasty experienced greater blood loss than those who were treated with internal fixation (weighted mean difference = 176.4 mL, 95% CI 132.4–220.4, p < 0.05). Similarly, surgical time in the arthroplasty-treated patients was greater than the patients treated with internal fixation (weighted mean difference = 29.0 minutes, 95% CI 23.2–34.8, p < 0.05).

Recommendations
• Arthroplasty significantly reduces the risk of revision surgery at 1 year compared to internal fixation [overall quality: moderate]
• Arthroplasty does not increase the risk of mortality at 1 year compared to internal fixation [overall quality: low]
• Arthroplasty significantly increases the risk of infection, blood loss, and operating time at 1 year compared to internal fixation [overall quality: moderate]

Question 2: What is the optimal implant for fixing femoral neck fractures?

Case clarification
In considering internal fixation you need to determine whether cancellous screws or sliding hip screws will result in the best outcome for your patient.

Relevance
As much of the focus in the literature is concerned with comparing internal fixation to arthroplasty, the question of which method of fixation generates superior results is less well understood. It is suggested that bias in certain study designs has caused outcomes for arthroplasty to fair better. For this reason, internal fixation cannot be overruled and further scrutiny of fixation methods is in order.[9]

Current opinion
Current opinion suggests that the majority of surgeons are using internal fixation with cancellous screws in undisplaced hip fractures. When internal fixation is chosen for displaced fractures, cancellous screws are also the preferred option.[9]

Finding the evidence
• Search terms: "hip OR femoral neck fracture" AND "internal fixation"

Quality of the evidence
Level I
• 2 systematic reviews/meta-analyses

Level II
• 28 randomized trials with methodologic limitations

Findings
Sliding hip screw (SHS) vs. screw fixation A review by Bhandari et al. summarized results for five randomized trials comparing SHS to screw fixation (Table 55.2).[9]

A Cochrane review of internal fixation (using screws, pins and/or plates) in intracapsular hip fractures included 28 trials (N = 5547).[10] The authors concluded that, due to the variability in study designs, outcomes, lack of methodological rigor, and small sample sizes, no definitive statements can be made to support the use of certain types or methods of fixation over others. While several studies did find significant results for certain outcomes, these results are questionable because of the multiple analyses performed.

Pooled results from trials comparing SHS to cancellous screws are shown in Table 55.3. Note that point estimates for AVN (avascular necrosis) favor SHS.

Table 55.2 Comparing outcomes between SHS and screw fixation

Fracture	Outcome	N	Trials	RRR[a]	95% CI	p value
Displaced	Revision surgery	516	4	27%	48 to −4	0.08
Undisplaced	Revision surgery	33	1	87%	99 to −142	>0.05

CI, confidence interval; N, total sample size pooled; RRR, relative risk reduction.
[a]The relative risk reduction of revision with SHS compared to screw fixation.

Table 55.3 Comparing outcomes in SHS vs. cancellous screw fixation

Outcome	N	Trials	SHS	Cancellous	RR[a]	95% CI	p value
Nonunion	462	4	62/226	64/236	1.02	0.76–1.37	0.88
AVN	565	5	23/227	39/288	0.62	0.38–1.01	0.053
Complications	772	6	107/378	131/394	0.86	0.70–1.05	0.13
Reoperations (arthroplasty)	565	5	65/277	69/288	0.99	0.74–1.33	0.96
Reoperations (implant removal)	565	5	20/277	25/288	0.81	0.46–1.42	0.46
Mortality	671	5	43/328	36/343	1.25	0.83–1.89	0.28
Deep wound infections	492	4	6/242	2/250	2.66	0.63–11.25	0.18

CI, confidence interval; N, total sample size pooled; RR, relative risk.
[a]The relative risk of outcome with SHS compared to cancellous screws. Values>1.0 favor cancellous screws, values<1.0 favor SHS.

Recommendations

• Sliding screws have a tendency towards decreased rates of AVN compared to cancellous screws [overall quality: low]

• Current studies comparing different implants for fixation of femoral neck fractures lack methodological rigor. The superiority of one method of fixation over others cannot be concluded [overall quality: low]

Question 3: What is the optimal approach to fixing femoral neck fractures?

Case clarification

You consider managing your patient's fracture using internal fixation. You want to know if there is a superior surgical approach for this procedure.

Relevance

In addition to selecting the optimal implant for fixation of femoral neck fractures, the surgical approach and technique may influence outcome. More specifically, certain methods applied in internal fixation may enhance stability and reduction and thereby decrease rates of AVN and nonunion.[11]

Current opinion

Opinions about compression and impaction during femoral neck fracture fixation are divergent.

Finding the evidence

• Search terms: "Femoral neck fractures" AND "internal fixation"

Level I
• 1 systematic review/meta-analysis

Level II
• 4 randomized trials with methodological limitations:

Table 55.4 Comparing femoral head vascularity in hip fracture impaction

Fracture type	Intervention	Isotope uptake	p value
Undisplaced	Impaction	1.49 ± 0.58	>0.05
	No impaction	1.67 ± 0.48	
Displaced	Impaction	1.08 ± 0.36	<0.05
	No impaction	1.34 ± 0.48	

Findings

A Cochrane review[11] found only four randomized controlled trials (RCTs) comparing different surgical approaches and ancillary techniques for internal fixation of intracapsular hip fractures. Due to the statistical heterogeneity of the studies, the data was not pooled. Results from individual trials are described below.

Impaction of the fracture One trial (n = 103) compared femoral head blood supply (presurgery and at 10 days postsurgery) using bone scintigraphy in femoral neck fractures randomized to impaction (with a 1 kg mallet) or no impaction (Table 55.4).

Compression of the fracture A single trial (n = 220 patients) compared compression of displaced intracapsular hip fractures with a compression screw using a sliding screw plate to no fracture compression (Table 55.5). Fracture nonunion was significantly greater in the compression group compared to the noncompression group.

Open vs. closed reduction Two trials compared outcomes in patients randomized to either closed or open internal fixation. Both studies found operating times to be significantly longer in the open reduction groups. Rates of nonunion, AVN, postoperative blood transfusions, mortality, and wound infections were not significantly different between groups in either study.[11]

Table 55.5 Comparing outcomes in compression vs. no compression

Outcome	Compression	No compression	RR[a]	95% CI	p value
Mortality	27/112	37/108	0.75	0.46–1.07	>0.05
Fracture nonunion	28/85	13/71	1.80	1.01–3.20	<0.05
Avascular necrosis	9/37	7/36	1.25	0.52–3.00	>0.05

CI, confidence interval; RR, relative risk.
[a] The relative risk of outcome with fracture compression compared to no compression. Values>1.0 favor no compression, values<1.0 favor compression.

Recommendations

• Impaction may decrease femoral head vascularity in fixation of displaced intracapsular fractures [overall quality: low]
• Compression may increase nonunion in fixation of displaced intracapsular fractures [overall quality: low]
• Operating times are significantly higher in open compared to closed internal fixation of femoral neck fractures [overall quality: low]

Question 4: What is the optimal approach to replacing femoral neck fractures?

Case clarification

You have decided to treat the fracture with arthroplasty and want to ensure that you are selecting the implant most appropriate for your patient's age and functional status.

Relevance

In making operative decisions about arthroplasty, it is important, for example, to know whether bipolar compared to unipolar hemiarthroplasty does in fact decrease acetabular wear and improve function. Also, what patient and implant risk factors should be considered when choosing between hemiarthroplasty and total hip arthroplasty (THA)?

Current opinion

THA is generally considered a better option for older, more active patients. Hemiarthroplasty is thought to be better for patients with low mobility because of the higher risk of hip dislocation in these implants.

Finding the evidence

• Search terms: "femoral neck fractures" OR "hip fractures" OR "intracapsular hip fractures" AND "arthroplasty"

Quality of the evidence

Level I
• 3 systematic reviews/meta-analyses
• 7 randomized trials

Level II
• 13 randomized trials with methodologic limitations

Findings

A Cochrane review of 19 trials (n = 2115) of arthroplasties in hip fractures provided the highest level of evidence shown below.[12]

Unipolar vs. bipolar hemiarthroplasty Seven clinical trials (n = 857) compared outcomes following unipolar and bipolar hemiarthroplasty (Table 55.6).

Cemented vs. uncemented arthroplasty Six clinical trials (n = 549 patients) compared cemented to uncemented arthroplasty in adults with hip fractures. The results revealed decreased risk of pain and failure to regain mobility in the cemented group (Table 55.7).

Hemiarthroplasty vs. THA Two trials (n = 232 patients) compared uncemented hemiarthroplasty to THA (Table 55.8).

Cemented hemiarthroplasty was compared to THA in 4 trials (n = 415 patients) (Table 55.9).

Recommendations

• There is no difference in the risk of complications, acetabular erosion, return to function, or mortality between unipolar and bipolar hemiarthroplasty in femoral neck fractures [overall quality: moderate]
• The risk of postoperative pain at 1 year after surgery is significantly increased in uncemented compared to cemented arthroplasty [overall quality: moderate]
• The risk of failure to regain mobility is increased in patients with uncemented compared to cemented arthroplasty prostheses [overall quality: low]
• No significant risk differences were found between uncemented hemiarthroplasty compared to THA for any outcome [overall quality: low]
• Patients with the Moore implant were significantly more at risk for residual pain compared to those with THA [overall quality: low]

Table 55.6 Comparing outcomes in unipolar and bipolar hemiarthroplasty

Outcome	N	Trials	Unipolar	Bipolar	RR[a]	95% CI	p value
Dislocation	668	5	6/333	6/335	1.09	0.36–3.31	0.88
Acetabular erosion (requiring revision)	505	3	4/258	1/247	2.97	0.47–18.85	0.25
Reoperations	370	3	10/186	7/184	1.41	0.54–3.69	0.49
Mortality (6 mo)	336	3	34/183	28/183	1.13	0.73–1.76	0.58
Mortality (1–2 yr)	433	3	49/228	49/205	0.90	0.64–1.26	0.54

CI, confidence interval; N, total sample size pooled; RR, relative risk.
[a]The relative risk of outcome with unipolar compared to bipolar hemiarthroplasty. Values>1.0 favor bipolar, values<1.0 favor unipolar.

Table 55.7 Comparing outcomes in cemented and uncemented arthroplasty

Outcome	N	Trials	Cemented	Uncemented	RR[a]	95% CI	p value
Postoperative pain (1–2 yrs)	97	2	16/52	24/45	0.51	0.31–0.81	0.0049
Failure to regain mobility	147	3	33/89	40/58	0.60	0.44–0.82	0.00050
Dislocation	390	4	7/205	2/185	2.00	0.55–7.26	0.29
Reoperation(minor)	141	2	2/175	1/66	0.97	0.13–7.50	0.98
Mortality(1–3 mo)	308	3	27/159	20/149	1.29	0.76–2.20	0.35
Mortality (1 yr)	393	4	48/195	51/198	0.95	0.67–1.34	0.76

CI, confidence interval; N, total sample size pooled; RR, relative risk.
[a]The relative risk of outcome with cemented compared to uncemented arthroplasty (Values>1.0 favor uncementedl, values<1.0 favor cemented)

Table 55.8 Comparing outcomes in uncemented hemiarthroplasty vs. THA

Outcome	N	Trials	Hemi	THA	RR[a]	95% CI	p value
Dislocation	232	2	11/113	17/119	0.70	0.33–1.51	0.36
Reoperations	232	2	25/113	22/119	0.94	0.24–3.67	0.93
Mortality (3–4 mo)	180	1	15/100	8/80	1.50	0.67–3.36	>0.05
Mortality (1 yr)	180	1	27/100	18/80	1.20	0.71–2.02	>0.05
Residual pain[b]	135	1	20/73	0/62	34.91	2.15–565.58	0.012
Failure to regain mobility	187	2	20/86	20/101	1.66	0.31-8.92	0.56

CI, confidence interval; N, total sample size pooled; RR, relative risk.
[a]The relative risk of outcome with uncemented hemiarthroplasty compared to THA. Values>1.0 favor THA, values<1.0 favor hemiarthroplasty.
[b]The Austin Moore hemiarthroplasty was compared to THA in this study. A trial by Ravikumar et al.[13] also reported high rates of pain in patients with the Moore implant (27% at 1yr; 45% at 13yrs) compared to hemiarthroplasty (0% at 1yr; 6% at 13yrs).

• No significant risk differences were found between cemented hemiarthroplasty compared to THA for any outcome [overall quality: low]
• The risk of dislocation is greater in THA compared to cemented hemiarthroplasty [overall quality: low]
• The risk of minor reoperation is higher in THA compared to cemented hemiarthroplasty [overall quality: low]
• Pain and function scores were better in patient with THA compared to cemented hemiarthroplasty [overall quality: low]

Question 5: What is the optimal perioperative care in patients with femoral neck fractures?

Case clarification

You know that perioperative factors may influence mortality in your patient and you look to the current literature on how to best care for your patient.

Table 55.9 Comparing outcomes in cemented hemiarthroplasty vs. THA

Outcome	N	Trials	Hemi	THA	RR[a]	95% CI	p value
Dislocation	4	415	4/207	13/208	0.34	0.12–0.96	**0.042**
Reoperations (all)	4	415	13/207	22/208	0.61	0.32–1.15	0.13
Reoperations (minor)	3	277	2/138	12/139	0.24	0.07–0.08	**0.0020**
Mortality (3–4 mo)	1	138	5/69	2/69	2.50	0.50–12.45	0.26
Mortality (1 yr)	2	258	9/129	8/129	1.13	0.45–2.83	0.80
Residual pain (1 yr)	1	121	30/60	29/61	1.05	0.73–1.52	0.79
Failure to regain mobility	1	76	6/37	7/39	0.90	0.33–2.44	0.84

CI, confidence interval; N, total sample size pooled; RR, relative risk.
[a]The relative risk of outcome with cemented hemiarthroplasty compared to THA. Values>1.0 favor THA, values<1.0 favor hemiarthroplasty.

Relevance

Perioperative management, particularly in the elderly population, requires optimal attention as certain factors may significantly impact morbidity and mortality among these patients. Anesthesia choices, deep vein thrombosis (DVT) prophylaxis, and antibiotic use may influence these outcomes.

Current opinion

Opinions concerning optimal perioperative care for elderly hip fracture patients are varied. The three topics with the highest level of evidence are considered here.

Finding the evidence

• Search terms: "femoral neck fractures" OR "hip fractures" AND "perioperative" OR "anesthesia" OR "deep vein thrombosis" OR "pulmonary embolism" OR "antibiotics"

Anesthesia in hip fractures
Level I
• 1 meta-analysis
• 7 randomized trials

Level II
• 15 randomized trials with methodologic limitations

Antibiotics in hip fractures
Level I
• 1 meta-analysis
• 7 randomized trials

Level II
• 15 randomized trials with methodologic limitations

Thromboprophylaxis in hip fractures
Level I
• 1 meta-analysis
• 8 randomized trials

Level II
• 23 randomized trials with methodologic limitations

Findings

Anesthesia A review of 22 trials (n = 2567 patients) compared outcomes of mortality and morbidity in patients randomized to either regional (spinal or epidural) or general anesthesia during operative hip fracture repair (Table 55.10).[14] It must be noted that 1 month mortality was not found to be significant when a trial from 1978 was removed, and this may reflect changes in anesthesia practices over the years (RR 0.79, 95% CI 0.56–1.12).

The risks of DVT and postoperative confusion were significantly reduced in the regional anesthesia group (Table 55.10). However, the authors caution the reader about the DVT risk results as this group may have been subject to selection bias.

Antibiotics A review of 22 trials (n = 8307 patients) evaluated the effects of antibiotic prophylaxis for surgery in proximal femoral and other closed long-bone fractures.[15] The effectiveness of a single antibiotic dose compared to placebo in closed fractures is shown in Table 55.11.

Four studies (n = 526) showed a significant risk reduction in deep wound infection for multiple-dose antibiotics compared to placebo in hip fracture fixation (RR 0.22, 95% CI 0.07–0.75, p = 0.015).

The results of single short-acting vs. multiple-dose antibiotics were not significant. Additionally, no significant risk reduction was found for operative day vs. longer antibiotic prophylaxis, or for oral vs. parenteral route.

Thromboprophylaxis A review of 31 trials compared the effects of unfractionated (U) heparin, low molecular weight (LMW) heparin, and mechanical pumping devices in patients with hip fractures (Table 55.12).[16] All three interventions were found to be significantly effective in the prevention of DVT.

Table 55.10 Comparison of outcomes in regional and general anesthesia

Outcome	N	Trials	Regional	General	RR[a]	95% CI	p value
Mortality 1 month	1668	8	56/811 (6.9%)	86/857 (10.0%)	0.69	0.50–0.95	0.021
Mortality 3 months	1491	6	86/726 (11.8%)	98/765 (12.8%)	0.92	0.71–1.21	0.55
Mortality 6 months	1264	3	103/613 (16.8%)	115/651 (16.1%)	1.04	0.81–1.33	0.76
Mortality 12 months	726	2	80/354 (22.6%)	78/372 (21.0%)	1.07	0.82–1.41	0.61
DVT	259	4	39/129 (30.0%)	61/130 (47%)	0.64	0.48–0.86	0.0029
Acute postoperative confusion	237	5	11/117 (9.4%)	23/120 (19.2%)	0.50	0.26–0.95	0.0034

CI, confidence interval; DVT, deep vein thrombosis; N, total sample size pooled; RR, relative risk.
[a]The relative risk of outcome with regional compared to general anesthesia. Values>1.0 favor general, values<1.0 favor regional.

Table 55.11 Comparison of effect of a single antibiotic dose vs. placebo or no treatment

Outcome	N	Trials	Treatment	Placebo	RR[a]	95% CI	p value
Deep wound infections							
All	3500	7	20/1745	51/1755	0.40	0.24–0.67	<0.001
Unspecified hip procedure	1251	5	7/615	11/636	0.68	0.28–1.66	0.40
Superficial infections	3500	7	59/1745	87/1755	0.69	0.50–0.95	0.023
Urinary tract infections	2975	4	131/1493	212/1482	0.63	0.53–0.76	<0.001
Respiratory Infections	2975	4	41/1493	92/1482	0.46	0.33–0.65	<0.001

CI, confidence interval; N, total sample size pooled; RR, relative risk.
[a]The relative risk of outcome with single dose antibiotics compared to placebo/no treatment. Values>1.0 favor placebo, values<1.0 favor treatment.

Recommendations

• Regional compared to general anesthesia may reduce short-term postoperative mortality, DVT and postoperative confusion in adult patients treated for hip fracture [overall quality: moderate]
• A single prophylactic dose of antibiotics significantly reduces postoperative deep and superficial wound infection, UTI, and respiratory infections in hip fracture patients [overall quality: moderate]
• Heparin (U and LMW) and physical devices are effective in reducing DVT in hip fracture patients [overall quality: moderate]
• The superiority of U heparin vs. LMW heparin in preventing adverse thromboembolic events is indeterminate [overall quality: moderate]

• Physical devices are effective in reducing overall risk of PE in postoperative hip fracture patients [overall quality: moderate]
• No conclusive evidence was found to show which form of thromboprophylaxis was most effective in reducing mortality and fatal PE [overall quality: moderate]

Question 6: What is the effect of surgical delay on morbidity and mortality after a femoral neck fracture?

Case clarification

Your elderly patient is on the trauma waiting list for surgery and you are concerned about the harmful effect that delaying surgery may have.

Table 55.12. Comparing the effects of U heparin, LMW heparin, and physical devices

Outcome	Intervention	N	Trials	Treatment	Control	RR	95% CI	p value
DVT	Heparin (U or LMW) vs. placebo	993	13	124/474	219/519	0.60	0.50–0.71	<0.001
	Physical device vs. placebo	450	5	16/221	52/229	0.31	0.19–0.51	<0.001
	LMW heparin vs. U heparin	479	5	47/252	64/227	0.67	0.48-0.94	0.02
PE	Heparin (U or LMW) vs. placebo	858	10	13/404	14/454	1.0	0.49-2.02	1.0
	Physical device vs. placebo	487	5	5/238	16/249	0.40	0.17–0.96	0.041
	LMW heparin vs. U heparin	354	4	7/189	1/165	0.094	0.82–13.32	0.094
Mortality	Heparin (U or LMW) vs. placebo	730	8	42/356	38/374	1.16	0.77–1.74	0.47
	Physical device vs. placebo	256	4	7/128	15/128	0.50	0.22–1.14	0.099
	LMW heparin vs. U heparin	242	3	6/122	7/120	0.85	0.31–2.36	0.76

CI, confidence interval; DVT, deep vein thrombosis; N, total sample size pooled; PE, pulmonary embolism; RR, relative risk.
[a]The relative risk of outcome with treatment vs. control. Values>1.0 favor control, values<1.0 favor treatment. Note: LMW vs U heparin intervention: LMW heparin is allocated to treatment column.

Relevance

It has been suggested in the literature that delaying surgery in elderly hip fracture patients is associated with increased risk of morbidity and mortality. However, other studies have contradicted this finding.[17]

Current opinion

The effect of time to surgery on morbidity and mortality in elderly hip fracture patients remains an issue of controversy.

Finding the evidence

• Search terms: "femoral neck fractures" OR "hip fractures" OR "intracapsular hip fractures" AND "surgical delay" OR "operative delay"

Quality of the evidence

Level I
• 1 systematic review/meta-analysis

Level III and IV
• 16 prospective and retrospective cohort studies

Findings

There were no randomized trials evaluating surgical delay in hip fractures patients. This is largely a result of the unethical nature inherent in such studies. A recent systematic review and meta-analysis included 16 historical and prospective observational studies.[18] Though data was significantly heterogeneous between the studies, the authors pooled the data for mortality odds ratios following "early" and "delayed" surgery. The effect of delaying surgery by more than 48 hours (cut-off used in the majority of studies) is significant for mortality within 30 days of surgery and at 1 year (Table 55.13).

Recommendations

• The risk of mortality (at 30 days and 1 year) is decreased in patients with hip fracture who undergo early (<48 hours) surgery compared to delayed [overall quality: low]

Summary of recommendations

• Arthroplasty significantly reduces the risk of revision surgery at one year compared to internal fixation
• Arthroplasty does not increase the risk of mortality at 1 year compared to internal fixation
• Arthroplasty significantly increases the risk of infection, blood loss and operating time at 1 year compared to internal fixation
• Sliding screws have a tendency towards decreased rates of AVN compared to cancellous screws
• Current studies comparing different implants for fixation of femoral neck fractures lack methodological rigor. The superiority of one method of fixation over others cannot be concluded
• Impaction may decrease femoral head vascularity in fixation of displaced intracapsular fractures
• Compression may increase nonunion in fixation of displaced intracapsular fractures
• Operating times are significantly higher in open compared to closed internal fixation of femoral neck fractures
• There is no difference in the risk of complications, acetabular erosion, return to function or mortality between unipolar and bipolar hemiarthroplasty in femoral neck fractures
• The risk of postoperative pain at 1 year post surgery is significantly increased in uncemented compared to cemented arthroplasty

Table 55.13 Comparison of effect early and delayed surgery on mortality

Outcome	N	Trials	Delayed	Early	OR[a]	95% CI	p value	Heterogeneity p value
Mortality(at 30 days)	236,179	13	5438/54,988	12,580/181, 191	1.44	1.33–1.55	<0.001	0.009
Prospective studies[b]	4396	3	259/1280	183/3116	1.34	0.94-1.92		0.22
Retrospective studies[c]	231,783	10	5179/53,708	12,259/178,075	1.44	1.33–1.56		0.006
Mortality(at 1 year)	93,391	9	5,991/21,773	16,547/71,618	1.33	1.22–1.44	<0.001	0.02
Prospective studies[b]	3995	2	43/274	266/3721	2.11	1.46–3.04		0.85
Retrospective studies[c]	89,396	7	5948/21,499	16,281/67,897	1.33	1.22–1.44		0.09

CI, confidence interval; N, total sample size pooled; RR, relative risk.

[a] The risk of outcome with delayed vs. early surgery. Values>1.0 favor delayed, values<1.0 favor early surgery). "Delayed" for most studies is >48 hours.

[b] A single study in this group used a cut-off of 24 hours for delay.

[c] A single study in this group used a cut-off of 72 hours for delay.

- The risk of failure to regain mobility is increased in patients with uncemented compared to cemented arthroplasty prostheses
- No significant risk differences were found between uncemented hemiarthroplasty compared to THA for any outcome
- Patients with the Moore implant were significantly more at risk for residual pain compared to those with THA
- No significant risk differences were found between cemented hemiarthroplasty compared to THA for any outcome
- The risk of dislocation is greater in THA compared to cemented hemiarthroplasty
- The risk of minor reoperation is higher in THA compared to cemented hemiarthroplasty
- Pain and function scores were better in patient with THA compared to cemented hemiarthroplasty
- Regional compared to general anesthesia may reduce short-term postoperative mortality, DVT and postoperative confusion in adult patients treated for hip fracture
- A single prophylactic dose of antibiotics significantly reduces postoperative deep and superficial wound infection, UTI, and respiratory infections in hip fracture patients
- Heparin (U and LMW) and physical devices are effective in reducing DVT in hip fracture patients
- The superiority of U heparin vs. LMW heparin in preventing adverse thromboembolic events is indeterminate
- Physical devices are effective in reducing overall risk of PE in postoperative hip fracture patients
- No conclusive evidence was found to show which form of thromboprophylaxis was most effective in reducing mortality and fatal PE
- The risk of mortality (at 30 days and 1 year) is decreased in patients with hip fracture who undergo early (<48 hours) surgery compared to delayed surgery

Conclusions

The incidence of hip fractures is increasing as the population ages, and controversies concerning the optimal treatment of intracapsular hip fractures continue to exist. It is therefore crucial that surgeons look to the current literature and seek out the evidence for the most optimal care of their patients. This chapter provides an overview of the best evidence on several of the top issues in hip fracture management. However, the need for trials with enough power and methodological rigor to answer the questions that are still inconclusive remains a priority in this patient population.

References

1. Cooper C, Campion G, Melton LJ. Hip fractures in the elderly: a world-wide projection. Osteoporos Int 1992;2:285–9.
2. Cummings SR, Rubin SM, Black D. The future of hip fractures in the United States. Numbers, costs, and potential effects of postmenopausal estrogen. Clin Orthop Relat Res 1990;252:163–6.
3. Johnell O, Kanis JA. An estimate of the worldwide prevalence, mortality and disability associated with hip fracture. Osteoporos Int 2004;15:897–902.
4. Bhandari M, Devereaux PJ, Tornetta P 3rd, et al. Operative management of displaced femoral neck fractures in elderly patients. An international survey. J Bone Joint Surg Am 2005;87:2122–30.
5. Papadimitropoulos EA, Coyte PC, Josse RG, et al. Current and projected rates of hip fracture in Canada. CMAJ 1997;157:1357–63.
6. Lu-Yao GL, Keller RB, Littenberg B et al. Outcomes after displaced fractures of the femoral neck: A meta analysis of 106 published reports. J Bone Joint Surg 1994;76A:15–25.
7. Masson M, MJ Parker, S Fleischer. Internal fixation versus arthroplasty for intracapsular proximal femoral fractures in adults. Cochrane Database Syst Rev 2002;2.

8. Bhandari M, Devereaux PJ, Swiontkowski M, et al. Internal fixation compared with arthroplasty for displaced fractures of the femoral neck. J Bone Joint Surg Am 2003;85:1673–81.

9. Bhandari M, Tornetta P 3rd, Hanson B, et al. Optimal internal fixation for femoral neck fractures: multiple screws or sliding hip screws? J Orthop Trauma 2009;23:403–7.

10. Parker MJ, Stockton G, Gurusamy KS. Internal fixation implants for intracapsular proximal femoral fractures in adults. Cochrane Database Syst Rev 2001;4.

11. Parker MJ, Banerjee A. Surgical approaches and ancillary techniques for internal fixation of intracapsular proximal femoral fractures. Cochrane Database Syst Rev 2005;2.

12. Parker MJ, Gurusamy K. Arthroplasties (with and without bone cement) for proximal femoral fractures in adults. Cochrane Database Syst Rev 2006;3.

13. Ravikumar K J, Marsh G. Internal fixation vs. hemiarthroplasty vs. total hip arthroplasty for displaced subcapital fractures of femur—13 year results of a prospective randomized study. Injury 2000;31:793–7.

14. Parker MJ, Handoll HH, Griffiths R. Anaesthesia for hip fracture surgery in adults. Cochrane Database Syst Rev 2004;18.

15. Gillespie WJ, Walenkamp G. Antibiotic prophylaxis for surgery for proximal femoral and other closed long bone fractures. Cochrane Database Syst Rev 2001;1.

16. Handoll HH, Farrar MJ, McBirnie J, et al. Heparin, low molecular weight heparin and physical methods for preventing deep vein thrombosis and pulmonary embolism following surgery for hip fractures. Cochrane Database Syst Rev 2002;4.

17. Beaupre LA, Jones CA, Saunders LD et al.. Best practices for elderly hip fracture patients. A systematic overview of the evidence. J Gen Intern Med 2005;11:1019–25.

18. Shiga T, Wajima Z, Ohe Y. Is operative delay associated with increased mortality of hip fracture patients? Systematic review, meta-analysis, and meta-regression. Can J Anaesth 2008;55:146–54.

56 Intertrochanteric Fractures

Ole Brink and Lars C. Borris
Department of Orthopaedics, Trauma Research Unit, Århus University Hospital, Århus, Denmark

Case scenario

A 83 year old woman lives with her husband of the same age in a large house. One evening she falls and is unable to get up. Her husband has already gone to bed and does not hear her calling for help. The next morning she is found by the housekeeper and immediately brought to the hospital. The left leg is externally rotated and shortened and she feels great pain. Radiographic examination of the left hip showed an intertrochanteric fracture (Figure 56.1). Operative fixation was conducted on the day after admission.

Relevant anatomy

Hip fractures are anatomically classified in relation to the hip capsule as intracapsular fractures (femoral neck fractures) or extracapsular fractures (intertrochanteric and subtrochanteric fractures). This chapter will focus on management options for intertrochanteric fractures (also called pertrochanteric fractures). These fractures may be either stable (two-fragment fractures) or unstable (three or four main fragments). One of the commonly used classification systems for intertrochanteric fractures (see box) is the Evans–Jensen classification system.[1] Another much used classification system is the AO/OTA classification system,[2] which divides the intertrochanteric fractures into three groups with each group further divided into three subgroups. This classification system is very well suited for research and documentation.

Classification of intertrochanteric fractures

Evans–Jensen classification
- I: stable, no comminution
- Type II: stable, minimally comminuted, but displaced
- Type III: unstable due to lack of lateral support
- Type IV: unstable due to lack of medial support
- Type V: unstable due to lack of medial and lateral support

AO/OTA classification
- Group 1: simple (two-part) and stable, with a single extension into the medial cortex, but with intact lateral cortex of greater trochanter
- Group 2: multifragmentary and unstable, involving the greater and lesser trochanter
- Group 3: involvement of both the medial and lateral cortices with differing fracture direction in the subgroups

---

Importance of the problem

Intertrochanteric fractures represent about 50% of all hip fractures in elderly people and therefore are very common. The number per year in Europe and the United States is about 300,000, with the majority in women. All these fractures need operative treatment, some of them more than once, so they place a major economic burden on society. For the patient, impaired walking ability and leg shortening are common and may influence quality of life. A substantial mortality (around 25%) is also observed following these fractures.

Evidence-Based Orthopedics, First Edition. Edited by Mohit Bhandari.
© 2012 Blackwell Publishing Ltd. Published 2012 by Blackwell Publishing Ltd.

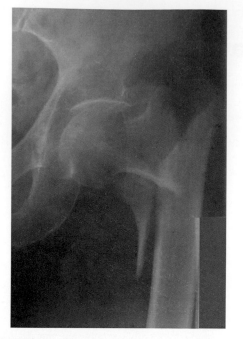

Figure 56.1 Left-sided intertrochantric fracture with involvement of the lesser trochanter.

Top five questions

1. How can surgeons reliably establish when an intertrochanteric fracture is unstable?
2. Should operative treatment take place within 24 hours of admission?
3. What is the best treatment option for this fracture type?
4. In patients with unstable intertrochanteric fractures, is a long intramedullary (IM) nail better than a short nail?
5. How can shortening of the leg be avoided after intertrochanteric fracture?

Question 1: How can surgeons reliably establish when an intertrochanteric fracture is unstable?

Case clarification

The radiograph of the patient's left hip shows an intertrochanteric fracture with involvement of the lesser trochanter and displacement at the fracture site (Figure 56.1). According to the Evans–Jensen classification it is a type IV fracture because there is lack of medial support; this means it is an unstable fracture.

Relevance

Whether an intertrochanteric fracture is stable or unstable is clinically important in terms of choosing the right method of stabilization and is related to the risk of complications and the overall outcome of treatment. A valid classification system for intertrochanteric fractures is an important tool for this purpose.

Current opinion

It is believed that the existing fracture classification systems can be used to discriminate between stable and unstable fracture patterns.

Finding the evidence

- Cochrane Database, with search term: "hip fracture"
- PubMed (www.ncbi.nlm.nih.gov/pubmed/) clinical queries search/systematic reviews: "hip fracture or intertrochanteric fracture"
- MEDLINE search identifying the population (hip fracture or intertrochanteric fracture) and the methodology (clinical trials). Keywords: "intertrochanteric fracture" and "classification," "hip fracture" and "classification"
- PubMed (www.ncbi.nlm.nih.gov/pubmed/) sensitivity search using keywords "intertrochanteric fracture" AND "classification" AND "intertrochanteric fracture" AND "classification" and "reliability"

Quality of the evidence

Level III
- 6 studies with consecutive and nonconsecutive patients without consistently applied reference gold standard

Findings

A number of studies have evaluated the observer agreement with focus on the reliability to classify fractures in accordance with the AO/OTA and/or Evans–Jensen fracture classification systems. Four of these studies comprising a total of 234 radiographs evaluated by a total of 32 reviewers found poor reproducibility and reliability of both classification systems, with kappa values ranging from 0.33 to 0.56.[3–6] Some evidence suggests, however, that the AO/OTA system without subgroups has a higher level of agreement and reproducibility compared with Evans–Jensen and in general should be used in preference to other classification systems.[3,4]

When the question whether a fracture is stable or unstable has to be answered, agreement between surgeons is also relatively poor. Thus, in 2 studies 10 surgeons evaluated a total of 101 radiographs and agreement on stability or instability was reported in only 57% and 65% of cases, respectively.[7,8] Another study with 12 reviewers who assessed 56 radiographs achieved fair agreement on fracture instability (intraclass correlation coefficient 0.38, 95% CI 0.28–0.50),[9] but the inter- and intraobserver agreement on fracture stability was poor in a study with 10 observers evaluating 50 radiographs.[10]

Recommendations

- There is no classification system that can be used to reliably discriminate between stable and unstable intertrochanteric fractures

• The AO/OTA classification without subgroups should be used in preference to other systems

Question 2: Should operative treatment take place within 24 hours of admission?

Case clarification
This patient fractured her hip late in the evening and was not admitted to hospital until the next morning. Surgery was performed on the following day; thus, the time delay from fracture to surgery in this case was more than 24 hours.

Relevance
Surgery for hip fracture is frequently delayed as a result of time spent on blood sampling and analyses, preoperative medical evaluation, and optimization, but also due to unavailability of surgeons, anesthesiologists, or operating rooms.

Current opinion
Delay to surgery increases mortality and morbidity after hip fracture due to associated medical complications, i.e., thromboembolic events or cardiopulmonary complications.

Finding the evidence
• See Question 1
• Additional keywords used: "delay," "timing of surgery"

Quality of the evidence
• Level I–II: 1
• Level III: 4

Findings
A systematic review and meta-analysis of 16 prospective and retrospective studies (257,357 patients) with a cut-off of 48 hours delay from hospital admission to surgery reported an increased 30 day mortality of 41% (OR 1.41, 95% CI 1.29–1.54) and an OR for 1 year mortality of 1.32 (95% CI 1.21–1.43).[11] In the analysis one large study accounted for 19% of all patients, but exclusion of this study had no significant effect on the overall results.[11,12] Another review on 52 published studies (291,413 hip fracture patients) was not able to identify a clear relation between delayed surgery, mortality, and morbidity.[13] Many of the studies included, however, represented a mixture of retrospective and unadjusted prospective studies with conflicting results, while studies with careful methodology were more likely to show a positive relation between early surgery and lower morbidity and mortality. A prospective study including 3,707 hip fracture patients found significantly increased mortality within 6 months when surgery was delayed more than 48 hours (OR 1.63, CI 1.16–2.3).[14]

Most studies have focused on the time delay from hospital admission until surgery, without considering the time delay from the fracture itself until surgery. A register study of 3,754 hip fracture patients analyzed the difference between the time delay from fracture until surgery and the time delay from hospital admission until surgery, and the influence on mortality.[15] The study concluded that the time delay from hospital admission until surgery can be used as a surrogate for the time delay from fracture until surgery.

Recommendation
• We recommend that operation is not delayed more than 48 hours from admission to hospital

Question 3: What is the best treatment option for this fracture type?

Case clarification
There are basically two different methods for fixation of intertrochanteric fractures: sliding hip screw (SHS) or intramedullary (IM) nails. Our patient was treated with closed reduction and internal fixation, and insertion of an IM nail locked distally with a single screw.

Relevance
The method of fixation used for intertrochanteric fractures is relevant because it may be related to the treatment outcome in terms of fracture healing, patient function, and quality of life.

Current opinion
The current opinion among orthopedic surgeons is that unstable fractures should be operated with an IM device because it is believed that this gives a more stable fixation and a reduced risk of secondary displacement and functional impairment.

Finding the evidence
• See Question 1
• Additional keywords used: "internal fixation," "nail," "hip screw"

Quality of the evidence
Level I
• 3 meta-analysis

Findings
The latest Cochrane review concludes that the SHS appears to be a better implant than IM nails for the more common types of intertrochanteric fractures.[16] The conclusions are based on results from 30 randomized controlled trials (RCTs) comparing sliding hip screw with either the Gamma nail (22 trials and 3,871 patients), IMHS (5 trials and 623 patients), or PFN (3 trials and 394 patients). The authors

found higher complication rates for the IM nails, with increased frequency of operative and postoperative fracture of the femur and more reoperation. Another meta-analysis of 24 studies and 3,279 fractures comparing short IM nails with SHS showed significantly more complications in the IM group, and the majority of complications occurred in unstable fractures.[17] The same study found no evidence of fewer complications when using newer-generation IM nails. Conversely, a more recent meta-analysis reported that there seems to be a trend towards fewer implant-related fractures with newer-generation nails, but no firm conclusion about the potential advantages of these implants can be drawn at the present time due to lack of properly dimensioned randomized clinical studies.[18] Nevertheless, a change towards more use of IM devices compared with SHS to fix intertrochanteric fractures from 3% in 1999 to 67% in 2006 has been demonstrated, especially among younger surgeons, and the change seems to be based on clinical outcome evidence factors.[19,20] Several explanations for this have been suggested in terms of a change in training to focus more on IM fixation rather than on fixation with SHS, an attraction towards new devices, concerns about medical liability in case of failure of fixation with SHS, and finally a higher resource value unit (RVU) with IM fixation relative to fixation with SHS.[19,20] In general it could be an advantage to use the same device to fix all intertrochanteric fractures because it will result in more experienced surgeons, however, the scientific evidence does not support superiority of IM nails over SHS for the time being.

Recommendation

• SHS and IM nails seem to be equally effective for surgical fixation of unstable intertrochanteric fractures based on the current evidence and can be chosen by the individual surgeon based on personal preference. We recommend using newer-generation nails

Question 4: In patients with unstable intertrochanteric fractures, is a long IM nail better than a short nail?

Case clarification

The patient was treated with a long IM nail (IMHS Smith & Nephew) locked distally with a single screw.

Relevance

The choice of a long vs. a short IM nail has an implication for the operative procedure and the experience of the surgeon.

Current opinion

Long nails are preferred by a number of surgeons in order to avoid the occurrence of secondary fractures at the tip of the nail and to obtain better stability.

Finding the evidence

• See Question 1
• Additional keywords used: "long nail," "short nail"

Quality of the evidence

• No evidence found

Findings

A short IM nail has a working length of around 150 mm whereas long nails have working lengths of 350–400 mm depending on the brand. Biomechanical data suggest that for unstable subtrochanteric fractures with comminution or segmental bone loss, treatment with long IM nails reduces fracture site motion which may allow early weightbearing.[21] Most surgeons prefer to use long nails for unstable subtrochanteric fractures, intertrochanteric fractures with a subtrochanteric extension, inverse oblique intertrochanteric fractures, and cases with combined fractures of the proximal femur and the femoral shaft. Long IM nails have performed acceptably with low complication rates when used to treat subtrochanteric and proximal femoral shaft fractures.[22,23] However, no comparative studies have been conducted to answer the question whether intertrochanteric fractures are best treated with short or long IM nails.

Recommendation

• We cannot recommend using long nails instead of short nails to treat unstable intertrochanteric fractures due to the sparse clinical evidence

Question 5: How can shortening of the leg be avoided after intertrochanteric fracture?

Case clarification

Our patient was a 83 year old woman with known osteoporosis and an unstable intertrochanteric fracture and was treated with an IM nail.

Current opinion

Current opinion among surgeons is that leg shortening is of minor clinical significance and is not related to the implant used.

Finding the evidence

• See Question 1
• Additional keywords used: "leg shortening"

Quality of evidence

Level I
• 2 systematic reviews/meta-analyses
• 2 randomized trials

Level II
• 2 randomized trials with methodological limitations

Level III
- 1 study

Findings

Leg shortening due to secondary fracture collapse with lateral displacement of the proximal fragment is common after unstable intertrochanteric fractures and among elderly patients with poor bone quality.[16] The consequence of leg shortening is not only cosmetic, but the fracture collapse results in a weakening of the muscles around the hip joint causing prolonged postoperative disability and decreased patient mobility.[24,25]

A retrospective study by Platzer (57 nongeriatric patients) reported that the degree of leg shortening was rather low and depended mainly on the fracture type,[26] but in case of unstable fractures the shortening was significantly less in patients treated with a IM nail.

The latest Cochrane review included 3 studies comparing Gamma nail with SHS and 1 study comparing IMHS with SHS with respect to leg shortening.[16] Overall there was no difference between the two treatment groups but there was a tendency towards a reduced leg shortening in favor of the nail No study has been identified any comparing PFN with SHS with respect to postoperative leg shortening, and studies comparing different nailing systems in this respect are also lacking.

Recommendation

- Unstable fractures may be better treated with IM nails, but the evidence is sparse

Summary of recommendations

- Classification systems cannot be used to identify stable and unstable fractures [overall quality: low]
- Operative treatment should not be delayed more than 48 hours from the patient's admission to hospital [overall quality: low]
- Stable intertrochanteric fractures can be treated with SHS without an increased risk of functional impairment [overall quality: moderate]
- Unstable intertrochanteric fractures can be treated with SHS or IM nails based on the current evidence and can be chosen by the individual surgeon based on personal preference [overall quality: low]
- We cannot recommend using long nails instead of short nails due to the lacking evidence [overall quality: low]
- Unstable fractures may be better treated with IM nails because of a tendency towards a decreased risk of secondary displacement and leg shortening [overall quality: low]

Conclusion

Intertrochanteric fractures are very frequent injuries in the elderly population. The diagnosis is made by clinical and radiographic examination. The existing fracture classification systems can be used to assess the type but are not useful to assess stability. There is some evidence to suggest that the operative treatment of these fractures should be carried out within 48 hours after hospital admission. Stable intertrochanteric fractures can be treated with SHS. Unstable fractures can be treated with SHS or IM nails, based on the current evidence. It cannot be evaluated whether long nails have better results compared with short nails. Overall, we need more studies to be able to make more valid conclusions.

In unstable fractures treatment may be better with newer-generation IM nailing compared with dynamic hip screw in order to avoid fracture collapse and secondary leg shortening.

References

1. Jensen JS, Michaelsen M. Trochanteric femoral fractures treated with McLaughlin osteosynthesis. Acta Orthop Scand 1975;46: 795–803.
2. Müller ME, Rea AMS. The Comprehensive Classification of Fractures of Long Bones. Springer-Verlag, New York, 1990.
3. Jin WJ, Dai LY, Cui YM, Zhou Q, Jiang LS, Lu H. Reliability of classification systems for intertrochanteric fractures of the proximal femur in experienced orthopaedic surgeons. Injury 2005;36: 858–61.
4. Pervez H, Parker MJ, Pryor GA, Lutchman L, Chirodian N. Classification of trochanteric fracture of the proximal femur: a study of the reliability of current systems. Injury 2002;33: 713–15.
5. Schipper IB, Steyerberg EW, Castelein RM, van Vugt AB. Reliability of the AO/ASIF classification for pertrochanteric femoral fractures. Acta Orthop Scand 2001;72:36–41.
6. van ED, Rhemrev SJ, Meylaerts SA and Roukema GR. The comparison of two classifications for trochanteric femur fractures:The AO/ASIF classification and the Jensen classification. Injury 2009.
7. Gehrchen PM, Nielsen JO, Olesen B, Andresen BK. Seinsheimer's classification of subtrochanteric fractures. Poor reproducibility of 4 observers' evaluation of 50 cases. Acta Orthop Scand 1997;68:524–6.
8. Andersen E, Jorgensen LG, Hededam LT. Evans' classification of trochanteric fractures: an assessment of the interobserver and intraobserver reliability. Injury 1990;21:377–8.
9. Fung W, Jonsson A, Buhren V, Bhandari M. Classifying intertrochanteric fractures of the proximal femur:does experience matter? Med Princ Pract 2007;16:198–202.
10. van ED, Rhemrev SJ, Meylaerts SA, Roukema GR. The comparison of two classifications for trochanteric femur fractures: the

AO/ASIF classification and the Jensen classification. Injury 2010;41:377–81.

11. Shiga T, Wajima Z, Ohe Y. Is operative delay associated with increased mortality of hip fracture patients? Systematic review, meta-analysis, and meta-regression. Can J Anaesth 2008;55: 146–54.

12. Bottle A, Aylin P. Mortality associated with delay in operation after hip fracture: observational study. BMJ 2006;332:947–51.

13. Khan SK, Kalra S, Khanna A, Thiruvengada MM, Parker MJ. Timing of surgery for hip fractures: a systematic review of 52 published studies involving 291,413 patients. Injury 2009;40: 692–7.

14. Maggi S, Siviero P, Wetle T, Besdine RW, Saugo M, Crepaldi G. A multicenter survey on profile of care for hip fracture:predictors of mortality and disability. Osteoporos Int 2010;21:223–31.

15. Vidal EI, Moreira-Filho DC, Coeli CM, Camargo KR, Jr., Fukushima FB, Blais R. Hip fracture in the elderly: does counting time from fracture to surgery or from hospital admission to surgery matter when studying in-hospital mortality? Osteoporos Int 2009;20:723–9.

16. Parker MJ, Handoll HH. Gamma and other cephalocondylic intramedullary nails versus extramedullary implants for extracapsular hip fractures in adults. Cochrane Database Syst Rev 2008:CD000093.

17. Jones HW, Johnston P, Parker M. Are short femoral nails superior to the sliding hip screw? A meta-analysis of 24 studies involving 3,279 fractures. Int Orthop 2006;30:69–78.

18. Bhandari M, Schemitsch E, Jonsson A, Zlowodzki M, Haidukewych GJ. Gamma nails revisited: gamma nails versus compression hip screws in the management of intertrochanteric fractures of the hip: a meta-analysis. J Orthop Trauma 2009;23:460–4.

19. Anglen JO, Weinstein JN. Nail or plate fixation of intertrochanteric hip fractures: changing pattern of practice. A review of the American Board of Orthopaedic Surgery Database. J Bone Joint Surg Am 2008;90:700–7.

20. Forte ML, Virnig BA, Eberly LE, et al. Provider factors associated with intramedullary nail use for intertrochanteric hip fractures. J Bone Joint Surg Am 2010;92:1105–14.

21. Roberts CS, Nawab A, Wang M, Voor MJ, Seligson D. Second generation intramedullary nailing of subtrochanteric femur fractures: a biomechanical study of fracture site motion. J Orthop Trauma 2002;16:231–8.

22. Hotz TK, Zellweger R, Kach KP. Minimal invasive treatment of proximal femur fractures with the long gamma nail: indication, technique, results. J Trauma 1999;47:942–5.

23. Hamilton RJ, Kelly IG. Evaluation of the long intra-medullary hip screw. Injury 2004;35:1264–9.

24. Pajarinen J, Lindahl J, Savolainen V, Michelsson O, Hirvensalo E. Femoral shaft medialisation and neck-shaft angle in unstable pertrochanteric femoral fractures. Int Orthop 2004;28:347–53.

25. Gotfried Y. The lateral trochanteric wall: a key element in the reconstruction of unstable pertrochanteric hip fractures. Clin Orthop Relat Res 2004:82–6.

26. Platzer P, Thalhammer G, Wozasek GE, Vecsei V. Femoral shortening after surgical treatment of trochanteric fractures in nongeriatric patients. J Trauma 2008;64:982–9.

57 Subtrochanteric Fractures

Steven Papp, Wade Gofton, and Allan S.L. Liew
University of Ottawa, Ottawa, ON, Canada

Case scenario

A 75 year old patient, currently ambulatory and living independently, presents to the Emergency Department after a fall at home. In the Emergency Department, she is found to have an isolated injury to the left lower extremity. She has hip pain and a shortened, externally rotated lower extremity. Radiographs show a proximal femur fracture (Figure 57.1). There is significant varus, abduction and flexion deformity of the proximal fragment in relation to the distal fragment. The OTA classification is an OTA 31 A3.1.

Relevant anatomy

In subtrochanteric femur fractures, the deformity of the fracture is determined by the deforming forces of muscular action on the proximal and distal fragments (Figure 57.2).

When dealing with subtrochanteric femur fractures, it is also important to understand the local bony anatomy and its relevance. It has been shown that as much as 1200 psi of force ($8 \, MN \, m^{-2}$) are present in the femur with weightbearing in an average 200 lb (90 kg) man.[1] These forces are seen along the medial side of the femur approximately 1–3 inches (2.5–7.5 cm) below the lesser trochanter. Therefore, fixation used to manage these fractures may see significant loads during the healing period (even if a patient is toe-touch weightbearing). A simple fracture pattern in which an anatomic reduction is achieved will likely have a much lower failure rate (due to bony contact) than a more medially comminuted fracture or a fracture in which an anatomic reduction is not achieved.

Importance of the problem

Subtrochanteric femur fractures are not as common as femoral neck fractures or intertrochanteric hip fractures. However, early studies showed high failure rates (20%) when treating these fractures and have therefore generated interest in improving outcomes with improved treatment.[2,3]

Top four questions

1. Which is the better starting point for nailing a subtrochanteric femur fracture: the trochanteric fossa or the tip of the trochanter?
2. Does anatomic reduction lead to lower failure rates than nonanatomic reduction?
3. When nailing a subtrochanteric fracture, does open reduction increase the nonunion rate in comparison to closed reduction?
4. Which device leads to the lowest failure device clinically: an extramedullary or intramedullary (IM) implant?

Finding the evidence

- PubMed and Ovid (1950–2010), search terms: "subtrochanteric femur fractures" AND "extramedullary implants" and "intramedullary implants" AND "open reduction" with limits: "Humans" and "English Language"
- Cochrane Review, search terms: "fracture" and "subtrochanteric femur fracture"

Evidence-Based Orthopedics, First Edition. Edited by Mohit Bhandari.
© 2012 Blackwell Publishing Ltd. Published 2012 by Blackwell Publishing Ltd.

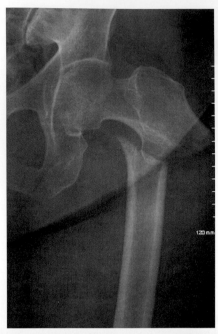

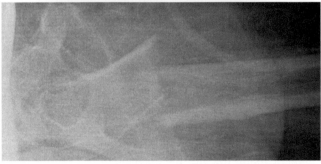

Figure 57.1 AP and lateral xray of a proximal femur fracture. This is a OTA 31 A3.1 type femur fracture with typical noted deformity. A/B.

• OTA meeting abstracts search (subtrochanteric fractures) 1996–2009

Question 1: Which is the better starting point for nailing a subtrochanteric femur fracture: the trochanteric fossa or the tip of the trochanter?

Case clarification

If an IM nail is chosen as the fixation device, there has been debate over different aspects of the surgical technique, including the starting point.

Relevance

The insertion site for anterograde nailing of subtrochanteric femur fractures may be the trochanteric fossa (many refer to this as a pirifomis starting point) or the tip of the trochanter. The trochanteric fossa starting point will offer "in line" access to reaming, straight nail insertion, and possibly improved fracture reduction. Fracture reduction is important when dealing with a subtrochanteric femur fracture.

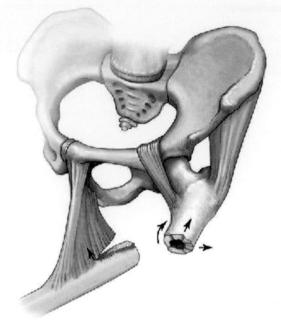

Figure 57.2 Schematic diagram of the muscular forces that deform a typical subtrochanteric femur fracture.

However, this insertion site may involve more soft tissue damage than a starting point at the tip of the trochanter. Starting at the tip of the trochanter may be easier, especially in an obese patient, and operative time and fluoroscopic time may be decreased. In addition, modern nails designed for insertion at the tip of the trochanter have a proximal lateral bend to fit this insertion site.

Current opinion

A trochanteric fossa starting point leads to less varus angulation in treatment of subtrochanteric femur fractures.

Quality of the evidence
• Level II: 1
• Level IV: 7

Reduction

In 4 studies there was a total of 153 cases in which the subtrochanteric fracture was stabilized with a nail that was started at the tip of the trochanter (level IV).[4-7] Seven cases were reported to be in more than 5° varus, and 4 out of 153 patients were reported to have clinical failures. In 2 studies in which the trochanteric fossa starting point was used, varus deformity occurred in 31 of 82 cases (level IV),[8,9] and 4 out of 82 patients had a clinical failure. However, the trochanteric fossa studies were more recent and evaluated alignment more carefully. In the only randomized study to date, 2 of 17 patients in the trochanteric fossa group and 4 of 17 patients in the trochanteric tip group had varus malaligment on follow-up radiographs (level II).[10] This was not found to be statistically significant, but the study was underpowered for this outcome.

The type of nail used may have an impact on the reduction when considering the starting point. In one study, five nails with differing lateral bends were studied and the amount of displacement in a cadveric subtrochanteric femur fracture model was studied. It was found that a starting point at the tip of the trochanter gave the best reduction in most cases, but the results were dependent on the lateral bend in the nail. Insertion through a laterally based (very lateral) trochanteric starting point always led to varus malreduction (level IV).[11]

Outcome

In the retrospective reviews that were available, there were 6 out of 153 failures in the trochanteric tip starting point group and 4 out of 82 in the trochanteric fossa group (level IV). In the only randomized trial, there was no statistically different outcome with respect to blood loss, incision length, or duration of surgery (level II). There were no nonunions is this study.

Recommendations

• Either starting point can be used, and varus malalignment is relatively common with both [overall quality: moderate]
• There is no conclusive evidence that one starting point leads to a better outcome with respect to blood loss, duration of surgery, healing of fracture, or assessment of hip function [overall quality: moderate]

Question 2: Does anatomic reduction lead to lower failure rates than nonanatomic reduction?

Relevance

Because of the difficulty of treating this fracture and the relatively high failure rate of fixation in early studies, there has been focus on trying to improve these results. There has also been some focus on the importance of fracture reduction.

Current opinion

Complete stripping of bony fragments to achieve perfect anatomic reduction may be detrimental to fracture healing. But there has also been a focus on alignment. Currently, it is felt that varus malalignment and flexion malalignment should be corrected, or the fixation has an increased chance of failure.

Quality of the evidence

• Level II: 3 studies
• Level IV: 24 studies

Findings

The level IV studies inconsistently reported on quality of fracture reduction. In the studies that reported on fracture reduction, there was heterogeneity in reporting style. Some studies reported on anatomic vs. nonanatomic reduction. Others calculated neck–shaft angles and some even compared the injured leg to the normal contralateral leg. In most studies, nonanatomic referred to a varus deformity greater than 5°, flexion deformity greater than 10°, or the presence of a significant gap. In a total of 312 fractures that were reported as having an anatomic reduction, 6 (2%) failures were found. In 86 patients with a nonantomic reduction, (26%) 22 patients had failure of fixation (level IV).

There were two studies that best documented correlation of reduction and outcomes. In the study by Haidukewych et al. there were 23 hips that were judged to be anatomic and 4 failed. In 24 fractures that were reduced nonanatomically, there were 11 failures (level IV).[12] Similarly, Shukla et al. found 3 of 19 failures when more than 10° of varus was present but no failures in anatomically reduced fractures. They recommended surgeons pay particular attention to alignment during reduction and that converting a closed to open nailing is necessary if an acceptable reduction cannot be achieved (level IV).[13] In the three randomized trials, very little data was available on fracture reduction.[14–16]

Recommendation

• Anatomic reduction decreases failure rates (2%) in comparison to poorly reduced fractures (26%) [overall quality: low]

Question 3: When nailing a subtrochanteric fracture, does open reduction increase the nonunion rate in comparison to closed reduction?

Case clarification

Closed reduction on the fracture table is unable to achieve a satisfactory reduction. Proceeding with closed nailing may improve the reduction but may not completely reduce the fracture, resulting in a malreduction. An open reduction would be needed to obtain a more accurate reduction.

Relevance

Varus malreduction is associated with higher nonunion rates and hardware failure. (see Question 2) Open reduction can improve the reduction to acceptable parameters; however, it has been suggested that open reduction techniques may be associated with increased nonunion rates secondary to soft tissue stripping, as well as increased infection rates.

Current opinion

Current opinion suggests that most surgeons use an open reduction technique for the IM nailing of subtrochanteric femur fractures.

Quality of the evidence

Level III
- 1 case-control study

Level IV
- 1 case series

Findings

Nonunion Limited publications specifically address the effects of open reduction techniques with subsequent IM nailing of subtrochanteric fractures with adequate stratification of the complications of infection, malreduction/ malunion, and nonunion by open or closed reduction technique. In two studies in which this was specifically addressed, no infection developed.

Nonunion was reported in 1/44 cases (2.3%) in one series in which an open reduction was performed for all cases.[17] In another study by Ziran et al., using cerclage cable (4/10) and cerclage wire (0/14), 4 of 24 had nonunions. In this same study, closed nailing had a nonunion rate of 14.3% (8/56) and malunion rate of 16.1% (9/56). Overall there was a nonunion or malunion in 16.7% (4/24) with an open reduction technique compared with 30.4% (17/56) for closed reduction (level IV).[18]

Recommendation

In patients with displaced subtrochanteric fractures where closed manipulation does not achieve a satisfactory reduction, evidence suggests:
- Open reduction reduces the risk of malunion [overall quality: very low]
- Open reduction does not increase the risk of nonunion [overall quality: very low]
- Open reduction does not increase the risk of infection [overall quality: very low]

Question 4: Which device leads to the lowest failure device clinically: an extramedullary or IM implant?

Case clarification

In this case, the patient has a subtrochanteric fracture. The OTA classification is an OTA 31 A3.1

Relevance

IM nail fixation and extramedullary plate and screw treatment have been advocated. Nail treatment is challenging in these fractures.

Current opinion

IM nailing is the most common treatment for subtrochanteric femur fractures and leads to a lower reoperation rate when compared to extramedullary plating.

Quality of the evidence

- Level II: 3 studies
- Level IV: 24 studies

Findings

Reoperation/failure of construct Restricting consideration to the use of more modern implants, we found 24 level IV articles and 3 level II studies. Retrospective reviews included 10 nail articles,[4–6,8,9,13,17, 19–21] 11 plate articles,[22–32] and 3 comparative reviews (Table 57.1).[12,33,34]. There was considerable variability in the sample population among the 23 level IV articles. Plate studies looked at the DCS, the angled blade plate, or a locking plate. The nailing articles investigated the Gamma nail, the Russell Taylor nail, the proximal femoral nail or the intramedullary hip screw. The heterogeneity of the devices used also makes it difficult to interpret pooled data. In these studies, an extramedullary implant was used in 340 patients and there were 17 failures for an overall failure rate of 5%. In a group of 1094 IM nails used for these fractures, there were 64 failures for a failure rate of 6%. It appears in more recent retrospective reviews that either nail or plate fixation is able to treat this fracture successfully, with a failure rate around 5%. However, failure rates may be higher in more comminuted fractures (Seinsheimer III–V) and one implant may be superior to the other when dealing with the more comminuted subtrochanteric femur fracture.

There are three randomized trials that compare extramedullary and IM implants for the treatment of subtrochanteric femur fractures (level II).[14–16] In all three of these studies the patient population involved elderly patients with low-energy falls, so this data may not apply to the younger patient with the higher-energy fracture pattern which makes up a significant portion of patients with this injury. In two of three studies, the subtrochanteric femur fractures were only a subset of a bigger population of patients with pertrochanteric hip fractures. All three studies had a small number of patients randomized. An evidence- based review of these studies has been published by Kuzyk et al.[35] Pooled data found a reduced relative risk for reoperation but this did not reach statistical significance (0.287; 95% CI 0.062–1.327). The majority of failures in the extramedullary group came in the study by Sadowski et al.[14] in which the device used was the Dynamic Compression Plate. Based on their assessment, Kuzyk made a grade B recommendation that IM fixation reduces the rate of postoperative fixation failure (Figure 57.3).

Table 57.1 Summary of studies and failure rates documented

Paper	Level of study	Implant	No. of patients	Mean age	Failure
Kang et al. 1995	IV	RT recon	13	55	2
Barquet et al. 2000	IV	Gamma	51	47	1
Cheng et al. 2004	IV	Gamma	64	61.6	1
Pervez et al. 2001	IV	Gamma	30	69	2
Robinson et al. 2005	IV	Gamma	302	78	27
French 1998	IV	RT recon	45	39	1
Afsari 2009	IV	Recon nail	55	na	0
Shukla 2007	IV	IMHS	102	75	3
Van Doorn 2000	IV	Gamma	329		17
Honkonen 2004	IV	Recon	77%	77	na
Yoo et al. 2005		Blade Plate	39	na	1
Vaidya et al. 2003	IV	DCS	31	32.6	0
Pai 1996	IV	DCS	16	36	1
Sanders et al. 1989	IV	DCS	32	64	5
Nungu 1993	IV	DCS	15	70	3
Chang-Wug 2009	IV	Locking Plate	20	49	0
Celebi 2006	IV	DCS/ Blade	33	39	0
Ceder 1998	IV	Medoff	32	77	1
Neher 2003	IV	DCS	20	37	0
Kinast 1987 Group 1	IV	DCS	24	47	4
Kinast 1987 Group 2	IV	DCS	23	47	0
Siebenrock et al. 1998	IV	Blade Plate	15	49	1
Haidukewych 2001	III	SHS	16		9
		Blade	15		2
		DCS	10		3
		IMHS	3		1
Pakuts 2004	III	Gamma	11	70	0
		DCS	15	70	1
Parker1997		DHS	80	73	9
		Recon/Gamma	12	74	3
Sadowski 2002	II	DCS	19	77	7
		PFN	20	80	1
Miedel 2004	II	Gamma	16	84	0
		Medoff plate	12	82	2
Ekstrom 2007	II	PFN	18	82	2
		Medoff	13	82	2

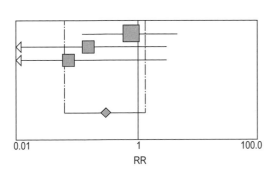

	RR	(95% CI)
Ekstrom 2007	0.76	(0.12 - 4.73)
Miedel 2005	0.15	(0.01 - 2.92)
Sadowski 2002	0.07	(0.00 - 1.20)

Random Effects Model
Pooled RR = 0.29 (0.06 to 1.33)
Cochran-Q = 2.42; df = 2 (p = 0.2986)
Inconsistency (I-square) = 17.3%
Tau-squared = 0.3367

Figure 57.3 Forest plot of relative risk (RR) for failure of fixation for intramedullary compared with extramedullary implants. (Squares represent the RR for individual studies and the diamond represents the pooled RR.) (Reproduced from Kuzyk et al. Intramedullary versus extramedullary fixation for subtrochanteric femur fractures. J Orthop Trauma. 2009 Jul;23(6):465–70 with permission from Wolters Kluwer Health.)

Recommendations

• There is a reduced relative risk of fixation failure with IM fixation over extramedullary fixation when dealing with elderly patients with osteoporotic fractures [overall quality: low]

• In younger patients with a high-energy fracture, fixation failure is equivalent for both IM fixation and extramedullary fixation. Further study is needed [overall quality: very low]

Summary of recommendations

• Both starting points can be used and varus malalignment is relatively common with both

• There is no conclusive evidence that one starting point leads to a better outcome with respect to blood loss, duration of surgery, healing of fracture or assessment of hip function

• Anatomic reduction decreases failure rates (2%) in comparison to poorly reduced fractures (26%)

• In patients with displaced subtrochanteric fractures where closed manipulation does not achieve a satisfactory reduction, evidence that open reduction reduces the risk of malunion and does not increase the risk of nonunion or infection

• There is a reduced relative risk of fixation failure with intramedullary fixation over extramedullary fixation when dealing with elderly patients with osteoporotic fractures

• In younger patients with a high-energy fracture, fixation failure is equivalent for both IM and extramedullary fixation

References

1. Koch J. The laws of bony architecture. Am J Anatomy 1917;21: 177–298.
2. Waddell. Subtrochanteric fractures of the femur. J Trauma 1978;19:582–92.
3. Valasco RU, Comfort TH. Analysis of treatment problems in subtrochanteric fractures of the femur. J Trauma 1978;18: 513–22.
4. Pervez H, Parker MJ. Results of the long Gamma nail for complex proximal femoral fractures. Injury 2001;32(9):704–7.
5. Cheng MT, Chiu FY, Chuang TY, Chen CM, Chen TH, Lee PC. Treatment of complex subtrochanteric fracture with the long gamma AP locking nail: a prospective evaluation of 64 cases. J Trauma 2005;58(2):304–11.
6. Barquet A, Francescoli L, Rienzi D, Lopez L. Intertrochanteric-subtrochanteric fractures: treatment with the long Gamma nail. J Orthop Trauma 2000;14(5):324–8.
7. Papagiannopoulos G, Stewart HD, Lunn PG. Treatment of sub-trochanteric fractures of the femur: a study of intramedullary compression nailing. Injury 1989;20(2):106–10.
8. Kang S, McAndrew MP, Johnson KD. The reconstruction locked nail for complex fractures of the proximal femur. J Orthop Trauma 1995;9(6):453–63.
9. French BG, Tornetta P, 3rd. Use of an interlocked cephalomedullary nail for subtrochanteric fracture stabilization. Clin Orthop Relat Res 1998;348:95–100.
10. Starr AJ, Hay MT, Reinert CM, Borer DS, Christensen KC. Cephalomedullary nails in the treatment of high-energy proximal femur fractures in young patients: a prospective, randomized comparison of trochanteric versus piriformis fossa entry portal. J Orthop Trauma 2006;20(4):240–6.
11. Ostrum RF, Marcantonio A, Marburger R. A critical analysis of the eccentric starting point for trochanteric intramedullary femoral nailing. J Orthop Trauma 2005;19(10):681–6.
12. Haidukewych GJ, Israel TA, Berry DJ. Reverse obliquity fractures of the intertrochanteric region of the femur. J Bone Joint Surg Am 2001;83(5):643–50.
13. Shukla S JP, Ahmad MA, Wynn-Jones H, Patel AD, Walton NP. Outcomes of traumatic subtrochanteric femoral fractures fixed using cephalo-medullary nails. Injury 2007;38:1286–93.
14. Sadowski C, Lubbeke A, Saudan M, Riand N, Stern R, Hoffmeyer P. Treatment of reverse oblique and transverse intertrochanteric fractures with use of an intramedullary nail or a 95 degrees screw-plate: a prospective, randomized study. J Bone Joint Surg Am 2002 Mar;84(3):372–81.
15. Miedel R, Ponzer S, Tornkvist H, Soderqvist A, Tidermark J. The standard Gamma nail or the Medoff sliding plate for unstable trochanteric and subtrochanteric fractures. A randomised, controlled trial. J Bone Joint Surg Br 2005;87(1):68–75.
16. Ekstrom W, Karlsson-Thur C, Larsson S, Ragnarsson B, Alberts KA. Functional outcome in treatment of unstable trochanteric and subtrochanteric fractures with the proximal femoral nail and the Medoff sliding plate. J Orthop Trauma 2007;21(1): 18–25.
17. Afsari A, Liporace F, Lindvall E, Infante A Jr., Sagi HC, Haidukewych GJ. Clamp-assisted reduction of high subtrochanteric fractures of the femur. J Bone Joint Surg Am 2009;91(8): 1913–18.
18. Ziran BH, Hull TF, Barrette-Grischow MK, Mace DM, Shaer JA. Are subtrochanteric cerclage wires really the work of the devil? OTA 2007.
19. Robinson CM, Houshian S, Khan LA. Trochanteric-entry long cephalomedullary nailing of subtrochanteric fractures caused by low-energy trauma. J Bone Joint Surg Am 2005;87(10): 2217–26.
20. van Doorn R, Stapert JW. The long gamma nail in the treatment of 329 subtrochanteric fractures with major extension into the femoral shaft. Eur J Surg 2000;166(3):240–6.
21. Honkonen SE, Vihtonen K, Jarvinen MJ. Second-generation cephalomedullary nails in the treatment of reverse obliquity intertrochanteric fractures of the proximal femur. Injury 2004; 35(2):179–83.
22. Yoo MC, Cho YJ, Kim KI, Khairuddin M, Chun YS. Treatment of unstable peritrochanteric femoral fractures using a 95 degrees angled blade plate. J Orthop Trauma 2005;19(10): 687–92.
23. Vaidya SV, Dholakia DB, Chatterjee A. The use of a dynamic condylar screw and biological reduction techniques for subtrochanteric femur fracture. Injury 2003;34(2):123–8.

24. Pai CH. Dynamic condylar screw for subtrochanteric femur fractures with greater trochanteric extension. J Orthop Trauma 1996;10(5):317–22.

25. Sanders R, Regazzoni P. Treatment of subtrochanteric femur fractures using the dynamic condylar screw. J Orthop Trauma 1989;3(3):206–13.

26. Nungu KS, Olerud C, Rehnberg L. Treatment of subtrochanteric fractures with the AO dynamic condylar screw. Injury 1993;24(2): 90–2.

27. Oh CW, Kim JJ, Byun YS, et al. Minimally invasive plate osteosynthesis of subtrochanteric femur fractures with a locking plate: a prospective series of 20 fractures. Arch Orthop Trauma Surg 2009;129(12):1659–65.

28. Celebi L, Can M, Muratli HH, Yagmurlu MF, Yuksel HY, Bicimoglu A. Indirect reduction and biological internal fixation of comminuted subtrochanteric fractures of the femur. Injury 2006;37(8):740–50.

29. Ceder L, Lunsjo K, Olsson O, Stigsson L, Hauggaard A. Different ways to treat subtrochanteric fractures with the Medoff sliding plate. Clin Orthop Relat Res 1998;348:101–6.

30. Neher C, Ostrum RF. Treatment of subtrochanteric femur fractures using a submuscular fixed low-angle plate. Am J Orthop (Belle Mead NJ) 2003;32(9 Suppl):29–33.

31. Kinast C, Bolhofner BR, Mast JW, Ganz R. Subtrochanteric fractures of the femur. Results of treatment with the 95 degrees condylar blade-plate. Clin Orthop Relat Res 1989;238:122–30.

32. Siebenrock KA, Muller U, Ganz R. Indirect reduction with a condylar blade plate for osteosynthesis of subtrochanteric femoral fractures. Injury 1998;29(Suppl 3):C7–15.

33. Pakuts AJ. Unstable subtrochanteric fractures—gamma nail versus dynamic condylar screw. Int Orthop 2004;28(1):21–4.

34. Parker MJ, Dutta BK, Sivaji C, Pryor GA. Subtrochanteric fractures of the femur. Injury 1997;28(2):91–5.

35. Kuzyk PR, Bhandari M, McKee MD, Russell TA, Schemitsch EH. Intramedullary versus extramedullary fixation for subtrochanteric femur fractures. J Orthop Trauma 2009;23(6):465–70.

58 Femoral Shaft Fractures

Costas Papakostidis and Peter V. Giannoudis

University of Leeds, Leeds General Infirmary, Leeds, UK

Case scenario

A 30 year old man is transferred to the Emergency Department after being involved in a motorcycle accident. He complains of severe pain in his right thigh. On examination his right thigh is swollen, while the entire right leg is abnormally deviated and shortened. He is neurovascularly intact.

Relevant anatomy and biomechanics of the femoral shaft

A femoral shaft fracture is easily diagnosed clinically by the presence of severe local pain, axial deviation, and shortening and abnormal function of the injured limb. As the femur is the largest and strongest tubular bone of the human skeleton, significant forces are required in order for it to be fractured. Consequently, femoral fractures, especially in young individuals, are the result of high-energy trauma. Associated injuries are often present and dictate the treatment plan. The bulky soft tissue envelope surrounding the femoral bone protects from open injuries in most cases. However, the high amount of energy dissipated by the thigh in case of femoral shaft fracture can sometimes result in various degrees of injury to the soft tissue envelope, including various grades of open fractures and even closed subcutaneous degloving injuries. Therefore, neurovascular assessment should be an integral part of the clinical examination.

Importance of the problem

Very few epidemiological studies regarding diaphyseal femoral fractures exist in the literature. In one study, conducted in the population of Rochester, Minnesota (USA) over a 20 year period (1965–1984) the overall incidence of diaphyseal femoral fractures was 18.9 per 100,000 person-years.[1] Severe trauma accounted for the majority of diaphyseal femoral fractures in young patients, and showed a male preponderance.[1] In a more recent epidemiological study conducted in Finland over a 10 year period (1985–1994), the documented incidence of diaphyseal femoral fractures was 9.9 per 100,000 person-years.[2] The highest incidences with regard to age and gender were seen in males 15–24 years old and females above 75 years of age, and 75% of the fractures were the result of high-energy trauma.[2]

From the above studies, it is clear that femoral shaft fractures present a bimodal distribution. The first peak incidence is associated with high-energy trauma occurring in young men; another peak incidence is observed in elderly women and is associated with low-energy trauma within the context of osteoporosis. The two distinct patient population groups should be considered separately when comparing treatment options, complications, and outcome. High-energy femoral shaft fractures present a high incidence of associated injuries, including chest, head, pelvis, and ipsilateral leg injuries in pedestrians, and pelvic and ipsilateral leg injuries in motorcyclists.[3]

The internet is teeming with an enormous amount of information regarding femoral shaft fractures. A Google

Evidence-Based Orthopedics, First Edition. Edited by Mohit Bhandari.
© 2012 Blackwell Publishing Ltd. Published 2012 by Blackwell Publishing Ltd.

search for "femoral shaft fractures" returns over 694,000 hits. However, the treating surgeon cannot easily draw useful information for optimal decision-making from this heterogenous material, and there is a pressing need for pre-evaluated evidence-based guidelines.

Top ten questions

Diagnosis

1. What are the implications of concomitant fractures of the ipsilateral neck of femur or distal end of femur?

Therapy

2. What is the optimal entry point in antegrade nailing?
3. Do unreamed nails have the same clinical success as reamed ones?
4. Does retrograde femoral nailing yield equivalent results to antegrade nailing?
5. Is the use of manual traction on a standard table more advantageous over the fracture table in intramedullary (IM) nailing of femoral shaft fractures?
6. What is the optimal timing for IM nailing of femoral shaft fractures in patients with chest trauma?
7. What is the optimal timing for IM nailing of femoral shaft fractures in patients with head injury?
8. Is the damage control orthopedics (DCO) approach a safer alternative to early total care (ETC) in polytrauma patients with femoral shaft fractures?
9. Is femoral plating preferable to reamed IM nailing in polytrauma patients with femoral shaft fractures and concomitant head or chest injury?

Prognosis

10. Is there a functional impairment after isolated femoral shaft fracture?

Question 1: What are the implications of concomitant fractures of the ipsilateral neck of femur or distal end of femur?

Case clarification

The patient's radiographs reveal a fracture of the femoral diaphysis and a concomitant fracture of the ipsilateral neck of femur. The combination of ipsilateral hip and femoral shaft fractures has been reported in 0.8–8.6% of femoral shaft fractures.[4] This represents a high-energy injury with a 44% prevalence of associated multiple trauma. A high index of suspicion is required for early diagnosis and appropriate treatment, as ipsilateral femoral neck fracture may be initially missed in one third of cases of femoral

shaft fractures.[4] Treatment options include: (1) IM nail with additional screws, (2) cephalomedullary nail, and (3) plate and screws for the fracture of the femoral diaphysis and additional screws for the fracture of the neck of femur. Although an anatomic reduction of the femoral neck fracture is considered of paramount importance, the best treatment option for this combined skeletal injury is controversial.

Finding the evidence

A systematic literature search was conducted in order to delineate the effect of the alternate treatment options of ipsilateral femoral neck and shaft fractures on union, malunion, deep infection, avascular necrosis (AVN) of the femoral head, and reoperation.
* Cochrane Database, with search term "femur fracture"
* PubMed (www.ncbi.nlm.nih.gov/pubmed/) clinical queries search/ systematic reviews: "femoral neck" AND "femoral shaft fracture" PubMed (www.ncbi.nlm.nih.gov/pubmed/): sensitivity search using keywords: "("ipsilateral femoral neck" AND "shaft fracture") OR ("concurrent femoral neck" AND "shaft fracture")
* Review of references of eligible studies

Quality of the evidence
Level III
* 1 case-control study[5]

Level IV
* 1 meta-analysis of case series studies[6]

Findings

A retrospective comparison between two methods of fixation—compression plate and hip screws (n = 15 patients) vs. reconstruction IM nailing (n = 12 patients)—failed to document any statistically significant difference between the two treatment methods with respect to nonunion, delayed union, loss of reduction of the femoral neck, osteonecrosis of the femoral head, and functional outcome.[5] Although the use of a single implant was associated with a higher reoperation rate compared with the combination of compression plate and hip screws (4/12 for the reconstruction nail vs. 0/15 for the plate and hip screws), the difference did not reach statistically significant levels (p = 0.06) (Table 58.1).

Evidence from the meta-analysis of case series studies suggests that customary locked IM nails in combination with hip screws and cephalomedullary nails (reconstruction nails) may result in better union rates for the femoral shaft fracture than plate fixation. On the other hand, separate neck and shaft implants (IM nails with hip screws or femoral shaft plates with hip screws) may result in fewer reoperations than single implants (reconstruction nails) (Table 58.2).

Table 58.1 Outcomes of a retrospective comparative study (Singh et al.[5]) of two treatment options for concomitant femoral shaft and ipsilateral femoral neck fractures: femoral shaft plating with additional hip screw vs. reconstruction intramedullary nail

	Age (mean, years)	Nonunion		Delayed union		AVN	Reoperation	Good outcome
		Neck	Shaft	Neck	Shaft			
Group 1 (n = 15): Hip:screws Shaft: plate	33.2 ± 6.2	0/15	0/15	nd	2/15	0/15	0/15	13/15
Group 2 (n = 12): Recon IMN	37.9 ± 11.6	1/12	0/12	nd	3/12	1/12	4/12	10/12
P value	0.18	0.9	0.78		0.78	0.9	0.06	1.0

AVN, avascular necrosis; IMN, intramedullary nail; nd, not determined.

Table 58.2 Outcomes of various treatment methods for ipsilateral femoral neck and shaft fractures, as documented in a systematic review of the literature (n = 659 patients)[6]

	Age (mean, years)	Nonunions		Reoperation		Malunion		AVN
		Neck	Shaft	Neck	Shaft	Neck	Shaft	
Neck: screws Shaft: plate	34	nd	8/82 (10%)	0/82 (0%)	5/82 (6%)	1/82 (1.2%)	3/82 (4%)	1/82 (1.2%)
Neck: screws Shaft: IMN	34	nd	2/73 (3%)	5/72 (7%)	1/73 (1.3%)	1/72 (1.4%)	6/72 (8%)	2/72 (3%)
Cephalomedullary nail (single implant)	34	nd	0/38 (0%)	6/38 (16%)	2/38 (5%)	2/38 (5%)	1/38 (3%)	2/38 (5%)

AVN, avascular necrosis; IMN, intramedullary nail; nd, not determined.

Recommendations
• It is doubtful whether the use of a single implant (ceplalomedullary nail) could result in increased likelihood for reoperation compared to the combined use of compression plate and hip screws [overall quality: low]
• Better union rates for the femoral shaft fracture may result from the use of intramedullary implants (locked intramedullary nails combined with hip screws or cephalomedullary nails) [overall quality: low]

Question 2: What is the optimal entry point in antegrade nailing?

Case clarification
Assuming, in our previous case scenario, that the patient had sustained an isolated fracture of the femoral shaft, then the treatment of choice would be antegrade IM nailing. The selection of entry point is important in antegrade nailing, since nail insertion through a wrong portal may lead to intraoperative complications.[7]

Current opinion
IM nail fixation constitutes the gold standard in femoral shaft fracture treatment. However, there still exist controversial issues related to the optimal management of these fractures. Many orthopedic surgeons prefer the piriformis fossa as the standard entry point because of its collinear relation with the long axis of the femoral shaft, while others utilize the tip of greater trochanter, although it is located more laterally with respect to the proximal projection of the medullary canal. Potential advantages of the use of the trochanteric tip as starting entry portal include less operative time, less intraoperative fluoroscopy, and a reduced risk of complications, such as AVN of the femoral head and iatrogenic fracture of the neck of femur.

Finding the evidence
In order to provide evidence as for the optimal entry portal in antegrade IM nailing we undertook a systematic literature search:

- Cochrane Database, with search terms "femur fracture," "intramedullary nail," "entry point"
- PubMed (www.ncbi.nlm.nih.gov/pubmed/) clinical queries search/ systematic reviews: "femoral shaft fracture," "intramedullary nailing," and "entry point"
- PubMed (www.ncbi.nlm.nih.gov/pubmed/):sensitivity search using the following keywords and Boolean operators: "femoral nailing" AND "entry point"
- Review of references of eligible studies

Quality of the evidence
Level II
- 2 randomized trials with methodologic limitations[8,9]

Findings
Pooled estimates of the key results are as follows.

Union rate Two trials (n = 125 patients) provided data regarding union rate.[8,9] The choice of entry portal in antegrade nailing (piriformis vs. greater trochanter entry) did not seem to affect union rate (risk ratio 1.01, CI 0.94–1.07, p = 0.82, homogeneity not applicable).

Malunion rate Both eligible trials (N = 125 patients) provided data with regard to malunion.[8,9] No statistically significant risk of malunion was documented with either technique using different entry portals (risk ratio 0.43, 95% CI 0.11–1.76, p = 0.24, homogeneity p = 0.68).

Operative time Although both trials provided data with regard to operative time, a pooled estimate of the effect size could not be estimated due to lack of standard deviation (SD) values of the mean operative time. Consequently, the results of each study were interpreted individually. In one study[8] the above two groups (piriformis fossa and greater trochanter) did not show statistically significant difference with respect to operative time (p = 0.26). In the other study[9] the piriformis fossa (PF) group showed a longer mean operative time compared to the greater trochanter (GT) group, although this difference did not reach statistically significant levels (p = 0.08). This difference, however, was magnified in obese patients, where the operative time was 30% greater in the PF group than in the GT group (p < 0.05).

Fluoroscopy time Only one trial provided relevant data regarding fluoroscopy time.[9] The PF group showed a 61% increase in fluoroscopy time with respect to the GT group and this difference was statistically significant (p < 0.05). Moreover the difference was further intensified in the subgroup of obese patients, where the fluoroscopy time was 73% higher in the PF group (p < 0.02).

Recommendations
- The union process or the risk of malunion of femoral shaft fractures does not depend on the choice of the entry

portal (piriformis or trochanteric) of the IM nail that is used for its treatment [overall quality: moderate]
- The use of piriformis entry portal in obese patients is associated with significant increase of both operative and fluoroscopy time compared with greater trochanter entry [overall quality: moderate]

Question 3: Do unreamed nails have the same clinical success as reamed ones?

Case clarification
In our case scenario the patient had a grade II open femoral shaft fracture. In addition he had suffered a chest contusion. An unreamed femoral nail is considered a more appropriate treatment option for such a situation.

Although the use of reamed IM nails for the management of femoral shaft fractures has been associated with overall excellent clinical results, concerns about the biological consequences of reaming have increased interest in the femoral nailing technique without reaming. Femoral nailing with reaming has been associated with high union and low implant failure rates, but the reaming process has been thought to generate bone marrow embolization phenomena, disrupt of cortical blood flow, and theoretically increase the risk of infection, particularly in open fractures. On the other hand, the use of smaller-diameter unreamed nails has raised concerns about rates of fracture healing and implant failure.

Finding the evidence
In order to evaluate reliably the merits of one technique over the other, we conducted a systematic literature search, using the following databases and references of retrieved articles:
- Cochrane Database, with search terms "femur fracture" AND "intramedullary nail"
- PubMed (www.ncbi.nlm.nih.gov/pubmed/) clinical queries search/ systematic reviews: "femur fracture" AND "intramedullary nail"
- PubMed (www.ncbi.nlm.nih.gov/pubmed/): sensitivity search using the following keywords and Boolean operators: "femur fracture" AND "reamed nails", "femur fracture" AND "unreamed nails" OR "nonreamed nails"
- Review of references of eligible studies

Quality of the evidence
Level I
- 7 randomized trials[10–16]

Level III
- 1 case-control study[17]

Our conclusions were based on the evidence available from higher-quality studies, i.e., randomized controlled trials (RCTs).

Study or Subgroup	rIMNs Events	Total	non rIMNs Events	Total	Weight	Risk Ratio M-H, Random, 95% CI	Year	Risk Ratio M-H, Random, 95% CI
Clatworthy, 98	3	22	3	23	42.2%	1.05 [0.24, 4.64]	1998	
Tornetta 2000	0	83	0	89		Not estimable	2000	
Selvakumar, 01	0	52	4	50	16.8%	0.11 [0.01, 1.94]	2001	
Can OTS, 03	2	121	8	107	41.0%	0.22 [0.05, 1.02]	2003	
Total (95% CI)		**278**		**269**	**100.0%**	**0.38 [0.10, 1.40]**		
Total events	5		15					

Heterogeneity: Tau² = 0.48; Chi² = 3.10, df = 2 (P = 0.21); I² = 36%
Test for overall effect: Z = 1.46 (P = 0.14)

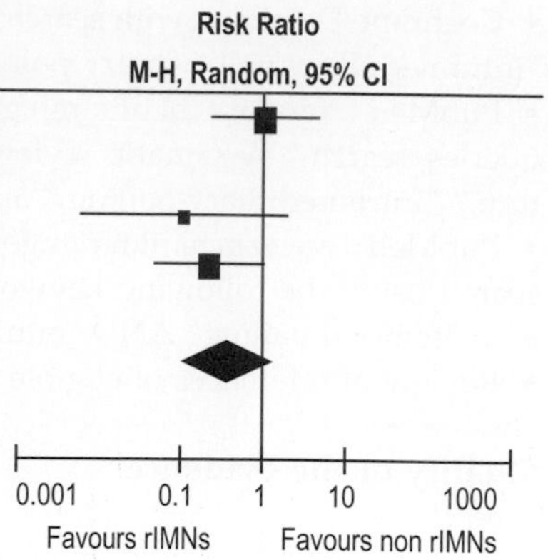

Figure 58.1 Forest plot of nonunion rates between reamed and nonreamed femoral nails.

Study or Subgroup	rIMNs Events	Total	non rIMNs Events	Total	Weight	Risk Ratio M-H, Random, 95% CI	Year	Risk Ratio M-H, Random, 95% CI
Tornetta 2000	0	83	4	89	20.6%	0.12 [0.01, 2.18]	2000	
Selvakumar, 01	2	52	9	50	79.4%	0.21 [0.05, 0.94]	2001	
Total (95% CI)		**135**		**139**	**100.0%**	**0.19 [0.05, 0.71]**		
Total events	2		13					

Heterogeneity: Tau² = 0.00; Chi² = 0.13, df = 1 (P = 0.72); I² = 0%
Test for overall effect: Z = 2.47 (P = 0.01)

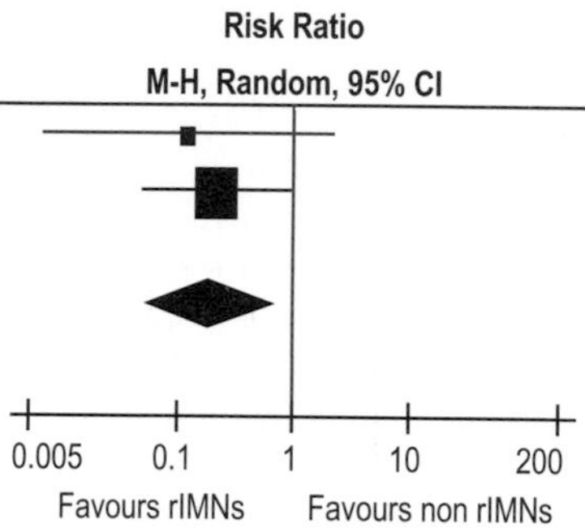

Figure 58.2 Forest tree of delayed union rates, between reamed and nonreamed femoral nails.

Study or Subgroup	rIMNs Events	Total	non rIMNs Events	Total	Weight	Risk Ratio M-H, Random, 95% CI	Risk Ratio M-H, Random, 95% CI
Clatworthy, 98	3	22	3	23	67.8%	1.05 [0.24, 4.64]	
Selvakumar, 01	0	52	3	50	17.4%	0.14 [0.01, 2.60]	
Tornetta 2000	0	83	1	87	14.8%	0.35 [0.01, 8.45]	
Total (95% CI)		**157**		**160**	**100.0%**	**0.62 [0.18, 2.13]**	
Total events	3		7				

Heterogeneity: Tau² = 0.00; Chi² = 1.71, df = 2 (P = 0.43); I² = 0%
Test for overall effect: Z = 0.75 (P = 0.45)

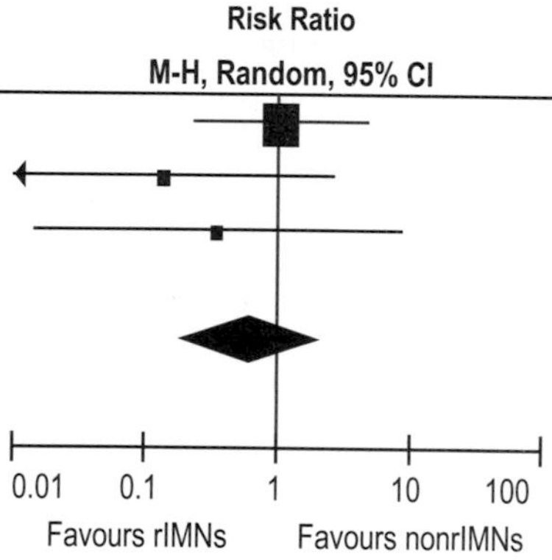

Figure 58.3 Forest plot of implant failure rates between reamed and nonreamed femoral nails.

Findings

Union complications

- Nonunion: Four trials[10,11,13,15] (N = 547 patients) provided relevant data. Reamed IM nails showed a tendency for fewer nonunions compared to nonreamed nails, although this difference did not reach statistically significant levels (relative risk 0.38, 95% CI 0.10–1.40, p = 0.14, homogeneity p = 0.21) (Figure 58.1).
- Delayed union: Two trials[10,15] (n = 274 patients) provided data regarding delayed union. Reamed IM nailing was associated with a statistically significant risk for delayed

union compared with nonreamed nails (risk ratio 0.19, 95% CI 0.05–0.71, p = 0.01, homogeneity p = 0.72) (Figure 58.2).

Implant failure Three trials[10,13,15] (N = 317 patients) provided data regarding implant failure. The reamed nails were associated with a lower risk (but not statistically significant) of implant failure compared to nonreamed nails (relative risk 0.62, 95% CI 0.18–2.13), p = 0.45, homogeneity p = 0.43) (Figure 58.3).

Pulmonary complications Three trials[10,12,16] (N = 569 patients) provided data on pulmonary complications. Reamed nails

Study or Subgroup	rIMNs Events	Total	non rIMNs Events	Total	Weight	Risk Ratio M-H, Random, 95% CI	Year	Risk Ratio M-H, Random, 95% CI
Tornetta 2000	1	83	1	89	10.6%	1.07 [0.07, 16.87]	2000	
Anwar, 04	8	41	4	41	64.0%	2.00 [0.65, 6.13]	2004	
Can OTS, 06	3	168	2	147	25.4%	1.31 [0.22, 7.75]	2006	
Total (95% CI)		292		277	100.0%	1.68 [0.69, 4.12]		
Total events	12		7					

Heterogeneity: Tau² = 0.00; Chi² = 0.27, df = 2 (P = 0.87); I² = 0%

Test for overall effect: Z = 1.14 (P = 0.25)

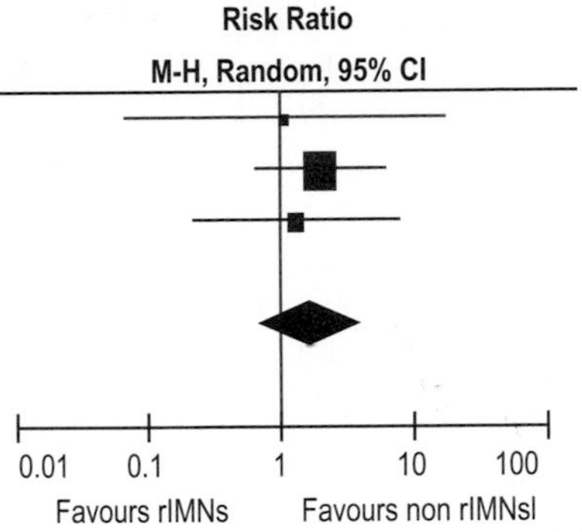

0.01 0.1 1 10 100
Favours rIMNs   Favours non rIMNsl

Figure 58.4 Forest plot of pulmonary complications between reamed and nonreamed femoral nails.

appeared to have a greater tendency towards developing pulmonary complications than nonreamed nails, but not to a statistically significant level (relative risk 1.68, 95% CI 0.69–4.12, p = 0.25, homogeneity p = 0.87) (Figure 58.4).

Recommendations
• The use of unreamed femoral nails is associated with a significant risk of delayed union compared with reamed nails [overall quality: high]
• With respect to other union complications (non union, implant failure), no significant superiority of the reamed over nonreamed nails was proven [overall quality: moderate]
• Reamed femoral nails were not associated with a significantly higher risk of developing pulmonary complications compared with nonreamed nails [overall quality: moderate]

Question 4: Does retrograde femoral nailing yield equivalent results to antegrade nailing?

Case clarification
In our initial case scenario the patient had suffered a femoral shaft fracture accompanied by an ipsilateral femoral neck fracture. One treatment option for the femoral shaft fracture is retrograde femoral nailing, so as to avoid interference with the fixation of the concomitant fracture of the ipsilateral femoral neck.

Antegrade nailing is the standard technique for operative management of femoral shaft fractures. It has yielded high union rates and low infection and malunion rates. However, as antegrade nail insertion in essence violates the abductor musculature; it can potentially cause abductor weakness and limp. Moreover, in certain situations retrograde nailing has appeared as a viable alternative. Such conditions include floating knee injury (as both femoral and tibial fractures can be addressed through the same skin incision), ipsilateral acetabular or pelvic fractures (where the incision for antegrade nailing is inappropriate for the fixation of the pelvic or acetabular fracture), ipsilateral frac-

ture of femoral neck (retrograde nailing of femoral shaft does not interfere with cannulated screw fixation of the concomitant fracture of the ipsilateral neck of femur), obesity, or pregnancy (retrograde nailing is associated with reduced exposure of fetus to radiation).

Finding the evidence
In order to provide a direct comparison of these two techniques in terms of clinical outcome, we undertook a systematic literature search using the following strategy:
• Cochrane Database, with search terms "femur fracture," "retrograde nailing," "antegrade nailing"
• PubMed (www.ncbi.nlm.nih.gov/pubmed/) clinical queries search/systematic reviews: "femur fracture" AND "antegrade" OR "retrograde nailing"
• PubMed (www.ncbi.nlm.nih.gov/pubmed/): sensitivity search using the following keywords and Boolean operators: "femur fracture" AND "antegrade nailing" and "femur fracture" AND "retrograde nailing"
• Review of references of eligible studies

Quality of the evidence
Level II
• 2 RCTs with methodologic limitations[18,19]

Level III
• 2 case-control studies[20,21]

Level IV
• 1 systematic review of case series studies[22]

Findings
The two RCTs (level II)[18,19] and one case-control study (level III)[20] were analyzed together and a pooled estimate of effect size for each outcome of interest was obtained. Another case-control study evaluating antegrade and retrograde nailing techniques in two distinct patient populations, obese and nonobese, was analyzed separately.[21] Lastly, the systematic review of literature provided summarized pooled estimates of various key outcomes of interest.[22]

Union complications
- Nonunion: Data regarding nonunion were available in all three trials (N = 353 patients).[18,19,20] A pooled estimate of effect size did not reveal any difference between antegrade and retrograde nailing with regard to union rate (relative risk 0.99, 95% CI 0.37–2.69, p = 0.99, homogeneity p = 0.65, $I^2 = 0\%$). One systematic review of literature[22] documented a combined union rate of 94.2% and a mean time to union of 3.2 ± 0.4 months for femoral shaft fractures treated with retrograde nailing.
- Malunion: Two studies provided relevant data with regard to axial malalignment (N = 267 patients).[18,20] The risk of axial malalignment did not differ significantly between the two evaluated nailing techniques (relative risk 0.85, 95% CI 0.20–3.68, p = 0.83, homogeneity p = 0.18, $I^2 = 45\%$). Two studies provided relevant data with regard to rotational malalignment.[18,20] Although antegrade nailing showed a clear advantage on controlling correct rotational alignment of the lower limb over retrograde nailing, the respective difference was not statistically significant (relative risk = 0.57, 95CI = 0.20–1.59, p = 0.28, homogeneity p = 0.72, $I^2 = 0\%$). The systematic review of literature documented an overall malunion rate of 7.4% for femoral shaft fractures treated with retrograde nailing.

Long-term pain at the entry portals Two studies reported on long-term hip pain (N = 256 patients),[19,20] and all three studies gave information about knee pain (N = 299).[18–20] The risk of long-term hip pain was quadruple with antegrade over retrograde technique (relative riskm 4.02, 95% CI 1.27–12.70, p = 0.02, homogeneity p = 0.46, $I^2 = 0\%$) (Figure 58.5). As for long-term knee pain, a clear conclusion could not be reached due to the presence of significant statistical heterogeneity (homogeneity p = 0.08, $I^2 = 60\%$). The systematic review of literature documented a 24.5% rate of knee pain in femoral shaft fractures treated with retrograde nailing. This was significantly greater compared to the prevalence of knee pain in distal femoral fractures treated with retrograde nailing (16.5%), (p = 0.014, odds ratio 1.65, 95% CI 1.11–2.45).

With regard to the role of either (retrograde vs. antegrade) technique in association with increased body mass index (BMI), one comparative study provided relevant data.[21] Antegrade technique in the obese group of patients (OG) was associated with 53% greater average operative time than in the nonobese group (NOG) (p < 0.003). As for the retrograde nailing technique, there was no statistically significant difference in terms of mean operative time between OG and NOG. Antegrade technique in the OG was associated with 79% greater average radiation exposure time compared with the same technique in the NOG (p < 0.003). For retrograde technique, mean fluoroscopy time was similar between OG and NOG. Within the OG, antegrade technique was proved more time consuming, requiring 40% greater average operative time compared with the retrograde technique (p < 0.02). As for radiation exposure time, within the same group of obese patients, antegrade technique required three times more average fluoroscopy time than retrograde nailing (p < 0.002).

Recommendations
- Current literature does not suggest any superiority of either technique over the other in the general population with regards to union complications [overall quality: moderate]
- The risk of long-term hip pain appears to be significantly more frequent with antegrade than retrograde technique [overall quality: low]
- Existing evidence cannot document any potential association of either of these techniques with long-term knee pain [overall quality: low]
- In obese patients, antegrade technique is associated with significantly greater operative and radiation exposure times compared with nonobese patients [overall quality: low]

Question 5: Is the use of manual traction on a standard table advantageous over the fracture table in IM nailing of femoral shaft fractures?

Case clarification
The patient in our case scenario was multiply injured with concomitant abdominal injury. An exploratory laparotomy was performed and, when completed, he was hemody-

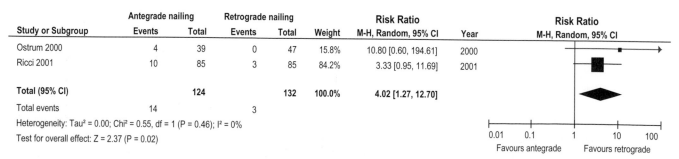

| Study or Subgroup | Antegrade nailing | | Retrograde nailing | | Weight | Risk Ratio | Year | Risk Ratio |
	Events	Total	Events	Total		M-H, Random, 95% CI		M-H, Random, 95% CI
Ostrum 2000	4	39	0	47	15.8%	10.80 [0.60, 194.61]	2000	
Ricci 2001	10	85	3	85	84.2%	3.33 [0.95, 11.69]	2001	
Total (95% CI)		124		132	100.0%	4.02 [1.27, 12.70]		
Total events	14		3					

Heterogeneity: Tau² = 0.00; Chi² = 0.55, df = 1 (P = 0.46); I² = 0%
Test for overall effect: Z = 2.37 (P = 0.02)

0.01 0.1 1 10 100
Favours antegrade   Favours retrograde

Figure 58.5 Forest plot of antegrade vs. retrograde nailing with respect to the outcome: "long-term hip pain."

namically stable and fit for having his femur fracture fixed. In order to avoid transfer of the patient to a fracture table for a standard femoral nailing procedure, it was decided to perform the operation on the standard table.

Closed IM nailing has become the standard procedure for the management of femoral shaft fractures. The technique is usually performed on a fracture table that exerts controlled longitudinal traction to facilitate fracture reduction and nail insertion. However, the use of a fracture table presents various disadvantages, such as prolonged time for setup, and is not practical for polytrauma patients (who often require transfer to a standard table to treat other injuries). In addition, use of a fracture table has been related to certain complications such as pudendal nerve palsy, well-leg compartment syndrome, and perineal skin sloughing. As an alternative, another technique has been described for IM nailing of femoral shaft fractures, using manual traction on a standard radiolucent table.

Finding the evidence

In order to compare the above two techniques in terms of quality of reduction, operative time, complications, and functional outcome we conducted a systematic literature review using the following search strategy:

- Cochrane Database, with search term: "femur fracture"
- PubMed (www.ncbi.nlm.nih.gov/pubmed/) clinical queries search/systematic reviews: "femur fracture" AND "fracture table" OR "manual traction"
- PubMed (www.ncbi.nlm.nih.gov/pubmed/): sensitivity search using the following keywords and Boolean operators: "femur fracture" AND "fracture table" and "femur fracture" AND "manual traction"
- Review of references of eligible studies

Quality of the evidence
Level I
- 1 study[23]

Level III
- 2 studies[24,25]

Findings
Quality of reduction In a level I study (N = 87 patients),[23] quality of reduction was evaluated by CT measurements, using the controlateral intact femur as reference. The fracture table group (FT) was characterized by a significantly greater risk of internal malrotation (>10°) compared with the manual traction group (MT) (relative risk 0.77, 95% CI 0.62–0.94, p = 0.007). The number needed to treat (NNT) was 4.6; this means that in every 5 patients treated with manual traction on a radiolucent table, 1 excessive internal malrotation (>10°) could have been prevented. The two groups did not differ significantly with respect to leg length

discrepancy greater than 10 mm (relative risk 0.31, 95% CI 0.03–2.88).

Operative time In a level I study (N = 87 patients),[23] operative time was significantly shorter in the MT group (mean 119 min, range 65–180 min) than in the FT group (mean 139 min, range 100–212 min), p < 0.05. Two other level III studies, including N1 = 83 patients and N2 = 720 patients respectively, reported on operative time,[24,25] but pooling of their results was not possible because of missing SD values. Both these studies also documented a significantly shorter operative time in the MT group compared to the FT group (p < 0.05).

Blood loss One level I study (N = 87 patients) provided relevant data. Although estimated blood loss was significantly higher in the FT group (p = 0.004), the observed mean difference (159 mL) was not of clinical importance.

Functional outcome Functional outcome (using Short Form-36[26] and Musculoskeletal Function Assessment Instrument[27]) was reported in one level I study.[23] No statistically significant difference was detected between the two groups with regard to functional status at 6 months and 1 year postoperatively.

Recommendations
Current evidence suggests that:
- The use of manual traction instead of a fracture table during IM nailing of femoral shaft fractures significantly reduces the risk of internal malrotation in excess of 15°, and shortens operative time [overall quality: high]
- The FT technique was associated with significantly higher blood losses than the MT technique, but the mean quantity of blood loss is perhaps of no clinical significance [overall quality: high]
- No statistically significant difference was documented between FT and MT with respect to functional outcome [overall quality: high]

Question 6: What is the optimal timing for IM nailing of femoral shaft fractures in patients with chest trauma?

Case clarification
Our patient, in addition to the abdominal injury, was suffering from lung contusions. What is the existing evidence in literature regarding optimal timing of femur fracture fixation?

It is well established that expeditious fixation of isolated femoral shaft fractures decreases the risk of severe pulmonary complications, allows prompt mobilization of the injured patient, and shortens hospital stay. However, femur fractures frequently occur within the context of multiple trauma. In such situations the optimal timing of femoral fracture fixation should weigh the benefits of early fracture stabilization against the detrimental effects of an operation that may decompensate an acutely injured and potentially incompletely resuscitated patient. Concomitant thoracic injury poses additional concerns for even fatal complications, particularly when reamed IM nailing is contemplated.

Finding the evidence

In order to investigate the impact of timing of femoral shaft fracture fixation on the outcome of polytrauma patients with concomitant chest injury, we undertook a systematic literature search. Our aim was to investigate whether early (<24 hours) femoral shaft fracture fixation in polytrauma patients with concomitant chest trauma resulted in more complications compared to delayed fracture fixation. Our search strategy was conducted according to the following steps:

- Cochrane Database, with search term: "femur fracture"
- PubMed (www.ncbi.nlm.nih.gov/pubmed/) clinical queries search/systematic reviews: "femur fracture" AND "timing of fixation"
- PubMed (www.ncbi.nlm.nih.gov/pubmed/): sensitivity search using the following keywords and Boolean operators: "femur fracture" AND "chest trauma" and "femur fracture" AND "pulmonary injury"
- Review of references of eligible studies

Quality of the evidence

Level I
- 1 study[28]

Level III
- 6 studies[29–34]

Findings

We pooled the results of the above studies, including both randomized and nonrandomized trials, in the absence of significant statistical heterogeneity. We used relative risk estimates for each outcome of interest and random effects model to estimate confidence intervals for relative risks.

Mortality Mortality rates were available in 6 studies reporting on N = 686 patients.[28–33] Early fixation (<24 hours) of femoral shaft fractures seemed to predispose to increased mortality compared to late fracture fixation (>24 hours), although the difference was not statistically significant (relative risk 1.66, 95% CI 0.69–4.00, p = 0.26, homogeneity p = 0.35, I^2 = 10%).

Acute respiratory distress syndrome (ARDS) Four studies (N = 298 patients) provided data on ARDS rates.[28,30,33,34] A pooled estimate of effect size could not be obtained due to the presence of significant statistical heterogeneity (homogeneity p = 0.01, I^2 = 73%). Three studies favored early (<24 hours) fracture fixation for minimizing the risk of ARDS,[28,33,34] while another one favored late (>24 hours) fracture fixation[30] (Figure 58.6).

Major pulmonary complications Five studies including 571 patients reported on major pulmonary complications (i.e., at least one of the following: ARDS, pneumonia, fat embolism, pulmonary embolism). A pooled estimate of effect size could not be obtained due to the presence of significant statistical heterogeneity (homogeneity p = 0.0001, I^2 = 83%). The results of three studies[28,29,33] favored early fixation for reducing the risk of major pulmonary complications, whereas another two studies[30,31] favored late fracture fixation (Figure 58.7).

Recommendation

- Current literature is unable to provide clear guidelines with regard to the optimal timing of IM nailing of femoral shaft fractures in multiply injured patients suffering from concomitant lung injuries [overall quality: moderate]

Study or Subgroup	Early fixation Events	Early fixation Total	Late fixation Events	Late fixation Total	Weight	Risk Ratio M-H, Random, 95% CI	Year	Risk Ratio M-H, Random, 95% CI
Bone 1989	1	46	6	37	22.3%	0.13 [0.02, 1.06]	1989	
Pape 1993	8	24	2	26	27.3%	4.33 [1.02, 18.41]	1993	
Charash 1994	2	57	2	25	23.6%	0.44 [0.07, 2.94]	1994	
Boulanger 1997	3	68	3	15	26.8%	0.22 [0.05, 0.99]	1997	
Total (95% CI)		**195**		**103**	**100.0%**	**0.52 [0.10, 2.69]**		
Total events	14		13					

Heterogeneity: Tau² = 2.01; Chi² = 11.07, df = 3 (P = 0.01); I² = 73%
Test for overall effect: Z = 0.78 (P = 0.44)

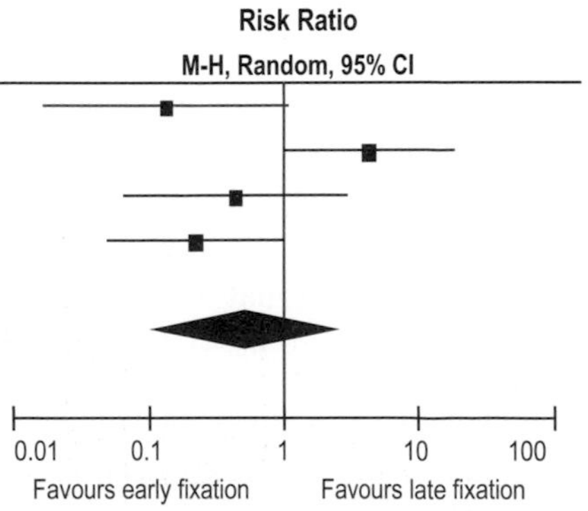

Figure 58.6 Forest plot of ARDS rate in two compared groups of patients: early IMN vs. late IMN.

| Study or Subgroup | Early fixation | | Late fixation | | Weight | Risk Ratio | Year | Risk Ratio |
	Events	Total	Events	Total		M-H, Random, 95% CI		M-H, Random, 95% CI
Bone 1989	1	46	11	37	11.7%	0.07 [0.01, 0.54]	1989	
Pape 1993	13	24	5	26	22.1%	2.82 [1.18, 6.72]	1993	
Charash 1994	9	57	14	25	23.9%	0.28 [0.14, 0.56]	1994	
Reynolds 1995	3	35	3	70	15.2%	2.00 [0.43, 9.40]	1995	
Brundage 2002	64	186	36	65	27.1%	0.62 [0.46, 0.83]	2002	
Total (95% CI)		348		223	100.0%	0.67 [0.27, 1.64]		
Total events	90		69					

Heterogeneity: Tau² = 0.75; Chi² = 23.19, df = 4 (P = 0.0001); I² = 83%

Test for overall effect: Z = 0.88 (P = 0.38)

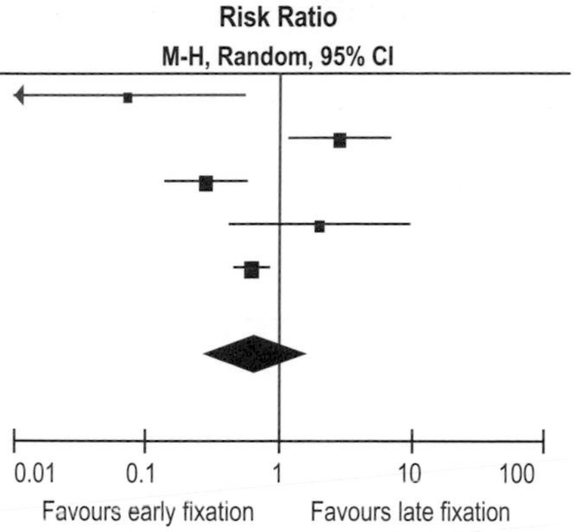

Favours early fixation   Favours late fixation

Figure 58.7 Forest tree of major pulmonary complication in two compared groups: early IMN vs. late IMN.

Question 7: What is the optimal timing for IM nailing of femoral shaft fractures in patients with head injury?

Case clarification

Assuming that the polytrauma patient, in our case scenario was additionally suffering from head injury with a Glasgow Coma Scale (GCS) of 10 points, the question that arises is: What is the optimal timing for femoral shaft fracture fixation to avoid further brain injury?

The presence of significant head injury in patients with femoral shaft fractures poses a therapeutic challenge. Inadvertent early definitive fracture fixation may cause increased blood loss, hypotension, and hypoxia, bringing about decreased cerebral perfusion and, ultimately, additional brain injury. This risk of secondary brain injury could potentially outweigh the benefits of early stabilization of a long bone fracture. Consequently, the issue of optimal timing of femoral shaft fixation in the presence of significant head trauma is of great clinical importance.

Finding the evidence

In order to find the best evidence that could provide reliable guidelines concerning the optimal timing of definitive treatment (preferably with IM nails) of femoral shaft fractures in patients with concomitant head trauma, a systematic literature search was conducted. The search strategy was as follows:

• Cochrane Database, with search terms: "femur fracture" AND "head injury"
• PubMed (www.ncbi.nlm.nih.gov/pubmed/) clinical queries search/ systematic reviews: "femur fracture" AND "timing of fixation"
• PubMed (www.ncbi.nlm.nih.gov/pubmed/): sensitivity search using the following keywords and Boolean operators: "femur fracture" AND "head injury" and "femur fracture" AND "cerebral injury"

• Review of references of eligible studies
Studies reporting on various long bone or pelvic fractures and not focusing exclusively on femoral fractures were excluded.

Quality of the evidence
Level III
• 4 studies[29,31,32,35]

Findings

Mortality All four eligible studies (N = 598 patients) provided data regarding mortality rates. In the presence of head injury, early fixation (<24 hours) of femoral fractures with IM nails is probably associated with increased mortality compared to late (>24 hours) fixation, but this difference did not reach statistical significance (risk ratio 1.60, 95% CI 0.51–5.01, p = 0.42, homogeneity p = 0.29, I² = 18%).

Pulmonary complications Three studies (N = 511 patients) provided data regarding pulmonary complications.[29,31,35] A pooled estimate of the effect size could be obtained due to moderate degree of statistical heterogeneity (I² = 52%). Early (<24 hours) fracture fixation showed a trend towards fewer pulmonary complications compared to late (>24 hours) fixation. Again, the documented difference was not statistically significant (risk ratio 0.59, 95% CI 0.21–1.62, p = 0.30, homogeneity p = 0.12).

CNS complications Two studies (N = 133 patients) provided relevant data.[31,35] The available data documented a trend of early fracture fixation towards more frequent CNS complications, but the wide confidence interval of the pooled estimate of effect size does not document statistical significance of the result (risk ratio 1.40, 95% CI 0.21–9.49, p = 0.73, homogeneity p = 0.72, I² = 0%).

Recommendation

• No clear conclusion could be drawn from the existing literature regarding optimal timing of IM nailing of femoral shaft fractures in patients with concomitant head trauma [overall quality: low]

Question 8: Is the DCO approach a safer alternative to ETC in polytrauma patients with femoral shaft fractures?

Case clarification

The polytrauma patient, suffering from femoral shaft fracture, bilateral lung contusions, intra-abdominal injuries and closed head injury is, in addition, haemodynamically unstable. What is the best treatment approach in such a scenario? Should the patient be stabilized haemodynamically first, and also have his long bone fracture provisionally fixed by a means of external fixation with the plan of converting it to an IM nail at a later stage, or should he be treated definitively in one stage, through a marathon surgery approach?

Expeditious, definitive fixation of all long bone fractures represents the optimal management of the patient suffering from multiple orthopedic injuries. The benefits of such an approach are well documented in literature.[28] However, this early total care (ETC) principle may not be applicable in polytrauma patients with high injury severity score (ISS), suffering from significant head, chest, or abdominal injuries in addition to the musculoskeletal trauma and presenting to the Emergency Department with signs of hemodynamic compromise (borderline patients). In this particular subgroup of polytrauma patients, an attempt at early aggressive and definitive treatment of all musculoskeletal injuries could result in fatal complications, such as acute lung injury (ALI), ARDS, and multiple organ failure (MOF). For these patients, an alternative management concept, consisting of initial temporary stabilization of long bone fractures and secondary conversion to a definitive fixation (preferably, internal fixation) has been advocated. The term "damage control orthopedic surgery" (DCO) was coined to describe this treatment approach.[36] In polytrauma patients with femoral shaft fractures, DCO is translated into initial temporary external fracture fixation and later conversion to IM nailing, when the patient's condition is deemed stable.

Finding the evidence

In order to elucidate whether DCO is preferable to ETC in the polytrauma setting, in terms of reducing the risk of systemic complications (pulmonary and MOF), and also to define the subgroup of polytrauma patients in which application of the staged approach is appropriate, we undertook a systematic literature search to isolate comparative studies

of these two treatment protocols (DCO vs. ETC). We conducted a literature search according to the following steps

• Cochrane Database, with search terms: "femur fracture" AND "damage control orthopedics," or "femur fracture" AND "early total care" or "femur fracture" AND "polytrauma"

• PubMed (www.ncbi.nlm.nih.gov/pubmed/) clinical queries search/ systematic reviews: "femur fracture" AND "damage control orthopedics"

• PubMed (www.ncbi.nlm.nih.gov/pubmed/): sensitivity search using the following keywords and Boolean operators: "femur fracture" AND "damage control orthopedics," or "femur fracture" AND "early total care" or "femur fracture" AND "polytrauma," or "femur fracture" AND "external fixation"

• Review of references of eligible studies

The studies considered eligible were comparative ones (DCO vs. ETC, with or without randomization), reporting on at least one outcome of interest (mortality, ALI, ARDS, sepsis, MOF, pneumonia).

Quality of the evidence

Level I
• 2 RCTs[37,38]

Level III
• 3 studies[36,39,40]

Findings

In most studies, the DCO group consisted of polytrauma patients with significantly higher ISS and longer stay in the intensive care unit (ICU) compared to the ETC group (Table 58.3). This reflects a trend towards applying the DCO protocol in more severe polytrauma patients and is responsible for methodological heterogeneity in our analysis which, in turn, could influence the results of pooling.

Pneumonia Three studies (N = 374 patients) reported on pneumonia.[37,38,40] Patients in the DCO group ran a statistically significant higher risk of developing pneumonia vs. patients in the ETC group (risk ratio 1.93, 95% CI 1.28–2.92, p = 0.002, homogeneity p = 0.77, I^2 = 0%) (Figure 58.8).

ARDS Four studies (N = 552 patients) provided relevant data on this outcome.[37–40] Although patients in the DCO group had a higher ISS than patients in the ETC group, application of the DCO principle did not result in statistically significant higher risk of developing ARDS compared to the ETC principle (risk ratio 1.11, 95% CI 0.66–1.84, p = 0.70, homogeneity p = 0.28, I^2 = 21%) (Figure 58.9).

MOF Two studies (N = 343 patients) reported on MOF rates.[38,39] Although the DCO group showed an increased risk for developing MOF vs. the ETC group, the docu-

Table 58.3 Descriptive characteristics of studies included in the pooled analysis

Study		Scalea [36]	Pape [37]	Pape [38]	Pape [39]	Harwood [40]
Type		RC	RCT	RCT	RC	RC
Year of publication		2000	2003	2007	2002	2005
Compared groups:						
DCO	n-pts	43	18	71	68	97
	Mean age	30.4	36.3	32.1	nd	32.3
	ISS (mean)	26.8 (p = 0.001)	23.2	29 (p < 0.001)	39.1	36.2 (p < 0.0001)
	ICU LOS (days, mean)	11	12.4	12.4	nd	21.5 (p < 0.05)
ETC	n-pts	281	17	94	110	77
	Mean age	30.5*	31.5	32.9	nd	33.3
	ISS (mean)	16.8 (p = 0.001)	21.7	23.3 (p < 0.001)	35.8	25.4 (p < 0.0001)
	ICU LOS (days, mean)	8	8.2	8.2	nd	10.2 (p < 0.05)

DCO, damage control orthopedics; ETC, early total care; ICU LOS, intensive care unit, length of stay; ISS, injury severity score; nd, not documented; RC, retrospective comparative; RCT, randomized controlled trial.

	DCO		ETC			Risk Ratio			Risk Ratio
Study or Subgroup	Events	Total	Events	Total	Weight	M-H, Random, 95% CI	Year		M-H, Random, 95% CI
Pape 2003	1	18	1	17	2.4%	0.94 [0.06, 13.93]	2003		
Harwood 2005	33	97	12	77	49.2%	2.18 [1.21, 3.93]	2005		
Pape 2007	20	71	15	94	48.4%	1.77 [0.97, 3.20]	2007		
Total (95% CI)		**186**		**188**	**100.0%**	**1.93 [1.28, 2.92]**			
Total events	54		28						

Heterogeneity: Tau² = 0.00; Chi² = 0.53, df = 2 (P = 0.77); I² = 0%
Test for overall effect: Z = 3.12 (P = 0.002)

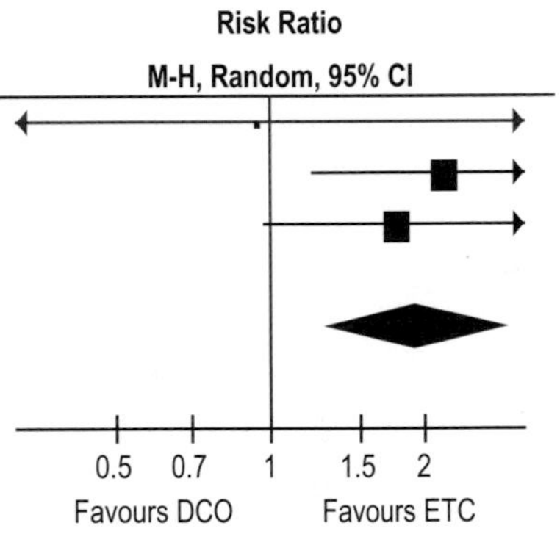

0.5 0.7 1 1.5 2
Favours DCO   Favours ETC

Figure 58.8 Forest plot of pneumonia rates for DCO vs. ETC.

	DCO		ETC			Risk Ratio			Risk Ratio
Study or Subgroup	Events	Total	Events	Total	Weight	M-H, Random, 95% CI	Year		M-H, Random, 95% CI
Pape 2002	15	68	29	110	54.3%	0.84 [0.49, 1.44]	2002		
Pape 2003	0	18	0	17		Not estimable	2003		
Harwood 2005	13	97	5	77	22.4%	2.06 [0.77, 5.54]	2005		
Pape 2007	7	71	8	94	23.3%	1.16 [0.44, 3.05]	2007		
Total (95% CI)		**254**		**298**	**100.0%**	**1.11 [0.66, 1.84]**			
Total events	35		42						

Heterogeneity: Tau² = 0.05; Chi² = 2.54, df = 2 (P = 0.28); I² = 21%
Test for overall effect: Z = 0.39 (P = 0.70)

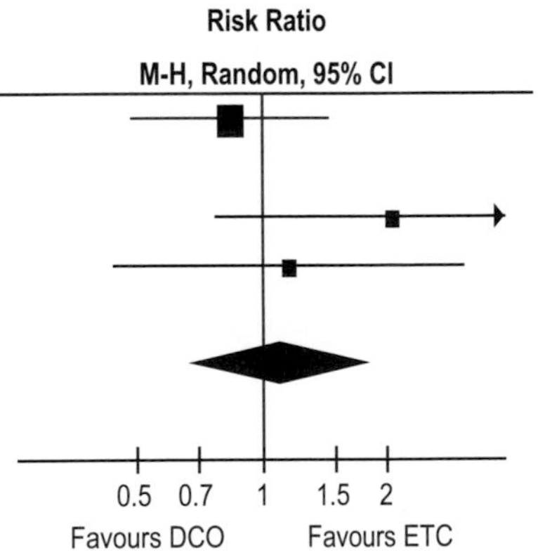

0.5 0.7 1 1.5 2
Favours DCO   Favours ETC

Figure 58.9 Forest plot of ARDS rates for DCO vs. ETC.

Study or Subgroup	DCO Events	DCO Total	ETC Events	ETC Total	Weight	Risk Ratio M-H, Random, 95% CI	Year	Risk Ratio M-H, Random, 95% CI
Scalea 1999	4	43	1	281	48.0%	26.14 [2.99, 228.41]	1999	
Harwood 2005	7	97	1	77	52.0%	5.56 [0.70, 44.20]	2005	
Total (95% CI)		**140**		**358**	**100.0%**	**11.68 [2.44, 55.98]**		
Total events	11		2					

Heterogeneity: Tau² = 0.11; Chi² = 1.09, df = 1 (P = 0.30); I² = 9%

Test for overall effect: Z = 3.07 (P = 0.002)

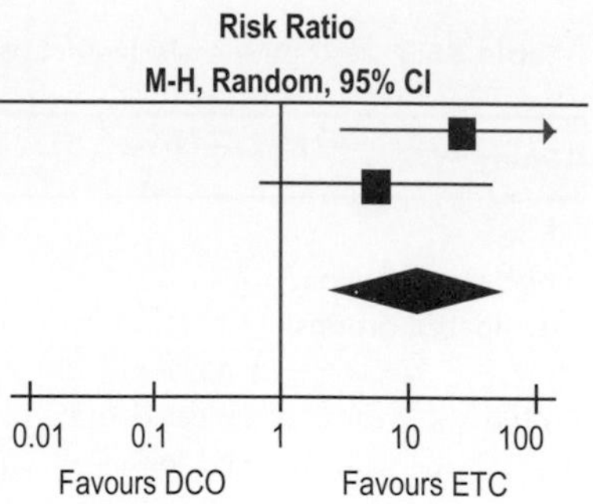

0.01 0.1 1 10 100
Favours DCO   Favours ETC

Figure 58.10 Forest plot of mortality rates for DCO vs. ETC.

Table 58.4 Outcomes of DCO vs. ETC in two subgroups of multiply injured patients (stable and borderline patients)[38]

Outcomes	Stable condition DCO (%)	ETC (%)	Regression analyses OR	p	Borderline condition DCO (%)	ETC (%)	Regression analyses OR	p
Pneumonia	23.8	6.5	0.40 (0.11–1.50)	0.176	38.9	45	1.00 (0.22–4.59)	0.995
ALI	28.6	12.9	0.39 (0.14–1.08)	0.170	16.7	52.4	6.69 (1.01–44.08)	0.048
ARDS	9.5	6.3	0.73 (0.15–3.53)	0.700	11.1	16.7	2.01 (0.13–31.91)	0.618
MOF	0	0			16.7	22.2	0.78 (0.13–4.75)	0.791

ALI, acute lung injury; ARDS, acute respiratory distress syndrome; DCO, damage control orthopedics; ETC, early total care; MOF, multiple organ failure; OR, odds ratio.

mented difference was not statistically significant (risk ratio 1.14, 95% CI 0.74–1.75, p = 0.56, homogeneity p = 0.91, I² = 0%).

Mortality Two studies (N = 498 patients) reported on mortality.[36,40] Mortality rates were significantly higher in the DCO group than in the ETC group (risk ratio 11.68, 95% CI 2.44–55.98, p = 0.002, homogeneity p = 0.30, I² = 0%) (Figure 58.10).

One prospective RCT conducted further analyses on two distinct subgroups of multiply injured patients, namely stable and borderline patients.[38] In addition, regression analyses were used to control for differences between the two treatment groups (DCO vs ETC) in terms of initial injury severity. The results of this study are presented in Table 58.4. The odds of developing ALI were 6.69 times greater in borderline patients who had received ETC treatment compared to those in the DCO group.

Recommendations

• In the multiply injured patient population, in general, implementation of the DCO principle is associated with increased mortality and pneumonia rates compared with the ETC principle. This difference may, however, reflect the inherent heterogeneity of the two groups of patients in terms of severity of initial injury, as more severely injured patients are recruited into the DCO group [overall quality: moderate]

• Treatment of femoral shaft fractures, within the context of polytrauma, according to the DCO principle does not seem to result in increased risk of developing ARDS or MOF compared with the ETC principle, even in the presence of more severe injuries in the DCO group [overall quality: moderate]

• In borderline patients, the ETC principle is associated with a significantly higher risk of developing ALI compared with the DCO principle [overall quality: high]

Question 9: Is femoral plating preferable to reamed IM nailing in polytrauma patients with femoral shaft fractures and concomitant head or chest injury?

Relevance
Although reamed IM nailing has been universally recognized as the treatment of choice for femoral shaft fractures, concerns have been raised that reamed nails could potentiate additional brain or pulmonary injury when used in polytrauma patients with concomitant head or chest trauma. For this particular patient population the use of plate fixation has been advocated as a viable alternative to IM nailing.

Finding the evidence
In order to compare the above methods with respect to certain outcomes of interest, such as mortality, pulmonary complications, CNS complications, and infection, we undertook a systematic literature search aiming to isolate relevant studies comparing directly these two methods, preferably within the context of multiple trauma. The literature search was conducted as follows:
- Cochrane Database, with search terms "femur fracture" AND "plate fixation," and "femoral plating"
- PubMed (www.ncbi.nlm.nih.gov/pubmed/) clinical queries search/systematic reviews: "femoral plating"
- PubMed (www.ncbi.nlm.nih.gov/pubmed/): sensitivity search using the following keywords and Boolean operators: "femur fracture" AND "plate fixation")
- Review of references of eligible studies

Quality of the evidence
Level III
- 2 studies[41,42]

Findings
Mortality Both studies[41,42] provided relevant data regarding mortality. A pooled estimate of effect size for mortality showed no statistically significant difference between the two treatment options (IM nailing vs. plating) for femoral shaft fractures (risk ratio 0.82, 95% CI 0.30–2.21, p = 0.69, homogeneity p = 0.56, I^2 = 0%).

Pulmonary complications Both included studies reported on pulmonary complications.[41,42] IM femoral nailing appeared equivalent to femoral plating with regards to the risk of developing pulmonary complications (risk ratio 1.38, 95% CI 0.88–2.16, p = 0.16, homogeneity p = 0.45, I^2 = 0%).

CNS complications and infection One study (N = 50 patients) documented 3.4% and 0% CNS complication rate in the femoral plating and IM nailing groups, respectively.[42] The same study documented 4.8% and 0% deep infection rates

in IM nailing and femoral plating groups, respectively. Both differences were not statistically significant.

Recommendation
- No convincing evidence exists in current literature supporting the use of plates over IM nails for the treatment of femoral shaft fractures within the context of multiple trauma [overall quality: low]

Question 10: Is there a functional impairment after isolated femoral shaft fracture?

The majority of femoral shaft fractures occur in young, otherwise healthy individuals, as a result of high-energy injury. Due to the high-energy nature of this injury and the operative intervention, resultant soft tissue trauma is common. In addition, iatrogenic muscle injury (abductor musculature) from antegrade nail insertion may further aggravate soft tissue injury. This combined soft tissue injury may predispose to impaired functional recovery even in the absence of postoperative complication such as nonunion, malunion, reoperation, or infection.

Finding the evidence
In order to assess the long-term functional consequences of femoral shaft fractures treated with antegrade IM nails, we conducted a systematic literature search using "femoral shaft fracture" and "functional outcome" as keywords. In order to avoid bias from concomitant multiple injuries or serious postoperative complications that could affect the eventual functional outcome of a femoral shaft fracture, we limited our search, posing certain inclusion and exclusion criteria. Consequently, eligible studies were those reporting on isolated femoral shaft fractures in adult population that had been treated with IM nails and healed with normal alignment, no residual leg length discrepancy, and no major complications or repeat operations in the postoperative period. Our search strategy followed these steps:
- Cochrane Database
- PubMed (www.ncbi.nlm.nih.gov/pubmed/) clinical queries search/systematic reviews
- PubMed (www.ncbi.nlm.nih.gov/pubmed/): sensitivity search
- Review of references of eligible studies

Quality of the evidence
Level III
- 1 study[43]

Level IV
- 5 studies[44–48]

Findings
Table 58.5 summarizes the basic results.

Table 58.5 Current evidence on functional outcome of isolated femur fractures

Study	Type of study	Inter-vention	No. of patients	Outcome measure	Control group	Follow-up	Results
Archdeacon et al. 2008[43]	P	a IMN	8	Dynamic hip abductor weakness at 2 time intervals: (1) independent ambulation without aid (~2 mo) (2) complete bone healing (~7 mo) S-MFA at 3 mo and at latest follow-up	Opposite limb	>12 mo (mean 21.6 mo)	Dynamic hip abductor weakness resolved at 7 mo S-MFA: significant improvement (p = 0.008)
Helmy et al. 2008[44]	R	a-IMN	21	Isokinetic muscle test of: Hip abductors, Hip extensors Knee extensors S-MFA	Controlateral uninjured limb	>12 mo (mean: 70 mo)	Muscle strength: -Hip abductors: reduced p < 0.05 -Hip extensors: reduced, p < 0.05 SF-36 / S-MFA: similar to population norms Residual pain (mild–moderate): Hip: 10/21 Knee: 9/21 Thigh: 17/21
Kapp et al. 2000[45]	R	a-IMN	17	BMD Muscle function	Controlateral uninjured limb	>18 mo	BMD, reduction (p < 0.05) Quadriceps strength: reduced (p < 0.05)
Bain et al. 2007[46]	R	a-IMN	32	Subjective complaints (trochanter pain, thigh pain, hip stiffness) Abduction strength	Asymptomatic controls	>24 mo (mean: 47 mo)	Trochanter pain: 13/32 Thigh pain: 3/32 Abduction strength: reduced (p < 0.05)
Bednar and Ali 1993[47]	R	a-IMN	47	Reoperation Return to work (41 pts available for analysis)	-	Mean 34.5 mo	Implant related pain: 20/47 (43%) [Implant removal: 17/20 (85%)] Return to original work: 33/41 (80%) Other full-time employment: 4/41 (10%) Part time employment: 3/41 (7%) Unable to work: 1/41 (2%)
Sanders et al. 2008[48]	R	a-IMN	40	VAS for pain: groin, buttock, thigh, knee WOMAC S-MFA	-	>12 mo	Functional recovery and pain relief within 6 mo No difference between 6 and 12 mo Residual functional impairment at 12 mo Knee pain most common and severe source of discomfort at 12 mo

a-IMN, antegrade intramedullary nail; BMD, bone mineral density; P, prospective; R, retrospective; SF-36, short form 36; S-MFA, short musculoskeletal functional assessment; VAS, visual analog scale; WOMAC, Western Ontario and McMaster Universities Osteoarthritis index.

Recommendation

Current evidence, though incomplete and of poor quality, may indicate that persistent reduced strength of certain muscle groups (hip abductors, knee extensors) and residual pain (in the knee, thigh, or hip region) could contribute to the presence of impaired functional capacity of the injured limb even in cases of successful treatment of femoral shaft fractures. Significant soft tissue trauma partly imparted by the initial injury and partly during surgery may be responsible. Carefully conducted large prospective cohort studies could provide strong evidence for possible causes and effects [overall quality: low]

Summary of recommendations

- It is doubtful whether the use of a single implant (ceplalomedullary nail) could result in increased likelihood for reoperation compared to the combined use of compression plate and hip screws
- In concomitant ipsilateral femoral neck and shaft fractures, the use of a single implant for addressing both injuries (cephalomedullary nails) is probably associated with better union rates of the femoral shaft fracture over the combined use of compression plate and hip screws
- The union process or the risk of malunion of femoral shaft fractures does not depend on the choice of the entry portal (piriformis or trochanteric) of the IM nail that is used for its treatment
- In obese patients, the use of greater trochanter entry portal appears more advantageous over piriformis entry portal as the latter is associated with significantly increased both operative and fluoroscopy times
- Unreamed femoral nails are associated with significant risk of delayed union compared with reamed nails
- Current literature does not suggest any superiority of either technique over the other in the general population with regards to union complications
- Antegrade nailing technique may be associated with significantly more frequent hip pain and, in obese patients, greater operative and radiation exposure times compared with retrograde technique
- Existing evidence cannot document any potential association of either of these techniques with long-term knee pain
- The use of manual traction instead of fracture table during nailing procedure significantly reduces the risk of internal malrotation (>15°) and shortens operative time
- The FT technique was associated with significantly higher blood losses than the MT technique, but the mean
- No statistically significant difference was documented between FT and MT with respect to functional outcome
- Current literature is unable to provide clear guidelines with regard to the optimal timing of IM nailing of femoral

shaft fractures in multiply injured patients suffering from concomitant lung injuries
- Contradictory evidence exists in current literature with regard to optimal timing of IM nailing of femoral shaft fractures in patients with concomitant chest or head trauma
- In borderline multiply injured patients, the ETC approach is associated with significantly higher risk of developing ALI than the DCO principle
- No convincing evidence exists in current literature supporting the use of plates over IM nails for the treatment of femoral shaft fractures within the context of multiple trauma
- Long-term functional impairment may persist after isolated femur fractures and may be due to soft tissue injury occurring during initial trauma and operative procedure

Conclusions

High-quality evidence from current literature supports the following conclusions with regard to IM nailing of femoral shaft fractures:
- Use of unreamed femoral nails will probably result in increased risk of delayed union compared with reamed nails
- Performing the procedure on a standard radiolucent operative table using manual traction instead of the classical fracture table will probably protect against excessive internal malrotation and will shorten operative time
- In borderline multiply injured patients, implementation of DCO principle significantly reduces the risk of developing ALI compared with ETC.

The current literature is lacking high-quality, clear evidence with regard to the optimal timing of IM nailing in patients with femoral shaft fractures and concomitant chest or head trauma. Similarly, no substantial evidence exist supporting substitution of femoral nails with plates and screws in multiply injured patients.

References

1. Arneson TJ, Melton LJ III, Lewallen DG, et al. Epidemiology of diaphyseal and distal femoral fractures in Rochester, Minnesota, 1965–1984. Clin Orthop 1988;234:188–94.
2. Salminen ST, Pihlajamaki HK, Avikainen VJ, et al. Population based epidemiologic and morphologic study of femoral shaft fractures. Clin Orthop Relat Res 2000;372:241–9.
3. Taylor MT, Banerjee B, Alpar EK. Injuries associated with a fractured shaft of the femur. Injury 1994;25(3):185–7.
4. Alho A. Concurrent ipsilateral fractures of the hip and shaft of the femur. A systematic review of 722 cases. Ann Chir Gynaecol 1997;86(4):326–36.

5. Singh R, Rohilla R, Magu NK et al. Ipsilateral femoral neck and shaft fractures: a retrospective analysis of two treatment methods. J Orthop Traumatol 2008;9,141–7.

6. Alho A. Concurrent ipsilateral fractures of the hip and femoral shaft: a meta-analysis of 659 cases. Acta Orthop Scand 1996; 67(1):19–28.

7. Browner BD. Pitfalls, errors and complications in the use of locking Kuntcher nails. Clin Orthop Relat Res 1986;212:192–208.

8. Starr AJ, Hay MT, Reinert CM, et al. Cephalomedullary nails in the treatment of high-energy proximal femur fractures in young patients: a prospective, randomized comparison of trochanteric vs. piriformis fossa entry portal. J Orthop Trauma 2006;20: 240–46.

9. Ricci WM, Schwappach J, Tucker M, et al. Trochanteric versus piriformis entry portal for the treatment of femoral shaft fractures. J Orthop Trauma 2006;20(10):663–7.

10. Tornetta P III, Tiburzi D. Reamed versus nonreamed antegrade femoral nailing. J Orthop Trauma 2000;14(1):15–19.

11. Canadian Orthopaedic Trauma Society. Nonunion following intramedullary nailing of the femur with and without reaming. Results of a multicenter randomized clinical trial. J Bone Joint Surg Am 2003;85:2093–96.

12. Canadian Orthopaedic Trauma Society. Reamed versus undreamed intramedullary nailing of the femur: comparison of the rate of ARDS in multiple injured patients. J Trauma 2006;20:384–7.

13. Clatworthy MG, Clark DI, Gray DH, et al. Reamed versus undreamed femoral nails. J Bone Joint Surg Br 1998;80: 485–9.

14. Shepherd LE, Shean CJ, Gelalis ID, et al. Prospective randomized study of reamed vs. unreamed femoral intramedullary nailing: an assessment of procedures. J Orthop Trauma 2001;15: 28–33.

15. Selvakumar K, Saw KY, Fathima M. Comparison study between reamed and undreamed nailing of closed femoral fractures. Med J Malaysia 2001;56(Suppl D):24–8.

16. Anwar IA, Battistella FD, Neiman R, et al. Femur fractures and lung complications: a prospective randomized study of reaming. Clin Orthop Relat Res 2004;422:71–6.

17. Giannoudis PV, Furlong AJ, MacDonald DA, et al. Reamed against unreamed nailing of the femoral diaphysis: a retrospective study of healing time. Injury 1997;28:15–18.

18. Tornetta PIII, Tiburzi D. Antegrade or retrograde reamed femoral nailing. A prospective randomized trial. J Bone Joint Surg Br 2000;82:652–4.

19. Ostrum RF, Agarwal A, Lakatos R, et al. Prospective comparison of retrograde and antegrade femoral intramedullary nailing. J Orthop Trauma 2000;14(7):496–501.

20. Ricci WM, Bellabarba C, Evanoff B, et al. Retrograde versus antegrade nailing of femoral shaft fractures. J Orthop Trauma 2001;15(3):161–9.

21. Tucker MC, Schwappach JR, Leighton RK, et al. Results of femoral intramedullary nailing in patients who are obese versus those who are not obese: a prospective multicenter comparison study. J Orthop Trauma 2007;21:523–29.

22. Papadokostakis G, Papakostidis C, Dimitriou R, Giannoudis PV. The role and efficacy of retrograde nailing for the treatment of diaphyseal and distal femoral fractures: a systematic review of the literature. Injury 2005;36(7):813–22.

23. Stephen DJG, Kreder HJ, Schemitsch EH, et al. Femoral intramedullary nailing: comparison of fracture-table and manual traction. A prospective, randomized study. J Bone Joint Surg Am 2002;84: 1514–21.

24. Sirkin MS, Berhens F, McCracken K, et al. Femoral nailing without a fracture table. Clin Orthop Relat Res 1996;332: 119–25.

25. Wollinski PR, McCarty EC, Shyr Y, et al. Length of operative procedures: reamed femoral intramedullary nailing performed with and without a fracture table. J Orthop Trauma 1998;12(7): 485–495.

26. Hopman WM, Towheed T, Anastassiades T, et al. Canadian normative data for the SF-36 health survey. Canadian Multicentre Osteoporosis Study Research Group. CMAJ 2000;163:265–71.

27. Engelberg R, Martin DP, Agel J, et al. Musculoskeletal Function Assessment instrument: criterion and construct validity. J Orthop Res 1996;14:182–92.

28. Bone LB, Johnson KD, Weigelt J, et al. Early versus delayed stabilization of femoral shaft fractures. J Bone Joint Surg Am 1989;71:336–40.

29. Brundage SI, McGhan R, Jurkovich G, et al. Timing of femur fracture fixation: effect on outcome in patients with thoracic and head injuries. J Trauma 2002;52(2):299–307.

30. Pape HC, Auf'm'Kolk M, Paffrath T, et al. Primary intramedullary femur fixation in multiple trauma patients with associated lung contusion—a cause of posttraumatic ARDS? J Trauma 1993;34(4):540–7.

31. Reynolds MA, Richardson DJ, Spain DA, et al. Is the timing of fracture fixation important for the patient with multiple trauma? Annals Surg 1995;222:470–81.

32. Fakhry SM, Rutledge R, Dahners LE, et al. Incidence, management, and outcome of femoral shaft fracture: a statewide population-based analysis of 2805 adult patients in a rural state. J Trauma 1994;37(2):255–261.

33. Charash WE, Fabian TC, Croce MA. Delayed surgical fixation of femur fractures is a risk factor for pulmonary failure independent of thoracic trauma. J Trauma 1994;37(4): 667–72.

34. Boulanger BR, Stephen D, Brenneman F. Thoracic trauma and early intramedullary nailing of femur fractures: are we doing harm? J Trauma 1997;43(1):24–28.

35. Starr AJ, Hunt JL, Chason DP, et al. Treatment of femur fracture with associated head injury. J Orthop Trauma 1998;12(1): 38–45.

36. Scalea TM, Boswell SA, Scott JD, et al. External fixation as a bridge to intramedullary nailing for patients with multiple injuries and with femur fractures: Damage Control Orthopedics. J Trauma 2000;48(4):613–23.

37. Pape HC, Grimme K, van Griensven M, et al. Impact of intramedullary instrumentation versus damage control for femoral fractures on immunoinflammatory parameters: prospective randomized analysis by the EPOFF study group. J Trauma 2003; 55(1):7–13.

38. Pape HC, Rixen D, Morley J, et al. Impact of the method of initial stabilization for femoral shaft fractures in patients with multiple injuries at risk of complications (borderline patients). Ann Surg 2007;246:491–501.

39. Pape HC, Hildebrand F, Pertschy S, et al. Changes in the management of femoral shaft fractures in polytrauma patients: from

early total care to damage control orthopedic surgery. J Trauma 2002;53:452–462.

40. Harwood PJ, Giannoudis PV, van Griensven M, et al. Alterations in the systemic inflammatory response after early total care and damage control procedures for femoral shaft fracture in severely injured patients. J Trauma 2005;58:446–54.

41. Bosse MJ, MacKenzie EJ, Riemer BL, et al. Adult respiratory distress syndrome, pneumonia, and mortality following thoracic injury and a femoral fracture treated either with intramedullary nailing with reaming or with a plate. A comparative study. J Bone Joint Surg Am 1997;79:799–809.

42. Banhari M, Guyatt GH, Khera V, et al. Operative management of lower extremity fractures in patients with head injuries. Clin Orthop Rel Res 2003;407:187–98.

43. Archdeacon M, Ford KR, Wyrick J, et al. A prospective functional outcome and motion analysis evaluation of the hip abductors after femur fracture and antegrade nailing. J Orthop Trauma 2008;22(1):3–9.

44. Helmy N, Jando VT, Lu T, et al. Muscle function and functional outcome following standard antegrade reamed intramedullary nailing of isolated femoral shaft fractures. J Orthop Trauma 2008;22:10–15.

45. Kapp W, Lindsey RW, Noble PC, et al. Long-term residual musculoskeletal deficits after femoral shaft fractures treated with intramedullary nailing. J Trauma 2000;49:446–9.

46. Bain GI, Zacest AC, Paterson DC, et al. Abduction strength following intramedullary nailing of the femur. J Orthop Trauma 1997;11(2):93–97.

47. Bednar DA, Ali P. Intramedullary nailing of femoral shaft fractures: reoperation and return to work. Can J Surg 1993;36(5):464–6.

48. Sanders DW, MacLeod M, Charyk-Stewart T, et al. Functional outcome and persistent disability after isolated fracture of the femur. Can J Surg 2008;51(5):366–70.

59

Distal Femur Fractures

Matthijs R. Krijnen¹, J. Carel Goslings², and Rudolf W. Poolman¹

¹Onze Lieve Vrouwe Gasthuis, Amsterdam, The Netherlands
²Academic Medical Center, Amsterdam, The Netherlands

Case scenario

Case 1

A 20 year old tourist was involved in a traffic accident in Amsterdam. The front wheel of his bicycle was trapped in the tram rails, after which he was hit by the tram on his right leg. He did not lose consciousness. Directly after the accident he was unable to bear weight with his right leg. There were no other obvious injuries. On examination the knee was swollen and painful. The skin was intact and the neurovascular examination was normal. Radiographs showed a distal femur fracture in the right leg.

Case 2

The patient is a 75 year old woman who had a total knee replacement 5 years ago. She has now had a fall on the sidewalk. Her radiographs show a distal femoral fracture above a total knee replacement.

Relevant anatomy

Fractures of the distal femur tend to follow the weakest planes in the femur. The main zones of weakness are first the transition from diaphysis to metaphysis, secondly the sagittal plane through the intercondylar notch, where the patella can act as a wedge, and finally the junction between the trochlear groove and medial or lateral condyle.[1] Due to high-energy trauma or osteoporosis, distal femoral fractures can be significantly comminuted.

As in every fracture, muscles play a major role in the dislocation of the fracture fragments. The most common dislocation is posterior angulation and displacement of the distal fragment with femoral shortening. The dislocating forces are produced by the quadriceps, hamstrings, and gastrocnemius muscles. The muscle pull of the quadriceps and posterior hamstrings results in shortening of the femur. The gastrocnemius pulls posteriorly, displacing and angulating the condyles posteriorly as the shaft overrides anteriorly. In intercondylar fractures, the heads of the gastrocnemius can cause a rotational malalignment and separation of the fracture. Adductor muscles may produce a varus deformity or even valgus when the fracture is located distally of the adductor tubercle.

The femoral and popliteal arteries are at risk of injury due to the close relation to the distal femur. Although a posteriorly angulated fracture could cause damage to the artery, this is a rare phenomenon.

The anatomy of the distal femur is complex and needs to be understood before restoration of the distal femur can be achieved. The cranial part of the trochlea is a shallow depression between the condyles. The patella predominantly articulates with the surface area of the lateral condyle. The lateral condyle is broader than the medial condyle. The medial condyle is longer and extents farther distally than the lateral condyle. The distal femur is trapezoidal when viewed from distal to proximal. The lateral metaphyseal surface is angulated approximately 10° while the medial surface is angulated approximately 25°. When using a lateral plate it is important to realize that the central axis of the femoral shaft normally aligns with the anterior half of the femoral condyles viewed lateral to medial (Figure 59.1).

Evidence-Based Orthopedics, First Edition. Edited by Mohit Bhandari.
© 2012 Blackwell Publishing Ltd. Published 2012 by Blackwell Publishing Ltd.

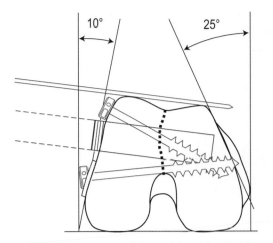

Figure 59.1 Caudal-cranial view of the condyles of the distal femur. The lateral metaphyseal surface is angulated approximately 10° while the medial surface is angulated approximately 25°.

Classification

The classification system commonly used for distal femur fractures is the AO/OTA system.[2] Fractures are arranged in order of increasing severity according to the complexity of the fracture, difficulty of treatment, and worsening prognosis. Each bone segment is numbered, followed by the fracture pattern and degree of comminution. In this system the distal femur fracture is numbered 33 and the fracture is subsequently classified based on the amount of articular involvement and comminution. Type 33 A describes an extra-articular fracture whereas type 33 B is partial articular involving one of the femoral condyles, and type 33 C is a complete articular fracture (Figure 59.2).

Importance of the problem

Fractures of the distal femur represent 4–7% of all femur fractures.[3,4] In Sweden this corresponds to an incidence of 51 per million habitants older than 16 years.[3] The occurrence of distal femur fractures shows a bimodal pattern with a marked variation in relation to gender and age. Low-energy trauma occurs in the elderly osteoporotic female patient (>50 years), while high-energy trauma primarily occurs in young men involved in traffic or sport accidents.[4]

Although the social and financial impact of proximal femur fractures is widely reported, this is not the case for the less common distal femur fracture. Increased life expectancy, greater participation in high-risk sports and more motor vehicle traffic will most likely lead to higher incidence. Distal femur fractures are not very forgiving and can lead to severe impairment and loss of quality of life.

Nonoperative treatment may be chosen for non- or minimally displaced fractures in low-demand elderly patients. In general, however, nonoperative treatment does not work well for displaced fractures and is reserved for those patients who cannot tolerate surgery.[5]

Top five questions

Diagnosis

1. Is there a role for standard CT scanning in choosing a treatment strategy in patients with distal femur fractures?

Therapy

2. What is the optimal type of osteosynthesis for distal femur fractures: plate or nail?
3. What is the best type of plate fixation for a distal femur fracture?
4. What is the optimal approach for operative fixation of a distal femur fracture above or around a total knee replacement?

Harm

5. What are the most important complications associated with internal fixation of distal femur fractures?

Question 1: Is there a role for standard CT scanning in choosing a treatment strategy in patients with distal femur fractures?

Case 1 clarification
The patient's radiographs show an undisplaced supracondylar fracture with possibly (inter)condylar involvement. You are trying to decide between an AO, A1, or C1 fracture, or maybe a Hoffa (B3) fracture.

> Unicondylar fractures are rare and usually occur in the sagittal plane. A unicondylar fracture oriented in the coronal plane is called a Hoffa fracture.

Relevance
In planning the surgery one should not underestimate the complexity of the fracture, potentially leading to unwanted surprises during surgery. Does that imply that it is necessary to perform standard CT scanning of every distal femur fracture?

Current opinion
The *AO Principles of Fracture Management*[6] states that AP and lateral radiographs of both the femur and the tibia should be taken, in combination with focused views of the

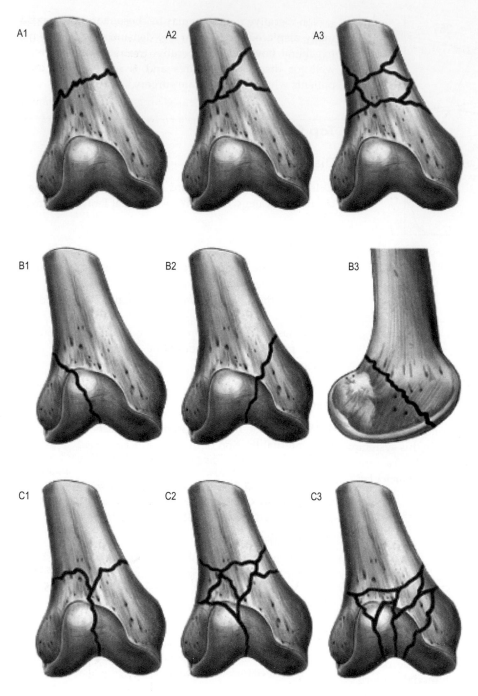

A1 A2 A3

B1 B2 B3

C1 C2 C3

Figure 59.2 AO/OTA classification system for distal femur fractures.

knee joint. CT scans or MRI, as well as 3D reconstructions, offer additional information but are rarely essential.[6] Browner and Levine, as well as Schatzker, conclude that if in doubt about intra-articular involvement CT scans help in planning the surgical approach, especially in minimally invasive techniques.[7,8] Therefore, preoperative CT scanning is currently widely advised and used.

Finding the evidence

• Cochrane Database: no reviews available

• PubMed: no reports on the use of CT scans in planning treatment strategies in distal femur fractures

Quality of the evidence

Level V
• 3 expert opinions

Recommendation

• The use of CT scanning can be considered for standard use in the treatment planning of distal femur fractures [overall level: very low]

Question 2: What is the optimal type of osteosynthesis for distal femur fractures: plate or nail?

Case 1 clarification
You present two options to your patient: plate fixation or retrograde nailing. Your patient wants to know what the best option is.

Relevance
The articular fracture component is usually treated with closed or open reduction, followed by lag screw fixation. However, there is no consensus on the type of implant for the fixation of the metaphyseal–diaphyseal fracture component.

Current opinion
Most surgeons use an osteosynthesis technique based on their own experience.

Finding the evidence
- Cochrane Database: no reviews available
- PubMed: 47 case reports, 2 nonrandomized comparative studies, 1 randomized controlled trial (RCT), 1 prospective cohort study, 1 review, 1 systematic review on the operative treatment of distal femur fractures.

Quality of the evidence
Level I
- 1 systematic reviews/meta-analyses/randomized trial

Level II
- 3 randomized trials with methodological limitations

Level III
- 2 case-control studies/retrospective comparative studies

Level IV
- 47 case series

Recommendation
- The use of either a nail or plate construct can be guided by surgeon experience [overall level: low]

Question 3: What is the best type of plate fixation for a distal femur fracture?

Case 1 clarification
After discussing the options of retrograde nailing and plate fixation with your patient, you both decide to use a plate fixation technique. Your patient now asks if you use the best kind of plate fixation. What is your answer?

Relevance
In addition to traditional compression plating and dynamic condylar screws, locking internal fixation plates have been developed in the last decade. These plates have screws that lock into the plate. The plate/screw construction has the possibility of minimally invasive application.

Current opinion
Internal fixation plates are used with increasing frequency since the development of plates with locking screws.

Finding the evidence
- Cochrane Database: no reviews available
- PubMed: 47 case reports, 2 nonrandomized comparative studies, 1 RCT, 2 prospective cohort studies, 1 review, 1 systematic review on the operative treatment of distal femur fractures

Quality of the evidence
Level I
- 1 systematic review/meta-analysis/randomized trial

Level II
- 4 randomized trials with methodologic limitations

Level III
- 2 case-control studies/retrospective comparative studies

Level IV
- 47 case series

   Despite the numerous cohort studies, there are few that compare different surgical options. Presently there are no reports on prospective, randomized trials comparing different surgical procedures for distal femoral fractures.[9]

Recommendation
- The rates of nonunion fixation failure and deep infection are not significantly different when comparing locking plate IMN or traditional plate constructs (e.g., blade plate, DCS etc.) [overall level: low]

Question 4: What is the optimal approach for operative fixation of a distal femur fracture above or around a total knee replacement?

Case 2 clarification
The patient's radiographs show a distal femoral fracture above a total knee replacement.

Relevance
With an increase in life expectancy and a growing number of total knee replacements all over the world, the incidence of a periprosthetic fracture above a total knee will increase.

Current opinion
- There is no consensus on the best treatment of periprosthetic supracondylar fractures.

Finding the evidence

- Cochrane Database: no reviews available
- PubMed: 29 case series, 1 systematic review

Quality of the evidence

Level I

- 1 systematic review/meta-analyses/randomized trial

Level IV

- 32 case series

Recommendation

- Surgical treatment is superior to nonoperative treatment. Retrograde intramedullary nailing and locking plates appear to be more successful than conventional (nonlocking) plating methods.[11] [overall level: very low]

Question 5: What are the most important complications associated with internal fixation of distal femur fractures?

Relevance

Improvement of current or future techniques should be focused on present failures (hardware failure), complications (nonunion, infection) and functional impairment in the treatment of distal femur fractures.

Current opinion

The reported evidence on the treatment of distal femur fractures consists of a large number of case series, a few comparative studies, and three reviews.[9–13] Unfortunately no RCTs have been performed directly comparing two or more different implants. Although the outcomes including complication rates and differences in complications are not comparable, no extreme differences in complications with respect to nonunions, fixation failure, deep infection, or secondary procedures between different treatment options have been reported. Present research should not be limited to case series and cohort studies; (large) RCTs, possibly multicentered, are necessary to assess the success of current treatment options and its flaws.

Finding the evidence

- Cochrane Database: no reviews available
- PubMed: no reports on complications and treatment of distal femur fractures

Summary of recommendations

- Standard CT scan of a distal femur fracture may be considered, but is not mandatory
- No evidence is available for a superior implant for surgical treatment of a distal femur fracture

- Surgical treatment is superior to nonoperative treatment. Retrograde intramedullary nailing and locking plates appear to be more successful than conventional (nonlocking) plating methods.[11]

Conclusions

The lack of RCTs or even direct (retrospective) comparative studies on the treatment of patients with distal femur fractures deprives the answers to the key questions regarding distal femoral fractures.

References

1. Aglietti P, Buzzi R. Fractures of the femoral condyles. In: Insall JN, Windsor RE, Scott WN, Kelly MA, Aglietti P, eds., Surgery of the Knee, 2nd ed. Churchill Livingstone, New York, 1993.
2. Marsh JL, Slongo TF, Agel J, et al. Fracture and dislocation classification compendium—2007: Orthopaedic Trauma Association classification, database and outcomes committee. J Orthop Trauma 2007;21(10 Suppl):S1–133.
3. Kolmert L, Wulff K. Epidemiology and treatment of distal femoral fractures in adults. Acta Orthop Scand 1982;53(6):957–62.
4. Martinet O, Cordey J, Harder Y, Maier A, Buhler M, Barraud GE. The epidemiology of fractures of the distal femur. Injury 2000;31(Suppl 3):C62–3.
5. Butt MS, Krikler SJ, Ali MS. Displaced fractures of the distal femur in elderly patients. Operative versus nonoperative treatment. J Bone Joint Surg Br 1996;78(1):110–14.
6. Kinzl L. Femur: Distal. In: Ruedi TP, Murphy WM, eds. AO Principles of Fracture Management. Thieme, New York, 2000.
7. Krettek C, Helfet DL. Fractures of the distal femur. In: Browner BD, Levine AM, eds. Skeletal Trauma, 3rd ed. Elsevier Science, Philadelphia, PA, 2003.
8. Schatzker J. Supracondylar fractures of the femur. In: Schatzker J, Tile M, eds., The Rationale of Operative Fracture Care, 3rd ed. Springer, New York, 2005.
9. Zlowodzki M, Bhandari M, Marek DJ, Cole PA, Kregor PJ. Operative treatment of acute distal femur fractures: systematic review of 2 comparative studies and 45 case series (1989 to 2005). J Orthop Trauma 2006;20(5):366–71.
10. Forster MC, Komarsamy B, Davison JN. Distal femoral fractures: a review of fixation methods. Injury 2006;37(2):97–108.
11. Herrera DA, Kregor PJ, Cole PA, Levy BA, Jonsson A, Zlowodzki M. Treatment of acute distal femur fractures above a total knee arthroplasty: systematic review of 415 cases (1981–2006). Acta Orthop 2008;79(1):22–7.
12. Schutz M, Muller M, Regazzoni P, et al. Use of the less invasive stabilization system (LISS) in patients with distal femoral (AO33) fractures: a prospective multicenter study. Arch Orthop Trauma Surg 2005;125(2):102–8.
13. Kao FC, Tu YK, Su JY, Hsu KY, Wu CH, Chou MC. Treatment of distal femoral fracture by minimally invasive percutaneous plate osteosynthesis: comparison between the dynamic condylar screw and the less invasive stabilization system. J Trauma 2009;67(4):719–26.

60 Knee Dislocations

James P. Stannard¹ and Allan Hammond²

¹University of Missouri Hospital, Columbia, MO, USA
²University of Manitoba Health Science Centre, Winnipeg, MB, Canada

Case scenario

A 32 year old male construction worker is involved in a motor vehicle collision on the way home from work. He sustains a right femur fracture and is noted to have mild swelling around the right knee as well. After intramedullary (IM) nailing of the femur the next day, it is noted that the patient has gross knee instability in all directions. He has a normal vascular exam with 2+ pulses bilaterally for both the dorsalis pedis and posterior tibial arteries.

Top eight questions

Diagnosis

1. How accurate is the diagnosis of knee dislocation? Are they easily missed?
2. What diagnostic tests or physical examination tests are necessary to exclude popliteal artery injuries?

Therapy

3. Should knee dislocation be treated surgically, or with casts or braces?
4. Should torn collateral ligaments be repaired or reconstructed?

Prognosis

5. What is the incidence of arthrofibrosis and motion problems following reconstructive surgery?
6. What is the likelihood of instability following reconstruction?
7. What yields better results, reconstruction of the knee acutely (3–4 weeks after injury) or delayed reconstruction?

8. Are patients able to return to work and/or sports and recreation following a knee dislocation?

Question 1: How accurate is the diagnosis of knee dislocation and is it easily missed?

Case clarification

It is extremely difficult to examine the knee when the patient has an ipsilateral long bone fracture, prior to stabilization of the fracture.

Clinical relevance

Missed knee dislocations can result in limb-threatening complications.

Current opinion

Vigilance is key, and orthopedic surgeons must realize that knee dislocations frequently present reduced, or have associated injuries, which can cause the dislocation to be missed.

Finding the evidence

- PubMed: English language articles, 1969–2010, with the following search terms: "knee" AND "multi-ligament" OR "multiligamentous" OR "multiple ligament" OR "dislocation" AND "epidemiology" OR "incidence" OR "diagnosis"

Quality of the evidence

- Level II: 1[1]
- Level IV: 1[2]

Findings

Although many current textbooks and reviews acknowledge the problem of diagnosis, there are no articles that can be identified in a literature search that directly address this topic. In the past it was believed that three or four ligament

Evidence-Based Orthopedics, First Edition. Edited by Mohit Bhandari.
© 2012 Blackwell Publishing Ltd. Published 2012 by Blackwell Publishing Ltd.

disruptions were required for knee dislocation to occur; however, Cooper presented a series of four cases (level IV) where only two ligaments were disrupted,[3] and single-ligament injuries resulting in dislocation have been documented as far back as 1969 (level IV).[4] A retrospective MRI study by Bui[2] (level IV) showed that in their review of 20 knee dislocations, only 25% presented with abnormal alignment on initial radiographs, and that in nearly one third of cases dislocation was not even suspected at the time the MRI was ordered. A prospective outcome study (level II) by Twaddle et al.[1] demonstrated that only one third of dislocated knees presented in the Emergency Department unreduced.

Recommendation

• Great vigilance is required to avoid missing knee dislocations in trauma patients. All patients with lower extremity trauma and pain or swelling around the knee should be carefully evaluated for knee instability [overall quality: low]

Question 2: What diagnostic tests or physical examination tests are necessary to exclude popliteal artery injury?

Case clarification

The diagnosis of a knee dislocation was not made until nearly 24 hours following the injury, when the femur fracture was stabilized.

Clinical relevance

A missed popliteal artery injury can lead to an above-knee amputation.

Current opinion

A selective arteriography protocol that employs a good vascular examination as the screening method is currently standard care. Any abnormality in the examination requires additional studies to document the integrity of the artery.

Finding the evidence

• PubMed: English language articles, 1969–2010, with the following search terms: "knee" AND "multi-ligament" OR "multiligamentous" OR "multiple ligament" OR "dislocation" AND "vascular"

Quality of the evidence

• Level II: 3[5–7]
• Level III: 1[8]
• Level IV: 10[9,10–18]

Findings

No prospective randomized trials have been published on this topic. However, one meta-analysis (level III),[8] four pro-spective studies (three level II,[5–7] one level VI[9]) and nine retrospective studies (level IV)[10–18] have been published regarding the use of physical examination as the primary screening tool for arterial injury. Physical examination was sufficient to rule out vascular injury in all but one study,[17] and in this study ankle brachial indices were not used and even angiography had a false-negative rate of more than 40%.

Recommendation

• All patients should be carefully screened for arterial injury with serial vascular physical examinations following knee dislocation. Any abnormality should be evaluated with additional testing [overall quality: moderate]

Question 3: Should knee dislocations be treated surgically or nonoperatively?

Relevance

Surgical treatment is complex and expensive, often requiring multiple procedures. Older treatment protocols advocated cast or brace treatment, but outcomes were frequently poor.

Current opinion

Knee dislocations should be treated surgically in the vast majority of patients.

Finding the evidence

• PubMed: English language articles, 1969–2010, with the following search terms: "knee" AND "multi-ligament" OR "multiligamentous" OR "multiple ligament" OR "dislocation" OR "anterior cruciate" AND "posterior cruciate" OR "posterolateral corner"

Quality of the evidence

• Level III: 5[19,20–23]
• Level IV: 11[3,4,24–32]

Findings

There are no prospective randomized trials in the literature, but there is one meta-analysis with methodological flaws[19] (level III), and 18 comparative studies with operatively and nonoperatively treated patients with published outcome data.[3,4,20–34] Ten of the 18 studies, all level IV, had either too few patients or presented their data in such a manner that no conclusions could be made.[3,4,24–31] The remaining studies, four level III[20–23] and one level IV,[32] found the Lysholm, Tegner, and IKDC outcome measures to be statistically superior in operative patients compared to those treated nonoperatively. Regarding range of motion (ROM), only two of eight studies (one level III and one level VI), showed decreased ROM in operatively treated patients, and in neither did it reach statistical significance.[21,35] In no study was instability, either by physical exam or via KT1000, found to be greater or more frequent in operative cases.

Recommendations

• Operative treatment of knee dislocations results in superior functional outcomes and stability with little risk of stiffness when compared to nonoperative treatment [overall quality: low]

Question 4: Should torn collateral ligaments be repaired or reconstructed?

Clinical relevance

Traditional teaching has been that the corners should be repaired if good quality tissue is present and the repair is accomplished within 3 weeks.

Current opinion

The failure rate is lower for both the posteromedial corner (PMC) and posterolateral corner (PLC) with reconstruction of the ligaments when compared with repair.

Finding the evidence for the treatment of PMC injury

• PubMed: English language articles, 1969–2010, using the search terms: "knee" AND "multi-ligament" OR "multiligamentous" OR "multiple ligament" OR "dislocation" AND "mcl" OR "medial collateral ligament" OR "posteromedial corner" OR "pmc"

Quality of the evidence for the treatment of PMC injury

• Level II: 1[36]
• Level III: 3[22,37,38]
• Level IV: 21[24,28,29,39–55]

Findings

There are currently no published studies in the literature directly comparing PMC reconstruction with repair. A systematic review was recently published on this topic (level III).[37] There is one level II study,[36] and three level VI studies which performed PMC reconstruction exclusively without synthetics,[53–55] as well as two level III studies,[22,38] and 18 level VI studies[24,28,29,39–52] which performed medial collateral ligament (MCL) repair, either with or without synthetic or biologic augmentation, in the management of knee dislocation. Of the four studies in which the PMC was reconstructed, only three had interpretable data. Combined, these three studies demonstrated a very low failure rate (<2%) for PMC reconstruction (1/72).[36,53,54] Regarding PMC/MCL repair with knee dislocation, of the 20 studies only 13 were suitable for analysis (1 level III [22] and 12 level VI[22,39–41,43–49,51]). Combining these studies gave an overall

failure rate for MCL repair of 17%. While no direct comparisons were made in the studies regarding acute vs. chronic MCL repair, analysis of individual studies suggests that acute repair may have lower failure rates (0, 11%, 16%)[36,41,45] than chronic repair (29%, 57%, 66%).[44–46]

Recommendations for the treatment of PMC injury

• PMC reconstruction has a low failure rate compared to repair. Acute PMC repair may have lower failure rates than chronic repair [overall quality: low]

Finding the evidence for the treatment of PLC injury

• PubMed: English language articles,1969–2010, using the search terms: "knee" AND "multiligament" OR "multiligamentous" OR "multiple ligament" OR "dislocation" AND "PLC" OR "posterolateral corner" OR "LCL" OR "lateral collateral"

Quality of the evidence for the treatment of PLC injury

• Level II: 1[56]
• Level III: 4 [20,22,46,57]
• Level IV: 16[31,36,39–41,43–45,47–49,58–62]

Findings

One level II study[56] and one level III study[57] directly compared PLC repair with reconstruction, while there were 3 level III studies[20,22,46]and 16 level VI studies [31,36,39–41,43–45,47–49,58,59–62] in which the PLC was managed surgically. The vast majority did not distinguish between repair, augmentation, or reconstruction, except for Stannard et al. and Levy et al. who found statistically significant higher failure rates in repair over reconstruction, 9% vs. 5% (p = 0.03)[56] and 40% vs. 6% (p = 0.04).[57] The overall combined failure rate for the surgical management of PLC injuries in knee dislocations in the literature, either by repair or reconstruction, is 89/406 (22%).

Recommendation for the treatment of PLC injury

• PLC reconstruction appears to have lower failure rate than repair [overall quality: low]

Question 5: What is the incidence of arthrofibrosis following knee dislocation?

Relevance

Many surgeons consider arthrofibrosis and painful loss of motion to be the biggest problem associated with knee dislocations.

Current opinion

Arthrofibrosis is a common complication that is decreasing as surgeons adopt more aggressive postoperative rehabilitation protocols.

Finding the evidence
- PubMed: English language articles, 1969–2010, using the search terms: "knee" AND "multiligament" OR "multiligamentous" OR "multiple ligament" OR "dislocation" AND "arthrofibrosis" OR "stiffness" OR "manipulation" OR "arthrolysis"

Quality of the evidence
- Level II: 1[56]
- Level III: 1[63]
- Level IV: 18 [3,30,33,36,39–43,45,50–52,61,62,64–66]

Findings
No comparative studies have been performed which have looked to minimize the incidence or severity of arthrofibrosis after knee dislocation. Twenty studies have been published that report on the incidence of arthrofibrosis; except for one level II and one level III study,[63] they are retrospective studies with level IV evidence.[3,30,33,36,39–43,45,50–52,61,62,64–66] The cumulative incidence of arthrofibrosis is 19% (76/403), although three recent studies[39–41] show current rates to be much lower (8%).

Recommendation
- Arthrofibrosis is common (about 19%) but decreasing due to modern reconstruction and rehabilitation techniques [overall quality: low]

Question 6: What is the likelihood of recurrent instability following reconstruction of a dislocated knee?

Relevance
Although many surgeons state that arthrofibrosis and motion loss is the greatest problem following knee dislocation, recurrent instability is a major problem.

Current opinion
Recurrent instability is the most common complication following the repair or reconstruction of knee dislocations.

Finding the evidence
- PubMed: English language articles, 1969–2010, using the search terms: "knee" AND "multiligament" OR "multiligamentous" OR "multiple ligament" OR "dislocation" AND "laxity" OR "instability" OR "failure"

Quality of the evidence
- Level II: 1[36]
- Level III: 4 [20,22,46,63]
- Level IV: 19[31,34,39–41,43–45,48–50,58,59,61,62,66–69]

Findings
There have been 24 published studies: one level II, four level III,[20,22,46,63] and 19 level IV,[31,34,39–41,43–45,48–50,58,59,61,62,66–69]

which document rates of ligamentous laxity, either by physical examination or KT1000, after surgical management of knee dislocations. By pooling all the data from these studies, surgical management of anterior cruciate ligament (ACL) and posterior cruciate ligament (PCL) disruption results in recurrent instability in 19% of cases, while there is recurrent instability of the MCL/PMC and PLC respectively 17% and 22% of the time.

Recommendation
- Recurrent instability is the most common complication following dislocation reconstruction. Patients should be counseled regarding the risk, and surgeons should continue to look for strategies that decrease the problem of recurrent instability [overall quality: low]

Question 7: What yields better results, reconstruction of the knee acutely (3–4 weeks after injury) or delayed reconstruction?

Relevance
Reconstruction during the acute phase after the injury allows patients to recover from fractures and knee reconstruction simultaneously. However, the risk of skin breakdown and arthrofibrosis may be higher during the inflammatory phase immediately following the injury.

Current opinion
Outcome results are somewhat more favorable for patients who have surgical reconstruction initiated within 1 month after the injury.

Finding the evidence
- PubMed: English language articles, 1969–2010, using the search terms: "knee" AND "multiligament" OR "multiligamentous" OR "multiple ligament" OR "dislocation" AND "acute" OR "chronic"

Quality of the evidence
- Level III: 1[38]
- Level IV: 2 [45,46]

Findings
Only three published studies have directly compared acute to chronic management of knee dislocations.[38,45,46] All three report superior Lysholm scores in the acute group, but statistical significance was not reached. Meyers, IKDC and Knee Outcome Survey scores were also found to be superior in acute management, but these scores also never reached statistical significance.

Recommendation
- If the patient's condition allows, knee reconstruction should be started acutely [overall quality: low]

Question 8: Are patients able to return to work and/or sports and recreation following a knee dislocation?

Clinical relevance

Reconstructing dislocated knees often requires multiple operations in order to maximize function. It is important for patients to know if they will be able to resume careers or leisure activities after completion of their care.

Current opinion

Most patients are able to return to employment following reconstruction of a knee dislocation. However, only about half of them are able to resume the same level of sporting activities.

Finding the evidence

• PubMed: English language articles, 1969–2010, using the search terms: "knee" AND "multiligament" OR "multiligamentous" OR "multiple ligament" OR "dislocation" AND "sport" OR "work"

Quality of the evidence

• Level II: 1[70]
• Level III: 2[21,61]
• Level IV: 18 [22,27,34,42,44,48–51,58,59,62,63,66,71–73]

Findings

There are 21 studies presenting data on these questions, with the vast majority being retrospective level VI studies.[21,22,27,34,42,44,48–51,58,59,61–63,66,70–73] Due to the ambiguity of the terminology in the literature, it is difficult to combine all these studies into an analysis. However, by selecting studies that use similar or specific phrases, some conclusions can be made. Of the seven studies that used the term "return to work," the combined data shows that 88% (189/215) of patients returned to work (range 75–100%).[22,42,44,50,58,62,70] Data on return to athletic activities is even more difficult to assess, due to variability in the definition and individual activity levels. However, when the terms "same level," "preinjury level," or "previous level" of sport are used as the outcome measure, nine studies show a combined rate of 40/158 or 25% (range 0–81%).[21,24,34,48,49,59,61,66,71]

Recommendation

• Patients are highly likely to be able to return to employment. Return to the same level of sporting activity is unlikely, but possible [overall quality: low]

Summary of recommendations

• Great vigilance is required to avoid missing knee dislocations in trauma patients. All patients with lower extremity trauma and pain or swelling around the knee should be carefully evaluated for knee instability
• All patients should be carefully screened for arterial injury with serial physical examinations following knee dislocation. Any abnormality should be evaluated with additional testing
• In the vast majority of instances, knee dislocations should be treated with surgical stabilization
• The failure rate of reconstruction of the PLC and PMC will be lower than the failure rate of repair
• Arthrofibrosis occurs in nearly 1/5 patients but recent literature suggests that the rate is decreasing
• If the patient's condition allows, knee reconstruction should be started acutely
• Recurrent instability is common following dislocation reconstruction. Patients should be counseled regarding the risk, and surgeons should continue to look for strategies that decrease the problem of recurrent instability
• Patients are very likely to be able to return to their previous employment. The probability of returning to the same level of preinjury athletics is unpredictable but unlikely.

Conclusion

No level I studies have been published regarding knee dislocations. Many questions regarding the ideal treatment of these challenging patients remain unanswered. However, good guidelines can be developed by combining the data from a large number of small level IV studies.

References

1. Twaddle BC, Bidwell TA, Chapman JR. Knee dislocations: where are the lesions? A prospective evaluation of surgical findings in 63 cases. J Orthop Trauma 2003;17:198–202.
2. Bui KL, Ilaslan H, Parker RD, Sundaram M. Knee dislocations: a magnetic resonance imaging study correlated with clinical and operative findings. Skeletal Radiol 2008;37:653–61.
3. Cooper DE, Speer KP, Wickiewicz TL, Warren RF. Complete knee dislocation without posterior cruciate ligament disruption. A report of four cases and review of the literature. Clin Orthop Relat Res 1992:228–33.
4. Shields L, Mital M, Cave EF. Complete dislocation of the knee: experience at the Massachusetts General Hospital. J Trauma 1969;9:192–215.
5. Stannard JP, Sheils TM, Lopez-Ben RR, McGwin G, Jr., Robinson JT, Volgas DA. Vascular injuries in knee dislocations: the role of physical examination in determining the need for arteriography. J Bone Joint Surg Am 2004;86:910–15.
6. Mills WJ, Barei DP, McNair P. The value of the ankle-brachial index for diagnosing arterial injury after knee dislocation: a prospective study. J Trauma 2004;56:1261–5.

7. Miranda FE, Dennis JW, Veldenz HC, Dovgan PS, Frykberg ER. Confirmation of the safety and accuracy of physical examination in the evaluation of knee dislocation for injury of the popliteal artery: a prospective study. J Trauma 2002;52:247–51; discussion 51–2.

8. Barnes CJ, Pietrobon R, Higgins LD. Does the pulse examination in patients with traumatic knee dislocation predict a surgical arterial injury? A meta-analysis. J Trauma 2002;53:1109–14.

9. Boisrenoult P, Lustig S, Bonneviale P, et al. Vascular lesions associated with bicruciate and knee dislocation ligamentous injury. Rev Chir Orthop Traumatol 2009;95:621–6.

10. Abou-Sayed H, Berger DL. Blunt lower-extremity trauma and popliteal artery injuries: revisiting the case for selective arteriography. Arch Surg 2002;137:585–9.

11. Dennis JW, Jagger C, Butcher JL, Menawat SS, Neel M, Frykberg ER. Reassessing the role of arteriograms in the management of posterior knee dislocations. J Trauma 1993;35:692–5; discussion 5–7.

12. Hollis JD, Daley BJ. 10-year review of knee dislocations: is arteriography always necessary? J Trauma 2005;59:672–5; discussion 5–6.

13. Kaufman SL, Martin LG. Arterial injuries associated with complete dislocation of the knee. Radiology 1992;184:153–5.

14. Kendall RW, Taylor DC, Salvian AJ, O'Brien PJ. The role of arteriography in assessing vascular injuries associated with dislocations of the knee. J Trauma 1993;35:875–8.

15. Klineberg EO, Crites BM, Flinn WR, Archibald JD, Moorman CT 3rd. The role of arteriography in assessing popliteal artery injury in knee dislocations. J Trauma 2004;56:786–90.

16. Martinez D, Sweatman K, Thompson EC. Popliteal artery injury associated with knee dislocations. Am Surg 2001;67:165–7.

17. McDonough EB, Jr., Wojtys EM. Multiligamentous injuries of the knee and associated vascular injuries. Am J Sports Med 2009;37:156–9.

18. Treiman GS, Yellin AE, Weaver FA, et al. Examination of the patient with a knee dislocation. The case for selective arteriography. Arch Surg 1992;127:1056–62; discussion 62–3.

19. Dedmond BT, Almekinders LC. Operative versus nonoperative treatment of knee dislocations: a meta-analysis. Am J Knee Surg 2001;14:33–8.

20. Plancher KD, Siliski J. Long-term functional results and complications in patients with knee dislocations. J Knee Surg 2008;21:261–8.

21. Wong C-H, Tan J-L, Chang H-C, Khin L-W, Low C-O. Knee dislocations—a retrospective study comparing operative versus closed immobilization treatment outcomes. Knee Surg Sports Traumatol Arthrosc 2004;12:540–4.

22. Richter M, Bosch U, Wippermann B, Hofmann A, Krettek C. Comparison of surgical repair or reconstruction of the cruciate ligaments versus nonsurgical treatment in patients with traumatic knee dislocations. Am J Sports Med 2002;30:718–27.

23. Montgomery TJ, Savoie FH, White JL, Roberts TS, Hughes JL. Orthopedic management of knee dislocations. Comparison of surgical reconstruction and immobilization. Am J Knee Surg 1995;8:97–103.

24. Shelbourne KD, Porter DA, Clingman JA, McCarroll JR, Rettig AC. Low-velocity knee dislocation. Orthop Rev 1991;20:995–1004.

25. Meyers MH, Moore TM, Harvey JP. Traumatic dislocation of the knee joint. J Bone Joint Surg Am 1975;57:430–3.

26. Taylor A, Arden G, Rainey H. Traumatic dislocation of the knee: A report of forty-three cases with special reference to conservative treatment. J Bone Joint Surg Br 1972;54:96.

27. King JJ, Cerynik DL, Blair JA, Harding SP, Tom JA. Surgical outcomes after traumatic open knee dislocation. Knee Surg Sports Traumatol Arthrosc 2009;17:1027–32.

28. Giannoudis PV, Roberts CS, Parikh AR, Agarwal S, Hadjikouti-Dyer C, Macdonald DA. Knee dislocation with ipsilateral femoral shaft fracture: a report of five cases. J Orthop Trauma 2005;19:205–10.

29. Gu M-q, Deng L, Liu Y. Posterolateral dislocation of the knee joints: analysis of 9 cases. Chin J Traumatol 2004;7:210–6.

30. Schenck RC, McGanity PL, Heckman JD. Femoral-sided fracture-dislocation of the knee. J Orthop Trauma 1997;11:416–21.

31. Thomsen PB, Rud B, Jensen UH. Stability and motion after traumatic dislocation of the knee. Acta Orthop Scand 1984;55:278–83.

32. Demirağ B, Oztürk C, Bilgen OF, Durak K. Knee dislocations: an evaluation of surgical and conservative treatment. Ulus Travma Acil Cerrahi Derg 2004;10:239–44.

33. Ríos A, Villa A, Fahandezh H, de José C, Vaquero J. Results after treatment of traumatic knee dislocations: a report of 26 cases. J Trauma 2003;55:489–94.

34. Almekinders LC, Logan TC. Results following treatment of traumatic dislocations of the knee joint. Clin Orthop Relat Res 1992:203–7.

35. Roman PD, Hopson CN, Zenni EJ. Traumatic dislocation of the knee: a report of 30 cases and literature review. Orthop Rev 1987;16:917–24.

36. Stannard JP, Sheils TM, Mcgwin G, Volgas DA, Alonso JE. Use of a hinged external knee fixator after surgery for knee dislocation. Arthroscopy 2003;19:626–31.

37. Kovachevich R, Shah JP, Arens AM, Stuart MJ, Dahm DL, Levy BA. Operative management of the medial collateral ligament in the multi-ligament injured knee: an evidence-based systematic review. Knee Surg Sports Traumatol Arthrosc 2009;17:823–9.

38. Tzurbakis M, Diamantopoulos A, Xenakis T, Georgoulis A. Surgical treatment of multiple knee ligament injuries in 44 patients: 2–8 years follow-up results. Knee Surg Sports Traumatol Arthrosc 2006;14:739–49.

39. Engebretsen L, Risberg MA, Robertson B, Ludvigsen TC, Johansen S. Outcome after knee dislocations: a 2–9 years follow-up of 85 consecutive patients. Knee Surg Sports Traumatol Arthrosc 2009;17:1013–26.

40. Lo Y-P, Hsu K-Y, Chen L-H, et al. Simultaneous arthroscopic reconstruction of the anterior and posterior cruciate ligament using hamstring and quadriceps tendon autografts. J Trauma 2009;66:780–8.

41. Ibrahim SAR, Ahmad FHF, Salah M, Al Misfer ARK, Ghaffer SA, Khirat S. Surgical management of traumatic knee dislocation. Arthroscopy 2008;24:178–87.

42. Owens BD, Neault M, Benson E, Busconi BD. Primary repair of knee dislocations: results in 25 patients (28 knees) at a mean follow-up of four years. J Orthop Trauma 2007;21:92–6.

43. Bin S-I, Nam T-S. Surgical outcome of 2-stage management of multiple knee ligament injuries after knee dislocation. Arthroscopy 2007;23:1066–72.

44. Karataglis D, Bisbinas I, Green MA, Learmonth DJA. Functional outcome following reconstruction in chronic multiple ligament

deficient knees. Knee Surg Sports Traumatol Arthrosc 2006;14: 843–7.

45. Harner C, Waltrip R, Bennett C, Francis K, Cole B, Irrgang J. Surgical management of knee dislocations. J Bone Joint Surg Am 2004;86:262.

46. Liow R, Mcnicholas M, Keating J, Nutton R. Ligament repair and reconstruction in traumatic dislocation of the knee. J Bone Joint Surg Br 2003;85:845.

47. Fanelli GC, Edson CJ. Arthroscopically assisted combined anterior and posterior cruciate ligament reconstruction in the multiple ligament injured knee: 2- to 10-year follow-up. Arthroscopy 2002;18:703–14.

48. Mariani PP, Margheritini F, Camillieri G. One-stage arthroscopically assisted anterior and posterior cruciate ligament reconstruction. Arthroscopy 2001;17:700–7.

49. Mariani PP, Santoriello P, Iannone S, Condello V, Adriani E. Comparison of surgical treatments for knee dislocation. Am J Knee Surg 2000;12:214–21.

50. Yeh WL, Tu YK, Su JY, Hsu RW. Knee dislocation: treatment of high-velocity knee dislocation. J Trauma 1999;46:693–701.

51. Wascher DC, Becker JR, Dexter JG, Blevins FT. Reconstruction of the anterior and posterior cruciate ligaments after knee dislocation. Results using fresh-frozen nonirradiated allografts. Am J Sports Med 1999;27:189–96.

52. Walker D, Hardison R, Schenck RC. A baker's dozen of knee dislocations. Am J Knee Surg 1994;7:117–24.

53. Yoshiya S, Kuroda R, Mizuno K, Yamamoto T, Kurosaka M. Medial collateral ligament reconstruction using autogenous hamstring tendons: technique and results in initial cases. Am J Sports Med 2005;33:1380–5.

54. Lind M, Jakobsen BW, Lund B, Hansen MS, Abdallah O, Christiansen SE. Anatomical reconstruction of the medial collateral ligament and posteromedial corner of the knee in patients with chronic medial collateral ligament instability. Am J Sports Med 2009;37:1116–22.

55. Hayashi R, Kitamura N, Kondo E, Anaguchi Y, Tohyama H, Yasuda K. Simultaneous anterior and posterior cruciate ligament reconstruction in chronic knee instabilities: surgical concepts and clinical outcome. Knee Surg Sports Traumatol Arthrosc 2008;16:763–9.

56. Stannard JP, Brown SL, Farris RC, Mcgwin G, Volgas DA. The posterolateral corner of the knee: repair versus reconstruction. Am J Sports Med 2005;33:881–8.

57. Levy BA, Dajani KA, Morgan JA, Shah JP, Dahm DL, Stuart MJ. Repair versus reconstruction of the fibular collateral ligament and posterolateral corner in the multiligament-injured knee. Am J Sports Med 2010;38:804–9.

58. Ibrahim SA. Primary repair of the cruciate and collateral ligaments after traumatic dislocation of the knee. J Bone Joint Surg Br 1999;81:987–90.

59. Shelbourne KD, Haro MS, Gray T. Knee dislocation with lateral side injury: results of an en masse surgical repair technique of the lateral side. Am J Sports Med 2007;35:1105–16.

60. Stannard JP, Brown SL, Robinson JT, Mcgwin G, Volgas DA. Reconstruction of the posterolateral corner of the knee. Arthroscopy 2005;21:1051–9.

61. Noyes FR, Barber-Westin SD. Reconstruction of the anterior and posterior cruciate ligaments after knee dislocation. Use of early protected postoperative motion to decrease arthrofibrosis. Am J Sports Med 1997;25:769–78.

62. Shapiro MS, Freedman EL. Allograft reconstruction of the anterior and posterior cruciate ligaments after traumatic knee dislocation. Am J Sports Med 1995;23:580–7.

63. Martinek V, Steinbacher G, Friederich NF, Müller WE. Operative treatment of combined anterior and posterior cruciate ligament injuries in complex knee trauma: can the cruciate ligaments be preserved? Am J Knee Surg 2001;13:74–82.

64. Zhao J, He Y, Wang J. Simultaneous arthroscopic reconstruction of the anterior and posterior cruciate ligaments with autogenous hamstring tendons. Arthroscopy 2006;22:497–504.

65. Talbot M, Berry G, Fernandes J, Ranger P. Knee dislocations: experience at the Hôpital du Sacré-Coeur de Montréal. Can J Surg 2004;47:20–4.

66. Sisto DJ, Warren RF. Complete knee dislocation. A follow-up study of operative treatment. Clin Orthop Relat Res 1985: 94–101.

67. Fanelli GC, Edson CJ. Combined posterior cruciate ligament-posterolateral reconstructions with Achilles tendon allograft and biceps femoris tendon tenodesis: 2- to 10-year follow-up. Arthroscopy 2004;20:339–45.

68. Frassica FJ, Sim FH, Staeheli JW, Pairolero PC. Dislocation of the knee. Clin Orthop Relat Res 1991:200–5.

69. Meyers MH, Harvey JP. Traumatic dislocation of the knee joint. A study of eighteen cases. J Bone Joint Surg Am 1971;53:16–29.

70. Stannard JP, Riley RS, Sheils TM, Mcgwin G, Volgas DA. Anatomic reconstruction of the posterior cruciate ligament after multiligament knee injuries. A combination of the tibial-inlay and two-femoral-tunnel techniques. Am J Sports Med 2003;31: 196–202.

71. Ross AE, Taylor KF, Kirk KL, Murphy KP. Functional outcome of multiligamentous knee injuries treated arthroscopically in active duty soldiers. Mil Med 2009;174:1113–7.

72. Lughi M, Vaienti E. Traumatic dislocation of the knee. A review of the literature and our experience. Chir Organi Mov 1999; 84:79–86.

73. Baker CL, Norwood LA, Hughston JC. Acute combined posterior cruciate and posterolateral instability of the knee. Am J Sports Med 1984;12:204–8.

61 Proximal Tibia

Richard J. Jenkinson and Hans J. Kreder
University of Toronto, Toronto, ON, Canada

Case scenario

A 48 year old man is injured in a fall from a ladder, from a height of 2m. He has sustained an isolated injury to his right proximal tibia. Clinical examination shows that there is no open wound, his compartments are soft, and his swelling is minimal. Radiographic examination shows a displaced bicondylar proximal tibia fracture.

Relevant anatomy

Fractures of the proximal tibia are also known as tibial plateau fractures. They are classified by the OTA classification, as described in Table 61.1. Another commonly used classification is that described by Schatzker,[1] as outlined in Table 61.2.

Case clarification

Careful inspection of radiographs and a CT scan show that this patient has suffered a Schatzker type 6 fracture involving both medial and lateral plateaus with metaphyseal/diaphyseal discontinuity. In terms of the OTA classification he has sustained a 41-3C injury, implying significant articular comminution.

Top five questions

Therapy

1. This patient will require surgical treatment. Are the functional outcomes different between patients treated with external fixation compared to open reduction and internal fixation (ORIF) with plates and screws?

2. I anticipate a metaphyseal bone void after reduction. Should I fill this with iliac crest autograft or a bone graft substitute.
3. How early should I allow range of motion postoperatively?

Prognosis

4. What is the effect of imperfect articular reduction on functional outcomes?
5. What is the effect of limb instability, malalignment and meniscus cartilage damage on functional outcomes?

Finding the evidence

The following general searches were undertaken to identify the best evidence (meta-analyses, systematic reviews and clinical trials). When level I evidence was lacking, studies at a lower level of evidence were reviewed.
- Cochrane Database: search term "proximal tibia fractures" and "tibial plateau fractures"
- PubMed: clinical queries search/systematic reviews: "tibial plateau fractures," "proximal tibial fractures"
- PubMed: "tibial plateau fracture" OR "proximal tibia fracture"

Question 1: This patient will require surgical treatment. Are the complication rates and functional outcomes different between patients treated with external fixation compared to ORIF with plates and screws?

Relevance
There are a number of treatment options for complex proximal tibia fractures. External fixation, combined with limited open techniques can potentially reduce complications but

Evidence-Based Orthopedics, First Edition. Edited by Mohit Bhandari.
© 2012 Blackwell Publishing Ltd. Published 2012 by Blackwell Publishing Ltd.

Table 61.1 OTA Classification of proximal tibia (41) fractures

Type	Group	Description
41-A Extra-articular	41-A1	Avulsion
	41-A2	Metaphyseal simple
	41-A3	Metaphyseal multifragmentary
41-B Partial articular	41-B1	Pure split
	41-B2	Pure depression
	41-B3	Split depression
41-C Complete articular	41-C1	Articular simple Metaphyseal simple
	41-C2	Articular simple Metaphyseal multifragmentary
	41-C3	Articular multifragmentary

Table 61.2 Schatzkter classification of tibial plateau fractures

Type	Description
1	Lateral plateau pure split fracture
2	Lateral plateau split and depression
3	Lateral plateau pure depression
4	Fracture of the medial plateau
5	Fracture of both medial and lateral plateau Some metaphyseal/diaphyseal continuity
6	Fracture of both medial and lateral plateau Metaphyseal/diaphyseal discontinuity

potentially limit the ability to obtain optimal reductions. Open plating techniques can allow a more precise reduction, but risk complications. When performing an ORIF, the surgeon must consider choice of incision and approach(es) to achieve surgical goals while limiting complications as well as considering the need for future procedures.

Current opinion

Treatment with ORIF with two plates inserted via an anterior or two incisions may have a higher complication and reoperation rate than limited ORIF with circular external fixator. There is insufficient evidence to definitively guide choice between open reduction and internal fixation, hybrid external fixation, and unilateral locked plating in proximal tibia fractures.

Quality of the evidence

Level I
- 1 randomized trial

Level II
- 1 randomized trial with methodologic limitations

Levels III and IV
- 6+ retrospective cohort studies or case series

Findings

A straight or modified midline anterior knee incision has historically been described to treat proximal tibia fractures.[1–3] This has recently fallen out of favor due to reported high rates of deep infection (13–88%) in high-energy bicondylar fractures.[3–5] This is thought to be due to the large amount of soft tissue dissection required to expose the proximal tibia for traditional techniques. In response to this, there has been a trend to consider the soft tissue more carefully with the introduction of less invasive surgical strategies. The literature describing these techniques consists almost entirely of retrospective and single-center cohort studies. For each technique, authors describe their surgical methods and report satisfactory results in terms of obtaining and maintaining reduction along with their low complication rates.

Two prospective comparative trials were identified in the literature. A trial from the Canadian Orthopaedic Trauma Society(COTS) compared closed/limited open reduction and circular external fixation with ORIF via midline or two-incision methods using nonlocking implants.[6] The patients were limited to high-energy fractures classified as Schatzker 5/6 injuries (AO 41-C). The authors identified HSS knee scores at 2 years postoperatively as their primary outcome. with an a-priori power calculated to predict a 25% difference with their sample size of 82 patients. There was no significant difference in HSS knee scores at 2 years (primary outcome) between groups (p = 0.31). However, the external fixation group was found to have a trend to earlier functional recovery with better HSS knee scores at 6 months postoperatively (p = 0.064). The ORIF group was found to have a 17%(8/40) infection rate vs. 4.7% (2/43) in the external fixation group (p = 0.032). The ORIF group was found to have a larger number of unplanned procedures (37 vs. 16, p = 0.001) which were often of significant magnitude, including one above-knee amputation. Other secondary outcomes of WOMAC scores, quality of reduction, development of osteoarthritis, and SF-36 scores were similar between groups.

Jiang et al. randomized 84 patients with bicondylar tibial plateau fractures to either double plating through 2 incisions or lateral locked plating with the LISS device.[7] Some limitations of this study include concerns that details of the randomization process were not clear and that a-priori primary and secondary outcomes were not discussed. However, a power calculation for HSS scores was presented, which is presumably the primary outcome. This group found no significant difference in HSS score at 12 or 24 months postoperatively (p = 0.215 and p = 0.84). They also found no significant difference in infection rate (5.9% overall (5/84), p = 0.96) or other complications.

Recommendations
• Midline anterior exposure should be avoided when two plates are required in high-energy proximal tibia fractures [overall quality: low]
• There is insufficient evidence to recommend between ORIF, hybrid/circular external fixation, and unilateral locked plating in proximal tibia fractures [overall quality: low]

Question 2: I anticipate a metaphyseal bone void after reduction. Should I fill this with iliac crest autograft or a bone graft substitute?

Relevance
Proximal tibia fractures often are associated with a component of joint surface depression.[1] Elevation of the joint surface to its anatomic location leaves behind a metaphyseal bone void of variable size. It is common practice to fill this resultant void with supportive material to augment internal fixation and support elevated articular bone fragments. Autograft bone, usually from the iliac crest, has been used historically.[1-3] Several bone graft substitute materials have been introduced recently, in part due to the known morbidity of bone graft harvest.

Quality of the evidence
Level I
• 1 systematic review/meta-analysis
• 1 randomized controlled trial (RCT)

Level II
• 2 RCTs with methodologic limitations

Findings
An RCT was published comparing calcium phosphate bone substitute (alpha-BSM) to iliac crest bone graft (ICBG) in tibial plateau fractures.[8] The authors of this study conducted a multicenter trial with patients requiring tibial plateau fracture surgery randomized to either ICBG or alpha-BSM. The primary outcome was joint subsidence as measured on follow-up radiographs. The authors defined significant articular subsidence as greater than 2 mm. They found the ICBG-treated patients to have a subsidence rate of 30% compared to a subsidence rate of 6% in the alpha-BSM treated group (p = 0.009). An unpublished study presented at the Orthopaedic Trauma Association meeting[9]

compared injectable calcium phosphate cement (Norian SRS™) to ICBG. The authors utilized radiostereometry with tantalum bead markers. They found less articular displacement and better functional knee scores in the group treated with bone graft substitute. These studies were included in a meta-analysis exploring the use of calcium phosphate cement in fracture surgery at multiple anatomic sites including the wrist, hip, tibial plateau, and calcaneus.[10] This article described a systematic literature review and analysis of level I studies comparing calcium phosphate cements to bone graft or no grafting. They found calcium phosphate cements to be associated with less pain at the fracture site and with less loss of reduction, especially in tibial plateau patients. Calcium sulfate graft substitutes are also available, but there is minimal evidence supporting their use in tibial plateau fractures. Two case series[11,12] describe the use of calcium sulfate products in tibial plateau fractures, and Kelly et al.[13] describe its use in a mixed group of patients with bone defects. They report radiographic resorption of the material by 3 months; however, complications of sterile drainage (4–8%) and loss of reduction (8–12.5%) are also reported. A randomized trial of grafting anterior cruciate ligament tunnels with calcium sulfate pellets vs. no grafting was reported.[14] They examined pellet resorption and bone growth with CT scans at up to 6 months after surgery. They found that resorption of the calcium sulfate pellets occurred by 6 weeks and that no significant bone growth differences were observed at any point between the treatment groups.

In fractures of the tibial plateau, level I evidence supports the use of calcium phosphate bone graft substitutes instead of ICBG to reduce harvest site related symptoms and to minimize articular collapse of the tibial plateau after surgery. Limited, inconclusive evidence is present regarding use of calcium sulfate bone graft substitutes. No data exists comparing functional outcome of patients treated with ICBG vs. bone graft substitutes. However, the relationship with residual joint incongruity and functional outcome suggests that improved maintenance of anatomic reduction with calcium phosphate bone graft substitute would also lead to a better outcome.

Recommendation
• Calcium phosphate bone substitutes, rather than ICBG or calcium sulfate, should be used when it is desirable to fill a metaphyseal bone void [overall quality: moderate–high]

Question 3: How early should I allow range of motion postoperatively?

Quality of the evidence
Levels III and IV
• 4+ retrospective cohort studies or case series

Findings

Modern fracture treatment principles prescribe early range of motion (ROM).[15] The series by Lucht and Pilgaard[16] noted patients have better clinical results when knee immobilization was less than 8 weeks before initiation of ROM exercises. Rasmussen[17] noted a better ROM among patients immobilized for less than 6 weeks. Volpin[18] showed similar results with better functional ratings and less pain in patients treated with less than 6 weeks of immobilization. Unfortunately, there is no data comparing immediate ROM with a short period of immobilization, so that it is not possible to state whether any immobilization is required at all. While these studies are limited by their retrospective design and lack of validated outcomes, the consistent finding of improved results with decreasing duration of immobilization allows us to recommend joint ROM as early as possible and preferably before 6 weeks.

Recommendation

- Joint ROM should begin as early as possible and preferably before 6 weeks [overall quality: low–moderate]

Question 4: What is the effect of imperfect articular reduction on functional outcomes?

Quality of the evidence

Level II

- 12 prospective studies with limitations and retrospective studies

Relevance

General principles of treatment for articular fractures demand anatomic reduction and stable fixation to permit early motion of the injured joint.[15] This is somewhat controversial in the proximal tibia, as several authors have suggested this joint may tolerate higher ° of articular displacement than other joints.[16,17,19–21]

Findings

Table 61.3 lists the published series which comment on a relationship between accurate joint reduction and clinical outcome. No level I prognostic studies exist (prospective cohort with >80% follow-up).[22] Among the several retrospective series, comparison is difficult due to lack of consistent definitions of malreduction and varied, often nonvalidated, clinical outcome measures. One often-quoted study by Blokker et al.[23] used a composite outcome including a clinical impression and radiographic parameters (residual displacement <5 mm) for their acceptable result. This meant it was impossible for a patient to have an acceptable result if they had residual displacement, regardless of their clinical outcome. Among the other studies, the majority (6 studies including 670 patients)[2,3,24–27] suggest a

relationship between some amount of residual displacement and functional outcome. This includes three modern studies[3,26,27] that use validated outcome measures. Five studies reporting on 562 patients showed no relationship clinical outcome and articular displacement.[16,17,19–21] Unfortunately, the two more recent studies with validated outcomes[20,21] were limited by the small number of patients with a malreduction, thus limiting their statistical ability to show a difference in functional outcomes. Among the more recent series using modern measurement methods,[20,21] there is a consistent finding that residual articular displacement is associated with deterioration in clinical and functional results. However, there is insufficient evidence to support a particular threshold of displacement as an indication for surgical intervention.

Recommendations

- Articular incongruity negatively affects outcomes and should be considered in combination with other injury factors when determining the need for surgical intervention [overall quality: low–moderate]
- When surgery is undertaken the best achievable reduction should be sought but balanced against the potential complications of achieving that reduction [overall quality: low–moderate]

Question 5: What is the effect of limb instability, malalignment, and meniscus cartilage damage on functional outcomes?

Quality of the evidence

Level II

- 12 prospective studies with limitations and retrospective studies

Findings

Joint instability, particularly in the coronal plane, has been suggested to be an important predictor of outcome and thus an indication for surgical stabilization.[17] Many of the studies listed in Table 61.3 regarding articular malreduction also comment on joint instability as a predictor of outcome. However, the modern series using validated outcomes[20,21,25,27] either do not comment on joint instability or have very few patients with significant instability. The classic studies[2,17,19] defined joint stability as less than 10° excess motion in the coronal plane in the extended knee. Instability in the sagittal and rotational planes has not been evaluated scientifically. Restoration of coronal plane stability, by bone elevation/reduction and/or ligament repair, improved clinical results and/or reduced post-traumatic osteoarthritis.[2,11,26] A study exploring post-traumatic osteoarthritis[28] showed a high risk of developing osteoarthritis (69%) was associated with residual knee instability. A limitation of these findings is that all patients with radiographic

Table 61.3 Summary of studies exploring relationship of residual articular displacement on clinical outcome

Reference (publication year)	No. of patients (no.assessed/ total no.)	Association of outcome to accurate reduction (Yes/No)	Reduction threshold suggested	Outcome measure(s)	Comments
Rademakers et al. 2007	109/222	No	2 mm or 5 mm	Neer and HSS knee scores	Neither reduction threshold associated with outcome Few malreductions for comparison
Barei et al. 2006	42/83	Yes	2 mm	MFA	Regression analysis <2 mm associated with better MFA scores
Weigel et al. 2002	23/30	Yes	Linear correlation (r = 0.51;p = 0.01)	SF-36 and Iowa Knee score	Association of residual displacement with bodily pain subscale of SF-36 but not other measures
Stevens et al. 2001	46	No	4 mm	SF-36 and WOMAC	Low numbers and few malreductions for comparison
Kumar and Whittle 2000	54	Yes	Not defined	Knee society score	Better Knee society score in patients with anatomic vs. non-anatomic reduction
Moore et al. 1994	320/988	Yes	Linear correlation Objective: r = 0.42 ; p < 0.001 Subjective: r = 0.26; p < o.001	"arbitrary" objective and subjective knee score	Nonvalidated outcomes Raw data shows similar outcomes until 5–10 mm of residual displacement
Honkonen 1994	131/212	Yes	4 mm	Vague surgeon defined grading as acceptable or not	Proportion of acceptable results lower with residual displacement >4 mm
Duwelius and Connely 1988	96	No	Not defined	Rasmussen's criteria	Vague description and nonvalidated outcomes
Lansinger et al. 1986	102/204	Yes	10 mm	Vague surgeon defined grading of acceptable or not	Longer follow-up of Rasmussen et al. Poorer results in those with >10 mm of joint depression
Blokker et al. 1984	60/64	Yes	5 mm	Vague surgeon defined grading as acceptable or not based on radiographs and clinical criteria	Defined a residual displacement of 5 mm as an unacceptable result therefore impossible for patient to have >5 mm of displacement and acceptable result
Rasmussen 1973	204/260	No	5 mm	Surgeon defined grading system	Insensitive outcome measure
Lucht et al. 1971	107	No	3 and 10 mm	Vague surgeon defined grading of acceptable or not	Insensitive outcome measure

osteoarthritis do not necessarily have severe functional problems. However, based on these retrospective studies, there is consistent level II evidence that joint instability is a significant predictor of worse outcome. Joint instability of more than 10° is an indication for surgery, and joint stabilization by articular elevation/reduction and fixation should be a goal of surgical treatment. If instability persists, ligament repair should be considered.

Proximal tibial malunion resulting in malalignment of the weightbearing axis of the lower extremity has been correlated with worse clinical results.[16,17,19–21,24,28] Unfortunately, there are no series that use validated outcome measures to evaluate the relationship of malalignment and worse function. However, several older studies[17,18,21,28] show increased rates of osteoarthritis in patients with residual coronal plane malalignment. Clinical results were worse in malaligned patients in the series by Honkonen.[24] Each of these studies shows less tolerance of varus malalignment compared to valgus malalignment. Clinical outcomes and rates of osteoarthritis worsen with even small amounts of varus, while valgus malalignment is tolerated up to 5–10°.[17,21,24] Osteoarthritis rates increase in the setting of malalignment and meniscectomy.[28,29] The consistency of these retrospective studies allows us to recommend articular malalignment of greater than 10° of valgus or any varus as indications for surgery, with a goal of reducing this malalignment via the surgical procedure. The meniscus is now recognized as an important structure, especially in the traumatized knee, and should be repaired when possible and not be removed.

Recommendation

- Joint instability or more than 10° is an indication for surgery and joint stabilization should be a goal of surgical treatment [overall quality: moderate]
- Articular malalignment of greater than 10° of valgus or any varus are indications for surgery with a goal of reducing this malalignment during the surgical procedure [overall quality: moderate]
- Menisci should be repaired when possible and not removed [overall quality: moderate]

Summary of recommendations

- Midline anterior exposure should be avoided when two plates are required in high-energy proximal tibia fractures
- There is insufficient evidence to recommend between open reduction internal fixation, hybrid/circular external fixation, and unilateral locked plating in proximal tibia fractures
- Calcium phosphate bone substitutes, rather than ICBG or calcium sulfate, should be used when it is desirable to fill a metaphyseal bone void

- Joint ROM should begin as early as possible and preferably before 6 weeks
- Articular incongruity negatively affects outcomes should be considered in combination with other injury factors when determining the need for surgical intervention
- When surgery is undertaken the best achievable reduction should be sought but balanced against the potential complications of achieving that reduction
- Joint instability or more than 10° is an indication for surgery and joint stabilization should be a goal of surgical treatment
- Articular malalignment of more than 10° of valgus or any varus are indications for surgery with a goal of reducing this malalignment during the surgical procedure
- Menisci should be repaired when possible and not be removed

References

1. Schatzker J, McBroom R, Bruce D. The tibial plateau fracture. The Toronto experience 1968–1975. Clin Orthop Relat Res 1979;138:94–104.
2. Lansinger O, Bergman B, Komer L, Andersson GB. Tibial condylar fractures. A twenty year follow-up. J Bone Joint Surg Am 1986;68:13–19.
3. Moore TM, Patzakis MJ, Harvey JP. Tibial plateau fractures: definition, demograpics, treatment rationale, and long-term results of closed traction management or operative reduction. J Orthop Trauma 1987;1(2):97–119.
4. Young MJ, Barrack RL. Complications of internal fixation of tibial plateau fractures. Orthop Rev 1994;23(2) 149–154.
5. Tscherne H, Lobenhoffer P. Tibial plateau fractures: management and expected results. Clin Orthop Relat Res 1993;292:87–100.
6. Canadian Orthopaedic Trauma Society. Open reduction and internal fixation compared with circular fixator application for bicondylar tibial plateau fractures. Results of a multicenter, prospective, randomized clinical trial. J Bone and Joint Surg Am 2006;88(12):2613–23.
7. Jiang R, Luo CF, Wang MC, Yang TY, Zeng BF. A comparative study of Less Invasive Stabilization System (LISS) fixation and two-incision double plating for the treatment of bicondylar tibial plateau fractures. Knee 2008;15:139–43.
8. Russell TA, Leighton RK. Alpha-BSM tibial plateau study group. Comparison of autogenous bone graft and endothermic calcium phosphate cement for defect augmentation in tibial plateau fractures. A multicenter, prospective randomized study. J Bone Joint Surg Am 2008;90:2057–61.
9. Larsson S, Berg P, Sagerfors M. Augmentation of tibial plateau fractures with calcium phosphate cement: a randomized study using radiostereometry. http://www.hwbf.org/ota/am/ota04/otapa/OTA04210.htm. Accessed December 31, 2009.
10. Bajammal SS, Zlowdski M, Lelwica A, et al. The use of calcium phosphate bone cement in fracture treatment. a meta-analysis of randomized trials. J Bone Joint Surg 2008;90:1186–96.
11. Lobenhoffer P, Gerich T, Witte F, Tscherne H. Use of calcium phosphate bone cement in the treatment of tibial plateau

fractures: a prospective study of twenty-six cases with twenty month mean follow-up. J Orthop Trauma 2002;16(3):143–49.

12. Watson JT. The use of an injectable bone graft substitute in tibial metaphyseal fractures. Orthopedics 2004;27(1 Suppl): s103–7.

13. Kelly CM, Wilkins RM, Gitelis S, Hartjen C, Watson JT, Kim PT. The use of a surgical grade calcium sulfate as a bone graft substitute: results of a multicenter trial. Clin Orthop Relat Res 2001;382:42–50.

14. Petruskevicius J, Nielsen S, Kaalund S, Knudsen PR, Overgaard S. No effect of Osteoset, a bone graft substitute, on bone healing in humans: a prospective randomized double-blind study. Acta Orthop Scand 2002;73(5):575–8.

15. Mueller ME, Allgower M, Schneider R, Willneger H, Perren SM. Manual of Internal Fixation: Techniques Recommended by the AO-ASIF group. Springer, New York, 1995.

16. Lucht U, Pilgaard S. Fractures of the tibial condyles. Acta Orthop Scand 1971;42(4):366–76.

17. Rasmussen P, Tibial condylar fractures: impairment of knee joint stability as an indication for surgical treatment. J Bone Joint Surg Am 1973;55:1331–50.

18. Volpin G, Dowd GSE, Stein H, Bentley G. Degenerative arthritis after intra-articular fractures of the knee. Long term results. J Bone Joint Surg Br 1990;72(4):634–8.

19. Duwelius PJ, Connoly JF. Closed reduction of tibial plateau fractures: a comparison of functional and roentgenographic end results. Clin Orthop Relat Res 1988;230:116–26.

20. Stevens DG, Beharry R, McKee MD, Waddell JP, Schemitsch EH. The long term functional outcome of operatively treated tibial plateau fractures. J Orthop Trauma 2001;15:312–20.

21. Rademakers MV, Kerkhoffs GMMJ, Sierevelt IN, Raamakers ELFB, Marti RK. Operative treatment of 109 tibial plateau fractures: Five to 27 year follow-up results. J Orthop Trauma 2007; 21(1):5–10.

22. Bhandari M, Joensson A. Clinical Research for Surgeons. Thieme, New York, 2009.

23. Blokker CP, Rorabeck CH, Bourne RB. Tibial plateau fractures: an analysis of results of treatment in 60 patients. Clin Orthop Relat Res 1984;182:193–9.

24. Honkonen SE. Indications for surgical treatment of tibial condyle fractures. Clin Orthop Relat Res 1994;302:199–205.

25. Kumar A, Whittle AP. Treatment of complex (Schatzker Type VI) fractures of the tibial plateau with circular wire external fixation: retrospective case review. J Orthop Trauma 2000;14(5): 339–44.

26. Weigel DP, Marsh JL. High energy fractures of the tibial plateau. Knee function after longer term follow-up. J Bone Joint Surg Am 2002;84(9):1541–51.

27. Barei DP, Nork SE, Mills WJ, Henley MB, Benirschke SK. Complications associated with internal fixation of high-energy bicondylar tibial plateau fractures utilizing a two-incision technique. J Orthop Trauma 2004;18(10):649–657.

28. Honkonen SE. Degenerative arthritis after tibial plateau fractures. J Orthop Trauma 1995;9(4):273–277.

29. Jensen D, Rude C, Duus B, Bjerg-Nielsen A. Tibial Plateau Fractures. A comparison of conservative and surgical treatment. J Bone Joint Surg Br 1990;72:49–52.

62 Tibial Shaft

Jennifer A. Klok
University of Ottawa, Ottawa, ON, Canada

Case scenario

A 29 year old man is brought to the Emergency Department following a motor vehicle collision. On examination the right lower leg is swollen and deformed and an open wound is noted. He is neurovascularly intact and there are no signs of compartment syndrome on initial clinical evaluation.

Relevant anatomy

Fractures of the tibial shaft (diaphysis) are defined by the Orthopedic Trauma Association as simple, wedge, and complex.[1] A detailed classification is presented in Table 62.1. Open fractures are generally described using the Gustilo classification (Table 62.2).[2]

Importance of the problem

Tibial shaft fractures are one of the most common long bone fractures presenting to the Emergency Department each year. The incidence of tibial and fibular fractures is approximately 500,000 per year in the United States.[3,4] The management of tibial fractures can be complex and complication rates high. Thus, knowledge of the evidence in current literature with respect to care of patients with these fractures is paramount.

Intramedullary (IM) nailing has become the generally accepted standard of management for displaced tibial fractures, but controversy concerning optimal treatment for these injuries continues to exist. This is largely due to the variations in degree of trauma and extent of soft tissue damage which have an impact on overall outcome. The nature of injury to the tibia may result in inadequacy of vascular supply and tissue coverage, and can make these diaphyseal fractures particularly prone to poor healing and infection.[4] It is the intention of this chapter to explore the best available research on areas of controversy in the management of tibial shaft fractures and provide the reader with recommendations for patient care.

Top six questions

Therapy

1. Is there any difference in outcomes between reamed and unreamed IM nails?
2. What is the best management of open tibial shaft fractures?
3. What is the best management for closed tibial shaft fractures?
4. Does low-intensity pulsed ultrasound (LIPUS) aid in the healing of tibial shaft fractures?

Prognosis

5. Is dissection of the patellar tendon in IM nailing of the tibia associated with chronic anterior knee pain?
6. What is the relative effect of reaming and intraoperative traction on the risk of compartment syndrome (CS)?

Finding the evidence

The following general searches were undertaken to identify the best evidence (meta-analyses, systematic reviews, and clinical trials) on tibial shaft fractures. More detailed search terms are outlined under each question.
- Cochrane Database: search term "tibial fractures"

Evidence-Based Orthopedics, First Edition. Edited by Mohit Bhandari.
© 2012 Blackwell Publishing Ltd. Published 2012 by Blackwell Publishing Ltd.

Table 62.1 Classification of tibial shaft fractures

Type	Fracture pattern	Description
A	Simple	A1: Spiral A2: Oblique (≥30°) A3: Transverse (<30°)
B	Wedge	B1: Spiral B2: Bending B3: Fragmented
C	Complex (comminuted)	C1: Spiral C2: Segmented C3: Irregular

Table 62.2 Gustilo classification of open tibial shaft fractures

Grade	Description
I	Skin opening: <1 cm
	Fracture pattern: short oblique or transverse
II	Skin opening: >1 cm
	Fracture pattern: short oblique or transverse, minimal comminution
III	General: high energy injury with extensive soft tissue damage (including neurovascular structures)
	Grade IIIA: 10 cm skin opening; soft tissue coverage of bone adequate
	Grade IIIB: tissue damage includes periosteal stripping and typically requires flap repair
	Grade IIIC: Requires vascular repair

- PubMed: (www.ncbi.nlm.nih.gov/pubmed/) clinical queries search/systematic reviews: "tibial fractures" OR "tibial shaft fractures" OR "tibial shaft"
- PubMed: advanced search/type of article/randomized control trials: "tibial fractures" OR "tibial shaft fractures"
- MEDLINE search: population ("tibial fracture" or "tibial shaft fractures"); methodology (clinical trial)

Question 1: Is there any difference in outcomes between reamed and unreamed IM nails?

Case clarification

The patient has an open fracture of the right tibia. The fracture will be treated with IM nailing and you consider whether reaming will be beneficial for your patient.

Relevance

Controversy about the superiority of the reamed over the unreamed technique in IM nailing of the tibia has been ongoing for many years. The reamed procedure has the advantage of creating space for a larger nail, which improves overall stability of the fracture. However, the process of reaming may destroy endosteal blood supply, thereby decreasing healing and increasing risk of infection.

Current opinion

IM nailing of the tibia is the preferred surgical method of treatment for displaced diaphyseal fractures. Opinions about whether or not to ream remain varied.

Finding the evidence

- Terms: "tibial fracture," "tibial shaft fractures," "intramedullary nailing"

Quality of the evidence

Level I

- 2 systematic reviews/meta-analyses
- 4 randomized trials

Level II

- 7 randomized trials with methodologic limitations

Findings

The pooled results of a meta-analysis comparing reamed to unreamed nails in long bone fractures of the lower extremity[5] are shown in Table 62.3. No risk differences were found for the rates of malunion, pulmonary embolism, CS, or infection.

Results of a systematic review of three trials evaluating effects of reamed and unreamed nails in tibial shaft fractures are also shown in Table 62.3 (n = 291).[6]

A large multicentere trial (n = 1319 patients) randomized patients to reamed or unreamed IM nailing of the tibia.[7] Results are provided in Table 62.4. Note that the significant findings for the closed fracture subgroup analysis may reflect the higher rates of dynamization in this group.

Recommendations

- Reamed IM nailing reduces the risk of reoperation at 1 year in closed tibial shaft fractures compared to unreamed IM nailing [overall quality: high]
- There is no difference in reoperation risk between reamed and unreamed IM nailing of tibial shaft fractures (open and closed) [overall quality: high]
- The risk of nonunion and implant failure is higher in unreamed compared to reamed IM nailing [overall quality: moderate]

Table 62.3 Effect of reamed vs. unreamed IM nailing of the tibia

Study	Outcome	N	Trials	Risk	95% CI	p value
Bhandari et al. 2000	Nonunion	646	9	RR 0.33	0.16–0.68	0.0019
	Implant failure*	358	4	RR 0.30	0.16–0.58	<0.001
Forster et al. 2005	Nonunion	291	3	OR 2.83	1.16–6.68	0.02
	Implant failure	291	3	OR 3.57	1.92–6.66	<0.001
Bhandari et al. 2008	Reoperation at 12 months (all fractures)	1319	1	RR 0.90	0.71–1.15	0.40
	Reoperation at 12 months (closed fractures)	826	1	RR 0.67	0.47–0.96	0.03

OR, odds ratio; RR, relative risk.

Table 62.4 Comparison of risk of reoperation in treatment of open tibial fractures

Intervention	N	Trials	RR[a]	95% CI	p value
External fixator vs. plate	56	1	0.13	0.03–0.54	<0.01
External fixator vs. unreamed nails	396	5	0.51	0.37–0.69	<0.001
Reamed vs. unreamed nails	132	2	0.75	0.43–1.32	0.32
Reamed nails vs. external fixators (indirect analysis)	—	—	0.56	0.19–0.95	<0.05

95%CI, confidence interval; N, total sample size pooled; RR, relative risk.
[a]The relative risk of reoperation when first listed intervention compared to second intervention Values<1.0 favor first intervention, values>1.0 favor second intervention.

Question 2: What is the best management of open tibial shaft fractures?

Case clarification
Your patient has an open tibial shaft fracture. Recognizing the complex nature of these fractures, you want to know the optimal treatment for decreasing complications and minimizing undesirable outcomes such as reoperation, nonunion, malunion, infection, and implant failure.

Relevance
There are several options for treatment of open tibial fractures. These include plate fixation, external fixation, unreamed IM nail, and reamed IM nails. The main concerns with open tibial shaft fractures are adequate blood supply and soft tissue coverage necessary for fracture union and infection reduction.

Current opinion
IM nailing of the tibia has been generally accepted for treatment of open tibial shaft fractures, although there are proponents of external fixation (EF).

Finding the evidence
- Search terms: "open tibial fracture," "open tibial shaft fractures"

Quality of the evidence
Level I
- 1 systematic review/meta-analysis
- 4 randomized trials

Level II
- 4 randomized trials with methodological limitations

Findings
Bhandari et al. conducted a meta-analysis primarily evaluating rates of reoperation with different methods of treatment for open tibial shaft fractures.[8] Eight trials were included in the analysis. Results are shown in Table 62.4 and Figure 62.1.

Secondary outcomes of nonunion, malunion, superficial and deep infection, and implant failure were also evalu-

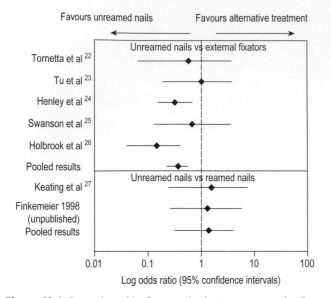

Figure 62.1 Comparing odds of reoperation between unreamed nails and external fixators, unreamed and reamed nails. Reproduced with permission and copyright © of the British Editorial Society of Bone and Joint Surgery. Bhandari M, Guyatt GH, Swiontkowski MF, Schemitsch EH. Treatment of open fractures of the shaft of the tibia: a systematic overview and meta-analysis. J Bone Joint Surg [Br] 2001;83-B:62–8.

ated. No significant differences were found between plate and EF for these outcomes. However, point estimates for all outcomes favored EF. Results of five trials revealed that risk of malunion (RR 0.42, 95% CI 0.25–0.71) and superficial infection (RR 0.24, 95% CI 0.08–0.73) were significantly less in unreamed nails compared to EF. Two trials comparing reamed to unreamed IM nails (n = 156) showed the risk of implant failure to be less in reaming of the tibia (RR 0.32, 95% CI 0.17–0.89, p < 0.025).

Grade IIIB fractures The meta-analysis[8] reported outcomes comparing EF with unreamed IM nailing in grade IIIB fractures (n = 45 patients). The results did not reveal significant differences between unreamed nails and EF with respect to nonunion (RR 0.70, 95% CI 0.24–2.43) or deep infection (RR 1.95, 95% CI 0.39–9.89). Additionally, when reamed and unreamed IM nailing was compared in grade IIIB fractures (n = 11 patients), the risks of nonunion (RR 1.14, 95% CI 0.15–8.99) and deep infection (RR 1.88, 95% CI 0.09–37.63) did not significantly differ between groups.

Two-stage management With respect to two-stage management, a systematic review[9] included a single randomized controlled trial (RCT)[10] which compared outcomes in patients who had been randomized to cast or IM nailing treatment following EF. The rate of union was significantly higher in the IM nailing group (94% vs. 64%, RR 4.8, p = 0.02). Weighted estimates from this trial and 21 case series (n = 504) in the review revealed that infection rates

were reduced when the interval between removal of the external fixator to IM nailing was shorter (≤14 days, RRR = 85%, 95% CI 68–93%, p < 0.001). Additionally, short EF periods (≤28 days) decreased risk of infection (RRR = 83%, 95% CI 62–93%, p < 0.001).

Recommendations

• The risk of reoperation with EF is lower than plate fixation in open tibial shaft fractures [overall quality: low]
• The risks of reoperation, malunion, and superficial infection in unreamed nailing of open fractures is less than EF [overall quality: moderate]
• The risks of implant failure in reamed IM nails is less than unreamed IM nails [overall quality: moderate]
• The risks of reoperation is reduced in reamed IM nailing of open tibial shaft fractures compared to EF [overall quality: low]
• The is no significant difference in the risk of nonunion or deep infection in grade IIIB tibial fractures when EF is compared to unreamed IM nailing, or in the comparison of reamed to unreamed nailing [overall quality: low–moderate]
• When EF is used as a preliminary step to IM nailing, shortening the EF duration and the period between EF removal and IM nailing reduces risk of infection. Well-designed prospective clinical trials are necessary for confirmation [overall quality: low–moderate]

Question 3: What is the best management for closed tibial shaft fractures?

Case clarification
Although your patient has an open tibial shaft fracture, you are interested in knowing if current evidence supports interventions such as casting, plating, and IM nailing in the treatment of closed tibial fractures.

Relevance
Closed tibial fractures may be treated with casting, IM nailing, or plating. Results in recent literature may challenge historical management of these fractures.

Current opinion
IM nailing is becoming the preferred method of fixation for closed tibial shaft fractures.[4]

Finding the evidence
• Search terms: "closed tibial fracture," "closed tibial shaft fracture"

Quality of the evidence
Level I
• 2 systematic reviews/meta-analyses
• 3 randomized trials

Level II
- 3 randomized trials with methodologic limitations

Findings

Littenberg et al. conducted a meta-analysis evaluating three different methods of treating closed tibial shaft fractures (casting, ORIF, IM rod).[11] There were few studies fitting the inclusion criteria; because of the lack of randomized trials, several nonrandomized trials and case series were included in the analysis. The review found the risk of superficial infections to be lower in casting compared to ORIF (OR 0.20, 95% CI 0.08–0.50, RD –5.81, $p = 0.02$). Casting was associated with a lower rate of union at 20 weeks compared to ORIF (OR 0.21, 95% CI 0.06–0.68, RD –18.07, $p = 0.008$). No significant differences (i.e., where $p < 0.05$) were found in mortality rates, "deep infection", reoperation, or nonunion following cast treatment.

The results of the meta-analysis by Coles et al. presented average values for the outcomes of the various closed reduction treatments.[12] Mean time to union was lowest in plate fixation (14.9 weeks) compared to IM nailing (19.5 weeks unreamed; 20.2 weeks reamed). Rates of delayed union and nonunion (combined) were lower in plate fixation (2.6%) compared to IM nailing (16.7% unreamed; 8.0% reamed). Reoperation rates were as follows: 4.7% plate fixation; 8.3% casting; 12.4% reamed nailing; 23.1% unreamed nailing.

Recommendations

- Treatment of closed tibial shaft fractures with casting has a lower risk of superficial infections compared to ORIF [overall quality: low]
- ORIF of closed tibial fractures has a higher rate of union compared to casting [overall quality: low]
- Evidence on the best method of closed tibial shaft fracture treatment is poor [overall quality: low]

Question 4: Does LIPUS aid in the healing of tibial shaft fractures?

Case clarification

You would like to optimize the healing process for your patient as much as possible and are interested in the efficacy of LIPUS in the management of tibial shaft fractures.

Relevance

The use of bone stimulators in fracture healing has received increasing attention over the past decade. LIPUS has been found to enhance the four stages of fracture healing (inflammation, soft callus formation, hard callus formation, remodeling) in laboratory studies.[13] However, studies to date are conflicting and scrutiny of the current literature is required before this method can be employed in the regular management of tibial fractures.

Current opinion

LIPUS is used by 21% of orthopedic surgeons in Canada in the management of tibial shaft fractures.[4]

Finding the evidence

- Search terms: "tibial fracture," "tibial shaft fracture," "fractures," "ultrasound," "low intensity pulsed ultrasound"

Quality of the evidence

Level I
- 4 systematic reviews/meta-analyses
- 4 randomized trials

Level II
- 3 randomized trials with methodologic limitations

Findings

A systematic review of trials evaluating healing time in fractures reported results for several studies on tibial shaft fractures.[14] The pooled effect of LIPUS in healing of tibial shaft fractures managed operatively was nonsignificant. Significant results in the study of conservatively managed tibial fractures supported the use of LIPUS in fracture healing (Table 62.5).

This same study was used in a meta-analysis of three trials comparing healing time in patients (n = 158) with fractures (tibial, distal radius, and scaphoid) treated with LIPUS or placebo.[17] The results for radiographic healing (3 of 4 cortices) were significant and revealed a decrease in healing time of 64 days in patients treated with LIPUS (effect size = 6.41, 95% CI 1.01–11.81). A trial evaluating healing time in tibial and radius fracture (n = 158) found that in tibial fractures, healing time was decreased in smokers treated with LIPUS by 41% ($p < 0.006$) and in non-smokers by 26% ($p < 0.05$).[17]

Table 62.5 Comparison of tibial shaft fracture healing with LIPUS

Method of fracture treatment	N	Trials	% reduction in healing time	95% CI
Operative (pooled)	62	2	16.6	76.8–60.7
Emami[15]	32	1	–24.0	–71.9 to 10.6
Leung[16]	30	1	42.5	31.7–51.6
Conservative	67	1	46.3	33.8–56.5

95%CI, confidence interval; N, total sample size pooled.

The results of two other systematic reviews[13,18] reported similarly on the studies discussed above. The conflicting outcomes are suggested to be the result of variations in the initiation and duration of LIPUS or the type and treatment of the fractures studied.

Recommendation
- The evidence supporting the use of LIPUS in the healing of tibial shaft fractures is conflicting and inconclusive [overall quality: low]

Question 5: Is dissection of the patellar tendon in IM nailing of the tibia associated with chronic anterior knee pain?

Case clarification
You will fix the tibial shaft fracture with an IM nail, but recognize that chronic anterior knee pain may be a residual effect of the procedure. You consider a paratendinous approach in anticipation that this will reduce painful outcomes in your patient.

Relevance
While current operative management of tibial shaft fractures is through IM nailing, anterior knee pain is recognized as an adverse outcome associated with this procedure. The reasons for this outcome are not well understood and are thought to be multifactorial. Dissection of the patellar tendon in IM nailing may risk factor for the development of chronic anterior knee pain.[19–21]

Current opinion
The causes of postoperative knee pain in IM nailing of the tibia are undetermined, and surgical approach varies among surgeons.

Finding the evidence
- Search terms: "tibial fracture," "tibial shaft fracture," "knee pain," "anterior knee pain," "intramedullary nailing"

Quality of the evidence
Level II
- 1 randomized trials with methodologic limitations

Findings
A randomized trial (n = 50 patients) comparing paratendinous (incision medial to the patellar tendon) to transtendinous (incision through the patellar tendon) in IM nailing reported outcomes at 3 and 8 years following surgery.[20] Anterior knee pain was evaluated in multiple ways, including a pain and impairment visual analog scale (VAS), simple functional tests, thigh muscle strength, and the Iowa knee scoring system.

No significant differences in knee pain were found between the two surgical approaches at either 3 or 8 years.[20,21] In both groups, the prevalence of knee pain decreased from 75% (at 3 years) to 29% (at 8 years). The number of patients in this study is small may not have enough power to show the true effect of patellar dissection in IM nailing.

Recommendations
- Evidence regarding the association between anterior knee pain and dissection of the patellar tendon in IM nailing of the tibia is limited. It cannot be said that one approach has greater risks than another [overall quality: low]
- The prevalence of anterior knee pain after IM nailing of the tibia decreases with time [overall quality: low]

Question 6: What is the relative effect of reaming and intraoperative traction on the risk of CS in patients undergoing IM nailing of the tibia?

Case clarification
You are concerned about the development of postoperative CS in your patient and would like to know if intraoperative steps can be taken to reduce the risk of this complication.

Relevance
CS has been reported to have a higher incidence following intraoperative traction. Additionally, concern exists about the risks associated with reaming of the tibia and the development of CS.[20,21]

Current opinion
Current practice is divided about the use of intraoperative traction and reaming in the treatment of tibial shaft fractures.

Finding the evidence
- Search terms: "tibial fracture," "tibial shaft fracture," "compartment syndrome"

Quality of the evidence
Level II
- 2 randomized trials with methodologic limitations

Findings
Does intraoperative traction increase the risk of CS? A single trial randomized patients (n = 30) with Tscherne CI fractures to traction or no traction during reamed IM nailing of the tibial shaft.[20] Pressures were measured in all four compartments immediately before and after surgery. Postoperative measurements in all compartments

were significantly (p < 0.05) higher in the traction group (6.8–8.5 mmHg).

Does reaming increase risk of CS? A small (n = 48) trial recorded compartment pressures preoperatively, intraoperatively, and for 24 hours postoperatively in patients who had been randomized to reamed or unreamed IM nailing of the tibia (no fracture tables or skeletal traction used).[21] Though no patients developed CS, peak average pressures in the deep posterior compartment were significantly higher (p < 0.05) in the unreamed group at 10–24 hours postoperatively. Measurements at 24 hours were provided (reamed 9.5 mmHg, unreamed 19.8 mmHg, p = 0.0143). ΔP was significantly higher (i.e., compartment pressure was lower) in the reamed group at 14 hours (reamed 64.4 mmHg, unreamed 48.0 mmHg, p = 0.0012) and at 18 hours (reamed 62.mmHg, unreamed 52.1 mmHg, p = 0.04).

Recommendations

• Acute (≤3 days) reamed IM nailing of closed, displaced tibia fractures does not increase the risk of CS [overall quality: low]
• Intraoperative traction increases the risk of compartment syndrome in IM nailing of the tibial shaft [overall quality: low]

Summary of recommendations

• Reamed IM nailing in closed tibial shaft fractures reduces the risk of reoperation at 1 year compared to unreamed IM nailing
• There is no difference in risk of reoperation between reamed and unreamed IM nailing of tibial shaft fractures (open and closed)
• The risk of nonunion and implant failure is higher in unreamed compared to reamed IM nailing
• The risk of reoperation with EF is lower than plate fixation in open tibial shaft fractures
• The risk of reoperation, malunion, and superficial infection in unreamed nailing of open fractures is less than EF
• The risk of implant failure in reamed IM nails is less than unreamed IM nails
• The risk of reoperation is reduced in reamed IM nailing of open tibial shaft fractures compared to EF
• There is no significant difference in the risk of nonunion or deep infection in grade IIIB tibial fractures when EF is compared to unreamed IM nailing, or in the comparison of reamed to unreamed nailing
• When EF is used as a preliminary step to IM nailing, shortening the EF duration and the period between EF removal and IM nailing reduces risk of infection. Well-designed prospective clinical trials are necessary for confirmation

• Treatment of closed tibial shaft fractures with casting has a lower risk of superficial infections compared to ORIF
• ORIF of closed tibial fractures has a higher rate of union compared to casting
• Evidence on the best method of closed tibial shaft fracture treatment is poor
• Evidence supporting the use of LIPUS in the healing of tibial shaft fractures is inconclusive
• No strong association between anterior knee pain and surgical approach in IM nailing of the tibia has been shown
• The prevalence of anterior knee pain after IM nailing of the tibia decreases with time
• Acute (≤3 days) reamed IM nailing of closed, displaced tibia fractures does not increase the risk of CS
• Intraoperative traction increases the risk of compartment syndrome in IM nailing of the tibial shaft

Conclusions

Management of tibial shaft fractures continues to be a complex and controversial issue. Levels of evidence in this area have improved over the years, but high-quality studies are still in their infancy. Certain topics have been adequately explored and have enough strength to change clinical practice. In particular, IM nailing has been shown to be the treatment of choice for tibial shaft fractures. Additionally, the use of reamed vs. unreamed nails has been an issue of controversy over the years, but there is strong evidence to support the use of reamed over unreamed nails in closed tibial shaft fractures. More large and methodologically rigorous randomized trials are required to bring clarification to the questions that still remain.

References

1. Orthopedic Trauma Association. Fracture and Dislocation Classification Compendium 2007. Orthopaedic Trauma Association/Classification, Database & Outcomes Committee. Available at http://www.ota.org/compendium/compendium.html. Accessed Jan 1, 2010.
2. Gustilo RB, Anderson JT. Prevention of infection in the treatment of one thousand and twenty-five open fractures of long bones: retrospective and prospective analyses. J Bone Joint Surg Am 1976;58:453–8.
3. Bhandari M, Guyatt GH, Tornetta P 3rd, et al. Current practice in the intramedullary nailing of tibial shaft fractures: an international survey. J Trauma 2002;53:725–32.
4. Busse JW, Morton E, Lacchetti C, Guyatt GH, Bhandari M. Current management of tibial shaft fractures: a survey of 450 Canadian orthopedic trauma surgeons. Acta Orthop 2008;79:689–94.

5. Bhandari M, Guyatt GH, Tong D, Adili A, Shaughnessy SG. Reamed versus non-reamed intramedullary nailing of lower extremity long bone fractures: a systematic overview and meta-analysis. J Orthop Trauma 2000;14:2–9.

6. Forster MC, Bruce AS, Aster AS. Should the tibia be reamed when nailing? Injury 2005;36:439–44.

7. Bhandari M, Guyatt G, Tornetta P 3rd, et al. Randomized trial of reamed and unreamed intramedullary nailing of tibial shaft fractures. J Bone Joint Surg Am 2008;90:2567–78.

8. Bhandari M, Guyatt GH, Swiontkowski MF, Schemitsch EH. Treatment of open fractures of the shaft of the tibia. J Bone Joint Surg Br 2001;83:62–8.

9. Bhandari M, Zlowodzki M, Tornetta P 3rd, Schmidt A, Templeman DC. Intramedullary nailing following external fixation in femoral and tibial shaft fractures. J Orthop Trauma 2005;19:140–4.

10. Antich-Adrover P, Marti-Garin D, Murias-Alvarez J, et al. External fixation and secondary intramedullary nailing of open tibial fractures. A randomised, prospective trial. J Bone Joint Surg Br 1997;79:433–7.

11. Littenberg B, Weinstein LP, McCarren M, et al. Closed fractures of the tibial shaft. A meta-analysis of three methods of treatment. J Bone Joint Surg Am 1999;80:174–83.

12. Coles CP, Gross M. Closed tibial shaft fractures: management and treatment complications. A review of the prospective literature. Can J Surg 2000;43:256–62.

13. Mundi R, Petis S, Kaloty R, Shetty V, Bhandari M. Low-intensity pulsed ultrasound: Fracture healing. Indian J Orthop 2009;43:132–40.

14. Busse JW, Kaur J, Mollon B, Bhandari M, et al. Low intensity pulsed ultrasonography for fractures: systematic review of randomised controlled trials. BMJ 2009;338, b351.

15. Emami A, Petren-Mallmin M, Larsson S. No effect of low-intensity ultrasound on healing time of intramedullary fixed tibial fractures. J Orthop Trauma 1999;13:252–7.

16. Leung KS, Lee WS, Tsui HF, Liu PP, Cheung WH. Complex tibial fracture outcomes following treatment with low-intensity pulsed ultrasound. Ultrasound Med Bio 2004;30:389–395.

17. Walker NA, Denegar CR, Preische J. Low-intensity pulsed ultrasound and pulsed electromagnetic field in the treatment of tibial fractures: a systematic review. J Athl Train 2007;42:530–5.

18. Busse JW, Bhandari M, Kulkarni AV, Tunks E. The effect of low-intensity pulsed ultrasound therapy on time to fracture healing: a meta-analysis. CMAJ 2002;166:437–41.

19. Lefaivre KA, Guy P, Chan H, Blachut PA. Long-term follow-up of tibial shaft fractures treated with intramedullary nailing. J Orthop Trauma 2008;22:525–9.

20. Toivanen JA, Väistö O, Kannus P, Latvala K, Honkonen SE, Järvinen MJ. Anterior knee pain after intramedullary nailing of fractures of the tibial shaft. A prospective, randomized study comparing two different nail-insertion techniques. J Bone Joint Surg Am 2002;84:580–5.

21. Väistö O, Toivanen J, Kannus P, Järvinen M. Anterior knee pain after intramedullary nailing of fractures of the tibial shaft: an eight-year follow-up of a prospective, randomized study comparing two different nail-insertion techniques. J Orthop Trauma 2008;64:1511–16.

22. Tornetta P III, Bergman M, Watnik N, Berkowitz G, Steuer J. Treatment of grade IIIB open tibial fractures: a prospective randomized comparison of external rotation and non-reamed locked nailing. J Bone Joint Surg Br 1994;76-B:13–9.

23. Tu YK, Lin CH, Su JI, Hsu DT, Chen RJ. Unreamed interlocking nail versus external fixator for open type III tibia fractures. J Trauma 1995;39:361–7.

24. Henley MB, Chapman JR, Agel J, et al. Treatment of II, IIIA and IIIB open fractures of the tibial shaft: a prospective comparison of unreamed interlocking intramedullary nails and half-pin external fixators. J Orthop Trauma 1998;12:1–7.

25. Swanson TV, Spiegel JD, Sutherland TB, Bray TJ, Chapman MW. A prospective evaluation of the lottes nail versus external fixation in 100 open tibial fractures. Orthop Trans 1990;14:716.

26. Holbrook JL, Swiontkowski MF, Sanders R. Treatment of open fractures of the tibial shaft: Ender nailing versus external fixation: a randomised, prospective comparison. J Bone Joint Surg Am 1989;71-A:1231–8.

27. Keating JF, O'Brien PJ, Blachut PA, Meek RN, Broekhuyse HM. Locking intramedullary nailing with and without reaming for open fractures of the tibial shaft: a prospective, randomized study. J Bone Joint Surg Am 1997;79-A:334–41.

Hossein Pakzad and Peter J. O'Brien
University of British Columbia, Vancouver, BC, Canada

Case scenario

The patient is a 30-year-old man who was involved in a motor vehicle accident. He suffered an isolated injury to his right ankle. He presented to the Emergency Department with pain, swelling, and inability to bear weight.

Relevant anatomy

The distal tibial articular surface is known as the plafond, which along with the medial and lateral malleoli forms the mortise to articulate with the talar dome. The plafond is concave in the sagittal plane and flat, or more often slightly convex, in the coronal plane. It is wider in the anterior plane to provide stability, especially while weightbearing. Ligaments providing support about the distal tibia include the tibiofibular ligament (anterior, posterior, and transverse portions), the interosseous ligament, and the strong deltoid ligament (divided into superficial and deep portions).

Pilon or plafond fractures are nonmalleolar distal tibia intra-articular fractures. They commonly occur either as a result of a high-energy axial compression load (a fall from height or motor vehicle accident) or as a result of rotational forces.

Axial compression type fractures typically have greater metaphyseal and articular comminution, greater soft tissue injury, swelling, and articular cartilage damage.

Fractures resulting from rotational forces typically have a spiral shape with minimal to moderate displacement of the fracture fragments and minimal soft tissue injury, although significant swelling may occur.

Traditionally, plafond fractures have been classified by Ruedi and Allgower[1] (level III) to three different types (Figure 63.1).

Traditional classification of plafond fractures
- Type I: simple fracture pattern without intra-articular displacement
- Type II: displaced intra-articular fracture with minimal comminution
- Type III: displaced intra-articular fracture with articular and metaphyseal comminution

The comprehensive AO/OTA classification[2] (level V) for long bone fractures permits more detailed information. In this classification type A is a nonarticular fracture (A1, A2, A3), type B is a partial articular fracture (B1, B2, B3), and type C is a total articular fracture (C1, C2, C3) (Figure 63.2).

AO/OTA classification of plafond fractures

Type A: Distal tibial metaphyseal injuries without intra-articular extension
- A1: simple
- A2: wedged or comminuted
- A3: complex or severely comminuted

Type B: Partial articular fractures
- B1: pure split
- B2: split-depression
- B3: multifragmentary depression

Type C: Fracture involves the entire joint surface
- C1: simple split in articular surface and metaphysis
- C2: articular simple split with a multifragmentary metaphyseal fracture
- C3: fracture with multiple fragments of the articular surface and the metaphysis

Evidence-Based Orthopedics, First Edition. Edited by Mohit Bhandari.
© 2012 Blackwell Publishing Ltd. Published 2012 by Blackwell Publishing Ltd.

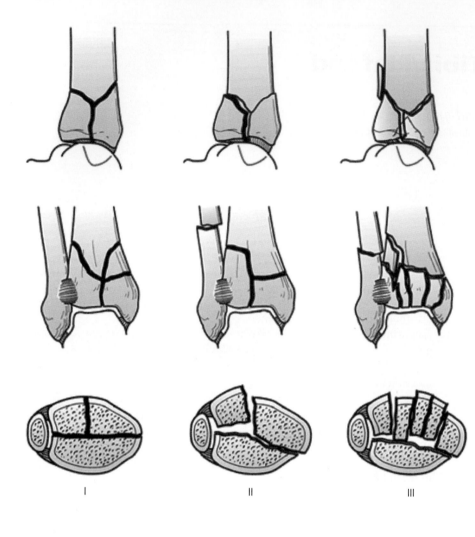

Figure 63.1 Ruedi and Allgower classification of plafond fractures.

Importance of the problem

Pilon fractures are uncommon, accounting for only approximately 10% of lower extremity fractures and are more common in men than women (level V).[3] With operative treatment, high-energy pilon fractures will take 4 months on average to heal and the total time of disability will be longer. Pilon fractures have a long-lasting negative effect on ankle function, work, recreation, and health-related quality of life. Patients frequently use pain medication, change jobs, and are unable to participate in all recreational activities (level IV).[4]

Top ten questions

Diagnosis

1. How important is the history and clinical examination in the diagnosis of pilon fractures?

2. What is the role of CT scanning in the diagnosis and treatment of pilon fractures?

Treatment

3. Is there any role for nonsurgical treatment in pilon fractures?
4. When is the optimum time for surgical intervention?
5. What is the role of external fixation in the treatment of pilon fractures?
6. Is ankle-sparing external fixation superior to ankle-spanning external fixation in the treatment of pilon fracture?
7. What are the common surgical approaches for pilon fracture reduction and fixation?
8. What is appropriate postoperative care and rehabilitation after pilon fractures?

Complications and outcome

9. What are the common early and late complications of pilon fracture, and what outcome is expected?

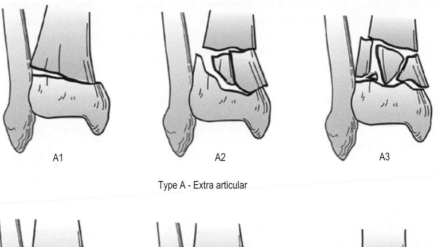

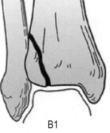 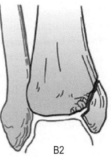 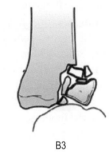

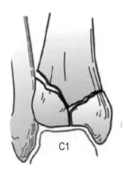 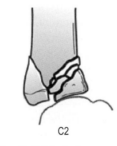 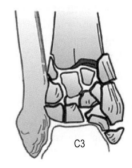

Figure 63.2 AO/OTA classification of plafond fractures.

Question 1: How important is history and clinical examination in the diagnosis of pilon fractures?

Case clarification

Clinical examination demonstrates that the patient's right foot and ankle is markedly swollen and deformed and there are tenderness and crepitus in palpation. There is no open wound injury. Neurovascular examination of his foot and ankle is normal. Radiographs in the AP, lateral and oblique views show a displaced comminuted intra-articular fracture of the distal tibia and a fracture of the distal fibula.

Relevance

Assessment starts with a careful history and a through physical examination along with good-quality radiographs.

Careful assessment of both the soft tissue injury and the fracture pattern are essential for successful treatment planning.

Current opinion

There are two different groups of mechanism of injury. High-energy fractures generally have a poorer outcome than do low-energy pilon fractures.

Finding the evidence

• Cochrane Database, with search terms: "plafond fracture," "pilon fracture," "distal tibia fracture," "mechanism of injury" and "physical examination"
• PubMed (www.ncbi.nlm.nih.gov/pubmed/) clinical queries search/ systematic reviews: "plafond fracture" OR

"pilon fracture" OR "distal tibia fracture" AND "mechanism of injury" AND "physical examination"
- MEDLINE search using keywords: "plafond fracture" OR "pilon fracture" OR "distal tibia fracture" AND "mechanism of injury" AND "physical examination"
- *Journal of the American Academy of Orthopaedic Surgeons*
- *Journal of Bone and Joint Surgery* (American and British volumes)

Quality of the evidence
Level II
- 2 prospective studies

Findings
Since soft tissue injury is an important component of a pilon fracture, a thorough lower extremity skin and soft tissue assessment should be performed to identify swelling, skin blister, or an open wound. Open tibial plafond fractures present with traumatic wounds typically over the medial aspect of the distal tibia or at the level of the fibular fracture (level II).[5] Finding fracture blisters, especially bloody blisters, demonstrates the magnitude of soft tissue trauma and usually indicates a full-thickness dermal injury. A clear-filled blister usually indicates superficial epidermal injury. Blood-filled blisters are more troublesome than clear-filled blister, usually have higher rate of infection, and leave scars after recovery (level II).[6]

Assessment of the neurovascular status of the limb must also be done and documented. Alignment of deformed foot and ankle needs to be corrected especially if there is any evidence of impaired foot perfusion. Patients need to be carefully assessed for associated injuries.

Recommendation
- A thorough physical examination of the lower extremity including neurovascular examination must be done in the Emergency Department. Attention to careful assessment of the soft tissue envelope is critical [overall quality: moderate]

Question 2: What is the role of CT scan in the diagnosis and treatment of pilon fractures?

Case clarification
The patient's radiographs revealed a multifragmentary distal tibia fracture with involvement of articular surface (type C pilon fracture) with proximal displacement of talus.

> A type C pilon fracture usually represents high-energy trauma with involvement of the entire joint surface.

Relevance
AP, mortise, and lateral ankle radiographs are usually sufficient for the diagnosis. Radiographs of the entire tibia and fibula are essential for detecting extension of the fracture into the diaphysis but should not be used alone to evaluate the tibial plafond.

Current opinion
CT of the injured extremity is essential in identifying the number of articular fragments, the amount of displacement (step, gap) between the fragments, and the presence of articular and subarticular impaction.

Finding the evidence
See Question 1.

Quality of the evidence
Level II
- 1 prospective cohort study

Level IV
- 3 case series

Level V
- 1 expert opinion

Findings
CT is used to guide operative treatment to minimize soft tissue stripping while allowing articular reduction and fixation, and is essential for understanding and planning definitive treatment (level V).[7] In one study the addition of an axial CT scan led to a change in the operative plan in 64% of patients (level IV).[8] In a recent study (level IV),[9] CT anatomy of 126 pilon fractures (85% type C) in 122 patients was reviewed. The authors categorized fracture patterns to be primarily coronal in 55% and primarily sagittal in 33%.

If a staged protocol is planned for a complex pilon fracture with soft tissue swelling, a distraction CT scan can be done after open reduction and internal fixation (ORIF) of fibula and length restoration with application of external fixator using the ligamentotaxis effect.[7]

The amount of information achieved in CT imaging is more precise in terms of restored length compared to a collapsed multifragmentary fracture.

In a recent prospective cohort study (level II),[10] the authors intraoperatively evaluated 248 consecutive patients with intra-articular fractures including 41 tibial plafond fractures. Standard fluoroscopy and 3D imaging (Iso-C3D system) intraoperatively were performed and compared for all patients. Based on intraoperative image analysis, 19% of all cases had immediate adjustment of the reduction or hardware exchange. These revisions were based on Iso-C3D views of the articular surface that were not visible using fluoroscopy.

Recommendation
- CT scan is essential in the assessment of pilon fractures and will help surgeons to understand the anatomy of the

fracture and select the best treatment [overall quality: moderate]

Question 3: Is there any role for nonsurgical treatment in pilon fractures?

Case clarification
The patient's radiographs demonstrate a complex comminuted intra-articular distal tibia fracture. There is an associated fibular fracture. The family asks if the fracture can be managed without surgery.

Relevance
Casting is commonly used to treat stable ankle fractures but only applies to nondisplaced plafond fractures.

Current opinion
If patient medical comorbidity is not a contraindication for surgical intervention, nonsurgical intervention or casting is only appropriate for AO type A1, B1, and C1 fractures with less than 2mm of articular displacement. When in doubt, CT or plain tomography can aid in determining articular congruity.[3]

Finding the evidence
See Question 1.

Quality of the evidence
Level IV
- 3 case series

Level V
- 1 expert opinion

Findings
In one study (level IV)[11] nonoperative treatment produced good functional results in all type I fractures, poor results in type II, and was not applicable to type III fractures.

Plaster immobilization may be used acutely for minimally or nondisplaced intra-articular fractures (level IV).[12]

In one study(level IV),[13] the authors demonstrated fair to poor outcomes in 73% (22/30) of their patients who were treated with nonoperative management. They reported 13 patients with type I fractures, 9 type II, and 8 type III fractures. Follow-up examinations were performed from 4 months to 4 years. Long-term results (mean 3 years) were good in 8 cases, fair in 12, and poor in 10; 23 cases showed early ankle osteoarthritis. In 16 cases there were deviations of bone axis (15° of varus). The range of movement was limited in all patients.

The primary indications for surgical intervention are articular fragment displacement of 2mm or more, joint instability resulting from the fracture, unacceptable axial alignment of the limb, and presence of open fractures (level

V).[14] Therefore, most pilon fractures are not amenable to nonoperative treatment.

Recommendation
- If the patient's medical condition is not a contraindication for surgery, nonsurgical treatment is only an option in nondisplaced plafond fractures [overall quality: low]

Question 4: What is the optimum time for surgical intervention?

Case clarification
The patient's ankle is very swollen and he has a few small amber-colored blisters anterior and medial to his ankle.

Relevance
The timing of definitive surgery depends on the condition of the soft tissues. Good surgical timing decreases the risk of wound complications, including skin slough and infection. Surgical intervention during maximum soft tissue swelling will lead to a higher risk of wound necrosis and infection. Early surgical intervention or delayed surgery as part of two-stage management is carried out when the soft tissue envelope is ready. Specific clinical signs that help the surgeon decide if the soft tissue is ready include resolution of edema and fracture blisters and the return of skin wrinkling.

Current opinion
Current treatment recommendations for pilon fractures involve a two-stage protocol in which an ankle-spanning external fixation with or without fibular reduction and fixation is used to stabilize the fracture until the soft tissue injury resolves.

Finding the evidence
See Question 1.

Quality of the evidence
Level II
- 1 prospective study

Level IV
- 4 case series

Level V
- 2 expert opinions

Findings
The decision on whether to operate and when to operate depends on multiple factors such as age, general health, soft tissue condition, current medical status, or other injuries that influence the safe administration of anesthesia. It

also depends on the time has elapsed between the injury and the definitive evaluation of the patient (level V).[15]

In 1986, Mast [15] stated that if surgery cannot be done before 8–12 hours have elapsed since the injury, the definitive procedure must be delayed for 7–10 days. Helfet (level IV)[16] retrospectively reported the outcomes of 34 (26 type II and 8 type III) pilon fractures, including 18 open fractures with average 7.3 days from injury to operation (range 0–25 days). He concluded that the timing of pilon fracture surgery is dependent on the status of the soft tissues. Immediate postinjury swelling represents fracture hematoma. However, within 8–12 hours, the soft tissues become edematous and definitive surgery should then be delayed for 7–12 days to allow soft tissue swelling and edema to subside. If not, skin closure without undue tension will not be possible, increasing the risk of soft tissue slough and infection.

The approach most commonly used to treat high-energy pilon fractures is a two-stage procedure involving initial reduction and application of external fixator followed by definite fixation about 10–21 days later when the soft tissue envelope is ready (level IV–V).[17–19]

Sirkin et al.[17] reported on 56 fractures, including group I with 34 closed fractures and group II with 22 open fractures. The treatment protocol included immediate (<24 hours) ORIF of the fibula and application of an external fixator spanning the ankle joint followed by ORIF of the tibia with plates and screws. ORIF was performed on an average of 12.7 days after injury in group I, and 14 days after injury in group II. In the closed fracture group, 5/34 patients (15%) with closed fractures had partial skin necrosis that healed with local wound care and 1 patient had a chronic draining sinus from osteomyelitis that resolved after fracture healing. In the open fracture group, 4/22 patients (18%) had complications, with 2 only having partial skin necrosis that resolved with local wound care. One of the remaining 2 patients required a below-knee amputation.

Patterson (level IV)[18] retrospectively reported the outcomes of 22 type C3 pilon fractures at 22 months treated with a two-stage procedure. He reported no infections or soft tissue complications. Objective outcome measurements were reported as 77% good and excellent results, 14% fair, and 9% poor results.

In a prospective study, Conroy et al. (level II)[20] reported the results of early ORIF in 32 patients who suffered from type B (21 patients) and type C pilon fractures (11 patients). They followed a "fix and flap" protocol by managing pilon fractures with early bone stabilization and flap coverage at the same time. In this study 28 patients were managed with early ORIF and early coverage using free muscle flaps (25 latissimus dorsi, 3 gracilis, 3 rectus abdominis, 1 latissimus dorsi and rectus abdominis) and split skin graft, and 4 patients were managed with application of external fixa-

tion. As a result there were 2 amputations (6.2%), 2 deep infections (6.2%), and 3 malunions (9.3%). After exclusion of the 2 amputees, all 30 remaining patients progressed to clinical and radiological union. Mean time to union was 35 weeks (range 12–78 weeks). Six patients had loss of joint congruity and demonstrated evidence of osteoarthritis on radiographs at final follow-up. They concluded their "aggressive protocol" showed excellent union rate, low rate of infection, and good functional outcome.

A recent cohort study done by Guy et al. (level IV)[21] presented results of early primary ORIF of 95 patients with type C pilon fractures (21 open and 74 closed fractures). Primary ORIF was performed within 24 hours in 70% and within 48 hours in 88% of patients. They reported six patients with deep wound infection that required surgical irrigation and debridement, including four patients who had presented with open fractures initially. Five patients developed delayed/nonunion who subsequently had revision with ORIF and bone grafting. The authors demonstrated an acceptable deep infection rate of 2.7% for closed fractures and 19% for open fractures, with satisfactory quality of reduction in 90% of cases. Although they demonstrated a good result on those who had surgery within 48 hours after injury they did not propose a golden surgical window for ORIF of pilon fractures, but concluded that type C pilon fractures can be stabilized effectively by primary ORIF with relatively low rate of deep wound complications, a high quality of reduction, and long-term outcome comparable with all other modalities of treatment.

Recommendation

• Surgical timing is dictated by patient medical status, soft tissue envelope condition and surgeon's experience. For most centers, a two-stage approach is appropriate. Definite internal fixation is not recommended between 2–7 days after injury [overall quality: low]

Question 5: What is the role of external fixation in the treatment of pilon fractures?

Case clarification

The patient's ankle is now severely swollen and there are a few big bloody blisters anterior and medial to his ankle.

Relevance

In high-energy pilon fractures, the soft tissue envelope has been damaged by the injury. A second insult from surgical dissection may increase soft tissue complications. Handling of the delicate thin soft tissue envelope in tibial pilon fractures is one of the greatest challenges in the treatment of these injuries. Maintenance of fracture length and stability decreases soft tissue swelling by helping to maintain vascular flow (level V).[22]

Current opinion

Fracture reduction through ligamentotaxis will maintain fracture length, provide fracture stabilization, and eventually promote soft tissue healing. With minimal dissection, the surgeon will avoid more insult to the vulnerable soft tissue envelope. The portability of the external fixator makes subsequent imaging studies easier to obtain and more informative. The fixator also provides stability for patient transfers. It is possible to use external fixation as definitive treatment for tibial plafond fractures.

Finding the evidence

See Question 1.

Quality of the evidence

Level II

• 1 randomized control trial without blinding

Level IV

• 4 case series

Findings

Historically, poor outcomes have been reported with primary ORIF of high-energy pilon fractures (level II–V),[1,12,19,23,24] and external skeletal fixation therefore became a popular treatment alternative. Limited ORIF of the joint surface was utilized for articular fragments not anatomically reduced by ligamentotaxis.

This was well demonstrated by Bonar et al. (level IV)[25] in their retrospective result with the use of a unilateral external fixator for the treatment of severe pilon fractures. This retrospective review of 21 patients included two distinct treatment groups. The first group (n = 5) consisted of patients who underwent only external fixation without attempted articular reduction. The second group (n = 16) included patients who underwent limited internal fixation combined with external fixation. Four of the five patients in the first group went on to an arthrodesis, while the fifth received a late amputation. Each of the fractures in the second group healed without evidence of wound infection, skin slough, or osteomyelitis. Reflecting on the results of the patients in the second group, the authors concluded that less extensive tissue dissection, in an area prone to wound complications, may have accounted for the low rate of infection, wound complication, and nonunions.

In a randomized prospective study, Wyrsch et al. (level II)[26] compared 18 patients who were treated with ORIF with 20 patients who were treated with external fixation with limited internal fixation. There were 15 major complications in 7 patients who had ORIF that necessitated 28 additional operations. In the external fixation group there were 4 major complications in 4 patients, necessitating 5 additional operations. The authors found no significant difference in post-traumatic arthritis and concluded that external fixation with limited internal fixation was a satisfactory method of treatment of pilon fractures and was associated with fewer complications than early ORIF.

In a prospective study, Watson et al. (level IV)[27] treated 107 pilon fractures according to a staged protocol from 1991 to 1997. All closed pilon fractures underwent stabilization with definitive fixation when patients' general health and soft tissues were ready, at an average of 5 days. They treated 26 type A, 29 type B, and 39 type C fracture patterns, 30 of which were open fractures. They treated 36 patients with ORIF and 58 patients with application of external fixation.

Clinical and radiographic evaluations were performed at an average 4.9 years after injury. For all fracture types (AO classification), 81% of the patients who were treated with external fixation and 75% of the patients who were treated with open plating had good or excellent results. The patients in the open plating group had a significantly higher rate of nonunion, malunion, and severe wound complications compared with the patients who received external fixation for type C fracture patterns. For severe fracture patterns (type C), patients in both groups had significantly poorer results than patients with type A and B fractures. They concluded that the worse the initial soft tissue injury, the poorer the overall function tended to be, regardless of the initial fracture pattern.

Recommendation

• External fixation with limited internal fixation is a widely accepted mode of definitive treatment in pilon fracture management. The existing literature suggests that the outcome is better with external fixation than with primary ORIF. There is not enough evidence to conclude whether two-stage ORIF or definitive management with an external fixator is superior [overall quality: low]

Question 6: Is ankle-sparing external fixation superior to ankle-spanning external fixation in the treatment of pilon fracture?

Case clarification

The soft tissue of the patient's ankle is not ready for definitive ORIF. His surgeon has decided to use external fixation as the definitive treatment.

Relevance

Loss of ankle range of motion (ROM) and post-traumatic osteoarthritis are common complications after pilon fractures with disrupted articular surface. Prolonged joint immobility is associated with permanent joint stiffness.

Current opinion

Early passive and active ROM is considered beneficial to restore preinjury ROM.

Finding the evidence
See Question 1.

Quality of the evidence
Level I
- 1 randomized controlled trial without blinding

Level III
- 1 systematic review of level III studies

Level IV
- 2 case series

Findings
Early ROM provides better overall scoring and improves ROM (level IV).[28] Salter (level IV)[29] demonstrated early motion was the most important factor in promoting cartilage nutrition and healing in his animal model.

Three categories of fixator design are available: (1) joint-spanning rigid fixator, (2) joint-spanning articulated fixator, and (3) non-joint-spanning fixator.

In a systematic review (level III),[30] the outcomes of the use of external fixation devices for spanning or sparing the ankle joint in the treatment of fractures of the tibial plafond were compared, focusing on the complications and the rates of healing. Although there was a statistically significant difference between spanning and sparing fixation systems regarding the rates of minor infections (pin track and superficial wound infection) there were no statistically significant differences regarding the rates of deep infection, nonunion, and the time to union. Patients treated with spanning frames had a significantly greater incidence of malunion compared with patients treated with sparing frames.

Marsh et al. (level II)[31] in a prospective multicenter study randomized pilon fractures to have either early postoperative ankle movements through a mobile articulated hinge or to have an immobile ankle with a locked hinge. All patients were treated with a uniform surgical technique, including application of a hinged transarticular external fixator with limited internal fixation. In the 31 patients (14 nonmobile and 17 mobile) who completed a 2-year follow-up, no significant differences were found between the 2 groups in any of the outcomes. The authors concluded that there was no detectable benefit of moving the ankle joint in the first 8–12 weeks after a tibial plafond fracture treated with articulated external fixation.

Recommendation
- The type of external fixation device employed is dictated by the fracture anatomy and surgeon experience. Nonspanning fixation requires large articular fragments. Use of hinged spanning external fixator has no benefit over nonhinged fixators [overall quality: moderate]

Question 7: What are the surgical approaches for pilon fracture reduction and fixation?

Case clarification
The patient's CT scan revealed a pilon fracture with a centrally depressed fragment and about a 5 mm step. The line of fracture starts laterally and passes through the central fragment and extends medially anterior and posterior to the medial fragment (V family). There is a fibular fracture 4 cm proximal to the syndesmosis.

Relevance
The ankle soft tissue envelope is thin and vulnerable to wound complications. Extensive soft tissue dissection may result in wound breakdown. The approach that results in the least amount of dissection should be chosen.

Current opinion
The surgical approach to a pilon fracture is primarily dictated by the fracture pattern and soft tissue status. The CT scan must be reviewed carefully as part of surgical planning for both reduction and fixation strategies. The goal is to achieve anatomic reduction of the joint surface, restoration of axial alignment of the nonarticular component and application of appropriate fixation with meticulous soft tissue handling.

Finding the evidence
See Question 1.

Quality of the evidence
Level IV
- 1 case series

Level V
- 4 expert opinions

Findings
The classic approaches to distal tibia and fibula are: (1) anteromedial (1 cm lateral to the anterior tibial crest), (2) anterolateral (between the peroneal and extensor muscles), (3) posterolateral (Harmon), (4) posteromedial, (5) anterior, and (6) direct lateral.

The traditional surgical approach, described by the AO Group (level V),[32] is the *anteromedial approach* for the tibia and lateral for the fibula. A 7 cm skin bridge between the lateral incision over the fibula and the medial approach for the tibial plafond was recommended by AO pioneers (level V)[33] and others[3,15] to avoid skin necrosis and wound complications.

A recent prospective study (level IV)[34] reported a low rate of wound complications in 46 pilon fractures with less than a 7 cm skin bridge between two or three skin incisions.

The authors concluded that with careful attention to soft tissue management and surgical timing, incisions for tibial plafond fractures may be placed less than 7 cm apart, allowing the surgeon to optimize exposures on the basis of the injury pattern.

Soft tissue injury or fracture pattern commonly necessitate the *anterolateral approach*. One study reported 131 pilon fractures treated with ORIF through an anterolateral surgical exposure (level V).[7] A satisfactory reduction (<2 mm of articular incongruity) was obtained in 92% of the patients. There were 3 wound infections that required further operative treatment and no nonunions.

The well-known *posterolateral approach* is commonly used for partial articular fractures that involve the posterolateral aspect of the tibia. The posteromedial approach is occasionally useful in some fracture patterns.

There is a wide choice of implants available for ORIF of pilon fractures. The fibula fracture is generally managed with standard open reduction and fixation with a small fragment compression plate. Precontoured plates are available for the medial and anterolateral surfaces of the distal tibia. These implants reduce surgical time by eliminating the need for extensive plate contouring and facilitate minimally invasive plating techniques. There is no evidence that locked plates are superior to nonlocked plates in this application.

Wound closure is extremely important. It should be accomplished with an atraumatic technique and without soft tissue tension.

Recommendation

- The surgical approach is dictated by anatomy of fracture and the status of the soft tissue. Careful physical examination and review of the CT scan will help the surgeon to choose the most appropriate surgical approach. Most fractures can be adequately stabilized with precountoured nonlocked plates [overall quality: low]

Question 8: What is appropriate postoperative care and rehabilitation after pilon fractures?

Case clarification

The patient was discharged home 5 days after ORIF of his pilon fracture. He wants to know if he needs physiotherapy and when he is going to walk again.

Relevance

Postoperative wound care and close follow-up are necessary following treatment of pilon fractures. Wound infection and skin necrosis need to be addressed appropriately before deep infection develops. Normally weightbearing is delayed for 12 weeks following ORIF of these fractures.

Current opinion

Most patients with pilon fracture will be observed closely after discharge for development of injury-related or postsurgical complications. If their course is uneventful they generally need to maintain non-weight-bearing status for at least 12 weeks.

Finding the evidence

See Question 1.

Quality of the evidence

Level IV

- 1 expert opinion

Findings

Patients are maintained toe-touch weightbearing (TTWB) and discharged home when comfortable. The ankle is often splinted for the first week or two. Active ROM of the ankle is allowed following wound healing at approximately 2 weeks after surgery. Physiotherapy is used for ROM exercises until full motion is regained. Typically the fracture is healed by 12 weeks postoperatively and the patient can be advanced to full weightbearing.[14]

Recommendation

- Patients must be followed closely. Postoperatively TTWB is recommended for 10–12 weeks. Non-weight-bearing ROM exercises are recommended after the surgical incision is healed. Weightbearing status will be increased when evidence of bone healing is observed in imaging studies [overall quality: low]

Question 9: What are the common early and late complications of pilon fracture, and what outcome is expected?

Case clarification

The patient comes back to clinic after a year for follow-up. He walks with a subtle limp and had to discontinue many of his recreational activities, including tennis. Examination demonstrates decreased ankle ROM. His radiograph reveals grade II ankle arthrosis. He wants to know if he might get more clinical improvement.

Relevance

Despite progress in techniques and hardware technology, pilon fractures are associated with high rates of complications and disability.

Current opinion

Depending on the severity of their pilon fracture, patients may experience a variety of early and late complications. A fair to poor outcome is expected in at least one third of C type pilon fractures.

Finding the evidence
See Question 1.

Quality of the evidence
Level II
- 1 prognostic study

Level IV
- 9 case series

Findings

In the 1990s, case series of early ORIF of pilon fractures reported complication rates as high as 70%.[23,24] Early local complications were mostly related to wound dehiscence and infection. The late complications included malunion, nonunion, osteomyelitis, ankle stiffness, osteomyelitis, and osteoarthritis.

The risk of complication following the currently accepted staged treatment strategy of reduction and external fixation followed by definitive ORIF on a delayed basis has been reported.[17,18] The technique is associated with a low risk of deep infection (0–4%), malunion, and nonunion in closed fractures.

In open fractures the risk of complication is higher. However, recently the two-stage protocol has been reported to have a low risk of complication (overall 8% infection, 8% delayed/nonunion) even in open fractures (level IV).[35]

Pollak et al. (level II)[36] reported mid-term outcomes (average 3.2 year follow-up) on 80 patients with pilon fracture treated with either ORIF or external fixation. General health, as measured with the Short Form-36 (SF-36), was significantly poorer than age- and gender-matched norms. Of the 65 participants who were employed at the time of injury, 28 (43%) were not working at the time of follow-up. Approximately one third of the participants reported notable difficulty with ankle stiffness (35%), swelling (29%), or pain (33%). The only injury or treatment characteristic that was significantly related to several of the selected outcomes was treatment method. Participants treated with external fixation with or without limited internal fixation had more overall ROM impairment and reported more pain and ambulatory dysfunction than did participants treated with ORIF (p < 0.05).

Between 1988 and 1994, Marsh et al.(type IV)[4] treated 56 pilon fractures (types B3, C1, C2, and C3) with a hinged external fixator with limited internal fixation. Their 5 year follow-up of 29 patients showed significantly reduced SF-36 scores compared to norms. Patients were generally satisfied with the results of treatment and perceived that they had improved for a long time after the injury. The patients reported improvement for an average of 2.4 years. Almost all patients had radiographic evidence of osteoarthritis in the ankle.

Surprisingly, radiological evidence of arthrosis had only weak correlations with clinical outcome, as measured with the Iowa Ankle Score, the Ankle Osteoarthritis Scale, and the SF-36.

Chen et al. (level IV)[37] published a 10 year follow-up of 128 pilon fractures treated with ORIF. Clinical outcomes were better in simple fracture patterns than they were in complex fractures, and this is a consistent finding of most studies.

Williams et al. (level IV)[38] found that injury severity and the quality of reduction were less important predictors of outcome than patient demographic factors (gender, age, level of education) and whether or not the injury was work related. This is not confirmed by other studies.[35]

Recommendation
- Complications after pilon fracture treatment are common and need to be addressed accordingly [overall quality: moderate]:
  ° Wound healing problems, including infection, are the commonest early local complications
  ° Delayed union and nonunion can occur, especially after high-energy open fractures
  ° Ankle osteoarthritis is a very common late complication
- Patients need to be advised that mid- to long-term outcomes of pilon fractures are associated with some degree of disability in most patients, especially in high-grade comminuted fractures

Summary of recommendations

- The diagnosis of a tibial pilon fracture requires a thorough history and physical examination with particular attention to careful assessment of the soft tissue envelope
- Plain radiographs are important for diagnosis and high-quality CT images are essential for operative planning
- Almost all tibial plafond fractures require surgical management
- Surgical timing is dictated by the patient's medical status, the condition of the soft tissue envelope, and the surgeon's experience. For most centers, a two-stage approach (closed reduction and external fixation ± ORIF of the fibula followed by delayed definitive internal fixation) is appropriate. Definite internal fixation is not recommended between 2 and 7 days after injury
- External fixation with limited internal fixation is a widely accepted mode of definitive treatment in pilon fracture management and is an alternative to ORIF in some settings
- The type of external fixation device employed is dictated by the fracture anatomy and surgeon experience. The use

of a hinged spanning external fixator has not been shown to have a benefit over nonhinged fixators

• For definitive ORIF, the surgical approach is dictated by the anatomy of the fracture and the status of the soft tissue. Careful physical examination and review of the CT scan will help the surgeon to choose the most appropriate surgical approach. Most fractures can be adequately stabilized with precountoured nonlocked plates

• Postoperative care involves early ankle ROM exercises. Weightbearing should be delayed until the fracture has healed (usually at about 12 weeks)

• Complications are common after pilon fractures. Early local complications often involve difficulties with wound healing and infection. Post-traumatic ankle osteoarthritis is a common late local complication

• The mid- and long-term outcome following high-energy tibial plafond fractures is guarded, with a high incidence of some degree of residual disability

Conclusions

High-energy tibial pilon fractures are challenging injuries for orthopedic surgeons to treat. Despite advances in the assessment and treatment of these complex injuries, complications do occur. The outcome is often associated with some degree of disability. Modern strategies for management that respect the soft tissue injury and provide restoration of the anatomy of the bone and joint are however, associated with lower risks of serious complication and better outcomes than have been reported historically.

References

1. Ruedi TP, Allgower M. The operative treatment of intraarticular fractures of the lower end of tibia. Clin Orthop 1979;136: 105–10.

2. Orthopaedic Trauma Association Committee for Coding and Classification. Fracture and dislocation compendium. J Orthop Trauma 1996;10(V–IX):56–60.

3. Bonar SK, Marsh JL. Tibial plafond fractures: changing principles of treatment. J Am Acad Orthop Surg 1994;2(6):297–305.

4. Marsh JL, Weigel DP, Dirschl DR. Tibial plafond fractures; How do these ankles function over time? J Bone Joint Surg Am 2003;85(2):287–95.

5. Gustilo RB, Anderson JT. Prevention of infection in the treatment of one thousand and twenty five open fractures of long bones. J Bone Joint Surg 1976;58:453–8.

6. Giordano CP, Koval KJ. Treatment of fracture blisters: a prospective study of 53 cases. J Orthop Trauma 1995;9:171–6.

7. Nork SE, Barei, DP, Gardner MJ, et al. Anterolateral approach for pilon fractures. Tech Foot Ankle Surg 2009;8(2):53–59.

8. Tornetta P 3rd. Axial computed tomography of pilon fractures. Clin Orthop 1996;323:273–6.

9. Topliss CJ, Jackson M, Atkins RM. Anatomy of pilon fracture of the distal tibia. J Bone Joint Surg Br 2005;87(5):692–7.

10. Kendoff D, Citak M, Gardner MJ. et al. Intraoperative 3D imaging: value and consequences in 248 cases. J Trauma 2009;66:232–8.

11. Ayeni JP. Pilon fractures of the tibia: a study based on 19 cases. Injury 1988;19(2):109–14.

12. Ovadia DN, Beals RK. Fractures of the tibial plafond. J. Bone Joint Surg Am. 1986;68:543–51.

13. Othman M, Strzelczyk P. Results of conservative treatment of "pilon" fractures. Ortop Traumatol Rehabil 2003;5(6):787–94.

14. Borrelli JJ, Ellis E. Pilon fractures: assessment and treatment. Orthop Clin North Am 2002;33(1):231–45.

15. Mast JW, Spiegel PG, Pappas JN. Fractures of the tibial pilon. Clin Orthop 1988;230:68–82.

16. Helfet DL, Koval K, Pappas J, et al. Intraarticular "pilon" fracture of the tibia. Clin Orthop Relat Res 1994;298:221–8.

17. Sirkin M, Sanders R, DiPasquale T, et al. A staged protocol for soft tissue management in the treatment of complex pilon fractures. J Orthop Trauma 1999;13(2):78–84.

18. Patterson MJ, Cole JD. Two-staged delayed open reduction and internal fixation of severe pilon fractures. J Orthop Trauma 1999;13(2):85–91.

19. Wade AM, Crist BD, Khazzam M, et al. Pilon fractures. Curr Orthop Pract 2008; 19(3):242–8.

20. Conroy J, Agarwal M, Giannoudis PV, et al. Early internal fixation and soft tissue cover of severe open tibial pilon fractures. Int Orthop 2003;27(6):343–7.

21. Guy P, White T, Cooke C, et al. The results of early primary open reduction and internal fixation for treatment of AO C-type tibial pilon fractures: a cohort study. J Orthop Trauma 2010;24(12): 757–63.

22. Bartlett CS 3rd, D'Amato MJ, Weiner LS. Fractures of the tibial pilon. In: Browner BD, Jupiter JB, Levine AM, et al., eds., Skeletal Trauma, 2nd edn, pp.2295–325. WB Saunders, Philadelphia, 1998.

23. McFerran MA, Smith SW, Boulas HJ et al. Complications encountered in the treatment of pilon fractures. J Orthop Trauma 1992;6:195–200.

24. Teeny SM, Wiss DA. Open reduction and internal fixation of tibial plafond fractures: variables contributing to poor results and complications. Clin Orthop 1993;292:108–17.

25. Bonar SK, Marsh JL. Unilateral external fixation for severe pilon fractures. Foot Ankle 1993;14:57–64.

26. Wyrsch B, McFerran MA, McAndrew M, et al. Operative treatment of fractures of the tibial plafond. J Bone Joint Surg Am 1996;78A:1646–57.

27. Watson JT, Moed BR, Karges DE, et al. Pilon fractures: treatment protocol based on severity of soft tissue injury. Clin Orthop Relat Res 2000;375:78–90.

28. Kellam JF, Waddell JP. Fractures of the distal tibia metaphysis with intra-articular extension: the distal tibial explosion fracture. J Trauma 1979;19:593–609.

29. Salter RB, Simmonds DF, Malcom BW. The biologic effect of continuous passive motion on the healing of full thickness defects in articular cartilage. An experimental investigation in the rabbit. J Bone Joint Surg Am 1980;62:1232–51.

30. Papadokostakis G, Kontakis G, Giannoudis P, et al. External fixation devices in the treatment of fractures of the tibial plafond:

a systematic review of the literature. J Bone Joint Surg Br 2008;90(1):1–6.

31. Marsh JL, Muehling V, Dirschl D et al. Tibial plafond fractures treated by articulated external fixation: a randomized trial of postoperative motion versus nonmotion. J Orthop Trauma 2006;20(8):536–41.

32. Summer C, Ruedi T. Tibia: distal (pilon). In: Ruedi T, Murphy W, eds., AO Principles of Fracture Management, pp.539–56. Thieme, Boston, 2000.

33. Muller ME, Allgower M, Schneider R, et al. Fractures of the shaft of the tibia. In: Manual of Internal Fixation: Techniques Recommended by the AO Group, p.278. Springer-Verlag, Heidelberg, 1979.

34. Howard JL, Agel J, Barei DP et al. A prospective study evaluating incision placement and wound healing for tibial plafond fractures. J Orthop Trauma 2008;22:299–306.

35. Boraiah S, Kemp TJ, et al. Outcome following open reduction and internal fixation of open pilon fractures. J Bone Joint Surg Am 2010;92(2):346–52.

36. Pollak AN, McCarthy ML, Bess RS, et al. Outcomes after treatment of high-energy tibial plafond fractures. J Bone Joint Surg Am 2003;85(10):1893–900.

37. Chen SH, Wu PH, Lee YS. Long-term results of pilon fractures. Arch Orthop Trauma Surg 2007;127:55–60.

38. Williams TM, Nepola JV, DeCoster TA et al. Factors affecting outcome in tibial plafond fractures. Clin Orthop 2004;423:93–8.

64 Malleolar Fractures

David W. Sanders and Ajay Manjoo

London Health Sciences Centre and the University of Western Ontario, London, ON, Canada

Case scenario

An active 23 year old man employed as a laborer sustains a rotational injury to his right ankle. He is unable to bear weight and is tender over the posterior aspect of his lateral malleolus.

Importance of the problem

The ankle is the most commonly injured weightbearing joint. The incidence of fractures has doubled since the 1960s. This is believed to be due to a rise in the elderly demographic as well as the increase in the popularity of high-energy sports. The highest incidence is seen in elderly women. Unimalleolar injuries are most common (68%), followed by bimalleolar fracture (25%). Trimalleolar and open fractures are a minority.

Top five questions

Diagnosis

1. Which ankle injuries require a radiograph for diagnosis?

Treatment

2. How do you assess ankle fracture stability?
3. How are syndesmosis injuries identified and managed?
4. What is the significance of posterior malleolar injuries?

Prognosis

5. What is the role of early postoperative mobilization?

Question 1: Which ankle injuries requires a radiograph for diagnosis?

Case clarification

The patient has sustained an inversion injury to his right ankle. He is unable to bear weight and is tender over the posterior aspect of his lateral malleolus. The patient asks whether he needs a radiograph of his ankle.

Relevance

Ankle injuries are among the most common reasons for visits to the Emergency. Department. Many patients do not require radiographic imaging, yet it is preferable to avoid "missed" fractures. A screening tool may help determine which injuries are at high risk for fractures and will require radiological investigation.

Current opinion

The most widely used screening tool to determine which ankle injuries require investigation is the Ottawa ankle rules (see box).

Ottawa ankle rules[1]

Ankle radiographs are indicated if there is pain in the malleolar area and any of the following:
- Bone tenderness along the distal 6 cm of the posterior edge of the tibia or tip of the medial malleolus
- Bone tenderness along the distal 6 cm of the posterior edge of the fibula or tip of the lateral malleolus
- An inability to bear weight, both immediately and in the Emergency Department, for 4 steps

---

Finding the evidence
- PubMed (www.ncbi.nlm.nih.gov/pubmed/) clinical queries search/ systematic reviews: "Ottawa ankle rules"

Evidence-Based Orthopedics, First Edition. Edited by Mohit Bhandari.

Quality of evidence
Level I
- 2 systematic reviews
- 1 randomized trial

Level II
- 1 prospective study

Findings
Various ankle rules have been validated in a number of prospective studies and systematic review. For the Ottawa ankle rules, a pooled analysis of 3,130 patients from 12 studies identified 671 fractures.[1] The overall sensitivity was 98.5% (95% CI 97.3–99.2). There were 10 missed fractures, of which several were deemed "insignificant." The rate of radiographic reduction was 24.8% (95% CI 23.3–26.3%). In a prospective study of 750 patients with acute ankle injuries, a simplified version of the Ottawa ankle rules was used.[2] Patients who had pain near the malleoli and were age 55 years or more, or had localized bone tenderness of the posterior edge or tip of either malleolus, or were unable to bear weight both immediately after the injury and in the Emergency Department, underwent radiography. This rule was 100% sensitive and 40.1% specific for detecting malleolar fractures and would allow a reduction of 36.0% of ankle radiographic series ordered.

Recommendation
- The Ottawa ankle rules are a reliable tool to exclude fractures in patients more than 5 years of age presenting with ankle injuries. These rules decrease use of radiography with a low likelihood of missing a fracture [overall quality: high]

Question 2: How do you assess ankle fracture instability?

Case clarification
The patient's radiographs show a fracture of the lateral malleolus at the level of the syndesmosis with no fracture of the medial malleolus and no obvious disruption of the mortise. The patient wants to know if he needs surgery.

Relevance
For rotational ankle fractures, once the fibula is fractured, the medial restraints (i.e., the deep deltoid and medial malleolus) act as important secondary stabilizers of the ankle joint.

Current opinion
Clinical signs of medial injury are unreliable. Injury films should be examined for signs of ankle subluxation including talar shift (widening of the medial clear space >4 mm).

In cases of isolated fractures of the fibula, a manual external rotation or gravity stress test can assess for medial ligamentous disruption.

Finding the evidence
- PubMed (clinical queries: systematic review), using search terms: "ankle fracture" OR "ankle injury" AND "stability" OR "operative stabilization" OR "intraoperative stress test"

Quality of the evidence
Level II
- 6 diagnostic studies (development of diagnostic criteria on the basis of consecutive patients)

Findings
A total of 152 patients (in 2 studies) with isolated Weber B ankle fractures (see box) were assessed for medial-sided ankle tenderness, and subsequently had an external rotation stress test performed.[3,4] There was no statistical correlation between medial-sided tenderness, ecchymoses or swelling, and deltoid ligament incompetence.

Weber classification of ankle fractures
This refers to the level of the fibula fracture:
Weber A: fracture distal to the ankle joint **Weber B:** fracture at the level of the syndesmosis **Weber C:** fracture proximal to the syndesmosis

Stress testing In a cadaveric study, ankles were destabilized according to the Lauge–Hansen mechanism for supination–external rotation (SER) injuries. Stress views taken in dorsiflexion and external rotation were most predictive of deep deltoid disruption.[5] A second cadaveric study tested intact ankles, then added a Weber B fibula osteotomy, and finally with transection of the superficial or deep deltoid ligament and the fibula osteotomized or plated.[6] The authors concluded that the gravity stress test was able to reliably diagnosed deltoid disruption.

In a pooled analysis of 54 ankle fractures there were no statistical differences in medial clear space (MCS) between the manual and the gravity stress test in either the SER II or SER IV fractures.[7,8]

Recommendation
- Clinical signs of medial-sided injury are unreliable. External rotation and gravity stress tests are an accurate and reliable method for differentiating SER II and SER IV injuries [overall quality: moderate]

Question 3: How are syndesmosis injuries identified and managed?

Case clarification

The patient's radiographs show a fracture of his lateral malleolus at the level of the syndesmosis with no fracture of the medial malleolus, with talar shift on stress views. Your patient wants to know what fixation will be needed to stabilize his ankle.

Relevance

The distal tibiofibular syndesmosis is a primary stabilizer of the ankle joint. Instability of this articulation has been shown to significantly increase joint contact pressures and thus predispose to secondary arthrosis and poor functional outcomes. Adequate reduction and stabilization improves functional outcome.

Current opinion

An intraoperative external rotation stress test or modified Cotton test can reliably diagnose syndesmosis instability. There is no consensus with regards to the use of 3.5 mm vs. 4.5 mm screws, bioabsorbable vs. metallic screws, or quadricortical vs. tricortical fixation for syndesmosis stabilization.

Finding the evidence

• PubMed clinical queries/systematic review: "syndesmosis injuries" or "syndesmosis stabilization"

Quality of the evidence

Level I
• 5 randomized trials

Level II
• 1 prospective cohort study

Level III
• 1 retrospective case control study

Findings

Intraoperative diagnosis of syndesmosis injury The static radiographs of 38 skeletally mature ankles were analyzed for signs of syndesmosis injury and medial instability. Intraoperatively an external rotation stress test was performed after stabilization of lateral and medial malleolar fractures.[9] Intraoperative stress tests predicted syndesmosis injuries in 37% of patients not thought to have syndesmosis injuries on the basis of preoperative films. Rigid bimalleolar fixation did not always stabilize the syndesmosis adequately.

Size of screws A number of clinical and biomechanical studies have not detected clinically important differences between 3.5 and 4.5 mm screws.[10]

Number of cortices In one study, 120 ankle fractures with syndesmosis injury were randomized to stabilization with a single 3.5 mm tricortical screw (59 patients) or with a single 3.5 mm quadricortical screw (61 patients).[11] There were no differences between the groups with respect to hardware failure and irritation requiring screw removal at a mean follow-up of 150 days. A second study randomly assigned 64 ankles to fixation with either a single 4.5 mm cortical quadricortical screw (30 patients) or with two 3.5 mm tricortical screws (34 patients).[12] At 1 year there was no difference in functional outcome or pain scores.

Metal vs. bioabsorbable screws In one study of 38 patients, patients with bioabsorbable screws demonstrated a faster return to preinjury activity and less swelling.[13]

Functional outcome A retrospective review of 106 patients followed up for an average of 21 months, found that patients in whom the screws were either loosened, broken, or removed had a better functional outcome than those in whom the screw was intact.[14] The authors theorized that restoration of normal mechanics occurs once the screw is no longer intact.

Recommendations

• Intraoperative stress tests are accurate in diagnosing syndesmosis injuries. There is no consensus with regard to the use of 3.5 mm vs. 4.5 mm screws, tricortical or quadricortical fixation, and the use of bioabsorbable implants [overall quality: high]

Question 4: What is the significance of posterior malleolar injuries?

Case clarification

The patient's radiographs show a fracture of his medial and lateral malleolus at the level of the syndesmosis with a fracture of the posterior malleolus (PM) involving 5% of the articular surface on the lateral radiographs. Your patient wants to know if he needs surgery and what fixation will be needed to stabilize his ankle.

Relevance

It is generally accepted that fractures involving the posterior malleolus have a worse prognosis than those with intact posterior malleoli. The literature remains divided with respect to the indications for surgical intervention.

Current opinion

Fractures involving more than 25% of the articular surface should be treated with operative reduction and internal fixation (ORIF). Fractures involving less than 10% of the articular cartilage are generally not addressed operatively. There remains controversy with respect to the optimal management of intermediate-sized posterior fragments.

Finding the evidence
• PubMed clinical queries/systematic review: "posterior malleolus fractures"

Quality of the evidence
Level I
• 1 individual inception prognostic cohort study

Level II
• 2 prospective cohort studies

Findings
In a cadaveric study, the posterior malleolus was sequentially resected to include 25%, 33%, and 50% of the articular surface.[15] Contact area decreased with increasing size of the resected fragment and normal congruency of the tibiotalar joint was lost. Authors recommended that fragments greater than 25% be addressed with operative stabilization.

A prospective study of 142 ankle fractures with an average of 5.7 years follow-up demonstrated that the presence of posterior malleolar fractures resulted in decreased functional scores regardless of the size of the fragment.[16] Larger fragments were more likely to develop osteoarthritis. In the case of the larger fragments, patients fared better with operative stabilization.

A second retrospective study of 57 trimalleolar fractures followed for a mean of 6.9 years determined that ankles with posterior fragments of 10% or more had better functional outcome scores if joint congruity was restored.[17] Restoration of congruity to fragments less than 10% did not affect outcome.

Recommendations
• Fragments less than 10% of the articular surface generally do not require fixation. Fragments greater than 25% may benefit from surgical stabilization. Fragments between 10% and 25% should be assessed on an individual basis when deciding whether surgical fixation is required [overall quality: moderate]

Question 5: What is the role of early postoperative mobilization?

Case clarification
The patient has sustained a Weber B bimalleolar fracture and undergoes ORIF. He asks about your plan for postoperative rehabilitation and how soon he could expect to go back to work.

Relevance
Early mobilization of ankle fractures should theoretically prevent postoperative stiffness and allow earlier return to work. However, early mobilization may increase wound complications. The orthopedic surgeon must weigh the risks and benefits of early mobilization when determining the optimal choice for postoperative rehabilitation.

Current opinion
Young healthy patients with high functional expectations may be ideally suited for early mobilization, whereas elderly patients with poor bone quality and those at risk for postoperative infection (i.e., diabetics, patients with rheumatoid arthritis) may benefit from longer cast immobilization.

Finding the evidence
• PubMed clinical queries/systematic review: "early mobilization" OR "early motion" AND "ankle injury" OR "ankle fracture"

Quality of the evidence
Level I
• 4 randomized controlled trials

Level II
• 1 nonrandomized control trial

Findings
In one study, 100 with isolated Weber A or B ankle fractures were randomized to either early postoperative mobilization or a conventional below-knee cast.[18] Functional scores at 2 years and the time to return to work were equivalent in the two groups. However the early mobilization group had a significantly higher wound complication rate (24 patients) compared to the conventional cast immobilization group (4 patients).

In another study, 53 patients with ORIF of ankle fractures were randomized to weightbearing in either an orthosis or a walking cast. There was no difference in overall ankle function, range of motion, and pain scores at 18 months.

Following ORIF, 55 ankle fractures were randomized to either a short-leg cast (28 patients) or a removal functional brace (27 patients).[19] All patients were kept non-weight-bearing for 6 weeks. They were no wound complications in either group. Patients who underwent early mobilization had a faster return to work (53.3 days) compared to those who were immobilized in the cast (106.5 days). There was a tendency for higher functional scores in the braced group but this difference was only significant at 6 weeks.

In another study, 59 operatively stabilized ankle fractures were assigned to cast immobilization (19 patients) or an ankle–foot orthosis (AFO) (32 patients). There was no difference in range of motion or complication rates between the two groups, nor was there any loss of reduction in any of the AFO patients.

Following ORIF, 62 ankle fractures were randomized to immobilization in a cast (29 patients) or to early mobilization in a custom made removable splint (33 patients).[20] Range of motion and functional scores were similar at 12 weeks. The early mobilization group had a faster return to work/preinjury level of function (67 days vs. 94.9 days) but demonstrated an increase in wound complication rate (9.1% vs. 0%) compared to the cast immobilization group.

Recommendations

- At 1 year there was no difference in outcome in any trial with early mobilization compared to cast immobilization. Early mobilization may allow a faster return to work/preinjury function, but may be associated with increased complication rates. The surgeon should weigh the risks and benefits individually for each patient when determining the optimal rehabilitation protocol [overall quality: high]

Summary of recommendations

- The Ottawa ankle rules are a reliable tool to exclude fractures in patients more than 5 years of age presenting with ankle and midfoot injuries. Use of the Ottawa ankle rules would significantly decrease use or radiography with a low likelihood of missing a fracture
- Clinical signs of medial-sided injury are unreliable, but external rotation and gravity stress tests are an accurate and reliable method for differentiating SER II and SER IV injuries
- Intraoperative stress tests are accurate in diagnosing syndesmosis injuries
- There is no consensus with regarding the ideal screw size, number, and material for stabilization of the tibiofibular syndesmosis
- Posterior malleolar fragments less than 10% of the articular surface generally do not require fixation, while fragments greater than 25% may benefit from surgical stabilization
- At 1 year there are no differences in outcome with early mobilization compared to cast immobilization. Early mobilization may allow a faster return to work/preinjury function, but early mobilization may be associated with increased complication rates

Conclusions

Ankle fractures are common orthopedic injuries. The ability to recognize injuries with a high probability for fracture is important in minimizing unnecessary radiography. One must be methodical in the assessment of ankle fractures in order to identify all injuries that may contribute to ankle instability. It is important to have an organized approach to the management of these injuries and to understand the indications and the techniques available for surgical stabilization. Postoperative rehabilitation should be individually tailored for each patient.

References

1. Stiell IG, Greenberg GH, McKnight RD, Nair RC, McDowell I, Reardon M. Decision rules for the use of radiography in acute ankle injuries. Refinement and prospective validation. JAMA 1993;269(9):1127–32.
2. Bachmann LM, Kolb E, Koller MT, Steurer J, ter Riet G. Accuracy of Ottawa ankle rules to exclude fractures of the ankle and midfoot: systematic review. BMJ 2003;326(7386):417.
3. Stiell IG, Greenberg GH, McKnight RD, Nair RC, McDowell I, Worthington JR. A study to develop clinical decision rules for the use of radiography in acute ankle injuries. Ann Emerg Med 1992;21(4):384–90.
4. DeAngelis NA, Eskander MS, French BG. Does medial tenderness predict deep deltoid ligament incompetence in supination-external rotation type ankle fractures? J Orthop Trauma 2007;21(4):244–7.
5. McConnell T, Creevy W, Tornetta P 3rd. Stress examination of supination external rotation-type fibular fractures. J Bone Joint Surg Am 2004;86(10):2171–8.
6. Park SS, Kubiak EN, Egol KA, Kummer F, Koval KJ. Stress radiographs after ankle fracture: the effect of ankle position and deltoid ligament status on medial clear space measurements. J Orthop Trauma 2006;20(1):11–18.
7. Michelson JD, Varner KE, Checcone M. Diagnosing deltoid injury in ankle fractures: the gravity stress view. Clin Orthop Relat Res 2001;387:178–82.
8. Gill JB, Risko T, Raducan V, Grimes JS, Schutt RC Jr. Comparison of manual and gravity stress radiographs for the evaluation of supination-external rotation fibular fractures. J Bone Joint Surg Am 2007;89(5):994–9.
9. Schock HJ, Pinzur M, Manion L, Stover M. The use of gravity or manual-stress radiographs in the assessment of supination-external rotation fractures of the ankle. J Bone Joint Surg Br 2007;89(8):1055–9.
10. Jenkinson RJ, Sanders DW, Macleod MD, Domonkos A, Lydestadt J. Intraoperative diagnosis of syndesmosis injuries in external rotation ankle fractures. J Orthop Trauma 2005;19(9):604–9.
11. Moore JA Jr, Shank JR, Morgan SJ, Smith WR. Syndesmosis fixation: a comparison of three and four cortices of screw fixation without hardware removal. Foot Ankle Int 2006;27(8):567–72.
12. Høiness P, Strømsøe K. Tricortical versus quadricortical syndesmosis fixation in ankle fractures: a prospective, randomized study comparing two methods of syndesmosis fixation. J Orthop Trauma 2004;18(6):331–7.
13. Kaukonen JP, Lamberg T, Korkala O, Pajarinen J. Fixation of syndesmotic ruptures in 38 patients with a malleolar fracture: a randomized study comparing a metallic and a bioabsorbable screw. J Orthop Trauma 2005;19(6):392–5.

14. Manjoo A, Sanders DW, Tieszer C, Macleod MD. Functional and radiographic results of patients with syndesmotic screw fixation: implications for screw removal. J Orthop Trauma 2010;24(1): 2–6.

15. Macko VW, Matthews LS, Zwirkoski P, Goldstein SA. The joint-contact area of the ankle. The contribution of the posterior malleolus. J Bone Joint Surg Am 1991;73(3):347–51.

16. Jaskulka RA, Ittner G, Schedl R.Fractures of the posterior tibial margin: their role in the prognosis of malleolar fractures. J Trauma 1989;29(11):1565–70.

17. Langenhuijsen JF, Heetveld MJ, Ultee JM, Steller EP, Butzelaar RM. Results of ankle fractures with involvement of the posterior tibial margin. J Trauma 2002;53(1):55–60.

18. Lehtonen H, Järvinen TL, Honkonen S, Nyman M, Vihtonen K, Järvinen M. Use of a cast compared with a functional ankle brace after operative treatment of an ankle fracture. A prospective, randomized study. J Bone Joint Surg Am 2003;85(2):205–11.

19. Egol KA, Dolan R, Koval KJ. Functional outcome of surgery for fractures of the ankle. A prospective, randomised comparison of management in a cast or a functional brace. J Bone Joint Surg Br 2000;82(2):246–9.

20. Vioreanu M, Dudeney S, Hurson B, Kelly E, O'Rourke K, Quinlan W. Early mobilization in a removable cast compared with immobilization in a cast after operative treatment of ankle fractures: a prospective randomized study. Foot Ankle Int 2007;28(1):13–19.

65 Talus Fractures

Gregory K. Berry
McGill University, Montreal, QC, Canada

Case scenario

A healthy 25 year old woman is involved in a motor vehicle collision. She presents to the Emergency Department with a painful and deformed right hindfoot as an isolated injury. The skin and neurovascular examinations are normal.

Relevant anatomy

Two related anatomic concerns arise in the care and outcome of talar body and talar neck fractures: blood supply and cartilage coverage. The talus shares these characteristics with the carpal scaphoid bone. The intactness of the blood supply to the talus has long been recognized as a key determinant in the outcome following these injuries,[1] with osteonecrosis (ON) of the body being a frequent complication following fracture. Given that over half of the surface of the talus is covered in cartilage and that it has no tendinous or muscular insertions, direct perfusion of the neck and body by the extraosseous blood supply is limited.

Importance of the problem

Fractures of the talar body and neck are dreaded injuries for a number of reasons: they are infrequent, representing less than 0.1–0.85% of all fractures (level IV),[2] limiting the experience of the general orthopedic surgeon in treating them; they typically occur in a young, active patient population (level IV);[3–7] surgical reduction and fixation is technically challenging; and outcomes remain unfavorable in a significant percentage of patients. The viability of the talus following injury has a major impact on functional outcome given its key role in hindfoot function.

Top eight questions

Diagnosis

1. Differentiating between talar body and neck fracture—does it matter in treatment strategy or outcome?
2. Does classification help in treatment or prognostication?

Therapy

3. Is the reduction and fixation of a displaced talar neck fracture a surgical emergency?
4. Should one or two incisions be used to reduce and fix talar neck fractures?
5. What is the optimal fixation construct: plates or screws; medial or lateral implants; anterior-to-posterior or posterior-to-anterior screws?
6. Talar extrusion: to keep or to discard?
7. Weightbearing in the face of ON: to protect or not?

Prognosis

8. What are the expected outcomes following fractures of the talar body and talar neck?

Question 1: Differentiating between talar body and neck fracture—does it matter in treatment strategy or outcome?

Case clarification
The patient's radiographs show a displaced type 3 talar neck fracture (Figure 65.1).

Relevance
Differentiation between body and neck fractures is important in choice of surgical approach and prognosis.

Evidence-Based Orthopedics, First Edition. Edited by Mohit Bhandari.

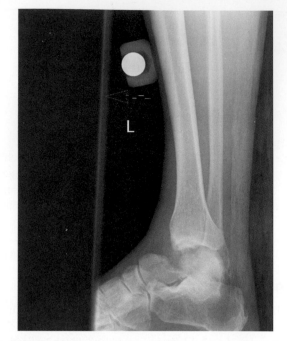

Figure 65.1 Lateral radiograph showing displaced type 3 talar neck fracture.

Finding the evidence

• Cochrane Database, with search term "talus fracture": no systematic reviews nor randomized trials; a single review on talus osteochondral injuries
• PubMed (www.ncbi.nlm.nih.gov/pubmed/) clinical queries search/systematic reviews: "talus neck and talus body fracture"

Quality of the evidence
Level IV
• 60 studies

Findings

Talar body fractures are rarer injuries than those of the neck, representing 6–40% of talus fractures, depending on the series. The two fractures differ in the position of the coronal plane fracture relative to the lateral process of the talus, as described by Inokuchi (level IV).[8] Given the fracture occurs through or posterior to the lateral process in body fractures, it by definition involves the articular surface of both the tibiotalar joint and posterior facet of the subtalar joint. Thus, any displacement will compromise load-bearing properties of both of these major weightbearing joints. Given the retrograde nature of the perfusion to the talar body from the soft tissue attachments on the talar neck, the same risks regarding ON apply to fractures of the body and the neck. In fact, in a recent review of these fractures, 40% of body fractures were associated with neck fractures (level IV).[5] Malleolar osteotomy, more commonly

medial, is more likely to be required in body fractures to reduce and fix all fracture components.

Recommendation
• Careful attention should be paid to preoperative imaging studies to clearly define the talar injury. In particular, the differentiation between neck and body fractures is important in the choice of approach, affecting overall quality of reduction and long-term prognosis [overall quality: low]

Question 2: Does classification help in treatment or prognostication?

Relevance
Fracture classification systems often lack clinical utility. A sound classification system should help guide treatment choice and inform overall prognosis.

Finding the evidence
• Cochrane Database: see Question 1
• PubMed (www.ncbi.nlm.nih.gov/pubmed/) clinical queries search/ systematic reviews: "fracture talus neck" AND "classification"

Quality of the evidence
Level IV
• 32 studies

Findings
The most commonly used classification system in talar neck fractures is that of Hawkins (level IV);[9] see box.

Hawkins classification of talar neck fractures

• Type I: undisplaced fracture
• Type II: displacement with subluxation or dislocation of the subtalar joint
• Type III: dislocation of ankle and subtalar joints
• Type IV: type III plus talonavicular subluxation or dislocation

---

The utility of classification relates to understanding fracture displacement as well as to prognosis with regards to ON. A proper appreciation of the classification scheme helps the surgeon to understand the displacement(s) involved in the fracture, which in turn will contribute to choice of approach (see below). Numerous studies have confirmed Hawkins' original correlation between displacement (or fracture grade) and incidence of ON (level IV).[3,4,10–12] This information can be transmitted to the patient early on, as the onset of ON is related to a greater number of subsequent surgeries as well as worse overall outcome.

Recommendation

• Classifying the talar neck fracture using the Hawkins classification is helpful in preoperative planning and in providing prognostic information to the patient [overall quality: low]

Question 3: Is the reduction and fixation of a displaced talar neck fracture a surgical emergency?

Relevance

Traditionally, the treatment of a displaced talar neck fracture was considered a surgical emergency.

Finding the evidence

• Cochrane Database: see Question 1
• PubMed (www.ncbi.nlm.nih.gov/pubmed/) clinical queries search/ systematic reviews: "fracture talus neck" AND "timing to surgery"

Quality of the evidence

Level IV
• 4 studies

Findings

Another way of formulating this question is: "Is there an association between the interval from injury to reduction and the incidence of ON?" Traditionally, the answer was yes, with many authors advocating urgent restoration of anatomy to limit the risk and extent of ON (level IV).[11,13,14] More recent data, however, has found no such correlation (level IV).[3,4] Thus, the indications for emergent of surgery have been modified; no longer is the isolated displaced talar neck fracture, in the absence of other factors, considered a surgical emergency. Reasons for urgent operation do exist and include open fracture, impending skin necrosis, and neurovascular compromise due to tension or compression of the posteromedial neurovascular bundle.

Recommendation

• Emergent reduction of talar neck fractures does not reduce the incidence of post-traumatic ON. Indications still remain for the emergent surgical care of these injuries, however [overall quality; low]

Question 4. Should one or two incisions be used to reduce and fix talar neck fractures?

Relevance

Soft tissue attachments to the talar neck, including perforating arteries, provide most of the blood supply to the talar body in a retrograde manner. Controversy exists whether a single or double incisions are preferable to optimize reduction quality while maintaining perfusion.

Finding the evidence

• Cochrane Database: see Question 1
• PubMed: see Question 1

Quality of the evidence

Level IV
• 60 studies

Findings

Displaced talar neck fractures typically approached through combined anteromedial and anterolateral approaches (level IV).[3,4,7,13,15–17] This strategy limits dissection on the anterior and posterior surfaces of the talar neck, thereby minimizing disruption of the critical blood supply to the talar body.

Each approach provides visual access to key components of displaced fractures. The anteromedial approach, in the interval between the tibialis posterior and anterior tendons, exposes the medial neck where comminution is usually greatest, permitting direct reduction and screw (and more rarely, plate) fixation. Cancellous and strut bone grafting are performed as needed. Extension proximally can be carried to an anteromedial ankle arthrotomy or a medial malleolar osteotomy to address an associated talar body fracture.

The anterolateral approach exposes the lateral neck and can be extended proximally to visualize the lateral ankle joint or the lateral talar process. The subtalar joint can also be cleared of fracture debris. Rarely, a lateral malleolar osteotomy is required to deal with lateral body fractures. Plate fixation, if required, is more often performed on the lateral side of the neck as the anatomy is more conducive than the medial side. Fixed angle plates such as 2.0 and 2.7 mm blade or locked plates applied to the lateral neck provide adequate stability despite there being more comminution on the medial neck.

Recommendation

• For displaced talar neck fractures, two incisions are preferable to optimize the accuracy of fracture reduction while minimizing soft tissue dissection on the anterior and posterior surfaces of the talar neck [overall quality: low]

Question 5: What is the optimal fixation construct: plates or screws; medial or lateral implants; anterior-to-posterior or posterior-to-anterior screws?

Case clarification

The patient above underwent surgery. Her surgeon had to choose one of three fixation strategies (Figure 65.2).

Relevance

A number of fixation strategies and implants are available to the surgeon for talar neck fractures.

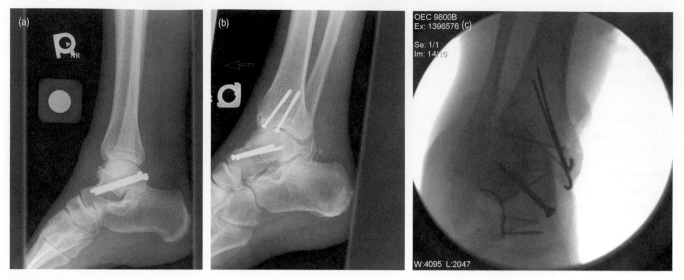

Figure 65.2 (a) Posterior-to-anterior screw fixation. (b) Anterior-to-posterior screw fixation. (c) Plate-and-screw construct.

Finding the evidence

• Cochrane Database: see Question 1
• PubMed (www.ncbi.nlm.nih.gov/pubmed/) clinical queries search/ systematic reviews: "talus neck fracture and implant," "talus neck fracture and implant fixation," "talus neck fracture and fixation"

Quality of the evidence

• Only two level IV studies exist to answer the clinical question

Findings

The aim of fixation is the maintenance of anatomic alignment while permitting range of motion exercises during the healing period. Malunion results in uneven load distribution on the articular surfaces and perturbed motion of the hindfoot complex (level IV).[18,19] Controversy exists as to the optimal choice of implants and their direction in talar neck fractures. Options include anterior-to-posterior screws, posterior-to-anterior screws, and plate fixation. Kirchner wires alone provide insufficient rigidity to withstand physiologic shear forces generated during active motion (level IV).[20]

In general, in simple (noncomminuted) fracture patterns, compression provided by screws provides adequate fixation stability. Screws directed from the posterior talus (entry at the posterolateral process) toward the talar head provide superior stability when compared to screws directed in the opposite direction (level IV).[20] This is likely due the perpendicularity of the screws relative to the coronal plane fracture line with the former technique. However, the insertion of these screws is technically more demanding.

In comminuted fractures, posterior-to-anterior screws, and medial neck plate fixation outperformed anterior-to-

posterior screws in a biomechanical study using a comminuted fracture model. However, the differences were not statistically significant and all three techniques provided enough stability to withstand the physiologic loads of active motion (level IV).[21] The authors concluded that all techniques provide sufficient stability to maintain reduction while permitting motion during healing, which has been borne out in clinical cohort outcomes (level IV).[3,4,6]

Recommendation

• Simple fracture patterns can be successfully fixed with compressive lag-screw fixation using either anterior-to-posterior or posterior-to-anterior directions. In comminuted neck fractures, plate-and-screw fixation montages on the medial or lateral neck provide favorable clinical outcomes in terms of maintenance of reduction. Biomechanical data suggests screws alone, especially when directed from posterior-to-anterior, should provide adequate stability to resist physiologic loads [overall quality: low]

Question 6: Talar extrusion: to keep or to discard?

Relevance

Faced with an extruded talar body, the surgeon must balance risk of reinsertion and attendant risk of infection vs. discarding the body and dealing with a significant bone defect (Figure 65.3).

Finding the evidence

• Cochrane Database: see Question 1
• PubMed (www.ncbi.nlm.nih.gov/pubmed/) clinical queries search/ systematic reviews: "extrusion of the talus"

Quality of the evidence
Level IV
• 24 studies

Findings
On the spectrum of injury severity, the most severe and dramatic scenario in talus fractures is that of talar body extrusion. The decision the surgeon faces is between discarding a significant portion (if not all) of the talus and being faced with a large bony deficit, and the risk of infection posed by an open wound and often extensive soft tissue stripping if the talus is reinserted. Recent evidence would support the latter strategy. In a cohort study of 19 cases of extrusion in which the talus was preserved following irrigation, debridement, reduction and rigid internal fixation, only 2 cases (10%) suffered deep infection and 12 of the 19 (63%) underwent a single surgery. Outcomes were significantly worse in those patients with talar neck fractures, with ON, collapse, and osteoarthritis (OA) occurring frequently (level IV).[22]

Recommendation
• Irrigation and debridement followed by reduction of the talar body provides favorable results considering the severity of the injury, with acceptable incidences of infection and

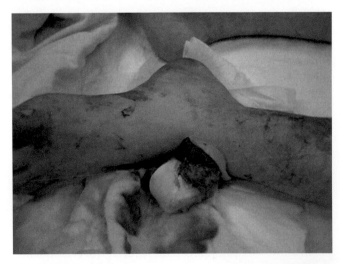

Figure 65.3 Extruded talus.

ON/OA. The talar body should not be routinely discarded [overall quality: low]

Question 7: Weightbearing in the face of ON: to protect or not?

Relevance
When faced with a case of ON of the body following talar neck fracture (Figure 65.4), the surgeon must decide whether to recommend weightbearing as tolerated vs. protected weightbearing.

Finding the evidence
• Cochrane Database: see Question 1.
• PubMed (www.ncbi.nlm.nih.gov/pubmed/) clinical queries search/ systematic reviews: "talus neck fracture", "osteonecrosis", "weightbearing"

Quality of the evidence
Level IV
• 8 studies

Findings
ON results from disruption of the retrograde blood supply from the anterior and posterior talar neck to the talar body. The degree of compromise is related to amount of displacement, as supported in nearly all outcome studies, which have consistently shown a correlation between Hawkins grade and rate of ON. The revascularization process weakens support for the articular surface(s), resulting in collapse, deformity and, eventually osteoarthrosis.

The patient who suffers ON following talus fracture represents a conundrum for the surgeon: allow weightbearing to simplify function and risk collapse, or limit weightbearing to minimize risk of collapse but impair function for up to 2 years. Unfortunately, no good evidence exists to guide the choice of strategies, and advocates exist both for[13,23,24] and against[3,25,26] (all level IV).

Recommendation
• In the case of ON following talar neck fracture, no good evidence exists to recommend protected weightbearing over weightbearing as tolerated

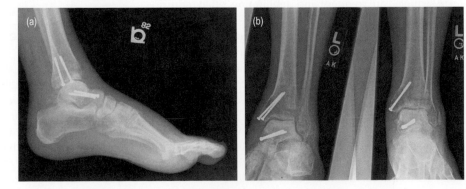

Figure 65.4 Lateral (a), mortice and AP (b) radiographs of patient at 6 months following her injury demonstrating osteonecrosis of the talar body.

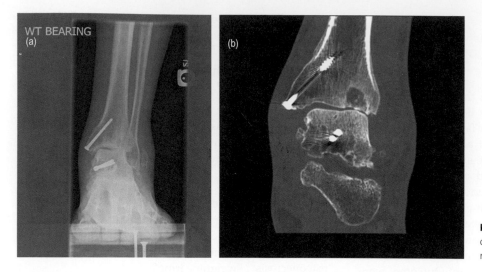

Figure 65.5 Osteonecrosis with subsequent osteoarthritis of the ankle joint. (a) AP radiograph (b) coronal plane CT scan.

Question 8: What are the expected outcomes following fractures of the talar body and talar neck?

Relevance

Displaced talar neck fractures are associated with significant functional limitations due to a high incidence of complications (Figure 65.5).

Finding the evidence

- Cochrane Database: see Question 1.
- PubMed (www.ncbi.nlm.nih.gov/pubmed/) clinical queries search/ systematic reviews: "talus neck fracture," "clinical outcome"

Quality of the evidence

Level IV
- 17 studies

Findings

In general, talar neck and body fractures are life-altering injuries, especially if they occur following high-energy mechanisms such as a motor vehicle accident. Although perioperative complications occur at acceptable rates, long-term sequelae are frequent and debilitating, often requiring further surgical management.

In recent reports of the surgical care of talar neck fractures, employing dual approaches as needed, rigid internal fixation with screws and/or plates, and early range of motion rehabilitation, superficial and deep infection occurred in 3–5% of cases, and wound dehiscence in 3% (level IV).[3,4] Late complications of delayed union (1.7%) and nonunion (3.3%) were associated with inexact reduction and open fractures in the same series.

Late sequelae were more frequent and more difficult to manage. ON occurred in 20–64% of patients and was correlated with degree of initial displacement (Hawkins grade), fracture comminution, and open fracture (level IV).[3,4] To reiterate, in neither series was delay to reduction associated with increased risk of ON. Post-traumatic osteoarthritis was a common finding and occurred at the ankle (0–18%), subtalar joint (15–40%), or both (0–57%), limiting function considerably. Lastly, pain of a mild or moderate intensity was present in 80% of patients who had suffered a talar neck fracture (level IV).[4]

As for talar body fractures, long-term sequelae occur at similar or increased rates. ON rates of 38% in isolated body fractures rise to 55% when combined with neck fractures (level IV).[3] Ankle (65%) and subtalar (35%) arthritis rates are higher than following neck fractures. Open fractures are associated with higher rates of ON and arthritis, and worse functional outcome can be expected in any patient experiencing ON, arthritis, open fracture, and comminution (level IV).[3,4]

Recommendation

- Patients who have suffered a talar body and/or neck fracture should be made aware of the significant risk of postfracture complications and sequelae [overall quality: low]

Summary of recommendations

- Careful attention should be paid to preoperative imaging studies to clearly define the talar injury. In particular, the differentiation between neck and body fractures is important in the choice of approach, affecting overall quality of reduction and long-term prognosis
- Classification of the talar neck fracture using the Hawkins classification is helpful in preoperative planning and in providing prognostic information to the patient

- Emergent reduction of talar neck fractures does not reduce the incidence of post-traumatic ON. Indications still remain for the emergent surgical care of these injuries, however
- For displaced talar neck fractures, two incisions are preferable to optimize the accuracy of fracture reduction while minimizing soft tissue dissection on the anterior and posterior surfaces of the talar neck
- Simple fracture patterns can be successfully fixed with compressive lag-screw fixation using either anterior-to-posterior or posterior-to-anterior directions. In comminuted neck fractures, plate-and-screw fixation montages on the medial or lateral neck provide favorable clinical outcomes in terms of maintenance of reduction. Biomechanical data suggests screws alone, especially when directed from posterior-to-anterior, should provide adequate stability to resist physiologic loads
- Irrigation and debridement followed by reduction of the talar body provides favorable results considering the severity of the injury, with acceptable incidences of infection and ON/OA. The talar body should not be routinely discarded
- No good evidence exists to recommend protected weightbearing over weightbearing as tolerated in the case of ON following talar neck fracture
- Patients who have suffered a talar body and/or neck fracture should be made aware of the significant risk of postfracture complications and sequelae

Conclusions

Fractures of the talar body and neck remain challenging injuries for the orthopedic surgeon. The level of quality of the evidence in the literature is in general poor, consisting primarily of case series and case reports. These do, however, provide some useful information to guide the surgical and postoperative care of these injuries.

References

1. Mulfinger GL, Trueta J The blood supply of the talus. J Bone Joint Surg 1970;52:160–7.
2. Santavirta S, Seitsalo S, et al. Fractures of the talus. J Trauma 1984;24:986–9.
3. Vallier HA, Nork SE, Barei DP, Benirschke SK, Sangeorzan B. Talar neck fractures: Results and outcomes. J Bone Joint Surg Am 2004;86:1616–24.
4. Lindvall E, Haidukewych G, DiPasquale T, Herscovici D, Sanders R. Open reduction and stable fixation of isolated, displaced talar neck and body fractures. J Bone Joint Am 2004;86:2229–34.
5. Vallier HA, Nork SE, Benirschke SK, Sangeorzan B. Surgical treatment of talar body fractures J Bone Joint Surg Am 2003;85:1716–24.
6. Fleuriau Chateau PB, Brokaw DS, Jelen BA, Scheid DK, Weber TG. Plate fixation of talar neck fractures: preliminary review of a new technique in twenty-three patients. J Orthop Trauma 2002;16:213–19.
7. Sanders DW, Busam M, Hattwick E, Edwards JR, McAndrew MP, Johnson K, Functional outcomes following displaced talar neck fractures. J Orthop Trauma 2004;18:265–70.
8. Inoguchi S, Ogawa K, Usami N. Classification of fractures of the talus: clear differentiation between neck and body fractures. Foot Ankle Int 1996;17:748–50.
9. Hawkins LG. Fractures of the neck of the talus. J Bone Joint Surg Am 1970;52:991–1002.
10. Canale ST, Kelly FB Jr. Fractures of the neck of the talus. Long-term evaluation of seventy-one cases. J Bone Joint Surg Am 1978;60:143–56.
11. Elgafy H, Ebraheim NA, Tile M, Stephen D, Kase J. Fractures of the talus: experience of two level 1 trauma centers. Foot Ankle Int 2000;21:1023–9.
12. Pearse MF, Fowler JL, Bracey DJ. Fracture of the body of the talus. Injury 1991;22:155–6.
13. Berlet GC, Lee TH, Massa EG. Talar neck fractures. Orthop Clin North Am 2001;32:53–64.
14. Frawley PA, Hart JA, Young DA. Treatment outcome of major fractures of the talus. Foot Ankle Int 1995;16:339–45.
15. Mayo KA. Fractures of the talus. principles of management and techniques of treatment. Tech Orthop 1987;2:42–54.
16. Sangeorzan BJ, Mayo KA, Hansen ST. Intraarticular fractures of the foot. Talus and lesser tarsals. Clin Orthop 1993;292:135–4.
17. Canale ST. Fractures of the neck of the talus. Orthopedics 1990;13:1105–15.
18. Daniels TR, Smith JW, Ross TI. Varus malalignment of the talar neck: its effect on the position of the foot and on subtalar motion. J Bone Joint Surg Am 1996;78:1559–67.
19. Sangeorzan BJ, Wagner UA, Harrington RM, et al. Contact characteristics of the subtalar joint: the effect of talar neck misalignment. J Orthop Res 1992;10:544–51.
20. Swanson TV, Bray TJ, Holmes GB Jr. Fractures of the talar neck: a mechanical study of fixation. J Bone Joint Surg Am 1992;74:544–51.
21. Attiah M, Sanders D, Valdivia G, Cooper I, Ferreira L, MacLeod M, Johnson A. Comminuted talar neck fractures: a mechanical comparison of fixation techniques J Orthop Trauma 2007;21:47–51.
22. Smith C, Nork S, Sangeorzan BJ. The extruded talus: the results of reimplantation. J Bone Joint Surg Am 2006;88:2418–24.
23. Pajenda G, Vecsei V, Reddy B, Heinz T. Treatment of talar neck fractures: clinical results of 50 patients. J Foot Ankle Surg 2000;39:365–75.
24. Mindell ER, Cisek EE, Kartalian G, Dziob JM. Late results of injuries to the talus. Analysis of forty cases. J Bone Joint Surg Am 1963;45:221–45.
25. Grob D, Simpson LA, Weber BG, Bray T. Operative treatment of displaced talus fractures. Clin Orthop. 1985;199:88–96.
26. Gilquist J, Oretop N, Stenstrom A, Rieger A, Wennberg E. Late results after vertical fracture of the talus. Injury. 1974;6:173–9.

66 Calcaneus Fractures

Stephen J. McChesney and Richard E. Buckley

University of Calgary, Calgary, AB, Canada

Case scenario

A 35 year old male construction worker is brought to the Emergency Department following a 3m fall at work. He complains of left heel pain and is unable to bear weight on the left. Initial trauma workup reveals an isolated injury to the left calcaneus, with no spinal or ipsilateral lower limb fractures. His left foot is very swollen and tender posteriorly, with a few blisters.

Relevant anatomy

The calcaneus is the largest of the tarsal bones. It has two articulations (comprised of three facets) with the talus superiorly, and a single saddle-shaped articulation with the cuboid anteriorly. The anterior and middle facets are frequently contiguous with one another forming one articulation, and are separated from the larger posterior articulation/facet (which is the major weightbearing surface) by the floor of the tarsal canal. The sustentaculum tali is the dense bone beneath the middle facet and it is medial to the calcaneal body. The medial aspect of the calcaneus contains thicker bone than the thin lateral wall. The area posterior to the posterior facet is the tuberosity which has two processes (lateral and medial) on its plantar surface and the insertion of the Achilles tendon on the inferior two thirds of its posterior surface.[1]

The soft tissue envelope surrounding the calcaneus has been problematic in the past. It is important to recognize that the lateral calcaneal artery, the lateral hindfoot artery, and the lateral tarsal artery contribute to the vascularity of the lateral skin and soft tissues of the foot. The lateral calcaneal artery is responsible for most of the blood supply to the corner of the flap in the extensile lateral approach.[2]

Importance of the problem

Fractures of the calcaneus are common, accounting for approximately 1.2–2% of all fractures[3] and 60% of all tarsal injuries.[1] In a study from the United Kingdom using data from the year 2000 their incidence has been estimated at 13.7/100,000 of population.[3] Only 5% of calcaneal fractures occur in children, and 80–90% occur in men aged 30–45 years.[4]

The displaced intra-articular fracture, which occurs in 75% of patients with calcaneal fractures, has been recognized as a fracture with poor functional outcome despite various treatment methods. Patients with this injury frequently have a significant period of time off work and away from normal recreation. One study showed that the mean time off work following a displaced intra-articular calcaneal fracture was 230 days or 7.5 months. The estimated average cost per patient was between $32,000 and $51,000 (Canadian) indicating a significant economic burden to society.[5]

The internet provides a significant volume of information on all medical topics and calcaneal fractures are no exception. A Google search for "calcaneal fractures" returns 500,000 hits. Given the highly variable nature of internet content, the assimilation and publication of appropriate evidence-based information to guide management of calcaneal fractures is a necessity.

Top six questions

Therapy

1. In skeletally mature patients with displaced intra-articular calcaneal fractures, is there a significant difference in outcome between nonoperative and operative treatment?

Evidence-Based Orthopedics, First Edition. Edited by Mohit Bhandari.
© 2012 Blackwell Publishing Ltd. Published 2012 by Blackwell Publishing Ltd.

2. What preoperative factors predict outcome with nonoperative vs. operative treatment of calcaneus fractures?

3. What is the effect of minimally invasive treatment on outcome and complications compared with current established treatment techniques?

4. What is the effect of using bone graft or bone-graft substitute vs. no graft on outcome in the operative management of intra-articular calcaneal fractures?

5. In patients with severely displaced intra-articular calcaneal fractures, what is the effect of acute subtalar fusion on outcome compared to current established treatment techniques?

Harm

6. What complications are associated with nonoperative vs. operative treatment of displaced intra-articular calcaneal fractures?

Question 1: In skeletally mature patients with displaced intra-articular calcaneal fractures is there a significant difference in outcome between nonoperative and operative treatment?

Case clarification

Plain radiographs and CT scan reveal a comminuted displaced intra-articular calcaneus fracture (Figure 66.1).

Relevance of the question

Operative treatment of calcaneal fractures is associated with a significant risk of serious complications. As such, it is important that both the treating surgeon and the

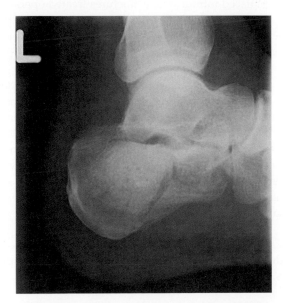

Figure 66.1 Comminuted displaced intra-articular fracture of the calcaneus.

patient are aware of the expected outcome of operative treatment and nonoperative treatment so that this can be accurately balanced against the risk involved in the chosen treatment.

Current opinion

Most trauma surgeons would currently suggest operative treatment of a displaced intra-articular calcaneal fracture in an otherwise healthy young male manual worker.

Finding the evidence

• Cochrane Database, with search terms: "(calcaneus OR calcaneal OR os calcis) AND fractures"

• PubMed (www.ncbi.nlm.nih.gov/pubmed/) clinical queries search/systematic reviews: "(calcaneus OR calcaneal OR os calcis) AND fractures"

• PubMed (www.ncbi.nlm.nih.gov/pubmed/): "(calcaneus OR calcaneal OR os calcis) AND fractures"

Quality of the evidence

Level II

• 4 randomized trials with methodologic limitations[5–16]

• 2 meta-analyses (NB: a Cochrane Review was published in 2000 but withdrawn in 2008 and is thus excluded)[17,18]

Findings

In 2005 Bajammal et al. performed a meta-analysis utilizing the results of four randomized trials with a total of 534 patients. These studies remain the best level of evidence available in the literature to date. Analysis of these studies fails to reveal a significant difference in pain or functional outcome between patients treated operatively or nonoperatively. Operative treatment may offer an advantage regarding earlier return to work and the patient's ability to continue wearing the same shoes. Subgroup analysis in the largest of these randomized trials revealed statistically significant differences in outcome between operative and nonoperative treatment in selected subgroups. These findings need to be interpreted with caution and are discussed in the following section.[6,13,14,16,18]

Ibrahim et al. reported on the longer-term follow-up of surviving patients from Parmar et al.'s original cohort.[15] This study also found no significant difference in functional outcome for those patients treated operatively vs. those treated nonoperatively. The authors concluded that 15 year follow-up demonstrated findings similar to those at 1 year; however, there were serious methodologic limitations.[14,15] No new randomized trials have been reported in the literature since 2005.

Subtalar arthrodesis has been used as a surrogate endpoint for subtalar arthritis. It has been shown that those treated nonoperatively have a six times greater risk of requiring subtalar arthrodesis than those treated nonoperatively.[6,7]

Recommendations

In patients with displaced intra-articular calcaneal fractures there is insufficient evidence to determine definitively if operative treatment is superior to nonoperative treatment. Current evidence shows:

• No statistically significant difference in pain or functional outcome between operative treatment modalities and nonoperative treatment [overall quality: moderate]

• Return to work may be improved with operative treatment [overall quality: moderate]

• Subtalar arthrodesis rates are significantly decreased with operative treatment [overall quality: moderate]

Question 2: What preoperative factors predict outcome with nonoperative vs. operative treatment of calcaneus fractures?

Case clarification

Careful history, physical examination, and radiologic examination allow the surgeon to get to know the patient. Usually the patient has 7–14 days for limb settling and soft tissue to be appropriate for surgery. Patient compliance seems most important to optimize results and minimize complications.

Relevance of the question

Only patients with appropriate variables for surgery should have surgery; other patients should have nonoperative care. Both patient and fracture variables are important when deciding on a course of treatment for an individual with a calcaneal fracture. Correctly identifying patient variables that could influence management should positively affect outcome in the individual undergoing treatment.

Current opinion

Surgeons hope to minimize complications, and by choosing patients appropriately for surgery they will predictably have the best results for the patients whether they operate or not.

Finding the evidence

• Cochrane Database, with search term: "(calcaneus OR calcaneal OR os calcis) AND fractures"

• PubMed (www.ncbi.nlm.nih.gov/pubmed/) clinical queries search/systematic reviews: "(calcaneus OR calcaneal OR os calcis) AND fractures"

• PubMed (www.ncbi.nlm.nih.gov/pubmed/): "(calcaneus OR calcaneal OR os calcis) AND fractures"

Quality of the evidence

Level II

• 4 randomized trials with methodologic limitations[5–16]

• 3 meta-analyses: (NB: A Cochrane Review was published in 2000 but withdrawn in 2008 and is thus excluded)[17–19]

• 1 prospective cohort study[20]

Level III

• 1 retrospective cohort study[21]

• 1 case-control study[22]

Findings

There are no well-designed studies on calcaneal fractures in which patient variables are incorporated in the main study question. Caution must be exercised when interpreting the results of subgroup analysis as sample size can often become small. It should also be noted that almost all studies relate only to displaced intra-articular calcaneal fractures. There is no level I or II evidence relating to extra-articular calcaneal fractures.

Age In skeletally immature patients, most calcaneal fractures are extra-articular and respond well to nonoperative treatment. Patients who are skeletally immature (<14 years) with displaced intra-articular calcaneal fractures do well regardless of whether they have operative or nonoperative care. Calcaneal fractures in adolescents behave much like those in adults and should be treated similarly.[21]

Once skeletal maturity is reached Tufescu reported that age did not alter outcome regardless of whether the treatment was operative or nonoperative. However, Buckley et al. demonstrated that patients less than 30 years of age had a statistically significant better outcome with operative treatment (odds ratio 20.0; relative risk 9.14). Their subgroup analysis also showed a trend towards poorer outcome with operative treatment in those more than 50 years of age, although this was not statistically significant.[6,20]

Gender Gender is not commonly analysed as a separate variable but it has been demonstrated that female patients with displaced intra-articular fractures treated operatively had a significantly better outcome compared to those treated nonoperatively. Young (<30 years) male patients also demonstrated a similar trend.[6,9]

Work type Patients with a light workload were significantly more likely to report a high outcome scores when treated operatively compared to nonoperative management. Patients with a heavy workload showed poor outcome scores, with no difference noted between those treated operatively and those treated nonoperatively. However, patients with a heavy workload treated operatively show a quicker return to work and a decreased incidence of subtalar arthrodesis.[6,20]

Smoking history Smoking has not been specifically correlated with outcome but does increase the risk of complications, as discussed below.

Insurance claim Patients with a pending insurance claim have been reported to have worse outcome results regard-

Table 66.1 Treatment of displaced intra-articular calcaneal fractures

Factors	Grade of evidence	Surgery recommended	Results equivocal	Nonoperative care
Patient factors				
Age[6,18]	Moderate	Adolescent	Middle age (50 yr)	>60 yr
Sex[6,18]	Moderate	Adult female; young male	Middle-aged male	Older male and female
Smoking history[8]	Poor	—	—	Recommended
Chronic medical illness[6]	Poor	—	—	Recommended
Insurance claim[6]	Moderate		+	
Workload[6,22]	Moderate	Any patient without insurance claim	Insurance claim pending	Light or sedentary work
Fracture factors				
Bilateral injury[6,10]	Moderate	—	+	—
Bohler's angle[6]	Moderate	>0°	<0°	—
Fracture classification[6]	Moderate	Sanders types II, III, IV	Type IV fractures ORIF or primary fusion	Extra-articular

less of treatment method. This group also has a higher incidence of late subtalar arthrodesis following calcaneus fracture, whether treated operatively or nonoperatively.[6,7,22]

Bohler's angle Patients with an initial Bohler's angle less than 0° show equivocal results with operative treatment. At least one study[13] has suggested better results with operative treatment compared to nonoperative. Those with a Bohler's angle greater than 15° at presentation tend to do better with operative intervention; however, they also do well with nonoperative treatment when compared to those with a Bohler's angle less than 0°.[6] Patients with a flat or negative initial Bohler's angle are significantly more likely to require subtalar arthrodesis than those with a higher initial Bohler's angle.

Sanders classification Simple fracture patterns such as Sanders II have better functional outcomes with operative treatment when compared to nonoperative treatment. Patients with a higher Sanders classification (Sanders IV) showed no difference in outcome whether treated operatively or nonoperatively.[6] However, patients with a Sanders IV fracture are 5.5 times more likely to require subtalar arthrodesis than those with a Sanders II fracture.[7]

Bilateral injury Patients with bilateral calcaneal injuries have worse outcomes than those with unilateral injuries but there is no significant difference between operative or nonoperative treatment in this group.[6,10]

Institutional fracture load A recent systematic review of operatively treated calcaneal fractures has demonstrated a significant inverse correlation between late subtalar arthrodesis (used as surrogate for post-traumatic subtalar arthritis) and institutional fracture load. This review suggests that an institutional fracture load of less than one calcaneus fracture per month jeopardizes the outcome of operatively treated calcaneal fractures.[19]

Recommendations

Due to a lack of good evidence it is only possible to give recommendations with moderate to low grades.

Current evidence suggests that treatment of displaced intra-articular calcaneal fractures be tailored to the individual, as summarized in Table 66.1.

• Institutional fracture load of less than one calcaneus fracture per month jeopardizes the outcome of operatively treated calcaneal fractures [overall quality: moderate]

Question 3: What is the effect of minimally invasive treatment on outcome and complications compared with current established treatment techniques?

Case clarification

The patient's cousin had a tibial fracture treated using "keyhole surgery." He asks if his fracture can be treated in a similar fashion.

Relevance of the question

Although minimally invasive reduction and fixation techniques are becoming widely accepted in orthopedic trauma practice, the role of this technique in calcaneal fracture fixation is unclear.

Current opinion

Currently very few surgeons are routinely using minimally invasive techniques for the treatment of displaced intra-articular calcaneal fractures.

Finding the evidence

- Cochrane Database, with search term "(calcaneus OR calcaneal OR os calcis) AND fractures AND (percutaneous OR minimally invasive)"
- PubMed (www.ncbi.nlm.nih.gov/pubmed/) clinical queries search/systematic reviews: "(calcaneus OR calcaneal OR os calcis) AND fractures AND (percutaneous OR minimally invasive)"
- PubMed (www.ncbi.nlm.nih.gov/pubmed/): "(calcaneus OR calcaneal OR os calcis) AND fractures AND (percutaneous OR minimally invasive)"

Quality of the evidence

Level III
- 1 study[23]

Level IV
- 1 systematic review[24]
- 21 studies[25–45]

Findings

There are no level I or II studies comparing minimally invasive techniques to any other form of treatment. We identified 22 level III or IV studies, but these cover a heterogeneous group of procedures. It is not possible to perform a meta-analysis of these studies because of their heterogeneity and poor study designs.

Weber et al. compared a series of percutaneously treated patients with Sanders II and III fractures to another group who had undergone open reduction and internal fixation (ORIF). They found no difference in radiologic or clinical outcome.[29] Frohlich reported on a retrospective series of percutaneously treated patients compared to a retrospective series of patients treated with open reduction, showing a favorable outcome and low complication rate for the percutaneously treated group.[23] Tornetta has reported on the successful use of percutaneous techniques for tongue fractures (OTA 73 C1,C2) using an Essex–Lopresti maneuver, and it is these fractures that are perhaps currently most applicable for minimally invasive fixation techniques.[43,44] Forgon has the largest series, consisting of 265 fractures with 90% good or excellent results.[45]

Recommendations

- At present there is insufficient evidence to make recommendations regarding the use of minimally invasive techniques for calcaneal fracture fixation

Question 4: What is the effect of using bone graft or bone-graft substitute vs. no graft on outcome in the operative management of intra-articular calcaneal fractures?

Case clarification

Following reduction of the fracture there is a significant void below the posterior facet.

Relevance of the question

It has been suggested that bone graft or bone graft substitute adds mechanical strength or post-fixation constructs and bone graft enhances bone healing in skeletally mature patients. However, bone graft has also been reported to increase complications, including wound breakdown and infection.

Current opinion

Currently opinion is divided on whether or not it is necessary to use some form of graft material to fill the void frequently found after reduction of an intra-articular calcaneal fracture.

Finding the evidence

- Cochrane Database, with search term "(calcaneus OR calcaneal OR os calcis) AND fractures AND (bone graft OR bone substitute OR bone cement)"
- PubMed (www.ncbi.nlm.nih.gov/pubmed/) clinical queries search/systematic reviews: "(calcaneus OR calcaneal OR os calcis) AND fractures AND (bone graft OR bone substitute OR bone cement)"
- PubMed (www.ncbi.nlm.nih.gov/pubmed/): "(calcaneus OR calcaneal OR os calcis) AND fractures AND (bone graft OR bone substitute OR bone cement)"

Quality of the evidence

Level I
- 1 meta-analysis[46]
- 1 randomized controlled trial[47]

Levels III–IV
- 6 studies[48–53]

Findings

The best-designed studies showed benefits with the use of calcium phosphate bone cement to fill the void left after reduction of a displaced intra-articular calcaneus fracture in terms of functional and radiologic outcomes.[46,47] Thordarson's group demonstrated in a cadaveric biomechanical study that calcium phosphate cement was superior to bone graft.[53] Longino showed no difference in functional or radiographic outcome when using iliac crest bone graft compared to no bone graft.[51]

Recommendations

• Use of calcium phosphate cement to fill a void after reduction of a displaced intra-articular calcaneal fracture improves functional and radiologic outcome [overall quality: moderate]

Question 5: In patients with severe displaced intra-articular calcaneal fractures, what is the effect of acute subtalar fusion on outcome compared to current established treatment techniques?

Case clarification

CT scan reveals a Sanders IV calcaneal fracture (Figure 66.2).

Relevance of the question

It is difficult to obtain an anatomic reduction in this type of fracture. Thus some surgeons would recommend immediate subtalar arthrodesis, given that that this fracture pattern is associated with poor functional results and a high rate of late subtalar arthrodesis.

Current opinion

Acute primary fusion is a single operation to deal with a difficult fracture. It may be reasonable to proceed with ORIF, but late fusion after nonoperative treatment is difficult.

Finding the evidence

• Cochrane Database, with search term "(calcaneus OR calcaneal OR os calcis) AND fractures AND subtalar arthrodesis"
• PubMed (www.ncbi.nlm.nih.gov/pubmed/) clinical queries search/systematic reviews: "(calcaneus OR calcaneal OR os calcis) AND fractures AND (subtalar arthrodesis or subtalar fusion)"
• PubMed (www.ncbi.nlm.nih.gov/pubmed/): "(calcaneus OR calcaneal OR os calcis) AND fractures AND (subtalar arthrodesis or subtalar fusion)"

Quality of the evidence

Level IV
• 7 retrospective case series[54-60]

Findings

There are no studies that compare reconstruction and primary subtalar arthrodesis with reconstruction for severe (Sanders IV) fractures. Seven level IV studies were identified that suggest favorable results for primary subtalar arthrodesis in patients with severe displaced intra-articular calcaneal fractures.

A multicenter randomized trial is currently in progress in Canada to evaluate this issue.

Recommendations

• There is insufficient evidence to tell if acute subtalar arthrodesis is an appropriate treatment for severe displaced intra-articular calcaneal fractures

Question 6: What complications are associated with nonoperative vs. operative treatment of displaced intra-articular calcaneal fractures?

Case clarification

Infection and hardware issues are common after operative care. Foot morphology problems and need for late subtalar fusion are common with nonoperative care.

Relevance of the question

Both operative and nonoperative treatments carry risk. It is important that both the treating surgeon and the patient are aware of what risks are involved in a course of treatment.

Current opinion

In most healthy young patients with displaced intra-articular calcaneal fractures the risks of operative treatment are justified given improved outcomes and a decreased

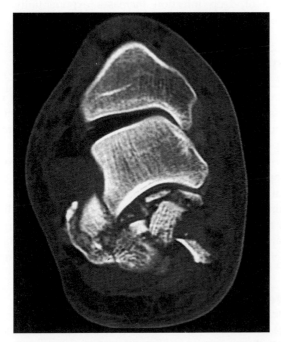

Figure 66.2 Sanders IV calcaneal fracture.

need for late surgical intervention when compared to non-operative care.

Finding the evidence

- Cochrane Database, with search term "(calcaneus OR calcaneal OR os calcis) AND fractures AND complications"
- PubMed (www.ncbi.nlm.nih.gov/pubmed/) clinical queries search/systematic reviews: "(calcaneus OR calcaneal OR os calcis) AND fractures AND complications"
- PubMed (www.ncbi.nlm.nih.gov/pubmed/) search:" (calcaneus OR calcaneal OR os calcis) AND fractures AND complications"

Quality of the evidence

Level II

- 4 randomized trials with methodologic limitations[5-16]
- 3 meta-analyses: (NB: A Cochrane Review was published in 2000 but withdrawn in 2008 and is thus excluded)[17-19]

Findings

Numerous studies have reported complications following treatment of calcaneal fractures; however, most of these are case series that do not compare treatment groups. Complications reported include poor wound healing/infection, pain, thromboembolism, neurologic complications, compartment syndromes, peroneal tendon problems, and shoe wear problems. Subsequent operative procedures have included arthrodesis, reoperations, fasciotomies, ostectomies, operative intervention for infection, and subsequent hardware removal.

The best evidence available comes from a large randomized controlled trial where complications of operative and nonoperatively treated patients were assessed. This study showed that complications occur regardless of the treatment. Complications caused significant morbidity, and patients who developed a complication had worse outcomes than those who did not develop complications, regardless of treatment. At least one major complication developed in 18% of fractures treated nonoperatively and in 25% of those treated operatively. Superficial wound slough was seen in 16% of patients treated operatively and there was a deep infection rate of 4.4%.[6-8] One recent systematic review demonstrated an exponential increase in the incidence of deep infection in operatively treated fractures with decreasing institutional fracture load, and suggests that an institutional load of less than one fracture per month jeopardizes the outcome of operatively treated displaced intra-articular fractures.[19] In Buckley et al.'s study the need for subsequent surgery was the most common complication in both groups (19% for nonoperatively treated patients and 18% for operatively treated patients), with the most common operation in the ORIF group being implant removal which occurred in 15%. The rate of late subtalar arthrodesis was significantly increased in the non-operatively treated group (16% vs. 3%). Footwear modification is often discussed as a minor complication and this study showed no difference in the incidence of footwear modification between the two groups.[6-8]

Recommendations

- At this time there is insufficient evidence to calculate relative risk for complications in those treated operatively vs. nonoperatively.
- Rate of deep infection increases exponentially with decreasing institutional fracture load [overall quality: moderate]

Summary of recommendations

- No statistically significant difference in pain or functional outcome between operative treatment modalities and nonoperative treatment
- Return to work may be improved with operative treatment
- Subtalar arthrodesis rates are significantly decreased with operative treatment
- Current evidence suggests that treatment of displaced intra-articular calcaneal fractures be tailored to the individual
- Institutional fracture load of less than one calcaneus fracture per month jeopardizes the outcome of operatively treated calcaneal fractures
- Use of calcium phosphate cement to fill a void after reduction of a displaced intra-articular calcaneal fracture improves functional and radiologic outcome
- Rate of deep infection increases exponentially with decreasing institutional fracture load

Conclusions

This difficult fracture in trauma surgery is best dealt with by institutions that perform this type of surgery commonly. Complications must be avoided with either nonoperative or operative care. With careful patient/limb selection and patient compliance, operative care is the standard. However, nonoperative care is common in patients at risk for complications or with medical illness or at extremes of age. Minimally invasive surgery is possible in patients or limbs that are amenable, to minimize complications. Surgeon experience is of significance. Young skeletally mature patients benefit from surgery. It is costly to suffer this injury.

References

1. Nork SE, Buckley RE. Hindfoot: calcaneus and talus. In: Ruedi TP, Buckley RE, Moran CG, eds. AO Principles of Fracture

Management, 2nd expanded edn, pp. 898–916. Thieme, New York, 2007.

2. Borrelli J Jr, Lashgari C. Vascularity of the lateral calcaneal flap: a cadaveric injection study. J Orthop Trauma 1999;13(2):73–7.

3. Court-Brown CM, Caesar BC. The epidemiology of fractures. In: Bucholz RW, Heckman JD, Court-Brown CM, eds., Rockwood and Green's Fractures in Adults, 6th edn, pp.96–143 Lippincott Williams & Wilkins, Philadelphia, 2006.

4. Barei DP, Bellabarba C, Sangeorzan BJ, et al. Fractures of the calcaneus. Orthop Clin North Am 2002;33:263–85.

5. Brauer CA, Manns BJ, Ko M, et al. An economic evaluation of operative compared with nonoperative management of displaced intra-articular calcaneal fractures. J Bone Joint Surg Am 2005;87(12):2741–9.

6. Buckley R, Tough S, McCormack R, et al. Operative compared with nonoperative treatment of displaced intra-articular calcaneal fractures: a prospective, randomized, controlled multicenter trial. J Bone Joint Surg Am 2002;84:1733–44.

7. Csizy M, Buckley R, Tough S, et al. Displaced intra-articular calcaneal fractures: variables predicting late subtalar fusion. J Orthop Trauma 2003;17:106–12.

8. Howard JL, Buckley R, McCormack R, et al. Complications following management of displaced intra-articular calcaneal fractures: a prospective randomized trial comparing open reduction internal fixation with nonoperative management. J Orthop Trauma 2003;17:241–9.

9. Barla J, Buckley R, McCormack R, et al. Displaced intraarticular calcaneal fractures: long-term outcome in women. Foot Ankle Int. 2004;25:853–6.

10. Dooley P, Buckley R, Tough S, et al. Bilateral calcaneal fractures: operative versus nonoperative treatment. Foot Ankle Int 2004;25:47–52.

11. Kingwell S, Buckley R, Willis N. The association between subtalar joint motion and outcome satisfaction in patients with displaced intraarticular calcaneal fractures. Foot Ankle Int 2004;25:666–73.

12. O'Brien J, Buckley R, McCormack R, et al. Personal gait satisfaction after displaced intraarticular calcaneal fractures: a 2–8 year follow-up. Foot Ankle Int 2004;25:657–65.

13. Thordarson D, Krieger L. Operative vs. nonoperative treatment of intraarticular fractures of the calcaneus: a prospective randomized trial. Foot Ankle Int 1996;17:2–9.

14. Parmar H, Triffitt P, Gregg P. Intra-articular fractures of the calcaneum treated operatively or conservatively. A prospective study. J Bone Joint Surg Br 1993;75:932–7.

15. Ibrahim T, Rowsell M, Rennie W, et al. Displaced intra-articular calcaneal fractures: 15 year follow-up of a randomised controlled trial of conservative versus operative treatment. Injury 2007;38:848–55.

16. O'Farrell DA, O'Byrne JM, McCabe JP, et al. Fractures of the os calcis: improved results with internal fixation. Injury 1993;24:263–5.

17. Bridgman SA, Dunn KM, McBride DJ, Richards PJ. Interventions for treating calcaneal fractures. Cochrane Database Syst Rev 2000;CD001161.

18. Bajammal S, Tornetta P, Sanders M et al. Displaced intra-articular calcaneal fractures. J Orthop Trauma 2005;19:360–5.

19. Poeze M, Verbruggen J, Brink P. The relationship between the outcome of operatively treated calcaneal fractures and institutional fracture load. A Systematic Review of the Literature. J Bone Joint Surg Am 2008;90:1013–21.

20. Tufescu T, Buckley R. Age, gender, work capability, and worker's compensation in patients with displaced intraarticular calcaneal fractures. J Orthop Trauma 2001;15:275–9.

21. Ceccarelli F, Fatdini C, Piras F et al. Surgical versus non-surgical treatment of calcaneal fractures in children: A long-term results comparative study. Foot Ankle Int 2000;21:825–32.

22. Buckley R, Meek R. Comparison of open versus closed reduction of intraarticular calcaneal fractures: a matched cohort in workmen. J Orthop Trauma 1992;6:216–22.

23. Frohlich P, Zakupszky Z, Csomor L. [Experiences with closed screw placement in intra-articular fractures of the calcaneus: Surgical technique and outcome]. Unfallchirurg 1999;102:359–364.

24. Schepers T, Patka P. Treatment of displaced intra-articular calcaneal fractures by ligamentotaxis: current concepts review. Arch Orthop Trauma Surg 2009;129(12):1677–83.

25. Rammelt S, Amlang M, Barthel S, Gavlik JM, Zwipp H. Percutaneous treatment of less severe intraarticular calcaneal fractures. Clin Orthop Relat Res 2010;468(4):983–90.

26. Demcoe AR, Verhulsdonk M, Buckley RE. Complications when using threaded K-wire fixation for displaced intra-articular calcaneal fractures. Injury 2009;40(12):1297–301.

27. Schuberth JM, Cobb MD, Talarico RH. Minimally invasive arthroscopic-assisted reduction with percutaneous fixation in the management of intra-articular calcaneal fractures: a review of 24 cases. J Foot Ankle Surg 2009;48:315–22.

28. Pezzoni M, Salvi AE, Tassi M et al. A minimally invasive reduction and synthesis method for calcaneal fractures: the "Brixian bridge" technique. J Foot Ankle Surg 2009;48:85–8.

29. Weber M, Lehmann O, Sägesser D, Krause F. Limited open reduction and internal fixation of displaced intra-articular fractures of the calcaneum. J Bone Joint Surg Br 2008;90:1608–16.

30. Hospodar P, Guzman C, Johnson P, et al. Treatment of displaced calcaneus fractures using a minimally invasive sinus tarsi approach. Orthopedics 2008;31:1112.

31. Walde TA, Sauer B, Degreif J, et al. Closed reduction and percutaneous Kirschner wire fixation for the treatment of dislocated calcaneal fractures: surgical technique, complications, clinical and radiological results after 2–10 years. Arch Orthop Trauma Surg 2008;128:585–91.

32. Schepers T, Vogels LM, Schipper IB, et al. Percutaneous reduction and fixation of intraarticular calcaneal fractures. Oper Orthop Traumatol 2008;20:168–75.

33. Schepers T, Van der Stoep A, Van der Avert H, et al. Plantar pressure analysis after percutaneous repair of displaced intraarticular calcaneal fractures. Foot Ankle Int 2008;29:128–35.

34. Schepers T, Schipper IB, Vogels LM, et al. Percutaneous treatment of displaced intra-articular calcaneal fractures. J Orthop Sci 2007;12:22–7.

35. Stulik J, Stehlik J, Rysavy M et al. Minimally-invasive treatment of intra-articular fractures of the calcaneum. J Bone Joint Surg Br 2006;88:1634–41.

36. Magnan B, Bortolazzi R, Marangon A, et al. External fixation for displaced intra-articular fractures of the calcaneum. J Bone Joint Surg Br 2006;88:1474–9.

37. McGarvey WC, Burris MW, Clanton TO, et al. Calcaneal fractures: indirect reduction and external fixation. Foot Ankle Int 2006;27:494–499.

38. Talarico LM, Vito GR, Zyryanov SY. Management of displaced intraarticular calcaneal fractures by using external ring fixation, minimally invasive open reduction, and early weightbearing. J Foot Ankle Surg 2004;43:43–50.

39. Stein H, Rosen N, Lerner A, et al. Minimally invasive surgical techniques for the reconstruction of calcaneal fractures. Orthopedics 2003;26:1053–6.

40. Gavlik JM, Rammelt S, Zwipp H. Percutaneous, arthroscopically-assisted osteosynthesis of calcaneus fractures. Arch Orthop Trauma Surg 2002;122:424–8.

41. Schildhauer TA, Sangeorzan BJ. Push screw for indirect reduction of severe joint depression-type calcaneal fractures. J Orthop Trauma 2002;16:422–4.

42. Levine DS, Helfet DL. An introduction to the minimally invasive osteosynthesis of intra-articular calcaneal fractures. Injury 2001; 32(Suppl 1):SA51–4.

43. Tornetta P 3rd. Percutaneous treatment of calcaneal fractures. Clin Orthop Relat Res 2000;375:91–6.

44. Tornetta P 3rd. The Essex-Lopresti reduction for calcaneal fractures revisited. J Orthop Trauma 1998;12:469–73.

45. Forgon M Closed reduction and percutaneous osteosynthesis: technique and results in 265 calcaneal fractures. In: Tscherne H, Schatzker J, eds., Major Fractures of the Pilon, the Talus, and the Calcaneus, pp. 207–213. Springer-Verlag, New York, 1993.

46. Bajammal SS, Zlowodzki M, Lelwica A, et al. The use of calcium phosphate bone cement in fracture treatment. A meta-analysis of randomized trials. J Bone Joint Surg Am 2008;90 1186–96.

47. Johal H, Buckley R, Le I, et al. A prospective randomized controlled trial of a bioresorbable calcium phosphate paste (α-BSM) in treatment of displaced intra-articular calcaneal fractures. J Trauma 2009;67(4):875–82.

48. Bibbo C, Patel DV. The effect of demineralized bone matrix-calcium sulfate with vancomycin on calcaneal fracture healing and infection rates: a prospective study. Foot Ankle Int 2006; 27:487–93.

49. Elsner A, Jubel A, Prokop A, et al. Augmentation of intraarticular calcaneal fractures with injectable calcium phosphate cement: densitometry, histology, and functional outcome of 18 patients. J Foot Ankle Surg 2005;44:390–5.

50. Thordarson DB, Bollinger M. SRS cancellous bone cement augmentation of calcaneal fracture fixation. Foot Ankle Int 2005; 26:347–52.

51. Longino D, Buckley RE. Bone graft in the operative treatment of displaced intraarticular calcaneal fractures: is it helpful? J Orthop Trauma 2001;15:280–6.

52. Schildhauer TA, Bauer TW, Josten C, et al. Open reduction and augmentation of internal fixation with an injectable skeletal cement for the treatment of complex calcaneal fractures. J Orthop Trauma 2001;14:309–17.

53. Thordarson DB, Hedman TP, Yetkinler DN et al. Superior compressive strength of a calcaneal fracture construct augmented with remodelable cancellous bone cement. J Bone Joint Surg Am 1999;81:239–46.

54. Gagała J, Guzik G, Modrzewski K. [Long-term results comparison of simultaneous open reduction and subtalar arthrodesis with the efficacy of closed reduction in the treatment of fresh fractures of calcaneus] Chir Narzadow Ruchu Ortop Pol 2007;72: 408–414. Polish.

55. Huefner T, Thermann H, Geerling J et al. Primary subtalar arthrodesis of calcaneal fractures. Foot Ankle Int 2001;22:9–14.

56. Buch BD, Myerson MS, Miller SD. Primary subtaler arthrodesis for the treatment of comminuted calcaneal fractures. Foot Ankle Int 1996;17:61–70.

57. Myerson MS. Primary subtalar arthrodesis for the treatment of comminuted fractures of the calcaneus. Orthop Clin North Am 1995;26:215–27.

58. Noble J, McQuillan WM. Early posterior subtalar fusion in the treatment of fractures of the os calcis. J Bone Joint Surg Br 1999;61:90–3.

59. Mignot P, Champetier J. [Results of primary reconstructive arthrodesis of the calcaneus (study of a homogenous series of 55 fractures of the medical surface of the calceneus)] J Chir (Paris) 1995;110:61–70. French.

60. Harris RI. Fractures of the os calcis. Treatment by early subtalar arthrodesis. Clin Orthop Relat Res 1993;30:100–10.

Midfoot/Metatarsal Fractures

Robin R. Elliot and Terence S. Saxby
Brisbane Foot and Ankle Centre, Brisbane, QLD, Australia

Case scenario

During a game of football, player A has to quickly turn and change direction in order to make a tackle on player B: he twists, and in doing so he sustains an injury to his right foot. Nevertheless, he makes a good tackle but lands with his body weight on the foot of player B. Both players are injured and unable to continue with the game. Both players attend the Emergency Department for a radiograph; player A is told he has a fracture of his 5th metatarsal, but player B is reassured that there is no bony injury.

Relevant anatomy

The proximal metatarsals and the cuneiform bones of the midfoot are trapezoidal shaped and together they form a Roman arch structure, the keystone being the base of the 2nd metatarsal (Figure 67.1). The 2nd tarsometatarsal joint is recessed proximally, locking the midfoot and protecting the area against medial and lateral shear forces. The arch protects the neurovascular and tendinous structures running underneath during weightbearing. The metatarsals function as supports in the stance phase of the gait cycle and as a lever during propulsion.

In assessing for a Lisfranc injury, key radiological alignments should be assessed in all cases (Figure 67.2 and Figure 67.3). Careful attention should be paid to the distances between the 1st and 2nd metatarsals and the medial and middle cuneiform and for the presence of avulsion fractures (fleck sign).[1] A weightbearing view is more sensitive in demonstrating tarsometatarsal instability, but this is often not practical in the acute setting.

Importance of the problem

Metatarsal fractures are relatively common injuries with fractures of the 5th metatarsal occurring most frequently.[2] A study of trauma in motorcyclists showed that metatarsal fractures were the most common injuries to the foot.[3] Metatarsal fractures may be caused by inversion/avulsion injuries, direct crushing forces to the foot, and overuse injuries. These injuries can be a cause of prolonged disability and lost work productivity.[4]

Lisfranc joint injuries are uncommon, with reported incidence of 1 per 55,000 per year, accounting for approximately 0.2% of all fractures.[5] These injuries have traditionally been associated with high-energy trauma, but it is now recognized that there is a spectrum of injuries involving this area of the foot, ranging from sprains to complete dislocations. Unfortunately, Lisfranc injury is a commonly missed diagnosis and this type of injury has the potential to lead to significant morbidity.[6]

Finding the evidence

A search of the literature was undertaken using available databases at our institution. These include MEDLINE through PubMed (citations 1950 to present), the Cochrane Database of Systematic Reviews, and CINAHL. Specific search details are listed below.
- PubMed: searches built using MeSH database contolled vocabulary. Combined searches: "Fractures, Bone" [Mesh] AND "Metatarsal Bones" [Mesh], "Fractures, Bone" [Mesh] AND Lisfranc. Word searches using "Lisfranc" AND "fracture," "metatarsal" AND "fracture"

Evidence-Based Orthopedics, First Edition. Edited by Mohit Bhandari.
© 2012 Blackwell Publishing Ltd. Published 2012 by Blackwell Publishing Ltd.

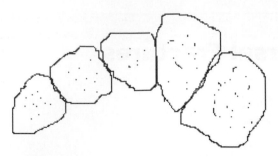
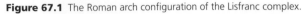

Figure 67.1 The Roman arch configuration of the Lisfranc complex.

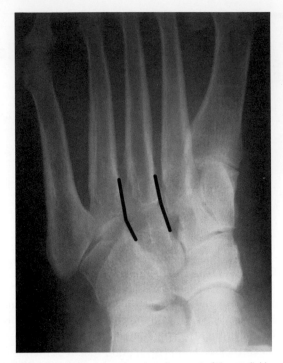

Figure 67.3 30° oblique view showing alignment of the medial borders of third metatarsal and the lateral cuneiform as well as the medial borders of the fourth metatarsal and the cuboid bone.

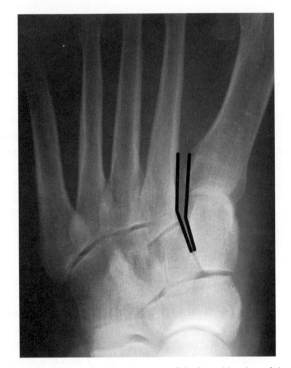

Figure 67.2 AP view showing alignment of the lateral borders of the first metatersal and the medial cuneiform as well as the medial borders of the 2nd metatarsal and the middle cuneiform.

• Cochrane Database: using text words "metatarsal," "Lisfranc," ("metatarsal" AND "fracture"), ("Lisfranc" AND "fracture")
• CINAHL: Combined searches "Fractures, Bone" [Mesh] AND "Metatarsal Bones" [Mesh], "Fractures, Bone" [Mesh] AND Lisfranc

---

Top six questions

Diagnosis

1. What are the different types of proximal 5th metatarsal fractures?
2. What is the role of further investigations in the diagnosis of Lisfranc fractures?

Therapy

3. What is the role of operative vs. nonoperative management of proximal 5th metatarsal fractures?
4. In a patient with a Lisfranc injury, does an anatomic reduction and fixation result in better outcomes than conservative treatment and how does this compare to primary fusion?

Prognosis

5. What is the chance of each of these players returning to their preinjury level of sport?

Harm

6. What are the potential problems with delayed or misdiagnosis of Lisfranc injuries, and what are the long-term complications associated with this injury?

Question 1: What are the different types of proximal 5th metatarsal fractures?

Case clarification

Player A presents with plain radiographs that reveal a fracture in the proximal part of the 5th metatarsal diaphysis with associated periosteal new bone formation and some sclerotic bone within the medullary canal. He reports that he has had some discomfort over the lateral border of his foot for many months prior to this acute injury.

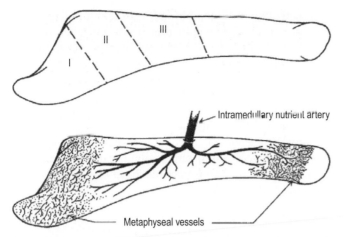

Figure 67.4 (Top) Dameron's three zones of the proximal 5th metatarsal. Zone I injuries are avulsion fractures of the tuberosity. Zone II injuries are fractures involving the intermetatarsal facet (as described by Jones). Zone III injuries are proximal diaphyseal fractures. (Bottom) Blood supply. (©1995 American Academy of Orthopaedic Surgeons. Reprinted with permission from Dameron TB. Fractures of the proximal fifth metatarsal: selecting the best treatment option. J Am Acad Orthop Surg 1995;3(2):110–14.)[8]

Relevance

This patient has a proximal diaphyseal stress fracture. The classification and description of fractures of the proximal 5th metatarsal can be confusing and central to this has been the regular misuse of the term "Jones fracture."

> Sir Robert Jones was one of the forefathers of British Orthopaedics and founder of the British Orthopaedic Association. In 1902 he wrote on six cases of fractures of the proximal 5th metatarsal.[7]

The use of a clear and practical classification system such as that provided by Dameron[8] can help in this respect (Figure 67.4).

Current opinion

Treatment should be individualized according to the type of fracture and the demands of the patient. Most zone 1 injuries heal with simple conservative management; zone 2 injuries can take longer to heal and are more likely to refracture if full activity is resumed too quickly. It is well recognized that zone 3 fractures are prone to delayed or nonunion.

Quality of the evidence

Level IV
• 3 case series

Findings

Clapper published a series of 100 patients with 5th meta-tarsal fractures which were followed prospectively to determine outcomes of their injuries: three distinct subgroups were identified depending on fracture location (level IV).[9] Dameron reported a case series of 100 tuberosity fractures treated conservatively, all but one healed clinically within 3 weeks (level IV).[10] In Kavanaugh's series of 22 "Jones" fractures delayed healing was observed in 2/3 of those cases treated conservatively (level IV).[11]

Recommendations

• For zone 1 (avulsion) fractures conservative, symptomatic treatment is sufficient and patients may resume normal activities as their symptoms permit irrespective of radiological appearance [overall quality: high]
• Zone 2 (Jones) fractures are slower to heal and more prone to refracture. A short-leg cast or a functional brace may be used and surgical fixation could be considered in the high-level athlete [overall quality: moderate]
• Zone 3 injuries (diaphyseal stress fractures) are prone to nonunion and surgical fixation results in a quicker time to union and return to sport and this may be beneficial in selected patients (see Question 5) [overall quality: moderate]

Question 2: What is the role of further investigations in the diagnosis of Lisfranc fractures?

Case clarification

Player B rests at home with his foot elevated for a week. Despite this, his foot remains swollen and he is unable to weight bear. He returns to the Emergency Department where the attending doctor notes significant swelling and an area of plantar ecchymosis. His initial radiographs are re-examined and once again no obvious malalignment of the tarsometatarsal joints is noticed. Nevertheless, there is high clinical suspicion of a midfoot injury and he is referred to the orthopedic clinic for further investigation.

Relevance

The initial mechanism of injury, the ongoing swelling and the plantar ecchymosis all raise the suspicion of a Lisfranc injury.

> Jacques Lisfranc (1787–1847) was a field surgeon in the Napoleonic wars. He described an amputation performed through the midfoot because of gangrene that developed after an injury incurred when a soldier fell off a horse with his foot caught in the stirrup.

Current opinion

In suspected midfoot injuries with apparently normal plain radiographs, no widely agreed imaging algorithm exists beyond the recommendation that weightbearing views should be obtained. Weightbearing or stress radiographs are favored because of the dynamic nature of the investigation and their ability to demonstrate instability. CT, MRI, bone scans, and ultrasound have also been reported as further investigations.[1,12,13]

Findings

A cadaver study showed that in comparison to weightbearing radiographs, injury-specific manual stress radiographs showed qualitatively greater displacement when used to evaluate Lisfranc instability (level V).[14]

A study examined plain radiographs and stress radiographs in 40 normal volunteer feet and compared these with images taken in cadaveric feet, which had undergone sectioning of the Lisfranc and dorsal tarsometatarsal ligaments. Disruption of a line tangential to the medial aspect of the navicular and medial cuneiform intersecting the base of the first metatarsal (medial column line) was found to be a simple and valuable diagnostic tool for determining significant ligamentous injury (level V).[15]

One study of 21 feet compared MRI findings with intraoperative findings to determine whether conventional MRI is a reliable diagnostic tool; 19 (90%) of the feet were correctly diagnosed with one false positive and one false negative (level III).[16]

A cadaver study showed the increased sensitivity of CT scanning vs. plain radiographs in revealing minor malalignments of the metatarsal cuneiform joints (level V).[17]

A prospective clinical study investigated midfoot hyperextension injuries in 75 consecutive patients. All patients had plain radiographs, stress radiographs, CT, and MRI. Their findings showed that both CT and MRI were more sensitive in identifying tarsal and metatarsal fractures and malalignments than plain radiographs and stress radiographs (level IV).[18]

Recommendation

• Plain radiographs and weightbearing/stress radiographs are appropriate initial investigations in patients with suspected Lisfranc injuries. If these investigations are normal or equivocal and there is ongoing clinical suspicion of a Lisfranc injury then further investigation in the form of bone scans, CT or MRI should be requested depending on which imaging modality is most readily available locally [overall quality: moderate]

Question 3: What is the role of operative vs. nonoperative management of proximal 5th metatarsal fractures?

Case clarification

Player A has sustained an acute injury to his metatarsal but his history and radiographic findings suggest that he had an underlying proximal diaphyseal stress fracture. He

reports that he is the captain of his team and they have an important game in 12 weeks' time. He wants to know what treatment would offer him the best chance of playing in that game. In discussing the treatment options with player A, he asks what the alternatives are to surgery.

Relevance

The majority of 5th metatarsal fractures heal with conservative management.[9,10] There is a small group that are prone to delayed healing and nonunion: diaphyseal stress fractures (zone 3). These fractures have been further subclassified by Torg (see box).[19]

Torg classification of diaphyseal stress fractures

• Torg I (acute fracture): no previous injury, no intramedullary sclerosis or cortical hypertrophy, sharp fracture margins
• Torg II (delayed union): previous injury, periosteal new bone, widened fracture line, some intramedullary sclerosis
• Torg III (nonunion): repetitive trauma, wide fracture line, periosteal new bone, obliteration of medullary canal with sclerotic bone

---

Current opinion

Zone 1 tuberosity fractures and distal metatarsal fractures are commonly treated symptomatically. Zone 2 and 3 proximal metatarsal injuries, when treated conservatively, should be put in an aircast boot or plaster and weightbearing can be allowed as tolerated. Prolonged absence of weightbearing may be counterproductive. In a high-demand athlete with an acute zone 2 (Jones fracture) or zone 3 fracture, most specialists would advise operative fixation to achieve a more rapid time to union and return to sport. Most surgeons use an intramedullary screw to fix these fractures. Guidelines for treatment should be individualized depending upon type of fracture and sporting demands.

Quality of the evidence (treatment methods)

The frequent, and often incorrect, use of the term Jones fracture makes interpretation of the literature difficult.

Level IIb
• 2 prospective randomized trials

Level IV
• 6 case series

Findings

A prospective randomized trial showed a significantly quicker (p < 0.01) time to union (7.5 weeks) and return to sport (8 weeks) in the surgical group when compared to conservative treatment (14.5 weeks and 15 weeks). The failure rate was also noticeably higher in the conservative group (44% vs. 5%) (level II).[20]

These findings are in keeping with the results of the various case series. Portland et al. showed time to union of 6.2 weeks for surgically treated Jones fractures (level IV)[21] and Leumann et al. found union in 64% of patients at 6 weeks, the remainder uniting by 12 weeks with one partial union. All patients returned to their previous levels of sporting activity (level IV).[22] Kavanaugh found delayed union (>6 months) in 66% patients treated conservatively, 50% having had refractures, whereas all 4 surgically treated patients united and returned to sport at 6–8 weeks (level IV).[11] De Lee achieved union (mean 7.5 weeks) in all patients in his series (10 patients) with screw fixation (level IV).[23] Mindrebo reports 9 patients fixed surgically with mean time to return to running of 5.5 weeks, all fractures clinically and radiologically united (level IV).[24]

A prospective randomized study included 60 patients comparing short-leg cast and soft dressings in the treatment of tuberosity fractures. All fractures healed however those treated in a soft dressing returned to preinjury levels of activity faster (average 33 days vs. 46 days) (level II).[25]

A case series of 38 patients with zone 1 (tuberosity) fractures showed that the most significant predictor of poor functional outcome was prolonged absence of weightbearing. Gender, age, and fracture type did not affect outcome (level IV).[26]

Quality of the evidence (fixation methods)
• Only two clinical studies (level IV) were found, the rest relying on cadaveric models to test different fixation methods

Findings
One clinical study and one cadaveric study compared the use of 4.5 mm and 5.5 mm screws to fix proximal 5th metatarsal fractures and neither was unable to show a significant difference between the two. In the clinical study, three bent screws were noted in the 4.5 mm group (level IV–V).[27,28]

Reese et al. cautioned against the use of screws of 4 mm and less due to the low number of cycles to failure in their cadaveric models fixed with these screws. They also found that solid screws displayed twice the number of cycles to failure when compared to cannulated screws (level V).[29]

Sides et al. compared bending stiffness and pull-out strength of tapered variable-pitch screws and 6.5 mm cancellous screws in acute Jones fractures using a cadaveric model. There was no demonstrable difference in bending stiffness between metatarsals fixed with the two types of screws (p = 0.688) (level V).[30] The 6.5 mm screw provided significantly higher resistance to pull-out (p = 0.001), a finding replicated in Kelly et al.'s cadaveric study (level V).[31]

The importance of torsional restraint was suggested by the findings of a cadaveric study by Vertullo et al. (level V).[32] Horst et al. tested torsional resistance of 5 mm and 6.5 mm screws used to fix simulated Jones fractures in cadaveric models. They found that both 5.0 mm or 6.5 mm screws provided equal torsional rigidity, but 5.0 mm screws needed to be longer to achieve stability and this could potentially cause problems in patients with curved metatarsals (level V).[33]

Moshirfar et al. studied strength of fixation comparing a bicortical lag screw with an intramedullary screw. The lag screw technique resulted in a significantly greater mean (± SD) load to failure (150 ± 90 N) (level V).[34]

Sarimo et al. present a series of zone 3 injuries treated successfully with a tension band wire construct. There were no refractures or hardware failures in their series (level IV).[35]

Recommendations
• Zone 1 injuries can be treated symptomatically. Consideration should be given to operative fixation of zone 2 and zone 3 injuries leads to a quicker time to union and return to sport and this may be beneficial in selected patients [overall quality: moderate]
• A solid screw of adequate size such that the threads gain purchase in the cortical diaphyseal bone should be used (Figure 67.5). Care should be taken not to oversize the screw as complications such as stress fracture and distal cortical penetration may occur.[36] Use of screws smaller than 4 mm risks failure/bending of the screw and refracture [overall quality: moderate]
• If Zone 2 and 3 injuries are treated conservatively they should be treated with support in a plaster or boot, and weightbearing should be encouraged as tolerated [overall quality: moderate]

Question 4: In a patient with a Lisfranc injury, does an anatomic reduction and fixation result in better outcomes than conservative treatment and how does this compare to primary fusion?

Case clarification
Player B has weightbearing radiographs of his foot taken at his outpatient follow-up. These clearly show instability of the tarsometatarsal joints and the radiographs indicate a homolateral pattern of Lisfranc injury (Figure 67.6).

Quenu and Kuss descibed the original classification of these injuries and this remains the most widely used today. They described three types, dependent upon the radiographic findings: homolateral, isolated, and divergent.[37]

Relevance

Anatomical reduction and rigid internal fixation has been shown to be an important factor in the eventual outcome (level IV).[38] Key to this is the reduction of the articulation between the 2nd metatarsal and the middle cuneiform and fixation, which replicates the function of the Lifranc ligament, tying the medial cuneiform to the 2nd metatarsal.

Current opinion

Lisfranc injuries require prompt anatomical reduction and surgical fixation with screws. There is some debate regarding the effectiveness of primary arthrodesis as treatment for these injuries, but this has not become mainstream treatment.

Quality of the evidence

Level II

• 2 prospective randomized studies have investigated primary arthrodesis

Level IV

• Numerous case series can be found relating to this topic

Findings

In Myerson's case series of 55 patients the major determinant of unacceptable results was identified as the quality of the initial reduction (level IV).[38] Goossens' case series of 20 patients showed that 70% of patients who were treated conservatively in an unreduced position had a poor outcome, compared with only 18% of those who had reduc-

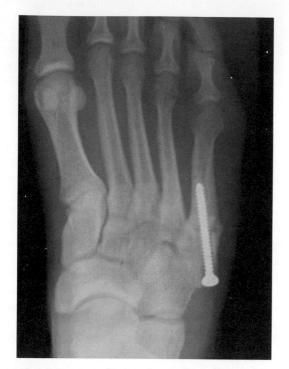

Figure 67.5 4.5 mm screw fixation of proximal 5th metatarsal fracture.

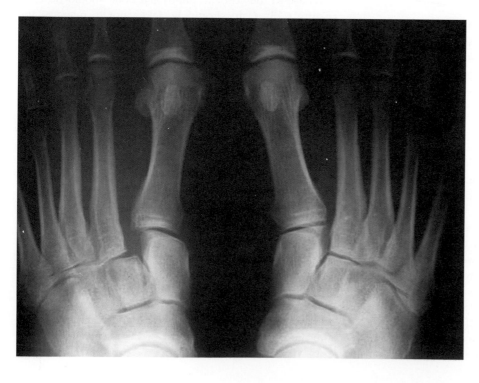

Figure 67.6 Weightbearing views showing instability of the left 1st and 2nd tarsometatarsal joints and widening of the space between the 1st and 2nd rays.

tion and pinning (level IV).[39] Arntz showed in a consecutive series of 40 patients that good or excellent results were obtained in 95% of patients with an anatomical reduction but only 20% of those in whom the reduction was nonanatomical (level IV).[40] One case series suggested that anatomical reduction was not a guarantee of satisfactory outcome: Teng et al. reported that the subjective functional outcome in their series of 11 patients was not very good despite successful restoration of normal anatomy (level IV).[41]

Coetzee reported favorable outcomes for patients treated with a primary arthrodesis with a significant improvement in midfoot American Orthopaedic Foot & Ankle Society (AOFAS) scores in the arthrodesis group at 2 years (level II).[42] These finding were not replicated by a similar study of 40 patients by Henning et al. which showed no significant difference in Short Form-36 (SF-36) and short musculoskeletal function assessment (SMFA) scores (level II).[43]

Recommendation

- In treating Lisfranc injuries, restoration of normal anatomy and surgical fixation gives the best chance of a favorable long-term outcome [overall quality: high]

Question 5: What is the chance of each of these players returning to their preinjury level of sport?

Case clarification

Both players attend follow-up and ask for insurance forms to be completed in relation to their injuries. One question asks whether they will be able to return to their preinjury level of function.

Relevance

Managing expectations is an important aspect of treating surgical patients and a thorough knowledge of prognosis helps in this respect.

Current opinion

Return to a preinjury level of sporting activity can almost always be expected after a 5th metatarsal injury, but the outcome is less certain after a Lisfranc injury.

Quality of the evidence

Level IV
- 5 case series

Findings

Lisfranc injury Chilvers published a case series including 5 gymnasts with Lisfranc injuries: only 1 returned to full competition (level IV).[44] Curtis et al. report that 3 of 19 patients with Lisfranc injury were unable to return to their sports (level IV).[45]

Nunley and Vertullo describe 15 patients with Lisfranc injuries sustained playing sport. Seven of these injuries were diagnosed as sprains (stage 1 injuries—see box) and treated conservatively. All patients in their series returned to sport (average 15.2 weeks) (level IV).[1] Nunley and Vertullo have proposed a classification system for the low-energy Lisfranc injury typically sustained playing sport.[1]

Classification system for low-energy Lisfranc injuries
Stage 1 (bone scan positive): a sprain of the Lisfranc ligament with no diastasis between the medial cuneiform and the base of the 2nd metatarsal
Stage 2: diastasis 1–5 mm
Stage 3: diastasis >5 mm and loss of arch height

Proximal 5th metatarsal Porter et al. report a case series of 23 athletes treated with internal fixation of the 5th metatarsal, all of whom returned to sport (mean 7.5 weeks) (level IV).[46]

Portland et al. surgically treated 22 patients with Jones fractures or proximal diaphyseal stress fractures, all fractures united (mean 6.25 weeks) with none to rare pain reported during athletic activity (level IV).[21]

Recommendation

- Patients with 5th metatarsal injuries can be reassured that they should be able to return to their preinjury sport. The outcome of Lisfranc injuries is less predictable, the recovery is slower and caution must be taken to avoid giving an overoptimistic prognosis [overall quality: moderate]

Question 6: What are the potential problems with delayed or misdiagnosis of Lisfranc injuries, and what are the long-term complications associated with this injury?

Case clarification

Player B attends his orthopedic follow-up clinic. He is unhappy that he was not referred immediately after his first attendance at the Emergency Department. He asks what effect the potential delay in diagnosing his injury might have and asks about his prognosis and possible complications.

Relevance

We live in an era where litigation is commonplace. Lisfranc injury is a commonly missed diagnosis in the acute setting,[47,48] and although it is a rare injury the potential for a poor outcome is significant, especially if mismanaged.

Current opinion

In this case the diagnosis was not significantly delayed: surgical intervention would not be recommended before the swelling had settled and the only evidence in the literature is that a significant delay (6 months) in treatment would affect outcome (level IV).[49] Nevertheless, clinicians who regularly attend to patients with acute foot trauma should always be alert to the possibility of a Lisfranc injury in order to expedite prompt further investigation and management. Lisfranc injuries usually occur with significant trauma to the foot. Most specialists would advocate a period of elevation, icing, and observation in the initial 24–48 hours. At the same time further investigations should be arranged, if necessary, to assess tarsometatarsal stability.

Long-term follow-up should be arranged because of the high number of delayed problems encountered.

Quality of the evidence (delayed diagnosis)
Level III
• 1 comparative cohort study

Level IV
• 1 retrospective case series

Findings
A retrospective study (46 patients) found that there was a worse outcome in terms of return to work when there was delay in diagnosis of more than 6 months (p = 0.01) (level IV).[49]

A comparative cohort study (44 patients) compared primary open reduction with delayed, corrective arthrodesis (mean 22 months) and found that the primary fixation leads to improved functional results, earlier return to work, and greater patient satisfaction than secondary corrective arthrodesis (p = 0.03) (level III).[50]

Quality of the evidence (complications)
• Most of the literature relating to complications consists of case reports and small case series (level IV)

Findings
Vascular injury The terminal part of the dorsalis pedis artery may be damaged as it dives down between the 1st and 2nd ray to join the plantar arterial arch (level IV).[51] Gossens desceibes three cases in his series which were found to have vascular compromise; two of these were also open injuries and eventually required amputation due to the development of gas gangrene (level IV).[39]

Compartment syndrome Compartment syndrome is a rare complication after Lisfranc injury sustained playing sport, and is more commonly seen in high-energy crushing type injuries. Nevertheless, Lisfranc injury is a common cause of compartment syndrome, implicated in a third of cases of foot compartment syndrome in a series reported by Myerson (level IV).[52]

Stiffness Loss of range of movement in the midfoot is well recognized after this injury. Wilson found that almost all patients in his series displayed some degree of stiffness and this was related to the quality of the initial reduction (level IV).[53]

Complex regional pain syndrome (CRPS) Goossens reported CRPS in 25% of the patients in his series: missed or delayed diagnosis was thought to be an important factor in many of those cases (level IV).[39]

Deformity Disruption of the Lisfranc complex can result in a planovalgus deformity. There is conflicting evidence as to whether this is significant in terms of outcome. Aitken and Poulson report good functional outcomes in their case series despite obvious residual deformity (level IV).[54] This is contrary to the findings of Faciszewski who reports that maintenance of the longitudinal arch is a major determinant of outcome (level IV).[55]

Post-traumatic arthritis Arthritis is the most common long-term complication in Lisfranc injuries. In many series this is reported to occur in a significant number of cases and is a significant cause of long-term morbidity (level IV).[38,56]

Recommendations
• Lisfranc injuries are best treated acutely to avoid potential problems associated with missed or delayed diagnosis [overall quality: high]
• Awareness of the immediate and late complications of these injuries is essential [overall quality: high]

Summary of recommendations

• Careful attention should be paid to the anatomy and alignment of the tarsometatarsal joints when reviewing foot radiographs
• It should be appreciated that there are three types of proximal 5th metatarsal fracture that may require different treatments and which have different prognoses
• Weightbearing or stress radiographs should be obtained to assess tarsometatarsal stability if there is ongoing clinical concern of Lisfranc injury after apparently normal initial radiographs
• Lisfranc injuries are best treated acutely to avoid potential problems associated with missed or delayed diagnosis
• Operative fixation of zone 2 and zone 3 proximal metatarsal injuries leads to a quicker time to union and return to sport and this may be beneficial in selected patients
• When fixing proximal 5th metatarsal fractures, use a solid screw of adequate size such that the threads gain purchase in the cortical diaphyseal bone

• When conservatively treating proximal 5th metatarsal fractures treat zone 1 injuries symptomatically and zone 2/3 injuries in a plaster or boot: weightbearing should be encouraged as tolerated

• In treating Lisfranc injuries, restoration of normal anatomy and surgical fixation gives the best chance of a favorable long-term outcome

• The prognosis of proximal 5th metatarsal fractures is good; the prognosis of Lisfranc injuries is significantly worse and less predictable

• Awareness of the immediate and late complications of Lisfranc injuries is essential

Conclusions

This chapter has provided an insight into the investigation and management of two important injuries to the midfoot: the proximal 5th metatarsal fracture and the Lisfranc injury. Proximal 5th metatarsal fractures are common but vary in their management according to the type of patient and the fracture location. The outcome is usually satisfactory. Lisfranc injuries are rare and have the ability to deceive unsuspecting clinicians. The outcome, if misdiagnosed or mismanaged, may be extremely poor.

Acknowledgement

R.R. Elliot would like to thank the HCA international foundation for their scholarship grant for his fellowship year.

References

1. Nunley JA, Vertullo CJ. Classification, investigation, and management of midfoot sprains: Lisfranc injuries in the athlete. Am J Sports Med 2002;30(6):871–8.

2. Shuen WM, Boulton C, Batt ME, Moran C. Metatarsal fractures and sports. Surgeon 2009;7(2):86–8.

3. Jeffers RF, Tam HB, Nicolopoulos C, Kamath R, Giannoudis PV. Prevalence and patterns of foot injuries following motorcycle trauma. J Orthop Trauma 2004;18:87–91.

4. Egol K, Walsh M, Rosenblatt K, Capla E, Koval KJ. Avulsion fractures of the fifth metatarsal base: a prospective outcome study. Foot Ankle Int 2007;28(5):581–3.

5. English TA. Dislocations of the metatarsal bone and adjacent toe. J Bone Joint Surg Br 1994;46:700–4.

6. Coetzee JC. Making sense of Lisfranc injuries. Foot Ankle Cli 2008;13(4):695–704, ix.

7. Jones R. Fracture of the base of the fifth metatarsal bone by indirect violence. Ann Surg 1992;35(6):697–700.

8. Dameron TB. Fractures of the proximal fifth metatarsal: selecting the best treatment option. J Am Acad Orthop Surg 1995;3(2):110–14.

9. Clapper MF, O'Brien TJ, Lyons PM. Fractures of the fifth metatarsal. Analysis of a fracture registry. Clin Orth Rel Res 1995;315:238–41.

10. Dameron TB. Fractures and anatomic variations of the proximal portion the fifth metatarsal. J Bone Joint Surg Am 1995;57·788–92.

11. Kavanaugh JH, Brower TD, Mann RV. The Jones fracture revisited. J Bone Joint Surg Am 1998;60:776–82.

12. Woodward S, Jacobson JA, Femino JE, Morag Y, Fessell DP, Dong Q. Sonographic evaluation of Lisfranc ligament injuries. J Ultrasound Med 2009;28(3):351–7.

13. Groshar D, Alperson M, Mendes DG, Barsky V, Liberson A. Bone scintigraphy findings in Lisfranc joint injury. Foot Ankle Int 1995; 16(11):710–11.

14. Kaar S, Femino J, Morag Y. Lisfranc joint displacement following sequential ligament sectioning. J Bone Joint Surg Am 2007; 89(10):2225–32.

15. Coss HS, Manos RE, Buoncristiani A, Mills WJ. Abduction stress and AP weightbearing radiography of purely ligamentous injury in the tarsometatarsal joint. Foot Ankle Int 1998;19(8):537–41.

16. Raikin SM, Elias I, Dheer S, Besser MP, Morrison WB, Zoga AC. Prediction of midfoot instability in the subtle Lisfranc injury. Comparison of magnetic resonance imaging with intraoperative findings. J Bone Joint Surg Am 2009; 91(4):892–9.

17. Lu J, Ebraheim NA, Skie M, Porshinsky B, Yeasting RA. Radiographic and computed tomographic evaluation of Lisfranc dislocation: a cadaver study. Foot Ankle Int 1997;18(6):351–5.

18. Peicha G, Preidler KW, Lajtai G, Seibert FJ, Grechenig W. Diagnostic value of conventional roentgen image, computerized and magnetic resonance tomography in acute sprains of the foot. A prospective clinical study. Unfallchirurg 2001;104(12):1134–9.

19. Torg JS, Balduini FC, Zelko RR, Pavlov H, Peff TC, Das M. Fractures of the base of the fifth metatarsal distal to the tuberosity. Classification and guidelines for non-surgical and surgical management. J Bone Joint Surg Am 1994;66(2):209–14.

20. Mologne TS, Lundeen JM, Clapper MF, O'Brien TJ. Early screw fixation versus casting in the treatment of acute Jones fractures. Am J Sports Med 2005;33(7):970–5.

21. Portland G, Kelikian A, Kodros S. Acute surgical management of Jones' fractures. Foot Ankle Int 2003;24(11):829–33.

22. Leumann A, Pagenstert G, Fuhr P, Hintermann B, Valderrabano V. Intramedullary screw fixation in proximal fifth-metatarsal fractures in sports: clinical and biomechanical analysis. Arch Orthop Trauma Surg 2008;128(12):1425–30.

23. DeLee JC, Evans JP, and Julian J. Stress fracture of the fifth metatarsal. Am J Sports Med 1993;11:349–53.

24. Mindrebo N, Shelbourne KD, Van Meter CD, Rettig AC. Outpatient percutaneous screw fixation of the acute Jones fracture. Am J Sports Med 1993;21:720–3.

25. Wiener BD, Linder JF, Giatti JF. Treatment of fractures of the fifth metatarsal: a prospective study. Foot Ankle Int 1997;18:267–9.

26. Vorlat P, Achtergael W, Haentjens P. Predictors of outcome of non-displaced fractures of the base of the fifth metatarsal. Int Orthop 2007;31(1):5–10.

27. Porter DA, Rund AM, Dobslaw R, Duncan M. Comparison of 4.5- and 5.5-mm cannulated stainless steel screws for fifth metatarsal Jones fracture fixation. Foot Ankle Int 2009;30(1):27–33.

28. Shah SN, Knoblich GO, Lindsey DP, Kreshak J, Yerby SA, Chou LB. Intramedullary screw fixation of proximal fifth metatarsal fractures: a biomechanical study. Foot Ankle Int 2001;22(7): 581–4.

29. Reese K, Litsky A, Kaeding C, Pedroza A, Shah N. Cannulated screw fixation of Jones fractures: a clinical and biomechanical study. Am J Sports Med 2004;32(7):1736–42.

30. Sides SD, Fetter NL, Glisson R, Nunley JA. Bending stiffness and pull-out strength of tapered, variable pitch screws, and 6.5-mm cancellous screws in acute Jones fractures. Foot Ankle Int 2006; 27(10):821–5.

31. Kelly IP, Glisson RR, Fink C, Easley ME, Nunley JA. Intramedullary screw fixation of Jones fractures. Foot Ankle Int 2001;22(7):585–9.

32. Vertullo CJ, Glisson RR, Nunley JA. Torsional strains in the proximal fifth metatarsal: implications for Jones and stress fracture management. Foot Ankle Int 2004;25(9):650–6.

33. Horst F, Gilbert BJ, Glisson RR, Nunley JA. Torque resistance after fixation of Jones fractures with intramedullary screws. Foot Ankle Int 2004;25(12):914–19.

34. Moshirfar A, Campbell JT, Molloy S, Jasper LE, Belkoff SM. Fifth metatarsal tuberosity fracture fixation: a biomechanical study. Foot Ankle Int 2003;24(8):630–3.

35. Sarimo J, Rantanen J, Orava S, Alanen J. Tension-band wiring for fractures of the fifth metatarsal located in the junction of the proximal metaphysis and diaphysis. Am J Sports Med 2006; 34(3):476–80.

36. Glasgow MT, Naranja RJ, Glasgow SG, Torg JS. Analysis of failed surgical management of fractures of the base of the fifth metatarsal distal to the tuberosity: the Jones fractures. Foot Ankle Int 1996;17(8):449–57.

37. Quenu E, Kuss G. Etude sur les luxations du metatarse (luxations metatarsotarsiennes) du diastasis entre le 1er et 2e metatarsien. Rev Chir 1999;39:281–336, 720–91, 1093–34.

38. Myerson MS, Fisher RT, Burgess AR, Kenzora JE. Fracture dislocations of the tarsometatarsal joints: end results correlated with pathology and treatment. Foot Ankle 1996;6: 225–42.

39. Goossens M, De Stoop N. Lisfranc's fracture-dislocations: etiology, radiology, and results of treatment. A review of 20 cases. Clin Orthop Relat Res 1993; 176:154–62.

40. Arntz CT, Veith RG, Hansen ST. Fractures and fracture-dislocations of the tarsometatarsal joint. J Bone Joint Surg Am 1998;70:174–82.

41. Teng AL, Pinzur MS, Lomasney L, Mahoney L, Havey R. Functional outcome following anatomic restoration of tarsal-metatarsal fracture dislocation. Foot Ankle Int 2002;23(10): 922–6.

42. Ly TV, Coetzee JC. Treatment of primarily ligamentous Lisfranc joint injuries: primary arthrodesis compared with open reduction and internal fixation. A prospective, randomized study. J Bone Joint Surg Am 2006;88(3):514–20.

43. Henning JA, Jones CB, Sietsema DL, Bohay DR, Anderson JG. Open reduction internal fixation versus primary arthrodesis for Lisfranc injuries: a prospective randomized study. Foot Ankle Int 2009;30(10):913–22.

44. Chilvers M, Donahue M, Nassar L, Manoli A 2nd. Foot and ankle injuries in elite female gymnasts. Foot Ankle Int 2007; 28(2): 214–18.

45. Curtis MJ, Myerson M, Szura B. Tarsometatarsal joint injuries in the athlete. Am J Sports Med 1993;21:497.

46. Porter DA, Duncan M, Meyer SJ. Fifth metatarsal Jones fracture fixation with a 4.5-mm cannulated stainless steel screw in the competitive and recreational athlete: a clinical and radiographic evaluation. Am J Sports Med 2005;33(5):726–33.

47. Moore MN. Orthopedic pitfalls in emergency medicine. South Med J 1998;81(3):371–8.

48. Englanoff G, Anglin D, Hutson HR. Lisfranc fracture-dislocation: a frequently missed diagnosis in the emergency department. Ann Emerg Med 1995;26(2):229–33.

49. Calder JD, Whitehouse SL, Saxby TS. Results of isolated Lisfranc injuries and the effect of compensation claims. J Bone Joint Surg Br 2004;86(4):527–30.

50. Rammelt S, Schneiders W, Schikore H, Holch M, Heineck J, Zwipp H. Primary open reduction and fixation compared with delayed corrective arthrodesis in the treatment of tarsometatarsal (Lisfranc) fracture dislocation. J Bone Joint Surg Br 2008; 90(11):1499–506.

51. Gissane W. A dangerous type of fracture of the foot. J Bone Joint Surg Br 1991;33:535–8.

52. Myerson MS. Management of compartment syndromes of the foot. Clin Orthop Relat Res 1991;271:239–48.

53. Wilson DW. Injuries of the tarso-metatarsal joints: etiology, classification and results of treatment. J Bone Joint Surg Br 1992;54: 677–86.

54. Aitken AP, Poulson D. Dislocations of the tarsometatarsal joint. J Bone Joint Surg Am 1993;45:246–60.

55. Faciszewski T, Burks RT, Manaster BJ. Subtle injuries of the Lisfranc joint. J Bone Joint Surg Am 1990;72:1519–22.

56. Jeffreys TE. Lisfranc's fracture-dislocation. J Bone Joint Surg Br 1993;45:546–51.

68 Pelvis

G. Yves Laflamme, Stephane Leduc, and Dominique M. Rouleau
University of Montreal, Montreal, QC, Canada

Case scenario

A 37 year old woman is severely injured in a motor vehicle accident and is brought to the Emergency Department with complaints of pain to the pelvis. She is unresponsive to the initial volume resuscitation. On examination, her left and right thighs are swollen and bruised. A sheet is immediately wrapped around the pelvis in the Emergency Department. Her blood pressure improves to 90/60 with tachycardia of 130/min. The neurological examination, the chest radiograph, and the abdominal ultrasound are negative. An AP radiograph of the pelvis is shown in Figure 68.1.

Relevant anatomy

This chapter focuses on the initial management of pelvic fractures associated with hemodynamic instability and on the definitive management of pelvic fractures that are mechanically unstable. Pelvic fractures are classified in relation to the mechanism of injury (Table 68.1) and in relation to the instability patterns (Table 68.2).

Importance of the problem

Fractures of the pelvis are the third most commonly encountered injury in motor vehicle accident fatalities (level IV).[1] Pelvic fractures account for 3–8% of all fractures seen in the Emergency Department but are present in up to 25% of multiply injured patients. Life-threatening hemorrhage is a frequent complication of major pelvic fractures and extensive bleeding is the leading cause of death in these patients, with a mortality rate as high as 50% for patients with open pelvic fractures.

The forces needed to create a pelvic ring disruption in a young patient are extreme and often life threatening. The priority is saving the patient's life and then managing the pelvic fracture in order to reduce the high morbidity associated with pelvic ring injuries. A significant number of survivors will suffer major chronic disability with long-term problems.

Top five questions

1. What is the role of angiography in an unstable patient? Should it be performed first, before external fixation?
2. Is there any evidence to support the use of an external fixator over noninvasive stabilization (sheets or belts)?
3. Is prophylactic inferior vena cava (IVC) filter insertion recommended in pelvic trauma patients in whom surgery is likely to be delayed?
4. What is the optimal thromboprophylaxis strategy in pelvic fracture patients?
5. What is the prognosis of patients with pelvic fractures?

Question 1: What is the role of angiography in an unstable patient? Should it be performed first before external fixation?

Case clarification

Blood pressure improves to 90/60 with tachycardia of 130/min. Should the patient be sent to the operating room for emergent external fixation or to the angiography suite?

Relevance

Bleeding pelvic fractures carry mortality as high as 60%, yet controversy remains over their optimal initial management. Some surgeons prefer immediate external fixation

Evidence-Based Orthopedics, First Edition. Edited by Mohit Bhandari.
© 2012 Blackwell Publishing Ltd. Published 2012 by Blackwell Publishing Ltd.

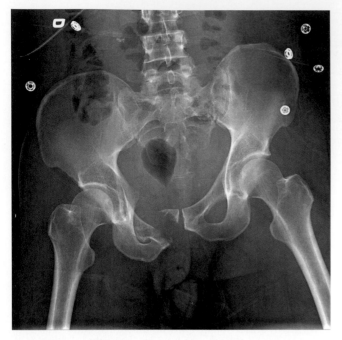

Figure 68.1 AP radiograph of fractured pelvis.

aimed at controlling venous bleeding. Others feel ongoing hemodynamic instability indicates arterial bleeding, and prefer early angiography before external fixation.

Current opinion

The establishment of standardized clinical treatment algorithms for patients with a bleeding pelvic injury increases the probability of rapid stabilization and survival. Two different families of algorithms can be found in the literature: fixation and packing first (level IV)[2,3] or angiography first (level IV, III).[4,5]

Finding the evidence

- Cochrane Database: search term: "pelvic fracture" AND "embolization"
- PubMed (www.ncbi.nlm.nih.gov/pubmed/) clinical queries search/systematic reviews search for "pelvic fracture" AND "thromboembolism (pulmonary embol*, thrombosis, pelvi$ fracture, embolization)"

Quality of the evidence

Level III
- 1 case-control study
- 2 retrospective comparative studies

Level IV
- 3 case series with 20 or more patients

Findings

All results are from retrospective studies using variable treatment algorithm and reporting results in different

Table 68.1 The Young–Burgess classification system, based on mechanism of injury

Category	Distinguishing characteristics
LC	Transverse fracture of pubic rami, ipsilateral or contralateral to posterior injury
LC I	Sacral compression on side of impact
LC II	Crescent (iliac wing) fracture on side of impact
LC III	LC-1 or LC-II injury on side of impact; contralateral open-book (APC) injury
APC	Symphyseal diastasis or longitudinal rami fractures
APC I	Slight widening of pubic symphysis; stretched but intact anterior SI, sacrotuberous, and sacrospinous ligaments; intact posterior SI ligaments
APC II	Widened anterior SI joint; disrupted anterior SI, sacrotuberous, and sacrospinous ligaments; intact posterior SI ligaments
APC III	Complete SI joint disruption with lateral displacement, disrupted anterior SI, sacrotuberous, and sacrospinous ligaments; disrupted posterior SI ligaments
VS	Symphyseal diastasis or vertical displacement anteriorly and posteriorly, usually through the SI joint, occasionally through the iliac wing or sacrum
CM	Combination of other injury patterns, LC/VS being the most common

SI, sacroiliac.

Table 68.2 Tile's classification system, based on the instability pattern

Category	Distinguishing characteristics
Type A	Stable
A1	Fractures of the pelvis not involving the ring
A2	Stable, minimally displaced fractures of the ring
Type B	Rotationally unstable, vertically stable
B1	Open book
B2	Lateral compression: ipsilateral
B3	Lateral compression: contralateral (bucket-handle)
Type C	Rotationally and vertically unstable
C1-	Rotationally and vertically unstable
C2-	Bilateral
C3	Associated with an acetabular fracture

ways. Some patients got angiography after external fixator or pelvis packing. Data specific to cases where angiography was done first were impossible to extract from these series. The only study comparing angiography to another treatment, i.e., pelvic packing, was a case-control study with two groups of 20 patients showing no significant difference

Table 68.3 Efficacy of arterial angiography for stopping bleeding in unstable patient with pelvis fracture

Author	N angio	Type	N embolization	BP (mmHg)		Average delay (min)	Angio time (min)	Success to stop bleeding visible in angio
				Pre angio	Post angio			
Fangio et al.[6]	32	Selective	25	Average. 69 + − 12	Average:108 + − 35	283 + − 372	93 + − 26	24/25 (96%)
Velmahos et al.[4]	73	IIA	30	Systolic:118	Systolic :128	?	?	27/30 (90%)
Tötterman et al.[7]	46	Selective	31	?	?	540	130	29/31 (94%)
Osborn et al.[2]	20	Selective	13	Average:76	Average: 87	276	?	?
Cook et al.[3]	23	Both	18	?	?	222	?	18/18 (100%)

IIA, internal iliac artery; Selective, arterial branch with active bleeding.

Table 68.4 Rate of unit of packed red blood cells transfusion before and after angiography

Author	N angio	Type	N embolization	Transfusion		Average delay (min)
				Pre angio	Post angio	
Fangio et al[6]	32	Selective	25	2.3/h	0.1/h (on 48h)	283
Tötterman et al.[7]	46	Selective	31	1.9/h	0.3 /h	540
Osborn et al.[2]	20	Selective	13	2/h	0.4/h (on 24h)	276

Table 68.5 Mortality in unstable patient with pelvic fracture going to embolization

Author	N angio	Average age	ISS	N patient unstable	Type	N embolization	Mortality	Mortality acute exsanguinations
Fangio et al.[6]	32	37	39	32	Selective	25	10/32 (31%)	4/32
Velmahos et al.[4]	73	43	25	25	IIA	30	10/30 (33%)	0/30
Tötterman et al.[7]	41	40	41	20	selective	31	5/31 (16%)	0/31
Osborn et al.[2]	20	40	46	20	selective	13	6/20 (30%)	2/20
Cook et al.[3]	23	38	34	23	both	18	10/23 (43%)	2/23
Sarin et al.[5]	37	45	35	37	?	37	13/37 (35%)	?

ISS, Injury Severity Score.

between both groups. However, in the pelvic packing group, three patients (15%) also required embolization.[2]

Efficacy to stop pelvic bleeding A total of 5 cohorts with comprehensive results were identified for a total of 194 unstable patients with pelvic fracture having angiography. Of them 117 (60%) received embolization and 90–100% of them were successful (Table 68.3 and Table 68.4).

Revision intervention Fangio et al.[6] showed that on 140 patients with pelvic fracture, 26 (18.6%) required repeat embolization for recurrent bleeding; an odds ratio of 3.22

of revision rate for superselective arterial (SSA) embolization compared to internal iliac artery embolization (IIAE) with a higher mortality rate (35% vs. 15%).

Mortality Mortality ranged from 16% to 43%, but the majority of death were secondary to the other injuries (brain, respiratory, etc.) (Table 68.5).

Recommendations
• Angiography is an effective option for bleeding control in hemodynamic unstable patients with pelvis fracture [overall quality low]

- A multidisciplinary standardized treatment algorithm must be established for unstable patients with a pelvic fracture
- The timing of angiography remains controversial and should be decided in collaboration with the trauma team
- Pelvic packing is a rapid method for controlling pelvic fracture-related hemorrhage and an alternative to emergent angiography

Question 2: Is there any evidence to support the use of an external fixator over noninvasive stabilization (sheets or belts)?

Case clarification

A few hours after successful embolization, the sheet wrapped around the patient's pelvis is carefully removed but a drop in the blood pressure is observed. The sheet is retightened over her pelvis and thighs.

Relevance

The anterior frame external fixator has gained widespread acceptance in the management of these injuries as a stabilizing frame, in the belief that this controls the fracture and reduces hemorrhage.

Current opinion

Experimental studies have shown that reduction in volume is much smaller than previously assumed,[1] and that a 'tamponade effect' of the pelvis is minimal. The external fixator will only adequately control a rotationally unstable pelvis, and may worsen a posterior injury.

Quality of the evidence

Level II
- 1 randomized trial with methodologic limitations

Level III
- 1 case-control study
- 1 systematic review (level III and IV studies)

Level IV
- 1 prospective cohort study

Findings

Immediate stabilization of unstable pelvic fractures to delayed stabilization with simple external fixation was studied by Waikakal et al. (level II).[8] A parallel trial with 2 year follow-up included 112 patients who were allocated randomly into 2 groups (acute fixation vs. delayed fixation). Blood transfusion, postoperative pain, need for reconstructive surgery of the pelvic fractures, and late deformities were less in the delayed fixation group.

A systematic review of literature was recently published on the effectiveness of pelvic circumferential compression

Table 68.6 Retrospective case-control study on transfusion requirements in patients with exsanguinating pelvic fracture[10]

Variable	POD (n = 93)	EPF (n = 93)	p value
24 h, Tx	4.9	17.1	0.008
48 h, Tx	5.6	18.6	0.008
Mortality, %	26	37	0.11

EPF, external pelvic fixation; POD, pelvic orthotic device; Tx, units of blood transfused.

devices (PCCDs) for unstable pelvic fractures (level III).[9] The authors included 17 articles with only one level III study (level III) (Table 68.6)[10] and concluded that PCCDs seem to be effective but prospective data was lacking. Krieg et al. (level IV)[11] were the only ones to investigate prospectively the effectiveness of a PCCD in 13 patients. In the external rotation group, the PCCD closely approximated the $10.0 \pm 4.1\%$ reduction in pelvic width achieved by definitive stabilization.

Recommendations

In the hemodynamically unstable pelvic fracture, evidence suggests [overall quality: low]:
- Emergent stabilization of the pelvis is beneficial
- External fixation is not superior to noninvasive stabilization devices. We therefore recommend the immediate application of a pelvic binder in resuscitation from life-threatening hypovolemic shock in patients with unstable pelvic injuries
- A pelvic binder can effectively reduce pelvic ring injuries with minimal risk for overcompression in lateral compression injuries

Question 3: Is prophylactic IVC filter insertion recommended in pelvic trauma patients?

Case clarification

The patient's hemodynamic status has been stabilized but the CT scan shows a large retroperitoneal hematoma. The surgery to fix her pelvis has been scheduled in 5 days.

Relevance

Patients with pelvic fractures are believed to be at very high risk for venous thromboembolisms (VTEs) such as spinal cord injuries. Prophylactic IVC filter insertion prior to the definitive surgical fixation procedure has been recommended by some clinicians for patients in whom early thromboprophylaxis has not been possible.

Current opinion

With current insertion techniques performed by experienced clinicians, the short-term complication rates associated with IVC filter use are very low and we should expand our indications.

Quality of the evidence
Level I
- 3 systematic reviews/meta-analyses

Level III
- 4 case-control studies

Level IV
- 1 case series

Findings
Two meta-analysis of prospective studies in trauma patients found no statistically significant difference in the rates of pulmonary embolism (PE) among patients with and without prophylactic IVC filters (level I).[12,13] Both PE and fatal PE still occur despite the presence of an IVC filter (level I, level II);[13,14] see Table 68.7 and Table 68.8.

Only one small prospective cohort study reported on a subgroup of 23 pelvic fracture patients (level III).[21] Another prospective cohort on acetabular fractures was published

by Webb et al. (level III).[22] The short-term complication rates associated with an IVC filter are lower than previously reported, but very little is known about the long-term follow-up (level III).[23] Retrievable IVC filters have recently become available but the majority are never removed (level IV).[24]

Recommendation
- For pelvic trauma patients, evidence suggests that prophylactic IVC filters do not significantly reduces the risk of pulmonary embolism or mortality. The use of an IVC filter as thromboprophylaxis is therefore not recommended [overall quality: low]

Question 4: What is the optimal thromboprophylaxis strategy in pelvic fracture patients?

Case clarification
The patient's pelvis was stabilized on the fifth day after trauma with an anterior plate and iliosacral screws. No complications occurred during surgery and bleeding was minimal.

Table 68.7 Pulmonary embolism after thromboprophylactic trials involving IVC filters after major trauma

Study	Type of injury	Pulmonary embolism		p value
		Control	With IVC filter	
Wilson et al.[15]	Major trauma	6.3% (7/111)	0%(0/15)	NA
Khansarinia et al.[16]	Major trauma	6.0% (13/216)	0% (0/108)	<0.009
Rodriguez et al.[17]	Major trauma	17.5% (14/80)	2.5% (1/40)	0.02
Gosin et al.[18]	Major trauma	4.8% (12/249)	0% (0/99)	<0.02
Rogers et al.[19]	Major trauma	0.9% (11/1150)	2.9% (1/35)	<0.05
Webb et al.[20]	Acetabular fracture	7.4% (2/27)	0% (0/24)	NA
Rogers et al.[21]	Pelvic fracture	2.9% (5/168)	4.3% (1/23)	NA

IVC, inferior vena cava; NA, not available.

Table 68.8 Relative risks of PE after thromboprophylactic trials involving IVC filters after trauma

Type of injury	Pulmonary embolism		RR	95% CI
	Control	IVC filter		
Pelvic fracture studies	3.6% (7/195)	2.1% (1/47)	0.6	0.10–4.09
Major trauma studies[a]	9.1% (27/296)	0.7% (1/148)	0.11	0.02–0.74

CI, confidence interval; IVC, inferior vena cava; NNT, number needed to treat; RR, relative risk.
[a]Required that two clearly identified groups be studied, one receiving prophylactic IVC filters and the other not, and that these two groups be matched for age and risk for VTE disease.[16,17]

Relevance

Without thromboprophylaxis, patients with a pelvic fracture have a DVT risk that exceeds 50%, and PE is the third-leading cause of death in those who survive beyond the first day (level I).[25]

Current opinion

Current prophylaxis guidelines for thromboprophylaxis are directed towards major trauma patients but their effectiveness, especially in the patient with an injured pelvis, is still debated.

Quality of the evidence

Level I
• 2 systematic reviews/meta-analyses

Level II
• 2 randomized trials with methodologic limitations

Level III
• 1 case-control study

Findings

A systematic review of thromboprophylaxis for pelvic fracture was conducted by Slobogean et al. in 2009 (level I).[26] Many limitations were encountered, including small sample sizes, with only one study of more than 200 patients, and the inability to extract injury-specific data from several eligible studies that did not stratify theirs results. In the pelvic fracture population, the early (<24 hours) administration of low molecular weight heparin (LMWH) was the only reviewed intervention that demonstrated a clear reduction in DVT and PE (level III).[27]

Two randomized trials (level II) were available comparing different mechanical compression devices (Table 68.9).[28,29] Important limitations of mechanical devices include their inability to be used in many trauma patients (due to lower extremity injuries), and evidence of poor compliance with proper use of these devices. According to the American College of Chest Physicians (ACCP) guidelines,[25] mechanical devices are recommended in patients with a contraindication to anticoagulant thromboprophylaxis, such as those with active bleeding or with a high risk for bleeding (grade 1A).

Recommendations

• For major trauma patients with a pelvic fracture, early administration of LMWH demonstrated a clear reduction in DVT and PE [overall quality: low]
• LMWH prophylaxis significantly protects against DVT in the major trauma patient [overall quality: moderate]
• Mechanical prophylaxis is less effective than LMWH

Question 5: What is the functional outcome of patients with pelvic injuries?

Case clarification

Two years after her injury, the patient comes back to clinic complaining of posterior back pain. She has yet to return to full-time work and has significant restrictions in her recreational activities.

Relevance

Pelvic ring injuries result in significant long-term functional disability and chronic pain. Even today, with modern management and early stabilization of the pelvic ring, morbidity remains high.

Current opinion

Patients with residual deformity and malunion seem to have the worst outcome. The literature supports the concept that the outcome depends on the fracture type and fracture stability. Restoration of a near-anatomic reduction in order to achieve a stable pelvic ring offers the best chance to return to a functional life. Improved techniques of reduction and fixation should improve outcomes and reduce complications.

Quality of the evidence

Level II
• 3 prognostic cohort studies

Table 68.9 Thromboprophylactic trials

Study	Intervention	Deep venous thrombosis			Pulmonary embolism		
		Control	Experimental	p value/RR	Control	Experimental	p value
Fisher et al.[28]	No prophylaxis/ postop PSLCD	7.9% (3/38)	2.9% (1/35)	0.24ᵃ/0.5	2.6% (1/38)	5.7% (2/35)	1.0ᵃ
Stannard et al.[29]	SCD/calf–foot pulsatile pump	18.5% (10/54)	9.4% (5/53)	0.16/0.5	1.9% (1/54)	0% (0/53)	NA
Steele et al.[27]	LMWH >24h /LMWH <24h	22.2% (8/36)	3% (2/64)	<0.01/0.3	13.9% (5/36)	0% (0/64)	0.01

LMWH, low molecular weight heparin; NA, not available; PSLCD, pneumatic sequential leg compression device; SCD, sequential compression device.
ᵃ Fisher's 2 × 2 exact test.

Table 68.10 Long-term outcomes of three basic treatment approaches from reviewed studies

Outcome	Nonoperative	Anterior fixation only	Posterior internal fixation	p value
Malunion rate	30.3% (23–37.5)	42% (9–64)	7% (0–44)	0.02*
Incidence of severe pain	27% (7–50)	5% (0–7)	1% (0–12)	0.06
Undisturbed gait	68% (55–70)	84% (75–91)	84.5% (77–100)	0.04[a]
Return to work	75.5% (62–89)	69.5% (55–84)	66% (45–77)	0.54
Functional outcome				
SF-36 PCS	NA	71.7	64 (55.5–75.3)	0.56
Majeed score (excellent to good results)	NA	51% (48–100)	81.3% (78.6–84)	0.77

NA, not available; PCS, Physical Component Score of the SF-36.
[a] Statistically significant p value.
From Papakostidis et al.[30]

Level III
- 1 systematic review of case series
- 1 case-control study

Findings

A systematic review (level III)[30] investigated the correlation of the clinical outcome of different types of pelvic ring injuries (27 case-series with 1,641 patients) to the method of treatment (Table 68.10). Few studies used validated outcome instruments, and prospective outcome studies are needed to better understand the relationship between fracture type, residual displacement, treatment modalities, and outcome.

Suzuki et al. evaluated the long-term functional outcome of patients with unstable pelvic ring fractures in 57 patients (level II).[31] The Majeed score, the Iowa pelvic score, and the physical component summary of the SF-36 correlated with the presence of neurological injury.

Tiles' C-type injuries of the pelvis are mechanically the worst injuries and may also have the worst functional outcome. According to a prospective clinical study evaluating 40 patients with Tile C-type fractures (level II),[32] 72% had returned to their original jobs at the time of the last follow-up visit. There was an inverse correlation between ability to work and depression and anxiety (r = –0.551, r = –0.391). Rommens et al. found that functional outcome was worse in C-type than in B-type lesions (level III).[33] Within the B-type group, B1 lesions had a worse functional end result than B2/B3 fractures. This finding was also supported by Kreder's prospective cohort of 366 patients (level II) using validated functional outcome tools (SF-36, MFA),[34] and by many other case series.

Recommendations

In unstable pelvic ring fractures, evidence suggests [overall quality: low]:

- Fixation of all the injured elements of the pelvic ring yields better anatomical results.
- Functional outcome is associated with neurological injury and fracture type, C-type injuries being the worst.
- No clear relationship can be found between quality of reduction/residual displacement of the pelvis and functional outcome.

Summary of recommendations

- Angiography is an effective option for bleeding control in hemodynamic unstable patients with pelvis fracture
- The timing of angiography remains controversial and should be decided in collaboration with the trauma team
- Pelvic packing is a rapid method for controlling pelvic fracture-related hemorrhage and an alternative to emergent angiography.
- In the hemodynamic unstable pelvic fracture, emergent stabilization of the pelvis is beneficial
- External fixation is not superior to noninvasive stabilization devices. We therefore recommend the immediate application of a pelvic binder in resuscitation from life-threatening hypovolemic shock in patients with unstable pelvic injuries. A pelvic binder can effectively reduce pelvic ring injuries with minimal risk for overcompression in lateral compression injuries.
- For pelvic trauma patients, evidence suggests prophylactic IVC filters do not significantly reduces the risk of pulmonary embolism or mortality. The use of an IVC filter as thromboprophylaxis is not recommended
- For major trauma patients (with a pelvic fracture), early administration of LMWH demonstrates a clear reduction in DVT and PE and LMWH prophylaxis significantly protects against DVT in the major trauma patient
- Mechanical prophylaxis is less effective than LMWH.

• In unstable pelvic ring fractures, evidence suggests that fixation of all the injured elements of the pelvic ring yields better anatomic results

• Functional outcome is associated with neurological injury and fracture type; C-type injuries being the worst

• No clear relationship can be found between quality of reduction/residual displacement of the pelvis and function outcome.

Conclusions

The priority is saving the patient's life and then managing the pelvic fracture in order to reduce the high morbidity associated with pelvic fractures. Every Emergency Department must create and apply a simple algorithm with the onsite surgical and radiological team following available resources for unstable patient with pelvic fracture to prevent confusion and loss of precious time in life-threatening pelvic injury.

References

1. Moss MC, Bircher MD. Volume changes within the true pelvis during disruption of the pelvic ring—where does the haemorrhage go? Injury 1996;27(Suppl 1):S-A21–3.

2. Osborn PM, Smith WR, Moore EE, et al. Direct retroperitoneal pelvic packing versus pelvic angiography: A comparison of two management protocols for haemodynamically unstable pelvic fractures. Injury 2009;40(1):54–60.

3. Cook RE, Keating JF, Gillespie I. The role of angiography in the management of haemorrhage from major fractures of the pelvis. J Bone Joint Surg Br 2002;84(2):178–82.

4. Velmahos GC, Chahwan S, Hanks SE, et al. Angiographic embolization of bilateral internal iliac arteries to control life-threatening hemorrhage after blunt trauma to the pelvis. Am Surg 2000;66(9):858–62.

5. Sarin EL, Moore JB, Moore EE, et al. Pelvic fracture pattern does not always predict the need for urgent embolization. J Trauma 2005;58(5):973–7.

6. Fangio P, Asehnoune K, Edouard A, Smail N, Benhamou D. Early embolization and vasopressor administration for management of life-threatening hemorrhage from pelvic fracture. J Trauma 2005;58(5):978–84.

7. Tötterman A, Dormagen JB, Madsen JE, Kløw NE, Skaga NO, Røise O. A protocol for angiographic embolization in exsanguinating pelvic trauma: a report on 31 patients. Acta Orthop. 2006;77(3):462–8.

8. Waikakul S, Harnroongroj T, Vanadurongwan V. Immediate stabilization of unstable pelvic fractures versus delayed stabilization. J Med Assoc Thai 1999;82(7):637–42.

9. Spanjersberg WR, Knops SP, Schep NW, van Lieshout EM, Patka P, Schipper IB. Effectiveness and complications of pelvic circumferential compression devices in patients with unstable pelvic fractures: a systematic review of literature. Injury. 2009;40(10):1031–5.

10. Croce MA, Magnotti LJ, Savage SA, Wood GW 2nd, Fabian TC. Emergent pelvic fixation in patients with exsanguinating pelvic fractures. J Am Coll Surg. 2007;204(5):935–9.

11. Krieg JC, Mohr M, Ellis TJ, Simpson TS, Madey SM, Bottlang M. Emergent stabilization of pelvic ring injuries by controlled circumferential compression: a clinical trial. Trauma 2005;59(3):659–64.

12. Velmahos GC, Kern J, Chan LS, et al. Prevention of venous thromboembolism after injury: an evidence-based report; part II. Analysis of risk factors and evaluation of the role of vena caval filters. J Trauma 2000;49:140–4.

13. Girard TD, Philbrick JT, Fritz Angle J, et al. Prophylactic vena cava filters for trauma patients: a systematic review of the literature. Thromb Res 2003;112:261–7.

14. McMurty AL, Owings JT, Anderson JT, et al. Increased use of prophylactic vena cava filters in trauma patients failed to decrease overall incidence of pulmonary embolism. J Am Coll Surg 1999;189:314–320.

15. Wilson JT, Rogers FB, Wald SL, Shackford SR, Ricci MA. Prophylactic vena cava filter insertion in patients with traumatic spinal cord injury: preliminary results. Neurosurgery 1994;35(2):234–9; discussion 239.

16. Khansarinia S, Dennis JW, Veldenz HC, Butcher JL, Hartland L. Prophylactic Greenfield filter placement in selected high-risk trauma patients. J Vasc Surg 1995;22(3):231–5; discussion 235–6.

17. Rodriguez JL, Lopez JM, Proctor MC, et al. Early placement of prophylactic vena caval filters in injured patients at high risk for pulmonary embolism. J Trauma 1996;40(5):797–802; discussion 802–4.

18. Gosin JS, Graham AM, Clocca RG, Hammond IS. Efficacy of prophylactic vena cava filters in high-risk trauma patients. Ann Vasc Surg. 1997;11(1):100–5.

19. Rogers FB, Shackford SR, Ricci MA, Huber BM, Atkins T. Prophylactic vena cava filter insertion in selected high-risk orthopaedic trauma patients. J Orthop Trauma 1997;11(4):267–72.

20. Webb LX, Rush PT, Fuller SB, Meredith JW. Greenfield filter prophylaxis of pulmonary embolism in patients undergoing surgery for acetabular fracture. J Orthop Trauma 1992;6(2):139–45.

21. Rogers FB, Shackford Sr, Ricci MA, et al. Routine prophylactic vena cava filter insertion in severely injured trauma patients decreases the incidence of pulmonary embolism J Am Coll Surg 1995;180:641–7.

22. Webb LX, Rush PT, Fuller SB, et al. Greenfield filter prophylaxis of pulmonary embolism in patients undergoing surgery for acetabular fractures. J Orthop Trauma 1992;6:139–45.

23. Patton JH, Fabian TC, Croce MA, et al. Prophylactic Greenfield filters: acute complications and long-term followup. J Trauma 1996;41:231–6.

24. Karmy-Jones R, Jurkovich GJ, Velmahos GC, et al. Practice patterns and outcomes of retrievable vena cava filters in trauma patients: an AAST multicenter study. J Trauma 2007;62:17–25.

25. Geerts WH, Bergqvist D, Pineo GF, et al. American College of Chest Physicians evidence-based clinical practice guidelines (8th edition). Chest 2008;133(Suppl 6):381S–453S.

26. Slobogean GP, Lefaivre KA, Nicolaou S, O'Brien PJ. A Systematic review of thromboprophylaxis for pelvic and acetabular fractures. J Orthop Trauma 2009;23:379–84.

27. Steele N, Dodenhoff RM, Ward AJ, et al. Thromboprophylaxis in pelvic and acetabular trauma surgery. The role of early treatment with low-molecular-weight-heparine. J Bone Joint Surg Br 2005;87:209–12.

28. Fisher CG, Blachut PA, Salvian AJ, et al. Effectiveness of pneumatic leg compression devices for prevention of thromboembolism disease in orthopaedic trauma patients. J Orthop Trauma 1995;9:1–7.

29. Stannard JP, Riley RS, McClenney MD, et al. Mechanical prophylaxis against deep-vein-thrombosis after pelvic and acetabular fractures. J Bone Joint Surg Am 2001;83:1047–51.

30. Papakostidis C, Kanakaris NK, Kontakis G, Giannoudis PV. Pelvic ring disruptions: treatment modalities and analysis of outcomes Int Orthop, 2009;33:329–38.

31. Suzuki T, Shindo M, Soma K, et al. Long-term functional outcome after unstable pelvic ring fracture. J Trauma 2007;63: 884–8.

32. Kabak S, Halici M, Tuncel M, Avsarogullari L, Baktir A, Basturk M. Functional outcome of open reduction and internal fixation for completely unstable pelvic ring fractures (type C): a report of 40 cases. J Orthop Trauma 2003;17(8):555–62.

33. Rommens PM, Hessmann MH. Staged reconstruction of pelvic ring disruption: differences in morbidity, mortality, radiologic results, and functional outcomes between B1, B2/B3, and C-type lesions. J Orthop Trauma 2002;16:92–8.

34. Kreder HJ. Outcome after pelvic injuries in adults. Chapter 23 in: Tile M, et al., Fractures of the Pelvis and Acetabulum, 3rd edn, p. 410. Lippincott, Williams and Wilkins Baltimore, MD, 2003.

69 Acetabulum

Kelly A. Lefaivre[1] and Adam J. Starr[2]
[1]University of British Columbia, Vancouver, BC, Canada
[2]University of Texas Southwestern Medical Center, Dallas, TX, USA

Case scenario

A 26 year old manual laborer is brought to the Emergency Department after a 20 ft (6 m) fall at work, with complaints of left pain. He is unable to weight bear, and has diffuse bruising and swelling around his left hip. The trauma team has cleared him otherwise, and this is an isolated left acetabulum fracture.

Relevant anatomy

Acetabulum fractures involve the "hip joint" portion of the pelvis—the socket side of the ball and socket hip joint. Acetabulum fractures are anatomically classified based on the parts of the bone involved in the injury. These parts are comprised of the anterior and posterior columns (structural attachments of the acetabulum to the remainder of the axial skeleton) and the anterior and posterior walls (rims that contribute to congruence of the hip joint). These structures can be seen in Figure 69.1.

Based on these anatomic components, Judet and Letournel described a widely used classification system, which divides injuries into two main categories, elementary and associated, each with subtypes.[1] Elementary fracture patterns are posterior wall, posterior column, anterior wall, anterior column and transverse (Figure 69.2a–e) Associated fracture patterns are posterior column/posterior wall, transverse posterior wall, t-type, anterior column posterior hemi-transverse and associated both column (Figure 69.2f–j).

Importance of the problem

Acetabular fractures are rare and few studies have examined their epidemiology. Laird et al. reported the experience from Edinburgh in the UK, where they noted 3 fractures per 100,000 population per year.[2] In practice, the relative scarcity of these fractures means that few will be encountered at individual community hospitals. Usually they are managed at trauma centers, but even at a busy trauma center they are infrequent. In the authors' opinion, 100 operative cases in a year represents a considerable caseload for a trauma center. This rarity makes it difficult to conduct research to guide treatment. To date, most of the literature on acetabular fractures consists of small retrospective series. Pioneers in the field published larger retrospective series with detailed analyses of fracture types, and more complete follow-up.[3–5] Recent well-conducted prospective series have examined aspects of particular fracture types, and biomechanical studies have improved our understanding of the hip socket's function.[6–10] However, despite the number of studies, most of the treatment recommendations in the literature consist of advice from experts. Sadly, the results obtained by experts in the field—who have years or even decades of experience, and who benefit from working with teams dedicated to acetabular fracture management—may not be reproduced by less experienced surgeons. To the contrary, there is evidence that surgeons who perform acetabular fracture repair infrequently will experience higher complication rates and inferior results.[11]

Evidence-Based Orthopedics, First Edition. Edited by Mohit Bhandari.
© 2012 Blackwell Publishing Ltd. Published 2012 by Blackwell Publishing Ltd.

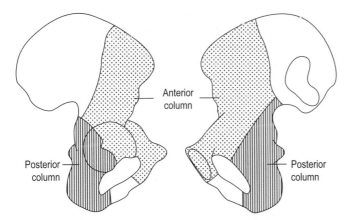

Figure 69.1 Anterior and posterior columns of the acetabulum.

It is fortunate that acetabular fractures are rare, because they can lead to devastating outcomes for patients. Post-traumatic arthritis of the hip can have a profound negative impact on a patient's life. It seems clear that operative restoration of the articular surface offers the best chance of avoiding arthritis, but the surgery to achieve joint restoration is difficult, risky, and requires dedication to master.[2–5] These facts, combined with the nature of acetabular fracture research as it exists today, make these fractures among the most complex and least well understood injuries that orthopedic trauma surgeons face. As stated by Tile in the first edition of his book, published in 1984, and repeated in the latest edition, "Fractures of the acetabulum remain an enigma to the orthopaedic surgeon."[5] Although many advances have been made in the management of these complex and disabling injuries in the last 25 years, many questions about their treatment remain.

Acetabulum fractures remain an injury with variable results and a significant complication rate.[4,5] Important questions remain about which patients and patterns to treat surgically. Similarly, the selection of surgical approach and the use of methods to avoid complications, such as heterotopic ossification (HO) or deep vein thrombosis (DVT) remain controversial. Clearly, the treatment of acetabulum fractures has become its own specialty within orthopedics, and is best undertaken by those with subspecialty training and expertise.

DVT is the development of a blood clot in the veins of the leg, an event that trauma patients in general are at risk for. The propagation of these clots to the arteries is a significant cause of death in otherwise healthy trauma patients.

HO refers to the nonmalignant overgrowth of bone, frequently occurring after a fracture, which can lead to pain, stiffness, and compromised outcome.

Given the relative youth of this area of orthopedic trauma surgery, evidence-based practice is in evolution. Further, surgeons and patients are inundated with an ever-increasing, easily accessible body of information about acetabulum fractures. To this end, as noted above, a Google search for "acetabular fractures" returns over 867,000 hits. The variable quality of this information mandates development of evidence-based guides.

Top seven questions

Diagnosis

1. How accurate are plain radiographs vs. CT scan in the characterization of acetabulum fractures?

Therapy

2. What are the indications for surgical management of acetabulum fractures in a young person?
3. What are the treatment options in elderly patients?
4. What is the optimal deep vein thrombosis/pulmonary embolus (DVT/PE) prophylaxis in patients with acetabulum fractures?
5. What is the optimal HO prophylaxis in patients with acetabulum fractures?

Prognosis

6. What is the expected long-term functional outcome in acetabulum fractures?
7. What are the important non-surgeon-related factors that determine prognosis in acetabulum fractures?

Question 1: How accurate are plain radiographs vs. CT scan in the characterization of acetabulum fractures?

Case clarification

The patient's AP pelvis and Judet views reveal a comminuted fracture involving the anterior column and posterior column, and apparent discontinuity of the entire weight-bearing dome from the axial skeleton (an associated both column acetabulum fracture). You are faced with the question of whether CT will be helpful in definitive characterization of the fracture type and properties, and subsequently planning for surgical approach.

Judet views of the acetabulum are obtained by turning the X-ray beam 45° away from the affected side (iliac oblique view) and towards the affected side (obturator oblique view). These views each give an advantageous view of a column and a wall (iliac oblique: posterior column and anterior wall; obturator oblique: anterior column and posterior wall).

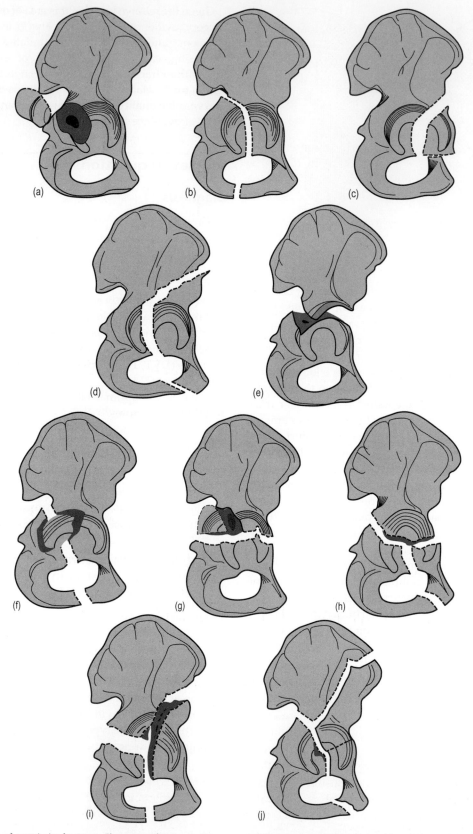

Figure 69.2 Patterns of acetabular fractures. Elementary fracture patterns: posterior wall (a), posterior column (b), anterior wall (c), anterior column (d) and transverse (e). Associated fracture patterns: posterior column/posterior wall (f), transverse posterior wall (g), t-type (h), anterior column posterior hemi-transverse (i) and associated both column (j). (Reprinted with kind permission from Springer Science+Business Media: Fractures of the Acetabulum, 1993, Letournel E, Judet R, figure 4.1).

Relevance

The accepted classification system for acetabulum fractures was based on multiplanar plain films (AP and Judet views)[1]. However, current discussions of classification and surgical planning most frequently involve CT information, as well as reformats of this information.

Current opinion

Current opinion suggests that the majority of surgeons find CT to be more accurate in fracture classification, identification of additional lesions, and for surgical planning.

Finding the evidence

- Cochrane Database, with search term: "acetabul$ fracture"
- PubMed (www.ncbi.nlm.nih.gov/pubmed/) clinical queries search/ systematic reviews: "acetabulum" and "acetabular"
- PubMed (www.ncbi.nlm.nih.gov/pubmed/): sensitivity search using keywords "acetabulum fracture OR acetabular fracture" AND "radiography" "acetabulum fracture OR acetabular fracture" AND "CT"
- MEDLINE search keywords: "acetabulum fracture" or "acetabular fracture" AND "tomography"

Quality of the evidence

Level II

- 4 studies developing diagnostic criteria on basis of consecutive patients (with universally applied reference gold standard)

Level III

- 1 study of nonconsecutive patients (without consistently applied reference gold standard)

Level IV

- 1 case-control study

Findings

The best research comparing plain films and CT scans in the classification of acetabular fractures, and in the preoperative detection of fracture characteristics, represents a heterogeneous group of papers that cannot be combined to synthesize results. A review of the work is below.

Fracture classification Beaule et al. reported on 65 cases of acetabulum fractures selected from a database, evaluated by three surgeons trained by Letournel (group 1), three acetabular specialists (group 2), and three general trauma surgeons (group 3). The interobserver reliability without and with CT during the first session was 0.70 and 0.74,

respectively, for group 1, 0.71 and 0.69 for group 2, and 0.51 and 0.51 for group 3. The overall agreement of the radiographic observation with the fracture pattern observed at surgery was 74%.[12]

Ohashi et al. reported on 101 sets of imaging reviewed by 2 musculoskeletal radiologists, first multiplanar CT followed by standard radiographs. Interobserver agreement on Letournel classification with plain films was 0.42, and 0.70 with reformatted and axial CT scans. Standard Judet films resulted in a change in classification in one case for each observer.[13]

Hufner et al. found an improvement in "correct diagnosis" of fracture type in plain films vs. 2-D CT scan 10 trainees (11–30%) 10 junior attendings (32–55%) and 10 acetabular experts (61–76%) in the review of 10 cases. The use of 3-D CT reformats increased this diagnosis rate to 65%, 64%, and 83% respectively. The diagnosis rate of additional lesions was universally based on CT (marginal impaction, head fractures, etc.), and was accurate vs. intraoperative findings in 73% of cases by acetabular experts.[14]

Fracture characteristics Borrelli et al. reported on 20 operatively treated acetabular fractures, and performed standardized assessment of step and gap at the articular surface using three observers (a senior resident, a junior resident, and a traumatologist). Compared to CT scan, plain films showed a sensitivity of 25% in detecting step deformity overall, and a sensitivity of 0% in fractures involving a single column of the acetabulum.[15]

Lang et al. used 12 sets of imaging and 3 independent observers to compare plain films and CT scans in quantifying fracture gaps, using a nonstandardized and a standardized method. The kappa statistic for interobserver (0.30 vs. 0.27) and intraobserver (0.43 vs. 0.36) agreements were superior for CT scans vs. radiographs.[16]

St. Pierre et al. used 67 consecutive cases, and evaluated the classification of fracture type as well as the presence of additional lesions. Although the CT information resulted in the alteration of classification in one case, the treatment plan was altered in 28 cases secondary to intra-articular fragments (20) and articular impaction (8).[17]

Recommendations

In surgical planning for acetabular fractures:

- While neither form of imaging is perfect when intraoperative findings are used as the gold standard, CT scan appears to offer little additional information over three plain film views in acetabular fracture classification [overall quality: moderate]
- The importance of CT in appropriate fracture classification appears to be inversely related to level of experience in acetabular fracture surgery [overall quality: moderate]
- CT imaging of acetabulum fractures is necessary to delineate additional fracture features such as impaction,

articular gap and step, and intra-articular loose bodies [overall quality: moderate]

Question 2: What are the indications for surgical management of acetabulum fractures in a young person?

Case clarification

The patient's CT scan confirms an associated both column fracture, with displacement visible on many of the CT scan cuts. You need to explain clearly to the trainees working with you what the absolute indications are for surgical treatment of acetabulum fractures are with patients this age, and apply them to this case.

> Surgical indications are considered based on demand as well as life expectancy of the patient. "Young person" in this context refers to a patient in whom preservation of the native hip joint is very important.

Relevance

The decision to intervene in order to provide reduction and fixation of an acetabular fracture is one that needs to be made in the acute phase, as the results from delayed reconstruction revision of late malunions are far inferior to acute anatomic open reduction and internal fixation (ORIF).[18–20] Although a significant number of biomechanical and cadaveric studies are available to help guide clinical decision-making, solid clinical evidence has been more difficult to gather in these uncommon and complex injuries.[21–24]

Current opinion

Articular displacement of greater than 3 mm, nonconcentric reduction of the hip joint (incongruence), and instability of the hip joint are indications for surgical management.

Finding the evidence

- Cochrane Database, with search term: "acetabul$ fracture"
- PubMed (www.ncbi.nlm.nih.gov/pubmed/) clinical queries search/systematic reviews: "acetabulum" and "acetabular"
- PubMed (www.ncbi.nlm.nih.gov/pubmed/): sensitivity search using keywords "acetabulum fracture OR acetabular fracture" AND "surgery"
- MEDLINE search keywords: "acetabulum fracture" or "acetabular fracture" AND "surgery"

Quality of the evidence

Level III
- 4 case-control studies

Level IV
- 2 case series

Findings

Much of what guides current standards of care is based largely on retrospective case series, retrospective comparative studies, and expert opinion in these rare injuries. Although much of the evidence is of low quality by today's standards, the most compelling of it has been included below.

Displacement Matta et al. described follow-up in a retrospective case series of 64 patients, with 21 nonoperatively treated cases (traction) and 43 operatively treated cases. Overall, there were 24% good or excellent clinical results in the nonoperative group and 40% in the operative group (author generated outcome measure and radiographic measurement technique). They found 91% good or excellent clinical results in all patients with less than 3 mm displacement at the weightbearing dome and congruence of the femoral head (all operative p < 0.001).[25]

Recently, a series of nonoperatively treated displaced acetabulum fractures involving the weightbearing dome were reported at 2 years after injury. In these patients treated in traction, 18/32 were considered to have an adequate reduction in traction (≤3 mm), and 14 were considered inadequate. Those with an adequate reduction had 77.8% good or excellent results rated by the Aubigné score, and the inadequate reductions had 14.3% good or excellent results.[26]

Incongruence In the often cited series by Rowe et al., which pre-dates the classification by Letournel, the idea of the importance of the weightbearing dome as an indication was coined. Displacement at the superior dome resulting in incongruence universally produced poor or fair radiographic and clinical outcomes exclusively in fractures involving the weightbearing dome.[27]

In the same series described above, Matta et al. delineated the "roof arc angle" as an assessment for risk for loss of congruence. The roof arc angle is measured from the geometric center of the acetabulum to the fracture line. Matta pointed out that it can be indicated by fracture displacement, but that loss of congruence between the weightbearing dome and femoral head carries special significance. In the series of 64 patients, subluxation occurred in 69% of cases with a medial roof arc of 30° or less.[25]

Olson and Matta again addressed the issue of roof arc measurements, and operative indications, with CT scan in 1993. This measurement does not apply to associated both column and posterior wall fractures. They describe the 10 mm of axial cuts caudad to the roof of the acetabulum as being intact equivalent to a roof arc measurement of greater than 45°. They report 82% good or excellent results overall when using these criteria to decide operative vs. nonoperative treatment.[28]

Instability Calkins et al. described the acetabular fracture index (percentage of intact acetabulum remaining) in posterior wall fractures as an assessment of stability in 31 patients. All hips with less than 34% remaining intact were unstable, and all those with 55% or greater were stable. Seven out of ten unstable hips showed at least 0.5 mm of subluxation on axial CT scan.[29]

Tornetta reported his experience with the use of dynamic stress views under anesthetic in all acetabulum patients meeting criteria for nonoperative management (roof arc angles of at least 45°, subchondral CT arc of 10 mm, and displacement of less than 50% in posterior wall fractures). Of 41 patients, one had a transverse fracture with a posterior dislocation and a roof arc measurement of 45°, and two were posterior wall fractures (one with a dislocation involving 15% of the surface, one without dislocation involving 33% of the articular surface).[30]

Recommendations

In surgical planning for acetabular fractures:
- Displacement is poorly tolerated in the weightbearing dome, and greater than 3 mm is a relative operative indication [overall quality: low]
- Incongruence at the hip joint is an indication for surgical reduction in acetabulum fractures, and can be predicted by the roof arc angle [overall quality: low]
- Clinical series support cadaveric data that instability in posterior wall fractures is predicted by greater than 50% involvement, and dynamic testing can offer additional information in those with 25–50% involvement. [overall quality: low]

Question 3: What are the treatment options in elderly patients?

Case clarification

The patient was working on the roof of a private home when he fell. During the commotion of the incident, and the arrival of the ambulance, the owner of the home lost his footing, and fell 2 ft (0.6 m) from a step, landing on his side. He also suffered an acetabulum fracture, which appears to be a T-type, and has similar displacement and incongruence to the 26 year old, but more comminution. This patient is 78 years old, has a history of coronary artery disease and type 2 diabetes mellitus, and two low-energy fractures in the last two years. You need to consider the options for this very different patient subgroup, and apply them to this case.

> Injuries in this "elderly" age group bring up important issues and goals. Decreased bone density, medical comorbidity, surgical morbidity, and life expectancy all play a role.

Relevance

In the treatment of injuries in the elderly patient one has to consider and balance the risks involved. It has been clearly outlined in the hip fracture literature that treatment with bed rest and surgical delay can be very dangerous in elderly patients, and efforts to facilitate early mobilization in these patients should therefore be made.[31-33] In addition, bone quality in this population can be poor, and physiologic reserve for prolonged surgery may also be poor. Consideration of the entire patient, not just the acetabular injury, is paramount.

Current opinion

The options for treatment of acetabulum fractures in elderly patients include nonoperative management, ORIF, acute total hip replacement, and delayed total hip replacement.

Finding the evidence

- Cochrane Database, with search term "acetabul$ fracture"
- PubMed (www.ncbi.nlm.nih.gov/pubmed/) clinical queries search/ systematic reviews: "acetabulum" and "acetabular"
- PubMed (www.ncbi.nlm.nih.gov/pubmed/): sensitivity search using keywords "acetabulum fracture OR acetabular fracture" AND "treatment"
- MEDLINE search keywords: "acetabulum fracture" or "acetabular fracture" AND "treatment"

Quality of the evidence

Level III
- 3 case control studies

Level IV
- 4 case series

Findings

Conservative management Spencer reported on 25 acetabular fractures treated in traction in patients over 65 years of age. Of 23 survivors, 7 had an unacceptable functional result (able to walk only with severe pain).[34]

ORIF Anglen et al. reported on a retrospective series of 48 patients over 60 years of age with an operatively treated acetabulum fracture. They reported 60% good or excellent radiographic results, and 40% fair, poor or, early arthroplasty. Ten patients were found to have superomedial impaction at the time of injury (Gull sign) and all had a fair or poor radiographic result. However, the functional outcomes of the group overall based on the Short Form 36 (SF-36) and Short Musculoskeletal Function Assessment (SMFA) were within a standard deviation of population age-matched norms.[35]

Helfet et al. reported a series of 18 patients 60 or older treated with ORIF. He reported concentric reductions in all, articular gap up to 3 mm. One patient had an early failure, and the remainder had Harris hip scores (HHS) of more than 90 at 2 years follow-up.[36]

Early total hip replacement Mears et al. published a series of 57 patients with a mean age of 69 years treated with acute total hip replacement for severely displaced acetabulum fractures. The mean HHS at 2–12 year follow-up was 89, with 79% of patients having good or excellent results (level IV).[37]

A series of 121 acetabular fractures by Sermon et al. published in 2008 were all treated with total hip replacement. These were 64 in the acute setting, and for failed primary treatment in 57 cases. The former group had a mean age of 78, and the later was 53. There was no statistical difference in HHS, but the primary group had a lower heterotopic ossification rate (28 vs. 41%) and revision rate (8 vs. 22%).[38]

Late total hip replacement Weber et al. reported on the Mayo clinic experience in 66 total hip replacements following ORIF for acetabular fracture, although the age group was diverse, and the results of the patients over 60 were not reported separately. The 10 year survival of the components was 78%, with age being protective for need for revision.[39]

Bellabarba compared post-traumatic arthritis treated with late total hip replacement in 30 patients to a matched cohort treated for nontraumatic osteoarthritis. The clinical results were similar, with a HHS of 88 vs. 90. Similarly, the survival of the acetabular component at 10 years was 97% (vs. 99% for the nontraumatic group).[40]

Recommendation

• Management of acetabulum fractures in elderly patients requires careful consideration of patient demands and risk of surgery. Reasonable functional results after operative treatment can be obtained with ORIF, early arthroplasty, and delayed arthroplasty [overall quality: low]

Question 4: What are the optimal DVT/PE prophylaxis and screening in patients with acetabulum fractures?

Case clarification

The 26 year old patient was taken to the operating room on postinjury day 2 and underwent ORIF of the acetabulum fracture through an extensile approach. Postoperatively, you wish to make an evidence-based decision about the use of prophylaxis or screening for DVT and/or PE.

DVT is the development of a blood clot in the veins of the leg, an event that trauma patients in general are at risk for. The propagation of these clots to the arteries is a significant cause of death in otherwise healthy trauma patients.

Relevance

Pelvic and acetabulum fractures are a few of the previously identified risk factors for embolic complications among trauma patients.[41–43] The identification of potential risk factors for venous thromboembolism has not solved the issue of prevention. Several strategies are in practice to prevent and detect venous thrombosis, and their effectiveness has been evaluated in other populations. The American College of Chest Physicians (ACCP) provides the most comprehensive thromboprophylaxis guidelines, but very few recommendations were directed toward the prophylaxis of trauma patients—specifically, patients with pelvic or acetabular fracture.[44] For major trauma patients, the ACCP authors recommend the routine use of low molecular weight heparin (LMWH) (grade 1A) or the use of mechanical prophylaxis alone if LMWH is contraindicated (grade 1B). They recommend against the routine use of duplex ultrasound for screening for asymptomatic DVT (grade 1B); however, screening of high-risk patients (including those with pelvic fractures) who had received suboptimal or no prophylaxis received a grade 1C recommendation. They also recommend against the use of inferior vena cava (IVC) filters as a method of prophylaxis (grade 1C).

Current opinion

Pelvic and acetabulum fracture patients should be receiving prophylaxis with LMWH when possible and otherwise with mechanical compression devices. Many centers routinely use IVC filters, as well as screening protocols.

Finding the evidence

• Cochrane Database, with search term "acetabul$ fracture"
• PubMed (www.ncbi.nlm.nih.gov/pubmed/) clinical queries search/ systematic reviews: "acetabulum" and "acetabular"
• PubMed (www.ncbi.nlm.nih.gov/pubmed/): sensitivity search using keywords "acetabulum fracture OR acetabular fracture" AND "thromboembolism"
• MEDLINE search keywords: "acetabulum fracture" or "acetabular fracture" AND "thromboembolism"

Quality of the evidence

Level II
• 1 systematic reviews[2] of 11 level II studies or level I studies with inconsistent results

Findings

Systematic reviews Slobogean et al. published a systematic review of the literature on this topic in 2009, with a goal of outlining practice guidelines. They found 11 studies with 1760 cases that met inclusion criteria, in the categories of mechanical compression, LMWH, IVC filters, ultrasound screening, and magnetic resonance venography screening. Quantitative pooling was not possible due to heterogeneity, and only LMWH demonstrated a clear reduction in DVT and PE.[45] The studies included in this review are summarized in Table 69.1.

Recommendation

• The recommendations of the ACCP chest guidelines for trauma patients in the use of LMWH are supported in pelvis and acetabulum fractures [overall quality: moderate]

Question 5: What is the optimal HO prophylaxis in patients with acetabulum fractures?

Case clarification

In addition to the postoperative decision about DVT prophylaxis, the trainees want to know if you plan to use either nonsteroidal anti-inflammatories (NSAIDs) or irradiation for prophylaxis against HO.

Relevance

The occurrence of, and subsequent surgical treatment of, acetabular fractures is known to be associated with HO. Although there have been reports of increasing risk with increasingly extensile approaches, the relationship between approach and HO is unclear.[57–60] Disabling forms of the condition occur in nonoperatively treated patients, but much more commonly in operatively treated patients. A meta-analysis founds the rate in operatively treated cases to be 25.6%.[61] The two widely accepted methods of prophylaxis for this are irradiation and indomethacin treatment. Both have disadvantages—burden, transport, and cost for irradiation; bleeding, gastrointestinal complications, and nonunion for NSAIDs.[62,63]

Current opinion

There is no difference between indomethacin and irradiation in the prevention of HO in acetabular fractures, ad choice is based on surgeon preference.

Finding the evidence

• Cochrane Database, with search term: "acetabul$ fracture"
• PubMed (www.ncbi.nlm.nih.gov/pubmed/) clinical queries search/ systematic reviews: "acetabulum" and "acetabular"
• PubMed (www.ncbi.nlm.nih.gov/pubmed/) -sensitivity search using keywords "acetabulum fracture OR acetabular fracture" AND "heterotopic ossification"
• MEDLINE search keywords: "acetabulum fracture" or "acetabular fracture" AND "heterotopic ossification"

Quality of the evidence

Level I
• 1 high-quality randomized controlled trial (RCT)

Level II
• 4 systematic reviews[2] of 3 level II studies or level I studies with inconsistent results

Findings

Systematic review Blokhuis et al. published a systematic review in 2009, evaluating all RCTs comparing these treatments either to each other, or no treatment. With synthesis of data, they found a rate of 5/160 in those treated with irradiation, and 20/224 in those treated with indomethacin (p = 0.034).[64–68]

Indomethacin Karunakar et al. published the only level I study in the above reviewed systematic review. They compared the rate of HO with indomethacin vs. placebo after a posterior approach to the acetabulum. They found no significant different (p = 0.722) with Brooker III or IV in 9/59 indomethacin patients and 12/62 placebo patients.[67,69]

Irradiation Childs et al. reported on a prospective series of 152 patients irradiated on day 1, 2, or 3. They found no statistically significant increase in HO with delay of up to 3 days in treatment. They also compared their prospective series to a retrospective cohort, and found a rate of 5.3% in those treated with radiation, and 60% in those treated without it.

Recommendation

• Irradiation is superior to indomethacin in the prevention of HO in surgically treated acetabulum fractures [overall quality: moderate]

Question 6: What is the expected long-term functional outcome in acetabulum fractures?

Case clarification

When the patient returns to your clinic 2 weeks after the surgery, he wants some clarification of what he can expect as a functional result from this injury and surgery.

Functional outcomes were classically surgeon generated, and reported as "good" or "fair" as we would in natural dialogue. In an effort to move toward the scientific, modern reports of outcomes involve the use of "outcome instruments" designed to collect relevant data and provide an "objective" basis for outcome reporting.

Relevance

Historically, the endpoint of orthopedic studies, or outcome reported, was radiographic. Over time, it was apparent that

Table 69.1 Summary of studies included in the systematic review by Slobogean et al.[45]

Study, Year	Method of diagnosis	Intervention		DVT		PE	
		Control	Experimental	Control	Experimental	Control	Experimental
Mechanical compression devices							
Fisher et al., 1995[46]	Duplex U/S, V/Q scan	No prophylaxis	PSLCD postop until ambulating	3/38	1/35	1/38	2/35
Stannard et al., 2001[47]	Duplex U/S & pelvic/leg MRV	Thigh–calf SCD	Calf–foot pulsatile pump	10/54	5/53	1/54	0/53
Low molecular weight heparin							
Steele et al., 2005[48]	Duplex U/S, V/Q scan, autopsy	Enoxaparin >24 h from injury	Enoxaparin <24 h from injury	8/36	2/64	5/36	0/64
Trials involving ultrasound screening							
White et al., 1990[51]	Duplex U/S, impedance plethysmography, contrast venography, V/Q scan	None;	Serial U/S 7d postop, weekly ×4, biweekly until discharge	N/A	8/60[†]	N/A	1/60
Fishmann et al., 1994[52]	Duplex U/S, V/Q scan, PA, contrast venography	None	Preop U/S, TEDs, PSLCD, warfarin	N/A	Preop: 11/197 Postop: 4/197	N/A	2/197
Magnetic resonance venography							
Montgomery et al., 1995[53]	Contrast venogram, MRV	Contrast venogram	MRV	7/45	15/45	0/45	0/45
Montgomery et al., 1997[54]	MRV	None	MRV	N/A	34/101	N/A	1/101
Stover et al., 2002[55]	Contrast venogram	MRV	CT venogram	4/30	2/30	n/a	n/a
Borer et al., 2005[56]	U/S, MRV, PA, V/Q scan, CT scan, or autopsy	No screening protocol	U/S & MRV of pelvis	n/a	19/316	7/487	10/486
Inferior vena cava filters							

		Intervention		PE	
		Control	Experimental	Control	Experimental
Webb et al., 1992[49]	Venography, duplex U/S, V/Q scan, or PA	Subjects with <2 risk factors	Subjects with ≥2 risk factors	2/27	0/24
Rogers et al., 1995[50]	Impedance plethysmography, duplex U/S, V/Q scan, or PA	Retrospective comparison of no IVC filter insertion	IVC filter if identified as high-risk trauma at admission	5/168	1/23

CT, spiral computed tomography; DVT, deep vein thrombosis; IVC, inferior vena cava; MRV, magnetic resonance venography; PA, pulmonary arteriography; PE, pulmonary embolism; PSLCD, pneumatic sequential leg compression device; SC, subcutaneous; SCD, sequential compression device; TEDs, thromboembolic stockings; U/S, ultrasound; V/Q, ventilation/perfusion.

radiographic outcome did not necessarily correspond to how patients actually felt. As such, authors began reporting functional result as reported by patients. In its most basic form, this is a simple author-generated outcome. In an attempt to move away from this to more objective measures, it is now considered standard practice to report some type of patient-reported validated functional instrument. For the hip joint, these can be generic or specific.[70] Most commonly in medicine overall, generic outcome is measured using the SF-36.[71] In orthopedics, generic musculoskeletal function is often measured using the SMFA.[72] In the hip specifically, the most common outcome measures reported for acetabulum fractures have been the HHS (pain, function deformity, and range of motion) and the Merle d'Aubigné–Postel hip score (pain, mobility, ability to walk). Both of these were designed for hip arthroplasty patients, and neither has been validated for the acetabulum fracture population.[70,73,74]

Current opinion

The majority of patients attain good to excellent functional results after acetabulum fracture with appropriate treatment.

Finding the evidence

• Cochrane Database, with search term "acetabul$ fracture"
• PubMed (www.ncbi.nlm.nih.gov/pubmed/) clinical queries search/systematic reviews: "acetabulum" and "acetabular"
• PubMed (www.ncbi.nlm.nih.gov/pubmed/): sensitivity search using keywords "acetabulum fracture OR acetabular fracture" AND "outcome"
• MEDLINE search keywords: "acetabulum fracture" or "acetabular fracture" AND "outcome"

Quality of the evidence

Level II
• 2 studies

Level III
• 4 studies

Findings

Systematic review In 2005, Giannoudis et al. published a systematic review of displaced acetabulum fractures in adults, treated within 4 weeks, with a follow-up of at least 12 weeks. They reviewed 160 articles, and included 34 with 3639 patients.[61] These were 5 prospective and 29 retrospective reviews; 16 of these studies reported functional outcome based on Merle d'Aubigné score (1610), and 5 reported functional outcome using the HHS (600). Using the former, a good or excellent clinical result was reported 79.4% of the time. With the HHS, a good

Table 69.2 Systematic review of displaced acetabulum fractures

	Satisfactory reduction Patients (%)	Unsatisfactory reduction Patients (%)
Merle d'Aubigné score		
Excellent	543 (62.4)	53 (48.2)
Good	203 (23.4)	28 (25.4)
Fair	46 (5.3)	11 (10.0)
Poor	77 (8.9)	18 (16.4)
Harris hip score		
Excellent	52 (56.5)	3 (18.8)
Good	26 (28.3)	1 (6.2)
Fair	4 (4.3)	4 (25.0)
Poor	10 (10.9)	8 (50.0)

Satisfactory, ≤2 mm; unsatisfactory, >2 mm.

or excellent functional outcome was reported 73.2% of the time. There was a correlation between outcome and radiographic outcome, when considering postoperative displacement of 2 mm or less as satisfactory (Table 69.2).

Individual reports Matta published his often cited prospective series in the *Journal of Bone and Joint Surgery* in 1996.[3] He reported on 262 displaced acetabulum fractures in 259 patients. Using the Merle d'Aubigné score for clinical outcome, he reported 76% good or excellent results, fair in 8%, and poor in 6%. There was a statistically significant relationship between quality of reduction (excellent, good, fair, poor) and quality of clinical outcome (excellent, good, fair, poor).

Since the publication of the meta-analysis in 2005, there have been several additional reports. Ovre et al. presented a prospective cohort of 176 fractures in 2008.[75] They reported a mean modified HHS of 99.9 (good). A multiple regression analysis was performed to delineate the independent relationship between articular step, articular gap, and roof arc angle. The strongest predictor was roof arc score (p = 0.02), and there was no relationship between diastasis and HHS. Articular step of 2 mm approached clinical significance (p = 0.08).

Moed et al. published two series in the *Journal of Bone and Joint Surgery* (American volume) highlighting weaknesses in currently used functional outcome scores for these injuries. In 2003, a series of 150 patients with all types of acetabulum fractures treated with surgery.[76] In this series they reported a modified Merle d'Aubigné score of 16.8 (good–excellent) and a SMFA of 24.9. There was a significant ceiling effect with the former. Despite good correlation, the SMFA score were significantly worse than population norms (p < 0.001), indicating that the Merle d'Aubigné score may not be capturing the functional level in these patients. This performance of the Merle d'Aubigné score was reiterated in 2007 with a series of 46 patients, in whom the Merle score was 17 (good–excellent) and the SMFA was 23.17.[77] Again here, there was a ceiling effect in the merle score, and a failure of this score to capture loss of function as captured on the SMFA.

In 2006, Kreder et al. described a series of simple posterior wall fractures compared to associated patterns with posterior wall fractures (128 patients);[78] 84 of these had functional outcome follow-up with SF-36 and SMFA. The mean SMFA score was 35.75 for the group overall, and was significantly worse in the associated patterns (p = 0.036). The mean scores in all SF-36 domains were worse than matched population norms (p < 0.001). There was a trend to worse functional outcome with residual displacement of greater than 2 mm (0.05 > p < 0.08).

Recommendations

- Despite largely good–excellent clinical scores on frequently used hip-related outcome measures reported, expected general functional outcome after acetabulum fracture is below population age matched norms [overall quality: moderate]
- Complexity of fracture and quality of reduction are important predictors of functional outcome [overall quality: moderate]

Question 7: What are the important non-surgeon-related factors that determine prognosis in acetabulum fractures?

Case clarification

Your patient continues to have some pain and disability after 6 months, and has been unable to return to his previous employment. There is a subtle loss of joint space on plain films, and a diagnostic local anesthetic block of the hip confirms that his hip joint is the source of his pain. The trainees ask whether this outcome could have been predicted in this patient.

> A diagnostic block with local anaesthetic involves injection of local anaesthetic into a particular anatomic space, and subsequent evaluation of the patient's symptoms. Resolution of symptoms indicates that the area is the source of the pain.

Relevance

As early as Rowe's review in 1961, it was becoming very apparent that there were particular factors that were important in determining patient outcomes in acetabulum fractures.[27] Those with articular cartilage damage, older patients with poor bone quality, more severe fractures, appear to be less likely to have a favorable outcome.[1,4,5] However, as with many areas of orthopedic surgery, this opinion has been largely based on expert opinion and experience, with scientific evidence being a more recent development.

Current opinion

Age, fracture type, damage to the femoral head, marginal impaction, and posterior dislocation are all important factors in determining outcome in acetabulum fractures, regardless of the quality of surgical reduction.

Finding the evidence

- Cochrane Database, with search term "acetabul$ fracture"
- PubMed (www.ncbi.nlm.nih.gov/pubmed/) clinical queries search/ systematic reviews: "acetabulum" and "acetabular"
- PubMed (www.ncbi.nlm.nih.gov/pubmed/) -sensitivity search using keywords "acetabulum fracture OR acetabular fracture" AND "prognosis"
- MEDLINE search keywords: "acetabulum fracture" or "acetabular fracture" AND "prognosis"

Quality of the evidence

Level II
- 2 studies

Level III
- 4 studies

Findings

Age Matta's series reported 81 percent good or excellent results in those less than 40, and 68% good or excellent results in those over 40 (p = 0.02).[3] This same age cut-off used to create a binary age variable was found to be statistically significant by Liebergall et al. in their review of 60 patients.[79]

Murphy et al.'s paper in injury in 2003 was aimed at determining the importance of prognostic factors on outcome (Merle d'Aubigné) using a logistic regression models in 201 patients. An increase in age of 1 year was associated with an odds ratio of having a worse outcome of 1.02 per year of increase in age (p = 0.036). Put simply, this means that even an increase in 1 year in age is statistically significant.[80]

Fracture type The Giannoudis et al. systematic review addressed the issue of fracture type (Table 69.3). Seven of the included studies with 906 patients correlated the results of the Merle d'Aubigné score with the Letournel fracture classification. The worst outcomes were seen in fractures of the anterior wall (16 patients) and of the posterior column (27 patients) with 48% and 37% fair and poor results, respectively. The best prognostic fracture types were anterior column and transverse fractures with nearly 90%

Table 69.3 Outcome and fracture types

Fracture type	Patients	Incidence (%)	Excellent/ good (%)	Fair/poor (%)
PW	204	22.2	82.4	17.6
PC	27	2.7	63.0	37.0
Anterior wall	16	1.7	56.2	47.8
AC	37	4.0	89.2	10.8
Transverse	51	5.6	86.3	13.7
All simple fracture types	**335**	**36.6**	**80.9**	**19.1**
T-shaped	128	14.0	71.1	28.9
PC–PW	47	5.1	83.0	17.0
Transverse–PW	136	14.8	71.3	28.7
AC–posterior hemitransverse	43	4.7	72.1	27.9
Associated both columns	227	24.8	71.4	28.6
All associated fracture types	**581**	**63.4**	**72.3**	**27.7**

AC, anterior column; PC, posterior column; PW, posterior wall.

of excellent and good results. As a group simple fractures showed a better functional outcome than associated fractures, with 80.9% and 72.3%, excellent and good results respectively (p = 0.07).[61]

Femoral head damage Liebergall's study outlined above found damage to the femoral head to be the strongest predictor of poor outcome, with only 35.7% of patients in the series with femoral head damage having a favorable outcome (p = 0.001).[79]

In a review of the experience with the T-extensile modified extended iliofemoral approach, Starr et al.[81] reported 14/43 "failures" with a HHS of less than 70, or total hip replacement. Ten of these patients had femoral head damage at surgery, one had known osteoarthritis, and in two the capsule was not opened. Only one patient with a poor outcome had visibly normal cartilage at surgery (p = 0.004).[81]

Dislocation Giannoudis's meta-analysis also addressed avascular necrosis (AVN) and posterior dislocation. In 18 studies with 2010 patients, the overall AVN rate was 5.6%. In patients with a posterior dislocation, this rate was 9.2% (28/303). This was statistically higher than the 5% in

those without posterior dislocation in the meta-analysis (85/1707) (p = 0.003).[61]

Moed et al. described the outcome of 108 fracture dislocation of the hip with posterior wall fractures 2 years from surgery, using the Merle d'Aubigné–Postel hip score. They found a highly significant relationship between time to reduction and fair/poor outcomes, with a progressively worse outcome at 12 hours, 12–24 hours and more than 24 hours (p < 0.0001). Of the 10 patients who had a poor result in this study, 5 had delayed reduction and development of osteonecrosis.[77]

Recommendations

• Younger patients have a more favorable prognosis in acetabulum fractures [overall quality: moderate]
• With a few exceptions of rare simple fracture types, the prognosis of simple fractures is better than that of complex fracture types [overall quality: moderate]
• Femoral head damage is a poor prognostic indicator in acetabulum fractures [overall quality: moderate]
• The presence of posterior dislocation increases risk of AVN. Reduction should be performed as soon as possible [overall quality: moderate]

Summary of recommendations

• CT scan appears to offer little additional information over three plain film views in acetabular fracture classification, and is inversely related to level of experience in acetabular fracture surgery
• CT scan imaging of acetabulum fractures is necessary to delineate additional fracture features such as impaction, articular gap and step, and intra-articular loose bodies
• Displacement is poorly tolerated in the weightbearing dome, and greater than 3 mm is a relative operative indication
• Incongruence at the hip joint is an indication for surgical reduction in acetabulum fractures, and can be predicted by the roof arc angle
• Clinical series support cadaveric data that instability in posterior wall fractures is predicted by greater than 50% involvement, and dynamic testing can offer additional information in those with 25–50% involvement
• In elderly patients, reasonable functional results after operative treatment can be obtained with open reduction and internal fixation, early arthroplasty, and delayed arthroplasty
• The recommendations of the ACCP chest guidelines for trauma patients in the use of LMWH for thromboprophylaxis are supported in pelvis and acetabulum fractures
• Irradiation is superior to indomethacin in the prevention of HO in surgically treated acetabulum fractures

- Despite largely good–excellent clinical scores on frequently used hip related outcome measures reported, expected general functional outcome after acetabulum fracture is below population age-matched norms
- Complexity of fracture and quality of reduction are important predictors of functional outcome
- Younger patients have a more favorable prognosis in acetabulum fractures
- With a few exceptions of rare simple fracture types, the prognosis of simple fractures is better than that of complex fracture types
- Femoral head damage is a poor prognostic indicator in acetabulum fractures
- The presence of posterior dislocation increases risk of AVN. Reduction should be performed as soon as possible

References

1. Judet R, Judet J, Letournel E. Fractures of the acetabulum. Classification and surgical approaches for open reduction. J Bone Joint Surg Am 1964;46:1615–46.
2. Laird A, Keating JF. Acetabular fractures. A 16-year prospective epidemiological study. J Bone Joint Surg Br 2005;87:969–73.
3. Matta JM. Fractures of the acetabulum: accuracy of reduction and clinical results in patients managed operatively within three weeks after the injury. J Bone Joint Surg Am 1996;78:1632–45.
4. Letournel E, Judet R. Fractures of the Acetabulum. Springer-Verlag, Berlin, 1981.
5. Tile M, Helfet DL, Kellam JF. Fractures of the Pelvis and Acetabulum, 3rd edn. Lippincott Williams and Wilkins, Philadelphia, 2003.
6. Moed BR, McMichael JC. Outcomes of posterior wall fractures of the acetabulum: surgical technique. J Bone Joint Surg Am 2002;90(Suppl 2):87–107.
7. Moed BR, Willson-Carr SE, Watson JT Results of Operative Treatment of Fractures of the Posterior Wall of the Acetabulum. J Bone Joint Surg Am 2002;84:752–8.
8. Hak DJ, Hamel AJ, Bay BK, et al. Consequences of transverse acetabular fracture malreduction on load transmission across the hip joint. J Orthop Trauma 1998;12:90–100.
9. Konrath G, Hamel A, Sharkey N, et al. Biomechanical consequences of anterior column fractures of the acetabulum. J Orthop Trauma 1998;12:547–552.
10. Olson SA, Bay BK, Chapman MW, et al. Biomechanical consequences of fracture and repair of the posterior wall of the acetabulum. J Bone Joint Surg Am 1995;77:1184–92.
11. Kaempffe FA, Bone LB, Border JR. Open reduction and internal fixation of acetabular fractures: heterotopic ossification and other complications of treatment. J Orthop Trauma 1991;5:439–45.
12. Beaule PE, Dorey FJ, Matta JM. Letournel classification for acetabular fractures: Assessment of interobserver and intraobserver reliability. J Bone Joint Surg Am 2003;85:1704–9.
13. Ohashi K, El-Khoury GY, Abu-Zahra KW, Berbaum KS. Interobserver agreement for Letournel acetabular fracture classification with multidetector CT: are standard Judet radiographs necessary? Radiology 2006;241(2):386–91.
14. Hufner T, Pohlemenn T, Gansslen A, Assassi P, Prokop M Tscherne H. The value of CT in classification and decision making in acetabulum fractures. A systematic analysis. Unfallchirurg 1999;102(2):124–31.
15. Borrelli J Jr, Goldfarb C, Catalano L, Evanoff BA. Assessment of articular fragment displacement in acetabular fractures: a comparison of computerized tomography and plain radiographs. J Orthop Trauma 2002;16(7):449–56.
16. Lang JE, Cothran RL, Pietrobon R, Olson SA. Observer variability in assessing articular surface displacement in acetabular fractures using a standardized measurement technique. J Surg Orthop Adv 2009;18(1):9–12.
17. St Pierre RK, Oliver T, Somoygi J, Whitesides T, Fleming LL. Computerized tomography in the evaluation and classification of fractures of the acetabulum. Clin Orthop Relat Res 1984;188:234–7.
18. Mayo KA, Letournel E, Matta JM, Mast JM, Johnson EE, Martimbeau CL. Surgical revision of malreduced acetabular fractures. Clin Orthop Relat Res 1994;305:47–52.
19. Johnson EE, Matta JM, Mast JW, Letournel E. Delayed reconstruction of acetabular fractures 21–120 days following injury. Clin Orthop Relat Res 1994;305:20–30.
20. Letournel E. Diagnosis and treatement of nonunions and malunions of acetabular fractures. CLin Orthop North Am 1990;21:769–88.
21. Hak DJ, Hamel AJ, Bay BK, Sharkey NA, Olson SA. Consequences of transverse acetabular fracture malreduction on load transmission across the hip joint. J Orthop Trauma 1998;12:90–100.
22. Olson SA, Bay BK, Pollak AN, Sharkey NA, Lee T. The effect of variable size posterior wall acetabular fractures on contact characteristics of the hip joint. J Orthop Trauma 1996;10:395–402.
23. Keith JE, Brashear HR, Guilford WB. Stability of posterior fracture dislocations of the hip. J Bone Joint Surg Am 1998;70:711–14.
24. Vailas JC, Hurwitz S, Wiesel SW. Posterior acetabular fracture-dislocations: fragment size, joint capsule, and stability. J Trauma 1989;29:1494–6.
25. Matta JM, Anderson LM, Epstein HC, Hendricks P. Fractures of the acetabulum: a retrospective analysis. Clin Orthop Relat Res 1986;205:230–40.
26. Sen RK, Veerappa LA. Long term outcome of conservatively managed displaced acetabular fractures. J Trauma 2009;67:155–9.
27. Rowe CR, Lowell JD. Prognosis of fractures of the acetabulum. J Bone Joint Surg Am 1961;43:30–59.
28. Olson SA, Matta JM. The computerized tomography subchondral arc: a new method of assessing acetabular continuity after fracture. J Orthop Trauma 1993;7:402–13.
29. Calkins MS, Zych G, Latta L, Borja FJ, Mnaymneh W. Computed tomography evaluation of stability in posterior fracture dislocation of the hip. Clin Orthop 1998;227:152–63.
30. Tornetta P III. Nonoperative management of acetabular fractures: The use of dynamic stress views. J Bone Joint Surg Br 1999;81:67–70.
31. Cree M, Soskolne CL, Belseck E, et al. Mortality and institutionalization following hip fracture. J Am Geriatr Soc 2000;48:283–8.

32. Weller I, Wai EK, Jaglal S, Kreder HJ. The effect of hospital type and surgical delay on mortality after surgery for hip fracture. J Bone Joint Surg Br 2005;87:361–6.

33. Lefaivre KA, Macadam SA, Davidson DJ, Gandhi R, Chan H, Broekhuyse HM. Length of stay, mortality, morbidity and delay to surgery in hip fractures. J Bone Joint Surg 2009;91:922–7.

34. Spencer RF. Acetabular fractures in older patients. J Bone Joint Surg Br 1989;71:774–6.

35. Anglen JO, Burd TA, Hendricks KJ, Harrison P. The "gull sign" a harbinger of failure for internal fixation of geriatric acetabular fractures. J Orthop Trauma 2003;17:625–34.

36. Helfet DL, Borrelli J Jr, DiPasquale T, Sanders R. Stabilization of acetabular fractures in elderly patients. J Bone Joint Surg 1992; 74:753–65.

37. Mears DC, Velyvis JH. Acute total hip arthroplasty for selected displaced acetabular fractures: two to twelve-year results. J Bone Joint Surg Am 2002;84:1–9.

38. Sermon A, Broos P, Vanderschot P. Total hip replacement for acetabular fractures: Results in 121 patients operated between 1983 and 2003. Injury 2008;39:914–921.

39. Weber M, Berry DJ, Harmsen WS. Total hip arthroplasty after operative treatment of an acetabular fracture. J Bone Joint Surg 1998;80:1295–1305.

40. Bellabarba C, Berger RA, Bentley CD, et al. Cementless acetabular reconstruction after acetabular fracture. J Bone Joint Surg Am 2001;83:868–76.

41. Velmahos GC, Nigro J, Tatevossian R, et al. Inability of an aggressive policy of thromboprophylaxis to prevent deep venous thrombosis (DVT) in critically injured patients: are current methods of DVT prophylaxis insufficient? J Am Coll Surg 1998;187:529–33.

42. Buerger PM, Peoples JB, Lemmon GW, et al. Risk of pulmonary emboli in patients with pelvic fractures. Am Surg 1993;59: 505–8.

43. Geerts WH, Code KI, Jay RM, et al. A prospective study of venous thromboembolism after major trauma. N Engl J Med 2008;331:1601–6.

44. Geerts WH, Bergqvist D, Pineo GF, et al. American College of Chest Physicians. Prevention of venous thromboembolism: American College of Chest Physicians evidence-based clinical practice guidelines (8th edition). Chest 2008;133(Suppl 6), 381S–453S.

45. Slobogean GP, Lefaivre KA, Nicolaou S, O'Brien PJ. A systematic review of thromboprophylaxis for pelvic and acetabular fractures. J Orthop Trauma 2009;23:379–84.

46. Fisher CG, Blachut PA, Salvian AJ, et al. Effectiveness of pneumatic leg compression devices for the prevention of thromboembolic disease in orthopaedic trauma patients: a prospective, randomized study of compression alone versus no prophylaxis. J Orthop Trauma 1995;9:1–7.

47. Stannard JP, Riley RS, McClenney MD, et al. Mechanical prophylaxis against deep-vein thrombosis after pelvic and acetabular fractures. J Bone Joint Surg Am 2001;83:1047–51.

48. Steele N, Dodenhoff RM, Ward AJ, et al. Thromboprophylaxis in pelvic and acetabular trauma surgery. The role of early treatment with lowmolecular- weight heparin. J Bone Joint Surg 2005;87: 209–12.

49. Webb LX, Rush PT, Fuller SB, et al. Greenfield filter prophylaxis of pulmonary embolism in patients undergoing surgery for acetabular fracture. J Orthop Trauma 1992;6:139–45.

50. Rogers FB, Shackford SR, Ricci MA, et al. Routine prophylactic vena cava filter insertion in severely injured trauma patients decreases the incidence of pulmonary embolism. J Am Coll Surg 1995;180:641–7.

51. White RH, Goulet JA, Bray TJ, et al. Deep-vein thrombosis after fracture of the pelvis: assessment with serial duplex-ultrasound screening. J Bone Joint Surg Am 1990;72:495–500.

52. Fishmann AJ, Greeno RA, Brooks LR, et al. Prevention of deep vein thrombosis and pulmonary embolism in acetabular and pelvic fracture surgery. Clin Orthop Relat Res 1994;305:133–7.

53. Montgomery KD, Potter HG, Helfet DL. Magnetic resonance venography to evaluate the deep venous system of the pelvis in patients who have an acetabular fracture. J Bone Joint Surg Am 1995;77:1639–49.

54. Montgomery KD, Potter HG, Helfet DL. The detection and management of proximal deep venous thrombosis in patients with acute acetabular fractures: a follow-up report. J Orthop Trauma 1997;11:330–6.

55. Stover MD, Morgan SJ, Bosse MJ, et al. Prospective comparison of contrast enhanced computed tomography versus magnetic resonance venography in the detection of occult deep pelvic vein thrombosis in patients with pelvic and acetabular fractures. J Orthop Trauma 2002;16:613–21.

56. Borer DS, Starr AJ, Reinert CM, et al. The effect of screening for deep vein thrombosis on the prevalence of pulmonary embolism in patients with fractures of the pelvis or acetabulum: a review of 973 patients. J Orthop Trauma 2005;19:92–5.

57. Alonso JE, Davila R, Bradley E. Extended iliofemoral versus triradiate approaches in management of associated acetabular fractures. Clin Orthop Relat Res 1994;305:81–7.

58. Chiu FY, Chen CM, Lo WH. Surgical treatment of displaced acetabular fractures: 72 cases followed for 10 (6–14) years. Injury 2003;31:181–5.

59. Matityahu A, Bruck N, Miclau T. Heterotopic ossification and acetabular fractures. Curr Opin Orthop 2006;17:34.

60. Routt ML Jr, Swiontkowski MF. Operative treatment of complex acetabular fractures: combined anterior and posterior exposures during the same procedure. J Bone Joint Surg Am 1990;72: 897–904.

61. Giannoudis PV, Grotz MR, Papakostidis C, Dinopoulos H. Operative treatment of displaced fractures of the acetabulum: a meta-analysis. J Bone Joint Surg Br 2005;87:2–9.

62. Anglen JO, Moore KD. Prevention of heterotopic bone formation after acetabular fracture fixation by single-dose radiation therapy: a preliminary report. J Orthop Trauma 1996;10:258–63.

63. Burd TA, Hughes MS, Anglen JO. Heterotopic ossification prophylaxis with indomethacin increases the risk of long-bone nonunion. J Bone Joint Surg Br 2003;85:700–5.

64. Blokhuis TJ, Frolke JP. Is radiation superior to indomethicin to prevent heterotopic ossification in acetabular fractures?: a systematic review. Clin Orthop Rel Res 2009;467:526–30.

65. Childs HA 3rd, Cole T, Falkenberg E, et al. A prospective evaluation of the timing of postoperative radiotherapy for preventing heterotopic ossification following traumatic acetabular fractures. Int J Radiat Oncol Biol Phys 2000;47:1347–52.

66. Matta JM, Siebenrock KA. Does indomethacin reduce heterotopic bone formation after operations for acetabular fractures? A prospective randomised study. J Bone Joint Surg Br 1997;79: 959–63.

67. Karunakar MA, Sen A, Bosse MJ, Sims SH, Goulet JA, Kellam JF. Indometacin as prophylaxis for heterotopic ossification after the operative treatment of fractures of the acetabulum. J Bone Joint Surg Br 2006;88:1613–17.

68. Iotov A. Heterotopic ossification in surgically treated patients with acetabular fractures and indomethacin prophylaxis for its prevention. Ortoped Travmatol. 2000;36:367–73.

69. Brooker AF, Bowerman JW, Robinson RA, Riley LH Jr. Ectopic ossification following total hip replacement: incidence and a method of classification. J Bone Joint Surg Am 1973;55:1629–32.

70. Suk M, Hanson BP, Norvell DC, Helfet DL. AO Handbook: Musculoskeletal Outcomes Measures and Instruments. AO Publishing: Davos, Switzerland, 2005.

71. Ware JE Jr, Shelbourne CD. The MOS 36-item short-form health survey (SF-36) I: conceptual Framework and item selection. Med Care 1992;30:473–83.

72. Swiontkowski MF, Engelberg R, Martin DP, Agel J. Short muscu-loskeletal function assessment questionnaire: validity, reliability, and responsiveness. J Bone Joint Surg Am 1999;81(9):1245–60.

73. D'Aubigné RM, Postel M. Functional results of hip arthroplasty with acrylic prosthesis. J Bone Joint Surg Am 1954;36:451–75.

74. Harris WH. Traumatic arthritis of the hip after dislocation and acetabular fractures: treatment by mold arthroplasty. An end-result study using a new method of result evaluation. J Bone Joint Surg Am 1969;51:737–55.

75. Ovre S, Madsen JE, Roise O. Acetabular fracture displacement, roof arc angles and 2 years outcome. Injury 2008;39:922–31.

76. Moed BR, Yu PH, Gruson KI. Functional outcomes of acetabular fractures. J Bone Joint Surg Am 2008;85:1879–83.

77. Moed BR, McMichael J. Outcomes of posterior wall fractures of the acetabulum. J Bone Joint Surg Am 2007;89:1170–6.

78. Kreder HJ, Rozen N, Borkhoff CM, et al. Determinants of functional outcome after simple and complex acetabular fractures involving the posterior wall. J Bone Joint Surg 2006;88: 776–82.

79. Liebergall M, Mosheiff R, Low J, et al. Acetabular fractures: clinical outcome of surgical treatment. Clin Orthop 1999;366: 205–16.

80. Murphy D, Kaliszer M, Rice J, McElwain JP. Outcome after acetabular fracture: prognostic factors and their inter-relationships. Injury 2003;34:512–17.

81. Starr AJ, Watson JT, Reinert CM, et al. Complications following the "T extensile" approach: a modified extensile approach for acetabular fracture surgery: report of forty-three patients. J Orthop Trauma 2002;16:535–42.

70

Open Fractures

*Atul F. Kamath[1], John G. Horneff[1], John L. Esterhai, Jr.[1,2],
Wesley G. Lackey[3], Kyle J. Jeray[3], and J. Scott Broderick[3]*

[1]Hospital of the University of Pennsylvania, Philadelphia, PA, USA
[2]Veterans Affairs Hospital, Philadelphia, PA, USA
[3]Greenville Hospital System University Medical Center, Greenville, SC, USA

Case scenario

A 28 year old man is involved in a serious motorcycle accident. His injuries include a closed head injury, an anterior–posterior compression (APC) type 1 pelvic ring injury, and an open comminuted tibial shaft fracture with associated fibula fracture. He is intubated in the trauma bay and is actively undergoing resuscitation. His distal pulses are normal and he has adequate capillary refill.

Relevant anatomy

An "open" fracture involves any injury pattern in which a breach in the soft tissue envelope has occurred, resulting in direct communication between the bone and the environment. Open fractures are more susceptible to wound infection or deeper bone infection, termed osteomyelitis. In general, the anatomic goal in open fracture care is to debride any nonviable tissue (including bone), while preserving as much of the perfused tissue as possible.

Open fractures are most commonly classified according to the Gustilo and Anderson system (see box), which considers wound size, fracture pattern, and degree of soft tissue compromise/contamination (level II, level III)[1,2] The classification of open fractures accounts for both soft tissue and bone injury, and predicts eventual prognosis, including rates of infection (level II).[1] Open fracture classification

can be estimated in the Emergency Department but should be definitively classified in the operating room once wound/fracture exploration and debridement have been completed.

Gustilo and Anderson classification of open fractures

- **Type I** Clean (minimally contaminated) wound smaller than 1 cm and simple fracture pattern; no skin crushing
- **Type II** Wound >1 cm but without significant soft tissue crushing; fracture pattern may be more complex but with minimal periosteal stripping
- **Type III** Segmental fracture or a single fracture with extensive soft tissue injury; subdivided into three subtypes:
- **Type IIIA** Adequate soft tissue coverage of the fracture despite high-energy trauma or extensive soft tissue damage
- **Type IIIB** Inadequate soft tissue coverage with periosteal stripping; requires soft tissue reconstruction
- **Type IIIC** Open fracture associated with arterial injury requiring repair

---

Importance of the problem

Data from Europe demonstrate an approximate 4% rate of open fractures,[3,4] which is likely similar to rates in other developed nations. As extrapolated in other reviews (level II),[5] this amounts to approximately 3,400 open fractures in Canada or 250,000 open fractures in the United States every year.

Although much has been written about open fractures, very little of the literature is level I quality. Many of the

---

No grants or external sources of funding were used for this study. Authors report no conflicts of interest related to the subject matter.

treatment recommendations that are ingrained in our everyday treatment of open fractures are based on retrospective data with low numbers of patients or simply on opinion-based literature.

Top five questions

1. What is the initial management of open fractures?
2. How soon does an open fracture need to get to the operating room?
3. What irrigation techniques afford the best results with open fractures?
4. Is there evidence for the use of negative pressure wound closure therapy (e.g., V.A.C.®) vs. antibiotic bead pouch placement in open fracture care?
5. What factors should be considered when performing a soft tissue closure in an open fracture?

Question 1: What is the initial management of open fractures?

Case clarification
The patient's tibia fracture is displaced and comminuted. The wound size is 10 cm, and there appears to be some soft tissue loss. The wound is not grossly contaminated, but some foreign debris is noted.

Relevance
Initial management of the open fracture wound includes antibiotics, a sterile dressing, appropriate splinting, and tetanus toxoid administration.

Current opinion
Prompt antibiotic administration and a tetanus shot are priority. A sterile gauze dressing moistened with normal saline may be an appropriate choice for a wound dressing, accompanied by temporary skeletal stabilization for patient comfort.

Finding the evidence
• Cochrane Database (http://www.cochrane.org/reviews), using search terms: "initial management open fracture" and "open fractures antibiotics"
  ° 1 review article
• PubMed, using search terms: "open fracture initial management" and "open fracture antibiotics"

Quality of the evidence
Level I
• 4 studies

Level II
• 5 studies

Level III
• 6 studies

Level IV
• 4 studies

Level V
• 1 study

Findings
Few articles on open fractures address the management of wounds in the field or Emergency Department. Simple debridement of any gross contamination is encouraged if possible, as well as direct pressure on active bleeding. Temporary splinting of any fracture is highly recommended. As experiments have suggested that antiseptics (such as povidone-iodine) may be toxic to the host cells (level V, level I),[6,7] a gauze dressing moistened with normal saline may be the safest, least destructive choice for short-term coverage.

The administration of systemic antibiotics for open fractures has been the standard of care since 1974 (level I).[8] A review by Gosselin et al. showed that antibiotics given for an open fracture reduces the infection risk by 59% (level III).[9] The current antibiotic recommendations stem from the original Gustilo and Anderson articles,[1,2] and no article since has challenged the basic antimicrobial approach, even with the plethora of broad-spectrum antibiotics now available. Several studies agree that the single most important factor in reducing infection is early administration of the appropriate antibiotics (level I–III).[7–12] In current protocols a first-generation cephalosporin (usually cefazolin) is given for type I and II fractures, while an aminoglycoside (usually gentamicin) is often added for type III fractures. In a prospective randomized double-blind trial, Patzakis et al. showed that ciprofloxacin alone was as effective as cefamandole plus gentamicin for type I and II injuries but not as effective in type III injuries (level I).[10] In wounds that are severely contaminated or have poor oxygenation (vascular injuries), penicillin is added for adequate anaerobic coverage (level II).[1]

Some exceptions exist to the early antibiotic rule. For example, a randomized placebo-controlled trial found that flucloxacillin did not add to the prevention of infection in conjunction with routine treatment of open distal phalanx fractures with irrigation and debridement (level II).[11]

Few articles give length of dosing recommendations for antibiotic therapy, although most surgeons agree that antibiotics should be continued for at least 24 hours after the final irrigation and debridement, similar to antibiotic prophylaxis recommendations for elective surgery (level I).[12]

Recommendations
Present recommendations for initial open fracture management are as follows [overall quality: moderate]:

- Systemic antibiotic administration is the most important factor in the initial management of open fractures
- A cephalosporin is appropriate for type I and II open fractures
- An aminoglycoside should be added for type III injuries and penicillin should be given for severely contaminated wounds
- Tetanus toxoid should be administered when appropriate
- A sterile dressing moistened with normal saline and temporary stabilization should be applied

Question 2: How soon does an open fracture need to get to the operating room?

Case clarification

The extremity is sterilely dressed and splinted. Appropriate antibiotics are administered, and a dose of tetanus toxoid is given. Full evaluation is completed by the trauma surgery team by midnight. The patient is hemodynamically and neurologically stable. The case is posted for surgery, but the operating room charge nurse reports that a room will not be available for at least 4–5 hours.

Relevance

As open fractures are at increased risk for infection, these injuries must be addressed promptly. However, the need for urgent surgical debridement must be balanced with the patient's overall physiological status, operating room availability, and reasonable demands on the surgeon.

Current opinion

Open fractures were long considered orthopedic emergencies requiring immediate debridement and fixation. Many trauma centers now reserve an operating room dedicated to orthopedic trauma. This room affords time for adequate patient workup and resuscitation, and allows the surgeon to operate during daytime hours with well-trained surgical support staff. More recent evidence supports the notion that many late-night open fractures can wait until morning with no increased risk to the patient (see below).

Finding the evidence

- PubMed (www.ncbi.nlm.nih.gov/pubmed/), using search term: "debridement open fracture"
  - Limits: English
- EMBASE (www.embase.com; excluding MEDLINE duplicates), using search term: "urgency delay timing debridement open fracture"
  - Limits: English
  - 78 results

Quality of the evidence

Level II
- 5 studies

Level III
- 2 studies

Level V
- 1 study

Findings

Based on the Gustilo–Anderson articles, open fractures have been considered emergent cases that need to be operatively debrided within 6 hours of injury. Time to initial surgical debridement—the traditional "6 hour rule"—is rooted in both historical animal studies (level V)[13] and more modern microbiologic analysis citing a theoretical open-fracture inoculum of 10^5 organisms (level II).[14] Only one recent human study supports the idea of debriding open fractures within 6 hours of injury; Kindsfater and Jonassen reviewed 47 high-energy open tibial fractures and found a significant increase in infection rate in fractures that were delayed greater than 5 hours (level III).[15] On the contrary, many are skeptical, based on the limited data, over the improved long-term outcomes with surgical intervention within 6 hours of injury (level II),[16] and some have even suggested that no debridement is necessary for isolated type I open injuries (level III).[17] The literature refuting the "the 6 hour rule" is summarized by Crowley et al. in their review article (level II).[18] Pollak concluded in a review article that, within the modern era of antibiotics, timing to debridement is not an independent predictor of postinjury infection (level II).[19] He later demonstrated, in a 2010 paper based on data from the Lower Extremity Assessment Program (LEAP), that there was no difference in development of infection outcomes when debridement occurred within the first 24 hours (level II).[20] This is the current thought process most often adopted at most level 1 trauma centers.

Recommendations

Present recommendations for timing of open fracture management are as follows [overall quality: high]:
- The patient should not be taken to the operating room until medically stabilized
- If possible, the patient should be taken to the operating room within 24 hours of injury

Question 3: What irrigation techniques afford the best results with open fractures?

Case clarification

The patient is admitted to the intensive care unit, resuscitation is continued, and the patient is scheduled to be first case in the dedicated trauma operating room. He goes to the operating room at 7:30 a.m. for irrigation and debridement of the open wound and stabilization of his tibial shaft fracture.

Relevance

The need for surgical debridement of open fractures to prevent infection is well established. Along with antimicrobial chemoprophylaxis and treatment, irrigation must be employed to decrease bacterial cell counts and to flush foreign matter and microorganisms from the wound.

Current opinion

Specific variables associated with the irrigation of open fractures remain controversial, including volume of irrigation, pressure of lavage, type of diluents, and any additional additives to lavage solution.

Finding the evidence

- Cochrane Database (http://www.cochrane.org/ reviews), using search terms: "irrigation open fracture lavage"
  - 9 results
- PubMed (www.ncbi.nlm.nih.gov/pubmed/) using search terms: "irrigation open fracture lavage"
  - Limits: English
  - 99 results, 20 reviews
- EMBASE (www.embase.com; excluding Medline duplicates) using search terms: "irrigation open fracture lavage"
  - Limits: English, EMBASE only
  - 82 results

Quality of the evidence

Level I
- 1 study

Level II
- 2 studies

Level III
- 1 study

Level IV
- 13 studies

Level V
- 17 studies

Findings

No consensus currently exists for the choice of irrigation solution or method of administration during the initial or subsequent procedures. A recent international survey found 70.5% of respondents favored normal saline as an irrigation solution, 71% of surgeons used low-pressure systems, and only 1.3% of the surgeons routinely used a soap additive (level V).[21] Experimental data suggest some toxicity to the host cells from antiseptic solutions. Other concerns for solutions other than normal saline include allergic reactions, additional cost, promotion of resistance, and unproven efficacy.

Volume of irrigation The volume of solution used to irrigate a wound after adequate debridement has not been studied in humans, but is somewhat rooted in tradition (level II).[5] One animal study showed increased bacterial removal with increased volume of irrigation but the correlation plateaued for normal saline alone (level V).[22] The traditionally accepted minimum volume is 3 L for type I, 6 L for type II, and 9 L for type III injuries.

Irrigation additives The efficacy of antiseptic additives in eliminating bacterial loads must be weighed against the potentially toxic side effects to normal host cells in the wound bed. For example, although povidone-iodine solution has demonstrated efficacy in reducing infection in surgical wounds (level 2),[23] undiluted povidone-iodine is toxic to bone cells (level V).[6] Furthermore, there is continued concern over local antibiotic resistance (level II)[24] and anaphylactic reactions (level IV).[25,26] Bhandari et al. showed cell density decrease in vitro with solutions of 10% ethanol, 10% povidone-iodine, 10% antimicrobial wash, and 4% chlorhexidine gluconate (level V).[27] He found the only solutions that did not significantly decrease cell count were soap solution and normal saline alone.

Animal models have shown that irrigation with an antibiotic reduces the rate of infection compared with the use of saline solution alone (level II, level V).[28–30]

Anglen reported the results of a prospective randomized controlled trial of 398 lower extremity open fractures comparing castile soap with bacitracin solution (level I).[31] Despite equivalent infection and bone-healing rates, bacitracin was more problematic in terms of wound-healing issues (9.5% vs. 4%; p = 0.03). Although this study provides some support for soap as the irrigation solution, it was a single-surgeon, single-site study with a relatively small sample size. Soap solutions were more effective than normal saline in removing bacteria from stainless steel screws, while antibiotic solutions showed no advantage (p > 0.05) (level II).[28]

Other potential additives not systematically studied in well-controlled controls include hydrogen peroxide, hexachlorophene (pHisoHex®), sodium hypochlorite (Dakin's solution), benzalkonium chloride (Zephiran®), and various alcohol-containing solutions (level I).[8]

Method of irrigation delivery Multiple studies have promoted the superior mechanical properties of high-pressure irrigation, while many others have addressed the more tissue-friendly approach of low-pressure methods. While high-pressure lavage systems may be more effective in reducing bacterial cell counts and protective biofilm barriers (level V, level V),[32,33] macro- and microscopic damage to both host soft tissues and bone occurs (level V)[34–36] and may result in deeper seeding of bacterial colonies (level V).[37,38] This data is limited by lack of human in-vivo testing of lavage systems. In general, the bulk of experimental evidence suggests an inverse relationship between efficacy of removal of contamination and potential tissue damage with the various methods of wound irrigation.

While the pendulum has swung towards lower-pressure lavage systems, newer innovations, such as the Versajet™ claim to provide controlled surgical debridement of tissues.[39] A purported Venturi effect creates a local vacuum on the surface of the debridement area. Recent studies have suggested that it produces a lower bacterial load in burns (level IV).[40,41] Manufacturers claim that it also prevents the diffusion of microbial contamination deeper into the wound. While applied to total joint infections and wound care, the Versajet system has yet to be systematically tested in the debridement of open fractures. Other techniques, such as tissue sonication to break up bacterial glycocalyx, are still relatively nascent technologies.

Recommendations

There is a clear lack of well-controlled human clinical studies to guide clinical practice recommendations (level II, level V),[24,42] despite decades of interest in systemic, local, and topical antibiotic wound prophylaxis (level III, level II).[43,44] Practicing orthopedic surgeons' opinions are clearly mixed, as demonstrated in the aforementioned survey, and rightly so, based on the inconclusive literature. The Fluid Lavage of Open Wounds (FLOW) study is an ongoing, multicenter study comparing multiple variables (normal saline with or without castile soap, and high-pressure vs. low-pressure vs. gravity flow) in a prospective randomized fashion.

Recommendations

Present recommendations for open fracture management are as follows [overall quality: moderate]:
- normal saline irrigation solution
- low-pressure (generally less than 50 psi, 345 kPa) lavage system
- additives have not demonstrated clear benefit and have additional risks to host tissue

Question 4: Is there evidence for the use of negative pressure wound closure therapy (e.g., V.A.C.) vs. antibiotic bead pouch placement in open fracture care?

Case clarification

After initial debridement of nonviable and highly contaminated soft tissue in the wound bed, a large soft tissue defect remains. The surgeon has performed stabilization of the patient's tibial shaft fracture with an external fixation device and has a discussion with his surgical colleagues, the patient, and his family regarding options for eventual wound coverage.

Relevance

Temporary coverage for wounds between procedures can include a simple mesh-gauze dressing, an antibiotic bead pouch, or negative pressure therapy. The use of negative pressure wound closure therapy (NPWCT) has gained momentum since its inception and routine clinical use in the early 1990s (level V),[45] with early applications for both soft tissue closure due to trauma and in secondary wound coverage after debridement for infection (level V, level III).[34,46]

Negative pressure wound closure therapy

Use of a sponge or foam placed over the wound bed connected to a closed suction system or vacuum device.

Antibiotic bead pouch

Polymethylmethacrylate (PMMA, a cement) mixed with powdered antibiotics; beads are fashioned while the cement is still in a doughy consistency. These beads are usually strung along a heavy suture or 24-gauge wire in a string-of-pearls configuration. The bead string or pouch may then be placed directly into the wound. Example ratio of antibiotics to cement: 3.6 g tobramycin to 40 g PMMA.

Current opinion

Negative pressure therapy and antibiotic bead pouches have proven to be effective in managing the initial soft tissue defects after high-energy injuries. Use of vacuum therapy vs. antibiotic beads may be surgeon- or institutional-based; no well-designed (level I) studies have directly compared these two treatment modalities, and there is limited data—often anecdotal evidence based on small case series—for combined modalities of therapy.

Finding the evidence

Vacuum-assisted closure
- Cochrane Database (http://www.cochrane.org/reviews), using search term: "vacuum-assisted closure orthopedic, V.A.C."
  - 0 results
- PubMed (www.ncbi.nlm.nih.gov/pubmed/), using search term: "vacuum-assisted closure orthopedic, V.A.C."
  - Limits: English
  - 54 results, 13 reviews
- EMBASE (www.embase.com; excluding MEDLINE duplicates), using search term: "vacuum-assisted closure orthopedic, V.A.C."
  - Limits: English, EMBASE only
  - 21 results

Bead pouch
- Cochrane Database (http://www.cochrane.org/reviews) , using search term: "bead pouch orthopedic"
  - 0 results

- PUBMED (www.ncbi.nlm.nih.gov/pubmed/), using search term: "bead pouch orthopedic"
  - Limits: English
  - 1 result, 1 review
- EMBASE (www.embase.com; excluding Medline duplicates) , using search term: "bead pouch orthopedic"
  - Limits: English, EMBASE only
  - 1 results

Quality of the evidence

Vacuum-assisted closure
Level I
- 2 studies

Level II
- 3 studies

Level III
- 4 studies

Level IV
- 10 studies

Level V
- 11 studies

Bead pouch
Level II
- 2 studies

Level V
- 2 studies

Findings

Negative pressure wound therapy Several reports have documented favorable results with the use of NPWCT, also known as vacuum-assisted closure (after the brand-name device V.A.C.,® in the management of orthopedic wounds (level II–III).[47-50] NPWCT aims to reduce tissue edema, to shrink wound size, and to stimulate granulation tissue formation. This modality is also thought to increase blood flow and perhaps stimulate angiogenesis (level I).[51] After each irrigation and debridement procedure, NPWCT is typically applied until the wound is considered clean; it may be changed in the operating room or at the bedside every 2–3 days. Originally used in the management of chronic wounds, its application has been extended to acute and contaminated wounds, large soft tissue defects, and even fasciotomy sites.

A retrospective analysis comparing this negative pressure technique to simple saline dressings for fasciotomy wounds of the leg demonstrated several advantages of the V.A.C technique: more rapid resolution of edema, earlier definitive closure/coverage, and higher rate of primary closure vs. skin grafting (level III).[52] Superior healing rates, decreased wound depths, and improved histologic profile (i.e., granulation tissue vs. inflammatory tissue/fibrosis) were all seen with NPWCT in a randomized prospective trial comparing V.A.C. to saline dressings in chronic non-healing wounds (level I).[53] Significant decrease in wound size with NPWCT has been demonstrated elsewhere (level IV).[54]

In type IIIB open fractures, NPWCT has been shown to be safe and reliable for wound protection until definitive coverage (level III),[55] given that wound coverage occurs within 7 days. While vacuum-assisted closure appears to be a promising modality in the management of musculoskeletal wounds, additional studies are required before definitive recommendations can be made regarding the nuances of NPWCT.

Antibiotic bead pouch Local/topical antibiotics have been shown to generate high bactericidal concentrations within the wound, while maintaining low systemic concentrations (level II)[56] and resultant systemic side effects. Candidate antibiotic agents include heat-stable, powderized formulations that properly target suspected pathogens. Aminoglycosides may be preferred over vancomycin because of concerns about resistance to vancomycin.

The bead pouch technique may attain local antibiotic concentrations up to 20 times greater than systemic formulations, which may decrease the need for systemic therapy. Like NPWCT, the bead pouch affords a sealant between the environment and wound bed. Moreover, a bead pouch may elute adequate antibiotic levels for at least 1 month, decreasing the need for replacement (level V).[57]

Ostermann et al. retrospectively looked at 1,085 open fractures. Patients treated with tobramycin antibiotic beads had lower infection rates than controls (3.7% vs. 12.1%; p < 0.001) (level III).[58] When results were stratified according to open fracture type, the reduction of infection was statistically significant in only the type III fractures (6.5% vs. 20%; p < 0.001). In a smaller patient group, Keating et al. conducted a retrospective analysis of 81 open tibial fractures and found tobramycin bead pouch use associated with fewer infections (4% vs. 16%) without reaching statistical significance (level II).[59]

Some authors have investigated the use of local antibiotic therapy alone. Moehring et al. conducted a prospective randomized controlled trial comparing local and systemic therapy in open type II, IIIA, and IIIB fractures (level V).[60] Patients were randomized after initial treatment in the Emergency Department and preoperatively, which included prophylactic (systemic) antibiotic treatment. Similar rates of infection were reported in the two groups; the study was limited by small study size and cross-treatment effects.

Recommendations

NPWCT has a demonstrated track record for wound management after high-energy orthopedic trauma (level V, level II).[37,39,61] There are no well-controlled human studies comparing results with V.A.C. vs. antibiotic bead pouch in open fracture wound management.[62]

Recommendations

Recommendations for wound coverage [overall quality: moderate]:
• There is insufficient data to make a recommendation for antibiotic bead pouch over negative pressure wound therapy
• Both V.A.C. therapy and antibiotic beads are adjunctive modalities in the management of open wounds associated with fractures
• The V.A.C. method is not a substitute for adequate wound debridement

Question 5: What factors should be considered when performing a soft tissue closure in an open fracture?

Case clarification

The patient is now at postinjury day 5 and has undergone two debridements of the wound. The orthopedic surgeon, in consultation with his plastic surgery colleagues, would like to perform definitive fixation and soft tissue reconstruction for wound coverage. He plans to place an intramedullary nail; afterwards, the plastic surgeon plans to transpose a local flap for wound coverage.

For soft tissue coverage of open tibial fractures, flaps are harvested/transposed based on the location of the tibial fracture:
• For proximal-third fractures, a **medial gastrocnemius muscle flap** is used.
• For middle-third fractures, a **soleus muscle flap** is used.
• For distal-third fractures, **free tissue transfer** is often used.

Relevance

Despite controversy surrounding the appropriate time to initial debridement, the need for definitive wound coverage to prevent infection is universally accepted. After a wound is initially irrigated and debrided and the fracture stabilized, there remains an important window of time in which the wound must be covered definitively with soft tissue to prevent the sequelae of late infection.

Current opinion

Definitive soft tissue coverage is best undertaken within 5–7 days by an experienced surgeon using orthoplastic reconstructive techniques.

There are a number of methods for achieving closure, including direct suturing, skin grafting, and the use of free or local muscle flaps. Treatment and choice of definitive coverage must be tailored to the individual patient.

Finding the evidence

• Cochrane Database (http://www.cochrane.org/reviews), using search term: "soft tissue closure orthopedic infection"
  ° 0 results
• PubMed (www.ncbi.nlm.nih.gov/pubmed/), using search term: "soft tissue closure orthopedic infection"
  ° Limits: English
  ° 27 results, 7 reviews
• EMBASE (www.embase.com; excluding Medline duplicates) , using search term: "soft tissue closure orthopedic infection"
  ° Limits: English, EMBASE only
  ° 0 results

Quality of the evidence

Level II
• 3 studies

Level III
• 5 studies

Level IV
• 2 studies

Level V
• 3 studies

Findings

Several studies have documented significantly better outcomes with early closure (within 7 days) than with late closure (p < 0.05) (level II–III).[63–66] Also, a number of studies have demonstrated excellent outcomes with closure performed within 3 days after injury (level III–IV).[67,68]

Delayed wound closure (within 3–7 days) affords the opportunity to do second-look debridements at 24- to 48-hour intervals. Any tissue of questionable viability may be removed in the interim. It may be difficult to evaluate muscle/ soft tissue viability in the acute setting or at initial debridement. Concern for clostridial infection from severe contamination is another contraindication to early closure and resulting entrapment of anaerobic bacteria.[69]

The management of high-energy open fractures requires both skeletal stability and adequate soft tissue coverage. Delays beyond 7 days have been associated with increased complications related to the flap or subflap tissues (level II).[59] When comparing free muscle flaps performed within 72 hours of injury vs. 72 hours to 90 days after injury, Godina reported a failure rate of less than 1% vs. 12%, respectively (level II).[62] Infection rates were 1.5% vs. 17.4%, respectively. Gopal et al. examined an aggressive wound coverage protocol in type IIIB and IIIC open fractures: comparing coverage within 72 hours with that of greater than 72 hours, infection rates were 6% vs. 29%, respectively (level III).[70]

Recommendations

The optimal method of closure depends on a number of host and injury factors, including wound size and location, and patient functional status and expectations.

Recommendations for definitive soft tissue wound coverage [overall quality: moderate]:
- Current trend toward earlier coverage and closure of open fracture wounds
- Exceptions to early coverage include concern for anaerobic infection or incomplete debridement of nonviable tissue
- Type IIIB and IIIC defects should be managed in a concerted effort by subspecialist teams

Summary of recommendations

- Prompt intravenous antibiotics should be given at the time of initial presentation to treat wound contamination in most open fractures
- Tetanus toxoid should be given if indicated, based on patient's immunization history
- Initial wound management should include a sterile dressing moistened with normal saline and temporary skeletal stabilization
- The timing of irrigation and debridement is not as important as the prompt administration of antibiotics but should occur within 24 hours of injury
- The wound should be irrigated with normal saline
- Additives have not demonstrated clear benefit and have additional risks to host tissue
- Pulsed lavage should not exceed 50 psi (345 kPa)
- There is insufficient data to make a recommendation for an antibiotic bead pouch over negative pressure wound therapy
- Both V.A.C. therapy and antibiotic beads are adjunctive modalities in the management of open wounds associated with fractures
- The V.A.C. method is not a substitute for adequate wound debridement
- There is a current trend toward coverage or closure of open fracture wounds within 5–7 days
- Exceptions to early coverage include concern for anaerobic infection or incomplete debridement of nonviable tissue
- Type IIIB and IIIC defects should be managed in a concerted effort by subspecialist teams

Conclusions

The factors that are of paramount importance in the treatment of open fractures are early administration of antibiotics and surgical irrigation with meticulous wound debridement. All interventions should lead toward the eradication of contamination from the wound and preservation of blood flow to the site of injury. Early fracture stabilization and wound closure/coverage are beneficial. Much of the information quoted in the orthopedic literature for open fractures, however, has inadequate scientific support and deserves further prospective investigation with appropriate sample sizes.

References

1. Gustilo RB, Anderson JT. Prevention of infection in the treatment of 1,025 open fractures of long bones: retrospective and prospective analyses. J Bone Joint Surg Am 1976;58:453–8.
2. Gustilo RB, Mendoza RM, Williams DN. Problems in the management of type III (severe) open fractures: a new classification of type III open fractures. J Trauma 1984;24:742–6.
3. Court-Brown CM, McQueen MM, Quaba AA. Management of Open Fractures.: Martin Dunitz, London 1996.
4. Court-Brown C, McQueen M, Tornetta P III. Trauma., Lippincott Williams & Wilkins, Philadelphia 2006.
5. Anglen JO. Wound irrigation in musculoskeletal injury. J Am Acad Orthop Surg 2001;9:219–26.
6. Kaysinger KK, Nicholson NC, Ramp WK, Kellam JF. Toxic effects of wound irrigation solutions on cultured tibiae and osteoblasts. J Orthop Trauma 1995;9:303–11.
7. Patzakis MJ, Harvey JP Jr, Ivler D. The role of antibiotics in the management of open fractures. J Bone Joint Surg Am 1974;56: 532–41.
8. Gosselin RA, Roberts I, Gillespie WJ. Antibiotics for preventing infection in open limb fractures. Cochrane Database Syst Rev 2004;1:CD003764.
9. Patzakis MJ, Wilkins J. Factors influencing infection rate in open fracture wounds. Clin Orthop Relat Res 1989;243:36–40.
10. Patzakis MJ, Bains RS, Lee J, et al. Prospective, randomized, double-blind study comparing single-agent antibiotic therapy, ciprofloxacin, to combination antibiotic therapy in open fracture wounds. J Orthop Trauma 2000;14:529–33.
11. Stevenson J, McNaughton G, Riley J. The use of prophylactic flucloxacillin in treatment of open fractures of the distal phalanx within an accident and emergency department: a double-blind randomized placebo-controlled trial. J Hand Surg Br 2003;28: 388–94.
12. Prokuski L. Prophylactic antibiotics in orthopaedic surgery. J Am Acad Orthop Surg 2008;16:283–93.
13. Friedrich PL. Die aseptische Versorgung frischer Wundern. Arch Klin Chir 1898;57:288–310.
14. Robson MC, Duke WF, Krizek TJ. Rapid bacterial screening in the treatment of civilian wounds. J Surg Res 1973;14: 426–30.

15. Kindsfater K, Jonassen EA. Osteomyelitis in grade II and III open tibia fractures with late debridement. J Orthop Trauma 1995;9:121–7.

16. Okike K, Bhattacharyya T. Trends in the management of open fractures. A critical analysis. J Bone Joint Surg Am 2006;88:2739–48.

17. Yang EC, Eisler J. Treatment of isolated type I open fractures: is emergent operative debridement necessary? Clin Orthop Relat Res 2003;410:289–94.

18. Crowley DJ, Kanakaris NK, Giannoudis PV. Debridement and wound closure of open fractures: the impact of the time factor on infection rates. Injury 2007;38:879–89.

19. Pollak AN. Timing of débridement of open fractures. J Am Acad Orthop Surg 2006;14:S48–51.

20. Pollak AN, Jones AL, Castillo RC, et al. The relationship between time to surgical debridement and incidence of infection after open high-energy lower extremity trauma. J Bone Joint Surg Am 2010;92:7–15.

21. Petrisor B, Jeray K, Schemitsch E, et al. FLOW Investigators. Fluid lavage in patients with open fracture wounds (FLOW): an international survey of 984 surgeons. BMC Musculoskelet Disord 2008;23:7.

22. Gainor BJ, Hockman DE, Anglen JO, et al. Benzalkonium chloride: a potential disinfecting irrigation solution. J Orthop Trauma 1997;11:121–5.

23. Gilmore OJ, Sanderson PJ. Prophylactic interparietal povidone-iodine in abdominal surgery. Br J Surg 1975;62:792–9.

24. Crowley DJ, Kanakaris NK, Giannoudis PV. Irrigation of the wounds in open fractures. J Bone Joint Surg Br 2007;89:580–5.

25. Sprung J, Schedewie HK, Kampine JP. Intraoperative anaphylactic shock after bacitracin irrigation. Anesth Analg 1990;71:430–3.

26. Antevil JL, Muldoon MP, Battaglia M, Green R. Intraoperative anaphylactic shock associated with bacitracin irrigation during revision total knee arthroplasty: a case report. J Bone Joint Surg Am 2003;85:339–42.

27. Bhandari M, Adili A, Schemitsch EH. The efficacy of low-pressure lavage with different irrigating solutions to remove adherent bacteria from bone. J Bone Joint Surg Am 2001;83:412–19.

28. Dirschl DR, Wilson FC. Topical antibiotic irrigation in the prophylaxis of operative wound infections in orthopaedic surgery. Orthop Clin North Am 1991;22:419–26.

29. Conroy BP, Anglen JO, Simpson WA, et al. Comparison of castile soap, benzalkonium chloride, and bacitracin as irrigation solutions for complex contaminated orthopaedic wounds. J Orthop Trauma 1999;13:332–7.

30. Rosenstein BD, Wilson FC, Funderburk CH. The use of bacitracin irrigation to prevent infection in postoperative skeletal wounds: an experimental study. J Bone Joint Surg Am 1989;71:427–30.

31. Anglen JO. Comparison of soap and antibiotic solutions for irrigation of lower limb open fracture wounds. A prospective, randomized study. J Bone Joint Surg Am 2005;87:1415–22.

32. Anglen JO, Apostoles S, Christensen G, Gainor B. The efficacy of various irrigation solutions in removing slime-producing staphylococcus. J Orthop Trauma 1994;8:390–6.

33. Bhandari M, Schemitsch EH, Adili A, et al. High and low pressure pulsatile lavage of contaminated tibial fractures: an in vitro study of bacterial adherence and bone damage. J Orthop Trauma 1999;13:526–33.

34. Boyd JI 3rd, Wongworawat MD. High-pressure pulsatile lavage causes soft tissue damage. Clin Orthop Relat Res 2004;427:13–17.

35. Adili A, Bhandari M, Schemitsch EH. The biomechanical effect of high pressure irrigation on diaphyseal fracture healing in vivo. J Orthop Trauma 2002;16:413–17.

36. Dirschl DR, Duff GP, Dahners LE, et al. High pressure pulsatile lavage irrigation of intraarticular fractures: effects on fracture healing. J Orthop Trauma 1998;12:460–3.

37. Hassinger SM, Harding G, Wongworawat MD. High-pressure pulsatile lavage propagates bacteria into soft tissue. Clin Orthop Relat Res 2005;439:27–31.

38. Bhandari M, Adili A, Lachowski RJ. High pressure pulsatile lavage of contaminated human tibiae: an in vitro study. J Orthop Trauma 1998;12:479–84.

39. Smith & Nephew. Versajet Hydrosurgery System. http://wound.smith-nephew.com/uk/node.asp?NodeId=3089. Site accessed August 22, 2009.

40. Klein MB, Hunter S, Heimbach DM, et al. The Versajet water dissector: a new tool for tangential excision. J Burn Care Rehabil 2005;26:483–7.

41. Rennekampff HO, Schaller HE, Wisser D, Tenenhaus M. Debridement of burn wounds with a water jet surgical tool. Burns 2006;32:64–9.

42. Roth RM, Gleckman RA, Gantz NM, Kelly N. Antibiotic irrigations. A plea for controlled clinical trials. Pharmacotherapy 1985;5:222–7.

43. Maguire WB. The use of antibiotics, locally and systemically, in orthopaedic surgery. Med J Aust 1964;2:412–14.

44. Nachamie BA, Siffert RS, Bryer MS. A study of neomycin instillation into orthopaedic surgical wounds. JAMA 1968;204:687–9.

45. Morykwas MJ, Argenta LC, Shelton-Brown EI, McGuirt W. Vacuum-assisted closure: a new method for wound control and treatment: animal studies and basic foundation. Ann Plast Surg 1997;38:553–62.

46. Fleischmann W, Lang E, Russ M. Treatment of infection by vacuum sealing. Unfallchirurg 1997;100:301–4.

47. Mooney JF 3rd, Argenta LC, Marks MW, et al. Treatment of soft tissue defects in pediatric patients using the V.A.C. system. Clin Orthop Relat Res 2000;376:26–31.

48. Herscovici D Jr, Sanders RW, Scaduto JM, Infante A, DiPasquale T. Vacuum assisted wound closure (VAC therapy) for the management of patients with high energy soft tissue injuries. J Orthop Trauma 2003;17:683–8.

49. Labler L, Keel M, Trentz O. Vacuum-assisted closure (V.A.C.) for temporary coverage of soft-tissue injury in type III open fracture of the lower extremities. Eur J Trauma 2004;30:305–12.

50. DeFranzo AJ, Argenta LC, Marks MW, et al. The use of vacuum-assisted closure therapy for the treatment of lower-extremity wounds with exposed bone. Plast Reconstr Surg 2001;108:1184–91.

51. Stannard JP, Robinson JT, Anderson ER, McGwin G Jr, Volgas DA, Alonso JE. Negative pressure wound therapy to treat hematomas and surgical incisions following high-energy trauma. J Trauma 2006;60(6):1301–6.

52. Yang CC, Chang DS, Webb LX. Vacuum-assisted closure for fasciotomy wounds following compartment syndrome of the leg. J Surg Orthop Adv 2006;15:19–23.

53. Joseph E, Hamori CA, Bergman S, et al. A prospective randomized trial of vacuum-assisted closure versus standard therapy of chronic non-healing wounds. Wounds 2000;12:60–7.

54. Wongworawat MD, Schnall SB, Holtom PD, Moon C, Schiller F. Negative pressure dressings as an alternative technique for the treatment of infected wounds. Clin Orthop Relat Res 2003;414: 45–8.

55. Bhattacharyya T, Mehta P, Smith M, Pomahac B. Routine use of wound vacuum-assisted closure does not allow coverage delay for open tibia fractures. Plast Reconstr Surg 2008;121(4):1263–6.

56. Eckman JB Jr, Henry SL, Mangino PD, Seligson D. Wound and serum levels of tobramycin with the prophylactic use of tobramycin-impregnated polymethylmethacrylate beads in compound fractures. Clin Orthop Relat Res 1988;237:213–15.

57. Greene N, Holtom PD, Warren CA, et al. In vitro elution of tobramycin and vancomycin polymethylmethacrylate beads and spacers from Simplex and Palacos. Am J Orthop 1998; 27:201–5.

58. Ostermann PA, Seligson D, Henry SL. Local antibiotic therapy for severe open fractures. A review of 1085 consecutive cases. J Bone Joint Surg Br 1995;77:93–7.

59. Keating JF, Blachut PA, O'Brien PJ, et al. Reamed nailing of open tibial fractures: does the antibiotic bead pouch reduce the deep infection rate? J Orthop Trauma 1996;10:298–303.

60. Moehring HD, Gravel C, Chapman MW, Olson SA. Comparison of antibiotic beads and intravenous antibiotics in open fractures. Clin Orthop Relat Res 2000;372:254–61.

61. Webb LX. New techniques in wound management: Vacuum-assisted wound closure. J Am Acad Orthop Surg 2002;10: 303–11.

62. Pape HC, Webb LX. History of open wound and fracture treatment. J Orthop Trauma 2008;22(10 Suppl):S133–4.

63. Cierny G 3rd, Byrd HS, Jones RE. Primary versus delayed soft tissue coverage for severe open tibial fractures. A comparison of results. Clin Orthop Relat Res 1983;178:54–63.

64. Caudle RJ, Stern PJ. Severe open fractures of the tibia. J Bone Joint Surg Am 1987;69:801–7.

65. Fischer MD, Gustilo RB, Varecka TF. The timing of flap coverage, bone grafting, and intramedullary nailing in patients who have a fracture of the tibial shaft with extensive soft-tissue injury. J Bone Joint Surg Am 1991;73:1316–22.

66. Byrd HS, Spicer TE, Cierney G 3rd. Management of open tibial fractures. Plast Reconstr Surg 1985;76:719–30.

67. Sinclair JS, McNally MA, Small JO, Yeates HA. Primary free-flap cover of open tibial fractures. Injury 1997;28:581–7.

68. Godina M. Early microsurgical reconstruction of complex trauma of the extremities. Plast ReconstrSurg 1986;78:285–92.

69. Patzakis MJ. Clostridial myonecrosis. Instr Course Lect 1990;39:491–3.

70. Gopal S, Majumder S, Batchelor AG, et al. Fix and flap: The radical orthopaedic and plastic treatment of severe open fractures of the tibia. J Bone Joint Surg Br 2000;82:959–66.

71

Acute Compartment Syndrome

Andrew H. Schmidt

University of Minnesota, Minneapolis, MN, USA

Case scenarios

Case 1

A 45 year old man is brought to the Emergency Department with injuries that occurred when he was struck by an automobile moving at less than 5 miles per hour (8 km/h). He is not intoxicated and has a normal mental status examination. He has no injuries other than those to his legs. He is normotensive with a blood pressure of 140/85 mmHg. His right leg has a transverse laceration over the medial leg with exposed bone and an unstable fracture, with minimal soft-tissue swelling. His left leg has no wounds and is firmly swollen (much more so than the right leg), with pain over the middle of the leg but no obvious instability of the limb.

Case 2

A 24 year old man is brought in by paramedics after a high-speed motorcycle accident. He smells of alcohol, was not wearing a helmet, and was combative at the scene of the accident. The patient had swelling and deformity of the right thigh, and his left lower leg was swollen and obviously fractured with instability of the tibia. The patient had a Glasgow Coma Score of 12 at the time of admission. He was intubated immediately upon arrival in order to protect his airway. His blood pressure was 125/75. A CT of his head showed a frontal lobe contusion and punctate hemorrhage in the right hemisphere. The patient was taken to the operating room by neurosurgery for placement of a ventriculostomy. An orthopedic consult was requested just before the patient was taken to the operating room.

Relevant anatomy

Compartment syndrome is a complication of trauma or other conditions and circumstances that alter perfusion to an extremity, and can potentially involve any myofascial compartment of the extremities or trunk. It most often occurs following a fracture or a crush injury to the limb.[1] When limb swelling occurs following fracture, a crush injury, or reperfusion following a period of ischemia, the mass of the myofascial compartment increases due to accumulation of blood and fluid (which may be extra- and/or intracellular). Due to the inelastic nature of muscle fascia and other connective tissues, this accumulation of mass leads to increased pressure within the compartment. This pressure is transmitted to the thin-walled venous system, which in turn collapses, causing venous hypertension.[2] Progressive tissue ischemia ensues, with increasing amounts of cellular necrosis with time. Cell lysis releases osmotically active cell contents into the interstitial space, causing further accumulation of fluid and further increase in intracompartment pressure. After about 8 hours, irreversible ischemic injury to myoneural tissues within the compartment has occurred.

Importance of the problem

Although the existence of compartment syndrome is well known and most clinicians are familiar with its pathophysiology and understand its potential limb-threatening nature, there is no clear definition of when compartment syndrome is actually present and considerable variation in its clinical management is the inevitable consequence.[3-5]

Evidence-Based Orthopedics, First Edition. Edited by Mohit Bhandari.
© 2012 Blackwell Publishing Ltd. Published 2012 by Blackwell Publishing Ltd.

Clinical signs and symptoms as well as direct measurements of intramuscular pressure are inaccurate as screening tests for compartment syndrome and have significant pitfalls as a means of diagnosis.[6-14] Not surprisingly, compartment syndrome is one of the most common causes of litigation against orthopedic surgeons.[15]

The only established treatment for acute compartment syndrome is immediate surgical fasciotomy, wherein the skin and muscle fascia of the involved compartment are generously incised to release the constricting soft tissues and increase the volume of the muscle compartment, thereby effecting immediate reduction of compartment pressure. Although intramuscular pressure varies in a continuum, given the lack of specific diagnostic criteria as well as reliable methods to prevent or reduce the occurrence of compartment syndrome, compartment syndrome is presently an "all or none" diagnosis, and patients who are considered to have compartment syndrome typically receive emergent fasciotomy. It is recognized that performing early fasciotomy is critical to achieving the best possible outcomes when compartment syndrome occurs,[16-21] and it is generally accepted that performing unnecessary fasciotomy is better than missing a true case of compartment syndrome, given the potential systemic risks and functional loss associated with rhabdomyolysis and myonecrosis.

Unfortunately, fasciotomy is associated with its own set of complications, including the need for further surgery for delayed wound closure or skin grafting, pain, cosmetic problems, nerve injury, permanent muscle weakness, and chronic venous insufficiency.[9,19,22-27]

In order to minimize morbidity and optimize treatment of a patient at risk for compartment syndrome, clinicians need a clear understanding of the pathophysiology, means (and problems) of diagnosis, and treatment of compartment syndrome.

Top five questions

Risk factors

1. What factors increase the risk of compartment syndrome?

Diagnosis

2. What are the clinical signs and symptoms of compartment syndrome? Which can I rely on for diagnosis?
3. Is measurement of compartment pressure always necessary?

Treatment

4. When should fasciotomy be done in the face of positive clinical signs and symptoms?

5. Is there a pressure threshold above which fasciotomy should always be done?

Question 1: What factors increase the risk of compartment syndrome?

Case 1 clarification

Our patient is a relatively young, active man, with a potentially high-energy bumper injury. Radiographs of the right leg show transverse fractures of the tibia and fibula at the junction of the middle and distal thirds of the tibia. Radiographs of the left leg show a nondisplaced bending-wedge fracture of the midshaft of the tibia with an intact fibula.

Case 2 clarification

The patient had an associated long bone injury, which increases the risk of hypotension, although at the time of admission his vital signs remained stable.

Relevance

The only accepted treatment for compartment syndrome is immediate fasciotomy, which if performed commits the patient to further surgery, a prolonged hospital stay, increased cost of care, and increased morbidity. Understanding the risk factors for compartment syndrome will allow the surgeon to modify his or her assessment of the a-priori risk of compartment syndrome for a given patient, and potentially raise or lower the threshold for fasciotomy in a given clinical scenario.

Current opinion

Young individuals sustaining high-energy trauma, especially of the lower leg, are considered to be the most at risk for compartment syndrome. The risk of compartment syndrome in other types of patients, and in other anatomic locations, is less-well understood.

Finding the evidence

- PubMed Search: "acute compartment syndrome risk factor"
  - limited to English
  - 81 results (only results relevant to the question are shown)

Quality of the evidence

Level II
- 2 prognostic studies[1,28]

Level IV
- 2 retrospective case series[29,30]

Level V
- 3 case reports, 11 review papers

Findings

The published literature documents both the demographics and risk factors for acute compartment syndrome (ACS). McQueen et al. documented 164 cases treated in their trauma unit.[1] Most patients were men younger than age 35, and fractures were present in 69% of cases. Slightly more than half of the fractures (52%) were of the tibia, and fractures of the forearm (radius and ulna shaft, plus distal radius) accounted for one quarter of the total cases. Isolated soft-tissue injuries were reasonably common, accounting for 23% of the total cases, and occurred in the leg, thigh, forearm, hand, and foot. It should be noted that this series excluded cases of postischemic ACS, which is another well-known etiology of ACS. In a later publication, the same investigators specifically studied the patients in this series who developed compartment syndrome without fracture and compared them to the patients who had ACS after fracture.[17] Patients who developed ACS in the absence of fracture were older and had more medical comorbidities than those with a fracture. Importantly, in the cohort of patients with ACS without fracture the time to fasciotomy was delayed, and a greater proportion of patients had myonecrosis, suggesting a significant delay in diagnosis (possibly due to the lack of a fracture). Park et al. evaluated 414 acute tibial fractures and looked at the rate of compartment syndrome requiring fasciotomy according to fracture location.[28] Compartment syndrome was most common in diaphyseal tibia fractures, occurring in 8% of cases, compared to less than 2% in proximal and distal metaphyseal fractures, respectively. In the diaphyseal group, patient and injury risk factors were examined; younger age was the only potential risk factor that was independently associated with the development of compartment syndrome. Several series report an appreciable incidence of compartment syndrome in patients with tibial plateau fractures,[29] and these fractures must also be considered in the high-risk category. Compartment syndrome of the thigh can also occur, often (but not necessarily) associated with a fracture of the femur, and in one series led to significant morbidity.[30]

Recommendations

• Younger age (25–35 years), male gender, and trauma are consistent risk factors for compartment syndrome in patients with fractures of the tibia and forearm [overall quality: moderate]

Question 2: What are the clinical signs and symptoms of compartment syndrome? Which can I rely on for diagnosis?

Case 1 clarification

The patient is able to actively flex and extend his great toe, lesser toes, and ankle bilaterally, although with some pain. He has mild pain with passive plantarflexion and dorsiflexion of the ankle and great toe. He reports completely normal sensation in his first web space and over the dorsum of the foot, lateral border of the foot, and bottom of the foot, bilaterally.

Relevance

Compartment syndrome is an entity without a definitive diagnostic test. The consequences of missed diagnosis are severe for the patient, the physician, and the hospital. As a result, overtreatment (surgical fasciotomy) is common, but contributes to morbidity as well. An understanding of the value of specific clinical findings and the meaning of elevated intramuscular pressure will aid the clinician in diagnosing and managing patients at risk for compartment syndrome.

Current opinion

The diagnosis of ACS is best made on the basis of the presence of specific clinical findings that include the tenseness or firmness of the involved compartment, motor weakness and pain with passive stretch of the involved muscle, increasing pain, pain that is out of proportion to that expected, and loss of sensation in a specific neuronal distribution for a given compartment (such as the deep peroneal nerve for the anterior compartment of the leg). However, all of these clinical findings are imprecise, subjective, and easily attributable to other aspects of the injury.

Finding the evidence

• PubMed search: "diagnosis acute compartment syndrome"
  ◦ limited to English
  ◦ 661 results (only results relevant to the question are shown)

Level I
• 1 therapeutic study[31]
• 4 diagnostic studies[13,32–34]

Level II
• 1 diagnostic study[35]

Level III
• 2 diagnostic studies[36,37]
• 1 therapeutic systematic review[38]

Level IV
• 20 therapeutic case series

Level V
• 150 case reports, 59 review papers, 2 surveys,[3,5] 2 editorials, 1 letter

Findings

The literature documents that ACS can occur in almost any muscle of the body, either following fracture, crush injury, muscle injury, overexertion, ischemia-reperfusion injury, or even without apparent provocation (acute deep vein thrombosis, spontaneous hemorrhage, etc.). The generally accepted clinical signs of compartment syndrome are worsening pain (out of proportion to what is otherwise expected), pain with passive stretch, paresthesias, and paresis. However, the published literature makes it clear that these clinical signs and symptoms are unreliable, both when they are present[12,39] and when they are absent.[40,41] Robinson et al. reviewed 208 consecutive patients treated with reamed nailing of a tibia fracture; 5% of the patients developed dysfunction of the common or deep peroneal nerve, with most of them exhibiting isolated weakness of the extensor hallucis longus (the "dropped hallux") with associated numbness in the first web space. All of these patients had continuous compartment pressure monitoring and none developed compartment syndrome.[39] Three patients were documented as having neurologic deficits before surgery.[39] Ulmer performed a methodical review of the published literature through 2001 and evaluated all four of these clinical signs.[12] Of 1,932 studies found in a literature search, only 4 had adequate data with which to calculate the sensitivity and specificity of these findings in patients with lower leg injuries. The sensitivity and positive predictive value of all four clinical signs of compartment syndrome was less than 20%. In contrast, the specificity and negative predictive value were above 97%. False-positive findings were present more often than true positive findings. Using the concept of likelihood ratios, Ulmer did demonstrate that there is increasing clinical utility when multiple findings are present; if three of the four signs were present the odds of compartment syndrome are increased to above 90% (given a pretest probability of 5%).[12]

Despite these problems, careful clinical monitoring appears to be useful for minimizing morbidity due to compartment syndrome.[31-33] Use of a specific checklist may help to formalize the clinical monitoring of patients.[33]

Given the emphasis on clinical findings that exists, it is not surprising that one are of concern has been the issue of analgesia. Several case reports exist of alert, adult patients who developed compartment syndrome without pain.[6,7,11,41] Mar et al. performed a systematic review of the literature, identifying 28 articles discussing the influence of analgesic technique on the diagnosis of compartment syndrome in 35 patients.[38] These authors concluded, on the basis of their review, that there is no convincing evidence that intravenous opioids or regional anesthetic blocks delays the diagnosis of compartment syndrome in "adequately monitored" patients.

Recommendations

• Due to the myriad causes of ACS, clinicians must consider this diagnosis in any patient with swelling of the limb. In an alert patient, careful and frequent (every 1–2 hour) clinical monitoring of pain (both at rest and with passive muscle stretching), limb swelling, and neurologic status is usually sufficient to make the diagnosis. The clinical findings are of greatest utility when several findings are present together. Clinicians should remember that clinical findings are positive more often in patients without ACS than in patients with compartment syndrome. The clinical diagnosis is not reliable if done infrequently, in children, or in unconscious patients in whom pain cannot be assessed. The influence of anesthetic technique on the clinical examination is uncertain; one systematic review of the topic contained mostly single case reports and a very small number of patients, such that definitive conclusions cannot be drawn. The highest available evidence is level I, but it is impossible to make conclusive statements because of the inherent nature of the treatment of compartment syndrome, in which the incidence of unneeded fasciotomy (false-positive diagnosis) and missed compartment syndrome (false-negative diagnosis) is impossible to know [overall level: low]

Question 3: Is measurement of intracompartment pressure always necessary?

Case 1 clarification

This patient has an isolated injury and a reliable physical examination.

Case 2 clarification

This patient does not have a reliable physical examination because he has been intubated; due to his traumatic brain injury this is likely to remain true for at least the next several days. Therefore all that can be used for diagnosis are serial (or continuous) measurements of intracompartment pressure.

Relevance

Recent literature has documented that the clinical findings typically associated with ACS are not reliable as a screening test (e.g., have poor sensitivity), and many patients considered to be at risk (or to have) ACS are not clinically evaluable due to head injury, intubation/sedation, or altered mental status. Making the diagnosis on the basis of clinical findings can also be particularly challenging in children.[18] In these instances, measurement of intramuscular pressure is another diagnostic option, and the accuracy and reliability of such measurements should be understood by anyone treating patients at risk for ACS. The potential benefit of continuous vs. intermittent pressure monitoring remains an area of clinical controversy.

Current opinion

Measurement of intracompartment pressure is of value in patients with clinically equivocal findings or in patients who cannot be evaluated clinically. Routine continuous pressure monitoring may lead to increased rate of fasciotomy, and is of unproven benefit in centers that are accustomed to careful clinical monitoring. When measurement of intramuscular pressure is done, using a threshold for fasciotomy based on a perfusion pressure (diastolic blood pressure minus intramuscular pressure) of at least 30 mmHg will avoid missed compartment syndrome.

Finding the evidence

- PubMed Search: "pressure monitoring acute compartment syndrome"
  - ° limited to English
  - ° 54 results (only results relevant to the question are shown)

Quality of the evidence

Level I
- 2 diagnostic studies[13,32]
- 1 therapeutic study[31]

Level II
- 1 diagnostic study[35]

Level III
- 2 diagnostic studies[36,37]

Level IV
- 3 case series

Level V
- 8 review papers, 3 case reports, 1 survey,

Other
- 1 animal study

Findings

Although compartment syndrome may be diagnosed in an alert adult patient on the basis of positive clinical findings, many experts have recommended routine measurement of intramuscular pressure in one or more compartments.[13,35,42,43]. It has been estimated that muscle necrosis may occur within 2 hours of injury in as many as 35% of patients with ACS.[44] Therefore, early diagnosis of compartment syndrome is key to avoiding morbidity,[16–18,21,36] and delay in diagnosis occurs often.[9] The incidence of delayed diagnosis appears to be lessened by use of frequent or continuous measurement of intramuscular pressure.[9,36] On the other hand, routine monitoring of intramuscular pressure could lead to increased use of fasciotomy, depending on what pressure threshold is used.[8,45]

Whenever the clinical examination is not reliable, direct measurement of intramuscular pressure in a patient at risk is a necessity. The proper role of compartment pressure monitoring in an alert patient is unknown.[4,8,10] There are several well-done studies that both support[13,36,42,43] and refute[10,31,32] the value of pressure monitoring. At issue is whether pressure monitoring improves the diagnosis of compartment syndrome (i.e., identifies cases that clinical monitoring would miss), and whether it leads to earlier diagnosis and therefore contributes to a reduction in morbidity from delayed diagnosis. The answer to these questions clearly depend on what pressure threshold is used to diagnose compartment syndrome, and this too remains a topic of controversy.[8,10,45]

With respect to the accuracy of diagnosis, several case series report that there is little difference in the rate of fasciotomy in groups of patients who are monitored clinically compared to those that have continuous measurement of intramuscular pressure.[31,32] However, careful review of these reports reveals that the patients that were monitored clinically were in fact followed very closely. For example, Al-Dadah et al. reported similar rates of fasciotomy and time to diagnosis of compartment syndrome in two sets of patients treated before and after adopting a protocol of continuous monitoring of anterior compartment pressure.[32] However, patients in both groups were assessed by trained nurses every hour.[31] It might be surmised that monitoring of compartment pressure would be of more value if such careful clinical monitoring were not possible, and that these results may not be generalizable to institutions that cannot offer that level of care. Harris et al. performed a trial in which 200 consecutive patients with tibia fracture were randomized to continuous monitoring for 36 hours or clinical assessment alone.[31] There were no cases of compartment syndrome in the monitored group, and five in the nonmonitored group, leading the authors to conclude that clinical monitoring alone is adequate. However, this report did not describe how the patients were assessed clinically, and included a mixture of both postoperative cases and patients monitored after admission but before surgery, as well as alert and unconscious patients. Data regarding the distribution of these patient groups in the study is not provided in the paper, making it difficult to draw conclusions.

Recommendations

- Frequent clinical assessment of the patient considered to be at risk for developing compartment syndrome, ideally using a structured checklist, remains the cornerstone of diagnosis. When a patient is unconscious or otherwise not able to be clinically assessed, then measurement of intramuscular pressure within the anterior is of benefit. It is difficult to recommend a specific absolute measure of pressure at which fasciotomy should be done. Performing fasciotomy whenever the intramuscular pressure is within 30 mmHg of the diastolic blood pressure is not likely to result in any missed cases of compartment syndrome, but will likely lead to overtreatment if used routinely. Further research is needed to provide more sensitive and specific means to diagnose compartment syndrome. The highest available evidence is level I, but the results are conflicting and the studies showing benefit to each modality may not be generalizable [overall quality: low]

Question 4: When should fasciotomy be done in the face of positive clinical signs and symptoms?

Relevance

As a surgical procedure, fasciotomy has its own set of potential complications, and at the very least, commits the patient to a large open wound that requires a second (or more) surgical procedure to close, and increases hospital stay and costs. When facing a patient with compartment syndrome, it is important to know if there are nonoperative medical interventions that might be done, and how to understand the urgency of when to do fasciotomy (what is the relative risk of waiting vs. early intervention).

Current opinion

There are no clinically relevant medical therapies for ACS, and immediate fasciotomy is warranted as soon as the diagnosis is considered to be present.

Finding the evidence

- PubMed Search: "fasciotomy acute compartment syndrome",
  - limited to English
  - 179 results (only results relevant to the question are shown)

Quality of the evidence

Level III
- 1 diagnostic study[36]

Level IV
- 3 therapeutic case series[18,46,47]

Findings

Experimental animal models indicate that irreversible muscle necrosis can occur in 8 hours or less as a consequence of elevated intramuscular pressure; the tolerance of muscle to ischemia depends on both the absolute pressure, the duration of elevated pressure, associated muscle injury, and differences in muscle metabolic demands between individuals. In one clinical series in which operative reports and pathologic specimens from fasciotomy were scrutinized, the authors concluded that appreciable muscle

necrosis can occur in over one third of patients in as little as 3 hours.[44]

Numerous series document the efficacy of early fasciotomy[18,27,46–48] and the complications associated with late fasciotomy.[17,47] Although all are level IV studies, it clearly would not be ethical to undertake any sort of prospective study of the effects of delayed fasciotomy in patients with compartment syndrome. Despite the universal acceptance that compartment syndrome is an "orthopedic emergency," Vaillancourt et al. documented frequent delays both in the time from initial assessment to diagnosis and in the time from diagnosis to surgery.[21] Interestingly, one study that specifically evaluated time from diagnosis to fasciotomy in two hospitals could not determine any statistical correlation between the time from diagnosis to fasciotomy and residual functional defects.[49]

Sheridan and Matsen found that fasciotomy performed within 12 hours of the onset of compartment syndrome, as defined by the first appearance of any clinical sign (motor weakness, stretch pain, or hyperesthesia in the appropriate nerve), resulted in normal function in 68% of patients, compared to only 8% of those who had delayed fasciotomy.[47] In addition, patients undergoing late fasciotomy had a 10-fold increase in the rate of complications (4.5% vs. 54%).[47] In a series of pediatric upper extremity compartment syndromes, a statistically significant difference in outcomes were found if surgery was delayed more than 6 hours.[18]

Recommendation

- When compartment syndrome is going to occur, early fasciotomy can avoid myonecrosis or ischemic neuropathy. However, the challenges in diagnosis, and the fact that compartment syndrome does not begin at a well-defined point in time, make it impossible to make draw specific conclusions about when fasciotomy is needed that apply to every case [overall quality: low]

Question 5: Is there a pressure threshold above which fasciotomy should always be done?

Case 2 clarification

While the patient was in surgery, his intracompartment pressures were measured in the left leg and found to be: anterior compartment, 77 mmHg; lateral compartment, 55 mmHg; deep posterior compartment, 35 mmHg; superficial posterior compartment, 15 mmHg.

Relevance

It is not clear how accurate recommended thresholds for fasciotomy are, and how such thresholds should be applied in a given clinical situation.

Current opinion

The use of a pressure threshold for fasciotomy that is based on an assessment of perfusion pressure rather than an absolute intracompartment pressure is more relevant physiologically, and less likely to lead to unnecessary fasciotomy. The best indicator of the need for fasciotomy is the perfusion pressure (also referred to as the "Delta-P"), which is defined as the difference between the patient's diastolic blood pressure and the intracompartment pressure. Fasciotomy may be safely avoided as long as the perfusion pressure remains greater than 30 mmHg.

Finding the evidence
- PubMed Search: "threshold fasciotomy acute compartment syndrome"
  ° limited to English
  ° 7 results (only results relevant to the question are shown)

Quality of the evidence
- No new articles identified.

Findings
Decisions for fasciotomy may be based on absolute compartment pressure,[37,45] or the so-called differential pressure (also called perfusion pressure or "Delta-P"), which represents the difference between the intramuscular pressure and some measure of the patient's blood pressure.[50] Although many definitions of perfusion pressure have been considered, the one proposed by McQueen et al. is most commonly used:

$$\text{perfusion pressure} = \text{diastolic blood pressure} - \text{intramuscular pressure}$$

with a threshold for fasciotomy when the perfusion pressure (so defined) is less than 30 mmHg when averaged over a 12-hour period.[13,35,43] Multiple studies demonstrate that perfusion pressure is a better diagnostic criteria for compartment syndrome than absolute pressure,[13,43] and that fasciotomy can be safely avoided whenever the limb perfusion pressure is greater than 30 mm Hg.[13,34,35,43] Typically, the anterior compartment is monitored since the pressures within it are typically highest.[47]

The difficulty in using specific thresholds for fasciotomy was highlighted by Prayson et al, who carefully followed blood pressure and compartment pressure in 19 patients with isolated lower extremity fractures who did not have compartment syndrome by clinical criteria, or at follow-up.[10] In this series, 84% of the patients had at least one reading in which their perfusion pressure was within 30 mmHg of their diastolic blood pressure, and 58% had a reading within 20 mmHg. Thus, single pressure measurements alone are not representative, and serial or continuous measurements demonstrating rising compartment pressure or falling perfusion pressure are likely to be more specific for patients that truly have compartment syndrome. Similar findings were noted by Janzing and Broos,

who reviewed 95 patients treated with continuous pressure monitoring, and after reviewing their patients at follow-up, could not identify a threshold that was both sensitive and specific for diagnosing compartment syndrome.[8]

There are several potential pitfalls with use of pressure measurements for decision-making in patients suspected of compartment syndrome. First, it has been shown that there is spatial variation in the pressure within a given compartment, with pressures being highest within 5 cm of the fracture[51] and more centrally in the muscle.[52] It is not known whether one should obtain pressures near the fracture to obtain the highest pressure, or measure further away (outside the zone of injury) to obtain a pressure that may be more representative of the compartment as a whole.[31] Another source of uncertainty when calculating perfusion pressure is what blood pressure value to use, especially if the patient is under general anesthesia. Tornetta and colleagues evaluated 242 patients undergoing tibial nailing, and recorded preoperative, intraoperative, and postoperative blood pressures.[53] During surgery, there was a statistically significant decrease in diastolic blood pressure comparing intraoperative to preoperative values (average decrease 18 mmHg), whereas postoperative diastolic pressure was within 2 mmHg of the preoperative value. Thus, use of intraoperative diastolic blood pressure measurements for calculation of perfusion pressure may give a spuriously low perfusion pressure and lead to unnecessary fasciotomy. These authors recommend using preoperative blood pressure values when calculating perfusion pressure in a patient under general anesthesia, except when the patient is going to remain under anesthesia for several more hours.[53]

Recommendations
- The concept of perfusion pressure has reduced the need for fasciotomy by avoiding unnecessary fasciotomy in patients with high absolute pressures but maintained perfusion. Setting the threshold for fasciotomy at a perfusion pressure of 30 mmHg, as defined by McQueen et al.,[36] can be considered to be safe, but still may lead to overtreatment if used routinely [overall quality: moderate]
- Transient intraoperative hypotension should be considered when making decisions about perfusion pressure.[53] The current literature does not contain recommendations for fasciotomy based on any measurement of pressure that can be relied upon in every situation [overall quality: low]

Summary of recommendations

- Younger age (25–35 years), male gender, and trauma are consistent risk factors for compartment syndrome in patients with fractures of the tibia and forearm.

- Careful and frequent (every 1–2 hour) clinical monitoring of pain (both at rest and with passive muscle stretching), limb swelling, and neurologic status is usually sufficient to make the diagnosis.
- Clinical diagnosis is not reliable if done infrequently, in children, or in unconscious patients in whom pain cannot be assessed. The influence of anesthetic technique on the clinical examination is uncertain.
- Performing fasciotomy whenever the intramuscular pressure is within 30 mmHg of the diastolic blood pressure is not likely to result in any missed cases of compartment syndrome, but will likely lead to overtreatment if used routinely.
- The concept of perfusion pressure has reduced the need for fasciotomy. Setting the threshold for fasciotomy at a perfusion pressure of 30 mmHg can be considered safe, but still may lead to overtreatment if used routinely.

References

1. McQueen MM, Gaston P, Court-Brown CM. Acute compartment syndrome. Who is at risk? J Bone Joint Surg Br 2000;82:200–3.
2. Matsen FA. Compartment syndrome. A unified concept. Clin Orthop Rel Res 1975;113:8–14.
3. Davis ET, Harris A, Keene D, Porter K, Manji M. The use of regional anaesthesia in patients at risk of acute compartment syndrome. Injury 2006;37:128–33.
4. O'Toole RV, Whitney A, Merchant N, Hui E, Higgins J, Kim TT, Sagebien C. Variation in diagnosis of compartment syndrome by surgeons treating tibial shaft fractures. J Trauma 2009;67:735–41.
5. Wall CJ, Richardson MD, Lowe AJ, Brand C, Lynch J, de Steiger RN. Survey of management of acute, traumatic compartment syndrome of the leg in Australia. J Trauma. 2007;63:268–75.
6. Badhe S, Baiju D, Elliott R, Rowles J, Calthorpe D. The "silent" compartment syndrome. Injury 2009;40:220–2.
7. Harrington P, Bunola J, Jennings AJ, Bush DJ, Smith RM. Acute compartment syndrome masked by intravenous morphine from a patient-controlled analgesia pump. Injury 2000;31:387–9.
8. Janzing HMJ, Broos PLO. Routine monitoring of compartment pressure in patients with tibial fractures: beware of overtreatment! Injury 2001;32:415–21.
9. Kashuk JL, Moore EE, Pinski S, et al. Lower extremity compartment syndrome in the acute care surgery paradigm: safety lessons learned. Patient Saf Surg 2009;3:11–16.
10. Prayson MJ, Chen JL, Hampers D, Vogt M, Fenwick J, Meredick R. Baseline compartment pressure measurements in isolated lower extremity fractures without clinical compartment syndrome. J Trauma 2006;60:1037–40.
11. Richards H, Langston A, Kulkarni R, Downes EM. Does patient controlled analgesia delay the diagnosis of compartment syndrome following intramedullary nailing of the tibia? Injury 2004;35:296–8.
12. Ulmer T. The clinical diagnosis of compartment syndrome of the lower leg: are clinical findings predictive of the disorder? J Orthop Trauma 2002;16:572–7.
13. White TO, Howell GED, Will EM, Court-Brown CM, McQueen MM. Elevated intramuscular pressures do not influence outcome after tibial fracture. J Trauma 2003;55:1133–8.
14. Williams PR, Russell ID, Mintowt-Czyz WJ. Compartment pressure monitoring—current UK orthopaedic practice. Injury 1998;29:229–32.
15. Bhattacharyya T, Vrahas MS. The medical-legal aspects of compartment syndrome. J Bone Joint Surg Am 2004;86:864–8.
16. Finkelstein JA, Hunter GA, Hu RW. Lower limb compartment syndrome: course after delayed fasciotomy. J Trauma 1996;40:342–4.
17. Hope MJ, McQueen MM. Acute compartment syndrome in the absence of fracture. J Orthop Trauma 2004;18: 220–4.
18. Prasarn ML, Ouellette EA, Livingstone A, Giuffrida AY. Acute pediatric upper extremity compartment syndrome in the absence of fracture. J Pediatr Orthop 2009;29:263–8.
19. Ritenour AE, Dorlac WC, Fang R, et al. Complications after fasciotomy revision and delayed compartment release in combat patients. J Trauma 2008;64:S153–62.
20. Shadgan B, Menon M, O'Brien PJ, Reid WD. Diagnostic techniques in acute compartment syndrome of the leg. J Orthop Trauma 2008;22:581–7.
21. Vaillancourt C, Shrier I, Falk M, Rossignol M, Vernec A, Somogyi D. Quantifying delays in the recognition and management of acute compartment syndrome. CEJM 2001;3:26–30.
22. Bermudez K, Knudson MM, Morabito D, Kessel O. Fasciotomy, chronic venous insufficiency, and the calf muscle pump. Arch Surg 1998;133:1356–61.
23. Frink M, Klaus AK, Kuther G, et al. Long term results of compartment syndrome of the lower limb in polytraumatised patients. Injury 2007;38:607–613.
24. Garfin SR, Tipton CM, Mubarak SJ, Woo Sl-Y, Hargens AR, Akeson WH. Role of fascia in maintenance of muscle tension and pressure. J Appl Physiol 1981;51:317–20.
25. Giannoudis PV, Nicolopoulos C, Dinopoulos H, Ng A, Adedapo S, Kind P. The impact of lower leg compartment syndrome on health related quality of life. Injury 2002;33: 117–21.
26. Heemskerk J, Kitslaar P. Acute compartment syndrome of the lower leg: retrospective study on prevalence, technique, and outcome of fasciotomies. World J Surg 2003;27:744–7.
27. Mithoefer K, Lhowe DW, Vrahas MS, Altman DT, Erens V, Altman GT. Functional outcome after acute compartment syndrome of the thigh. J Bone Joint Surg Am 2006;88:729–37.
28. Park S, Ahn J, Gee AO, Kuntz AF, Esterhai JL. Compartment syndrome in tibial fractures. J Orthop Trauma 2009;23:514–18.
29. Chang YH, Tu YK, Yeh WL, Hsu RW. Tibial plateau fracture with compartment syndrome: a complication of higher incidence in Taiwan. Chang Gung Med J 2000;23(3):149–55.
30. Schwartz JT Jr, Brumback RJ, Lakatos R, Poka A, Bathon GH, Burgess AR. Acute compartment syndrome of the thigh. A spectrum of injury. J Bone Joint Surg Am 1989;71:392–400.
31. Harris IA, Kadir A, Donald G. Continuous compartment pressure monitoring for tibia fractures: does it influence outcome? J Trauma 2006;60:1330–5.
32. Al-Dadah OQ, Darrah C, Cooper A, Donell ST, Patel AD. Continuous compartment pressure monitoring vs. clinical monitoring in tibial diaphyseal fracture. Injury 2008;39:1204–9.
33. Kosir R, Moore FA, Selby JH, et al. Acute lower extremity compartment syndrome (ALECS) screening protocol in critically ill trauma patients. J Trauma 2007;63:268–75.

34. Ogunlusi JD, Oginni LM, Ikem IC. Compartment pressure in adults with tibial fractures. Int Orthop 2005;29:130–3.

35. McQueen MM, Court-Brown CM. Compartment monitoring in tibial fractures. The pressure threshold for decompression. J Bone Joint Surg Br 1996;78:99–104.

36. McQueen MM, Christie J, Court-Brown CM. Acute compartment syndrome in tibial diaphyseal fractures. J Bone Joint Surg Br 1996;78:95–8.

37. Mubarak SJ, Owen CA, Hargens AR, Garetto LP, Akeson WH. Acute compartment syndromes: diagnosis and treatment with the aid of the wick catheter. J Bone Joint Surg Am. 1978;60:1091–5.

38. Mar GJ, Barrington MJ, McGuirk BR. Acute compartment syndrome of the lower limb and the effect of postoperative analgesia on diagnosis. Br J Anaesth 2009;102:3–11.

39. Robinson CM, O'Donnell J, Will E, Keating JF. Dropped hallux after the intramedullary nailing of tibial fractures. J Bone Joint Surg Br 1999;81:481–4.

40. Marcu D, Dunbar WH, Kaplan LD. Footdrop without significant pain as late presentation of acute peroneal compartment syndrome in an intercollegiate football player. Am J Orthop. 2009;38:241–4.

41. O'Sullivan MJ, Rice J, McGuinness AJ. Compartment syndrome without pain! Irish Med J 2002;95:22.

42. Allen MJ, Stirling AJ, Crawshaw CV, Barnes MR. Intra-compartmental pressure monitoring of leg injuries. An aid to management. J Bone Joint Surg Br 1985;67:53–7.

43. Ozkayin N, Aktuglu K. Absolute compartment pressure versus differential pressure for the diagnosis of compartment syndrome in tibial fractures. Int Orthop 2005;29:396–401.

44. Vaillancourt C, Shrier I, Vandal A, et al. Acute compartment syndrome: How long before muscle necrosis occurs? CJEM 2004;6:147–54.

45. Øvre S, Hvaal K, Holm I, Strømsøe K, Nordsletten L, Skjeldal S. Compartment pressure in nailed tibial fractures. A threshold of 30 mmHg for decompression gives 29% fasciotomies. Arch Orthop Trauma Surg 1998;118:29–31.

46. Rorabeck CH. The treatment of compartment syndromes of the leg. J Bone Joint Surg Br 1984;66:93–7.

47. Sheridan GW, Matsen FA. Fasciotomy in the treatment of the acute compartment syndrome. J Bone Joint Surg Am 1976;58:112–15.

48. Lagerstrom CF, Reed RL II, Rowlands BJ, Fischer RP. Early fasciotomy for acute clinically evident posttraumatic compartment syndrome. Am J Surg 1989;158:36–9.

49. Cascio BM, Pateder DB, Wilckens JH, Frassica FJ. Compartment syndrome: time from diagnosis to fasciotomy. J Surg Orthop Adv 2005;14:117–21.

50. Whitesides TE, Haney TC, Morimoto K. Tissue pressure measurements as a determinant for the need for fasciotomy. Clin Orthop Relat Res 1975;113:43–51.

51. Heckman MM, Whitesides TE, Grewe SR, Rooks MD. Compartment pressure in association with closed tibial fractures: the relationship between tissue pressure, compartment, and the distance from the site of the fracture. J Bone Joint Surg Am 1994;76:1285–92.

52. Nakhostine M, Styf JR, van Leuven S, Hargens AR, Gershuni DH. Intramuscular pressure varies with depth. The tibialis anterior muscle studied in 12 volunteers. Acta Orthop Scand 1993;64:377–81.

53. Kakar S, Firoozabadi R, McKean J, Tornetta P III. Diastolic blood pressure in patients with tibia fractures under anesthesia: implications for the diagnosis of compartment syndrome. J Orthop Trauma 2007;21:99–103.

72 Noninvasive Technologies for Fracture Repair

Yoshinobu Watanabe, Makoto Kobayashi, and Takashi Matsushita
Teikyo University School of Medicine, Tokyo, Japan

Case scenario

A 32 year old man, who was otherwise healthy, sustained a comminuted open tibial shaft fracture as a result of a motor vehicle accident. After initial debridement and irrigation, the fracture was fixed by an unreamed interlocking nail. Radiographs showed no sign of callus formation 6 months after surgery (Figure 72.1). There was no clinical, biochemical, or radiographic evidence of deep infection or osteomyelitis.

Relevant anatomy

Fracture healing of locked tibial nailing is controlled by many factors such as stability, gap, and vascularity of fracture site (level II–V).[1-4] Therefore comminuted open tibial shaft fractures are potentially at risk of developing delayed healing (level II).[1,5]

Importance of the problem

Of the estimated 5.6 million fractures occurring annually in the United States, it is believed that 5–10% demonstrated delayed union or nonunion (level II).[6] Acceleration of fracture healing is important to reduce the socioeconomic loss by shortening the period of fracture treatment.

Top five questions

1. What are the predictors of nonunion?
2. What kinds of noninvasive biophysical technologies can be available for noninfected delayed union and nonunion?

3. Does low-intensity pulsed ultrasound (LIPUS) accelerate fracture healing and improve the patient's health-related quality of life (QOL)?
4. Does pulsed electromagnetic fields (PEMF) accelerate fracture healing and improve the patient's health-related QOL?
5. Does extracorporeal shock wave therapy (ESWT) accelerate fracture healing and improve the patient's health-related QOL?

Question 1: What are the predictors of nonunion?

Case clarification

The patient's radiograph reveals a comminuted tibial shaft fracture fixed by a relatively small unreamed intramedullary (IM) nail. Subsequent radiographs showed no bridging callus with existence of visible fracture line (Figure 72.1). If we know the probability of this open tibial fracture developing to established nonunion, this information will help us to determine when additional treatment or therapy is needed to achieve union.

Relevance

Evaluation of predictors for nonunion will help us to recognize the risk of delayed union or nonunion earlier, and early treatment can help patients avoid prolonged periods of pain and disability.

Current opinion

Predictors of nonunion of open tibial fracture treated by using IM nail are Gustilo grades, postoperative fracture gap, unreamed IM nailing, and dynamization.

Finding the evidence

• PubMed (www.ncbi.nlm.nih.gov/pubmed/) advanced search with meta-analysis, clinical trial, randomized

Evidence-Based Orthopedics, First Edition. Edited by Mohit Bhandari.
© 2012 Blackwell Publishing Ltd. Published 2012 by Blackwell Publishing Ltd.

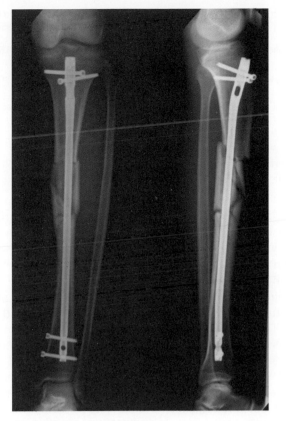

Figure 72.1 Delayed union or nonunion?

clinical trial, and review: search term: "(tibia*) AND (fracture*)"

• PubMed (www.ncbi.nlm.nih.gov/pubmed/) advanced search with meta-analysis, clinical trial, randomized clinical trial, and review: search term "((tibia*) AND (fracture*)) AND ((nonunion*) OR (delay*))"

• PubMed (www.ncbi.nlm.nih.gov/pubmed/) advanced search with meta-analysis, clinical trial, randomized clinical trial, and review: search term "((fracture*) AND ((nonunion*) OR (delay*))) AND ((ultrasound*) OR (electromag*) OR (shock wave*) OR (LIPUS) OR (PEMF) OR (ESW*))"

Quality of the evidence

Level I

• 1 meta-analysis for reaming
• 5 randomized clinical trials (RCTs) for reaming

Level II

• 3 cohort studies for postoperative fracture gap, and 1 for dynamization

Level IV (case series) or II (cohort)

• There are over 500 case series for Gustilo grades of open fracture. Among these articles some one-group cohort studies must be included, but the exact numbers of these

could not be determined because of the inadequate description

Findings

Court-Brown et al. have analyzed the mean time to union for different Gustilo grades of open fracture. These results indicated that the risk of nonunion increased with Gustilo grades (level II).[5,7,8]

Drosos et al. studied factors affecting fracture healing after tibial nailing for closed and grade I open fractures, and reported that the risk of failure of union increased by 2.38 times for highly comminuted fractures, by 3.14 times when nail dynamization was applied, and by 1.65 times when the locking screws failed (level II).[1] They also showed that the risk of nonunion increased if the postreduction gap was 3mm or more in fractures with no or only minimal comminution (level II).[1] Bhandari et al. identified that postoperative fracture gap is one of the predictors of reoperation following operative treatment of tibial shaft fracture (level II).[9]

Meta-analyses of prospective RCTs have suggested large reductions in the risk of nonunion in association with the use of reamed IM nailing (RR 0.44; 95% CI 0.21–0.93) (level I– II).[10-13] A well-designed randomized trial with a large number of participants demonstrated that overall nonunion rate was 4.6% and there is a possible benefit for reamed IM nailing in patients with closed fractures (RR 0.67; 95% CI 0.47–0.96) (level I).[14]

Recommendations

• Risk factors for nonunion in tibial shaft fractures include: (1) open fractures with high-grade Gustilo classification [overall quality: moderate]; (2) fixation with unreamed nails [overall quality: moderate]; and (3) fixation with large fracture gap between main fragments [overall quality: moderate]

• In these situations, some sort of additional intervention would be needed to avoid nonunion [overall quality: moderate

Question 2: What kinds of noninvasive biophysical technologies can be available for noninfected delayed union and nonunion?

Case clarification

Some noninvasive technologies would be worth trying before surgical interventions for delayed union and nonunion.

Relevance

Some type of bone growth stimulation can be widely applied for acceleration of fracture healing as an adjuvant therapy and/or alternative therapy.

Current opinion

LIPUS, PEMF, and ESWT have been widely used to enhance fracture healing.

Finding the evidence

See Question 1.

Quality of the evidence

Level I
- 3 meta-analyses (2 for LIPUS and 1 for PEMF)
- 1 RCT for ESWT

Findings

LIPUS and PEMF have been most popular devices for the adjuvant and/or alternative treatment of choice for surgical intervention to enhance fracture healing (level I–III).[15–17] Currently the effectiveness of ESWT for hypertrophic nonunions has been confirmed by RCT.

Recommendation

- Noninvasive biophysical stimulation may be available for possible tibial nonunion, and LIPUS, PEMF, and ESWT are recommended methods

Question 3: Does LIPUS accelerate fracture healing and improve the patient's health-related QOL?

Case clarification

Before surgical intervention is considered for delayed or nonunion after tibial fracture, there is a chance to achieve union by LIPUS.

Relevance

How much is fracture healing accelerated by using LIPUS? What is the overall union rate for delayed union/nonunion by LIPUS? Does LIPUS improve QOL of the patient with a tibial fracture?

Current opinion

The use of LIPUS is considered to augment fracture healing in those fracture types at risk for nonunion such as open or comminuted fracture and/or compromised patients with smoking and malnutrition.

Finding the evidence

See Question 1.

Quality of the evidence

Level I
- 7 meta-analyses

Findings

Most meta-analyses included several kinds of bone and fractures, not focusing on tibial nonunion. Heckman et al.

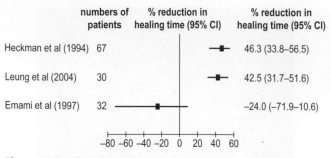

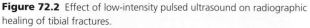

	numbers of patients	% reduction in healing time (95% CI)	% reduction in healing time (95% CI)
Heckman et al (1994)	67		46.3 (33.8–56.5)
Leung et al (2004)	30		42.5 (31.7–51.6)
Emami et al (1997)	32		–24.0 (–71.9–10.6)

Figure 72.2 Effect of low-intensity pulsed ultrasound on radiographic healing of tibial fractures.

concluded that LIPUS shortened the time to healing fracture by 38% and significantly reduced the incidence of delayed union for the relatively simple closed or Gustilo I open tibial shaft fracture immobilized by a cast (level I).[18] Leung et al. investigated the effect of LIPUS on fracture healing for open and/or severely comminuted tibial shaft fractures immobilized by IM nail or external fixator (level I).[19] They concluded that the LIPUS-treated group showed statistically significant better healing, as demonstrated by all assessments. Emami et al., however, concluded that LIPUS did not shorten healing time in fresh tibial fractures treated with a reamed and statically locked IM nail (level I).[20] Limited information for tibial shaft fracture from these three RCTs suggested that LIPUS probably enhances or accelerates fracture healing in tibial fracture (Figure 72.2), although the results of these three trials were heterogeneous (level I).[17]

The benefits of LIPUS for delayed and nonunion were also investigated by cohort studies, which revealed that the overall success rate of LIPUS for delayed union and nonunions of tibia/tibia-fibula or fibula is approximately 88% (Table 72.1) (level II).[21–24] Unfortunately, there is little literature that studies the improvement of health-related QOL of the patient (level II).[25]

Recommendation

- LIPUS is likely to accelerate fracture healing in a fresh fracture as well as in delayed union or nonunion [overall quality: high]

Question 4: Does PEMF accelerate fracture healing and improve the patient's health-related QOL?

Case clarification

Before surgical intervention is considered for delayed or nonunion after tibial fracture, there is a chance to achieve union by PEMF.

Relevance

How much does the use of PEMF accelerate fracture healing? What is the overall union rate for delayed union/

Table 72.1 Success rate of LIPUS for long bone fractures

Study	Delayed or nonunion	Overall of long bones		Humerus		Radius/ radius-ulna		Femur		Tibia/tibia-fibula or fibula	
		Success rate	%	Success rate	%	Success rate	%	Success rate	%	Success rate	%
Mayr et al. 2000	Delayed	(525/584)	90	(41/54)	76	(49/52)	94	(85/98)	87	(350/380)	92
Rubin et al. 2001	Nonunion	(216/256)	84	(33/48)	69	(21/22)	95	(57/66)	86	(105/120)	88
Nolte et al. 2001	Nonunion	(779/959)	B1	(102/148)	69	(60/69)	87	(213/259)	82	(404/483)	84
Gebauer et al. 2005	Nonunion	(19/21)	91	(1/1)	100	(4/5)	80	(4/5)	80	(10/10)	100
Subtotal	Nonunion	(41/46)	89	(2/3)	67	(5/6)	83	(11/12)	92	(23/25)	92
		(1580/1856)	85	(179/254)	70	(139/154)	90	(370/440)	84	(892/1018)	88

nonunion by PEMF? Does PEMF improve QOL of the patient with tibial fractures?

Current opinion

The use of PEMF is considered to augment fracture healing in those fracture types at risk for nonunion such as open or comminuted fractures and/or compromised patients with smoking and malnutrition.

Finding the evidence

See Question 1.

Quality of the evidence

Level I
- 4 meta-analyses

Findings

For fracture healing, three types of electrical stimulation are available: (1) direct current stimulation using electrodes; (2) electromagnetic stimulation by inductive coupling; (3) capacitive coupling stimulation (level II).[26]

Sharrard (level I)[27] and Simonis et al. (level I),[28] in a placebo-controlled randomized trial, examined the efficacy of PEMF on tibial delayed or nonunions. Both reports indicated that a greater proportion of patients in the treatment group achieved union (Table 72.2), and PEMF increased the chance of union by 3.8 or 1.8 times. However, the 95% confidence interval suggested that the increase could be as low as 1.1-fold (level III).[29] Baker et al., in a placebo-controlled randomized trial, showed a negative effect of PEMF for tibial nonunion conservatively treated by cast (Table 72.2) (level II);[30] however, the number of participants seemed to be too small.

Cohort studies or case series without control group showed that PEMF showed a high union rate (87–93%) of long-bone nonunions with non-weight-bearing treatment (level IV).[31,32]

No evidence was available for improvement of the patient's QOL.

Table 72.2 Effect of pulsed electromagnetic fields on increasing chance of union for tibial nonunion

	Active		Placebo		Increased chance of union	
	United	Not united	United	Not united	Times	95% CI
Sharrard 1990	9	11	3	22	3.8	1.09–16.2
Simonis 2003	16	2	8	8	1.8	1.06–2.98
	Active		Placebo		Decreased chance of union	
	United	Not united	United	Not united	Times	95% CI
Barker 1984	5	4	5	2	1.2	0.61–2.72

Recommendation

- PEMF is likely to improve healing rate in delayed union or nonunion [overall quality: high], but no evidence was available for acceleration of fracture healing in fresh fracture

Question 5: Does ESWT accelerate fracture healing and improve the patient health-related QOL?

Case clarification

Before surgical intervention is considered for delayed or nonunion after tibial fracture, there is a chance to achieve union by ESWT.

Relevance

How much is fracture healing accelerated by using ESWT? What is the overall union rate for delayed union/nonunion by ESWT? Does ESWT improve QOL of the patient with tibial fractures?

Current opinion

Predictors of open tibial fracture treated by IM nailing are Gustilo grades, postoperative fracture gap, unreamed IM nailing, and dynamization.

Finding the evidence

See Question 1.

Quality of the evidence

Level II

- 1 systematic review of case series

Findings

A shock wave is defined as a sonic pulse characterized by a high peak pressure (500 bar = 100 kPa), a short life cycle (10 ms), fast pressure rise (<10 ns), and broad frequency spectrum (16–20 MHz) (level IV).[33]

Elster et al. currently reported the result of 192 tibial nonunions treated by ESWT coupled with post-treatment immobilization, external fixation, or ESWT alone (level IV).[34] They stated that 138 of 172 (80.2%) patients demonstrated complete fracture healing at the time of last follow-up, and that mean time from first shock wave therapy to complete healing of the tibia nonunion was 4.8 ± 4.0 months.

Cacchio et al. prospectively compared the results of ESWT produced by two different devices (with 4000 impulses of shock waves with an energy flux density of $0.40 \, mJ/mm^2$ (group 1) or $0.70 \, mJ/mm^2$ (group 2) with those of surgical treatment for long-bone hypertrophic nonunions (group 3) (level IV).[35] At 6 months, 70% of the nonunions in group 1, 71% of the nonunions in group 2, and 73% of the nonunions in group 3 had healed. They concluded that ESWT is as effective as surgery in stimulating union of long-bone hypertrophic nonunions.

Zelle et al. reviewed 10 case series and reported that the overall union rate in patients with delayed union/nonunion was 76% (95% CI 73–79%) and ranged from 41% to 85%. The union rate in atrophic nonunions was 29% as compared with 76% in hypertrophic nonunions (RR 2.6; 95% CI 1.6–4.7; $p < 0.0001$).

Recommendation

- ESWT is likely to be the alternative treatment of choice for hypertrophic long-bone nonunion [overall quality: low]

Summary of recommendations

- Risk factors for nonunion in tibial shaft fractures include (1) open fractures with high-grade Gustilo classification, (2) fixation with unreamed nails, and (3) fixation with large fracture gap between main fragments. In these situations, some sort of additional intervention would be needed to avoid nonunion
- Noninvasive biophysical stimulation may be available for possible tibial nonunion, and LIPUS, PEMF, and ESWT are among the recommended methods
- LIPUS is likely to accelerate fracture healing in fresh fracture as well as in delayed union or nonunion
- PEMF is likely to improve healing rate in delayed union or nonunion, but no evidence was available for acceleration of fracture healing in fresh fracture
- ESWT is likely to be the alternative treatment of choice for hypertrophic long-bone nonunion

References

1. Drosos GI, Bishay M, Karnezis IA, Alegakis AK. Factors affecting fracture healing after intramedullary nailing of the tibial diaphysis for closed and grade I open fractures. J Bone Joint Surg Br 2006;88(2):227–31.
2. Audige L, Griffin D, Bhandari M, Kellam J, Ruedi TP. Path analysis of factors for delayed healing and nonunion in 416 operatively treated tibial shaft fractures. Clin Orthop Relat Res 2005;438:221–32.
3. Claes L, Augat P, Suger G, Wilke HJ. Influence of size and stability of the osteotomy gap on the success of fracture healing. J Orthop Res 1997;15(4):577–84.
4. Dickson KF, Katzman S, Paiement G. The importance of the blood supply in the healing of tibial fractures. Contemp Orthop 1995;30(6):489–93.
5. Court-Brown CM, McQueen MM, Quaba AA, Christie J. Locked intramedullary nailing of open tibial fractures. J Bone Joint Surg Br 1991;73(6):959–64.
6. Einhorn TA. Enhancement of fracture-healing. J Bone Joint Surg Am 1995;77(6):940–56.
7. Court-Brown CM, Christie J, McQueen MM. Closed intramedullary tibial nailing. Its use in closed and type I open fractures. J Bone Joint Surg Br 1990;72(4):605–11.
8. Court-Brown CM, Keating JF, Christie J, McQueen MM. Exchange intramedullary nailing. Its use in aseptic tibial nonunion. J Bone Joint Surg Br 1995;77(3):407–11.
9. Bhandari M, Tornetta P, 3rd, Sprague S, Najibi S, Petrisor B, Griffith L, et al. Predictors of reoperation following operative management of fractures of the tibial shaft. J Orthop Trauma 2003;17(5):353–61.
10. Bhandari M, Guyatt GH, Tong D, Adili A, Shaughnessy SG. Reamed versus nonreamed intramedullary nailing of lower extremity long bone fractures: a systematic overview and meta-analysis. J Orthop Trauma 2000;14(1):2–9.
11. Forster MC, Bruce AS, Aster AS. Should the tibia be reamed when nailing? Injury 2005;36(3):439–44.

12. Littenberg B, Weinstein LP, McCarren M, Mead T, Swiontkowski MF, Rudicel SA, et al. Closed fractures of the tibial shaft. A meta-analysis of three methods of treatment. J Bone Joint Surg Am 1998;80(2):174–83.

13. Coles CP, Gross M. Closed tibial shaft fractures: management and treatment complications. A review of the prospective literature. Can J Surg 2000;43(4):256–62.

14. Bhandari M, Guyatt G, Tornetta P, 3rd, Schemitsch EH, Swiontkowski M, Sanders D, et al. Randomized trial of reamed and unreamed intramedullary nailing of tibial shaft fractures. J Bone Joint Surg Am 2008;90(12):2567–78.

15. Brighton CT, Shaman P, Heppenstall RB, Esterhai JL, Jr., Pollack SR, Friedenberg ZB. Tibial nonunion treated with direct current, capacitive coupling, or bone graft. Clin Orthop Relat Res 1995(321):223–34.

16. Romano CL, Romano D, Logoluso N. Low-intensity pulsed ultrasound for the treatment of bone delayed union or nonunion: a review. Ultrasound Med Biol 2009;35(4):529–36.

17. Busse JW, Kaur J, Mollon B, Bhandari M, Tornetta P, 3rd, Schunemann HJ, et al. Low intensity pulsed ultrasonography for fractures: systematic review of randomised controlled trials. BMJ 2009;338:b351.

18. Heckman JD, Ryaby JP, McCabe J, Frey JJ, Kilcoyne RF. Acceleration of tibial fracture-healing by non-invasive, low-intensity pulsed ultrasound. J Bone Joint Surg Am 1994;76(1):26–34.

19. Leung KS, Lee WS, Tsui HF, Liu PP, Cheung WH. Complex tibial fracture outcomes following treatment with low-intensity pulsed ultrasound. Ultrasound Med Biol 2004;30(3):389–95.

20. Emami A, Petren-Mallmin M, Larsson S. No effect of low-intensity ultrasound on healing time of intramedullary fixed tibial fractures. J Orthop Trauma 1999;13(4):252–7.

21. Mayr E, Frankel V, Ruter A. Ultrasound–an alternative healing method for nonunions? Arch Orthop Trauma Surg 2000; 120(1–2):1–8.

22. Rubin C, Bolander M, Ryaby JP, Hadjiargyrou M. The use of low-intensity ultrasound to accelerate the healing of fractures. J Bone Joint Surg Am 2001;83(2):259–70.

23. Nolte PA, van der Krans A, Patka P, Janssen IM, Ryaby JP, Albers GH. Low-intensity pulsed ultrasound in the treatment of non-unions. J Trauma 2001;51(4):693–702; discussion 02–3.

24. Gebauer D, Mayr E, Orthner E, Ryaby JP. Low-intensity pulsed ultrasound: effects on nonunions. Ultrasound Med Biol 2005; 31(10):1391–402.

25. Watanabe Y, Matsushita T, Bhandari M, Zdero R, Schemitsch EH. Ultrasound for fracture healing: current evidence. J Orthop Trauma 2010;24 Suppl 1:S56–61.

26. Ryaby JT. Clinical effects of electromagnetic and electric fields on fracture healing. Clin Orthop Relat Res 1998(355 Suppl): S205–15.

27. Sharrard WJ. A double-blind trial of pulsed electromagnetic fields for delayed union of tibial fractures. J Bone Joint Surg Br 1990;72(3):347–55.

28. Simonis RB, Parnell EJ, Ray PS, Peacock JL. Electrical treatment of tibial non-union: a prospective, randomised, double-blind trial. Injury 2003;34(5):357–62.

29. Bhandari M, Schemitsch EH, Emil H. Clinical advances in the treatment of fracture nonunion: the response to mechanical stimulation. Curr Opin Orthop 2000;11(5):372–77.

30. Barker AT, Dixon RA, Sharrard WJ, Sutcliffe ML. Pulsed magnetic field therapy for tibial non-union. Interim results of a double-blind trial. Lancet 1984;1(8384):994–6.

31. Bassett CA, Mitchell SN, Gaston SR. Treatment of ununited tibial diaphyseal fractures with pulsing electromagnetic fields. J Bone Joint Surg Am 1981;63(4):511–23.

32. Bassett CA, Mitchell SN, Schink MM. Treatment of therapeutically resistant non-unions with bone grafts and pulsing electromagnetic fields. J Bone Joint Surg Am 1982;64(8):1214–20.

33. Zelle BA, Gollwitzer H, Zlowodzki M, Buhren V. Extracorporeal shock wave therapy: current evidence. J Orthop Trauma 2010;24(Suppl 1):S66–70.

34. Elster EA, Stojadinovic A, Forsberg J, Shawen S, Andersen RC, Schaden W. Extracorporeal shock wave therapy for nonunion of the tibia. J Orthop Trauma 2010;24(3):133–41.

35. Cacchio A, Giordano L, Colafarina O, et al. Extracorporeal shock-wave therapy compared with surgery for hypertrophic long-bone nonunions. J Bone Joint Surg Am 2009;91(11): 2589–97.

73 Calcium Phosphate Cements in Fracture Repair

Ross K. Leighton[1], Kelly Trask[1], Thomas A. Russell[2], Mohit Bhandari[3], and Richard E. Buckley[4]

[1]Queen Elizabeth II Health Sciences Centre, Halifax, NS, Canada
[2]Campbell Clinic, University of Tennessee, Memphis, TN, USA
[3]McMaster University, Hamilton, ON, Canada
[4]Foothills Medical Centre, University of Calgary, Calgary, AB, Canada

Case scenarios

Case 1

A 54 year old woman presents with a fractured tibial plateau following a low-energy injury at home. The patient's radiographs indicate a split depression injury laterally, with an associated medial condylar injury with a posterior medial split (Schatzker V) (Figure 73.1).

Case 2

A 42 year old man presents with a significant tibial plateau fracture (Figure 73.2).

Case 3

A 72 year old woman presents with a fracture of the distal radius with significant posterior comminution (Figure 73.3).

Importance of the problem

Metaphyseal fractures are among the most difficult fractures to treat. Depressed articular fragments can crush the underlying weak subchondral cancellous bone, leaving a void when the articular segments are reduced surgically. Potential long-term problems including pain, post-traumatic arthritis, and limitation of motion and function may occur if joint surface subsidence cannot be prevented or at least limited.

Definitions
• **Articular:** bone close to and including the joint surface • **Metaphyseal:** bone adjacent to the joint consisting of cancellous bone with a weak cortical layer and extending to the shaft of the long bone • **Diaphyseal:** bone located in the narrow part of the long bone, generally consists of hard cortical bone with a narrow medullary canal

Top five questions

Diagnosis

1. What types of fractures lend themselves to fixation with calcium phosphate bone substitutes?

Therapy

2. What type of bone graft should be used to treat subchondral contained defects: autograft, allograft, or a calcium phosphate bone substitute?
3. What are the features of calcium phosphate that make it suitable as a bone substitute?

Prognosis

4. When does the calcium phosphate resorb?
5. Are there any other benefits to using calcium phosphate?

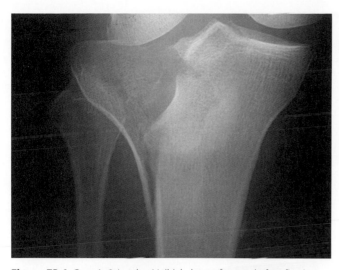

Figure 73.1 Case 1: Schatzker V tibial plateau fracture before fixation.

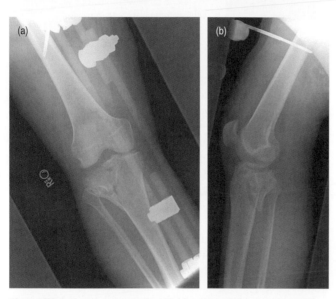

Figure 73.2 Case 2: preoperative AP (a) and lateral (b) views of a Schatzker V fracture.

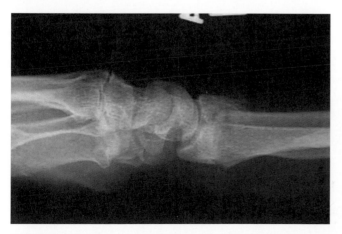

Figure 73.3 Case 3: distal radius fracture with dorsal comminution.

Finding the evidence

Bajammal et al. employed a comprehensive search strategy for a 2008 meta-analysis,[1] which we expanded to locate articles published more recently. We selected the most relevant articles for this review.

Quality of the evidence

Level I
- 4 randomized trials and meta-analyses[1–4]

Level II
- 7 retrospective reviews and prospective cohorts[5–11]

Level IV
- Case reports, review articles, animal and laboratory studies

Question 1: What types of fractures lend themselves to fixation with calcium phosphate bone substitutes?

Case 1 clarification

Provisional fixation of this patent's fracture is obtained with wires (Figure 73.4). Open reduction with a lateral locking plate plus the use of calcium phosphate (alpha-BSM) allowed for rigid fixation (Figure 73.5).

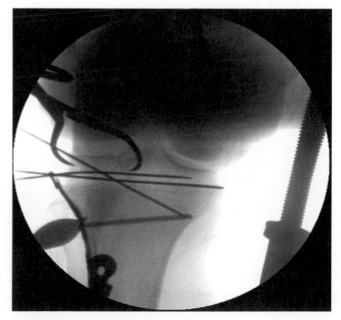

Figure 73.4 Case 1: provisional fixation with wires.

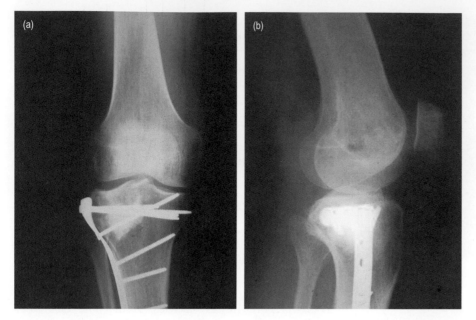

Figure 73.5 Case 1: postoperative AP (a) and lateral (b) views of postoperative fixation with calcium phosphate in place.

Relevance

Periarticular fractures are common injuries that result from indirect coronal and/or direct axial compressive forces. As the patient ages, the fracture pattern is usually a split depression type without associated ligamentous injury. Surgical guidelines advocate anatomic reduction, re-establishment of the long bone alignment, subchondral bone grafting to support the articular cartilage, and stable internal fixation.[2]

Findings

Two recent prospective, randomized, multicenter trials have studied the use of calcium phosphate bone substitutes in periarticular fractures. Russell et al. compared the treatment of subarticular bone defects in tibial plateau fractures with conventional autogenous iliac bone graft (AIBG) to bioabsorbable calcium phosphate paste (alpha-BSM, Etex Corporation).[2] All fractures united in both groups within the same time periods.

There was an unexpected statistically significant (p = 0.009, Fisher's exact two-tailed test) higher rate of articular subsidence in the AIBG group compared to the alpha-BSM group. Subsidence of 2 mm or more on the AP radiographs was found in 31% of patients in the AIBG group compared to 8% in the alpha-BSM group in the final evaluation. This provided level I evidence that bioabsorbable calcium phosphate material, such as alpha-BSM, appeared to be a better choice for treatment of subarticular defects than AIBG in tibial plateau fractures.

Johal et al. performed a similar randomized controlled trial (RCT) on os calcis fractures comparing open reduction and internal fixation (ORIF) plus alpha-BSM to ORIF alone in the treatment of calcaneal bone voids encountered after operative treatment of displaced intraarticular fractures of the calcaneus.[3] There was no difference between the groups in the degree of collapse of Bohler's angle at 6 weeks and 3 months when compared to initial postoperative values. However, at 6 months the mean collapse of the alpha-BSM and ORIF group was 5.6° and ORIF alone was 10.6°. This was statistically significant (p < 0.01).

Recommendations

- For a subarticular defect in metaphyseal bone, ORIF plus calcium phosphate provides better support for the elevated subarticular bone and prevents late subsidence [overall quality: high]
- There is no evidence to support the use of calcium phosphate in acute diaphyseal fractures or nonunions

Question 2: What type of bone graft should be used: autograft, allograft, or a calcium phosphate bone substitute?

Autogenous bone graft, typically from the iliac crest, has been stated in the past to be the gold standard of bone grafting. However, it is associated with donor site morbidity, including chronic pain and wound complications.[5–9,12,13] Alternative grafting materials for filling fracture voids include allograft and synthetic bone materials. Although using allograft avoids the donor site morbidity associated with autograft, it also can lead to complications including potential disease transmission, histoincompatibility, and possibly lower union rates.[10,14,15] Synthetic bone materials, such as calcium phosphate bone cement therefore appear to be an attractive alternative. They perform better acutely and over the first year, and lack the disadvantage of bone site morbidity or the potential for infection and disease transmission associated with allograft.

There are several narrative review articles that address the use of bone grafting in fractures and trauma situations.[16–19] In addition Bajammal et al. have completed a meta-analysis of studies comparing calcium phosphate bone cement to bone graft.[1] The meta-analysis included 15 RCTs. The studies had documented outcomes that included pain, maintenance of fracture reduction, infection, and functional outcomes.

The meta-analysis suggested that the use of calcium phosphate bone cement in treatment of factures in adult patients is associated with lower incidences of pain and loss of fracture reduction; lower infection rates in radius fractures; and likely improved functional outcomes.

Recommendation

• Calcium phosphate avoids the need for a second incision to harvest autograft and results in a reduction in assessed pain and better maintenance of subarticular reduction

Question 3: What are the features of calcium phosphate that make it suitable as a bone substitute?

Findings

Calcium phosphate synthetic bone substitutes have been investigated as devices by the U.S. Food and Drug Authority (FDA) and by industry over the last number of years. Initially animal studies were done with critical defects in rats, dogs, and sheep.[20] Biomechanical studies were then undertaken, such as Trenholm et al.'s paper,[21] indicating that calcium phosphate (alpha-BSM) in proximal tibias was stronger than the cancellous bone graft used to repair periarticular fractures (Figure 73.6).

Similar substances such as calcium sulfate and calcium phosphate resins have not been as successful. A study by Petruskevicius looking at Osteoset (Wright Medical) vs. no bone graft showed no difference in the amount of bone in the defect.[4] The Osteoset pellets were almost resorbed after 6 weeks. A study looking at the use of calcium sulfate in nonunions demonstrated no improvement in bone healing, an increased infection rate, and increased wound drainage.[11] Calcium sulfate cement does not perform in the same way as calcium phosphate cement. Because of its early resorption it has also been noted to cause an early drainage in the wound that resembles very liquid white fluid. This has been confused with pus in some cases, so it has to be evaluated very carefully if used in cases prone to infection.

Kryptonite (Doctor's Research Group, Inc.), a calcium phosphate resin, has been mostly evaluated in the spine. It

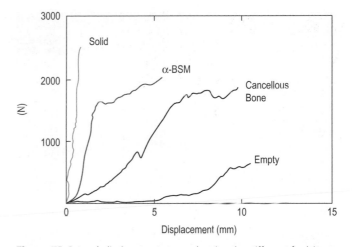

Figure 73.6 Load–displacement curves showing the stiffness of calcium phosphate (alpha-BSM) compared to solid bone, cancellous bone, and a tibial plateau defect with no fill. Reproduced with permission from Trenholm A, Landry S, McLaughlin K, et al. Comparative fixation of tibial plateau fractures using a-BSM, a calcium phosphate cement, versus cancellous bone graft. J Orthop Trauma 2005;19:698–702.[21]

seems to work as an adhesive material. Unfortunately, for subarticular fractures it does not resorb at all. Bone does seem to grow around it and perhaps into the pores, but very little if any resorption occurs. Its use therefore appears to be in those areas where one might normally use polymethylmethacrylate cement. There are many ongoing on- and off-label studies, but no compelling level I information to date. This substance should only be used in acute fractures where prospective studies are being performed at this time.

Recommendations

• Calcium sulfate is not recommended for nonunions or periarticular fractures [overall quality: high]
• Osteoset T may be used carefully to allow a depot of tobramycin in the local area [overall quality: high]
• There is not enough evidence to support the use of calcium phosphate resins; therefore, these should only be used for acute fractures as part of a clinical trial.

Question 4: When does the calcium phosphate resorb?

Case 2 clarification

Initial management consists of plating the posterior medial plateau fragment to buttress it in place. This is followed by a lateral approach with a plate and the use of calcium phosphate to prevent late collapse (Figure 73.7). Beta-BSM putty was placed into the subarticular defect (Figure 73.8). The final radiographs illustrate resorption of the calcium phosphate (Figure 73.9). Figure 73.10 illustrates the correct position for the skin incisions for this simultaneous approach.

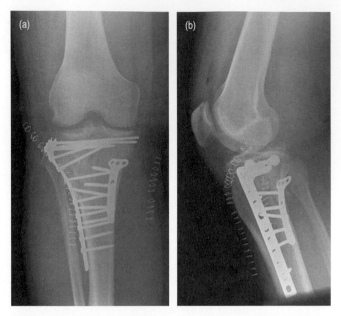

Figure 73.7 Case 2: postoperative AP (a) and lateral (b) views showing fixation and the graft in place laterally.

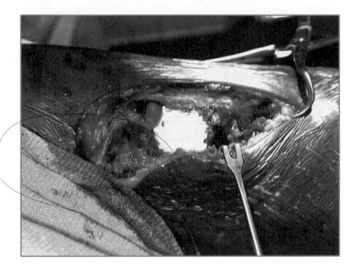

Figure 73.8 Case 2: insertion of calcium phosphate into the lateral defect.

Findings

According to Russell et al., gradual reduction in density of alpha-BSM was observed on successive radiographs, but approximately 10% of the material was still visible at 1 year in the majority of patients.[2] At 2 years it is no longer visible on plain radiographs. However, CT scans were not done on these patients so it could still be present in a microscopic sense.

Recommendation

• Calcium phosphate is clinically resorbed by 1 year [overall quality: high]

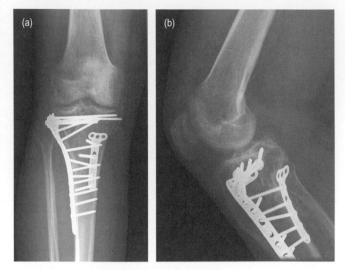

Figure 73.9 Case 2: postoperative AP (a) and lateral (b) views showing the graft nearly resorbed.

Question 5: Are there any other benefits to using calcium phosphate?

Case 3 clarification

A closed reduction was performed and the radius pinned with two crossed Kirchner wires (K-wires). Gamma-BSM putty was injected into the dorsal comminuted area (Figure 73.11).

Findings

According to the meta-analysis by Bajammal et al., the use of calcium phosphate reduces the risk of infection in distal radius fractures.[1] This is in addition to better maintenance of the articular reduction. Calcium phosphate by itself will not provide stability. It must be only used as addition to the usual fixation.

The cost of autogenous bone graft harvesting was investigated in a study by St. John et al.[22] The direct and indirect costs involved in harvesting iliac crest were gathered from a cross-section of hospitals in the United States by means of a questionnaire completed by both finance and surgical staff. The study concluded the mean cost of autologous bone graft is estimated to be $4,154, assuming a hospital stay extended by 1 day. In comparison, 10 mL of alpha-BSM, an amount commonly used in Russell's trial,[2] has an average cost of US$1270. Additional cost savings include no additional tray instrumentation and a reduction in operating time.

Recommendations

• Calcium phosphate reduces infection risk in distal radius fractures when used in addition to fixation [overall quality: moderate]

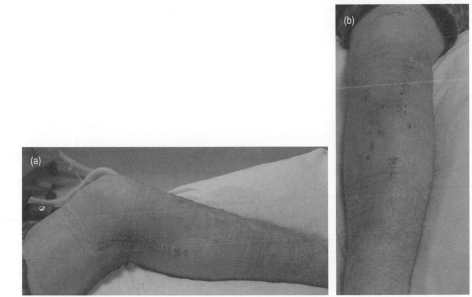

Figure 73.10 Case 2: location of the skin incision for the posterior medial approach (a) and the lateral approach (b).

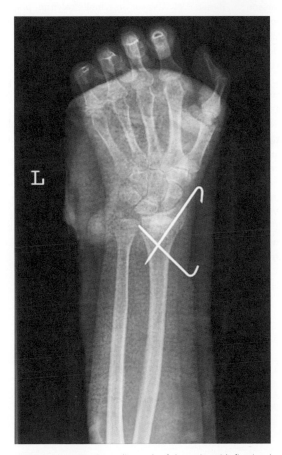

Figure 73.11 Postoperative radiograph of the wrist with fixation (crossed Kirschner wires) and calcium phosphate to fill the dorsal defect.

• Inclusive healthcare costs are actually less with calcium phosphate than iliac crest autograft if it saves the patient a day or more in hospital [overall quality: moderate]

Summary of recommendations

• For a subarticular defect in metaphyseal bone, using fixation plus calcium phosphate provides better support for the elevated bone and prevents late subsidence
• There is no evidence to support the use of calcium phosphate in acute diaphyseal fractures or nonunions
• Calcium phosphate avoids the need for a second incision to harvest autograft and results in less pain and less loss of fracture reduction
• Calcium sulfate is not recommended for nonunions or peri-articular fractures
• Osteoset T may be used carefully to allow a depot of tobramycin in the local area
• There is not enough evidence to support the use of calcium phosphate resins; therefore, these should only be used for acute fractures as part of a clinical trial
• Calcium phosphate is clinically resorbed by 1 year
• Calcium phosphate reduces infection risk in distal radius fractures when used in addition to fixation
• Inclusive healthcare costs are actually less with calcium phosphate than iliac crest autograft if it saves the patient a day or more in hospital

Conclusion

When dealing with a fresh periarticular fracture with a contained defect in the metaphysis of the bone, it appears that the literature would support the following: if two techniques are equally successful, it seems logical that the simpler procedure should be the surgeon's first choice. Bone grafting for subarticular defects in periarticular fractures should be discouraged in favor of bioresorbable calcium phosphate material in order to improve the early maintenance of the subchondral reduction, improve pain and prevent late collapse.

References

1. Bajammal SS, Zlowodzki M, Lelwica A, et al. The use of calcium phosphate bone cement in fracture treatment. A meta-analysis of randomized trials. J Bone Joint Surg Am 2008;90:1186–96.

2. Russell TA, Leighton RK. Comparison of autogenous bone graft and endothermic calcium phosphate cement for defect augmentation in tibial plateau fractures. A multicenter, prospective, randomized study. J Bone Joint Surg Am 2008;90:2057–61.

3. Johal HS, Buckley RE, Le IL, et al. A prospective randomized controlled trial of a bioresorbable calcium phosphate paste (alpha-BSM) in treatment of displaced intra-articular calcaneal fractures. J Trauma 2009;67:875–82.

4. Petruskevicius J, Nielsen S, Kaalund S, et al. No effect of Osteoset, a bone graft substitute, on bone healing in humans: a prospective randomized double-blind study. Acta Orthop Scand 2002;73:575–8.

5. Silber JS, Anderson DG, Daffner SD, et al. Donor site morbidity after anterior iliac crest bone harvest for single-level anterior cervical discectomy and fusion. Spine 2003;28:134–9.

6. Goulet JA, Senunas LE, DeSilva GL, et al. Autogenous iliac crest bone graft. Complications and functional assessment. Clin Orthop Relat Res, 1997;339:76–81.

7. Arrington ED, Smith WJ, Chambers HG, et al. Complications of iliac crest bone graft harvesting. Clin Orthop Relat Res, 1996;329:300–9.

8. Summers BN, Eisenstein SM. Donor site pain from the ilium. A complication of lumbar spine fusion. J Bone Joint Surg Br 1989;71:677–80.

9. Younger EM, Chapman MW. Morbidity at bone graft donor sites. J Orthop Trauma 1989;3:192–5.

10. Abidi NA, Dhawan S, Gruen GS, et al. Wound-healing risk factors after open reduction and internal fixation of calcaneal fractures. Foot Ankle Int 1998;19:856–61.

11. Ziran BH, Smith WR, Lahti Z, et al. Use of calcium-based demineralized bone matrix/allograft product for nonunions and posttraumatic reconstruction of the appendicular skeleton: preliminary results and complications. J Trauma 2007;63(6):1324–8.

12. Auleda J, Bianchi A, Tibau R, et al. Hernia through iliac crest defects. A report of four cases. Int Orthop 1995;19:367–9.

13. Kurz LT, Garfin SR, Booth RE, Jr. Harvesting autogenous iliac bone grafts. A review of complications and techniques. Spine 1989;14:1324–31.

14. Stevenson S. Biology of bone grafts. Orthop Clin North Am 1999;30:543–52.

15. Boyce T, Edwards J, Scarborough N. Allograft bone. The influence of processing on safety and performance. Orthop Clin North Am 1999;30:571–81.

16. Ladd AL, Pliam NB. Use of bone-graft substitutes in distal radius fractures. J Am Acad Orthop Surg 1999;7:279–90.

17. Larsson S, Bauer TW. Use of injectable calcium phosphate cement for fracture fixation: a review. Clin Orthop Relat Res 2002;395:23–32.

18. Moore WR, Graves SE, Bain GI. Synthetic bone graft substitutes. Aust N Z J Surg 2001;71:354–61.

19. Szpalski M, Gunzburg R. Applications of calcium phosphate-based cancellous bone void fillers in trauma surgery. Orthopedics 2002;25:s601–9.

20. Welch RD, Zhang H, Bronson DG. Experimental tibial plateau fractures augmented with calcium phosphate cement or autologous bone graft. J Bone Joint Surg Am 2003;85:222–31.

21. Trenholm A, Landry S, McLaughlin K, et al. Comparative fixation of tibial plateau fractures using a-BSM, a calcium phosphate cement, versus cancellous bone graft. J Orthop Trauma 2005;19:698–702.

22. St John TA, Vaccaro AR, Sah AP, et al. Physical and monetary costs associated with autogenous bone graft harvesting. Am J Orthop 2003;32:18–23.

74 Damage Control Orthopedics

Philipp Kobbe and Hans-Christoph Pape
University Hospital, Aachen, Germany

Case scenario

A young man was involved in a severe motor vehicle accident. Rescue time was approximately 65 minutes. Upon admission the patient is mechanically ventilated, hemodynamically unstable with a systolic blood pressure of 85 mmHg and has a core body temperature of 33 °C. Obvious findings are diminished ventilation of the right thorax, an extended abdomen, an unstable pelvis, a bilaterally displaced femur, and a displaced right tibia.

Relevant definitions

Polytrauma

The term polytrauma defines a patient with multiple injuries of which at least one injury or the combination of several injuries is life-threatening. When scoring systems are used, patients with an Injury Severity Score (ISS) of 16 points or more are classified as polytrauma.[1]

Definitions

- Injury Severity Score (ISS): an anatomical scoring system that provides an overall score for patients with multiple injuries
- New Injury Severity Score (NISS): a modification of the ISS. In contrast to the ISS, which considers at most one injury per body region, the NISS takes the three most severe injuries regardless of the body region into account

---

- Early total care (ETC): a concept implying the primary definitive management of all major injuries within 24 hours after trauma
- Damage control orthopedics (DCO): minimally invasive surgical techniques are used for the primary stabilization of all major fractures. Based upon the patient's physiological status, temporary stabilization with external fixation for certain fractures is used.

Patient's condition determined by physiology

- *Stable patients* have no immediately life-threatening injuries and respond to initial therapy.
- *Borderline patients* have stabilized in response to initial resuscitative attempts but sustained injuries that put them at risk of rapid deterioration (Table 74.1).
- *Unstable patients* remain hemodynamically unstable despite initial intervention and are at high risk for clinical complications.
- *Patients in extremis* have ongoing uncontrolled blood loss despite resuscitation and may succumb if blood loss is not immediately stopped.

Importance of the problem

During the last decade there has been a debate on whether severely injured patients should be managed by definitive operative care or whether a staged management is favorable. In patients under 45 years of age, trauma is the leading cause of death worldwide, with about 5.8 million deaths/year.[2] Today, motor vehicle accidents account for approximately 1.2 million deaths/year[3] and it has been estimated that this will increase to 8.4 million deaths/year by 2020.[4]

Evidence-Based Orthopedics, First Edition. Edited by Mohit Bhandari.
© 2012 Blackwell Publishing Ltd. Published 2012 by Blackwell Publishing Ltd.

Table 74.1 Clinical features or injuries defining the borderline patient[28]

ISS >40
Hypothermia below 35°C
Patients with bilateral femoral fracture
Multiple injuries (ISS >20) in association with thoracic trauma (AIS >2)
Multiple injuries in association with severe abdominal or pelvic injury and hemorrhagic shock at presentation (systolic BP <90 mmHg)
Radiographic evidence of pulmonary contusion
Patients with moderate or severe head injuries (AIS ≥3)
Initial mean pulmonary arterial pressure >24 mmHg or a >6 mmHg rise in pulmonary artery pressure during intramedullary nailing or other operative intervention

AIS, Abbreviated Injury Scale; BP, blood pressure; ISS, Injury Severity Score.

Severe traumatic injuries have a higher socioeconomic impact in the age group under 45 years than cardiovascular or neoplastic diseases.[5]

Top four questions

1. Does DCO reduce primary operation time and blood loss?
2. Does DCO reduce systemic complications and mortality in the severely injured patient?
3. Does DCO influence the posttraumatic inflammatory response?
4. Is DCO associated with an increased risk of local infection?

Question 1: Does DCO reduce primary operation time and blood loss?

Case clarification
The question arises whether this patient's fractures should be managed with definitive operation right away or whether they should be stabilized with external fixation and minimally invasive techniques.

Relevance
Lengthy operations with increased blood loss after trauma are a heavy burden for the polytraumatized patient.

Current opinion
DCO reduces initial operation time and blood loss.

Finding the evidence
- PubMed (www.ncbi.nlm.nih.gov/pubmed/) advanced search using [Text Word]: "damage control" AND "blood loss" as well as "damage control" AND "operation time"

Quality of the evidence
Level II
- 1 prospective controlled trial[6]

Level III
- 2 retrospective cohorts[7,8]

Findings
In their retrospective study, Scalea et al. compared blood loss and operation time in patients with fractures of the femur either managed with ETC (n = 284) or DCO (n = 43).[7] Median operating room time for patients managed with DCO was 35 minutes with an estimated blood loss of 90 mL. In patients managed with ETC the median operating room time was 135 minutes with an estimated blood loss of 400 mL. Similar results have been reported by Tuttle et al., who found a significantly reduced operation time (22 minutes vs. 125 minutes) and blood loss (37 mL vs. 330 mL) in patients with femoral shaft fractures managed with DCO (n = 55) as compared to ETC (n = 42).[8]

These findings have been confirmed by Taeger et al. who managed 75 patients with DCO of which they converted 57 patients in the course of surgery (hypothetical ETC).[6] Operation time for DCO was 62 ± 30 minutes as compared to a significantly higher mean operation time for conversion (hypothetical ETC) of 233 ± 19 minutes. Also, blood loss was significantly reduced for DCO (<50 mL) as compared to hypothetical ETC (472 mL).

Recommendation
- In critical patients DCO is useful to perform fracture stabilization faster and less bloodily than ETC [overall quality: moderate]

Question 2: Does DCO reduce systemic complications and mortality in the severely injured patient?

Case clarification
The patient is managed according to DCO principles. Although severely injured, he survives and develops no signs of organ failure.

Relevance
A subset of polytraumatized patients does not tolerate ETC right after trauma and dies during the lengthy primary surgery.

Current opinion

The trauma population is a very heterogenic group and the application of the DCO concept does not make sense in all patients. Most patients (~85%) can be treated with ETC without complications; however, a subset of severely injured patients, especially those with severe thoracic and head injuries, appears to benefit from DCO.

Finding the evidence

• PubMed (www.ncbi.nlm.nih.gov/pubmed/) advanced search using time interval from 1990 to present in English language with the following [Text Word]:
  ◦ "timing of stabilization" OR "timing of fixation" AND "mortality" OR "morbidity"
  ◦ "damage control" AND "mortality" OR "morbidity"
  ◦ "delayed stabilization" OR "delayed fixation" AND "mortality" OR "morbidity"
  ◦ "early stabilization" OR "early fixation" AND "mortality" OR "morbidity"

Quality of the evidence

Level I
• 1 study investigating systemic complications[9]

Level III
• Several retrospective studies[7,10–21]

Findings

Including all suitable studies in the analysis it appears that DCO principles have no benefit in terms of mortality as compared to ETC; however, several included studies have major limitations, e.g., a significantly higher ISS in the DCO group (Figure 74.1).[7,10,13,16,19] Analyzing the effect of DCO

without these biased studies shows a trend towards a reduced mortality in the overall trauma population managed with DCO as compared to ETC (Figure 74.2). The benefit of DCO becomes even more obvious once the heterogenic trauma population is divided into subgroups (stable, borderline, unstable, in extremis). This is supported by Morshed et al. with their retrospective study including 3,069 patients and by the only available prospective study investigating the incidence of acute lung injury, showing that ETC is fine in stable patients but has a higher risk of mortality and acute lung injury (ALI) in more severely injured patients (borderline patients) than DCO.[9,17] Prospective randomized clinical trials (RCTs) for the management of femur fractures in polytraumatized patients are listed in Table 74.2.

Nonetheless, the evidence for DCO is difficult to establish since most studies are retrospective cohorts which are not matched for ISS. Further, the impact of several studies is limited due to selection bias: in many countries the patient is cleared for surgery either by the Emergency Department or intensive care unit (ICU) physician, thus these studies only investigate the method of primary stabilization in stable patients who usually do not benefit from DCO; some studies even equate DCO with plaster stabilization of long-bone fractures.

Recommendation

• So far there is no evidence that the concept of DCO reduces mortality in the overall polytrauma population; however, there is growing evidence that severely injured patients (categorized as borderline, unstable, or in extremis) benefit from DCO [overall quality: moderate]

Study	Major Limitations	ETC Events	Total	DCO Events	Total	Weight	Odds Ratio M-H, Fixed, 95% CI
Brundage et al. 2002	ISS significantly higher in DCO group	15	399	6	117	9.3%	0.72 [0.27, 1.91]
Charash et al. 1994	none	4	105	3	33	4.6%	0.40 [0.08, 1.87]
Fakhry et al. 1994	none	8	212	2	120	2.6%	2.31 [0.48, 11.08]
Hofman et al. 1991	restricted Fx stabilization in DCO group	2	15	20	43	9.4%	0.18 [0.04, 0.88]
Jaicks et al. 1997	none	2	19	0	14	0.5%	4.14 [0.18, 93.36]
Kalb et al. 1998	none	8	84	3	39	3.9%	1.26 [0.32, 5.05]
Kotwika et al. 1990	no Fx stabilization in DCO group	7	51	11	49	10.1%	0.55 [0.19, 1.56]
Morshed et al. 2009	none	65	1759	43	1310	49.6%	1.13 [0.76, 1.67]
Poole et al. 1992	none	2	46	0	26	0.6%	2.98 [0.14, 64.41]
Reynolds et al. 1995	ISS significantly higher in DCO group	2	35	0	70	0.3%	10.52 [0.49, 225.34]
Scalea et al. 2000	ISS significantly higher in DCO group	1	284	4	43	7.2%	0.03 [0.00, 0.32]
Starr et al. 2001	none	0	14	0	14		Not estimable
Velmahos et al. 1998	none	1	22	2	25	1.9%	0.55 [0.05, 6.49]
Total (95% CI)			**3045**		**1903**	**100.0%**	**0.91 [0.69, 1.22]**
Total events		117		94			

Heterogeneity: Chi^2 = 21.45, df = 11 (P = 0.03); I^2 = 49%
Test for overall effect: Z = 0.61 (P = 0.54)

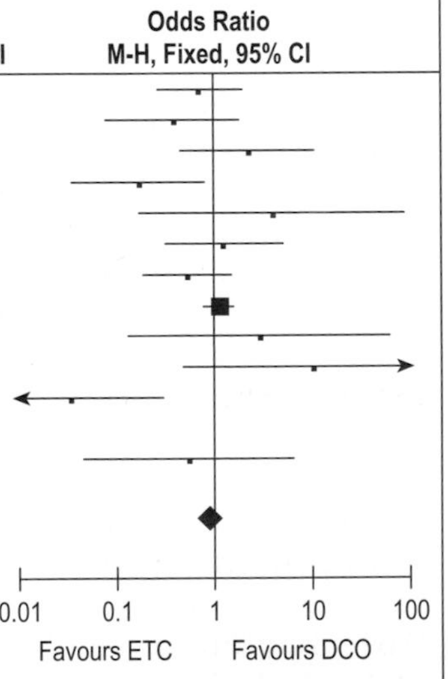

Odds Ratio M-H, Fixed, 95% CI — scale 0.01 0.1 1 10 100 — Favours ETC / Favours DCO

Figure 74.1 Overview of cohort studies investigating the incidence of mortality depending on the initial surgical approach (ETC vs. DCO).

Study or Subgroup	ETC Events	Total	DCO Events	Total	Weight	Odds Ratio M-H, Fixed, 95% CI
Charash et al. 1994	4	105	3	33	7.2%	0.40 [0.08, 1.87]
Fakhry et al. 1994	8	212	2	120	4.0%	2.31 [0.48, 11.08]
Jaicks et al. 1997	2	19	0	14	0.8%	4.14 [0.18, 93.36]
Kalb et al. 1998	8	84	3	39	6.1%	1.26 [0.32, 5.05]
Morshed et al. 2009	65	1759	43	1310	77.9%	1.13 [0.76, 1.67]
Poole et al. 1992	2	46	0	26	1.0%	2.98 [0.14, 64.41]
Starr et al. 2001	0	14	0	14		Not estimable
Velmahos et al. 1998	1	22	2	25	2.9%	0.55 [0.05, 6.49]
Total (95% CI)		2261		1581	100.0%	1.16 [0.82, 1.64]
Total events	90		53			

Heterogeneity: Chi² = 3.98, df = 6 (P = 0.68); I² = 0%
Test for overall effect: Z = 0.84 (P = 0.40)

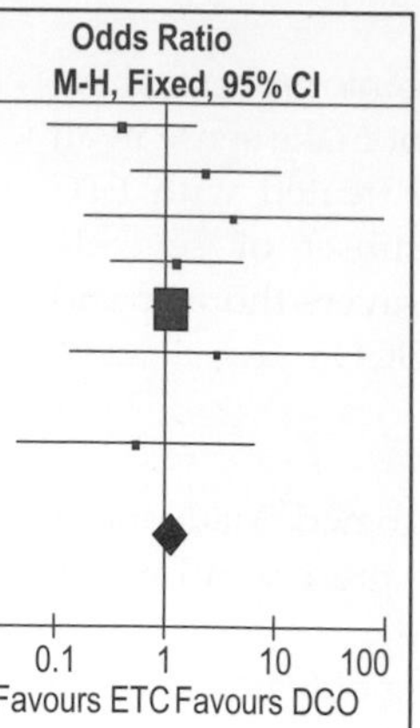

Figure 74.2 Exclusion of studies with major limitations shows a trend towards a favorable DCO treatment in the overall trauma population.

Table 74.2 Prospective randomized trials for the management of femur fractures in severely injured patients[23,29,30]

Study	Year	Level of evidence
Bone et al.	1989	II (moderate)
Pape et al.	2003	I (high)
Can. Orthop. Trauma Soc.	2006	I (high)

Question 3: Does DCO influence the posttraumatic inflammatory response?

Case clarification
A major risk factor for systemic complications is an overwhelming posttraumatic inflammatory response.

Relevance
The systemic inflammatory response after trauma is recognized as a part of the physiologic reaction and called the "first-hit" phenomenon.[22] The "second hit" is observed to be compounded by factors such as the type of surgical procedure, blood loss, sepsis, and ischemia, all of which can increase the inflammatory response.[22] The overriding principle of damage control surgery is therefore to minimize subsequent stresses imposed upon unstable patients with high risk of posttraumatic complications.

Current opinion
The DCO concept reduces the second-hit phenomenon and lowers the inflammatory response.

Finding the evidence
• PubMed (www.ncbi.nlm.nih.gov/pubmed/) advanced search using [Text Word]: "inflammation" AND "fracture stabilization" as well as "inflammatory response" AND "damage control orthopedics" OR "early total care"

Quality of the evidence
Level I
• 1 prospective randomized multicenter study[23]

Level III
• 1 retrospective clinical investigation[24]

Findings
In a prospective randomized multicenter study, 35 polytraumatized patients (ISS >16) with long-bone shaft fractures were included.[23] Patients were either managed with ETC (n = 17) or with DCO (n = 18) and serum inflammatory markers were measured pre-, peri-, and postoperatively. The main findings are that a sustained increase in the inflammatory burden was only obvious in the patients managed with ETC, but not after initial external fixation and secondary conversion to an intramedullary implant. These data are supported by a cohort of 174 patients with femoral shaft fractures and a NISS of 20 or more.[24] Patients in the DCO group (n = 97) had a significantly higher NISS than those in the ETC group (n = 77), but patients managed with ETC showed a significantly higher systemic inflammatory response.

Recommendation
• There is some evidence that DCO minimizes the second-hit phenomenon, and these findings may become clinically relevant in patients at high risk of developing systemic complications [overall quality: moderate]

Question 4: Is DCO associated with an increased risk of local infection?

Case clarification
The patient's fractures were converted to intramedullary implants between days 8–20 after trauma. The patient developed osteomyelitis of his right tibia, resulting in lower leg amputation.

Relevance

Pin tract infection can be the source of severe complications, such as osteomyelitis and sepsis.

Current opinion

We perform a conversion to definitive implants once the systemic inflammatory response has been resolved, which is usually around days 5–7 after trauma. In cases of an unknown inflammatory status, inflammatory mediators such as serum interleukin-6 (IL-6) can be measured.

Finding the evidence

- PubMed (www.ncbi.nlm.nih.gov/pubmed/) advanced search using [Text Word]: "damage control" OR "external fixation" AND "infection"

Quality of the evidence

Level III

- 3 retrospective studies directly comparing the incidence of infection between groups of early vs. delayed definitive care[7,25,26]
- Several studies reporting on the incidence of infection following external fixation in polytrauma patients

Findings

Van den Bossche et al. showed that external fixation for femoral shaft fractures in severely injured patients is a safe option in terms of infectious complications (neither superficial nor deep infections).[27]. Harwood et al. showed that the risk of infection following DCO was equivalent as compared with primary definitive care (~4.5%).[25] Equivalent results have been reported by Scalea et al. and Nowotarski et al., who found no significant differences in infectious complications comparing DCO with ETC.[7,26] Although no increased risk of infection following external fixation could be shown, contamination of pin sites was significantly more likely when conversion to intramedullary nailing occurred later than 14 days after trauma.[25]

Recommendation

- There is some evidence that DCO is associated with an increased risk of local infection. In view of the inflammatory burden, conversion to a definitive, biomechanical superior implant should not be performed before days 5–7 after trauma. However, due to an increased risk of local pin site contamination it is recommended that the conversion should be performed before day 14 [overall quality: low]

Summary of recommendations

Overall there is a moderate level of evidence for the following recommendations:

- DCO should be applied in patients who fail to tolerate primary lengthy operations with an associated increase of intraoperative inflammation and blood loss. Typically, these are patients who have been defined as unstable or in extremis
- Patients defined as borderline should be re-evaluated during surgery
- When in doubt about the patient's condition, treat according to DCO principles, because DCO is a safer initial approach, significantly decreasing the initial operative exposure and blood loss

---

Conclusions

DCO reduces the primary operative burden by reducing intraoperative inflammation, blood loss, and operation time. This is of minor importance in stable patients but has clinical relevance for critical patients in the initial treatment phase. These patients should be managed with external fixators which should be converted to a definitive fixation method within 14 days after trauma.

References

1. Long WB, Bachulis BL, Hynes GD. Accuracy and relationship of mechanisms of injury, trauma score, and injury severity score in identifying major trauma. Am J Surg 1986; 151(5):581–4.

2. Hauser CJ. Preclinical models of traumatic, hemorrhagic shock. Shock 2005;24(Suppl 1):24–32.

3. Oestern HJ. Polytrauma—Preclinical and Clinical Management. Elsevier, Philadelphia, 2007.

4. Murray CJ, Lopez AD. Alternative projections of mortality and disability by cause 1990–2020: Global Burden of Disease Study. Lancet 1997;349(9064):1498–504.

5. Westhoff J, Hildebrand F, Grotz M, Richter M, Pape HC, Krettek C. Trauma care in Germany. Injury 2003;34(9):674–83.

6. Taeger G, Ruchholtz S, Waydhas C, Lewan U, Schmidt B, Nast-Kolb D. Damage control orthopedics in patients with multiple injuries is effective, time saving, and safe. J Trauma 2005;59(2):409–16.

7. Scalea TM, Boswell SA, Scott JD, Mitchell KA, Kramer ME, Pollak AN. External fixation as a bridge to intramedullary nailing for patients with multiple injuries and with femur fractures: damage control orthopedics. J Trauma 2000;48(4):613–21.

8. Tuttle MS, Smith WR, Williams AE, et al. Safety and efficacy of damage control external fixation versus early definitive stabilization for femoral shaft fractures in the multiple-injured patient. J Trauma 2009;67(3):602–5.

9. Pape HC, Rixen D, Morley J, et al. Impact of the method of initial stabilization for femoral shaft fractures in patients with multiple injuries at risk for complications (borderline patients). Ann Surg 2007;246(3):491–9.

10. Brundage SI, McGhan R, Jurkovich GJ, Mack CD, Maier RV. Timing of femur fracture fixation: effect on outcome in patients with thoracic and head injuries. J Trauma 2002;52(2):299–307.

11. Charash WE, Fabian TC, Croce MA. Delayed surgical fixation of femur fractures is a risk factor for pulmonary failure independent of thoracic trauma. J Trauma 1994;37(4):667–72.

12. Fakhry SM, Rutledge R, Dahners LE, Kessler D. Incidence, management, and outcome of femoral shaft fracture: a statewide population-based analysis of 2805 adult patients in a rural state. J Trauma 1994;37(2):255–60.

13. Hofman PA, Goris RJ. Timing of osteosynthesis of major fractures in patients with severe brain injury. J Trauma 1991;31(2): 261–3.

14. Jaicks RR, Cohn SM, Moller BA. Early fracture fixation may be deleterious after head injury. J Trauma 1997;42(1):1–5.

15. Kalb DC, Ney AL, Rodriguez JL, et al. Assessment of the relationship between timing of fixation of the fracture and secondary brain injury in patients with multiple trauma. Surgery 1998;124(4):739–44.

16. Kotwica Z, Balcewicz L, Jagodzinski Z. Head injuries coexistent with pelvic or lower extremity fractures–early or delayed osteosynthesis. Acta Neurochir (Wien) 1990;102(1–2):19–21.

17. Morshed S, Miclau T, III, Bembom O, Cohen M, Knudson MM, Colford JM, Jr. Delayed internal fixation of femoral shaft fracture reduces mortality among patients with multisystem trauma. J Bone Joint Surg Am 2009;91(1):3–13.

18. Poole GV, Miller JD, Agnew SG, Griswold JA. Lower extremity fracture fixation in head-injured patients. J Trauma 1992;32(5): 654–9.

19. Reynolds MA, Richardson JD, Spain DA, Seligson D, Wilson MA, Miller FB. Is the timing of fracture fixation important for the patient with multiple trauma? Ann Surg 1995;222(4):470–8.

20. Starr AJ. Timing of femoral fracture stabilization. J Bone Joint Surg Am 2001;83 (2):293–4.

21. Velmahos GC, Arroyo H, Ramicone E, et al. Timing of fracture fixation in blunt trauma patients with severe head injuries. Am J Surg 1998;176(4):324–9.

22. Giannoudis PV. Current concepts of the inflammatory response after major trauma: an update. Injury 2003;34(6):397–404.

23. Pape HC, Grimme K, van Griensven M, et al. Impact of intramedullary instrumentation versus damage control for femoral fractures on immunoinflammatory parameters: prospective randomized analysis by the EPOFF Study Group. J Trauma 2003;55(1):7–13.

24. Harwood PJ, Giannoudis PV, van Griensven M, Krettek C, Pape HC. Alterations in the systemic inflammatory response after early total care and damage control procedures for femoral shaft fracture in severely injured patients. J Trauma 2005;58(3): 446–52.

25. Harwood PJ, Giannoudis PV, Probst C, Krettek C, Pape HC. The risk of local infective complications after damage control procedures for femoral shaft fracture. J Orthop Trauma 2006;20(3): 181–9.

26. Nowotarski PJ, Turen CH, Brumback RJ, Scarboro JM. Conversion of external fixation to intramedullary nailing for fractures of the shaft of the femur in multiply injured patients. J Bone Joint Surg Am 2000;82(6):781–8.

27. Van den Bossche MR, Broos PL, Rommens PM. Open fractures of the femoral shaft, treated with osteosynthesis or temporary external fixation. Injury 1995;26(5):323–5.

28. Pape HC, Giannoudis PV, Krettek C, Trentz O. Timing of fixation of major fractures in blunt polytrauma: role of conventional indicators in clinical decision making. J Orthop Trauma 19(8): 2005;551–62.

29. Reamed versus unreamed intramedullary nailing of the femur: comparison of the rate of ARDS in multiple injured patients. J Orthop Trauma 2006;20(6):384–7.

30. Bone LB, Johnson KD, Weigelt J, Scheinberg R. Early versus delayed stabilization of femoral fractures. A prospective randomized study. J Bone Joint Surg Am 1989;71(3):336–40.

75 Mangled Extremity

Ted V. Tufescu
University of Manitoba, Winnipeg, MB, Canada

Case scenario

A motorcyclist collides with a car at highway speed. He is brought to the Emergency Department with a severe open injury of his leg.

Relevant anatomy

Any extremity may be mangled. At least three out of four tissue groups are affected (integument/soft tissue, nerve, vessels and bone).[1] Lower extremities are more commonly involved, with 63% tibia and 23% femur fractures.[2]

Arterial injuries can determine the prognosis of the limb,[3] while nerve injury is less important.[4] The most frequent vascular injury is to the popliteal artery,[2,5] which enters the popliteal fossa via the adductor canal, at the distal femur. Here it travels immediately posterior to the knee. It then exits the popliteal fossa and enters the posterior compartment of the leg under the origin of the soleus muscle. The popliteal artery is therefore fixed at the adductor canal and soleus origin. This places it at risk of being torn with displaced fractures and dislocations about the knee.

Importance of the problem

Although uncommon, this is the most severe limb injury short of traumatic amputation. It frequently results in severe disability and loss of work.[6,7]

In addition, the physician is faced with one of the toughest decisions in medicine: whether the limb should undergo salvage or amputation. Salvage may require multiple, costly procedures,[6] and may result in failure rates as high as 40%.[8–11] Patients with failed salvage would not do it again;[8,11] however, at the time of injury 92% prefer an attempt at salvage.[9] This chapter reviews factors that influence the decision to salvage or amputate the mangled extremity.

Top five questions

Diagnosis

1. When does an open fracture (Gustilo–Anderson grade III) become a mangled extremity?

Therapy

2. What is the expected resource investment for salvage vs. amputation?
3. What patient factors affect success of therapy and return to work?
4. What is the utility of scoring systems in choosing between salvage and amputation?

Prognosis

5. What is the outcome after salvage and amputation?

Question 1: When does an open fracture (Gustilo–Anderson grade III) become a mangled extremity?

Gustilo graded open fractures I through III based on increasing involvement of soft tissue and bone[2]. Grade III fractures are subdivided, with III B requiring soft tissue reconstruction and III C requiring vascular bypass[12].

Evidence-Based Orthopedics, First Edition. Edited by Mohit Bhandari.
© 2012 Blackwell Publishing Ltd. Published 2012 by Blackwell Publishing Ltd.

Case clarification

The emergency physician diagnoses a Gustilo–Anderson IIIB open tibia fracture. He counsels the patient that with current technology, there is little risk of amputation.

Relevance

Understanding when in the spectrum of open fractures amputation becomes a real possibility allows better management decisions.

Current opinion

Current opinion suggests Gustilo–Anderson grade IIIB and IIIC injuries have substantial amputation rates.

Finding the evidence

The search strategy employed was based on a recent systematic review.[12]

- MEDLINE: "leg injuries" AND "(amputation OR limb salvage OR reconstructive surgical procedures)"
- CINAHL: "leg injuries" AND "(amputation OR limb salvage OR reconstructive surgical procedures)"
- EMBASE: "leg injuries" AND "(amputation OR limb salvage OR reconstructive surgical procedures)"

Quality of the evidence

Level III

- 8 studies[3,9,10,13–17]

Findings

Gustilo reported overall amputation rates of 0% for IIIA, 16% for IIIB, and 42% for IIIC fractures.[12]

Primary amputation rate Amputation is primary when it is the planned initial treatment. Data was pooled from five studies.[3,14,15,16,18] The average primary amputation rate was 0% for IIIA fractures (0 of 82), 7% for IIIB (11 of 149) and 44% for IIIC (28 of 63). See Table 75.1.

Delayed amputation rate Delayed amputation follows attempted salvage. Depending on follow-up duration, it is possible that some delayed amputations were missed. Data was pooled from seven studies.[3,9,10,14–17] The average delayed amputation rate was 1% for IIIA fractures (1 of 93), 9% for IIIB (23 of 256), and 36% for IIIC (23 of 64). See Table 75.2.

Recommendations

- Gustilo IIIA fractures are unlikely to require amputation [overall quality: low]
- Gustilo IIIB and IIIC fractures may require amputation [overall quality: low]

Table 75.1 Primary amputation rate (raw data and calculated averages)

	Gustilo–Anderson grade			Reference
	IIIA	IIIB	IIIC	
Primary amputation rate	0% (0 of 42)	7% (5 of 67)		14
	0% (0 of 40)	0% (0 of 18)	45% (10 of 22)	16
		2% (1 of 43)		15
		24% (5 of 21)	72% (13 of 18)	17
			22% (5 of 23)	3
Average primary amputation rate	0% (0 of 82)	7% (11 of 149)	44% (28 of 63)	

Table 75.2 Delayed amputation rate (raw data and calculated averages)

	Gustilo–Anderson grade			Reference
	IIIA	IIIB	IIIC	
Delayed amputation rate	0% (0 of 42)	3% (2 of 67)		14
	0% (0 of 11)	16% (7 of 43)	78% (7 of 9)	15
	2.5% (1 of 40)	6% (1 of 18)	14% (3 of 22)	16
		9% (2 of 22)	60% (3 of 5)	10
		10% (4 of 41)	20% (1 of 5)	9
		11% (7 of 65)		18
			39% (9 of 23)	3
Average delayed amputation rate	1% (1 of 93)	9% (23 of 256)	36% (23 of 64)	

Question 2: What is the expected resource investment for salvage vs. amputation?

Case clarification

This man lives in a remote location 8 hours from the hospital. He would prefer a short hospitalization time so he can rejoin his family.

Relevance

Salvage and amputation place different requirements on the patient and the surgeon. This should be considered before initiating treatment.

Current opinion

Current opinion suggests that limb salvage requires greater resource investment.

Finding the evidence

See Question 1.

Quality of the evidence

Level II
- 1 study[19]

Level III
- 4 studies[9,10,16,20]

Findings

Cost Georgiadis reported a lower acute hospitalization charge ($65,624) for amputation than for salvage ($109,044) (p < 0.006).[10] Hertel reported equal mean annual hospital cost, based on 4 years, for amputation (15,112 Swiss francs) and salvage (17,365 Swiss francs).[16] MacKenzie reported equal long-term hospital costs for amputation ($78,221) and salvage ($81,091).[19] Hertel reported a higher total cost, including pension and loss of wage benefits for amputation (64,000 Swiss francs) than salvage (33,000 Swiss francs) (p < 0.01).[16] Including lifetime prosthesis-related costs, amputation is three times more costly ($509,275) than salvage ($163,282).[19]

Hospitalization and rehabilitation time Georgiadis reported a shorter acute hospitalization for amputation (48 days) than salvage (71 days) (p < 0.05).[10] Dagum reported equal stays for amputation (28 days) and salvage (25 days).[9] Georgiadis reported shorter readmission for amputation (5 days) than for salvage (18 days).[10] Hutchins reported equal total hospital stays, including readmission, for amputation (14 weeks) and for salvage (14.8 weeks).[20] Hertel emphasized the importance of rehabilitation center admission.[16] Total acute and rehabilitation admission times were equal for amputation (101 days) and for salvage (129 days).[20] Hutchins reported shorter outpatient rehabilitation time for amputation (12 months) than for salvage (30 months), although this was self-reported by patients (p < 0.009).[20]

Recommendation

- The cost of salvage and amputation is:
  - probably equal, for in-hospital charges [overall quality: low]

  - higher for amputation, when considering lost wages, pension, and lifetime prosthesis-related charges [overall quality: moderate]
- The duration of hospitalization for salvage and amputation is probably equal [overall quality: low]
- The duration of rehabilitation for salvage and amputation is equal for inpatient and probably shorter for outpatient rehabilitation of amputation patients [overall quality: low]

Question 3: What patient factors affect success of therapy and return to work?

Case clarification

The physician inquires whether the patient's family should be notified. This man divorced after his family business failed. He was unable to find other employment due to poor education, and has no other social support.

Relevance

Patient factors are often overshadowed by the urgency of the situation, but they have an important influence on success of therapy, and may guide necessary counseling.

Current opinion

Current opinion suggests that certain patient factors, such as education level and presence of social support, can affect success of therapy.[6]

Finding the evidence

See Question 1.

Quality of the evidence

Level I
- 2 studies[6,21]

Level II
- 1 study[7]

Level III
- 2 studies[9,20]

Findings

Predictors of outcome Dagum reported patient involvement with legal action was not associated to SF-36 mental component scores or WOMAC pain scores,[9] in a small study. The LEAP (Lower Extremity Assessment Project) studies analyzed a large body of prospectively collected data and measured outcome with the Sickness Impact Profile (SIP).[6,7] The following patient characteristics predicted poor outcome at 2 years:[6] less than high school education, household income below poverty level, being nonwhite, lack of insurance, poor social support network, low level of self-efficacy (confidence in one's ability to resume chief life activities), smoking, and involvement with the legal system for injury compensation. The following predicted poor outcome at 7 years:[7] low education level, older age, female gender, being nonwhite, household income below poverty line, smoking, low self-efficacy, poor self-reported health status before injury, and involvement with the legal system for injury compensation. Success of salvage and amputation was equally influenced.

Predictors of return to work Hutchins reported older age to be inversely related to return to work (RTW).[20] The LEAP study found the following predictors of RTW:[21] age less than 55, being white, high school or college education, being a nonsmoker, average to high self-efficacy and motivation (high job involvement and being in a preinjury job for one or more years). Involvement with the legal system for compensation predicted lower RTW.[21]

Recommendation

• Patient characteristics predicting poor outcome and difficulty with RTW are: older age, being nonwhite, lack of education, poverty, smoking, involvement in disability-compensation litigation, and low self-efficacy [overall level: moderate]

Question 4: What is the utility of scoring systems in choosing between salvage and amputation?

Case clarification

A junior physician calculates a Mangled Extremity Severity Score (MESS) greater than 7.[22] She suggests amputation is warranted.

Scoring systems grade the injury based on physical findings. A score higher than a set threshold is predictive of amputation. MESS is based on injury findings, ischemia time, shock, and age. The threshold for amputation is 7.

Relevance

A limb may be inappropriately amputated if a scoring system is applied without understanding the supporting evidence and its role in clinical practice.

Current opinion

Current opinion suggests that scoring systems should not be considered in isolation, but rather in combination with clinical judgment.

Finding the evidence

See Question 1.

Quality of the evidence

Level I
• 4 studies[22,25,29,30]

Level II
• 6 studies[1,23,24,26,27,28]

Findings

The Mangled Extremity Syndrome Index (MESI) was created in 1985. The authors reported 100% accuracy,[1] but Bonanni reported only 6% sensitivity and 90% specificity.[23] The Predictive Salvage Index (PSI) was created in 1987. The authors reported 78% sensitivity and 100% specificity,[24] while Bonanni reported only 33% sensitivity and 70% specificity.[23] The MESS was created in 1990. Multiple studies reported 100% sensitivity and 100% specificity,[22,25–27] but Bonanni reported only 22% sensitivity and 53% specificity.[23] The Limb Salvage Index (LSI) was created in 1991. The authors reported 100% sensitivity and 100% specificity,[28] while Bonanni reported only 61% sensitivity and 43% specificity.[23] The Nerve injury, Ischemia, Soft tissue injury, Skeletal injury, Shock and Age of patient score (NISSSA) was created in 1994. The authors reported improved sensitivity and specificity compared to the MESS, at the cost of increased complexity.[27] The LEAP study looked at all scoring systems prospectively and found that low scores predicted salvage,[29] but high scores did not predict amputation, as some of these limbs were successfully salvaged.[29] The LEAP group also showed that scoring systems are not predictive of function after salvage.[30]

Recommendation

• Scoring systems predict limb salvage [overall level: high]
• Scoring systems do not predict amputation [overall level: high]
• Scoring systems do not predict function of salvaged limbs [overall level: high]

Question 5: What is the outcome after salvage and amputation?

Case clarification

At 2 year follow-up the patient has ongoing pain and has not returned to work. He wonders if further recovery is expected.

Relevance

Ultimately, patients and physicians must be aware of the outcomes of both limb salvage and amputation. The longest prospective record and measure of outcome is provided by the LEAP study.

Current opinion

Current opinion suggests that patients suffer significant disability after a mangled extremity, regardless of treatment type.[6]

Finding the evidence

See Question 1.

Quality of the evidence
Level I
• 2 studies[4,6]

Level II
• 2 studies[7,31]

Level III
• 5 studies[3,8–11]

Findings
Outcome At 2 years the SIP was the same for salvage and amputation;[6] 42% of all patients had a SIP greater than 10, indicating severe disability.[6] RTW was 49% after salvage and 53% after amputation.[6] At 7 years, 49.4% of all patients had a SIP greater than 10.[7] Between 2 year and 7 year follow-up, rehospitalization was 39.4% for salvage and 33.3% for amputation patients.[7] Through-the-knee amputees had a worse outcome.[7] Most studies support these findings,[8–11] with minor exceptions.[3,9,10] Dagum reported better SF-36 physical function scores after salvage.[9] Georgiadis reported longer time to weightbearing, and more interference of health on work and recreation for salvage.[10] Lange reported greater walking distances after salvage.[3]

Outcome after insensate foot At 2 year follow-up, 55% of patients with an insensate foot had normal plantar sensation.[4] An insensate foot did not lead to worse function at 2 years.[4]

Complications The most common complication after salvage is nonunion (31.5%), usually diagnosed at 6 months.[31] The most common complication after amputation is wound infection (34.2%), which usually occurs at 3 months.[31] Salvage patients have more complications, longer time to complication, and require more interventions.[31]

Recommendation
• Outcome of salvage and amputation is equal [overall level: high]
• Outcome does not improve from 2 to 7 years after injury [overall level: high]
• Lack of plantar sensation is not predictive of long-term sensory status or function [overall level: high]
• Salvage patients have a higher risk of complications [overall level: moderate]

Summary of recommendations

• Gustilo IIIA fractures are unlikely to require amputation, while Gustilo IIIB and IIIC fractures may require amputation

• The cost of salvage and amputation is probably equal for in-hospital charges, but higher for amputation, when considering lost wages, pension and lifetime prosthesis-related charges
• The duration of hospitalization for salvage and amputation is probably equal
• The duration of rehabilitation for salvage and amputation is equal for inpatient and probably shorter for outpatient rehabilitation of amputation patients
• Patient characteristics predicting poor outcome and difficulty with RTW are: older age, being nonwhite, lack of education, poverty, smoking, involvement in disability-compensation litigation, and low self-efficacy
• Scoring systems predict limb salvage but they do not predict amputation or function of salvaged limbs
• Outcome of salvage and amputation is equal, and outcome does not improve from 2 to 7 years after injury
• Lack of plantar sensation is not predictive of long-term sensory status or function
• Limb salvage patients have a higher risk of complications

Conclusions

The decision to salvage or amputate remains difficult. Outcomes are poor with both options. Patient characteristics are not helpful in choosing treatment, and scoring systems provide little guidance. Amputation is more costly, due to prosthesis-related charges, and salvage leads to more complications.

References

1. Gregory RT, Gould RJ, Peclet M, et al. The mangled extremity syndrome (M.E.S.): a severity grading system for multisystem injury of the extremity. J Trauma 1985;25:1147–50.
2. Gustilo RB, Anderson JT. Prevention of infection in the treatment of one thousand and twenty-five open fractures of long bones: retrospective and prospective analyses. J Bone Joint Surg Am 1976;58:453–8.
3. Lange RH, Bach AW, Hansen ST Jr., et al. Open tibial fractures with associated vascular injuries. Prognosis for limb salvage. J Trauma 1985;25:203–8.
4. Bosse MJ, McCarthy ML, Jones AL, et al. Lower Extremity Assessment Project (LEAP) study group: The insensate foot following severe lower extremity trauma: An indication for amputation? J Bone Joint Surg Am 2005;87:2601–8.
5. DeBakey ME, Simeone FA. Battle injuries of the arteries in World War II: an analysis of 2471 cases. Ann Surg 1946;123:534–79.
6. Bosse MJ, MacKenzie EJ, Kellam J, et al. An analysis of outcomes of reconstruction or amputation of leg threatening injuries. N Engl J Med 2002;347:1924–31.

7. MacKenzie EJ, Bosse MJ, Pollak AN, et al. Long-term persistence of disability following severe lower limb trauma: results of a seven year follow-up. J Bone Joint Surg Am 2005;87:1801–9.

8. Dahl B, Andersson AP, Andersen M, et al. Functional and social long term results after free tissue transfer to the lower extremity. Ann Plast Surg 1995;34:372–5.

9. Dagum AB, Best AK, Schemitsch EH, et al. Salvage after severe lower-extremity trauma: Are the outcomes worth the means? Plast Reconstr Surg 1999;103:1212–20.

10. Georgiadis GM, Behrens FF, Joyce MJ, et al. Open tibial fractures with severe soft-tissue loss: limb salvage compared with below-the-knee amputation. J Bone Joint Surg Am 1993;75:1431–41.

11. Fairhurst MJ. The function of below-knee amputee versus the patient with salvaged grade III tibial fracture. Clin Orthop 1994;301:227–32.

12. Busse JW, Jacobs CL, Swiontkowski, et al. Complex limb salvage or early amputation for severe lower-limb injury: a meta-analysis of observational studies. J Orthop Trauma 2006;21:70–76.

13. Gustilo RB, Mendoza RM, Williams DN. Problems in the management of type III (severe) open fractures: a new classification of type III open fractures. J Trauma 1984;24:742–6.

14. Rajasekaran S, Naresh Babu J, Dheenadhayalan J, et al. A score for predicting salvage and outcome in Gustilo type-IIIA and type-IIIB open tibial fractures. J Bone Joint Surg Br 2006;88: 1351–60.

15. Caudle RJ, Stern PJ. Severe open fractures of the tibia. J Bone Joint Surg Am 1987;69:801–7.

16. Hertel R, Strebel N, Ganz R. Amputation versus reconstruction in traumatic defects of the leg: outcome and costs. J Orthop Trauma 1996;10:223–9.

17. Choudry U, Moran S, Karacor Z. Soft-tissue coverage and outcome of Gustilo grade IIIB midshaft tibia fractures: a 15-year experience. Plast Reconstr Surg 2008;122:479–85.

18. Gustilo RB, Gtuninger RP, Davis T. Classification of type III (severe) open fractures relative to treatment and results. Orthopedics 1987;10:1781–8.

19. MacKenzie EJ, Snow Jones A, Bosse MJ, et al. Health-care costs associated with amputation or reconstruction of a limb-threatening injury. J Bone Joint Surg 2007;89:1685–92.

20. Hutchins PM. The outcome of severe tibial injury. Injury 1981;13:216–19.

21. MacKenzie EJ, Bosse MJ, Kellam JF. Early predictors of long-term work disability after major limb trauma. J Trauma 2006; 61:688–94.

22. Helfet DL, Howey T, Sanders R, et al. Limb salvage versus amputation: Preliminary results of the Mangled Extremity Severity Score. Clin Orthop 1990;256:80–6.

23. Bonanni F, Rhodes M. Peclet The futility of predictive scoring of mangled lower extremities. J Trauma 1993;34:99–140.

24. Howe HR Jr., Poole GV Jr., Hansen ST Jr., et al. Salvage of lower extremities following combined orthopaedic and vascular trauma: a predictive salvage index. Am Surg 1987;53:205–8.

25. Johansen K, Daines M, Howey T, et al. Objective criteria accurately predict amputation following lower extremity trauma. J Trauma 1990;30:568–73.

26. Robertson PA. Prediction of amputation after severe lower limb trauma. J Bone Joint Surg Br 1991;73:816–18.

27. McNamara MG, Heckman JD, Corley FG. Severe open fractures of the lower extremity: A retrospective evaluation of the Mangled Extremity Severity Score (MESS). J Orthop Trauma 1994;8:81–7.

28. Russell WL, Sailors DM, Whittle TB, et al. Limb salvage versus traumatic amputation: A decision based on a seven-part predictive index. Ann Surg 1991;213:473–81.

29. Bosse MJ, MacKenzie EJ, Kellam JF, et al. A prospective evaluation of the clinical utility of lower extremity injury severity scores. J Bone Joint Surg Am 2001;83:3–14.

30. Ly TV, Travison TG, Castillo RC, et al. Ability of lower-extremity injury severity scores to predict functional outcome after limb salvage. J Bone Joint Surg Am 2008;90:1738–1743.

31. Harris AM, Althausen PL, Kellam J, et al. Complications following limb- threatening lower extremity trauma. J Orthop Trauma 2009;23:1–6.

V Adult Spine

Adult Spine

76 Mechanical Neck Pain

Gabrielle van der Velde

Toronto Health Economics and Technology Assessment (THETA) Collaborative, University of Toronto, and Institute for Work & Health, Toronto, ON, Canada

Case scenario

A 50 year old woman presents with acute neck pain which she attributes to sleeping in an awkward position. The pain is sharp and tight, and located over the right posterolateral aspect of her neck. The patient also describes a generalized ache involving her right upper back and arm.

Relevant anatomy

Nonspecific (mechanical) neck pain is a symptom-based diagnosis of exclusion that is assigned once serious, observable cervical spinal pathology has been ruled out. In the United States, patients presenting with neck pain are assigned symptom-based rather than pathology-based diagnoses in 64% of physician office or hospital outpatient visits.[1]

The Bone and Joint Decade 2000–2010 Task Force on Neck Pain and Its Associated Disorders (Neck Pain Task Force) has proposed a clinical grading system for neck pain (Table 76.1), similar to the severity grading for whiplash-associated disorders proposed by the Québec Task Force on Whiplash-associated Disorders.[2,3] In most settings, a simple descriptive clinical diagnosis is preferable to a speculative assignment of causation with respect to the origin of pain (e.g., cervical facet irritation, cervical facet joint dysfunction), since there is no definitively identifiable tissue lesion associated with nonspecific neck pain. This chapter focuses on the nonoperative management of acute neck pain without structural pathology or radiculopathy: grade I–II neck pain.

Importance of the problem

Neck pain is common: 30–50% of adults in the general population experience neck pain in any given year.[4] Neck pain prevalence rises with increasing age and peaks in middle-aged individuals.[4] On average, women are affected twice as often as men.[4] The incidence of self-reported neck pain in the general population is estimated to be 146–213 per 1,000 persons.[4] During 2000 and 2001 in the United States, 10.2 million visits for neck pain were made to physician offices and hospital Outpatient/Emergency Departments.[1] These numbers underestimate the total number of visits to all practitioners because visits to complementary and alternative medicine providers (e.g., chiropractors, massage therapists, physiotherapists) were not included.

Top five questions

History

1. What are the "red flags" that are used during history-taking to rule out serious pathology underlying neck pain?

Treatment

2. Have physical electro-modalities been demonstrated to be effective compared to placebo, or other treatments, for nonspecific neck pain?
3. Has acupuncture been demonstrated to be effective compared to placebo, or other treatments, for nonspecific neck pain?

Evidence-Based Orthopedics, First Edition. Edited by Mohit Bhandari.

Table 76.1 The Bone and Joint 2000–2010 Task Force on Neck Pain and Its Associated Disorders clinical grading system for neck pain[2]

Grade	Clinical presentation
I	No signs of major pathology. No or little interference with daily activities. This is frequently the case. Reassurance is typically all that is required
II	No signs of major pathology, but interference with daily activities. This occurs less frequently (<10% of people report having experienced this severity of pain during the previous year). Clinical intervention may be provided to decrease symptoms
III	Neck pain with neurological signs[a] or symptoms (radiculopathy). This is uncommon, but may require specific tests and treatments
IV	Neck pain with signs of major pathology (e.g., serious instability or spinal infection). Rare, but might require urgent tests and treatments

[a] Neurologic signs include decreased or absence of deep tendon reflexes, weakness, and sensory deficits.

Table 76.2 System of "red flags" for triage of neck pain patients seeking care in nonemergency settings suggested by the Bone and Joint Decade 2000–2010 Task Force on Neck Pain and Its Associated Disorders[8]

Suggested red flag	Definition
Trauma	Minor or no trauma, but potential for bone loss due to osteoporosis or corticosteroid treatment
Tumour, cancer, malignancy	Previous history of cancer, unexplained weight loss, failure to improve after a month of therapy
Spinal cord compromise	Cervical myelopathy (where about half of patients with cervical myelopathy have pain in their neck or arms, most have symptoms of arm, leg or, uncommonly bowel and bladder dysfunction)
Systemic diseases	Ankylosing spondylitis, inflammatory arthritis or other
Infections	Intravenous drug abuse, urinary tract infection or skin infection
Pain	Intractable pain, tenderness over vertebral body
Prior medical history	Previous neck surgery

4. Have nonsteroidal anti-inflammatories (NSAIDs), muscle relaxants, or analgesics been demonstrated to be effective compared to placebo, or other treatments for non-specific neck pain?

Harm

5. What is the risk of stroke associated with cervical manipulation?

Question 1: What are the "red flags" that are used during history-taking to rule out serious pathology underlying neck pain?

Case clarification
During history-taking, the patient states that she was previously diagnosed with melanoma in situ 7 years ago, which was successfully excised. She was monitored for 5 years following surgical resection with no recurrence.

Relevance
The presence of red flags raise the suspicion of serious underlying spinal pathology; their absence rules out the need for special investigations.

Current opinion
Clinicians who treat neck pain should use a collection of red flags during assessment similar to those formally pro-

posed for the examination of acute low back pain by professional organizations worldwide.[5–7]

Finding the evidence
• MEDLINE: suggested search terms: "neck pain" (MesH term, exploded), combined with "assessment" or "examination" or "history" or "guideline" (search as keywords), combined with "red flags" (search as keyword), and limited to "English" (publication language).

Quality of the evidence
• 1 best-evidence synthesis[8]

Findings
There are currently no formal systems of red flags for the assessment of neck pain as there are for the assessment of low back pain.[5–8] The Neck Pain Task Force has therefore suggested a list of red flags for patients with no exposure to blunt trauma, similar to those currently used in the assessment of low back pain (Table 76.2).

Recommendations
• Serious underlying pathology must be considered during assessment of neck pain
• A suggested system of red flags can be used during patient history until a formal system is validated for neck pain

Question 2: Have physical electro-modalities been demonstrated to be effective compared to placebo, or other treatments, for nonspecific neck pain?

Case clarification
The patient denies symptoms suggestive of radiculopathy. Active cervical range of motion is mildly reduced. She is neurologically intact. The clinical presentation is consistent with grade II neck pain (Table 76.1). She would like maintain her usual work activities and asks whether she should buy a transcutaneous electrical nerve stimulation (TENS) unit to provide relief while she works at her sedentary job.

Relevance
There are numerous electro-modalities available for neck pain treatment. It is important to select treatments with demonstrated effectiveness.

Current opinion
The effectiveness of physical electro-modalities remains unclear and opinions are mixed regarding their effectiveness.

Finding the evidence
- Cochrane Library: "by topic" > "back" > "cervical spine" > "nonspecific neck pain"
- MEDLINE: suggested search terms: "neck pain" (MesH term, exploded), combined with "electric stimulation therapy" (MeSH term, exploded), or "physical modalities" (search as keyword), and limit to "English" (publication language) and 1) "review" (publication type), and 2) "clinical trial" (publication type).

Quality of the evidence
- 1 systematic review[9]
- 1 best-evidence synthesis[10]

Findings
The preponderance of evidence does not support the effectiveness of physical electro-modalities for neck pain, nor has their effectiveness been demonstrated in high-quality trials.[9,10] A 2009 Cochrane review concluded that there is very low-quality evidence that pulsed electromagnetic field therapy, repetitive magnetic stimulation, and TENS are more effective than placebo.[9] The review also concluded that there is low-quality evidence that necklace magnets, modulated galvanic current, iontophoresis, and electric muscle stimulation are not more effective than placebo. The Neck Pain Task Force concluded that physical modalities have not been proven effective for nonspecific neck pain.[10] Note that the Neck Pain Task Force only considered evidence provided by studies that were judged to be scientifically admissible.[10]

Recommendation
- Physical electro-modalities are not more effective than placebo [overall quality: low]

Question 3: Has acupuncture been demonstrated to be effective compared to placebo, or other treatments, for nonspecific neck pain?

Case clarification
After you advise that physical electro-modalities do not have demonstrated effectiveness, the patient asks whether she should consult with a Chinese traditional medicine practitioner for acupuncture to relieve her neck pain.

Relevance
Visits to complementary and alternative medicine providers for neck pain are common. A 1997 United States survey estimated that 42.1% of adults (83 million persons) reported complementary–alternative medicine use.[11]

Current opinion
There are conflicting opinions on the effectiveness of acupuncture for nonspecific neck pain.

Finding the evidence
- Cochrane Library: "by topic" > "back" > "cervical spine" > "nonspecific neck pain"
- MEDLINE: suggested search terms: "neck pain" (MeSH term, exploded), combined with "acupuncture therapy" (MesH term, exploded) or "acupuncture" (MeSH term, exploded), and limit to "English" (publication language) and 1) "review" (publication type), and 2) "clinical trial" (publication type).

Quality of the evidence
- 1 systematic review[12,13]
- 1 best-evidence synthesis[10]
- 2 randomized trials[14,15]

Findings
The search identified two systematic reviews,[12,13] a best-evidence synthesis,[10] and two randomized trials[14,15] published subsequent to the reviews and best-evidence synthesis. The Neck Pain Task Force accepted six trials as scientifically admissible for its best-evidence synthesis, and concluded that the evidence was conflicting on the effectiveness of acupuncture compared to placebo.[10] A Cochrane review accepted 10 trials and found moderate evidence that acupuncture was more effective than sham treatments, and limited evidence that acupuncture was more effective than massage, both at short-term follow-up.[12] One trial, published subsequent to these reviews, found acupuncture to be more effective than deactivated TENS.[14] Another,

large trial concluded that acupuncture added to routine care was more effective than routine care alone in patients with chronic neck pain.[15]

Recommendations

• There is conflicting evidence that acupuncture provides short-term relief of neck pain compared to placebo

• Limited evidence suggests that acupuncture may be superior to massage

• A single trial supports the use of acupuncture in addition to primary care in patients with chronic neck pain

Question 4: Have NSAIDs, muscle relaxants, or analgesics been demonstrated to be effective compared to placebo, or other treatments for nonspecific neck pain?

Case clarification

The patient expresses concern that her neck pain will interfere with her work-related activities. She asks whether an analgesic would be helpful.

Relevance

Interventions that provide symptomatic relief are widely recommended for neck pain. To justify their use, these interventions should allow patients to maintain activities related to work and daily living.

Current opinion

NSAIDs, muscle relaxants, and analgesics are considered effective treatments and are widely prescribed.

Finding the evidence

• Cochrane Library: "by topic" > "back" > "cervical spine" > "nonspecific neck pain"

• MEDLINE: suggested search terms: "neck pain" (MeSH term, exploded), combined with "anti-inflammatory agents, nonsteroidal" (MesH term, exploded) or "analgesics, non-narcotic" (MeSH, exploded) or "analgesics (MeSH, exploded) or "analgesics, opioid" (MeSH, exploded) or "NSAIDS" or "muscle relaxants" (search as keywords), and limit to "English" (publication language) and 1) "review" (publication type), and 2) "clinical trial" (publication type).

Quality of the evidence

• 1 systematic review[16]
• 1 best-evidence synthesis[10]
• 1 randomized trial[17]

Findings

A Cochrane review concluded that muscle relaxants, opioid analgesics, and NSAIDs have limited evidence and unclear benefits for nonspecific neck pain.[16] The Neck Pain Task

Force found no evidence to suggest that one medication is superior to any other medication or nonmedication intervention.[10] Based on six clinical trials considered to be scientifically admissible, the Neck Pain Task Force concluded that the short-term management of symptoms with non-narcotic analgesics may be helpful for grade II neck pain.[2]

A subsequent trial found that oxycodone (an opioid analgesic) was effective for recurrent episodes of neck pain.[17] However, the use of oxycodone for noncancer pain is controversial due to limited evidence for long-term efficacy, side effects, and potential for abuse and addiction.[18]

Recommendation

• A short course of nonopioid analgesics or NSAIDs may be helpful for the short-term management of grade II neck pain symptoms

Question 5: What is the risk of stroke associated with cervical manipulation?

Case clarification

The patient advises that another clinician has suggested that she consider a short course of mobilization or manipulation for symptomatic relief. The patient expresses concern about the risk of stroke associated with neck manipulation.

Relevance

Current evidence suggests that mobilization or manipulation are likely to be helpful for in decreasing symptoms in grade II neck pain;[2] however, there is concern about the risk of vertebrobasilar artery (VBA) stroke associated with neck manipulation.

Current opinion

Opinions are mixed on the risk of stroke associated with neck manipulation, with widely varying judgments on the magnitude of risk.

Finding the evidence

• MEDLINE: suggested search terms: "stroke" (MeSH term, exploded), combined with "manipulation, orthopedic" (MesH term, exploded) or "manipulation, chiropractic" (MesH term, exploded), or "manipulation, spinal" (MesH term, exploded) or "manipulation, osteopathic" (MeSH, exploded), and limit to "English" (publication language).

Quality of the evidence

One ranking system for prognostic studies distinguishes between types of studies that provide increasing strength of evidence (see box).[19–21]

Ranking of prognostic studies

- *Phase I* studies are exploratory, hypothesis-generating studies characterized by descriptive exploration and demonstration of crude (unadjusted) associations
- *Phase II* studies are also exploratory, but use multivariable techniques/stratification to identify risk factors related to the outcome of interest, while adjusting for other factors
- *Phase III* studies are hypothesis-driven and confirmatory. The goal is to confirm or refute the independence of a relationship between a prognostic factor and outcome of interest, after adjusting for confounding[4,22]

Best evidence
- 2 systematic reviews[10,23]
- 2 case-control studies (phase III)[24,25]
- 1 case-crossover study (phase III)[24]

Findings

Trials of neck manipulation are too small to evaluate the risk of rare, treatment-related complications. There are three phase III population-based studies that have investigated the risk of VBA stroke following neck manipulation.[10,23] Rothwell et al. showed an increased risk of vertebrobasilar dissection within a week of a chiropractic visit in patients <45 years of age (OR 5.03; 95% CI 1.32,43.87).[25] No significant associations were found for patients aged 45 years or more. Cassidy et al. extended these findings using a case-control and a case-crossover design.[24] There was a strong association between chiropractic visits and subsequent stroke, but also a similar increase in the risk of stroke after visiting a primary care physician for neck pain.[24] The authors proposed that a plausible explanation for the increased risk of VBA stroke associated with chiropractic and physician visits is that patients with VBA dissection-related neck pain and headache consult with chiropractors and physicians during the prodromal stage of a VBA stroke.[24]

Recommendation

- Since several nonoperative treatments seem to be roughly equivalent in efficacy and the overall risk of serious side effects is minimal, patient preference should be an important guide in choice of treatment for the short-term relief of neck pain

Summary of recommendations

- A suggested system of red flags should be used to screen for serious pathology underlying a complaint of neck pain
- The preponderance of evidence does not support the effectiveness of physical electro-modalities

- There is conflicting evidence on the effectiveness of acupuncture for neck pain
- A course of nonopioid analgesics may be helpful for short-term management of neck pain symptoms
- Since several nonoperative treatments seem roughly equivalent in efficacy and the overall risk of significant side effects is minimal, patient preference should be an important guide in choice of treatment for short-term relief of neck pain

Conclusions

Once serious underlying pathology has been reasonably ruled out, it is preferable to use a simple, descriptive clinical diagnosis (such as the grading system proposed by the Bone and Joint Decade 2000–2010 Task Force on Neck Pain), rather than a speculative assignment of causation, for nonspecific neck pain. For grade I–II nonspecific neck pain, the patient should be reassured about the absence of serious pathology. A short course of treatment using an intervention shown to provide some degree of short-term relief (e.g., exercise training, nonopioid analgesics, or mobilization) is appropriate. This approach will assist patients to adhere to their clinician's encouragement to maintain activities related to work and daily living.

References

1. Riddle DL, Schappert SM. Volume and characteristics of inpatient and ambulatory medical care for neck pain in the United States: data from three national surveys. Spine 2007;32:132–40; discussion 141.
2. Guzman J, Haldeman S, Carroll LJ, et al. Clinical practice implications of the Bone and Joint Decade 2000–2010 Task Force on Neck Pain and Its Associated Disorders: from concepts and findings to recommendations. Spine 2008;33(4:Suppl):S199–213.
3. Spitzer WO, Skovron ML, Salmi LR, et al. Scientific Monograph of the Quebec Task Force on Whiplash-Associated Disorders: Redefining "Whiplash" and its Management. Spine 1995;20(8S): 73S.
4. Hogg-Johnson S, van der Velde G, Carroll LJ, et al. The burden and determinants of neck pain in the general population: results of the Bone and Joint Decade 2000–2010 Task Force on Neck Pain and Its Associated Disorders. Spine 2008;33(4:Suppl):S51.
5. European Guidelines for Low Back Pain. http://www.backpaineurope.org/web/files/WG1_Guidelines.pdf. 2004.
6. Royal College of General Practitioners. Clinical Guidelines for the Management of Acute Low Back Pain. Royal College of General Practitioners, London, 1999.
7. Materson RS. The AHCPR practice guidelines for low back pain. Bull Rheum Dis 1996;45:6–8.
8. Nordin M, Carragee EJ, Hogg-Johnson S, et al. Assessment of neck pain and its associated disorders: results of the Bone and

Joint Decade 2000–2010 Task Force on Neck Pain and Its Associated Disorders. Spine 2008;33(4:Suppl):S-22.

9. Kroeling P, Gross A, Goldsmith CH, et al. Electrotherapy for neck pain. Cochrane Database Syst Rev 2009;4:CD004251.

10. Hurwitz EL, Carragee EJ, van der Velde G, et al. Treatment of neck pain: noninvasive interventions: results of the Bone and Joint Decade 2000–2010 Task Force on Neck Pain and Its Associated Disorders. Spine 2008;33(4:Suppl):S52.

11. Eisenberg DM, Davis RB, Ettner SL, et al. Trends in alternative medicine use in the United States, 1990–1997: Results of a follow-up national survey. JAMA 1998;280:1569–75.

12. Trinh K, Graham N, Gross A, et al. Acupuncture for neck disorders. Spine 2007;32:236–43.

13. Trinh KV, Graham N, Gross AR, et al. Acupuncture for neck disorders. Cochrane Database Syst Rev 2006;3:CD004870.

14. Vas J, Perea-Milla E, Mendez C, et al. Efficacy and safety of acupuncture for chronic uncomplicated neck pain: a randomised controlled study. Pain 2006;126:245–55.

15. Witt CM, Jena S, Brinkhaus B, Liecker B, Wegscheider K, Willich SN. Acupuncture for patients with chronic neck pain. Pain 2006;125:98–106.

16. Peloso P, Gross A, Haines T, et al. Medicinal and injection therapies for mechanical neck disorders. Cochrane Database Syst Rev 2007;3:CD000319.

17. Ma K, Jiang W, Zhou Q, Du DP. The efficacy of oxycodone for management of acute pain episodes in chronic neck pain patients. Int J Clin Pract 2008;62:241–7.

18. Manchikanti L, Singh A. Therapeutic opioids: a ten-year perspective on the complexities and complications of the escalating use, abuse, and nonmedical use of opioids. Pain Physician 2008;11(2:Suppl):S88.

19. Côté P, Cassidy JD, Carroll L, Frank JW, Bombardier C. A systematic review of the prognosis of acute whiplash and a new conceptual framework to synthesize the literature. Spine 2001;26:E445–58.

20. Altman DG, Lyman GH. Methodological challenges in the evaluation of prognostic factors in breat cancer. Breast Cancer Res Treat 1998;52:289–303.

21. Carroll L, Cassidy JD, Peloso P, et al. Prognosis for mild traumatic brain injury: results of the WHO Collaborating Centre Task Force on Mild Traumatic Brain Injury. J Rehab Med 2004;43(Suppl):84–105.

22. Carroll LJ, Hogg-Johnson S, van der Velde G, et al. Course and prognostic factors for neck pain in the general population: results of the Bone and Joint Decade 2000–2010 Task Force on Neck Pain and Its Associated Disorders. Spine 2008;33(4S):S75–82.

23. Gouveia LO, Castanho P, Ferreira JJ. Safety of chiropractic interventions: a systematic review. Spine 2009;34:E405–13.

24. Cassidy JD, Boyle E, Côté P, et al. Risk of vertebrobasilar stroke and chiropractic care: results of a population-based case-control and case-crossover study. Spine 2008;33(4:Suppl):S83.

25. Rothwell DM, Bondy SJ, Williams JI. Chiropractic manipulation and stroke: a population-based case-control study. Stroke 2001;32:1054–60.

Gabrielle van der Velde

Toronto Health Economics and Technology Assessment (THETA) Collaborative, University of Toronto, and Institute for Work & Health, Toronto, ON, Canada

Case scenario

A 45 year old man presents to your office with a complaint of neck pain following a traffic accident the previous day. He describes generalized pain and stiffness in the neck and upper back. He denies radiating pain into the upper limbs.

Relevant anatomy

Whiplash defined by the Québec Task Force on Whiplash-associated Disorders is an "acceleration-deceleration mechanism of energy transferred to the neck that results in soft tissue injury that may lead to a variety of clinical manifestations including neck pain and associated symptoms".[1] "Whiplash-associated disorder" (WAD) describes the clinical syndrome characterized by neck pain and clusters of physical and psychological symptoms, and is classified into five grades of severity (Table 77.1). This chapter focuses on the nonoperative management of the most prevalent grades of WAD in nonemergency settings: grade I–II.

Importance of the problem

Whiplash affects 83% of individuals involved in traffic accidents.[2] Most Western countries have seen a rise in the annual cumulative incidence of emergency visits for traffic-related WAD. A Dutch study found a 10-fold increase, from an average annual incidence of 3.4 visits per 100,000 inhabitants in 1970–1974 to 40.2 visits per 100,000 in 1990–1994.[3] An American study reported the weighted annual incidence of Emergency Department visits to be 328 visits per 100,000 inhabitants, based on the population of the United States in 2000.[4] WAD represents a significant burden in terms of pain, disability, and healthcare utilization,[1,2,5,6] and increases the risk of future health complaints.[2,7,8]

Top five questions

Assessment

1. When is it appropriate to use radiography when assessing whiplash injury in nonemergency settings?

Course

2. What is the expected rate of recovery for acute whiplash injury?

Prognosis

3. Is initial pain severity and WAD grading predictive of a patient's recovery?

Treatment

4. What is the most effective nonoperative treatment for grade I–II WAD?
5. What is the appropriate frequency and duration of treatment?

Question 1: When is it appropriate to use radiography when assessing whiplash injury in nonemergency settings?

Case clarification

The patient describes being involved in a traffic collision in which his vehicle was rear-ended by another vehicle travelling at approximately 60 km/hour. He was not

Evidence-Based Orthopedics, First Edition. Edited by Mohit Bhandari.
© 2012 Blackwell Publishing Ltd. Published 2012 by Blackwell Publishing Ltd.

Table 77.1 The Québec classification of whiplash-associated disorders[1]

Grade	Clinical presentation
0	No neck symptoms, no physical sign(s)
I	Neck pain, stiffness or tenderness only, no physical sign(s)
II	Neck symptoms and musculoskeletal sign(s)[a]
III	Neck symptoms and neurologic sign(s)[b]
IV	Neck symptoms and fracture or dislocation

[a]Musculoskeletal signs include decreased range of motion and point tenderness.
[b]Neurologic signs include decreased or absence of deep tendon reflexes, weakness, and sensory deficits.
Symptoms and disorders that can be manifested in all grades include deafness, dizziness, tinnitus, headache, memory loss, dysphagia, and temporomandibular pain.

Table 77.2 The NEXUS low-risk criteria[12]

Cervical spine radiography is indicated for patients with trauma unless they meet all of the following criteria:
1. No posterior midline cervical spine tenderness
2. No evidence of intoxication
3. A normal level of alertness
4. No focal neurologic deficit
5. No painful distracting injuries

intoxicated and did not lose consciousness. Active cervical range of motion is moderately decreased by pain and stiffness; rotation is 70° right and left. There is generalized tenderness in the neck and upper back and the patient is neurologically intact.

Relevance

Even in nonemergency settings, cervical instability can be a concern in patients with secondary trauma to the neck.

Current opinion

Current opinion is divergent. While many practitioners believe that the majority of patients presenting with WAD I or WAD II do not require radiographic assessment in nonemergency settings, there is considerable variation among clinicians with respect to the use of radiography to rule out cervical instability.

Finding the evidence

• MEDLINE: suggested search terms: "cervical vertebrae" (MeSH term, exploded) and "blunt trauma" (search as keyword), combined with "screening" or "criteria" or "decision" or "rule" (search as keywords), and limit to "English" (publication language).

Quality of the evidence

Sackett and Haynes proposed a ranking system for studies that provide evidence for diagnostic tests (see Chapter 76).[9] In this system, phase III studies establish the validity of a test by answering the question: "Do test results distinguish patients with and without the target disorder among those in whom it is clinically sensible to suspect the disorder?" and are required for the widespread adoption of a test. Phase IV studies provide evidence of the test's utility (i.e., a test may be valid, but have not impact on outcome).

Best evidence

• 1 best-evidence synthesis[10]
• 3 cohort studies (phase III)[11–13]

Findings

There are no formal screening criteria for determining the appropriateness of diagnostic imaging of patients with secondary trauma to the neck in nonemergency settings.[10,14,15] In the emergency setting, there are two decision rules for identifying low-risk patients that do not require imaging: the National Emergency X-Radiography Utilization Study (NEXUS) low-risk criteria (NLC) (Table 77.2),[11,12] and the Canadian C-spine rule (CCR) (Figure 77.1).[13] Both rules are validated by phase III studies and widely used. Although developed for emergency settings, they also inform the need for radiography in nonemergency settings.

Although the American College of Radiology does not take a stand on their relative merits,[17] a recent comparison of the NLC and CCR concluded that for alert patients with trauma who are in stable condition, the CCR is superior to the NLC with respect to sensitivity and specificity.[16]

Recommendation

• In adults with an acute whiplash injury presenting to nonemergency settings, the NLC and/or CCR can be used to provide clues of significant cervical trauma in low-risk WAD patients that should be followed up with acquisition of plain films.

Question 2: What is the expected rate of recovery for acute whiplash injury?

Case clarification

The patient's presentation based on history and physical examination is consistent with grade II WAD. He would like to know when he will recover.

Relevance

The likelihood of recovery from whiplash injury is of essential interest to patients, and their families and employers.

Current opinion

Opinions are widely divergent on the rate of recovery from WAD.

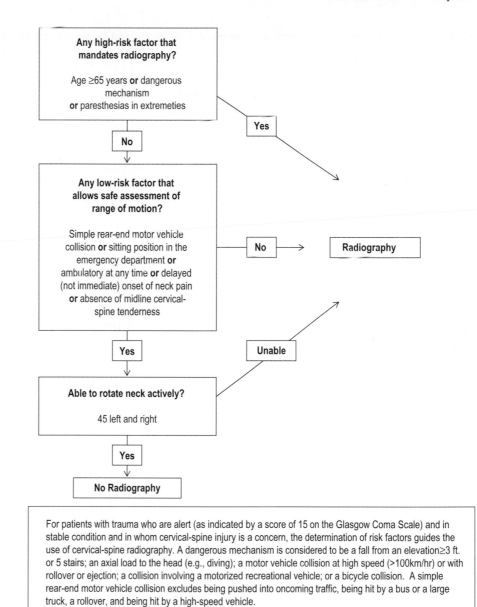

Figure 77.1 The Canadian C-spine rule.[13,16]

For patients with trauma who are alert (as indicated by a score of 15 on the Glasgow Coma Scale) and in stable condition and in whom cervical-spine injury is a concern, the determination of risk factors guides the use of cervical-spine radiography. A dangerous mechanism is considered to be a fall from an elevation≥3 ft. or 5 stairs; an axial load to the head (e.g., diving); a motor vehicle collision at high speed (>100km/hr) or with rollover or ejection; a collision involving a motorized recreational vehicle; or a bicycle collision. A simple rear-end motor vehicle collision excludes being pushed into oncoming traffic, being hit by a bus or a large truck, a rollover, and being hit by a high-speed vehicle.

Finding the evidence

• MEDLINE: suggested search terms: "whiplash injuries" (MeSH term, exploded), combined with "course" or "recovery" (search as keywords), and limit to "English" (publication language) and 1) "review" (publication type), and 2) "2007-current" (publication year).

Quality of the evidence

• 1 systematic review[18]
• 1 best-evidence synthesis[19]
• 1 cohort study[20]

Findings

The preponderance of evidence identified by a recent review and a best-evidence synthesis suggests that recovery from WAD is prolonged. Approximately 40–56% of individuals with acute whiplash injury recover in 3 months.[18,19] The proportion recovering then declines over time, with 50–71% recovering by 12 months.[18,19] However, these estimates should be interpreted with two points in mind. First, 20–40% of the general population report neck pain in the previous month.[21] Second, sampling frames in half of the studies accepted by one review were emergency departments.[19] Patients in these studies likely had more severe whiplash injuries, and therefore a poorer prognosis for recovery. A recent cohort study, published subsequent to these reviews, reported estimates within the above ranges.[20]

Recommendations

• A substantial proportion of patients with acute whiplash injuries recover within 3 months after injury

• Most patients will have recovered at 1 year, though periodic symptoms may persist

Question 3: Are initial pain severity and WAD grading predictive of a patient's rate of recovery?

Case clarification

The patient's neck pain intensity, measured on a 10-point visual analog scale, is 5. WAD severity grading is II. Neck pain-related disability, measured by the Neck Disability Index, is 45%.[22]

Relevance

Clinicians should understand the role of initial symptom severity on recovery, in order to guide the expectations of patients, and their families and employers.

Current opinion

Patients with more severe initial symptoms recover more slowly.

Finding the evidence

• MEDLINE: suggested search terms: "whiplash injuries" (MeSH term, exploded), combined with "prognosis" (MeSH term, exploded) or "prognosis" (search as a keyword), and limit to "English" (publication language) and 1) "review" (publication type), and 2) "2007-current" (publication year).

Quality of the evidence

A ranking system for prognostic studies distinguishes between studies that provide increasing strength of evidence and ranks them as phase I–IV (see Chapter 76).[23–25]

Best evidence
• 2 systematic reviews[18,26]
• 1 best-evidence synthesis[19]
• 1 cohort study (phase II)[27]

Findings

On average, patients with more severe symptoms have a poorer prognosis. An association between high initial neck pain intensity and poor outcome was reported in 7 of 10 cohort studies identified by one review.[18] Similarly, high initial neck pain intensity and disability were associated with late whiplash syndrome.[26] The Bone and Joint Decade 2000–2010 Task Force on Neck Pain identified three cohorts (one phase I, two phase II) that examined WAD grading as a prognostic factor.[19] Individuals with more severe WAD grades were more likely to report work or leisure limitations at long-term follow-up.[19] Results of a prospective cohort (phase II) published subsequent to these reviews

and best-evidence synthesis found that higher initial pain was associated with delayed recovery.[27]

Recommendation

• Recovery from whiplash injury is slower in patients with greater initial symptom severity
• Recovery is delayed with increasing WAD severity grading

Question 4: What is the most effective nonoperative approach for grade I–II WAD?

Case clarification

There are numerous noninvasive WAD treatments that are commonly provided to patients, including heat and ice, traction, massage, exercise, manual therapies, electromodalities, and combined approaches.

Relevance

Clinicians should choose treatments with demonstrated effectiveness, based on the best available evidence.

Current opinion

Opinions are conflicting about the most effective treatment approaches.

Finding the evidence

• Cochrane Library: "by topic" > "back" > "cervical spine" > "whiplash-associated disorders"
• MEDLINE: Suggested search terms: "whiplash injuries" (MeSH term, exploded), combined with "therapeutics" (MeSH term, exploded) or "treatment" (search as a keyword), and limit to "review" (publication type) and "English" (publication language).

Quality of the evidence

• 1 systematic review[28]
• 1 best-evidence synthesis[29]

Findings

Both the Cochrane review by Verhagen (2007) and the best-evidence synthesis by the Bone and Joint Decade 2000–2010 Task Force on Neck Pain concluded that evidence is limited and conflicting.[28,29] The reviews did not statistically pool effectiveness estimates due to clinical and statistical heterogeneity. The Neck Pain Task Force found support for the short-term effectiveness of interventions that involve mobilization and exercises, or supervised training and rehabilitation. Educational videos that included exercises and recommendations to return to work and activities of daily living were also effective.[29] In contrast, the Cochrane review did not draw conclusions about the most effective therapy for grade I–II WAD given methodological limitations of the identified studies. The authors did note a trend that suggested active treatments, such as exercise, may be more effective than passive treatments.[28]

Recommendations
• Patients should be encouraged to a timely return to work and activities of daily living
• Active treatment should be used rather than passive treatments such as electro-modalities, neck collars, or traction

Question 5: What is the appropriate frequency and duration of treatment?

Case clarification
The patient's employer is flexible with respect to time off for treatment visits, but would like to know how often the patient will be treated and for how long.

Relevance
Deciding on the frequency and duration of treatment is complicated. Besides uncertainty of the impact of patterns of care on recovery, there is much at stake, including time and resources of stakeholders (patients, clinicians, employers).

Current opinion
There is considerable divergence in opinion, as demonstrated by wide variations in patterns of care; however, it is broadly believed that early, aggressive, intervention leads to faster recovery.

Finding the evidence
• MEDLINE: suggested search terms: "whiplash injuries" (MeSH term, exploded), combined with "patterns of care" or "frequency" or treatment" or "duration" (search as keywords), and limit to "English" (publication language).

Quality of the evidence
• 1 best-evidence synthesis[19]
• 3 cohort studies (phase III)[30,31]

Findings
Contrary to current opinion, on average, frequent, early healthcare utilization leads to delayed recovery.[19] Two phase III prognostic studies found that more frequent healthcare visits were associated with slower recovery.[31,32] Patients who increased their frequency of care beyond two visits to general practitioners and six visits to chiropractors, or added chiropractic to medical care, had slower recovery. High healthcare utilization also appears to be associated with poorer recovery from WAD. A phase III prognostic cohort found that attendance at a community-based multidisciplinary rehabilitation program did not enhance patients' recovery.[19,30] Attendees of these programs recovered 30–50% more slowly than those who did not attend.[30]

Recommendation
• The optimal frequency and duration of care has not been determined, but clinicians should avoid intensive treatment of patients after whiplash injury

Summary of recommendations

• Radiographic assessment is not necessary for most grade I–II WAD
• The NEXUS LRC or CCS rule can be used to identify clues of serious cervical trauma
• Recovery from acute whiplash injury is slower in patients with more severe symptoms and higher WAD grade
• Clinicians should promote a timely return to work and resumption of activities of daily living
• Active rather than passive treatments appear to be more effective for treating grade I–II WAD
• Intensive treatment shortly after whiplash injury should be avoided

Conclusions

The evidence suggests that grade I–II WAD requires less healthcare intervention (including radiographic assessment and early intensive treatment) than has been the standard of care in many jurisdictions. It is important to promote a timely return to work and activities of daily living, and to provide active rather than passive approaches to treatment.

References

1. Spitzer WO, Skovron ML, Salmi LR, et al. Scientific Monograph of the Quebec Task Force on Whiplash-Associated Disorders: Redefining "Whiplash" and its Management. Spine 1995;20[8S]:1–73S.
2. Cassidy JD, Carroll LJ, Côté P, Lemstra M, Berglund A, Nygren A. Effect of eliminating compensation for pain and suffering on the outcome of insurance claims for whiplash injury. N Engl J Med 2000; 342:1179–86.
3. Versteegen GJ, Kingma J, Meijler WJ, ten Duis HJ. Neck sprain in patients injured in car accidents: a retrospective study covering the period 1970–1994. Eur Spine J 1998;7:195–200.
4. Quinlan KP, Annest JL, Myers B, Ryan G, Hill H. Neck strains and sprains among motor vehicle occupants—United States, 2000. Accid Anal Prevent 2004; 36:21–7.
5. Côté P, Hogg-Johnson S, Cassidy JD, Carroll L, Frank JW, Bombardier C. Early aggressive care and delayed recovery from whiplash: isolated finding or reproducible result? Arthritis Rheum 2007;57:861–8.
6. Holm L, Cassidy JD, Sjogren Y, Nygren A. Impairment and work disability due to whiplash injury following traffic collisions. An

analysis of insurance material from the Swedish Road Traffic Injury Commission. Scand J Public Health 1999;27:116–23.

7. Berglund A, Alfredsson L, Jensen I, Cassidy JD, Nygren A. The association between exposure to a rear-end collision and future health complaints. J Clin Epidemiol 2001;54:851–6.

8. Côté P, Cassidy JD, Carroll L. Is a lifetime history of neck injury in a traffic collision associated with prevalent neck pain, headache and depressive symptomatology? Accid Anal Prevent 2000;32:151–9.

9. Sackett DL, Haynes RB. The architecture of diagnostic research. BMJ 2002;24:539–41.

10. Nordin M, Carragee EJ, Hogg-Johnson S, et al. Assessment of neck pain and its associated disorders: results of the Bone and Joint Decade 2000–2010 Task Force on Neck Pain and Its Associated Disorders. Spine 2008;33:S22.

11. Hoffman JR, Wolfson AB, Todd K, Mower WR. Selective cervical spine radiography in blunt trauma: methodology of the National Emergency X-Radiography Utilization Study (NEXUS). Ann Emerg Med 1998;32:461–9.

12. Panacek EA, Mower WR, Holmes JF, Hoffman JR, NEXUS Group. Test performance of the individual NEXUS low-risk clinical screening criteria for cervical spine injury. Ann Emerg Med 2001;38:22–5.

13. Stiell IG, Wells GA, Vandemheen KL, et al. The Canadian C-spine rule for radiography in alert and stable trauma patients. JAMA 2001;286:1841–8.

14. Scholten-Peeters GG, Bekkering GE, Verhagen AP, et al. Clinical practice guideline for the physiotherapy of patients with whiplash-associated disorders. Spine 2002;27:412–22.

15. Binder A. The diagnosis and treatment of nonspecific neck pain and whiplash. Eur Medicophys 2007;43:79–89.

16. Stiell IG, Clement CM, McKnight RD, et al. The Canadian C-spine rule versus the NEXUS low-risk criteria in patients with trauma. N Engl J Med 2003; 349:2510–18.

17. Daffner RH, Hackney DB. ACR Appropriateness Criteria on suspected spine trauma. J Am Coll Radiol 2007;4:762–75.

18. Kamper SJ, Rebbeck TJ, Maher CG, McAuley JH, McAuley JH, Sterling M. Course and prognostic factors of whiplash: a systematic review and meta-analysis. Pain 2008;138:617–29.

19. Carroll LJ, Holm LW, Hogg-Johnson S, et al. Course and Prognostic Factors for Neck Pain in Whiplash-Associated Disorders (WAD): Results of the Bone and Joint Decade 2000–2010 Task Force on Neck Pain and Its Associated Disorders. Spine 2008;33(4S):S83–92.

20. Buitenhuis J, de Jong PJ, Jaspers JP, Groothoff JW. Work disability after whiplash: a prospective cohort study. Spine 2009; 34(3):262–7.

21. Hogg-Johnson S, van der Velde G, Carroll LJ, et al. The burden and determinants of neck pain in the general population: results of the Bone and Joint Decade 2000–2010 Task Force on Neck Pain and Its Associated Disorders. Spine 2008;33(4:Suppl):S51.

22. Vernon H, Mior S. The Neck Disability Index: a study of reliability and validity. J Manipulative Physiol Ther 1991;14:409–15.

23. Altman DG, Lyman GH. Methodological challenges in the evaluation of prognostic factors in breat cancer. Breast Cancer Res Treat 1998;52:289–303.

24. Carroll L, Cassidy JD, Peloso P, et al. Prognosis for mild traumatic brain injury: results of the WHO Collaborating Centre Task Force on Mild Traumatic Brain Injury. J Rehab Med 2004;43(Suppl):84–105.

25. Côté P, Cassidy JD, Carroll L, Frank JW, Bombardier C. A systematic review of the prognosis of acute whiplash and a new conceptual framework to synthesize the literature. Spine 2001;26:E445–58.

26. Williams M, Williamson E, Gates S, Lamb SE, Cooke M. A systematic literature review of physical prognostic factors for the development of late whiplash syndrome. Spine 2007;32:E764–80.

27. Dufton JA, Kopec JA, Wong H, et al. Prognostic factors associated with minimal improvement following acute whiplash-associated disorders. Spine 2006;31:E759–65.

28. Verhagen AP, Scholten-Peeters GG, van WS, de Bie RA, Bierma-Zeinstra SM. Conservative treatments for whiplash. Cochrane Database Syst Rev 2007;2:CD003338.

29. Hurwitz EL, Carragee EJ, van der Veld G, et al. Treatment of neck pain: noninvasive interventions: results of the Bone and Joint Decade 2000–2010 Task Force on Neck Pain and Its Associated Disorders. Spine 2008;33(4:Suppl):S52.

30. Cassidy JD, Carroll LJ, Côté P, Frank J. Does multidisciplinary rehabilitation benefit whiplash recovery?: results of a population-based incidence cohort study. Spine 2007;32:126–31.

31. Côté P, Hogg-Johnson S, Cassidy JD, Carroll L, Frank JW, Bombardier C. Initial patterns of clinical care and recovery from whiplash injuries: a population-based cohort study. Arch Intern Med 2005;165:2257–63.

32. Côté P, Hogg-Johnson S, Cassidy JD, Carroll L, Frank JW, Bombardier C. Early aggressive care and delayed recovery from whiplash: isolated finding or reproducible result? Arthritis Rheum 2007;57:861–8.

78 Mechanical Low Back Pain: Operative Treatment—Fusion

Rahul Basho[1], Alex Gitelman[1], and Jeffrey C. Wang[2]

[1]UCLA Medical Center, Santa Monica, CA, USA
[2]UCLA School of Medicine, Los Angeles, CA, USA

Case scenario

A 60 year old man with a 2 year history of lower back pain presents to your clinic. He describes the pain as being located entirely in his lower back, with no symptoms of leg pain. Sitting for long periods of time exacerbates his pain, as does prolonged standing. He is most comfortable when he is lying down. The pain has gradually worsened over the course of the past few months. He has tried multiple conservative treatment modalities, including physical therapy and epidural steroid injections, each with minimal benefit. He indicates that he recently had a discogram performed by his pain management specialist, the results of which show concordant pain at L5–S1 with normal controls at L3–L4 and L4–L5. Physical examination shows the patient has slightly decreased motion in flexion and extension, normal gait, and a normal neurovascular examination in his lower extremities

Relevant anatomy

In order to understand the changes occurring in a degenerative disc, one must understand the relevant anatomy of a normal, healthy disc. Intervertebral discs which make up approximately 30% of the height of the lumbar spine, are composed of three primary structures: the cartilaginous endplates, the annulus fibrosus, and the nucleus pulposus. The outer layer, known as the annulus fibrosus, has a sparse vascular supply along its periphery. It is composed of type I collagen fibrils arranged in concentric lamellae. Each lamina has fibrils arranged obliquely relative to the vertebral endplates, with the direction of the fibrils alternating from one lamina to the next. This arrangement con-

tributes to the tensile strength of a spinal unit. The inner gelatinous layer, known as the nucleus pulposus, is composed primarily of type II collagen, proteoglycans, and mucopolysaccharides. The compressive strength of the spinal unit is conferred by the proteoglycans within the nucleus pulposus. They provide an osmotic gradient for water to enter the disk. Axial loading of the disk due to a patient's upright posture, forces water out of the disc, creating a cycle of flow seen in normal disks.[1] Hyaline cartilage connects the endplates of the vertebral bodies to the disks and permits diffusion between the two. Because the disk is a relatively avascular structure, this is the major mechanism of providing nutrition to the disk.

Importance of the problem

Chronic low back pain places a tremendous burden on the patient, society, and resources allocated to health care. Data indicates that 70–85% of all people experience an episode of back pain at some point in their lifetime, and that patients with back pain for a period of more than 3 months use health services more often than most patient groups.[2] Patients suffering from low back pain who have not been able to return to work for a period of 2 years are unlikely ever to return.[2] In addition, a large percentage of healthcare resources are used to treat chronic low back pain. European studies estimate the cost of low back pain to be 1.7% of the gross national product, and in the United States the figure is between 0.5% and 6%.[2] There is a huge amount of literature available to both practitioners and patients regarding to low back pain. In fact, an internet search for "chronic low back pain" results in 51 million hits. Even with all of this data, there is unfortunately only a handful of randomized, prospective, multicenter studies comparing treatment options for low back pain. These studies themselves are not perfect, but they provide the most scientific data available and they assist clinicians in making evidence-based decisions.

Top question

1. Does lumbar fusion provide improved pain relief for patients with mechanical low back compared to nonoperative treatment?

Question 1: Does lumbar fusion provide improved pain relief for patients with mechanical low back compared to nonoperative treatment?

Case clarification
The presenting patient has clinical and radiographic findings consistent with degenerative disk disease. He has exhausted conservative measures and wishes to know if a fusion can reliably improve his lower back pain.

Relevance
There is a great deal of controversy among orthopedic surgeons regarding treatment of mechanical low back pain. Whether the intervertebral disk is the true pain generator and the efficacy of an operative fusion for treating mechanical low back remain controversial in both the literature and in clinical practice.

Current opinion
Current opinion suggests that operative fusion for the treatment of mechanical low back pain is one of the less reliable surgical options in spine surgery.

Finding the evidence
- Cochrane Database, with search term: "lumbar fusion"
- PubMed clinical queries search/systematic reviews "lumbar operative fusion"
- MEDLINE search for "low back pain" with subheading "surgical"

Quality of the evidence
Level I
- 1 systematic review/meta-analysis[3]
- 4 randomized trials

Findings
Oswestry Disability Index The common measurement outcome amongst the four randomized trials was the Oswestry Disability Index (ODI), a validated outcome measure specific for lumbar degenerative disorders.[8] This index is measured from 1 to 100, with higher scores

indicating a higher level of disability. The developers of the ODI indicate that a clinically relevant change is 4 points, whereas other studies have suggested thresholds of up to 18 points corresponding to a clinically relevant change.[4]

All four of the randomized trials compared surgical treatment of mechanical low back pain with nonoperative treatment. Of the four randomized trials reviewed, three had structured nonoperative regimens.[5–7] The Fritzell 2002 study[2] did not have a structured regimen of physical therapy, instead using physical therapy as the main component, which could be supplemented with "information and education, TENS, acupuncture, injections, cognitive and functional training, and coping strategies."[2]

All four studies showed a similar improvement in the surgical arm of patients, with improvement from baseline ranging from 8.9 to 15.6 points (percentage improvement 18.9–37.1%).[3] In the nonoperative arm, improvements ranged from 2.8 to 12.8 (percentage improvements from baseline were 5.8–30.1%). Only in the Fritzell et al. study was the improvement in nonoperative treatment below the clinically relevant threshold of 4 points on the ODI, whereas in the other three studies the improvement seen in the nonoperative patients was similar to that of the operative patients. These three studies used a structured nonoperative treatment regimen incorporating cognitive behavioral therapy, whereas the Fritzell et al study did not.

The greatest improvement in surgical patients when compared to their nonsurgical counterparts was seen in the Fritzell et al. study (ΔODI surgery group – ΔODI nonsurgical group) at 8.8. The Fairbank et al. study showed improvement in the surgical group of patients as well, with a lesser improvement at 4.1 (95% CI 0.1–8.1), but this value was not considered statistically significant.[5] Neither Brox et al.[6,7] study showed a statistically significant difference between surgical and nonsurgical intervention for the ODI. The first study, looking at patients without prior surgery, the improvement seen with surgery for this study was 2.3 (95% CI –6.8 to 11.4).[6] In the second Brox et al study, looking at patients with a prior discectomy, greater improvements in the ODI were seen with nonsurgical treatment. When adjusted for gender and treatment expectations, this value was –9.7 (95% CI –21.7 to 1.7).[7]

Recommendations
- Compared with an unstructured nonoperative treatment regimen, lumbar fusion can be expected to reduce pain by about 63% and improve ODI by about 25% [overall quality: moderate]
- Structured nonoperative treatment regimens that incorporate cognitive behavioral therapy can provide pain relief and improvements in the ODI that are comparable if not better than lumbar fusion [overall quality: moderate]
- Nonoperative treatment for mechanical back pain should be strongly considered [overall quality: high]

Conclusions

The studies discussed above are not without limitations: Fritzell et al. did not use a structured nonoperative treatment regimen, Fairbanks et al. had a high crossover rate and included patients with spondylolisthesis, and both Brox et al. studies had wide confidence intervals. However, these studies provide the best available data for surgeons to make clinical decisions in regards to lower back pain. Though these studies are not standardized and contain different treatment arms, time points, and patient populations, their conflicting results indicate that lumbar fusion for chronic low back pain should be recommended only as a last resort in a group of well-informed patients with realistic expectations.

References

1. Biyani A, Haman S, Anderssson G. Lumbar disc disease. In: Herkowitz H, Garfin S, eds, The Spine, 5th edn, Vol. II, pp. 930–44. Saunders; Philadelphia, 2006.
2. Fritzell P, Hagg O, Wessberg P, et al. 2001 Volvo Award Winner in Clinical Studies: Lumbar fusion versus nonsurgical treatment for chronic low back pain: A multicenter randomized controlled trial from the Swedish Lumbar Spine Study Group. Spine 2002; 26:2521–32.
3. Gibson JNA, Waddell G. Surgery for degenerative lumbar spondylosis. Cochrane Database Syst Rev 2005;4:CD001352.
4. Mirza S, Deyo R. Systematic review of randomized trials comparing lumbar fusion surgery to nonoperative care for treatment of chronic back pain. Spine 2007;32:816–23.
5. Fairbank J, Frost H, Wilson-MacDonald J, et al. Randomised controlled trial to compare surgical stabilization of the lumbar spine with an intensive rehabilitation programme for patients with chronic low back pain: the MRC spine stabilization trial. BMJ 2005;330:1233.
6. Brox JI, Sorensen R, Friis A, et al. Randomized clinical trial of lumbar instrumented fusion and cognitive intervention and exercises in patients with chronic low back pain and disc degeneration. Spine 2003;28:1913–21.
7. Brox JI, Reikeras O, Nygaard O, et al. Lumbar instrumented fusion compared with cognitive intervention and exercises in patients with chronic back pain after previous surgery for disc herniation: A prospective randomized controlled study. Pain 2006;122:145–55.
8. Carreon L, Glassman S, Howard J. Fusion and nonsurgical treatment for symptomatic lumbar degenerative disease: a systematic review of Oswestry Disability Index and MOS Short Form-36 outcomes. Spine J 2008;8:747–55.

79 Mechanical Low Back Pain: Nonoperative Management

Andrea D. Furlan[1,2,3], *Victoria Pennick*[1,3], *Jill A. Hayden*[4], *and Carlo Ammendolia*[1,3,5]

[1]Institute for Work & Health, Toronto, ON, Canada
[2]Toronto Rehabilitation Institute, Toronto, ON, Canada
[3]University of Toronto, Toronto, ON, Canada
[4]Dalhousie University, Halifax, NS, Canada
[5]Mount Sinai Hospital, Toronto, ON, Canada

Case scenario

A 45 year old man is brought to the Emergency Department with a 2 day history of insidious and incapacitating low back pain (LBP). Because of his pain, he has been unable to return to work at the post office where he works as a mail handler. On examination, the range of motion of the lumbar spine is difficult to examine because of severe pain; deep tendon reflexes are present and symmetrically equal, and straight leg raise is full to 90° bilaterally. Babinski reflexes are down-going bilaterally.

Relevant anatomy

Low back pain is defined as pain localized from the costal margin or 12th rib to the inferior gluteal fold. "Nonspecific" indicates that objective causes for symptoms, such as infection, neoplasm, metastasis, osteoporosis, fracture, inflammatory process, or radicular syndrome have been ruled out.

Importance of the problem

Low back pain affects 70–85% of people at some point in their lives.[1] A national telephone survey of the United States workforce found that the 2-week period prevalence of back pain was 15.1%; the cost to employers was esti-mated as $7.4 billion/year.[2] A recent review of cost of illness identified 27 studies reporting data from Australia, Belgium, Japan, Korea, the Netherlands, Sweden, the UK, and the US. They found that the largest proportion of direct medical costs for LBP was spent on physical therapy (17%) and inpatient services (17%), followed by pharmacy (13%) and primary care (13%). Among studies providing estimates of total costs, indirect costs resulting from lost work productivity represented a majority of overall costs associated with LBP.[3]

Patients are inundated with a variety of potential treatment modalities, all claiming efficacy in the treatment of LBP. Haldeman and Dagenais termed this situation the "supermarket approach."[4] They presented a partial list of treatment options available to patients with chronic LBP that contained 96 options divided into "supermarket aisles": storefront window shopping (activity modification, coping and acceptance, reassurance, rest, etc.), pharmacological, manual therapies, exercise, physical modalities, educational and psychological therapies, treatment and interventions, injections, minimally invasive interventions, surgery, lifestyle therapies, and complementary and alternative therapies.[4]

Approximately 63 million hits appear on Google when the search term "low back pain" is entered, and 19,834 citations are identified in PubMed. One of the goals of the Cochrane Back Review Group (established in 1996) is to synthesize the evidence from randomized trials of interventions for neck and LBP. As of the Cochrane Library 2011, issue 8, this group has published 50 reviews, including 1

Evidence-Based Orthopedics, First Edition. Edited by Mohit Bhandari.
© 2012 Blackwell Publishing Ltd. Published 2012 by Blackwell Publishing Ltd.

review of diagnostic test accuracy and 13 protocols. (www.cochrane.iwh.on.ca) Fifty-two reviews were co-published in peer-reviewed journals.

Top five questions

Diagnosis

1. What is the role of lumbar imaging studies in the diagnosis of LBP?

Therapy 1

2. What is the optimal nonoperative approach for the treatment of acute LBP?

Prognosis

3. Are there prognostic indicators for the development of chronic LBP?

Therapy 2

4. What is the optimal nonoperative approach for the treatment of chronic LBP?

Harm

5. What are the complications associated with epidural injections and facet blocks for the treatment of LBP?

Question 1: What is the role of lumbar imaging studies in the diagnosis of LBP?

Case clarification

The patient presents with an episode of acute LBP.

LBP is usually classified according to duration:

- **Acute LBP:** duration of 4 weeks or less
- **Subacute LBP:** duration between 4 and 12 weeks
- **Chronic LBP:** constant pain for 12 weeks or longer
- **Recurrent LBP:** recurrent episodes of acute LBP with asymptomatic periods between episodes

Relevance

The use of imaging (radiography, CT scan and MRI) in patients with LBP should be judicious and discriminating. Decisions should be based on the presence of clinical features (risk factors) in the history and physical examination that significantly raise the suspicion of underlying serious

conditions. Serious disease is rare in patients with LBP. Once serious disease is ruled out, the patient is considered to have nonspecific LBP. However, making the diagnosis of nonspecific LBP is often challenging in the acute care setting or during a single visit to a specialist.

Finding the evidence

- Cochrane Database of Systematic Reviews (April 2010) for reviews published by the Cochrane Back Review Group (query: hm-back in 'all text')
- PubMed (www.pubmed.com) query: "(low back pain) AND (imaging) AND (systematic review OR meta-analysis)"

Quality of the evidence
Level I
- 1 systematic review/meta-analysis[5]

Findings

Immediate lumbar imaging (radiography, CT scan or MRI) was compared to usual care without immediate imaging in six randomized trials (1,804 patients). Most patients had acute or subacute LBP and all trials were conducted in primary care or urgent care settings. These trials were summarized in a meta-analysis[5] and no significant differences were found between the two groups at either 3 month follow-up (standardized mean difference 0.19, 95% CI −0.01 to 0.39 for pain; and 0.11, 95% CI −0.29 to 0.50 for function) or 6–12 month follow-up (SMD−0.04, 95% CI −0.15 to 0.07 for pain and 0.01, 95% CI −0.17 to 0.19 for function).

Adults with LBP should be assessed by taking a focused history and conducting a physical examination, evaluating the duration of symptoms, risk factors for potentially serious conditions, symptoms suggesting radiculopathy or spinal stenosis, presence and severity of neurological deficits, and psychosocial risk factors. If potentially serious conditions are suspected, then the clinician should perform diagnostic studies to identify the cause. In the absence of symptoms or signs suggesting a serious condition, the clinician should avoid ordering diagnostic imaging tests. The indicators of a serious underlying condition in patients with LBP were summarized in a systematic review conducted for the American Pain Society for the development of the clinical practice guidelines for diagnosis and treatment of LBP.[6] Figure 79.1 shows the diagnostic workup to rule out possible serious underlying conditions recommended by the American Pain Society.

Recommendations

- Lumbar imaging for LBP without indications of serious underlying conditions does not improve clinical outcomes [overall quality: high]
- Clinicians should refrain from routine, immediate lumbar imaging in patients with acute or subacute LBP

Diagnostic Work-up

Possible cause	key features on history or physical examination	Imaging*	Additional studies*
Cancer	History of cancer with new onset of LBP	MRI	ESR
	Unexplained weight loss Failure to improve after 1 month Age >50 years	Lumbosacral plain radiography	
	Multiple risk factors present	Plain radiography or MRI	
Vertebral infection	Fever Intravenous drug use Recent infection	MRI	ESR and/or CRP
Cauda equina syndrome	Urinary retention Motor deficits at multiple levels Fecal incontinence Saddle anesthesia	MRI	None
Vertebral compression fracture	History of osteoporosis Use of corticosteroids Older age	Lumbosacral plain radiography	None
Ankylosing spondylitis	Morning stiffness Improvement with exercise Alternating buttock pain Awakening due to back pain during the second part of the night Younger age	Anterior-posterior pelvis plain radiography	ESR and/or CRP, HLA-B27
Severe/ progressive neurologic deficits	Progressive motor weakness	MRI	Consider EMG/NCV
Herniated disc	Back pain with leg pain in an L4, L5, or S1 nerve root distribution Positive straight-leg-raise test or crossed straight-leg-raise test	None	None
	Symptoms present >1 month	MRI	Consider EMG/NCV
Spinal stenosis	Radiating leg pain Older age (Pseudoclaudication a weak predictor)	None	None
	Symptoms present >1 month	MRI	Consider EMG/NCV

Figure 79.1 Diagnostic workup. Reproduced with permission from Chou R, Qaseem A, Snow V, Casey D, Cross JT, Jr, Shekelle P, Owens DK. Diagnosis and treatment of low back pain: a joint clinical practice guideline from the American College of Physicians and the American Pain Society. Ann Intern Med, 2007; 147: 478–491.

without features suggesting a serious underlying condition [overall quality: high]

Question 2: What is the optimal nonoperative approach for the treatment of acute LBP?

Case clarification

The patient's focused history and physical examination did not reveal signs of radiculopathy, spinal stenosis, or any specific spinal cause, therefore there is no need to order imaging studies. The patient receives the diagnosis of "acute nonspecific LBP."

LBP can be classified according to the underlying cause:[6]

- **Nonspecific low back pain:** more than 85% of patients who present to primary care have LBP that cannot reliably be attributed to a specific disease or spinal abnormality.[10]
- In a minority of patients presenting for initial evaluation in a primary care setting, LBP is **caused by a specific disorder**, such as cancer (0.7%), compression fracture (4%), spinal infection (0.01%), ankylosing spondylitis (0.3–5%), spinal stenosis (3%), and symptomatic herniated disc (4%). Cauda equina syndrome is most commonly associated with a massive midline disc herniation but is rare, with an estimated prevalence of 0.04% among patients with LBP.[7–9]

The goal of therapy is to help the patient manage their symptoms with minimal disruption in their normal life.

Finding the evidence

• Cochrane Database of Systematic Reviews (April 2010) for reviews published by the Cochrane Back Review Group (query: hm-back in 'all text')
• PubMed (www.pubmed.com) query: "(low back pain) AND (intervention OR treatment OR therapy) AND (systematic review OR meta-analysis OR guideline)"

Quality of the evidence

Level I
• 5 systematic reviews/meta-analyses

Findings

A Cochrane review of individual patient education strategies found 24 randomized trials.[10] The results showed that intensive patient education (lasting 2 hours) seems to be effective for pain relief and global improvement for patients with acute or subacute LBP. Providing the patient with pamphlets, booklets, or a 20-minute session resulted in little or no difference compared to no intervention.

A Cochrane review of bed rest included 10 randomized trials.[11] They found high-quality evidence that people with acute LBP who are advised to rest in bed have more pain (standardized mean difference 0.22; 95% CI 0.02–0.41) and less functional recovery (SMD 0.31; 95% CI 0.06–0.55) than those advised to stay active.

A Cochrane review of nonsteroidal anti-inflammatory drugs (NSAIDs) for LBP included 65 randomized trials (11,237 patients); 28 trials were considered to have a low risk of bias.[12] The authors found 11 trials comparing NSAIDs with placebo for acute LBP, and statistical pooling was possible for 6 of the 11 trials: the mean difference (MD) in pain reduction was −8.39 (95% CI −12.68 to −4.10), indicating an effect in favor of NSAIDs. Six trials compared some type of NSAID with acetaminophen (paracetamol). The statistical pooling showed an SMD of −0.21 (95% CI −0.43 to 0.02) which indicates that NSAIDS and acetaminophen are equally effective for pain relief and global improvement for acute nonspecific LBP. However, NSAIDS were associated with more adverse effects than paracetamol (relative risk [RR] 1.76; 95% CI 1.12–2.76).

A Cochrane review of muscle relaxants for LBP included 24 trials of acute LBP.[13] Results showed that muscle relaxants were more effective than placebo on short-term pain relief, but adverse effects were also more prevalent, (especially dizziness and drowsiness) with an RR of 2.04 (95% CI 1.23–3.37). The various muscle relaxants were found to be similar in performance.

A meta-analysis of 76 trials reporting on 34 different treatments for LBP was conducted to estimate the treatment effects in placebo-controlled trials. Fifty percent of the investigated treatments had statistically significant effects, but for most the effects were small or moderate: 47% had point estimates of effects of less than 10 points on a 100-point scale, 38% had point estimates of 10–20 points, and 15% had point estimates of more than 20 points. Treatments reported to have large effects (>20 points) had only been investigated in a single trial (electroacupuncture, immunoglobulins, infrared, vitamin B_{12}, and neuroreflexotherapy) (Figure 79.2). This meta-analysis found that the analgesic effects of many treatments for nonspecific LBP are small and that they do not differ in populations with acute or chronic symptoms.

Recommendations

Based on systematic reviews[10–13] and existing clinical practice guidelines,[6,14] practitioners should start with the following, when treating patients with acute nonspecific low back pain:
• Provide patient education and reassurance [overall quality: high]
• Avoid bed rest as a treatment [overall quality: high]
• Advise patients to stay active and continue normal daily activities, including work if possible [overall quality: high]
• Prescribe medications as necessary for pain relief; preferably to be taken at regular intervals; first choice paracetamol, second choice NSAIDs [overall quality: high]
• Consider adding a short course of muscle relaxants on its own or added to NSAIDs, if paracetamol or NSAIDs fail to reduce pain and promote functional gains [overall quality: high]

Question 3: Are there prognostic indicators for the development of chronic LBP?

Case clarification

The patient is seen again at 6 months: he now has constant daily pain and is on long-term disability leave from his job. This patient has progressed from an acute episode of nonspecific LBP to chronic nonspecific LBP.

There are flags in the acute and subacute phases that may have indicated that this patient was at risk of developing chronic pain. "Yellow flags" are psychosocial factors that may be associated with delayed recovery.[15]

Yellow flags

Psychosocial "yellow flags" are factors associated with increased risk of developing, or perpetuating chronic pain and long-term disability (including) work-loss associated with LBP. Identification of 'yellow flags' should lead to appropriate cognitive and behavioral management. Examples of yellow flags are:
• Inappropriate attitudes and beliefs about back pain
• Inappropriate pain behavior
• Work related problems or compensation issues
• Emotional problems (depression, anxiety, stress, withdrawal from social interactions)

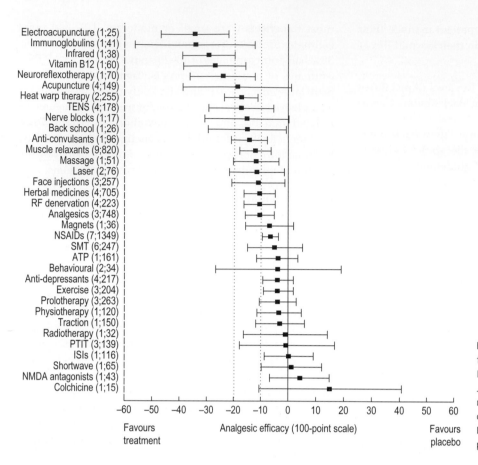

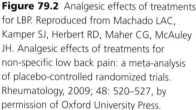

Figure 79.2 Analgesic effects of treatments for LBP. Reproduced from Machado LAC, Kamper SJ, Herbert RD, Maher CG, McAuley JH. Analgesic effects of treatments for non-specific low back pain: a meta-analysis of placebo-controlled randomized trials. Rheumatology, 2009; 48: 520–527, by permission of Oxford University Press.

Finding the evidence

• Cochrane Database of Systematic Reviews (April 2010) for reviews published by the Cochrane Back Review Group (query: hm-back in 'all text')
• PubMed (www.pubmed.com) query: "(low back pain) AND (broad prognosis clinical query) AND (systematic review OR meta-analysis)"

Quality of the evidence

Level I
• 1 systematic review

Findings

Chou and Shekelle systematically reviewed the usefulness of individual prognostic factors or outcome prediction tools for identifying patients more likely to develop persistent disabling LBP.[16] This review identified 20 studies evaluating 10,842 patients. Considering evidence from these studies, the following factors are identified as predictors of persistent LBP.

Demographic and work-related factors Age, sex, educational level, smoking status, and being overweight did not predict worse outcomes. Receiving compensation at baseline was associated with a slightly increased likelihood of worse

outcomes at 1 year (median likelihood ratio (LR) 1.4; range 1.2–0.8). Higher work dissatisfaction and higher physical work demands did not predict worse outcomes at 3 months, but did at 1 year (median LR 1.4; range 1.2–1.7).

Health status at the onset of LBP Worse general health status before the onset of LBP was associated with worse outcomes at 3–6 months (median LR 1.6; range 1.1–1.7) and at 1 year (median LR 1.8; range 1.1–2.0). Higher psychiatric comorbidity was associated with worse outcomes at 3–6 months (median LR 1.9; range 1.4–2.1) and at 1 year (median LR 2.2; range 1.9–2.3). A history of previous LBP was not associated with persistent disabling LBP at 3–6 months or 1 year.

LBP episode signs and symptoms High baseline pain intensity was found to be associated with worse outcomes at 3–6 months (median LR 1.7; range 1.1–3.7), but was less useful at 1 year. High baseline functional impairment was associated with increased likelihood of poor outcome at 3–6 months (median LR 1.4; range 1.3–3.5) and at 1 year (median LR 2.1; range: 1.2–2.7). Radiculopathy or leg pain was associated with worse outcomes at 3–6 months (median LR 1.4; range 1.1–1.7) and 1 year (median LR 1.4; range 1.2–2.4). Patients with maladaptive pain coping behaviors, such as fear-avoidance beliefs had more persistent LBP at 3–6 months (median LR 2.2; range 1.5–4.9) and 1 year (median LR 2.5; range 2.2–2.8). High somatization/nonorganic signs (exaggerated pain symptoms) were associated with poor work outcomes at 1 year (median LR 3.0; range 1.7–4.6).

Recommendations

Current evidence on the prognosis of acute nonspecific LBP supports the following:

• The majority of patients with acute nonspecific LBP will recover, although recurrences are common [overall quality: low]

• Helpful characteristics for predicting persistent disabling LBP are maladaptive pain coping behaviors, somatization/nonorganic signs, increased functional impairment, poor general health status, and presence of psychiatric comorbidities [overall quality: high]

Question 4: What is the optimal nonoperative approach for the treatment of chronic LBP?

Case clarification

The patient's LBP is severe and debilitating.

Severity of pain is usually measured with a numerical pain rating scale from 0 (no pain) to 10 (most severe pain).
• **Mild pain** is when the average pain is 4 or less
• **Moderate pain** is between 5 and 7
• **Severe pain** is 8 or greater

Finding the evidence

• Cochrane Database of Systematic Reviews (April 2010) for reviews published by the Cochrane Back Review Group (query: hm-back in 'all text')

• PubMed (www.pubmed.com) query: "(low back pain) AND (intervention OR treatment OR therapy) AND (systematic review OR meta-analysis OR guideline)"

Quality of the evidence

Level I
• 5 systematic reviews/meta-analyses

Findings

In 2007, the American Pain Society's clinical practice guideline[17] found the following interventions for chronic LBP that were of moderate or small benefit and supported by at least fair-quality evidence: advice to remain active, patient education, acetaminophen, NSAIDs, antidepressants, benzodiazepines, tramadol (opioid), spinal manipulation, exercise therapy, massage, acupuncture, yoga, cognitive-behavioral therapy, progressive relaxation, and intensive interdisciplinary rehabilitation. They found no intervention that was supported by high-quality evidence (Figure 79.3).

Interventions

	Low Back Pain	Acute	Subacute or Chronic
	Duration	< 4 Weeks	> 4 Weeks
Self-care	Advice to remain active	•	•
	Books, handout	•	•
	Application of superficial heat	•	
Pharmacologic therapy	Acetaminophen	•	•
	NSAIDs	•	•
	Skeletal muscle relaxants	•	
	Antidepressants (TCA)		•
	Benzodiazepines	•	•
	Tramadol, opioids	•	•
Nonpharmacologic therapy	Spinal manipulation	•	•
	Exercise therapy		•
	Massage		•
	Acupuncture		•
	Yoga		•
	Cognitive-behavioral therapy		•
	Progressive relaxation		•
	Intensive interdisciplinary rehabilitation		•

• Interventions supported by grade B evidence (at least fair-quality evidence of moderate benefit, or small benefit but no significant harms, costs, or burdens). No intervention was supported by grade A evidence (good-quality evidence of substantial benefit).

Figure 79.3 Conservative interventions for LBP. Reproduced with permission from Chou R, Qaseem A, Snow V, Casey D, Cross JT, Jr, Shekelle P, Owens DK. Diagnosis and treatment of low back pain: a joint clinical practice guideline from the American College of Physicians and the American Pain Society, Ann Intern Med 2007; 147: 478–491.

Henschke et al reviewed 27 RCTs, 14 on injection therapy and 13 on denervation procedures.[18] Eighteen (66%) of the studies were determined to have a low risk of bias. Because of clinical heterogeneity, only two comparisons could be pooled. Overall, there is only low to very low quality evidence to support the use of injection therapy and denervation procedures over placebo or other treatments for patients with chronic LBP.

A Cochrane review of injection therapies for LBP included 18 trials (1179 patients).[19] Statistical pooling was not possible due to clinical heterogeneity amongst the trials. Overall the results indicate that there is no strong evidence for or against the use of any type of injection therapy for subacute or chronic LBP. The injection sites varied from epidural and facet joints to local sites (tender and trigger points). The drugs injected were corticosteroids, local anesthetics, and a variety of other drugs.

In 2004, the European guidelines for chronic LBP systematically reviewed the evidence for various treatment options.[20] They found no evidence to support epidural steroids, intra-articular injections of steroids or facet nerve blocks in patients with nonspecific chronic LBP.[20]

In 2009, the American Pain Society published a clinical practice guideline on the use of interventional therapies for chronic nonspecific LBP.[5] They concluded that there is no convincing evidence from randomized trials that injections and other interventional therapies are effective for nonradicular LBP. Facet joint steroid injection, prolotherapy, and intradiscal steroid injections were no more effective than sham therapies. For local injections, there was insufficient evidence to accurately judge the benefits because available trials were small, had a high risk of bias, and evaluated heterogeneous populations and interventions.

Recommendations
• The following nonoperative treatments for chronic nonspecific LBP have been found to show some evidence of benefit with minimal risk of harm: advice to remain active, patient education, acetaminophen, NSAIDS, antidepressants, spinal manipulation, exercise, massage, acupuncture, yoga, cognitive-behavioral therapy, and intensive interdisciplinary rehabilitation [overall quality: low to moderate]
• Tramadol and benzodiazepines have some evidence of benefit, but are also associated with adverse events [overall quality: low to moderate]

Question 5: What are the complications associated with epidural injections and facet blocks for the treatment of LBP?

Relevance
Although the use of epidural steroids and facet blocks for nonspecific LBP is not supported by current evidence, many patients end up receiving these interventions. Patients should be aware of the potential complications of these procedures.

Finding the evidence
• Cochrane Database of Systematic Reviews (April 2010) for reviews published by the Cochrane Back Review Group (query: hm-back in 'all text')
• PubMed (www.pubmed.com) query: "(low back pain) AND (epidural steroids OR facet blocks)"

Quality of the evidence
Level I
• 2 systematic reviews/meta-analyses

Findings
In the Cochrane review of injections for LBP, adverse effects such as headache, dizziness, transient local pain, paresthesia, and nausea were reported in a small number of patients in 9 of the 18 included trials.

The American Pain Society guideline development panel found insufficient evidence from randomized trials to reliably judge harms of these interventional therapies for LBP.

Rare complications are usually not reported in randomized trials due to the small sample sizes and relatively short follow-up duration. As such, a review of case reports and epidemiological studies is necessary. The 2004 European guidelines for LBP used this approach to summarize the evidence regarding complications and harms of these interventions:
• Technical complications: accidental dural puncture (5% of the cases) with consequent postdural puncture headache; and epidural hematoma (very rare)
• Infectious complications: several cases of epidural abscess after epidural steroid injection have been documented, most of which occurred in diabetic patients; however, the incidence is very rare
• Neurological complications: neurological sequelae (chemical meningitis) can occur after intrathecal application of steroids. Arachnoiditis after epidural injection of steroids is very rare
• There is one report of septic facet joint arthritis after facet injection,[21] but the rate of such an event is unknown and seems likely to be rare

Recommendation
• Epidural steroid injections, intra-articular injections and facet blocks have potential complications, but the incidence is rare [overall quality: very low]

Summary of recommendations

• Clinicians should refrain from routine, immediate lumbar imaging in patients with acute or subacute LBP and without features suggesting a serious underlying condition
• Avoid bed rest as a treatment
• Advise patients to stay active and continue normal daily activities including work if possible. Provide information on back-care and self-care
• Prescribe medications, if necessary for pain relief; preferably to be taken at regular intervals; first choice paracetamol, second choice NSAIDs
• Consider adding a short course of muscle relaxants on its own or added to NSAIDs, if acetaminophen or NSAIDs have failed to reduce pain and promote function
• Patients with acute nonspecific LBP will likely recover although recurrences are common
• Helpful characteristics for predicting persistent disabling LBP are maladaptive pain coping behaviors, somatization/nonorganic signs, increased functional impairment, poor general health status, and presence of psychiatric comorbidities

- The following nonoperative treatments for chronic non-specific LBP have been found to show some evidence of benefit with minimal risk of harm: advice to remain active, patient education, acetaminophen, NSAIDS, antidepressants, spinal manipulation, exercise, massage, acupuncture, yoga, cognitive-behavioral therapy, and intensive interdisciplinary rehabilitation
- Tramadol and benzodiazepines also have shown some evidence of effectiveness, but are associated with adverse events
- Use of epidural steroid injections, intra-articular injections and facet blocks is not evidence-based and these therapies have potential complications, but the incidence is rare.

References

1. Andersson HI, Ejlertsson G, Leden I, Schersten B. Musculoskeletal chronic pain in general practice. Studies of health care utilisation in comparison with pain prevalence. Scand J Prim Health Care 1999;17:87–92.
2. Ricci JA, Stewart WF, Chee E, Leotta C, Foley K, Hochberg MC. Back pain exacerbations and lost productive time costs in United States workers. Spine 2006;31:3052–60.
3. Dagenais S, Caro J, Haldeman S. A systematic review of low back pain cost of illness studies in the United States and internationally, Spine J 2008;8:8–20.
4. Haldeman S, Dagenais S A supermarket approach to the evidence-informed management of chronic low back pain. Spine J 2008;8:1–7.
5. Chou R, Fu R, Carrino JA, Deyo RA. Imaging strategies for low back pain: systematic review and meta-analysis. Lancet 2009;373: 463–72.
6. Chou R, Qaseem A, Snow V, Casey D, Cross JT, Jr, Shekelle P, Owens DK. Diagnosis and treatment of low back pain: a joint clinical practice guideline from the American College of Physicians and the American Pain Society, Ann Intern Med 2007; 147:478–91.
7. Deyo RA, Rainville J, Kent DL. What can the history and physical examination tell us about low back pain? JAMA 1992;268: 760–765.
8. Jarvik JG, Deyo RA. Diagnostic evaluation of low back pain with emphasis on imaging. Ann Intern Med 2002;137:586–597.
9. Underwood MR, Dawes P. Inflammatory back pain in primary care. Br J Rheumatol 1995;34:1074–1077.
10. Engers A, Jellema P, Wensing M, van der Windt DA, Grol R, van Tulder MW. Individual patient education for low back pain. Cochrane Database Syst Rev 2008, issue 1:CD004057.
11. Dahm KT, Brurberg KG, Jamtvedt G, Hagen KB. Advice to rest in bed versus advice to stay active for acute low back pain and sciatica, Cochrane Database Syst Rev 2010, issue 6:CD007612.
12. Roelofs PD, Deyo RA, Koes BW, Scholten RJ, van Tulder MW. Non-steroidal anti-inflammatory drugs for low back pain. Cochrane Database Syst Rev 2008, issue 1:CD000396.
13. van Tulder MW, Touray T, Furlan AD, Solway S, Bouter LM. Muscle relaxants for non-specific low back pain. Cochrane Database Syst Rev 2003, issue 2:CD004252.
14. van Tulder MW, Assendelft WJ, Koes BW, Bouter LM. Spinal radiographic findings and nonspecific low back pain. A systematic review of observational studies. Spine 1997;22:427–34.
15. ACC and the National Health Committee. New Zealand Acute Low Back Pain Guide. Wellington, New Zealand, 1997.
16. Chou R, Shekelle P. Will this patient develop persistent disabling low back pain? JAMA 2010;303:1295–302.
17. Chou R, Loeser JD, Owens DK, et al. Interventional therapies, surgery, and interdisciplinary rehabilitation for low back pain: an evidence-based clinical practice guideline from the American Pain Society. Spine 2009;34:1066–77.
18. Henschke N, Kuijpers T, Rubinstein SM, et al. Injection therapy and denervation procedures for chronic low back pain: a systematic review. Eur Spine J 2010;19(9):1425–49.
19. Staal JB, de Bie R, de Vet HC, Hildebrandt J, Nelemans P. Injection therapy for subacute and chronic low back pain. Cochrane Database Syst Rev 2008, issue 3:CD001824.
20. Airaksinen O, Brox JI, Cedraschi C, et al. On behalf of the COST B13 Working Group on Guidelines for Chronic Low Back Pain. European guidelines for the management of chronic non-specific low back pain http://www.backpaineurope.org/web/html/wg2_results.html.
21. Orpen NM, Birch NC. Delayed presentation of septic arthritis of a lumbar facet joint after diagnostic facet joint injection. J Spinal Disord Tech 2003 Jun;16(3):285–7.

80 Neurogenic Claudication—Operative Management (Decompression and Fusion)

Hormuzdiyar H. Dasenbrock, Reza Yassari, and Timothy F. Witham
Johns Hopkins University, Baltimore, MD, USA

Case scenario

A 59 year old woman presented with buttock and leg pain that developed upon ambulation. Her pain appeared after walking a distance of one block (200m) or more, was accompanied by lower extremity numbness, and was relieved by sitting down. The patient also noted that she did not normally experience this pain while grocery shopping. Neurological examination was normal but MRI of the lumbar spine revealed severe spinal stenosis (Figure 80.1). Flexion and extension radiographs demonstrated evidence of instability with spondylolithesis (Figure 80.2). After failure to improve with conservative therapy (including physical therapy and epidural steroid injections), surgery was recommended. The patient underwent L3–4 and L4–5 decompression and interbody arthrodesis with transpedicular instrumentation from L3 to L5 (Figure 80.3). The patient noted significant reduction in her pain at 1 year follow-up.

Relevant anatomy and pathophysiology

Spinal stenosis describes a spinal canal with a diminished caliber causing compression of neural structures, including the thecal sac and the nerve roots.[1–2] Coexisting foraminal stenosis and/or spinal instability may further exacerbate neural compression. Patients may have pre-existing narrowing of the spinal canal due to congenital stenosis with short pedicles, excessive lordosis, or scoliosis.[3] Superimposed upon any pre-existing narrowing of the canal that may be present are degenerative and arthritic changes associated with aging, including the development of osteophytes, hypertrophy of the ligamentum flavum, degeneration of the intervertebral disc (with bulging and/or herniation), and hypertrophy of the facet joint and its capsule.[4] The narrowed diameter of the spinal canal leads to compression of the neural structures and the microvasculature. Symptoms are hypothesized to be due to direct neural compression as well as to ischemia from microvascular compression.[5–6]

Spinal stenosis may be accompanied by degenerative spondylolisthesis, which describes the anterior slippage of one vertebral body relative to the adjacent one and is indicative of an unstable spinal unit.[7] Although displacement can occur posteriorly or laterally, spondylolisthesis is synonymous with anterior slippage.[8] Degenerative spondylolisthesis is due to a combination of arthritic and degenerative changes in the disc and facet joints that leads to spinal stenosis and vertebral body displacement.[9]

Importance of the problem

The importance of the surgical treatment of lumbar spinal stenosis was evaluated in a study of more than 1000 patients in South Korea. The authors compared those who underwent surgical decompression to age- and sex-matched controls in the general population. Using a Cox multivariable regression analysis, the authors calculated standardized mortality ratios for different age groups: patients treated surgically had lower mortality compared to the general population. The mortality ratios were 0.53 for patients who were aged 60–69 and 0.45 for patients who were aged 70–79 at the time of the operation.[10] The authors concluded that the improvement in mortality may be due to superior mobility and the ability to exercise regularly.

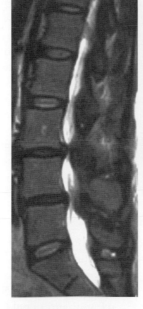
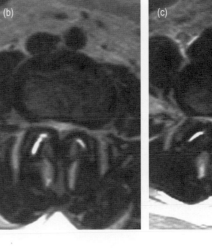
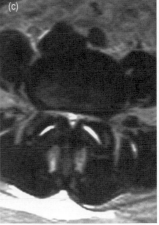

Figure 80.1 A 59 year old woman presented with neurogenic claudication. Sagittal T2-weighted MRI images (a) reveals severe spinal stenosis at the levels of the L3–4 and L4–5 intervertebral discs. Axial T2-weighted MRI images at the level of the L3–4 (b) and L4–5 (c) discs also demonstrate severe stenosis with impingement of the thecal sac, as well as low epidural fat and cerebrospinal fluid (CSF) signal.

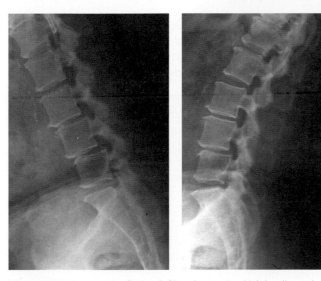

Figure 80.2 Preoperative flexion (left) and extension (right) radiographs reveal low-grade spondylolisthesis at L3–4 and L4–5 that is visible on flexion, but reduces upon extension. Because of the evidence of instability, the patient underwent a fusion operation: decompression with interbody arthrodesis and adjunct L3–L5 transpedicular instrumentation was performed.

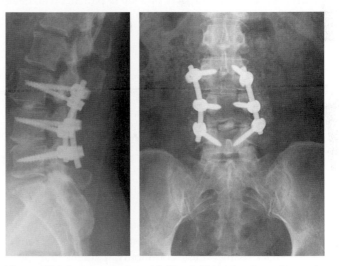

Figure 80.3 Postoperative lateral (left) and AP (right) radiographs reveal appropriate placement of the transpedicular instrumentation, with no progression of the spondylolisthesis.

Top 6 questions

Diagnosis

1. What are the typical presentation, examination findings, and imaging characteristics of patients with lumbar spinal stenosis?

Therapy

2. What is the evidence for surgical treatment compared to conservative management for patients with lumbar spinal stenosis *without* spondylolisthesis?

3. What is the evidence that there is a benefit to surgical treatment compared to conservative management for patients with lumbar spinal stenosis *with* spondylolisthesis?

4. What is the evidence for lumbar fusion with decompression compared to decompression alone for patients with lumbar spinal stenosis *without* spondylolisthesis?

5. What is the evidence for lumbar fusion with decompression compared to decompression alone for patients with lumbar spinal stenosis *with* accompanying spondylolithesis?

Harm

6. What are the perioperative and long-term complications associated with decompression alone or decompression and fusion for patients with spinal stenosis?

Question 1: What are the typical presentation, examination findings, and imaging characteristics of patients with lumbar spinal stenosis?

Relevance

An understanding of the presentation and findings of spinal stenosis is important in order to evaluate patients who may benefit from treatment.

Current opinion

Neurogenic claudication may be seen in patients who have underlying spinal stenosis with or without accompanying spondylolisthesis.

Finding the evidence

• MEDLINE, with search terms: "lumbar spinal stenosis," as well as "lumbar spinal stenosis" AND "magnetic resonance imaging" OR "computed tomography"

Quality of the evidence

Level I
• 1 meta-analysis

Findings

Patients with lumbar spinal stenosis typically present with neurogenic claudication, radiculopathy, paresthesias, and/or low back pain.[11] Less commonly, patients may also present with sensory deficits, lower extremity weakness, or bowel and bladder dysfunction. Neurogenic claudication describes pain in the buttocks and along the proximal thigh that occurs when standing or walking. The pain may be accompanied by paresthesias or weakness in the lower extremities and it is typically relieved by resting, sitting down, or assuming a flexed position of the spine (such as leaning on a shopping cart). Neurological examination may be normal, although radicular signs, including a positive straight leg raise test, may be elicited.[12-13] Signs and symptoms may be exacerbated if the examination is repeated after a brief period of exercise.[14]

Patients with symptoms consistent with neurogenic claudication should have a thorough evaluation performed to exclude other conditions that may present similarly, including peripheral vascular disease. Vascular claudica-

tion is due to atherosclerosis of the pelvofemoral vasculature leading to hypoperfusion of the lower extremities upon ambulation. Patients with claudication will typically describe pain that is produced by walking but not by standing; the pain will not be relieved by flexion of the spine.

The accuracy of different imaging modalities to diagnose lumbar stenosis was evaluated in a 2006 systematic review: the authors concluded that the literature does not permit strong conclusions about the diagnostic accuracies of MRI or CT, primarily because of the heterogeneity and overall poor quality of the studies.[15] However, MRI may be useful to visualize neural compression, and CT may determine the presence of additional bony pathology, such as osteophytes.[16] Dynamic flexion-extension radiographs will demonstrate spondylolisthesis or subtle instability.

Recommendation

• Patients who have a presentation concerning for spinal stenosis should also be evaluated for peripherial vascular disease and their spinal anatomy imaged by MRI with or without additional CT [overall quality: very low]

Question 2: What is the evidence for surgical treatment compared to conservative management for patients with lumbar spinal stenosis without spondylolisthesis?

Relevance

The quality of life of patients with lumbar spinal stenosis may be improved with surgery. However, operative intervention should be reserved for patients who are likely to experience a greater benefit from the procedure then they would from conservative treatment.

Current opinion

Surgery is generally preferred for patients with spinal stenosis whose symptoms have persisted despite a reasonable trial of conservative therapy or who have evidence of neurological motor deficits.

Finding the evidence

• MEDLINE, using the search term: "lumbar spinal stenosis" AND "surgery"

Quality of the evidence

Level I
• 2 randomized controlled trials (RCTs)

Findings

The role of conservative therapy for patients with lumbar spinal stenosis is debated.[17-18] A trial of nonsurgical management is typically attempted, which may consist of nonsteroidal anti-inflammatory drugs (NSAIDs), activity modification, and physical therapy—including core muscle and lower extremity stretching and strengthening exercises. Operative treatment is pursued in patients who continue to remain symptomatic despite a reasonable trial of conservative management (typically defined as at least 3 months). Surgery is the preferred treatment for patients with neurological motor deficits. The goals of surgery include pain relief, improved mobility, prevention of the development of neurological deficits, or restoration of neurological function.[19]

The Spine Patient Outcomes Research Trial (SPORT) was a large prospective randomized multicenter trial (with an additional observational cohort) that compared surgical decompression (with or without fusion) to usual nonsurgical care. The study included 289 randomized (and 356 observational) patients from 13 centers in 11 US states. The primary inclusion criteria were at least 12 weeks of symptoms that persisted despite conservative treatment and evidence of spinal stenosis without spondylolisthesis on imaging.[20]

At the 2 year follow-up, there was a significant crossover between cohorts: only 67% of those assigned to surgery had undergone an operation, while 43% of patients who had been assigned to nonsurgical care had surgery performed. The intention-to-treat analysis found a significant improvement in one primary outcome measure favoring surgery—SF-36 bodily pain score. However, the associated measure of precision included both clinically relevant and clinically unimportant differences (mean increase in 7.8 points, 95% CI 1.5–14.1 points), and there was no significant difference in scores on the two other primary outcome measures assessing disability—SF-36 physical function or Oswestry Disability Index (ODI) scores. The as-treated analysis, which negated the benefits of randomization, showed a significant improvement in all outcome measures at both 2 year and 4 year follow-up.[20–21]

Another RCT that compared surgical decompression to standard nonoperative care for 94 patients with lumbar spinal stenosis was conducted by the Finnish lumbar spine research group. At 1 year follow-up the study found a statistically significant benefit to surgery for their primary outcome measure, the ODI (mean improvement 11.3 points, 95% CI 4.3–18.4 points) and the associated measure of precision included both clinically important and trivial changes. However, at 2 year follow-up this difference failed to meet the minimal important difference—the smallest change in ODI score that patients perceive is important—of 10 points[22] (mean improvement 7.8; 95% CI 0.8–14.9).[23]

Recommendation

• Surgery may lead to a significant improvement in pain in patients with symptomatic spinal stenosis who have not substantially improved despite a reasonable trial (at least 3 months) of conservative therapy. The effect of surgery on disability is uncertain [overall quality: moderate]

Question 3: What is the evidence that there is a benefit to surgical treatment compared to conservative management for patients with lumbar spinal stenosis with spondylolisthesis?

Relevance

Operative intervention should be reserved for patients who are likely to have a greater benefit from the procedure than from nonsurgical care.

Current opinion

Surgery is generally preferred for patients with lumbar spondylolisthesis with spinal stenosis whose symptoms have persisted despite a reasonable trial of conservative therapy or who have evidence of neurological deficits.

Finding the evidence

• MEDLINE, with search term: "lumbar spondylolisthesis" AND "surgery"

Quality of the evidence

Level I

• 1 RCT

Findings

The optimal treatment for patients with degenerative spondylolisthesis was examined by a different arm of the SPORT trial, which compared surgical to usual nonoperative care. Inclusion criteria were persistent symptoms (neurogenic claudication or radiculopathy) for more than 12 weeks and evidence of degenerative spondylolisthesis on lateral static radiographs. Enrollment was in either a randomized cohort (304 patients) or an observational cohort (303 patients), outcomes were evaluated quantitatively using the ODI and SF-36, and patients were followed for 2 years.[24]

As was the case with the SPORT trial evaluating patients with lumbar spinal stenosis, there was substantial crossover from the initial assignment: 66% of those randomized to receive surgery and 54% of those randomized to conservative treatment had an operation performed within 4 years. The intention-to-treat analysis for the randomized cohort showed no statistically significant effects for the primary outcomes. However, the as-treated analysis showed a substantial and significant benefit to surgery that was sustained 4 years later in the three primary outcome measures: ODI (mean improvement 14.3 points, 95% CI 11.1–17.5 points), SF-36 bodily pain (mean increase 15.3 points, 95% CI 11–19.7 points), and SF-36 physical function (mean increase 18.9 points, 95% CI 14.8–23.0 points).[24–25]

Recommendation

• Surgery may lead to a greater improvement in pain and disability than usual nonsurgical care alone in patients with symptomatic lumbar spinal stenosis with spondylolisthesis who have failed to substantially improve with conservative management [overall quality: moderate]

Question 4: What is the evidence for lumbar fusion with decompression compared to decompression alone for patients with lumbar spinal stenosis without spondylolisthesis?

Relevance
While a fusion operation may be important for patients who have evidence of instability, its utility for patients with spinal stenosis without spondylolisthesis is debated.

Current opinion
A fusion operation is not routinely added to a decompression for patients with lumbar spinal stenosis. However, in certain situations—such as coexisting spinal deformity or where there are concerns about postoperative iatrogenic instability—a posterolateral fusion may be preferred.

Finding the evidence
• MEDLINE, using the search term: "lumbar spinal stenosis" AND "fusion"

Quality of the evidence
Level II
• 1 prospective nonrandomized study

Findings
The benefit to the addition of a (primarily posterolateral) fusion to a decompressive surgery in patients with spinal stenosis has been debated.[26] Patients with evidence of preoperative instability,[27–28] concerns for the development of postoperative instability (due to extensive resection of the facet joints),[19] or coexisting spinal deformity (including degenerative scoliosis or loss of lordosis)[29–31] may benefit from a fusion operation. However, a fusion may increase operative times, blood loss, complication rates, and cost.[32]

One prospective (but nonrandomized) study examined 272 patients undergoing laminectomy with or without non-instrumented arthrodesis for lumbar spinal stenosis. Primary outcomes were health status, walking capacity, back and leg pain, and satisfaction with surgery was assessed 6 and 24 months postoperatively. Loss to follow-up was 13% at 6 months and 27% at 24 months. Adjusted models showed that arthrodesis was associated with greater improvement in back pain at 6 months (p = 0.05) and 24 months (p = 0.02), and in walking capacity at 6 months (p = 0.02) and 24 months (p = 0.03); however, the authors noted that given the adjustment for multiple comparisons, these results are of borderline statistical significance. For all other outcome measures, there was no benefit to the addition of a fusion and total hospital cost was sig-

nificantly greater for a fusion procedure (p = 0.0001).[33] Moreover, recent guidelines on the management of patients with spinal stenosis without spondylolisthesis recommend decompression without additional fusion in patients who do not have evidence of instability.[2]

Recommendation
• When operative treatment of lumbar spinal stenosis without spondylolisthesis is pursued, a decompression and fusion may not lead to superior outcomes compared with decompression alone [overall quality: low]

Question 5: What is the evidence for lumbar fusion with decompression compared to decompression alone for patients with lumbar spinal stenosis with accompanying spondylolithesis?

Relevance
Decompression without a fusion may exacerbate the instability of patients with spinal stenosis and accompanying spondylolisthesis postoperatively.

Current opinion
When surgical treatment is pursued for patients with lumbar spinal stenosis with accompanying spondylolisthesis, a fusion is typically performed.

Finding the evidence
• MEDLINE, using the search term: "lumbar spondylolisthesis" AND "fusion"

Quality of the evidence
Level I
• 1 systematic review

Findings
The utility of spinal fusion (compared with decompression alone) to improve clinical outcomes in patients with degenerative spondylolisthesis has also been investigated.[34] While some retrospective studies have reported good outcomes in patients treated with decompression alone,[35–36] a laminectomy is likely to further destabilize an already unstable spinal segment.[37–38] A 2007 systematic review found that decompression and fusion is significantly more likely to produce a satisfactory clinical outcome than decompression alone (relative risk 1.40, CI 1.04–1.89).[9]

Recommendation
• When surgery is performed for symptomatic lumbar spondylolisthesis, a fusion procedure may lead to superior clinical outcomes than decompression alone [overall quality: low]

Question 6: What are the perioperative and long-term complications associated with decompression alone or decompression and fusion for patients with spinal stenosis?

Relevance

A number of perioperative and long-term complications may occur after decompression and fusion of the lumbar spine.

Current opinion

Perioperative mortality after lumbar fusion is rare, but surgical site infections and neurologic injury can occur.

Finding the evidence

• Medline, using the search term: "lumbar fusion" OR "lumbar laminectomy" AND "complications"

Quality of the evidence

Level III

• Many retrospective studies

Findings

Perioperative mortality after posterior lumbar decompression with or without additional fusion is rare.[39–41] Data from the national inpatient sample (NIS) from 1993–2002 on 66,601 hospitalizations across America for patients undergoing a fusion operation where degenerative spondylolisthesis was the primary admitting diagnosis showed in-hospital mortality as 0.15%. Complication rates were also low (5.4%), of which more than half were cardiac, pulmonary, or renal in nature, manifesting in patients with chronic comorbidities.[42]

Surgical site infections are one of the most common complications, especially after a fusion: reported rates range from 0.65% to 12%.[43–48] Risk factors include obesity (especially morbid obesity),[43,45,47,49] diabetes,[45,47] a prior surgical site infection,[45,47] alcohol abuse,[47] greater operative blood loss,[45] longer operation times,[45,49] and the use of instrumentation.[49] Other known complications include nerve root injury due to instrumentation misplacement, incidental durotomy leading to the development of a cerebrospinal fluid leak,[50] spinal epidural hematoma (and other postoperative causes of cauda equina syndrome),[51–52] rhabdomyolysis,[53] venous thromboembolic events[54] and sudden visual loss.[55] Long-term complications after spinal fusion include sacral stress fractures,[56–58] adjacent level disease,[59–61] pseudoarthrosis,[62] sexual dysfunction,[63] and chronic donor allograft site pain.[64]

Recommendation

• Patients with recurrent postoperative pain who have undergone a fusion should be examined with imaging for the possibility of sacral stress fractures, adjacent level disease, or instrumentation complications [overall quality: very low]

Summary of recommendations

• Patients who have a presentation consistent with spinal stenosis should be evaluated for the presence of peripheral vascular disease and their spinal anatomy imaged by MRI
• Patients with spinal stenosis (with or without accompanying spondylolisthesis) who remain symptomatic despite a trial of conservative management may have a greater improvement with surgical treatment than with continued nonsurgical care
• If there is no evidence of spondylolisthesis, deformity, preoperative instability, or concern about postoperative iatrogenic instability, there may be no benefit to the addition of a fusion to decompression
• When there is evidence of spinal stenosis and spondylolisthesis, patients may have a greater degree of pain relief with a decompression and fusion

Conclusions

Neurogenic claudication is a common presenting symptom for patients with lumbar spinal stenosis. Those who fail an adequate trial (typically at least 3 months) of nonsurgical therapy may be considered for surgical intervention. The standard surgical approach supported by the literature is decompression alone. Patients who have concomitant spondylolisthesis or instability, spinal deformity, or concerns for iatrogenic postoperative instability (due to extensive resection of the fact joints) should be considered for decompression with fusion.

References

1. Zak PJ. Surgical management of spinal stenosis. Phys Med Rehabil Clin N Am 2003;14:143–55.
2. Watters WC, Baisden J, Gilbert TJ, et al. Degenerative lumbar spinal stenosis: an evidence-based clinical guideline for the diagnosis and treatment of degenerative lumbar spinal stenosis. Spine J 2008;8:305–10.
3. Suzuki H, Endo K, Kobayashi H, Tanaka H, Yamamoto K. Total sagittal spinal alignment in patients with lumbar canal stenosis accompanied by intermittent claudication. Spine 2010;35: E344–6.
4. Djurasovic M, Glassman SD, Carreon LY, Dimar JR. Contemporary management of symptomatic lumbar spinal stenosis. Orthop Clin North Am 2010;41:183–91.
5. Chosa E, Sekimoto T, Kubo S, Tajima N. Evaluation of circulatory compromise in the leg in lumbar spinal canal stenosis. Clin Orthop Rel Res 2005;431:129–33.

6. Morishita Y, Hida S, Naito M, Arimizu J, Takamori Y. Neurogenic intermittent claudication in lumbar spinal canal stenosis: the clinical relationship between the local pressure of the intervertebral foramen and the clinical findings in lumbar spinal canal stenosis. J Spinal Disord Tech 2009;22:130–4.

7. Hu SS, Tribus CB, Diab M, Ghanayem AJ. Spondylolisthesis and spondylolysis. J Bone Joint Surg Am 2008;90:656–71.

8. Metz LN, Deviren V. Low-grade spondylolisthesis. Neurosurg Clin N Am 2007;18:237–48.

9. Martin CM, Gruszcynski AT, Braunsfurth HA, Fallatah SM, O'Neil J, Wai EK. The surgical management of degenerative lumbar spondylolisthesis: a systematic review. Spine 2007;32: 1791–8.

10. Kim HJ, Lee HW, Kim HS, et al. Life expectancy After lumbar spine surgery: one- to eleven-year follow-up of 1015 patients. Spine 2008;33:2116–21.

11. Kleinstück FS, Grob D, Lattig F, et al. The influence of preoperative back pain on the outcome of lumbar decompression surgery. Spine 2009;34:1198–203.

12. Siebert E, Prüss H, Klingebiel R, Failli V, Einhäupl KM, Schwab JM. Lumbar spinal stenosis: syndrome, diagnostics and treatment. Nat Rev Neurol 2009;5:392–403.

13. Genevay S, Atlas SJ. Lumbar spinal stenosis. Best Pract Res Clin Rheumatol 2010;24:253–65.

14. Okoro T, Qureshi A, Sell B, Sell P. The accuracy of assessment of walking distance in the elective spinal outpatients setting. Eur Spine J 2010;19:279–82.

15. Graaf Id, Prak A, Zeinsta SB, Thomas S, Peul W, Koes B. Diagnosis of lumbar spinal stenosis: a systematic review of the accuracy of diagnostic tests. Spine 2006;31:1168–76.

16. Morita M, Miyauchi A, Okuda S, Oda T, Iwasaki M. Comparison between MRI and myelography in lumbar spinal canal stenosis for the decision of levels of decompression surgery. J Spinal Disord Tech 2010.

17. Athiviraham A, Yen D. Is spinal stenosis better treated surgically or nonsurgically? Clin Orthop Rel Res 2007;458:90–3.

18. Gibson JN, Waddell G. Surgery for degenerative lumbar spondylosis: updated Cochrane Review. Spine 2005;30:2312–20.

19. Atlas SJ, Delitto A. Spinal stenosis: surgical versus nonsurgical treatment. Clin Orthop Rel Res 2006;443:198–207.

20. Weinstein JN, Tosteson TD, Lurie JD, et al. Surgical versus non-surgical therapy for lumbar spinal stenosis. N Engl J Med 2008;358:794–810.

21. Weinstein JN, Tosteson TD, Lurie JD, et al. Surgical versus non-operative treatment for lumbar spinal stenosis four-year results of the Spine Patient Outcomes Research Trial. Spine 2010;35: 1329–38.

22. Ostelo RWJG, Deyo RA, Stratford P, et al. Interpreting change scores for pain and functional status in low back pain. Spine 2008;33:90–4.

23. Malmivaara A, Slatis P, Heliovaara M, et al. Surgical or nonoperative treatment for lumbar spinal stenosis? a randomized controlled trial. Spine 2007;32:1–8.

24. Weinstein JN, Lurie JD, Tosteson TD, et al. Surgical versus non-surgical treatment for lumbar degenerative spondylolisthesis. N Engl J Med 2007;356:2257–70.

25. Weinstein JN, Lurie JD, Tosteson TD, et al. Surgical compared with nonoperative treatment for lumbar degenerative spondylolisthesis. J Bone Joint Surg Am 2009;91:1295–304.

26. Ausman JI. Spinal stenosis—what is the best treatment? Surg Neurol 2007;68:486.

27. Hansraj KK, O'Leary PF, Cammisa FP, et al. Decompression, fusion, and instrumentation surgery for complex lumbar spinal stenosis. Clin Orthop Rel Res 2001;384:18–25.

28. Iguchi T, Kurihara A, Nakayama J, Sato K, Kurosaka M, Yamasaki K. Minimum 10-year outcome of decompressive laminectomy for degenerative lumbar spinal stenosis. Spine 2000;25:1754–9.

29. Fraser JF, Huang RC, Girardi FP, Cammisa FP. Pathogenesis, presentation, and treatment of lumbar spinal stenosis associated with coronal or sagittal spinal deformities. Neurosurg Focus 2003;14:E6.

30. Simmons ED. Surgical treatment of patients with lumbar spinal stenosis with associated scoliosis. Clin Orthop Rel Res 2001;384:45–53.

31. Bridwell KH, Lenke LG, Lewis SJ. Treatment of spinal stenosis and fixed sagittal imbalance. Clin Orthop Rel Res 2001;384: 35–44.

32. Deyo RA, Mirza SK, Martin BI, Kreuter W, Goodman DC, Jarvik JG. Trends, major medical complications, and charges associated with surgery for lumbar spinal stenosis in older adults. JAMA 2010;303:1259–65.

33. Katz JN, Lipson SJ, Lew RA, et al. Lumbar Laminectomy alone or with instrumented or noninstrumented arthrodesis in degenerative lumbar spinal stenosis: patient selection, costs, and surgical outcomes. Spine 1997;22:1123–31.

34. Watters WC, Bono CM, Gilbert TJ, et al. An evidence-based clinical guideline for the diagnosis and treatment of degenerative lumbar spondylolisthesis Spine J 2009;9:609–14.

35. Kristof RA, Aliashkevich AF, Schuster M, Meyer B, Urbach H, Schramm J. Degenerative lumbar spondylolisthesis-induced radicular compression: nonfusion-related decompression in selected patients without hypermobility on flexion-extension radiographs. J Neurosurg 2002;97:281–6.

36. Epstein NE. Decompression in the surgical management of degenerative spondylolisthesis: advantages of a conservative approach in 290 patients. J Spinal Disord 1998;11:116–22.

37. Resnick DK, Choudhri TF, Dailey AT, et al. Guidelines for the performance of fusion procedures for degenerative disease of the lumbar spine. Part 9: fusion in patients with stenosis and spondylolisthesis. J Neurosurg Spine 2005;2:679–85.

38. Bassewitz H, Herkowitz H. Lumbar stenosis with spondylolisthesis: current concepts of surgical treatment. Clin Orthop Rel Res 2001;384:54–60.

39. Fu KM, Smith JS, Polly DW, et al. Morbidity and mortality in the surgical treatment of 10,329 adults with degenerative lumbar stenosis. J Neurosurg Spine 2010;12:443–6.

40. Cloyd JM, Acosta FL, Cloyd C, Ames AP. Effects of age on perioperative complications of extensive multilevel thoracolumbar spinal fusion surgery. J Neurosurg Spine 2010;12:402–8.

41. Wang MY, Green BA, Shah S, Vanni S, Levi AD. Complications associated with lumbar stenosis surgery in patients older than 75 years of age. Neurosurg Focus 2003;14:E7.

42. Kalanithi PS, Patil CG, Boakye M. National complication rates and disposition after posterior lumbar fusion for acquired spondylolisthesis. Spine 2009 34:1963–9.

43. Olsen MA, Mayfield J, Lauryssen C, et al. Risk factors for surgical site infection in spinal surgery. J Neurosurg Spine 2003;2: 149–55.

44. Lietard C, Thebaud V, Besson G, Lejeune B. Risk factors for neurosurgical site infections: an 18-month prospective survey. J Neurosurg 2008;109:729–34.

45. Gunne AF, Cohen DB. Incidence, prevalence, and analysis of risk factors for surgical site infection following adult spinal surgery. Spine 2009;34:1422–8.

46. Weinstein MA, McCabe JP, Cammisa FP. Postoperative spinal wound infection: a review of 2,391 consecutive index procedures. J Spinal Disord 2000;13:422–26.

47. Fang A, Hu SS, Endres N, Bradford DS. Risk factors for infection after spinal surgery. Spine 2005;30:1460–65.

48. Beiner JM, Grauer J, Kwon BK, Vaccaro AR. Postoperative wound infections of the spine. Neurosurg Focus 2003;15:A14.

49. Maragakis LL, Cosgrove SE, Martinez EA, Tucker MG, Cohen DB, Perl TM. Intraoperative fraction of inspired oxygen is a modifiable risk factor for surgical site infection after spinal surgery. Anesthesiology 2009;110:556–62.

50. Khong P, Day MJ. Spontaneous cerebellar haemorrhage following lumbar fusion. J Clin Neurosci 2009;16:1673–5.

51. Ogilvie JW. Complications in spondylolisthesis surgery. Spine 2005;30:S97–101.

52. Podnar S. Cauda equina lesions as a complication of spinal surgery. Eur Spine J 2010;19:451–7.

53. Papadakis M, Sapkas G, Tzoutzopoulos A. A rare case of rhabdomyolysis and acute renal failure following spinal surgery. J Neurosurg Spine 2008;9:387–9.

54. Epstein NE. Efficacy of pneumatic compression stocking prophylaxis in the prevention of deep venous thrombosis and pulmonary embolism following 139 lumbar laminectomies with instrumented fusions. J Spinal Disord Tech 2006;19:28–31.

55. Gill B, Heavner JE. Postoperative visual loss associated with spine surgery. Eur Spine J 2006;15:479–84.

56. Vavken P, Krepler P. Sacral fractures after multi-segmental lumbosacral fusion: a series of four cases and systematic review of literature. Eur Spine J 2008;17:S285–S90.

57. Fourney DR, Prabhu SS, Cohen ZR, Gokaslan ZL, Rhines LD. Early sacral stress fracture after reduction of spondylolisthesis and lumbosacral fixation: case report. Neurosurgery 2002;51:1507–11.

58. Papadopoulos EC, Cammisa FP, Girardi FP. Sacral fractures complicating thoracolumbar fusion to the sacrum. Spine 2008;33:E699–E707.

59. Ghiselli G, Wang JC, Bhatia NN, Hsu WK, Dawson EG. Adjacent segment degeneration in the lumbar spine. J Bone Joint Surg Am 2004;86:1497–503.

60. Cheh G, Bridwell KH, Lenke LG, et al. Adjacent segment disease following lumbar/thoracolumbar fusion with pedicle screw instrumentation: a minimum 5-year follow-up. Spine 2007;32:2253–7.

61. Ekman P, Moller H, Shalabi A, Yu YX, Hedlund R. A prospective randomized study on the long-term effect of lumbar fusion on adjacent disc degeneration. Eur Spine J 2009;18:1175–86.

62. Kornblum MB, Fischgrund JS, Herkowitz HN, Abraham DA, Berkower DL, Ditkoff JS. Degenerative lumbar spondylolisthesis with spinal stenosis: a prospective long-term study comparing fusion and pseudoarthrosis. Spine 2004;29:726–34.

63. Berg S, Fritzell P, Tropp H. Sex life and sexual function in men and women before and after total disc replacement compared with posterior lumbar fusion. Spine J 2009;9:987–94.

64. Kim DH, Rhim R, Li L, Martha J, et al. Prospective study of iliac crest bone graft harvest site pain and morbidity. Spine J 2009;9:886–92.

81 Neurogenic Claudication: Nonoperative Management

Carlo Ammendolia

Mount Sinai Hospital, University of Toronto and Institute for Work & Health, Toronto, ON, Canada

Case scenario

A 71 year old woman presents with a 5 month history of insidious lower back pain with radiating pain and numbness bilaterally into the buttock and lateral thighs. The pain comes on after several minutes of standing. When she tries to walk, the pain becomes progressive worse and she needs to stop after walking no more than a block (200 m). Sitting reduces the pain significantly. On examination, she has a stooped posture with moderate limitation of lumbar spine extension. There is decreased sensation to light touch over the dorsum of the feet and large toes.

Relevant anatomy

Lumbar spinal stenosis (LSS) causing neurogenic claudication is one of the most commonly diagnosed and treated pathological spinal conditions and frequently afflicts the elderly population.[1] It is characterized by narrowing of the lateral and central vertebral canals with concomitant neural compression and clinical symptoms. Symptoms include pain, parasthesias and/or weakness of the back, buttock, and legs usually precipitated by walking and/or prolonged standing.[2] Degenerative changes in the spine are the most common cause of LSS characterized by osteoarthritic thickening of the articulating facet joints, infolding of the ligamentum flavum, and degenerative bulging of the intervertebral discs.[3]

Importance of the problem

Neurogenic claudication can have a significant impact on functional ability, quality of life, and independence in elderly people. Those afflicted have greater physical limitations than patients with congestive heart failure, chronic obstructive pulmonary disease, or systemic lupus erythematosus.[4]

In primary care 3–4% of low back pain (LBP) patients are diagnosed with LSS. This prevalence increases to 13–14% among LBP patients seeking care from specialists.[5] In the general population LSS is estimated to affect up to 6% of individuals over the age of 65.[6]

Currently in Canada individuals over the age of 65 represent 13% of the population. In 2031 this proportion is expected to rise to 23–25%.[7] This will significantly impact future healthcare resources, and new cases of LSS are expected to increase dramatically over the next 20 years.

Top nine questions

Diagnosis

1. How accurate is the history and clinical examination in the diagnosis of neurogenic claudication?
2. What is the role of imaging in the diagnosis of neurogenic claudication?
3. What are the key differential diagnoses of neurogenic claudication?

Therapy

4. What is the effectiveness of epidural steroid injections for the treatment of neurogenic claudication?
5. What is the effectiveness of other nonoperative treatment for neurogenic claudication?
6. What medications have been found to be effective for patients with neurogenic claudication?

Evidence-Based Orthopedics, First Edition. Edited by Mohit Bhandari.
© 2012 Blackwell Publishing Ltd. Published 2012 by Blackwell Publishing Ltd.

Harms

7. What are the complications related to epidural injections for neurogenic claudication?

Prognosis

8. What is the long-term prognosis of patients with neurogenic claudication treated nonoperatively, and what factors are prognostic in these patients

Cost

9. How does the cost of nonsurgical treatment compare to that of surgical treatment?

Question 1: How accurate is the history and clinical examination in the diagnosis of neurogenic claudication?

Question 2: What is the role of imaging in the diagnosis of neurogenic claudication?

Question 3: What are the key differential diagnoses of neurogenic claudication?

Case clarification

On examination, our patient walks with a wide stance gait. Standing lumbar spine extension reproduces her symptoms, whereas lumbar flexion provides immediate relief. MRI reveals moderate to severe central and bilateral lateral canal stenosis at the levels L4–L5 and L5–S1. Making a diagnosis of neurogenic claudication is often challenging in elderly patients because other comorbidities are often present, some of which give rise to similar symptoms.

Finding the evidence

- PubMed (www.ncbi.nlm.nih.gov/pubmed/) clinical queries search/diagnosis and sensitive: "neurogenic claudication AND lumbar spinal stenosis," "neurogenic claudication," and "lumbar spinal stenosis"
- PubMed (www.ncbi.nlm.nih.gov/pubmed/) sensitivity search using terms "diagnosis AND lumbar spinal stenosis," "diagnosis AND neurogenic claudication" as well as "imaging OR magnetic resonance imaging OR computerized tomography OR myelography AND lumbar spinal stenosis"

Quality of the evidence

Level I

- 3 systematic reviews[8,10,15]

Findings

A systematic review on the accuracy of diagnostic tests for LSS identified 12 diagnostic imaging studies and 7 studies evaluating clinical tests.[8] Firm conclusions about the accuracy of diagnostic tests could not be made because of the overall poor quality and high heterogeneity of studies. This review highlighted one study that found 21% of asymptomatic subjects over the age of 60 years to have evidence of LSS on MRI.[9] The systematic review by Kent et al. emphasized the importance of corroborating both clinical and imaging findings in order to make an accurate diagnosis.[10]

Diagnostic accuracy is typically expressed using values of sensitivity, specificity, and likelihood ratios. Sensitivity is the proportion of patients with the disorder of interest who have a positive diagnostic test, and specificity is the proportion of patients without the condition of interest who have a negative diagnostic test result.[11]

A likelihood ratio (LR) combines the information contained within sensitivity and specificity values into a concise and meaningful expression of diagnostic usefulness.[11] A positive LR (sensitivity/[1 − specificity]) expresses the odds that a positive test result would be expected in a patient with the disorder of interest. A negative LR ([1 − sensitivity]/specificity) expresses the odds that a negative test result would be expected in a patient with the disorder of interest.[12] LRs close to 1 indicate a test which does little to alter diagnostic probability. A high positive LR (e.g., >5.0) indicates a test in which a positive result is helpful for ruling in the diagnosis, whereas a small negative LR (e.g., <0.30) is associated with tests in which a negative result is helpful in ruling out the diagnosis.[13]

Fritz et al. compared studies evaluating the diagnostic accuracy of myelography, CT scan, and MRI for the diagnosis of LSS. These authors demonstrated that MRI had the largest positive LR, ranging from 8.1 to 16.2, and lowest negative LR, ranging from 0.03 to 0.19, and concluded that MRI is the diagnostic imaging of choice for suspected LSS. Similarly, these authors compared the LRs of findings from the history and physical examination and concluded that findings from the history were most useful. Specifically, the absence of pain when seated (positive LR = 6.6), improvement of pain when sitting (positive LR = 3.1), sitting being the best posture for reducing symptoms (negative LR = 0.28), and standing/ walking being the worse postures for symptoms (negative LR = 0.33) were the most useful diagnostic factors.[14] Patients with signs and symptoms highly suggestive of LSS require imaging only if they are possible candidates for surgery or other invasive interventions or if the patient presents with clinical features ("red flags") suggestive of other underlying pathology.[15]

Other potential causes of our patient's symptoms include peripheral vascular insufficiency, osteoarthritis of the hips, trochanteric bursitis, and peripheral neuropathy.[3,14]

Recommendations

- Findings in the history are most important in the diagnosis of neurogenic claudication. Key diagnostic features include the presence of lower extremity symptoms that worsen when standing and/or walking and improve with sitting and forward flexion
- Imaging (MRI) should be restricted to patients with neurogenic claudication who are potential candidates for invasive procedures or have signs and symptoms suggestive of other underlying serious disease. The use of imaging alone without corroborating the findings with presenting clinical features poses a considerable risk for inaccurate diagnosis

Question 4: What is the effectiveness of epidural steroid injections for the treatment of neurogenic claudication?

Question 5: What is the effectiveness of other nonoperative treatment for neurogenic claudication?

Question 6: What medications have been found to be effective for patients with neurogenic claudication?

Relevance

Although surgery may be a therapeutic option, evidence-based reviews suggest an initial course of conservative treatment prior to surgical intervention.[16,17] An epidural steroid injection introduces a mixture of corticosteroids into the epidural space with the aim of reducing inflammation at the level of neural compression. Various approaches are used to access the epidural space including interlaminar, caudal, and transforaminal. The use of epidural steroid injections is a rapidly growing treatment in the elderly population for spine-related leg pain,[18] and approximately a quarter of all epidural steroid injections are administered for symptoms ascribed to LSS.[15] Other common nonoperative treatments include analgesic and anti-inflammatory medication, patient education, spinal manipulation and mobilization, therapeutic exercises, and the use of therapeutic modalities.[19–21] Exercises and instruction in body repositioning techniques are aimed at improving back and lower limb strength and flexibility and teaching patients how to position their body to reduce symptoms.[20] Commonly prescribed medications include acetaminophen (paracetamol), narcotic analgesics, and anti-inflammatory drugs.[3,16]

Finding the evidence

- Cochrane Database of Systematic Reviews (www.cochrane.org) using search terms: "neurogenic claudication" and "lumbar spinal stenosis"

- Cochrane Database of Clinical Trials (www.cochrane.org) using search terms "neurogenic claudication" and "lumbar spinal stenosis"
- PubMed (www.ncbi.nlm.nih.gov/pubmed/) clinical queries search/therapy and sensitive: "neurogenic claudication AND lumbar spinal stenosis", "neurogenic claudication" and "lumbar spinal stenosis"
- PubMed (www.ncbi.nlm.nih.gov/pubmed/) clinical queries/systematic reviews (including meta-analysis, evidence-based reports, reviews of clinical trials, consensus development conferences and guidelines) using the search term: "neurogenic claudication OR lumbar spinal stenosis"

Quality of the evidence

Level I
- 3 systematic reviews[15,25,32]
- 4 randomized controlled trials (RCTs)[30,31,38,39]

Findings

Epidural steroid injections Three RCTs[22–24] were identified from one systematic review[25] that included only patients with neurogenic claudication with confirmatory lumbar stenosis on imaging. Table 81.1 summarizes the trials and Table 81.2 provides GRADE evidence profiles for the trials.

Cuckler et al. compared the proportion of patients who self-reported at least 75% improvement from preinjection status among 37 patients randomized to receive either a translaminar steroid injection or placebo injection. The investigators found no differences in self-reported improvement in symptoms among the two groups 24 hours after the injection or after a mean of 21 months.[22]

Zahaar used similar outcome measures and randomized 33 patients to receive either a prone caudal epidural steroid injection or a placebo injection. There were no differences in treatment outcomes between the groups 24 hours after the injection or after a mean of 20 months.[24]

Fukusaki et al. evaluated walking distance among 53 patients randomized to receive an epidural block, an epidural block with methylprednisolone, or an epidural saline injection. At 1 week after the injection the groups who received either the epidural block or epidural block with methylprednisolone had a greater proportion of patients with good or excellent walking distance (55.5% and 63.2% respectively) compared to the group receiving the placebo injection (12.5%, p < 0.05) . However, at one and 3 months post injection there were no differences in walking distance among the three groups.[23]

Other medications There are no placebo controlled RCTs evaluating anti-inflammatory medication or narcotics for treatment of LSS. A pilot RCT (n = 55) assessed the effectiveness of gabapentin plus physiotherapy compared to physiotherapy alone and demonstrated positive benefit in

Table 81.1 Description of studies on epidural injections for neurogenic claudication due to lumbar spinal stenosis

Study	Participants	Intervention	Control	Outcomes	Results
Fukusaki 1998	53 patients with pseudoclaudication, all of the patients in the three groups had unilateral or bilateral pseudoclaudication with less than 20 m in walking distance because of intolerable leg pain	Gr 1-Epidural injection with 8 mL of 1% mepivacaine. The same epidural injection was repeated twice during the first 1-week period in all groups Gr 2-Epidural injection with a mixture of 8 mL of 1% mepivacaine and 40 mg of methylprednisolone. The same epidural injection was repeated twice during the first 1-week period in all groups	Gr 3- Epidural injection with 8 mL of saline. The same epidural injection was repeated twice during the first 1-week period in all groups	Walking distance was evaluated as follows: excellent effect, more than a mean of 100 m in walking distance; good effect, mean of 20–100 m in walking distance; poor effect, less than a mean of 20 m in walking distance	At 1 week Gr 2 and Gr 3 significantly greater number of patients with good or excellent results compared to Gr 1. At 1 and 3 months no difference in the groups
Cuckler 1985	73 patients from private clinic practice with clinical features (neurogenic claudication or sciatica) and confirmatory imaging for either spinal stenosis (n = 37) or herniated disc (n = 36)	2 mL of sterile water containing 80 mg of methylprednisolone acetate combined with 5 mL of 1% procaine was injected into the epidural space in the region between the 3rd and 4th lumbar vertebrae with the patient in the lateral decubitus position lying on the side of the painful limb	2 mL of saline with 5 mL of 1% procaine was injected into the epidural space in the region between the 3rd and 4th lumbar vertebrae with the patient in the lateral decubitus position lying on the side of the painful limb	Short-term successful result was defined as subjective improvement of 75% or more 24 hours after injection. Short-term failure was defined as less than 75% improvement during this time. Long-term success was defined as improvement of 75% or more in the preinjection symptoms at 13–36 months (mean 20.85 months) Other outcomes were re-injection rates and need for surgery	No significant difference in the short or long term between the steroid or control group
Zahaar 1991	63 patients with clinical features of neurogenic claudication (n = 30) or sciatica (n = 33) and confirmatory imaging for either acute herniated nucleus pulposus or spinal stenosis	Using a caudal route with patient prone, 2 mL of carbocaine, 4% were injected into the epidural after infiltration at the site of injection. This was immediately followed by injection of one ampule of 5 mL of hydrocortisone acetate suspension, combined with another ampule (2 mL) of carbocaine, 4%: the volume was completed with sterile saline to 30 mL	Using a caudal route with patient prone, 2 mL of carbocaine, 4% were injected into the epidural after infiltration at the site of injection. This was immediately followed by injection of one ampule (2 mL) of carbocaine, 4%: the volume was completed with sterile saline to 30 mL	Short-term successful result was defined as subjective improvement of 75% or more 24 hours after injection. Short-term failure was defined as less than 75% improvement during this time. Long-term success was defined as improvement of 75% or more in the preinjection symptoms at 13–36 months (mean 20.85 months)	No significant difference in the short or long term between the steroid or control group

Table 81.2 Epidural injections for neurogenic claudication due to lumbar spinal stenosis—GRADE table

No of studies	Design	Limitations	Inconsistency	Indirectness	Imprecision	Other considerations	No of patients		Difference Quality in proportions (95% CI)	
							Intervention	Control		

Translaminar epidural steroid injection vs. placebo injection

Outcome: proportion of subjects reporting >75% preinjection improvement after 24 hours (short term)

| 1 (22) | RCT | Serious limitations[a] | No important inconsistencies | Direct | Imprecise | None | 20 | 17 | +0.07 (−0.19 to 0.34) | Low |

Outcome: proportion of subjects reporting >75% preinjection improvement after 13–30 months (long term)

| 1 (22) | RCT | Serious limitations[a] | No important inconsistencies | Direct | Imprecise | None | 20 | 17 | −0.19 (−0.45 to 0.06) | Low |

Caudal epidural steroid injection vs. placebo injection

Outcome: proportion of subjects reporting >75% preinjection improvement after 24 hours (short term)

| 1 (24) | RCT | Serious limitations[a] | No important inconsistencies | Direct | Imprecise | None | 18 | 12 | +0.06 (−0–31 to 0.42) | Low |

Outcome: proportion of subjects reporting >75% preinjection improvement after 13–30 months (long term)

| 1 (24) | RCT | Serious limitations[a] | No important inconsistencies | Direct | Imprecise | None | 18 | 12 | +0.06 (−0.29 to 0.40) | Low |

Translaminar epidural steroid injection plus epidural block vs. placebo injection

Outcome: proportion of subjects with excellent (mean >100 m), good (mean 20–100 m), or poor (mean <20 m) walking ability at 1 week post treatment

| 1 (23) | RCT | Serious limitations[a] | No important inconsistencies | Direct | Imprecise | None | 19 | 16 | +0.51 (0.24 to 0.78) | Low |

Outcome: proportion of subjects with excellent (mean >100 m), good (mean 20–100 m), or poor (mean <20 m) walking ability at 1 month post treatment

| 1 (23) | RCT | Serious limitations[a] | No important inconsistencies | direct | Imprecise | None | 19 | 16 | +0.10 (−0.11 to 0.30) | Low |

Outcome: proportion of subjects with excellent (mean >100 m), good (mean 20–100 m), or poor (mean <20 m) walking ability at 3 month post treatment

| 1 (23) | RCT | Serious limitations[a] | No important inconsistencies | Direct | Imprecise | None | 19 | 16 | −0.01 (−0.17 to 0.15) | Low |

Translaminar epidural steroid injections plus epidural block vs. epidural block

Outcome: proportion of subjects with excellent (mean >100 m), good (mean 20–100 m), or poor (mean <20 m) walking ability at 1 week post treatment

| 1 (23) | RCT | Serious limitations[a] | No important inconsistencies | Direct | Imprecise | None | 19 | 18 | −0.07 (−0.24 to 0.39) | Low |

Outcome: proportion of subjects with excellent (mean >100 m), good (mean 20–100 m), or poor (mean <20 m) walking ability at 1 month post treatment

| 1 (23) | RCT | Serious limitations[a] | No important inconsistencies | Direct | Imprecise | | 19 | 18 | +0.01 (−0.25 to 0.23) | Low |

Outcome: proportion of subjects with excellent (mean >100 m), good (mean 20–100 m), or poor (mean <20 m) walking ability at 3 month post treatment

| 1(23) | RCT | Serious limitations[a] | No important inconsistencies | Direct | Imprecise | None | 19 | 18 | +0.003 (−0.15 to 0.1) | Low |

CI, confidence interval; RCT, randomized controlled trial.

[a]High risk of bias (unsure of method of randomization or concealment, blinding of patient and care provider and cointerventions).

walking distance (p < 0.001), pain scores (p < 0.006), and recovery of sensory deficits (p < 0.04) over a 4 month period.[31] One RCT (n = 79), demonstrated that prostaglandin E1 is more effective than etodolac in improving walking distance (p < 0.01) and leg numbness (p < 0.01) at eight weeks follow-up. [Matsudaira 2009][38]. Another single RCT (n = 152) showed that Vitamin B12 when added to conservative treatment improved walking ability (p < 0.05) compared to conservative treatment alone at six months, 12 months and 18 months follow-up. [Waikakul 2000][39]. In a recent systematic review of RCTs, the use of calcitonin was found to be of no benefit for neurogenic claudication in patients with LSS.[32]

Other conservative care Various conservative treatments have been used as controls for surgical trials; however, the type, frequency, treatment combination, and provider varied significantly among the trials, limiting the ability to make conclusions about effectiveness.[29]

Whitman et al. randomized 58 patients with neurogenic claudication and LSS to receive either flexion exercises, manual therapy (thrust and nonthrust manipulation of the spine and lower extremity joints) and body-supported treadmill walking or flexion exercises, treadmill walking, and subtherapeutic ultrasound. After 12 treatment sessions, over 6 weeks, both groups achieved clinically important improvements at the completion of each treatment program and at 1 year. However, the group that included manual therapy showed significantly greater self-reported improvement in perceived recovery (79% vs. 41%, p = 0.0015) and on the Satisfaction Subscale of the Spinal Stenosis Scale at 6 weeks (1.57; 95% CI 1.36–1.78 vs. 2.03; 95% CI 1.8–2.31) but not at 1 year or long-term follow-up (a mean of 29 months).[30] There were no significant differences in other outcomes: Oswestry Disability Index, treadmill walking distance, and Numeric Pain Rating Scale for lower extremity symptoms.

Recommendations

• Low-quality evidence does not support the use of epidural steroid injections for neurogenic claudication. Manual therapy with exercise may provide short-term (up to 6 weeks) improvement in perceived recovery and patient satisfaction over exercise alone [overall quality: low];[30] however, there is insufficient evidence to support the use of other conservative care including analgesics or anti-inflammatory drugs. Gabapentin may be helpful; however the benefits noted were based on pilot data.[31] Any potential benefit of gabapentin should be weighed against potential risk for adverse effects, including dizziness and drowsiness [overall quality: low]. Vitamin B12 and Prostaglandin E1 may be useful in improving walking ability. [overall quality: low]
• Although high-quality evidence is lacking to guide specific self-management strategies, providing patients with neurogenic claudication advice to keep active and perform regular nonaggravating exercise, and use acetaminophen or anti-inflammatory medication, similar to advice for nonspecific LBP, may be a reasonable initial approach. This is the position of a recent clinical practice guideline from the American College of Physicians and the American Pain Society with the rationale that recommendations from high-quality systematic reviews for nonspecific LBP include RCTs that enrolled patients with low back related leg symptoms.[15] With respect to which types of exercise are likely to be helpful, evidence from observational studies suggest that body repositioning techniques and performing flexion exercises including stationary cycling and abdominal strengthening exercises may be beneficial in reducing symptoms of neurogenic claudication.[3,20,33–36]

Question 7: What are the complications related to epidural injections for neurogenic claudication?

Finding the evidence
See Questions 4–6.

Findings
Only one of the included trials on epidural steroid injection[23] provided information on adverse events following the intervention. This trial reported no incidence of dural puncture, hypotension, or subarachnoid injection. There have been case reports of serious adverse events including paralysis and infection following epidural steroid injection.[26–28]

Recommendation
• There is insufficient evidence to provide a recommendation.

Question 8: What is the long-term prognosis of patients with neurogenic claudication treated nonoperatively, and what factors are prognostic in these patients?

Case clarification
We want to inform our patient on the long-term prognosis of nonoperative treatment. We also want to examine factors that may impact success of nonoperative treatment.

Finding the evidence
• PubMed: we repeated the search for therapy replacing the word "therapy" with "prognosis"

Quality of the evidence
Level II
• 1 prospective cohort study[37]

Findings

Atlas et al. followed 148 patients with lumbar spinal stenosis over an 8–10 year period managed either surgically (n = 81) or non-surgically (n = 67) in a community-based setting.[37] Nonsurgical treatment varied and included epidural steroid (18%), spinal manipulation (23%), physical therapy (23%), bed rest (29%), exercises (39%), narcotics (21%), and other modalities, such as TENS, traction, and bracing (39%). When surgical intervention was compared to nonsurgical treatment, improvement in predominant symptom (lower back or leg pain) from baseline was reported by 77% and 44% of patients at 1 year (p < 0.05), 70% and 52% of patients at 4 years (p < 0.05), and 54% and 42% of patients at 8–10 year follow-up (p > 0.05), respectively. Symptoms of nonsurgical patients were unchanged in 36%, 18%, and 22% of patients at year 1, 4, and 8–10 years respectively. Follow-up rates at 1, 4, and 8–10 years were 87.8%, 80.4%, and 65.5% respectively. It was not possible to identify predictors of outcome among nonsurgical patients in this study because of the limited number of individuals at long-term follow-up.

Recommendation

• A large proportion of patients receiving nonoperative management either improve or remain stable, making this a reasonable initial management option for our patient. It is unknown what patient factors predict favourable nonoperative outcomes

Question 9: How does the cost of nonsurgical treatment compare to that of surgical treatment?

There are no cost-effectiveness studies evaluating nonoperative treatment for neurogenic claudication.[13]

Summary of recommendations

• Findings in the history are most important in the diagnosis of neurogenic claudication. Key diagnostic features include the presence of lower extremity symptoms that worsen when standing and/or walking and improve with sitting and forward flexion
• Imaging (MRI) should be restricted to patients with neurogenic claudication who are potential candidates for invasive procedures or have signs and symptoms suggestive of other underlying serious disease
• Low-quality evidence does not support the use of epidural steroid injections for neurogenic claudication. Low quality evidence suggests that manual therapy with exercise may provide short-term improvement in perceived recovery and patient satisfaction over exercise alone; low quality evidence suggests that gabapentin, prostaglandins and Vitamin B12 may improve walking ability. There is

insufficient evidence to support the use of other conservative care including analgesics or anti-inflammatory drugs
• Although low quality evidence limits the ability to provide recommendations for clinical practice, advising patients to keep active and perform regular nonaggravating exercise, and use acetaminophen or anti-inflammatory medication, may be a reasonable initial approach
• Body repositioning techniques and flexion exercises including stationary cycling and abdominal strengthening exercises may be beneficial in reducing symptoms of neurogenic claudication
• A large proportion of patients receiving nonoperative management either improve or remain stable, making this a reasonable initial management option

Conclusions

A comprehensive history is essential in the diagnosis of neurogenic claudication. Advanced imaging should be restricted to patients with persistent symptoms who may be candidates for invasive procedures. Low-quality evidence suggests that epidural steroid injections are ineffective, and that gabapentin, prostaglandins, Vitamin B12 and manual therapy in addition to exercise may provide improvement. High-quality randomized controlled studies are needed to further evaluate nonoperative treatment for neurogenic claudication. Most patients do not have progressive deterioration of symptoms and a conservative approach that includes self-management strategies is a reasonable first step in the treatment of neurogenic claudication. Large studies on the natural history of neurogenic claudication are needed to enable early identification of high-risk patients who may require more aggressive interventions.

References

1. Kalichman L, Cole R, Kim DH, et al. Spinal stenosis prevalence and association with symptoms: the Framingham Study. Spine J 2009;9(7):545–50.
2. Katz JN, Dalgas M, Stucki G, et al. Degenerative lumbar spinal stenosis: diagnostic value of the history and physical examination. Arthritis Rheum 1995;38(9):1236–41.
3. Katz JN, Harris MB. Clinical practice. Lumbar spinal stenosis. N Engl J Med 2008;21;358(8):818–25.
4. Fanuele JC, Birkmeyer NJ, Abdu WA, Tosteson TD, Weinstein JN. The impact of spinal problems on the health status of patients: have we underestimated the effect? Spine 2000;25(12):1509–14.
5. Hart LG, Deyo RA, Cherkin DC. Physician office visits for low back pain: Frequency, clinical evaluation, and treatment patterns from a U.S. National survey. Spine 1995;20(1):11–19.
6. De Villiers PD, Booysen EL. Fibrous spinal stenosis. A report on 850 myelograms with a water-soluble contrast medium. Clin Orthop Relat Res 1976;115:140–4.

7. Government of Canada. Statistics Canada. Statistics Canada 2006 June 11. Available from: URL: www.statcan.gc.ca/bsolc/olc-cel/olc-cel?lang=eng&catno=11–008-X

8. de Graaf, I, Prak A, Bierma-Zeinstra S, Thomas S, Peul W, Koes B. Diagnosis of lumbar spinal stenosis: a systematic review of the accuracy of diagnostic tests. Spine 2006;31(10):1168–76.

9. Boden SD, Davis DO, Dina TS, Patronas NJ, Wiesel SW. Abnormal magnetic-resonance scans of the lumbar spine in asymptomatic subjects. A prospective investigation. J Bone Joint Surg Am 1990;72(3):403–8.

10. Kent DL, Haynor DR, Larson EB, Deyo RA. Diagnosis of lumbar spinal stenosis in adults: a metaanalysis of the accuracy of CT, MR, and myelography. AJR Am J Roentgenol 1992;158(5):1135–44.

11. Sackett DL, Richardson WS, Rosenberg W, Haynes RB. Evidence Based Medicine. How to Practice and Teach EBM. Churchill Livingstone, New York, 1997.

12. Sackett DL, Haynes RB, Guyatt GB, Tugwell R Clinical Epidemiology. A Basic Science for Clinical Medicine, 2nd ed. Little, Brown, Boston, 1992.

13. Riegelman RK, Hirsch RP. Studying a Study and Testing a Test: How to Read the Health Science Literature, 3rd ed. Little, Brown, Boston, 1996.

14. Fritz JM, Delitto A, Welch WC, Erhard RE. Lumbar spinal stenosis: a review of current concepts in evaluation, management, and outcome measurements. Arch Phys Med Rehabil 1998;79(6): 700–8.

15. Chou R, Qaseem A, Snow V, et al. Diagnosis and treatment of low back pain: a joint clinical practice guideline from the American College of Physicians and the American Pain Society. Ann Intern Med 2007;147(7):478–91.

16. Agency for Healthcare Research and Quality. Treatment of Degenerative Lumbar Spinal Stenosis. Evidence Report/Technology Assessment No.32. Report No. AHRQ01-E048. Rockville, MD, Jan 6, 2001.

17. Fritz JM, Erhard RE, Vignovic M. A nonsurgical treatment approach for patients with lumbar spinal stenosis. Phys Ther 1997;77(9):962–73.

18. Friedly J, Chan L, Deyo R. Increases in lumbosacral injections in the Medicare population: 1994 to 2001.[see comment]. Spine 2007;32(16):1754–60.

19. Comer CM, Redmond AC, Bird HA, Conaghan PG. Assessment and management of neurogenic claudication associated with lumbar spinal stenosis in a UK primary care musculoskeletal service: a survey of current practice among physiotherapists. BMC Musculoskelet Disord 2009;10:121.

20. Whitman JM, Flynn TW, Fritz JM. Nonsurgical management of patients with lumbar spinal stenosis: a literature review and a case series of three patients managed with physical therapy. Phys Med Rehabil Clin North Am 2003;14(1):77–101.

21. Stuber K, Sajko S, Kristmanson K. Conservative treatments for lumbar spinal stenosis: a systematic review of randomized controlled trials. J Chiropractic Ed 2009;23(1):96–7.

22. Cuckler JM, Bernini PA, Wiesel SW, Booth RE, Jr., Rothman RH, Pickens GT. The use of epidural steroids in the treatment of lumbar radicular pain. A prospective, randomized, double-blind study. J Bone Joint Surg Am 1985;67(1):63–6.

23. Fukusaki M, Kobayashi I, Hara T, Sumikawa K. Symptoms of spinal stenosis do not improve after epidural steroid injection. Clin J Pain 1998;14(2):148–51.

24. Zahaar M. The value of caudal epidural steroid in the treatment of lumbar neurogenic syndromes. J Neurol Orthop Med Surg 1991;12:181–4.

25. Chou R, Loeser JD, Owens DK, et al. Interventional therapies, surgery, and interdisciplinary rehabilitation for low back pain: an evidence-based clinical practice guideline from the American Pain Society. Spine 2009;34(10):1066–77.

26. Glaser SE, Falco F. Paraplegia following a thoracolumbar transforaminal epidural steroid injection. Pain Physician 2005;8(3): 309–14.

27. Hooten WM, Hogan MS, Sanemann TC, Maus TJ. Acute spinal pain during an attempted lumbar epidural blood patch in congenital lumbar spinal stenosis and epidural lipomatosis. Pain Physician 2008;11(1):87–90.

28. Huntoon MA, Martin DP. Paralysis after transforaminal epidural injection and previous spinal surgery [see comment]. Reg Anesth Pain Med 2004 Sep;29(5):494–5.

29. Chou R, Baisden J, Carragee EJ, Resnick DK, Shaffer WO, Loeser JD. Surgery for low back pain: a review of the evidence for an American Pain Society Clinical Practice Guideline. Spine 2009;34(10):1094–109.

30. Whitman JM, Flynn TW, Childs JD, Wainner RS, Gill HE, Ryder MG, et al. A comparison between two physical therapy treatment programs for patients with lumbar spinal stenosis: a randomized clinical trial [see comment]. Spine 2006;31(22):2541–9.

31. Yaksi A, Ozgonenel L, Ozgonenel B. The efficiency of gabapentin therapy in patients with lumbar spinal stenosis. Spine 2007;32(9): 939–42.

32. Coronado-Zarco R, Cruz-Medina E, Arellano-Hernandez A, Chavez-Arias D, Leon-Hernandez SR. Effectiveness of calcitonin in intermittent claudication treatment of patients with lumbar spinal stenosis: a systematic review. Spine 2009;34(22):E818–22.

33. Bodack MP, Monteiro M. Therapeutic exercise in the treatment of patients with lumbar spinal stenosis. Clin Orthop Relat Res 2001;144–52.

34. Chung SS, Lee CS, Kim SH, Chung MW, Ahn JM. Effect of low back posture on the morphology of the spinal canal. Skeletal Radiol 2000;29:217–23.

35. Madsen R, Jensen TS, Pope M, Sorensen JS, Bendix T. The effect of body position and axial load on spinal canal morphology: an MRI study of central spinal stenosis. Spine 1976;2008;33:61–7.

36. Takahashi K, Kagechika K, Takino T, Matsui T, Miyazaki T, Shima I. Changes in epidural pressure during walking in patients with lumbar spinal stenosis. Spine 1976;1995;20:2746–9.

37. Atlas SJ, Keller RB, Wu YA, Deyo RA, Singer DE. Long-term outcomes of surgical and nonsurgical management of lumbar spinal stenosis: 8 to 10 year results from the Maine lumbar spine study. Spine 2005;30(8):936–43.

38. Matsudaira K, Seichi A, Kunogi J, Yamazaki T, Kobayashi A, Anamizu Y, et al. The efficacy of prostaglandin E1 derivative in patients with lumbar spinal stenosis. Spine 2009 Jan 15;34(2): 115–20.

39. Waikakul W, Waikakul S. Methylcobalamin as an adjuvant medication in conservative treatment of lumbar spinal stenosis. Journal of the Medical Association of Thailand 2000 Aug;83(8): 825–31.

82 Adolescent Idiopathic Scoliosis—Nonoperative Management

Calvin T. Hu and James O. Sanders
University of Rochester Medical Center, Rochester, NY, USA

Case scenario

An asymptomatic 12 year-old Risser 0 premenarchal girl presents with a spinal deformity. Radiographs demonstrate a right thoracic curve measuring 32° Cobb angle from T6 to T12. Her examination is normal with the exception of a right thoracic deformity on forward flexion.

Relevant anatomy

Idiopathic scoliosis is a deforming condition of the spine with coronal plane deviation typically associated with apical rotation. Progression during adolescence can be marked. The Cobb angle is a radiographic measurement of severity. Curves can appear in several areas of the spine but are stereotypic in their location and direction. Detection is usually by trunk asymmetry on forward bend. The Risser iliac apophyseal ossification sign is a common maturity measurement.

Risser iliac apophyseal ossification sign

- Stage 0: No ossification of iliac crest apophysis
- Stage 1: Up to 25% ossification
- Stage 2: 25–50% ossification
- Stage 3: 50–75% ossification
- Stage 4: 75–100% ossification
- Stage 5: Fusion of apophysis to iliac crest

Importance of the problem

The prevalence of scoliosis is 1–3% in the United States. Adolescent onset scoliosis is not life threatening, but consequences to the patient may include deformity and pain.

A Google search in August 2010 for "scoliosis" returned more than 17 million results. In 1995, there were 602,884 visits[1] in the U.S. for adolescent idiopathic scoliosis (AIS), with more than 4,500 surgeries performed in 2000. A functional outcome measurement, the Scoliosis Research Society (SRS) instrument was developed from the Short Form 50 (SF-50) and several scoliosis-specific issues. It has been well tested in adults[2,3] but, like other deforming conditions in childhood where the treatment goal is prevention of presumed long-term effects, outcome instruments show a significant ceiling effect in the short run.

Top six questions

Diagnosis

1. Are school scoliosis screening programs beneficial to children?

Therapy

2. Do exercise programs prevent curve progression?
3. Does bracing prevent curve progression?

Prognosis—curve progression

4. Is it possible to predict which curves will progress markedly during the adolescent growth spurt?

Prognosis—functional outcomes

5. What is the association between nonoperatively managed scoliosis and back pain or functional impairment?
6. What is the association between nonoperatively managed scoliosis and pulmonary compromise?

Evidence-Based Orthopedics, First Edition. Edited by Mohit Bhandari.
© 2012 Blackwell Publishing Ltd. Published 2012 by Blackwell Publishing Ltd.

Question 1: Are school scoliosis screening programs beneficial to children?

Case clarification
School screening programs are commonly used to identify children with potential scoliosis.

Relevance
The benefits of scoliosis school screening are controversial.

Current opinion
The U.S. Preventive Services Task Force (USPSTF) recommends against schools screening, but several physician groups recommend the contrary.

Finding the evidence
- Cochrane Database: "scoliosis"
- PubMed Clinical Queries:
  ○ Systematic Reviews: "(adolescent idiopathic scoliosis anterior posterior) AND systematic[sb]"
  ○ MeSH: "mass screening"[Majr] AND ("scoliosis/diagnosis"[Mesh] OR "scoliosis/epidemiology"[Mesh] OR "scoliosis/therapy"[Mesh])

Quality of the evidence
Level III
- 2 case-control studies

Findings
In 2004, the USPSTF[4] recommended against school scoliosis screening, finding poor accuracy of the forward bending test, poor follow-up from screening programs, and poor evidence that screening detects scoliosis at an earlier age than without screening. They found fair evidence that treatment leads to health benefits in only a small proportion of cases, since few progress to require aggressive treatment, such as surgery, and these subjects are likely to be detected without screening. The USPSTF also found fair evidence that screening leads to moderate harms, including unnecessary brace wear and specialty care referral. Several physician societies issued a statement[5,6] supporting school screening, as earlier referral can identify those who are at high risk for progression, allowing earlier nonoperative treatment. Only one recent higher-evidence study evaluated the efficacy of scoliosis screening[7] and found an 86% probability that screening did not prevent surgery.

The utility of school screening depends upon identifying those most likely to have scoliosis and relies on proxies rather than radiographs. The sensitivity and specificity of the simple tests are low, making multistage screening more effective. However, this increases cost.[8–11] Various ages have been recommended for school screening. Potentially, screening at age 10 will identify all patients with high curve progression potential.[12] In order to justify school screening programs, children who screen positive should derive some benefit, such as improved treatment outcomes or a reduced likelihood of surgery. Likewise, screening should minimize harms such as unnecessary radiation exposure, costs, and misdiagnosis. Ultimately, schools may not be the proper place for screening since proper follow-up is problematic.[13]

Recommendations
- Until the completion of studies evaluating the effectiveness of bracing for adolescent idiopathic scoliosis, we are unable to identify substantial benefit from current school screening programs [overall quality: low]

Question 2: Does exercise prevent curve progression?

Case clarification
Bracing is confining, and exercise makes sense to many patients as a potential treatment or adjunct for scoliosis.

Relevance
Many patients are hesitant to wear a brace to school or do not tolerate wearing a brace at night.

Current opinion
Exercise is ineffective in preventing scoliosis progression.

Finding the evidence
- Cochrane Database: 1 protocol for review
- PubMed Clinical Queries:
  ○ Clinical Studies Category: "(adolescent idiopathic scoliosis exercise) AND (Therapy/Broad[filter])"
  ○ Systematic Reviews: "(adolescent idiopathic scoliosis exercise) AND systematic[sb]"

Quality of the evidence
Level III
- 3 systematic reviews
- 1 comparative study

Findings
Exercises used in the treatment of AIS are diverse and can be classified into four program types (Table 82.1). A recent systematic review[14] found the overall methodological quality of existing studies low. Most had no controls and heterogeneity prevented a meta-analysis. Overall, decreased Cobb angle progression was seen primarily near the beginning of the adolescent growth spurt, while Cobb angle improvement was seen after growth completion. We identified one level III study[15] showing a statistically significant difference in progression between an exercise-treated group (Schroth method) and observed patients. The

Table 82.1 Exercises used in the treatment of adolescent idiopathic scoliosis

Program type	Definition
Scoliosis inpatient or outpatient rehabilitation (Schroth method)	Uses exercises to correct scoliotic posture through elongation and realignment of trunk segments, positioning of the arms, as well as the use of specific breathing patterns. Proprioceptive and exteroceptive stimulation and mirror control is used
Extrinsic autocorrection (side-shift method)	Introduced by Mehta, uses a lateral trunk shift exercise which is then incorporated into the activities of daily living
Intrinsic autocorrection	Based on auto-elongation exercises, intrinsic autocorrection utilizes the intrinsic back muscles to correct spinal alignment. These principles are now taught as a three-dimensional autocorrection in the SEAS (Scientific Exercises Approach to Scoliosis) program. Also known as active self-correction
No autocorrection, asymmetric exercises	Studies classified in this category used a particular fitness machine to strengthen torso muscles. This machine is also marketed for general resistance training

patients were controlled for age but not physiological maturity. Closer examination of the systematic reviews shows the reported studies were not properly stratified by maturity in conjunction with curve magnitude and pattern. Although it is plausible that exercise may improve scoliosis, absent properly designed studies, evidence is weak that exercise therapy alters the natural history.

Recommendations

In patients with adolescent idiopathic scoliosis who are treated primarily with exercises, the evidence suggests:
• Only weak evidence exists that exercise therapy alters the natural history of idiopathic scoliosis [overall quality: very low]

Question 3: Does bracing prevent curve progression?

Case clarification

The patient's parents ask if a brace will keep their daughter's curve from worsening.

Relevance

A real benefit (stabilization of curve, avoidance of surgery) should be attainable if a patient is to commit to brace treatment.

Current opinion

Bracing is recommended for curves of 25–40° in patients Risser 2 or less, or in curves 20° or more with documented progression.

Finding the evidence

• Cochrane Database: 1 protocol filed
• PubMed Clinical Queries:
  ° Systematic Reviews: "((scoliosis braces) AND systematic[sb]) OR ((scoliosis bracing) AND systematic[sb])"
  ° Clinical Studies Category: "scoliosis AND brace AND 'clinical trial'"

Quality of the evidence

Level II
• 2 systematic reviews/meta-analyses
• 1 prospective study with treatment determined by individual centers
• 1 prospective study with results compared by compliance with bracing

Level III
• 1 systematic review/meta-analysis
• 1 retrospective cohort comparison

Findings

A 1995 multicenter prospective study[16] is often considered the definitive study showing brace effectiveness. This study compared observation and bracing for girls with curve apices T8–L1 and Cobb angles 25–35°. With progression defined as 6° change or more, 74% of braced patients and 34% of observed patients did not progress. Danielsson, et al.[17] used some of this earlier study's subjects and compared longer-term follow-up of two sites, one bracing all eligible patients and the other only bracing progressing curves. None of 41 initially braced patients progressed 6°, while 26 of 65 (40%) initially observed patients progressed with 6 (10%) of them undergoing surgery. There was no difference in progression between the two groups after maturity (5.7° for braced and 7.0° for observed patients). Assuming these results are generalizable, bracing prevents surgery in 10% of eligible patients.

Of two systematic reviews, one[18] found overall methodologically poor-quality studies without strong evidence that bracing was effective and the other[1] found no difference in surgical rates between braced and observed patients.

A recent observational study[19] examined the dose response curve of patients with idiopathic scoliosis based upon the amount of time the brace was worn, the Risser sign, and the status of the triradiate cartilage. Again, curve progression was defined by 6° change. The authors found that more time wearing the brace resulted in less likelihood of curve progression more than 6°. Less mature patients (open tririadiate cartilage) required more time in the brace for the same effect. Methodologically, the study has important limitations including not documenting the specific curve pattern, using the orthotist to measure radiographs, lack of a functional endpoint such as surgery, and inability to distinguish whether compliance led to better results or vice versa.

A basic critique of prior studies is that different curve patterns behave differently and that far better maturity assessments exist than the Risser sign. Future studies must stratify by curve pattern, magnitude and sex, and use quality maturity indicators. Understanding whether bracing prevents progression to a surgical range and which patients are likely to benefit must await higher level studies which are currently in progress.[20]

Recommendations
- There is weak evidence that bracing can prevent curve progression of 6° or more in adolescent idiopathic scoliosis curves [overall quality: low]
- There is no evidence that bracing can prevent curve progression to a surgical range in moderate-sized adolescent idiopathic scoliosis curves [overall quality: low]

Question 4: Is it possible to predict which curves will progress markedly during the adolescent growth spurt?

Case clarification
The patient's mother knows of other children whose curves increased significantly despite bracing and required surgery and is concerned about this risk for her daughter.

Relevance
With knowledge that curves tend to progress more rapidly during the adolescent growth spurt, it is helpful to know which patients can be observed and which patients may require intervention.

Current opinion
Scoliosis progresses primarily during the adolescent growth spurt centered about the timing of maximum growth velocity (peak height velocity, PHV). Small curves at the PHV tend to remain small, while larger curves can progress substantially.

Finding the evidence
- Cochrane Database: "scoliosis"
- PubMed Clinical Queries:
  ° Clinical Studies Category: "(idiopathic scoliosis progression adolescence) AND (Prognosis/Narrow[filter]), and (idiopathic scoliosis progression growth) AND (Prognosis/Narrow[filter])"
  ° Systematic Reviews: "scoliosis progression"

- PubMed sensitivity search: "Scoliosis"[Mesh] AND (Prognosis/Broad[filter])

Quality of the evidence
Level I
- 3 studies (2 of same series)

Level II
- 14 studies (2 of same series)

Findings
A number of primarily retrospective level II studies[21–32] examining prognostic factors for scoliosis consistently show:
- curve progression is more common in patients with larger curves and less skeletal maturity
- thoracic and thoracic predominant double curves progress more than thoracolumbar curves or lumbar curves[21,24,27,28,30–32]
- the timing of progression is during the adolescent growth spurt and then slows markedly as maturity is reached

Most of these studies have important weaknesses, including not controlling for the important variables of curve pattern, magnitude, and maturity, and defining progressive curves as a change of 5 or 6° rather than functional endpoints.

The most commonly used maturity indicators in the literature are the Risser sign and chronological maturity. Several other indicators have been proposed which correlate more highly with scoliosis progression. One indicator is curve magnitude at the time of the growth spurt, with curves of les sthan 30° at the peak growth highly unlikely to progress to surgery and conversely for larger curves.[22,23] Skeletal maturity also highly correlates with curve progression and is a superior maturity indicator to Risser sign, chronological age, menarche, and other commonly used maturity indicators.[33] Both the hand[34] and the elbow[35,36] have useful maturity markers. Studies of curve progression using nonphysiological endpoints provide very little information to the clinician. It is quite clear that the studies must also separate curves based upon their pattern, since differing curve patterns behave quite differently.

Recent presentations have identified potential genetic markers as highly indicative of scoliosis progression.[37] At this time, there is too little literature to assess whether this is a viable alternative to the combination of maturity, curve pattern, and curve magnitude.

Recommendations
- Studies looking at skeletal maturity in conjunction with pattern and magnitude provide a reasonable method of ascertaining curve prognosis for progression. Larger studies must be completed before clinicians have accurate predictive value for many curve types [overall quality: moderate]

- There is insufficient evidence on genetic predictors to make recommendations for or against their use [overall quality: very low]

Question 5: What is the association between nonoperatively managed scoliosis and back pain or functional impairment?

Case clarification
Many people believe scoliosis looks as if it should become painful.

Relevance
With back pain common and sometimes debilitating in the general population, patients may be concerned that their future quality of life will be diminished by chronic back pain due to untreated scoliosis.

Current opinion
Patients with adolescent idiopathic scoliosis experience chronic back pain at a higher rate, but without any higher rate of disability.

Finding the evidence
- Cochrane Database: "scoliosis"
- PubMed Clinical Queries
  ° Clinical Studies Category: "(adolescent idiopathic scoliosis back pain) AND (Prognosis/Broad[filter])"
  ° Systematic Reviews: "(adolescent idiopathic scoliosis back pain) AND systematic[sb]"
- PubMed sensitivity search: "Scoliosis"[Mesh] AND "Back Pain"[Mesh]

Quality of the evidence
Level III
- 6 comparative studies

Level IV
- 1 case series

Findings
Untreated Weinstein, et al.[38] reported on 117 AIS patients with minimum follow-up of 50 years compared to matched controls. Sixty-one percent of patients reported chronic back pain at any level compared to 35% of controls (p = 0.003) with no correlation between pain scores and thoracic or lumbar spine radiographic osteoarthritis. Cordover et al.[39] studied 34 patients with average follow-up of 22 years and average age of 36 years, compared to controls. The rate of back pain in this cohort was 65% in scoliosis patients compared to 32% of controls. Ascani et al.[40] studied a cohort of 187 untreated patients with 15–47 year follow-up without a control group. The rate of back pain was 61%, similar to the other studies.

Brace-treated Danielsson and Nachemson[41] reported on 127 Swedish brace-treated patients with an average 22 year follow-up compared to controls. Seventy-six percent of patients reported back pain in the last year compared to 58% of controls (p = 0.0076). Functional outcome measures (Oswestry Disability Index and Short Form-36) demonstrated that back pain had a minimal effect on daily life and function. Other studies of this Swedish cohort indicated that pain intensity correlated with reduced lumbar range of motion[42] and was a minor reason for limitation in social activities, compared to physical difficulties or self-consciousness.[43]

Recommendations
- Scoliosis patients are more likely than controls to experience back pain over the long term [overall quality: high]
- Back pain for most untreated patients with scoliosis is typically neither disabling nor restricts daily activities [overall quality: moderate]

Question 6: What is the association between nonoperatively managed scoliosis and pulmonary compromise?

Case clarification
The patient asks if she will end up like her aunt with scoliosis, who was unable to walk up a flight of stairs without becoming short of breath.

Relevance
Thoracic curves can affect the geometry of the thoracic cage and possibly pulmonary function.

Current opinion
While infantile and juvenile curves may affect pulmonary development and function, only severe cases of adolescent idiopathic scoliosis impact on long-term pulmonary function.

Finding the evidence
- Cochrane Database: "scoliosis"
- PubMed Clinical Queries
  ° Clinical Studies Category: "(adolescent idiopathic scoliosis pulmonary) AND (Prognosis/Broad[filter])"
  ° Systematic Reviews: "(adolescent idiopathic scoliosis pulmonary) AND systematic[sb]"
- PubMed sensitivity search: "adolescent idiopathic scoliosis pulmonary"

Quality of the evidence
Level III
- 4 comparative studies

Findings

Weinstein et al.[38] in 51 year follow-up compared to controls found no significant difference in rates of shortness of breath (SOB) with daily activities or walking. Among patients with large curves (defined as >80° thoracic or >50° lumbar), those with thoracic curves had greater odds of SOB than patients with lumbar curves (OR 9.75, 95% CI 1.15–82.98). Those with curves >50° at maturity had greater odds of SOB at all three time-points in the study (OR 3.67 in 1992, 95% CI 1.11–12.12). Correlation was found between pulmonary function test (PFT) results and curve angles only for patients with single thoracic curves, and severe pulmonary impairment in a nonsmoker occurred only in patients with curve angles greater than 120°.[44] Pehrsson et al.[45] compared 141 surgically treated patients and 110 brace-treated patients with 100 randomly selected controls at mean follow-up of 25 years. There were no significant differences in dyspnea or wheezing among all groups. The authors also found 20 year unchanged mean vital capacity (VC) in untreated patients (65% predicted in 1968, 64% predicted in 1988), despite curves progressing from 79° to 86°, although six patients developed respiratory failure, and two had died.[46] Multivariate analysis indicated that low VC (<45% predicted) and large curve angle (>110°) were the strongest predictors of respiratory failure.

Recommendations

In patients with adolescent idiopathic scoliosis who are treated nonoperatively, evidence suggests:

• Untreated and braced scoliosis patients report no statistically significant increased rate of SOB or dyspnea when compared to controls [overall quality: moderate]

• In untreated patients with thoracic curves, VC is inversely related to curve angle, but only patients with severe thoracic curves (>110°) will experience severe impairment [overall quality: high]

• In moderate-sized curves, braced patients do not have statistically significant differences in PFTs when compared to surgically treated patients or controls [overall quality: low]

Summary of recommendations

• Until the completion of studies evaluating the effectiveness of bracing for adolescent idiopathic scoliosis, we are unable to identify substantial benefit from current school screening programs

• Only weak evidence exists that exercise therapy alters the natural history of idiopathic scoliosis

• Although there is weak evidence that bracing can prevent some curve progression, there is no evidence that bracing can prevent curve progression to a surgical range

in moderate-sized adolescent idiopathic scoliosis curves during immaturity

• The studies looking at skeletal maturity in conjunction with pattern and magnitude provide a reasonable method of ascertaining curve prognosis for progression. Larger studies must be completed before clinicians have accurate predictive value for many curve types

• There is insufficient evidence on genetic predictors to make recommendations for or against their use

• Scoliosis patients are more likely than controls to experience back pain over the long term

• Back pain for most untreated scoliosis patients is typically neither disabling nor restricts daily activities

• Untreated and braced patients report no statistically significant increased rate of SOB or dyspnea when compared to controls

• In untreated patients with thoracic curves, VC is inversely related to curve angle, but only patients with severe thoracic curves (>110°) will experience severe impairment

Conclusions

Limited high-quality evidence relevant to nonoperative treatment of scoliosis precludes strong recommendations. Large trials of high methodological quality focusing on patient-important outcomes such as quality of life and risk of surgery are urgently needed to better inform the diagnosis, treatment, and prognosis of conservatively managed scoliosis.

References

1. Dolan LA, Weinstein SL. Surgical rates after observation and bracing for adolescent idiopathic scoliosis: an evidence-based review. Spine 2007;32(19 Suppl):S91–100.

2. Bridwell KH, Berven S, Glassman S, et al. Is the SRS-22 instrument responsive to change in adult scoliosis patients having primary spinal deformity surgery? Spine 2007;32(20):2220–5.

3. Berven S, Deviren V, Demir-Deviren S, Hu SS, Bradford DS. Studies in the modified Scoliosis Research Society Outcomes Instrument in adults: validation, reliability, and discriminatory capacity. Spine 2003;28(18):2164–9; discussion 69.

4. U.S. Preventive Services Task Force Report on Screening for Idiopathic Scoliosis in Adolescents. Screening for Idiopathic Scoliosis in Adolescents, Topic Page 2004. http://www.uspreventiveservicestaskforce.org/uspstf/uspsaisc.htm

5. Richards BS, Beaty JH, Thompson GH, Willis RB. Estimating the effectiveness of screening for scoliosis. Pediatrics 2008;121(6): 1296–97.

6. Richards BS, Vitale MG. Screening for idiopathic scoliosis in adolescents. An information statement. J Bone Joint Surg Am 2008;90(1):195–98.

7. Bunge EM, de Koning HJ, brace trial g. Bracing patients with idiopathic scoliosis: design of the Dutch randomized controlled treatment trial. BMC Musculoskelet Disord 2008;9:57.

8. Yawn BP, Yawn RA. The estimated cost of school scoliosis screening. Spine 2000;25(18):2387–91.

9. Bunnell WP. Selective screening for scoliosis. Clin Orthop Relat Res 2005;434:40–5.

10. Grivas TB, Vasiliadis ES, O'Brien JP. Suggestions for improvement of school screening for idiopathic scoliosis. Stud Health Technol Inform 2008;140:245–8.

11. Karachalios T, Sofianos J, Roidis N, Sapkas G, Korres D, Nikolopoulos K. Ten-year follow-up evaluation of a school screening program for scoliosis. Is the forward-bending test an accurate diagnostic criterion for the screening of scoliosis? Spine 1999;24(22):2318–24.

12. Bremberg S, Nilsson-Berggren B. School screening for adolescent idiopathic scoliosis. J Pediatr Orthop 1986;6(5):564–7.

13. Velezis MJ, Sturm PF, Cobey J. Scoliosis screening revisited: findings from the District of Columbia. J Pediatr Orthop 2002;22(6):788–91.

14. Negrini S, Fusco C, Minozzi S, Atanasio S, Zaina F, Romano M. Exercises reduce the progression rate of adolescent idiopathic scoliosis: results of a comprehensive systematic review of the literature. Disabil Rehabil 2008;30(10):772–85.

15. Weiss HR, Weiss G, Petermann F. Incidence of curvature progression in idiopathic scoliosis patients treated with scoliosis in-patient rehabilitation (SIR): an age- and sex-matched controlled study. Pediatr Rehabil 2003;6(1):23–30.

16. Nachemson AL, Peterson LE. Effectiveness of treatment with a brace in girls who have adolescent idiopathic scoliosis. A prospective, controlled study based on data from the Brace Study of the Scoliosis Research Society. J Bone Joint Surg Am 1995;77(6):815–22.

17. Danielsson AJ, Hasserius R, Ohlin A, Nachemson AL. A prospective study of brace treatment versus observation alone in adolescent idiopathic scoliosis: a follow-up mean of 16 years after maturity. Spine 2007;32(20):2198–207.

18. Lenssinck ML, Frijlink AC, Berger MY, Bierman-Zeinstra SM, Verkerk K, Verhagen AP. Effect of bracing and other conservative interventions in the treatment of idiopathic scoliosis in adolescents: a systematic review of clinical trials. Phys Ther 2005;85(12):1329–39.

19. Katz DE, Herring JA, Browne RH, Kelly DM, Birch JG. Brace wear control of curve progression in adolescent idiopathic scoliosis. J Bone Joint Surg Am 2010;92(6):1343–52.

20. Weinstein SL, Dolan LA. BrAIST: the bracing in adolescent idiopathic scoliosis trial. US National Institute of Health 2007; www.clinicaltrials.gov/ct/show/NCT00448448.

21. Charles YP, Daures JP, de Rosa V, Dimeglio A. Progression risk of idiopathic juvenile scoliosis during pubertal growth. Spine 2006;31(17):1933–42.

22. Song KM, Little DG. Peak height velocity as a maturity indicator for males with idiopathic scoliosis. J Pediatr Orthop 2000;20(3):286–8.

23. Little DG, Song KM, Katz D, Herring JA. Relationship of peak height velocity to other maturity indicators in idiopathic scoliosis in girls. J Bone Joint Surg Am 2000;82(5):685–93.

24. Robinson CM, McMaster MJ. Juvenile idiopathic scoliosis. Curve patterns and prognosis in one hundred and nine patients. J Bone Joint Surg Am 1996;78(8):1140–8.

25. Upadhyay SS, Nelson IW, Ho EK, Hsu LC, Leong JC. New prognostic factors to predict the final outcome of brace treatment in adolescent idiopathic scoliosis. Spine 1995;20(5):537–45.

26. Peterson LE, Nachemson AL. Prediction of progression of the curve in girls who have adolescent idiopathic scoliosis of moderate severity. Logistic regression analysis based on data from The Brace Study of the Scoliosis Research Society. J Bone Joint Surg Am 1995;77(6):823–7.

27. Duval-Beaupere G, Lamireau T. Scoliosis at less than 30 degrees. Properties of the evolutivity (risk of progression). Spine 1985;10(5):421–4.

28. Lonstein JE, Carlson JM. The prediction of curve progression in untreated idiopathic scoliosis during growth. J Bone Joint Surg Am 1984;66(7):1061–71.

29. Urbaniak JR, Schaefer WW, Stelling FH, 3rd. Iliac apophyses. Prognostic value in idiopathic schliosis. Clin Orthop Relat Res 1976;116:80–5.

30. Zaoussis AL, James JIP. The iliac apophysis and the evolution of curves in scoliosis. J Bone Joint Surg Br 1958;40(3):442–53.

31. James JI. Idiopathic scoliosis; the prognosis, diagnosis, and operative indications related to curve patterns and the age at onset. J Bone Joint Surg Br 1954;36(1):36–49.

32. Ponseti IV, Friedman B. Prognosis in idiopathic scoliosis. J Bone Joint Surg Am 1950;32(2):381–95.

33. Sanders JO, Browne RH, McConnell SJ, Margraf SA, Cooney TE, Finegold DN. Maturity assessment and curve progression in girls with idiopathic scoliosis. J.Bone Joint Surg Am 2007;89(1):64–73.

34. Sanders JO, Khoury JG, Kishan S, et al. Predicting scoliosis progression from skeletal maturity: a simplified classification during adolescence. J Bone Joint Surg Am 2008;90(3):540–53.

35. Charles YP, Dimeglio A, Canavese F, Daures JP. Skeletal age assessment from the olecranon for idiopathic scoliosis at Risser grade 0. J Bone Joint Surg Am 2007;89(12):2737–44.

36. Dimeglio A, Charles YP, Daures JP, de RV, Kabore B. Accuracy of the Sauvegrain method in determining skeletal age during puberty. J Bone Joint Surg Am. 2005;87(8):1689–96.

37. Ogilvie J. Adolescent idiopathic scoliosis and genetic testing. Curr Opin Pediatr 2010;22(1):67–70.

38. Weinstein SL, Dolan LA, Spratt KF, Peterson KK, Spoonamore MJ, Ponseti IV. Health and function of patients with untreated idiopathic scoliosis: a 50-year natural history study. JAMA 2003;289(5):559–67.

39. Cordover AM, Betz RR, Clements DH, Bosacco SJ. Natural history of adolescent thoracolumbar and lumbar idiopathic scoliosis into adulthood. J.Spinal Disord 1997;10(3):193–96.

40. Ascani E, Bartolozzi P, Logroscino CA, et al. Natural history of untreated idiopathic scoliosis after skeletal maturity. Spine 1986;11(8):784–89.

41. Danielsson AJ, Nachemson AL. Back pain and function 22 years after brace treatment for adolescent idiopathic scoliosis: a case-control study-part I. Spine 2003;28(18):2078–85; discussion 86.

42. Danielsson AJ, Romberg K, Nachemson AL. Spinal range of motion, muscle endurance, and back pain and function at least 20 years after fusion or brace treatment for adolescent idiopathic scoliosis: a case-control study. Spine 2006;31(3):275–83.

43. Danielsson AJ, Wiklund I, Pehrsson K, Nachemson AL. Health-related quality of life in patients with adolescent idiopathic sco-

liosis: a matched follow-up at least 20 years after treatment with brace or surgery. Eur Spine J 2001;10(4):278–88.

44. Weinstein SL, Zavala DC, Ponseti IV. Idiopathic scoliosis: long-term follow-up and prognosis in untreated patients. J Bone Joint Surg Am 1981;63(5):702–12.

45. Pehrsson K, Danielsson A, Nachemson A. Pulmonary function in adolescent idiopathic scoliosis: a 25 year follow up after surgery or start of brace treatment. Thorax 2001;56(5): 388–93.

46. Pehrsson K, Bake B, Larsson S, Nachemson A. Lung function in adult idiopathic scoliosis: a 20 year follow up. Thorax 1991;46: 474–78.

83 Adolescent Idiopathic Scoliosis— Operative Management

Calvin T. Hu and James O. Sanders
University of Rochester Medical Center, Rochester, NY, USA

Case scenario

A 14-year-old boy presents with a Risser 1 spinal deformity associated with a 75° left thoracic curve and a 45° right lumbar curve. His neurological examination shows slight asymmetry in his abdominal reflexes.

Relevant anatomy

Absence of the superficial abdominal reflex is a risk factor for spinal cord abnormalities such as syringomyelia.

Importance of the problem

The issues involved with idiopathic scoliosis are outlined in the introduction to the previous chapter on nonoperative treatment. Once the curve reaches a surgical range (50° at skeletal maturity), other questions assume importance, and some of the major questions are discussed in this chapter.

Top six questions

Diagnosis

1. Which patients with presumed adolescent idiopathic scoliosis (AIS) should have MRI imaging preoperatively?

Therapy

2. When do patients with AIS benefit from anterior surgery compared to posterior surgery?

3. What are the criteria for determining the cranial/caudal extent of fusion?
4. Does the amount of curve correction correlate with patient satisfaction?
5. Does the type of bone graft material affect fusion rates?
6. Is intraoperative neuromonitoring effective in preventing neurologic injury?

Question 1: Which patients with presumed AIS should have MRI imaging preoperatively?

Case clarification

The patient above has been followed for scoliosis and is referred to you for surgical evaluation.

Relevance

There is controversy regarding the necessity of routine preoperative MRI for patients with presumed AIS. Some surgeons have reported neurological complications in patients with spinal cord abnormalities (e.g., syringomyelia) who undergo surgery for curve correction.[1–3] These spinal cord abnormalities may be subclinical. With this in mind, several case series have reported on the results of screening MRI of the spine for patients with normal physical examination who are about to undergo spinal fusion for AIS (Table 83.1). Combining the results of these studies, there is an overall 4% rate (33 of 791) of spinal cord abnormalities, with 9% of these patients (0.4% of all patients) requiring neurosurgical procedures to treat the abnormality (e.g., decompression of syringomyelia). But, both the highest rate of spinal cord abnormalities (8%) and the only neurosurgical procedures required came from a single study. No neurological complications were reported in any of the studies.

Evidence-Based Orthopedics, First Edition. Edited by Mohit Bhandari.
© 2012 Blackwell Publishing Ltd. Published 2012 by Blackwell Publishing Ltd.

Table 83.1 Summary of studies reporting on the use of routine preoperative MRI

Reference	AIS, normal physical exam?	Number of patients	Number of abnormalities (%)	Type of abnormality found (n)	Number requiring neurosurgical procedure	Neurological complications
Ozturk et al.[8]	Yes	249	20 (8%)	Syrinx (15) Arnold–Chiari type I with syrinx (3) Arnold–Chiari type I (2)	3 (those with Arnold–Chiari type I with syrinx)	0
Do et al.[9]	Yes	327	7 (2%)	Syrinx (2) Arnold–Chiari type I (4) Vertebral body anomaly (1)	0	0
Maiocco et al.[10]	Yes	45	2 (2%) (one patient was juvenile onset)	Syrinx (1) Arnold–Chiari type I with syrinx (1)	0	0
Winter et al.[11]	Yes	140	4 (3%)	Syrinx (3) Arnold–Chiari type I (1)	0	0
O'Brien et al.[12]	Yes, with curve >70°	30	0 (0%)	n/a	n/a	0

Current opinion

At the time of initial evaluation, if a patient is male, has a left thoracic curve, thoracic kyphosis, or any abnormality on neurologic exam, MRI should be obtained. Routine MRI is not necessary.

Finding the evidence

- Cochrane Database, with search term: "scoliosis"
- PubMed clinical queries:
  - Clinical Studies category, with search term: "(scoliosis magnetic resonance imaging) AND (Diagnosis/Broad[filter])"
  - Systematic Reviews, with search term: "(scoliosis magnetic resonance imaging) AND systematic[sb]"
- PubMed sensitivity search, with search term: "scoliosis magnetic resonance imaging"

Quality of the evidence

Level III
- 1 observational study
- 2 case-control studies

Level IV
- 6 case series

Findings

Left thoracic curve Davids et al.[4] studied 1,280 patients with presumed AIS who had MRI performed based on the examination findings listed in Table 83.2 and found no association between curve direction and MRI abnormality. Goldberg et al.[5] reviewed 666 cases of AIS and found no correlation between left-sided curves and CNS abnormal-

Table 83.2 Examination findings that were tested for an association with preoperative abnormal MRI findings

Pain	Neurological findings	Atypical curve pattern
Back	Clonus	Left thoracic
Neck	Abnormal abdominal reflexes	Short segment (4–6 levels)
Radicular	Weakness	Decreased vertebral rotation
Headache	Urinary dysfunction (urinary tract infection)	Absence of thoracic apical segment lordosis
	Hyperreflexia	Rapid progression
	Asymmetric deep tendon reflexes	
	Paresthesias	
	Diminished rectal tone	
	Cavus foot deformity	
	Skin lesions	

ity. In contrast, Loder et al.[6] in a much smaller study compared radiographic findings of 30 patients with Arnold–Chiari I malformation with or without syringomyelia to 26 patients with normal MRI and found a positive relationship with left-sided curves (40% vs. 0%, p = 0.0002).

Thoracic kyphosis on sagittal plain radiograph In the study by Davids et al.,[4] of all the atypical curve pattern findings listed as an indication for MRI, the absence of apical segment lordosis (or hyperkyphosis, as defined by sagittal plane thoracic kyphosis ≥20°) was associated most frequently with abnormal findings on MRI. Ouellet et al.[7] conducted a case-control study comparing radiographs of 30 patients with syringomyelia to 54 patients with normal MRI to examine the importance of apical segment lordosis and found apical segment lordosis present in 97% of those with normal MRI but only 25% of those with syringomyelia (p < 0.00001).

Abnormality on neurological exam In the study by Davids et al.,[4] clonus (7 of 42 patients), weakness (7 of 46 patients), and abnormal abdominal reflexes (5 of 42 patients) were the abnormal neurological findings most frequently associated with MRI abnormalities. The presence of more than one abnormal finding on neurological examination did not increase the frequency of MRI abnormalities. However, the combination of a neurological abnormality and an atypical curve pattern was associated with a higher rate of MRI abnormalities.

Male sex Loder et al.[6] found that 37% of cases vs. 8% of controls (p = 0.01) were males, suggesting an association. But the much larger study by Davids et al.[4] failed to confirm a relationship between gender and preoperative MRI abnormalities.

Pain Davids et al.[4] found that when pain alone was used as an indication for MRI, no MRI abnormalities were found.

Recommendations

Only a small proportion of AIS patients have been found to have spinal cord abnormalities. In patients with presumed AIS, evidence suggests:
• Absence of apical segment lordosis or abnormality on neurological exam are indicators for MRI [overall quality: low]
• Pain, left thoracic curve, and male sex are not indicators for MRI [overall quality: low]
    There is low-quality information arguing for the use of a preoperative MRI in the case of our patient.

Question 2: When do patients with AIS benefit from anterior surgery compared to posterior surgery?

Case clarification

Consider a patient with a single structural 80° thoracic curve with considerable clinical deformity. Supine lateral bending films demonstrate only 20° correction of the curve.

Frontal radiograph of the patient's pelvis reveals closed triradiate cartilage.

Relevance

Anterior surgery involving thoracotomy and disc excision has several purposes. If used in lieu of a posterior approach for instrumentation and fusion, anterior surgery may spare motion segments. In large curves, anterior discectomy may enhance correction. Or, it may prevent the crankshaft phenomenon,[13] which is deforming anterior growth in younger children following a posterior fusion.[14,15] However, anterior surgery may cause adverse pulmonary effects, and combined anterior–posterior surgery takes longer than posterior-only surgery.

Current opinion

Anterior surgery for thoracic curve correction has decreased due to reports of long-term adverse effects on pulmonary function and improved curve correction with pedicle screw instrumentation compared to older techniques.

Finding the evidence

• Cochrane Database, with search term: "scoliosis"
• PubMed Clinical Queries:
    ○ Clinical Studies Categories, with search term: "(adolescent idiopathic scoliosis anterior posterior) AND (Therapy/Narrow[filter])" and "scoliosis surgery anterior posterior Limits Activated: Clinical Trial, Meta-Analysis, Randomized Controlled Trial"
    ○ Systematic Reviews, with search term: "(adolescent idiopathic scoliosis anterior posterior) AND systematic[sb]"
• PubMed sensitivity search, with search term: "adolescent idiopathic scoliosis anterior posterior"

Quality of the evidence

Level I
• 2 prospective cohort studies

Level II
• 1 prospective cohort study

Level III
• 6 comparative studies

Findings

Very skeletally immature patients, defined as those with open triradiate cartilages of the pelvis at the time of surgery, treated with either an isolated anterior or posterior instrumentation and fusion rather than a combined procedure, experience a higher incidence of adding more levels to the curve or of main curve progression postoperatively (8 of 28 patients vs. 0 of 16 patients).[16] The results are mixed for curve correction and maintenance. A level II study of 32 patients comparing single rod anterior instrumentation with posterior pedicle screw instrumentation[17] found the anterior approach superior in terms of blood loss (also seen in a level I study[18]) and curve correction. However, a larger level III study[19] of 62 patients found worse curve correction and maintenance of correction with dual rod anterior instrumentation compared to posterior pedicle screw instrumentation. Several level III studies[20–22] found posterior pedicle screw constructs as effective as anterior–posterior fusions for curve correction.

No studies compare functional outcomes based upon surgical approach. A level I[23] and a level III[24] study each documented decreased pulmonary function in patients treated with anterior surgery when compared to patients treated with posterior procedures. The previously mentioned level I study[23] found surgical approach to be only a small contributor to decreased pulmonary function, with preoperative pulmonary function test (PFT) results being a stronger predictor of decreased postoperative function. Unfortunately, the minimal clinically important difference (MCID) for PFTs is not well delineated, making this information difficult to interpret.

Recommendations

• For most cases of AIS, including large curves, posterior pedicle screw instrumentation and fusion alone is as effective as anterior–posterior surgery [overall quality: low]
• Anterior fusion in conjunction with posterior fusion results in a lower incidence of adding on and curve progression in patients with open triradiate cartilages [overall quality: low]
• Pulmonary function is adversely affected by an anterior approach, but its clinical significance is uncertain [overall quality: moderate]

There is low-quality evidence that posterior pedicle screw instrumentation would be best for this patient.

Question 3: What are the criteria for determining the cranial/caudal extent of fusion?

Case clarification

A patient has a 65° right thoracic, 50° left lumbar curve, and a 30° left upper thoracic curve with even shoulders. She has elected to have posterior surgery, but the specific spinal vertebra to include in the fusion must be decided upon.

Relevance

The selection of fusion levels is of importance because the more levels included in the fusion, the straighter and more centered the spine can become. However, more levels included in the fusion may also lead to stress on the remaining open spinal segments.

Current opinion

The selection of fusion levels is generally based upon expert opinion, originally with the goal to provide a harmoniously "balanced" spine, improving both appearance and curvature. Early evidence in the late 1960s indicated fusion into the lumbar spine might be associated with early degenerative arthritis of the lower spine, with subsequent recommendations to limit the amount of lumbar spine fusion. Another concern arose with the development of powerful posterior correction systems in whether or not to include upper thoracic curves, or lower lumbar curves in the fusion. Upper thoracic curves are typically included if they are likely to cause poor appearance if not included.

A number of terms require definition to properly discuss fusion levels. These terms are used freely here, and we recommend consulting the *Spinal Deformity Study Group Radiographic Measurement Manual*[25] or the Scoliosis Research Society (SRS) website (http://www.srs.org/professionals/glossary/) for term definitions. Fusion recommendations typically relate to the curve's end vertebra (EV), neutrally rotated vertebra (NV), and the stable vertebra (SV), which is that vertebra bisected by the center sacral vertical line (CSVL). Recommendations typically are to fuse entire structural curves and leave secondary curves alone. Defining these secondary curves has been problematic, with several classification schemes devised for this purpose, particularly the King and Lenke classifications.

King[26] described follow-up of patients treated with fusion using Harrington instrumentation from the neutral vertebra above to the SV below. For double major curves with the lumbar curve larger than the thoracic spine, the fusion extended to L4. If the lumbar curve is smaller, it was not included in the fusion which was stopped at the SV above. Following the development of multiple hook implants, some patients were found to "decompensate" by shifting to the side if the lumbar curve was not included. Suggested reasons included "overcorrection" in the thoracic spine, which the lumbar spine could not accommodate or persistent obliquity of L4 leading to this shift.[27] Lenke developed his classification in an attempt to define which curves required fusion.[28] The Lenke classification has become widely used. In this classification, only curves defined as structural require fusion. Other criteria, such as those by Burton and Asher[29] or Suk,[30–32] also attempt to straighten the spine while retaining lumbar motion segments.

Finding the evidence

• Cochrane Database, with search term: "scoliosis"
• PubMed Clinical Queries:
  ○ Clinical Studies Category, with search term: "(adolescent scoliosis fusion levels) AND (Therapy/Broad[filter])"
  ○ Systematic Reviews, with search term: "(adolescent scoliosis fusion levels) AND systematic[sb]"

• PubMed sensitivity search, with search term: "Scoliosis/surgery"[Mesh] AND "Spinal Fusion/adverse effects"[Mesh]

Quality of the evidence

Level III
• 5 comparative studies

Level IV
• 8 case series

Level V
• 3 opinion studies

Findings

One level III study[33] compared patients treated by surgeon judgment to those treated using the Lenke criteria and found superior radiographic outcomes in those treated according to the Lenke criteria. Three studies[34–36] compared what different surgeons would do for various curve patterns and patient scenarios and found marked variation between surgeons in the selection of fusion levels. Although a few studies have attempted to address the upper level of fusion, they are uncontrolled.[37–39]

We performed a systematic review of the effects of fusion into the lower lumbar spine and found a marked degree of heterogeneity in the length of follow-up, the outcomes measured, and the use of controls. No studies compared fused and unfused scoliosis patients, and all controls were nonscoliotic adults. Most studies used an early, non-validated measure to determine pain;[40] however, recent studies have used validated outcomes measures. All except a few studies report Harrington instrumentation results. There is only one report[41] of later-generation (CD) instrumentation with short follow-up. We performed a meta-analysis of those studies with sufficient data to determine odds ratios of severe back pain for fusion into the lower lumbar spine compared to stopping at L3 or above[41–48] which excluded many well-known studies.[40,49–60] When several articles were found from the same cohort, only the most complete data set was used. Our meta-analysis (Figure 83.1) and the highest-quality study[48] found no significant difference in severe lumbar pain between patients fused to L3 or above compared to L4 or below. This same higher-quality series found no substantial difference in back pain or disc degeneration based upon the amount of residual lumbar lordosis.[61] We found that disc degeneration was most severe at the lowest lumbar motion segment rather than just below the instrumentation. Unfortunately, the lack of controls in this literature is problematic because without comparing untreated scoliosis controls to similar scoliosis patients, it is not possible to say that the fusion level rather than the scoliosis itself caused the disc degeneration.

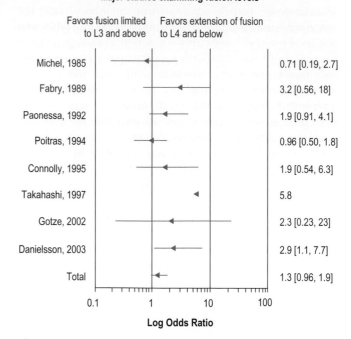

Major studies examining fusion levels

Favors fusion limited to L3 and above | Favors extension of fusion to L4 and below

Study	Log Odds Ratio
Michel, 1985	0.71 [0.19, 2.7]
Fabry, 1989	3.2 [0.56, 18]
Paonessa, 1992	1.9 [0.91, 4.1]
Poitras, 1994	0.96 [0.50, 1.8]
Connolly, 1995	1.9 [0.54, 6.3]
Takahashi, 1997	5.8
Gotze, 2002	2.3 [0.23, 23]
Danielsson, 2003	2.9 [1.1, 7.7]
Total	1.3 [0.96, 1.9]

0.1   1   10   100

Log Odds Ratio

Figure 83.1 Major studies examining fusion levels.

Recommendations

There is considerable variation in recommendations for fusion levels in idiopathic scoliosis. Established criteria for instrumentation are based upon expert opinion (level V evidence) with weak support from level IV evidence. Because these types of studies are very difficult to randomize and require evaluating function several decades after instrumentation with controls consisting of either patients with similar curves fused to different levels or unfused scoliosis, it is likely that recommendations for instrumentation and fusion levels will continue to be based upon expert opinion for the foreseeable future. That is, unless nonfusion treatments replace instrumentation and fusion.

• There is very weak evidence that extending instrumentation and fusion into the lower lumbar spine for scoliosis results in long-term disability compared to fusion into the thoracic or upper lumbar spine [overall quality: very low]

Based on the available evidence, extending instrumentation into the lower lumbar spine is not contraindicated.

Question 4: Does the amount of curve correction correlate with patient satisfaction?

Case clarification

Your AIS patient asks if his back will look straight after surgery.

Relevance

There is evidence that successful radiographic outcomes do not always correlate with patient-centered outcomes. The patient's responses on quality of life measures may correlate more strongly with physical appearance as opposed to radiographic parameters.

Current opinion

Current opinion suggests that the magnitude of curve correction correlates to patient satisfaction.

Finding the evidence

- Cochrane Database, with search term: "scoliosis"
- PubMed Clinical Queries:
  - Clinical Studies Category, with search term: "(adolescent scoliosis surgery quality of life) AND (Therapy/Broad[filter])"
  - Systematic Reviews, with search term: "adolescent scoliosis surgery quality of life"
- PubMed sensitivity search, with search terms: "adolescent idiopathic scoliosis curve correction patient outcomes surgical," "adolescent scoliosis surgery quality of life surgery"

Quality of the evidence

Level II

- 4 prospective comparative studies

Level III

- 7 retrospective comparative studies

Level IV

- 1 case series

Findings

There are few studies that investigate the relationship between curve correction and patient-important outcome measures. The most commonly used patient based outcome measure in scoliosis surgery is the SRS Patient Questionnaire. Studies have shown that patients' self-image scores on the SRS Patient Questionnaire are affected by curve severity.[62–67] Four prospective studies compared SRS measurements both before and after surgery and found improvements, particularly in the self-image domain from preoperatively to postoperatively[68–71], with the largest of these studies[71] finding more improvement in self-image scores in patients with greater curve correction (correlation coefficient 0.288, p = 0.000). It should be noted that the MCID for the SRS instrument has not been reported. From these studies, it is apparent that patients who have surgical treatment of scoliosis generally improve their self-image but the association with curve correction is not clear at this time.

Other factors may play a role in patients' self-image and satisfaction with surgery. Patients treated with different surgical approaches or instrumentation but with similar magnitudes of curve correction can have differences in SRS scores.[69,72,73] So, although patient self-image and satisfaction will likely improve after surgery, the improvement is likely multifactorial and cannot be attributed solely to the postoperative curve magnitude.

Recommendations

- Patient self-image and satisfaction will likely improve after surgery, but the improvement is multifactorial and cannot be solely attributed to the postoperative magnitude of the curve [overall quality: low]

The patient can be told that his back will look straighter after surgery, but his parents should be informed that there are other factors that determine a patient's satisfaction with the outcome of surgery for AIS.

Question 5: Does the type of bone graft material affect fusion rates?

Case clarification

Your patient's mother states she had iliac crest bone graft harvest performed for her scoliosis surgery, and that she still has bothersome pain at the donor site. She inquires about alternatives to iliac crest bone graft.

Relevance

Iliac crest bone graft is the gold standard for bone grafting, but donor site morbidity can affect a patient's quality of life. Thus, alternatives to iliac crest bone graft deserve consideration if they offer advantages.

Current opinion

Adolescent patients can achieve high rates of fusion when cancellous allograft is used. There is no consensus regarding synthetic bone graft substitutes.

Finding the evidence

- Cochrane Database, using search term: "scoliosis"
- PubMed Clinical Queries
  - Clinical Studies Categories, using search term: "(scoliosis bone graft substitute) AND (Therapy/Broad[filter]), (scoliosis allograft) AND (Therapy/Broad[filter])"
  - Systematic Reviews: none
- PubMed sensitivity search, using search terms: "scoliosis AND allograft," "Scoliosis"[Mesh] AND "Bone Substitutes"[Mesh]

Quality of the evidence

Level I

- 3 randomized trials

Level III
• 8 case-control studies

Findings

The interpretation of these studies is difficult for many reasons. The definition of pseudoarthrosis is not universally agreed upon, with several different definitions being used in the literature. Also, because it is a relatively rare complication often not becoming clinically evident until prolonged follow-up, randomized controlled trials (RCTs) or observational studies require large sample sizes and long follow-up periods to detect this complication. Case-control studies are therefore a reasonable study design to explore factors associated with pseudoarthrosis. One recent systematic review of pedicle screw instrumentation reported the incidence of pseudoarthrosis at 0.5%.[74] Because pseudarthrosis may be related to surgical technique, surgeon ability and experience as well as the bone graft material may be important variables.

Iliac crest autograft vs. allograft Five retrospective studies directly compared the use of iliac crest autograft to bone bank allograft.[75–79] The instrumentation techniques varied from Harrington–Luque to Cotrel–Dubousset to Texas Scottish Rite Hospital systems. Follow-up ranged from 6 to 24 months. The combined rate of pseudoarthrosis was similar, with 5 pseudoarthroses in 269 patients receiving autograft, compared to 6 in 274 patients receiving allograft. Two studies reported that operative times (141 vs. 176 minutes, $p < 0.001$ and 221 vs. 259 minutes, $p < 0.01$) and were less with allograft than autograft,[78,79] while one of these showed blood loss was less with allograft compared to autograft (1,485 vs. 1,815 mL, $p < 0.01$).[79] A randomized prospective trial by Betz et al.[80] compared allograft to no bone graft material, including local bone, and failed to detect a significant difference between groups.

Bone substitutes Two randomized prospective trials[81,82] compared the use of beta-tricalcium phosphate (β-TCP) to iliac crest autograft, with one study supplementing β-TCP with hydroxyapatite. A range of instrumentation systems were used. At minimum 18 month follow-up, there was one pseudoarthrosis in 190 patients receiving β-TCP, while none were reported in 191 patients receiving iliac crest. The authors claimed inadequate instrumentation as the cause of the pseudoarthrosis. Two smaller retrospective studies compared β-TCP to allograft, finding no pseudoarthroses in either group.[83,84]

Demineralized bone matrix (DBM) was compared with allograft and iliac crest autograft in a 88 consecutive patients.[75] One pseudoarthrosis each was reported in the allograft and iliac crest groups, with none in the DBM group during an average follow-up period ranging from 35 to 56 months. When loss of correction of 10° was used to define "possible pseudoarthrosis," the rates in each group were 24%, 12%, and 11% respectively. Unfortunately, no statistical analysis was performed in this study. Finally, another consecutive series of 88 patients[85] evaluated the use of bioactive glass compared to iliac crest autograft and found three reported cases of pseudoarthrosis in the iliac crest group and none with the bioglass group at mean 40 month follow-up.

Recommendations

• To date, there are no clear differences in the rates of pseudoarthrosis for various bone graft materials [overall quality: low]

In the case of our patient, the mother can be informed that because there is no clear evidence to support the use of iliac crest autograft or its alternatives over one another, an alternative is a reasonable choice, especially given her concerns about postoperative iliac crest pain

Question 6: Is intraoperative neuromonitoring effective in preventing neurologic injury?

Case clarification

The patient asks what the chances are he will become paralyzed as a result of surgery and what you can do minimize the risk.

Relevance

While the risk of spinal cord injury during scoliosis surgery is relatively rare, the consequences can be devastating.

Current opinion

Multimodality neuromonitoring with both sensory and motor evoked potentials is effective in detecting impending injury to the spinal cord during curve correction.

Finding the evidence

• Cochrane Database, using search term: "scoliosis"
• PubMed Clinical Queries:
  ○ Clinical Studies Category, using search term: "scoliosis neuromonitoring"
  ○ Systematic Reviews, using search term: "neuromonitoring"
• PubMed sensitivity search, using search term: "Scoliosis"[Mesh] AND "Monitoring, Intraoperative"[Mesh]

Quality of the evidence

Level I
• 1 systematic review
• 1 cohort study

Findings

Curve correction can place traction on the spinal cord and lead to changes in neuromonitoring. Reversal of the curve correction by removal of the rod can potentially reverse the onset of a permanent spinal cord injury. In contrast, screw misplacement into the spinal cord or nerve root is likely to cause irreversible damage. A recent systematic review of level II and level III studies[86] focused on the use of intraoperative neuromonitoring primarily in adult spine surgery. High-level evidence supported the use of multimodal (somatosensory evoked potentials, or SSEP and motor evoked potentials, or MEP) neuromonitoring as a sensitive and specific means to detect potentially reversible intraoperative neurological injury. High-level evidence also confirmed that if used alone, MEPs are more sensitive than SSEPs; however, these two tests are similar in specificity. This recommendation included one study evaluating MEP and SSEP monitoring in AIS, whose results were in agreement.[87] The systematic review also found low-level evidence that intraoperative neuromonitoring could reduce the rate of neurological injury during curve correction

Recommendations

• SSEP and MEP neuromonitoring is a sensitive and specific means to detect intraoperative neurological injury. MEPs are more sensitive than SSEPs in detecting injury, but the two modalities should continue to be used together [overall quality: high]
• Intraoperative neuromonitoring can reduce the rate of neurological injury [overall quality: low]

The patient is told there is low probability that he will become paralyzed as a result of scoliosis surgery and that there is low-quality evidence that the use of intraoperative neuromonitoring can help detect potentially reversible neurological injury.

Summary of recommendations

• MRI is recommended for patients with atypical curves, particularly with kyphosis rather than lordosis at the apex as well as in patients with abnormal neurological evaluations
• For most AIS, including large curves, posterior pedicle screw instrumentation and fusion alone is as effective as anterior–posterior surgery
• Anterior fusion in conjunction with posterior fusion results in a lower incidence of adding on and curve progression in patients with open triradiate cartilages
• Pulmonary function is adversely affected by an anterior approach, but clinical significance is uncertain
• There is very weak evidence that extending instrumentation and fusion into the lower lumbar spine for scoliosis results in long-term disability compared to fusion into the thoracic or upper lumbar spine
• Patient self-image and satisfaction will likely improve after surgery, but the improvement is multifactorial and cannot be solely attributed to the postoperative magnitude of the curve

• There are no published differences in the rates of pseudoarthrosis for various bone graft materials
• SSEP and MEP neuromonitoring is a sensitive and specific means to detect intraoperative neurological injury. MEPs are more sensitive than SSEPs in detecting injury, but the two modalities should continue to be used together
• Intraoperative neuromonitoring can reduce the rate of neurological injury

Conclusions

High-quality evidence to inform clinical decision making for scoliosis surgery is currently limited, which precludes strong recommendations. The long-term follow-up required to assess patient outcomes and rare complications, and difficulty randomizing patients are methodological challenges in this area of study.

References

1. Huebert HT, MacKinnon WB. Syringomyelia and scoliosis. J Bone Joint Surg Br 1969;51:338–43.
2. Noordeen MH, Taylor BA, Edgar MA. Syringomyelia. A potential risk factor in scoliosis surgery. Spine 1994;19:1406–9.
3. Nordwall A, Wikkelsø C. A late neurologic complication of scoliosis surgery in connection with syringomyelia. Acta Orthop Scand 1979;50:407–10.
4. Davids JR, Chamberlin E, Blackhurst DW. Indications for magnetic resonance imaging in presumed adolescent idiopathic scoliosis. J Bone Joint Surg Am 2004;86:2187–95.
5. Goldberg CJ, Moore DP, Fogarty EE, et al. Left thoracic curve patterns and their association with disease. Spine (Phila Pa 1976) 1999;24:1228–33.
6. Loder RT, Stasikelis P, Farley FA. Sagittal profiles of the spine in scoliosis associated with an Arnold-Chiari malformation with or without syringomyelia. J Pediatr Orthop 2002;22:483–91.
7. Ouellet JA, LaPlaza J, Erickson MA, et al. Sagittal plane deformity in the thoracic spine: a clue to the presence of syringomyelia as a cause of scoliosis. Spine 2003;28:2147–51.
8. Ozturk C, Karadereler S, Ornek I, et al. The role of routine magnetic resonance imaging in the preoperative evaluation of adolescent idiopathic scoliosis. Int Orthop 2009;34:543–6.
9. Do T, Fras C, Burke S, et al. Clinical value of routine preoperative magnetic resonance imaging in adolescent idiopathic scoliosis: a prospective study of three hundred and twenty-seven patients. J Bone Joint Surg Am 2001;83:577–9.
10. Maiocco B, Deeney VF, Coulon R, et al. Adolescent idiopathic scoliosis and the presence of spinal cord abnormalities. Preoperative magnetic resonance imaging analysis. Spine 1997;22:2537–41.
11. Winter RB, Lonstein JE, Heithoff KB, et al. Magnetic resonance imaging evaluation of the adolescent patient with idiopathic scoliosis before spinal instrumentation and fusion. A prospective, double-blinded study of 140 patients. Spine (Phila Pa 1976) 1997;22:855–8.

12. O'Brien MF, Lenke LG, Bridwell KH, et al. Preoperative spinal canal investigation in adolescent idiopathic scoliosis curves > or = 70 degrees. Spine (Phila Pa 1976) 1994;19:1606–10.

13. Dubousset J, Herring JA, Shufflebarger H. The crankshaft phenomenon. J Pediatr Orthop 1989;9:541–50.

14. Sanders JO, Little DG, Richards BS. Prediction of the crankshaft phenomenon by the peak height velocity. Spine 1997;22:1352–7.

15. Sanders JO, Herring JA, Browne RH. Posterior arthrodesis and instrumentation in the immature (Risser-grade-0) spine in idiopathic scoliosis. J Bone Joint Surg Am 1995;77:39–45.

16. Sponseller PD, Betz R, Newton PO, et al. Differences in curve behavior after fusion in adolescent idiopathic scoliosis patients with open triradiate cartilages. Spine (Phila Pa 1976) 2009; 34:827–31.

17. Wang Y, Fei Q, Qiu G, et al. Anterior spinal fusion versus posterior spinal fusion for moderate lumbar/thoracolumbar adolescent idiopathic scoliosis: a prospective study. Spine (Phila Pa 1976) 2008;33:2166–72.

18. Carreon LY, Puno RM, Lenke LG, et al. Non-neurologic complications following surgery for adolescent idiopathic scoliosis. J Bone Joint Surg Am 2007;89:2427–32.

19. Geck MJ, Rinella A, Hawthorne D, et al. Comparison of surgical treatment in Lenke 5C adolescent idiopathic scoliosis: anterior dual rod versus posterior pedicle fixation surgery: a comparison of two practices. Spine (Phila Pa 1976) 2009;34:1942–51.

20. Dobbs MB, Lenke LG, Kim YJ, et al. Anterior/posterior spinal instrumentation versus posterior instrumentation alone for the treatment of adolescent idiopathic scoliotic curves more than 90 degrees. Spine 2006;31:2386–91.

21. Luhmann SJ, Lenke LG, Kim YJ, et al. Thoracic adolescent idiopathic scoliosis curves between 70 degrees and 100 degrees: is anterior release necessary? Spine (Phila Pa 1976) 2005;30: 2061–7.

22. Potter BK, Kuklo TR, Lenke LG. Radiographic outcomes of anterior spinal fusion versus posterior spinal fusion with thoracic pedicle screws for treatment of Lenke Type I adolescent idiopathic scoliosis curves. Spine (Phila Pa 1976) 2005;30:1859–66.

23. Newton PO, Perry A, Bastrom TP, et al. Predictors of change in postoperative pulmonary function in adolescent idiopathic scoliosis: a prospective study of 254 patients. Spine (Phila Pa 1976) 2007;32:1875–82.

24. Kim YJ, Lenke LG, Bridwell KH, et al. Pulmonary function in adolescent idiopathic scoliosis relative to the surgical procedure. J Bone Joint Surg Am 2005;87:1534–41.

25. O'Brien MF Kuklo TR, Blanke KM, Lenke LG, eds. Spinal Deformity Study Group Radiographic Measurement Manual. Medtronic Sofamor Danek, Memphis, 2004.

26. King HA, Moe JH, Bradford DS, et al. The selection of fusion levels in thoracic idiopathic scoliosis. JBone Joint SurgAm 1983;65:1302–13.

27. Richards BS. Lumbar curve response in type II idiopathic scoliosis after posterior instrumentation of the thoracic curve. Spine (Phila Pa 1976) 1992;17:S282–6.

28. Lenke LG, Betz RR, Harms J, et al. Adolescent idiopathic scoliosis: a new classification to determine extent of spinal arthrodesis. J Bone Joint Surg Am 2001;83:1169–81.

29. Burton DC, Asher MA, Lai SM. The selection of fusion levels using torsional correction techniques in the surgical treatment of idiopathic scoliosis. Spine 1999;24:1728–39.

30. Suk SI, Kim WJ, Lee CS, et al. Indications of proximal thoracic curve fusion in thoracic adolescent idiopathic scoliosis: recognition and treatment of double thoracic curve pattern in adolescent idiopathic scoliosis treated with segmental instrumentation. Spine 2000;25:2342–9.

31. Suk SI, Lee SM, Chung ER, et al. Selective thoracic fusion with segmental pedicle screw fixation in the treatment of thoracic idiopathic scoliosis: more than 5-year follow-up. Spine 2005;30: 1602–9.

32. Suk SI, Lee SM, Chung ER, et al. Determination of distal fusion level with segmental pedicle screw fixation in single thoracic idiopathic scoliosis. Spine (Phila Pa 1976) 2003;28:484–91.

33. Puno RM, An KC, Puno RL, et al. Treatment recommendations for idiopathic scoliosis: an assessment of the Lenke classification. Spine (Phila Pa 1976) 2003;28:2102–14; discussion 2114–15.

34. Robitaille M, Aubin CE, Labelle H. Intra and interobserver variability of preoperative planning for surgical instrumentation in adolescent idiopathic scoliosis. Eur Spine J 2007;16:1604–14.

35. Aubin CE, Labelle H, Ciolofan OC. Variability of spinal instrumentation configurations in adolescent idiopathic scoliosis. Eur Spine J 2007;16:57–64.

36. Sanders JO, Haynes R, Lighter D, et al. Variation in care among spinal deformity surgeons: results of a survey of the Shriners hospitals for children. Spine (Phila Pa 1976) 2007;32:1444–9.

37. Lenke LG, Bridwell KH, O'Brien MF, et al. Recognition and treatment of the proximal thoracic curve in adolescent idiopathic scoliosis treated with Cotrel-Dubousset instrumentation. Spine (Phila Pa 1976) 1994;19:1589–97.

38. Wilson PL, Newton PO, Wenger DR, et al. A multicenter study analyzing the relationship of a standardized radiographic scoring system of adolescent idiopathic scoliosis and the Scoliosis Research Society outcomes instrument. Spine (Phila Pa 1976) 2002;27:2036–40.

39. Ilharreborde B, Even J, Lefevre Y, et al. How to determine the upper level of instrumentation in Lenke types 1 and 2 adolescent idiopathic scoliosis: a prospective study of 132 patients. J Pediatr Orthop 2008;28:733–9.

40. Moskowitz A, Moe JH, Winter RB, et al. Long-term follow-up of scoliosis fusion. J Bone Joint Surg Am 1980;62:364–76.

41. Takahashi S, Delecrin J, Passuti N. Changes in the unfused lumbar spine in patients with idiopathic scoliosis. A 5- to 9-year assessment after Cotrel-Dubousset instrumentation. Spine 1997;22:517–23.

42. Gotze C, Liljenqvist UR, Slomka A, et al. Quality of life and back pain: outcome 16.7 years after Harrington instrumentation. Spine (Phila Pa 1976) 2002;27:1456–63; discussion 1463–4.

43. Poitras B, Mayo NE, Goldberg MS, et al. The Ste-Justine Adolescent Idiopathic Scoliosis Cohort Study. Part IV: Surgical correction and back pain. Spine 1994;19:1582–8.

44. Paonessa KJ, Engler GL. Back pain and disability after Harrington rod fusion to the lumbar spine for scoliosis. Spine (Phila Pa 1976) 1992;17:S249–53.

45. Connolly PJ, Von Schroeder HP, Johnson GE, et al. Adolescent idiopathic scoliosis. Long-term effect of instrumentation extending to the lumbar spine. J Bone Joint Surg Am 1995;77: 1210–16.

46. Michel CR, Lalain JJ. Late results of Harrington's operation. Long-term evolution of the lumbar spine below the fused segments. Spine (Phila Pa 1976) 1985;10:414–20.

47. Fabry G, Van Melkebeek J, Bockx E. Back pain after Harrington rod instrumentation for idiopathic scoliosis. Spine (Phila Pa 1976) 1989;14:620–4.

48. Danielsson AJ, Nachemson AL. Back pain and function 22 years after brace treatment for adolescent idiopathic scoliosis: a case-control study-part I. Spine (Phila Pa 1976) 2003;28:2078–85; discussion 2086.

49. Dickson JH, Erwin WD, Rossi D. Harrington instrumentation and arthrodesis for idiopathic scoliosis. A twenty-one-year follow-up. J Bone Joint Surg Am 1990;72:678–83.

50. Hayes MA, Tompkins SF, Herndon WA, et al. Clinical and radiological evaluation of lumbosacral motion below fusion levels in idiopathic scoliosis. Spine (Phila Pa 1976) 1988;13:1161–7.

51. Luk KD, Lee FB, Leong JC, et al. The effect on the lumbosacral spine of long spinal fusion for idiopathic scoliosis. A minimum 10-year follow-up. Spine (Phila Pa 1976) 1987;12:996–1000.

52. Edgar MA, Mehta MH. Long-term follow-up of fused and unfused idiopathic scoliosis. J Bone Joint Surg Br 1988;70:712–716.

53. Grouw AV, Nadel CI, Weierman RJ, et al. Long term follow-up of patients with idiopathic scoliosis treated surgically: a preliminary subjective study. Clin Orthop Relat Res 1976;117:197–201.

54. Bartie BJ, Lonstein JE, Winter RB. Long-term follow-up of adolescent idiopathic scoliosis patients who had Harrington instrumentation and fusion to the lower lumbar vertebrae: is low back pain a problem? Spine (Phila Pa 1976) 2009;34:E873–8.

55. Perez-Grueso FS, Fernandez-Baillo N, Arauz de Robles S, et al. The low lumbar spine below Cotrel-Dubousset instrumentation: long-term findings. Spine (Phila Pa 1976) 2000;25:2333–41.

56. Padua R, Padua S, Aulisa L, et al. Patient outcomes after Harrington instrumentation for idiopathic scoliosis: a 15- to 28-year evaluation. Spine (Phila Pa 1976) 2001;26:1268–73.

57. Helenius I, Lamberg T, Osterman K, et al. Scoliosis research society outcome instrument in evaluation of long-term surgical results in spondylolysis and low-grade isthmic spondylolisthesis in young patients. Spine 2005;30:336–41.

58. Helenius I, Remes V, Lamberg T, et al. Long-term health-related quality of life after surgery for adolescent idiopathic scoliosis and spondylolisthesis. J Bone Joint Surg Am 2008;90:1231–9.

59. Helenius I, Remes V, Yrjonen T, et al. Comparison of long-term functional and radiologic outcomes after Harrington instrumentation and spondylodesis in adolescent idiopathic scoliosis: a review of 78 patients. Spine 2002;27:176–80.

60. Remes V, Helenius I, Schlenzka D, et al. Cotrel-Dubousset (CD) or Universal Spine System (USS) instrumentation in adolescent idiopathic scoliosis (AIS): comparison of midterm clinical, functional, and radiologic outcomes. Spine 2004;29:2024–30.

61. Danielsson AJ, Cederlund CG, Ekholm S, et al. The prevalence of disc aging and back pain after fusion extending into the lower lumbar spine. A matched MR study twenty-five years after surgery for adolescent idiopathic scoliosis. Acta Radiol 2001;42:187–97.

62. Asher M, Lai SM, Burton D, et al. The influence of spine and trunk deformity on preoperative idiopathic scoliosis patients' health-related quality of life questionnaire responses. Spine 2004;29:861–8.

63. Parent EC, Hill D, Mahood J, et al. Discriminative and predictive validity of the scoliosis research society-22 questionnaire in management and curve-severity subgroups of adolescents with idiopathic scoliosis. Spine 2009;34:2450–7.

64. Tsutsui S, Pawelek J, Bastrom T, et al. Dissecting the effects of spinal fusion and deformity magnitude on quality of life in patients with adolescent idiopathic scoliosis. Spine 2009;34:E653–8.

65. Watanabe K, Hasegawa K, Hirano T, et al. Use of the scoliosis research society outcomes instrument to evaluate patient outcome in untreated idiopathic scoliosis patients in Japan: part I: comparison with nonscoliosis group: preliminary/limited review in a Japanese population. Spine 2005;30:1197–201.

66. Bunge EM, Juttmann RE, de KM, et al. Health-related quality of life in patients with adolescent idiopathic scoliosis after treatment: short-term effects after brace or surgical treatment. Eur Spine J 2007;16:83–9.

67. Helenius I, Remes V, Yrjonen T, et al. Harrington and Cotrel-Dubousset instrumentation in adolescent idiopathic scoliosis. Long-term functional and radiographic outcomes. J Bone Joint Surg Am 2003;85:2303–9.

68. Merola AA, Haher TR, Brkaric M, et al. A multicenter study of the outcomes of the surgical treatment of adolescent idiopathic scoliosis using the Scoliosis Research Society (SRS) outcome instrument. Spine 2002;27:2046–51.

69. Koch KD, Buchanan R, Birch JG, et al. Adolescents undergoing surgery for idiopathic scoliosis: how physical and psychological characteristics relate to patient satisfaction with the cosmetic result. Spine 2001;26:2119–24.

70. Sanders JO, Harrast JJ, Kuklo TR, et al. The Spinal Appearance Questionnaire: results of reliability, validity, and responsiveness testing in patients with idiopathic scoliosis. Spine (Phila Pa 1976) 2007;32:2719–22.

71. Sanders JO, Carreon LY, Sucato DJ, et al. Preoperative and perioperative factors effect on adolescent idiopathic scoliosis surgical outcomes. Spine (Phila Pa 1976) 2010;35:1867–71.

72. Lonner BS, Kondrachov D, Siddiqi F, et al. Thoracoscopic spinal fusion compared with posterior spinal fusion for the treatment of thoracic adolescent idiopathic scoliosis. J Bone Joint Surg Am 2006;88:1022–34.

73. Kim YJ, Lenke LG, Kim J, et al. Comparative analysis of pedicle screw versus hybrid instrumentation in posterior spinal fusion of adolescent idiopathic scoliosis. Spine 2006;31:291–8.

74. Hicks JM, Singla A, Shen FH, et al. Complications of pedicle screw fixation in scoliosis surgery: a systematic review. Spine 2010;35:E465–470.

75. Price CT, Connolly JF, Carantzas AC, et al. Comparison of bone grafts for posterior spinal fusion in adolescent idiopathic scoliosis. Spine 2003;28:793–798.

76. Recht J, Bayard F, Delloye C, et al. Freeze-dried allograft versus autograft bone in scoliosis surgery. A retrospective comparative study. Eur Spine J 1993;2:235–8.

77. Fabry G. Allograft versus autograft bone in idiopathic scoliosis surgery: a multivariate statistical analysis. J Pediatr Orthop 1991;11:465–8.

78. Dodd CA, Fergusson CM, Freedman L, et al. Allograft versus autograft bone in scoliosis surgery. J Bone Joint Surg Br 1988;70:431–4.

79. Aurori BF, Weierman RJ, Lowell HA, et al. Pseudarthrosis after spinal fusion for scoliosis. A comparison of autogeneic and allogeneic bone grafts. Clin Orthop Relat Res 1985;199:153–8.

80. Betz RR, Petrizzo AM, Kerner PJ, et al. Allograft versus no graft with a posterior multisegmented hook system for the treatment of idiopathic scoliosis. Spine 2006;31:121–7.

81. Lerner T, Bullmann V, Schulte TL, et al. A level-1 pilot study to evaluate of ultraporous beta-tricalcium phosphate as a graft extender in the posterior correction of adolescent idiopathic scoliosis. Eur Spine J 2009;18:170–9.

82. Ransford AO, Morley T, Edgar MA, et al. Synthetic porous ceramic compared with autograft in scoliosis surgery. A prospective, randomized study of 341 patients. J Bone Joint Surg Br 1998;80:13–18.

83. Muschik M, Ludwig R, Halbhübner S, et al. Beta-tricalcium phosphate as a bone substitute for dorsal spinal fusion in adolescent idiopathic scoliosis: preliminary results of a prospective clinical study. Eur Spine J 2001;10(Suppl 2):S178–84.

84. Le Huec JC, Lesprit E, Delavigne C, et al. Tri-calcium phosphate ceramics and allografts as bone substitutes for spinal fusion in idiopathic scoliosis as bone substitutes for spinal fusion in idiopathic scoliosis: comparative clinical results at four years. Acta Orthop Belg 1997;63:202–11.

85. Ilharreborde B, Morel E, Fitoussi F, et al. Bioactive glass as a bone substitute for spinal fusion in adolescent idiopathic scoliosis: a comparative study with iliac crest autograft. J Pediatr Orthop 2008;28:347–51.

86. Fehlings MG, Brodke DS, Norvell DC, et al. The evidence for intraoperative neurophysiological monitoring in spine surgery: does it make a difference? Spine (Phila Pa 1976) 2010;35:S37–46.

87. Schwartz DM, Auerbach JD, Dormans JP, et al. Neurophysiological detection of impending spinal cord injury during scoliosis surgery. J Bone Joint Surg Am 2007;89:2440–9.

84 Metastatic/Myeloma Disease— Operative Management

Harsha Malempati[1], Erion Qamirani[1], and Albert J.M. Yee[2]
[1]University of Toronto, Toronto, ON, Canada
[2]Sunnybrook Health Sciences Centre, Toronto, ON, Canada

Case scenario

A 65 year old man presents to the Emergency Department with significant back pain that has been progressively worsening over the past 3 months. He has a history of prostate cancer. An MRI reveals multiple spinal lesions.

Relevant anatomy

General indications for surgical management of spinal metastases include: (1) establishing a tissue diagnosis, (2) failure of radiation therapy, (3) spinal instability, and (4) neurological deficits. One proposed scoring system was developed by Tokuhashi et al.,[1] whereby six different parameters are scored from 0 to 2 points with a maximum of 12. Aggressive surgery is recommended for patients having a score of greater than 9 and palliative surgery is reserved for those with scores less than 5. The six parameters are: (1) general condition of the patient, (2) number of extraspinal metastases, (3) number of vertebral metastases, (4) metastases to internal organs, (5) the primary tumor site, and (6) severity of neurological deficits.

Some authors have attempted to use the three-column model originally proposed by Denis[2] for thoracolumbar trauma to assess stability in the setting of spinal metastases.[3] For spine metastasis, each of the three columns of the spine (anterior, middle, and posterior) is divided into two halves, creating a total of six zones. Instability is then defined as destruction of three or more zones by the tumor. Other authors have proposed a number of criteria that contribute to spinal instability in the setting of spinal metastases: (1) anterior and middle-column involvement or more than 50% loss of vertebral height, (2) middle and posterior-column or shearing deformity, (3) three-column involvement, (4) involvement of the same column in two or more adjacent vertebrae, and (5) iatrogenic, defined as laminectomy in the setting of anterior and/or middle-column disease or resection of more than 50% of the vertebral body.[4]

Importance of the problem

Metastatic tumors are the most common spinal tumors. The most common sites of origin for spinal metastases are breast, lung, prostate, and the hematopoietic system. In most clinical series, these primary sites alone account for 50–66% of all metastases to the spine.[5] Although most patients with spinal metastases present with pain as their chief complaint, the natural history of untreated spinal metastasis in generally one of relentless progression towards paralysis and loss of bowel and bladder function.[6] Therefore, early diagnosis and appropriate treatment are necessary. The surgical management of spinal metastasis has gone through an extensive evolution over the past few decades.

Top five questions

1. What is the role of corticosteroids in the initial management of spinal metastases causing cord compression?
2. What is the efficacy of kyphoplasty in the management of spinal metastases?
3. What is the role of vertebroplasty in the management of spinal metastases? Is it more efficacious than kyphoplasty?
4. Does surgical decompression followed by radiotherapy have better outcomes than radiotherapy alone for the management of spinal metastases causing cord compression?
5. Is there a role for en-bloc tumor resection for spinal metastases?

Evidence-Based Orthopedics, First Edition. Edited by Mohit Bhandari.
© 2012 Blackwell Publishing Ltd. Published 2012 by Blackwell Publishing Ltd.

Systematic reviews and meta-analyses that were relevant to the topic in question were referenced in isolation for the purpose of this review. Randomized controlled trials (RCTs) and other important studies pertinent to the topic that were published after (or not included in) systematic reviews were evaluated and discussed separately.

Question 1: What is the role of corticosteroids in the initial management of spinal metastases causing cord compression?

Case clarification

The patient complains of progressive muscle weakness and decreased sensation of the lower extremities. MRI confirms metastatic spinal cord compression.

Relevance

Although this chapter is devoted to the operative management of spinal cord metastases, a discussion of the use of corticosteroids is warranted because they have been shown to improve outcomes when administered before surgery in other cases involving spinal cord compression.

Finding the evidence

• Cochrane Database, search term: "corticosteroids AND spine"
• PubMed (www.ncbi.nlm.nih.gov/pubmed/) clinical queries search/systematic reviews: "spinal metastasis AND steroids"
• PubMed (www.ncbi.nlm.nih.gov/pubmed/): sensitivity search using keywords "spinal metastasis AND steroids"

Quality of the evidence

Level I
• 2 systematic reviews of RCTs

Findings

A systematic review found that although corticosteroids have been used for the treatment of metastatic epidural spinal cord compression (MESCC) for many years, there were only three inadequately powered RCTs designed to determine clinical benefit and optimal dosage.[6] The review of these three RCTs did not show significant benefit for high-dose corticosteroids in improving patient ambulation (total patients 105, RR 0.91, 95% CI 0.68–1.23). The trials also showed no difference between high-dose vs. moderate or no corticosteroids for 2 year survival, pain relief, or urinary incontinence.[6] Furthermore, there was a significant increase in the incidence of serious drug-related adverse events such as perforated gastric ulcers, psychoses, and deaths due to infection in patients who received high-dose corticosteroids.[6] The results are summarized in Table 84.1. The authors concluded that the extent of benefit from corticosteroids, and the optimal dosage, is unclear. The three RCTs evaluated in this systematic review were underpowered given their low number of enrolled patients; therefore the grade of recommendation is moderate.

Another systematic review included two RCTs, one phase II study, and an observational study.[7] One of the randomized trials included 57 patients with MESCC and found that 81% of the patients were ambulatory 3 months after receiving radiation and high-dose dexamethasone, while only 63% of the patients treated with radiation alone

Table 84.1 High-dose corticosteroids vs. no or moderate-dose corticosteroids

Parameters	Results
Overall ambulatory rates (short term)	RR 0.91; 95% CI 0.68–1.23 (n = 105, three trials)
Proportion of pretreatment ambulant participants maintaining ambulation (short term)	17/17 (100%) vs. 17/19 (90%) RR 0.90; 95% CI 0.75–1.08 (n = 36, one trial)
Proportion of pretreatment nonambulant participants regaining ambulation (short term)	5/10 (50%) vs. 2/11 (18%) RR 0.36; 95% CI 0.09–1.47 (n = 21, one trial)
Survival (long term)	5/10 (50%) vs. 2/11 (18%) RR 0.36; 95% CI 0.09–1.47 (n = 21, one trial)
Pain relief	11/14 (79%) vs. 10/11 (91%) RR 1.16; 95% CI 0.83–1.61 (n = 25, one trial)
Urinary continence	12/19 (63%) vs. 8/15 (53%) RR 0.84; 95% CI 0.47–1.52 (n = 34, one trial)
Adverse effects	High-dose corticosteroids vs. no or moderate-dose corticosteroids RR 0.12; 95% CI 0.02–0.97 (n = 77, two trials)
	High-dose vs. no corticosteroids RR 0.10; 95% CI 0.01–1.78) (n = 57, one trial)
	High-dose vs. moderate-dose corticosteroids RR 0.17; 95% CI 0.01–3.08 (n = 20, one trial)
Outcomes not reported	Quality of life, participant rated and caregiver satisfaction

Adapted from George R, Jeba J, Ramkumar G, et al. Interventions for the treatment of metastatic extradural spinal cord compression in adults. Cochrane Database Syst Rev 2010;1.

were ambulatory (p = 0.046). However, 11% of patients treated with dexamethasone had significant adverse events including psychoses and gastric ulcers requiring surgery.[7] The other RCT in this systematic review included 37 patients and found no difference in improvement of neurological status in patients with MESCC receiving high vs. moderate corticosteroids (25% vs. 8% respectively, p = 0.22). Although these RCTs had good randomization and follow-up, the low number of patients makes the grade of recommendation moderate at best.

Recommendations

• There is no significant benefits of using corticosteroids for improving patient ambulation in patients with MESCC [overall quality: moderate]
• Treatment with corticosteroids for MESCC can result in severe adverse effects [overall quality: moderate]
• When combined with radiation treatment, corticosteroid therapy can result in modest improvement in patient ambulatory rates [overall quality: moderate]
• High-dose corticosteroids do not improve patient outcomes compared to moderate-dose corticosteroids in the setting of MESCC [overall quality: moderate]

Question 2: What is the efficacy of kyphoplasty in the management of spinal metastases?

Case clarification

The patient does not have any neurological deficits but MRI confirms a pathologic fracture. He asks if there are any surgical options for his condition.

Relevance

Kyphoplasty is a percutaneous cement augmentation technique that involves inflation of a balloon within the vertebral body to create a cavitary space and potentially reduce the fracture deformity before injection of polymethylmethacrylate cement under fluoroscopy. The cement reinforces and stabilizes the fracture. This percutaneous procedure has been used to treat hemangiomas, osteoporotic fractures, and lytic spinal tumors including multiple myeloma and lytic spinal metastases.

Finding the evidence

• Cochrane Database, search term "kyphoplasty"
• PubMed (www.ncbi.nlm.nih.gov/pubmed/) clinical queries search/systematic reviews: "spinal metastasis AND kyphoplasty"

Quality of the evidence

Level II
• 1 systematic review of prospective observational studies

Level III
• 1 systematic review of retrospective observational studies, 1 retrospective study

Findings

A systematic review of 26 studies (including both controlled prospective and observational studies) that evaluated kyphoplasty for treatment of vertebral compression fractures found that there was a significant reduction in pain measured on a visual analog scale (VAS) postoperatively (weighted mean difference (WMD) −5.11, 95% CI −5.72 to −4.49, p = 0.000; based on 0–10 VAS scores from 11 studies), at 1 year (WMD −6.10, 95% CI −7.47 to −4.48, p = 0.000; based on 0–10 VAS scores from 5 studies), and 2 years (WMD −9.3, 95% CI −10.65 to −7.94, p = 0.000; based on 0–20 VAS scores from 1 study) as compared with baseline.[8] There was also a significant percentage increase in vertebral height compared to baseline in all three regions (anterior, middle, and posterior) of the spine. Compared to baseline, there was a significant percentage reduction in Cobb's angle after balloon kyphoplasty (WMD −7.68, 95% CI −9.34 to −6.03, p = 0.00; based on 7 studies). Finally, there was a significant improvement in quality of life and functional capacity, measured by the Oswestry Disability Index as compared to baseline after balloon kyphoplasty (WMD −23.8, 95% CI −34.0 to −13.55, p = 0.00; based on 4 studies). The majority of patients in the included studies were women over 65 years with painful vertebral compression fracture secondary to osteoporosis, metastases, or multiple myeloma between levels T4 and L5. Although these results suggest that kyphoplasty improves pain associated with metastatic spine fractures, the grade of recommendation is low because of the nonrandomized nature of the studies reviewed and the fact that pathologies other than metastatic disease were also included in the analysis.

Another systematic review of kyphoplasty for the treatment of pathologic fractures in patients with spinal tumors included 12 prospective and retrospective observational studies with a total of 333 patients and 481 treated levels.[9] The review found statistically significant success rates in terms of pain relief and functional outcome for kyphoplasty. However, since other pathologies (multiple myeloma, hemangioma) were also included in the final analysis for 9 of the 12 studies, these findings are indirect. Therefore the grade of recommendation from this systematic review is low given the indirect findings and observational nature of the studies reviewed.

Recommendation

• Balloon kyphoplasty is effective in providing pain relief and improving functional outcome in patients with vertebral compression fractures due to spinal metastases [overall quality: low]

Question 3: What is the role of vertebroplasty in the management of spinal metastases? Is it more efficacious than kyphoplasty?

Case clarification

You explain to the patient that one of the treatment options available includes a minimally invasive procedure called kyphoplasty/vertebroplasty. He then asks if one is better than the other.

Relevance

Vertebroplasty is a percutaneous technique where radiopaque polymethylmethacrylate cement is injected under fluoroscopy. It is commonly employed in treating osteoporotic fractures and is now increasingly used for pain management in patients with lytic spine tumors.

Finding the evidence

- Cochrane Database, search term: "vertebroplasty"
- PubMed (www.ncbi.nlm.nih.gov/pubmed/) clinical queries search/systematic reviews: "spinal metastasis AND vertebroplasty"
- PubMed (www.ncbi.nlm.nih.gov/pubmed/): sensitivity search using keywords "spinal metastasis AND vertebroplasty AND kyphoplasty"

Quality of the evidence

Level II
- 1 systematic review of prospective observational studies

Level III
- 1 systematic review of retrospective observational studies, 1 observational retrospective study

Level IV
- 1 systematic review of case series studies

Findings

No studies that prospectively compared kyphoplasty to vertebroplasty for the treatment of spinal metastase resulting in pathologic fractures were found. A retrospective review of 56 patients with painful pathologic vertebral fractures that compared balloon kyphoplasty and vertebroplasty demonstrated no significant difference between these two treatments in terms of pain (OR 0.89, 95% CI 0.29–2.67) or functional improvement.[10] Balloon kyphoplasty resulted in a significant increase in vertebral height (4.5 mm) and significant improvement in local kyphosis (WMD –5.2, 95% CI –9.71, –0.89, $p = 0.02$) from baseline; however this change was not compared to vertebroplasty.[10] The spine tumors evaluated in this retrospective study included both multiple myeloma and other metastatic spine tumors, thus making the findings indirect in regards

to the topic of this question. Therefore the grade of recommendation is low.

A systematic review of 18 case series studies for tumor vertebral compression fractures found that vertebroplasty and kyphoplasty results in less pain, less disability, and greater improvement in general health compared with optimal medical management within the first 3 months after the procedure; however, no significant differences were found by 2 years after the intervention.[11] The grade of recommendation from this review is very low, based on the low level of the studies.

Another systematic review that performed an indirect comparison of vertebroplasty and kyphoplasty for the treatment of all vertebral compression fractures (osteoporotic and pathologic) from four observational comparative studies found that both balloon kyphoplasty and vertebroplasty provided similar levels of pain relief after surgery.[12] In 70 noncomparative case series studies, the same systematic review found a significant reduction in the pooled level of pain ($p < 0.0001$) following both balloon kyphoplasty and vertebroplasty. Lastly, they reported a significantly higher rate of cement leakages for vertebroplasty compared to balloon kyphoplasty ($p < 0.0001$). No leaks were reported to be symptomatic with balloon kyphoplasty, while some 3% of leaks with vertebroplasty were reported to be symptomatic. The grade of recommendation from this systematic review is very low given the indirect findings in relation to spine metastases combined with the observational nature of the studies reviewed.

Finally, a systematic review of 11 prospective observational studies that evaluated percutaneous techniques in the treatment of spine tumors found that both vertebroplasty and balloon kyphoplasty were successful at providing pain relief.[9] For vertebroplasty, the rate of radiologic extravasation was 9.2–139% (multiple areas of extravasations occurred per level), whereas the range was 0–26.3% in kyphoplasty. The reported range of symptomatic extravasation in vertebroplasty was 0–13.5%, while there was none in kyphoplasty. Complications for vertebroplasty and kyphoplasty are summarized in Table 84.2. The grade of recommendation from this systematic review is low since the nonrandomized studies reviewed here also included non-metastatic spine tumors in their evaluation.

Recommendations

- Vertebroplasty is as effective as balloon kyphoplasty in providing pain relief and improved functional outcome for patients with metastatic spine disease [overall quality: low]
- Vertebroplasty has a higher rate of surgical complications (such as symptomatic cement extravasation) as compared to kyphoplasty [overall quality: low]

Table 84.2 Summary of prospective studies using vertebroplasty and kyphoplasty for symptomatic spine tumors

Prospective studies	Vertebroplasty	Kyphoplasty
No. of studies	5	6
No. of tumor patients	98	204
No. of tumor levels	152	330
Tumor types per patient		
Metastases	73 (74.5%)	91 (44.6%)
Multiple myeloma	23 (23.5%)	113 (55.4%)
Hemangioma	2 (2.0%)	0
Complications		
Medical	0	1/204 (0.5%)
Neurological	4 (4.1%)	0
Corrective surgery	3 (3.1%)	0
Extravasation		
Total per level	59/101 (58.4%)	12/239 (12.1%)
Symptomatic patients	3/98 (3.1%)	0
Adjacent vertebral fracture	0	6/204 (2.9%)
Corrective surgery	0	3/204 (1.5%)

Adapted with permission from Mendel E, Bourekas E, Gerszten P, et al. (2009) Percutaneous techniques in the treatment of spine tumors. Spine 34, S93–100.

Question 4: Does surgical decompression followed by radiotherapy have better outcomes than radiotherapy alone for the management of spinal metastases causing cord compression?

Case clarification

The patient does have neurological compromise on presentation to the Emergency Department. He states that he has noticed a rapid progression in the loss of strength to his legs and decreased sensation in the lower extremities. After initiating corticosteroids, a decision has to be made whether the patient should be given radiation or have surgical decompression.

Relevance

MESCC can lead to pain, progressive motor and sensory loss, incontinence, and disability (including paraplegia). Corticosteroids, radiotherapy, and surgical options have all been used to treat this problem.

Finding the evidence

- Cochrane Database, search term: "spinal cord compression"
- PubMed (www.ncbi.nlm.nih.gov/pubmed/) clinical queries search/systematic reviews: "metastatic epidural spinal cord compression"
- PubMed (www.ncbi.nlm.nih.gov/pubmed/): sensitivity search using keywords "metastatic epidural spinal cord compression"

Quality of the evidence

Level I
- 1 RCT

Level II
- 3 systematic reviews of prospective observational studies

Level III
- 1 meta-analysis of prospective and retrospective observational studies

Findings

A randomized, multi-institutional, nonblinded trial of patients with spinal metastases causing spinal cord compression assigned patients to either decompressive surgery followed by radiotherapy (n = 50) or radiotherapy alone (n = 51).[13] The study found that significantly more patients were able to ambulate after surgery compared to radiotherapy alone (84% vs. 57% respectively, OR 6.2, 95% CI 2.0–19.8, p = 0.001). Also, those patients treated with surgery retained the ability to walk significantly longer than those with radiotherapy alone (median 122 days vs. 13 days, p = 0.003). For those patients who were unable to walk initially, significantly more patients who received surgery regained the ability to walk than those who received radiotherapy alone (62% vs. 19%, p = 0.01). In the patients who could walk initially, 94% in the surgery group continued to walk compared to 74% in the radiation-alone group (p = 0.024). The grade of recommendation based on this well-conducted RCT is high.

A meta-analysis of 28 observational (both prospective and retrospective in nature) studies that evaluated surgical decompression (24 studies) vs. conventional radiotherapy (4 studies) for the treatment of metastatic epidural spinal cord compression found that surgical patients were 1.3 times more likely to be ambulatory after treatment and twice as likely to regain ambulatory function (RR 1.28, 95% CI 1.20–1.37).[14] Overall the ambulatory success rates for surgery and radiation were 85% and 64% respectively. The study therefore concludes that surgery should usually be the primary treatment, with radiation given as adjuvant therapy for metastatic disease causing spinal cord compression. However, since all studies evaluated in this meta-analysis were observational, the grade of recommendation is moderate.

Lastly, systematic reviews of other prospective observational studies have also found that, with respect to ambulation and preservation of neurological function, operative decompression followed by adjuvant radiation is superior to radiotherapy alone.[15,16]

Recommendation

- In patients with symptomatic spinal cord compression from metastatic disease, surgical decompression should be performed, followed by adjuvant radiotherapy [overall quality: high]

Question 5: Is there a role for en-bloc tumor resection for spinal metastases?

Case clarification
The patient's MRI shows only a single metastasis to the spine. He asks if you can remove the metastasis surgically.

Relevance
In some situations, particularly in the case of a solitary spine metastasis from certain primary tumors, en-bloc tumor evacuation has been advocated.

Finding the evidence
- Cochrane Database, search term: "spine metastasis"
- PubMed (www.ncbi.nlm.nih.gov/pubmed/) clinical queries search/systematic reviews: "spinal metastasis AND surgery"
- PubMed (www.ncbi.nlm.nih.gov/pubmed/): sensitivity search using keywords "spinal metastasis AND surgery"

Quality of the evidence
Level IV
- 1 systematic review of retrospective/case-control observational studies

Findings
A systematic review of solitary spine metastatic renal cell carcinoma revealed 15 patients among 6 retrospective observational studies.[15] Local recurrence was observed in 2 patients (13%) at 9 and 24 months after en-bloc resection. The remaining 13 patients had no local recurrence of disease with follow-up ranging from 2 to 84 months. The review also cites unpublished data in 25 patients undergoing en-bloc resection with a 4% recurrence at a median follow-up of 30 months. Given the retrospective nature of these studies and the low number of patients, the grade of recommendation is very low.

Recommendation
- There is insufficient evidence to recommend en-bloc tumor resection as a surgical option to prevent disease progression of solitary spine metastasis [overall quality: very low]

Summary of recommendations

- There is no significant benefits of using corticosteroids for improving patient ambulation in patients with MESCC
- Treatment with corticosteroids for MESCC can result in severe adverse effects

- When combined with radiation treatment, corticosteroid therapy can result in modest improvement in patient ambulatory rates
- High-dose corticosteroids do not improve patient outcomes compared to moderate-dose corticosteroids in the setting of MESCC
- Balloon kyphoplasty is effective in providing pain relief and improving functional outcome in patients with vertebral compression fractures due to spinal metastases
- Vertebroplasty is as effective as balloon kyphoplasty in providing pain relief and improved functional outcome for patients with metastatic spine disease
- Vertebroplasty has a higher rate of surgical complications (such as symptomatic cement extravasation) as compared to kyphoplasty
- In patients with symptomatic spinal cord compression from metastatic disease, surgical decompression should be performed, followed by adjuvant radiotherapy
- There is insufficient evidence to recommend en-bloc tumor resection as a surgical option to prevent disease progression of solitary spine metastasis

Conclusions

Balloon kyphoplasty and vertebroplasty are effective therapeutic options in patients with pathological fractures and painful spinal metastases. Corticosteroids have a limited role in the treatment of patients with neurological compromise from spinal metastases. In patients with significant neurological deficits, surgical decompression should be performed before radiotherapy.

References

1. Tokuhashi Y, Matsuzaki H, Toriyama S, et al. Scoring system for the preoperative evaluation of metastatic spine tumor prognosis. Spine 1990;15:1110–13.
2. Denis F. Spinal instability as defined by the three-column spine concept in acute spinal trauma. Clin Orthop 1984;189:65–76.
3. Kostuik JP, Weinstein JN. Differential diagnosis and surgical treatment of metastatic spine tumors. In: Frymoyer JW. The Adult Spine Principles and Practice, pp.861–888. Raven Press, New York, 1991.
4. Siegal T, Siegal T. Current consideration in the management of neoplastic spinal cord compression. Spine 1989;14:223–8.
5. Marazano E, Latini P, Checcaglini F, et al. Radiation therapy in metastatic spinal cord compression: A prospective analysis of 105 consecutive patients. Cancer 1991;67:1311–17.
6. George R, Jeba J, Ramkumar G, et al. Interventions for the treatment of metastatic extradural spinal cord compression in adults. Cochrane Database Syst Rev 2010;1.
7. Loblaw DA, Perry J, Chambers A, et al. Systematic review of the diagnosis and management of malignant extradural spinal cord compression: the Cancer Care Ontario Practice Guidelines

Initiative's Neuro-Oncology Disease Site Group. J Clin Oncol 2005;23:2028–37.

8. Bouza C, Lopez T, Magro A, et al. Efficacy and safety of balloon kyphoplasty in the treatment of vertebral compression fractures: a systematic review. Eur Spine J 2006;15:1050–67.

9. Mendel E, Bourekas E, Gerszten P, et al. Percutaneous techniques in the treatment of spine tumors. Spine 2009;34:S93–100.

10. Fourney DR, Schomer DF, Nader R, et al. Percutaneous vertebroplasty and kyphoplasty for painful vertebral body fractures in cancer patients. J Neurosurg 2003;98:21–30.

11. McGirt MJ, Parker SL, Wolinsky JP, et al. Vertebroplasty and kyphoplasty for the treatment of vertebral compression fractures: an evidene-based review of the literature. Spine 2009;9:501–8.

12. Taylor RS, Taylor RJ, Fritzell P. Balloon kyphoplasty and vertebroplasty for vertebral compression fractures: a comparative systematic review of efficacy and safety. Spine 2006;31:2747–55.

13. Patchell RA, Tibbs PA, Regine WF, et al. Direct decompressive surgical resection in the treatment of spinal cord compression caused by metastatic cancer: a randomized trial. Lancet 2005;366:643–8.

14. Klimo P, Thompson CJ, Kestle J, et al. A meta-analysis of surgery versus conventional radiotherapy for the treatment of metastatic spinal epidural disease. Neuro Oncol 2005;7:64–76.

15. Bilsky MH, Laufer I, Burch S. Shifting paradigms in the treatment of metastatic spine disease. Spine 2009;34:S101–7.

16. Jeba GR, Ramkumar G, Chacko AG et al. Interventions for the treatment of metastatic extradural spinal cord compression in adults. Cochrane Database Syst Rev 2010;1.

85 Metastatic/Myeloma Disease—Nonoperative Management

Harsha Malempati[1], Erion Qamirani[1], and Albert J.M. Yee[2]

[1]University of Toronto, Toronto, ON, Canada
[2]Sunnybrook Health Sciences Centre, Toronto, ON, Canada

Case scenario

A 50-year-old woman with a history of metastatic breast cancer is referred to the office. She presents with a recent MRI that shows multiple lytic lesions in the vertebral bodies of the thoracic and lumbar spine.

Relevant anatomy

There are four potential pathways for bone metastases: venous, arterial, direct extension, and lymphatic. The venous system is the most common pathway for spinal metastases via Batson's plexus, a network of veins located in the epidural space, situated between the bony spinal column and the dura mater covering the spinal cord. This plexus is connected to the major veins that return blood to the heart via the inferior and superior vena cavae. This plexus has no blood flow control valves, and any increased pressure in the vena cavae system results in increased flow backwards into Batson's plexus, leading to spread of metastases along the axial skeleton.

Importance of the problem

Over the past decade approximately 1 million people per year were diagnosed with cancer in the United States alone,[1] with metastases developing in approximately two-thirds of patients.[2] The skeletal system is the third most common site of cancer metastases, after the lung and liver, and metastatic lesions of the spine represent the most common site of skeletal involvement.[3–5]

Top five questions

1. What is the efficacy of bisphosphonates in the treatment of spinal metastases?
2. Do radiopharmaceuticals play a role in the treatment of metastatic spine disease?
3. Can radiation alone play a role in the palliative management of myeloma/metastatic disease of the spine?
4. Do different radiation schedules affect outcomes in the treatment of myeloma/metastatic disease of the spine?
5. What is the efficacy of stereotactic radiosurgery in treating symptomatic spinal metastases?

Systematic reviews and metanalyses that were relevant to the topic in question were referenced in isolation for the purpose of this review. Randomized controlled trials (RCTs) and other important studies pertinent to the topic that were published after (or not included in) systematic reviews were evaluated and discussed separately.

Question 1: What is the efficacy of bisphosphonates in the treatment of spinal metastases?

Case clarification

The patient complains of pain in her back but is otherwise asymptomatic. She asks if there are any "anticancer" medications that would help her spine.

Relevance

Axial pain is a common clinical presentation of spinal metastases. It is often progressive and can occur both at rest and with weightbearing, and may be related to pathologic fractures caused by loss of the structural integrity of the vertebrae due to a lytic lesion.

Evidence-Based Orthopedics, First Edition. Edited by Mohit Bhandari.
© 2012 Blackwell Publishing Ltd. Published 2012 by Blackwell Publishing Ltd.

Finding the evidence

- Cochrane Database, search term: "spinal metastasis AND bisphosphonates"
- PubMed (www.ncbi.nlm.nih.gov/pubmed/) clinical queries search/systematic reviews: "spinal metastasis AND bisphosphonates"
- PubMed (www.ncbi.nlm.nih.gov/pubmed/): sensitivity search using keywords "bisphosphonates AND spinal metastasis"

Quality of the evidence

Level I
- 1 meta-analysis of RCTs, 3 RCTs

Level II
- 1 meta-analysis of observational studies, 2 observational studies

Findings

Several studies have examined the use of bisphosphonates in the treatment of metastatic disease.[6–10] Pavlakis et al.[6] conducted a meta-analysis of randomized studies comparing bisphosphonates and placebo, or different bisphosphonates, in women with metastatic breast cancer. In nine studies of women with advanced metastatic breast cancer and existing bone metastases, bisphosphonates reduced risk of skeletal events such as pathologic fracture by 17% (RR 0.83; 95% CI 0.78–0.89; p < 0.00001).[6] Furthermore, women with advanced breast cancer and clinically evident bone metastases had improved bone pain and significant delays in median time to pathologic fractures. Overall strength of evidence from this study is high. Another meta-analysis of randomized trials comparing the effectiveness of bisphosphonates to placebo in metastatic prostate cancer found that bisphosphonates decreased the risk of skeletal events (OR 0.79; 95% CI 0.62–1.00; p = 0.05); however, the associated measure of precision includes no effect.[7] There was also a trend towards improved pain relief, but this was not statistically significant. Overall strength of evidence from this study is moderate.

A guideline by the American Society of Clinical Oncology on the role of bisphosphonates in controlling pain resulting from breast cancer bony metastases recommends that there is insufficient evidence to support the use of intravenous bisphosphonates alone for pain control.[8] Although multiple trials of bisphosphonates compared to placebo have shown modest pain control benefit with bisphosphonates, many of these results were not statistically significant.[9–11] For example, one randomized study of intravenous clondronate vs. placebo found a mean difference in pain score of 0.89 (95% CI 1.43 to −0.35) in favor of clondronate.[9] These are well-conducted studies, therefore the grade of recommendation is high.

Lastly, bisphosphonate therapy does increase bone mineral density (BMD) in the spine. One study of oral clondronate on BMD of the lumbar spine showed statistically significant increases in the clondronate-treated group compared to placebo at multiple intervals after initiation of treatment (Table 85.1).[12] However, due to the significant loss to follow-up of patients in both treatment group and the minimal increase on BMD in the lumbar spine, the grade of recommendation from this study is low. Multiple trials have shown significant increases in lumbar spine BMD after initiation of bisphosphonate treatment; however, BMD is a surrogate for the patient-important outcome of fracture, and the improvements in BMD are associated with estimates of precision that include clinically trivial effects (Table 85.2). Another study showed a palliative benefit of significantly increased bone density (+19.6 Hounsfield Units, 95% CI: +0.685 to +38.4) and osteoblastic volume (+6.49 cm^3, 95% CI +1.20 to +11.8) when switching

Table 85.1 Changes in lumbar spine bone mineral density in patients with metastatic breast cancer (% of baseline)

Follow-up time (months)		10.5 ± 0.4	17.3 ± 0.9	24.7 ± 1.4
Number of patients	Placebo	18	15	12
	Clondronate	20	12	9
Bone mineral density changes (%)	Placebo	+7.1 ± 5.4	+4.5 ± 3.2	+0.5 ± 1.9
	Clondronate	+8.2 ± 3.2	+7.8 ± 4.6	+0.8 ± 2.9

BMD, bone mineral density.
Reprinted from Bone, 18, Rizzoli R, Forni M, Schaad MA, et al, Effects of oral clondronate of bone mineral density in patients with relapsing breast cancer,531–37, Copyright 1996, with permission from Elsevier.

Table 85.2 Results of bone mineral density studies of bisphosphonate therapy

Study	Description	No. of patients (No. included at last follow-up)	Follow-up	Change in BMD at the spine (%)
Delmas et al.[30]	Randomized trial	53 (53)	2 years	2.5% (95% CI 0.2–4.9)
Powles et al.[31]	Randomized trial	414 (311)	2 years	1.7% (95% CI 0.12–3.34)
Saarto et al.[32]	Randomized trial	93 (89)	2 years	2.9% (no measure of precision reported)

BMD, bone mineral density.

from first-line bisphosphonates to more potent agents such as zoledronic acid.[13] Even though there was no loss to follow-up, this non-randomized prospective observational study had a small numbers of patients (15).Therefore, the grade of recommendation is moderate at best.

Recommendations

With respect to the use of bisphosphonates for the treatment of metastatic disease of the spine:

• There is good evidence that supports bisphosphonate therapy to prevent adverse outcomes such as pathologic fractures in breast cancer patients with metastatic vertebral lesions [overall quality: high]
• Limited evidence exists to suggest that similar benefits of bisphosphonate therapy may be realized in patients with metastatic prostate cancer [overall quality: moderate]
• Bisphosphonates are not effective for pain control in patients with metastatic disease of the spine [overall quality: high]
• Bisphosphonate therapy increases lumbar BMD in patients with metastatic disease of the spine as determined by multiple well-conducted RCTs [overall quality: moderate]

Question 2: Do radiopharmaceuticals play a role in the treatment of metastatic spine disease?

Case clarification

The patient states that she has tried chemotherapy and pain medications including opiates. She asks if there are any new medications that might improve her pain.

Relevance

In patients with metastatic disease, systemic radiopharmaceutical therapy (RPT) has increasingly been recognized as an important contributor to the improvement of quality of life. Using this modality, all painful osseous sites can be addressed simultaneously with little long-term toxicity.

Finding the evidence

• Cochrane Database, search term: "radiopharmaceutical AND metastasis"
• PubMed (www.ncbi.nlm.nih.gov/pubmed/) clinical queries search/systematic reviews: "radiopharmaceutical AND metastasis"
• PubMed (www.ncbi.nlm.nih.gov/pubmed/): sensitivity search using keywords "radiopharmaceutical AND metastasis"

Quality of the evidence

Level I
• 1 RCT, 2 systematic reviews of RCTs

Findings

Radionuclides have so far been used mainly as an adjuvant to external beam radiation for the management of metastatic disease. We were unable to find studies of radionuclides used for treatment of spine metastasis specifically, but there have been several studies evaluating the use of radionuclides for management of bone metastases.[14-17] An RCT comparing the effectiveness of strontium-89 to placebo as an adjunct to local field radiotherapy in patients with metastatic prostate cancer to bone found a statistically significant improvement in quality of life ($p = 0.006$), alleviation of pain ($p < 0.05$), and physical activity ($p < 0.05$).[14] No estimate of effect was calculated for any of these parameters. A systematic review of three RCTs studying the role of strontium-89 in palliative pain relief for patients with stage D endocrine-refractory prostate cancer and multiple bone metastases (including but not specific to spine) found that strontium-89 demonstrated palliative efficacy compared to placebo ($p < 0.01$) in two of the three studies.[15] None of the studies mentioned showed any significant difference in patient survival. Hemotoxicity was found to be mild, and limited evidence suggested a decrease in treatment costs. Finally, a thorough systematic review of nine RCTs studying the role of radiopharmaceuticals in the palliation of bone pain in adults with uncomplicated, multifocal painful bone metastases from breast, prostate, and lung cancer found that single-agent radiopharmaceuticals (strontium-89 and samarium-153, whether used alone or in conjunction with radiation) provided significantly greater pain relief (30–40% strontium-89 vs. 20–23% placebo, and 31–73% samarium-153 vs. 14% placebo, $p < 0.05$) and a decreased need for opiates (17% decrease for strontium-89 vs. 2% placebo, and 37–60% decrease for samarium-153 vs. 26% increase for placebo, $p < 0.05$).[16] Although the quality of studies evaluating the effects of strontium-89 and samarium-153 on pain relief from bony metastases was good (appropriate randomization, acceptable follow-up), none of these studies specifically evaluated spine metastases. Therefore, the evidence presented in these studies is limited due to indirect findings.

Recommendation

• Radiopharmaceuticals (strontium-89 and samarium-153) should be considered as an option for palliation of multiple sites of bone pain from metastatic disease involving the spine [overall quality: moderate]

Question 3: Can radiation alone play a role in the palliative management of spinal metastases?

Case clarification

In addition to the chemotherapy suggested above, the patient would like to know if radiation might help her current condition.

Table 85.3 Summary of results from a systematic review for conventional radiotherapy as a stand-alone therapy for spinal metastases

Author	N	Ambulatory status	Pain status	Median patient survival	Quality of evidence
Patchell et al.	51	74% remained ambulatory/19% regained ambulation		3 months	High
Maranzano et al.	276	67% remained ambulatory/26% regained ambulation	57% improved	4 months	High
Young et al.	13	60% remained ambulatory/33% regained ambulation	46% improved	5 months	High

Modified from the systematic review by Nair N. (1999) Relative efficacy of 32P and 89Sr in palliation in skeletal metastases. J Nucl Med 40(2), 256–61.[17]

Relevance

Radiation therapy is an important modality in the management of both primary and metastatic tumors involving the spine and spinal cord. Radiation therapy has evolved with better pretreatment imaging, improved dosing regimens, and more flexible treatment schedules.

Finding the evidence

- Cochrane Database, search term: "spine metastasis"
- PubMed (www.ncbi.nlm.nih.gov/pubmed/) clinical queries search/therapy, narrow specific search: "radiation AND metastasis"
- PubMed (www.ncbi.nlm.nih.gov/pubmed/) clinical queries search/systematic reviews: "radiation AND metastasis"

Quality of the evidence

Level I
- 2 systematic reviews of RCTs

Level III
- 1 systematic review of observational studies

Findings:

Several systematic reviews have examined the use radiotherapy for palliative pain management, local pain control, and improved quality of life in patients with metastatic disease and myeloma of the spine.[18–21] A systematic review of 16 RCTs comparing single- vs. multiple-fraction radiotherapy for bone metastases demonstrated that overall response to pain was 58% for single-fraction and 59% for multiple-fraction therapy (measures of precision not reported).[18] This is a well-conducted review of good quality RCTs, therefore the grade of recommendation regarding radiotherapy for pain control in bony metastases is high. This finding has been confirmed by other studies as well.[19,20] Unfortunately, no uniform method of reporting pain has been used and the length of follow-up varied from one study to another. Despite these shortcomings, the data suggests that palliative radiotherapy is an important treatment modality for spine metastases. Local control of metastases, defined as the absence of recurrent cord compression after conventional radiotherapy, has been achieved at rates of 61–89% in one systematic review of several observational studies.[20] However, given the observational nature of these studies, the grade of recommendation regarding radiotherapy for local control of spine metastases is low.

With respect to ambulatory status, a systematic review of three well-designed RCTs demonstrated that 60–74% of patients remain ambulatory after conventional radiation in the setting of cord compression, whereas 19–33% of nonambulatory patients are able to walk after radiation.[21] Several other observational studies (both prospective and retrospective in nature) were evaluated in the same systematic review but are not included here because of their lower quality. A selected summary of the three RCTs included in this systematic review demonstrating an improvement in ambulatory status and pain control is shown in Table 85.3. Given the good quality of evidence presented in these three RCTs, the overall grade of recommendation is high.

There will be variation in radiotherapy response based on the histology of the primary tumor. In general, lymphomas, myelomas, seminomas, breast cancer, and prostate cancer are considered radiosensitive, whereas sarcomas, melanomas, renal cell carcinomas, gastrointestinal carcinomas, and non-small-cell lung cancer (NSCLC) are considered radioresistant.[21]

Recommendations

- Conventional radiotherapy alone is beneficial for the treatment of spinal metastases. It is particularly effective in palliative pain management [overall quality: high]
- Conventional radiotherapy is effective in achieving local control of radiosensitive spinal metastases [overall quality: low]
- Conventional radiotherapy is effective in maintaining ambulatory function in a select group of patients with spinal metastases [overall quality: high]

Question 4: Do different fractionation schedules of radiotherapy affect efficacy in the management of spinal metastases?

Case clarification

The patient would like to go ahead with radiation for the treatment of her painful spine metastases. She would like to know if she will be receiving one or multiple doses of radiation.

Relevance

There has been much interest in investigating radiotherapy fractionation schedules for bone metastases. Several patterns-of-practice studies suggest that physician training or bias, resource availability, and/or reimbursement system are some of the factors that can influence the choice of fractionation prescribed.[18]

Finding the evidence

- Cochrane Database, search term "spine metastasis"
- PubMed (www.ncbi.nlm.nih.gov/pubmed/) clinical queries search/therapy, narrow specific search: "radiation AND metastasis"
- PubMed (www.ncbi.nlm.nih.gov/pubmed/) clinical queries search/systematic reviews: "radiation AND metastasis"

Quality of the evidence

Level I
- 2 meta-analyses of RCTs, 6 RCTs

Level II
- 3 systematic reviews

Findings

A meta-analysis of 8 RCTs by Wu et al.[22] including 3260 randomized patients with painful bone metastases showed similar overall pain response rates for single-fraction and multifraction radiotherapy at 72.7% and 72.5% respectively (risk ratio 1.00; 95% CI 0.95–1.04). Furthermore, exploratory analyses by biologic effective dose did not reveal any dose–response relationship among fractionation schedules used (single 8 Gy to 40 Gy in 15 fractions) and only the reirradiation rates were consistently different between the treatment arms (more frequent reirradiation in lower-dose arms among trials reporting reirradiation rates).[22] In addition, a systematic review of 11 RCTs including 3435 patients with bone metastases demonstrated no difference in pain response rates between single-fraction and multiple-fraction radiotherapy (OR 1.03, 95% CI 0.89–1.19).[23] Other RCTs and systematic reviews also confirm these findings.[18,24–29] The studies listed above are of good quality, but the site of metastases is not exclusively limited to spine, thus making the findings indirect with regard to the topic of this question. The grade of recommendation based on these studies is therefore moderate. The rates of pathologic fractures were shown to be significantly higher with single-fraction treatment in only one study,[23] while reirradiation rates were higher in the single-fraction group as compared to the multiple-fraction group across multiple studies.[18,23,24] Therefore, the grade of recommendation regarding pathologic fractures in single- vs. multiple-fraction radiotherapy is low, given that the findings are not directly related to spine and differences were found in only one study. In contrast, multiple studies found a significant difference between single and multiple fractions with regards to reirradiation rates, thus the grade of recommendation is moderate (lack of spine-specific metastases prevents a higher grade recommendation). The findings of some of these studies are summarized in Table 85.4.

Recommendations

- For the purposes of pain relief in the palliation of spinal metastases, there is no significant difference among different fractionation schedules for localized radiotherapy [overall quality: moderate]
- Single-fraction radiotherapy for spinal metastases results in higher reirradiation rates [overall quality: moderate] and higher rates of pathological fractures [overall quality: low]

Question 5: What is the efficacy of stereotactic radiosurgery in treating symptomatic spinal metastases?

Case clarification

The patient states that she has read on the internet about a new type of radiation surgery. She asks whether this would help with her condition.

Table 85.4 Effects of radiotherapy on bone metastases

	Single-dose radiotherapy			Fractionated radiotherapy		
	Sze et al.	Chow et al.	Arnalot et al.	Sze et al.	Chow et al.	Arnalot et al.
Pain reduction (%)	60	58	75	59	59	86
Complete pain remission (%)	34	23	15	32	24	13
Reirradiation (%)	21.5[a]	20[a]	28[a]	7.4[a]	8[a]	2[a]
Pathologic fractures (%)	3[a]	3.2	Not stated	1.6[a]	2.8	Not stated

[a]Statistically significant

Reproduced with kind permission from Springer Science+Business Media: Strahlenther Onkol, DEGRO practice guidelines for palliative radiotherapy of metastatic breast cancer-bone metastases and metastatic spinal cord compression, 185, 2009,417–24, Souchon R, Wenz F, Sedlmayer F, et al.

Relevance

With new advances in radiotherapy techniques, greater doses of radiation can be administered to the tumor with fewer side effects on the surrounding structures including the spinal cord.

Finding the evidence

- Cochrane Database, search term: "spine metastasis"
- PubMed (www.ncbi.nlm.nih.gov/pubmed/) clinical queries search/therapy, narrow specific search: "radiosurgery AND metastasis"
- PubMed (www.ncbi.nlm.nih.gov/pubmed/) clinical queries search/systematic reviews: "radiosurgery AND metastasis"

Quality of the evidence

Level III
- 2 systematic reviews of observational studies

Findings

A systematic review of 29 observational studies (1655 patients, only 27 of the studies assessed clinical outcomes measures) that included prospective cohort, retrospective reviews, and case series found that radiosurgery was highly effective at decreasing pain associated with symptomatic spine metastases regardless of prior treatment with conventional fractionated radiotherapy, with an overall reported improvement rate of approximately 85% (no measures of precision reported).[21] Although this improvement rate is slightly higher than that of conventional radiotherapy (reported as 50–70% in the same systematic review, no measures of precision given), the overall low quality of studies reviewed makes the grade of recommendation low. Durable pain improvement of spinal metastases was demonstrated in metastatic breast cancer, melanoma, lung cancer, and renal cell carcinoma. Pain was reported to decrease within weeks of treatment and quality of life was maintained up to 48 months after treatment.[21] Another systematic review of 3 studies (retrospective reviews) of patients with renal cell metastases found a radiographic tumor control rate of approximately 87% with pain control being achieved in 89% of patients presenting with axial or radicular pain (no measures of precision reported).[20] Again, given the observational nature of the studies reviewed, the overall grade of recommendation is low.

Recommendations

- Radiosurgery is effective in achieving symptomatic response and local control for radioresistant histologies, regardless of prior fractional radiotherapy. [overall quality: low]
- Radiosurgery achieves slightly higher pain improvement rates for spine metastases as compared to conventional radiotherapy [overall quality: low]

Summary of recommendations

- There is good evidence that supports bisphosphonate therapy to prevent adverse outcomes such as pathologic fractures in breast cancer patients with metastatic vertebral lesions, but limited evidence exists to suggest that similar benefits may be realized in patients with metastatic prostate cancer
- Bisphosphonates are not effective for pain control in patients with metastatic disease of the spine
- Bisphosphonate therapy increases lumbar BMD in patients with metastatic disease of the spine as determined by multiple well-conducted RCTs
- Radiopharmaceuticals (strontium-89 and samarium-153) should be considered as an option for palliation of multiple sites of bone pain from metastatic disease involving the spine
- Conventional radiotherapy alone is beneficial for the treatment of spinal metastases. It is particularly effective in palliative pain management
- Conventional radiotherapy is effective in achieving local control of radiosensitive spinal metastases
- Conventional radiotherapy is effective in maintaining ambulatory function in a select group of patients with spinal metastases
- For the purposes of pain relief in the palliation of spinal metastases, there is no significant difference among different fractionation schedules for localized radiotherapy
- Single-fraction radiotherapy for spinal metastases results in higher reirradiation rates and higher rates of pathological fractures
- Radiosurgery is effective in achieving symptomatic response and local control for radioresistant histologies, regardless of prior fractional radiotherapy
- Radiosurgery achieves slightly higher pain improvement rates for spine metastases as compared to conventional radiotherapy

Conclusions

Bisphosphonates, radiopharmaceuticals, and radiotherapy play an important role in the nonsurgical management of metastatic disease of the spine. Radiosurgery is a relatively new therapeutic modality that shows promising preliminary results but requires further investigation to assess its true treatment effect and potential limitations.

References

1. National Cancer Institute. Web site: http://www.cancer.gov. Accessed March 2011.

2. Shaw B, Mansfield FL, Borges L. One-stage posterolateral decompression and stabilization for primary and metastatic vertebral tumors in the thoracic and lumbar spine. J Neurosurg 1989;70:405–10.

3. Boland PJ, Lane JM, Sundaresan N. Metastatic disease of the spine. Clin Orthop 1982;169:95–102.

4. Harrington KD. Metastatic disease of the spine. In: Harrington KD, Orthopaedic Management of Metastatic Bone Disease, pp.309–383. Mosby, St. Louis, 1988.

5. Berrettoni BA, Carter JR. Mechanisms of cancer metastasis to bone. J Bone Joint Surg Am 1986;68:308–12.

6. Pavlakis N, Schmidt RL, Stockler MR. Bisphosphonates for breast cancer. Cochrane Database Syst Rev 2008;3.

7. Yuen KK, Shelley M, Sze WM, et al. Bisphosphonates for advanced prostate cancer. Cochrane Database Syst Rev 2006;4.

8. Hillner BE, Ingle JN, Benson JR, et al. American Society of Clinical Oncology guideline on the role of bisphosphonates in breast cancer. J Clin Oncol 2000;18:1378–91.

9. Ernst DS, MacDonald RN, Paterson AH, et al. A double-blind, crossover trial of intravenous clodronate in metastatic bone pain. J Pain Symptom Manage 1992;7:4–11.

10. Ernst DS, Brasher P, Hagen N, et al. A randomized, controlled trial of intravenous clodronate in patients with metastatic bone disease and pain. J Pain Symptom Manage 1997;13:319–26.

11. Coleman RE, Purohit OP, Vinholes JJ, et al. High dose pamidronate: Clinical and biochemical effects in metastatic bone disease. Cancer 1997;80:1686–90.

12. Rizzoli R, Forni M, Schaad MA, et al. Effects of oral clondronate of bone mineral density in patients with relapsing breast cancer. Bone 1996;18:531–7.

13. Amir E, Whyne C, Freedman OC, et al. Radiological changes following second-line zoledronic acid treatment in breast cancer patients with bone metastases. Clin Exp Metastases 2009;26:479–84.

14. Porter AT, McEwan AJ, Powe JE, et al. Results of a randomized phase-III trial to evaluate the efficacy of strontium-89 adjuvant to local field external beam irradiation in the management of endocrine resistant metastatic prostate cancer. Int J Radiat Oncol Biol Phys 1993;25(5):805–13.

15. Brundage MD, Crook JM, Lukka H. Use of strontium-89 in endocrine-refractory prostate cancer metastatic to bone. Cancer Prev Control 1998;2(2):79–87.

16. Bauman G, Charette M, Reid R et al. Radiopharmaceuticals for the palliation of painful bone metastasis-a systematic review. Radiother Oncol 2005;75(3):258–70.

17. Nair N. Relative efficacy of ^{32}P and ^{89}Sr in palliation in skeletal metastases. J Nucl Med 1999;40(2):256–61.

18. Chow E, Harris K, Fan G, et al. Palliative radiotherapy trials for bone metastases: a systematic review. J Clin Oncol 2007;25(11):1423–36.

19. Hoegler D. Radiotherapy for palliation of symptoms in incurable cancer. Curr Probl Cancer 1997;21:132–83.

20. Bilsky MH, Laufer I, Birch S. Shifting paradigms in the treatment of metastatic spine disease. Spine 2009;34:S101–7.

21. Gerszten PC, Mendel E, Yamada Y. Radiotherapy and radiosurgery for metastatic spine disease. Spine 2009;34:S78–92(21).

22. Wu JS, Wong R, Johnston M et al. Meta-analysis of dose-fractionation radiotherapy trials for the palliation of painful bone metastases. Int J Radiat Oncol Biol Phys 2003;55:594–604.

23. Sze WM, Shelley M, Held I, et al. Palliation of metastatic bone pain: single fraction versus multifraction radiotherapy—a systematic review of randomized trials. Cochrane Database Syst Rev 2004;2.

24. Foro Arnalot P, Fontanals AV, Galcerán JC, et al. Randomized clinical trial with two palliative radiotherapy regimens in painful bone metastases: 30 Gy in 10 fractions compared with 8 Gy in single fraction. Radiother Oncol 2008;89(2):150–5.

25. Roos DE, Turner SL, O'Brien PC, et al. Randomized trial of 8 Gy in 1 versus 20 Gy in 5 fractions of radiotherapy for neuropathic pain due to bone metastases. J Eur Soc Therapeut Radiol Oncol 2005;75:54–63.

26. Steenland E, Leer JW, van Houwelingen H, et al. The effect of a single fraction compared to multiple fractions on painful bone metastases: a global analysis of the Dutch Bone Metastasis Study. J Eur Soc Therapeut Radiol Oncol 1999;52:101–9.

27. Roos DE, O'Brien PC, Smith JG, et al. A role of radiotherapy in neuropathic bone pain: preliminary response rates from a prospective trial. Int J Radiat Oncol Biol Phys 2000;46:975–81.

28. Amouzegar-Hashimi F, Behrouzi H, Kazemian A, et al. Single versus multiple fractions of palliative radiotherapy for bone metastases: a randomized clinical trial in Iranian patients. Curr Oncol 2008;15:36–9.

29. Hamouda WE, Roshdy W, Teema M. Single versus conventional fractionated radiotherapy in the palliation of painful bone metastases. Gulf J Oncol 2007;1:35–41.

30. Delmas PD, Balena R, Confravreaux E, et al. Bisphosphonate risedronate prevents bone loss in women with artificial menopause due to chemotherapy of breast cancer: a double-blind, placebo-controlled study. J Clin Oncol 1997;15:955–62.

31. Powles TJ, McCloskey E, Paterson AH, et al. Oral clondronate and reduction in loss of bone mineral density in women with operable primary breast cancer. J Natl Cancer Inst 1998;90:704–8.

32. Saarto T, Blomqvist C, Valimaki M, et al. Clondronate improves bone mineral density in postmenopausal breast cancer patients treated with adjuvant antiestrogens. Br J Cancer 1997;75:602–5.

33. Souchon R, Wenz F, Sedlmayer F, et al. DEGRO practice guidelines for palliative radiotherapy of metastatic breast cancer-bone metastases and metastatic spinal cord compression. Strahlenther Onkol 2009;185:417–24.

VI Sports Medicine

86

Treatment of the First Shoulder Dislocation

Charles L. Cox and John E. Kuhn
Vanderbilt University School of Medicine, Nashville, TN, USA

Case scenario

A 21 year old collegiate athlete sustains an injury to his dominant shoulder and reports a sudden forceful, posteriorly directed force on his forearm while his arm was in a position of abduction and external rotation. On examination, he holds the affected arm at his side and refuses any attempts at range of motion assessment. He is neurovascularly intact distally.

Relevant anatomy

The diagnosis of shoulder instability represents a broad range of injury patterns to the glenohumeral joint. Injuries are frequently classified on the basis of several clinical factors including frequency (initial vs. recurrent event), etiology (traumatic vs. nontraumatic mechanism), direction (anterior vs. posterior instability), and severity (joint dislocation vs. subluxation). Anatomical evaluation generally reveals an injury to the labrum and the adjacent joint capsule, and treatment options are based upon attempts to restore preinjury tension and alignment of injured structures.

Importance of the problem

Based upon previous studies, shoulder instability rates range from 8.2–23.9/100,000 person-years in the general population with a prevalence of 1.7%, but these values are based upon presentation to medical facilities and are there-fore likely low estimates due to failure to capture subtle events such as subluxations.[1-3] These values are also representative of the general population, leading to a decreased external validity when extrapolating these estimates to predict numbers for younger individuals. In analyzing a younger subset of the population, the United States Military Academy followed over 4,100 students for 9 months capturing 117 events for an incidence of 2.8%. The vast majority of these injuries were subluxations (85%) and anterior in orientation (80%). In evaluating etiology, 44% were related to contact injuries.[4] This data again indicates that frank glenohumeral dislocation likely represents only a small subset of the actual instability injury patterns seen in relation to the glenohumeral joint.

At present, definitive recommendations are lacking regarding optimal treatment strategies for those presenting with first-time dislocation events as published recurrence rates are extremely variable across broad levels of study quality, and risk factors for repeat injury are unclear. Owens et al. queried the United States Defense Medical Epidemiology Database for ICD-9 codes related to shoulder instability for a period from 1998 to 2006 determining risks factors for recurrence were male gender, age less than 30 years, being white, junior enlisted rank, and army postion.[5] Although this data assists the treating clinician when counseling a patient with a first-time shoulder dislocation, numerous questions remain surrounding treatment options ranging from choice of method of joint reduction to position of initial immobilization to decision for operative vs. nonoperative management. Knowledge of current published literature offers insight into maximizing clinical outcomes and can be used to individualize treatment for each patient.

Top five questions

Therapy

1. What premedication regimen works best for reducing a glenohumeral dislocation?
2. Is there an ideal reduction method?
3. Does position of the extremity in immobilization reduce recurrence rates?
4. Does surgical treatment reduce recurrence compared with nonoperative management for patients with a first-time dislocation?

Prognosis

5. What is the long-term prognosis for the patient with a first-time glenohumeral dislocation?

Question 1: What premedication regimen works best for reducing a glenohumeral dislocation?

Case clarification

The athlete's radiographs reveal an anterior dislocation of the glenohumeral joint. He is in obvious discomfort and resists any attempts at closed reduction of the extremity due to pain. You must decide upon the best method of premedication to achieve a successful reduction.

Relevance

The treating clinician must decide upon the best method of sedation to maximize patient safety while achieving reduction and minimizing complications. In the medical care setting, current options range from intravenous sedation to intra-articular anesthetic to regional block.

Current opinion

At present, intravenous sedation is the most commonly utilized strategy to alleviate pain allowing for closed reduction.

Finding the evidence

- Cochrane Database, with search term "shoulder reduction"
- PUBMED (www.ncbi.nlm.nih.gov/pubmed/) clinical queries search/systematic reviews: "shoulder OR glenohumeral reduction"
- PUBMED (www.ncbi.nlm.nih.gov/pubmed/): sensitivity search using keywords "shoulder" AND "reduction" as well as "glenohumeral" AND "reduction"

Quality of the evidence

Level I
- 2 systematic reviews/meta-analyses[6-7]
- 6 randomized trials[8-13]

Findings

The included trials compared various outcome measures amongst two techniques: intravenous sedation vs. intra-articular lidocaine injection. Trial outcomes can be compared based upon reduction success, complications, pain level, time to reduction, and overall time in the Emergency Department (Table 86.1). No differences were seen in rates of reduction amongst the techniques with 92% (103/111) overall success reported for intra-articular lidocaine vs. 92% (101/110) for intravenous sedation. This was found despite slight differences between the trials in patient population and utilized manual reduction techniques. Regarding complications, the intra-articular technique resulted in a 0.9% (1/111) overall rate compared with 16.4% (18/110) in the intravenous sedation group. The most common complication associated with intravenous sedation was respiratory depression. No significant differences were noted in any of the trials regarding pain level associated with each technique. Three of the studies compared time to reduction, with 2/3 significantly favoring intravenous sedation as the quicker method for achieving reduction. Three trials compared overall time spent in the Emergency Department, with 2/3 trials significantly favoring intra-articular lidocaine as the preferred method.

Recommendations

In patients with glenohumeral dislocations, evidence pertaining to premedication prior to reduction suggests:
- No difference exists between the two techniques regarding success rate for reduction and patient pain level [overall quality: high]

Table 86.1 Comparison of premedication techniques

	Success rate	Complication rate	Pain	Time to reduction	Time in Emergency Department
Intra-articular lidocaine	92%	0.9%	NS	2/3 significantly favored intravenous sedation	2/3 significantly favored intra-articular lidocaine
Intravenous sedation	92%	16.4%			

NS, not significant.

• Intra-articular lidocaine significantly reduces the risk of complications, mainly in the form of respiratory depression associated with intravenous sedation [overall quality: high]

• Data is variable amongst the two techniques regarding time required for reduction (2/3 in favor of intravenous sedation) and time spent in the Emergency Department (2/3 in favor of intra-articular lidocaine) [overall quality: high]

Question 2: Is there an ideal reduction method?

Case clarification

The athlete clearly has a dislocated glenohumeral joint. The standard of care is expeditious reduction. You must decide upon the best technique to achieve reduction.

Relevance

Numerous described techniques for achieving reduction exist. Many utilize different strategies to overcome muscular forces and allow the humeral head to slide back into the face of the glenoid. It is important to avoid potential iatrogenic injury to the anatomic structures as reduction is attempted.

Current opinion

At present, there is no consensus as to the best technique for reduction, and many regional variations exist.

Finding the evidence

• Cochrane Database, with search term "shoulder reduction"

• PUBMED (www.ncbi.nlm.nih.gov/pubmed/) clinical queries search/systematic reviews: "shoulder OR glenohumeral reduction"

• PUBMED (www.ncbi.nlm.nih.gov/pubmed/): sensitivity search using keywords "shoulder" AND "reduction" as well as "glenohumeral" AND "reduction"

Quality of the evidence

Level I

• 2 randomized trials[14–15]

Findings

Both trials compare various reduction techniques for success rate without the use of analgesia or sedation. The first trial involves a comparison of the Milch and Kocher techniques for reduction.[14] No difference in success rate was noted amongst the two techniques. The second trial compares the hippocratic, Kocher, and FARES (Fast, Reliable, and Safe) methods of reduction and includes patient visual analog pain ratings as an outcome measure (Table 86.2).[15] The FARES method was significantly more successful, quicker, and less painful to the patients than the other two techniques.

Table 86.2 Comparison of the FARES, hippocratic, and Kocher reduction methods

	Success rate	Complication rate	Visual analog pain score	Time to reduction (min)
FARES	88.7%	NS	1.57	2.36
Hippocratic	72.5%		4.88	5.55
Kocher	68%		5.44	4.32

NS, not significant.

Recommendations

In patients with glenohumeral dislocations, evidence pertaining to choice of reduction technique in a patient without sedation or analgesia suggests:

• No difference exists in success rate between the Milch and Kocher techniques [overall quality: high]

• The FARES technique is associated with a significantly higher success rate, quicker time to reduction, and lower visual analog pain score than the hippocratic and Kocher techniques [overall quality: high]

• Despite a large number of described techniques for reducing the dislocated glenohumeral joint, only two high-level studies were identified. Therefore, it is recommended that the clinician obtain experience with multiple techniques [overall quality: low]

Question 3: Does the position of the extremity in immobilization reduce recurrence rates?

Case clarification

Once the reduction has been achieved, the arm must be placed in a position of relative stability to maintain anatomical congruence and avoid redislocation. You must decide upon the position of the arm in immobilization.

Relevance

Classically the arm was placed in a sling in a position of glenohumeral joint internal rotation, but some now advocate immobilization in external rotation to place tension upon the anterior capsulolabral structures and thereby reapproximate the areas of injury. This is theorized to improve restoration of preinjury anatomy and decrease likelihood of recurrence.

Current opinion

At present, most acute care settings employ a sling and/or swathe following reduction maintaining the arm in a position of internal rotation.

Finding the evidence

• Cochrane Database, with search term "shoulder dislocation"
• PUBMED (www.ncbi.nlm.nih.gov/pubmed/) clinical queries search/ systematic reviews: "shoulder OR glenohumeral dislocation"
• PUBMED (www.ncbi.nlm.nih.gov/pubmed/): sensitivity search using keywords "shoulder" AND "dislocation" as well as "glenohumeral" AND "dislocation"

Quality of the evidence

Level I
• 1 systematic review/meta-analysis[16]
• 5 randomized trials[17–21]

Level II
• 1 observational cohort study[22]
• 2 randomized trials with methodologic limitations[23–24]

Findings

Internal rotation In comparing length of time immobilized in internal rotation for over 500 patients combined, no significant differences in recurrence were noted amongst the various studies.[17–20,22] Hovelius et al. followed the same cohort of patients over a 25-year period in a level I prognosis study and reported that recurrence rates progressively increased with time (29% at 2 years, 45% at 5 years, 48% at 10 years) but plateau at approximately 5 years after the initial injury.[17–20] Younger age at initial dislocation and the presence of a Hill Sachs lesion were noted to be risk factors for recurrence.

External rotation Finestone et al. compared a cohort of 51 patients immobilized for 4 weeks in internal or external rotation for an average of 33 months and found no significant difference in rates of recurrence amongst the groups (42% internal rotation group vs. 37% external rotation group).[21] This is in contrast to two level II studies (representing the same cohort) that found a decreased recurrence rate in the external rotation group as compared to the internal rotation group (26% vs. 42%, respectively).[23–24]

Recommendations

In patients with initial glenohumeral dislocations, evidence pertaining to length and method of immobilization (internal vs. external) on recurrence rate suggests:
• No significant difference exists in recurrence rate between immobilization for several weeks in internal rotation vs. early motion [overall quality: high]
• Immobilization for several weeks in external rotation compared with internal rotation revealed no significant difference in recurrence in the level I study but did find a significant difference in the level II studies [overall quality: moderate]

Question 4: Does surgical treatment reduce recurrence compared with nonoperative management for patients with a first-time dislocation?

Case clarification

After reduction, the athlete inquires as to the best method to prevent future recurrence. Specifically, he inquires as to whether surgery is necessary to reduce risk in a clinically significant manner.

Relevance

Definitive treatment strategy generally requires a choice between a variable period of immobilization vs. surgical intervention in the setting of a first-time dislocation. Current opinion is mixed based upon high recurrence rates reported across the literature when nonoperative management is chosen.

Current opinion

At present, surgery is felt to decrease the overall risk of recurrence.

Finding the evidence

• Cochrane Database, with search term "shoulder dislocation"
• PUBMED (www.ncbi.nlm.nih.gov/pubmed/) clinical queries search/ systematic reviews: "shoulder OR glenohumeral dislocation"
• PUBMED (www.ncbi.nlm.nih.gov/pubmed/): sensitivity search using keywords "shoulder" AND "dislocation" as well as "glenohumeral" AND "dislocation"

Quality of the evidence

Level I
• 1 systematic review/meta-analysis[25]
• 5 randomized trials[26–32]

Level II
• 1 observational cohort study[33]

Findings

Three of the level I studies and the included level II cohort compare surgical stabilization to nonoperative treatment (immobilization or sling or early motion) and report a significant decrease in recurrence rates in the operatively stabilized group.[26–28,33] Two of the included level I studies compare initial arthroscopic lavage to nonoperative treatment and display a significant decrease in recurrence rates in the lavage group.[29–30] Two of the level I studies utilize initial arthroscopic diagnosis followed by nonoperative treatment or surgical stabilization and again report a significant decrease in recurrence in the surgically repaired group.[31–32] In the systematic review by Handoll et al., results were pooled among included trials revealing a significant decrease in recurrence in the operative group compared to the nonoperative group (RR 0.20; 95% CI 0.11–0.33).[25] Of note, the systematic review included an abstract rated as level I evidence although it was not available as a published trial.

Recommendations

In patients with initial glenohumeral dislocations, evidence pertaining to the effect of operative vs. nonoperative treatment on recurrence rate suggests:

• Surgical stabilization results in a decreased risk of recurrence compared with arthroscopic lavage alone or nonoperative management techniques [overall quality: high]

• Arthroscopic lavage alone displays a decreased risk of recurrence compared with strictly nonoperative management strategies [overall quality: high]

Question 5: What is the long-term prognosis for the patient with a first-time glenohumeral dislocation?

Case clarification

The athlete inquires about the future ramifications for shoulder function later in life as a result of this primary dislocation event.

Relevance

The bulk of the current literature is focused upon strategies to reduce recurrence and restore preinjury anatomical integrity. However, most of the published data is centered on relatively short-term results (1–10 years after treatment). Long-term outcomes and effects of initial dislocation on future function are generally unknown.

Current opinion

At present, dislocation of the glenohumeral joint is presumed to increase the risk of future arthritis and resultant dysfunction.

Finding the evidence

• Cochrane Database, with search term "shoulder dislocation"

• PUBMED (www.ncbi.nlm.nih.gov/pubmed/) clinical queries search/ systematic reviews: "shoulder OR glenohumeral dislocation"

• PUBMED (www.ncbi.nlm.nih.gov/pubmed/): sensitivity search using keywords "shoulder" AND "dislocation" as well as "glenohumeral" AND "dislocation"

Quality of the evidence

Level I
• 1 randomized trials[20]

Findings

In reviewing the available published literature, only one high-level study was found that followed patients on average for more than 10 years. Hovelius et al. followed 227 patients for 25 years after an initial glenohumeral dislocation event treated nonoperatively, many of which went on to display recurrence and opt for surgical intervention. In comparing scores on the Disabilities of the Arm, Shoulder and Hand (DASH) outcome questionnaire at the end of this time period, values were similar for shoulders classified as nonrecurrent, stable over time, or surgically stabilized, but patients with persistent, recurrent dislocations fared statistically worse than the aforementioned groups. Women also displayed statistically worse scores as compared to men.[20]

Recommendations

In patients with an initial glenohumeral dislocation, evidence pertaining to long-term outcome suggests:

• Long-term DASH scores are comparable amongst groups regardless of treatment as long as stability is displayed over time, manifested by a lack of persistent recurrence. Women tend to score statistically worse than men over time [overall quality: high]

Summary of recommendations

• Intra-articular lidocaine significantly reduces the risk of complications during shoulder reduction compared with intravenous sedation, but no difference exists between the two techniques regarding success rate for reduction and patient pain level

• Despite a large number of described techniques for reducing the dislocated glenohumeral joint, only two high-level studies were identified. Therefore, it is recommended that the clinician obtain experience with multiple techniques. Evidence exists suggesting that the FARES technique is superior to the hippocratic and Kocher techniques

• The highest-level evidence indicates that there is no difference in recurrence rate amongst choice of initial immobilization in internal vs. external rotation following a first-time shoulder dislocation

• Surgical treatment results in a decreased risk of recurrence compared with nonoperative management of first-time shoulder dislocations

• 25 year DASH score outcomes following a primary dislocation event are comparable amongst treatment strategies as long as shoulder stability is achieved over time

Conclusions

Shoulder dislocation is a relatively common clinical event, and review of the best available evidence provides guidelines for management ranging from initial encounter with the patient (premedication decisions prior to reduction, choice of reduction technique, method of immobilization) to definitive treatment decision (operative vs. nonoperative management) to counseling on long-term prognosis.

References

1. Simonet WT, Melton LJ III, Cofield RH, et al. Incidence of anterior shoulder dislocation in Olmstead County, Minnesota. Clin Orthop Relat Res 1984;186:186–91.

2. Nordqvist A, Petersson CJ. Incidence and causes of shoulder girdle injuries in an urban population. J Shoulder Elbow Surg 1995;4:107–12.

3. Hovelius L. Incidence of shoulder dislocation in Sweden. Clin Orthop Relat Res 1982;166:127–31.

4. Owens BD, Duffey ML, Nelson BJ, et al. The incidence and characteristics of shoulder instability at the United States Military Academy. Am J Sports Med 2007;35:1168–73.

5. Owens BD, Dawson L, Burks R, Cameron KL. Incidence of shoulder dislocation in the United States military: demographic considerations from a high-risk population. J Bone Joint Surg Am 2009;91:791–6.

6. Fitch RW, Kuhn JE. Intraarticular lidocaine versus intravenous procedural sedation with narcotics and benzodiazepines for reduction of the dislocated shoulder: a systematic review. Acad Emerg Med 2008;15:703–8.

7. Ng VK, Hames H, Millard WM. Use of intra-articular lidocaine as analgesia in anterior shoulder dislocation: a review and meta-analysis of the literature. Can J Rural Med 2009;14:145–9.

8. Suder PA, Mikkelsen JB, Hougaard K, Jensen PE. Reduction of traumatic primary anterior shoulder dislocation under local analgesia. Ugeskr Laeger 1995;157:3625–9.

9. Kosnik J, Shamsa F, Raphael E, Huang R, Malachias Z, Georgiadis GM. Anesthetic methods for reduction of acute shoulder dislocations: a prospective randomized study comparing intraarticular lidocaine with intravenous analgesia and sedation. Am J Emerg Med 1999;17:566–70.

10. Matthews DE, Roberts T. Intraarticular lidocaine versus intravenous analgesic for reduction of acute anterior shoulder dislocations. A prospective randomized study. Am J Sports Med 1995;23:54–8.

11. Miller SL, Cleeman E, Auerbach J, Flatow EL. Comparison of intra-articular lidocaine and intravenous sedation for reduction of shoulder dislocations: a randomized, prospective study. J Bone Joint Surg Am 2002;84:2135–9.

12. Orlinsky M, Shon S, Chiang C, Chan L, Carter P. Comparative study of intra-articular lidocaine and intravenous meperidine/diazepam for shoulder dislocations. J Emerg Med 2002;22:241–5.

13. Suder PA, Mikkelsen JB, Hougaard K, Jensen PE. Reduction of traumatic secondary shoulder dislocations with lidocaine. Arch Orthop Trauma Surg 1995;114:233–6.

14. Beattie TF, Steedman DJ, McGowan A, Robertson CE. A comparison of the Milch and Kocher techniques for acute anterior dislocation of the shoulder. Injury 1986;17:349–52.

15. Sayegh FE, Kenanidis EI, Papavasiliou KA, Potoupnis ME, Kirkos JM, Kapetanos GA. Reduction of acute anterior disloca-

tions: a prospective randomized study comparing a new technique with the hippocratic and Kocher methods. J Bone Joint Surg Am 2009;91:2775–82.

16. Handoll HH, Hanchard NC, Goodchild L, Feary J. Conservative management following closed reduction of traumatic anterior dislocation of the shoulder. Cochrane Database Syst Rev 2006;1:CD004962.

17. Hovelius L, Eriksson K, Fredin H, et al. Recurrences after initial dislocation of the shoulder. Results of a prospective study of treatment. J. Bone Joint Surg Am 1983;65:343–9.

18. Hovelius L. Anterior dislocation of the shoulder in teen-agers and young adults. Five-year prognosis. J Bone Joint Surg Am 1987;69:393–9.

19. Hovelius L, Augustini BG, Fredin H, et al. Primary anterior dislocation of the shoulder in young patients. A ten-year prospective study. J Bone Joint Surg Am 1996;78:1677–84.

20. Hovelius L, Olofsson A, Sandström B, et al. Nonoperative treatment of primary anterior shoulder dislocation in patients forty years of age and younger. A prospective twenty-five-year follow-up. J Bone Joint Surg Am 2008;90:945–52.

21. Finestone A, Milgrom C, Radeva-Petrova DR, et al. Bracing in external rotation for traumatic anterior dislocation of the shoulder. J Bone Joint Surg Br 2009;91:918–21.

22. Kiviluoto O, Pasila M, Jaroma H, et al. Immobilization after primary dislocation of the shoulder. Acta Orthop Scand 1980;51:915–19.

23. Itoi E, Hatakeyama Y, Kido T, et al. A new method of immobilization after traumatic anterior dislocation of the shoulder: a preliminary study. J Shoulder Elbow Surg 2003;12:13–415.

24. Itoi E, Hatakeyama Y, Sato T, et al. Immobilization in external rotation after shoulder dislocation reduces the risk of recurrence. A randomized controlled trial. J Bone Joint Surg Am 2007;89:2124–31.

25. Handoll HH, Almaiyah MA, Rangan A. Surgical versus non-surgical treatment for acute anterior shoulder dislocation. Cochrane Database Syst Rev 2004;1:CD004325.

26. Bottoni CR, Wilckens JH, DeBerardino TM, et al. A prospective, randomized evaluation of arthroscopic stabilization versus non-operative treatment in patients with acute, traumatic, first-time shoulder dislocations. Am J Sports Med 2002;30:576–80.

27. Kirkley A, Griffin S, Richards C, et al. Prospective randomized clinical trial comparing the effectiveness of immediate arthroscopic stabilization versus immobilization and rehabilitation in first traumatic anterior dislocations of the shoulder. Arthroscopy 1999;15(5):507–14.

28. Kirkley, A, Werstine, R, Ratjek, A, et al. Prospective randomized clinical trial comparing the effectiveness of immediate arthroscopic stabilization versus immobilization and rehabilitation in first traumatic anterior dislocations of the shoulder: long-term evaluation. Arthroscopy 2005;21(1):55–63.

29. Wintzell, G, Haglund-Akerlind, Y, Tidermark, J, et al. A prospective controlled randomized study of arthroscopic lavage in acute primary anterior dislocation of the shoulder: one-year follow-up. Knee Surg Sports Traumatol Arthrosc 1996;4(1):43–7.

30. Wintzell G, Haglund-Akerlind Y, Nowak J, Larsson S. Arthroscopic lavage compared with nonoperative treatment for traumatic primary anterior shoulder dislocation: a 2-year follow-up of a prospective randomized study. J Shoulder Elbow Surg 1999;8:399–402.

31. Robinson CM, Jenkins PJ, White TO, et al. Primary arthroscopic stabilization for a first-time anterior dislocation of the shoulder. A randomized, double-blind trial. J Bone Joint Surg Am 2008; 90(4):708–21.

32. Jakobsen BW, Johannsen HV, Suder P, et al. Primary repair versus conservative treatment of first-time traumatic anterior dislocation of the shoulder: a randomized study with 10-year follow-up. Arthroscopy 2007;23(2):118–23.

33. Arciero RA, Wheeler JH, Ryan JB, et al. Arthroscopic Bankart repair versus nonoperative treatment for acute, initial anterior shoulder dislocations. Am J Sports Med 1994;22(5):589–94.

87 Chronic Shoulder Instability

Joost I.P. Willems[1] and W. Jaap Willems[2]

[1]Free University, Amsterdam, The Netherlands
[2]Onze Lieve Vrouwe Gasthuis, Amsterdam, The Netherlands

Case scenario

A 35 year old man presents in the clinic with a history of shoulder instability. He had frequent dislocations until the age of 25, followed by a period without recurrence after adaptation of his lifestyle. Recently he started windsurfing and again experienced a sensation of instability. He is now looking for advice about his shoulder problem and a possible treatment for his instability.

Relevant anatomy

The majority (>90%) of traumatic shoulder dislocations occur in the anterior–inferior direction. A small minority of shoulders dislocate in posterior direction. Dislocation in the superior direction is extremely rare. Multidirectional instability is also extremely rare, unlike multidirectional laxity.

In nearly all anterior cases a disruption of the labrum takes place, the so-called Bankart lesion (Figure 87.1). Other eponyms are Perthes or anterior labro-periosteal sleeve avulsion (ALPSA) lesion. Sometimes this occurs in combination with a tear of the capsule; sometimes an isolated lesion of the capsule is the only soft tissue defect. When the capsule is detached from the humeral head, the acronym HAGL (humeral avulsion of the glenohumeral ligaments) is used.

In most cases of chronic instability a posterolateral impression fracture of the head, the so-called Hill–Sachs lesion, is seen (Figure 87.2). At the glenoid side an erosion of the glenoid frequently arises, either due to impaction of bone or due to avulsion of a bony fragment at the anterior glenoid together with the labrum avulsion, a so-called bony Bankart lesion (Figure 87.3). In posterior instability sometimes a posterior Bankart lesion, a reversed Hill–Sachs on the anterior aspect of the head, or a posterior erosion of the glenoid can be seen.

Top six questions

1. Which clinical tests are accurate and necessary to perform in the diagnosis of chronic shoulder instability?
2. What is the role of imaging in the diagnosis of chronic shoulder instability?
3. What is the best surgical approach to treat chronic shoulder instability?
4. What is the role of bone defects in the treatment of chronic unstable shoulder?
5. What is the role of rehabilitation in chronic shoulder instability?
6. What is the natural history in chronic unstable shoulders?

Question 1: Which clinical tests are accurate and necessary to perform in the diagnosis of chronic shoulder instability?

Finding the evidence

We performed a literature search of literature published between 1990 and December 2009 in the online resources MEDLINE and Embase with combinations of the following search terms:
- "Clinical tests," "apprehension test," "clunk test," "load and shift test," "drawer test," "relocation test," "release test," "hyperabduction test," "jerk test," "crank test," "posterior drawer test," "Kim test," "sensitivity," "specificity," "diagnosis," "chronic," "recurrent," "shoulder instability,"

Evidence-Based Orthopedics, First Edition. Edited by Mohit Bhandari.

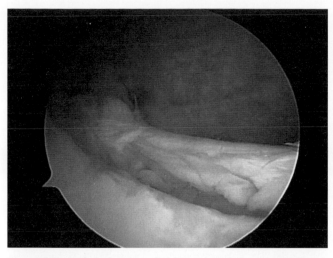

Figure 87.1 Arthroscopic view of a labrum avulsion from the glenoid.

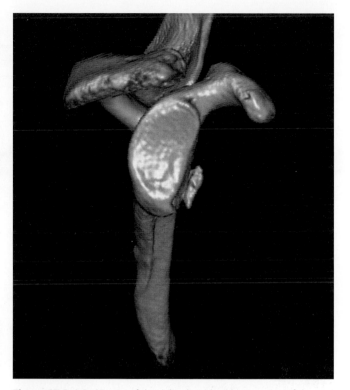

Figure 87.3 3-D CT scan of the right glenoid, with an erosion of the anterior aspect of the glenoid with a detached bony fragment.

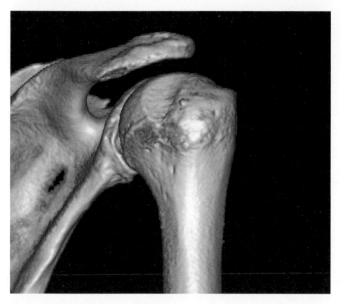

Figure 87.2 3-D CT scan of the right humeral head with an impression fracture on the postero-superior aspect, a so-called Hill–Sachs lesion.

"glenohumeral instability," "shoulder dislocation," "shoulder subluxation"

Quality of the evidence
See Tables 87.1 and 87.2.

Findings
Chronic anterior instability In the past many tests have been developed to diagnose anterior shoulder instability. We have reviewed the tests that have been evaluated and rated them for their evidence in proving anterior instability (Table 87.1). As shown in Table 87.1, only Farber et al.[4] and

Guanche et al.[5] reported publications with good evidence of level Ib and IIb respectively. Considering these studies, we can conclude that the relocation test is the only test providing a sensitivity and specificity higher than 80%, making it a clinically important test. Although specificity is high for the apprehension, release, and clunk tests, they do not give reliable results.

Chronic posterior instability Posterior instability is far less frequent than anterior instability. This explains why only a small number of tests have been developed to diagnose posterior instability (Table 87.2). The evidence of tests in chronic posterior instability is very sparse. This is most likely due to its low occurrence in daily practice. Results show a high sensitivity and specificity for the Kim test, which makes this test clinically relevant. Only Kim et al.[12] have published an evaluation of this test, making it more susceptible to bias.

Recommendations
- The relocation test is the only test providing a sensitivity and specificity higher than 80% for chronic anterior instability [overall quality: moderate]
- The Kim test for chronic posterior instability is clinically relevant although it is susceptible to bias [overall quality: moderate]

Table 87.1 The evidence of tests for anterior glenohumeral instability

Studies	N	Sensitivity (%)	Specificity (%)	PPV	NPV	LR+ (95% CI)	LR− (95% CI)	Level of evidence/grade
Load and shift test								
T'Jonck et al.[1]	72	54	78			2.5 (1.5–3.8)	0.59 (0.38–0.92)	IIIb/Moderate
Apprehension test								
Speer et al.[2]	100	68	**100**	**100**	78			IIIb/Low
T'Jonck et al.[1]	72	**88**	50			1.8 (1.3–2.5)	0.23 (0.08–0.69)	IIIb/Moderate
Lo et al.[3]	46	53	**99**	**98**	73			IIIb/Low
Farber et al.[4]	363	72	**96**	75	**96**	20.2		Ib/High
Relocation test								
Speer et al.[2]	100	57	**100**	**100**	73			IIIb/Low
T'Jonck et al.[1]	72	**85**	87			6.5 (3.0–14.0)	0.18 (0.07–0.45)	IIIb/Moderate
Guanche and Jones[5]	61	44	87					IIb/Moderate
Lo et al.[3]	46	46	54	44	56			IIIb/Low
Farber et al.[4]	363	**81**	92	53	**98**	10.4		Ib/High
Release test								
Gross and Distefano[6,a]	100	**92**	89	87	93	8.2(3.6–19)	0.09(0.03–0.27)	IIIb/Low
T'Jonck et al.[1]	72	**85**	87					IIIb/Moderate
Lo et al.[3]	46	64	**99**	**98**	77			IIIb/Low
Clunk test								
T'Jonck et al.[1]	72	35	**98**			16 (2.1–110)	0.67 (0.5–0.89)	IIIb/Moderate
Crank test								
Liu et al.[7,a]	62	**91**	**93**	**94**	**90**	14 (3.5–52.0)	0.1 (0.03–0.29)	IV/Very low
Stetson and Templin[8]	65	46	56	41	61	1.1 (0.6–1.9)	0.95 (0.61–1.50)	IIIb/Low
Guanche and Jones[5]	61	40	73	**82**	29			IIb/Moderate
Walsworth et al.[9]	55	61	55			1.35 (0.68–2.69)	0.71 (0.37–1.36)	IIIb/Low
Drawer test								
Cuellar et al.[10]	300	**98**	63	35	**99**			IIIb/Low
Farber et al.[4]	363	53	**85**	35	**92**	3.6		Ib/High
Hyperabduction test								
Gagey and Gagey[11,b]	290							n/a

LR+, positive likelihood ratio, LR−, negative likelihood ratio; NPV, negative predictive value, PPV, positive predictive value.

All numbers are taken from the studies described.

Specificity, sensitivity, PPV and NPV values higher than 80% are shown in **bold.**

[a]Studies that developed and evaluated the test mentioned.

[b]Gagey and Gagey[11] developed the hyperabduction test but did not evaluate it.

Table 87.2 Evidence of tests for posterior glenohumeral instability

Tests	Studies	N	Sensitivity (%)	Specificity (%)	PPV	NPV	LR+ (95% CI)	LR− (95% CI)	Level of evidence/grade
Jerk test	Kim et al.[12]	172	73	98	88	95			IIb/Moderate
Posterior drawer test	None found								
Kim test	Kim et al.[12]	172	80	94	73	96			IIb/moderate

Question 2: What is the role of imaging in the diagnosis of chronic shoulder instability?

Finding the evidence

We performed a literature search of literature published between 1980 and December 2009 in the online resources MEDLINE and Embase with combinations of the following search terms:

- "diagnosis," "imaging," "radiology," "MRI," "MRA," "arthrography," "CT," "conventional radiographs," "ABER," "chronic," "recurrent," "shoulder instability," "glenohumeral instability," "shoulder dislocation," "shoulder subluxation"

Quality of the evidence

Level II
- 4 studies[16,18,19,20]

Level III
- 3 studies[14,15,17]

Level IV
- 1 study[21]

Level V
- 2 studies[13,22]

Findings

Radiography In the chronic unstable shoulder, conventional radiographs are useful in the acute phase of a recurrence or if the patient had no previous experience of total dislocation. They are useful in detecting bony lesions such as Hill–Sachs lesions, an impression fracture in the posterolateral humerus, and bony Bankart lesions, an avulsion of the anterior inferior part of the glenoid, or other bony abnormalities, such as fractures of the greater tuberosity.[13]

MRI For two decades, MRI and MRA have been the gold standard in diagnosing any soft tissue abnormalities in chronic shoulder instability. Cartilage, rotator cuff, ligamentous and labral status can be detected by MRI. MRI can also be used to evaluate the acuteness of bony lesions, because of its ability to identify edema. Studies have shown sensitivity of 44–100% and specificity of 66–100% of MRI in identification of labral tears associated with anterior shoulder instability.[14]

MRA is used to increase the performance of detecting labral lesions. Two types of arthrography are available: MRA using direct contrast injection in the joint, or MRA using indirect contrast injection intravenously. In a comparison of MRI and MRA findings with surgical findings, Chandnani et al.[15] found the two techniques to be roughly equivalent in ability to detect labral tears, at 96% and 93%, respectively. However, MRA was significantly more accurate in detecting detached labral fragments (96% vs. 46%) and correctly identifying labral degeneration (56% vs. 11%). Waldt et al.[16] found the accuracy of direct MRA to be 89% in detection, and 84% in classification of all labroligamentous pathology compared with arthroscopic findings. Overall, 80% of Bankart lesions, 77% of ALPSA lesions, and 50% of Perthes lesions were correctly identified. In studies by Palmer[17,18] MRA demonstrated sensitivity of 91% and 92%, and specificity of 93% and 92%, respectively, in detection of labral pathology associated with anterior shoulder instability.[15] Accurate quantification of glenoid defects by MRI has been demonstrated by Huijsmans et al.[19] when compared with CT and direct measurement in cadavers. As MRI is usually performed in the workup of symptomatic instability, this should obviate the need to obtain a CT for this purpose.

ABER view Imaging in the ABER position (abduction external rotation) improves the accuracy of labral interpretation and recognition of undersurface cuff tears (Figure 87.4). Cvitanic et al.,[20] in a study comparing MR and operative findings in 92 patients, demonstrated 89% sensitivity and 95% specificity in the diagnosis of anterior labral injuries

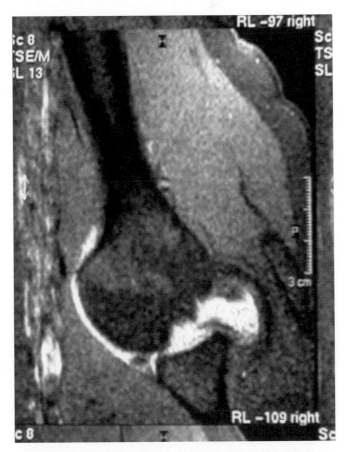

Figure 87.4 MRI-A with ABER view, showing a detached labrum, a glenoid erosion, and a Hill–Sachs lesion.

with MRA in the ABER position, compared with 48% sensitivity and 91% specificity with MRA in the conventional position. Using both in conjunction increased sensitivity to 96% and specificity to 97%.[20] In a cadaver study, Kwak[21] found that MRA in the ABER position achieved the best visualization of the inferior glenohumeral ligament. Clinicians should consider obtaining MRA in the ABER position for patients who are suspected to having a lesion of the anterior capsulolabral complex.

CT CT imaging provides a good view of bony defects as well as small glenoid fractures, glenoid version, intra-articular bodies, and the cartilage surface. It also provides the possibility to create a 3-D image of the bone. CT imaging alone is not sufficient for detection of soft tissue lesions.

An approach using contrast-injected CT arthrography (CTA) shows it to be useful in identifying labral lesions. In 1983, Shuman et al.[22] were the first to describe a good result in double-contrast CTA of the shoulder. CTA can also show lesions of the labrum, making this a good second choice when MRI is not available.

Recommendations

In the chronic unstable shoulder:
- Conventional radiography can detect bony lesions but does not supply quantitative information on the size of these lesions. It is not useful for detecting concomitant soft tissue lesions [overall quality: high]
- MRI/MRA is useful for soft tissue lesions but not for bony lesions [overall quality: high]
- The accuracy of MRA is improved in the ABER view [overall quality: high]
- CT is useful for bony lesions but not for soft tissue lesions [overall quality: high]

Question 3: What is the best surgical approach to treat chronic shoulder instability?

Finding the evidence

We performed a literature search of literature published between 2000 and December 2009 in the online resources MEDLINE and Embase with combinations of the following search terms:
- "treatment," "therapy," "surgical technique," "chronic," "recurrent," "shoulder instability," "glenohumeral instability," "shoulder dislocation," "shoulder subluxation," "open treatment," "arthroscopic"

Quality of the evidence

Level III
- 2 studies[23,24]

Findings

No consensus has so far been achieved on the surgical approach to chronic shoulder instability. Whether the tech-

nique should be open or arthroscopic has been the subject of many recent studies. Even within those two types of surgery there seems to be no consensus. For the treatment of anterior instability Hobby et al.[23] published a systematic review including a meta-analysis involving 62 studies, of which only 19 were comparative and of the comparative studies only 2 were randomized controlled trials (RCTs). Nine studies compared an open Bankart repair with or without capsular shift with arthroscopic stabilization using suture anchors or bioabsorbable tacks. There was no significant heterogeneity (p = 0.72). The meta-analysis provided a risk ratio estimate of 1.3 in favor of open surgery (95% CI 0.8–2.1) which was not statistically significant (p = 0.33). Six studies compared open techniques with arthroscopic stabilization using transglenoid sutures. The studies did not show significant heterogeneity (p = 0.42). Meta-analysis showed a statistically significant risk ratio estimate of 2.9 in favor of open surgery (95% CI 1.6–5.2; p < 0.01). The other four comparisons were of arthroscopic stabilization using transglenoid sutures with that using suture anchors. No significant heterogeneity was reported (p = 0.64), and meta-analysis showed a statistically significant risk ratio estimate of 2.0 (95% CI 1.3–3.1; p < 0.01) in favor of the use of anchors. On the basis of this meta-analysis, it appears that arthroscopic stabilization with suture anchors or bioabsorbable tacks may be as effective as open surgery, whereas transglenoid sutures should be avoided.[23]

Also for anterior instability, Lenters et al.[24] published a systematic review consisting of 4 RCTs, 10 controlled clinical trials, and 4 other comparative studies. His meta-analysis revealed that, compared with open methods, arthroscopic repairs were associated with significantly higher risks of recurrent instability (RR 2.37; 95% CI 1.66–3.38; p < 0.00001), recurrent dislocation (RR 2.74: 95% CI 1.75–4.28; p < 0.0001), and a reoperation (RR 2.32; 95% CI 1.35–3.99; p = 0.002). When considered alone, arthroscopic suture anchor techniques were associated with significantly higher risks of recurrent instability (RR 2.25; 95% CI 1.21–4.17; p = 0.01) and recurrent dislocation (RR 2.57; 95% CI 1.35–4.92; p = 0.004) than were open methods. Arthroscopic approaches were also less effective than open methods with regard to enabling patients to return to work and/or sports (RR 0.87; 95% CI 0.77–0.99; p = 0.03).

On the other hand, analysis of the randomized clinical trials indicated that arthroscopic repairs were associated with higher Rowe scores (standardized mean difference 0.43; 95% CI 0.16–0.70; p = 0.002) than were open methods. Similarly, analysis of the arthroscopic suture anchor techniques alone showed the Rowe scores to be higher (standardized mean difference 0.29, 95% CI 0.01–0.56; p = 0.04) than those associated with open methods. Although the higher Rowe scores in the arthroscopic repairs suggest a better function and motion of the shoulder, this is not proven in this review.[24]

The conclusion of these meta-analyses is that at the present state the open methods provide better results with respect to recurrence compared to all possible arthroscopic methods. However, at present anchors are mostly used and the results of arthroscopic repair with anchors can compete with the standard open methods. In these meta-analyses the influence of other aspects, like the extent of bony lesions at the glenoid or humeral side are not considered.

Recommendation
• The results of arthroscopic repair with anchors are comparable to the standard open methods [overall quality: moderate]

Question 4: What is the role of bone defects in the treatment of chronic unstable shoulder?

Finding the evidence
We performed a literature search of literature published between 2000 and December 2009 in the online resources MEDLINE and Embase with combinations of the following search terms:
• "bone defect," "bony lesion," "bone avulsion," "bony Bankart," "glenoid," "humeral," "chronic," "recurrent," "shoulder instability," "glenohumeral instability," "shoulder dislocation," "shoulder subluxation"

Quality of the evidence
Level II
• 2 studies[27,28]

Level III
• 5 studies[25,26,29–31]

Findings
Since Burkhart et al.[25] showed an important role of the glenoid defect on the results of arthroscopic repair there has been an ongoing discussion about the limit of soft tissue repair in chronic instability.

The incidence of bone defects varies widely in the literature. The reported prevalence of fracture or erosion of the anteroinferior part of the glenoid rim among shoulders with recurrent anterior dislocation has been reported to range from 8% to 73%.[26] The prevalence of a Hill–Sachs lesion in patients with recurrent anterior dislocation of the shoulder ranges from 47% to 100%.[27]

There are now adequate ways to measure the glenoid defect, following the finding that the inferior part of the glenoid is circular,[28,29] but the only precise and quantitative way is with CT or MRI. Humeral head defects are measured in different ways, focusing on either the depth or the width of the defect. The interplay of the defects at either side of the joint is also under investigation.[30]

Recommendation
• No studies are available showing the relation of the results of soft tissue repair, either arthroscopically or open, with an exactly measured defect of either the humeral head or the glenoid cavity[31] [overall quality: low]

Question 5: What is the role of rehabilitation in chronic shoulder instability?

Finding the evidence
We performed a literature search of literature published between 1990 and December 2009 in the online resources MEDLINE and Embase with combinations of the following search terms:
• "rehabilitation," "physiotherapy," "conservative treatment," "nonsurgical treatment," "chronic," "recurrent," "shoulder instability," "glenohumeral instability," "shoulder dislocation," "shoulder subluxation"

Quality of the evidence
Level II
• 1 study[34]

Level III
• 1 study[32]

Level IV
• 1 study[33]

Findings
In a systematic review of 14 studies (3 RCTs, 3 moderate quality cohorts, 5 poor quality cohorts and 3 case series) Gibson has shown that evidence is weak for the statement that physical therapy enables the athlete to return to premorbid activity level.[32] Physiotherapy plays no role in prevention of recurrences in chronic shoulder instability.[33]

After repair of a chronic unstable shoulder, a protocol is generally recommended that includes immobilization and exercises in a restricted range of motion during 6 weeks, especially regarding external rotation. This is based on the presumption that soft tissue heals to bone in about this period of time.

One level IIb study, comparing a group of patients after arthroscopic instability repair with either immobilization or accelerated rehabilitation postoperatively with a follow-up of a mean of 31 months shows that an accelerated program, including immediate staged exercises and strengthening, does not influence the results.[34]

Recommendation
• Physiotherapy plays no role in prevention of recurrences in chronic shoulder instability, and an accelerated rehabilitation program, including immediate staged exercises and

strengthening, does not influence the results [overall quality: low]

Question 6: What is the natural history in chronic unstable shoulders?

Finding the evidence
We performed a literature search of literature published between 1990 and December 2009 in the online resources MEDLINE and Embase with combinations of the following search terms:
- "natural history," "conservative treatment," "non-surgical treatment," "prognosis," "chronic," "recurrence," "shoulder instability," "glenohumeral instability," "shoulder dislocation," "shoulder subluxation"

Quality of the evidence
Level I
- 2 studies[35,36]

Findings
Few studies are available to demonstrate the natural history of a chronic unstable shoulder. Hovelius[35] showed, that at 25 years, the total number of shoulders that became stable over time had increased, when compared with the 10 year follow-up, from 49% to 65%.

In another study by Hovelius[36] with a 25 year follow-up it was shown that, among other factors, recurrence is associated with the development of arthropathy. Shoulders without a recurrence were also associated with arthropathy. Thirty-nine per cent of the shoulders that redislocated once or more (without surgery) and 26% of the surgically stabilized shoulders showed moderate to severe arthropathy after 25 years of follow-up after the first dislocation.

Recommendation
- Recurrence is associated with the development of arthropathy, but shoulders without a recurrence were also associated with arthropathy [overall quality: moderate]

Summary of recommendations

- The relocation test is the only test providing a sensitivity and specificity higher than 80% for chronic anterior instability
- The Kim test for chronic posterior instability is clinically relevant although it is susceptible to bias
- Conventional radiography can detect bony lesions but does not supply quantitative information on the size of these lesions. It is not useful for detecting concomitant soft tissue lesions
- MRI/MRA is useful for soft tissue lesions but not for bony lesions

- The accuracy of MRA is improved in the ABER view
- CT is useful for bony lesions but not for soft tissue lesions
- The results of arthroscopic repair with anchors are comparable to the standard open methods
- No studies are available showing the relation of the results of soft tissue repair, either arthroscopically or open, with an exactly measured defect of either the humeral head or the glenoid cavity
- Physiotherapy plays no role in prevention of recurrences in chronic shoulder instability, and an accelerated rehabilitation program, including immediate staged exercises and strengthening, does not influence the results
- Recurrence is associated with the development of arthropathy, but shoulders without a recurrence were also associated with arthropathy

References

1. T'Jonck L, Staes F, Smet L de, Lysens R. The relationship between clinical shoulder tests and the findings in arthroscopic examination. Geneeskunde Sport 2001;34:15–24.
2. Speer KP, Hannafin JA, Altchek DW, Warren RF, An evaluation of the shoulder relocation test. Am J Sports Med 1994;22(2):177–83.
3. Lo IKY, Nonweiler B, Woolfrey M, Litchfield R, Kirkley A. An evaluation of the apprehension, relocation, and surprise tests for anterior shoulder instability. Am J Sports Med 2004;32(2):301–307.
4. Farber AJ, Castillo R, Clough M, Bahk M, McFarland EG Clinical assessment of three common tests for traumatic anterior shoulder instability. J Bone Joint Surg Am 2006;88(7):1467–74.
5. Guanche CA, Jones DC. Clinical testing for tear of the glenoid labrum. Arthroscopy 2003;19(5):517–23.
6. Gross ML, Distefano MC Anterior release test: a new test for occult shoulder instability. Clin Orthop Relat Res 1997;339:105–8.
7. Liu SH, Henry MH, Nuccion SL. A prospective evaluation of a new physical examination in predicting glenoid labral tears. Am J Sports Med 1996;24(6):721–5.
8. Stetson WB, Templin K. The crank test, the O'Brien test, and routine magnetic resonance imaging scans in the diagnosis of labral tears. Am J Sports Med 2002;30(6):806–9.
9. Walsworth MK, Doukas WC, Murphy KP, Mielcarek BJ, Michener LA. Reliability and diagnostic accuracy of history and physical examination for diagnosing glenoid labral tears. Am J Sports Med 2008;36(1):162–8.
10. Cuéllar R, González J, Herrán G de la, Usabiaga J. Exploration of glenohumeral instability under anesthesia: the shoulder jerk test. Arthroscopy 2005;21(6):672–9.
11. Gagey OJ, Gagey N. The hyperabduction test: an assessment of the laxity of the inferior glenohumeral ligament. J Bone Joint Surg Br 2000;83(1):69–74.
12. Kim S-H, Park J-S, Jeong W-K, Shin S-K. The Kim test: a novel test for posteroinferior labral lesion of the shoulder—a comparison to the jerk test. Am J Sports Med 2005;33(8):1188–92.

13. Goud A, Segal D, Hedayati P, Pan JJ, Weissman BN. Radiographic evaluation of the shoulder. Eur J Radiol 2008;68:2–15.

14. Murray PJ, Shaffer BS Clinical update: MR imaging of the shoulder. Sports Med Arthrosc Rev 2009;17(1):40–8.

15. Chandnani VP, Yeager TD, DeBerardino T, et al. Glenoid labral tears: prospective evaluation with MR imaging, MR arthrography, and CT arthrography. Am J Roentgenol 1993;161:1229–35.

16. Waldt S, Burkart A, Imhoff AB, et al. Anterior shoulder instability: accuracy of MR arthrography in the classification of anteroinferior labroligamentous injuries. Radiology 2005;237:578–83.

17. Palmer WE, Brown JH, Rosenthal DI. Labral-ligamentous complex of the shoulder: evaluation with MR arthrography. Radiology 1994;190:645–51.

18. Palmer WE, Caslowitz PL. Anterior shoulder instability: diagnostic criteria determined from prospective analysis of 121 MR arthrograms. Radiology 1995;197:819–25.

19. Huijsmans PE, Haen PS, Kidd M, Hulst VP van der, Willems WJ. Quantification of a glenoid defect with three-dimensional computed tomography and magnetic resonance imaging: a cadaveric study. J Shoulder Elbow Surg 2007;16:803–9.

20. Cvitanic O, Tirman PF, Feller JF. Using abduction and external rotation of the shoulder to increase the sensitivity of MR arthrography in revealing tears of the anterior glenoid labrum. Am J Roentgenol 1997;169(3):837–44.

21. Kwak SM, Brown RR, Trudell D. Glenohumeral joint: comparison of shoulder positions at MR arthrography. Radiology 1998;208:375–80.

22. Shuman WP, Kilcoyne RF, Matsen FA, Rogers JV, Mack LA. Double-contrast computed tomography of the glenoid labrum. Am J Roentgenol 1983;141(3):581–4.

23. Hobby J, Griffin D, Dunbar M, Boileau P. Is arthroscopic surgery for stabilisation of chronic shoulder instability as effective as open surgery? A systematic review and meta-analysis of 62 studies including 3044 arthroscopic operations. J Bone Joint Surg Br 2007;89,1188–96.

24. Lenters TR, Franta AK, Wolf FM, Leopold SS, Matsen FA 3rd. Arthroscopic compared with open repairs for recurrent anterior shoulder instability: A systematic review and meta-analysis of the literature. J Bone Joint Surg Am 2007;89:244–54.

25. Burkhart SS, De Beer JF Traumatic glenohumeral bone defects and their relationship to failure of arthroscopic Bankart repairs: significance of the inverted-pear glenoid and the humeral engaging Hill-Sachs lesions. Arthroscopy 2000;16(7):677–94.

26. Itoi E, Lee S-B, Berglund LJ, Berge LL, An K-N. The effect of a glenoid defect on anteroinferior stability of the shoulder after Bankart repair: a cadaveric study. J Bone Joint Surg Am 2000;82(1):35–46.

27. Saito H, Itoi E, Minagawa H, Yamamoto N, Tuoheti Y, Seki, N. Location of Hill-Sachs lesion in shoulders with recurrent dislocation. Arch Orthop Trauma Surg 2009;129:1327–34.

28. Sugaya H, Moriishi J, Dohi M, Kon Y, Tsuchiya A. Glenoid rim morphology in recurrent anterior glenohumeral instability. J Bone Joint Surg Am 2003;85:878–84.

29. Huysmans PE, Haen PS, Kidd M, Dhert WJ, Willems WJ. The shape of the inferior part of the glenoid: a cadaveric study. J Shoulder Elbow Surg 2006;15:759–63.

30. Yamamoto N, Itoi E, Abe H, Minagawa H, Seki N, Shimada Y, Okada K. Contact between the glenoid and the humeral head in abduction, external rotation and horizontal extension: a new concept of glenoid track. J Shoulder Elbow Surg 2007;16:649–56.

31. Balg F, Boileau P. The instability severity index score. A simple pre-operative score to select patients for arthroscopic or open shoulder stabilisation. J Bone Joint Surg Br 2007;89(11):1470–7.

32. Gibson K, Growse A, Korda L, Wray E, Macdermid JC. The effectiveness of rehabilitation for non-operative management of shoulder instability: a systematic review. J Hand Therap 2004;17:229–42.

33. Brostrom LA, Kronberg M, Nemeth G, Oxelback U. The effect of shoulder muscle training in patients with recurrent shoulder dislocations. Scan J Rehabil Med 1992;24:11–15.

34. Kim SH, Ha KI, Jung MW, Lim MS, Kim YM, Park JH. Accelerated rehabilitation after arthroscopic Bankart repair for selected cases: a prospective randomized clinical study. Arthroscopy 2003;19:722–31.

35. Hovelius L, Olofsson A, Sandstrom B, et al. Nonoperative treatment of primary anterior shoulder dislocation in patients forty years of age and younger. a prospective twenty-five-year follow-up. J Bone Joint Surg Am 2008;90:945–52.

36. Hovelius L, Saeboe M. Arthropathy after primary anterior shoulder dislocation—223 shoulders prospectively followed up for twenty-five years. J Shoulder Elbow Surg 2009;18:339–47.

88   Rotator Cuff Injury

John E. Kuhn

Vanderbilt University School of Medicine, Nashville, TN, USA

Case scenario

A 75 year old woman presents to the office with a complaint of right shoulder pain of insidious onset. She describes difficulty sleeping at night, pain with activity, and crepitus in the shoulder. Physical examination demonstrates full active range of motion except in external rotation with the arm at the side, atrophy in the supraspinatus and infraspinatus fossae, pain with supraspinatus strength testing, and weakness in external rotation.

Relevant anatomy

The rotator cuff consists of four muscles (subscapularis, supraspinatus, infraspinatus, and teres major) whose origins are on the scapular body and insertions are on the lesser (subscapularis) and greater (supra and infraspinatus, teres major) tuberosities. The upper two thirds of the subscapularis is mostly tendon—much more so than the other rotator cuff muscles. The suprascapular nerve innervates the supraspinatus and infraspinatus. The tendon has layers with different mechanical properties—the articular side of the rotator cuff is more like glenohumeral joint capsule, whereas the middle portion is more like tendon. Tears generally start in the supraspinatus, and propagate posterior to involve the infraspinatus.

Importance of the problem

Rotator cuff disease is a common cause of disability and pain. Approximately one third of subjects over the age of 65 report shoulder pain with some degree of disability,[1,2] and in the workplace, rotator cuff disease is common and seen in 54.0 per 10,000 full time employees in Washington State worker's compensation claims,[3] second only to carpal tunnel syndrome for upper extremity disorders.[4]

Rotator cuff tears are extremely prevalent in symptomatic and asymptomatic individuals[5] (Table 88.1), but are more common in symptomatic people[5] and older people,[6] and are often bilateral.[7]

Between 1998 and 2004 over 5 million physician visits in the United States were attributed to rotator cuff problems,[8] a figure that will increase as the population ages. In New York State, rotator cuff repairs increased by 50% over a 5 year span.[9]

Most rotator cuff repairs are performed in an outpatient setting, and although accurate numbers are not available, estimates for outpatient rotator cuff repair range from 75,000/year[4] to 250,000/year.[10]

Although the cost per patient for rotator cuff repairs in US averaged $17,427 in 2004,[11] rotator cuff repair is considered a cost-effective procedure by Health Utility Index ($13,092.84/QALY) and by the EuroQol (3,091.90/QALY)—values that compare favorably with other common interventions, and reach cost-effective benchmarks currently in use.[12]

Top five questions

Diagnosis

1. What are the best physical examination tests to identify a rotator cuff tear?
2. What is the best way to image the rotator cuff tear?

Evidence-Based Orthopedics, First Edition. Edited by Mohit Bhandari.
© 2012 Blackwell Publishing Ltd. Published 2012 by Blackwell Publishing Ltd.

Table 88.1 Prevalence of rotator cuff tears[5]

	Asymptomatic		Symptomatic	
	Partial thickness tears (%)	Full thickness tears (%)	Partial thickness tears (%)	Full thickness tears (%)
Cadaver studies	10.39	12.68	NA	
Ultrasound	17.2	21.7	6.7	34.7
MRI	15.87	10.33	49.38	40.8

NA, data not available.

Treatment

3. Does nonoperative treatment have a role?
4. What are the best techniques for rotator cuff repair?

Harm

5. What are the complications of rotator cuff surgery?

Question 1: What are the best physical examination tests to find a rotator cuff tear?

Case clarification

The patient has night pain, crepitus, and full motion. Does this patient have a rotator cuff tear?

Relevance

Some physical examination tests may be helpful to identify if a rotator cuff tear exists, which may prompt the healthcare provider to consider imaging or other measures before initiating treatment.

Current opinion

Most physicians consider the physical examination to be only moderately helpful in finding rotator cuff tears.

Finding the evidence

The following literature databases were searched using the search terms "(rotator cuff tear AND physical exam$)":
- Cochrane Database of Systematic Reviews
- ACP Journal Club
- DARE
- PubMed (clinical queries and systematic reviews)
- PubMed 1950–April 2010
- Embase

   This produced 67 potential references. Of these 51 were excluded as they did not study physical examination techniques, 2 were excluded as they were not studies of rotator cuff disease, and 8 were excluded as they were review

papers. This left 6 articles for thorough review; an additional 13 were found using the references cited in these manuscripts, to give a total of 19 on which this review is based.

Quality of evidence

Level I
- 8 studies[13–20]

Level II
- 1 study[21]

Level III
- 7 studies[22–28]

Level IV
- 2 systematic reviews/meta-analyses[29,30]
- 1 study[31]

Findings

Surprising variation is noted when different researchers evaluate the same test (Table 88.2). This may relate to problems in reproducibility of physical examination tests for rotator cuff disease.[32,33] One of the best tests for identifying rotator cuff tears is the "rent test" where the defect in the supraspinatus is palpated through the deltoid muscle. This test has a positive likelihood ratio (+LR) approaching that of MRI imaging. Lag signs, when present, are also helpful to identify rotator cuff tears. Unfortunately, as evidenced by negative likelihood ratio (–LR) close to 1.0, a rotator cuff tear may still be present if the test is negative (Table 88.2).

Recommendation

- When examining patients with suspected rotator cuff tears, lag signs and the rent test, when positive, are helpful to diagnose a rotator cuff tear. If the history suggests a rotator cuff tear when these tests are negative, imaging modalities may be required [overall quality: moderate]

Question 2: What is the best imaging study to diagnose rotator cuff tears?

Case clarification

The patient has a full range of motion, pain with supraspinatus strength testing, a positive rent test, and a negative lag sign. You suspect a rotator cuff tear. What imaging test should you order?

Relevance

A number of imaging tests are available to identify rotator cuff tears. Some patients with advanced cuff disease have radiographs that can identify cuff tears. MRI is used commonly, but is expensive. MRI arthrogram may improve accuracy. Ultrasound is gaining in popularity.

Table 88.2 Data from level I studies of physical examination techniques to diagnose full thickness rotator cuff tears

Test	Authors	N	Sens	Spec	PPV	NPV	LR+	LR–
Drop test	Miller 2008	37	0.73	0.77	0.61	0.85	3.2	0.3
Jobe–pain	Itoi 1999	143	0.63	0.55	0.31	0.82	1.4	0.7
Jobe–pain	Kim2006	200	0.939	0.939	0.462	0.939	15.39	0.065
Jobe–weakness	Itoi 1999	143	0.77	0.68	.44	.90	2.4	0.3
Jobe–weakness	Kim 2006	200	0.757	0.709	0.562	0.855	2.60	0.343
Full can–pain	Itoi 1999	143	0.66	0.64	0.37	0.85	1.8	0.5
Full can–pain	Kim 2006	200	0.712	0.679	0.552	0.827	2.218	.424
Full can–weakness	Itoi 1999	143	0.77	0.74	0.49	0.91	3.0	0.3
Full can–weakness	Kim 2006	200	0.773	0.679	0.543	0.858	2.408	.334
Supraspinatus test	Holtby 2004	50	0.411	0.697	0.411	0.697	1.37	0.84
External rotation lag sign	Miller 2008	37	0.46	0.94	0.77	0.78	7.2	0.6
Neer	MacDonald 2000	85	0.833	0.508	.400	0.886	1.693	0.329
Hawkins	MacDonald 2000	85	0.875	0.426	0.375	0.897	1.524	0.293
Rent test (trans deltoid palpation)	Wolf 2001	109	0.957	0.968	0.957	0.968	30.1	0.0

LR, likelihood ratio; NPV, negative predictive value; PPV, positive predictive value; Sens, sensitivity; Spec, specificity.

Current opinion

Plain radiographs can identify rotator cuff tears by superior humeral head migration. MRI is very useful, but ultrasound is gaining in popularity.

Finding the evidence

The following literature databases were searched using the search terms: "(rotator cuff tear AND (imaging or magnetic resonance imaging OR arthrography OR arthrogram OR ultrasound OR ultrasonography)":

- Cochrane Database of Systematic Reviews
- ACP Journal Club
- DARE
- PubMed (clinical queries: systematic reviews)
- PubMed 1950–April 2010
- Embase

This search produced 648 references. Of these 265 were excluded for not dealing with rotator cuff tears; 190 were excluded for not studying imaging techniques; 57 were review papers or abstracts; 12 were excluded for imaging of postoperative shoulders. This left 124 articles for review. Of this group 20 were excluded for not involving rotator cuff tears; 13 were excluded as they were comparisons of different MRI techniques; 18 were excluded as they were studies of cadavers or normal subjects; 23 were excluded as they were published before 1995; 19 were excluded as they were not in English. This left 30 manuscripts for thorough review which were broken down as follows.

Quality of evidence

Level I
- 16 studies[34–49]

Level II
- 3 studies[50–52]

Level III
- 2 systematic reviews/meta-analysis[53–54]
- 5 studies[55–59]

Level IV
- 4 case control studies[60–63]

Findings

AP radiographs used to measure superior humeral head migration are accurate compared to CT imaging.[47] When superior humeral head migration is seen it has been associated with multiple tendon rotator cuff tears[60,62,63] and fatty degeneration of the rotator cuff muscle.[51] A decreased acromiohumeral interval is also seen in patients with impingement when compared to normal subjects.[61]

Arthrography, or digital subtraction arthrography may be helpful to diagnose a full thickness tear,[55] but cannot accurately determine the size of the tear.[36]

CT arthrography has sensitivities and specificities above 95% for diagnosis of supraspinatus and infraspinatus tears.[50] MRI sensitivities and specificities are generally above 85%.[46,49,52,59] Ultrasound sensitivities and specificities are generally above 85% for full thickness tears,[35,42,43,45] with some variation.[58] Ultrasound is less sensitive or specific for the diagnosis of partial thickness tears.[40,43–45,54,57]

Studies that compare different imaging techniques have shown that double contrast arthrography cannot diagnose or determine the size of a rotator cuff tear as well as ultrasound or CT arthrography.[37] Ultrasound compares well to

CT arthrography[37] in evaluating the size and site of rotator cuff tears.

MRI and ultrasound are not very different in their ability to diagnose full thickness rotator cuff tears and determine the size of the tear.[34,38–41,45,53,56] MRI arthrography is more sensitive and specific than MRI or ultrasound in diagnosing a full or partial thickness rotator cuff tear.[53]

Recommendations

• When superior humeral head migration is seen on AP radiographs it usually is diagnostic for a large rotator cuff tear with fatty infiltration. MRI or ultrasound may be used for identification of smaller tears and to assess the size of the rotator cuff tear equally well. MRI arthrography may add information, particularly when a partial rotator cuff tear is suspected [overall quality: moderate]

Question 3: Does nonoperative treatment have a role in rotator cuff tears?

Case clarification

The patient has a rotator cuff tear. How should you manage it? What is the role of nonoperative treatment?

Relevance

There is great geographic variation in how rotator cuff tears are managed.[64] The indications for surgical intervention are not agreed upon or clear.[65,66]

A conservative estimate of prevalence suggests that 10% of people over the age of 60 have rotator cuff tears.[5] Using data from the 2006 US census, this equates to more than 5 million people. In the USA approximately 75,000 rotator cuff surgeries are performed each year.[12] This means that over 98% of the population with rotator cuff tears do not have surgery, suggesting very few are symptomatic.

In addition, patients who undergo surgery often fail their repairs (Table 88.3), yet report satisfaction and pain relief after treatment.[67] This data suggests that there is a role for nonoperative treatment of patients with rotator cuff tears.

Table 88.3 Failure of repair

Author	Failures (%)	Features related to failures
Galatz 2004	94	All massive tears
Boileau 2005	25	Age, size of tear
Liu 1994	24	Size of tear
Cole 2007	22	Age, size of tear
Levy 2008	18.6	Age
Fuchs 2006	13	Not reported
Paulos 1994	5.5	Size of tear

Current opinion

Rotator cuff repairs should be performed in select patients.

Finding the evidence

The following literature databases were searched using the search terms: "(rotator cuff tear AND non-operative OR physical therapy OR rehabilitation)"

• Cochrane Database of Systematic Reviews
• ACP Journal Club
• DARE
• PubMed (clinical queries: systematic reviews)
• PubMed 1950–April 2010
• Embase

This search produced 378 hits. Of these 366 were excluded: 66 were review manuscripts; 170 did not related to rotator cuff tears; 98 involved surgical treatment; 11 were in-vitro or outcome tool development studies; 12 were imaging studies; 5 assessed comorbidities, indications for surgery, or surgeons' perceptions; and 4 assessed topical or injectable treatments for shoulder pain, leaving 12 studies for more thorough review.

Quality of the evidence

Level I

• 1 study[68]

Level III

• 1 study[69]

Level IV

• 1 systematic review/meta-analysis[70]
• 9 studies[71–79]

Findings

Multiple case series report success with nonoperative treatment to range between 59–85%; however, these studies are subject to selection bias and generally include only those patients with massive tears in whom surgery cannot be performed, and data was collected retrospectively.[70]

One randomized trial compared open surgery (N = 52) to physical therapy (N = 51) in patients with traumatic and atraumatic tears less than 3 cm.[68] ASES and Constant scores were significantly different after 6 months, favoring surgery (suggesting the improvement in strength influences scores). Interestingly 24% of repairs did not heal completely, and only 9 of 51 (18%) of the physical therapy group decided to have surgery.

A level IV systematic review of the literature suggests that acute rotator cuff tears with functional loss and weakness may benefit from earlier surgical intervention.[65]

Rotator cuff tears may progress after nonoperative treatment, with increases in size, and fatty infiltration.[80–83] It is unknown if these increases in disease produce patient difficulties later; however, asymptomatic tears may progress and become symptomatic.[84]

Recommendations

• Currently the evidence is weak to make recommendations regarding indications for surgery, and deciding who would do well with nonoperative treatment. Low-level evidence suggests that traumatic tears with loss of function, or weakness are reasonable indications for surgery. Other patients may be managed nonoperatively, but should be counseled that their tear may progress in size [overall quality: low]

Question 4: What surgical treatments are best?

Case clarification

The patient has a rotator cuff tear. She would like to have surgery. What approaches might work best?

Relevance

Rotator cuff repairs are common and technology is evolving

Current opinion

Rotator cuff repairs should be performed in select patients; opinions vary on indications and technical aspects of the approach.

Finding the evidence

The following literature databases were searched using the search terms: "(rotator cuff repair)" and a separate search for "(rotator cuff trial)"

• Cochrane Database of Systematic Reviews
• ACP Journal Club
• DARE
• PubMed (clinical queries: systematic reviews)
• PubMed 1950–April 2010
• Embase

This search produced 273 hits. Of these, 120 were not comparative trials and were excluded, 55 were not pertaining to rotator cuff tears, 24 were not clinical studies, 24 were not in English, and 14 were reviews or abstracts, 2 systematic reviews were withdrawn as they were not up to date, leaving 34 for thorough review.

Quality of the evidence

Level I
• 16 studies[68,85–99]

Level II
• 6 studies[100–105]

Level III
• 2 systematic reviews/meta-analysis[106,107]
• 9 studies[108–116]

Level IV
• 1 systematic review/meta-analysis[117]

Findings

Evidence on comparative effectiveness for different surgical treatments is limited and somewhat inconclusive,[107] and it may not be appropriate to generalize the results of single-site studies of technical aspects of surgery to other surgeons; however, comparative trials have concluded the following.

Patients who have failed rotator cuff repairs report outcome scores that are not significantly different than patients whose repairs have healed,[95,112,117] unless the outcome score includes a large component for strength (e.g., the Constant score), in which case healed repairs have better scores.[68,117]

With regard to the approach used, open repairs improve strength, function, and outcome scores compared to arthroscopic debridement of rotator cuff tears, but patient satisfaction does not differ.[104] Patients with massive tears who undergo a partial repair have better Constant scores than tears that are debrided.[85] Mini-open rotator cuff repair has similar outcome scores[107,110] and improved active forward elevation compared to open repair.[110] Mini-open rotator cuff repairs have improved short-term scores (3 months), but scores at 28 months or 2 years are comparable to open repairs.[98] Arthroscopic repairs (with both knot tying and knotless systems) have improved outcomes compared to open repairs;[114] however, rotator cuff repair failure is more common for large tears repaired arthroscopically compared to open repair.[102] Arthroscopic rotator cuff repair techniques produce similar outcome scores[107,111,113,115] and healing rates[113] when compared to mini-open repairs.

With regard to open techniques, transosseous repair using No. 3 Ethibond and modified Mason-Allen sutures had similar Constant scores, failure rates, and complications compared to transosseous repair with 1.0 mm polydioxanone cord and modified Kessler sutures.[87] Porcine small intestine submucosa augmentation of large and massive rotator cuff tear repairs produced lower outcome scores,[94] greater strength deficits,[116] and did not improve healing rates[94] compared to controls.

With regard to arthroscopic techniques, arthroscopic subacromial decompression has not been shown to improve outcome scores after rotator cuff repair.[92,97,107] Rotator cuff repairs using a suture anchor to the greater tuberosity have better Constant scores and strength than repairs performed side to side without fixation to the tuberosity.[86] Double row repairs do not seem to improve outcomes over single row repairs;[101,103,105–107] however, healing rates[103] and improvements in strength for larger tears[105] may favor double row techniques. Failures of single row repairs were more likely to occur at the repair site than with the suture bridge technique, which failed at the musculotendinous junction.[108] A massive cuff stitch method of arthroscopic rotator cuff repair had significantly improved healing rates compared to an arthroscopic simple stitch repair.[112]

Patients with rotator cuff repairs have outcomes similar to patients who have rotator cuff repairs and concomitant SLAP (superior labrum from anterior to posterior) lesion repairs,[109] but patients with concomitant rotator cuff repairs and SLAP lesions have better outcomes and motion if the SLAP tear is debrided than if it is repaired.[89,100]

There is conflicting evidence regarding continuous passive motion compared to passive self-assisted range of motion exercises for 4 weeks, with some studies suggesting continuous passive motion may reduce pain and improve range of motion,[91] and others finding no differences.[96]

Recommendations

- The data suggests that rotator cuff repairs can improve patient reported outcomes, even if the repairs fail. Strength and functional improvements are greater if the repair heals [overall quality: high]
- Open, mini-open, and arthroscopic approaches are similar, but patients who have open approaches may have lower outcome scores at 3 months [overall quality: high]
- Arthroscopic approaches should include anchor fixation to the greater tuberosity. However, the double row technique does not seem to affect outcome scores, but may improve healing, especially for larger tears [overall quality: high]
- Acromioplasty has not been shown to affect outcome scores, but has not been studied to see if it has an effect on healing [overall quality: high]
- Porcine small intestine mucosa should not be used to augment repairs [overall quality: high]

Question 5: What are the complications after rotator cuff repair?

Case clarification

The patient is interested in undergoing surgery. What are the risks of rotator cuff repair surgery?

Relevance

Patient should understand risks of rotator cuff repair surgery.

Current opinion

Risks are small.

Finding the evidence

The following literature databases were searched using the search terms "(rotator cuff repair AND (complications OR risk))"

- Cochrane Database of Systematic Reviews
- ACP Journal Club
- DARE
- PubMed (clinical queries: systematic reviews)
- PubMed 1950–April 2010
- Embase

418 hits were reviewed. Of these, 49 were reviews, editorials, or letters; 39 were in-vivo studies or technical reports; 59 were describing surgeries other than rotator cuff repair for cuff tears; 23 were reports for subscapularis tears, partial tears, tendonosis, or revision repairs; 15 were not in English; 151 were reports on conditions other than the treatment of rotator cuff tears; leaving 82 manuscripts for more thorough review. Of these, 23 offered data on complications after rotator cuff repair.

Quality of the evidence

Level III
- 2 studies[118–119]

Level IV
- 21 studies[120–140]

Findings

Complications included failure of repair (Table 88.3), and infection, stiffness, hardware failure, nerve injury, deltoid disruption (Table 88.4), and technical aspects such as the creation of dog-ear deformity using suture bridge technique.[132] Case reports included anchor penetration through

Table 88.4 Complications after rotator cuff repair

Complication	Prevalence (%)	Reference
Technical—dog ear deformity	47	132
Heterotopic ossification[1]	20.7	124
Stiffness	13.6	119
	8.7	121
	4.9	131
	0.5	136
Deltoid detachment open repair	8	127
	0.5	136
Infection	Superficial 4.3	134
	Superficial 3.4	136
	Deep 1.9	129
	Deep 1.7	136
	Deep 0.9	128
	Deep 0.8	120
	Deep 0.4	121
Hardware anchor failure	2.4	122
	2.3	137
Nerve injury	1.1	136
	0.9	128
Suture granuloma	0.5	136
Wound hematoma	0.4	136
Reflex sympathetic dystrophy	0.4	121
	0.1	136
Deep venous thrombosis	0.4	121
Pulmonary embolism	0.86	136
	0.26	130

articular cartilage,[140] unrecognized breakage of nitinol needle in shoulder,[138] heterotopic ossification,[124,133] and persistent fistula.[125,139] Patients with diabetes are at higher risk for failure and infection.[118]

Recommendations

• Patients who are considering surgery to treat rotator cuff tears should be made aware of all complications, including failure, stiffness, infection, and failure of hardware, all of which have been reported to occur in more than 1% of rotator cuff repairs. Failure is the highest complication [overall quality: low]

Summary of recommendations

• When evaluating a patient with a suspected rotator cuff tear, the rent test and lag signs can identify a torn rotator cuff, but when these signs are absent imaging in the form of ultrasound or MRI may be indicated.
• Nonoperative treatment may be effective for relief of pain, but high-level evidence is lacking in the literature
• Weakness or loss of function, and acute injuries are indications for repair, but even if repairs fail, patient outcomes are improved and may be difficult to distinguish from healed repairs
• A variety of repair techniques have been described in the literature. Acromioplasty at the time of rotator cuff repair does not seem to change outcomes. The tendon should be anchored to the tuberosity, yet double row techniques do not seem to improve outcomes compared to single row techniques, except perhaps for larger tears where healing may be better with double row techniques. Porcine submucosa graft should not be used to augment rotator cuff repair. Many complications have been described, but failure of the repair is most common

Conclusions

Rotator cuff tears are extremely common and most are presumably asymptomatic. The evidence suggests that physical examination tests may detect tears, but cannot rule out tears. Ultrasound and MRI are fairly equivalent in detecting full thickness tears. More work is needed to identify who would be treated best with surgery, and which surgical techniques improve healing rates.

References

1. Chakravarty K, Webley M. Shoulder joint movement and its relationship to disability in the elderly. J Rheumatol 1993;20: 1359–61.

2. Chard MD, Hazleman R, Hazleman BL, et al. Shoulder disorders in the elderly: a community survey. Arthritis Rheum 1991;34:766–9.

3. Silverstein B, Welp E, Nelson N, et al. Claims incidence of work-related disorders of the upper extremities: Washington state, 1987 through 1995. Am J Public Health 1998;88:1827–33.

4. Silverstein B, Viikari-Juntura E, Kalat J. Use of a prevention index to identify industries at high risk for work-related musculoskeletal disorders of the neck, back, and upper extremity in Washington state, 1990–1998. Am J Ind Med 2002;41: 149–69.

5. Reilly P, Macleod I, Macfarlane R, Windley J. Dead men and radiologists don't lie: a review of cadaveric and radiological studies of rotator cuff tear prevalence. Ann R Coll Surg Engl 2006;88:116–21.

6. Tempelhof S, Rupp S, Seil R. Age-related prevalence of rotator cuff tears in asymptomatic shoulders. J Shoulder Elbow Surg 1999;8(4):296–9.

7. Yamaguchi K, Ditsios K, Middleton WD, Hildebolt CF, Galatz LM, Teefey SA. The demographic and morphological features of rotator cuff disease. J Bone Joint Surg 2006;88:1699–704.

8. American Academy of Orthopaedic Surgeons, Research Statistics on Rotator Cuff Repairs, National Ambulatory Medical Care Survey, 1998–2004. Data obtained from: U.S. Department of Health and Human Services; Centers for Disease Control and Prevention; National Center for Health Statistics. Retrieved on May 9, 2007 from http://www.aaos.org/Researh/stats/patientstats.asp

9. Sherman SL, Lyman S, Koulouvaris P, Willis A, Marx RG. Risk factors for readmission and revision surgery following rotator cuff repair. Clin Orthop Relat Res 2008;466:608–13.

10. McCormick H. ArthroCare closes opus medical acquisition, Orthopaedic and Dental Industry News, Healthpoint Capital, NY, NY, November 22, 2004.

11. American Academy of Orthopaedic Surgeons, Research Statistics on Rotator Cuff Repairs, National Inpatient Sample, 1998–2004. Data obtained from: The Agency for Healthcare Research and Quality, 2007.

12. Vitale MA, Vitale MG, Zivin JG, Braman JP, Bigliani LU, Flatow EL. Rotator cuff repair: an analysis of utility scores and cost-effectiveness. J Shoulder Elbow Surg 2006;16:181.

13. Holtby R, Razmjou H. Validity of the supraspinatus test as a single clinical test in diagnosing patients with rotator cuff pathology. J Orthop Sports Phys Ther 2004;34(4):194–200.

14. Itoi E, Kido T, Sano A, Urayama M, Sato K. Which is more useful, the "full can test" or the "empty can test," in detecting the torn supraspinatus tendon? Am J Sports Med. 1999; 27(1):65–8.

15. Kim E, Jeong HJ, Lee KW, Song JS Interpreting positive signs of the supraspinatus test in screening for torn rotator cuff. Acta Med Okayama 2006;60(4):223–8.

16. Leroux JL, Thomas E, Bonnel F, Blotman F. Diagnostic value of clinical tests for shoulder impingement syndrome. Rev Rheum Engl Ed. 1995;62(6):423–8.

17. MacDonald PB, Clark P, Sutherland K. An analysis of the diagnostic accuracy of the Hawkins and Neer subacromial impingement signs. J Shoulder Elbow Surg 2000;9(4):299–301.

18. Miller CA, Forrester GA, Lewis JS. The validity of the lag signs in diagnosing full-thickness tears of the rotator cuff: a prelimi-

nary investigation. Arch Phys Med Rehabil 2008;89(6): 1162–8.

19. Murrell GA, Walton JR. Diagnosis of rotator cuff tears. Lancet 2001;357(9258):769–70.

20. Wolf EM, Agrawal V. Transdeltoid palpation (the rent test) in the diagnosis of rotator cuff tears. J Shoulder Elbow Surg. 2001;10(5):470–3.

21. Castoldi F, Bionna D, Hertel R. External rotation lag sign revisited: accuracy for diagnosis of full thickness supraspinatus tear. J Shoulder Elbow Surg 2009;18(4):529–34.

22. Hertel R, Ballmer FT, Lombert SM, Gerber C. Lag signs in the diagnosis of rotator cuff rupture. J Shoulder Elbow Surg 1996; 5(4):307–13.

23. Itoi E, Minagawa H, Yamamoto N, Seki N, Abe H. Are pain location and physical examinations useful in locating a tear site of the rotator cuff? Am J Sports Med. 2006;34(2):256–64.

24. Kim HA, Kim SH, Seo YI. Ultrasonographic findings of painful shoulders and correlation between physical examination and ultrasonographic rotator cuff tear. Mod Rheumatol 2007;17(3): 213–19.

25. Litaker D, Pioro M, El Bilbeisi H, Brems J. Returning to the bedside: using the history and physical examination to identify rotator cuff tears. J Am Geriatr Soc 48(12):1633–7.

26. Lyons AR, Tomlinson JE. Clinical diagnosis of tears of the rotator cuff. J Bone Joint Surg Br 1992;74(3):414–5.

27. Park HB, Yokota A, Gill HS, El Rassi G, McFarland EG. Diagnostic accuracy of clinical tests for the different degrees of subacromial impingement syndrome. J Bone Joint Surg Am 2005;87(7):1446–55.

28. Yamamoto A, Takagishi K, Osawa T, Yanagawa T, Nakajima D, Shitara H, Kobayashi T. Prevalence and risk factors of a rotator cuff tear in the general population. J Shoulder Elbow Surg 2010;19(1):116–20.

29. Hegedus EJ, Goode A, Campbell S, Morin A, Tamaddoni M, Moorman CT 3rd, Cook C. Physical examination tests of the shoulder: a systematic review with meta-analysis of individual tests. Br J Sports Med. 2008;42(2):80–92.

30. Hughes PC, Taylor NF, Green RA. Most clinical tests cannot accurately diagnose rotator cuff pathology: a systematic review. Aust J Physiother 2008;54(3):159–70.

31. Walch G, Boulahia A, Calderone S, Robinson AH. The "dropping" and "hornblower's" signs in evaluation of rotator-cuff tears.; J Bone Joint Surg Br. 1998;80(4):624–8.

32. Nomden JG, Slagers AJ, Bergman GJ, Winters JC, Kropmans TJ, Dijkstra PU. Interobserver reliability of physical examination of shoulder girdle. Man Ther 2009;14(2):152–9.

33. Ostor AJ, Richards CA, Prevost AT, Hazleman BL, Speed CA. Interrater reproducibility of clinical tests for rotator cuff lesions. Ann Rheum Dis 2004;63(10):1288–92.

34. Bryant L, Shnier R, Bryant C, Murrell GA. A comparison of clinical estimation, ultrasonography, magnetic resonance imaging, and arthroscopy in determining the size of rotator cuff tears. J Shoulder Elbow Surg 2002;11(3):219–24.

35. Chiou HJ, Hsu CC, Chou YH, Tiu CM, Jim YF, Wu JJ, Chang CY. Sonographic signs of complete rotator cuff tears. Chung Hua i Hsueh Tsa Chih—Chin Med J 1996;58(6):428–34.

36. Farin PU, Jaroma H. Digital subtraction shoulder arthrography in determining site and size of rotator cuff tear. Invest Radiol 1995;30(9):544–7.

37. Farin PU, Kaukanen E, Jaroma H, Vaatainen U, Miettinen H, Soimakallio S. Site and size of rotator-cuff tear. Findings at ultrasound, double-contrast arthrography, and computed tomography arthrography with surgical correlation. Invest Radiol 1996;31(7):387–94.

38. Iannotti JP, Ciccone J, Buss DD, et al. Accuracy of office-based ultrasonography of the shoulder for the diagnosis of rotator cuff tears. J Bone Joint Surg Am 2005;87(6):1305–11.

39. Kluger R, Mayrhofer R, Kroner A, Pabinger C, Partan G, Hruby W, Engel A. Sonographic versus magnetic resonance arthrographic evaluation of full-thickness rotator cuff tears in millimeters. J Shoulder Elbow Surg 2003;12(2):110–16.

40. Martin-Hervas C, Romero J, Navas-Acien A, Reboiras JJ, Munuera L. Ultrasonographic and magnetic resonance images of rotator cuff lesions compared with arthroscopy or open surgery findings. J Shoulder Elbow Surg 2001;10(5):410–5.

41. Naqvi GA, Jadaan M, Harrington P. Accuracy of ultrasonography and magnetic resonance imaging for detection of full thickness rotator cuff tears. Int J Shoulder Surg 2009;3(4):94–7.

42. Olive RJ Jr, Marsh HO. Ultrasonography of rotator cuff tears. Clin Orthop Relat Res 2002;282:110–13.

43. Read JW, Perko M. Shoulder ultrasound: diagnostic accuracy for impingement syndrome, rotator cuff tear, and biceps tendon pathology. J Shoulder Elbow Surg 1998;7(3):264–71.

44. Takagishi K, Makino K, Takahira N, Ikeda T, Tsuruno K, Itoman M. Ultrasonography for diagnosis of rotator cuff tear. Skelet Radiol 1996;25(3):221–4.

45. Teefey SA, Hasan SA, Middleton WD, Patel M, Wright RW, Yamaguchi K. Ultrasonography of the rotator cuff. A comparison of ultrasonographic and arthroscopic findings in one hundred consecutive cases. J Bone Joint Surg Am 2000;82(4): 498–504.

46. Tuite MJ, Turnbull JR, Orwin JF. Anterior versus posterior, and rim-rent rotator cuff tears: prevalence and MR sensitivity. Skeletal Radiol 1998;27(5):237–43.

47. van de Sande M, Rozing P. Proximal migration can be measured accurately on standardized anteroposterior shoulder radiographs. Clin Orthop Relat Res 2006;443:260–5.

48. Wang YM, Shih TT, Jiang CC, et al. Magnetic resonance imaging of rotator cuff lesions. J Formosan Med Assoc 1994;93(3): 234–9.

49. Yamakawa S, Hashizume H, Ichikawa N, Itadera E, Inoue H. Comparative studies of MRI and operative findings in rotator cuff tear. Acta Med Okayama 2001;55(5):261–8.

50. Charousset C, Bellaiche L, Duranthon L, Grimberg J. Accuracy of CT arthrography in the assessment of tears of the rotator cuff. J Bone Joint Surg Br 2005;87(6):824–8.

51. Nove-Josserand L, Edwards T, O'Connor D, Walch G. The acromiohumeral and coracohumeral intervals are abnormal in rotator cuff tears with muscular fatty degeneration. Clin Orthop Relat Res 2005;433:90–6.

52. Toyoda H, Ito, Y, Tomo H, Nakao Y, Koike T, Kunio T. Evaluation of rotator cuff tears with magnetic resonance arthrography. Clin Orthop Relat Res 2005;439:109–115.

53. de Jesus JO, Parker L, Frangos AJ, Nazarian LN. Accuracy of MRI, MR arthrography, and ultrasound in the diagnosis of rotator cuff tears: a meta-analysis. AJR 2009;192(6):1701–7.

54. Dinnes J, Loveman E, McIntyre L, Waugh N. The effectiveness of diagnostic tests for the assessment of shoulder pain due to

soft tissue disorders: a systematic review. Health Technol Assessment (Winchester, England) 2003;7(29):iii, 1–166.

55. Blanchard TK, Bearcroft PW, Constant CR, Griffin DR, Dixon AK. Diagnostic and therapeutic impact of MRI and arthrography in the investigation of full thickness rotator cuff tears. Eur Radiol 1999;9(4):638–42.

56. Frei R, Chladek P, Trc T, Kopecny Z, Kautzner J. Arthroscopic evaluation of ultrasonography and magnetic resonance imaging for diagnosis of rotator cuff tear. Ortop Traumatol Rehabil 2008;10(2):111–14.

57. Masaoka S, Hashizume H, Senda M, Nishida K, Nagoshi M, Inoue H. Ultrasonographic analysis of shoulder rotator cuff tears. Acta Med Okayama 1999;53(2):81–9.

58. Vick CW, Bell SA. Rotator cuff tears: diagnosis with sonography. AJR 1990;154(1):121–3.

59. Yeu K, Jiang CC, Shih TT. Correlation between MRI and operative findings of the rotator cuff tear. J Formosan Med Assoc 1994;93(2):134–9.

60. Bezer M, Yildirim Y, Akgun U, Erol B, Guven O. Superior excursion of the humeral head: a diagnostic tool in rotator cuff tear surgery. J Shoulder Elbow Surg 2005;14(4):375–9.

61. Deutsch A, Altchek DW, Schwartz E, Otis JC, Warren RF. Radiologic measurement of superior displacement of the humeral head in the impingement syndrome. J Shoulder Elbow Surg 1996;5(3):186–93.

62. Kaneko K, De Mouy EH, Brunet ME. Massive rotator cuff tears. Screening by routine radiographs. Clin Imaging 1995;19(1):8–11.

63. Saupe N, Pfirrmann CW, Schmid MR, Jost B, Werner CM, Zanetti M. Association between rotator cuff abnormalities and reduced acromiohumeral distance. AJR.2006;187(2):376–82.

64. Vitale MG, Krant JJ, Gelijns AC, et al. Geographic variations in the rates of operative procedures involving the shoulder, including total shoulder replacement, humeral head replacement, and rotator cuff repair. J Bone Joint Surg Am 1999;81(6): 763–72.

65. Oh LS, Wolf BR, Hall MP, Levy BA, Marx RG. Indications for rotator cuff repair: a systematic review. Clin Orthop Relat Res 2007;455:52–63.

66. Wolf BR, Dunn WR, Wright RW Indications for repair of full-thickness rotator cuff tears. Am J Sports Med 2007;35(6): 1007–16.

67. Slabaugh MA, Nho SJ, Grumet RC, et al. Does the literature confirm superior clinical results in radiographically healed rotator cuffs after rotator cuff repair? Arthroscopy 2010;26(3): 393–403.

68. Moosmayer S, Lund G, Seljom U, Svege I, Hannig T, Tariq R, Smith HJ. Comparison between surgery and physiotherapy in the treatment of small and medium sized tears of the rotator cuff. J Bone Joint Surg Br 2010;92(1):83–91.

69. Yamada N, Hamada K, Nakajima T, Kobayashi K, Fukuda H. Comparison of conservative and operative treatments of massive rotator cuff tears. Tokai J Exp Clin Med 2000;25(4–6): 151–63.

70. Ainsworth R, Lewis JS. Exercise therapy for the conservative management of full thickness tears of the rotator cuff: a systematic review. Br J Sports Med 2007;41(4):200–10.

71. Ainsworth R. Physiotherapy rehabilitation in patients with massive irreparable rotator cuff tears. Musculoskel Care 2006; 4(3):140–51.

72. Bokor DJ, Hawkins RJ. Results of non-operative management of full thickness tears of the rotator cuff. Clin Orthop Relat Res 1993;294:103–10.

73. Goldberg BA, Nowinski RJ, Matsen FA 3rd. Outcome of non-operative management of full-thickness rotator cuff tears. Clin Orthop Relat Res 2001;382:99–107.

74. Hawkins RH, Dunlop R. Non-operative treatment of rotator cuff tears. Clin Orthop Relat Res 1995;321:178–88.

75. Heers G, Anders S, Werther M, Lerch K, Hedtmann A, Grifka J. [Efficacy of home exercises for symptomatic rotator cuff tears in correlation to the size of the defect]. Sportverletz Sportschaden 2005;19(1):22–7.

76. Itoi E, Tabata S. Conservative treatment of rotator cuff tears. Clin Orthop Relat Res 1992;275:165–73.

77. Koubaa S, Ben Salah FZ, Leviv S, Miri I, Ghorbel S, Dziri C. Conservative management of full-thicnkess rotator cuff tears. A prospective study of 24 patients. Ann Readapt Med Phys 2006;49(2):62–7.

78. Levy O, Mullett H, Roberts S, Copeland S. The role of anterior deltoid reeducation in patients with massive irreparable degenerative rotator cuff tears. J Shoulder Elbow Surg 2008;17(6): 863–70.

79. Vad V, Warren R, Altchek D, O'Brien D, Rose H, Wickiewicz T. Negative prognostic factors in managing massive rotator cuff tears. Clin J Sport Med 12(3):151–7.

80. Maman E, Harris C, White L, Tomlinson G, Shashank M, Boynton E. Outcome of non-operative treatment of symptomatic rotator cuff tears monitored by magnetic resonance imaging. J Bone Joint Surg Am 2009;91(8):1898–906.

81. Melis B, Wall B, Walch G. Natural history of infraspinatus fatty infiltration in rotator cuff tears. J Shoulder Elbow Surg 2010;19(5):757–63.

82. Melis B, DeFranco MJ, Chuinard C, Walch G. Natural history of fatty infiltration and atrophy of the supraspinatus muscle in rotator cuff tears. Clin Orthop Relat Res 2010;468(6):1498–505.

83. Zingg PO, Jost B, Sukthankar A, Buhler M, Pfirrmann CWA, Gerber C. Clinical and structural outcomes of non-operative management of massive rotator cuff tears. J Bone Joint Surg Am 2007;89(9):1928–34.

84. Yamaguchi K, Tetro AM, Blam O, Evanoff BA, Teefey SA, Middleton WD. Natural history of asymptomatic rotator cuff tears: a longitudinal analysis of asymptomatic tears detected sonographically. J Shoulder Elbow Surg 2001;10(3): 199–203.

85. Berth A, Neumann W, Awiszus F, Pap G. Massive rotator cuff tears: functional outcome after debridement or arthroscopic partial repair. J Orthop Traumatol. 2010;11(1):13–20.

86. Bigoni M, Gorla M, Guerrasio S, et al. Shoulder evaluation with isokinetic strength testing after arthroscopic rotator cuff repairs. J Shoulder Elbow Surg. 2009;18(2):178–83.

87. Boehm TD, Werner A, Radtke S, Mueller T, Kirschner S, Gohlke F. The effect of suture materials and techniques on the outcome of repair of the rotator cuff: a prospective, randomised study. J Bone Joint Surg Br 2005;87(6):819–23.

88. Burks RT, Crim J, Brown N, Fink B, Greis PE. A prospective randomized clinical trial comparing arthroscopic single- and double-row rotator cuff repair: magnetic resonance imaging and early clinical evaluation. Am J Sports Med. 2009;37(4): 674–82.

89. Franceschi F, Longo UG, Ruzzini L, Rizzello G, Maffulli N, Denaro V. No advantages in repairing a type II superior labrum anterior and posterior (SLAP) lesion when associated with rotator cuff repair in patients over age 50: a randomized controlled trial. Am J Sports Med 2008;36(2):247–53.

90. Franceschi F, Ruzzini L, Longo UG, et al. Equivalent clinical results of arthroscopic single-row and double-row suture anchor repair for rotator cuff tears: a randomized controlled trial. Am J Sports Med. 2007;35(8):1254–60.

91. Garofalo R, Conti M, Notarnicola A, Maradei L, Giardella A, Castagna A. Effects of one-month continuous passive motion after arthroscopic rotator cuff repair: results at 1-year follow-up of a prospective randomized study. Musculoskel Surg 2010; 94(Suppl 1):S79–83.

92. Gartsman GM, O'Connor DP. Arthroscopic rotator cuff repair with and without arthroscopic subacromial decompression: a prospective, randomized study of one-year outcomes. J Shoulder Elbow Surg. 2004;13(4):424–6.

93. Grasso A, Milano G, Salvatore M, Falcone G, Deriu I, Fabbriciani C. Single-row versus double-row arthroscopic rotator cuff repair: a prospective randomized clinical study. Arthroscopy 2009;25(1):4–12.

94. Iannotti JP, Codsi MJ, Kwon YW, Derwin K, Ciccone J, Brems JJ. Porcine small intestine submucosa augmentation of surgical repair of chronic two-tendon rotator cuff tears. A randomized, controlled trial. J Bone Joint Surg Am 2006;88(6):1238–44.

95. Klepps S, Bishop J, Lin J, Cahlon O, Strauss A, Hayes P, Flatow EL. Prospective evaluation of the effect of rotator cuff integrity on the outcome of open rotator cuff repairs. Am J Sports Med 2004;32(7):1716–22.

96. Lastayo PC, Wright T, Jaffe R, Hartzel J. Continuous passive motion after repair of the rotator cuff. A prospective outcome study. J Bone Joint Surg Am 1998;80(7):1002–11.

97. Milano G, Grasso A, Salvatore M, Zarelli D, Deriu L, Fabbriciani C. Arthroscopic rotator cuff repair with and without subacromial decompression: a prospective randomized study. Arthroscopy 2007;23(1):81–8.

98. Mohtadi NG, Hollinshead RM, Sasyniuk TM, Fletcher JA, Chan DS, Li FX. A randomized clinical trial comparing open to arthroscopic acromioplasty with mini-open rotator cuff repair for full-thickness rotator cuff tears: disease-specific quality of life outcome at an average 2-year follow-up. Am J Sports Med. 2008;36(6):1043–51.

99. Shinoda T, Shibata Y, Izaki T, Shitama T, Naito M. A comparative study of surgical invasion in arthroscopic and open rotator cuff repair. J Shoulder Elbow Surg 2009;18(4):596–9.

100. Abbot AE, Li X, Busconi BD. Arthroscopic treatment of concomitant superior labral anterior posterior (SLAP) lesions and rotator cuff tears in patients over the age of 45 years. Am J Sports Med 2009;37(7):1358–62.

101. Aydin N, Kocaoglu B, Guven O. Single-row versus double-row arthroscopic rotator cuff repair in smallto medium-sized tears. J Shoulder Elbow Surg 2010;19(5):722–5.

102. Bishop J, Klepps S, Lo IK, Bird J, Gladstone JN, Flatow EL. Cuff integrity after arthroscopic versus open rotator cuff repair: a prospective study. J Shoulder Elbow Surg 2006;15(3):290–9.

103. Charousset C, Grimberg J, Duranthon LD, Bellaiche L, Petrover D. Can a double-row anchorage technique improve tendon healing in arthroscopic rotator cuff repair? A prospective, non-randomized, comparative study of double-row and single-row anchorage techniques with computed tomographic arthrography tendon healing assessment. Am J Sports Med. 2007; 35(8):1247–53.

104. Ogilvie-Harris DJ, Demazière A. Arthroscopic debridement versus open repair for rotator cuff tears. A prospective cohort study. J Bone Joint Surg Br 1993;75(3):416–20.

105. Park JY, Lhee SH, Choi JH, Park HK, Yu JW, Seo JB. Comparison of the clinical outcomes of single- and double-row repairs in rotator cuff tears. Am J Sports Med 2008;36(7):1310–16.

106. Nho SJ, Slabaugh MA, Seroyer ST. et al. Does the literature support double-row suture anchor fixation for arthroscopic rotator cuff repair? A systematic review comparing double-row and single-row suture anchor configuration. Arthroscopy 2009;25(11):1319–28.

107. Seida JC, LeBlanc C, Schouten JR, et al. Systematic review: non-operative and operative treatments for rotator cuff tears. Ann Intern Med 2010:153(4):246–55.

108. Cho NS, Yi JW, Lee BG, Rhee YG. Retear patterns after arthroscopic rotator cuff repair: single-row versus suture bridge technique. Am J Sports Med 2010;38(4):664–71.

109. Forsythe B, Guss D, Anthony SG, Martin SD. Concomitant arthroscopic SLAP and rotator cuff repair. J Bone Joint Surg Am 2010;92(6):1362–9.

110. Hata Y, Saitoh S, Murakami N, Seki H, Nakatsuchi Y, Takaoka K. A less invasive surgery for rotator cuff tear: mini-open repair. J Shoulder Elbow Surg 2001;10(1):11–16.

111. Kim SH, Ha KI, Park JH, Kang JS, Oh SK, Oh I. Arthroscopic versus mini-open salvage repair of the rotator cuff tear: outcome analysis at 2 to 6 years' follow-up. Arthroscopy 2003;19(7): 746–54.

112. Ko SH, Friedman D, Seo DK, Jun HM, Warner JJ. A prospective therapeutic comparison of simple suture repairs to massive cuff stitch repairs for treatment of small- and medium-sized rotator cuff tears. Arthroscopy 2009;25(6):583–9.

113. Liem D, Bartl C, Lichtenberg S, Magosch P, Habermeyer P. Clinical outcome and tendon integrity of arthroscopic versus mini-open supraspinatus tendon repair: a magnetic resonance imaging-controlled matched-pair analysis. Arthroscopy 2007; 23(5):514–21.

114. Millar NL, Wu X, Tantau R, Silverstone E, Murrell GA. Open versus two forms of arthroscopic rotator cuff repair. Clin Orthop Relat Res 2009;467(4):966–78.

115. Pearsall AW 4th. Ibrahim KA, Madanagopal SG. The results of arthroscopic versus miniopen repair for rotator cuff tears at midterm follow-up. J Orthop Surg 2007;2:24.

116. Walton JR, Bowman NK, Khatib Y, Linklater J, Murrell GA. Restore orthobiologic implant: not recommended for augmentation of rotator cuff repairs. rotator cuff repairs. J Bone Joint Surg Am 2007;89(4):786–91.

117. Slabaugh MA, Nho SJ, Grumet RC, et al. Does the literature confirm superior clinical results in radiographically healed rotator cuffs after rotator cuff repair? Arthroscopy 2010;26(3): 393–403.

118. Chen AL, Shapiro JA, Ahn AK, Zuckerman JD, Cuomo F. Rotator cuff repair in patients with type I diabetes mellitus. J Shoulder Elbow Surg 2003;12(5):416–21.

119. Namdari S, Green A. Range of motion limitation after rotator cuff repair. J Shoulder Elbow Surg 2010;19(2):290–6.

120. Athwal GS, Sperling JW, Rispoli DM, Cofield RH. Deep infection after rotator cuff repair. J Shoulder Elbow Surg. 2007;16(3): 306–11.

121. Brislin KJ, Field LD, Savoie FH 3rd. Complications after arthroscopic rotator cuff repair. Arthroscopy 2007;23(2):124–8.

122. Benson EC, MacDermid JC, Drosdowech DS, Athwal GS. The incidence of early metallic suture anchor pullout after arthroscopic rotator cuff repair. Arthroscopy 2010;26(3):310–15.

123. Boileau P, Brassart N, Watkinson DJ, Carles M, Hatzidakis AM, Krishnan SG, Arthroscopic repair of full-thickness tears of the supraspinatus: Does the tendon really heal? J Bone Joint Surg Am 2005;87(6):1229–40.

124. Degreef I, Debeer P. Heterotopic ossification of the supraspinatus tendon after rotator cuff repair: case report. Clin Rheumatol 2006;25(2):251–3.

125. Dossche L, Naert PA, Van Bouwel S. Persistent aseptic fistula after rotator cuff repair: fistuloscopic approach. J Shoulder Elbow Surg 2002;11(1):86–7.

126. Fuchs B, Gilbart MK, Hodler J, Gerber C. Clinical and structural results of open repair of an isolated one-tendon tear of the rotator cuff. J Bone Joint Surg Am 2006:88(2):309–16.

127. Gumina, S. Di Giorgio G, Perugia D, Postacchini F. Deltoid detachment consequent to open surgical repair of massive rotator cuff tears. Int Orthop. 2008;32(1):81–4.

128. Grondel RJ, Savoie FH 3rd, Field LD. Rotator cuff repairs in patients 62 years of age or older. J Shoulder Elbow Surg 2001; 10(2):97–9.

129. Herrera MF, Bauer G, Reynolds F, Wilk RM, Bigliani LU, Levine WN. Infection after mini-open rotator cuff repair. J Shoulder Elbow Surg 2002;11(6):605–8.

130. Hoxie SC, Sperling JW, Cofield RH. Pulmonary embolism following rotator cuff repair. Int J Shoulder Surg 2008;2(3): 49–51.

131. Huberty DP, Schoolfield JD, Brady PC, Vadala AP, Arrigoni P, Burkhart SS. Incidence and treatment of postoperative stiffness following arthroscopic rotator cuff repair. Arthroscopy 2009; 25(8):880–90.

132. Kim KC, Rhee KJ, Shin HD. Deformities associated with the suture-bridge technique for full-thickness rotator cuff tears. Arthroscopy 2008;24(11):1251–7.

133. Kircher J, Martinek V, Mittelmeier W. Heterotopic ossification after minimally invasive rotator cuff repair. Arthroscopy 2007;23(12):1359.

134. Krishnan SG, Harkins DC, Schiffern SC, Pennington SD, Burkhead WZ. Arthroscopic repair of full-thickness tears of the rotator cuff in patients younger than 40 years. Arthroscopy 2008;24(3):324–8.

135. Levy O, Venkateswaran B, Even T, Ravenscroft M, Copeland S. Mid-term clinical and sonographic outcome of arthroscopic repair of the rotator cuff. J Bone Joint Surg Br 2008;90(10): 1341–7.

136. Mansat P, Cofield RH, Kersten TE, Rowland CM. Complications of rotator cuff repair. Orthop Clin N Am 1997;28(2):205–13.

137. Rizal E, Sarkhel T, Mok D. Loss of anchor fixation after arthroscopic rotator cuff repair. J Bone Joint Surg Br 2009;91(Suppl 2);258–9.

138. Song HS, Ramsey ML. Suture passing needle breakage during arthroscopic rotator cuff repair: a complication report. Arthroscopy 2008;24(12):1430–2.

139. Torres JA, Wright TW. Synovial cutaneous fistula of the shoulder after failed rotator cuff repair. Orthopedics 1999;22(11): 1095–7.

140. Wong AS, Kokkalis ZT, Schmidt CC. Proper insertion angle is essential to prevent intra-articular protrusion of a knotless suture anchor in shoulder rotator cuff repair. Arthroscopy 2010;26(2):286–90.

89

Shoulder Impingement Syndrome

Ron L. Diercks and Oscar Dorrestijn

University Medical Center Groningen, University of Groningen, The Netherlands

Case scenario

A 48 year old man employed in a hardware store has been suffering from progressive pain in his right shoulder for 5 months. The pain is located over the anterolateral part of his shoulder and radiates to the upper arm. There is no history of trauma. Overhead activities are painful and sleeping on the right shoulder is disturbed. At examination he experiences a painful arc during active abduction between 70 and 120°. Neer, Hawkins–Kennedy, and Jobe signs are positive. The impingement test, which is based on the Neer sign after subacromial injection with a local anesthetic, confirms the suspected diagnosis of subacromial impingement syndrome. Radiographs show a small calcification just proximal to the major tubercle. Ultrasound (US) examination shows an intact rotator cuff with tendinopathic changes at the insertion and small calcifications.

Relevant anatomy

Shoulder impingement syndrome (SIS) is characterized by pain, exacerbated by arm elevation or overhead activities. Neer was the first to describe the concept of impingement as mechanical impingement of the rotator cuff tendon beneath the anteroinferior acromion when the shoulder was placed in forward flexion and internal rotation.[1]

The impingement implies compression of the subacromial bursa and rotator cuff fibers. The syndrome includes cuff and/or biceps tendon tendinopathy, calcifying tendinosis, subacromial bursitis, and rotator cuff tears.[2] Overuse and overload induce microtraumas in the tendon. As rotator cuff tendinopathy is a degenerative process, the syndrome has an increasing prevalence in the adult population, and in people with overhead activities in work or sports.[3,4]

Importance of the problem

Shoulder pain is responsible for 16–21% of all musculoskeletal complaints in general practice. A recently published review has summarized 18 studies on the prevalence of shoulder complaints among the general population.[5] Prevalence figures ranged from 6.7% to 66.7% for lifetime prevalence. The cumulative incidence of shoulder problems was estimated at 19 per 1,000 person-years.[6] SIS is the most frequently recorded disorder (44%).[7]

This syndrome has been shown to have a substantial impact on the ability to work: 73% of SIS patients are unable to work at their usual job, and return to heavy overhand work is not common.[8] Also, differences in outcome are seen for patients on workers' compensation, therefore SIS has a high socioeconomic impact.[9]

Top nine questions

Diagnosis

1. How accurate is clinical examination in diagnosing SIS?
2. What is the role of imaging in the diagnosis of SIS?

Therapy (effectiveness assessed in terms of improvement of shoulder function or reduction of pain)

3. What is the effect of subacromial anesthetic and/or corticosteroid injections on SIS?

Evidence-Based Orthopedics, First Edition. Edited by Mohit Bhandari.
© 2012 Blackwell Publishing Ltd. Published 2012 by Blackwell Publishing Ltd.

4. What is the effect of physical therapy interventions on SIS?

5. Is there a place for extracorporeal shockwave therapy (ESWT), acupuncture, topical agents, or US in SIS?

6. What is the indication for surgery to treat SIS?

7. If surgery is chosen for SIS, what is the optimal surgical technique?

Prognosis

8. What is the effect of treatment on shoulder function and recovery?

Harm

9. What are the complications associated with interventions for SIS?

Question 1: How accurate is clinical examination in diagnosing SIS?

Case clarification

Upon examination, the patient experiences a painful arc during abduction between 70 and 120°. Hawkins and Jobe signs are positive. Neer sign with passive abduction is positive, and the impingement test, which is based on the Neer sign after a subacromial injection with a local anesthetic, confirms the suspected diagnosis of SIS.

Relevance

This is a clinical diagnosis of impingement syndrome. Numerous tests have been described since Neer's original publication.[10] The method of execution of most tests is not always clear, nor is the technique. Sensitivity, specificity, and reliability have been tested in recent years.

Current opinion

Pain with abduction of the arm, the "painful arc syndrome," and an abnormal rhythm of movement between glenohumeral and scapulothoracic motion between 60° and 120° of abduction is the foremost sign of impingement syndrome.

Finding the evidence

• Cochrane Database, search term: "shoulder tests"
• PubMed clinical queries search/ systematic reviews: "diagnostic test impingement shoulder"

Quality of the evidence

Level II

• 6 systematic reviews/meta-analyses

Findings

The sensitivity, specificity, positive predictive value, negative predictive value, and overall accuracy of the tests vary considerably. The pooled sensitivity and specificity for the Neer test were 0.79 (95% CI 0.75–0.82) and 0.53 (95% CI 0.48–0.58), respectively, and for the Hawkins–Kennedy test 0.79 (95% CI 0.75–0.82) and 0.59 (95% CI 0.53–0.64).[11] A recent systematic review concluded that some tests show good sensitivity with somewhat lower specificity when weakness is used to assess the test result.[12] Test reliability is poorer when pain is the response criterion. The right way to execute these tests differs essentially in some publications. This problem also has been addressed in a number of articles.[12–16]

The Neer test is performed with the examiner standing behind a seated or standing patient. The ipsilateral scapula should be fixated to prevent protraction. The test consists of passive forward elevation. If the patient experiences pain in the shoulder, the test is positive. The Hawkins–Kennedy test is performed with the examiner facing the seated or standing patient. The patient has his/her arm 90° in forward elevation in the scapular plane and 90° flexed in the elbow. The test consists of passive internal rotation until pain occurs.[17]

Recommendations

• The Hawkins–Kennedy test is a useful and reliable screening test for SIS [overall quality: moderate]
• The supraspinatus/empty can or infraspinatus test is as a confirmatory test for impingement [overall quality: moderate]
• The supine impingement test, when negative, is a valuable screen for any rotator cuff tear [overall quality: low]
• The hornblower's sign may be diagnostic of severe degeneration or absence of the teres minor muscle [overall quality: low]
• The external rotation lag sign may be diagnostic of an infraspinatus muscle tear [overall quality: low]

Question 2. What is the role of imaging in the diagnosis of SIS?

Case clarification

The patient's radiographs show a small calcification just proximal to the major tubercle. US examination shows an intact rotator cuff with tendinopathic changes at the insertion and small calcifications.

Relevance

As SIS is predominantly a soft tissue disorder, imaging of those structures is important in evaluating the problem and planning interventions.

Current opinion

US or MRI imaging of the integrity of the rotator cuff support clinical decision-making and choice of therapeutic intervention, and help establish a prognosis.

Finding the evidence
- Cochrane Database, with search term "impingement syndrome'
- PubMed: "imaging shoulder," "impingement syndrome shoulder," "imaging subacromial impingement syndrome"

Quality of the evidence
Level I
- 3 systematic reviews/meta-analyses

The value of US US combined with radiography is accepted as the primary investigation for shoulder impingement and suspected partial and full thickness rotator cuff tear. US is a cost-effective diagnostic tool for rotator cuff tears with a sensitivity of 94% and a specificity of 93%, but is operator-dependent. In experienced hands US of the rotator cuff is a reproducible diagnostic test (kappa > 0.60, p < 0.01), but agreement is poor when there is marked disparity between operators' experience levels.[18] There is only a 41% detection rate of partial thickness tears.[19]

The value of MRI A recent meta-analysis summarized 10 studies using conventional MRI for detection of rotator cuff tears.[20] Overall sensitivity and specificity were high for full thickness tears, 0.89 (95% CI 0.86–0.92) and 0.93 (95% CI 0.91–0.95) respectively. For detection of partial thickness tears, sensitivity rates were much lower (0.44, 95% CI 0.36–0.51) although specificity remained high (0.90, 95% CI 0.87–0.92). For full thickness tears MR arthrography (MRA) has a sensitivity of 0.95 (95% CI 0.82–0.98) and a specificity of 0.93 (95% CI 0.84–0.97). MRI offers the advantage of diagnosing concomitant abnormalities.

Three studies compared MRI and US to surgery prospectively and found higher sensitivity and accuracy rates for MRI. A negative MRI would rule out the presence of a tear with more certainty than a negative US.[20] MRI seems to be more accurate than US in detecting partial tears. Overall, MRI is a useful tool in the identification of shoulder pathology.[21–23]

Recommendations
- US may be the more cost-effective diagnostic method [overall quality: very low]
- MRI or US could be equally used for impingement syndrome and full thickness tears rotator cuff tears [overall quality: moderate]
- All imaging modalities were less accurate for partial thickness tears [overall quality: moderate]
- US has operator dependency, leading to variable results in daily practice [overall quality: low grade]
- The clinical correlation of imaging and the assessment of outcomes remains unknown [overall quality: very low]

Question 3: What is the effect of subacromial anesthetic and/or corticosteroid injections on SIS?

Case clarification
The impingement test, which is based on the Neer sign after subacromial injection with a local anesthetic, confirms the suspected diagnosis of SIS.

Relevance
By judging the effect of a subacromial anesthetic and corticosteroid injection, a definite diagnosis of SIS can be made.

Current opinion
Subacromial injections of corticosteroids are effective for SIS.

Finding the evidence
- PubMed clinical queries search/systematic reviews, with search terms: "subacromial injection," "local infiltration shoulder"

Quality of the evidence
- 1 level I meta-analysis
- 1 Cochrane Database entry
- 11 reviews and randomized controlled trials (RCTs)

Findings
Subacromial infiltration as a diagnostic procedure In the hands of experienced orthopedic surgeons, subacromial injections through standard approaches often fail to infiltrate the subacromial space.[24,25] This can create both false-positive and false-negative results. The evaluation of the effect appears to be time-dependent: rapid responders show more than 50% pain relief at 10 minutes, delayed responders after 10 minutes or more.[26]

Subacromial infiltration as a therapeutic intervention In a Cochrane review (three pooled trials), Buchbinder et al. state that subacromial steroid injections have a small benefit over placebo in some trials, but no benefit over NSAIDs was demonstrated.[27] There is some evidence that corticosteroid injections are superior to physical therapy. A recent meta-analysis (seven trials) by Arroll et al. underlines a significant benefit of steroid injections above placebos.[28] They found a large benefit, with a number needed to treat of 2.5, when compared with NSAIDs. The reported duration of the effect of subacromial corticosteroid injections is up to 32 weeks. Conflicting evidence was found about the benefit of adding corticosteroids to local anesthetics, and the doses that should be used. In the study that showed no effect, the lowest dose of corticosteroids was given.[29] Higher doses of corticosteroids (50 mg equivalent of prednisone or greater) may be more effective than lower doses. Pooling of three high-quality studies resulted in a relative risk of 5.9 (95% CI 2.8–12.6).[28]

All this evidence is put in a different light in a recent RCT by Ekeberg et al., showing no important differences in short-term outcomes for rotator cuff disease between local US-guided corticosteroid injections and systemic corticosteroid injections.[30]

Recommendations

• There is conflicting evidence on the benefit of subacromial corticosteroid injections above placebo, NSAIDs, and physical therapy [overall quality: low]
• Higher doses of corticosteroids seem to be more effective than lower doses [overall quality: high]
• The duration of the effect can be as long as 32 weeks [overall quality: high]
• As nonguided subacromial injections often fail to infiltrate the subacromial space, imaging-guided subacromial steroid injections are to be preferred [overall quality: high]
• There should be serious doubt about the placebo effect of "puncturing the painful area" vs. the systemic effect of corticosteroids [overall quality: moderate]

Question 4: What is the effect of physical therapy interventions on SIS?

Relevance
The first line of treatment for SIS in most cases is physical therapy.

Current opinion
Exercise and instruction can be helpful in the rehabilitation of SIS.

Finding the evidence
• PubMed clinical queries search/systematic reviews, with search terms: "physiotherapy interventions for shoulder pain"

Quality of the evidence
Level I
• 1 Cochrane systematic review
• 1 systematic review
• 3 RCTs

Findings
In a Cochrane review, including 26 trials, little evidence to guide treatment was found.[31] There is some evidence that exercise is effective in terms of short-term recovery for rotator cuff disease (RR 7.74, 1.97–30.32). Another systematic review, which included 16 RCTs, shows an equal effectiveness of physiotherapist-led exercises compared with surgery and of home-based exercises compared with physi-

otherapy.[32] An RCT showed that self-training after instruction showed no difference in outcomes with physiotherapist-supervised exercises.[33] Another RCT reported that addition of manual therapy resulted in an improvement at follow-up.[34]

A recent RCT comparing surgery with physical therapy found no clinically important effects in terms of subjective outcome at 24 months of follow-up.[35] The effect of eccentric training, used nowadays for a number of tendinopathies, has only been published as a pilot study.[36]

Recommendations
• Systematic reviews and RCTs show no differences in outcome between patients treated with physical therapy and surgery [overall quality: high]
• There is limited evidence that exercise is more effective than no intervention [overall quality: high]
• Combining manual therapy with exercises can have additional benefits [overall quality: moderate]
• No difference is noted between physiotherapist-supervised exercises and self-training after instruction [overall quality: moderate]
• The effect of eccentric training in SIS has not yet been shown [overall quality: very low]

Question 5: Is there a place for Extracorporeal Shockwave Therapy (ESWT), acupuncture, or ultrasound for the treatment of SIS?

Relevance
Shoulder complaints, including SIS, are often treated with different modalities.

Current opinion
ESWT can have an effect on acute calcific tendinosis; no other therapeutic modalities have been proven worthwhile.

Finding the evidence
• PubMed clinical queries search/systematic reviews, with search terms: "treatment modalities tendinopathy," "extracorporeal shockwave therapy and SIS"

Quality of the evidence
• 2 Cochrane systemic reviews
• 1 review

Findings
ESWT There is evidence for the effectiveness of ESWT in the treatment of calcific tendinosis compared with placebo, with a reported improvement in pain scores and a decrease in the size of calcific deposits.[37,38] Two RCTs report no major benefit with ESWT compared with placebo for the treatment of noncalcific tendinopathy of the supraspinatus.[39,40]

Supervised exercises were more effective than radial ESWT for short-term improvement in patients with subacromial shoulder pain.[41]

Acupuncture Acupuncture was of benefit over placebo in shoulder function (measured with Constant–Murley score) at 4 weeks. However, by 4 months the difference was not clinically significant.[42]

Topical glyceryl nitrate There is some evidence that topical glyceryl trinitrate is more effective than placebo for rotator cuff disease among patients with acute symptoms (<7 days duration). Any benefits of treatment need to be balanced against the risk of headaches.[43]

Ultrasound There is no evidence that US therapy has any effect on SIS.[44,45]

Recommendations

- ESWT has an effect on radiologic calcific tendinosis [overall quality: high]
- There is no reported effect of extracorporeal shockwave therapy on SIS without calcific tendinosis [overall quality: high]
- There is some effect described of acupuncture in SIS [overall quality: moderate]
- There could be a very short time effect of topical glyceryl nitrate on SIS [overall quality: low]
- There is evidence that US therapy has no effect on SIS [overall quality: moderate]

Question 6: What is the indication for surgery to treat SIS?

Relevance

Surgical therapy for SIS is a very common procedure. The indication is mostly persistent impingement syndrome after a period of conservative therapy.

Current opinion

Surgical therapy (arthroscopic or open subacromial decompression) is the therapy of choice after failed physical therapy and steroid injections.

Finding the evidence

- PubMed clinical queries search/systematic reviews, with search terms: "shoulder impingement syndrome," "subacromial impingement," "rotator cuff" AND "surgical procedures" OR "arthroscopy" AND "therapy" AND "nonoperative" OR "nonsurgical" OR "conservative"

Quality of the evidence

Level I
- 1 Cochrane review
- 1 systematic review/meta-analysis
- 2 RCTs

Findings

In a Cochrane review published in 2008,[46] a systematic review published in 2009,[47] and a recent RCT,[35] no differences in reduction of pain or improvement of shoulder function were found between surgery and nonsurgical treatments. Coghlan et al. found a "silver" level of evidence that there are no significant differences in outcome between subacromial decompression and active nonoperative treatment for impingement.[46] Dorrestijn et al. found four RCTs comparing effects of conservative and surgical treatment,[47–52] showing no difference in outcome. In an RCT, Ketola et al. found no clinically important effects in terms of self-reported pain when measured at 24 months of follow-up.[35] However, the mean healthcare costs in the combined treatment group (€2,961), which consisted of an arthroscopic acromioplasty followed by an exercise program, were considerably higher (160%) than those for the exercise group (€1,864) alone.

Recommendation

- Surgical treatment of patients with SIS is not superior to conservative treatment [overall quality: high]

Question 7: If surgery is chosen for SIS, what is the optimal surgical technique?

Relevance

Open vs. arthroscopic acromioplasty, bursectomy only, and whether to leave the coracoacromial ligament intact are issues much debated in shoulder surgery.

Current opinion

Arthroscopic subacromial decompression with resection of the coracoacromial ligament and abrasion of the anteroinferior part of the acromion is the current standard of surgical treatment.

Finding the evidence

- PubMed clinical queries search/systematic reviews, with search terms: "shoulder impingement syndrome," "subacromial impingement," "rotator cuff" AND "surgery" AND "open surgery" AND "arthroscopy"

Quality of the evidence

Level I
- 1 Cochrane review
- 1 systematic review/meta-analysis
- 2 RCTs

Findings

Coghlan et al. found a "silver" level of evidence from six trials that there are no significant differences in outcome between arthroscopic and open subacromial decompression, although four trials reported earlier recovery with arthroscopic decompression.[46] A more recent meta-analysis by Davis et al. (nine studies) came to the same conclusion.[53] Open arthroscopy, however, was associated with longer hospital stays (2.3 days, p = 0.05) and a greater length in time until return to work (65.1 days) compared with the arthroscopic technique (48.6 days, p < 0.05). In an RCT published by Henkus et al., arthroscopic subacromial bursectomy alone was compared with debridement of the subacromial bursa followed by acromioplasty. At a mean follow-up of 2.5 years no significant differences were found between the two treatments.[54] There was no significant difference in occurrence of adverse events between the various techniques. Only mobility was sometimes reported to return earlier after arthroscopic surgery.[55–61]

Recommendations
- There is no evidence supporting a difference in long-term outcome of arthroscopic over open subacromial decompression [overall quality: moderate]
- Arthroscopic subacromial decompression may lead to earlier recovery than open acromioplasty [overall quality: moderate]
- Bursectomy alone has an effect equal to decompression with acromioplasty [overall quality: moderate]

Question 8: What is the effect of treatment on shoulder function and recovery?

Relevance
SIS can have a profound impact on quality of life as well as on working ability. Many studies show a negative effect of workers' compensation on the outcome of interventions.

Current opinion
Pain and impairment diminish significantly after therapy for SIS, but heavy overhead work increases chances of recurrence.

Finding the evidence
- PubMed search: "shoulder", "rotator cuff", "impingement", "work", "sick leave", "disability"

Quality of the evidence
Level I
- 4 systematic reviews

Findings
Chronic shoulder impingement results in significant functional disability and a reduction in quality of life.[62] Many articles demonstrate that compensation status of individuals who underwent shoulder surgery continues to be a positive predictor of poor functional outcome. However, cohort studies of workers with shoulder complaints in occupational settings show strong evidence for predicting poorer outcome for the middle-aged (45–54 years).[63] Although 30% of all workers with shoulder pain reported sick leave during follow-up, for most workers the duration of sick leave was only a few days. There is limited evidence that arthroscopic acromioplasty is more effective than open acromioplasty in terms of time to return to work.[59] A systematic review summarizing 28 studies showed a strong link between workers' compensation status and poor outcome after shoulder surgery.[64] Faber et al. found a low correlation between functional outcomes and limitations for returning to work, and found that duration of sick leave was seldom included in the outcome scores.[45]

Recommendations
- The effect of workers' compensation on the outcome of interventions for SIS is influenced by countries' social security systems and outcome measures [overall quality: moderate][45]
- Studies with duration of sick leave or work status as outcome measures provide evidence with regard to effectiveness similar to studies using functional limitations as outcome measure [overall quality: moderate][45]
- There is a strong link between workers' compensation status and poor outcome after shoulder surgery [overall quality: moderate]

Question 9: What are the complications associated with interventions for SIS?

Relevance
As there is no evidence supporting the use of one therapy or intervention above another, the chances of adverse effects can be an important factor in choice of therapy.

Current opinion
Side effects of surgery include prolonged pain, infection, difficulty moving the shoulder after the operation, wasting of the shoulder muscle, and the need to have another surgical procedure. Side effects for subacromial steroid injections could be degeneration and rupture of the rotator cuff and septic arthritis.

Finding the evidence
- PubMed, using search terms: "septic arthritis shoulder", "glenohumeral joint", "adverse outcome impingement surgery"

Quality of the evidence
- 1 Cochrane review
- 1 meta-analysis

Findings

Complications of surgical therapy A Cochrane review summarized adverse events of three trials comparing open with arthroscopic acromioplasty (arthroscopy group n = 74, open group n = 75).[46] The most-reported adverse event was postoperative pain (12% each group, n = 9), followed by stiffness/capsulitis (12% arthroscopy group, n = 9) and 4% open group, n = 3). Atrophy of the deltoid muscle was reported for 3% of patients in the arthroscopy group (n = 2). One deep wound infection was reported for the arthroscopy group and one superficial wound infection for the open group. In a meta-analysis performed by Davis et al. (nine studies) no significant differences were found in complications between the open and arthroscopic acromioplasty groups.[53]

Other surgical pitfalls include not addressing the entire pathology and doing an incomplete or excessive decompression. Spangehl et al. published the results of a randomized controlled trial which compared arthroscopic (n = 32) with open (n = 30) acromioplasty.[60] Repeat (open) acromioplasty was performed in five patients (16%) in the unsuccessful arthroscopic group without improvement. Unsatisfactory results were reported up to 52% for arthroscopic subacromial decompression.[65] Inadequate decompression was noted in 14 of 20 failed patients. Rehabilitation pitfalls include prescribing the wrong exercises at the wrong time and omitting steps in the rehabilitation process.[66]

Complications of injection therapy It is probably not possible to identify safety issues such as tendon rupture in a series of clinical trials. Iatrogenic septic arthritis has an estimated incidence of 1 in 14,000–50,000 injections, with sometimes dramatic consequences.[67,68] Aseptic procedures are advised when injecting corticosteroids.

Recommendations

- There is only low evidence concerning the complications of surgical treatment of SIS [overall quality: low]
- A 4%–12% incidence of postoperative stiffness is mentioned in studies [overall quality: low]
- There is conflicting evidence of the complication rates in arthroscopic compared to open surgery [overall quality: low]
- Poor outcome or recurrence is mentioned most often (up to 52%) [overall quality: moderate]
- Septic arthritis after steroid injections has dramatic consequences [overall quality: low]
- An aseptic technique is advised [overall quality: very low grade]

Summary of recommendations

- The Hawkins–Kennedy test is a useful and reliable screening test for SIS

- US may be the most cost-effective diagnostic method
- MRI or US could be equally used for impingement syndrome and rotator cuff tears
- There should be serious doubt about the placebo effect of "puncturing the painful area" versus the systemic effect of corticosteroids
- ESWT can have an effect on radiologic calcific tendinosis
- Surgical treatment of patients with SIS is not superior to conservative treatment
- There is no evidence supporting a difference in outcome after arthroscopic over open subacromial decompression or arthroscopic bursectomy

Conclusions

SIS is a common disorder, with an impact on quality of life and ability to work. Although patients are offered different treatment modalities sequentially during the period of the disability, no evidence for a difference in outcome between those modalities, i.e., physical therapy, subacromial steroid injection, and surgery (acromioplasty), can be found. Although the association of workers' compensation cases with inferior outcomes can be influenced by the different outcome measures and different social systems, there seems to be no evidence for the effect of therapeutic interventions on return to work. From a cost-effectiveness perspective, steroid injections, and home exercises are to be preferred to physical therapy and surgery.

References

1. Neer CS. Anterior acromioplasty for the chronic impingement syndrome in the shoulder: a preliminary report. J Bone Joint Surg Am 1972;54(1):41–50.
2. Silva L, Andreu JL, Munoz P, et al. Accuracy of physical examination in subacromial impingement syndrome. Rheumatology (Oxford) 2008;47(5):679–83.
3. Bigliani LU, Levine WN. Subacromial impingement syndrome. J Bone Joint Surg Am 1997;79(12):1854–68.
4. Blevins FT. Rotator cuff pathology in athletes. Sports Med 1997;24(3):205–20.
5. Luime JJ, Koes BW, Hendriksen IJ, et al. Prevalence and incidence of shoulder pain in the general population; a systematic review. Scand J Rheumatol 2004;33(2):73–81.
6. Bot SD, van der Waal JM, Terwee CB, et al. Incidence and prevalence of complaints of the neck and upper extremity in general practice. Ann Rheum Dis 2005;64(1):118–23.
7. van der Windt DA, Koes BW, de Jong BA, Bouter LM. Shoulder disorders in general practice: incidence, patient characteristics, and management. Ann Rheum Dis 1995;54(12):959–64.
8. Diercks RL, Ham SJ, Ros JM. [Results of anterior shoulder decompression surgery according to Neer for shoulder

impingement syndrome; little effect on fitness for work]. Ned Tijdschr Geneeskd 1998;142(22):1266–9.

9. Holtby R, Razmjou H. Impact of work-related compensation claims on surgical outcome of patients with rotator cuff related pathologies: a matched case-control study. J Shoulder Elbow Surg 2010;19(3):452–60.

10. Neer CS. Impingement lesions. Clin Orthop Relat Res 1983;(173): 70–7.

11. Holtby R, Razmjou H. Validity of the supraspinatus test as a single clinical test in diagnosing patients with rotator cuff pathology. J Orthop Sports Phys Ther 2004;34(4):194–200.

12. Beaudreuil J, Nizard R, Thomas T, et al. Contribution of clinical tests to the diagnosis of rotator cuff disease: a systematic literature review. Joint Bone Spine 2009 Jan;76(1):15–9.

13. Dinnes J, Loveman E, McIntyre L, Waugh N. The effectiveness of diagnostic tests for the assessment of shoulder pain due to soft tissue disorders: a systematic review. Health Technol Assess 2003;7(29):iii, 1–166.

14. Hughes PC, Taylor NF, Green RA. Most clinical tests cannot accurately diagnose rotator cuff pathology: a systematic review. Aust J Physiother 2008;54(3):159–70.

15. Park HB, Yokota A, Gill HS, El Rassi G, McFarland EG. Diagnostic accuracy of clinical tests for the different degrees of subacromial impingement syndrome. J Bone Joint Surg Am 2005;87(7): 1446–55.

16. Tennent TD, Beach WR, Meyers JF. A review of the special tests associated with shoulder examination. Part I: the rotator cuff tests. Am J Sports Med 2003;31(1):154–60.

17. Moen MH, de Vos RJ, Ellenbecker TS, Weir A. Clinical tests in shoulder examination: how to perform them. Br J Sports Med 2010;44(5):370–5.

18. O'Connor PJ, Rankine J, Gibbon WW, Richardson A, Winter F, Miller JH. Interobserver variation in sonography of the painful shoulder. J Clin Ultrasound 2005;33(2):53–6.

19. Brenneke SL, Morgan CJ. Evaluation of ultrasonography as a diagnostic technique in the assessment of rotator cuff tendon tears. Am J Sports Med 1992;20(3):287–9.

20. Shahabpour M, Kichouh M, Laridon E, Gielen JL, De Mey J. The effectiveness of diagnostic imaging methods for the assessment of soft tissue and articular disorders of the shoulder and elbow. Eur J Radiol 2008;65(2):194–200.

21. Vander Maren C, Shahabpour M, Willems S, Vande Berg B, Handelberg F, Malghem J. [The value of MRI in the evaluation of lesions of the supraspinous muscle. Multicentric retrospective study of 66 records]. Acta Orthop Belg 1995;61 Suppl 1:8–13.

22. Teefey SA, Rubin DA, Middleton WD, Hildebolt CF, Leibold RA, Yamaguchi K. Detection and quantification of rotator cuff tears. Comparison of ultrasonographic, magnetic resonance imaging, and arthroscopic findings in seventy-one consecutive cases. J Bone Joint Surg Am 2004;86-A(4):708–16.

23. Mohtadi NG, Vellet AD, Clark ML, et al. A prospective, double-blind comparison of magnetic resonance imaging and arthroscopy in the evaluation of patients presenting with shoulder pain. J Shoulder Elbow Surg 2004;13(3):258–65.

24. Henkus HE, Cobben LP, Coerkamp EG, Nelissen RG, van Arkel ER. The accuracy of subacromial injections: a prospective randomized magnetic resonance imaging study. Arthroscopy 2006; 22(3):277–82.

25. Gruson KI, Ruchelsman DE, Zuckerman JD. Subacromial corticosteroid injections. J Shoulder Elbow Surg 2008;17 (1 Suppl):118S-30S.

26. Skedros JG, Pitts TC. Temporal variations in a modified Neer impingement test can confound clinical interpretation. Clin Orthop Relat Res 2007;460:130–6.

27. Buchbinder R, Green S, Youd JM. Corticosteroid injections for shoulder pain. Cochrane Database Syst Rev 2003;(1): CD004016.

28. Arroll B, Goodyear-Smith F. Corticosteroid injections for painful shoulder: a meta-analysis. Br J Gen Pract 2005;55(512):224–8.

29. Plafki C, Steffen R, Willburger RE, Wittenberg RH. Local anaesthetic injection with and without corticosteroids for subacromial impingement syndrome. Int Orthop 2000;24(1):40–2.

30. Ekeberg OM, Bautz-Holter E, Tveita EK, Juel NG, Kvalheim S, Brox JI. Subacromial ultrasound guided or systemic steroid injection for rotator cuff disease: randomised double blind study. BMJ 2009;338:a3112.

31. Green S, Buchbinder R, Hetrick S. Physiotherapy interventions for shoulder pain. Cochrane Database Syst Rev 2003;(2):CD004258.

32. Kromer TO, Tautenhahn UG, de Bie RA, Staal JB, Bastiaenen CH. Effects of physiotherapy in patients with shoulder impingement syndrome: a systematic review of the literature. J Rehabil Med 2009;41(11):870–80.

33. Walther M, Werner A, Stahlschmidt T, Woelfel R, Gohlke F. The subacromial impingement syndrome of the shoulder treated by conventional physiotherapy, self-training, and a shoulder brace: results of a prospective, randomized study. J Shoulder Elbow Surg 2004;13(4):417–23.

34. Bang MD, Deyle GD. Comparison of supervised exercise with and without manual physical therapy for patients with shoulder impingement syndrome. J Orthop Sports Phys Ther 2000;30(3): 126–37.

35. Ketola S, Lehtinen J, Arnala I, Nissinen M, Westenius H, Sintonen H, et al. Does arthroscopic acromioplasty provide any additional value in the treatment of shoulder impingement syndrome?: a two-year randomised controlled trial. J Bone Joint Surg Br 2009;91(10):1326–34.

36. Jonsson P, Wahlstrom P, Ohberg L, Alfredson H. Eccentric training in chronic painful impingement syndrome of the shoulder: results of a pilot study. Knee Surg Sports Traumatol Arthrosc 2006;14(1):76–81.

37. Andres BM, Murrell GA. Treatment of tendinopathy: what works, what does not, and what is on the horizon. Clin Orthop Relat Res 2008;466(7):1539–54.

38. Saithna A, Jenkinson E, Boer R, Costa ML, Drew S. Is extracorporeal shockwave therapy for calcifying tendinitis of the rotator cuff associated with a significant improvement in the Constant-Murley score? A systematic review. Curr Orthop Pract 2009; 20(5):566–71.

39. Schmitt J, Tosch A, Hunerkopf M, Haake M. [Extracorporeal shockwave therapy (ESWT) as therapeutic option in supraspinatus tendon syndrome? One year results of a placebo controlled study]. Orthopade 2002;31(7):652–7.

40. Speed CA, Nichols D, Wies J, Humphreys H, Richards C, Burnet S, et al. Extracorporeal shock wave therapy for plantar fasciitis. A double blind randomised controlled trial. J Orthop Res 2003;21(5):937–40.

41. Engebretsen K, Grotle M, Bautz-Holter E, Sandvik L, Juel NG, Ekeberg OM, et al. Radial extracorporeal shockwave treatment compared with supervised exercises in patients with subacromial pain syndrome: single blind randomised study. BMJ 2009;339:b3360.

42. Green S, Buchbinder R, Hetrick S. Acupuncture for shoulder pain. Cochrane Database Syst Rev 2005;(2):CD005319.

43. Cumpston M, Johnston RV, Wengier L, Buchbinder R. Topical glyceryl trinitrate for rotator cuff disease. Cochrane Database Syst Rev 2009;(3):CD006355.

44. Downing DS, Weinstein A. Ultrasound therapy of subacromial bursitis. A double blind trial. Phys Ther 1986;66(2):194–9.

45. Faber E, Kuiper JI, Burdorf A, Miedema HS, Verhaar JAN. Treatment of impingement syndrome: A systematic review of the effects on functional limitations and return to work. J Occup Rehabil 2006;16(1).7–25.

46. Coghlan JA, Buchbinder R, Green S, Johnston RV, Bell SN. Surgery for rotator cuff disease. Cochrane Database Syst Rev 2008;(1):CD005619.

47. Dorrestijn O, Stevens M, Winters JC, van der Meer K, Diercks RL. Conservative or surgical treatment for subacromial impingement syndrome? A systematic review. J Shoulder Elbow Surg 2009;18(4):652–60.

48. Brox JI, Staff PH, Ljunggren AE, Brevik JI. Arthroscopic surgery compared with supervised exercises in patients with rotator cuff disease (stage II impingement syndrome). BMJ 1993;307(6909): 899–903.

49. Haahr JP, Ostergaard S, Dalsgaard J, Norup K, Frost P, Lausen S, et al. Exercises versus arthroscopic decompression in patients with subacromial impingement: a randomised, controlled study in 90 cases with a one year follow up. Ann Rheum Dis 2005;64(5): 760–4.

50. Haahr JP, Andersen JH. Exercises may be as efficient as subacromial decompression in patients with subacromial stage II impingement: 4–8-years' follow-up in a prospective, randomized study. Scand J Rheumatol 2006;35(3):224–8.

51. Peters G, Kohn D. [Mid-term clinical results after surgical versus conservative treatment of subacromial impingement syndrome]. Unfallchirurg 1997;100(8):623–9.

52. Rahme H, Solem-Bertoft E, Westerberg CE, Lundberg E, Sorensen S, Hilding S. The subacromial impingement syndrome. A study of results of treatment with special emphasis on predictive factors and pain-generating mechanisms. Scand J Rehabil Med 1998;30(4):253–62.

53. Davis AD, Kakar S, Moros C, Kaye EK, Schepsis AA, Voloshin I. Arthroscopic versus open acromioplasty: a meta-analysis. Am J Sports Med 2010;38(3):613–8.

54. Henkus HE, de Witte PB, Nelissen RG, Brand R, van Arkel ER. Bursectomy compared with acromioplasty in the management of subacromial impingement syndrome: a prospective randomised study. J Bone Joint Surg Br 2009;91(4):504–10.

55. Husby T, Haugstvedt JR, Brandt M, Holm I, Steen H. Open versus arthroscopic subacromial decompression: a prospective, randomized study of 34 patients followed for 8 years. Acta Orthop Scand 2003;74(4):408–14.

56. Iversen T, Reikeras O, Solem OI. [Acromion resection for shoulder impingement syndrome. Results after an open and a percutaneous surgical method]. Tidsskr Nor Laegeforen 1996;116(16): 1879–82.

57. Lindh M, Norlin R. Arthroscopic subacromial decompression versus open acromioplasty. A two-year follow-up study. Clin Orthop Relat Res 1993;290:174–6.

58. Norlin R. Arthroscopic subacromial decompression versus open acromioplasty. Arthroscopy 1989;5(4):321–3.

59. Sachs RA, Stone ML, Devine S. Open vs. arthroscopic acromioplasty: A prospective, randomized study. 1994;10(3):248–54.

60. Spangehl MJ, Hawkins RH, McCormack RG, Loomer RL. Arthroscopic versus open acromioplasty: a prospective, randomized, blinded study. J Shoulder Elbow Surg 2002;11(2): 101–7.

61. T'Jonck L, Lysens R, De SL, et al. Open versus arthroscopic subacromial decompression: analysis of one-year results. Physiother Res Int 1997;2(2):46–61.

62. Chipchase LS, O'Connor DA, Costi JJ, Krishnan J. Shoulder impingement syndrome: preoperative health status. J Shoulder Elbow Surg 2000;9(1):12–5.

63. Kuijpers T, van der Windt DA, van der Heijden GJ, Bouter LM. Systematic review of prognostic cohort studies on shoulder disorders. Pain 2004;109(3):420–31.

64. Koljonen P, Chong C, Yip D. Difference in outcome of shoulder surgery between workers' compensation and nonworkers' compensation populations. Int Orthop 2009;33(2):315–20.

65. Hawkins RJ, Plancher KD, Saddemi SR, Brezenoff LS, Moor JT. Arthroscopic subacromial decompression. J Shoulder Elbow Surg 2001;10(3):225–30.

66. Ben Kibler BW, Sciascia A. What went wrong and what to do about it: pitfalls in the treatment of shoulder impingement. Instr Course Lect 2008;57:103–12.

67. Lossos IS, Yossepowitch O, Kandel L, Yardeni D, Arber N. Septic arthritis of the glenohumeral joint. A report of 11 cases and review of the literature. Medicine (Baltimore) 1998;77(3): 177–87.

68. Brinkman MJ, Diercks RL. [Septic arthritis after injection therapy in the shoulder]. Ned Tijdschr Geneeskd 2009;153(13):607–11.

90

Pathology of the Long Head of the Biceps

Paul W.L. ten Berg, Luke S. Oh, and David Ring

Massachusetts General Hospital, Boston, MA, USA

Case scenario

A 58 year old self-employed electrician who was diagnosed with long head of biceps brachii (LHB) tendinopathy 6 months ago on his dominant shoulder now presents with increased pain after putting together a swing set in his back yard. On examination, he is tender over the bicipital groove and has a positive Speed's test, Yergason's, O'Brien's, Neer, and Hawkins signs, and no lag signs or weakness of the rotator cuff.

Relevant anatomy

The LHB tendon originates from the posterosuperior labrum and the supraglenoid tubercle. The proximal portion of the LHB tendon is intra-articular but extrasynovial. It passes obliquely within the shoulder joint, arching anteriorly over the humeral head before entering the bicipital groove. The exact role of the LHB in the glenohumeral joint is debated. Some believe that the biceps muscle is an important depressor of the humeral head against proximal migration.

Importance of the problem

LHB tendinopathy is a common cause of shoulder pain, although its incidence remains unknown.[1] It is generally encountered in concert with rotator cuff tendinopathy in older individuals or overhead athletes.

Top seven questions

Diagnosis

1. How accurate are clinical examination maneuvers for the diagnosis of biceps tendinitis?
2. What is the role of images studies in the diagnosis of proximal biceps pathology?

Therapy

3. Is there a role for nonoperative treatment?
4. What are the indications for surgical treatment?
5. What is involved in the decision-making to perform a biceps tendon debridement vs. tenodesis vs. tenotomy?
6. Is there an advantage to arthroscopic over open biceps tenodesis?
7. Is any one operative technique superior to another?

Question 1: How accurate are clinical examination maneuvers for the diagnosis of biceps tendinitis?

Clinical examination maneuvers used in the office setting for the diagnosis of biceps tendinitis include bicipital groove palpation and the Speed, Yergason, and O'Brien tests (see box).

Evidence-Based Orthopedics, First Edition. Edited by Mohit Bhandari.
© 2012 Blackwell Publishing Ltd. Published 2012 by Blackwell Publishing Ltd.

Physical examination tests

- *Bicipital groove palpation:* In case of LHB pathology patients are usually tender directly over the biceps tendon, as it exits the intra-articular space, through the intertubercular groove, and down to a point approximately 7 cm below the acromion while the arm is internally rotated 10°.[2]
- *Speed test:* The externally rotated (supinated) arm with an extended elbow is forward elevated. The examiner resists this forward elevation of the arm while palpating the patient's biceps tendon over the anterior aspect of the shoulder. Pain felt in the bicipital groove indicates biceps tendon pathology.[3]
- *Yergason test:* A test for evaluation of biceps tendon pathology in which supination of the forearm is resisted. The elbow is flexed to 90° and the patient is asked to resist while externally rotating the arm. The test is considered positive if this resistance produces pain referred to the bicipital groove.[4]
- *O'Brien test:* O'Brien's active compression test is designed to maximally load and compress the acromioclavicular joint and bicipitallabral complex. The patient is instructed to flex their arm to 90° with the elbow fully extended and then adduct the arm 10–15° medial to the sagittal plane. The arm is then internally rotated (pronated) and the patient resists the examiner's downward force. The procedure is reiterated in supination. The test is positive if pain appears in maximal internal rotation, then disappears in external rotation. It is a common test for detecting acromioclavicular joint and superior labral pathology.[5]

Relevance

It can be difficult to isolate the precise cause of shoulder pain.

Current opinion

Most shoulder surgeons believe they can distinguish pain from the LHB from other types of shoulder pain.

Finding evidence

- Cochrane Database, with search term: "shoulder examination"
- PubMed (www.ncbi.nlm.nih.gov/pubmed/): sensitivity search using keywords: "biceps tendon" AND "tests", "biceps tendon" AND "speed"/"Yergason"/"O'Brien"/"groove test"
- Bibliography of eligible articles

Quality of the evidence

Level I
- 1 prospective blinded study of consecutive patients[11]

Level II
- 1 randomized cohort study[9]
- 3 prospective nonrandomized clinical trials[7,12,15]
- 4 cohort studies[6,8,13,14,16]

Level IV
- 1 diagnostic study with poor reference standard[10]

Findings

Table 90.1 summarizes the findings in the literature. For diagnosis of LHB pathology, tenderness in the bicipital groove has a sensitivity of 53 and a specificity of 54; Speed's test has a sensitivity from 32 to 69 (with one outlier of 90) and a specificity from 48 to 75 (with one outlier of 14); Yegerson's test has a sensitivity of 43 and a specificity of 79; and O'Brien's test has an average sensitivity of 48 and a specificity of 47.

Recommendation

- Physical examination maneuvers have limited ability to diagnose biceps pathology [overall quality: moderate]

Question 2: What is the role of imaging in the diagnosis of proximal biceps pathology?

Case clarification

The patient's MRI demonstrated fluid surrounding the biceps tendon in the bicipital groove, with signal changes interpreted as tendinopathy and possible partial tear. There was no evidence of rotator cuff tear.

Relevance

Ultrasound and MRI are often used to diagnose LHB tendinopathy.

Current opinion

Management decisions are often based on the findings of radiological tests.

Finding the evidence

- Cochrane Database, with search term: "shoulder" AND "imaging"
- PubMed (www.ncbi.nlm.nih.gov/pubmed/): sensitivity search using keywords "biceps tendon" AND "ultrasound"/ "MRI"/ "MRA"; "shoulder" AND "ultrasound"/ "MRI"/"MRA"
- Bibliography of eligible articles

Quality of the evidence

Level I
- 2 independent, blinded comparisons with a reference standard among consecutive patients with a defined clinical presentation[20,21]

Table 90.1 Shoulder trials with physical maneuver tests and sensitivity/specificity rates

Test, author, and year	Sample size	Sensitivity/ specificity (%)	Criterion standard	Positive by criterion standard
Bicipital groove tenderness				
LHB tendon pathology				
Gill 2007[6]	847 patients	53/54	Arthroscopy	40 LHB partial tear
Superior labrum pathology				
Nakagawa 2005[7]	54 patients	25/80	Arthroscopy	24 SLAP lesions
Guanche 2003[8]	60 shoulders	48/52	Arthroscopy	33 SLAP lesions
Speed test				
LHB tendon pathology				
Gill 2007[6]	847 patients	50/67	Arthroscopy	40 LHB partial tear
Ardic 2006[9]	36 patients	69/60	MRI	26 biceps pathology
Lafosse 2007[10]	200 patients	41/48	Arthroscopy/open surgery	46 Type I LHB lesions
		51/48		63 Type II LHB lesions
LHB tendon pathology combined with labrum pathology				
Holtby 2004[11]	152 patients	32/75	Arthroscopy	42 biceps pathology or SLAP lesions
Bennet 1998[12]	46 shoulders	90/14	Arthroscopy	10 biceps and labral complex pathology
Superior labrum pathology				
Parentis 2006[13]	132 patients	48/67	Arthroscopy	40 SLAP lesions
Guanche 2003[8]	60 shoulders	9/74	Arthroscopy	33 SLAP lesions
Morgan 1998[14]	102 patients	68/.	Arthroscopy	81 SLAP lesions
Rotator cuff pathology				
Park 2005[15]	552 patients	33/70	Arthroscopy	72 partial thickness rotator cuff tears
	552 patients	40/75	Arthroscopy	215 rotator cuff tears
Impingement syndrome				
Park 2005[15]	552 patients	38/83	Arthroscopy	359 SIS*
Calis 2000[16]	125 Shoulders	69/56	Subacromial injection test; MRI	89 SIS*
Yergason test				
LHB tendon pathology combined with superior labrum pathology				
Hotlby 2004[11]	152 patients	43/79	Arthroscopy	42 biceps pathology or SLAP lesions
Impingement syndrome				
Calis 2000[16]	125 Shoulders	37/86	Subacromial injection test; MRI	89 SIS*
Labrum pathology				
Parentis 2006[13]	132 patients	13/94	Arthroscopy	40 SLAP lesions
Guanche 2003[8]	60 shoulders	12/96	Arthroscopy	33 SLAP lesions
O'Briens test				
Lafosse 2007[10]	200 patients	45/46	Arthroscopy/open surgery	46 Type I LHB lesions (mild)
		51/48		63 Type II LHB lesions (severe)
Bicipital groove tenderness combined with speed test				
LHB tendon pathology				
Gill 2007[6]	847 patients	68/49	Arthroscopy	40 LHB partial tear
Speed combined with Yergason test				
LHB tendon pathology combined with superior labrum pathology				
Hotlby 2004[11]	152 patients	56/63	Arthroscopy	42 biceps pathology or SLAP lesions

LHB, long head of biceps; SIS, subacromial impingement syndrome; SLAP, superior labrum anterior–posterior.

Level II
• 7 independent blinded comparisons with a reference standard among nonconsecutive patients or confined to a narrow population of study patients[9,24–27,29,30]

Level IV
• 1 independent unblinded comparison with a reference standard[22]
• 1 independent unblinded comparison with poor reference standard[23]

Level V
• 3 expert opinions[17–19]

Findings

Table 90.2 summarizes the literature regarding imaging diagnosis of LHB pathology. Ultrasound has a sensitivity of 53–100% and a specificity of 97–100% for diagnosis of dislocation, subluxation, and rupture of the LHB tendon. Intracapsular partial tears of the LHB tendon are not detectable. Biceps tendon sheath effusions detected sonographically are not specific to LHB pathology.[17,18]

The oblique sagittal plane MRI gives the best image of the intra-articular portion of the biceps tendon in the rotator cuff interval. Ruptures are easier to detect than partial tears.[19] Mohtadi et al. (level I) found 60% of the patients whose findings were identified by arthroscopy and MRI as normal or abnormal and 38% of the patients in whom structures were identified exactly according to the classification of pathology on both MRI and arthroscopy.[20] MR arthrography has a sensitivity of 67–100% and a specificity of 56–100% for LHB pathology.

Recommendation

• Diagnostic imaging has limited and variable sensitivity and specificity for LHB tendon pathology [overall quality: moderate]

Question 3: Is there a role for nonoperative treatment?

Relevance

Physical therapy and selective cortisone injections are commonly used to treat LHB pathology.

Current option

Physical therapy and associated modalities may offer symptom relief as well as exercises and patient education regarding activity modification. Selective cortisone injections offer the advantage of providing useful diagnostic information regarding the location of pain as well as therapeutic benefit.

Finding the evidence

• Cochrane Database, with search term: "shoulder" and "physiotherapy"/"injections"

• PubMed (www.ncbi.nlm.nih.gov/pubmed/): sensitivity search using keywords as above

Quality of the evidence

Level II
• 2 reviews using randomized or pseudo-randomized controlled trials[31,32]

Level IV
• 1 case series[33]

Findings

There is no data on physical therapy or selective cortisone injections in the treatment of LHB tendon pathologies.

A review of the Cochrane collaboration (level II) using 26 trials of physiotherapy for shoulder conditions stated that there was some evidence for combining mobilization with exercise in rotator cuff disorders, but did not find any studies specific to LHB pathology.[31]

Another Cochrane review (Level II) including 26 trials showed some weak evidence for rotator cuff disease that corticosteroid injections were superior to physiotherapy.[32]

A case series (level IV) from 1979 reported seven LHB tendon ruptures in patients with an average age of 65 years after local steroid injection (triamcinolone hexacetonide) for bicipital tendinitis (average interval injection to rupture was 3 weeks). However, the author mentioned that it is likely that the tendons which ruptured were already in a state of degeneration that predisposed to their rupture.[33]

Recommendation

• There is no evidence of superiority of one nonoperative treatment over other treatment modalities [overall quality: very low]

Question 4: What are the indications for surgical treatment of a LHB rupture?

Relevance

There is no consensus regarding when to offer surgical treatment.

Current option

Tenodesis may be considered for an acute LHB rupture in an active individual

Finding the evidence

• PubMed (www.ncbi.nlm.nih.gov/pubmed/): sensitivity search using keywords "tenodesis" AND "biceps" AND "rupture"; "biceps" AND "rupture"
• Bibliography of eligible articles

Quality of the evidence

Level III
• 2 case-control studies[35,36]

Table 90.2 Imaging trials for tendon pathologies and sensitivity/specificity rates

Test, author, and year	Examiner/ overall	Sample size	Sensitivity/ specificity%	Criterion standard	Positive by criterion standard
Ultrasound in LHB tendon pathology					
Kayser 2005[21]	Average	239 patients	53/97		8 LHB dislocations, 15 LHB ruptures
Teefey 2000[22]		100 shoulders	64/99	Arthroscopy	11 LHB ruptures
			83/100		6 LHB dislocations
Read 1998[23]		42 patients	80/100	Open surgery / arthroscopy	10 LHB tendinitis (extracapsular)
			100/100		2 LHB dislocations
			75/100		4 LHB ruptures
Armstrong 2006[24]		71 patients	0.0/92	Arthroscopy	23 LHB partial tears (intracapsular)
		71 patients	100/94		7 LHB tendon complete ruptures
		60 patients	100/96		4 LHB tendon subluxations
Le Corroller 2008[25]	Average	65 patients	93/99	MR arthrography	7 LHB "abnormalities" (extracapsular)
Ardic 2006[9]		59 patients	100/100	MRI	2 LHB ruptures
			100/100		34 LHB effusion/ hypertrophy
MRI in LHB tendon pathology					
Mohtadi 2004[20]		53 patients	72.2/54.3	Arthroscopy	18 normal LHB tendons
			9.1/96.8		22 LHB tendon inflammations
			50.0/69.8		10 LHB partial-thickness tears
			0.0/94.0		3 nonretracted LHB tendon ruptures
MRA in LHB tendon pathology					
Zanetti 1998[26]	Observer 1	42 Patients	92/56	Arthroscopy	Overall 26 tendinopathies or ruptures
	Observer 2		89/81		
Jung 2009[27]	Observer 1	19 patients	67/78	Arthroscopy	Indirect MRA, partial tears
	Observer 1		100/100		Direct MRA, partial tears
	Observer 2		78/89		Indirect MRA, partial tears
	Observer 2		90/100		Direct MRA, partial tears
Guckel 1998[28]		27 patients	100/100	Arthroscopy	17 LHB tenosynovitis
MRI vs.MRA in general shoulder pathologies					
Flannigan 1990[29]		9 shoulders	33/100	Arthroscopy	MRI, 9 labral tears
					MRA, 9 labral tears
		14 shoulders	64/79		MRI, 14 rotator cuff tears
					MRA, 14 rotator cuff tears
Dinauer 2007[30]	Reader A	104 shoulders	85/75	Arthroscopy	MRI, 24 normal superior labrum
	Reader B		66/83		80 abnormal superior labral
	Reader A		91/71		MRA, 24 normal superior labrum
	Reader B		84/58		80 abnormal superior labral

LHB, long head of biceps; MRA, MR arthrography.

Level IV
- 1 case series[34]

Findings

Evaluation (level IV) of 25 patients (all >40 years of age) an average of 7.9 years after complete rupture of the LHB tendon found few differences between those treated non-operatively and those treated operatively.[34] Only one patient complained about a cosmetic deformity. Muscle examination (with the Cybex II testing machine) of 19 patients found no significant differences in supination or elbow flexion strength in the two groups.

A similar study (level III) investigated the strength difference by using the Cybex II testing machine in 10 conservatively treated patients and 5 surgically treated patients after LHB tendon rupture, compared to 20 healthy individuals.[35] Nonoperatively treated patients had an average of 16% less elbow flexion strength, 11% less supination strength, and 16% less shoulder abduction compared to the healthy controls. The surgically treated patients lost 8% elbow flexion strength, 7% supination strength, and 20% of shoulder abduction strength.

In third study (level III), 26 patients treated operatively were compared to 30 patients treated nonoperatively a mean of 13 and 4.6 years respectively after LHB tendon rupture.[36] Biomechanical testing was performed on 10 patients in the surgical group and 13 in the nonsurgical group. Residual subjective weakness at the elbow was reported in 15.4% (4) of the surgical group and in 66.7% (20) of the nonsurgical group. Of the nonsurgical patients 36.7% (11) were not able to return to full work capacity, vs. only 7.7% (2) in the surgical group. The nonsurgical group had lost a mean of 21% of supination strength and 8% of elbow flexion strength but had no weakness in grip, pronation, or elbow extension. The surgical group had lost no significant strength in any of these testing modes.

Recommendation

- The role of surgery for LHB rupture is unclear [overall quality: very low]

Question 5: When operative treatment is elected for LHB tendinosis, which is better: biceps tenotomy or tenodesis?

Relevance

The optimal treatment of tendinosis of the LHB is debated.

Current opinion

Tenotomy or tenodesis are considered when there is a partial tear, significant tenosynovitis, subluxation, or dislocation. Tenotomy is a good option in the less active patient and in those patients who would accept having a "Popeye" sign. Tenodesis is becoming a more popular option, particularly in the younger and more active patient population.

Finding the evidence

- PubMed (www.ncbi.nlm.nih.gov/pubmed/): sensitivity search using keywords "biceps" AND "tenotomy" AND "tenodesis"
- Bibliography of eligible articles

Quality of the evidence

Level III
- 3 case-control studies[40–42]

Level IV
- 4 case series[37–39,43]

Findings

Data from three retrospective case series that assessed tenotomy were pooled together (N = 377),with 73% of the patients achieving good/excellent outcome or satisfaction, but in 58% a Popeye sign (deformity of the biceps) was visible and 16% of the patients had a poor outcome.[37–39]

In case-control studies comparing both treatments, there were no significant differences between tenotomy and tenodesis in clinical assessment (N = 281, with mean follow-up interval >15 months) except for greater deformity in the tenotomy group.[40–42] Within a total group of 129 patients with tenotomy, 30% had a severe cosmetic deformity or noticeable Popeye sign vs. less than 5% in the tenodesis group (N = 152). However, Boileau (level III) mentioned that the Popeye sign was not a concern for any patient.[41]

In one case series (level IV) 40 patients were treated with tenotomy and the muscle force for elbow flexion-supination was decreased by 40% compared with age-, sex-, and dominance-matched controls. Nevertheless, 86% of the patients were satisfied with the outcome.[43]

Paulos and Franklin (level III) noted for 20% within the tenotomy group (N = 39) a near normal strength in the affected arm, and 64% within the tenodesis (N = 33) group.[41] Boileau et al. (Level III) compared the preoperative Constant strength score with the final Constant strength score and noticed no significant difference between both tenotomy and tenodesis groups.[42]

Recommendation

- There are insufficient data to determine the optimal operative treatment for LHB tendinopathy [overall quality: low]

Question 6: Is there an advantage to arthroscopic over open biceps tenodesis?

Relevance

The optimal tenodesis approach is debated, i.e., arthroscopic biceps tenodesis (proximal) vs. open biceps tenodesis (distal).

Current opinion

The surgical approach is based on the physician's preferences and skills.

Findings in evidence

- PubMed (www.ncbi.nlm.nih.gov/pubmed/): sensitivity search using keywords "biceps" and "tenodesis"
- Bibliography of eligible articles

Quality of the evidence

Level III
- 1 case-control study[41]

Level IV
- 4 case series[44-47]

Findings

Paulos and Franklin (level III) compared 22 patients treated with arthroscopic wedge tenodesis and 17 treated with open keyhole tenodesis. All patients were satisfied and 68% of the wedge group and 59% of the keyhole group had near normal strength. Tenderness to palpation in the proximal biceps groove was present in 23% and 6% of each group respectively.[41]

Case series of patients treated with arthroscopic tenodesis including bioabsorbable interference screw, suture, and subdeltoid transfer shows an overall rate for good results of 88%.[44-47] The highest rate of poor outcome is 5%.

Recommendation

- There are insufficient data regarding tenodesis techniques to determine the optimal approach [overall quality: low]

Question 7: Is one operative technique superior to another?

Relevance

The optimal tenodesis technique is debated: e.g., deltopectoral approach vs. subpectoral approach for an open biceps tenodesis; "keyhole" technique vs. soft tissue tenodesis vs. metal suture anchor vs. bioabsorbable suture anchor.

Current opinion

Several tenodesis techniques are described in the treatment of LHB pathologies and are related to the preference and skills of the surgeon.

Finding the evidence

- PubMed (www.ncbi.nlm.nih.gov/pubmed/)—sensitivity search using keywords "biceps tenodesis"; "bicep*" AND " tenodesis" AND "tendon"
- Bibliography of eligible articles

Quality of the evidence

Level III
- 2 case-control studies[44,48]

Level IV
- 6 case series[45-47,49-51]

Findings

A comparative study (level III) investigated the results after open subpectoral biceps tenodesis with either interference screw fixation (N = 34) or suture anchor fixation (N = 54) (mean follow-up interval 13 months). No significant difference between the two procedures was noted. There were no failures of fixation and no complications postoperatively.[48]

Franceschi et al. (level III) compared two cohorts: soft tissue tenodesis incorporated with rotator cuff suture (N = 11) and the same treatment with an extra resection of the remaining intra-articular tendon stump of the biceps from glenoid tubercle (N = 11). Both groups had a 100% good to excellent outcome and no significant difference in the total UCLA scores was found when comparing treatments performed with or without additional tenotomy.[44]

Two studies included respectively 40 and 15 patients for two different soft tissue tenodesis techniques: arthroscopic subdeltoid transfer of the LHB tendon to its conjoint tendon and arthroscopic stay suture integrated with the rotator cuff (mean interval of respectively 28 and 32 months). Good to excellent results were noted in over 80 % and poor outcomes in less than 5%.[46,47]

Mazzocca et al. and Boileau et al. both used bioabsorbable interference screws but different approaches: open subpectoral (N = 41, mean follow-up interval of 29 months) and arthroscopic (N = 43, mean follow-up interval of 17 months).[49,50] Mozzocca et al. (level IV) noticed one case of tendon pulled out from the bone tunnel. However of the 56% of patients who had completed preoperative and postoperative assessments, all clinical outcome measures demonstrated statistically significant improvement at follow-up when compared with the preoperative scores. Boileau et al. (level IV) observed an average significant postoperative improvement of the Constant score and only 5% of the patients had a poor result. There was no loss of elbow movement and biceps strength was 90% of the strength of the other side.

A study (level IV) including 10 patients investigated the suture anchor technique (mean follow-up interval of 24 months).[45] In this study 90% had good to excellent outcome and there was 100% satisfaction with cosmetic results.

With a relatively large mean follow-up interval of 84 months, Berlemann and Bayley (level IV) noticed a 60% rate of good to excellent outcome in 15 patients treated with keyhole tenodesis;[51] 13% had a poor outcome at final follow-up.

Recommendation

• Clinical data does not show large differences between attachments techniques [overall quality: low]

Summary of recommendations

• Physical examination maneuvers have limited ability to diagnose biceps pathology
• Diagnostic imaging has limited and variable sensitivity and specificity for LHB tendon pathology
• There is no evidence that any one nonoperative treatment modality is superior to any other
• The role of surgery for LHB rupture is unclear
• There are insufficient data to determine the optimal operative treatment for LHB tendinopathy
• There are insufficient data regarding tenodesis techniques to determine the optimal approach
• Clinical data does not show large differences between attachments techniques

Conclusions

Physical examination and imaging have low sensitivity in the detection of LHB tendon pathologies, and therefore have less diagnostic value. At present, there is a paucity of high-quality evidence with regard to surgical approach and treatment. Trials with long follow-up interval are desirable for decision-making about treatment. No significant differences can be found, except for the cosmetic deformity which is more likely to occur after tenotomy.

References

1. Murthi AM, Vosburgh CL, Neviaser TJ. The incidence of pathologic changes of the long head of the biceps tendon. J Shoulder Elbow Surg 2000;9:382–5.
2. Mazzocca AD, Rios CG, Romeo AA, Arciero RA. Subpectoral biceps tenodesis with interference screw fixation. Arthroscopy 2005;21:896.
3. Crenshaw AH, Kilgore WE. Surgical treatment of bicipital tenosynovitis. J Bone Joint Surg Am 1966;48:1496–502.
4. Yergason RM. Supination sign. J Bone Joint Surg 1931;13:160.
5. O'Brien SJ, Pagnani MJ, Fealy S, McGlynn SR, Wilson JB. The active compression test: a new and effective test for diagnosing labral tears and acromioclavicular joint abnormality. Am J Sports Med 1998;26:610–13.
6. Gill HSERG, Bahk MS, Castillo RC, McFarland EG. Physical examination for partial tears of the biceps tendon. Am J Sports Med 2007;35:1334–42.
7. Nakagawa S, Yoneda M, Hayashida K, Obata M, Fukushima S, Miyazaki Y. Forced shoulder abduction and elbow flexion test: a new simple clinical test to detect superior labral injury in the throwing shoulder. Arthroscopy 2005;21:1290–5.
8. Guanche CA, Jones DC. Clinical testing for tears of the glenoid labrum. Arthroscopy 2003;19:517–23.
9. Ardic F, Kahraman Y, Kacar M, Kahraman MC, Findikoglu G, Yorancioglu ZR. Shoulder impingement syndrome: relationships between clinical, functional, and radiologic findings. Am J Phys Med Rehabil 2006;85:53–60.
10. Lafosse L, Reiland Y, Baier GP, Toussaint B, Jost B. Anterior and posterior instability of the long head of the biceps tendon in rotator cuff tears: a new classification based on arthroscopic observations. Arthroscopy 2007;23:73–80.
11. Holtby R, Razmjou H. Validity of the supraspinatus test as a single clinical test in diagnosing patients with rotator cuff pathology. J Orthop Sports Phys Ther 2004;34:194–200.
12. Bennett WF. Specificity of the Speed's test: arthroscopic technique for evaluating the biceps tendon at the level of the bicipital groove. Arthroscopy 1998;14:789–96.
13. Parentis MA, Glousman RE, Mohr KS, Yocum LA. An evaluation of the provocative tests for superior labral anterior posterior lesions. Am J Sports Med 2006;34:265–8.
14. Morgan CD, Burkhart SS, Palmeri M, Gillespie M. Type II SLAP lesions: three subtypes and their relationships to superior instability and rotator cuff tears. Arthroscopy 1998;14:553–65.
15. Park HB, Yokota A, Gill HS, El Rassi G, McFarland EG. Diagnostic accuracy of clinical tests for the different° of subacromial impingement syndrome. J Bone Joint Surg Am 2005;87:1446–55.
16. Calis M, Akgun K, Birtane M, Karacan I, Calis H, Tuzun F. Diagnostic values of clinical diagnostic tests in subacromial impingement syndrome. Ann Rheum Dis 2000;59:44–7.
17. Middleton WD, Reinus WR, Totty WG, Melson CL, Murphy WA. Ultrasonographic evaluation of the rotator cuff and biceps tendon. J Bone Joint Surg Am 1986;68:440–50.
18. Farin PU. Sonography of the biceps tendon of the shoulder: normal and pathologic findings. J Clin Ultrasound 1996;24:309–16.
19. Tuckman GA. Abnormalities of the long head of the biceps tendon of the shoulder: MR imaging findings. AJR Am J Roentgenol 1994;163:1183–8.
20. Mohtadi NG, Vellet AD, Clark ML, et al. A prospective, double-blind comparison of magnetic resonance imaging and arthroscopy in the evaluation of patients presenting with shoulder pain. J Shoulder Elbow Surg 2004;13:258–65.
21. Kayser R, Hampf S, Pankow M, Seeber E, Heyde CE. [Validity of ultrasound examinations of disorders of the shoulder joint]. Ultraschall Med 2005;26:291–8.
22. Teefey SA, Hasan SA, Middleton WD, Patel M, Wright RW, Yamaguchi K. Ultrasonography of the rotator cuff. A comparison of ultrasonographic and arthroscopic findings in one hundred consecutive cases. J Bone Joint Surg Am 2000;82:498–504.
23. Read JW, Perko M. Shoulder ultrasound: diagnostic accuracy for impingement syndrome, rotator cuff tear, and biceps tendon pathology. J Shoulder Elbow Surg 1998;7:264–71.
24. Armstrong A, Teefey SA, Wu T, et al. The efficacy of ultrasound in the diagnosis of long head of the biceps tendon pathology. J Shoulder Elbow Surg 2006;15:7–11.
25. Le Corroller T, Cohen M, Aswad R, Pauly V, Champsaur P. Sonography of the painful shoulder: role of the operator's experience. Skeletal Radiol 2008;37:979–86.

26. Zanetti M, Weishaupt D, Gerber C, Hodler J. Tendinopathy and rupture of the tendon of the long head of the biceps brachii muscle: evaluation with MR arthrography. AJR Am J Roentgenol 1998;170:1557–61.

27. Jung JY, Yoon YC, Yi SK, Yoo J, Choe BK. Comparison study of indirect MR arthrography and direct MR arthrography of the shoulder. Skeletal Radiol 2009;38:659–67.

28. Guckel C, Nidecker A. MR arthrographic findings in tenosynovitis of the long bicipital tendon of the shoulder. Skeletal Radiol 1998;27:7–12.

29. Flannigan B, Kursunoglu-Brahme S, Snyder S, Karzel R, Del Pizzo W, Resnick D. MR arthrography of the shoulder: comparison with conventional MR imaging. AJR Am J Roentgenol 1990;155:829–32.

30. Dinauer PA, Flemming DJ, Murphy KP, Doukas WC. Diagnosis of superior labral lesions: comparison of noncontrast MRI with indirect MR arthrography in unexercised shoulders. Skeletal Radiol 2007;36:195–202.

31. Green S, Buchbinder R, Hetrick S. Physiotherapy interventions for shoulder pain. Cochrane Database Syst Rev 2003:CD004258.

32. Buchbinder R, Green S, Youd JM. Corticosteroid injections for shoulder pain. Cochrane Database Syst Rev 2003:CD004016.

33. Ford LT, DeBender J. Tendon rupture after local steroid injection. South Med J 1979;72:827–30.

34. Phillips BB, Canale ST, Sisk TD, Stralka SW, Wyatt KP. Ruptures of the proximal biceps tendon in middle-aged patients. Orthop Rev 1993;22:349–53.

35. Sturzenegger M, Beguin D, Grunig B, Jakob RP. Muscular strength after rupture of the long head of the biceps. Arch Orthop Trauma Surg 1986;105:18–23.

36. Mariani EM, Cofield RH, Askew LJ, Li GP, Chao EY. Rupture of the tendon of the long head of the biceps brachii. Surgical versus nonsurgical treatment. Clin Orthop Relat Res 1988;228:233–9.

37. Walch G, Nove-Josserand L, Boileau P, Levigne C. Subluxations and dislocations of the tendon of the long head of the biceps. J Shoulder Elbow Surg 1998;7:100–8.

38. Gill TJ, McIrvin E, Mair SD, Hawkins RJ. Results of biceps tenotomy for treatment of pathology of the long head of the biceps brachii. J Shoulder Elbow Surg 2001;10:247–9.

39. Kelly AM, Drakos MC, Fealy S, Taylor SA, O'Brien SJ. Arthroscopic release of the long head of the biceps tendon: functional outcome and clinical results. Am J Sports Med 2005;33:208–13.

40. Osbahr DC, Diamond AB, Speer KP. The cosmetic appearance of the biceps muscle after long-head tenotomy versus tenodesis. Arthroscopy 2002;18:483–7.

41. Paulos LE, Franklin JL. Arthroscopic shoulder decompression development and application. A five year experience. Am J Sports Med 1990;18:235–44.

42. Boileau P, Baque F, Valerio L, Ahrens P, Chuinard C, Trojani C. Isolated arthroscopic biceps tenotomy or tenodesis improves symptoms in patients with massive irreparable rotator cuff tears. J Bone Joint Surg Am 2007;89:747–57.

43. Maynou C, Mehdi N, Cassagnaud X, Audebert S, Mestdagh H. [Clinical results of arthroscopic tenotomy of the long head of the biceps brachii in full thickness tears of the rotator cuff without repair: 40 cases]. Rev Chir Orthop Reparatrice Appar Mot 2005;91:300–6.

44. Franceschi F, Longo UG, Ruzzini L, Papalia R, Rizzello G, Denaro V. To detach the long head of the biceps tendon after tenodesis or not: outcome analysis at the 4-year follow-up of two different techniques. Int Orthop 2007;31:537–45.

45. Nord KD, Smith GB, Mauck BM. Arthroscopic biceps tenodesis using suture anchors through the subclavian portal. Arthroscopy 2005;21:248–52.

46. Drakos MC, Verma NN, Gulotta LV, et al. Arthroscopic transfer of the long head of the biceps tendon: functional outcome and clinical results. Arthroscopy 2008;24:217–23.

47. Checchia SL, Doneux PS, Miyazaki AN, et al. Biceps tenodesis associated with arthroscopic repair of rotator cuff tears. J Shoulder Elbow Surg 2005;14:138–44.

48. Millett PJ, Sanders B, Gobezie R, Braun S, Warner JJ. Interference screw vs. suture anchor fixation for open subpectoral biceps tenodesis: does it matter? BMC Musculoskelet Disord 2008;9:121.

49. Mazzocca AD, Cote MP, Arciero CL, Romeo AA, Arciero RA. Clinical outcomes after subpectoral biceps tenodesis with an interference screw. Am J Sports Med 2008;36:1922–9.

50. Boileau P, Krishnan SG, Coste JS, Walch G. Arthroscopic biceps tenodesis: a new technique using bioabsorbable interference screw fixation. Arthroscopy 2002;18:1002–12.

51. Berlemann U, Bayley I. Tenodesis of the long head of biceps brachii in the painful shoulder: improving results in the long term. J Shoulder Elbow Surg 1995;4:429–35.

91

Ulnar Collateral Ligament Injury

Denise Eygendaal[1] and Laurens Kaas[2]

[1]Amphia Hospital, Breda, The Netherlands
[2]Orthopaedic Research Center Amsterdam, Academic Medical Center, Amsterdam, The Netherlands

Case scenario

A 23 year old professional athlete (baseball pitcher) has been complaining about his right elbow for 6 months. The pain is medial sided and the onset of the symptoms was gradual. A wrong pitch 5 months ago has severely increased the pain, resulting in an inability to pitch. At physical examination there is a slight extension deficit of 10°, a positive moving valgus test and a positive milking test.[1] This test can identify partial tears of the ulnar collateral ligament (UCL) by extending the elbow from the fully flexed position, while the examiner exerts a valgus moment by grasping the thumb and resisting extension. The patient has no neurovascular symptoms.

Relevant anatomy

Stability of the elbow is attained by dynamic and static constraints. Static or passive constraints are provided by both the bones and the soft tissues of the elbow. The role of the muscles as dynamic constraints is becoming increasingly clear and is probably larger than previously postulated. The relative role of the osseous and soft tissue restraints are shown in Table 91.1.

The UCL consists of an anterior and a posterior bundle, and a transverse ligament (also known as the Cooper ligament). The anterior and posterior bundles originate from a broad anteroinferior surface of the medial humeral epicondyle. The anterior bundle inserts the base of the coronoid process of the ulna and the posterior bundle inserts the medial part of the semilunar notch of the ulna. The mean length of the anterior UCL is 27.1 mm and that of

posterior UCL 24.2 mm, and the mean widths are about 4.7 mm and 5.3 mm respectively. The function of these ligaments is to restrain valgus stress during extension (anterior bundle) and during flexion (posterior bundle). Studies reveal that the anterior medial collateral ligament can be subdivided into three regions or bands according to their function (see Figure 91.1).[3-5]

Importance of the problem

Injury to the UCL was first recognized in 1946 in javelin throwers.[6] The injury has since become well recognized in baseball pitchers and other overhead throwing athletes. However, exact numbers or incidence of this injury in athletes or in the general population are not known. The three most common causes of UCL injury are elbow dislocation, chronic attenuation in athletes, or acute valgus injury. The elbow joint is the second most commonly dislocated major joint after the shoulder. In children it is the most commonly dislocated joint.[7] The incidence of this dislocation is estimated to be 6/100,000 in the general population, usually in the posterior or posterolateral direction.[8] Josefsson[9] showed that elbow dislocation induced injury in the lateral as well as the medial ligamentous structures, whereas O'Driscoll[10] demonstrated that the joint could be dislocated experimentally with preservation of the medial ligaments. During dislocation ligamentous injury occurs in a lateral to medial circle. In stage 1, the radial collateral ligament is disrupted; in stage 2, the other lateral ligamentous structures as well as the anterior and posterior capsule are disrupted. In stage 3, disruption of the medial collateral ligament can be partial with disruption of the posterior bundle only (3A) or complete (3B).[10] The UCL can therefore

Evidence-Based Orthopedics, First Edition. Edited by Mohit Bhandari.
© 2012 Blackwell Publishing Ltd. Published 2012 by Blackwell Publishing Ltd.

Table 91.1 Relative contribution to valgus stress resistance (%)[2]

	Extended	90° elbow flexion
MCL	31	56
Soft tissue, capsule	38	10
Osseous articulation	31	34

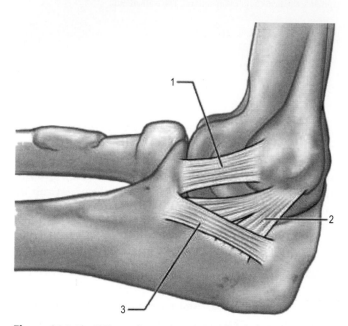

Figure 91.1 The UCL complex consists of an anterior (1) and a posterior (2) bundle, and a transverse ligament.

be disrupted after dislocation of the elbow joint. Persistent valgus instability after conservative treatment of elbow dislocation has been described in up to 50% of cases. It is related to degenerative changes of the elbow joint after an average follow-up of 9 years.[11]

Top five questions

Diagnosis

1. Is UCL insufficiency a problem frequently encountered in general orthopedic practice?
2. As the clinical instability of the elbow is underestimated in most cases, what is the gold standard for the evaluation of the UCL?

Treatment

3. Should (professional) athletes with an acute injury of the UCL always be treated surgically?
4. What are the surgical treatment options?

Prognosis

5. Does surgical reconstruction of the UCL prevent accelerated degeneration of the elbow joint?

Question 1: Is UCL insufficiency a problem frequently encountered in general orthopedic practice?

Case clarification

The patient was treated in an upper limb unit specializing in sports medicine. In a general orthopedic practice with a small number of sports-related injuries or post-traumatic deformities of the elbow, the incidence is low. In those situations the "doctor's delay," due to unfamiliarity with UCL injury, can be an issue.

Finding the evidence

- Cochrane Database: No reviews available
- PubMed: No reports on incidence on UCL injury of the elbow in the general population or in throwing athletes.

Findings

There are no scientific reports on the incidence of UCL injury in throwing athletes or the general population. One study found an incidence of UCL lesions in 33% of 490 baseball players who underwent rehabilitation for any kind of injury of the upper extremity.[12] As previously mentioned, persistent valgus instability after conservatively treated elbow dislocations has been described in up to 50% of cases.[11] In up to 54% of patients with a radial head fracture a UCL lesion is diagnosed with MRI, although the incidence of clinical relevant UCL injuries is much lower (1–8%).[13–16] Orthopedic surgeons should think of UCL insufficiency in patients with medial-sided elbow pain, especially in athletes and in patients with post-traumatic conditions of the elbow as a posterolateral dislocation.

Recommendations

- UCL insufficiency of the elbow has been mainly reported in athletes and in patients with post-traumatic conditions of the elbow as a posterolateral dislocation, although the incidence in the general (or athlete) population is unknown [overall quality very low]

Question 2: As the clinical instability of the elbow is underestimated in most cases, what is the gold standard for the evaluation of UCL injury?

Case clarification

In the case described above, the history was very suggestive for UCL injury. Apparently this athlete had ruptured the UCL 5 months ago, but this injury had subsided; after a new event, the "chronic rupture" of the UCL became symptomatic again. Physical examination revealed a positive milking maneuver; the MRI with arthrogram (MRA) revealed a detachment of the UCL on the humeral side.

Current opinion

AP, lateral, and axillary views of the elbow are assessed for degenerative changes such as joint space narrowing, ossification of the UCL, and loose bodies. A small bony avulsion fragment might be identified when a UCL bony avulsion exists.

Finding the evidence

• Cochrane Database: No reviews available
• PubMed: 7 reports on MRA in UCL pathology and 2 reports on CTA in UCL pathology

Quality of the evidence

Level IV
• 6 case series

Level V
• 2 expert opinion

Findings

Dynamic radiographs under valgus load have been described in the past as a useful diagnostic tool; however, mild valgus laxity has been observed in uninjured overhead athletes, and dynamic radiographs in symptomatic elbows seems to be inconsistent.[17,18] Another imaging modality is CT with arthrogram (CTA), with a sensitivity of 86% and a specificity of 91%.[19] However, the preferred imaging technique for UCL injuries of the elbow is MRA. MRI is capable of identifying full thickness tears, and MRA improves the diagnosis of partial tears.[18,20–23] Another advantage of MRI/MRA is the ability to identify associated pathology, such as medial epicondylitis and chondral lesions. The sensitivity of MRA is reported to be up to 97% in detecting UCL injury, including partial undersurface UCL tears, with a specificity of up to 100%.[19,24,25] No comparative studies of CTA and MRA are currently available.

Recommendation

• MRA is the preferred imaging technique for detection of UCL injuries of the elbow [overall quality: very low]

Question 3: Should (professional) athletes with an acute injury of UCL always be treated surgically?

Case clarification

Treatment of UCL of the elbow injuries is based on the patient's athletic demands and the degree of UCL injury.

In this case, initial conservative treatment consisted of rest, anti-inflammatory measures, and physical therapy.

Finding the evidence

• Cochrane Database: No reviews on conservative treatment of UCL available
• PubMed: 1 report on conservative treatment of UCL injury of the elbow

Quality of the evidence

Level IV
• 1 case series

Findings

Rettig et al.[26] was the first to report on the results of conservative treatment in throwing athletes. Phase I of the conservative treatment consisted of rest and modalities to treat symptoms for 2–3 months. If pain free, the athlete began with phase II which consisted of muscle strengthening and throwing. Thirteen of 31 athletes (42%) returned to same level of play, with an average return of 24 weeks after injury after conservative treatment. This rehabilitation period is shorter than the rehabilitation period after UCL reconstruction. No history or physical examination features are predictive for athletes who will respond to no nonoperative treatment.

Recommendations

• Treatment of UCL injuries is based on the patient's athletic demands and the degree of UCL injury. [overall quality: very low]

Question 4: What are the surgical treatment options?

Current opinion

Persistent symptomatic UCL instability after initial conservative treatment is an indication for reconstruction.

Finding the evidence

• Cochrane Database: Noreviews available on results of UCL reconstruction
• PubMed: 17 reports available on results of UCL reconstruction

Quality of the evidence

Level I
• 2 systematic reviews

Level IV
• 14 case series

Level V
• 1 expert opinion

Findings

The first successful UCL reconstruction was performed in 1974 by Dr. Frank Jobe and colleagues. They published their initial results in throwing athletes in 1986, using the palmaris longus tendon as an autograft, with detachment of the flexor–pronator musculature, submuscular transposition of the ulnar nerve, and a figure-of-eight graft fixation technique. In this fixation technique the autograft is placed through two drill holes in the ulna and three in the medial epicondyle in a figure-of-eight fashion, going through the posterior humeral cortex and suturing the graft to itself.[27] Several modifications of this original technique have been introduced over the past 35 years. Muscle splitting instead of detachment, and abandoning the obligatory ulnar nerve transposition, have improved clinical results and decreased the complication rate.[28,29] The introduction of the docking technique by Rohrbough et al.[30] allows easier graft passing, tensioning, and fixation. It uses the same ulnar tunnels as in the Jobe technique, but the humeral tunnels are created with one single inferior tunnel, with two small superior and one anterior exit tunnels. The graft is positioned in the inferior tunnel, and tensioned with sutures that exit the superior tunnels. The graft is fixated by tying the sutures over a bony bridge. Another graft fixation technique is interference screw fixation, where one or both graft endings are fixed with a bioabsorbable interference screw.[24,31] Different autografts have been described: the palmaris longus tendon, plantaris tendon, hamstrings tendon, tendon allografts, or triceps tendon can be used.[28,31] Ulnar decompression or transposition can be indicated in patients with symptoms of ulnar nerve irritation, which is present in more than 40% of patients with UCL insufficiency.[17] Additional diagnostic arthroscopy can be performed if intra-articular pathology is suspected.[24,30] After surgery a long-arm cast is applied for 1–2 weeks to allow wound healing. Some authors use an additional hinged brace during mobilization for 2–6 weeks. Strengthening exercises (with or without brace) are initiated after 4–6 weeks. Throwing is usually allowed after 2–5 months. Return to competition varies from "when ready" to 12 months after surgery.[24,32–36] The original report on UCL reconstruction by Jobe et al. reported excellent results in 63%.[27] With the improvement of the surgical technique, success rates increased: 74–95% of all athletes returned to their previous level of injury or higher.[17,35,37] Previous surgery for UCL insufficiency is associated with poorer results.[17,18] The most frequent reported complication is a transient ulnar neuropathy, which occurs in 1–21% of patients, with a mean of 6%. About 1% of patients experience graft site complications.[28] In this case UCL reconstruction is advised, if conservative treatment under supervision of a specialized physiotherapist for 3 months is not successful.

Recommendations

• Symptomatic UCL insufficiency is indication for reconstruction. Reconstruction of a nonsymptomatic UCL injury is not indicated [overall quality: very low]
• The preferred surgical techniques are the docking technique or interference screw fixation [overall quality: very low]
• Injury to the UCL of the elbow was once a career-ending injury in overhead athletes, but UCL reconstruction has made return to previous or higher level of athlete participation in sports likely [overall quality: very low]

Question 5: Does surgical reconstruction of the UCL prevent accelerated degeneration of the elbow joint?

Current opinion

Persistent valgus instability can be related to accelerated degeneration of the elbow joint. The question of whether surgical reconstruction of the UCL can prevent accelerated degeneration of the elbow has not yet been answered.

Finding the evidence

• Cochrane Database: No reviews available on prevention of degeneration with UCL reconstruction
• PubMed: No reports available on prevention of degeneration with UCL reconstruction

Findings

Symptomatic UCL insufficiency is indication for reconstruction; a reconstruction of UCL to prevent further damage to the joint in the future is not indicated. Reconstruction of a nonsymptomatic UCL injury is not indicated.[11]

Recommendations

• A reconstruction of the UCL to prevent further damage to the joint in the future is not indicated [Overall quality very low]

Summary of recommendations

• UCL insufficiency of the elbow has mainly been reported in athletes and in patients with post-traumatic conditions of the elbow as a posterolateral dislocation, although the incidence in the general (or athlete) population is unknown
• MRA is the preferred imaging technique for detection of UCL injuries of the elbow
• Treatment of UCL injuries is based on the patient's athletic demands and the degree of UCL injury
• Symptomatic UCL insufficiency is indication for reconstruction. Reconstruction of a nonsymptomatic UCL injury is not indicated

- The preferred surgical techniques are the docking technique or interference screw fixation
- Injury to the UCL of the elbow was once a career-ending injury in overhead athletes, but UCL reconstruction has made return to previous of higher level of athlete participation in sports likely
- A reconstruction of the UCL to prevent further damage to the joint in the future is not indicated

Conclusions

Research on diagnosis and treatment of UCL injury should continue to find higher levels of evidence. Prospective studies to determine preferable diagnostic technique, best graft fixation techniques, and long-term results of conservative and surgical treatment are in demand.

References

1. Veltri DM, O'Brien SJ, Field LD, Altchek DW, Warren RF. The milking maneuvre. In: 10th Open Meeting of the American Shoulder and Elbow Surgeons, New Orleans, 1994.
2. Morrey BF, An KN. Articular and ligamentous contributions to the stability of the elbow joint. Am J Sports Med 1983;11:315–19.
3. Callaway GH, Field LD, Deng XH, et al. Biomechanical evaluation of the medial collateral ligament of the elbow. J Bone Joint Surg Am 1997;79:1223–31.
4. Regan WD, Korinek SL, Morrey BF, An KN. Biomechanical study of ligaments around the elbow joint. Clin Orthop Relat Res 1991;271:170–9.
5. Eygendaal D, Olsen BS, Jensen SL, Seki A, Sojbjerg JO. Kinematics of partial and total ruptures of the medial collateral ligament of the elbow. J Shoulder Elbow Surg 1999;8:612–16.
6. Waris W. Elbow injuries in javelin throwers. Acta Chir Scand 1946;93:563–75.
7. Linscheid RL, Wheeler DK. Elbow dislocations. JAMA 1965;194:1171–6.
8. Josefsson PO, Nilsson BE. Incidence of elbow dislocation. Acta Orthop Scand 1986;57:537–8.
9. Josefsson PO, Johnell O, Wendeberg B. Ligamentous injuries in dislocations of the elbow joint. Clin Orthop Relat Res 1987:221–5.
10. O'Driscoll SW, Morrey BF, Korinek S, An KN. Elbow subluxation and dislocation. A spectrum of instability. Clin Orthop Relat Res 1992:280;186–97.
11. Eygendaal D, Verdegaal SH, Obermann WR, van Vugt AB, Poll RG, Rozing PM. Posterolateral dislocation of the elbow joint. Relationship to medial instability. J Bone Joint Surg Am 2000;82:555–60.
12. Han KJ, Kim YK, Lim SK, Park JY, Oh KS. The effect of physical characteristics and field position on the shoulder and elbow injuries of 490 baseball players: confirmation of diagnosis by magnetic resonance imaging. Clin J Sport Med 2009;19:271–6.
13. Itamura J, Roidis N, Mirzayan R, Vaishnav S, Learch T, Shean C. Radial head fractures: MRI evaluation of associated injuries. J Shoulder Elbow Surg 2005;14:421–4.
14. van Riet RP, Morrey BF, O'Driscoll SW, van Glabbeek F. Associated injuries complicating radial head fractures: a demographic study. Clin Orthop Relat Res 2005;441:351–5.
15. Kaas L, Turkenburg JL, van Riet RP, Vroemen J, Eygendaal D. Magnetic resonance imaging findings in 46 elbows with a radial head fracture. Acta Orthopaedica 2010;81:373–6.
16. Morrey BF. Current concepts in the treatment of fractures of the radial head, the olecranon, and the coronoid. Instr Course Lect 1995;44:175–85.
17. Conway JE, Jobe FW, Glousman RE, Pink M. Medial instability of the elbow in throwing athletes. Treatment by repair or reconstruction of the ulnar collateral ligament. J Bone Joint Surg Am 1992;74:67–83.
18. Thompson WH, Jobe FW, Yocum LA, Pink MM. Ulnar collateral ligament reconstruction in athletes: muscle-splitting approach without transposition of the ulnar nerve. J Shoulder Elbow Surg 2001;10:152–7.
19. Timmerman LA, Schwartz ML, Andrews JR. Preoperative evaluation of the ulnar collateral ligament by magnetic resonance imaging and computed tomography arthrography. Evaluation in 25 baseball players with surgical confirmation. Am J Sports Med 1994;22:26–31.
20. Cotten A, Jacobson J, Brossmann J, et al. Collateral ligaments of the elbow: conventional MR imaging and MR arthrography with coronal oblique plane and elbow flexion. Radiology 1997;204:806–12.
21. Munshi M, Pretterklieber ML, Chung CB, et al. Anterior bundle of ulnar collateral ligament: evaluation of anatomic relationships by using MR imaging, MR arthrography, and gross anatomic and histologic analysis. Radiology 2004;231:797–803.
22. Kijowski R, Tuite M, Sanford M. Magnetic resonance imaging of the elbow. Part II: Abnormalities of the ligaments, tendons, and nerves. Skeletal Radiol 2005;34:1–18.
23. Kaplan LJ, Potter HG. MR imaging of ligament injuries to the elbow. Radiol Clin North Am 2006;44:583–94, ix.
24. Azar FM, Andrews JR, Wilk KE, Groh D. Operative treatment of ulnar collateral ligament injuries of the elbow in athletes. Am J Sports Med 2000;28:16–23.
25. Schwartz ML, al-Zahrani S, Morwessel RM, Andrews JR. Ulnar collateral ligament injury in the throwing athlete: evaluation with saline-enhanced MR arthrography. Radiology 1995;197:297–9.
26. Rettig AC, Sherrill C, Snead DS, Mendler JC, Mieling P. Nonoperative treatment of ulnar collateral ligament injuries in throwing athletes. Am J Sports Med 2001;29:15–17.
27. Jobe FW, Stark H, Lombardo SJ. Reconstruction of the ulnar collateral ligament in athletes. J Bone Joint Surg Am 1986;68:1158–63.
28. Vitale MA, Ahmad CS. The outcome of elbow ulnar collateral ligament reconstruction in overhead athletes: a systematic review. Am J Sports Med 2008;36:1193–205.
29. Purcell DB, Matava MJ, Wright RW. Ulnar collateral ligament reconstruction: a systematic review. Clin Orthop Relat Res 2007;455:72–7.

30. Rohrbough JT, Altchek DW, Hyman J, Williams RJ, III, Botts JD. Medial collateral ligament reconstruction of the elbow using the docking technique. Am J Sports Med 2002;30:541–8.

31. Eygendaal D. Ligamentous reconstruction around the elbow using triceps tendon. Acta Orthop Scand 2004;75:516–23.

32. Paletta GA Jr., Wright RW. The modified docking procedure for elbow ulnar collateral ligament reconstruction: 2-year follow-up in elite throwers. Am J Sports Med 2006;34:1594–8.

33. Koh JL, Schafer MF, Keuter G, Hsu JE. Ulnar collateral ligament reconstruction in elite throwing athletes. Arthroscopy 2006;22:1187–91.

34. Nissen CW. Effectiveness of interference screw fixation in ulnar collateral ligament reconstruction. Orthopedics 2008;31:646.

35. Savoie FH III, Trenhaile SW, Roberts J, Field LD, Ramsey JR. Primary repair of ulnar collateral ligament injuries of the elbow in young athletes: a case series of injuries to the proximal and distal ends of the ligament. Am J Sports Med 2008;36:1066–72.

36. Bowers AL, Dines JS, Dines DM, Altchek DW. Elbow medial ulnar collateral ligament reconstruction: clinical relevance and the docking technique. J Shoulder Elbow Surg 2010;19:110–17.

37. Gibson BW, Webner D, Huffman GR, Sennett BJ. Ulnar collateral ligament reconstruction in major league baseball pitchers. Am J Sports Med 2007;35:575–81.

92 Tennis Elbow

Peter A.A. Struijs[1], Rachelle Buchbinder[2], and Sally E. Green[3]

[1]Academic Medical Centre, Amsterdam, The Netherlands
[2]Monash University, Malvern, VIC, Australia
[3]Monash Institute of Health Services Research, Clayton, VIC, Australia

Case scenario

Case 1

A 45 year old woman who generally works at a supermarket is unable to do her job any more. She comes to your orthopedic practice with complaints of pain at the lateral side of her right, dominant, elbow. The complaints have been present for 3 months and do not seem to decrease in intensity. The strength in her right arm seems decreased, possibly due to pain. At physical examination she has pain with pressure on the origin of the common extensor tendon of the wrist at the lateral epicondyle of the humerus. There is pain on active dorsiflexion of the wrist. She is neurovascularly intact.

Case 2

A 48 year old man presents to your orthopedic outpatient clinic with pain at the lateral side of his elbow.

Relevant anatomy

Tennis elbow is characterized by pain and tenderness over the lateral epicondyle of the humerus, and pain on resisted dorsiflexion of the wrist, middle finger, or both. Pain is located over the origin of common extensor tendon of the wrist, which is a combined origin of the extensor carpi radialis brevis, the extensor digitorum communis, the extensor digiti minimi, and the extensor carpi ulnaris muscles.

Importance of the problem

Lateral elbow pain is a common entity, with a population prevalence of 1–3%.[1] Its peak incidence occurs at 40–50 years of age. In women aged 42–46 years, incidence increases to 10%.[2,3] In the UK, the Netherlands, and Scandinavia the incidence of lateral elbow pain in general practice is 4–7/1,000 people per year.[3–5]

In approximately 10% of the patients the complaint will result in sick leave, for a mean period of 11 weeks.[6] Untreated, the complaint is estimated to last from 6 months to 2 years.[7–9] Several treatment options are available,[10] including an expectant policy, corticosteroid injections, orthotic devices, surgery, and physiotherapeutic modalities such as exercises, ultrasound, laser, massage, electrotherapy, and manipulations.

The number of Google hits for "tennis elbow" is over 2,500,000.

Top eight questions

Diagnosis

1. Is there a role for additional imaging in tennis elbow?

Therapy

2. What is the effect of a wait-and-see policy?
3. What is the effect of corticosteroid injections?

4. What is the effect of acupuncture?
5. What is the effect of physical therapy?
6. What is the effect of nonsteroidal anti-inflammatory drugs (NSAIDs)?
7. What is the effect of orthotic devices?
8. What is the effect of surgery?

Question 1: Is there a role for additional imaging in tennis elbow?

Case 2 clarification

A 48 year old man presents to your orthopedic outpatient clinic with pain at the lateral side of his elbow. When you tell him it is most likely a tennis elbow he asks you whether he needs a "scan."

Relevance

Patients in our clinics are becoming more demanding, and will more frequently ask for additional imaging when you confront them with a diagnosis. Knowledge of the usefulness of additional imaging is helpful for healthcare providers in this context. Additional imaging might have diagnostic, prognostic, or therapeutic implications.

Current opinion

No additional imaging is usually performed when a patient presents with tennis elbow.

Finding the evidence

• Cochrane Database of Systematic Reviews, with search term: "tennis elbow"
• PubMed: clinical queries: systematic reviews: "tennis elbow"
• PubMed, using keywords "tennis elbow" AND "ultrasound"; "tennis elbow" AND "MRI"

Quality of the evidence

Level I
• 1 systematic review[11]
• 5 descriptive studies[12–15]

Findings

MRI A systematic review[11] of 7 studies including 148 patients with epicondylitis comprehensively reviewed the literature to identify studies on MRI findings in epicondylitis. The MRI technique was divergent, and the observed pathological changes also varied. The most frequent alteration was a change in the common extensor tendon signal in 90% of the patients (95% CI 84–94%); 14% of the healthy volunteers and 50% of the contralateral elbows showed similar alterations.

One study compared MRI with ultrasound findings in 11 patients with clinically diagnosed tennis elbow.[12] Two readers compared the findings in two sessions, 1 week apart. Sensitivity for detecting epicondylitis ranged from 64% to 82% for sonography and from 90% to 100% for MRI. Sensitivity ranged from 67% to 100% for sonography and from 83% to 100% for MRI.

Ultrasound Four studies on ultrasound and tennis elbow were identified. The first compared the prognostic and diagnostic value of ultrasound in tennis elbow patients. This randomized controlled trial (RCT) compared the effectiveness of physical therapy, a brace, and a combination of both. No prognostic value was found and diagnostic value showed to be limited: abnormal findings were found in only 75% of the patients.[13]

The second study compared 37 elbows of 22 patients with a clinically diagnosed tennis elbow with 20 elbows of 10 healthy volunteers.[14] Three sonographers/skeletal radiologists performed two sessions. Sensitivity ranged from 72% to 88% and specificities from 36% to 48.5%. A third study[15] compared sonoelastography with clinical examination in 32 consecutively registered patients with symptoms of lateral epicondylitis and 44 asymptomatic elbows of 28 healthy volunteers. The sensitivity of real-time sonoelastography was 100%, the specificity 89%, and the accuracy 94%, with clinical examination as the reference standard. The fourth study compared 26 monosymptomatic, otherwise healthy patients with lateral elbow pain and a diagnosis of lateral epicondylitis and 16 asymptomatic controls. An investigator blinded to study group performed ultrasonography. A sensitivity of 95% (95% CI 73–100%) and a specificity of 88% (CI 54–99%) was found for diagnosing lateral epicondylitis.[16]

Recommendations

• MRI and ultrasound may support the clinical diagnosis of lateral epicondylitis [overall quality: low]

Question 2: What is the effect of a wait-and-see policy?

Case 1 clarification

A 52 year old female shop assistant presents with a tennis elbow at your orthopedic outpatient clinic. Her family doctor told her the complaint is self-limiting but the problem has now been bothering her for more than 3 months. She asks you if there is no treatment for the complaint that is more effective than her doctor's wait-and-see policy.

Relevance

Patients do not generally accept a wait-and-see policy and are usually willing to try anything that will relieve their complaints faster. As a physician, it is important to know what treatment option is best for treating the complaints and what the effectiveness of a certain treatment strategy is compared to other strategies.

Current opinion

Several treatment strategies can be used for tennis elbow complaints. Corticosteroid injections, physical therapy, and orthotic devices (braces) are the most commonly used. Newer and/or alternative strategies include acupuncture and extracorporeal shockwave treatment (ESWT). As tennis elbow is a self-limiting condition, a wait-and-see policy *could* be applied. However, if other treatment strategies have advantages for the patient, these *should* be applied.

Finding the evidence

• Cochrane Database, with search terms "tennis elbow," "epicondylitis," "epicondylalgia"
• PubMed (http://www.ncbi.nlm.nih.gov/pubmed/), clinical queries: "tennis elbow," "epicondylitis," "epicondylalgia"
• PubMed (http://www.ncbi.nlm.nih.gov/pubmed/): sensitivity search: "tennis elbow"; "epicondylitis"; "lateral humeral epicondylitis, " combined with AND treatment; AND corticosteroid; AND injections; AND brace; AND orthotic device; AND extracorporeal; AND ESWT; AND acupuncture; AND physical therapy; AND physiotherapy; AND surgery

Quality of the evidence

See question 3–8.

Findings

See question 3–8.

Recommendations

A wait-and-see policy can be applied, since tennis elbow is usually a self limiting disease. However, some treatment strategies might have advantages over the wait-and-see policy. For details per treatment: see question 3-8.

Question 3: What is the effect of corticosteroid injections?

We found two systematic reviews (search dates 1999[17] and 2003[18]) and three additional RCTs.[19–21] None of the RCTs evaluated the effects of corticosteroid injections on quality of life or return to work.

Finding the evidence

• See Question 2.

Quality of the evidence

Level I
• 2 RCTs
• 1 systematic review

Level II
• 1 RCT
• 1 systematic review

Findings

Corticosteroid injections vs. placebo/no treatment The first review identified two RCTs comparing corticosteroid injection (1 mL methylprednisoloneacetate) vs. injection of saline solution.[17] The first RCT (29 people in smallest group) found that corticosteroid injection significantly increased short-term global improvement compared with placebo (timescale not further specified; absolute numbers not reported; RR 0.11, 95% CI 0.04–0.33; RR <1 favors corticosteroid injections).[17] This RCT did not measure pain or grip strength. The second RCT (10 people in smallest group) found no significant difference in short-term pain, global improvement, or grip strength. The second review[18] identified one RCT (59 people in the smallest group),[22] which compared corticosteroid injection vs. watchful waiting vs. physiotherapy. It found that corticosteroid injection significantly improved people's "main complaint" and functional disability at 3 and 6 weeks compared with watchful waiting (mean difference in "main complaint" at 6 weeks: 24%, 95% CI 14–35%). It found no significant difference between groups at 12, 26, or 52 weeks (at 52 weeks, mean difference in "main complaint" –9%, 95% CI –19% to +2%).[22] The first additional RCT (39 people with symptoms for less than 4 weeks) compared corticosteroid injection vs. a control injection.[19] All patients received rehabilitation. It found that corticosteroid injection significantly improved pain compared with control from 8 weeks to 6 months (improvement on 100-point visual analogue scale was 24.3 with corticosteroid injection vs. 8.9 with control injection; p = 0.04; CI not reported). It found no significant difference in other pain outcomes or in grip strength.

Corticosteroid injections vs. physiotherapy We found one systematic review (search date 1999),[17] which included one RCT (53 people in the smallest group; see comment below) comparing corticosteroid injections (1 mL triamcinoloneacetate 1% plus 1 mL lidocaine) vs. physiotherapy (friction massage plus a manipulation technique). It found that corticosteroid injection significantly increased global improvement and pain scores at 6 weeks compared with physiotherapy (global improvement: RR 0.45, 95% CI 0.29–0.69; pain: RR 0.61, 95% CI 0.48–0.78), but found no significant difference in global improvement, pain, or grip strength at 52 weeks.[17] The second review[12] identified one RCT (59 people in the smallest group)[22] comparing corticosteroid injection vs. physiotherapy (consisting of nine sessions of ultrasound, deep friction massage, and an exercise program over 6 weeks) vs. no treatment. It found that corticosteroid injection significantly improved the "main complaint" and functional disability at 3 and 6 weeks compared with physiotherapy (at 6 weeks, mean difference in "main complaint" 20%, 95% CI 10–31%). However, there was no significant difference at 12 weeks. At 26 and 52 weeks, corticosteroid injections were significantly less effective at improving the "main complaint" compared with physiotherapy (at 52 weeks, mean difference in "main complaint" 15%, 95% CI 5–25%).[22]

Corticosteroid injections vs. orthoses A review[23] identified one RCT comparing orthoses with corticosteroid injections.[24] It found that corticosteroid injection significantly increased the proportion of people rating global improvement as "good" or "excellent" at 2 weeks, but found no significant difference at 6 or 12 months (global improvement rated as "good" or "excellent," at 2 weeks: 3/37 [8%] pooled results for splint and elbow band vs. 13/19 [68%] with injection, RR 2.9, 95% CI 1.8–5.7; 6 months: 19/37 [51%] vs. 14/19 [74%], RR 0.70, 95% CI 0.46–1.05; 12 months: 22/37 [59%] vs. 13/19 [68%], RR 0.90, 95% CI 0.60–1.03).

Corticosteroid injections vs. oral NSAIDs The review included three RCTs, but because of incomplete reporting of results, only two RCTs were included in the meta-analysis. The first of these RCTs compared naproxen 500 mg vs. methylprednisolone 20 mg plus lidocaine; and the second RCT compared naproxen 500 mg (initial high dose, then 250 mg) vs. betamethasone 6 mg plus pilocaine plus placebo tablets. Meta-analysis of self-reported perception of benefit found a significant difference at 4 weeks in favor of corticosteroid injection (2 RCTs, subjective assessment of improvement at 4 weeks: RR 3.06, 95% CI 1.55–6.06).[25] The third RCT, which was not included in the meta-analysis because of skewed data, found lower pain and functional impairment at 4 weeks in the corticosteroid injection group than in the NSAIDs group (median pain measured from 0 = lowest to 9 = highest [baseline]: 1 with corticosteroids vs. 4 with NSAIDs; significance not reported; median functional impairment measured from 0 = lowest to 9 = highest [baseline]: 0 with corticosteroids vs. 3 with NSAIDs; significance not reported).[26] The greater benefit of corticosteroid injection compared with NSAID (naproxen) was only found in the short term (up to 4 weeks). The largest RCT (53 people in smallest group; see comments) found significantly greater improvement in pain at 26 weeks with an NSAID (RR 1.71, 95% CI 1.17–2.51). It found no significant difference in grip strength, and results were not reported for global improvement.

Corticosteroid injections vs. ESWT The second review[18] identified one RCT (93 people),[27] which compared a single corticosteroid plus local anesthetic injection (20 mg triamcinolone made up to 1.5 mL with 1% lidocaine) vs. three sessions weekly of ESWT.[27] Self-reported pain was measured at 6 weeks and 3 months, and treatment success was defined as over 50% reduction in pain from baseline. It found that corticosteroid plus local anesthetic injections were significantly more effective at reducing pain at 6 weeks and at 3 months compared with ESWT (treatment success rates: 21/25 [84%] vs. 29/48 [60%] with ESWT; p < 0.05).[27]

Recommendations

Pain relief
- Corticosteroid injections may be more effective at improving pain at 8 weeks and 6 months in people who have had symptoms for less than 4 weeks compared to placebo treatment [overall quality: very low quality]
- Corticosteroid injection may be more effective than physiotherapy at improving pain scores at 6 weeks, but not at 52 weeks [overall quality: very low]
- Corticosteroid injection may be less effective than oral NSAIDs at improving pain at 26 weeks. It is unclear whether corticosteroid injection is more effective at improving pain at 4 weeks [overall quality: very low]
- A single corticosteroid injection plus local anesthetic injection may be more effective at improving pain at 6 weeks and 3 months compared to ESWT [overall quality: low]

Global improvement
- Corticosteroid injections may be more effective than placebo at increasing "short-term" global improvement (timescale not defined), and at improving people's "main complaint" at 3 and 6 weeks compared with watchful waiting. It is not clear whether injections are more effective than watchful waiting at improving people's "main complaint" in the longer term (12–52 weeks) [overall quality: very low]
- Corticosteroid injection may be more effective than physiotherapy at increasing global improvement scores at 6 weeks, but not at 52 weeks We don't know whether corticosteroid injection is more effective than physiotherapy at improving the "main complaint" [overall quality: very low]
- Corticosteroid injection may be more effective than orthoses at increasing the proportion of people who rate their global improvement as "good" or "excellent" at 2 weeks, but not at 6 or 12 months [overall quality: low]
- Corticosteroid injection may be more effective than oral NSAIDs at increasing self-reported perception of benefit at 4 weeks [overall quality: very low]

Functional improvement
- Corticosteroid injection may be more effective than no treatment at improving functional disability at 3 and 6 weeks, but not in the longer term (from 12–52 weeks). It is unclear whether it is more effective than placebo at improving grip strength [overall quality: very low]
- It is unclear whether corticosteroid injection is more effective than physiotherapy at improving functional disability at 12 weeks [overall quality: low]

Question 4: What is the effect of acupuncture?

Finding the evidence

We found three systematic reviews (search dates 2001,[28] 2003,[18] and 2004[29]) about the effects of acupuncture on tennis elbow. The systematic reviews did not pool results of the RCTs because of considerable heterogeneity among trials. We found no RCTs assessing the effects of acupuncture on quality of life, strength, or return to work.

Quality of the evidence

Level I
- 3 systematic reviews including 5 RCTs[25,30–33]

Findings

The first RCT (45 people) found that 10 acupuncture treatments significantly improved pain and functional outcomes at 2 weeks compared with sham treatment.[30] The second RCT (48 people) found that needle acupuncture significantly increased the duration of pain relief and the proportion of people with at least 50% reduction in pain after one treatment compared with sham acupuncture where needles were not inserted.[31] The third RCT (82 people) found that, compared with sham treatment, needle acupuncture significantly increased the proportion of self-reported "good" or "excellent" results, and the pain threshold on gripping after 10 treatments, but found no significant difference at 3 or 12 months.[25] A fourth RCT (49 people) found no significant difference in the proportion of people reporting either no improvement or a worsening of symptoms, after 10 sessions, and at 3 or 12 months, between laser acupuncture and sham treatment. It found a smaller proportion of "excellent" or "good" results in the laser group compared with the placebo group after 10 treatments, but not at 3 and 10 months; none of the differences was significant.[32] A fifth RCT found no significant difference in cure rate (definition of cure not reported) between vitamin B_{12} injection plus acupuncture and vitamin B_{12} injection alone.[33]

Recommendations

Pain relief
- Needle acupuncture may be more effective than sham treatment at increasing pain relief duration after one treatment, or at improving pain after 10 acupuncture sessions at 2 weeks, but may not be more effective at improving pain at 3 or 12 months [overall quality: low]

Global improvement
- It is not clear whether needle or laser acupuncture is more effective at increasing the proportion of people who report "good" or "excellent" results or "cure" at 3–12 months, or whether it is more effective at decreasing the proportion of people who report "no improvement" or "worse" outcome at 3–12 months [overall quality: very low]

Functional improvement
- Needle acupuncture may be more effective than sham treatment at improving functional impairment at 2 weeks [overall quality: low]

Question 5: What is the effect of physical therapy?

Finding the evidence
- See Question 2.

Quality of the evidence

Level I
- 2 RCTs [34,35]
- One systematic review[18] including 5 RCTs

Findings

Exercise vs. control We found one RCT (62 people) comparing eccentric exercises plus proprioceptive neuromuscular facilitation plus counseling vs. sham ultrasound plus counseling.[34] All participants were allowed to use an orthosis during painful activities. It found that exercise significantly improved pain and function scores after treatment and at 11 months compared with control (pain at end of treatment [baseline: 16 vs. 16]: 36.3 with exercise vs. 17.4 with placebo, p = 0.0001; pain at 11 months: 34.9 with exercise vs. 15.7 with placebo, p = 0.0001; function at end of treatment [baseline range: 14.4–14.9] 27.8 with exercise vs. 15.7 with placebo, p = 0.0001; function at 11 months: 26.7 with exercise vs. 14.9 with placebo, p = 0.0001).[34]

Exercise vs. ultrasound plus friction massage We found one systematic review (search date 2003, 1 RCT).[18] The small RCT (36 people) identified by the review found that exercise significantly improved pain at 6–8 weeks compared with ultrasound plus friction massage (SMD 0.66, 95% CI 0.01 to 1.31).[18]

Exercise plus massage plus ultrasound vs. no treatment We found one systematic review (search date 2003,1 RCT).[18] The RCT (183 people) included in the review was a three-arm trial comparing 6 weeks of combined physical intervention (exercise plus massage plus ultrasound) vs. corticosteroid injection vs. watchful waiting. It found no significant difference between combined physical intervention and watchful waiting at 6 weeks (global improvement: RR 1.46, 95% CI 0.93–2.29; pain: SMD 0.26, 95% CI −0.10 to +0.61) or at 52 weeks (global improvement: RR 1.09, 95% CI 0.95–1.25; pain: SMD 0.26, 95% CI −0.10 to +0.61).[18]

Eccentric strengthening with stretching vs. concentric strengthening with stretching vs. stretching alone We found one RCT (94 people, lateral elbow pain of more than 3 months) comparing eccentric strengthening plus stretching vs. concentric strengthening plus stretching vs. stretching alone.[35]

It found no significant difference between groups at 6 weeks in pain-free grip strength, pain, or function (difference from baseline to 6 weeks in pain-free grip strength, SD −4.2 ± 6.1 with eccentric strengthening plus stretching vs. −7.4 ± 8.3 with concentric strengthening plus stretching vs. −6.7 ± 7.0 with stretching alone, difference among groups p = 0.44; difference from baseline to 6 weeks in pain [visual analogue scale] SD 23 ± 24 with eccentric strengthening plus stretching vs. 14 ± 27 with concentric strengthening plus stretching vs. 23 ± 21 with stretching alone, difference among groups p = 0.33; difference from baseline to 6 weeks in Patient-rated Forearm Evaluation Questionnaire [PRFEQ] SD 1.2 ± 1.7 with eccentric strengthening plus stretching vs. 1.3 ± 1.8 with concentric strengthening plus stretching vs. 1.5 ± 1.6 with stretching alone, difference among groups p = 0.87; difference from baseline to 6 weeks in Disability of the Arm, Shoulder and Hand Scale [DASH] SD 9.3 ± 14 with eccentric strengthening plus stretching vs. 8.4 ± 10 with concentric strengthening plus stretching vs. 11 ± 12 with stretching alone, difference among groups p = 0.66).[35]

Different manipulation techniques for mobilization The review identified four small RCTs on cervical, wrist, and elbow manipulation, one of which (in 15 people) was too small to meet our inclusion criteria for this review.[18] Pooled results for two RCTs (total of 48 people) investigating elbow manipulation vs. control found a positive immediate effect on pain-free grip strength (SMD 1.28, 95% CI 0.84–1.73). One RCT (28 people) found no significant benefit from wrist manipulation vs. friction massage plus ultrasound plus exercise (pain-free grip strength: SMD 0.43, 95% CI −0.32 to +1.19).

Recommendations
Pain
• Exercise plus counseling may be more effective than sham ultrasound plus counseling at improving pain scores at 11 months [overall quality: very low]
• Exercise may be more effective than ultrasound and friction massage at improving pain at 6–8 weeks [overall quality: very low]
• Combined physical intervention (exercise plus massage plus ultrasound) may be no more effective than watchful waiting at improving pain at 6 weeks or at 52 weeks [overall quality: very low-quality]
• It is unclear whether eccentric strengthening with stretching is more effective at 6 weeks at improving pain-free grip strength or pain when compared to concentric strengthening with stretching and with stretching alone [overall quality: low]
• It is not clear whether manipulation (of wrist or elbow) is more effective than control at improving pain-free grip strength [overall quality: very low]

Global improvement
• Combined physical intervention (exercise plus massage plus ultrasound) may be no more effective than watchful waiting at increasing global improvement at 6 weeks or at 52 weeks [overall quality: very low]

Functional improvement
• Exercise plus counseling may be more effective at 11 months than sham ultrasound plus counseling at improving function scores [overall quality: very low]
• Eccentric strengthening with stretching, concentric strengthening with stretching, and stretching alone seem equally effective at improving function at 6 weeks [overall quality: moderate]

Question 6: What is the effect of NSAIDs?

Finding the evidence
We found one systematic review (search date 2001)[36] and no subsequent RCTs. None of the RCTs in the review evaluated the effect of NSAIDs on return to work or quality of life.

Quality of the evidence
Level I
• One systematic review[36] including two RCTs

Findings
The review[36] included two RCTs. The RCTs were not pooled, because one reported means and standard deviations and the other reported medians and ranges. One RCT (129 people) found limited evidence that an NSAID (diclofenac) improved pain in the short term compared with placebo, but did not assess long-term results (pain WMD −13.9, 95% CI −23.2 to −4.6 on 100-point scale).[36] The second RCT (164 people) found no significant difference between NSAIDs (naproxen) and vitamin C placebo in pain over 4 weeks, 6 months, or 1 year, or in functional impairment at 6 months or 1 year (median pain measured from 0 = lowest to 9 = highest [baseline], at 4 weeks: 4 with NSAIDs vs. 3.5 with placebo; 6 months: 1 with NSAIDs vs. 1 with placebo; 12 months: 0 with NSAIDs vs. 0 with placebo; median functional impairment measured from 0 = lowest to 9 = highest [baseline = 4 for both groups]: at 4 weeks: 3 with NSAIDs vs. 2 with placebo; at 6 months: 0 with NSAIDs vs. 0.5 with placebo; at 12 months: 0 with NSAIDs vs. 0 with placebo; significance not reported).[36]

Recommendations
Pain relief
• Oral NSAIDs may be more effective than placebo at improving pain in the short term, but it is unclear whether they are more effective at improving pain at 4 weeks, 6 months, or 1 year [overall quality: very low]

Functional improvement
- Oral NSAIDs may be no more effective than placebo at improving functional impairment [overall quality: very low]

Question 7: What is the effect of orthotic devices?

Finding the evidence
We found one systematic review (search date 1999)[37] and one additional RCT.[38]

Quality of the evidence
Level I
- One RCT[38]

Findings
We found one RCT (180 people), a three-arm trial comparing orthoses vs. physiotherapy (ultrasound plus friction massage plus exercise) vs. a combination of orthoses plus physiotherapy.[38] It found that, over the short term, orthosis was less effective at reducing pain among people with pain as their main complaint (34–45% of the study population at 6 weeks) compared with physiotherapy (mean pain score on a scale of 0 = no complaint to 100 = severe complaints among people with pain as main complaint at 6 weeks: mean difference in improvement 18 with orthosis vs. 31 with physiotherapy; mean difference 13, 95% CI 3–21), improving Pain Free Function Questionnaire[37] scores (mean improvement [scale of 0–100; baseline range 48–51]: mean difference in improvement 10 with orthoses vs. 17 with physiotherapy; mean difference 7, 95% CI 1–12), and improving patient satisfaction scores (mean improvement [scale of 0–100; baseline range not reported]: mean difference in improvement 66 with orthoses vs. 75 with physiotherapy; mean difference 9, 95% CI 1–18). However, it found that orthoses were more effective than physiotherapy at improving ability to perform daily activities (mean improvement [scale of 0–100; baseline range 59–64]: mean difference in improvement 26 with orthoses vs. 15 with physiotherapy; mean difference 11, 95% CI 1–21). It found no significant difference between orthoses and physiotherapy at 6 months and 12 months.[38]

Recommendations
Pain relief
- Orthoses may be less effective at 6 weeks than physiotherapy at improving pain in people who have pain as their main complaint [overall quality: very low]

Global improvement
- Orthoses may be less effective at improving patient satisfaction scores at 6 weeks compared with physiotherapy [overall quality: low]

Functional improvement
- Orthoses may be more effective than physiotherapy at improving the ability to perform daily activities at 6 weeks [overall quality: low]

Question 8: What is the effect of open vs. percutaneous release surgery?

Finding the evidence
We found one systematic review (search date 2001),[39] which identified no RCTs, and one subsequent RCT.[40]

Quality of the evidence
Level II
- 1 RCT with methodologic limitations[40]

Findings
The RCT (not blinded, 47 people who had failed 12 months of conservative treatment) compared open release surgery (removal of the damaged portion of the common extensor origin) vs. percutaneous release surgery (tenotomy).[40] The RCT measured function and pain using the DASH scale. It found that percutaneous release significantly improved DASH scores at 1 year compared with open release (improvement in median DASH score: 20 with percutaneous release vs. 17 with open release; p = 0.001).[40] The clinical importance of this 3-point difference has been questioned, because the minimum clinically important difference has been reported to be 10–15 points.[41] The RCT also found that percutaneous release significantly reduced median time to return to work compared with open release (2 weeks with percutaneous release vs. 5 weeks with open release; p = 0.0001) and significantly improved measures of subjective satisfaction (p = 0.012).[40]

Recommendations
Functional improvement
- Percutaneous release surgery may be more effective than open release at improving function at 1 year, and may be more effective at reducing the median time to return to work, in people who had not improved with 12 months of conservative treatment [overall quality: very low]

Summary of recommendations

- Tennis elbow affects up to 3% of the population, and is usually an overload injury that often follows minor trauma to extensor forearm muscles. Although usually self-limiting, symptoms may persist for over 1 year in up to 20% of people.
- MRI and ultrasound may be useful in confirming the diagnosis tennis elbow.

- Corticosteroid injections improve pain from tennis elbow in the short term compared with placebo, local anesthetic, orthoses , physiotherapy, and oral NSAIDs.
- It is not certain which corticosteroid regimen leads to greatest pain relief.
- Over the long term, physiotherapy or oral NSAIDs may be more effective than corticosteroid injections at reducingpain.
- Topical NSAIDs lead to short-term pain relief, but long-term effects are unknown.
- Extracorporeal shock wave therapy is unlikely to be more effective than placebo at improving pain, and may be less effective than corticosteroid injections.
- It is not sure whether acupuncture or exercise and mobilization reduce symptoms of tennis elbow as few studies have been found, and they gave conflicting results.
- It is not sure whether orthoses (braces) reduce symptoms compared with no treatment or other treatments, as few studies have been found.
- It is uncertain whether open or percutaneous surgical techniques improve pain and function, as no good-quality studies have been identified.

References

1. Allander E. Prevalence, incidence and remission rates of some common rheumatic diseases and syndromes. Scand J Rheumatol 1974;3:145–53.
2. Chard MD, Hazleman BL. Tennis elbow—a reappraisal. Br J Rheumatol 1989;28:186–90.
3. Verhaar J. Tennis elbow: anatomical, epidemiological and therapeutic aspects. Int Orthop 1994;18:263–7.
4. Hamilton P. The prevalence of humeral epicondylitis: a survey in general practice. J R Coll Gen Pract 1986;36:464–5.
5. Kivi P. The etiology and conservative treatment of lateral epicondylitis. Scand J Rehabil Med 1983;15:37–41.
6. Verhaar JA. Tennis elbow. Dissertation, University of Maastricht, 1992.
7. Cyriax JH. The pathology and treatment of tennis elbow. J Bone Joint Surg Am 1936;4:921–40.
8. Murtagh JE. Tennis elbow. Aust Fam Physician 1994;17:90–1.
9. Hudak PL, Cole DC, Haines AT. Understanding prognosis to improve rehabilitation: the example of lateral elbow pain. Arch Phys Med Rehabil 1996;77:586–93.
10. Ernst E. Conservative therapy for tennis elbow. Br J Clin Pract 1992;46:55–7.
11. Pasternack I, Tuovinen EM, Lohman M, Vehmas T, Malmivaara A. MR findings in humeral epicondylitis. A systematic review. Acta Radiol. 2001;42(5):434–40.
12. Miller TT, Shapiro MA, Schultz E, Kalish PE. Comparison of sonography and MRI for diagnosing epicondylitis. J Clin Ultrasound 2002;30(4):193–202.
13. Struijs PA, Spruyt M, Assendelft WJ, van Dijk CN. The predictive value of diagnostic sonography for the effectiveness of conservative treatment of tennis elbow. Am J Roentgenol 2005;185(5):1113–18.
14. Levin D, Nazarian LN, Miller TT, et al. Lateral epicondylitis of the elbow: US findings. Radiology 2005;237(1):230–4.
15. De Zordo T, Lill SR, Fink C, et al. Real-time sonoelastography of lateral epicondylitis: comparison of findings between patients and healthy volunteers. AJR 2009;193:180–5.
16. Torp-Pedersen T, Torp-Pedersen S, Bliddal H. Diagnostic value of ultrasonography in epicondylitis. Ann Intern Med 2002;136(10):781–2.
17. Smidt N, Assendelft WJJ, van der Windt DAWM, et al. Corticosteroid injections for lateral epicondylitis: a systematic review. Pain 2002;96:23–40.
18. Bisset L, Paungmali A, Vicenzino B, et al. A systematic review and meta-analysis of clinical trials on physical interventions for lateral epicondylalgia. Br J Sports Med 2005;39:411–22.
19. Newcomer K, Laskowski E, Idank DM, et al. Corticosteroid injection in early treatment of lateral epicondylitis. Clin J Sport Med 2001;11:214–22.
20. Bär C, Bias P, Rose P. [Dexamethasonepalmitate for the treatment of tennis elbow]. Dtsch Z Sportmed 1997;48:119–124.
21. Okcu G, Yercan HS, Özic U. [The comparison of single dose versus multidose local corticosteroid injections for tennis elbow]. J Arthroplasty Arthroscopic Surg 2002;13:158–63.
22. Smidt N, van der Windt D, Assendelft W, et al. Corticosteroid injections, physiotherapy, or a wait-and-see policy for lateral epicondylitis: a randomised controlled trial. Lancet 2002;359:657–62.
23. Struijs PAA, Smidt N, Arola H, et al. Orthotic devices for the treatment of tennis elbow. Cochrane Library Syst Rev 2006;3.
24. Haker E, Lundeberg T. Elbow-band, splintage and steroids in lateral epicondylalgia (tennis elbow). Pain Clin 1993;6:103–12.
25. Haker E, Lundberg T. Acupuncture treatment in epicondylalgia: a comparative study of two acupuncture techniques. Clin J Pain 1990;6:221–6.
26. Green S, Buchbinder R, Barnsley L, et al. Non-steroidal anti-inflammatory drugs (NSAIDs) for treating lateral elbow pain in adults. Cochrane Library Syst Rev 2006;3.
27. Crowther MAA, Bannister GC, Huma H, et al. A prospective randomised study to compare extracorporeal shock wave therapy and injection of steroid for the treatment of tennis elbow. J Bone Joint Surg Br 2002;84:678–79.
28. Green S, Buchbinder R, Barnsley L, et al. Acupuncture for lateral elbow pain. Cochrane Library Syst Rev 2006;3.
29. Trinh KV, Phillips S-D, Ho E, et al. Acupuncture for alleviation of lateral elbow pain: a systematic review. Rheumatology 2004;43:1085–90.
30. Fink M, Wolkenstein E, Karst M, et al. Acupuncture in chronic epicondylitis: a randomized controlled trial. Rheumatology 2002;41:205–9.
31. Molsberger A, Hille E. The analgesic effect of acupuncture in chronic tennis elbow pain. Br J Rheumatol 1994;33:1162–5.
32. Haker E, Lundeberg T. Laser treatment applied to acupuncture points in lateral humeral epicondylalgia. A double blind study. Pain 1990;40:243–7.
33. Wang LC. Thirty cases of tennis elbow treated by moxibustion. Shanghai J Acupunct Moxibust 1997;16:20.
34. Selvanetti A, Barrucci A, Antonaci A. [Eccentric exercise in the functional reeducation of epicondylitis] Med Sport 2003;56:103–13.

35. Martinez-Silvestrini JA, Newcomer KL, Gay RE. Chronic lateral epicondylitis: Comparative effectiveness of a home exercise program including stretching alone versus stretching supplemented with eccentric or concentric strengthening. J Hand Therapy 2005;18:411–20.

36. Green S, Buchbinder R, Barnsley L, et al. Non-steroidal anti-inflammatory drugs (NSAIDs) for treating lateral elbow pain in adults. Cochrane Library Syst Rev 2006;3.

37. Struijs PAA, Smidt N, Arola H, et al. Orthotic devices for the treatment of tennis elbow. Cochrane Library Syst Rev 2006;3.

38. Struijs PAA, Kerkhoffs GMMJ, Assendelft WJJ, et al. Conservative treatment of lateral epicondylitis: brace versus physical therapy. A randomised clinical trial. Am J Sports Med 2004;32: 462–9.

39. Buchbinder R, Green S, Bell S, et al. Surgery for lateral elbow pain. Cochrane Library Syst Rev 2006;3.

40. Dunkow PD, Jatti M, Muddu BN. A comparison of open and percutaneous techniques in the surgical treatment of tennis elbow. J Bone Joint Surg Br 2004;86:701–4.

41. Schmitt JS, Di Fabio RP. Reliable change and minimum important difference (MID) proportions facilitated group responsiveness comparisons using individual threshold criteria. J Clin Epidemiol 2004;57:1008–18.

Jaskarndip Chahal[1], Christopher Peskun[1], and Daniel B. Whelan[1,2]

[1]University of Toronto, Toronto, ON, Canada
[2]St. Michael's Hospital, Toronto, ON, Canada

Case scenario

A 25 year old female soccer player presents to your outpatient sports medicine clinic 2 days after sustaining a twisting injury to her right knee. A workup in the Emergency Department on the day of injury revealed no fractures.

Relevant anatomy

Most acute knee injuries with intra-articular pathology are associated with a hemarthrosis. The most common lesion causing a hemarthrosis is rupture of the anterior cruciate ligament (ACL). Other lesions include patellar dislocation, meniscal tears, chondral or osteochondral injuries, capsular tears, or rupture of the deep medial collateral ligament or other ligaments.

Importance of the problem

The annual incidence of knee injuries has been estimated to be 110 per 10,000 individuals, with 10% of these injuries leading to a surgical consultation.[1]

Top five questions

Diagnosis

1. What is the relative frequency of various injuries when patients present with a knee hemarthrosis?
2. What is the effectiveness of physical examination in diagnosing an ACL rupture in an acutely injured knee?

3. What is the role of MRI vs. arthroscopy in the diagnosis of acute knee injury?

Therapy

4. What is the role for aspiration in the acutely injured knee with hemarthrosis?
5. Is there evidence in favor of surgical reconstruction of an acute (<3 weeks) ACL injury?

Finding the evidence

Where there were recently published systematic reviews/meta-analyses that spoke directly to the questions above, those reviews were considered in isolation without referencing the index studies.

Question 1: What is the relative frequency of various injuries when patients present with a knee hemarthrosis?

Case clarification

The clinical examination of the knee initially reveals a hemarthrosis. The patient asks you what your differential diagnosis is.

Relevance

Given the relative frequency of acute knee injuries, it is important to have a grasp of the possible intra-articular pathoanatomy. Most experts would agree that the ACL is the most common presenting cause of an acute hemarthrosis in patients with athletic injuries. Other injuries that can present as hemarthrosis include meniscus tears, osteochon-

Evidence-Based Orthopedics, First Edition. Edited by Mohit Bhandari.
© 2012 Blackwell Publishing Ltd. Published 2012 by Blackwell Publishing Ltd.

dral defects, patellar dislocations, and medial collateral ligament injuries.

Finding the evidence
- Cochrane Database, with search term: "knee injury"
- PubMed (www.ncbi.nlm.nih.gov/pubmed/) clinical queries search/systematic reviews: "knee injury AND hemarthrosis"
- PubMed (www.ncbi.nlm.nih.gov/pubmed/) sensitivity search using keywords: "knee injury AND hemarthrosis AND arthroscopy OR MRI" Exclusions: <16 years old, atraumatic injury, road traffic accidents

Quality of the evidence
Level II
- 13 prospective diagnostic studies using arthroscopy or MRI

Level IV
- 1 retrospective study

Findings
O'Conner[2] and Jackson[3] initially reported that arthroscopy might be of value in acute injuries. Since then, many other investigators have conducted retrospective and prospective diagnostic studies using arthroscopy as a diagnostic modality to analyze acute patterns of pathoanatomy giving rise to traumatic hemarthrosis.[1,4-14] Based on our pooled statistical analyses of 12 diagnostic studies (n = 1468) from 1977 to 2002, it is evident that injuries to the ACL are the most common cause of an acute hemarthroses occurring in approximately in 57.5% (n = 844) of cases. This observation was consistent over time and across various studies. Meniscus injuries and medial collateral ligament injuries occurred in approximately 32.5% (n = 477) and 18.8% (n = 276) of cases, respectively. Osteochondral defects were observed in 13.0% (n = 191) of cases.[1,4-14] The results are presented in Table 93.1. The possibility of patellar dislocation leading to a hemarthrosis is unclear since most studies did not report this data. According to a recent review, this injury has been diagnosed in 4–23% of cases presenting with a hemarthrosis.[15]

A recent prospective MRI study conducted by LaPrade et al.[16] analyzed ligament injuries alone as a cause for hemarthrosis. The authors demonstrated that in the setting of an acute hemarthroses, 18.4% of patients have multiple-ligament injuries. Of patients with posterior cruciate ligament (PCL) and posterolateral corner injury (PLC), multiple ligaments were injured in 52% and 87% of cases, respectively. The most commonly observed combined patterns included ACL–MCL (medial collateral ligament) and ACL–PLC injuries.

Recommendations
- ACL injuries are the most common cause of an acute knee hemarthroses [overall quality: high]

- PCL and PLC injury should increase suspicion for a multiple-ligament knee injury [overall quality: moderate]

Question 2: What is the effectiveness of physical examination in diagnosing an ACL rupture in an acutely injured knee?

Case clarification
The patient would like to know the likelihood of her having an ACL rupture based on your physical examination findings.

Relevance
Knowledge of the diagnostic accuracy of the anterior drawer test, Lachman's test, and the pivot-shift test, has implications in terms of generating differential diagnoses, ordering imaging studies, and planning for operative intervention.

Finding the evidence
- Cochrane Datbase, with search term: "anterior cruciate ligament"
- PubMed (www.ncbi.nlm.nih.gov/pubmed/) clinical queries search: "anterior cruciate ligament injury AND diagnosis"
- PubMed (www.ncbi.nlm.nih.gov/pubmed/): sensitivity search using keywords: "anterior cruciate ligament injury AND diagnosis AND physical examination"

Quality of the evidence
Level I
- 5 meta-analyses

Findings
Several meta-analyses have examined the diagnosis of ACL rupture via physical examination.[17-21] These meta-analyses have included between 17 and 28 studies, the majority of which have included young patients with an average age of 28.6 years. Although most studies involved examination by a senior surgeon with experience in knee injury treatment, not all studies were explicit. In most of the studies the gold standard for diagnosis was arthroscopy, which may have selected for more severe knee injuries as the booking of the arthroscopic procedure was a determining factor for inclusion in most studies. The findings indicate that the Lachman test is the most sensitive test and the pivot-shift is the most specific test for diagnosis of an ACL injury. Benjaminse et al.[17] stratified patients based on the chronicity (acute or chronic) of the injury and whether or not the tests were performed with the benefit of anesthesia. In the acute setting, anesthesia drastically improves the sensitivity of the pivot-shift test and modestly improves the accuracy of the anterior drawer test (Table 93.2).[17] Anesthesia does not alter the diagnostic accuracy of the

Table 93.1 Pooled statistical analysis of 12 diagnostic studies

Study	Description	# pts	Age (ave)	Total ACL (%)	ACL	PCL	Meniscus	Osteochondral	MCL rupture
Maffuli et al.[11]	Prospective arthroscopic study	106	28.35	70%	28 partial, 43 complete	1 partial, 1 complete	17	14	
Sarimo et al.[1]	Prospective arthroscopic study	320	31	45%	144 total	11	68	57 (9 isolated)	68
Munshi et al.[12]	Prospective study (MRI, arthroscopy)	23	26	20/23	16 high grade partial or complete	5	10		9
Simonsen et al.[14]	Prospective study (arthroscopy arthrotomy)	117	27		75 total; 49 complete, 26 partial	16 total (4 isolated); 10 complete and 6 partial	25 total, 1 isolated		66 total; 29 isolated; 52 complete, 14 partial
DeHaven[6]	Prospective study, arthroscopy,	113		72%	81 total; 25 isolated, 56 combined	3 cases	17 cases isolated; 81 total	7 cases	
Noyes et al.[13]	Prospective	85	21	72%	61 total (partial 24, complete 37)	2 partial	5 isolated, 38 combined, 43 total	7 total	3 combined, none isolated; 13 medial capsule
Butler and Andrews[5]	Retrospective	80	22	62%	50 total (21 partial, 29 complete)		15 isolated, 29 combined; 44 total	9 total	
Jones and Allum[10]	Prospective	50	twenty six	66%	33 total (13 partial, 20 complete)	3	11	4 total	
Bomberg and McGinty[4]	Prospective	45	21	71%	32 total (26 complete, 6 partial)		21	6	7
Harilainen et al.[9] mixed series, includes patellar disloc	Prospective	328	29.6	41%	135 total	10	62	54	46
Gillquist et al.[7]	Prospective	69	15–60	45%	31 complete, 10 partial	2	16	7	41
Hardarker et al.[8]	Prospective	132	22	77%	101 total; 62% complete, 38% partial		17 isolated, 62 combined	11 isolated, 15 combined	36 combined
Total counts		1468		41%–77%	844	55	477	191	276
Total (%)					57.50%	3.75%	32.50%	13.00%	18.80%

ACL, anterior cruciate ligament; MCL, medial collateral ligament; PCL, posterior cruciate ligament.

Lachman test. The notion of combing the three tests into a composite assessment was examined by Solomon et al.[21] The combination of the three tests resulted in a positive likelihood ratio (LR+) of 25.0 (range 2.1–306.0) and a negative likelihood ratio (LR–) of 0.04 (range 0.01–0.50) for the diagnosis of ACL rupture. These results must be tempered by the fact that the pivot-shift examination lacks perfect reproducibility and is dependent on many patient factors.

Recommendations

• The Lachman test is the most sensitive test for ACL rupture in an acutely injured knee while the pivot-shift test is the most specific [overall quality: high]
• Anesthesia improves the diagnostic accuracy of the pivot-shift test in the acutely injured knee [overall quality: high]
• Composite physical examination improves the diagnostic accuracy of physical examination for ACL rupture in the acutely injured knee [overall quality: high]

Question 3: What is the role of MRI vs. arthroscopy in the diagnosis of acute knee injury?

Case clarification

The physical examination remains indeterminate due to pain and spasm. Although you suggest a MRI investigation to your patient, she would like to proceed with arthroscopy to clarify the diagnosis.

Relevance

In some institutions, the availability of MRI is limited and a patient may have to wait for weeks before an evaluation. In current practice, the majority of surgeons would order an MRI and decide whether or not to proceed with arthroscopy based its results. Although this is not a formal cost-effectiveness assessment, determining whether it is more practical to obtain an MRI or proceed with arthroscopy for diagnostic purposes would be of importance in the clinical realm.

Finding the evidence

• Cochrane Database, with search term: "knee injury"
• PubMed (www.ncbi.nlm.nih.gov/pubmed/): sensitivity search using keywords "knee injury AND hemarthrosis AND diagnosis"

Quality of the evidence

Level I
• 1 randomized trial

Level II
• 1 systematic review, 3 prospective studies

Findings

Crawford et al.[22] performed a systematic review of largely level II evidence (47 prospective studies of a total of 59 articles) to assess the difference between MRI and arthroscopy in the diagnosis of knee pathology. The findings indicate that MRI is highly accurate in diagnosing ligament and meniscal pathology. The results are presented in Table 93.3. Furthermore, performing an early MRI prior to diagnostic arthroscopy has been reported to avoid unnecessary surgical intervention in 22–51% of cases.[12,23–25] A randomized trial also demonstrated that there are no differences in functional outcome 1 year after comparing early (<48 hours) and delayed (3–21 days) arthroscopy for acute knee

Table 93.2 Pooled data for physical examination test with and without anesthesia

Test		No anesthesia	Anesthesia
Anterior drawer test	Sensitivity	49 (43–55)	78 (73–82)
	Specificity	58 (39–76)	75 (64–83)
Lachman test	Sensitivity	94 (91–96)	97 (95–99)
	Specificity	97 (93–99)	(82–97)
Pivot-shift test	Sensitivity	32 (25–38)	85 (80–90)
	Specificity	100 (48–100)	97 (91–100)

Modified from Benjaminse et al.[17]

Table 93.3 MRI in the diagnosis of knee pathology

Diagnosis	N	Sensitivity	Specificity	Accuracy	PPV	NPV
Medial meniscus	1207	91.4	81.1	86.4	83.2	90.1
Lateral meniscus	525	76	93.3	88.8	80.4	91.6
ACL	372	86.5	95.2	93.4	82.9	96.4
ACLL, MM, LM	2104	86.2	90.7	89.2	82.4	92.8
Other knee pathology	443	68.7	97.9	90.8	91.3	90.7
Total	2547	82.5	92.8	89.6	83.9	92.2

NPV, negative predictive value; PPV, positive predictive value.
Adapted from Crawford, R., et al., Magnetic resonance imaging versus arthroscopy in the diagnosis of knee pathology, concentrating on meniscal lesions and ACL tears: a systematic review. Br Med Bull, 2007. 84: p. 5–23, by permission of Oxford University Press.[22]

injuries.[26] Avoiding unnecessary arthroscopic procedures will help minimize associated complications such as ecchymoses, infection, deep venous thrombosis, iatrogenic cartilage injury, and the need for anesthesia.

Recommendations

• Early MRI is recommended to elucidate an equivocal physical exam as opposed to a diagnostic arthroscopy [overall quality: moderate]

• Routine MRI avoids unnecessary diagnostic arthroscopy in over 20% of cases [overall quality: moderate]

Question 4: What is the role for aspiration in the acutely injured knee with hemarthrosis?

Case clarification

The results of the MRI confirm the presence of an isolated ACL rupture. However, the patient is suffering from pain and a fixed flexion deformity due to the presence of a large hemarthrosis. You are considering an aspiration of the knee. The patient would like to know the associated risks and benefits.

Relevance

Aspiration of an acute hemarthrosis is a procedure which was initially used as a diagnostic aid. With the advent and availability of MRI, diagnostic aspiration has largely been supplanted, although many practitioners continue to rely on aspiration to offer their patients pain relief and increased function. However, the risks of iatrogenic infection and reaccumulation of the hemarthrosis must be considered before undertaking aspiration.

Finding the evidence

• Cochrane Database, with search term: "knee aspiration"

• PubMed (www.ncbi.nlm.nih.gov/pubmed/) clinical queries search: "knee aspiration AND hemarthrosis"

Quality of the evidence

Level IV

• 5 retrospective case series

Findings

Several studies have examined the diagnostic utility of aspiration for an acute hemarthrosis. However, to the authors' knowledge there are no known studies examining the utility of aspiration for pain relief or improved functionality. Five retrospective studies, with a total of 889 patients, have included routine aspiration of acutely injured knees as part of a larger management protocol.[11,27–30] None of these studies quantified the degree of pain relief or improved functionality after aspiration. The cumulative incidence of iatrogenic infection was zero, although this

was not always indicated as a study endpoint. One study (n = 510) consistently sent the aspirated fluid for culture.[27] This study returned nine positive aspirates, all of which were thought to be clinically insignificant in that no patient developed symptoms consistent with septic arthritis. Overall there is a paucity of literature to help guide the utility of aspiration in the acutely injured knee with hemarthrosis. This is highlighted by a recent short-cut review that returned zero relevant studies.[31] This remains an important issue which requires investigation to help clarify indications and safety.

Recommendations

• The available literature cannot recommend or dissuade the use of aspiration for symptomatic relief or functional improvement in the acutely injured knee with hemarthrosis

Question 5: Is there evidence in favor of surgical reconstruction of an acute (<3 weeks) ACL injury?

Case clarification

You have suggested an acute period of rehabilitation and quads strengthening, but the patient would like to proceed with surgery immediately so she can return to her activities before the upcoming skiing season.

Relevance

There has been some recent controversy on whether it is safe to proceed with an ACL reconstruction in the acute setting and whether early surgical reconstruction should be routinely offered to patients. Current opinion dictates that is preferable to initiate an early structured rehabilitation program to optimize range of motion and quadriceps strength in order to avoid arthrofibrosis, and to offer surgery to patients who experience symptomatic instability.

Finding the evidence

• Cochrane Database, with search term: "anterior cruciate ligament" AND "surgery" AND "timing"

• PubMed (www.ncbi.nlm.nih.gov/pubmed/) clinical queries search/systematic reviews: "early anterior cruciate ligament reconstruction"

Quality of the evidence

Level I

• 1 randomized controlled trial (2010)

Level II

• 1 systematic review (2009)

Findings

A recent systematic review by Smith et al.[32] compared outcomes following the ACL reconstruction in patients with early (<3 weeks) and delayed surgery (>6 weeks). There were 161 patients in the "early" group compared with 209 patients in the "delayed" group. There were no statistically significant differences with regard to various functional outcome measures or perceived patient satisfaction. One study also investigated return to sport; there was no difference between the early and delayed groups. There was also no difference between the two groups in instrumented laxity testing, range of motion, and rates of arthrofibrosis. One caveat made by the authors states that the quality of literature pertaining to ACL reconstruction is quite heterogeneous and that the cost–benefit analysis of early vs. delayed surgery requires further assessment.

In a recent randomized controlled trial (RCT) for acute ACL tears,[33] it was demonstrated that for young active adults, a strategy of rehabilitation plus early ACL reconstruction (<10 weeks) was not superior to a strategy of optional delayed reconstruction in those with symptomatic instability. The absolute change in the mean Knee Injury and Osteoarthritis Outcome Score (KOOS) from baseline to 2 years was equivalent in both groups. There were also no reported differences in Short Form-36, Tegner activity scores, and return to pre-injury activity at 2 years. Additionally, it was demonstrated that more than half of the ACL reconstructions can be avoided without adversely affecting outcomes. Nevertheless, further longitudinal follow-up is required to ascertain whether the comparable results in the intervention and control groups are maintained over time and to assess longer-term outcomes such as the risk of knee osteoarthritis.[33] Furthermore, since the participants in this study were not stratified according to activity level or age, these results may not be generalizable to professional athletes and young children as these groups have an exceptionally high risk of a pivoting episode (and resultant meniscal injury). Any treatment protocol which involves delayed optional reconstruction should caution patients about the potential risk to the menisci with pivoting.

Recommendations

• There is no difference in surgeon and patient-based outcomes when comparing early and delayed ACL reconstruction. Early structured rehabilitation and delayed optional reconstruction for the symptomatic patient is recommended for the acutely injured patient as opposed to *routine* early reconstruction [overall quality: high]

Summary of recommendations

• ACL injuries are the most common cause of an acute knee hemarthroses
• PCL and PLC injury should increase suspicion for a multiple-ligament knee injury

• The Lachman test is the most sensitive test for ACL rupture in an acutely injured knee while the pivot-shift test is the most specific
• Anesthesia improves the diagnostic accuracy of the pivot-shift test in the acutely injured knee
• Composite physical examination improves the diagnostic accuracy of physical examination for ACL rupture in the acutely injured knee
• Early MRI is recommended to elucidate an equivocal physical exam as opposed to a diagnostic arthroscopy
• Routine MRI avoids unnecessary diagnostic arthroscopy in over 20% of cases
• The available literature cannot recommend or dissuade the use of aspiration for symptomatic relief or functional improvement in the acutely injured knee with hemarthrosis
• There is no difference in surgeon and patient-based outcomes when comparing early and delayed ACL reconstruction. Early structured rehabilitation and delayed optional reconstruction for the symptomatic patient is recommended for the acutely injured patient as opposed to *routine* early reconstruction

Conclusions

While clinical examination, imaging and examination under anesthesia are able to accurately diagnosis acute traumatic knee injuries, there are many aspects of the management of these injuries that requires further investigation. Well-designed RCTs are required in order to elucidate the benefit of early stabilization of acute ACL injury as well the benefit of knee aspiration in the setting of acute traumatic knee hemarthroses.

References

1. Sarimo J, Rantanen J, Heikkilä J, Helttula I, Hiltunen A, Orava S. Acute traumatic hemarthrosis of the knee. Is routine arthroscopic examination necessary? A study of 320 consecutive patients. Scand J Surg 2002;91(4):361–4.
2. O'Connor RL. Arthroscopy in the diagnosis and treatment of acute ligament injuries of the knee. J Bone Joint Surg Am 1974; 56(2):333–7.
3. Jackson RW. The role of arthroscopy in the management of the arthritic knee. Clin Orthop Relat Res 1974;101:28–35.
4. Bomberg BC, McGinty JB. Acute hemarthrosis of the knee: indications for diagnostic arthroscopy. Arthroscopy 1990;6(3): 221–5.
5. Butler JC, Andrews JR. The role of arthroscopic surgery in the evaluation of acute traumatic hemarthrosis of the knee. Clin Orthop Relat Res 1988;228:150–2.
6. DeHaven KE. Diagnosis of acute knee injuries with hemarthrosis. Am J Sports Med 1980;8(1):9–14.

7. Gillquist J, Hagberg G, Oretorp N. Arthroscopy in acute injuries of the knee joint. Acta Orthop Scand 1977;48(2):190–6.

8. Hardaker WT Jr., Garrett WE Jr., Bassett FH 3rd. Evaluation of acute traumatic hemarthrosis of the knee joint. South Med J 1990;83(6):640–4.

9. Harilainen A, Myllynen P, Antila H, Seitsalo S. The significance of arthroscopy and examination under anaesthesia in the diagnosis of fresh injury haemarthrosis of the knee joint. Injury 1988;19(1):21–4.

10. Jones JR, Allum RL. Acute traumatic haemarthrosis of the knee: expectant treatment or arthroscopy? Ann R Coll Surg Engl 1989;71(1):40–3.

11. Maffulli N, Binfield PM, King JB, Good CJ. Acute haemarthrosis of the knee in athletes. A prospective study of 106 cases. J Bone Joint Surg Br 1993;75(6):945–9.

12. Munshi M, Davidson M, MacDonald PB, Froese W, Sutherland K. The efficacy of magnetic resonance imaging in acute knee injuries. Clin J Sport Med 2000;10(1):34–9.

13. Noyes FR, Bassett RW, Grood ES, Butler DL. Arthroscopy in acute traumatic hemarthrosis of the knee. Incidence of anterior cruciate tears and other injuries. J Bone Joint Surg Am 1980;62(5): 687–95; 757.

14. Simonsen O, Jensen J, Lauritzen J. Arthroscopy in acute knee injuries. Acta Orthop Scand 1986;57(2):126–9.

15. Shaerf D, Banerjee A. Assessment and management of posttraumatic haemarthrosis of the knee. Br J Hosp Med (Lond) 2008; 69(8):459–60; 462–3.

16. LaPrade RF, Wentorf FA, Fritts H, Gundry C, Hightower CD. A prospective magnetic resonance imaging study of the incidence of posterolateral and multiple ligament injuries in acute knee injuries presenting with a hemarthrosis. Arthroscopy 2007; 23(12):1341–7.

17. Benjaminse A, Gokeler A, van der Schans CP. Clinical diagnosis of an anterior cruciate ligament rupture: a meta-analysis. J Orthop Sports Phys Ther 2006;36(5):267–88.

18. Keating J. Physical examination can detect the presence or absence of cruciate ligament injury. Aust J Physiother 2002; 48(2):132.

19. Prins M. The Lachman test is the most sensitive and the pivot shift the most specific test for the diagnosis of ACL rupture. Aust J Physiother 2006;52(1):66.

20. Scholten RJ, Opstelten W, van der Plas CG, Bijl D, Deville WL, Bouter LM. Accuracy of physical diagnostic tests for assessing ruptures of the anterior cruciate ligament: a meta-analysis (structured abstract). J Fam Pract 2003;52:689–94.

21. Solomon DH, Simel DL, Bates DW, Katz JN, Schaffer JL. The rational clinical examination. Does this patient have a torn meniscus or ligament of the knee? Value of the physical examination. JAMA 2001;286(13):1610–20.

22. Crawford R, Walley G, Bridgman S, Maffulli N. Magnetic resonance imaging versus arthroscopy in the diagnosis of knee pathology, concentrating on meniscal lesions and ACL tears: a systematic review. Br Med Bull 2007;84:5–23.

23. Ruwe PA, Wright J, Randall RL, Lynch JK, Jokl P, McCarthy S. Can MR imaging effectively replace diagnostic arthroscopy? Radiology 1992;183(2):335–9.

24. Spiers AS, Meagher T, Ostlere SJ, Wilson DJ, Dodd CA. Can MRI of the knee affect arthroscopic practice? A prospective study of 58 patients. J Bone Joint Surg Br 1993;75(1):49–52.

25. Bui-Mansfield LT, Youngberg RA, Warme W, Pitcher JD, Nguyen PL. Potential cost savings of MR imaging obtained before arthroscopy of the knee: evaluation of 50 consecutive patients. AJR Am J Roentgenol 1997;168(4):913–8.

26. Wilson-MacDonald J, Dodd C, Cockin J. Arthroscopy in acute knee injuries: a prospective controlled trial. Injury 1990;21(3): 165–8.

27. Ansari MZ, Ahee P, Iqbal MY, Swarup S. Traumatic haemarthrosis of the knee. Eur J Emerg Med 2004;11(3):145–7.

28. Casteleyn PP, Handelberg F, Opdecam P. Traumatic haemarthrosis of the knee. J Bone Joint Surg Br 1988;70(3):404–6.

29. Jain AS, Swanson AJ, Murdoch G. Haemarthrosis of the knee joint. Injury 1983;15(3):178–81.

30. Mariani PP, Puddu G, Ferretti A. Hemathrosis treated by aspiration and casting. How to condemn the knee. Am J Sports Med 1982;10(6):343–5.

31. Wallman P, Carley S. Aspiration of acute traumatic knee haemarthrosis. Emerg Med J 2002;19(1):50.

32. Smith TO, Davies L, Hing CB. Early versus delayed surgery for anterior cruciate ligament reconstruction: a systematic review and meta-analysis. Knee Surg Sports Traumatol Arthrosc 2010; 18(3):304–11.

33. Frobell RB, Roos EM, Roos HP, Ranstam J, Lohmander LS. A randomized trial of treatment for acute anterior cruciate ligament tears. N Engl J Med 2010;363(4):331–42.

94

Meniscal Tears (Meniscectomy, Meniscopexy, Meniscal Transplants/Scaffolds)

Nicola Maffulli[1], Umile Giuseppe Longo[2], Stefano Campi[2], and Vincenzo Denaro[2]

[1]Barts and The London School of Medicine and Dentistry, London, UK
[2]Campus Bio-Medico University, Rome, Italy

Case scenario

A 28 year old soccer player comes to the Emergency Department with right knee pain after a trauma during a match. Clinical examination reveals effusion, locking, tenderness and painful flexo-extension of the knee. He has no neurovascular deficits.

Relevant anatomy

Meniscal tear patterns include vertical (longitudinal and radial), oblique, complex (or degenerative),[1–3] and horizontal[4,5] tears. Oblique and vertical longitudinal tears constitute about 80% of meniscal tears.[4] Degenerative complex tears occur in multiple planes and are more common in older age groups. They occur most commonly in the posterior horns.[2,3]

Importance of the problem

The mean annual incidence of meniscal tears is about 60–70 per 100,000,[6,7] with a male to female ratio ranging from 2.5:1 to 4:1. Meniscal pathology in younger patients is likely consequent to an acute traumatic event, while degenerative changes are more frequent at an older age.[5]

More than one third of all meniscal tears are associated with an anterior cruciate ligament (ACL) injury,[8] with a peak incidence in men 21–30 years old and in girls and women 11–20 years old. Degenerative types of meniscal tears commonly occur in men between 40 and 60.

A Google search for "meniscal injuries" returns over 1,200,000 hits.

Top six questions

Diagnosis

1. What is the accuracy of clinical examination in the diagnosis of meniscal tears?
2. What is the best diagnostic tool for meniscal lesions? MRI vs. arthroscopy

Therapy

3. Does the repair technique influence the surgical outcome?
4. Does meniscal transplantation prevent osteoarthritis development after total meniscectomy?
5. Is there a role for synthetic materials in meniscal reconstruction?
6. What is the best rehabilitation protocol?

Question 1: What is the accuracy of clinical examination in the diagnosis of meniscal tears?

Case clarification

At clinical examination, medial joint line tenderness is present. McMurray's test is positive. The Apley test elicits pain with rotation of the tibia in the flexed knee joint.

Evidence-Based Orthopedics, First Edition. Edited by Mohit Bhandari.
© 2012 Blackwell Publishing Ltd. Published 2012 by Blackwell Publishing Ltd.

Relevance

A variety of clinical diagnostic tests are available for meniscal tears. Therefore, clinicians need to select diagnostic tests that are the most specific to confirm meniscal tears and the most sensitive to establish that meniscal tears is unlikely.

Current opinion

Mosthealth care professionals use the joint line tenderness, McMurray's test, Apley test, and the Thessaly test as clinical diagnostic tests for meniscal tears.

Finding the evidence

- Cochrane Database, with search terms: "meniscus," "meniscal injury," "meniscal tears," "knee clinical examination," "McMurray's test," "Apley test," "Thessaly test"
- PubMed (www.ncbi.nlm.nih.gov/pubmed/) clinical queries search/systematic reviews: "meniscus," "meniscal injury," "meniscal tears," "knee clinical examination," "McMurray's test," "Apley test," "Thessaly test"
- MEDLINE search identifying the population (meniscal tears) and the methodology (diagnosis). We used the keywords "meniscus" AND "clinical examination" as well as "meniscal tears" AND "diagnosis"

Quality of the evidence

Level I
- 4 meta-analyses[9–12]
- 1 systematic reviews[13]
- 4 randomized trials[14–17]

Level II
- 1 systematic review[18]

Findings

Sensitivity and specificity Four trials[14–17] (n = 668 patients) provided the accuracy of clinical tests for assessing meniscal lesions of the knee (Table 94.1). According to a systematic review by Meserve[11] the overall average sensitivity for meniscal tears is 0.76 (95% CI 0.73, 0.80) for joint line tenderness, 0.55 (95% CI 0.50, 0.60) for McMurray's test, and 0.22 (95% CI 0.17, 0.28) for the Apley test (Table 94.1). According to a meta-analysis by Ockert,[12] the overall average sensitivity for meniscal tears is 0.91% (95% CI 0.98–0.94) for the Thessaly test.

The overall average specificity for meniscal tears is 0.76 (95% CI 0.64, 0.87) for joint line tenderness, 0.77 (95% CI 0.62, 0.87) for McMurray's test, 0.88 (95% CI 0.72, 0.96) for

Table 94.1 Accuracy of clinical tests for assessing meniscal lesions of the knee

Reference	Level of evidence	Total no. of patients studied	Age of patients mean (range)	Affected meniscus	Sensitivity	Specificity	LR+	LR−
Fowler[16]	I	161	33 (16–67)	M+L	JLT 0.850	JLT 0.296	1.21	0.506
					M 0.288	M 0.693	7.76	0.74
					A 0.156	A 0.800	0.78	1.06
Evans[15]	I	104	—	M+L	M 0.239	M 0.931	3.467	0.817
Manzotti[14]	I	130	32.4 (17–48)	M+L	M	M	M	M
					MM 0.88	MM 0.50	MM 1.760	MM: 0.240
					LM 0.795	LM 0.200	LM 0.994	LM 1.026
Karachalios[17]	I	213	29.4 (18–55)	M+L	JLT	JLT	JLT	JLT
					MM 0.71	MM 0.87	MM 5.46	MM 0.33
					LM 0.78	LM 0.90	LM 7.80	LM 0.24
					M	M	M	M
					MM 0.48	MM 0.94	MM 8.00	MM 0.55
					LM 0.65	LM 0.86	LM 4.64	LM 0.41
					A	A	A	A
					MM 0.41	MM 0.93	MM 5.85	MM 0.63
					LM 0.41	LM 0.86	LM 2.93	LM 0.69
					T 5°	T 5°	T 5°	T 5°
					MM 0.66	MM 0.96	MM 2.9	MM 11.4
					LM 0.81	LM 0.91	LM 8	LM 1.7
					T 20°	T 20°	T 20°	T 20°
					MM 0.89	MM 0.97	MM 2.2	MM 3.6
					LM 0.92	LM 0.96	LM 3.7	LM 0.73

A, Apley; JLT, joint line tenderness; LM, lateral meniscus; LR+, likelihood ratio of a positive test; LR−, likelihood ratio of a negative test; M, Mc Murray; MM, medial meniscus; T, Thessaly.

the Apley test, and 0.97 (95% CI 0.95, 0.99) for the Thessaly test.

Recommendations

• The most sensitive clinical diagnostic test for meniscal tears is joint line tenderness at 76% [overall quality: moderate]
• The McMurray and Apley tests could be considered high specificity but low sensitivity tests [overall quality: low]
• The Thessaly test in isolation is not useful for the detection of meniscal tears, but it helps to increase diagnostic certainty when combined with other standard tests[19] [overall quality: low]

Question 2: What is the best diagnostic tool for meniscal lesions? MRI vs. arthroscopy

Case clarification

Clinical examination suggests a meniscal tear. MRI should be useful to confirm the diagnosis before surgical management.

Relevance

Arthroscopy is the gold standard for the diagnosis of meniscal tears. However, this procedure carries an unquantifiable surgical risks.[20] MRI is a suitable noninvasive and safe alternative tool to establish a diagnosis of meniscal tear.

Current opinion

Current opinion suggests that most healthcare professionals consider MRI as an appropriate screening tool before therapeutic arthroscopy

Finding the evidence

• Cochrane Database, with search term "meniscus," "meniscal injury," "meniscal tears," "MRI," "magnetic resonance imaging," "arthroscopy"
• PubMed (www.ncbi.nlm.nih.gov/pubmed/) clinical queries search/systematic reviews: "meniscus," "meniscal injury," "meniscal tears," "MRI," "Magnetic resonance imaging," "arthroscopy"
• MEDLINE search identifying the population (meniscal tears) the intervention (diagnosis) and the methodology (MRI). We used the keywords "meniscus" AND "diagnosis" as well as "meniscal tears" AND "MRI"

Quality of the evidence
Level I
• 13 randomized trials[21–33]

Level II
• 2 systematic reviews[13,18]

Findings

Correlation between MRI and arthroscopy Thirteen trials (n = 1162 patients) provided correlation between MRI and arthroscopy (Table 94.2). According to the systematic review by Oei,[13] the overall average sensitivity for medial meniscal tears is 93.3 (95% CI 91.7, 95.0) and 79.3 (95% CI 74.3, 84.2) for lateral meniscal tears. The overall average specificity for medial meniscal tears is 88.4 (95% CI 85.4, 91.4) and 95.7 (95% CI 94.6, 96.8) for lateral meniscal tears.

Recommendation

• MRI is preferable to diagnostic arthroscopy in most patients because it avoids the surgical risks of arthroscopy with high accuracy in diagnosing meniscal and ACL tears[20] [overall quality: high]

Question 3: Does the repair technique influence the surgical outcome?

Case clarification

MRI shows an extended vertical longitudinal meniscal tear. Meniscal repair could represent an option for this patient. Arthroscopic meniscal repair surgery includes inside-out, outside-in, and all-inside techniques.

Relevance

Several techniques have been proposed to optimize the healing of a repairable meniscal tear. However, the long-term follow-up of the different techniques is not well defined. Also, the percentage of meniscal healing and its correlation with the clinical outcome is not clear.

Current opinion

All-inside meniscal repair devices are an attractive option owing to cosmesis, surgical time, and decreased risk of injury to neurovascular structures. However, the clinical outcome of the different devices has not been clarified. The newer self-adjusting suture device repairs do not have the length of follow-up of suture repair, but are showing promising initial results.

Finding the evidence

• Cochrane Database, with search term "meniscal repair," "arthroscopy," "meniscal sutures," "inside-out meniscal repair," "outside-in meniscal repair," "all-inside meniscal repair"
• PubMed (www.ncbi.nlm.nih.gov/pubmed/) clinical queries search/ systematic reviews: "meniscal repair," "arthroscopy," "meniscal sutures," "inside-out meniscal repair," "outside-in meniscal repair," "all-inside meniscal repair"
• MEDLINE search identifying the population (meniscal tears) the intervention (meniscal repair) and the methodology (clinical trial). We used the keywords "meniscal tear"

Table 94.2 Correlation between MRI and arthroscopy

Reference	Total no. of patients studied	Age of patients (mean)	Affected meniscus	Magnetic field strength (T)	Accuracy (%) M/L	Sensitivity (%) M/L	Specificity (%) M/L	PPV M/L	NPV M/L
Gluckert et al.[32]	80	33	M+L	1.5	95	97	93	92	98
					100	100	100	100	100
Grevitt et al.[31]	55	36	M+L	0.2	91	92	90	88	93
					96	89	98	89	98
Heron and Calvert[30]	100	38	M+L	1.5	—	98	95	—	—
						94	94		
Kinnunen[29]	33	36	M+L	0.1	—	87	80	—	—
						25	97		
La Prade et al.[28]	72	34	M+L	1.0	99	100	97	97	100
					90	70	98	93	89
Justice and Quinn[27]	561	—	M+L	1.5	—	96	91	—	—
						82	98		
Lundberg et al.[26]	69	26	M+L	1.5	68	74	66	45	89
					71	50	84	65	73
Bui-Mansfield et al.[25]	50	31	M+L	1.5	94	90	97	95	94
					88	60	100	100	85
Franklin et al.[24]	35	40	M+L	0.2	—	90	100	—	—
						89	100		
Rappeport et al.[23]	47	—	M+L	0.1	77	86	73	57	92
					91	40	98	67	93
Riel et al.[33]	244	36	M+L	0.2	95	93	94	97	94
					94	83	96	84	96
Cotten et al.[22]	90	34	M+L	0.2	—	88	100	—	—
						83	90		
				1.5	—	89	100	—	—
						86	95		
Winters and Tregonning[21]	67	—	M+L	1.5	92	87	92	89	90
					82	46	91	88	55

L, lateral; M, medial; NPV, negative predictive value; PPV, positive predictive value.

AND "meniscal repair," "meniscal suture," as well as "meniscal tear" AND "inside-out meniscal repair," "outside-in meniscal repair" and "all-inside meniscal repair"

Quality of the evidence
Level I
- 3 randomized trials[34–36]

Level II
- 2 systematic reviews[37,38]
- 2 randomized trials with methodologic limitations[39,40]

Findings
Clinical outcome In a randomized controlled trial (RCT) of 100 patients, Bryant[35] compared the effectiveness of inside-out suturing to bioabsorbable arrows. They reported 22 failed meniscal repairs (11 in each group), with no significant difference in the failure rate between the two groups (p = 0.92). There was no significant difference in mean quality of life scores and side-to-side differences in extension and flexion measurements. They concluded that, at intermediate follow-up, there are no statistically significant differences in measured outcomes between meniscal suturing and arrows.

According to a systematic review by Lozano et al.,[38] no substantial differences in failure rate were found among various meniscus devices. No substantial differences in failure rates were found with length of follow-up. Given the paucity of RCTs comparing different all-inside meniscal repairs, no definite conclusions could be made regarding the difference in clinical outcomes of various all-inside meniscal repair devices.[37]

Recommendation

• There is currently no scientifically substantiated reason to believe that the choice of a particular repair technique would improve the outcome [overall quality: low]

Question 4: What is the overall success of meniscal transplantation?

Case clarification

After a failed meniscal repair, the patient underwent a near complete meniscectomy. Meniscal allograft transplant could be an option to avoid development of osteoarthritis at long-term follow-up.

Relevance

Unfortunately, not all the meniscal lesions are reparable, and often a complete or near complete meniscectomy is required to alleviate the patient's symptoms. A complete or near complete meniscectomy predictably results in deterioration and subsequent degenerative joint disease.

Current opinion

Meniscal transplantation offers a potential alternative to the negative consequences of a total meniscectomy.

Finding the evidence

• Cochrane Database, with search term "meniscal allograft transplantation"
• PubMed (www.ncbi.nlm.nih.gov/pubmed/) clinical queries search/ systematic reviews: "meniscal tear," "meniscal transplantation," "meniscal allograft transplantation"
• MEDLINE search identifying the population (meniscal tears, complete meniscectomy) the intervention (meniscal allograft transplantation) and the methodology (clinical trial). We used the keywords "meniscectomy," "meniscal tear" AND "meniscal allograft transplantation"

Quality of the evidence

Level II
• Randomized trials with methodologic limitations 1[42]

Level III
• 1 systematic review/meta-analysis[41]

Findings

The available literature about meniscal allograft transplantation lacks prospective RCTs. A prospective clinical study on 101 patients showed an overall failure in 11 of 39 (28%) medial allograft and 10 on 61 (16%) lateral allograft. The cumulative survival rates at 10 years were 74.2% and 69.8% for the medial and lateral allografts respectively, producing a beneficial effect in approximately 70% of the patients at 10 years. Transplantation of a viable meniscal allograft can significantly relieve pain and improve function of the knee joint.[42]

According to a systematic review by Matava,[41] a meta-analysis of clinical studies evaluating meniscal transplantation is not feasible because of a lack of randomization, the absence of control groups, and variable outcome measures in the published studies. Most studies providing outcome data show that over 60% of patients exhibit a successful result. However, the range of "successful" results varied between 12.5% and 100%. Also, the more recent series utilizing modern methods of graft insertion with attention to associated pathology have described favorable outcomes in approximately 85% of their patient cohorts.

Recommendations

• Meniscal transplantation will likely provide short- or medium-term symptomatic improvement in knee function, based on subjective as well as objective measures, at least in the short term [overall quality: low]
• The ideal patient for this procedure would appear be a young to middle-aged adult with joint line pain and limited degenerative joint disease, following a complete or near complete meniscectomy [overall quality: low]

Question 5: Is there a role for synthetic materials in meniscal reconstruction?

Case clarification

The patient refuses to undergo cadaveric allograft meniscal transplantation. After searching the internet for treatment options, he requires the surgeon to perform a synthetic meniscal reconstruction.

Relevance

Synthetic materials could have low risk of transmission of infective diseases, and solve the problems with the availability of human cadaveric allograft. However, before using such modalities, clinicians must make sure of their effectiveness for meniscal reconstruction.

Current opinion

Synthetic materials are sometimes used as meniscal transplants.

Finding the evidence

• Cochrane Database, with search terms: "meniscal scaffold," "meniscus synthetic materials," "meniscus regeneration," "meniscus substitution"
• PubMed (www.ncbi.nlm.nih.gov/pubmed/) clinical queries search/ systematic reviews: "meniscal scaffold," "meniscus synthetic materials," "meniscus regeneration," "meniscus substitution"
• MEDLINE search identifying the population (complete meniscectomy) the intervention (meniscal substitution)

and the methodology (clinical trial). We used the keywords "meniscal substitution" AND "scaffold," "synthetic materials"

Quality of the evidence
Level I
- 1 randomized trial[43]

Level IV
- 2 case series[44,45]

Findings
Rodkey et al.[43] conducted a RCT to compare a collagen meniscus implant and partial medial meniscectomy alone. This study enrolled 311 patients with an irreparable injury of the medial meniscus or a previous partial medial meniscectomy. The collagen meniscus implants had resulted in significantly increased meniscal tissue compared with that seen after the original index partial meniscectomy. Only other small case series studies are available.[44,45]

Recommendation
- There is no evidence to justify a meniscal reconstruction [overall quality: low]

Question 6: What is the best rehabilitation after arthroscopic meniscectomy?

Case clarification
After undergoing arthroscopic partial meniscectomy, the patient asks for indications about the best way to recover knee function and muscle strength in the operated leg.

Relevance
An appropriate rehabilitation program is a key point for the overall success of surgery.

Current opinion
Home exercise under surgeon's indications is a satisfactory rehabilitation program to obtain the best recovery after arthroscopic partial meniscectomy.

Finding the evidence
- Cochrane Database, with search terms: "meniscal tear," "knee arthroscopy," "rehabilitation," "physiotherapy," "physical therapy"
- PubMed (www.ncbi.nlm.nih.gov/pubmed/) clinical queries search/ systematic reviews: "meniscus rehabilitation," "meniscus physiotherapy," "meniscus physical therapy"
- PubMed (www.ncbi.nlm.nih.gov/pubmed/): sensitivity search using keywords "meniscal tears" AND "rehabilitation" or "physiotherapy" or "physical therapy". as well as "knee arthroscopy" AND "rehabilitation" or "physiotherapy" or "physical therapy"

- MEDLINE search identifying the population (meniscal tears) the intervention (rehabilitation, physiotherapy, physical therapy) and the methodology (clinical trial). We used the keywords "meniscal tear," "knee arthroscopy" AND "rehabilitation," "physiotherapy," "physical therapy"

Quality of the evidence
Level I
- 9 RCTs[46–54]

Findings
Supervised physical therapy vs. home program Four randomized trials (n = 165)[48–50,52] compared supervised physical therapy and home programs. Goodwin[50] reported the results in 84 patients, indicating that the supervised physical therapy used in the study was not beneficial for patients in the early period after uncomplicated arthroscopic partial meniscectomy. In a prospective randomized study, Jokl[52] compared 30 patients assigned to a home exercise program or supervised physical therapy after arthroscopic partial medial meniscectomy. Evaluation was performed 2, 4, and 8 weeks after surgery. The two groups showed no statistically significant differences in strength at any evaluation time, and similar results were reported with regard to the patient's subjective evaluations of knee function and ability to resume usual activities. Nevertheless, in an RCT on 20 patients, Vervest[49] concludes that the physical therapy under the supervision of a physiotherapist led to high patient satisfaction and good functional rehabilitation after partial arthroscopic meniscectomy with regard to SARS score, hop test, and distance jumps. In another RCT on 31 patients, Moffet[48] compared supervised physical therapy plus home exercises to home exercises alone. Patients in the supervised physical therapy group had better recovery of the knee extensor strength than patients allocated to the home exercises group, highlighting the importance of an early intensive and supervised rehabilitation program.

NSAIDs Two RCTs (n = 207)[46,47] compared the use of nonsteroidal anti-inflammatory drugs (NSAIDs) in the postoperative period to no treatment (or placebo). In an RCT on 139 patients, Ogilvie-Harris[46] concluded that patients undergoing NSAID therapy after arthroscopic partial meniscectomy had significantly less pain, less synovitis, and less effusion. They had significantly more rapid return of movement and of quadriceps function, with a faster return to work and sport. In contrast, a randomized study by Birch[47] on 68 patients indicates no significant benefits from postoperative administration of diclofenac sodium compared with the control group. Complications attributable to the anti-inflammatory drug occurred in 9.6% of the patients, advising against the routine administration of NSAIDs after arthroscopy of the knee.

Electrical stimulation In an RCT on 21 patients, Williams[53] compared electrical stimulation and exercise to exercise alone in increasing quadriceps strength after arthroscopic meniscectomy. Twenty-one postmenisectomy patients were randomly assigned to one of the two groups. Electrical stimulation combined with a regular program of quadriceps exercise produces a significant beneficial effect in strengthening the quadriceps at four different contraction speeds. Jensen[54] performed a prospective study of the use of transcutaneous neural stimulation (TNS) in 90 arthroscopic knee surgery patients to determine whether TNS is as effective as traditional pain medication in postoperative knee pain, and whether patients that had received TNS regain preoperative motion and strength quicker than the control population. The use of a TNS unit is an effective adjunct in decreasing postoperative pain in 93% of patients. The TNS group regained isokinetic power in flexion and extension, range of motion, and leg volume sooner than the control group.

Recommendations

- There is no evidence to recommend supervised physical therapy vs. home program [overall quality: low]
- There is no evidence to prescribe NSAIDs postoperatively [overall quality: low]
- Electrical stimulation combined with a regular program of quadriceps exercise can have a significant effect in strengthening the quadriceps [overall quality: low]

Summary of recommendations

- The most sensitive clinical diagnostic test for meniscal tears is joint line tenderness at 76%
- The McMurray and Apley tests could be considered high specificity but low sensitivity tests
- The Thessaly test in isolation was not useful for the detection of meniscal tears but it helps to increase diagnostic certainty when combined with other standard tests
- MRI is preferable to diagnostic arthroscopy in most patients because it avoids the surgical risks of arthroscopy with high accuracy in diagnosing meniscal and ACL tears
- There is currently no scientifically substantiated reason to believe that the choice of a particular repair technique would improve the outcome
- Meniscal transplantation will likely provide short- or medium-term symptomatic improvement in knee function, based on subjective as well as objective measures, at least in the short term
- The ideal patient for this procedure would appear be a young to middle-aged adult with joint line pain and limited arthrosis, following a complete or near complete meniscectomy
- There is no evidence to justify a meniscal reconstruction

- There is no evidence to recommend supervised physical therapy vs. home program
- There is no evidence to prescribe NSAIDs postoperatively
- Electrical stimulation combined with a regular program of quadriceps exercise can have a significant effect in strengthening the quadriceps

---

Conclusions

Even though meniscal tears are frequent, and are responsible for high healthcare costs, the quality of the available studies is generally low, and, given methodologic limitations, pooling of data is almost always impossible. There is an urgent need for large, well-conducted RCTs to improve the science around meniscal injuries.

References

1. Maffulli N, Longo UG, Campi S, Denaro V. Meniscal tears. Open Access J Sports Med 2010;1:45–54.
2. Binfield PM, Maffulli N, King JB. Patterns of meniscal tears associated with anterior cruciate ligament lesions in athletes. Injury 1993;24(8):557–61.
3. Maffulli N, Chan KM, Bundoc RC, Cheng JC. Knee arthroscopy in Chinese children and adolescents: an eight-year prospective study. Arthroscopy 1997;13(1):18–23.
4. Metcalf RW, Burks RT, Metcalf MS, McGinty JB. Arthroscopic meniscectomy. In: McGinty JB, Caspari RB, Jackson RW, Poehling GG, eds, Operative Arthroscopy, 2nd edn, pp 263–97. Lippincott-Raven, Philadelphia, PA, 1996.
5. Greis PE, Bardana DD, Holmstrom MC, Burks RT. Meniscal injury: I. Basic science and evaluation. J Am Acad Orthop Surg 2002;10(3):168–76.
6. Hede A, Jensen DB, Blyme P, Sonne-Holm S. Epidemiology of meniscal lesions in the knee. 1,215 open operations in Copenhagen 1982–84. Acta Orthop Scand 1990;61(5):435–7.
7. Nielsen AB, Yde J. Epidemiology of acute knee injuries: a prospective hospital investigation. J Trauma 1991;31(12):1644–8.
8. Poehling GG, Ruch DS, Chabon SJ. The landscape of meniscal injuries. Clin Sports Med 1990;9(3):539–49.
9. Hegedus EJ, Cook C, Hasselblad V, Goode A, McCrory DC. Physical examination tests for assessing a torn meniscus in the knee: a systematic review with meta-analysis. J Orthop Sports Phys Ther 2007;37(9):541–50.
10. Scholten RJ, Deville WL, Opstelten W, Bijl D, van der Plas CG, Bouter LM. The accuracy of physical diagnostic tests for assessing meniscal lesions of the knee: a meta-analysis. J Fam Pract 2001;50(11):938–44.
11. Meserve BB, Cleland JA, Boucher TR. A meta-analysis examining clinical test utilities for assessing meniscal injury. Clin Rehabil 2008;22(2):143–61.
12. Ockert B, Haasters F, Polzer H, Grote S, Kessler MA, Mutschler W, Kanz KG. [Value of the clinical examination in suspected

meniscal injuries: A meta-analysis.]. Unfallchirurg 2010;113: 293–9.

13. Oei EH, Nikken JJ, Verstijnen AC, Ginai AZ, Myriam Hunink MG. MR imaging of the menisci and cruciate ligaments: a systematic review. Radiology 2003;226(3):837–48.

14. Manzotti A, Baiguini P, Locatelli A. Statistical evaluation of McMurray's test in the clinical diagnosis of meniscus injuries. J Sports Traumatol Relat Res 1997;19:83–9.

15. Evans PJ, Bell GD, Frank C. Prospective evaluation of the McMurray test. Am J Sports Med 1993;21(4):604–8.

16. Fowler PJ, Lubliner JA. The predictive value of five clinical signs in the evaluation of meniscal pathology. Arthroscopy 1989; 5(3):184–6.

17. Karachalios T, Hantes M, Zibis AH, Zachos V, Karantanas AH, Malizos KN. Diagnostic accuracy of a new clinical test (the Thessaly test) for early detection of meniscal tears. J Bone Joint Surg Am 2005;87(5):955–62.

18. Ryzewicz M, Peterson B, Siparsky PN, Bartz RL. The diagnosis of meniscus tears: the role of MRI and clinical examination. Clin Orthop Relat Res 2007;455:123–33.

19. Konan S, Rayan F, Haddad FS. Do physical diagnostic tests accurately detect meniscal tears? Knee Surg Sports Traumatol Arthrosc 2009;17(7):806–11.

20. Crawford R, Walley G, Bridgman S, Maffulli N. Magnetic resonance imaging versus arthroscopy in the diagnosis of knee pathology, concentrating on meniscal lesions and ACL tears: a systematic review. Br Med Bull 2007;84:5–23.

21. Winters K, Tregonning R. Reliability of magnetic resonance imaging of the traumatic knee as determined by arthroscopy. N Z Med J 2005;118(1209):U1301.

22. Cotten A, Delfaut E, Demondion X, et al. MR imaging of the knee at 0.2 and 1.5 T: correlation with surgery. AJR Am J Roentgenol 2000;174(4):1093–7.

23. Rappeport ED, Wieslander SB, Stephensen S, Lausten GS, Thomsen HS. MRI preferable to diagnostic arthroscopy in knee joint injuries. A double-blind comparison of 47 patients. Acta Orthop Scand 1997;68(3):277–81.

24. Franklin PD, Lemon RA, Barden HS. Accuracy of imaging the menisci on an in-office, dedicated, magnetic resonance imaging extremity system. Am J Sports Med 1997;25(3):382–8.

25. Bui-Mansfield LT, Youngberg RA, Warme W, Pitcher JD, Nguyen PL. Potential cost savings of MR imaging obtained before arthroscopy of the knee: evaluation of 50 consecutive patients. AJR Am J Roentgenol 1997;168(4):913–18.

26. Lundberg M, Odensten M, Thuomas KA, Messner K. The diagnostic validity of magnetic resonance imaging in acute knee injuries with hemarthrosis. A single-blinded evaluation in 69 patients using high-field MRI before arthroscopy. Int J Sports Med 1996;17(3):218–22.

27. Justice WW, Quinn SF. Error patterns in the MR imaging evaluation of menisci of the knee. Radiology 1995;196(3):617–21.

28. LaPrade RF, Burnett QM, 2nd, Veenstra MA, Hodgman CG. The prevalence of abnormal magnetic resonance imaging findings in asymptomatic knees. With correlation of magnetic resonance imaging to arthroscopic findings in symptomatic knees. Am J Sports Med 1994;22(6):739–45.

29. Kinnunen J, Bondestam S, Kivioja A, et al. Diagnostic performance of low field MRI in acute knee injuries. Magn Reson Imaging 1994;12(8):1155–60.

30. Heron CW, Calvert PT. Three-dimensional gradient-echo MR imaging of the knee: comparison with arthroscopy in 100 patients. Radiology 1992;183(3):839–44.

31. Grevitt MP, Pool CJ, Bodley RN, Savage PE. Magnetic resonance imaging of the knee: initial experience in a district general hospital. Injury 1992;23(6):410–12.

32. Gluckert K, Kladny B, Blank-Schal A, Hofmann G. MRI of the knee joint with a 3-D gradient echo sequence. Equivalent to diagnostic arthroscopy? Arch Orthop Trauma Surg 1992;112(1): 5–14.

33. Riel KA, Reinisch M, Kersting-Sommerhoff B, Hof N, Merl T. 0.2-Tesla magnetic resonance imaging of internal lesions of the knee joint: a prospective arthroscopically controlled clinical study. Knee Surg Sports Traumatol Arthrosc 1999;7(1):37–41.

34. Albrecht-Olsen P, Kristensen G, Burgaard P, Joergensen U, Toerholm C. The arrow versus horizontal suture in arthroscopic meniscus repair. A prospective randomized study with arthroscopic evaluation. Knee Surg Sports Traumatol Arthrosc 1999; 7(5):268–73.

35. Bryant D, Dill J, Litchfield R, Amendola A, Giffin R, Fowler P, Kirkley A. Effectiveness of bioabsorbable arrows compared with inside-out suturing for vertical, reparable meniscal lesions: a randomized clinical trial. Am J Sports Med 2007;35(6): 889–96.

36. Spindler KP, McCarty EC, Warren TA, Devin C, Connor JT. Prospective comparison of arthroscopic medial meniscal repair technique: inside-out suture versus entirely arthroscopic arrows. Am J Sports Med 2003;31(6):929–34.

37. Starke C, Kopf S, Petersen W, Becker R. Meniscal repair. Arthroscopy 2009;25(9):1033–44.

38. Lozano J, Ma CB, Cannon WD. All-inside meniscus repair: a systematic review. Clin Orthop Relat Res 2007;455:134–41.

39. Barber FA, Johnson DH, Halbrecht JL. Arthroscopic meniscal repair using the BioStinger. Arthroscopy 2005;21(6):744–50.

40. Choi NH, Kim TH, Victoroff BN. Comparison of arthroscopic medial meniscal suture repair techniques: inside-out versus all-inside repair. Am J Sports Med 2009;37(11):2144–50.

41. Matava MJ. Meniscal allograft transplantation: a systematic review. Clin Orthop Relat Res 2007;455:142–57.

42. Verdonk PC, Demurie A, Almqvist KF, Veys EM, Verbruggen G, Verdonk R. Transplantation of viable meniscal allograft. Survivorship analysis and clinical outcome of one hundred cases. J Bone Joint Surg Am 2005;87(4):715–24.

43. Rodkey WG, DeHaven KE, Montgomery WH, 3rd, et al. Comparison of the collagen meniscus implant with partial meniscectomy. A prospective randomized trial. J Bone Joint Surg Am 2008;90(7):1413–26.

44. Steadman JR, Rodkey WG. Tissue-engineered collagen meniscus implants: 5- to 6-year feasibility study results. Arthroscopy 2005;21(5):515–25.

45. Rodkey WG, Steadman JR, Li ST. A clinical study of collagen meniscus implants to restore the injured meniscus. Clinical Orthop Relat Res 1999; 367(Suppl):S281–292.

46. Ogilvie-Harris DJ, Bauer M, Corey P. Prostaglandin inhibition and the rate of recovery after arthroscopic meniscectomy. A randomised double-blind prospective study. J Bone Joint Surg Br 1985;67(4):567–71.

47. Birch NC, Sly C, Brooks S, Powles DP. Anti-inflammatory drug therapy after arthroscopy of the knee. A prospective, ran-

domised, controlled trial of diclofenac or physiotherapy. J Bone Joint Surg Br 1993;75(4):650–2.

48. Moffet H, Richards CL, Malouin F, Bravo G, Paradis G. Early and intensive physiotherapy accelerates recovery postarthroscopic meniscectomy: results of a randomized controlled study. Arch Phys Med Rehabil 1994;75(4):415–26.

49. Vervest AM, Maurer CA, Schambergen TG, de Bie RA, Bulstra SK. Effectiveness of physiotherapy after meniscectomy. Knee Surg Sports Traumatol Arthrosc 1999; 7(6):360–4.

50. Goodwin PC, Morrissey MC, Omar RZ, Brown M, Southall K, McAuliffe TB. Effectiveness of supervised physical therapy in the early period after arthroscopic partial meniscectomy. Phys Ther 2003;83(6):520–35.

51. St-Pierre DM. Rehabilitation following arthroscopic meniscectomy. Sports Med 1995;20(5):338–47.

52. Jokl P, Stull PA, Lynch JK, Vaughan V. Independent home versus supervised rehabilitation following arthroscopic knee surgery—a prospective randomized trial. Arthroscopy 1989;5(4):298–305.

53. Williams RA, Morrissey MC, Brewster CE. The effect of electrical stimulation on quadriceps strength and thigh circumference in menisectomy patients. J Orthop Sports Phys Ther 1986;8(3): 143–6.

54. Jensen JE, Conn RR, Hazelrigg G, Hewett JE. The use of transcutaneous neural stimulation and isokinetic testing in arthroscopic knee surgery. Am J Sports Med 1985;13(1):27–33.

95 Anterior Cruciate Ligament Injury

Verena M. Schreiber[1], Kenneth D. Illingworth[1], Hector A. Mejia[2], and Freddie H. Fu[1]

[1]University of Pittsburgh Medical Center, Pittsburgh, PA, USA
[2]Florida State University Medical School, Tallahassee, FL, USA

Case scenario

A 20 year old college student presents to the office complaining of right knee pain and instability after sustaining an injury while playing soccer 1 month ago. The patient describes how he planted his foot on the turf and sustained a twisting injury.

Relevant anatomy

The anterior cruciate ligament (ACL) is made up of the anteromedial (AM) and the posterolateral (PL) bundles, which are named for the orientation of their tibial insertion. In addition, two osseous structures can be found on the femoral side that delineate the location of the AM and PL bundles: the lateral intercondylar ridge and the lateral bifurcate ridge.[1-3]

Importance of the problem

Rupture of the ACL is one of the most frequent types of knee injuries, with a yearly incidence of 35 out of 100,000 people.[4] Its predominant occurrence is during sports activities, which can put extreme forces on the ACL.[5] Although recent studies have called into question the benefit of surgical management vs. conservative treatment for ACL injuries,[6] reconstruction of the ACL continues to be one of the most often performed orthopedic operations in the United States, with approximately 105,000 procedures performed each year, and can be performed with either single- or double-bundle reconstructions.

Top five questions

1. How accurate is the clinical examination in the diagnosis of ACL injury?
2. Which procedure provides the patient with the best clinical outcome, single- or double-bundle ACL reconstruction?
3. What is the better graft choice in ACL reconstruction, autograft vs. allograft?
4. Which autograft provides the better outcome, patellar tendon vs. hamstring tendons?
5. What influence does ACL rupture/ACL reconstruction have on the development of knee osteoarthritis?

Question 1: How accurate is the clinical examination in the diagnosis of ACL injury?

Case clarification

During the clinical exam, a Lachman and anterior drawer test of the patient shows signs of pathological laxity. The pivot shift test is inconclusive due to guarding by the patient. KT-1000 shows a side-to-side difference of 5 mm. No medial or lateral joint line tenderness or opening on varus and valgus stress can be appreciated. Posterior drawer test is negative.

Relevance

Often the knee clinical examination is the only method used to make the diagnosis of an ACL rupture and therefore the validity of these tests is of importance.

Current opinion

The diagnosis of ACL rupture by clinical examination is thought of as a reliable method; however secondary

Evidence-Based Orthopedics, First Edition. Edited by Mohit Bhandari.
© 2012 Blackwell Publishing Ltd. Published 2012 by Blackwell Publishing Ltd.

methods of diagnosis, such as MRI, continue to be commonplace.

Finding the evidence

• Cochrane Database of systematic reviews, search term: "(anterior cruciate ligament*) AND (injury*)"
• PubMed (www.ncbi.nlm.nih.gov/pubmed/) clinical queries search/ systematic reviews with search term: "(anterior cruciate ligament*) AND (injury*)"
• PubMed (www.ncbi.nlm.nih.gov/pubmed/) advanced search with meta-analysis, randomized clinical trial, and review: search terms "(anterior cruciate ligament*) AND (injury*)"
• PubMed (www.ncbi.nlm.nih.gov/pubmed/): search terms "(anterior cruciate ligament*) AND (injury*) AND (treatment*) OR (*outcome)

Articles that were not in the English language were excluded. Data from abstracts and book chapters were not included.

Quality of the evidence

Level I
• 3 systematic reviews/meta-analyses
• 1 randomized controlled trial (RCT)

Level II
• 8 prospective cohort studies
• 3 retrospective cohort studies
• 1 exploratory cohort study

Findings

Three systematic reviews/meta-analyses evaluated 53 studies in total, and all three of them concluded that the Lachman test seemed to be most accurate in diagnosing ACL tears in the clinical setting.[7–9]

Twelve level II cohort studies could be identified that matched the search criteria:[10–21] 6 studies (n = 355) provided data on the Lachman test preoperatively. The Lachman test was able to diagnose an ACL tear in 296 cases (sensitivity 83.3%, 95% CI 0.79–0.87). Six studies (n = 355) evaluated the use of the pivot shift test for the diagnosis of ACL tears and it was positive in 176 cases (sensitivity 49.4%, CI 0.34–0.55).The KT-1000 was evaluated in 5 studies (n = 352, Table 95.1). In addition, 5 studies also used the anterior drawer test when examining the ACL (n = 310). A positive anterior drawer test could be found in 177 cases (sensitivity 57.1%. CI 0.51–0.63).

Recommendation

• In comparison to arthroscopy as gold standard for diagnosing ACL tears, the Lachman test has been shown to be the most accurate of all the diagnostic clinical examinations [overall quality: moderate].

Question 2: Which procedure provides the patient with the best clinical outcome, single- or double-bundle ACL reconstruction?

Case clarification

As previously mentioned, the patient is a 20 year old college student who plays competitive soccer. The MRI shows a complete rupture of the ACL. The patient tells you that he would like to continue playing competitive sports after surgery.

Relevance

Single-bundle reconstruction is the traditional way of reconstructing the ACL. Double-bundle reconstruction has gained increased interest as it is theorized to more closely restore the native anatomy of the ACL.

Current opinion

Current opinion suggests that a double-bundle reconstruction better restores the native knee kinematics when compared to a traditional single-bundle reconstruction.

Finding the evidence

See Question 1.

Quality of the evidence

Level I
• 5 RCTs

Level II
• 5 cohort studies

Findings

Five RCTs and five level II cohort studies compared single- vs. double-bundle reconstruction by evaluating knee laxity exams, KT-1000 and, common knee score, i.e., International Knee Documentation Committee (IKDC) (Table 95.1).

Recommendations

• Double-bundle ACL reconstruction seems to restore rotation and laxity better than single-bundle ACL reconstruction [overall quality: moderate]
• Subjective knee scores seem to be overall equal for both reconstruction techniques [overall quality: moderate]

Question 3: Which is the better graft choice in ACL reconstruction, autograft vs. allograft?

Case clarification

The patient wishes to continue playing collegiate-level soccer and thus would like to proceed with an anterior cruciate ligament reconstruction. You present him with two options for choice of graft: allograft or autograft.

Table 95.1 Single-bundle vs. double-bundle RCTs

	N	Level of evidence	Treatment	Outcome SB vs. DB knee scores	Outcome SB vs. DB laxity test
Muneta et al.[31]	68	1	34 single 34 double	No significant difference between SB and DB for IKDC	KT-1000 SB: 2.4 ± 1.4 DB: 1.4 ± 1.4 Normal Pivot shift SB: 29/34 DB: 20/34
Jarvela[32]	65	1	30 single 35 double	No significant difference between SB and DB for IKDC	Normal Pivot shift SB: 16/25 DB: 29/30 (p = 0.002)
Siebold et al.[33]	70	1	35 single 35 double	Subj. IKDC SB: 90P DB: 88P Obj. IKDC SB: 24% A DB: 78% A	KT-1000 SB: 1.6 mm DB. 1.0 mm Normal Pivot shift SB: 71% DB: 97% (p = 0.01)
Streich et al.[34]	50	1	25 single 24 double	No significant difference between SB and DB for IKDC	KT-1000 SB: 0.94 ± 1.76, DB: 1.10 ± 1.57 (p = 0.839) Normal Pivot shift SB: 19/25 DB: 23/24
Aglietti et al.[35]	70	1	35 single 35 double	IKDC 2 Year F/U SB: 78 ± 13 DB: 83 ± 15 (Ns)	KT-1000 SB: 0.94 ± 1.76, DB: 1.10 ± 1.57 (p = 0.839) Normal Pivot shift SB: 19/25 DB: 23/24
Kanaya et al.[36]	26	1	18 single 15 double		AP displacement at 30° SB 3 mm DB 2 mm (NS)

Table 95.1 (*Continued*)

	N	Level of evidence	Treatment	Outcome SB vs. DB knee scores	Outcome SB vs. DB laxity test
Sastre et al.[37]	40	1	20 single 20 double	IKDC 2 Year F/U SB: 81 DB: 80 (NS)	
Kondo et al.[38]	328	2	157 single 171 double	No significant difference for SB and DB for IKDC	Anterior Laxity SB: 2.5 mm DB: 1.2 mm
Seon et al.[39]	40	2	20 single 20 double		Anterior laxity SB: 6.1 ± 1.2 DB: 5.1 ± 1.5 (p = 0.02) Rotation SB: 29.5 ± 3.8 DB: 23.3 ± 4.0 (p < 0.001)
Park et al.[40]	113	2	50 single 63 double	No significant difference for SB and DB for IKDC	No significant difference for DB and SB for KT-1000 and pivot shift
Tsuda et al.[41]	144	2	62 single 82 double	No significant difference for SB and DB for IKDC	No significant difference for DB and SB for KT-1000 and pivot shift
Hofbauer et al.[42]	55	2	27 single 28 double	IKDC SB: 91 (±11.3) DB: 95 (±4.8) (p = 0.034) Lysholm SB: 95 (±8.0) DB: 98 (±3.0) (p = 0.046)	Rotation SB: 20.3 (±0.2) DB: 12.3 (±0.3) (p = 0.029)
Sadoghi et al.[43]	92	2	41 single 51 double	No significant difference for SB and DB for IKDC	Equal pivot shift SB: 49% DB: 84% (p < 0.001)

DB, double bundle; IKDC, International Knee Documentation Committee; n, number of patients evaluated on particular outcome; SB, single bundle.

Relevance

The choice of graft can have important implications for outcome and function after ACL reconstruction. Both allograft and autograft have their respective advantages and disadvantages, which need to be discussed with the patient.

Current opinion

Current opinion suggests that the majority of surgeons choose autograft in ACL reconstruction for young active patients.

Finding the evidence

See Question 1.

Quality of the evidence

Level I

• 1 systematic review/meta-analysis

Level II

• 6 prospective cohort studies

Findings

One systematic review met the search criteria for a level I systematic review.[22] No statistical significant difference between allograft and autograft could be found in the majority of outcome measures (Table 95.2).

Six prospective cohort studies could be identified.[23–28] Five studies evaluated the outcome of allograft vs. autograft reconstruction with respect to long-term follow-up (Table 95.3). Another study by Greenberg et al. (n = 861) looked at the infection rate of allograft vs. autograft and could not show a significant difference in the rate of superficial infec-

tions between allograft and autograft (95% CI allograft group 0–0.57% and autograft group 0–1.66%).

Recommendation

• Graft choice does not appear to play a major role with respect to long-term outcome and infection in ACL reconstruction [overall quality: moderate]

Question 4: Which autograft provides the better outcome, patellar tendon vs. hamstring tendons?

Case clarification

If the patient decides to proceed with autograft ACL reconstruction, the two most commonly used tendons are the patellar tendon and the hamstring tendon.

Relevance

It is important to have options for the patient regarding graft choice and therefore both patellar tendon and hamstring tendon should be discussed with the patient.

Current opinion

Current opinion suggests that outcomes after patellar tendon and hamstring tendons are equivocal.

Finding the evidence

See Question 1.

Quality of the evidence

Level I

• 6 systematic reviews/meta-analyses

Table 95.2 Allograft vs. autograft systematic review functional outcome[22]

	N	Autograft	Allograft	p value
Lysholm mean	17	n = 1087	n = 137	>0.5 (Ns)
		92.4 ± 0.3	92.5 ± 0.5	
Failure rate	28	n = 2083	n = 137	>0.1 (Ns)
		4.5 ± 0.4/100 cases	8.3 ± 2.3/100 cases	
Abnormal pivot shift	19	n = 1271	n = 66	>0.1 (Ns)
		2.7% ± 0.5%	5.0% ± 2.7%	
KT-1000	21	n = 1768	n = 112	<0.02
		1.8 ± 0.1 mm	1.4 ± 0.2 mm	
Complication rate	27	n = 1793	n = 137	>0.1 (Ns)
		4.5 ± 0.5/100 cases	5.3 ± 2.1/100 cases	
IKDC = A rate	18	n = 1482	n = 82	<0.2
		28.2% ± 1.0%	43.9% ± 5.5%	

IKDC, International Knee Documentation Committee; N, number of studies reporting on particular outcome; n, number of patients evaluated on particular outcome; NS, not significant.

Table 95.3 Allograft vs. autograft prospective cohort studies

	Peterson et al.[23]	Kleipool et al.[24]	Sun et al.[25]	Edgar et al.[26]	Poehling et al.[27]
N	60	62	172	84	159
N allograft vs. autograft	30 vs. 30	36 vs. 26	86 vs. 86	47 vs. 37	41 vs. 118
Level of evidence	II	II	II	II	II
Mean length of F/U	63 months	46 months	5.6 years	52 months autograft 48 months allograft	4.2 years
Lachman					
Autograft	20 <3 mm	17 <3 mm	62 <3 mm	Not evaluated	64% <3 mm
Allograft	22 <3 mm	21 <3 mm	65 <3 mm		68.1% <3 mm
Pivot shift					
Autograft	27 normal	19 normal	71 normal		91.7% normal
Allograft	25 normal	28 normal	74 normal	Not evaluated	91% normal
Lysholm score					
Autograft	88.6	95	90	91.0	Not evaluated
Allograft	90.0	94	91	92.7	
Tegener score					
Autograft	6.1	6	7.8	6.8	Not evaluated
Allograft	5.4	5	7.6	6.9	
IKDC					
Autograft	Not evaluated	7 = A	27 = A	12 = A	At 2 year F/U 11 = A
Allograft		17 = A	30 = A	29 = A	33 = A
KT-1000					
Autograft	28 <5 mm translation	18 <3 mm translation	65 <3 mm	40 <3 mm	Anterior mean across time: 3 mm
Allograft	30 <5 mm translation	27 <3 mm translation	67 <3 mm	32 <3 mm	2.8 mm

F/U, follow-up; IKDC, International Knee Documentation Committee, N, number of patients evaluated on particular outcome.

Level II

• 1 systematic review

Findings

Six systematic reviews evaluated patellar tendon vs. hamstring tendon (Table 95.4). Two studies reported a significant increase in graft failure, anterior knee laxity, and increased pivot shift with hamstring tendon compared to patellar tendon.[28,29] A study by Poolman et al.[30] investigated the overlap of systematic reviews of ACL reconstruction comparing hamstring autograft with bone–patellar tendon–bone (BPTB) autograft to evaluate reviewed systematic reviews of ACL reconstruction in order to assess quality of reporting and internal validity. The authors came to the conclusion that hamstring autografts have better outcome regarding anterior knee pain when evaluating the best evidence. However, they also advise that these reviews can only be applied as a guide for clinical decision-making or policy-making if each review is looked upon critically with respect to its methodological quality.

Table 95.4 Subjective and objective outcome measures

Systematic review	Group	Graft failure	Anterior knee laxity	Anterior drawer	Lachman	Pivot shift	IKDC
Reinhardt et al.[44]	PT vs. HT	Increase with HT (p = 0.02)	Increase absolute laxity in HT group 3/5 studies (p < 0.05)	—	—	—	Higher score in 1/5 studies favoring PT (p = 0.02)
Samuelsson et al.[45]	PT vs. HT	—	NS	NS	NS	NS	NS
Biau et al.[29]	PT vs. HT	—	—	—	NS (p = 0.93)	Decrease Pivot shift in PT (p = 0.016)	—
Goldblatt et al.[46]	PT vs. HT	—	NS (p = 0.84)	—	NS (p = 0.22)	NS (p = 0.83)	—
Forster et al.[47]	PT vs. HT	NS	—	—	NS	NS (p = 0.12)	NS
Spindler et al.[48]	PT vs. HT	NS	NS	—	—	—	—

DB, double bundle; HT, hamstring tendon; IKDC, International Knee Documentation Committee; NS, not significant; PT, patellar tendon; SB, single bundle.

Recommendation
• Based on the following outcome measures (graft failure, anterior knee laxity, anterior drawer, Lachman, pivot shift, IKDC) no overall significant difference could be found between patellar tendon and hamstring tendon [overall quality: moderate]

Question 5: What influence does ACL rupture/ACL reconstruction have on the development of knee osteoarthritis?

Case clarification
There are two main goals after ACL reconstruction for the patient: the short-term goal of restoration of knee stability and return to athletic activity and the restoration of normal knee kinematics in order to prevent osteoarthritis (OA) and promote long-term knee health.

Relevance
The development of knee OA in both ACL reconstruction and ACL-deficient patients has been documented in the literature.

Current opinion
Current opinion suggests that there is an accelerated progression of OA after traditional single-bundle ACL reconstruction. The goal of long-term knee health following ACL injury should be the restoration of normal knee kinematics; which is hypothesized to be the biggest determining factor in prevention of OA progression.

Finding the evidence
See Question 1.

Quality of the evidence
Level I
• 5 systematic reviews/meta-analyses
• 4 RCTs

Level II
• 3 prospective cohort studies

Findings
The natural history of an isolated ACL-deficient knee shows development of OA in 0–16% of patients. Without taking into account graft choice, the development of OA after ACL reconstruction is 16–70% at 5–15 years. The literature showed an increase in OA in BPTB autografts when compared with hamstring tendon autografts (Tables 95.5 and 95.6)

Recommendations
• Current ACL reconstruction techniques lead to an accelerated progression of OA [overall quality: moderate]
• Concomitant meniscus injury leads to an accelerated progression of OA [overall quality: high]

Summary of recommendations

In the treatment of ACL injury, there is moderate or high evidence to support the following recommendations:
• Of the clinical examinations, the Lachman test has been shown to be the most accurate test to diagnose ACL tears in the clinic setting
• Double-bundle ACL reconstruction better restores rotation and anterior laxity. Overall, there is no difference in

Table 95.5 Systematic reviews on development of knee osteoarthritis after ACL injury/reconstruction

Systematic review	Result
Samuelson et al.[45]	BPTB vs. OA—possible correlation between BPTB and OA
Risberg[49]	Isolated ACL tear—OA prevalence (0–13%) ACL tear plus meniscus injury—OA prevalence (21–48%)
Andersson[50]	Isolated ACL tear—OA prevalence 50% ACL tear plus meniscus injury—increased risk of OA
Lewis[51]	SB ACL-R—tricompartmental disease at 5 years
Roos[52]	All ACL reconstructions—10–20 yr s/p ACL recon 50% prevalence OA

ACL, anterior cruciate ligament; ACL-R, ACL reconstruction; BPTP, bone–patellar tendon–bone; OA, osteoarthritis; SB, single bundle; s/p, status post.

subjective knee scores for single- and double-bundle reconstruction
• Successful long-term outcome in ACL reconstruction does not depend on the graft source
• No significant difference in outcome measures exists between hamstring tendon and patellar tendon in ACL reconstruction. Patellar tendon may decrease anterior knee laxity and pivot shift tests, but this is not clinically significant
• The currently studied ACL reconstruction techniques lead to an increased progression of knee OA, with concominant meniscal injuries leading to an even greater increase in progression

Conclusions

Numerous reports on the diagnosis, treatment and outcome of ACL tears have been published. However, only few recommendations for the management of ACL tears are supported by high-level evidence.

Table 95.6 Studies on development of knee osteoarthritis after ACL injury/reconstruction

Study	Design	Group(s)	OA classification	Results
Ahlden et al.[53]	RCT	BPTB vs. HT autografts	Ahlbäck and Fairbank rating system	Ahlbäck rating system 7 yr 16% OA (BPTB 19%; ST 13%; n.s.) Fairbank rating system 7 yr 68% OA (BPTB 67%; ST 70%; n.s.)
Sajovic et al.[54]	RCT	BPTB vs. HT autografts	IKDC	Grade B OA 50% BPTB, 17% grade B OA in HT (p = 0.012). 5 yr
Holm et al.[55]	RCT	BPTB vs. HT autografts	Kellgren and Lawrence grading system	2 or more OA 55% HT with contralateral knee 28%, 64% BPTB with contralateral knee 22% (p = 0.27) between reconstructed knee, (p = 0.62) between contralateral knees
Sun et al.[25]	PCS	Allograft vs. autograft	Kellgren classification	p < 0.05 prevalence OA both groups, p > 0.05 between groups 5.6 yr
Meunier et al.[56]	RCT	Primary repair vs. nonsurgical treatment	Ahlbäck and Fairbank rating system	p < 0.05 OA between groups, with menisectomy 2/3 OA. 10 yr
Neuman et al.[57]	PCS	ACL injury	Atlas of the Osteoarthritis Research Society International	16% prevalence PF OA. Increased PF OA with meniscal injury (p = 0.004) and ACL reconstruction (22 of 94 patients) (p = 0.002) at 15 yr
Neuman et al.[58]	PCS	ACL injury nonoperative treatment	Atlas of the Osteoarthritis Research Society International	35% received menisectomy of which 46% had OA. 0% of no menisectomy group had OA p < 0.0001

ACL, anterior cruciate ligament; BPTP, bone–patellar tendon–bone; IKDC, International Knee Documentation Committee; n.s., not significant; OA, osteoarthritis; PCS, prospective cohort study; PF, patellofemoral; RCT, randomized controlled trial; s/p, status post; SB, single bundle.

The authors did not receive any outside funding or grants in support of their research for or preparation of this work. They did not receive payments or other benefits from a commercial entity. No commercial entity paid or directed any benefits to any research or clinical organization with which the authors are affiliated or associated. The aforementioned also applies to the authors' immediate families.

References

1. Ferretti M, Ekdahl M, Shen W, et al. Osseous landmarks of the femoral attachment of the anterior cruciate ligament: an anatomic study. Arthroscopy 2007;23:1218–25.

2. Purnell ML, Larson AI, Clancy W. Anterior cruciate ligament insertions on the tibia and femur and their relationships to critical bony landmarks using high-resolution volume-rendering computed tomography. Am J Sports Med 2008;36:2083–90.

3. Fu FH, Jordan SS. The lateral intercondylar ridge—a key to anatomic anterior cruciate ligament reconstruction. J Bone Joint Surg Am 2007;89:2103–4.

4. Gianotti SM, Marshall SW, Hume PA, et al. Incidence of anterior cruciate ligament injury and other knee ligament injuries: a national population-based study. J Sci Med Sport 2009;12(6):622–7.

5. Prodromos CC, Han Y, Rogowski J, et al. A meta-analysis of the incidence of anterior cruciate ligament tears as a function of gender, sport, and a knee injury-reduction regimen. Arthroscopy 2007;23:1320–5 e6.

6. Frobell RB, Roos EM, Roos HP, et al. A randomized trial of treatment for acute anterior cruciate ligament tears. N Engl J Med 2010;363:331–42.

7. Malanga GA, Andrus S, Nadler SF, et al. Physical examination of the knee: a review of the original test description and scientific validity of common orthopedic tests. Arch Phys Med Rehabil 2003;84:592–603.

8. Scholten RJ, Opstelten W, van der Plas CG, et al. Accuracy of physical diagnostic tests for assessing ruptures of the anterior cruciate ligament: a meta-analysis. J Fam Pract 2003;52:689–94.

9. Benjaminse A, Gokeler A, van der Schans CP. Clinical diagnosis of an anterior cruciate ligament rupture: a meta-analysis. J Orthop Sports Phys Ther 2006;36:267–88.

10. Oberlander MA, Shalvoy RM, Hughston JC. The accuracy of the clinical knee examination documented by arthroscopy. A prospective study. Am J Sports Med 1993;21:773–8.

11. Kocabey Y, Tetik O, Isbell WM, et al. The value of clinical examination versus magnetic resonance imaging in the diagnosis of meniscal tears and anterior cruciate ligament rupture. Arthroscopy 2004;20:696–700.

12. Daniel DM, Stone ML, Sachs R, et al. Instrumented measurement of anterior knee laxity in patients with acute anterior cruciate ligament disruption. Am J Sports Med 1985;13:401–7.

13. Sernert N, Kartus JT, Jr., Ejerhed L, et al. Right and left knee laxity measurements: a prospective study of patients with anterior cruciate ligament injuries and normal control subjects. Arthroscopy 2004;20:564–71.

14. Monaco E, Labianca L, Maestri B, et al. Instrumented measurements of knee laxity: KT-1000 versus navigation. Knee Surg Sports Traumatol Arthrosc 2009;17:617–21.

15. Donaldson WF, 3rd, Warren RF, Wickiewicz T. A comparison of acute anterior cruciate ligament examinations. Initial versus examination under anesthesia. Am J Sports Med 1985;13:5–10.

16. Bach BR, Jr., Warren RF, Wickiewicz TL. The pivot shift phenomenon: results and description of a modified clinical test for anterior cruciate ligament insufficiency. Am J Sports Med 1988;16:571–6.

17. Robert H, Nouveau S, Gageot S, et al. A new knee arthrometer, the GNRB: experience in ACL complete and partial tears. Orthop Traumatol Surg Res 2009;95:171–6.

18. Anderson AF, Snyder RB, Federspiel CF, et al. Instrumented evaluation of knee laxity: a comparison of five arthrometers. Am J Sports Med 1992;20:135–40.

19. Katz JW, Fingeroth RJ. The diagnostic accuracy of ruptures of the anterior cruciate ligament comparing the Lachman test, the anterior drawer sign, and the pivot shift test in acute and chronic knee injuries. Am J Sports Med 1986;14:88–91.

20. Liu SH, Osti L, Henry M, et al. The diagnosis of acute complete tears of the anterior cruciate ligament. Comparison of MRI, arthrometry and clinical examination. J Bone Joint Surg Br 1995;77:586–8.

21. Peeler J, Leiter J, MacDonald P. Accuracy and reliability of anterior cruciate ligament clinical examination in a multidisciplinary sports medicine setting. Clin J Sport Med 2010;20:80–5.

22. Foster TE, Wolfe BL, Ryan S, et al. Does the graft source really matter in the outcome of patients undergoing anterior cruciate ligament reconstruction? An evaluation of autograft versus allograft reconstruction results: a systematic review. Am J Sports Med 2010;38:189–99.

23. Peterson RK, Shelton WR, Bomboy AL. Allograft versus autograft patellar tendon anterior cruciate ligament reconstruction: A 5-year follow-up. Arthroscopy 2001;17:9–13.

24. Kleipool AE, Zijl JA, Willems WJ. Arthroscopic anterior cruciate ligament reconstruction with bone-patellar tendon-bone allograft or autograft. A prospective study with an average follow up of 4 years. Knee Surg Sports Traumatol Arthrosc. 1998;6:224–30.

25. Sun K, Tian SQ, Zhang JH, et al. Anterior cruciate ligament reconstruction with bone-patellar tendon-bone autograft versus allograft. Arthroscopy 2009;25:750–9.

26. Edgar CM, Zimmer S, Kakar S, et al. Prospective comparison of auto and allograft hamstring tendon constructs for ACL reconstruction. Clin Orthop Relat Res 2008;466:2238–46.

27. Poehling GG, Curl WW, Lee CA, et al. Analysis of outcomes of anterior cruciate ligament repair with 5-year follow-up: allograft versus autograft. Arthroscopy 2005;21:774–85.

28. Greenberg DD, Robertson M, Vallurupalli S, et al. Allograft compared with autograft infection rates in primary anterior cruciate ligament reconstruction. J Bone Joint Surg Am 2010;92:2402–8.

29. Biau DJ, Katsahian S, Kartus J, et al. Patellar tendon versus hamstring tendon autografts for reconstructing the anterior cruciate ligament: a meta-analysis based on individual patient data. Am J Sports Med 2009;37:2470–8.

30. Poolman RW, Abouali JA, Conter HJ, et al. Overlapping systematic reviews of anterior cruciate ligament reconstruction com-

paring hamstring autograft with bone-patellar tendon-bone autograft: why are they different? J Bone Joint Surg Am 2007;89:1542–52.

31. Muneta T, Koga H, Mochizuki T, et al. A prospective randomized study of 4-strand semitendinosus tendon anterior cruciate ligament reconstruction comparing single-bundle and double-bundle techniques. Arthroscopy 2007;23:618–28.

32. Jarvela T. Double-bundle versus single-bundle anterior cruciate ligament reconstruction: a prospective, randomize clinical study. Knee Surg Sports Traumatol Arthrosc 2007;15:500–7.

33. Siebold R, Dehler C, Ellert T. Prospective randomized comparison of double-bundle versus single-bundle anterior cruciate ligament reconstruction. Arthroscopy 2008;24:137–45.

34. Streich NA, Friedrich K, Gotterbarm T, et al. Reconstruction of the ACL with a semitendinosus tendon graft: a prospective randomized single blinded comparison of double-bundle versus single-bundle technique in male athletes. Knee Surg Sports Traumatol Arthrosc 2008;16:232 8.

35. Aglietti P, Giron F, Losco M, et al. Comparison between single- and double-bundle anterior cruciate ligament reconstruction: a prospective, randomized, single-blinded clinical trial. Am J Sports Med 2010;38:25–34.

36. Kanaya A, Ochi M, Deie M, et al. Intraoperative evaluation of anteroposterior and rotational stabilities in anterior cruciate ligament reconstruction: lower femoral tunnel placed single-bundle versus double-bundle reconstruction. Knee Surg Sports Traumatol Arthrosc 2009;17:907–13.

37. Sastre S, Popescu D, Nunez M, et al. Double-bundle versus single-bundle ACL reconstruction using the horizontal femoral position: a prospective, randomized study. Knee Surg Sports Traumatol Arthrosc 2010;18:32–6.

38. Kondo E, Yasuda K, Azuma H, et al. Prospective clinical comparisons of anatomic double-bundle versus single-bundle anterior cruciate ligament reconstruction procedures in 328 consecutive patients. Am J Sports Med 2008;36:1675–87.

39. Seon JK, Park SJ, Lee KB, et al. Stability comparison of anterior cruciate ligament between double- and single-bundle reconstructions. Int Orthop 2009;33:425–9.

40. Park SJ, Jung YB, Jung HJ, et al. Outcome of arthroscopic single-bundle versus double-bundle reconstruction of the anterior cruciate ligament: a preliminary 2-year prospective study. Arthroscopy 2010;26:630–6.

41. Tsuda E, Ishibashi Y, Fukuda A, et al. Comparable results between lateralized single- and double-bundle ACL reconstructions. Clin Orthop Relat Res 2009;467:1042–55.

42. Hofbauer M, Valentin P, Kdolsky R, et al. Rotational and translational laxity after computer-navigated single- and double-bundle anterior cruciate ligament reconstruction. Knee Surg Sports Traumatol Arthrosc 2010;18:1201–7.

43. Sadoghi P, Muller PE, Jansson V, et al. Reconstruction of the anterior cruciate ligament: a clinical comparison of bone-patellar tendon-bone single bundle versus semitendinosus and gracilis double bundle technique. Int Orthop 2011;35(1):127–33.

44. Reinhardt KR, Hetsroni I, Marx RG. Graft selection for anterior cruciate ligament reconstruction: a level I systematic review comparing failure rates and functional outcomes. Orthop Clin North Am 2010;41:249–62.

45. Samuelsson K, Andersson D, Karlsson J. Treatment of anterior cruciate ligament injuries with special reference to graft type and surgical technique: an assessment of randomized controlled trials. Arthroscopy 2009;25:1139–74.

46. Goldblatt JP, Fitzsimmons SE, Balk E, et al. Reconstruction of the anterior cruciate ligament: meta-analysis of patellar tendon versus hamstring tendon autograft. Arthroscopy 2005;21: 791–803.

47. Forster MC, Forster IW. Patellar tendon or four-strand hamstring? A systematic review of autografts for anterior cruciate ligament reconstruction. Knee 2005;12:225–30.

48. Spindler KP, Kuhn JE, Freedman KB, et al. Anterior cruciate ligament reconstruction autograft choice: bone-tendon-bone versus hamstring: does it really matter? A systematic review. Am J Sports Med 2004;32:1986–95.

49. Oiestad BE, Engebretsen L, Storheim K, et al. Knee osteoarthritis after anterior cruciate ligament injury: a systematic review. Am J Sports Med 2009;37:1434–43.

50. Andersson D, Samuelsson K, Karlsson J. Treatment of anterior cruciate ligament injuries with special reference to surgical technique and rehabilitation: an assessment of randomized controlled trials. Arthroscopy 2009;25:653–85.

51. Lewis PB, Parameswaran AD, Rue JP, et al. Systematic review of single-bundle anterior cruciate ligament reconstruction outcomes: a baseline assessment for consideration of double-bundle techniques. Am J Sports Med 2008;36:2028–36.

52. Roos H, Adalberth T, Dahlberg L, et al. Osteoarthritis of the knee after injury to the anterior cruciate ligament or meniscus: the influence of time and age. Osteoarthritis Cartilage 1995;3: 261–7.

53. Ahlden M, Kartus J, Ejerhed L, et al. Knee laxity measurements after anterior cruciate ligament reconstruction, using either bone-patellar-tendon-bone or hamstring tendon autografts, with special emphasis on comparison over time. Knee Surg Sports Traumatol Arthrosc 2009;17:1117–24.

54. Sajovic M, Vengust V, Komadina R, et al. A prospective, randomized comparison of semitendinosus and gracilis tendon versus patellar tendon autografts for anterior cruciate ligament reconstruction: five-year follow-up. Am J Sports Med 2006;34: 1933–40.

55. Holm I, Oiestad BE, Risberg MA, et al. No difference in knee function or prevalence of osteoarthritis after reconstruction of the anterior cruciate ligament with 4-strand hamstring autograft versus patellar tendon-bone autograft: a randomized study with 10-year follow-up. Am J Sports Med 2010;38:448–54.

56. Meunier A, Odensten M, Good L. Long-term results after primary repair or non-surgical treatment of anterior cruciate ligament rupture: a randomized study with a 15-year follow-up. Scand J Med Sci Sports 2007;17:230–7.

57. Neuman P, Kostogiannis I, Friden T, et al. Patellofemoral osteoarthritis 15 years after anterior cruciate ligament injury—a prospective cohort study. Osteoarthritis Cartil 2009; 17:284–90.

58. Neuman P, Englund M, Kostogiannis I, et al. Prevalence of tibiofemoral osteoarthritis 15 years after nonoperative treatment of anterior cruciate ligament injury: a prospective cohort study. Am J Sports Med 2008;36:1717–25.

96 Posterior Cruciate Ligament Injury

Rune Bruhn Jakobsen[1,2] and Bent Wulff Jakobsen[3]

[1]Oslo Sports Trauma Research Center, Norwegian School of Sport Sciences, Oslo, Norway
[2]Norway Institute of Basic Medical Sciences, Faculty of Medicine, University of Oslo, Oslo, Norway
[3]Hamlet Private Hospital, Åarhus, Denmark

Case scenario

A 19-year-old man seeks medical help at the Emergency Department after a game of soccer. He is the team's goalkeeper and was injured when an opponent hit him on his left shinbone while he jumped forward on flexed knees trying to catch the ball. He felt a sudden onset pain in the hollow of the knee and could not continue playing. In the Emergency Department the trauma doctor reveals an effusion of the left knee with lack of full extension. Standard radiographs reveal no fractures, and the patient is scheduled for a follow-up appointment with the orthopedic department.

Relevant anatomy

The posterior cruciate ligament (PCL) is the main stabilizer in the knee against posterior translation of the tibia.[1] Secondarily it is a restraint to external rotation of the tibia.[2] Approximately 38 mm in length, the PCL consist of two main bundles, the anterolateral and the posteromedial, both originating from approximately 10 mm inferior to the posterior tibial joint line and running anteromedial to attach to the lateral aspect of the medial femoral condyle.[3] The anterolateral bundle is tight with the knee in flexion and the posteromedial when the knee is extended.[2] Injuries to the PCL are classified as either isolated or combined as part of a multiligament injury including the posterolateral or posteromedial corner (PLC or PMC). There may be either a total rupture of the ligament (most often the mid-

substance), a bony avulsion injury, or a partial tear. This chapter focuses on the evidence for diagnosis, treatment, and prognosis relating to isolated PCL tears.

Importance of the problem

There is great variability in the reported incidence of injury to the PCL with numbers ranging between 1% and 44% of all acute knee injuries depending on the population studied.[4-6] In a cohort study of 46,500 adolescents the incidence of cruciate ligament injury was found to be 60.9 per 100,000 life years, of which about 8% were likely to be PCL tears.[7] Arguably much less common than the ACL (anterior cruciate ligament) tear, the risk of sustaining an injury to the PCL is highly sport-specific with increasing incidence in contact sports. The incidence has been studied in hockey, team handball, soccer, wrestling, and rugby and has retrospectively been found to vary from 1% to 4% of the total number of injuries.[8-11] The archetypical injury mechanism is described as the dashboard injury, with a blow to the anterior of the tibia. In the sports setting a fall onto a flexed knee, hyperflexion, or hyperextension are typical mechanisms.[12] In patients with isolated PCL tears that are treated nonoperatively only about 50% return to sport at the same or higher level; however, in general the patients report good subjective knee function regardless of objective laxity.[13] It is generally believed that damage to the internal structures of the knee leads to progressive secondary osteoarthritis (OA), but whether this is the case with isolated PCL tears is still a matter of debate.[13-16] As with every subject in medicine, an increasing amount of information is readily avail-

Evidence-Based Orthopedics, First Edition. Edited by Mohit Bhandari.
© 2012 Blackwell Publishing Ltd. Published 2012 by Blackwell Publishing Ltd.

able online and a Google search for *posterior cruciate ligament injury* returns more than 134,000 hits. This stresses the need for guidelines based on critically appraised evidence.

Top five questions

Diagnosis

1. How accurate is clinical examination in the diagnosis of PCL injury, and is additional imaging needed?

Therapy

2. Should reconstruction be performed?
3. What is the optimal reconstruction technique?
4. Which type of graft should be used?

Prognosis

5. Does an isolated PCL tear lead to increased OA?

Question 1: How accurate is clinical examination in the diagnosis of PCL injury, and is additional imaging needed?

Case clarification

The patient is seen at the outpatient clinic the day after the injury. He is not able to fully bear weight without pain. He keeps his knee in slight flexion. Examination reveals a slight AP laxity without posterior sag sign and a slight effusion but is otherwise unremarkable.

Relevance

The ability to accurately diagnose a PCL tear in both the acute and the chronic setting is paramount for the orthopedic surgeon in guiding the further treatment. The finding that a PCL injury is often overlooked by both patient and clinician underlines the importance of using sensitive and specific tools in the diagnostic process.[17]

Current opinion

Current opinion suggests that clinical examination should be sufficient in diagnosing a PCL tear; however, a MRI is often needed to evaluate concomitant injury.

Finding the evidence

- Cochrane Database with search term: "knee examination"
- PubMed, with search terms: "clinical," "examination," "knee," "accuracy"

Quality of the evidence[18]

Level I
- 1 randomized trial

Level II
- 4 exploratory cohort studies
- 1 systematic review of level II or better

Level III
- 4 nonconsecutive studies

Level IV
- 2 studies not fulfilling criteria for level I–III

Clinical examination

We found a total of 11 studies and 1 systematic review reporting on the performance of clinical examination for PCL injuries (Table 96.1). Only one study, which focused entirely on chronic injuries, could be deemed to be of level I evidence. Due to heterogeneity, pooled statistical analysis is not presented. Summarizing, based on level I and II evidence: in chronic injuries the posterior drawer test has a satisfactory sensitivity and excellent specificity, and when combined with other tests the composite examination yields a sensitivity of 97–100% in chronic injuries. The specificity of the composite clinical examination for chronic injuries is approximately 100%. In acute injuries the sensitivity of the posterior drawer test drops substantially, to between 22% and 67%, and for the composite examination the sensitivity is reported to be between 44% and 100% (the latter study including only four PCL injuries), and a specificity of 90–98%. These findings indicate why PCL injuries are often overlooked in the acute phase.

Recommendations

- In acute injuries evidence suggests that clinical examination is not sufficient and if the trauma mechanism is compatible with injury to the PCL clinical re-evaluation and/or additional imaging with MRI is recommended [overall quality: moderate]
- In chronic injuries evidence suggests that clinical examination should be sufficient for diagnosing a rupture of the PCL [overall quality: moderate]
- Concomitant injury to the PLC should always be considered and evaluated when an injury to the PCL is considered [overall quality: moderate]

Question 2: Should reconstruction be performed?

Case clarification

A faculty-level orthopedic surgeon repeats the clinical examination 6 weeks later. The patient states that the pain is now manageable and he has actually started to walk without crutches. The effusion is reduced but he now has a grade III posterior laxity and shows a posterior sag sign.

Table 96.1 Sensitivity and specificity of clinical tests for PCL insufficiency

Test	Test performance	Comments	Level of evidence
Posterior sag sign	Rubinstein et al. 1994: Sensitivity 79% Specificity 100%	Double-blinded, randomized controlled study (39 subjects, 75 knees, chronic injuries)	Ib
	Staubli and Jakob. 1990: Sensitivity 83% Specificity N/A	Nonrandomized, unblinded, uncontrolled (24 PCL-deficient knees, acute injuries)	III
Posterior drawer test	Baker et al. 1984: Sensitivity 86% Specificity N/A	Nonrandomized, unblinded, uncontrolled (7 knees preanesthesia, acute injuries)	III
	Sensitivity 77% Specificity N/A	As above (13 knees, under anesthesia)	
	Staubli and Jakob 1990: Sensitivity 83% Specificity N/A	As above (under anesthesia)	III
	Rubinstein et al. 1994: Sensitivity 90% Specificity 99%	As above	Ib
	Loos et al. 1981: Sensitivity 51% Specificity N/A	Nonrandomized, unblinded, uncontrolled (59 knees, acute injuries)	III
	Hughston et al. 1976: Sensitivity 22% Specificity 100%	Nonrandomized, unblinded, controlled (68 knees, acute injuries, anesthesia unclear)	IIb
	Moore and Larson. 1980: Sensitivity 67% Specificity N/A	Nonrandomized, unblinded, uncontrolled (18 knees, acute)	IV
	Harilainen et al. 1987: Sensitivity 33% Specificity N/A	Nonrandomized, unblinded, uncontrolled (9 knees, acute)	III
	Sensitivity 100% Specificity N/A	As above (under anesthesia)	
	Clendenin et al. 1980: Sensitivity 100% Specificity N/A	Nonrandomized, unblinded, uncontrolled (10 knees)	IV
Abduction stress test	Hughston et al. 1976: Sensitivity 94% Specificity 100%	As above	III
Quadriceps active test	Daniel et al. 1988: Sensitivity 98% Specificity 100%	Nonrandomized, unblinded, controlled (92 knees, acute and chronic injuries)	IIb
	Rubinstein et al. 1994: Sensitivity 54% Specificity 97%	As above	Ib
Composite exam	Rubinstein et al. 1994: Sensitivity 97% Specificity 100%	As above (grade II and III)	Ib
	Simonsen et al. 1984: Sensitivity 44% Specificity 98%	Nonrandomized, unblinded, controlled (118 knees, acute, note: authors calculate predictive values, not sensitivity/specificity)	IIb
	O'Shea et al. 1996: Sensitivity 100% Specificity 90%	Nonrandomized, blinded, controlled (156 knees, acute and chronic)	IIb
	Solomon et al. 2001: Positive LR 25.0 Negative LR 0.04	Meta-analysis of 5 studies	IIa

Without anesthesia unless stated.

Adapted from Malanga et al. (2003), Arch Phys Med Rehabil 84(4):592–603, expanded and restructured with relevant studies from the present literature search.

A grade I posterior laxity measures 1–5 mm of posterior translation of the tibia as compared to the contralateral knee, grade II 6–10 mm, and grade III >10 mm.

Relevance

All surgical procedures pose a risk to the patient. The orthopedic surgeon needs relevant evidence-based data on long-term outcome and risks in order to determine whether the benefit of a reconstruction is greater than of conservative treatment and whether the risk/benefit ratio is justifiable.

Current opinion

The isolated posterior cruciate lesion with less than 10 mm side-to-side difference compared to the contralateral normal knee may be treated conservatively. Patients with grade III lesions (see box) or patients primarily treated conservatively who develop pain or instability are strong candidates for reconstruction.

Finding the evidence

The following search strategy was used for Questions 2–6.
• Cochrane Database with search term: "posterior cruciate ligament"
• PubMed search with search terms "posterior cruciate ligament" [MeSH Terms] OR ("posterior" [All Fields] AND "cruciate" [All Fields] AND "ligament" [All Fields]) OR "posterior cruciate ligament" [All Fields]

Quality of the evidence

Level I
• 1 prognostic cohort study

Level II
• 2 randomized trials with methodologic limitations
• 3 prospective comparative studies

Level III
• 14 retrospective comparative studies

Level IV
• 52 case series

Findings

We found and reviewed a total of 72 studies (N = 2552, median = 35 patients). Only one study could be classified as a level I prognostic study (N = 271 patients) and five studies were classified as level II (N = 215 patients). Twelve studies reported on conservatively treated patients, 57 reported on only surgically treated patients, and only two studies (level III) looked at surgically vs. conservatively treated patients. We found large variations in inclusion criteria, choice of surgical technique, and type of graft in the reviewed studies. This large variation and the lack of proper randomized controlled trials (RCTs) make it inappropriate to present pooled statistics. We base our recommendations primarily on the level I–III studies, which are briefly summarized in Table 96.2 and 96.3. Level IV studies are listed in Table 96.4 with only minimal details, acknowledging the fact that valuable information can be deduced from this type of study. The overall heterogeneity of included studies is reflected in the generally poor overall quality scores of each recommendation.

Recommendations

• Isolated grade I and II PCL injuries (<10 mm posterior laxity) should be treated conservatively [overall quality: moderate]
• Isolated acute grade III injuries may be treated conservatively with good results but in some patients without adequately defined characteristics at time of injury, instability persists which hinder sports and/or daily activities and reconstruction should be performed [overall quality: low]
• Dislocated tibial avulsion fractures should be reattached with anchors or screw fixation within 3 weeks; however, there is no clear evidence of what determines the minimum size of fragment for fixation to be an appropriate option [overall quality: low]
• Chronic isolated grade I and II injuries should be treated conservatively with physiotherapy and activity modification [overall quality: very low]
• Chronic isolated grade III injuries should be reconstructed if pain and instability persist after adequate rehabilitation with physiotherapy. It should be evaluated whether there is injury to the PLC [overall quality: low]

Question 3. What is the optimal reconstruction technique?

Case clarification

After 4 months of intensive physiotherapy and rehabilitation the patient has not been able to fully return to sport at his previous level, and returns to the clinic. Posterior laxity is still grade III and a reconstruction is planned. He has been surfing the web and asks questions about the double-bundle technique.

Relevance

Several techniques are used for reconstructing the PCL. It is necessary to be critically aware of the technical and biomechanical strengths and weaknesses of these techniques and, most importantly, know the documented outcome from each technique.

Current opinion

Expert opinions on PCL treatment suggest that reconstructions should be performed arthroscopically by a skilled

Table 96.2 Identified level I and level II studies with summary of intervention and results

Study	No. of patients	Surgery or conservative	Level of evidence	Treatment and results summary
Shelbourne and Muthukaruppan[19]	271	Conservative	I	Conservatively treated grade I and II, mean follow-up of 7,8 years (215 patients) with a modified Noyes score of 85,6 ± 15. Greater PCL laxity was not associated with poorer scores
Chen et al.[20]	49	Surgery	II	Prospective comparison between isolated grade III lesions treated with either hamstring og quadriceps autograft reconstruction. At mean follow-up of app. 28 months there was no significant difference between groups with Lysholm scores of 90,6 ± 7,7 and 91,44 ± 6,2 in quadriceps and hamstring groups respectively. 3 patients (14%) in the quadriceps group and 2 patients in the hamstring group (8%) showed radiographic changes, 1 in each group with joint space narrowing
Houe and Jørgensen[21]	16	Surgery	II	Prospective comparison between single-bundle patellar bone-tendon-bone or double-bundle hamstring autograft reconstructed isolated chronic grade III lesions. At median follow-up of 35 months there was no significant difference between group with median Lysholm scores of 100 and 95 in single- and double-bundle groups respectively
Wang et al.[22]	55	Surgery	II	Prospective comparison of subacute isolated grade III lesions treated with single-bundle reconstruction with either allo- (Achilles or anterior tibial tendon) or autograft (quadriceps or hamstring). At mean follow-up of 34 months there was no significant difference with Lysholm scores of 87.8 ± 9.6 and 92.3 ± 6.8 in the autograft and allograft groups respectively. More minor complications in the autograft group (7 patients) including 4 patients with donor site pain and 2 infections
Wang et al.[23]	35	Surgery	II	Prospective randomized (improperly described randomization procedure) comparison between single-bundle versus double-bundle reconstruction of subacute isolated grade III lesions with hamstring autografts. At mean follow-up of 41 months in the single-bundle and 28 months in the double-bundle group there was no significant difference between groups with Lysholm scores of 88 ± 10 and 89 ± 9 in the single- and double-bundle groups respectively
Wong et al.[24]	60	Surgery	II	Prospective randomized (less-than-optimal randomization procedure) comparison of isolated grade III lesion reconstructed with single-bundle hamstring autograft with either a transtibial anterolateral or anteromedial approach. At average follow-up of app. 45 months there was no significant difference with Lysholm scores of 88 ± 10 and 91 ± 8 in the anteromedial and anterolateral group respectively. In both groups ~60% showed radiographic stage 1 changes

knee surgeon with a considerable number of PCL procedures per year. Biomechanically the two-bundle technique is superior to the single-bundle technique,[39] but it is surgically more demanding, and has clinically not demonstrated superior results.

Recommendations

• Reconstruction may be performed arthroscopically using single- or double-bundle technique with tibial inlay or onlay/transtibial technique [overall quality: low]

• Fixation methods are numerous and none has shown superiority [overall quality: very low]

Question 4: Which type of graft should be used?

Case clarification

The surgery is scheduled a few weeks later. A week before surgery the surgical coordinator calls you and asks whether they need to order allograft for the surgery? And if so,

Table 96.3 Identified level III studies with summary of intervention and results

Study	No. of patients	Surgery or conservative	Treatment
Ahn et al.[25]	36	Surgery	Retrospective comparison of chronic isolated grade III lesions reconstructed with either single-bundle double-loop hamstring tendon autograft or Achilles tendon allograft. At mean follow-up of 35 months for the autograft group and 27 months for the allograft group there was no significant difference between IKDC scores but a significant difference between Lysholm scores of 90.1 and 85.8 in favor of the hamstring autograft
Hatayama et al.[26]	20	Surgery	Retrospective comparison of isolated and combined grade 3 lesions reconstructed with hamstring autograft either with single-bundle og double-bundle technique. At follow-up at 2 years there was no significant difference between groups neither in IKDC scores, nor in biomechanical measurements. 3 tears of posteromedial bundle at second-look arthroscopy at 1 year
Kim et al.[27]	60	Surgery	Retrospective comparison of subacute and chronic combined and isolated grade III lesions reconstructed via either an anteromedial (AM) or anterolateral (AL) tibial approach with a variety of grafts (Achilles and tibialis posterior allografts, patellar bone-tendon-bone autograft). At mean follow-up of 58.6 months in the AL group and 56.9 in the AM group there was no significant difference with Lysholm scores of 88.6 ± 7.1 and 88.4 ± 6.4 respectively
Kim et al.[28]	29	Surgery	Retrospective comparison of chronic isolated grade III lesions reconstructed with Achilles tendon allograft using either transtibial single-bundle, arthroscopic tibial inlay single-bundle or arthroscopic tibial inlay double-bundle technique. At mean follow-up of 46.4, 36.3 and 29,4 months respectively there was no clinical significant difference with Lysholms scores of 86.8 ± 7.5, 79.7 ± 11.7 and 84.3 ± 9.7, however biomechanically there was significantly less posterior translation in the double-bundle inlay vs. transtibial technique (3.6 vs. 5.6 mm)
Kim et al.[29]	55	Surgery	Retrospective comparison of isolated subacute and chronic grade III lesions reconstructed with patellar bone-tendon-bone auto- or allograft using either a one- or a two-incision technique. At a mean follow-up of 36 months and 45 months in the one-incision and the two-incision group respectively there was no significant difference with Lysholm scores of 90.6 and 90.0 respectively
Li et al.[30]	36	Surgery	Retrospective comparison of isolated chronic grade III lesions with either four-strand hamstring autograft or a LARS artificial ligament. At mean follow-up of 29 months and 26 months in the autograft and artificial ligament group respectively there was a significant difference in the Lysholm scores in favour of the artificial ligament (85 vs. 93)
MacGillivray et al.[31]	29	Surgery	Retrospective comparison of chronic isolated lesions (tibia flush with or offset posteriorly at 90°) reconstructed with either transtibial or tibial inlay single-bundle using a variety of grafts (patellar bone-tendon-bone auto- and allograft and Achilles tendon autograft). At mean follow-up of 75 months and 57 months in transtibial and inlay groups respectively there was no significant difference with Lysholm scores of 81 and 76 respectively
Noyes and Barber-Westin[32]	25	Surgery	Retrospective comparison of isolated acute and chronic grade III lesions reconstructed with either single-bundle allograft (Achilles tendon or patellar bone-tendon-bone) or a combined allograft-ligament augmentation device. At mean follow-up of 45 months there was no benefit of augmentation. Cartilage deterioration was noted in all patients with chronic lesions
Ohkoshi et al.[33]	51	Surgery	Retrospective comparison of subacute and chronic grade III lesions reconstructed with hamstring autografts using either a 2-incision technique or an endoscopic transtibial technique. At mean follow-up of 19.2 months there was no significant difference in the IKDC ratings, significantly shorter rehabilitation period in the endoscopic group
Patel et al.[34]	58	Conservative	Retrospective cohort prognosis study of nonoperatively treated isolated partial and complete lesions. Preinjury Tegner score was 7. At mean follow-up of 6.9 years the Lysholm score was 85.2, Tegner score was 6.6., on the IKDC form 6 patients had a nearly normal result, 50 patients had an abnormal result and 1 patient had a severely abnormal result, radiographic OA was seen in the medial compartment of 17% (grade I and II), in the patellafemoral joint of 7% (grade I) and in the lateral compartment of 5% of patients. No significant correlations existed between subjective and objective findings

(Continued)

Table 96.3 (Continued)

Study	No. of patients	Surgery or conservative	Treatment
Roth et al.[35]	39	Surgery/ Conservative	Retrospective comparison of combined and isolated grade III mainly chronic lesions treated either conservatively or with medial gastrocnemius tendon transfer. At mean follow-up of 53 months there were no significant changes biomechanically nor was there subjective improvement in the operated group as compared to the conservative group
Seon and Song[36]	43	Surgery	Retrospective comparison of chronic grade III lesions reconstructed with either transtibial hamstring autograft or tibial inlay patellar bone-tendon-bone autograft. At mean follow-up of 31.8 months there was no significant difference between groups with Lysholm scores of 91.3 and 92.8 in the transtibial and the tibial inlay groups respectively
Shirakura et al.[37]	40	Surgery/ conservative	Retrospective comparison of isolated grade III lesions (midsubstance tears) treated with either primary repair or nonoperatively. At mean follow-up of 80 months in the surgery group and 52 months in the conservative group the operated knees were significantly more stable though not on par with a group of un-injured controls. No significant change existed on a knee rating score with 92.9 ± 5.1 and 90.9 ± 2.8 respectively. Grade I degenerative radiographic findings in 3 patients in the operated group and 1 in the conservative group
Zhao and Huangfu[38]	51	Surgery	Retrospective comparison of isolated chronic grade III lesions reconstructed transtibially with either 4-strand or 7-strand hamstring autograft. At mean follow-up of 31 months in the 4-strand group and 30 months in the 7 strand group there was significant difference between the groups in favor of the 7-strand technique with Lysholm scores of 83 ± 4 and 92 ± 4

which type? You remember that it was discussed with the patient but you forgot to put it down on the note that was sent to the surgical coordinator.

Relevance

Several types of grafts are used for PCL reconstruction, both autografts and allografts. The chosen graft may have implications for surgical technique and time, donor site morbidity, risk of disease transmission, and, most important, outcome.

Current opinion

The most commonly used autografts are four-strand hamstring graft, quadriceps tendon or bone–patellar tendon–bone (BPTB) grafts. These are also commonly used as allografts with the addition of Achilles tendon grafts.

Recommendations

• Reliable results have been demonstrated with a variety of auto- and allograft choices including BPTB, hamstring tendons (quadruple and 7-double), quadriceps tendon, Achilles tendon. There are no data indicating superiority of any graft type [overall quality: low]
• Allografts have the advantage of shorter durations of surgery, no donor site morbidity, and potentially stronger grafts by choosing specific types of grafts. However, availability, potential risk of disease transmission, and tissue quality are essential factors that need to be considered and which may vary depending on geographical location [overall quality: low]

Question 5: Does an isolated PCL tear lead to increased osteoarthritis?

Case clarification

You see the patient at regular follow-ups and at 9 months he is doing very well subjectively, having been able to return to his previous level of activity. Posterior laxity is now grade I. Occasionally, he has a little aching from the knee after a hard game and he asks whether he is likely to develop OA.

Relevance

Knowledge of the longtime risk of developing secondary OA is important both in the decision process of opting for surgery or not, and in the long-term follow-up of PCL-deficient and/or reconstructed patients.

Current opinion

A cruciate ligament injury is generally believed to lead to secondary OA and there is conflicting evidence whether reconstruction of ligaments halts this development. Current opinion suggests that isolated PCL ruptures may be treated conservatively with minor risk of patellofemoral or medial compartment OA.

Table 96.4 Identified level IV studies

Author	Year	No. of patients	Type of treatment
Aglietti et al.	2002	18	Surgery
Ahn et al.	2006	61	Surgery
Boynton et al.	1996	30	Conservative
Cain et al.	2002	22	Surgery
Chan et al.	2006	20	Surgery
Chen et al.	2009	22	Surgery
Chen et al.	1999	12	Surgery
Chen et al.	2002	27	Surgery
Chen et al.	2004	29	Surgery
Chen et al.	2006	57	Surgery
Clancy et al.	1983	23	Surgery
Cooper et al.	2004	41	Surgery
Dandy et al.	1982	20	Conservative
Deehan et al.	2003	29	Surgery
Fanelli et al.	2004	41	Surgery
Fanelli et al.	1994	30	Surgery
Fowler et al.	1987	13	Conservative
Garofalo et al.	2006	15	Surgery
Goudie et al.	2009	23	Surgery
Gui et al.	2009	28	Surgery
Hermans et al.	2009	22	Surgery
Hughston et al.	1982	26	Surgery
Jackson et al.	2008	26	Surgery
Jenner et al.	2006	18	Surgery
Jung et al.	2008	17	Conservative
Jung et al.	2005	12	Surgery
Jung et al.	2006	89	Surgery
Keller et al.	1993	40	Conservative
Kim et al.	1999	37	Surgery
Lim et al.	2009	22	Surgery
Mariani et al.	1997	24	Surgery
Nicandri et al.	2008	16	Surgery
Noyes et al.	2005	19	Surgery
Noyes et al.	2005	15	Surgery
Nyland et al.	2002	19	Surgery
Ohkoshi et al.	2001	21	Surgery
Parolie et al.	1986	25	Conservative
Pournaras et al.	1991	20	Surgery
Richter et al.	1996	32	Surgery
Roolker et al.	2000	13	Surgery
Sekiya et al.	2005	21	Surgery
Shelbourne et al.	1999	133	Conservative
Shino et al.	1995	22	Conservative
Sun et al.	2007	49	Surgery
Torg et al.	1989	43	Conservative
Toritsuka et al.	2004	16	Conservative
Wang al.	2003	30	Surgery
Wu et al.	2007	22	Surgery
Yoon et al.	2005	26	Surgery
Zhang et al.	2006	11	Surgery
Zhao et al.	2006	29	Surgery
Zhao et al.	2008	18	Surgery

Recommendations

• An injury to the PCL is a significant injury to the knee and the index injury itself is likely to damage the cartilage [overall quality: moderate]

• In injuries to the PCL with concomitant injury to the cartilage progressive OA may occur, but early reconstruction has not been shown to have an impact on this development [overall quality: low]

• An isolated injury to the PCL without concomitant cartilage injury does not necessarily lead to progressive OA of the knee and there is no clear evidence that a reconstruction prevents OA from occurring [overall quality: low]

• Successfully conservatively treated knees do not show progressive OA at long-term follow-up [overall quality: low]

Summary of recommendations

• In acute injuries evidence suggests that clinical examination is not sufficient and if the trauma mechanism is compatible with injury to the PCL clinical re-evaluation and/or additional imaging with MRI is recommended

• In chronic injuries evidence suggests that clinical examination should be sufficient for diagnosing a rupture of the PCL

• Concomitant injury to the PLC should always be considered and evaluated when an injury to the PCL is considered

• Isolated grade I and II PCL injuries (<10 mm posterior laxity) should be treated conservatively

• Isolated acute grade III injuries may be treated conservatively with good results but in some patients without adequately defined characteristics at time of injury instability persists which hinder sports and/or daily activities and reconstruction should be performed

• Dislocated tibial avulsion fractures should be reattached with anchors or screw fixation within 3 weeks; however, there is no clear evidence of what determines the minimum size of fragment for fixation to be an appropriate option

• Chronic isolated grade I and II injuries should be treated conservatively with physiotherapy and activity modification

• Chronic isolated grade III injury should be reconstructed if pain and instability persist after adequate rehabilitation with physiotherapy. It should be evaluated whether there is injury to the PLC

• Reconstruction may be performed arthroscopically using single or double bundle with tibial inlay or onlay/transtibial technique

• Fixation methods are numerous and none has shown superiority

• Reliable results have been demonstrated with a variety of auto-and allograft choices including BPTB, hamstring tendons (quadruple and 7-double), quadriceps tendon, Achilles tendon. There are no data indicating superiority of any graft type

• Allografts have the advantage of shorter durations of surgery, no donor site morbidity, and potentially stronger grafts by choosing specific types of grafts. However, availability, potential risk of disease transmission, and tissue quality are essential factors that need to be considered and which may vary depending on geographical location

• An injury to the PCL is a significant injury to the knee and the index injury itself is likely to damage the cartilage

• In injuries to the PCL with concomitant injury to the cartilage progressive OA may occur, but early reconstruction has not been shown to have an impact on this development

• An isolated injury to the PCL without concomitant cartilage injury does not necessarily lead to progressive OA of the knee and there is not clear evidence that a reconstruction prevents OA from occurring

• Successfully conservatively treated knees do not show progressive OA at long-term follow-up

Conclusion

Unfortunately, the overall quality of the evidence for the diagnosis, treatment, and prognosis for PCL tears is poor, which is reflected in our recommendations.[40] There is a need for more studies on the management of PCL injuries. It is likely that a multicenter approach may be needed for RCTs with adequate statistical power to be feasible.

References

1. Veltri DM, Deng XH, Torzilli PA, et al. The role of the cruciate and posterolateral ligaments in stability of the knee. A biomechanical study. Am J Sports Med 1995;23(4):436–43.

2. Fu FH, Harner CD, Johnson DL, et al. Biomechanics of knee ligaments: basic concepts and clinical application. J Bone Joint Surg Am 1993;75(11):1716–27.

3. Harner CD, Baek GH, Vogrin TM, et al. Quantitative analysis of human cruciate ligament insertions. Arthroscopy 1999;15(7): 741–9.

4. Fanelli GC. Posterior cruciate ligament injuries in trauma patients. Arthroscopy 1993;9(3):291–4.

5. Hughston JC, Degenhardt TC. Reconstruction of the posterior cruciate ligament. Clin Orthop Relat Res 1982;164:59–77.

6. Majewski M, Susanne H, Klaus S. Epidemiology of athletic knee injuries: a 10-year study. Knee 2006;13(3):184–8.

7. Parkkari J, Pasanen K, Mattila VM, et al. The risk for a cruciate ligament injury of the knee in adolescents and young adults: a population-based cohort study of 46 500 people with a 9 year follow-up. Br J Sports Med 2008;42(6):422–6.

8. Arendt E, Dick R. Knee injury patterns among men and women in collegiate basketball and soccer. NCAA data and review of literature. Am J Sports Med 1995;23(6):694–701.

9. Petrigliano FA, McAllister DR. Isolated posterior cruciate ligament injuries of the knee. Sports Med Arthrosc 2006;14(4): 206–12.

10. Myklebust G, Maehlum S, Engebretsen L, et al. Registration of cruciate ligament injuries in Norwegian top level team handball. A prospective study covering two seasons. Scand J Med Sci Sports 1997;7(5):289–92.

11. Jarret GJ, Orwin JF, Dick RW. Injuries in collegiate wrestling. Am J Sports Med 1998;26(5):674–80.

12. Malone AA, Dowd GS, Saifuddin A. Injuries of the posterior cruciate ligament and posterolateral corner of the knee. Injury 2006;37(6):485–501.

13. Shelbourne KD, Davis TJ, Patel DV. The natural history of acute, isolated, nonoperatively treated posterior cruciate ligament injuries. A prospective study. Am J Sports Med 1999;27(3):276–83.

14. Boynton MD, Tietjens BR. Long-term followup of the untreated isolated posterior cruciate ligament-deficient knee. Am J Sports Med. 1996;24(3):306–10.

15. Clancy WG, Jr., Sutherland TB. Combined posterior cruciate ligament injuries. Clin Sports Med 1994;13(3):629–47.

16. Dejour H, Walch G, Peyrot J, et al. [The natural history of rupture of the posterior cruciate ligament]. Rev Chir Orthop Reparatrice Appar Mot 1988;74(1):35–43.

17. Simonsen O, Jensen J, Mouritsen P, et al. The accuracy of clinical examination of injury of the knee joint. Injury 1984;16(2): 96–101.

18. Oxford Centre for Evidence Based Medicine. Levels of Evidence. 2009 [updated March 2009; cited 2009 November 21.]; Available from http://www.cebm.net/index.aspx?o=1025.

19. Shelbourne KD, Muthukaruppan Y. Subjective results of nonoperatively treated, acute, isolated posterior cruciate ligament injuries. Arthroscopy. 2005;21(4):457–61.

20. Chen CH, Chen WJ, Shih CH. Arthroscopic reconstruction of the posterior cruciate ligament: a comparison of quadriceps tendon autograft and quadruple hamstring tendon graft. Arthroscopy 2002;18(6):603–12.

21. Houe T, Jørgensen U. Arthroscopic posterior cruciate ligament reconstruction: one- vs. two-tunnel technique. Scand J Med Sci Sports 2004;14(2):107–11.

22. Wang CJ, Chan YS, Weng LH, Yuan LJ, Chen HS. Comparison of autogenous and allogenous posterior cruciate ligament reconstructions of the knee. Injury 2004;35(12):1279–85.

23. Wang CJ, Weng LH, Hsu CC, Chan YS. Arthroscopic single- versus double-bundle posterior cruciate ligament reconstructions using hamstring autograft. Injury 2004;35(12):1293–9.

24. Wong T, Wang CJ, Weng LH, Hsu SL, Chou WY, Chen JM, Chan YS. Functional outcomes of arthroscopic posterior cruciate ligament reconstruction: comparison of anteromedial and anterolateral trans-tibia approach. Arch Orthop Trauma Surg 2009;129(3): 315–21.

25. Ahn JH, Yoo JC, Wang JH. Posterior cruciate ligament reconstruction: double-loop hamstring tendon autograft versus Achilles tendon allograft—clinical results of a minimum 2-year follow-up. Arthroscopy 2005;21(8):965–9.

26. Hatayama K, Higuchi H, Kimura M, Kobayashi Y, Asagumo H, Takagishi K. A comparison of arthroscopic single- and double-

bundle posterior cruciate ligament reconstruction: review of 20 cases. Am J Orthop (Belle Mead NJ) 2006;35(12):568–71.

27. Kim SJ, Chang JH, Kang YH, Song DH, Park KY. Clinical comparison of anteromedial versus anterolateral tibial tunnel direction for transtibial posterior cruciate ligament reconstruction: 2 to 8 years' follow-up. Am J Sports Med 2009;37(4):693–8.

28. Kim SJ, Kim TE, Jo SB, Kung YP. Comparison of the clinical results of three posterior cruciate ligament reconstruction techniques. J Bone Joint Surg Am 2009;91(11):2543–9.

29. Kim SJ, Shin SJ, Kim HK, Jahng JS, Kim HS. Comparison of 1- and 2-incision posterior cruciate ligament reconstructions. Arthroscopy 2000;16(3):268–78.

30. Li B, Wen Y, Wu H, Qian Q, Wu Y, Lin X. Arthroscopic single-bundle posterior cruciate ligament reconstruction: retrospective review of hamstring tendon graft versus LARS artificial ligament. Int Orthop 2009;33(4):991–6.

31. MacGillivray JD, Stein BE, Park M, Allen AA, Wickiewicz TL, Warren RF. Comparison of tibial inlay versus transtibial techniques for isolated posterior cruciate ligament reconstruction: minimum 2-year follow-up. Arthroscopy. 2006;22(3):320–8.

32. Noyes FR, Barber-Westin SD. Posterior cruciate ligament allograft reconstruction with and without a ligament augmentation device. Arthroscopy 1994;10(4):371–82.

33. Ohkoshi Y, Nagasaki S, Yamamoto K, Shibata N, Ishida R, Hashimoto T, Yamane S. Description of a new endoscopic posterior cruciate ligament reconstruction and comparison with a 2-incision technique. Arthroscopy 2003;19(8):825–32.

34. Patel DV, Allen AA, Warren RF, Wickiewicz TL, Simonian PT. The nonoperative treatment of acute, isolated (partial or complete) posterior cruciate ligament-deficient knees: an intermediate-term follow-up study. HSS J 2007;3(2):137–46.

35. Roth JH, Bray RC, Best TM, Cunning LA, Jacobson RP. Posterior cruciate ligament reconstruction by transfer of the medial gastrocnemius tendon. Am J Sports Med. 1988;16(1):21–8.

36. Seon JK, Song EK. Reconstruction of isolated posterior cruciate ligament injuries: a clinical comparison of the transtibial and tibial inlay techniques. Arthroscopy. 2006;22(1):27–32.

37. Shirakura K, Terauchi M, Higuchi H, Takagishi K, Kobayashi Y, Kimura M. Knee stability after repair of isolated midsubstance tears of the posterior cruciate ligament. J Orthop Surg (Hong Kong) 2001;9(2):31–6.

38. Zhao J, Huangfu X. Arthroscopic single-bundle posterior cruciate ligament reconstruction: Retrospective review of 4- versus 7-strand hamstring tendon graft. Knee 2007;14(4):301–5.

39. Race A, Amis AA. PCL reconstruction. In vitro biomechanical comparison of "isometric" versus single and double-bundled "anatomic" grafts. J Bone Joint Surg Br 1998;80(1):173–9.

40. Watsend AM, Osestad TM, Jakobsen RB, et al. Clinical studies on posterior cruciate ligament tears have weak design. Knee Surg Sports Traumatol Arthrosc 2009;17(2):140–9.

97

Operative vs. Nonoperative Treatment of Combined Anterior Cruciate Ligament and Medial Collateral Ligament Injuries

Rocco Papalia[1], Sebastiano Vasta[1], Vincenzo Denaro[1], and Nicola Maffulli[2]

[1]Campus Bio–Medico University, Rome, Italy
[2]Barts and The London School of Medicine and Dentistry, London, UK

Case scenario

A 27 year old woman came to the outpatient clinic describing symptoms of her left knee giving out from under her and pain.

Relevant anatomy

There are four major ligaments in the knee. Ligaments are elastic bands of tissue that connect bones to each other and provide stability and strength to the joint. The four main ligaments in the knee, connecting the femur to the tibia, are:

• *anterior cruciate ligament* (ACL): the ligament that controls rotation and forward movement of the tibia; located in the center of the knee

• *posterior cruciate ligament* (PCL): the ligament that controls backward movement of the tibia; located in the center of the knee

• *medial collateral ligament* (MCL): the ligament that gives stability to the inner knee. The MCL provides the primary restraint to valgus stress at both 5° and 25° of flexion from full hyperextension while the cruciate ligaments, primary the ACL, are important secondary restraints to lateral opening of the knee joint, especially at 5° of flexion[1]

• *lateral collateral ligament* (LCL): the ligament that gives stability to the outer knee

Importance of the problem

The incidence of knee ligament ruptures, primarily involving the ACL and MCL, is estimated to be 2 per 1,000 people per year in the general population.[2,3] The incidence of combined ACL–MCL tears range from 20%[4] to 38%[5] of all knee ligament injuries. From 60,000 to 175,000 ACL tears occur annually in the United States.[2,3] A Google search for "combined ACL MCL injuries" returned a total of 128,000 hits.

Top six questions

1. How does an ACL–MCL tear occur?
2. What are the risk factors?
3. What is the accuracy of clinical examination in the diagnosis of ACL–MCL tears?
4. What is the best diagnostic tool for ACL–MCL tears?
5. What is the treatment for ACL–MCL tears?
6. What about the use of prophylactic devices?

Question 1: How does an ACL–MCL tear occur?

Case clarification
The patient mentions having fallen while skiing 2 months before. At the time of the injury she heard a "pop" followed by about 4 days of knee pain and swelling, which forced her to remain immobile.

Relevance
The majority of ACL–MCL disruptions are sustained during sport activities.

Finding the evidence
• Cochrane Database, with search terms: "ACL–MCL injury mechanism," "ACL injury," "ACL–MCL rupture biomechanics"
• PubMed (www.ncbi.nlm.nih.gov/pubmed/) clinical queries search/systematic reviews: "ACL–MCL injury

Evidence-Based Orthopedics, First Edition. Edited by Mohit Bhandari.
© 2012 Blackwell Publishing Ltd. Published 2012 by Blackwell Publishing Ltd.

mechanism," "ACL injury," "ACL–MCL rupture biomechanics"

Quality of the evidence

Level I
- 1 clinical trial[6]
- 1 systematic review[7]
- 1 book[1]

Findings

Ligament injuries are closely related to sport traumas.[6] Combined ACL–MCL injuries are often the result of concomitant rotational and valgus stress. Combination injuries involving both the ACL and the MCL may occur during contact sports such as a football, soccer, or rugby tackle, or in noncontact situations, particularly in an athlete who is making an abrupt pivot in which the tibia goes into valgus relatively to the femur. This type of injury results from a deceleration maneuver in which the forces can be substantial.[1,7]

Recommendation

- A combined ACL–MCL lesion rather than an isolated ACL lesion should be suspected in patients playing sports that put them at risk of knee rotational and valgus stress maneuvers [overall quality: high]

Question 2: What are the risk factors?

Case clarification

Two weeks after the trauma, feeling good, the patient resumed playing sports, and while playing basketball she had the first episode of her knee giving out.

Relevance

Sport is an important risk factor for ACL–MCL injuries, but many recent studies have showed that sex and anatomical features can favor ligament rupture.

Finding the evidence

- Cochrane Database, with search term "ACL AND MCL AND risk factors," "sex AND ligament injury," "femoral notch stenosis AND ACL injuries"
- PubMed (www.ncbi.nlm.nih.gov/pubmed/) clinical queries search/systematic reviews: "ACL AND MCL AND risk factors," "sex AND ligament injury," "femoral notch stenosis AND ACL injuries"

Quality of the evidence

Level I
- 1 meta-analysis[8]

Level II
- 7 prospective comparative studies[9–12,14–16]

Level V
- 1 expert opinion[13]

Findings

High-risk sports for ACL injuries are basketball, soccer, alpine skiing, lacrosse, football, handball, Australian rules football, rugby, volleyball, and wrestling.[8]

Female athletes have a higher risk of tearing the ACL,[9–11] as a result of multiple factors such as biomechanical, neuromuscular, physiologic, hormonal, and anatomical mechanisms.[11,12] In particular, with maturity, women experience worsening of their neuromuscular joint control.[13]

Some studies have demonstrated a relation between a narrow femoral intercondylar notch, measured as a smaller notch width index (NWI) on radiographs and CT scans, and a higher risk of ACL injuries.[14–16]

Recommendation

- A combined ACL–MCL lesion should be suspected in female athletes, in patients playing sports that have a high risk for ligament injuries, and in patients with a previous diagnosis of narrow femoral intercondylar notch or in whom the radiographs or CT scans show a smaller NWI during the diagnostic process [overall quality: moderate]

Question 3: How can we diagnose ACL–MCL injury?

Case clarification

On examination, performing the anterior drawer and the Lachman tests on both knees, abnormal anterior laxity was detected in the injured left knee. Also, there was a grade III positive valgus stress test.

Relevance

Many clinical diagnostic tests are available to diagnose ligament injuries.

Finding the evidence

- Cochrane Database, with search terms: " clinical test ACL injury," "clinical test MCL injury," physical diagnostic tests ACL MCL injury," "accuracy ligament diagnostic test"
- PubMed (www.ncbi.nlm.nih.gov/pubmed/) clinical queries search/systematic reviews: " clinical test ACL injury," "clinical test MCL injury," physical diagnostic tests ACL MCL injury," "accuracy ligament diagnostic test"

Quality of the evidence

Level I
- 1 meta-analysis[24]

Level II
- 1 descriptive study[23]
- 1 book[22]

Findings

Generally the diagnostic process includes history-taking, physical examination, and MRI of the knee. Accurate history-taking must be done to investigate the symptoms and the mechanism of the injury. Physical examination follows, and includes the assessment of range of motion (ROM), the palpation of the bony structure to exclude associated tibial plateau fractures, palpation of the joint lines to evaluate a possible associated meniscal tear (the frequency of meniscal injuries range from 16% to 82% in acute ligament tears and 96% in knees with chronic ligament tears[17–21]), and finally tests to assess knee laxity. The most commonly used are the valgus stress test, Lachman's test, and the anterior drawer test.

The valgus stress test assesses the integrity of the MCL complex (superficial and deep MCL fibers), and makes it possible to establish the degree of the lesion (see box).[22] A study by Kastelein et al. evaluated the reliability of "pain valgus stress test (PVST)" and "laxity valgus stress test (LVST)" comparing them with MRI data. The sensitivity and specificity were 0.78 (0.64–0.92) and 0.67 (0.57–0.76) respectively for the PVST, and 0.91 (0.81–1.00) and 0.49 (0.39–0.59) respectively for the LVST.[23]

Classical method of grading MCL injuries using the valgus stress test[22]

- **Grade I:** The MCL is tender and swollen but exhibits no increased laxity, it signifies an injury without elongation of ligament
- **Grade II:** The MCL is elongated but not completely disrupted; there is increased laxity to the valgus stress test but with a firm endpoint
- **Grade III:** The MCL has lost all structural integrity so there is laxity without an endpoint

---

Lachman's test and the anterior drawer test are the two most basic tests for abnormal anterior knee laxity that is related to ACL injury.[22] A meta-analysis by Scholten et al. has shown good reliability of these tests in diagnosing ACL injuries. The Lachman's test sensitivity ranges from 0.63 to 0.93 and its specificity from 0.55 to 0.99. According to the bivariate random effects model, the pooled sensitivity is 0.86 and the specificity 0.91. The sensitivity of the anterior drawer test ranges from 0.18 to 0.92 and its specificity from 0.78 to 0.9. According to the bivariate random effects model, the pooled sensitivity is 0.62 and the specificity 0.88.[24]

The pivot shift test is a dynamic test that demonstrates the subluxation occurring when the ACL is nonfunctional.[22] The sensitivity of the pivot shift test ranges from 0.18 to 0.48 and its specificity from 0.97 to 0.99.[24]

Recommendations

In patients with suspected ACL–MCL injury, the evidence suggests [overall quality: high]:
- The diagnostic process should include accurate history-taking
- Physical examination should assess ROM
- Suspected MCL lesions should be addressed by the valgus stress test for the MCL
- Suspected ACL lesions should be addressed by the Lachman's test, the anterior drawer test, and the pivot shift test

Question 4: What is the best diagnostic tool for ACL–MCL tears?

Case clarification

An MRI was prescribed for a suspected diagnosis of ACL and MCL injury.

Relevance

A diagnostic tool is useful to confirm clinical suspicion of a ligament injury. MRI is a noninvasive and safe tool to establish the diagnosis.

Finding the evidence

- Cochrane Database, with search terms: "diagnosis MCL injury," "MRI AND MCL injury diagnosis"
- PubMed (www.ncbi.nlm.nih.gov/pubmed/) clinical queries search/systematic reviews: "diagnosis MCL injury," "MRI AND MCL injury diagnosis"

Quality of the evidence

Level II
- 2 descriptive studies[25,26]

Findings

MRI is an appropriate diagnostic tool for the evaluation of internal derangement of the knee. It is very useful in assessing the location and the severity of the injury (Table 97.1). A descriptive study by Halinen et al.[25] has shown MRI to have an accuracy and sensitivity of 93.2% for ACL tears and 86.4% for MCL tears.

Recommendation

- In patients with suspected ACL–MCL injury, MRI is a reliable diagnostic tool [overall quality: high]

Question 5: What is the treatment for ACL–MCL tears?

Case clarification

Because MRI confirmed the diagnosis of an ACL–MCL injury, the patient was surgically treated with an arthroscopic reconstruction of the ACL and MCL.

Table 97.1 Method of grading MCL injury by MRI[26]

Grade	MRI findings
I (minor tearing of ligament fibers)	Periligamentous swelling without complete disruption of superficial or deep layer
II (complete disruption of superficial layer)	Periligamentous swelling with complete disruption of superficial layer
III (complete disruption of superficial and deep layer)	Same as grade II but with fluid extravasating from the joint into the periligamentous tissue

Relevance

The management of combined ACL–MCL injuries is widely debated. The possible options are: full conservative MCL–ACL treatment, full surgical MCL–ACL treatment, combined surgical MCL and conservative ACL treatment, and combined conservative MCL and surgical ACL treatment (Table 97.2).

Finding the evidence

• Cochrane Database, with search terms: "ACL" and "MCL" in combination with "surgery treatment," "conservative treatment," "surgery management," "conservative management," "surgical treatment," and "surgical management"

Table 97.2 Relevant data of each study on ACL–MCL combined tears

Author	n	MCL		Treatment		Outcome
		Grade	Diagnosis	MCL injury	ACL injury	
Osti et al.[37]	22	II	MVST at 30° and valgus stress radiograph at 20°	Surgery	Surgery	After 24 months from surgery, clinical and functional variables were significantly improved and 90% of patients returns to preinjury sport activity level
Andersson et al.[42]	167	—	—	Combined	Combined	The score distributions showed that 82% of surgically treated groups of patients had a total score of 84 points or more, compared to 64% in the nonsurgically treated
Andersson and Gillquist[43]	107	II–III	MVST at 30°	Surgery	Combined	Patients who had primary ACL repair returned to a higher level of competitive sports than patients who had undergone conservative ACL treatment
Schierl et al.[53]	28	I–II	MVST at 30° and valgus stress radiograph	Conservative	Surgery	The mean Lyshom score was 95.0 ranging from 79 to 100. Subjective findings and functional outcome in patients with ACL instability or combined ACL–MCL lesions were the same
Shelbourne and Porter[44]	84	—	MVST at 30°	Conservative	Surgery	Patients regained ROM, strenght equal to uninjured leg and ligamentous instability
Zaffagnini et al.[35]	57	II	IKDC grading	Conservative	Surgery	Postoperative varus-valgus laxity at 30° of flexion was approximately 1° greater in patients with ACL–MCL combined lesions than in patients with ACL lesion
Hara et al.[36]	342	II	IKDC grading	Conservative	Surgery	No clinically significant difference regarding outcome between patient with ACL–MCL combined lesion and patients with isolated ACL lesion
Jokl et al.[32]	28	III	Medial joint opening at valgus stress radiograph	Conservative	Conservative	68% of patients returns to pre injury sport activity level and no significant change in the Hospital for Special Surgery Knee assessment form was noted with the passage of the time
Frolke et al.[41]	22	III	MVST at 25° (medial joint opening .10 mm)	Surgery	Conservative	After surgical treatment of MCL and conservative treatment of ACL a considerable improvement was observed in pivot shift, Lachman, and total AP translation
Robins et al.[45]	20	I		Surgery	Surgery	Patients with a distal lesion of MCL had a more rapid return to motion both for flexion and extension than patient with proximal MCL lesion

(Continued)

Table 97.2 (*Continued*)

Author	n	MCL		Treatment		Outcome
		Grade	Diagnosis	MCL injury	ACL injury	
Nakamura et al.[46]	17	II–III	MRI	Combined	Surgery	There was no significant difference between patients who underwent ACL surgical repair and patient who underwent ACL–MCL surgical group
Petersen and Laprell[40]	64	III	MVST without endpoint	Conservative	Surgery	The Lysholm score was significantily better in the group with late ACL reconstruction than in the group with early ACL reconstruction
Halinen[39]	47	III	—	Combined	Surgery	There were no significant differences in IKDC scores of the patients who underwent surgically repair of MCL and patient who underwent nonoperative treatment of MCL
Hillard et al.[47]	66	II–III	MVST at 20°(medial joint opening, 3–5 mm side to side difference for grade II)	Conservative	Surgery	There was no differences in stability or function
Lundberg and Messner[6]	40	I–III	Valgus stress test	Combined	Combined	There was no significant differences in Lysholm score among patients with isolated MCL tear and patients with combined ACL–MCL tear
Ballmer et al.[48]	14	—	Medial joint opening at valgus stress radiograph	Conservative	Surgery	Both clinical and radiological stability were almost normal and all patient had returned to their preinjury activities
Yoshiya et al.[34]	24	III	Medial joint opening at valgus stress radiograph	Surgery	Surgery	Statistically significant improvement in medial stability and ROM were observed in postoperative follow-up and they graded almost normal in all patients according to IKDC evaluation system
Shirakura et al.[54]	25	II–III	Manual valgus stess test at 0° and 30° Grade I–III)	Combined	Conservative	Higher functional levels were observed in patients treated with surgical MCL repair
Sankar et al.[49]	180	II–III	Medial joint opening at valgus stress test (5–10 mm Grade II)	Conservative	Surgery	No significant differences were shown in Lysholm score between patients with ACL/MCL combined injury and patients with isolated ACL injury. All patients returned to their preinjury sport activity level
Noyes and Barber-Westin[50]	46	I–III	MVST at 5° and 25° (medial joint opening, side to side difference)	Combined	Surgery	Overall rating was 58% excellent or good and 42% fair or poor for operatively treated MCL tear patients while it was 91% excellent or good and 9% fair for nonoperatively treated MCL tear patients
Hughston JC[38]	41	III	MVST at 30°	Surgery	Surgery	38 on 41 patients had good stability and normal ROM as well as little or no muscle atrophy and most of the patients had maintained a high level of physical fitness and athletic activity
Mok and Good[51]	25	III	—	Conservative	Conservative	All 25 patients had good or excellent results, with return to the preinjury level of sporting activities by 1 year and with restoration of medial stability
Millet et al.[52]	18	—	—	Conservative	Surgery	Patients showed a mean Lysholm score of 94.5 and a mean Tegner activity score of 8.4. Serial clinical examinations demonstrated good functional outcomes,ROM, and strength

IKDC, International Knee Documentation Committee score; MVST, manual valgus stress test; ROM, range of motion.

- PubMed (www.ncbi.nlm.nih.gov/pubmed/) clinical queries: "ACL" and "MCL" in combination with "surgery treatment," "conservative treatment," "surgery management," "conservative management," "surgical treatment," and "surgical management"

Quality of the evidence
Level I
- 23 clinical trials[3,32,34–52]

Current opinion
Isolated and partial injuries of the MCL can be treated nonoperatively given the good healing properties of this ligament.[27–34] In contrast, the management of MCL injuries combined with other ligaments is still controversial.

Grade II MCL lesions Zaffagnini et al.[35] showed that residual laxity remain in patients with injured ACL–MCL successively treated with operative ACL reconstruction, raising the question of addressing the MCL.

In the study by Hara et al.,[36] 90% of patients with ACL injury associated with grade II valgus laxity in whom the ACL was operatively reconstructed regained medial stability with nonoperative management of MCL. The authors believed that it was not necessary to implement a combined ACL–MCL operative treatment.

Osti et al.[37] treated operatively, in the same surgical setting, 22 patients with chronic ACL injury and chronic grade II valgus instability. After 24 months from surgery, clinical and functional variables were significantly improved, and 90% of patients returned to preinjury sport activity level. For these reasons, the authors recommend surgical management of both ACL and MCL as a safe and reliable option.

Grade III MCL lesions In the series of Hughston et al.,[38] of the 41 patients with grade III valgus instability managed surgically with repair of the posterior oblique ligament and the semimembranosus complex, only 3 continued to have mild or moderate instability which impaired function. In two of these patients, the original repair had been a technical failure. This technique provides good long-term results.

Yoshiya et al.[34] used autogenous hamstring tendons to surgically repair injured MCL on 24 patients. At follow-up, 20 patients were stable to valgus stress test, while 4 were mildly unstable.

Halinen et al.[39] treated 47 patients with combined ACL and grade III MCL injury. The follow-up data suggest that nonsurgical and surgical management of MCL tears leads to equivalent results, and that the MCL does not need to be surgically repaired when the ACL undergoes early reconstruction.

In the study of Petersen et Laprell,[40] on 64 patients with combined ACL–MCL injury, 37 patients had late operative ACL reconstruction and 27 had early operative ACL. All had nonoperative MCL treatment. At 22 months from surgery, no difference in the frequency of anterior or medial instabilities or in the loss of motion were seen, but a lower rate of motion complications in the early postoperative period, lower rate of rearthroscopies, and significantly better results in the Lysholm score were seen in the group treated with late ACL reconstruction. The authors prefer late ACL reconstruction in combined injuries of the ACL and the MCL.

Frolke et al.[41] undertook primary operative repair of the MCL and conservative management of the ACL injury on 22 patients. In a follow-up at 2.5 years, testing of the MCL showed a change from 22 severely abnormal knees to 17 normal and 5 nearly normal knees.

In the study of Jokl et al.,[32] 28 patients with an ACL–MCL combined injury were managed conservatively. After a mean follow-up of 3 years (ranging from 8 months to 11 years), 68% of patients had returned to preinjury sport activity levels, with significant changes in the Hospital for Special Surgery Knee assessment form with the passage of time. No data are available on valgus stability. The authors support conservative management as a valid therapeutic option.

Given the lack of standardization in the selection process of patients, outcome criteria, and outcome assessment, the question about which is the best treatment for ACL–MCL combined injuries still remains open.

Recommendations
- In patients with suspected ACL–MCL injury, isolated partial injuries of the MCL can be managed nonoperatively [overall quality: moderate]
- There are no differences in outcomes when an ACL injury associated with grade II valgus laxity is addressed by surgical reconstruction of ACL and conservative measures or surgical repair of MCL [overall quality: moderate]
- Comparable results are achieved with conservative measure or with surgical repair in combined ACL–MCL injuries with grade III valgus laxity. Early or late ACL reconstruction is still controversial [overall quality: moderate]

Question 6: What about the use of prophylactic devices?

Relevance
For the last 30 years, knee braces have been used to assist individuals with ACL deficiency and ACL-reconstructed knees. Knee bracing may have a prophylactic role in preventing knee ligament injuries.

Finding the evidence
- Cochrane Database, with search term "knee ligament injury prophylactic devices"

• PubMed (www.ncbi.nlm.nih.gov/pubmed/) clinical queries search/systematic reviews: knee ligament injury prophylactic devices"

Quality of the evidence

Level I

• 1 systematic review[55]

Findings

Rishiraj et al.[55] reviewed several studies with a protective effect of functional knee bracing (FKB) on knee ligaments injuries. However, the exact mechanism that may protect the knee ligaments is unknown, because of a lack of studies on FKB worn during competitive sport, probably because of the fear of performance hindrance.

Recommendation

• In patients with suspected ACL–MCL injury, there is evidence for a protective role of knee bracing devices but only in the noninjured population [overall quality: low]

Summary of recommendations

• A combined ACL–MCL lesion rather than an isolated ACL lesion should be suspected in patients playing sports that put them at risk of knee rotational and valgus stress maneuvers

• A combined ACL–MCL lesion should be suspected in female athletes, in patients playing sports that have a high risk for ligament injuries, and in patients with a previous diagnosis of narrow femoral intercondylar notch or in whom the radiographs or CT scans show a smaller NWI during the diagnostic process

• In patients with suspected ACL–MCL injury, the diagnostic process should include accurate history-taking and physical examination should assess ROM

• Suspected MCL lesions should be addressed by the valgus stress test for the MCL

• Suspected ACL lesions should be addressed by the Lachman's test, the anterior drawer test, and the pivot shift test

• MRI is a reliable diagnostic tool

• Isolated partial injuries of the MCL can be managed nonoperatively

• There are no differences in outcomes when an ACL injury associated with grade II valgus laxity is addressed by surgical reconstruction of ACL and conservative measures or surgical repair of MCL

• Comparable results are achieved with conservative measure or with surgical repair in combined ACL–MCL injuries with grade III valgus laxity. Early or late ACL reconstruction is still controversial

• In patients with suspected ACL–MCL injury, there is evidence for a protective role of knee bracing devices but only in the noninjured population

References

1. Siliski JM. Traumatic Disorders of the Knee, pp. 303–4. Springer, New York, 1994.
2. Spindler KP, Wright RW. Clinical practice. Anterior cruciate ligament tear. N Engl J Med 2008;359(20):2135–42.
3. Frank CB, Jackson DW. The science of reconstruction of the anterior cruciate ligament. J Bone Joint Surg Am 1997;79(10):1556–76.
4. Myasaka KC, Daniel D, Stone M, Hirschmann P. The incidence of knee ligament injuries in the general population. Am J Knee Surg 1991;4(4):3–8.
5. Duncan JB, Hunter R, Purnell M, Freeman J. Meniscal injuries associated with acute anterior cruciate ligament tears in alpine skiers. Am J Sports Med 1995;23(2):170–2.
6. Lundberg M, Messner K. Ten-year prognosis of isolated and combined medial collateral ligament ruptures. A matched comparison in 40 patients using clinical and radiographic evaluations. Am J Sports Med 1997;25(1):2–6.
7. Alentorn-Geli E, Myer GD, Silvers HJ, et al. Prevention of non-contact anterior cruciate ligament injuries in soccer players. Part 1: Mechanisms of injury and underlying risk factors. Knee Surg Sports Traumatol Arthrosc 2009;17(7):705–29.
8. Prodromos CC, Han Y, Rogowski J, Joyce B, Shi K. A meta-analysis of the incidence of anterior cruciate ligament tears as a function of gender, sport, and a knee injury-reduction regimen. Arthroscopy 2007;23(12):1320–25 e6.
9. Lim BO, Lee YS, Kim JG, An KO, Yoo J, Kwon YH. Effects of sports injury prevention training on the biomechanical risk factors of anterior cruciate ligament injury in high school female basketball players. Am J Sports Med 2009;37(9):1728–34.
10. Tanaka Y, Yonetani Y, Shiozaki Y, et al. Retear of anterior cruciate ligament grafts in female basketball players: a case series. Sports Med Arthrosc Rehabil Ther Technol;2:7.
11. Arendt E, Dick R. Knee injury patterns among men and women in collegiate basketball and soccer. NCAA data and review of literature. Am J Sports Med 1995;23(6):694–701.
12. Hewett TE, Myer GD, Ford KR. Decrease in neuromuscular control about the knee with maturation in female athletes. J Bone Joint Surg Am 2004;86-A(8):1601–8.
13. Hewett TE. Predisposition to ACL injuries in female athletes versus male athletes. Orthopedics 2008;31(1):26–8.
14. Shelbourne KD, Davis TJ, Klootwyk TE. The relationship between intercondylar notch width of the femur and the incidence of anterior cruciate ligament tears. A prospective study. Am J Sports Med 1998;26(3):402–8.
15. Anderson AF, Lipscomb AB, Liudahl KJ, Addlestone RB. Analysis of the intercondylar notch by computed tomography. Am J Sports Med 1987;15(6):547–52.
16. Stein V, Li L, Guermazi A, et al. The relation of femoral notch stenosis to ACL tears in persons with knee osteoarthritis. Osteoarthritis Cartilage;18(2):192–9.

17. Bellabarba C, Bush-Joseph CA, Bach BR, Jr. Patterns of meniscal injury in the anterior cruciate-deficient knee: a review of the literature. Am J Orthop (Belle Mead NJ) 1997;26(1):18–23.

18. Shoemaker SC, Markolf KL. The role of the meniscus in the anterior-posterior stability of the loaded anterior cruciate-deficient knee. Effects of partial versus total excision. J Bone Joint Surg Am 1986;68(1):71–9.

19. Thompson WO, Fu FH. The meniscus in the cruciate-deficient knee. Clin Sports Med 1993;12(4):771–96.

20. Warren RF, Levy IM. Meniscal lesions associated with anterior cruciate ligament injury. Clin Orthop Relat Res 1983 (172):32–7.

21. Wickiewicz TL. Meniscal injuries in the cruciate-deficient knee. Clin Sports Med 1990;9(3):681–94.

22. Reider B. Traumatic disorders of the knee. In: The Orthopaedic Physical Exam, pp. 227–32. Elsevier Saunders Philadelphia, 2005.

23. Kastelein M, Wagemakers HP, Luijsterburg PA, et al. Assessing medial collateral ligament knee lesions in general practice. Am J Med 2008;121(11):982–88 e2.

24. Scholten RJ, Opstelten W, van der Plas CG, Bijl D, Deville WL, Bouter LM. Accuracy of physical diagnostic tests for assessing ruptures of the anterior cruciate ligament: a meta-analysis. J Fam Pract 2003;52(9):689–94.

25. Halinen J, Koivikko M, Lindahl J, Hirvensalo E. The efficacy of magnetic resonance imaging in acute multi-ligament injuries. Int Orthop 2009;33(6):1733–8.

26. Rasenberg EI, Lemmens JA, van Kampen A, et al. Grading medial collateral ligament injury: comparison of MR imaging and instrumented valgus-varus laxity test-device. A prospective double-blind patient study. Eur J Radiol 1995;21(1):18–24.

27. Fetto JF, Marshall JL. Medial collateral ligament injuries of the knee: a rationale for treatment. Clin Orthop Relat Res 1978(132):206–18.

28. Indelicato PA. Non-operative treatment of complete tears of the medial collateral ligament of the knee. J Bone Joint Surg Am 1983;65(3):323–9.

29. Jones RE, Henley MB, Francis P. Nonoperative management of isolated grade III collateral ligament injury in high school football players. Clin Orthop Relat Res 1986(213):137–40.

30. Ballmer PM, Jakob RP. The nonoperative treatment of isolated complete tears of the medial collateral ligament of the knee. A prospective study. Arch Orthop Trauma Surg 1988;107(5):273–6.

31. Ellsasser JC, Reynolds FC, Omohundro JR. The non-operative treatment of collateral ligament injuries of the knee in professional football players. An analysis of seventy-four injuries treated non-operatively and twenty-four injuries treated surgically. J Bone Joint Surg Am 1974;56(6):1185–90.

32. Jokl P, Kaplan N, Stovell P, Keggi K. Non-operative treatment of severe injuries to the medial and anterior cruciate ligaments of the knee. J Bone Joint Surg Am 1984;66(5):741–4.

33. Kannus P. Long-term results of conservatively treated medial collateral ligament injuries of the knee joint. Clin Orthop Relat Res 1988(226):103–12.

34. Yoshiya S, Kuroda R, Mizuno K, Yamamoto T, Kurosaka M. Medial collateral ligament reconstruction using autogenous hamstring tendons: technique and results in initial cases. Am J Sports Med 2005;33(9):1380–5.

35. Zaffagnini S, Bignozzi S, Martelli S, Lopomo N, Marcacci M. Does ACL reconstruction restore knee stability in combined lesions? An in vivo study. Clin Orthop Relat Res 2007;454:95–9.

36. Hara K, Niga S, Ikeda H, Cho S, Muneta T. Isolated anterior cruciate ligament reconstruction in patients with chronic anterior cruciate ligament insufficiency combined with grade II valgus laxity. Am J Sports Med 2008;36(2):333–9.

37. Osti L, Papalia R, Del Buono A, Merlo F, Denaro V, Maffulli N. Simultaneous surgical management of chronic grade-2 valgus instability of the knee and anterior cruciate ligament deficiency in athletes. Knee Surg Sports Traumatol Arthrosc;18(3):312–6.

38. Hughston JC. The importance of the posterior oblique ligament in repairs of acute tears of the medial ligaments in knees with and without an associated rupture of the anterior cruciate ligament. Results of long-term follow-up. J Bone Joint Surg Am 1994;76(9):1328–44.

39. Halinen J, Lindahl J, Hirvensalo E, Santavirta S. Operative and nonoperative treatments of medial collateral ligament rupture with early anterior cruciate ligament reconstruction: a prospective randomized study. Am J Sports Med 2006;34(7):1134–40.

40. Petersen W, Laprell H. Combined injuries of the medial collateral ligament and the anterior cruciate ligament. Early ACL reconstruction versus late ACL reconstruction. Arch Orthop Trauma Surg 1999;119(5–6):258–62.

41. Frolke JP, Oskam J, Vierhout PA. Primary reconstruction of the medial collateral ligament in combined injury of the medial collateral and anterior cruciate ligaments. Short-term results. Knee Surg Sports Traumatol Arthrosc 1998;6(2):103–6.

42. Andersson C, Odensten M, Gillquist J. Knee function after surgical or nonsurgical treatment of acute rupture of the anterior cruciate ligament: a randomized study with a long-term follow-up period. Clin Orthop Relat Res 1991(264):255–63.

43. Andersson C, Gillquist J. Treatment of acute isolated and combined ruptures of the anterior cruciate ligament. A long-term follow-up study. Am J Sports Med 1992;20(1):7–12.

44. Shelbourne KD, Porter DA. Anterior cruciate ligament-medial collateral ligament injury: nonoperative management of medial collateral ligament tears with anterior cruciate ligament reconstruction. A preliminary report. Am J Sports Med 1992;20(3):283–6.

45. Robins AJ, Newman AP, Burks RT. Postoperative return of motion in anterior cruciate ligament and medial collateral ligament injuries. The effect of medial collateral ligament rupture location. Am J Sports Med 1993;21(1):20–5.

46. Nakamura N, Horibe S, Toritsuka Y, Mitsuoka T, Yoshikawa H, Shino K. Acute grade III medial collateral ligament injury of the knee associated with anterior cruciate ligament tear. The usefulness of magnetic resonance imaging in determining a treatment regimen. Am J Sports Med 2003;31(2):261–7.

47. Hillard-Sembell D, Daniel DM, Stone ML, Dobson BE, Fithian DC. Combined injuries of the anterior cruciate and medial collateral ligaments of the knee. Effect of treatment on stability and function of the joint. J Bone Joint Surg Am 1996;78(2):169–76.

48. Ballmer PM, Ballmer FT, Jakob RP. Reconstruction of the anterior cruciate ligament alone in the treatment of a combined instability with complete rupture of the medial collateral ligament. A prospective study. Arch Orthop Trauma Surg 1991;110(3):139–41.

49. Sankar WN, Wells L, Sennett BJ, Wiesel BB, Ganley TJ. Combined anterior cruciate ligament and medial collateral ligament injuries in adolescents. J Pediatr Orthop 2006;26(6):733–6.

50. Noyes FR, Barber-Westin SD. The treatment of acute combined ruptures of the anterior cruciate and medial ligaments of the knee. Am J Sports Med 1995;23(4):380–9.

51. Mok DW, Good C. Non-operative management of acute grade III medial collateral ligament injury of the knee: a prospective study. Injury 1989;20(5):277–80.

52. Millett PJ, Pennock AT, Sterett WI, Steadman JR. Early ACL reconstruction in combined ACL–MCL injuries. J Knee Surg 2004;17(2):94–8.

53. Schierl M, Petermann J, Trus P, Baumgartel F, Gotzen L. Anterior cruciate and medial collateral ligament injury. ACL reconstruction and functional treatment of the MCL. Knee Surg Sports Traumatol Arthrosc 1994;2(4):203–6.

54. Shirakura K, Terauchi M, Katayama M, Watanabe H, Yamaji T, Takagishi K. The management of medial ligament tears in patients with combined anterior cruciate and medial ligament lesions. Int Orthop 2000;24(2):108–11.

55. Rishiraj N, Taunton JE, Lloyd-Smith R, Woollard R, Regan W, Clement DB. The potential role of prophylactic/functional knee bracing in preventing knee ligament injury. Sports Med 2009; 39(11):937–60.

98 Posterolateral Corner Injury

Pankaj Sharma[1] and Daniel B. Whelan[2]
[1]University of Toronto, Toronto, ON, Canada
[2]St Michael's Hospital, Toronto, ON, Canada

Case scenario

A 32 year old hockey player injured his knee 8 months ago. He now complains of posterolateral knee pain, and is unable to play hockey. His knee hyperextends when going up and down stairs, and gives way with twisting and pivoting activities.

Relevant anatomy

Posterolateral corner (PLC) anatomy is complex, and has only recently been fully elucidated. Historically, confusion surrounded the anatomical relationship of PLC structures secondary to the use of inconsistent terminology.

Seebacher et al.[1] performed a cadaveric study of 35 knees, which helped delineate the complex structural arrangement of the PLC. They described a three-layered arrangement in which the most superficial layer is composed of the iliotibial band and the superficial portion of biceps femoris. The middle layer is made up of the patellomeniscal ligament along with the quadriceps retinaculum anteriorly and the two patellofemoral ligaments posteriorly. The third and deepest layer is divided into a superficial lamina composed of the lateral collateral ligament (LCL) and the fabellofibular ligament. The deep lamina contains the popliteofibular ligament (PFL), the arcuate ligament, and the popliteus muscle. However, significant anatomical variability exists, which confuses matters further. One study demonstrated that only 68% of 50 cadaveric knees had a fabellofibular ligament and the arcuate ligament was present in just 24% of cases.[2]

The main stabilizers of the PLC are the LCL, PFL, and the popliteus muscle–tendon unit. Injury to these structures results in increased varus laxity, increased external rotation laxity, and increased posterior tibial translation. More recent surgical techniques aim to anatomically reconstruct these three structures.

Importance of the problem

Injuries to the PLC are rare but severely debilitating. Isolated PLC injuries are even rarer. Delee[3] found that only 12 (1.6%) out of 735 knee ligament injury patients had acute isolated posterolateral instability. LaPrade found a similar incidence of 2.1%; only 4 out of 331 consecutive patients with an acute knee injury resulting in hemarthrosis had an isolated PLC injury.[4]

Surgeons should be aware of potential PLC injury, as it has been established that unrecognized or untreated posterolateral instability is the commonest cause for failure of cruciate ligament reconstruction. Noyes and coworkers found 17 of 76 patients undergoing anterior cruciate ligament (ACL) revision surgery had unrecognized PLC injury.[5]

Google searches for "knee posterolateral corner injury" and "knee posterolateral corner reconstruction" generate respectively 38,000 and 58,800 results. As these links are often of uncertain quality, there is need for high-quality, evidence-based guides.

Top five questions

Diagnosis

1. How reliable is clinical examination in the diagnosis of PLC injury?
2. How accurate is MRI for the evaluation of PLC injury?

Evidence-Based Orthopedics, First Edition. Edited by Mohit Bhandari.
© 2012 Blackwell Publishing Ltd. Published 2012 by Blackwell Publishing Ltd.

Therapy

3. What are the indications for nonoperative management for PLC injury?
4. Does acute surgical repair give better results than reconstruction for the management of PLC injury?
5. What is the best method of reconstruction for PLC injury?

Question 1: How reliable is clinical examination in the diagnosis of PLC injury?

Relevance

Accurate diagnosis of ligamentous injury of the knee allows an appropriate management plan to be formulated.

Current opinion

Several clinical tests have been described to evaluate PLC injury. However, limited data exists on the reliability of these tests and they rely on subjective assessment.

Finding the evidence

• Cochrane Database, with search term: "posterolateral corner injury"
• PubMed (www.ncbi.nlm.nih.gov/pubmed/) clinical queries search: "posterolateral knee instability and clinical tests"
• PubMed (www.ncbi.nlm.nih.gov/pubmed/): sensitivity search using keywords "posterolateral corner injury" AND "clinical evaluation"
• Citations from relevant articles captured by the search

Quality of the evidence

Level IV
• 3 case series[6–8]

Findings

Hughston et al.[6] found that 84% of 140 patients with chronic posterolateral rotatory instability of the knee had a positive external rotation recurvatum test, and 80% had a positive posterolateral drawer test. Overall, 72% of knees had a positive result for both tests.

In 71 patients, LaPrade et al.[7] found a positive result for the posterolateral external rotation test performed at 90° of knee flexion and external rotation recurvatum test in 54 (76%) and 52 (73%) knees respectively. However, a positive result was not associated with injury to any specific PLC structure (p > 0.05). The posterolateral external rotation test performed at 90° of knee flexion is a variation of Hughston and Norwood's posterolateral drawer test. Therefore, although these tests confirm injury to the PLC, they are unable to diagnose which structures are damaged.

More recently, LaPrade et al.[8] reported that only 10 out of 134 patients with grade III PLC injury had a positive external rotation recurvatum test. All 10 patients had a combined PLC and ACL injury, which was confirmed at the time of surgery. Overall the test was only positive in 30% of patients with a combined PLC and ACL injury (n = 33), and was not positive in any patients with isolated PLC injury or combined PLC and PCL injury. Therefore, in this study in which examination was performed in a clinical setting on conscious patients, the external rotation recurvatum test was shown to be very inaccurate in predicting a PLC injury.

Recommendations

• Clinical tests for assessing the PLC should be interpreted carefully as a significant number of patients with negative results may still have a PLC injury
• The overall evidence presented here is poor, as it is based on relatively small numbers of patients. In addition, there are also some conflicting findings from these studies

Question 2: How accurate is MRI for the evaluation of PLC injury?

Case clarification

Clinical examination reveals grade 3+ laxity on varus stress testing with the knee in 30° of flexion. In addition there is a positive external rotation recurvatum test. Plain radiographs of the knee demonstrate a small avulsion fracture of the fibular head. Ligament injury grading is based on the nomenclature described by DeLee et al.[3] in 1983 (see box).

> **Ligament injury grading[3]**
>
> • 1+: 0–5 mm with definite endpoint to stress
> • 2+: 5–10 mm with definite endpoint to stress
> • 3+: >10 mm of joint opening with no or soft endpoint to stress

Relevance

Accurate diagnosis of ligamentous injury of the knee allows an appropriate management plan to be formulated.

Current opinion

Routine MRI scan is sought in the evaluation of almost all knee ligament injuries, as clinical examination cannot reliably determine which component of the PLC has been damaged. A fibular head fracture (arcuate fracture) is considered to be pathognomonic for PLC injury.

Finding the evidence

• Cochrane Database, with search term "posterolateral corner injury"
• PubMed (www.ncbi.nlm.nih.gov/pubmed/) clinical queries search: "knee posterolateral AND MRI" and "arcuate fracture AND MRI"
• PubMed (www.ncbi.nlm.nih.gov/pubmed/): sensitivity search using keywords "posterolateral knee" AND "magnetic resonance imaging"
• Citations from relevant articles captured by the search

Quality of the evidence
Level IV
- 5 case series[9–13]

Findings
Miller and coworkers[9] found that 30 of 481 patients undergoing MRI for evaluation of internal derangement of the knee had injury to at least one PLC structure. Of these 30 patients the LCL was injured in 19 cases and popliteus in 16 cases. On the basis of clinical examination only 3 of these 30 patients were suspected to have a PLC injury.

Two studies (n = 20) have correlated MRI findings with examination under anesthesia or surgical findings. Ross et al.[10] found that they were able to accurately diagnose PLC injuries in all of their six cases. Theodorou et al.[11] reported 100% accuracy for diagnosing LCL and gastrocnemius tendon tears 93% for biceps tendon tears and 86% for popliteus tendon tears.

Two studies report on the MRI evaluation of patients found to have an arcuate fracture. Juhng et al.[12] (n = 18) found that in 16 cases there was an injury to at least one cruciate ligament (13 ACL injuries and 12 PCL injuries), and in 9 cases both cruciate ligaments were injured. The popliteus musculotendinous unit was injured in 6 cases. Huang et al.[13] (n = 13) found a popliteus injury in only 1 case, but a PCL injury was noted in all 13 cases; there were no cases of ACL injury. At surgery, 6 of 10 cases were found to have disruption of the arcuate complex. The arcuate complex was defined to consist of the arcuate, popliteofibular and fabellofibular ligaments; however, the authors were unable to assess the integrity of these structures on MRI scan.

Recommendations
- An MRI scan should be obtained in cases of suspected PLC injury, as clinical examination alone can miss injuries
- Clinicians should be aware that although an MRI scan can evaluate larger structures, the small ligaments cannot be confidently assessed
- In the presence of an arcuate fracture an MRI scan should be performed, as there is a high incidence of associated cruciate ligament injury
- The overall level of evidence presented here is low, as it is based on only a few studies with small numbers of patients

Question 3: What are the indications for nonoperative management for PLC injury?

Relevance
If some types of PLC injury have a satisfactory outcome with nonoperative management, then surgery can be avoided for certain patients.

Current opinion
Surgery should be reserved for symptomatic patients with significant instability on clinical examination

Finding the evidence
- Cochrane Database, with search term "posterolateral corner injury"
- PubMed (www.ncbi.nlm.nih.gov/pubmed/) clinical queries search: "posterolateral corner injury AND non operative management"
- PubMed (www.ncbi.nlm.nih.gov/pubmed/): sensitivity search using keywords "knee lateral ligament" AND "non operative management"
- Citations from relevant articles captured by the search

Quality of the evidence
Level IV
- 2 case series[14,15]

Findings
Kannus reported nonoperative management for 11 grade II and 12 grade III injuries of the lateral ligament compartment (Newcastle Ottawa Scale 3).[14] Kannus describes the lateral ligament compartment to consist of the middle third of the lateral capsular ligament and the arcuate complex, which in turn comprised the LCL, arcuate ligament, popliteus muscle, and the lateral head of gastrocnemius. Patients were immobilized for a variable period of time (grade II 2–5 weeks, grade III 2–7 weeks), followed by early rehabilitation which continued for at least 6 months. At follow-up (average 8.3 years) the grade II patients were found to have approximately the same level of laxity as at the time of initial injury (Table 98.1). Patients with grade III injuries fared more poorly and at follow-up the knees were still laterally unstable; 2 patients changed occupation and 2 received a partial pension.

Krukhaug et al. reported on the nonoperative management of 7 patients with primary lateral instability of 1+ (Newcastle Ottawa Scale 5).[15] Six patients were managed with early range of motion and 1 with a cylinder cast for 6 weeks. At follow-up (average 7.5 years), 6 patients had a completely stable knee on varus stressing, and 1 patient treated in cylinder cast had residual laxity of 1+. Median Lysholm score for the stable patients was excellent, at 95.

Recommendations
- In patients with isolated lateral laxity of 1+ or 2+, nonoperative management is likely to lead to a satisfactory result in terms of function and stability
- Patients with lateral laxity of 3+ or with evidence of other instability should be considered for surgery
- The overall level of evidence presented here is low, as it is based on only two studies with a small numbers of patients. Also there is no data on which structures of the PLC were damaged, as MRI scans were not performed

Table 98.1 Results reported by Kannus[14]

Injury grade	Lysholm score	Return to preinjury activity	Post-traumatic OA
Grade II (n = 11)	88 (good)	9	0
Grade III (n = 12)	65 (fair)	2	6

OA, osteoarthritis.

Question 4: Does acute surgical repair give better results than reconstruction for the management of PLC injury?

Relevance
Compelling data on acute repair vs. reconstruction will allow surgeons to perform the procedure which yields better results.

Current opinion
Acute repair is believed to lead to better results, although often a delay in patient presentation precludes repair in favor of surgical reconstruction.

Finding the evidence
• Cochrane Database, with search term "posterolateral corner injury"
• PubMed (www.ncbi.nlm.nih.gov/pubmed/) clinical queries search: "posterolateral corner reconstruction" and "posterolateral corner repair"
• PubMed (www.ncbi.nlm.nih.gov/pubmed/): sensitivity search using keywords "posterolateral corner injury" AND "surgery"
• Citations from relevant articles captured by the search

Quality of the evidence
Level II 1 prospective cohort study[16] (Newcastle Ottawa Scale 6)

Level III 1 retrospective cohort study[17] (Newcastle Ottawa Scale 4)

Level IV 1 case series[18] (Newcastle Ottawa Scale 5)

Findings
In 2005, Stannard et al. reported their prospective cohort study in which there were 57 cases of PLC injury.[16] However, 44 of these patients had sustained high-energy trauma resulting in multiligament knee injury. A total of 13 patients had isolated PLC injury, with or without single cruciate ligament injury. Of these 13 patients, 7 underwent acute repair within 3 weeks of injury; the remaining 6 underwent

reconstruction. None of the 6 reconstructions failed, but 2 of the 7 repairs failed. Although knee scores were reported in this study, they were not broken down according to isolated PLC injury or multiligament injury.

In 2006, Tzurbakis et al. reported follow-up of 44 patients with multiligament injury.[18] A subgroup in this study consisted of 11 patients with single cruciate ligament injury and total PLC rupture. Of these 11 patients 5 underwent acute repair, and 6 underwent reconstruction. Again in this study, results were reported as a composite for the whole group. In general acutely treated patients, scored better in a few areas of the International Knee Documentation Committee (IKDC) score, but this was not statistically significant.

Levy et al. have reported their results on patients with knee multiligament injuries who underwent either repair (n = 10) or reconstruction (n = 18) of the posterolateral structures.[17] The repair group underwent staged surgery; therefore whilst initial surgical repair took place on average 19 days after injury, subsequent cruciate ligament reconstruction occurred on average 132 days after the repair. There were 4 failures in the repair group and only 1 failure in the reconstruction group; this difference was found to be significant (p = 0.04). No statistical difference was found between the two groups in terms of IKDC or Lysholm scores. Multivariate regression analysis found that patient demographics, time to surgery, interval between stages (for the repair group), number of ligaments involved, and location of FCL/PLC tears did not affect final outcome.

Recommendation
• Surgical reconstruction should be performed for PLC injuries, as acute repair results in a higher failure rate

Question 5: What is the best method of reconstruction for PLC injury?

Relevance
Strong evidence to establish the optimal form of reconstruction for PLC injury will allow that particular technique to be used in the management of these complex cases.

Current opinion
There is no clear consensus as to the optimal technique for PLC reconstruction.

Finding the evidence
• Cochrane Database, with search term "posterolateral corner injury"
• PubMed (www.ncbi.nlm.nih.gov/pubmed/) clinical queries search: "posterolateral corner reconstruction"
• PubMed (www.ncbi.nlm.nih.gov/pubmed/): sensitivity search using keywords "posterolateral corner injury" AND "surgery"

- Citations from relevant articles captured by the search
- Studies with a minimum follow-up of 12 months and average follow-up of 24 months that employed validated knee scores for preoperative and postoperative analyses were included

Quality of the evidence

Level IV
- 9 case series[19–27]

Findings

Our search yielded seven studies that reported on a variety of techniques employed for PLC reconstruction,[19,20,22–24,26–27] summarized in Table 98.2. In four studies a limited reconstruction was performed, such as local augmentation, biceps tenodesis, or PFL reconstruction. In three studies a more extensive anatomic reconstruction was performed, whereby the LCL, PFL, and popliteus were reconstructed. In all studies the number of patients was small and the injuries sustained were varied. Therefore in three studies cases consisted of only PCL and PLC injury, but in three studies a variable combination of ligament injuries was included. All studies reported an improvement in knee specific scoring systems. In the most recent study on PLC reconstruction, LaPrade et al. employed an anatomic technique. They found an improvement in Cincinatti and IKDC scores.[19] A significant improvement was noted in IKDC scores for varus opening at 20°, external rotation at 30°, reverse pivot shift, and single leg hop (p < 0.001). However it can be seen from Table 98.2 that no specific technique yielded a clearly superior improvement in knee scores.

Two studies have compared clinical outcomes for different types of reconstruction technique. Jung and coworkers reported a retrospective cohort study of patients with PCL and grade II PLC (increased external rotation of >10° combined with grade 0–2 varus instability) injury.[21] In this study 19 patients underwent PLC reconstruction via a tran-

stibial sling procedure and 20 patients via a transfibular sling procedure. The fibular head tunnel technique led to a significantly better improvement in rotational stability (p = 0.007), although no significant difference was found for varus stability and clinical outcome scores. Yoon et al. retrospectively compared anatomic reconstruction (n = 21) with a PLC sling procedure (n = 25).[25] They found a significantly better improvement in external rotation laxity and varus laxity with anatomic reconstruction (p < 0.5). The Lysholm knee score improved significantly in both groups (p < 0.5) and no significant difference was found between the two groups.

Recommendations

- On the basis of available evidence no recommendation can be made
- The overall level of evidence presented here is low, as it is based on relatively small numbers of patients. In addition, there are also some conflicting findings from these studies

---

Summary of recommendations

- Clinical examination alone is inadequate to diagnose PLC injury
- A MRI scan should always be obtained in cases of suspected PLC injury, particularly in the presence of an arcuate fracture
- In patients with isolated lateral laxity of 1+ or 2+, nonoperative management is likely to lead to a satisfactory result in terms of function and stability
- Surgical reconstruction should be performed for PLC injuries, as acute repair results in a higher failure rate
- There is insufficient evidence to make a recommendation regarding the best technique for surgical reconstruction

Table 98.2 Summary of studies on reconstruction procedures

Study	NOS	No. of patients	Type of reconstruction	Av. age	Av F/U	Time to surgery(months)	Lysholm		IKDC(% normal/ near normal)		Tegner	
							Preop	Postop	Preop	Postop	Preop	Postop
LaPrade et al.[19]	4	54	Anatomic	32	52	53	NR	NR	NR	62.6	NR	NR
Zhang et al.[20]	4	22	PFL	34	42	Chronic	NR	NR	0	64	NR	NR
Noyes et al.[22]	4	7	Anatomic	37.8	50	20	NR	NR	0	71	NR	NR
Chang et al.[23]	3	12	Anatomic	30.6	37	18	39.5	78.1	NR	NR	1.9	3.9
Khanduja et al.[24]	3	19	Biceps tenodesis	29.6	66.8	27.3	41.2	76.5	0	89	2.6	6.4
Fanelli et al.[26]	5	41	Biceps tenodesis	15–40	2–10yr	4–240	65.48	91.67	NR	NR	2.71	4.92
Wang et al.[27]	4	25	Local augmentation	28	40	10	64	86	NR	NR	NR	3.72

F/U, follow-up; IKDC, International Knee Documentation Committee; NOS, Newcastle Ottawa Scale; NR, not recorded; PFL, popliteofibular ligament.

Conclusions

PLC injuries are both rare and complex; hence there is a shortage of high-quality evidence on which to base decision making. On the basis of available evidence, suspected PLC injuries should be investigated with an MRI scan. Isolated lateral laxity of grade 1+ or 2+ can be managed nonoperatively. However, more severe lateral laxity or combined posterolateral laxity should be managed with surgical reconstruction. The key PLC structures that require reconstruction are the LCL, the popliteofibular ligament, and the popliteus muscle–tendon unit. Various techniques have been described for PLC reconstruction, but at present there is insufficient evidence to recommend one specific technique.

References

1. Seebacher JR, Inglis AE, Marshall JL, Warren RF. The structure of the posterolateral aspect of the knee. J Bone Joint Surg Am 1982;64(4):536–41.

2. Sudasna S, Harnsiriwattanagit K. The ligamentous structures of the posterolateral aspect of the knee. Bull Hosp Jt Dis Orthop Inst 1990;50(1):35–40.

3. DeLee JC, Riley MB, Rockwood CA Jr. Acute posterolateral rotatory instability of the knee. Am J Sports Med 1983;11(4):199–207.

4. LaPrade RF, Wentorf FA, Fritts H, Gundry C, Hightower CD. A prospective magnetic resonance imaging study of the incidence of posterolateral and multiple ligament injuries in acute knee injuries presenting with a hemarthrosis. Arthroscopy 2007;23(12):1341–7.

5. Noyes FR, Barber-Westin SD, Roberts CS. Use of allografts after failed treatment of rupture of the anterior cruciate ligament. J Bone Joint Surg Am 1994;76(7):1019–31.

6. Hughston JC, Jacobson KE. Chronic posterolateral rotatory instability of the knee. J Bone Joint Surg Am 1985;67(3):351–9.

7. LaPrade RF, Terry GC. Injuries to the posterolateral aspect of the knee. Am J Sports Med 1997;25(4):433–8.

8. LaPrade RF, Ly TV, Griffith C. The external rotation recurvatum test revisited. Am J Sports Med 2008;36(4):709–12.

9. Miller TT, Gladden P, Staron RB, Henry JH, Feldman F. Posterolateral stabilizers of the knee: anatomy and injuries assessed with MR imaging. AJR 1997;169:1641–7.

10. Ross G, Chapman AW, Newberg AR, Scheller AD Jr. Magnetic resonance imaging for the evaluation of acute posterolateral complex injuries of the knee. Am J Sports Med 1997;25(4):444–8.

11. Theodorou DJ, Theodorou SJ, Fithian DC, Paxton L, Garelick DH, Resnick D. Posterolateral complex knee injuries: magnetic resonance imaging with surgical correlation. Acta Radiologica 2005;46(3):297–305.

12. Juhng SK, Lee JK, Choi SS, Yoon KH, Roh BS, Won JJ. MR Evaluation of the "arcuate" sign of posterolateral knee instability. AJR 2002;178:583–8.

13. Huang GS, Yu JS, Munshi M, Chan WP, Lee CH, Chen CY, Resnick D. Avulsion fracture of the head of the fibula (the "arcuate" sign): mr imaging findings predictive of injuries to the posterolateral ligaments and posterior cruciate ligament. AJR 2003;180:381–7.

14. Kannus P. Nonoperative treatment of grade II and III sprains of the lateral ligament compartment of the knee. Am J Sports Med 1989;17(1):83–87.

15. Krukhaug Y, Mølster A, Rodt A, Strand T. Lateral ligament injuries of the knee. Knee Surg Sports Traumatol Arthrosc 1998;6:21–25.

16. Stannard JP, Brown SL, Farris RC, McGwin G Jr, Volgas DA. The posterolateral corner of the knee. Repair versus reconstruction. Am J Sports Med 2005;33(6):881–8.

17. Levy BA, Dajani KA, Morgan JA, Shah JP, Dahm DL, Stuart MJ. Repair versus reconstruction of the fibular collateral ligament and posterolateral corner in the multiligament-injured knee. Am J Sports Med 2010;38(4):804–9.

18. Tzurbakis M, Diamantopoulos A, Xenakis T, Georgoulis A. Surgical treatment of multiple knee ligament injuries in 44 patients: 2–8 years follow-up results. Knee Surg Sports Traumatol Arthrosc 2006;14(8):739–49.

19. LaPrade RF, Johansen S, Agel J, Risberg MA, Moksnes H, Engebretsen L. Outcomes of an anatomic posterolateral knee reconstruction. J Bone Joint Surg Am 2010;92(1):16–22.

20. Zhang H, Feng H, Hong L, Wang XS, Zhang J. Popliteofibular ligament reconstruction for posterolateral external rotation instability of the knee. Knee Surg Sports Traumatol Arthrosc 2009;17:1070–1077.

21. Jung YB, Jung HJ, Kim SJ, Park SJ, Song KS, Lee YS, Lee SH. Posterolateral corner reconstruction for posterolateral rotatory instability combined with posterior cruciate ligament injuries: comparison between fibular tunnel and tibial tunnel techniques. Knee Surg Sports Traumatol Arthrosc 2008;16:239–248.

22. Noyes FR, Barber-Westin SD. Posterolateral knee reconstruction with an anatomical bone-patellar tendon-bone reconstruction of the fibular collateral ligament. Am J Sports Med 2007;35(2):259–73.

23. Chang CB, Seong SC, Lee S, Yoo JH, Park YK, Lee MC. Novel methods for diagnosis and treatment of posterolateral rotatory instability of the knee. J Bone Joint Surg Am 2007;89(Suppl 3):2–14.

24. Khanduja V, Somayaji HS, Harnett P, Utukuri M, Dowd GSE. Combined reconstruction of chronic posterior cruciate ligament and posterolateral corner deficiency. A two- to nine-year follow-up study. J Bone Joint Surg Br 2006;88(9):1169–72.

25. Yoon KH, Bae DK, Ha JH, Park SW. Anatomic reconstructive surgery for posterolateral instability of the knee. Arthroscopy 2006;22(2):159–65.

26. Fanelli GC, Edson CJ. Combined posterior cruciate ligament–posterolateral reconstructions with achilles tendon allograft and biceps femoris tendon tenodesis: 2- to 10-year follow-up. Arthroscopy 2004;20(4):339–45.

27. Wang CJ, Chen HS, Huang TW, Yuan LJ. Outcome of surgical reconstruction for posterior cruciate and posterolateral instabilities of the knee. Injury 2002;33:815–21.

99   Cartilage Injury

Joris E.J. Bekkers, Anika I. Tsuchida, and Daniël B.F. Saris
University Medical Center Utrecht, Utrecht, The Netherlands

Case scenario

A 25 year old patient presents with a torsion trauma of the knee. He complains of persistent pain and occasional catching and locking which prevents him from returning to his preinjury sports level. A mild effusion of the left knee is present, the knee ligaments are intact, and meniscus tests indicate medial meniscus pathology. In addition, an articular cartilage defect is suspected.

Relevant anatomy

Articular cartilage is a zonal-oriented tissue that promotes smooth articulation and conducts high impact forces to the subchondral bone.[1] In a healthy joint, there is a stable equilibrium between the synovium and cartilage matrix.[2] After cartilage injury this joint homeostasis can be disturbed, resulting in a cascade of intra-articular factors which negatively influence cartilage healing.[2]

Importance of the problem

The prevalence of trauma-related cartilage lesions ranges from 23% to 54%.[3] Most lesions are not detected at first evaluation and are likely to develop towards osteoarthritis (OA) at a young age, with subsequent decreased quality of life and increased medical costs. Adequate evaluation of cartilage injury, design of custom-made treatment plans, and identification of prognostic factors is essential to delay this progression and improve the functionality of patients after cartilage injury.

Top five questions

Diagnosis

1. How accurate is MRI in the diagnosis of focal cartilage lesions of the knee?

Therapy

2. What is the difference in clinical outcome between various surgical options to treat focal cartilage lesions of the knee?
3. What is the optimal rehabilitation protocol for patients after cartilage surgery?

Prognosis

4. Does a specific treatment perform better for specific patients?
5. What are prognostic factors that predict the outcome after articular cartilage surgery?

Question 1: What is the accuracy of MRI in the diagnosis of a focal cartilage lesion of the knee?

Case clarification
A meniscal tear is often accompanied by focal articular cartilage pathology. To evaluate the presence of a focal cartilage defect an additional MRI is obtained.

Relevance
Evaluation of cartilage pathology on MRI is important to inform the patient on possible treatment decisions during arthroscopy.

Evidence-Based Orthopedics, First Edition. Edited by Mohit Bhandari.
© 2012 Blackwell Publishing Ltd. Published 2012 by Blackwell Publishing Ltd.

Current opinion

The clinical suspicion of an articular cartilage defect and related surgical strategy is mainly based on clinical examination and MRI.

Finding the evidence

- PubMed, with search term: "((MRI[TiAB]) OR (magnetic resonance imaging[TiAB])) AND Arthroscopy[TiAB]"
- Quality of the evidence was appraised using the Cochrane Handbook for Systematic Reviews of Diagnostic Test Accuracy[4]

Quality of the evidence

Level I

- 3 validating cohort studies with good reference standard[5–7]

Level III

- 1 diagnostic study of nonconsecutive patients[8]

Findings

All studies included had a prospective character and compared a prearthroscopic MRI to the findings during arthroscopy. Overall the sensitivity ranged from 33% to 100%, the specificity from 86% to 100%, the negative predictive value from 86% to 95%, and the positive predictive value from 39% to 85%.[5–8] A pooled analysis, subcategorized to the defect grade (Figure 99.1), showed a good specificity (range 95–97%) and a sensitivity increasing with defect grade (Table 99.1).

Table 99.1 Specificity and sensitivity of MRI to detect articular cartilage lesions

Outerbridge grade	I	II	III	IV
Sensitivity	23%	22%	64%	70%
Specificity	95%	97%	97%	95%

Recommendation

- The MRI shows a moderate detection of clinically relevant (grade III and IV) articular cartilage defects (sensitivity 64–70%) [overall quality: moderate]

Question 2: What is the difference in clinical outcome between various surgical options to treat focal cartilage lesions of the knee?

Case clarification

The MRI showed a grade IV articular cartilage lesion at the medial femoral condyle. Several treatment options are available (see box).

Treatment options for focal articular cartilage lesions

- *Autologous chondrocyte implantation (ACI):* Chondrocytes are taken by biopsy, expanded in vitro and reinjected under a periosteal flap[9] that covers the defect. Newer generations of ACI use collagen covers (2nd generation) or seed chondrocytes onto matrices (3rd generation)[10]

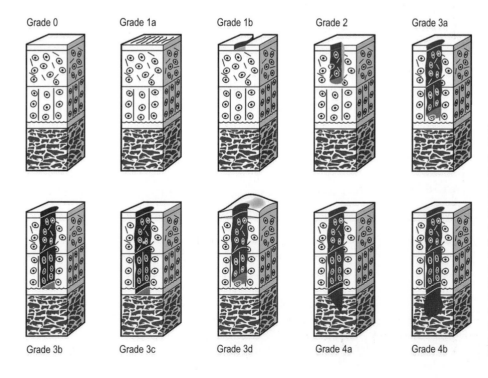

Grade 0 Grade 1a Grade 1b Grade 2 Grade 3a

Grade 3b Grade 3c Grade 3d Grade 4a Grade 4b

Figure 99.1 The International Cartilage Repair Society (ICRS) articular cartilage defect classification: Grade 0, macroscopically normal cartilage; Grade 1, nearly normal: superficial lesions, soft indentation (1a) and/or superficial fissures and cracks (1b); Grade 2, abnormal: lesions extending down to less than 50% of cartilage depth; Grade 3, severely abnormal: cartilage defects extending down to more than 50% of cartilage depth (3a), as well as down to the calcified layer (3b), and down to but not through the subchondral bone (3c) and cartilage defects with blisters (3d); Grade 4, severely abnormal: all cartilage defects into the subchondral bone. Permission to use this image was granted by the president of the ICRS, Professor Dr. D.B.F. Saris.

Treatment options for focal articular cartilage lesions (continued)

- *Osteochondral autologous transplantation (OAT):* Osteochondral autografts are harvested from less-weightbearing areas of the knee and transferred to the defect[11]
- *Microfracturing (MF):* A 1–2mm diameter awl is used to penetrate the subchondral plate creating access to the bone marrow filling the cartilage lesion with a clot populated with bone-marrow-derived stem cells, growth factors, and platelets[12]

Relevance

Adequate treatment is important for patients presenting with focal cartilage lesions of the knee, who are generally young, to prevent progression towards OA in middle age.

Current opinion

MF is a good first line treatment, but ACI and OAT provide better long-term clinical results.

Finding the evidence

- PubMed: several synonyms of the treatment options. See detailed description in Bekkers et al.[13]
- Quality appraisal as explained in the Cochrane Handbook[14]

Quality of the evidence

Level I

- 1 systematic review of randomized controlled trials (RCTs)[13]
- 6 randomized trials[15–20]

Findings

All studies included were of high quality, with Coleman scores ranging from 74 to 94.[13] The average defect size ranged from 2.4 to 5.1cm^2 and all defects were at least grade III (Figure 99.1). A pooled analysis of clinical outcome was not possible due to the heterogeneity of clinical outcome measures. After 1 year follow-up OAT showed clinical superior outcome compared to MF in both the Hospital for Special Surgery (p < 0.05) and International Cartilage Repair Society (p < 0.03) questionnaires.[16] After 3 years follow-up MF shows inferior clinical results when compared to characterized chondrocyte implantation (CCI) (p = 0.048) or OAT (p < 0.001).[16,20] After 19 months follow-up OAT and ACI did not differ (p = 0.227) on the modified Cincinnati score.[15] A randomized study of chronic articular cartilage lesions did not show any difference in clinical outcome between ACI and MF at 5 year follow-up.[18] An increase in clinical outcome after ACI or a decrease in MF is generally observed after 1 year follow-up, indicating a less stable regenerative product after MF.[16,20]

Recommendations

- Treatment of focal articular cartilage lesions by ACI or OAT provides better mid-term clinical results than MF [overall quality: high]

- ACI and OAT are both good treatment options for grade III and IV focal articular cartilage lesions, with similar clinical results

Question 3: What is the optimal rehabilitation protocol for patients after cartilage surgery?

Case clarification

Rehabilitation after cartilage surgery aims at resumption of previous function and activity levels.

Relevance

Rehabilitation is essential for optimal success after cartilage surgery.

Current opinion

Cartilage surgery requires extensive rehabilitation, which is currently primarily based on expert opinion.

Finding the evidence

- PubMed, with search term: "cartilage[TiAB] AND revalidation[TiAB]"

Quality of the evidence

Level I

- 2 RCTs[21,22]

Level II

- 1 cohort study[23]

Level V

- 1 expert opinion[24]

Findings

Time to weightbearing Two RCTs compared traditional weightbearing (full weightbearing after 8–10 or 11 weeks) vs. accelerated weightbearing (full weightbearing after respectively 6 or 8 weeks) after matrix-induced autologous chondrocyte implantation (MACI).[21,22] The accelerated group reported less pain at 3 months (p = 0.033) compared to the traditional group[21] and after 2 years both groups reported similar clinical outcome (p = 0.910) on the knee injury and osteoarthritis outcome (KOOS) score.[22]

Low-load activities An RCT reported on the effect of low-load activities during rehabilitation on functional outcome after CCI or MF.[23] Lack of postoperative low-load activities resulted in a significantly worse functional outcome (p < 0.05) compared to high levels of postsurgery low-load activities.

Principles of rehabilitation Currently, the rehabilitation protocols after cartilage surgery are mainly based on expert opinion and the hypothesis of graft maturation, which divides the rehabilitation into several phases (Table 99.2).[24]

Table 99.2 Phases of rehabilitation

Phase I	**Recovery and protection (weeks 0–4)**
	Protect graft from load and shear forces, weightbearing control
	Restore full passive knee extension, gradually increase pain-free knee flexion
Phase II	**Inauguration (weeks 4–8)**
	Increase pain-free ROM and weightbearing
	Gain quadriceps control in safe, multiangle CKC exercises
Phase III	**Maturation (weeks 8–12)**
	Full active pain-free ROM and gradual return to full weightbearing
	Regain optimal coordination for walking, stair climbing/descending
Phase IV	**Integration (weeks 12–26)**
	Increase lower limb strength and gradually increase training load and volume
	Ensure safe static postures with balance exercises
Phase V	**Functional adaptation (weeks 26–52+)**
	Unrestricted ADL
	Prevent future damage/injury
Phase VI	**Return to sports (weeks 26–78+)**
	Restore symmetry, including lower limb strength and flexibility
	Aim for unrestricted sport (at same or lower level)

ADL, activities of daily living; CKC, closed kinetic chain; ROM, range of motion.

Recommendations

• Accelerated weightbearing is safe and does not lead to inferior clinical results.[overall quality: high]
• Low-load activities increase functional outcome after both MF and CCI [overall quality: moderate]
• Cartilage therapies require careful rehabilitation guided by trained professionals [overall quality: low]

Question 4: Do specific patients achieve a higher clinical outcome after a specific articular cartilage surgery?

Case clarification

The nature of regenerated tissue and the theoretical basis of different cartilage surgeries vary.

Relevance

Selecting the optimal treatment, based on specific patient characteristics, leads to a tailor-made treatment strategy

leading to superior outcomes after articular cartilage surgery.

Current opinion

Current opinion suggests that large articular cartilage lesions should preferably be treated by ACI or OAT. For small articular cartilage lesions or (multiple) chronic lesions, MF is the first treatment option.

Finding the evidence

• See Question 2

Quality of the evidence

Level I
• 3 randomized trials[16,17,20]

Findings

Lesion size Lesions larger than $4\,cm^{2,17}$ or larger than $2\,cm^{2,16}$ perform clinically worse ($p < 0.05$) after MF treatment, while the influence of lesion size on clinical outcome was not present after ACI or OAT.[16,17]

Symptom duration CCI resulted in a better clinical outcome than MF ($p < 0.04$) for patients with a symptom duration of less than 3 years.[20]

Recommendations

• Large articular cartilage lesions ($>4\,cm^2$) should be treated with ACI or OAT [overall quality: high]
• Patients with duration of symptoms less than 3 years should preferably be treated with CCI [overall quality: high]

Question 5: What are patient-specific, prognostic factors that predict the clinical outcome after articular cartilage surgery?

Case clarification

The overall benefit from cartilage surgery is 70–95%.

Relevance

Identification of prognostic factors for the clinical outcome after cartilage surgery will improve surgical timing leading to optimal benefit from the surgery.

Current opinion

Increasing age is expected to negatively influence the clinical outcome after cartilage surgery.

Finding the evidence

• See Question 2

Quality of the evidence

Level I
• 6 individual inception cohort studies validated in a single population[25–29]

Level II
- 2 prospective cohort studies[30,31]

Findings

Patient age Four studies showed a statistically significant influence (p < 0.05) of patient age on treatment outcome;[26–28,32] increasing age is associated with inferior clinical results.

Duration of symptoms Treatment of articular cartilage lesions with a traumatic origin and symptoms for less than 1 year (p < 0.05) was more successful than those with symptoms for more than 1 year.[29] Similar results were shown for a symptom duration of 2 years (p = 0.03)[26] and patients with symptom duration less than 2 years are more likely to reach their age-matched healthy reference score.[32]

Defect location Superior clinical results were described for defects located at the lateral femoral condyle (p < 0.05)[26,28] while others report superiority (p < 0.05) of defects at the medial condyle.[32] Additionally, other cohorts did not identify defect location as a prognostic factor for the outcome after ACI.[25,27]

Recommendations
- Increasing age negatively influences the clinical outcome after cartilage surgery [overall quality: high]
- A shorter duration of symptoms favors the clinical outcome after cartilage surgery [overall quality: high]
- Location of the defect seems to influence the clinical outcome, however, results are conflicting [overall quality: low]

Summary of recommendations

- The MRI shows a moderate detection of clinically relevant (grade III and IV) articular cartilage defects (sensitivity 64–70%)
- The treatment of grade III and IV focal articular cartilage lesions by ACI or OAT provide better mid-term clinical results compared to MF
- ACI and OAT are both good treatment options for grade III and IV focal articular cartilage lesions with similar clinical results
- Accelerated weightbearing is safe and does not lead to inferior clinical results
- Low-load activities increase functional outcome after MF and CCI
- Cartilage therapies require careful rehabilitation guided by trained professionals
- Large grade III or IV articular cartilage lesions (>4 cm^2) should be treated with ACI or OAT
- Patients with symptoms duration less than 2 years should preferably be treated with CCI

- Increasing age negatively influences the clinical outcome after cartilage surgery
- A shorter duration of symptoms favors the clinical outcome after cartilage surgery
- Location of the defect seems to influence the clinical outcome, however, results are conflicting

Conclusions

MRI is the best available noninvasive diagnostic tool to detect high-graded focal articular cartilage lesions. Several surgical treatment options for focal articular cartilage lesions are available. Mid-term clinical outcomes favor cell therapy over other cartilage surgeries. However, globally accepted outcome measures of cartilage surgery would enhance the comparison between studies. In addition, treatment selection and timing, based on patient profiling and prognostic factors respectively, will be essential to reach optimal results from articular cartilage surgery. The recent increase in scientific publications on rehabilitation after cartilage surgery initiates a shift from expert opinion towards a more evidence-based approach in rehabilitation after cartilage surgery.

Acknowledgements
The authors gratefully acknowledge the support of the TeRM Smart Mix Program of the Netherlands Ministry of Economic Affairs and the Netherlands Ministry of Education, Culture and Science.

References

1. Buckwalter JA, Mankin HJ, Grodzinsky AJ. Articular cartilage and osteoarthritis. Instr Course Lect 2005;54:465–80.
2. Saris DB, Dhert WJ, Verbout AJ. Joint homeostasis. The discrepancy between old and fresh defects in cartilage repair. J Bone Joint Surg Br 2003;85(7):1067–76.
3. Indelicato PA, Bittar ES. A perspective of lesions associated with ACL insufficiency of the knee. A review of 100 cases. Clin Orthop Relat Res 1985;198:77–80.
4. Reitsma J, Rutjes A, Whiting P, Vlassov V, Leeflang M, Deeks J. Assessing methodological quality. In: Deeks J, Bossuyt P, Gatsonis C, eds. Cochrane Handbook for Systematic Reviews of Diagnostic Test Accuracy, 2009.
5. Friemert B, Oberlander Y, Schwarz W, et al. Diagnosis of chondral lesions of the knee joint: can MRI replace arthroscopy? A prospective study. Knee Surg Sports Traumatol Arthrosc 2004; 12(1):58–64.
6. Potter HG, Linklater JM, Allen AA, Hannafin JA, Haas SB. Magnetic resonance imaging of articular cartilage in the knee. An evaluation with use of fast-spin-echo imaging. J Bone Joint Surg Am 1998;80(9):1276–84.
7. von Engelhardt LV, Kraft CN, Pennekamp PH, Schild HH, Schmitz A, von Falkenhausen M. The evaluation of articular

cartilage lesions of the knee with a 3-Tesla magnet. Arthroscopy 2007;23(5):496–502.

8. Figueroa D, Calvo R, Vaisman A, Carrasco MA, Moraga C, Delgado I. Knee chondral lesions: incidence and correlation between arthroscopic and magnetic resonance findings. Arthroscopy 2007;23(3):312–5.

9. Brittberg M, Lindahl A, Nilsson A, Ohlsson C, Isaksson O, Peterson L. Treatment of deep cartilage defects in the knee with autologous chondrocyte transplantation. N Engl J Med 1994; 331(14):889–95.

10. Marlovits S, Zeller P, Singer P, Resinger C, Vecsei V. Cartilage repair: generations of autologous chondrocyte transplantation. Eur J Radiol 2006;57(1):24–31.

11. Hangody L, Kish G, Karpati Z, Szerb I, Udvarhelyi I. Arthroscopic autogenous osteochondral mosaicplasty for the treatment of femoral condylar articular defects. A preliminary report. Knee Surg Sports Traumatol Arthrosc 1997;5(4):262–7.

12. Steadman JR, Rodkey WG, Rodrigo JJ. Microfracture: surgical technique and rehabilitation to treat chondral defects. Clin Orthop Relat Res 2001;391 Suppl:S362–9.

13. Bekkers JEJ, Inklaar M, Saris DBF. Treatment selection in articular cartilage lesions of the knee: A systematic review. Am.J.Sports Med 2009;37(Suppl 1):S148–55.

14. Higgins JPT, Green S. Cochrane Handbook for Systematic Reviews of Interventions Version 5.0.1 [updated September 2008]. The Cochrane Collaboration, 2008; Available from www.cochrane-handbook.org.

15. Bentley G, Biant LC, Carrington RW, et al. A prospective, randomised comparison of autologous chondrocyte implantation versus mosaicplasty for osteochondral defects in the knee. J Bone Joint Surg Br 2003;85(2):223–30.

16. Gudas R, Kalesinskas RJ, Kimtys V, et al. A prospective randomized clinical study of mosaic osteochondral autologous transplantation versus microfracture for the treatment of osteochondral defects in the knee joint in young athletes. Arthroscopy 2005;21(9):1066–75.

17. Knutsen G, Engebretsen L, Ludvigsen TC, et al. Autologous chondrocyte implantation compared with microfracture in the knee. A randomized trial. J Bone Joint Surg Am 2004;86(3): 455–64.

18. Knutsen G, Drogset JO, Engebretsen L, et al. A randomized trial comparing autologous chondrocyte implantation with microfracture. Findings at five years. J Bone Joint Surg Am 2007; 89(10):2105–12.

19. Saris DB, Vanlauwe J, Victor J, et al. Characterized chondrocyte implantation results in better structural repair when treating symptomatic cartilage defects of the knee in a randomized controlled trial versus microfracture. Am J Sports Med 2008; 36(2):235–46.

20. Saris DB, Vanlauwe J, Victor J, et al. Treatment of symptomatic cartilage defects of the knee: characterized chondrocyte implantation results in better clinical outcome at 36 months in a randomized trial compared to microfracture. Am J Sports Med 2009;37(Suppl 1):S10–19.

21. Ebert JR, Robertson WB, Lloyd DG, Zheng MH, Wood DJ, Ackland T. Traditional vs accelerated approaches to postoperative rehabilitation following matrix-induced autologous chondrocyte implantation (MACI): comparison of clinical, biomechanical and radiographic outcomes. Osteoarthritis Cartilage 2008;16(10):1131–40.

22. Wondrasch B, Zak L, Welsch GH, Marlovits S. Effect of accelerated weightbearing after matrix-associated autologous chondrocyte implantation on the femoral condyle on radiographic and clinical outcome after 2 years: a prospective, randomized controlled pilot study. Am J Sports Med 2009;37(Suppl 1):S88–96.

23. Assche van D, Caspel van D, Vanlauwe J, et al. Physical activity levels after characterized chondrocyte implantation versus microfracture in the knee and the relationship to objective functional outcome with 2-year follow-up. Am J Sports Med 2009;37(Suppl 1):S42–9.

24. Hambly K, Bobic V, Wondrasch B, Van AD, Marlovits S. Autologous chondrocyte implantation postoperative care and rehabilitation: science and practice. Am J Sports Med 2006; 34(6):1020–38.

25. Bhosale AM, Kuiper JH, Johnson WE, Harrison PE, Richardson JB. Midterm to long-term longitudinal outcome of autologous chondrocyte implantation in the knee joint: a multilevel analysis. Am J Sports Med 2009;37(Suppl 1):S131–8.

26. Krishnan SP, Skinner JA, Bartlett W, et al. Who is the ideal candidate for autologous chondrocyte implantation? J Bone Joint Surg Br 2006;88(1):61–4.

27. McNickle AG, L'Heureux DR, Yanke AB, Cole BJ. Outcomes of autologous chondrocyte implantation in a diverse patient population. Am J Sports Med 2009;37(7):1344–50.

28. Niemeyer P, Steinwachs M, Erggelet C, et al. Autologous chondrocyte implantation for the treatment of retropatellar cartilage defects: clinical results referred to defect localisation. Arch Orthop Trauma Surg 2008;128(11):1223–31.

29. Pietschmann MF, Horng A, Niethammer T, et al. Cell quality affects clinical outcome after MACI procedure for cartilage injury of the knee. Knee Surg Sports Traumatol Arthrosc 2009;17(11):1305–11.

30. Minas T, Gomoll AH, Rosenberger R, Royce RO, Bryant T. Increased failure rate of autologous chondrocyte implantation after previous treatment with marrow stimulation techniques. Am J Sports Med 2009;37(5):902–8.

31. Zaslav K, Cole B, Brewster R, et al. A prospective study of autologous chondrocyte implantation in patients with failed prior treatment for articular cartilage defect of the knee: results of the Study of the Treatment of Articular Repair (STAR) clinical trial. Am J Sports Med 2009;37(1):42–55.

32. de Windt ThS, Bekkers JEJ, Creemers LB, Dhert WJA, Saris DBF. Patient profiling in cartilage regeneration: prognostic factors determining success of treatment for cartilage defects. Am J Sports Med 2009;37(Suppl 1):S58–62.

100 Runner's Knee

Ella W. Yeung and Simon S. Yeung
Department of Rehabilitation Sciences, Hong Kong Polytechnic University, Kowloon, Hong Kong

Case scenario

A 30 year old woman presented to the physiotherapy clinic with bilateral anterior knee pain. She is a keen runner and she stated that the pain began 3 months ago when she increased her weekly mileage in preparation for running a marathon. She continued to run through the pain until it got so bad that it was impossible to ignore. Activities such as going up and down stairs also aggravated her pain. She stopped running to rest the knee but pain recurred as soon as she resumed training. She has had an MRI taken which showed no abnormality. Her doctor says she has runner's knee and advices her to stop running and start doing some quadriceps strengthening exercise.

Finding the evidence

To identify relevant trials, we searched the following electronic database systems:
- Cochrane Database of Systematic Reviews
- Cochrane Central Register of Controlled Trials (Cochrane Library Issue 3, 2009)
- Ovid MEDLINE (1966 to October 2009).

A combination of MeSH headings and keywords relevant to runner's knee was used. These include the following terms:
- "runner or jogg* OR sprint* OR racer," "athletic injuries," "knee injuries," "patella," "patellofemoral pain," "patellofemoral syndrome," "anterior knee pain," "chondromalacia patellae," "tendinitis," "physiotherapy," "physical therapy," "rehabilitation," "exercise," "strength," stretch," "electrophysical," "orthoses," "orthotic," "brace," "splint," "strap," "taping," "massage," "manipulation," "mobilization"

Any systematic review, randomized controlled trial (RCT), or quasi-randomized trial of prevention or intervention for runners' knee in adolescent and adult subjects was considered.

Top seven questions

1. What is runner's knee and how commonly does it occur in runners?
2. What are the possible risk factors associated with patellofemoral pain syndrome (PFPS)?
3. What is the optimal training volume for a runner to remain injury free?
4. What are the best treatment options for patellofemoral pain, and is exercise therapy effective in alleviating or preventing it?
5. Is external support useful in preventing or alleviating patellofemoral pain?
6. Can other treatment modalities be used in the treatment of patellofemoral pain?
7. What is the prognosis for PFPS?

Question 1: What is runner's knee and how commonly does it occur in runners?

Case clarification

Runner's knee or PFPS is a common cause of anterior knee pain in young active individuals. Although it is common among runners, the condition is not unique to runners. In this chapter, we use the term PFPS to describe this condition.

Relevance

It has been reported that patellofemoral pain affects approximately 1 in 4 of the general population.[1] Both genders are affected but the incidence is reported to be higher in women.[2] Runners in particular are susceptible to PFPS, accounting for 20–25% of all new running injuries seen in sports medicine clinics.[2-4] Recreational runners tend to have a higher incidence of PFPS than experienced runners.[5] Besides runners, PFPS also occur in different athletes such as soccer, hockey and volleyball players and in military recruits.[6,7]

If not managed properly, this condition can be both painful and debilitating. If pain becomes severe, it can adversely affect both training and performance. The symptoms have an insidious onset with no history of trauma. The clinical presentation is characterized by pain behind and around the patella and is aggravated by knee loading activities such as running, squatting, ascending and descending stairs, and prolonged sitting.

Current opinion

The pathogenesis of PFPS is unclear; several anatomical sources of pain including lateral and medial retinaculae structures, subchondral bone and the synovium have been proposed.[8,9] The etiology of PFPS is multifactorial; causative factors such as overuse, malalignment, and muscle imbalance have been suggested. Diagnostic radiological imaging often failed to detect specific pathology. Thus diagnosis of PFPS is based on symptoms and physical examination after excluding intra-articular and peripatellar pathology. Symptoms can often be reproduced with palpation of the patella facet and patella compression tests.[10,11] Despite the uncertainty as to the underlying etiology, conservative management is generally accepted as the management approach in improving pain and function in the literature.

Question 2: What are the possible risk factors associated with PFPS?

Case clarification

The symptoms of PFPS are often characterized by slow insidious onset. The causation of this condition is multifactorial, involving both intrinsic and extrinsic factors. In the case study presented here, the extrinsic factor relating to training error may contribute to the onset of symptoms.

Relevance

To prevent injury, there is a need to identify the potential risk factors associated with PFPS.

Current opinion

Literature suggests that the causes of PFPS are multifactorial.

Quality of the evidence

Level I
- 1 systematic review[12]

Findings

Four categories of risk factors were identified that might predispose to the lower extremity running injuries:[12] systemic, lifestyle, health, and running/training related factors. The systemic, lifestyle, and health factors can broadly be grouped under intrinsic factors while running/training related factors are extrinsic causes.

It has frequently been suggested that excessive loading on the patellofemoral joint (PFJ) is the principal cause of PFPS.[13] The intrinsic factors influence the magnitude and distribution of the PFJ load when a runner lands on his/her feet during running. For instance, Thijs et al.[14] showed that runners who developed PFPS exerted a significantly higher vertical peak force underneath the lateral heel (2nd and 3rd metatarsal) during running. Distribution of the load at the knee joint is governed by how the patella moves into contact with the femoral trochlea during knee excursion. Structures around the knee joint that influence patella tracking include patella position, soft tissue tension, and control of the medial and lateral components of the vastus medialis obliquus (VMO) muscle.[15,16] Given the interaction between the kinematics of the lower extremities in functional activities, it has been also been suggested that patellar tracking is influenced by back posture, femoral internal rotation, knee valgus, tibial rotation, subtalar pronation, and muscle flexibility.[17-19]

For running/training related factors, several risk factors have been reported in the literature. These include weekly mileage, history of previous running injuries, number of years in running, training characteristics (running speed, frequency of training, training surface, weekly running mileage) and footwear.[19-22] Amongst them, increase in weekly running mileage has frequently been suggested.[19,22] These potential contributing factors have led to different treatment approaches. The efficacy of these treatment in relieving pain is addressed in the following sections.

Recommendation

- Intrinsic risk factors that influence the PFJ loading, including muscle imbalances and biomechanical alterations, are thought to contribute to the onset of pain. Extrinsic risk factors including training error and footwear are commonly reported [overall level: moderate]

Question 3: What is the optimal training volume for a runner to remain injury free?

Case clarification

One of the most common factors implicated in running injuries is errors in training methods. Often injury results because of increasing the training intensity too quickly and too soon without allowing the tissues to adapt to the stress.

Relevance

The training volume is a modifiable risk factor by which runners can prevent injury.

Current opinion

To avoid injuries, it has been suggested that total weekly running distance should not exceed 64 km.[12] One popular strategy in preventing injuries is the use of the 10% rule; i.e., increasing mileage by no more than 10% a week.

Quality of the evidence

Level I

- 1 systematic review[23] and 1 RCT[27]

Findings

A meta-analysis[23] revealed 20 RCTs related to the prevention of the running-related soft tissue lower limb injuries. Four studies[24-27] reported training schedule modifications. Pollock et al.[25] showed that modification of training frequency (RR 0.19; 95% CI 0.06–0.66) and duration (RR 0.41; 95% CI 0.21–0.79) can reduce injury, while another study of army recruits showed that reducing running distance[26] could reduce injury (RR 0.70; 95% CI 0.54–0.91). Thus there is strong evidence for an association between training volume and running-related lower limb injuries. However, direct evidence for quantifying the optimal training load for a runner preparing for a 10 km or marathon race is lacking.

Gradual increase in the volume of training over time has been a long-held belief in preventing overuse running injuries in novice runners. No significant reduction in injury was observed in a study that examined graduated running program in the prevention of shin splints.[24] The 10% running rule, which states that an athlete should not increase training volume (time or distance or intensity) by more than 10% per week, is a common practice among runners. However, an RCT[27] that examined novice runners training for a 4 mile (6.4 km) run reported that a graded 13-week training program that adhered to the 10% rule did not reduce the number of running-related injuries compared with a standard 8-week training program that increased training volume by 50% (RR 1.02, 95% CI 0.72–1.45).

Recommendations

- There is high quality evidence indicating an association of running-related lower limb injuries with training volume. However there is lack of data to quantify optimal training load for a runner in preparation for a 10 km or marathon race

Question 4: What are the best treatment options for patellofemoral pain, and how effective is exercise therapy in alleviating or preventing it?

Case clarification

Generalized quadriceps strengthening exercises may not be able to address patella maltracking caused by muscle imbalances.

Relevance

As discussed previously, weakness of the VMO relative to vastus lateralis muscle (VL) leading to patella maltracking has been suggested as a contributing risk factor to the development of PFPS.[30] A prospective cohort study[31] tested the onset timing of VMO-VL in healthy subjects subjected to 6 weeks of strenuous training and showed that those individuals who developed PFPS during training had a significant delayed onset of VMO activity. Thus it may suggest that individuals with a delayed onset of VMO activation are susceptible to developing PFPS. Furthermore, in a systematic review[32] of patients with PFPS, a delay in the activation of VMO relative to VL during functional activities (e.g., stair descent: pooled mean difference: 30.25 ms; 95% CI 16.68–43.81) has been demonstrated. Our study also demonstrated a lengthening of electromechanical delay in the VMO during fatiguing condition, which would affect the stabilizing effect on the patella during knee extension.[33]

Current opinion

Although the etiology of patellofemoral pain is uncertain, it is generally well accepted that nonoperative management is the treatment of choice. Long-term outcome results showed that up to 75% of the PFPS patents treated conservatively had good subjective and functional recovery and did develop patellofemoral osteoarthritis.[28,29] It is, therefore, important that the treatment decision for PFPS is built on the best research evidence. In the literature, treatment options include exercise therapy, use of external support, pharmacological intervention and electrical modalities. VMO retraining addressing the imbalance in VMO and VL has often been recommended as an essential component for treatment. This is often performed in combination with other physiotherapeutic interventions.

Quality of the evidence

Level I

- 5 RCTs,[40-44] 1 controlled clinical trial,[45] and a systematic review[46] were identified to compare the beneficial effects of open kinetic chain (OKC) vs. closed kinetic chain (CKC) quadriceps strengthening exercises
- 1 systematic review[49] was identified to assess whether VMO retraining is effective in the treatment of PFPS

Level II
• 1 systemic review,[34] 1 controlled clinical trial,[35] and 2 RCTs[36,37] were identified to examine the efficacy of exercise therapy for PFPS

Level III
• 2 systematic reviews[55,56] were identified to examine if hip musculature strengthening is beneficial in reducing symptoms associated with PFPS; the studies included in these reviews[50–54,57–59] are of low quality

Findings

A systematic review[34] of studies published between 1966 and 2001 concluded that there was limited evidence to support that exercise therapy reduces anterior knee pain in patients with PFPS. There is conflicting evidence of functional improvement after exercise therapy. Three trials (2 RCTs and 1 controlled clinical trial) were included,[35–37] with only one RCT[37] being assessed as high quality. In this study, the investigators[37] compared (6 treatments over 3 months) exercise therapy with a control group not receiving exercise therapy. The exercises consisted of eccentric quadriceps strengthening, stretching, and functional exercises. At the end of the intervention, improvements for pain (effect size = 0.10) and function (effect size = 0.11) were observed in both groups. At 12 month follow-up, patients in the exercise group showed significant improvements in pain compared to the nonexercise group. Although the large dropout rate (40%) at 12 months in this study[37] might have contributed to the significant difference, it has to be noted that more patients in the exercise group reported greater patient satisfaction and were discharged at 3 months (p = 0.001). An RCT conducted by Crossley et al.[38] compared physiotherapy intervention (6 treatments over 6 weeks; emphasizing VMO exercise retraining) in subjects with anterior knee pain with placebo treatment. Results indicated that the intervention group improved in pain (effect size = 0.80) and function (effect size = 0.91). A recent high-quality RCT[39] on 131 subjects provided further evidence to the positive effects of physiotherapy-supervised exercise therapy for improving pain and function in patients with PFPS at 3 (effect size = 0.47 for pain; 0.34 for function) and 12 months (effect size = 0.56 for pain) than usual care in general medical practice. The exercises included strengthening exercises for quadriceps, adductors and gluteal muscles, balance and stretching. Together, these three high-quality trials provide evidence that exercise therapy resulted in better clinical outcomes.

Quadriceps strengthening exercises can be either OKC or CKC. OKC exercises involve movement in which the distal segment is free to move in space, whereas CKC exercises are performed with the distal segment fixed (either on the ground or on a support surface). CKC exercises has been suggested to be more effective in the treatment of

anterior knee pain because of their close resemblance to daily activities and are also believe to produce less compressive stress to the PFJ. The benefits of both forms of exercises have been suggested in the literature. Five trials[40–45] were included in a systematic review[34] which compared the effects of OKC and CKC exercises in the treatment of subjects with PFPS, and showed that both exercises are effective in the short term (6–12 weeks) for pain reduction or functional improvement. In one trial,[43] a 5 year follow-up was undertaken to examine the long-term effects of an OKC or CKC program in subject with PFPS. The results demonstrated that both groups maintained equally good subjective and functional outcomes.[44] Another systematic review[46] on training methods also concluded that quadriceps strength training is beneficial, but no single approach (CKC or OKC; isometric or eccentric training mode) is superior to another. Thus there is strong evidence to support that both OKC and CKC exercises are effective in the short- and long-term management of PFPS.

To address VMO:VL imbalance in patients with patellofemoral pain, it has been proposed that VMO must be specifically strengthened to restore abnormal patella tracking. Is there evidence to suggest a specific VMO retraining exercise to be more effective? In the study by Crossley et al.,[38] the authors reported that exercises emphasizing VMO retraining resulted in less pain and better outcome. This same group of investigators conducted two subgroup RCTs[47,48] to show that VMO retraining significantly improved the timing of VMO activation onset, and this was not observed in the placebo group. However, it is important to note that in addition to specific VMO retraining, subjects were given other interventions (patella taping, stretching, and hip external rotator strengthening). The authors stated that these interventions were aimed at improving VMO function, but inevitably this claim is difficult to establish. Debate also arises as to whether VMO can be preferentially activated with limb position or cocontraction. A systematic review of studies (20 trials) published up to 2008 suggest that the evidence remain unclear.[49]

Hip muscle weakness (specifically abductors and external rotators) has been suggested to contribute to the development of PFPS. These muscles act eccentrically to control or resist excessive femoral adduction and internal rotation during activities, and strength deficits may result in increased dynamic Q-angle and PFJ contact area. Based on five cross-sectional studies,[50–54] Prins et al.[55] reported in their review that women with PFPS demonstrate a decrease in hip abduction, external rotation, and extension strength when compared with healthy controls. Is there any evidence to support the use of hip muscle strengthening for the treatment of PFPS? Based on a systematic review,[56] three studies (a case report, a cohort study, and a cross-sectional study)[57–59] published in 1998–2006 were identified. Currently there is limited evidence to suggest that hip musculature strengthening has any beneficial effect in reducing symptoms associated with PFPS.

Tightness of the iliotibial band,[60] hamstrings, and gastroncnemius muscles,[15,51] and reduced patellar mobility[61] have also been suggested to cause patella maltracking and are associated with subject with PFPS. Stretching has not been shown to be effective in preventing PFPS and running-related lower limb soft tissue injuries.[23] There is also no evidence to suggest that stretching these tight anatomical structures is beneficial to the treatment of PFPS.

Recommendations

• Moderate-quality evidence shows that physiotherapy-supervised exercise therapy is effective for PFPS
• High-quality evidence supports the use of OKC or CKC quadriceps strengthening in reducing pain and improving function in subjects with PFPS, both short- and long-term
• There is moderate quality evidence to suggest that VMO retraining is effective in the treatment of PFPS. However it is unclear if VMO can be preferentially activated
• There is low quality evidence to support hip muscle strengthening or stretching exercises in improving symptoms in individuals with PFPS

Question 5: Is external support useful in preventing or alleviating patellofemoral pain?

Relevance
Applying external supports such as patella tape, patellofemoral brace, or foot insoles/orthoses for prevention or reduction of PFPS has been suggested in the literature.

Current opinion
The rationale behind external support is to influence the intrinsic risk factors by (1) realigning the patella to improve tracking and to enhance the activation and/or timing of the VMO muscle; or (2) realigning the lower leg/foot alignment to reduce the PFJ contact pressure and improve shock impact.

Quality of the evidence
Level I
• 6 systematic reviews[62–66] published between 2001 and 2008 were identified to examine whether subjects receiving patella taping show an improvement in pain and knee function
• 3 systematic reviews[23,46,66] and 4 RCTs[74–77] examined the use of a knee brace
• 1 systematic review[23] examined whether the use of insoles protects against knee injuries

Findings
Many of the same studies were included in the six systematic reviews.[62–66] These studies assessed the effectiveness of patella taping for PFPS but have incorporated other interventions into the treatment program, making it difficult to ascertain treatment effectiveness. Four included RCT studies of high quality[37,38,67,68] examined the outcomes of patients who received patella taping. Only one trial[37] compared patella taping vs. no taping, which showed no significant improvement in pain and knee function at 3 and 12 months follow-up. Although taping alone has not been demonstrated to have significant benefits, positive effects were observed with combined treatment. The other three RCTs[38,67,68] incorporated different physical interventions (strengthening, stretching, biofeedback) with patella taping as a component. The results (n = 214, mean age 23 years) showed significant short-term (duration 4–6 weeks) improvement in pain and function compared to the control group. Although the effectiveness of taping alone cannot be determined, the findings nevertheless showed a clear advantage of a combined treatment approach addressing the multifactorial etiology of PFPS.

The effects of patella taping on patella position and in enhancing neuromuscular control (i.e., VMO activation pattern and/or timing) were also evaluated. Three controlled clinical trials[69–71] were identified in a systematic review[56] which examined the effect of taping on VMO activation. However, the results are conflicting and thus the evidence is inconclusive.

The use of a knee brace was examined in three systematic reviews,[23,46,66] with two RCTs[72,73] showing patellofemoral bracing to be an effective method in preventing the development of PFPS (n = 210; RR 0.33; 95% CI 0.17–0.65). Although the underlying mechanism of the positive effects is not known, it has to be noted that subjects (respectively athletes and army recruits) in these two trials had to participate in an unaccustomed strenuous training program with a minimal period of adaptation. The braces used in these trials purport to provide support or to correct the position of the patella. It may be possible that the brace facilitates quadriceps activity, which in turn helps stabilize the knee joint dynamically or decreases the loading to the PFJ.

Four RCTs[74–77] examined the use of a knee brace for the treatment of pain in subjects with PFPS. Different types of braces, all aiming to improve patella alignment, were used. The evidence is conflicting, with two trials[76,77] reporting improvement in pain and function while the other two[74,75] reported no significance difference. In fact, Lun et al.'s study[77] which compared the effectiveness of four treatment approaches (exercise alone, patella bracing alone, patella bracing and exercise, exercise and knee sleeve) showed that all groups showed subjective and functional improvement over time.

Our meta-analysis[23] indicated significant protection of overall lower limb injuries with the use of insoles (RR 0.80; 95% CI 0.66–0.98). However, no such protection was observed when only the incidence of knee injuries was analyzed (RR 0.99; 95% CI 0.73–1.33).

Recommendations

- There is moderate quality evidence that patella taping alone has no beneficial effect in the management of PFPS
- Moderate-quality evidence suggests that taping combined with other physiotherapeutic treatment approaches can improve pain and function in individuals with PFPS. The challenge is to find the optimal combination of physical interventions
- There is a moderate-high level of evidence to suggest the use of patellofemoral brace in the prevention of PFPS in individuals undertaking strenuous and intensive exercises with short adaptation period
- There is a low level of evidence to support the use of knee brace in reducing pain in individuals with PFPS
- There is very low quality evidence to suggest that insoles is effective in preventing PFPS

Question 6: Can other treatment modalities be used in the treatment of patellofemoral pain?

Current opinion

Other treatment options such as pharmacological intervention and electrical modalities have been suggested in the literature for the treatment of PFPS.

Quality of the evidence
Level I
- 2 systematic reviews[78,79]

Findings

The role of nonsteroidal anti-inflammatory drugs (NSAIDs) and glucocorticosteroids has been examined in a systematic review[78] which showed that there is limited evidence for short-term pain reduction in PFPS. Furthermore, the evidence for the effect of glucosamine polysulfate injection is contradictory. There is also insufficient evidence to show that therapeutic ultrasound therapy[79] is useful for pain relief in individuals with PFPS.

Recommendation

- There is very low quality evidence to suggest that pharmacological treatment or ultrasound therapy reduces pain in individuals with PFPS

Question 7: What is the prognosis for PFPS?

Relevance

The rehabilitation of PFPS can be slow, but understanding the natural history and prognosis of the condition can increase the individual's compliance with treatment recommendations.

Current opinion

Different management approaches to the treatment of PFPS have been suggested in the literature. There is a need for long-term follow-up to examine if the treatment is able to change the natural course of the condition.

Quality of evidence
Level II
- 4 follow-up studies[28,29,80,81] address the long-term outcome and prognosis for subjects with PFPS at different age groups; the duration of follow-up ranges from 7 to 20 years

Findings

In a cross-sectional study[81] which examined the long-term outcome of anterior knee pain developed in childhood (n = 22; mean age 10.5 years at first diagnosis), 91% of the subjects at follow-up (4–18 years) still had complaints of knee pain which affected their daily activities. However, the diagnosis of PFPS had not been so clearly defined, except that the subjects had anterior knee pain. This is also reflected in the fact that a high percentage of subjects developed other medical conditions such as psoriasis, arthritis, and pain in other joints. As such, the result may not be a true reflection of the prognosis of PFPS. In a long-term study[80] which examined the outcome of adolescent girls (mean age 15.5 years at entry into the study) with PFPS showed that 50% of the subjects improved spontaneously at 3.8 years follow-up. This natural history of recovery may be related to the musculoskeletal development in adolescents. At 16 years follow-up, 27% of subjects continued to have pain and disability though there was no evidence of structural pathology. This incidence of pain is much lower than that previously reported.[81] Prospective studies[28,29] that examined the outcome in subjects with PFPS (mean age 27 years at entry to the study) showed that 75% of subjects who received a 6-week intensive quadriceps muscle training had good subjective and functional recovery at 6-month and 7-year follow-up. Furthermore, the results showed that good quadriceps strength significantly predicted good long-term outcome, whereas radiologic and MRI changes showed no association.

Recommendations

- PFPS developed during adolescence has a better prognosis and tends to resolve spontaneously [overall level: moderate]
- In adults with PFPS, if symptoms do not spontaneously resolve, an intensive quadriceps rehabilitation program is likely to produce a favorable outcome [overall level: moderate]

Summary of recommendations

- Intrinsic risk factors that influence the PFJ loading, including muscle imbalances and biomechanical alterations, are thought to contribute to the onset of pain. Extrinsic risk factors including training error and footwear are commonly reported
- There is strong evidence for an association between training volume and running-related lower limb injuries
- Direct evidence for quantifying the optimal training load for a runner preparing for a 10km or marathon race is lacking
- Physiotherapy-supervised exercise therapy is effective for PFPS
- Either OKC or CKC quadriceps strengthening has beneficial effects in reducing pain and improving function in subjects with PFPS, short- and long-term
- There is moderate-quality evidence to suggest that VMO retraining is effective in the treatment of PFPS, but it is unclear if VMO can be preferentially activated
- There is insufficient evidence to suggest that hip muscle strengthening or stretching to be effective in improving symptoms in subjects with PFPS
- The efficacy of patella taping alone in the management of PFPS is unclear, but taping combined with other physiotherapeutic treatment approaches can improve pain and function in subjects with PFPS
- There is moderate-high quality evidence to suggest the use of patellofemoral brace in the prevention of PFPS in individuals undertaking strenuous and intensive exercises with short adaptation period
- The evidence that knee brace is effective in improving pain in subjects with PFPS is conflicting
- There is limited evidence that the use of insoles is effective in preventing PFPS
- PFPS developed during adolescence has a better prognosis and tends to resolve spontaneously
- In adults with PFPS, if symptoms do not spontaneously resolve, an intensive quadriceps rehabilitation program is likely to produce a favorable outcome

References

1. McConnell J. The management of chondromalacia patellae: A long-term solution. Aust J Physiother 1986;32:215–23.
2. Taunton JE, Ryan MB, Clement DB, et al. A retrospective case-control analysis of 2002 running injuries. Br J Sports Med 2002;36:95–101.
3. Pinshaw R, Atlas V, Noakes TD. The nature and response to therapy of 196 consecutive injuries seen at a runners' clinic. S Afr Med J 1984;65:291–8.
4. Ballas MT, Tytko J, Cookson D. Common overuse running injuries: diagnosis and management. Am Fam Physician 1997;55:2473–84.
5. Macintyre J, Taunton J, Clement D, et al. Running injuries: A clinical study of 4173 cases. Clin J Sport Med 1991;1:81–7.
6. Cichanowski HR, Schmitt JS, Johnson RJ, et al. Hip strength in collegiate female athletes with patellofemoral pain. Med Sci Sports Exerc 2007;39:1227–32.
7. Milgrom C, Finestone A, Eldad A, et al. Patellofemoral pain caused by overactivity. J Bone Joint Surg Am 1991;73:1041–3.
8. Biedert RM, Kernen V. Neurosensory characteristics of the patellofemoral joint: what is the genesis of patellofemoral pain? Sports Med Arthrosc 2001;9:295–300.
9. Dye SF. The pathophysiology of patellofemoral pain: a tissue homeostasis perspective. Clin Orthop Relat Res 2005;436:100–10.
10. LaBella C. Patellofemoral pain syndrome: evaluation and treatment. Prim Care 2004;31:977–1003.
11. Dixit S, DiFiori JP, Burton M, et al. Management of patellofemoral pain syndrome. Am Fam Physician 2007;75:194–202.
12. van Gent RN, Siem D, van Middelkoop M, et al. Incidence and determinants of lower extremity running injuries in long distance runners: a systematic review. Br J Sports Med 2007;41:469–80.
13. Hreljac A. Etiology, prevention, and early intervention of overuse injuries in runners: a biomechanical perspective. Phys Med Rehabil Clin N Am 2005;16:651–67.
14. Thijs Y, De Clercq D, Roosen P, et al. Gait-related intrinsic risk factors for patellofemoral pain in novice recreational runners. Br J Sports Med 2008;42:466–71.
15. Witvrouw E, Lysens R, Bellemans J, et al. Intrinsic risk factors for the development of anterior knee pain in an athletic population: a two-year prospective study. Am J Sports Med 2000;28:480–9.
16. Powers CM, Chen PY, Reischl SF, et al. Comparison of foot pronation and lower extremity rotation in persons with and without patellofemoral pain. Foot Ankle Int 2002;23:634–40.
17. Cowan DN, Jones BH, Frykman PN, et al. Lower limb morphology and risk of overuse injury among male infantry trainees. Medi Sci Sports Exerc 1996;28:945–52.
18. Duffey MJ, Martin DF, Cannon DW, et al. Etiologic factors associated with anterior knee pain in distance runners. Med Sci Sports Exerc 2000;32:1825–32.
19. Messier SP, Legault C, Schoenlank CR, et al. Risk factors and mechanisms of knee injury in runners. Med Sci Sports Exerc 2008;40:1873–9.
20. Marti B, Vader JP, Minder CE, et al. On the epidemiology of running injuries. The 1984 Bern Grand-Prix study. Am J Sports Med 1988;16:285–94.
21. Macera CA. Lower extremity injuries in runners. Advances in prediction. Sports Med 1992;13:50–7.
22. Taunton JE, Ryan MB, Clement DB, et al. A prospective study of running injuries: the Vancouver Sun Run "In Training" clinics. Br J Sports Med 2003;37:239–44.
23. Yeung EW, Yeung SS. Interventions for preventing lower limb soft-tissue injuries in runners. Cochrane Database Syst Rev 2001;3.
24. Andrish JT, Bergfeld JA, Walheim J. A prospective study on the management of shin splints. J Bone Joint Surg 1974;56:1697–700.
25. Pollock ML, Gettman LR, Milesis CA, et al. Effects of frequency and duration of training on attrition and incidence of injury. Med Sci Sports Exerc 1977;9:31–6.

26. Rudzki SJ. Injuries in Australian army recruits. Part I: Decreased incidence and severity of injury seen with reduced running distance. Part II: Location and cause of injuries seen in recruits. Mil Med 1997;162:472–6.

27. Buist I, Bredeweg SW, van Mechelen W, et al. No effect of a graded training program on the number of running-related injuries in novice runners. Am J Sports Med 2008;36:33–9.

28. Kannus P, Natri A, Paakkala T, et al. An outcome study of chronic patellofemoral pain syndrome. Seven-year follow-up of patients in a randomized, controlled trial. J Bone Joint Surg Am 1999;81:355–63.

29. Natri A, Kannus P, Järvinen M. Which factors predict the long-term outcome in chronic patellofemoral pain syndrome? A 7-yr prospective follow-up study. Med Sci Sports Exerc 1998;30: 1572–7.

30. Sakai N, Luo ZP, Rand JA, et al. The influence of weakness in the vastus medialis oblique muscle on the patellofemoral joint: an in vitro biomechanical study. Clin Biomech 2000;15:335–9.

31. van Tiggelen D, Cowan S, Coorevits P, et al. Delayed vastus medialis obliquus to vastus lateralis onset timing contributes to the development of patellofemoral pain in previously healthy men: a prospective study. Am J Sports Med 2009;37:1099–105.

32. Chester R, Smith TO, Sweeting D, et al. The relative timing of VMO and VL in the aetiology of anterior knee pain: a systematic review and meta-analysis. BMC Musculoskelet Disord 2008;9:64.

33. Yeung SS, Au AL, Chow CC. Effects of fatigue on the temporal neuromuscular control of vastus medialis muscle in humans. Eur J Appl Physiol Occup Physiol 1999;80:379–85.

34. Heintjes EM, Berger M, Bierma-Zeinstra SMA, et al. Exercise therapy for patellofemoral pain syndrome. Cochrane Database Syst Rev 2003;4.

35. McMullen W, Roncarati A, Koval P. Static and isokinetic treatments of chondromalacia patella: A comparative investigation. J Orthop Sports Phys Ther 1990;12:256–66.

36. Timm KE. Randomized controlled trial of Protonics on patellar pain, position, and function. Med Sci Sports Exerc 1998;30: 665–70.

37. Clark DI, Downing N, Mitchell J, et al. Physiotherapy for anterior knee pain: a randomised controlled trial. Ann Rheum Dis 2000;59:700–4.

38. Crossley K, Bennell KL, Green S, et al. Physical therapy for patellofemoral pain: A randomized, double-blinded, placebo-controlled trial. Am J Sports Med 2002;30:857–65.

39. van Linschoten R, van Middelkoop M, Berger MY, et al. Supervised exercise therapy versus usual care for patellofemoral pain syndrome: an open label randomised controlled trial. BMJ 2009;339, b4074.

40. Colón VF, Mangine R, McKnight C, et al. The pogo stick in rehabilitating patients with patellofemoral chondrosis. J Rehabil 1988;54:73–7.

41. Gaffney K, Fricker P, Dwyer T, et al. Patellofemoral joint pain: a comparison of two treatment programmes. Excel 1992;8:179–89.

42. Wijnen LCAM, Lenssen AF, Kuys-Wouters YMS, et al. McConnell therapy versus Coumans bandage for patellofemoral pain - a randomised pilot study. Nederlands Tijdschrift voor fysiotherapie Special, 1996;12–17.

43. Witvrouw E, Lysens R, Bellemans J, et al. Open versus closed kinetic chain exercises for patellofemoral pain. A prospective, randomized study. Am J Sports Med 2000;28:687–94.

44. Witvrouw E, Danneels L, Van Tiggelen D, et al. Open versus closed kinetic chain exercises in patellofemoral pain: a 5-year prospective randomized study. Am J Sports Med 2004;32: 1122–30.

45. Stiene HA, Brosky T, Reinking MF, et al. A comparison of closed kinetic chain and isokinetic joint isolation exercise in patients with patellofemoral dysfunction. J Orthop Sports Phys Ther 1996;24:136–41.

46. Bizzini M, Childs JD, Piva SR, et al. Systematic review of the quality of randomized controlled trials for patellofemoral pain syndrome. J Orthop Sports Phys Ther 2003;33:4–20.

47. Cowan SM, Bennell KL, Crossley KM, et al. Physical therapy alters recruitment of the vasti in patellofemoral pain syndrome. Med Sci Sports Exerc 2002;34:1879–85.

48. Cowan SM, Bennell KL, Hodges PW, et al. Simultaneous feed-forward recruitment of the vasti in untrained postural tasks can be restored by physical therapy. J Orthop Res 2003;21:553–8.

49. Smith TO, Bowyer D, Dixon J, et al. Can vastus medialis oblique be preferentially activated? A systematic review of electromyographic studies. Physiother Theory Pract 2009;25:69–98.

50. Ireland ML, Willson JD, Ballantyne BT, et al. Hip strength in females with and without patellofemoral pain. J Orthop Sports Phys Ther 2003;33:671–6.

51. Piva SR, Goodnite EA, Childs JD. Strength around the hip and flexibility of soft tissues in individuals with and without patellofemoral pain syndrome. J Orthop Sports Phys Ther 2005; 35:793–801.

52. Cichanowski HR, Schmitt JS, Johnson RJ, et al. Hip strength in collegiate female athletes with patellofemoral pain. Med Sci Sports Exerc 2007;39:1227–32.

53. Robinson RL, Nee RJ. Analysis of hip strength in females seeking physical therapy treatment for unilateral patellofemoral pain syndrome. J Orthop Sports Phys Ther 2007;37:232–8.

54. Bolgla LA, Malone TR, Umberger BR, et al. Hip strength and hip and knee kinematics during stair descent in females with and without patellofemoral pain syndrome. J Orthop Sports Phys Ther 2008;38:12–18.

55. Prins MR, van der Wurff P. Females with patellofemoral pain syndrome have weak hip muscles: a systematic review. Aust J Physiother 2009;55:9–15.

56. Fagan V, Delahunt E. Patellofemoral pain syndrome: a review on the associated neuromuscular deficits and current treatment options. Br J Sports Med 2008;42:789–95.

57. Mascal CL, Landel R, Powers C. Management of patellofemoral pain targeting hip, pelvis, and trunk muscle function: 2 case reports. J Orthop Sports Phys Ther 2003;33:647–60.

58. Boling MC, Bolgla LA, Mattacola CG, et al. Outcomes of a weight-bearing rehabilitation program for patients diagnosed with patellofemoral pain syndrome. Arch Phys Med Rehabil 2006;87:1428–35.

59. Tyler TF, Nicholas SJ, Mullaney MJ, et al. The role of hip muscle function in the treatment of patellofemoral pain syndrome. Am J Sports Med 2006;34:630–6.

60. Puniello MS. Iliotibial band tightness and medial patellar glide in patients with patellofemoral dysfunction. J Orthop Sports Phys Ther 1993;17:144–8.

61. Haim A, Yaniv M, Dekel S, et al. Patellofemoral pain syndrome: validity of clinical and radiological features. Clin Orthop Relat Res 2006;451:223–8.

62. Crossley K, Bennell K, Green S, et al. A systematic review of physical interventions for patellofemoral pain syndrome. Clin J Sport Med 2001;11:103–10.

63. Bizzini M, Childs JD, Piva SR, et al. Systematic review of the quality of randomized controlled trials for patellofemoral pain syndrome. J Orthop Sports Phys Ther 2003;33:4–20.

64. Overington M, Goddard D, Hing W. A critical appraisal and literature critique on the effect of patellar taping—is patellar taping effective in the treatment of patellofemoral pain syndrome? N Z J Physiother 2006;34:66–80.

65. Aminaka N, Gribble PA. Patellar taping, patellofemoral pain syndrome, lower extremity kinematics, and dynamic postural control. J Athl Train 2008;43:21–28.

66. Warden SJ, Hinman RS, Watson MA Jr, et al. Patellar taping and bracing for the treatment of chronic knee pain: a systematic review and meta-analysis. Arthritis Rheum 2008;59:73–83.

67. Harrison EL, Sheppard MS , McQuarrie AM. A randomized controlled trial of physical therapy treatment programs in patellofemoral pain syndrome. Physiother Can 1999;51:93–106.

68. Whittingham M, Palmar S, Macmillan F.: Effects of taping on pain and function in patellofemoral pain syndrome: A randomized controlled trial. J Orthop Sports Phys Ther 2004;34:504–10.

69. Cowan SM, Bennell KL, Hodges PW. Therapeutic patellar taping changes the timing of vasti muscle activation in people with patellofemoral pain syndrome. Clin J Sports Med 2002;12:339–47.

70. Cowan SM, Hodges PW, Crossley KM, et al. Patellar taping does not change the amplitude of electromyographic activity of the vasti in a stair stepping task. Br J Sports Med 2006;40:30–4.

71. Keet JHL, Gray J, Harley Y, et al. The effect of medial patellar taping on pain, strength and neuromuscular recruitment in subjects with and without patellofemoral pain. Physiotherapy 2007;93:42–52.

72. BenGal S, Lowe J, Mann G, et al. The role of the knee brace in the prevention of anterior knee pain syndrome. Am J Sports Med 1997;25:118–22.

73. Van Tiggelen D, Witvrouw E, Roget P, et al. Effect of bracing on the prevention of anterior knee pain — a prospective randomized study. Knee Surg Sports Traumatol Arthrosc 2004;12:434–9.

74. Finestone A, Radin EL, Lev B, et al. Treatment of overuse patellofemoral pain—prospective randomised controlled clinical trial in a military setting. Clin Orthop Relat Res 1993;293:208–10.

75. Miller MD, Hinkin DT, Wisnowski JW. The efficacy of orthotics for anterior knee pain in military trainees. A preliminary report. Am J Knee Surg 1997;10:10–13.

76. Timm KE. Randomized controlled trial of Protonics on patellar pain, position, and function. Med Sci Sports Exerc 1998;30:665–70.

77. Lun VM, Wiley JP, Meeuwisse WH, et al. Effectiveness of patellar bracing for treatment of patellofemoral pain syndrome. Clin J Sport Med 2005;15:235–40.

78. Heintjes EM, Berger M, Bierma-Zeinstra SMA, et al. Pharmacotherapy for patellofemoral pain syndrome. Cochrane Database Syst Rev 2004;3.

79. Brosseau L, Casimiro L, Welch V, et al. Therapeutic ultrasound for treating patellofemoral pain syndrome. Cochrane Database Syst Rev 2001;4.

80. Nimon G, Murray D, Sandow M, et al. Natural history of anterior knee pain: a 14- to 20-year follow-up of nonoperative management. J Pediatr Orthop 1998;18:118–22.

81. Stathopulu E, Baildam E. Anterior knee pain: a long-term follow-up. Rheumatology (Oxford) 2003;42:380–2.

101 Ankle Ligament Injury

Michel P.J. van den Bekerom[1], Rover Krips[2], and Gino M.M.J. Kerkhoffs[1]

[1]Academic Medical Centre, Amsterdam, The Netherlands
[2]Diaconessenhuis, Leiden, The Netherlands

Case scenario

A female patient twisted her right ankle because she jumped while playing basketball and landed awkwardly on the foot of an opponent. Later that day she went to the Emergency Department because her ankle was painful and swollen. The Ottawa rules indicated a possible fracture, which was excluded with standard radiographs. Physical examination (range of motion and stability tests) was difficult to perform because of pain. There was no evidence of redness or heat. However, there was considerable swelling and pain on palpation over the lateral side of the injured ankle.

Relevant anatomy

The lateral ankle ligaments consist of three ligaments: the anterior talofibular ligament (ATFL), the calcaneofibular ligament (CFL), and the posterior talofibular ligament (PTFL).[1] The most common mechanism of injury is supination and adduction (i.e., inversion) of the plantar-flexed foot. It is known that the ATFL is almost always the first or only ligament to sustain injury. Broström[2] found that combined ruptures of the ATFL and the CFL occurred in 20% of cases and that isolated rupture of the CFL was very rare. The PTFL is usually not injured unless there is a frank dislocation of the ankle.

Most authors use the term "sprain" to describe a morphologic condition representing a diversity of pathology, ranging from overstretching of the ligament to complete rupture with instability of the joint. To classify the severity of ankle sprains and injury to the lateral ligaments, a grading system has been introduced (see box).[3,4]

> Grading system for ankle sprains and injury to lateral ligaments
>
> - *Grade I:* mild stretching of the ligament with no instability
> - *Grade II:* partial rupture with mild instability of the joint (e.g., isolated rupture of the ATFL)
> - *Grade III:* complete rupture of the ligaments with instability of the joint

Importance of the problem

Acute ankle trauma is one of the most prevalent injuries of the musculoskeletal tract and it is the most frequently observed injury in the Emergency Department. It has been estimated that one ankle sprain occurs per 10,000 people each day.[5] Each year, approximately 1 million patients with acute lateral ankle ligament injury are seen by primary care physicians in the United States.[6] Inversion injuries are treated by emergency and primary healthcare physicians as well as by orthopedic and trauma surgeons.[4]

Inversion injuries involve about 25% of all injuries of the locomotor system, with over 20,000 patients in the US each day.[7] About 50% of these injuries are sport related.[2,8] Sports such as basketball, soccer, and volleyball have a particularly high incidence of ankle injuries.[9] Inversion injuries of the ankle, if not treated properly, may lead to late symptoms in 30–40% of patients.[7,10]

Although most physicians probably consider the clinical result as the most important outcome, the socioeconomic consequences of ankle sprains are impressive as well. The annual costs to society for ankle injuries have been estimated to be approximately US$35 million per 1 million people.[6] A Harvard study dating from 1983 estimated the annual costs for ankle ligament injuries in the US at approximately US$2 billion.[11] Apart from direct costs (materials, visits to Emergency Department and outpatient clinic, and consultant fees), these estimates include indirect costs, such as loss of income and incapacity to work during (part) of the rehabilitation period.

Care providers and patients are inundated with an ever-increasing and easily accessible body of information about lateral ankle ligament injuries. When the search term "ankle sprain" is entered into Google, over 5,000,000 hits appear. The variable quality and lack of filtering mandates the need for preappraised evidence-based guides.

Top ten questions

Diagnosis

1. How accurate is clinical examination in the diagnosis of acute lateral ankle ligament injuries?
2. When should the physical examination be performed?
3. Is there a role for additional examinations?

Therapy

4. Is rest, ice, compression, and elevation (RICE) therapy beneficial in the treatment of acute lateral ankle ligament injuries?
5. Is ultrasound beneficial in the treatment of acute lateral ankle ligament injuries?
6. Is functional treatment the optimal treatment compared with immobilization for acute lateral ankle ligament injuries?
7. What is the preferred type of functional treatment for acute lateral ankle ligament injuries?
8. Are the results of surgical treatment superior to conservative treatment for acute injuries of the lateral ligament complex of the ankle?

Prognosis

9. What are the long-term results of lateral ankle ligament injuries?

Prevention

10. What is the optimal prevention strategy to avoid acute lateral ankle ligament injuries?

Question 1: How accurate is clinical examination in the diagnosis of acute lateral ankle ligament injuries?

Case clarification

Our patient twisted her ankle while playing basketball. Which tests should be performed during physical examina-tion to be sure that she sustained lateral ankle ligament injury? What is the sensitivity and specificity of these tests?

Relevance

Standard radiographs including AP, lateral, and mortise views are sufficient to rule out fractures, severe osteoarthritis, and significant osteochondral defects. The Ottawa ankle rules are helpful to save unnecessary radiographic investigation, using bony tenderness and ability to bear weight as indicator for radiography.[12]

Current opinion

The most important features of physical examination are swelling, hematoma, discoloration, localized pain on palpation, and positive anterior drawer test. The site of the pain on palpation is important. If there is no pain on palpation on the ATFL, there is no acute lateral ankle ligament rupture.[13] Pain on palpation on the ALTL itself cannot differentiate a mild stretch from rupture.

Finding the evidence

- Cochrane Bone, Joint and Muscle Trauma Group Specialized Register
- Cochrane Controlled Trials Register
- Pubmed/MEDLINE
- Embase
- CINAHL
- PEDro—the Physiotherapy Evidence Database
- Reference lists of included articles

Quality of the evidence

Level III
- 2 studies[13,14]

Findings

Localized pain on palpation in combination with hematoma discoloration gives a 90% chance that there is an acute lateral ligament rupture.[15] A positive anterior drawer test by itself has a sensitivity of 73% and a specificity of 97%.[14] A positive anterior drawer test in combination with pain on palpation on the ATFL and hematoma discoloration has a sensitivity of 100% and specificity of 77%.

Recommendation

- The anterior drawer test in combination with pain on palpation on the ATFL and hematoma discoloration is very reliable in diagnosing acute lateral ankle ligament injury [overall quality: low]

Question 2: When should the physical examination be performed?

Case clarification

We know which tests we have to perform during physical examination, but when is this examination most reliable?

Relevance

The inconsistent outcome of physical examination within 48 hours of trauma is caused by the diffuse character of the pain; the swelling itself, which gives no information as to whether it is due to hematoma or edema formation; and the unreliability of the anterior drawer test, due to pain and swelling.

Current opinion

By waiting a few days and performing a delayed physical examination, the pain and swelling can be expected to have decreased. First, this decrease in pain and swelling facilitates the palpation of the separate ligaments. The presence or absence of pain on palpation of the ligaments indicates a ligament rupture. Secondly, it allows clearer interpretation of a positive anterior drawer test as an indicator of ligament rupture. Thirdly, we will gain more insight into the contents of the swelling—hematoma indicates a rupture, while the absence of hematoma discoloration is likely to be associated with intact ligaments.

Finding the evidence

See Question 1

Quality of the evidence

Level III
• 2 studies[13,14]

Findings

The specificity and sensitivity of delayed physical examination for the presence or absence of lateral ankle ligament rupture were 84% and 96% respectively.[13,14]

Recommendation

• Delayed physical examination (4–5 days after trauma) provides a diagnostic modality of high quality and is more reliable than physical examination within 48 hours after trauma [overall quality: low]

Question 3: Is there a role for additional examinations?

Case clarification

We performed the physical examination 5 days after our patient twisted her ankle. Is there a role for additional examinations (stress radiography, CT, MRI, or ultrasound)?

Relevance

For most injuries, after the physical examination is performed additional investigations are necessary in order to make the definite diagnosis. Is the reliability of physical examination with additional radiographic examinations higher than that of physical examination alone? Should we perform these investigations despite the costs, radiation exposure, and possible complications?

Current opinion

Today the golden standard in the diagnosis of acute lateral ligament injury is the delayed physical examination. Additional examinations could be useful in diagnosing and workup of chronic lateral ankle ligament instability.

Finding the evidence

See Question 1.

Quality of the evidence

Level III
• 12 studies[3,13,14–22]

Findings

Stress radiography has proven helpful with concerns about lateral ankle ligament laxity. Both talar tilt and the anterior drawer test are useful in assessment of ligament laxity in patients with chronic instability complaints. In the acutely injured ankle, a stress test is quite painful; also, because of the wide variation of normal values, the interpretation of stress radiographs if often difficult. There is also the disadvantage of the use of radiography itself. Nowadays stress radiography is merely of scientific interest and has a limited role in making the definite diagnosis in clinical practice.

Ankle arthrography provides a relatively simple method for investigating acute ankle ligament ruptures.[16,17] Since the ATFL is intimately associated with the joint capsule, a ligament tear will also result in a capsular tear, which can be demonstrated arthrographically. Capsular tears are rapidly sealed by clots and fibrin, so arthrography is only reliable within the first 24–48 hours after trauma. Arthrography has a high sensitivity with a lower specificity.[21,22] The reliability of arthrography for quantification of the severity of ligament damage is quite poor;[18] also, the test is invasive and thus a relative high burden for the patient.[18]

MRI is less suitable for differentiating between acute and chronic lateral ankle ligament injury. The primary use of MRI in the evaluation of acute ankle injuries therefore remains in the diagnosis and evaluation of tendon disorders and osteochondral lesions, although the latter can be diagnosed more reliably with a CT scan.[15]

Ultrasound investigation causes little discomfort to patients. The sensitivity and specificity of the ultrasound investigation are 92% and 64% respectively. The predictive value of a positive ultrasound investigation is 85% and of a negative ultrasound investigation 77%.[3,13,14] Ultrasound investigation can be useful in diagnosing additional (cartilage) damage in patients with acute lateral ankle ligament injury.[17]

Recommendation
- The high costs, high burden for the patient, availability, possible complications, and lack of reliability of the most diagnostic modalities, as well as the lack of a simple test, motivated the improvements in reliability of the physical examination as a diagnostic tool [overall level: low]

Question 4: Is RICE therapy beneficial in the treatment of acute lateral ankle ligament injuries?

Case clarification
Our patient is not yet diagnosed with an evident acute lateral ankle ligament injury, but we know she has a sprained ankle. Is RICE therapy beneficial for the first few days before making the definite diagnosis?

Relevance
The variation in treatment observed for the acutely injured lateral ankle ligament complex in the first week after the injury suggests a lack of evidence-based management strategies for this problem.

Current opinion
According to the Dutch Institute for Healthcare Improvement (CBO) consensus guidelines, RICE therapy is the treatment of choice for the first 4–5 days to reduce pain and swelling. After this period the physical examination provides a diagnostic modality of high quality.

Finding the evidence
See Question 1.

Quality of the evidence
Level I
- 1 systematic review[15]

Level II
- 11 randomized trials with methodological limitations

Findings
After removal of the overlaps between the different databases, evaluation of the abstracts, and contact with some authors, a final total of 24 potentially eligible trials remained. This resulted in the inclusion of 11 trials, involving 868 patients.

Pooling the results of the included studies was not realistic, mainly because of different outcome measures. Insufficient evidence is available from randomized controlled trials (RCTs) to determine the relative effectiveness of RICE therapy for acute ankle sprains in adults.[23]

Recommendations
Treatment decisions concerning RICE therapy must be made on an individual basis, carefully weighing the relative benefits and risks of each option.

- Rest should be interpreted as relative rest and not as complete immobilization without weightbearing [overall level: very low]
- There is little evidence to support the use of ice in the treatment of acute ankle sprains [overall level: low]
- There is very little evidence to support the use of compression in the treatment of acute ankle sprains [overall level: very low]
- There is no evidence to support the use of elevation in the treatment of acute ankle sprains

Question 5: Is additional ultrasound beneficial for patients with acute lateral ankle ligament injuries?

Case clarification
Our patient has an evident acute lateral ankle ligament injury and was treated with RICE for the first days. Thereafter treatment (operative or nonoperative) will be continued. Is additional ultrasound treatment beneficial for our patient?

Relevance
Ultrasound has been used in the treatment of musculoskeletal conditions for many years. Ultrasound equipment consists of a generator and transducer. The generator produces electromagnetic energy with a frequency of 0.5–3.5 MHz, which is converted by the transducer to mechanical energy with a similar frequency and intensity of up to $3 W/cm^2$.[24] Laboratory research has demonstrated that the application of ultrasound results in the promotion of cellular metabolic rate and increased viscoelastic properties of collagen.[25] In animal studies, an exposure to 1 MHz ultrasound at $50 J/cm^2$ is reported to be sufficient to increase tissue temperature.[26] This rise in temperature is assumed to be the mediating mechanism for tissue repair, the enhancement of soft tissue extensibility, promotion of muscle relaxation, augmentation of blood flow, and alleviation of inflammatory reactions of soft tissue.[25,27–29]

Current opinion
Based on these experimental findings, ultrasound is used in physical therapy to relieve pain, reduce swelling, and improve joint immobility in a wide variety of musculoskeletal disorders including ankle sprains. Despite the theoretical benefits and widespread use, conclusive evidence on the effectiveness of ultrasound therapy in patient care is not yet available.

Finding the evidence
See Question 1.

Quality of the evidence
Level I
- 1 meta-analysis[30]
- 4 randomized trials

Level II
- 2 randomized trials with methodologic limitations

Findings
Six trials were included, involving 572 participants. None of the four placebo-controlled trials (sham ultrasound) demonstrated statistically significant differences between true and sham ultrasound therapy for any outcome measure at 7–14 days of follow-up. The pooled relative risk for general improvement was 1.04 (random effects model, 95% CI 0.92–1.17) for active vs. sham ultrasound. The differences between intervention groups were generally small, 0–6% for most dichotomous outcomes. However, one trial reported relatively large differences for pain-free status (20%) and swelling (25%) in favor of ultrasound.

Recommendations
- The results of four placebo-controlled trials do not support the use of ultrasound in terms of symptom relief [overall level: high] and functional disability [overall level: moderate] in the treatment of ankle sprains
- Because of the limited amount of information on treatment parameters, no conclusions can be made regarding an optimal and adequate dosage schedule for ultrasound therapy, or whether such a schedule would improve on the reported effectiveness of ultrasound for ankle sprains

Question 6: Is functional treatment the optimal treatment compared with immobilization for acute lateral ankle ligament injuries?

Case clarification
We have chosen to treat our patient nonoperatively after the initial RICE treatment. Do we have to treat her with a period of immobilization, or is a functional treatment more beneficial?

Relevance
Different nonoperative options are available for the treatment of an acute ankle sprain. The two main modalities of treatment are: (1) treatment with plaster cast immobilization and (2) functional treatment with tape, elastic bandage, or (lace-up) brace. The latter is an early mobilization program and involves the use of an external support combined with coordination training. Both types of treatment should have a minimal duration of 4 weeks and should be considered as a different treatment from short-term immobilization in the early inflammatory phase (first 4–5 days). The variation in treatment practice identified for lateral ankle ligament complex injuries suggests a lack of evidence-based management strategies for this problem.[2,3]

Current opinion
Dehne first reported ankle injury treatment with immobilization below the knee.[31] Many studies presenting results of this type of immobilization have since been published.[32,33] Freeman introduced a new concept in the conservative treatment of ruptures of the lateral ligaments of the ankle by suggesting that the use of proprioceptive training using coordination exercises could reduce the proprioceptive deficit and symptoms of the ankle "giving way".[10,34] Consequently, many patients were treated functionally with supportive elastic bandage combined with coordination training. Functional treatment with tape bandage or orthotic support has become more popular since the 1980s.[35–39]

Finding the evidence
See Question 1.

Quality of the evidence
Level I
- 2 meta-analyses[40,41]
- 9 randomized trials

Level II
- 16 randomized trials with methodological limitations

Findings
Twenty-five trials involving 2587 participants were included. For the primary outcomes, statistically significant differences in favor of functional treatment when compared with immobilization were found. More patients returned to sport in the long term (RR 1.89; 95% CI 1.24–2.89); more patients had returned to work at short-term follow-up (RR 5.17; 95% CI 2.36–11.34); the time taken to return to work was shorter (WMD 12.47 days; 95% CI 10.74–14.20); fewer patients complained about persistent pain at short-term follow-up (RR 1.90; CI 1.34–2.68) as well as at intermediate-term follow-up (RR 1.53; CI 1.13–2.06); and fewer patients complained of subjective instability at intermediate-term follow-up (RR 1.91, CI 1.36–2.61). In all analyses performed, no results were significantly in favor of immobilization. No significant differences between varying types of immobilization, immobilization and physiotherapy, or no treatment were found, apart from one trial where patients returned to work sooner after treatment with a soft cast.

Recommendation
- Functional treatment appears to be the favorable strategy for treating acute ankle sprains when compared with a period of more than 4 weeks of immobilization, with regard to symptom relief [overall level: low], return to work [overall level: moderate], return to sport [overall level: low], and joint stability [overall level: low]

Question 7: What is the preferred type of functional treatment for acute lateral ankle ligament injuries?

Case clarification
We have chosen to treat our patient with an acute lateral ligament injury nonoperatively, and we know that a functional treatment is superior to immobilization. What is the best functional treatment?

Relevance
Freeman introduced a new concept in the conservative treatment of ruptures of the lateral ligaments of the ankle by suggesting that the use of proprioceptive training using coordination exercises could reduce the proprioceptive deficit and symptoms of the ankle "giving way".[10,34] Consequently, patients were treated with nonspecific elastic bandage combined with coordination training.

Current opinion
Functional treatment with tape bandage or orthotic support has become more popular since the 1980s.[35–39] The preferable type of functional treatment was not known until the review by Kerkhoffs et al.[42]

Finding the evidence
See Question 1.

Quality of the evidence
Level I
- 2 meta-analyses[40,42]
- 8 randomized trials

Level II
- 3 randomized trials with methodologic limitations

Findings
Eleven trials and 1235 participants were included. Lace-up ankle support had significantly better results for persistent swelling at short-term follow-up when compared with semi-rigid ankle support (RR 4.19; 95% CI 1.26–13.98), elastic bandage (RR 5.48; 95% CI 1.69–17.76), or tape (RR 4.07; 95% CI 1.21–13.68). Use of a semi-rigid ankle support resulted in a significantly faster to return to work when compared to an elastic bandage (WMD 4.24 days; 95% CI 2.42–6.06). One trial found the use of a semi-rigid ankle support a significantly quicker return to sport compared with elastic bandage (RR 9.60; 95% CI 6.34–12.86); another trial found fewer patients reported instability at short-term follow-up when treated with a semi-rigid support than with an elastic bandage (RR 8.00; 95% CI 1.03–62.07). A fourth trial found a semi-rigid brace to be better than an elastic bandage with regard to swelling in the short term (WMD 5.90; 95% CI 0.59–11.21). A semi-rigid device was also shown to be significantly better for pain in the intermediate (WMD 4.00; 95% CI 3.33–4.67) and long term (WMD 5.2; 95% CI 4.49; 5.91). Tape treatment resulted in significantly more complications, the majority being skin irritations, when compared to treatment with an elastic bandage (RR 0.11; 95% CI 0.01–0.86). No other comparisons showed statistically significant differences.

Recommendations
The most effective treatment, both clinically and in terms of cost, is unclear from currently available randomized trials. Definitive conclusions are hampered by the variety of treatments used, and the inconsistency of reported follow-up times.
- The use of an elastic bandage has fewer complications than taping [overall level: high] but appears to be associated with a slower return to work [overall level: high] and sport [overall level: high], and more reported instability than a semi-rigid ankle support [overall level: high]
- Lace-up ankle support appears to be effective in reducing swelling in the short-term compared with semi-rigid ankle support [overall level: high], elastic bandage [overall level: high] and tape [overall level: high]

Question 8: Are the results of surgical treatment superior to conservative treatment for acute injuries of the lateral ligament complex of the ankle?

Case clarification
Would surgical treatment be superior to nonoperative treatment for our patient?

Relevance
Ankle sprains are one of the most commonly treated musculoskeletal injuries. The three main treatment modalities for acute lateral ankle ligament injuries are (1) immobilization with plaster cast or splint, (2) functional treatment consisting of early mobilization and use of an external support (e.g., ankle brace), and (3) surgical repair or reconstruction.

Current opinion
Today, most patients with acute lateral ankle ligament injury are treated nonoperatively. Surgical repair is performed in patients with chronic lateral ankle ligament injury.

Finding the evidence
See Question 1.

Quality of the evidence
Level I
- 2 meta-analyses[43,44]
- 2 randomized trials

Level II
- 18 randomized trials with methodologic limitations

Findings

Twenty trials were included. These involved a total of 2562 mostly young active adult males. Almost all trials had methodologic weaknesses. Specifically, concealment of allocation was confirmed in only one trial. Data for pooling individual outcomes were only available for a maximum of 12 trials and less than 60% of participants. The findings of statistically significant differences in favor of the surgical treatment group for the four primary outcomes (nonreturn to preinjury level of sports; ankle sprain recurrence; long-term pain; subjective or functional instability) when using the fixed-effect model were not robust when using the random effects model, or when one low-quality (quasi-randomized) trial that had more extreme results was removed. A corresponding drop in the I^2 statistics showed the remaining trials to be more homogeneous. The functional implications of the statistically significantly higher incidence of objective instability in conservatively treated trial participants are uncertain. There was some limited evidence for longer recovery times, and higher incidences of ankle stiffness, impaired ankle mobility, and complications in the surgical treatment group.

Recommendations

- Insufficient evidence is available from RCTs to determine the relative effectiveness of surgical and conservative treatment for acute injuries of the lateral ligament complex of the ankle in adults with emphasis on joint stability [overall level: very low], symptom relief [overall level: very low), recurrence [overall level: very low], and return to sport [overall level: low]
- Treatment decisions must be made on an individual basis, carefully weighing the relative benefits and risks of each option. Given the risk of operative complications, the higher costs (including those of hospital admission) associated with surgery, and the good results of secondary anatomic reconstructions of the lateral ankle ligaments, the best available option for most patients would be conservative treatment for acute injuries and close follow-up to identify patients who may remain symptomatic

Question 9: What are the long-term results or prognosis of lateral ankle ligament injuries?

Case clarification

We have treated our patient according to the current evidence. What can we tell her to expect in the long term?

Relevance

In order to evaluate the effectiveness of therapeutic interventions and to guide management decisions, it is impor-tant to have clear insight into the course of recovery after an acute lateral ankle injury and to evaluate potential factors for nonrecovery and resprains.

Current opinion

van Rijn et al.[22] present a clear overview of the clinical course of acute lateral ankle sprains and an evaluation of prognostic factors for incomplete recovery and resprains.

Finding the evidence

See Question 1.

Quality of the evidence

Level I
- 1 meta-analysis[45]

Level III
- 24 high-quality observational studies

Level IV
- 7 low-quality observational studies

Findings

In total, 31 studies were included, from which 24 studies were of high quality. There was a rapid decrease in pain reporting within the first 2 weeks. After 1 year 5–33% of patients still experienced pain, while 36–85% reported full recovery within a period of 3 years. The risk of resprains ranged from 3% to 34% of the patients, and resprain was registered in periods ranging from 2 weeks to 96 months after the initial injury. There was a wide variation in subjective instability, ranging from 0% to 33% in the high-quality studies and from 7% to 53% in the low-quality studies. One study described prognostic factors and indicated that training more than three times a week is a prognostic factor for residual symptoms.

Recommendation

- A high percentage of patients still experienced pain and subjective instability after 1 year of follow-up, and within a 3 year period, as many as 34% of the patients reported at least one resprain. From 36% to 85% of the patients reported full recovery within a period of 3 years.

Question 10: What is the optimal prevention strategy to avoid acute lateral ankle ligament injuries?

Case clarification

We have treated our patient according to the current evidence and we have informed her about the long-term prognosis. How can she avoid recurrent lateral ankle ligament injuries?

Relevance

Prevention of ankle injuries has the potential to play an important role in maintaining health for people who engage in high-risk sports and those who have suffered a previous injury to the ankle ligament complex.

Current opinion

Methods of prevention of ankle ligament injuries include use of modified footwear and associated supports, ankle taping, adapted training regimens including ankle exercises, and injury awareness. Prevention of injury recurrence may include interventions such as ankle disk exercises aimed at enhancing coordination and retraining proprioception (sense of muscular position). Secondary prevention, the prevention of recurrence, is a common treatment goal for many studies of ankle sprain treatment.

Finding the evidence

See Question 1.

Quality of the evidence

Level I
- 1 meta-analysis[46]

Level III
- 4 high-quality observational studies

Level IV
- 10 low-quality observational studies

Findings

Fourteen randomized trials with data for 8,279 participants were included. Twelve trials involved active, predominantly young, adults participating in organized, generally high-risk, activities. The other two trials involved injured patients who had been active in sports before their injury. The prophylactic interventions under test included the application of an external ankle support in the form of a semi-rigid orthosis (three trials), air-cast brace (one trial), or high-top shoes (one trial); ankle disk training; taping; muscle stretching; boot inserts; a health education program, and controlled rehabilitation.

The main finding was a significant reduction in the number of ankle sprains in people allocated external ankle support (RR 0.53; 95% CI 0.40–0.69). This reduction was greater for those with a previous history of ankle sprain, but still possible for those without prior sprain. There was no apparent difference in the severity of ankle sprains or any change to the incidence of other leg injuries. The protective effect of high-top shoes remains to be established. There was limited evidence for reduction in ankle sprain for those with previous ankle sprains who did ankle disk training exercises. Various problems with data reporting limited the interpretation of the results for many of the other interventions.

Recommendation

- There is high-level evidence for the beneficial effect of ankle supports in the form of semi-rigid orthoses or air-cast braces to prevent ankle sprains during high-risk sporting activities (e.g., soccer, basketball) [overall level: high]. Participants with a history of previous sprain can be advised that wearing such supports may reduce the risk of incurring a future sprain. [overall level: high]. However, any potential prophylactic effect should be balanced against the baseline risk of the activity, the supply and cost of the particular device, and for some, the possible or perceived loss of performance

Summary of recommendations

- The anterior drawer test in combination with pain on palpation on the ATFL and hematoma discoloration is very reliable in diagnosing acute lateral ankle ligament injury. Delayed physical examination (4–5 days after trauma) provides a diagnostic modality of high quality and is more reliable than physical examination within 48 hours after trauma. The high costs, high burden for the patient, availability, possible complications and lack of reliability of the most diagnostic modalities as well as the lack of a simple test formed the motivation to examine how to improve the outcome of the physical examination as a diagnostic tool
- Rest should be interpreted as relative rest and not as complete immobilization without weightbearing. Mobilization and weightbearing as tolerated is the most optimal regime. There is little evidence to support the use of ice and compression in the treatment of acute ankle sprains, and no evidence to support the use of elevation
- The results of four placebo-controlled trials do not support the use of ultrasound in terms of symptoms relief and functional disability in the treatment of ankle sprains. Due to the limited amount of information on treatment parameters, no conclusions can be made regarding an optimal and adequate dosage schedule for ultrasound therapy or whether such a schedule would improve on the reported effectiveness of ultrasound for ankle sprains
- Functional treatment appears to be the favorable strategy (with regard to symptom relief, return to work, return to sport, and joint stability for treating acute ankle sprains when compared with a period of more than 4 weeks of immobilization
- The use of an elastic bandage has fewer complications than taping but appears to be associated with a slower return to work and sport, and more reported instability than a semi-rigid ankle support. Lace-up ankle support appears to be effective in reducing swelling in the short term compared with semi-rigid ankle support, elastic bandage, and tape

• There is insufficient evidence available from RCTs to determine the relative effectiveness of surgical and conservative treatment for acute injuries of the lateral ligament complex of the ankle in adults with emphasis on joint stability, symptom relief, recurrence, and return to sport. Given the risk of operative complications, the higher costs (including those of hospital admission) associated with surgery and the good results of secondary anatomic reconstructions of the lateral ankle ligaments, the best available option for most patients would be conservative treatment for acute injuries and close follow-up to identify patients who may remain symptomatic and may require operative intervention

• After 1 year of follow-up, a high percentage of patients still experienced pain and subjective instability, and within a period of 3 years as many as 34% of the patients reported at least one resprain. From 36% to 85% of the patients reported full recovery within a period of 3 years

• There is high-level evidence for the beneficial effect of ankle supports in the form of semi-rigid orthoses or air-cast braces to prevent ankle sprains during high-risk sporting activities (e.g., soccer, basketball). Participants with a history of previous sprain can be advised that wearing such supports may reduce the risk of incurring a future sprain. However, any potential prophylactic effect should be balanced against the baseline risk of the activity, the supply and cost of the particular device, and for some, the possible or perceived loss of performance

References

1. van den Bekerom MPJ, Oostra RJ, Golano Alvarez P, van Dijk CN. The anatomy in relation to injury of the lateral collateral ligaments of the ankle: a current concepts review. Clin Anat 2008;21(7):619–26.
2. Broström L: Sprained ankles. V. Treatment and prognosis in recent ligament ruptures. Acta Chir Scand 1966;132:537–50.
3. Van Dijk CN. On diagnostic strategies in patients with severe ankle sprain. Thesis, University of Amsterdam, the Netherlands, 1994.
4. Kannus P, Renstrom P. Current concept review. Treatment for acute tears of the lateral ligaments of the ankle. J Bone Joint Surg Am 1991;73:305–12.
5. Brooks SC, Potter BT, Rainey JB. Inversion injuries of the ankle: clinical assessment and radiographic review. Br Med J (Clin Res Ed) 1981;282:607–8.
6. Zeegers AVCM. The supination injury of the ankle. Thesis, University of Utrecht, The Netherlands, 1995.
7. Klenerman L. The management of sprained ankle. J Bone Joint Surg Am 1998;80:11–12.
8. Bosien WR, Staples OS, Russell SW. Residual disability following acute ankle sprains. J Bone Joint Surg Am 1955;37:1237–43.
9. Lindenfeld TN, Schmitt DJ, Hendy MP, et al. Incidence of injury in indoor soccer. Am J Sports Med 1994;22:364–71.
10. Freeman MAR. Instability of the foot after injuries to the lateral ligament of the ankle. J Bone Joint Surg Br 1965;47:669–77.
11. Soboroff SH, Papplus EM, Komaroff AL, et al. Benefits, risks, and costs of alternative approaches to the evaluation and treatment of severe ankle sprain. Clin Orthop 1984;183:160–8.
12. Stiell IG, McKnight RD, Greenberg GH, et al. Implementation of the Ottawa ankle rules. JAMA 1994;16;271(11):827–32.
13. van Dijk CN, Lim LS, Bossuyt PM, Marti RK. Physical examination is sufficient for the diagnosis of sprained ankles. J Bone Joint Surg Br 1996;78(6):958–62.
14. van Dijk CN, Mol BW, Lim LS, Marti RK, Bossuyt PM. Diagnosis of ligament rupture of the ankle joint. Physical examination, arthrography, stress radiography and sonography compared in 160 patients after inversion trauma. Acta Orthop Scand 1996;67(6):566–70.
15. Breitenseher MJ, Trattnig S, Kukla C, et al. MRI versus lateral stress radiography in acute lateral ankle ligament injuries. J Comput Assist Tomogr 1997;21:280–5.
16. van Dijk CN, Molenaar AH, Cohen RH, Tol JL, Bossuyt PM, Marti RK. Value of arthrography after supination trauma of the ankle. Skeletal Radiol 1998;27(5):256–61.
17. Broström L, Liljedahl SO, Lindval N. Sprained ankles. II. arthrographic diagnosis of recent ligament ruptures. Acta Chir Scand 1965;129:485–99.
18. Trnka HJ, Ivanic G, Trattnig S. Arthrography of the foot and ankle. Ankle and subtalar joint. Foot Ankle Clin 2000;5(1): 49–62.
19. Guillodo Y, Riban P, Guennoc X, Dubrana F, Saraux A. Usefulness of ultrasonographic detection of talocrural effusion in ankle sprains. J Ultrasound Med 2007;26:831–6.
20. Nikken JJ, Oei EH, Ginai AZ, et al. Acute ankle trauma: value of a short dedicated extremity MR imaging examination in prediction of need for treatment. Radiology 2005;234:134–42.
21. Spiegel PK, Staples OS. Arthrography of the ankle joint: problems in diagnosis of acute lateral ligament injuries. Radiology 1975;114:587–90.
22. Mayer F, Herberger U, Reuber H, Meyer U. Vergleich der Wertigkeit gehaltener Augnahmen und der Arthrographie des oberen Sprunggelenks bei Verletzungen des lateralen Bandkapselapparates. Unfallchirurg 1987;90:86–91.
23. van den Bekerom MPJ, Struijs PAA, Welling L, Blankevoort L, van Dijk CN, Kerkhoffs GMMJ: What is the evidence for RICE therapy in the treatment of ankle sprains? Systematic review of literature. Submitted for publication.
24. Ebenbichler G, Resch KL. Kritische Uberprufung des therapeutischen Ultraschalls [Critical evaluation of ultrasound therapy]. Wiener Med Wochenschr 1994;144(3):51–3.
25. Maxwell L. Therapeutic ultrasound. Its effects on the cellular and molecular mechanisms of inflammation and repair. Physiotherapy 1992;78:421–6.
26. Hykes DL, Hendrick WR, Starchman DE. Biological effects. In: Ultrasound Physics and Instrumentation, pp. 133–47. Churchill Livingstone, New York, 1985.
27. Falconer J, Hayes KW, Chang RW. Therapeutic ultrasound in the treatment of musculoskeletal conditions. Arthritis Care Res 1990;3:85–91.
28. Hayes KW. The use of ultrasound therapy to decrease pain and improve mobility. Crit Rev Phys Rehabil Med 1992;3:271–87.

29. Kitchen SS, Partridge J. A review of therapeutic ultrasound. Physiotherapy 1990;76:593–600.

30. van den Bekerom MPJ, van der Windt DAWM, ter Riet G, van der Heijden GJ, Bouter LM. Therapeutic ultrasound for acute ankle sprains. Cochrane Database of Systematic Reviews submitted.

31. Dehne E. Die Klinik der frischen und habituellen adduktion-supinations Distorsion des Fusses [Inversion injuries of the ankle.]. Dtsche Zeitschr Chir 1933;242:40–61.

32. Adler H. Therapie und Prognose der frischen Aussenknochel-bandlesion [Therapy and prognosis of fresh external ankle ligament lesions]. Unfallheilkunde 1976;79(3):101–4.

33. Leonard MH. Injuries of the lateral ligaments of the ankle. A clinical and experimental study. J Bone Joint Surg Am 1949;31:373–7.

34. Freeman MAR. The etiology and prevention of functional instability of the foot. J Bone Joint Surg Br 1965;47(4):678–85.

35. Jacob RP, Raemy H, Steffen R, Zeegers AVCM. Zur funktionellen behandlung des frischen aussenbaderrisses mit der Aircast-Schiene. Der Orthopäde 1986;14:434–40.

36. Lim LSL, van Dijk CN, Marti RK. De functionele behandeling van acute enkelbandrupturen. Nederlands Tijdschrift voor Traumatologie 1995;1:14–20.

37. Moller Larsen F, Wethelund JO, Jurik AG, de Carvalho A, Lucht U. Comparison of three different treatments for ruptured lateral ankle ligaments. Acta Orthop Scand 1988;59(5):564–6.

38. Stover CN. Air stirrup management of ankle injuries in the athlete. Am J Sports Med 1980;8(5):360–5.

39. Vaes P, de Boeck H, Handelberg F, Oxman AD. Comparative radiologic study of the infuence of ankle joint bandages on ankle stability. Am J Sports Med 1985;13:46–50.

40. Pijnenburg AC, Van Dijk CN, Bossuyt PM, Marti RK. Treatment of ruptures of the lateral ankle ligaments: a meta-analysis. J Bone Joint Surg Am 2000;82(6):761–73.

41. Kerkhoffs GM, van den Bekerom MP, Rowe BH, Assendelft WJ, Struijs PA, van Dijk CN. Immobilisation and functional treatment for acute lateral ankle ligament injuries in adults. Cochrane Database Syst Rev, submitted.

42. Kerkhoffs GM, van den Bekerom MP, Assendelft WJ, Blankevoort L, Struijs PA, van Dijk CN. Different functional treatment strategies for acute lateral ankle ligament injuries in adults. Cochrane Database Syst Rev, submitted.

43. Kerkhoffs GM, Handoll HH, de Bie R, Rowe BH, Struijs PA. Surgical versus conservative treatment for acute injuries of the lateral ligament complex of the ankle in adults. Cochrane Database Syst Rev 2007;18(2):CD000380.

44. Pijnenburg AC, Van Dijk CN, Bossuyt PM, Marti RK. Treatment of ruptures of the lateral ankle ligaments: a meta-analysis. J Bone Joint Surg Am 2000;82(6):761–73.

45. van Rijn RM, van Os AG, Bernsen RM, Luijsterburg PA, Koes BW, Bierma-Zeinstra SM. What is the clinical course of acute ankle sprains? A systematic literature review. Am J Med 2008;121(4):324–31.

46. Handoll HHG, Rowe BH, Quinn KM, de Bie R. Interventions for preventing ankle ligament injuries. Cochrane Database Syst Rev 2001;3:CD000018.

102 Achilles Tendinopathy

Nicola Maffulli[1], Umile Giuseppe Longo[2], Stefano Campi[2],
and Vincenzo Denaro[2]

[1]Barts and The London School of Medicine and Dentistry, London, UK
[2]Campus Bio-Medico University, Rome, Italy

Case scenario

A 41 year old male runner presents with a swelling 2.5 cm in diameter, 4 cm proximal to the insertion of the Achilles tendon. For 3 months he has felt pain at the beginning and at the end of a training session, with diminished discomfort in between. There is tenderness of the Achilles tendon. He has no neurovascular deficits.

Relevant anatomy

The confluence of the gastrocnemius and soleus muscles forms the Achilles tendon. The gastrocnemius is more superficial and originates from two heads above the knee. The soleus is anterior to the gastrocnemius and originates below the knee.[1] The Achilles tendon derives its sensory nerve supply from the nerves of the attaching muscles and cutaneous nerves, in particular the sural nerve.[1]

Achilles tendinopathy (AT) is characterized by pain, impaired performance, and swelling in and around the tendon.[2] It can be categorized as insertional and noninsertional, two distinct disorders with different underlying pathophysiology and management options.[3–5] Other terms used as synonymous of noninsertional tendinopathy include tendinopathy of the main body of the Achilles tendon and midportion AT.[2,6]

Importance of the problem

Although scientifically sound epidemiological data are lacking, AT is common in athletes, accounting for 6–17% of all running injuries.[7,8] However, it also presents in middle-aged, overweight, nonathletic patients without history of increased physical activity.[7] To date, the incidence and prevalence of AT in other populations has not been established, even though the condition has been correlated with seronegative arthropathies.[9]

Most studies include more men than women, although a definite greater prevalence in men has not been shown. Aging has not been shown to represent a risk factor for tendinopathy.[8] AT is not, by itself, a predisposing factor to rupture. Most series reporting the results of conservative or surgical management of an Achilles tendon rupture report that up to 5% of patients had a diagnosis of AT before rupture. The vast majority of ruptures occurs in patients who were otherwise asymptomatic before the tear.[10]

A Google search for "Achilles tendinitis" or "Achilles tendinopathy" returns over 900,000 hits.

Top seven questions

Diagnosis

1. What is the accuracy of clinical examination in the diagnosis of AT?

Treatment

2. What is the efficacy of a program of eccentric exercises vs. control?
3. What is the efficacy of eccentric exercises with or without heel brace?
4. What is the efficacy of eccentric exercises vs. shockwave therapy?
5. What is the efficacy of eccentric exercises vs. topical glyceryl trinitrate?

6. What is the efficacy of low-level laser therapy vs. a programme of eccentric exercises?

7. What is the efficacy of eccentric exercises vs. platelet-rich plasma injections plus eccentric exercises?

Question 1: What is the accuracy of clinical examination in the diagnosis of AT?

Case clarification

At clinical examination, palpation of the tendon is present. The painful arc sign and the Royal London Hospital test are positive.

Relevance

A variety of clinical diagnostic tests are available for AT. Therefore, clinicians need to select diagnostic tests that are the most specific to confirm AT and the most sensitive to establish that AT is unlikely.

Current opinion

Current opinion suggests that the majority of health professionals use pain and tenderness following performance of palpation, the painful arc sign, and the Royal London Hospital test as clinical diagnostic tests for AT.

Finding the evidence

• Cochrane Database, with search term "Achilles," "tendon," "tendinopathy," "Achilles clinical examination," "palpation," "arc sign," and "Royal London Hospital"
• PubMed (www.ncbi.nlm.nih.gov/pubmed/) clinical queries search/systematic reviews: "Achilles," "tendon," "tendinopathy," "Achilles clinical examination," "palpation," "arc sign," and "Royal London Hospital"
• MEDLINE search identifying the population (Achilles tendon) and the methodology (diagnosis), using keywords: "Achilles," "tendon," "tendinopathy," "Achilles clinical examination," "palpation," "arc sign," AND "Royal London Hospital"

Quality of the evidence
Level III
• 1 study[11]

Findings

Sensitivity and specificity One study[11] (n = 24 patients) investigated the accuracy of clinical tests for assessing AT. The overall average sensitivity for AT is 0.583 (95% CI 0.393, 0.752) for palpation, 0.525 (95% CI 0.347, 0.697) for the arc sign, and 0.542 (95% CI 0.345, 0.726) for the Royal London test. The overall average specificity for AT is 0.845 (95% CI 0.745, 0.911) for palpation, 0.833 (95% CI 0.717, 0.908) for the arc sign, and 0.912 (95% CI 0.858, 0.952) for the Royal London test.

Recommendation
• If a patient presents with a tender area of intratendinous swelling that moves with the Achilles tendon and whose tenderness significantly decreases or disappears when the tendon is put under tension, a clinical diagnosis of tendinopathy can be formulated [overall quality: low]

Question 2: What is the efficacy of eccentric exercise vs. control?

Case clarification

The physician makes a diagnosis of AT. Eccentric exercise could represent an option for this patient. However, the patient would like to apply a wait-and-see policy or a program of concentric exercises.

Relevance

Several management options have been proposed to allow recovery of patients with AT. However, the long-term follow-up of the different options is not well defined.

Current opinion

Current opinion suggests that the majority of health professionals consider eccentric exercises as an appropriate management tool for AT.

Finding the evidence

• Cochrane Database, with search term "Achilles," "tendon," "tendinopathy," "eccentric exercises," "training," "physiotherapy"
• PubMed (www.ncbi.nlm.nih.gov/pubmed/) clinical queries search/systematic reviews: "Achilles," "tendon," "tendinopathy," "eccentric exercises," "training," "physiotherapy"
• MEDLINE search identifying the population (Achilles tendinopathy), the intervention (diagnosis) and the methodology (MRI), using the keywords: "Achilles," "tendon," "tendinopathy," "eccentric exercises," "training," "physiotherapy"

Quality of the evidence
Level I
• 3 randomized trials[12–14]

Level II
• 3 systematic reviews[15–17]

Findings

Comparison of eccentric exercise vs. wait-and-see strategy Rompe et al.[12] conducted a randomized controlled trial (RCT) comparing the effectiveness of eccentric loading vs. repetitive low-energy shockwave therapy (SWT) vs. wait-and-see. At 4 month follow-up, eccentric loading and low-energy SWT showed comparable results. The wait-and-see strategy was ineffective for the management of AT.

Comparison of eccentric exercises vs. concentric exercises
Silbernagel et al.[14] compared eccentric and concentric exercises in 32 patients with proximal achillodynia. They found an overall better result for the eccentric group with significant improvements in plantar flexion, and reduction in pain on palpation, number of patients having pain during walking, having periods when asymptomatic, and having swollen Achilles tendon. The controls did not show such changes.

Mafi et al.[13] conducted a prospective randomized study to compare eccentric and concentric training regimen for 44 patients. After completion of the eccentric training regimen, 82% of the patients (18/22) were satisfied and had resumed their previous (preinjury)activity level, compared to 36% of the patients (8/22) who were treated with the concentric training regimen. The results after treatment with eccentric training were significantly better (p < 0.002) than after concentric training.

Recommendation

• Eccentric exercises are superior to wait-and-see treatment or concentric exercise [overall quality: good]

Question 3: What is the efficacy of eccentric exercises with or without heel brace?

Case clarification

The patient decides to go for a program of eccentric exercises, but he says that he would like to have a brace in addition to the exercises.

Relevance

Several braces have been proposed to optimize the healing of AT. However, the efficacy of these braces is not well defined.

Current opinion

Braces are an attractive option for patients with AT because they are associated with high compliance and do not require the patient to take medication. However, clinical results of the use of braces have not been clarified.

Finding the evidence

• Cochrane Database, with search term "Achilles," "tendon," "tendinopathy," "heel," "brace," "pad"
• PubMed (www.ncbi.nlm.nih.gov/pubmed/) clinical queries search/ systematic reviews: "Achilles," "tendon," "tendinopathy," "heel," "brace," "pad"
• MEDLINE search identifying the population (Achilles tendon) the intervention (Brace) and the methodology (clinical trial), using the keywords "Achilles," "tendon," "tendinopathy," "heel," "brace," "pad"

Quality of the evidence

Level I
• 7 randomized trials[18–24]

Findings

Roos et al.[23] showed that a program of eccentric exercises resulted in significantly lower pain scores after 12 weeks when compared with night splints alone. They did not find any difference in pain score when comparing those who performed eccentric exercises and wore night splints to patients who received eccentric exercises alone. Similarly, Mayer et al.[24] demonstrated no difference in pain score when comparing eccentric exercises with custom-fit insoles,[24] although the insole group was noted to have significantly better pain scores than controls.

In an RCT, Knobloch et al.[18,19] showed that the combination of eccentric training with the AirHeel brace can optimize tendon microcirculation, but these microcirculatory advantages do not translate into superior clinical performance when compared with eccentric training alone. On the other hand, Petersen et al.[20] found that the AirHeel brace was as effective as eccentric training in the treatment of chronic AT and that was no synergistic effect when both treatment strategies are combined.

De Vos et al.[21,22] concluded that night splint is not beneficial in addition to eccentric exercises in the treatment of chronic midportion AT.

Recommendation

• There is currently no scientifically substantiated reason to believe that splinting would improve the outcome over a program of eccentric exercises [overall quality: low]

Question 4: What is the efficacy of eccentric exercises vs. SWT?

Case clarification

After failed management with eccentric exercises and brace, the physician proposes to the patient that he should undertake SWT.

Relevance

Unfortunately, not all patients with AT respond well to a program of eccentric exercises, and often other management modalities are required. SWT may be a good option in these patients

Current opinion

SWT offers a potential alternative to other more invasive management modalities

Finding the evidence

• Cochrane Database, with search term: "shockwave therapy"

- PubMed (www.ncbi.nlm.nih.gov/pubmed/) clinical queries search/systematic reviews: "Achilles tendon," "shockwave therapy"
- MEDLINE search identifying the population (Achilles tendon) the intervention (shockwave therapy) and the methodology (clinical trial), using the keywords: "Achilles tendon," AND "shockwave therapy"

Quality of the evidence
Level I
- 4 randomized trials[12,25–27]

Findings
A prospective RCT showed comparable results of eccentric loading and low-energy SWT.[12] The same scientific team found in another RCT that, at 4-month follow-up, eccentric loading alone was less effective when compared with a combination of eccentric loading and repetitive low-energy SWT.[26] A prospective RCT on 48 patients comparing the effect of supplementing eccentric exercises with extracorporeal SWT or placebo showed similar results.[25]

No advantage of SWT was found in another RCT on 49 patients.[27]

Recommendations
- Comparable results can be obtained with eccentric loading or low-energy SWT [overall quality: good]
- Eccentric loading alone is less effective when compared with a combination of eccentric loading and repetitive low-energy SWT [overall quality: low]

Question 5: What is the efficacy of a program of eccentric exercises vs. topical glyceryl trinitrate?

Case clarification
After undergoing eccentric exercises, the patients asks for topical glyceryl trinitrate.

Relevance
A molecular link between the apparently disparate events of tendon degeneration and the subsequent orchestration of effective tendon healing may lie in the control of the production and persistence of reactive oxygen species within both the intra- and extracellular milieu of the tendon tissue.

Current opinion
Topical glyceryl trinitrate may enhance tendon healing.[28]

Finding the evidence
- Cochrane Database, with search terms: "Achilles," "tendon," "tendinopathy," "topical glyceryl trinitrate," "oxygen free radicals," "nitric oxide"

- PubMed (www.ncbi.nlm.nih.gov/pubmed/) clinical queries search/systematic reviews: "Achilles," "tendon," "tendinopathy," "topical glyceryl trinitrate," "oxygen free radicals," "nitric oxide"
- MEDLINE search identifying the population (Achilles tendon) the intervention (topical glyceryl trinitrate) and the methodology (clinical trial), using the keywords: "Achilles," "tendon," "tendinopathy," "topical glyceryl trinitrate," "oxygen free radicals," "nitric oxide"

Quality of the evidence
Level I
- 3 RCTs[29–31]

Findings
Paoloni et al. showed that topical glyceryl trinitrate significantly reduced pain with activity and at night, improved functional measures, and improved outcomes in patients with AT both in the short[29] and long term.[30] However, another RCT on 40 patients[31] did not produce the same results, failing to support the clinical benefit of topical glyceryl trinitrate patches.

Recommendation
- In patients with tendinopathy of the main body of the Achilles tendon, there is some evidence to recommend topical glyceryl trinitrate for the management of AT [overall quality: low]

Question 6: What is the efficacy of low-level laser therapy and a program of eccentric exercises?

Case clarification
The patient is still not well. He asks for laser therapy.

Relevance
Laser therapy is a widely available and frequently used electrophysical agent in sports medicine.

Current opinion
There is insufficient evidence to support a beneficial effect of laser therapy for AT.

Finding the evidence
- Cochrane Database, with search terms: "Achilles tendon," "laser therapy"
- PubMed (www.ncbi.nlm.nih.gov/pubmed/) clinical queries search/systematic reviews: "Achilles tendon," "laser therapy"
- MEDLINE search identifying the population (meniscal tears) the intervention (meniscectomy) and the methodology (clinical trial), using the keywords "Achilles tendon," "laser therapy"

- PubMed (www.ncbi.nlm.nih.gov/pubmed/): sensitivity search using keywords "Achilles tendon," AND "laser therapy"

Quality of the evidence
Level I
- 3 randomized trials[32–34]

Findings
Stergioulas[32] conducted an RCT on 52 recreational athletes with chronic AT randomized to either eccentric exercises plus low-level laser therapy (LLLT) or eccentric exercises plus placebo LLLT over 8 weeks in a blinded manner. The results of the intention-to-treat analysis for the primary outcome, pain intensity during physical activity on the 100 mm visual analog scale, were significantly lower in the LLLT group than in the placebo group.

Tumilty et al.[33] performed a similar study on 20 patients randomized into an active laser or placebo group. No conclusions were made regarding effectiveness because of the low statistical power of this pilot study.

Chester et al.[34] in a prospective randomized single-blind pilot study investigated the potential effectiveness of eccentric exercise compared with therapeutic ultrasound in subjects with relatively sedentary lifestyles. There were no statistically significant differences between groups or clear trends over time.

Recommendation
- There is no definitive evidence whether LLLT may lead to better clinical outcome in patients undergoing a program of eccentric exercise [overall quality: low]

Question 7: What is the efficacy of eccentric exercises vs. platelet-rich plasma injections?

Case clarification
After searching the internet, the patient asks the doctor to give him an injection of platelet-rich plasma (PRP).

Relevance
PRP is a bioactive component of whole blood, which is now being widely tested in different fields of medicine for its possibilities in aiding the regeneration of tissue with poor healing potential.[35] The rationale for the use of PRP to promote tendon healing is the high content of cytokines and cells in hyperphysiologic doses of PRP.

Current opinion
PRP can be used for the management of AT.

Finding the evidence
- Cochrane Database, with search terms: "Achilles tendon," "platelet-rich plasma," "growth factors"

- PubMed (www.ncbi.nlm.nih.gov/pubmed/) clinical queries search/systematic reviews: "Achilles tendon," "platelet-rich plasma," "growth factors"
- MEDLINE search identifying the population (complete meniscectomy) the intervention (meniscal substitution) and the methodology (clinical trial), using the keywords "Achilles tendon," "platelet-rich plasma," AND "growth factors"

Quality of the evidence
Level I
- 1 RCT[36]

Findings
De Vos[36] performed an RCT at a single center of 54 randomized patients with chronic AT. Patients were randomized to eccentric exercises (usual care) with either a PRP injection (PRP group) or saline injection (placebo group). The mean VISA-A score improved significantly after 24 weeks in the PRP group by 21.7 points (95% CI 13.0–30.5) and in the placebo group by 20.5 points (95% CI 11.6–29.4). The increase was not significantly different between both groups (adjusted between-group difference from baseline to 24 weeks, −0.9; 95% CI, −12.4 to 10.6). This confidence interval did not include the predefined relevant difference of 12 points in favor of PRP treatment.

Recommendation
- There is no evidence to justify a PRP injection in patients with AT [overall quality: good]

Summary of recommendations

- If a patient presents with Achilles tendon with a tender area of intratendinous swelling that moves with the tendon and whose tenderness significantly decreases or disappears when the tendon is put under tension, a clinical diagnosis of tendinopathy can be formulated
- Eccentric exercises are superior to wait-and-see treatment and concentric exercise
- There is currently no scientifically substantiated reason to believe that splinting would improve the outcome over a program of eccentric exercises
- Comparable results can be obtained with eccentric loading or low-energy SWT
- Eccentric loading alone or low-energy SWT are each less effective than a combination of eccentric loading and repetitive low-energy SWT
- There is some evidence to recommend topical glyceryl trinitrate for the management of AT
- There is no definitive evidence whether LLLT may lead to better clinical outcome in patients undergoing a program of eccentric exercise

- There is no evidence to justify a PRP injection in patients with AT

Conclusion

Even though AT is frequent and results in high healthcare costs, the quality of the available studies on its management is generally low, and, because of methodologic limitations, pooling of data is almost always impossible. There is an urgent need for large well-conducted RCTs to improve the evidence basis on the management of AT.

References

1. Maffulli N, Ajis A, Longo UG, Denaro V. Chronic rupture of tendo Achillis. Foot Ankle Clin 2007;12(4):583–96, vi.

2. Longo UG, Ronga M, Maffulli N. Achilles tendinopathy. Sports Med Arthrosc 2009;17(2):112–26.

3. Longo UG, Ramamurthy C, Denaro V, Maffulli N. Minimally invasive stripping for chronic Achilles tendinopathy. Disabil Rehabil 2008;30(20–22):1709–13.

4. Maffulli N, Longo UG. How do eccentric exercises work in tendinopathy? Rheumatology (Oxford) 2008;47(10):1444–5.

5. Maffulli N, Longo UG. Conservative management for tendinopathy: is there enough scientific evidence? Rheumatology (Oxford) 2008;47(4):390–1.

6. Longo UG, Ronga M, Maffulli N. Acute ruptures of the Achilles tendon. Sports Med Arthrosc 2009;17(2):127–38.

7. McLauchlan GJ, Handoll HH. Interventions for treating acute and chronic Achilles tendinitis. Cochrane Database Syst Rev 2001;2:CD000232.

8. Longo UG, Rittweger J, Garau G, et al. No influence of age, gender, weight, height, and impact profile in achilles tendinopathy in masters track and field athletes. Am J Sports Med 2009;37(7):1400–5.

9. Ames PR, Longo UG, Denaro V, Maffulli N. Achilles tendon problems: not just an orthopaedic issue. Disabil Rehabil 2008;30(20–22):1646–50.

10. Longo UG, Lamberti A, Maffulli N, Denaro V. Tendon augmentation grafts: a systematic review. Br Med Bull 2010;94:165–88.

11. Maffulli N, Kenward MG, Testa V, Capasso G, Regine R, King JB. Clinical diagnosis of Achilles tendinopathy with tendinosis. Clin J Sport Med 2003;13(1):11–15.

12. Rompe JD, Nafe B, Furia JP, Maffulli N. Eccentric loading, shock wave treatment, or a wait-and-see policy for tendinopathy of the main body of tendo Achillis: a randomized controlled trial. Am J Sports Med 2007;35(3):374–83.

13. Mafi N, Lorentzon R, Alfredson H. Superior short-term results with eccentric calf muscle training compared to concentric training in a randomized prospective multicenter study on patients with chronic Achilles tendinosis. Knee Surg Sports Traumatol Arthrosc 2001;9(1):42–7.

14. Silbernagel KG, Thomee R, Thomee P, Karlsson J. Eccentric overload training for patients with chronic Achilles tendon pain—a randomised controlled study with reliability testing of the evaluation methods. Scand J Med Sci Sports 2001;11(4):197–206.

15. Meyer A, Tumilty S, Baxter GD. Eccentric exercise protocols for chronic non-insertional Achilles tendinopathy: how much is enough? Scand J Med Sci Sports 2009;19(5):609–15.

16. Woodley BL, Newsham-West RJ, Baxter GD. Chronic tendinopathy: effectiveness of eccentric exercise. Br J Sports Med 2007;41(4):188–98; discussion 199.

17. Magnussen RA, Dunn WR, Thomson AB. Nonoperative treatment of midportion Achilles tendinopathy: a systematic review. Clin J Sport Med 2009;19(1):54–64.

18. Knobloch K, Schreibmueller L, Longo UG, Vogt PM. Eccentric exercises for the management of tendinopathy of the main body of the Achilles tendon with or without an AirHeel Brace. A randomized controlled trial. B: Effects of compliance. Disabil Rehabil 2008;30(20–22):1692–6.

19. Knobloch K, Schreibmueller L, Longo UG, Vogt PM. Eccentric exercises for the management of tendinopathy of the main body of the Achilles tendon with or without the AirHeel Brace. A randomized controlled trial. A: effects on pain and microcirculation. Disabil Rehabil 2008;30(20–22):1685–91.

20. Petersen W, Welp R, Rosenbaum D. Chronic Achilles tendinopathy: a prospective randomized study comparing the therapeutic effect of eccentric training, the AirHeel brace, and a combination of both. Am J Sports Med 2007;35(10):1659–67.

21. de Jonge S, de Vos RJ, van Schie HT, Verhaar JA, Weir A, Tol JL. One-year follow-up of a randomised controlled trial on added splinting to eccentric exercises in chronic midportion Achilles tendinopathy. Br J Sports Med 2010;44(9):673–7.

22. de Vos RJ, Weir A, Visser RJ, de Winter T, Tol JL. The additional value of a night splint to eccentric exercises in chronic midportion Achilles tendinopathy: a randomised controlled trial. Br J Sports Med 2007;41(7):e5.

23. Roos EM, Engstrom M, Lagerquist A, Soderberg B. Clinical improvement after 6 weeks of eccentric exercise in patients with mid-portion Achilles tendinopathy—a randomized trial with 1-year follow-up. Scand J Med Sci Sports 2004;14(5):286–95.

24. Mayer F, Hirschmuller A, Muller S, Schuberth M, Baur H. Effects of short-term treatment strategies over 4 weeks in Achilles tendinopathy. Br J Sports Med 2007;41(7):e6.

25. Rasmussen S, Christensen M, Mathiesen I, Simonson O. Shockwave therapy for chronic Achilles tendinopathy: a double-blind, randomized clinical trial of efficacy. Acta Orthop 2008;79(2):249–56.

26. Rompe JD, Furia J, Maffulli N. Eccentric loading versus eccentric loading plus shockwave treatment for midportion achilles tendinopathy: a randomized controlled trial. Am J Sports Med 2009;37(3):463–70.

27. Costa ML, Shepstone L, Donell ST, Thomas TL. Shock wave therapy for chronic Achilles tendon pain: a randomized placebo-controlled trial. Clin Orthop Relat Res 2005;440:199–204.

28. Longo UG, Oliva F, Denaro V, Maffulli N. Oxygen species and overuse tendinopathy in athletes. Disabil Rehabil 2008;30(20–22):1563–1571.

29. Paoloni JA, Appleyard RC, Nelson J, Murrell GA. Topical glyceryl trinitrate treatment of chronic noninsertional achilles tendinopathy. A randomized, double-blind, placebo-controlled trial. J Bone Joint Surg Am 2004;86(5):916–22.

30. Paoloni JA, Murrell GA. Three-year followup study of topical glyceryl trinitrate treatment of chronic noninsertional Achilles tendinopathy. Foot Ankle Int 2007;28(10):1064–8.

31. Kane TP, Ismail M, Calder JD. Topical glyceryl trinitrate and noninsertional Achilles tendinopathy: a clinical and cellular investigation. Am J Sports Med 2008;36(6):1160–3.

32. Stergioulas A, Stergioula M, Aarskog R, Lopes-Martins RA, Bjordal JM. Effects of low-level laser therapy and eccentric exercises in the treatment of recreational athletes with chronic achilles tendinopathy. Am J Sports Med 2008;36(5):881–7.

33. Tumilty S, Munn J, Abbott JH, McDonough S, Hurley DA, Baxter GD. Laser therapy in the treatment of achilles tendinopathy: a pilot study. Photomed Laser Surg 2008;26(1):25–30.

34. Chester R, Costa ML, Shepstone L, Cooper A, Donell ST. Eccentric calf muscle training compared with therapeutic ultrasound for chronic Achilles tendon pain—a pilot study. Man Ther 2008;13(6):484–491.

35. Forriol F, Longo UG, Concejo C, Ripalda P, Maffulli N, Denaro V. Platelet-rich plasma, rhOP-1 (rhBMP-7) and frozen rib allograft for the reconstruction of bony mandibular defects in sheep. A pilot experimental study. Injury 2009;40(Suppl 3):S44–49.

36. de Vos RJ, Weir A, van Schie HT, et al. 2010; Platelet-rich plasma injection for chronic Achilles tendinopathy: a randomized controlled trial. JAMA 303(2):144–9.

103 Labral Tears

Sanaz Hariri[1], Henk Eijer[2], and Marc R. Safran[1]

[1]Stanford University, Redwood City, CA, USA

[2]Regionalspital Emmental, Burgdorf, Switzerland

Case scenario

An athletic 38 year old woman presents with insidious-onset, moderately severe, groin pain that is activity related, especially when she is walking or pivoting on the right leg. Pain is worse going from sitting to standing. She also has night pain.[1]

Relevant anatomy

The acetabular labrum is triangular in cross-section. It is an incomplete ring composed primarily of type II collagen fibro-cartilage, attached to the acetabular rim peripherally (its base) with a free margin centrally (its apex).[2]

Importance of the problem

Magnetic resonance arthrography with intra-articular contrast (MRA) has recently greatly enhanced our ability to diagnosis labral tears. The relatively constrained anatomy of the hip joint (e.g., its shape, difficulty achieving sufficient distraction, relative depth, and surrounding thick soft tissue envelope) has only recently been addressed sufficiently to fuel the recent popularity of hip arthroscopy for treatment of labral tears.

One study reported a 22% prevalence of labral tear in young patients presenting with groin pain.[3] Cadaveric studies show an increasing prevalence of labral tears with age: 52% in those over age 48 and 96% in those over age 61.[4,5]

There is debate as to the predominant mechanism of injury resulting in labral tears. Ganz asserts that the labrum and cartilage undergo a degenerative process due to impingement between the femur and the acetabulum, specifically in internal rotation.[6–13] Alternatively, McCarthy theorizes that tears are largely caused by chronic repetitive stress by maneuvers such as twisting and pivoting which place high strains on the labrum even in positions not consistent with impingement.[4,14–16]

> **Impingement**
>
> - *Femoroacetabular impingement* (FAI) occurs when an osseous abnormality of the proximal femur (cam) and/or acetabulum (pincer) traps soft tissue between the two bony structures, damaging the labrum and/or articular cartilage
> - *Cam impingement* occurs when a nonspherical femoral head abuts against the anterior acetabulum (e.g., with hip flexion)
> - *Pincer impingement* is the result of femoral overcoverage by the acetabulum (e.g., retroversion, coxa profunda, and/or protrusio)

Searching the Cochrane Database of systemic reviews using the term "labrum," we found no studies of the hip acetabular labrum. A PubMed search for "shoulder labrum" yields 792 results while a search for "hip labrum" yields 316 results. We did not find a single randomized controlled trial (RCT) or meta-analysis investigating labral tears. The vast majority of studies are retrospective case series.

Because the focus of this chapter is sports medicine, we have primarily concentrated on arthroscopic treatment of hip pathology. However, it must be noted that FAI was originally treated with an open surgical dislocation and that the open approach is commonly used to address FAI anatomy, particularly in Europe.[17,18]

Evidence-Based Orthopedics, First Edition. Edited by Mohit Bhandari.

© 2012 Blackwell Publishing Ltd. Published 2012 by Blackwell Publishing Ltd.

Top ten questions

Background/diagnosis

1. What is the vascular supply of the labrum?
2. What is the function of the labrum?
3. How do patients with labral tears present clinically?
4. What is the sensitivity of MRI and MRA?

Therapy

5. What are the results of labral debridement (a.k.a. labrectomy)?
6. In patients with a labral tear in the presence of abnormal hip morphology, how are the results affected by surgically addressing the morphology?
7. What are the results of labral repair?

Prognosis

8. How does the presence of articular cartilage damage affect the prognosis of a patient with a labral tear?

Harm

9. What are the complications associated with labral debridement and repair?
10. What are the possible pitfalls of labral debridement in patients with acetabular dysplasia?

Question 1: What is the vascular supply of the labrum and how does that affect the choice of treatment options?

Case clarification

When inspecting a typical labral tear during surgery, it is found that the tear mostly involves the free edge of the labrum on its articular side.

Divivsions of the labrum

The labrum is considered to consist of two portions:
- the *articular portion* is the layer adjacent to the femoral head
- the *capsular portion* is the layer opposite to the articular side
The labrum is also divided as:
- the *free edge* or *apex*
- the *bony attachment* adjacent to the acetabulum[19,20]

Relevance

Since blood supply is important for a labral repair to heal, the location of the tear (and relative vascularity) are important in determining reparability

Current opinion

It has been shown that the periphery of the acetabular labrum is better vascularized than its more central (apex) portion.

Finding the evidence

- PubMed (www.ncbi.nlm.nih.gov/pubmed/) search, using keywords: "hip" AND "labrum" AND "vascularity" as well as "hip" AND "labrum" AND "vascularization"

Quality of the evidence

- 3 cadaver studies

Findings

The synovium surrounding the labrum is highly vascularized. The adjacent joint capsule supplies blood vessels to only the peripheral one third of the labrum. A group of small vessels travel circumferentially in the substance of the labrum at the labrum's attachment site on the outer surface of the bony acetabular extension.[2,19] The capsular portion is significantly better vascularized than the articular portion.[20]

Recommendation

- Labral tears in central, avascular zones should be debrided because they have limited capacity to heal, whereas those in the peripheral, vascular regions should be considered for repair [cadaver studies]

Question 2: What is the function of the labrum and how might that affect the choice of treatment?

Case clarification

During surgery, 1 cm of the labrum is found to be detached from the acetabular rim. The surgeon must decide whether to perform a partial labrectomy or a labral repair.

Relevance

When deciding how much labrum to debride and whether to repair the labrum, one should consider the function of the intact labrum and therefore the possible consequences of a partial or complete labrectomy.

Current opinion

The biomechanical functions of the acetabular labrum are not yet well understood.

Finding the evidence

- PubMed search, using keywords: "hip" AND "labrum" AND "biomechanics"

Quality of the evidence

- 8 biomechanical studies

Findings

The labrum significantly increases the surface area and volume of the acetabulum.[21] In the normal hip, the labrum does not have a significant load-sharing role in the single-leg stance phase.[22] Disruption of the labrum creates subtle joint instability.[23] In the dysplastic hip, the labrum may assume a load-sharing role and hypertrophy, helping to stabilize the femoral head within the acetabulum.[24]

The labrum acts as a seal against synovial fluid flow in and out of the hip central compartment. This seal may enhance joint lubrication and articular cartilage nutrition, maintain a protective fluid film between the articular surfaces, and unload the cartilage by limiting fluid expression from its matrix during loading.[25–28]

> Compartments of the hip joint
>
> - The *central compartment* is limited by the confines of the acetabulum and labrum
> - The *peripheral compartment* is the intra-articular region outside the confines of the acetabulum and labrum, i.e., the region along the femoral neck

Recommendation

- The labrum may play a significant role in articular cartilage health and hip stability. Therefore, the labrum should be conservatively debrided and/or repaired when possible [biomechanical studies]

Question 3: How does a patient with a labral tear present clinically on history and physical examination?

Case clarification

The patient reports having had groin pain for about 1.5 years and has seen two other physicians about this pain. They had diagnosed her with muscle strains and early osteoarthritis (OA). She has gone to about 20 physical therapy sessions without any pain relief.

Relevance

Labral tear as part of the differential diagnosis of hip pain has only recently achieved prominence in the lexicon of orthopedics.

Current opinion

As evidenced by the frequent delay in diagnosis, the signs and symptoms of labral tears are not yet well appreciated and therefore inadequately investigated.

Finding the evidence

- PubMed search using keywords "hip" AND "labrum tear" AND "diagnosis" as well as "hip" AND "labral tear" AND "presentation"

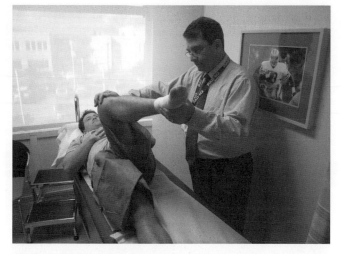

Figure 103.1 The impingement test (hip flexion, adduction and internal rotation) typically produces pain or a clicking sensation in the presence of an anterior-superior labral tear.

Quality of the evidence

Level IV
- 8 case series

Level V
- 1 expert opinion

Findings

Patients are on average in their late 30s. The onset of symptoms can be insidious or traumatic with pain predominantly in the groin, both sharp and dull, activity related, present at night, and exacerbated by sitting. Most have a painful mechanical locking. The average period between onset of symptoms and diagnosis is 21–35 months; patients see an average of 3.3 healthcare providers before diagnosis.[1,29]

Physical examination should include gait analysis, impingement test (Figure 103.1), Trendelenburg sign, flexion–abduction–external rotation test, flexion–internal rotation–adduction test, and palpation of the greater trochanter. Clinical examination maneuvers need improvement in accuracy, sensitivity, and interobserver reliability.[30–33] Radiographs should be examined to detect abnormalities in hip morphology—i.e., FAI (e.g. coxa profunda, Figure 103.2) or dysplasia—that may guide treatment.[34–38]

Recommendations

In patients presenting with nonarthritic hip pain:
- History should focus on location of pain, character of pain (sharp and/or dull), activities that induce pain, and whether they have pain at night [overall quality: low]
- Physical examination should include the impingement test [overall quality: low]

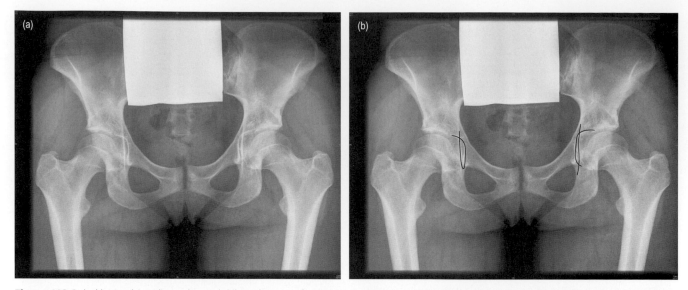

Figure 103.2 (a, b) AP pelvis radiograph reveals bilateral coxa profunda (i.e., the medial acetabular wall is medial to the ilioischial line).

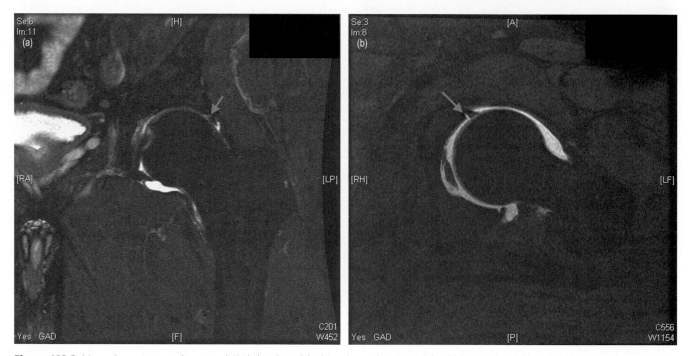

Figure 103.3 Magnetic resonance arthrograms (MRA) showing a labral tear (arrows) on T2 weighted (a) coronal and (b) axial images.

• Radiographs should be studied for the anatomy of impingement and dysplasia to help guide treatment [overall quality: low]

Question 4: What is the sensitivity of MRI vs. MRA?

Case clarification

The patient has an MRI of the hip without contrast that does not show a labral tear, but history and examination are very suspicious for a labral tear.

Relevance

Intra-articular injection of contrast has associated cost and morbidity. When evaluating a patient with history and examination consistent with a labral tear, clinicians must decide whether to order an MRI or an MRA.

Current opinion

Physicians order an MRA if the history and examination are consistent with a labral tear (Figure 103.3) These gadolinium injections are often combined with an intra-articular anesthetic injection to discern whether the pain generator

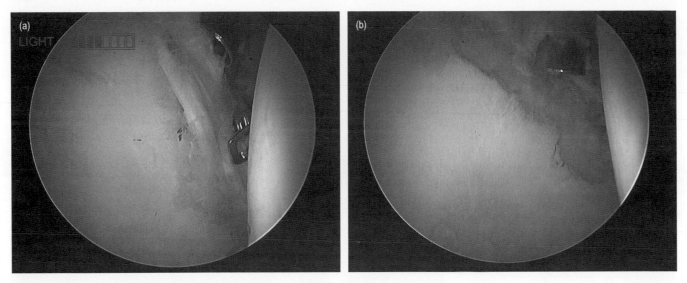

Figure 103.4 Intraoperative picture of a torn labrum (a) before and (b) after debridement.

is actually within the joint. However, patients are often referred with just a noncontrast MRI.

Finding the evidence

• PubMed search, using keywords: "magnetic resonance" AND "labral tear" AND "hip"

Quality of the evidence

Level IV

• 6 case series

Findings

Hip MRIs have been found to have an 8–95% sensitivity (lowest for those of the pelvis, highest for those focusing on the hip), 67% specificity, and 92% interobserver reliability for labral tears.[30,39,40] MRAs studies reported a 63–100% sensitivity and 71–96% specificity for detecting labral tears.[30,40–42] An intra-articular anesthetic can help identify patients with intra-articular pathology and can possibly identify labral tears that are asymptomatic.[30,32]

Recommendations

• Patients with history and physical examination suspicious for a labral tear should be sent for an MRA rather than a MRI [overall quality: moderate]

• Addition of an intra-articular anesthetic during contrast injection for the MRA is helpful in discerning whether the pain generator is intra-articular [overall quality: low]

Question 5: What are the results of labral debridement?

Case clarification

During arthroscopy, the anterolateral labrum is torn with evidence of mucoid degeneration.

Relevance

The labrum contains sensory nerve end organs, mostly in the superficial layer of the labrum, that presumably cause the hip pain associated labral tears.[43] With advances in hip arthroscopy, these tears are most commonly being debrided (partial limbectomy or partial labrectomy) (Figure 103.4).

Current opinion

Partial labrectomy is thought to alleviate the pain and mechanical symptoms associated with a labral tear.

Finding the evidence

• PubMed search, using keywords: "hip arthroscopy" AND "labral tear"

Quality of the evidence

Level IV

• 8 case series

Findings

Labral debridement studies report 46–100% satisfaction or good results, even at up to 10 years follow-up, with worse results in the context of OA.[29,44–48] Those with secondary gain also appear to have a poorer prognosis.[49] For those patients with symptoms during athletic activities, results of labral debridement are also good, with 87% returning to their sport.[50]

Recommendation

• Arthroscopic partial labrectomy for labral tears without bony work to address FAI anatomy, when present, yields an approximately 70% satisfaction rate overall [overall quality: low] (See Question 3, Chapter 104, Hip Impingement)

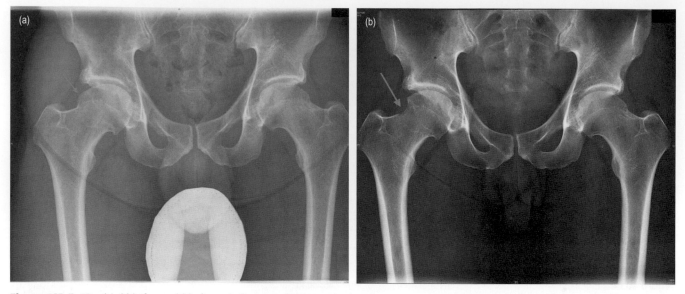

Figure 103.5 AP pelvis (a) before and (b) after a cheilectomy of cam-type impingement.

Question 6: In patients with the anatomy of FAI and a labral tear, how is prognosis affected by the addition of osteochondroplasty to the labral debridement/repair?

Case clarification

On preoperative radiographs it is apparent that the patient has a crossover sign (indicating relative cranial acetabular retroversion), coxa profunda, and loss of femoral offset anteriorly—consistent with mixed pincer and cam impingement.

Relevance

If indeed there is an anatomic predisposition to labral tears, addressing the symptoms (i.e., the tear) without the underlying pathology may doom the patient to recurrent tears or continued pain.

Current opinion

There is a growing sentiment that the anatomy of FAI can lead to labral and chondral lesions and that the underlying hip morphology should be addressed.

Finding the evidence

• PubMed search, using keywords: "hip arthroscopy" AND "femoroacetabular impingement" as well as "hip arthroscopy" AND "osteoplasty"

Quality of the evidence

Level IV
• 7 case series

Findings

Studies of FAI patients show better results when an arthroscopic osteochondroplasty supplements the labral/chondral debridement (Figure 103.5) In the context of cam impingement, osteochondroplasty patients improved more in their outcomes scores, were less likely to require a reoperation, and had a higher proportion of good/excellent results compared to those with labral debridement alone.[51–53] In FAI patients with chondral damage, there was no significant improvement in pain scores when a labral debridement was performed without an osteoplasty.[54]

Analyzing revision hip arthroscopies for persistent hip pain, 79–97% had FAI anatomy seen on radiographs at the time of revision.[55,56] Addressing the associated bony pathology at revision improved patients' pain and increased function and activity levels.[57]

Recommendation

• In patients with a labral tear and radiographically evident FAI anatomy, the FAI anatomy should be addressed to optimize pain relief [overall quality: low]

Question 7: Can the labrum be repaired, and what are the outcomes of labral repair?

Case clarification

Preoperative radiographs were consistent with pincer impingement: a crossover sign (indicating cranial acetabular retroversion) and coxa profunda. The patient is consented for an acetabuloplasty and labral debridement vs. repair. During arthroscopy, the anterosuperior labrum is not found to have any significant signs of intrasubstance degeneration, calcification, ossification, or tearing.

Relevance

When arthroscopically treating pincer type impingement with an intact labrum, the surgeon must decide whether to debride the overlying labrum or to detach it from the rim and reattach it after the acetabular rim trimming.

Current opinion

In general, one should preserve nonpathologic normal structures if possible. Therefore, repair or refixation of the labrum is being increasingly attempted if the labrum does not appear significantly degenerated or torn within its substance (Figure 103.6). A study on sheep demonstrated that labral repairs do heal.[58]

Finding the evidence

• PubMed search, using keywords: "hip arthroscopy" AND "labral tear"; "hip arthroscopy" AND "labral repair"; as well as "labral refixation"

Quality of the evidence

Level IV
• 2 case series

Level V
• 3 expert opinions

Findings

There are a couple of arthroscopic labral repair technique papers with only nonspecific reports on outcomes, noting that "nearly all" patients had marked symptomatic improvement with clinically "positive results."[59–61]

Larson published a detailed outcomes report comparing labral debridement with labral refixation in patients with pincer impingement at a minimum of 1 year follow-up and found the outcomes and proportion of good/excellent results were significantly higher in the labrum refixation group.[62]

Recommendation

• Labral repair should be attempted, if possible, when performing an acetabuloplasty or treating a torn labrum (particularly if the tissue is of good substance and tear occurs at the labral–chondral junction) [overall quality: low]

Question 8: How does the presence of articular cartilage damage affect the prognosis of a patient with a labral tear?

Case clarification

During arthroscopy, a 10 mm × 12 mm full thickness cartilage defect is found in the anterior-superior quadrant of the

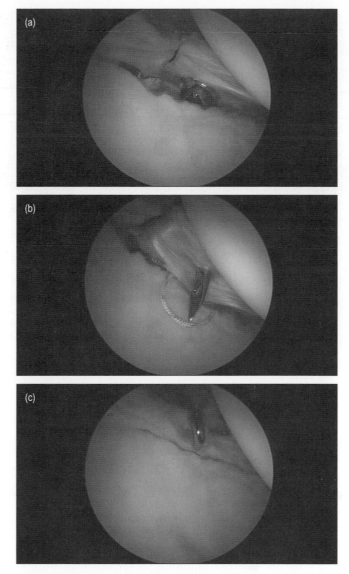

Figure 103.6 A labral repair. (a) Chondro-labral separation. The acetabular rim is prepared for the suture anchors. (b) The suture anchor has been placed, and a bird beak pierces through the labrum to create a vertical mattress stitch. (c) The labrum has been reattached to the acetabular rim.

acetabulum. When the arthroscopic photographs are reviewed with the patient postoperatively, she asks how this chondral lesion affects her prognosis.

Relevance

McCarthy et al. reported that, of those with both a labral lesion and chondral damage, 80% had both lesions located in the same acetabular zone. They theorized that labral tears may destabilize the adjacent acetabular cartilage, creating a weak point where joint fluid, under pressure during loading conditions, can furrow under the cartilage and create a lesion via a delamination mechanism. Subchondral cysts may eventually be formed when the fluid furrows under the subchondral bone.[4,16,63] The biomechanics of FAI can also explain the concurrence of chondral lesions and labral tears in similar locations.[53,64,65] The pattern of chondral and labral damage has been found to correlate with hip morphology (i.e., cam or pincer type FAI).[66]

Current opinion

Patients with radiographically moderate to severe OA may have concomitant labral pathology, but it is widely believed that those patients are best served by hip arthroplasty (THA) as the results of hip arthroscopy in the face of OA are poor.[48] The treatment decision-making for those patients with radiographically mild OA and the prognosis for those with normal radiographs but arthroscopically diagnosed chondral on the femoral head or acetabulum is less clear.

Finding the evidence

• PubMed search, using keywords: "hip arthroscopy" AND "labral tear"

Quality of the evidence

Level IV

• 7 case series

Findings

The data analyzing the influence of chondral damage on prognosis following a labral debridement is mixed, but several studies indicate that the presence of chondral damage is a poor prognostic indicator.[44,48,67]

Three other studies have not found a correlation between chondromalacia/OA and outcomes after labral debridement.[45,47,49] Byrd reported that their FAI patients who had microfracture had a similar improved modified Harris hip score (MHHS) compared to the overall average improvement in FAI patients following labral debridement and femoroplasty (Figure 103.7).[68]

Recommendation

• Patients with labral tears in the context of chondral damage should be cautioned that their prognosis is overall less favorable than those with intact articular cartilage [overall quality: low]

Question 9: What are the complications associated with labral debridement and repair?

Case clarification

Postoperatively, the patient has some numbness along her anterolateral thigh. She wonders how common this is and if it will resolve.

Relevance

Overall, the rate of complications for hip arthroscopy ranges from 0.5% to 6.4%.[69–71] The largest case series (1,054

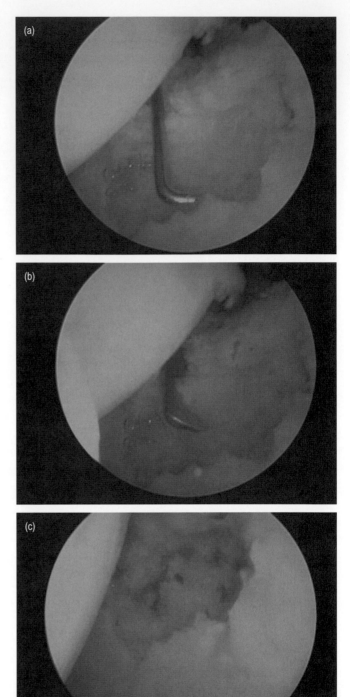

Figure 103.7 (a) Full thickness chondral lesion of the acetabular rim. (b) An awl is used to penetrate the subchondral bone. (c) Microfracture is completed.

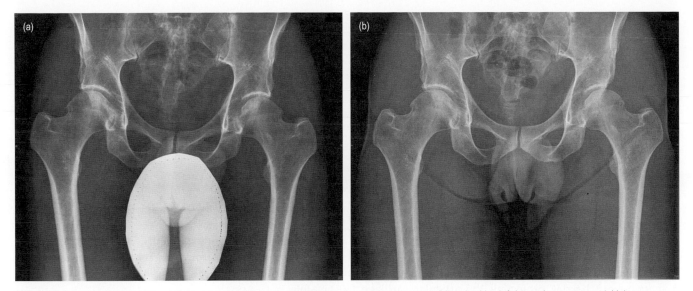

Figure 103.8 (a) A patient with a left hip labral tear presented to our clinic for a second opinion. (b) He had his left hip arthroscopy, partial labrectomy, acetabuloplasty, and cheilectomy elsewhere and returned to our clinic with persistent left hip pain. The radiograph shows a decreased center-edge angle now meeting the criteria for hip dysplasia.

arthroscopies) reported a 1.4% complication rate.[72] An understanding of the possible complications can help the surgeon take steps to minimize the patients' risk and to properly inform the patient during the consent process.

Current opinion

To minimize the risk of the most common complication—i.e., traction injuries—traction time should be as brief as possible (<2 hours is optimal), and traction force should be the minimum needed to distract the joint sufficiently. Neuropraxias are regarded as transient and due to stretch and/or pressure rather than direct nerve trauma.

Finding the evidence

• PubMed search, using keywords: "hip arthroscopy" AND "labral tear" as well as "hip arthroscopy" AND "complications"

Quality of the evidence

Level IV
• 7 case series
• 5 case studies

Nonclinical
• 1 cadaver study

Findings

Though likely under-reported, perhaps the most common complication is iatrogenic chondral scuffing and labral perforation, though it has been suggested that it may not affect outcomes.[73] The most commonly reported complication is transient neuropraxia of the pudendal, sciatic, peroneal, lateral femoral cutaneous nerve (LFCN), and femoral nerves due to traction.[74] Direct trauma to neurovascular structures may also occur, most commonly affecting the LFCN during establishment of the anterior portal (incidence of ~0.5%). Direct trauma to the sciatic nerve or femoral neurovascular structures can be catastrophic.[75]

Hip instability and even dislocation can occur with extensive debridement of the labrum, acetabular osteoplasty, and/or anterior hip capsulotomy, particularly in dysplastic hips (Figure 103.8).[71,76,77] Femoral neck fractures, though exceedingly rare, can occur after a cheilectomy.[71,75,78] A rare but potentially fatal complication is fluid extravasation into the retroperitoneal and intraperitoneal cavities.[79–81]

Other reported complications include inadequate access or observation, excessive portal bleeding and hematoma, instrument breakage, vaginal tear, trochanteric bursitis, and infection.[72]

Recommendation

• Preoperatively, hip arthroscopy patients should be counseled regarding the most common complications, particularly neuropraxias that are almost all transient [overall quality: low]

Question 10: What are the possible pitfalls of labral debridement in patients with hip dysplasia?

Case clarification

The patient comes back for follow-up at 6 months and reports pain in her other groin, with catching. An MRA shows a labral tear. Radiograph shows a center-edge angle of 18° (i.e., she has a dysplastic hip).

Center–edge angle (CEA)

The CEA is the angle formed by (1) a line drawn from the center of the femoral head to the lateral edge of the acetabulum and (2) a line straight up from the center of the femoral head. The CEA is measured on the AP pelvis radiograph.

Relevance

In acetabular dysplasia, the acetabulum does not provide adequate bony containment of the femoral head. In response, the labrum hypertrophies to accommodate increased load-bearing and is therefore subject to increased weightbearing stress and chronic shear stress. A tear of the labrum may be a sign of decompensation of the dysplastic hip. There is a high incidence of labral tears in dysplasics (up to 46%).[82] Tearing and/or debridement of the labrum may remove a barrier protecting the articular cartilage, instigating or accelerating the development of hip OA.

Current opinion

The labrum is debrided conservatively in patients with acetabular dysplasia and a labral tear. Overall, hip arthroscopy has a limited role in acetabular dysplasia.

Finding the evidence

• PubMed search, using keywords: "hip arthroscopy" AND "labral tear" as well as "hip arthroscopy" AND "dysplasia"

Quality of the evidence

Level IV
• 1 case study
• 3 case series

Findings

Addressing labral tears without regard to the underlying morphology (ranging from FAI to dysplasia) may predispose patients to failure.[83] Removing large pieces of the labrum in a patient with dysplasia can increase pain, accelerate OA, and result in lateral hip subluxation.[76] However, acetabular dysplasia is not necessarily a poor prognostic indicator in hip arthroscopy. In a series of patients with a CEA less than 25, patients with rupture of the ligamentum teres and loose bodies had the best results, those with labral and chondral issues had average results, and those with clinical evidence of arthritis had the poorest results.[24] Dysplastics can also develop symptomatic labral tears after pelvic osteotomies that can successfully be treated arthroscopically.[84]

Recommendations

• Labral debridement in classic acetabular dysplasia should be approached with caution as there is a risk of increased hip pain, chondral degeneration, and/or hip instability [overall quality: low]
• A labral tear may be the harbinger of accelerated OA in dysplastic patients [overall quality: low]

Summary of recommendations

• The central, articular portion of the labrum is the least vascular while the peripheral, capsular portion of the labrum is the most vascular region. Thus, those tears in avascular zones should be debrided due to the limited capacity to heal while those in the vascular regions should be considered for repair
• The labrum may play a significant role in articular cartilage health and hip stability. Therefore, the labrum should be conservatively debrided and/or repaired when possible
• In patients presenting with nonarthritic hip pain:
  ○ History should focus on location of pain, character of pain (sharp and/or dull), activities that induce pain, and whether they have pain at night
  ○ Physical examination should include the impingement test
  ○ Radiographs should be studied for the anatomy of impingement and dysplasia to help guide treatment
• Patients with history and physical examination suspicious for a labral tear should be sent for an MRA rather than a MRI
• Addition of an intra-articular anesthetic during contrast injection for the MRA is helpful in discerning whether the pain generator is intra-articular
• Arthroscopic partial labrectomy for labral tears without bony work to address FAI anatomy, when present, yields an approximately 70% satisfaction rate overall
• In patients with a labral tear and radiographically evident FAI anatomy, the FAI anatomy should be addressed to optimize pain relief
• Labral repair should be attempted, if possible, when performing an acetabuloplasty or treating a torn labrum (particularly if the tissue is of good substance and tear occurs at the labral–chondral junction)
• Patients with labral tears in the context of chondral damage should be cautioned that their prognosis is overall less favorable than those with intact articular cartilage
• Preoperatively, hip arthroscopy patients should be counseled regarding the most common complications, particularly neuropraxias that are almost all transient
• Labral debridement in classic acetabular dysplasia should be approached with caution as there is a risk of increased hip pain, chondral degeneration, and/or hip instability
• A labral tear may be the harbinger of accelerated OA in dysplastic patients

Conclusion

Advances in imaging (i.e., MRA) and treatment (i.e., hip arthroscopy) have only recently brought labral tears to the forefront of orthopedics, so the literature on this topic is limited. Patients with labral tears classically present with insidious onset of moderate/severe activity-related groin pain that is both sharp and dull, painful mechanical locking, and a positive impingement sign. Given that the function of the labrum is not yet fully understood, surgeons should be conservative in debriding a torn labrum and should consider labral repair if possible, particularly in the dysplastic hips. Currently, there is low-level evidence that addressing FAI anatomy during arthroscopy for a torn labrum enhances the prognosis. Chondral lesions are considered a poor prognostic indicator for recovery after hip arthroscopy.

References

1. Burnett RS, Della Rocca GJ, Prather H, Curry M, Maloney WJ, Clohisy JC. Clinical presentation of patients with tears of the acetabular labrum. J Bone Joint Surg Am 2006;88(7):1448–57.

2. Petersen W, Petersen F, Tillmann B. Structure and vascularization of the acetabular labrum with regard to the pathogenesis and healing of labral lesions. Arch Orthop Trauma Surg 2003;123(6):283–8.

3. Narvani AA, Tsiridis E, Kendall S, Chaudhuri R, Thomas P. A preliminary report on prevalence of acetabular labrum tears in sports patients with groin pain. Knee Surg Sports Traumatol Arthrosc 2003;11(6):403–8.

4. McCarthy JC, Noble PC, Schuck MR, Wright J, Lee J. The Otto E. Aufranc Award: The role of labral lesions to development of early degenerative hip disease. Clin Orthop Relat Res 2001;393:25–37.

5. Seldes RM, Tan V, Hunt J, Katz M, Winiarsky R, Fitzgerald RH, Jr. Anatomy, histologic features, and vascularity of the adult acetabular labrum. Clin Orthop Relat Res 2001; 382:232–40.

6. Giordano G, Lindsey DP, Gold G, Zaffagnini S, Safran MR. Poster 1182: Strains within the intact acetabular labrum during passive range of motion. Presented at the 55th Annual Meeting of the Orthopaedic Research Society, Las Vegas, NV, February 22–25, 2009.

7. Ito K, Leunig M, Ganz R. Histopathologic features of the acetabular labrum in femoroacetabular impingement. Clin Orthop Relat Res 2004;429:262–71.

8. Leunig M, Beaule PE, Ganz R. The concept of femoroacetabular impingement: current status and future perspectives. Clin Orthop Relat Res 2009;467(3):616–22.

9. Parvizi J, Leunig M, Ganz R. Femoroacetabular impingement. J Am Acad Orthop Surg 2007;15(9):561–70.

10. Ito K, Leunig M, Ganz R. Histopathologic features of the acetabular labrum in femoroacetabular impingement. Clin Orthop Relat Res 2004;429:262–71.

11. Beck M, Kalhor M, Leunig M, Ganz R. Hip morphology influences the pattern of damage to the acetabular cartilage: femoroacetabular impingement as a cause of early osteoarthritis of the hip. J Bone Joint Surg Br 2005;87(7):1012–18.

12. Ganz R, Leunig M, Leunig-Ganz K, Harris WH. The etiology of osteoarthritis of the hip: an integrated mechanical concept. Clin Orthop Relat Res 2008;466(2):264–72.

13. Wenger DE, Kendell KR, Miner MR, Trousdale RT. Acetabular labral tears rarely occur in the absence of bony abnormalities. Clin Orthop Relat Res 2004 Sep;426:145–50.

14. Dy CJ, Thompson MT, Crawford MJ, Alexander JW, McCarthy JC, Noble PC. Tensile strain in the anterior part of the acetabular labrum during provocative maneuvering of the normal hip J Bone Joint Surg Am 2008;90(7):1464–72.

15. McCarthy JC, Lee J. Hip arthroscopy: indications and technical pearls. Clin Orthop Relat Res 2005;441:180–7.

16. McCarthy J, Noble P, Aluisio FV, Schuck M, Wright J, Lee JA. Anatomy, pathologic features, and treatment of acetabular labral tears. Clin Orthop Relat Res 2003;406:38–47.

17. Ganz R, Gill TJ, Gautier E, Ganz K, Krugel N, Berlemann U. Surgical dislocation of the adult hip a technique with full access to the femoral head and acetabulum without the risk of avascular necrosis. J Bone Joint Surg Br 2001;83(8):1119–24.

18. Gautier E, Ganz K, Krugel N, Gill T, Ganz R. Anatomy of the medial femoral circumflex artery and its surgical implications. J Bone Joint Surg Br 2000;82(5):679–83.

19. Seldes RM, Tan V, Hunt J, Katz M, Winiarsky R, Fitzgerald RH, Jr. Anatomy, histologic features, and vascularity of the adult acetabular labrum. Clin Orthop Relat Res 2001;382:232–40.

20. Kelly BT, Shapiro GS, Digiovanni CW, Buly RL, Potter HG, Hannafin JA. Vascularity of the hip labrum: a cadaveric investigation. Arthroscopy 2005;21(1):3–11.

21. Tan V, Seldes RM, Katz MA, Freedhand AM, Klimkiewicz JJ, Fitzgerald RH, Jr. Contribution of acetabular labrum to articulating surface area and femoral head coverage in adult hip joints: an anatomic study in cadavers. Am J Orthop 2001;30(11):809–12.

22. Konrath GA, Hamel AJ, Olson SA, Bay B, Sharkey NA. The role of the acetabular labrum and the transverse acetabular ligament in load transmission in the hip. J Bone Joint Surg Am 1998;80(12):1781–8.

23. Crawford MJ, Dy CJ, Alexander JW, et al. The 2007 Frank Stinchfield Award. The biomechanics of the hip labrum and the stability of the hip. Clin Orthop Relat Res 2007;465:16–22.

24. Byrd JW, Jones KS. Hip arthroscopy in the presence of dysplasia. Arthroscopy 2003;19(10):1055–1060.

25. Ferguson SJ, Bryant JT, Ganz R, Ito K. An in vitro investigation of the acetabular labral seal in hip joint mechanics. J Biomech 2003;36(2):171–8.

26. Hlavacek M. The influence of the acetabular labrum seal, intact articular superficial zone and synovial fluid thixotropy on squeeze-film lubrication of a spherical synovial joint. J Biomech 2002;35(10):1325–35.

27. Ferguson SJ, Bryant JT, Ganz R, Ito K. The influence of the acetabular labrum on hip joint cartilage consolidation: a poroelastic finite element model. J Biomech 2000;33(8):953–60.

28. Takechi H, Nagashima H, Ito S. Intra-articular pressure of the hip joint outside and inside the limbus. Nippon Seikeigeka Gakkai Zasshi 1982;56(6):529–36.

29. Hase T, Ueo T. Acetabular labral tear: arthroscopic diagnosis and treatment. Arthroscopy 1999;15(2):138–41.

30. Byrd JW, Jones KS. Diagnostic accuracy of clinical assessment, magnetic resonance imaging, magnetic resonance arthrography, and intra-articular injection in hip arthroscopy patients. Am J Sports Med 2004;32(7):1668–74.

31. Martin RL, Sekiya JK. The interrater reliability of 4 clinical tests used to assess individuals with musculoskeletal hip pain. J Orthop Sports Phys Ther 2008;38(2):71–7.

32. Martin RL, Irrgang JJ, Sekiya JK. The diagnostic accuracy of a clinical examination in determining intra-articular hip pain for potential hip arthroscopy candidates. Arthroscopy 2008;24(9):1013–1018.

33. Martin RL, Kelly BT, Leunig M, et al. Reliability of clinical diagnosis in intraarticular hip diseases. Knee Surg Sports Traumatol Arthrosc 2010;18(5):685–90.

34. Cooperman DR, Wallensten R, Stulberg SD. Acetabular dysplasia in the adult. Clin Orthop Relat Res 1983;175:79–85.

35. Teratani T, Naito M, Kiyama T, Maeyama A. Periacetabular osteotomy in patients fifty years of age or older. J Bone Joint Surg Am 2010;92(1):31–41.

36. Troelsen A, Jacobsen S, Romer L, Soballe K. Weightbearing anteroposterior pelvic radiographs are recommended in DDH assessment. Clin Orthop Relat Res 2008;466(4):813–19.

37. Fadul DA, Carrino JA. Imaging of femoroacetabular impingement. J Bone Joint Surg Am 2009;91(Suppl 1):138–43.

38. Notzli HP, Wyss TF, Stoecklin CH, Schmid MR, Treiber K, Hodler J. The contour of the femoral head-neck junction as a predictor for the risk of anterior impingement. J Bone Joint Surg Br 2002;84(4):556–60.

39. Mintz DN, Hooper T, Connell D, Buly R, Padgett DE, Potter HG. Magnetic resonance imaging of the hip: detection of labral and chondral abnormalities using noncontrast imaging Arthroscopy 2005;21(4):385–93.

40. Toomayan GA, Holman WR, Major NM, Kozlowicz SM, Vail TP. Sensitivity of MR arthrography in the evaluation of acetabular labral tears. AJR Am J Roentgenol 2006;186(2):449–453.

41. Leunig M, Werlen S, Ungersbock A, Ito K, Ganz R. Evaluation of the acetabular labrum by MR arthrography. J Bone Joint Surg Br 1997;79(2):230–234.

42. Chan YS, Lien LC, Hsu HL, et al. Evaluating hip labral tears using magnetic resonance arthrography: a prospective study comparing hip arthroscopy and magnetic resonance arthrography diagnosis. Arthroscopy 2005;21(10):1250.

43. Kim YT, Azuma H. The nerve endings of the acetabular labrum. Clin Orthop Relat Res 1995;(320):176–181.

44. Farjo LA, Glick JM, Sampson TG. Hip arthroscopy for acetabular labral tears. Arthroscopy 1999;15(2):132–137.

45. Santori N, Villar RN. Acetabular labral tears: result of arthroscopic partial limbectomy Arthroscopy 2000;16(1):11–15.

46. O'Leary JA, Berend K, Vail TP. The relationship between diagnosis and outcome in arthroscopy of the hip. Arthroscopy 2001;17(2):181–8.

47. Potter BK, Freedman BA, Andersen RC, Bojescul JA, Kuklo TR, Murphy KP. Correlation of Short Form-36 and disability status with outcomes of arthroscopic acetabular labral debridement. Am J Sports Med 2005;33(6):864–70.

48. Byrd JW, Jones KS. Prospective analysis of hip arthroscopy with 10-year followup. Clin Orthop Relat Res 2010;468(3):741–6.

49. Kamath AF, Componovo R, Baldwin K, Israelite CL, Nelson CL. Hip arthroscopy for labral tears: review of clinical outcomes with 4.8-year mean follow-up. Am J Sports Med 2009 Jul 22.

50. Byrd JW, Jones KS. Hip arthroscopy in athletes: 10-year follow-up. Am J Sports Med 2009;37(11):2140–3.

51. Nepple JJ, Zebala LP, Clohisy JC. Labral disease associated with femoroacetabular impingement: do we need to correct the structural deformity? J Arthroplasty 2009;24(6 Suppl):114–19.

52. Bardakos NV, Vasconcelos JC, Villar RN. Early outcome of hip arthroscopy for femoroacetabular impingement: the role of femoral osteoplasty in symptomatic improvement. J Bone Joint Surg Br 2008;90(12):1570–5.

53. Tanzer M, Noiseux N. Osseous abnormalities and early osteoarthritis: the role of hip impingement. Clin Orthop Relat Res 2004;429:170–7.

54. Kim KC, Hwang DS, Lee CH, Kwon ST. Influence of femoroacetabular impingement on results of hip arthroscopy in patients with early osteoarthritis. Clin Orthop Relat Res 2007;456:128–32.

55. Philippon MJ, Schenker ML, Briggs KK, Kuppersmith DA, Maxwell RB, Stubbs AJ. Revision hip arthroscopy. Am J Sports Med 2007;35(11):1918–21.

56. Heyworth BE, Shindle MK, Voos JE, Rudzki JR, Kelly BT. Radiologic and intraoperative findings in revision hip arthroscopy. Arthroscopy 2007;23(12):1295–1302.

57. May O, Matar WY, Beaule PE. Treatment of failed arthroscopic acetabular labral debridement by femoral chondro-osteoplasty: a case series of five patients. J Bone Joint Surg Br 2007;89(5):595–8.

58. Philippon MJ, Arnoczky SP, Torrie A. Arthroscopic repair of the acetabular labrum: a histologic assessment of healing in an ovine model. Arthroscopy 2007;23(4):376–80.

59. Philippon MJ, Schenker ML. A new method for acetabular rim trimming and labral repair. Clin Sports Med 2006;25(2):293–7, ix.

60. Kelly BT, Weiland DE, Schenker ML, Philippon MJ. Arthroscopic labral repair in the hip: surgical technique and review of the literature. Arthroscopy 2005;21(12):1496–1504.

61. Murphy KP, Ross AE, Javernick MA, Lehman RA, Jr. Repair of the adult acetabular labrum. Arthroscopy 2006;22(5):567.e1–e3.

62. Larson CM, Giveans MR. Arthroscopic debridement versus refixation of the acetabular labrum associated with femoroacetabular impingement. Arthroscopy 2009;25(4):369–76.

63. Gdalevitch M, Smith K, Tanzer M. Delamination cysts: a predictor of acetabular cartilage delamination in hips with a labral tear. Clin Orthop Relat Res 2009;467(4):985–91.

64. Tannast M, Goricki D, Beck M, Murphy SB, Siebenrock KA. Hip damage occurs at the zone of femoroacetabular impingement. Clin Orthop Relat Res 2008;466(2):273–80.

65. Ganz R, Leunig M, Leunig-Ganz K, Harris WH. The etiology of osteoarthritis of the hip: an integrated mechanical concept. Clin Orthop Relat Res 2008;466(2):264–72.

66. Beck M, Kalhor M, Leunig M, Ganz R. Hip morphology influences the pattern of damage to the acetabular cartilage: femoroacetabular impingement as a cause of early osteoarthritis of the hip. J Bone Joint Surg Br 2005;87(7):1012–18.

67. Streich NA, Gotterbarm T, Barie A, Schmitt H. Prognostic value of chondral defects on the outcome after arthroscopic treatment of acetabular labral tears. Knee Surg Sports Traumatol Arthrosc 2009;17(10):1257–63.

68. Byrd JW, Jones KS. Arthroscopic femoroplasty in the management of cam-type femoroacetabular impingement. Clin Orthop Relat Res 2009;467(3):739–46.

69. Shetty VD, Villar RN. Hip arthroscopy: current concepts and review of literature. Br J Sports Med 2007;41(2):64–8; discussion 68.

70. Smart LR, Oetgen M, Noonan B, Medvecky M. Beginning hip arthroscopy: indications, positioning, portals, basic techniques, and complications. Arthroscopy 2007;23(12):1348–53.

71. Ilizaliturri VM, Jr. Complications of arthroscopic femoroacetabular impingement treatment: a review. Clin Orthop Relat Res 2009;467(3):760–8.

72. Clarke MT, Arora A, Villar RN. Hip arthroscopy: complications in 1054 cases. Clin Orthop Relat Res 2003;406:84–8.

73. Lo YP, Chan YS, Lien LC, Lee MS, Hsu KY, Shih CH. Complications of hip arthroscopy: analysis of seventy three cases. Chang Gung Med J 2006;29(1):86–92.

74. Sampson TG. Complications of hip arthroscopy. Clin Sports Med 2001;20(4):831–5.

75. Sampson TG. Complications of hip arthroscopy. Techn Orthop 2005;20(1):63–6.

76. Benali Y, Katthagen BD. Hip subluxation as a complication of arthroscopic debridement. Arthroscopy 2009;25(4):405–7.

77. Matsuda DK. Acute iatrogenic dislocation following hip impingement arthroscopic surgery. Arthroscopy 2009;25(4):400–4.

78. Mardones RM, Gonzalez C, Chen Q, Zobitz M, Kaufman KR, Trousdale RT. Surgical treatment of femoroacetabular impingement: evaluation of the effect of the size of the resection. Surgical technique. J Bone Joint Surg Am 2006;88(Suppl 1 Pt 1):84–91.

79. Haupt U, Volkle D, Waldherr C, Beck M. Intra- and retroperitoneal irrigation liquid after arthroscopy of the hip joint. Arthroscopy 2008;24(8):966–968.

80. Sharma A, Sachdev H, Gomillion M. Abdominal compartment syndrome during hip arthroscopy. Anaesthesia 2009;64(5):567–569.

81. Bartlett CS, DiFelice GS, Buly RL, Quinn TJ, Green DS, Helfet DL. Cardiac arrest as a result of intraabdominal extravasation of fluid during arthroscopic removal of a loose body from the hip joint of a patient with an acetabular fracture. J Orthop Trauma 1998;12(4):294–9.

82. Haene RA, Bradley M, Villar RN. Hip dysplasia and the torn acetabular labrum: an inexact relationship. J Bone Joint Surg Br 2007;89(10):1289–92.

83. Parvizi J, Bican O, Bender B, et al. Arthroscopy for labral tears in patients with developmental dysplasia of the hip: a cautionary note. J Arthroplasty 2009;24(6 Suppl):110–13.

84. Ilizaliturri VM, Jr., Chaidez PA, Valero FS, Aguilera JM. Hip arthroscopy after previous acetabular osteotomy for developmental dysplasia of the hip. Arthroscopy 2005;21(2):176–181.

104 Hip Impingement

Marc J. Philippon and Karen K. Briggs

Steadman Philippon Research Institute, Vail, CO, USA

Case scenario

A 19 year old man is the goaltender for his hockey team. He uses the butterfly stance and is complaining of significant right hip pain. The pain is worse when he is playing hockey. It also bothers him when he sits for a long period of time. He has tried conservative management with no resolution of symptoms.

Relevant anatomy

Recently, femoroacetabular impingement (FAI) has been documented as a common problem in the athletic population. FAI is thought to be the underlying cause of many tears and chondral injuries.[1-4] Anterosuperior labral and chondral injury has been described as a result of abnormal contact between the femoral head–neck junction and the anterior acetabulum during terminal hip flexion.[2] FAI has been classified into two distinct categories—cam impingement and pincer impingement—based upon the location of the deformity (femoral head–neck junction vs. acetabulum) and the patterns of labral and chondral injury.[5]

Cam impingement is the result of an abnormally shaped femoral head and neck that contacts a normal acetabulum. The femoral head–neck junction has an increased radius of curvature and is not spherical anteriorly. This bony abnormality contacts the anterior acetabulum as the hip flexes and internally rotates. Chondral injury and labral tears result from the shear forces produced by the contact.[4,6,7]

Pincer impingement is the result of contact from an abnormal anterior acetabular "overcoverage."[5] Repetitive contact between the acetabular rim and the femoral head–neck junction causes the labrum to become crushed, leading over time to degeneration. Additionally, the contact can also cause leverage of the femoral head out of the acetabulum posteriorly leading to a "contre-coup" injury to the posteroinferior labrum.[5]

Importance of the problem

As the emphasis on FAI is relatively new, few studies have documented the cost of the disease. In young patients with hip pain, the prevalence of FAI is very high. FAI may be a cause of early osteoarthritis in young patients.[4,5,7] The bony abnormalities associated with FAI expose the hip joint to excessive forces leading to labral tears and cartilage damage. If FAI and its sequelae go untreated, there may be rapid progression of joint degeneration, which has a large impact on the individual and society. With improved understanding of FAI and its treatment, it is possible that the prevalence of early osteoarthritis of the hip in the young patient could be reduced.

Top four questions

Diagnosis

1. What physical examination tests are used in the diagnosis of FAI?

Treatment

2. Is open or arthroscopic treatment of FAI the most effective in the sports medicine population?
3. Should a torn labrum be debrided or repaired?

Prognosis

4. Can athletes return to sport in a timely manner following treatment of FAI?

Question 1: What physical examination tests are used in the diagnosis of FAI?

Case clarification

The young hockey player had a positive anterior impingement sign and he had an increased FABER distance test on the painful hip.

> - **Anterior impingement:** To perform the anterior impingement test, the patient is placed supine on the examination table. The hip is passively flexed to 90°, followed by forced adduction and internal rotation. In this position, the anterior femoral neck approximated the anterosuperior acetabulum, the most frequent region of chondral and labral injury. Recreation of the patient's pain with this maneuver is considered to be a positive impingement sign.
> - **FABER distance test:** It is performed in the supine position by placing the affected extremity in the figure-4 position of flexion, abduction, and external rotation. A gentle downward force is then applied to the leg while stabilizing the pelvis. The vertical distance from the lateral aspect of the knee to the examination table is recorded. If the distance is greater for the painful hip, this is considered a positive test.

Relevance

A thorough physical examination is critical in order to determine the source of the patient's symptoms. The findings of the physical examination should guide the clinician in the ordering of further diagnostic investigations.

Current opinion

Current opinion suggests that use of the anterior impingement test, measured deficits of range of motion, and a positive FABER distance may provide good evidence that FAI is present.

Finding the evidence

- PubMed (www.ncbi.nlm.nih.gov/pubmed/), from 2005 to 2010, using the search terms: "(femoroacetabular impingement) AND (diagnosis OR physical examination OR tests) AND (radiographs)"

Quality of the evidence

Level II
- 4 studies developing diagnostic criteria with gold standard

Level III
- 4 nonconsecutive patient studies with no gold standard

Level IV
- 6 case control studies

Findings

Several studies have investigated the physical examination for diagnosis of hip pain.[8–11] Although surgeons do not use one specific battery of tests, there are a few tests that are commonly reported in the clinical presentation of FAI.[12–14] One study showed the ability to detect FAI is not dependent on the type of impingement. The FABER test was shown to have fair diagnostic ability and the impingement test was shown to have low diagnostic ability.[11] In several papers reporting clinical presentation of patients with FAI, the FABER test and the anterior impingement test are usually positive. The FABER test is used in two ways, and it is unclear which FABER test is more specific. The anterior impingement test is very examiner specific. It has been shown to be more specific when performed by physicians compared to physical therapists. When used in combination, these tests can be helpful in identifying patients who are at high risk for chondrolabral dysfunction due to FAI.

Several types of radiographs are used for analysis of the cam lesion.[4,15–18] However, one study showed a direct correlation between the alpha angle and chondrolabral damage in the hip. Reported reliability of the alpha angle varies widely.[15,16,18] Using the alpha angle as a dichotomous indicator of FAI has not been tested. It has been our experience that patients with an alpha angle over 55° are at high risk of pathologies associated with FAI. We have also shown the alpha angle to be associated with the FABER distance test as well. With a combination of tests, a screening program can be developed to identify those individuals who are at risk of intra-articular hip pathologies associated with FAI.

Recommendations

- A thorough clinical examination is necessary as there is no evidence to support the use of specific tests for the diagnosis of FAI [overall quality: moderate]
- It is our experience that the FABER distance test and the anterior impingement test are relatively specific for the diagnosis of FAI [overall quality: high]
- The alpha angle measured on radiographs is a helpful adjunct to the clinical examination in the diagnosis of FAI [overall quality: moderate]

Question 2: Is open or arthroscopic treatment of FAI the most effective in the sports medicine population?

Case clarification

The patient underwent hip arthroscopy for treatment of a labral tear with associated chondral delamination as a result of FAI.

Relevance

Several techniques are described to treat FAI. These include surgical dislocation, mini-open, and arthroscopy. The goal of these procedures is to return the patient to normal activities of daily living. In the sports medicine population, return to activity is the desired outcome following surgical intervention for injury. For many, activity is part of their work environment. The extent of surgical trauma, hospitalization, and rehabilitation differs between open and arthroscopic procedures. If arthroscopic intervention has similar or superior outcomes to open intervention, then hip arthroscopy would be the procedure of choice and would reduce the overall costs of treating FAI.

Current opinion

Current opinion suggests that hip arthroscopy allows the patient to return to activity sooner and is less likely to cause the patient to reduce their activity level and change their lifestyle.

Finding the evidence

• PubMed (www.ncbi.nlm.nih.gov/pubmed/), from 2005 to 2010, using the search terms: "(femoroacetabular impingement) AND (open OR arthroscopy OR arthroscopic)"

Quality of the evidence

Level IV
• 14 case control studies
• 1 therapeutic study

Findings

A recent systematic review of the literature concluded that treatment of FAI results in improvement in pain and function.[19] It further concluded that current literature is limited and there is no evidence to support one surgical technique over another.[19] In a review of six papers on the open surgical approach for the treatment of FAI, the failure rate was 16%.[20–25] This was based on each author's individual definition of failure. In a review of eight studies that reported on hip arthroscopy for FAI, the failure rate was 5%.[26–33] There was also a higher rate of major complications in the open studies. Comparison of two studies showed that longer rehabilitation is required after an open approach. Bizzini et al. reported on open treatment of FAI.[24] Their patients returned to hockey in 6.7 months. In another study, 29 hockey players were treated with arthroscopic decompression of FAI and returned to hockey at an average of 3.4 months.[32] The arthroscopic technique allowed for shorter rehabilitation and quicker return to sport. It is difficult to compare outcome scores between open and arthroscopic approaches. Most studies on open treatment report the Merle d'Aubigné score while most arthroscopic treatment papers report the modified Harris hip score (MHHS).

Recommendation

• An arthroscopic approach is preferred because of its lower failure rate, fewer major complications, and shorter rehabilitation time [overall quality: low]

Question 3: Should the torn labrum be debrided or repaired?

Case clarification

At arthroscopy, a large tear in the anterior–superior labrum was identified. The labrum was detached at the articular–fibrocartilage interface, consistent with a cam type pathology, and there was some flattening of the labrum consistent with pincer impingement. The tear was repaired with suture anchors. Three anchors were used to refix the labrum to its anatomic position.

Relevance

FAI is commonly associated with labral tears.[2,5,6,14,28] When the damaged labrum is debrided or resected, the goal is to eliminate the unstable labral flap which is causing pain and discomfort. However, removing the native labrum eradicates its functional role in the hip, which may lead to future degeneration.[34] A recent study showed increased cartilage strain after labral resection when compared to labral repair.[35] This increase in strain may lead to early development of osteoarthritis. Similar to the meniscus in the knee, efforts should be made to preserve healthy labral tissue to help protect the articular cartilage. Loss of labral tissue and labral function can also lead to hip instability.[34]

Current opinion

Preservation of healthy labral tissue is important when addressing labral pathology. Treatment should be based on the type of tear, the quality of tissue and the quantity of labral tissue. When feasible, repair should be the treatment of choice. There are instances when the tear is small and debridement is an acceptable option.

Finding the evidence

• PubMed (www.ncbi.nlm.nih.gov/pubmed/), from 2005 to 2010, using the search terms: "(acetabular OR acetabulum) AND (labral OR labrum tears) AND (hip arthroscopy)"

Quality of the evidence

Level III
• 1 case control study

Level IV
• 11 case series

Findings

One level III study provides the strongest evidence regarding arthroscopic labral debridement compared to labral repair.[36] A group of 36 patients with labral debridement was compared to a group of 39 patients with labral repair. The study showed that labral repair resulted in improved function, fewer poor results, and fewer degenerative changes.[36] The results of this study are supported by several level IV studies.[28,30,32,37] In one study, the choice of labral repair over labral debridement was an independent predictor of improved function.[28]

Recommendations

• If adequate tissue is available, a labral repair is the preferred treatment [overall quality: low]
• Labral debridement should be used judiciously and only when repair is not possible [overall quality: low]

Question 4: Can athletes return to sport in a timely manner following treatment of FAI?

Case clarification

Eight weeks following arthroscopy, this patient passed the hip sport test and was allowed to return to full activity. The patient returned to the ice at 8 weeks and completed full training sessions at 9 weeks.

> The **hip sport test** was developed to evaluate the patient's rehabilitation progress and determine if the patient can safely to return sport specific training. Instead of isolated measures of range of motion and single plane strength, the sport test uses combined coordinated movements of the entire involved extremity assessing muscle power (strength over time), ability to maintain correct form during exercises and presence of pain in common training situations.

Relevance

In the sports medicine population, return to activity is what patients expect following surgery. Many patients undergo surgery not because of the severity of symptoms, but because of inability to participate in their sport. In other populations, keeping people active is not only critical for muscle strength and weight control and to decrease the risk of osteoarthritis, but it is also a key element in the prevention of other chronic diseases.

Current opinion

Return to sport is possible following treatment of FAI.[26] However, there is no consensus on how long it will take the patient to return to sport. The rehabilitation program that patients are prescribed is critical in preparing the patient to return to sport in a timely manner. The patient must comply with the program.

Finding the evidence

• PubMed (www.ncbi.nlm.nih.gov/pubmed/), from 2005 to 2010, using the search terms: "(femoroacetabular impingement) AND (activity OR athlete OR sport) AND (arthroscopy OR arthroscopic)"

Quality of the evidence
Level IV
• 6 case series

Findings

Information on return to sport was available in four studies including a total of 228 athletes.[26,32,33,37,38] In these studies, 79% of the athletes returned to activities. However, in two studies involving professional athletes, there was a 96% return to sport in a total of 73 athletes.[26,32] One study documented the average time from surgery to return to activity: it showed that following hip arthroscopy, professional hockey players returned to skating/hockey drills at an average of 3.8 months with a range of 1–5 months.[32] As noted above, this is half the time that was required to return to hockey following open treatment of FAI.

Three studies reported on the symptoms and function of active patients.[30,33,38] Most active patients had improved symptoms and high function scores. It is difficult to interpret these studies together, as multiple outcome scores were used and these scores have not been validated in an active sports medicine population.

Recommendations
The evidence here is limited.
• Patients can expect to return to prior levels of activity [overall quality: low]
• Professional athletes will return to their professional sports [overall quality: low]
• A functional test should be used to determine if patients are ready to start sport specific training [overall quality: low]
• A new validated hip outcome score and activity scale is needed for the active sports medicine population [overall quality: low]

Summary of recommendations

• A thorough clinical examination is necessary as there is no evidence to support the use of specific tests for the diagnosis of FAI
• It is our experience that the FABER distance test and the anterior impingement test are relatively specific for the diagnosis of FAI
• The alpha angle measured on radiographs is a helpful adjunct to the clinical examination in the diagnosis of FAI
• In the active, sports medicine population, an arthroscopic approach is preferred due to shorter rehabilitation, lower complication rate, and lower failure rate

- If adequate tissue is available, a labral repair is the preferred treatment
- Labral debridement should be used judiciously and only when repair is not possible
- Active patients can expect to return to activities following hip arthroscopy
- A test of overall function should be used to determine if patients are ready to start sport specific training
- A new validated hip outcome score and activity scale is needed for the active sports medicine population

Conclusion

FAI is being seen more often in the sports medicine population. Early diagnosis and treatment of FAI is essential in avoiding degenerative changes in the joint. Arthroscopic treatment of bony abnormalities and associated pathologies can result in improvement in symptoms and function in the active population. These patients can also return to activity following a structured rehabilitation program.

References

1. Beck M, Leunig M, Parvizi J, Boutier V, Wyss D, Ganz R. Anterior femoroacetabular impingement: part II. Midterm results of surgical treatment. Clin Orthop Relat Res 2004;418:67–73.

2. Ferguson SJ, Bryant JT, Ganz R, Ito K. An in vitro investigation of the acetabular labral seal in hip joint mechanics. J Biomech 2003;36:171–8.

3. Ganz R, Parvizi J, Beck M, Leunig M, Notzli H, Siebenrock KA. Femoroacetabular impingement: a cause for osteoarthritis of the hip. Clin Orthop Relat Res 2003;417:112–20.

4. Johnston TL, Schenker ML, Briggs KK, Philippon MJ. Relationship between offset angle alpha and hip chondral injury in femoroacetabular impingement. Arthroscopy 2008;24:669–75.

5. Philippon MJ, Stubbs AJ, Schenker ML, Maxwell RB, Ganz R, Leunig M. Arthroscopic management of FAI: osteoplasty technique and literature review. Am J Sports Med 2007;3:1571–80.

6. Ferguson SJ, Bryant JT, Ito K. The material properties of the bovine acetabular labrum. J Orthop Res 2001;19:887–96.

7. Wagner S, Hofstetter W, Chiquet M, et al. Early osteoarthritic changes of human femoral head cartilage subsequent to femoroacetabular impingement. Osteoarthritis Cartilage 2003;11:508–18.

8. Martin RL, Kelly BT, Leunig M, et al. Reliability of clinical diagnosis in intraarticular hip diseases. Knee Surg Sports Traumatol Arthrosc 2010;18:685–90.

9. Martin HD, Kelly BT, Leunig M, et al. The pattern and technique in the clinical evaluation of the adult hip: the common physical examination tests of hip specialists. Arthroscopy 2010;26:161–72.

10. Martin RL, Mohtadi NG, Safran MR, et al. Differences in physician and patient ratings of items used to assess hip disorders. Am J Sports Med 2009;37:1508–12.

11. Martin RL, Sekiya JK. The interrater reliability of 4 clinical tests used to assess individuals with musculoskeletal hip pain. J Orthop Sports Phys Ther 2008;38:71–7.

12. Clohisy JC, Knaus ER, Hunt DM, Lesher JM, Harris-Hayes M, Prather H. Clinical presentation of patients with symptomatic anterior hip impingement. Clin Orthop Relat Res 2009;467:638–44.

13. Sink EL, Gralla J, Ryba A, Dayton M. Clinical presentation of femoroacetabular impingement in adolescents. J Pediatr Orthop 2008;28:806–11.

14. Philippon MJ, Maxwell RB, Johnston TL, Schenker M, Briggs KK. Clinical presentation of femoroacetabular impingement. Knee Surg Sports Traumatol Arthrosc 2007;15:1041–7.

15. Konan S, Rayan F, Haddad FS. Is the frog lateral plain radiograph a reliable predictor of the alpha angle in femoroacetabular impingement? J Bone Joint Surg Br 2010;92:47–50.

16. Clohisy JC, Carlisle JC, Trousdale R, et al. Radiographic evaluation of the hip has limited reliability. Clin Orthop Relat Res 2009;467:666–75.

17. Dudda M, Albers C, Mamisch TC, Werlen S, Beck M. Do normal radiographs exclude asphericity of the femoral head-neck junction? Clin Orthop Relat Res 2009;467:651–9.

18. Gosvig KK, Jacobsen S, Palm H, Sonne-Holm S, Magnusson E. A new radiological index for assessing asphericity of the femoral head in cam impingement. J Bone Joint Surg Br 2007;89:1309–16.

19. Clohisy JC, St John LC, Schutz AL. Surgical treatment of femoroacetabular impingement: a systematic review of the literature. Clin Orthop Relat Res 2010;468:555–64.

20. Beck M, Leunig M, Parvizi J, Boutier V, Wyss D, Ganz R. Anterior femoroacetabular impingement: part II. Midterm results of surgical treatment. Clin Orthop Relat Res 2004;418:67–73.

21. Murphy S, Tannast M, Kim YJ, Buly R, Millis MB. Debridement of the adult hip for femoroacetabular impingement: indications and preliminary clinical results. Clin Orthop Relat Res 2004;429:178–81.

22. Peters CL, Erickson JA. Treatment of femoro-acetabular impingement with surgical dislocation and débridement in young adults. J Bone Joint Surg Am 2006;88:1735–41.

23. Peters CL, Schabel K, Anderson L, Erickson J. Open treatment of FAI is associated with clinical improvement and low complication rate at short-term followup. Clin Orthop Relat Res 2010;468:504–10.

24. Bizzini M, Notzli HP, Maffiuletti NA. FAI in professional ice hockey players: a case series of 5 athletes after open surgical decompression of the hip. Am J Sports Med 2007;35:1955–9.

25. Beaulé PE, Le Duff MJ, Zaragoza E. Quality of life following femoral head-neck osteochondroplasty for FAI. J Bone Joint Surg Am 2007;89:773–9.

26. Philippon M, Schenker M, Briggs K, Kuppersmith D. FAI in 45 professional athletes: associated pathologies and return to sport following arthroscopic decompression. Knee Surg Sports Traumatol Arthrosc 2007;15:908–14.

27. Ilizaliturri VM Jr, Nossa-Barrera JM, Acosta-Rodriguez E, Camacho-Galindo J. Arthroscopic treatment of FAI secondary to paediatric hip disorders. J Bone Joint Surg Br 2007;89:1025–30.

28. Philippon MJ, Briggs KK, Yen YM, Kuppersmith DA. Outcomes following hip arthroscopy for FAI with associated chondrolabral

dysfunction: minimum two-year follow-up. J Bone Joint Surg Br 2009;91:16–23.

29. Bardakos NV, Vasconcelos JC, Villar RN. Early outcome of hip arthroscopy for FAI the role of femoral osteoplasty in symptomatic improvement. J Bone Joint Surg Br 2008;90:1570–5.

30. Philippon MJ, Yen YM, Briggs KK, Kuppersmith DA, Maxwell RB. Early outcomes after hip arthroscopy for FAI in the athletic adolescent patient: a preliminary report. J Pediatr Orthop 2008; 28:705–10.

31. Ilizaliturri VM Jr, Orozco-Rodriguez L, Acosta-Rodríguez E, Camacho-Galindo J. Arthroscopic treatment of cam-type FAI: preliminary report at 2 years minimum follow-up. J Arthroplasty 2008;23:226–34.

32. Philippon MJ, Weiss DR, Kuppersmith DA, Briggs KK, Hay CJ. Arthroscopic labral repair and treatment of FAI in professional hockey players. Am J Sports Med 2010;38:99–104.

33. Brunner A, Horisberger M, Herzog RF. Sports and recreation activity of patients with FAI before and after arthroscopic osteoplasty. Am J Sports Med 2009;37:917–22.

34. Crawford MJ, Dy CJ, Alexander JW, et al. The biomechanics of the hip labrum and the stability of the hip. Clin Orthop Relat Res 2007;465:16–22.

35. Greaves LL, Gilbart MK, Yung AC, Kozlowski P, Wilson DR. Effect of acetabular labral tears, repair and resection on hip cartilage strain: A 7T MR study. J Biomech 2010;43:858–63.

36. Larson CM, Giveans MR. Arthroscopic debridement versus refixation of the acetabular labrum associated with FAI. Arthroscopy 2009;25:369–76.

37. Larson CM, Giveans MR. Arthroscopic management of FAI: early outcomes measures. Arthroscopy 2008;24:540–6.

38. Kang C, Hwang DS, Cha SM. Acetabular labral tears in patients with sports injury. Clin Orthop Surg 2009;1:230–5.

105 Snapping Hip

Bas van Ooij and Matthias U. Schafroth
Academic Medical Center and Orthopedic Research Center Amsterdam, Amsterdam, The Netherlands

Case scenario

A 21 year old ballet dancer presented with an 18 month history of an audible and painful "snap" during particular hip movements. Initially, the "snap" was only audible, but after 8 months it became painful. Because of this pain, she could no longer fully participate in ballet dancing. As no specific event or trauma had occurred, she attributed her complaint to her training program. Six months of physiotherapy (strengthening exercises and general stretching) and avoidance of ballet activities did not result in pain reduction. She described the therapy as having little to no benefit.

Relevant anatomy

The snapping hip syndrome or coxa saltans represents several different pathologic processes of the hip. It is a symptom complex of an audible, palpable, or even visible "snap" during movement of the hip. The causes can be classified as external, internal, and intra-articular. Intra-articular snapping has different causes, including loose bodies, labral tears, or articular cartilage fragments. In this chapter, the external and internal types of snapping hip are discussed.

In the *external snapping hip*, structures over the trochanter major can cause snapping. Most often, the snapping is caused by thickening of the iliotibial band. Fibrosis of the posterior fibers of the gluteus maximus can also cause hip snapping.[1] This thickening is believed to be caused by microtrauma of these structures and could cause an inflamed trochanteric bursa.[2]

The *internal snapping hip* is caused by the iliopsoas tendon or underlying bursa. The iliopsoas muscle is the strongest

hip flexor. The exact mechanism that causes snapping, due to the iliopsoas tendon or bursa, is controversial. It has been shown that the iliopsoas tendon shifts laterally in relation to the center of the femoral head during flexion of the hip. The tendon slides medially across the femoral head during extension (Figure 105.1).[3,4] The iliopsoas bursa lies between the tendon and the anterior hip capsule and therefore could be involved and inflamed in iliopsoas snapping.

It has also been noted that in iliopsoas snapping, the prominence of the iliopectineal eminence or an exostosis of the lesser trochanter could be involved.[4] Recently, another mechanism has been described: sudden flipping of the iliopsoas tendon around the iliac muscle, allowing the tendon to contact the pubic bone.[5]

Importance of the problem

No exact numbers have been published concerning the prevalence of the snapping hip in the general population. It is often reported as an unusual condition, most common in people in the age range 15–40 years and more common in women.[6] The external snapping hip is the type most frequently encountered.[2] Snapping of the iliopsoas tendon as an asymptomatic sign is estimated to occur in approximately 5% of the population.[7]

However, the condition is very common in ballet dancers and athletes.[8–10] Winston et al. reported a snapping hip in 91% of elite ballet dancers, of whom 58% had significant pain associated with the snap. Only a small number of dancers had to take time off training because of their pain.[10]

As it is clear that the snapping hip is usually asymptomatic, treatment is rarely necessary. If treatment is necessary, most patients will respond to a conservative program. This includes resting the hip from activities that cause pain, taking nonsteroidal anti-inflammatory medication, and

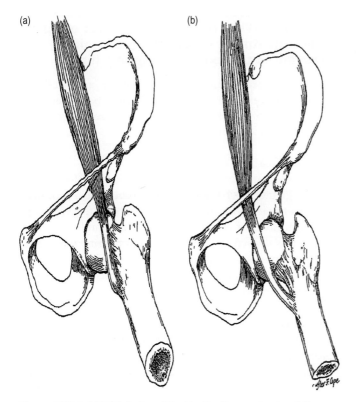

Figure 105.1 (a) With flexion of the hip, the iliopsoas tendon shifts laterally in relation to the center of the femoral head. (b) With extension of the hip, the iliopsoas tendon shifts medially in relation to the femoral head. (©1995 American Academy of Orthopaedic Surgeons. Reprinted from the Journal of the American Academy of Orthopaedic Surgeons, Volume 3(5), pp. 303–308, with permission.)

stretching and stimulating flexibility to reduce the tension on the tendinous structures.[7] Complete resolution of symptoms may take up to 1 year.[2] If conservative treatment fails and pain with snapping remains or becomes worse, surgical treatment should be considered.

Top four questions

Diagnosis

1. Which radiographic study is the most useful to diagnose the snapping hip?

Therapy

2. What is the relative effect of open surgical treatment vs. endoscopic surgical treatment in the external snapping hip?
3. What is the relative effect of open surgical treatment vs. endoscopic surgical treatment in the internal snapping hip?
4. What is the optimal approach in endoscopic surgical treatment of the internal snapping hip?

Question 1: Which radiographic study is the most useful to diagnose the snapping hip?

An external snapping hip can be readily diagnosed by clinical examination alone, but if it is not clinically evident, ultrasound could be helpful.[10,11]

Although no exact numbers of comparisons are published in literature concerning the internal snapping hip, a suitable question would be: What is the sensitivity and specificity of dynamic ultrasound compared to bursography in the internal snapping hip?

Case clarification

At clinical examination, the patient revealed pain along the inguinal crease and medial thigh. She reproduced the snap during active motion. In passive motion the snap occurred during adduction, internal rotation and extension, moved from an abducted, externally rotated, and flexed position. An internal snapping hip was suspected. Plain radiographs of the hip revealed no intra-articular loose bodies or bone spurs. To confirm the suspected diagnosis, we presented two options: a bursography or dynamic ultrasound of the iliopsoas bursa. Along with bursography or ultrasound examination, an injection of lidocaine and steroid would be administered.

Relevance

MRI with and without contrast is an excellent methodology for diagnosing intra-articular lesions or nondynamic iliopsoas diseases.[12,13] In the internal snapping hip, it is not yet clear if bursography or dynamic ultrasound is the most accurate method.

Current opinion

Current opinion suggests that bursography is the most useful radiographic study to differentiate between intra-articular and internal causes, with or without therapeutic injections.[4,14,15] Others consider ultrasound necessary to diagnose and confirm iliopsoas snapping.[5,10,16,17] Ultrasound-guided injections are also considered useful to confirm and treat iliopsoas snapping.[18,19]

Finding the evidence

- Cochrane Database, with search term: "snapping hip" OR "coxa saltans"
- PubMed clinical queries search/systematic reviews: "snapping hip" OR "coxa saltans"
- PubMed and Embase sensitivity search using keywords: ("snapping hip" OR "coxa saltans") AND "bursography," ("snapping hip" OR "coxa saltans") AND "bursa imaging," ("snapping hip" OR "coxa saltans") AND "ultrasound" as well as ("snapping hip" OR "coxa saltans") AND "sonography"

Quality of the evidence
Level III
- 1 cross-sectional study
- 5 studies of nonconsecutive patients

Findings
Bursography In 3 case series about bursography (n = 25), 18 patients (72%) revealed an abnormal motion of the iliopsoas musculotendinous unit during bursography.[14–16] Because no gold standard is determined, sensitivity and specificity could not be calculated. Of these 25 patients, 10 received a therapeutic bursa injection, resulting in relief of symptoms in 8 patients for 2 weeks up to 2 years. Two of these 8 patients returned for another injection because of limited symptom relief. In 1 patient, the injection of cortisone did not alleviate symptoms.

> In bursography of the iliopsoas bursa, the bursa is injected with contrast dye. After this injection, the hip is moved under fluoroscopy. In the case of an internal snapping hip, a sudden jerk of the iliopsoas muscle over the bursa is diagnostic.

Dynamic ultrasound In a cross-sectional study among elite ballet dancers, ultrasound was performed on 46 hips. In 27 (59%) of the hips, the iliopsoas tendon demonstrated an abnormal motion, but in this study, the snapping hips were also caused by the iliotibial band (in 2 hips, 4%) or by a possible intra-articular problem (in one-third of the hips, ultrasound did not identify the cause of the snap). It was concluded that ultrasound is helpful to diagnose an internal snapping hip.[10]

In two case series abnormal iliopsoas movement has been reported using dynamic ultrasound. One case series confirmed 100% of 10 patients,[16,20] while the second reported 22 hips of 20 patients as having snapping hips.[17] In contrast to these results, only 9 patients (23%) of 40 patients with a clinical confirmed internal snapping hip had documentation of an abnormal iliopsoas movement during ultrasound. These results possibly differed because the population could not reproduce the snap in a supine position. Sixteen of 18 patients (89%) had a good response to an iliopsoas bursa injection with steroids with an average of 4 months (range 2–10 months), so they concluded that even if the internal snapping hip was not visualized with ultrasound, a steroid injection could reduce symptoms.[18]

Recommendations
- Bursography and dynamic ultrasound are both useful to diagnose abnormal iliopsoas movement in the internal snapping hip with a higher sensitivity if the patient can reproduce the snap [overall quality: low]
- Both methods are useful to perform steroid injection in the iliopsoas bursa with variable results of the injection [overall quality: moderate]

Question 2: What is the relative effect of open surgical treatment vs. endoscopic surgical treatment in the external snapping hip?

Although no exact numbers of comparison are published in the literature, a suitable question would be: What is the relative effect of endoscopic iliotibial band release vs. open release in the external snapping hip?

Case clarification
At clinical examination, the patient revealed tenderness over the greater trochanter and a snap could be reproduced with repetitive flexion and extension. Ober's test was positive, indicative for a contracted iliotibial band. After two injections of corticosteroids with no improvement of symptoms, we presented two options for surgery: an open Z-plasty of the iliotibial band or an endoscopic release of the iliotibial band.

Relevance
Few surgical techniques have been described, often with disappointing results.[21–23] Different open approaches and endoscopic iliotibial band release have been introduced to improve the success rate in surgery of the external snapping hip.[1,24–29]

Current opinion
Current opinion suggests that the majority of surgeons use Z-plasty for surgical release of the iliotibial band in surgery of the external snapping hip.

Finding the evidence
- Cochrane Database, with search term: "snapping hip" OR "coxa saltans"
- PubMed clinical queries search/systematic reviews: "snapping hip" OR "coxa saltans"
- PubMed and Embase sensitivity search using keywords: "external snapping hip" OR "external coxa saltans" OR "snapping iliotibial band"

Quality of the evidence
Level IV
- 7 case series

Findings
Open release Four small case series described open Z-plasty of the iliotibial band in the external snapping hip.[1,24,25,27] The total number of patients was 30 (34 hips). Success rates, based on both snapping and pain, were 100%,[24] 88%,[1] 89%,[27] and 72%.[25] Complications occurred in 6 patients. One patient needed a second Z-plasty with good results.

Two other recently described open techniques are the "step cut iliotibial tract over greater trochanter" and the "multiple fibrous band release."[28,29] The first technique was performed in 16 patients (17 hips) with a success rate of 88% and patient satisfaction rate of 100%. Two patients needed a second release because of recurrent snapping; their symptoms resolved completely.[28]

The second technique was performed in 44 patients with a success rate of 89%. Five patients had recurrence of snapping, but without the need for second surgery. Ten patients reported some limping or weakness, but it did not interfere with their work.[29]

Endoscopic release Endoscopic iliotibial band release was performed in 11 patients (12 hips), with a success rate of 91%.[26] WOMAC scores were evaluated; the average preoperative score was 81 (range 78–87) and the average postoperative score at last follow-up was 94 points (range 89–96). One patient presented with recurrent snapping but without pain at the 2 year follow-up.

Recommendations
• Open release by use of Z-plasty, step cut iliotibial tract, and multiple fibrous band release has a reproducible high success rate, but attention has to be paid to recurrence and postoperative complications [overall quality: low]
• Endoscopic release of the iliotibial band is an effective and reproducible procedure in the external snapping hip [overall quality: low]

Question 3: What is the relative effect of open surgical treatment vs. endoscopic surgical treatment in the internal snapping hip?

Although no exact numbers for comparison are published in literature, a suitable question would be: What is the relative effect of endoscopic iliopsoas release vs. open iliopsoas release in the internal snapping hip?

Case clarification
The patient's clinical examination revealed an internal snapping hip. After conservative therapy without improvement of symptoms, we presented two options for surgical treatment: open iliopsoas release or endoscopic iliopsoas release.

Relevance
Complications from open procedures in the internal snapping hip have been reported to occur in 43–50% of patients.[2,3,30] Endoscopic treatment could reduce this complication rate.

Current opinion
Current opinion suggests that endoscopic release could reduce the complication rate of open procedures.

Finding the evidence
• Cochrane Database, with search term: "snapping hip" OR "coxa saltans"
• PubMed clinical queries search/systematic reviews: "snapping hip" OR "coxa saltans"
• PubMed and Embase sensitivity search using keywords: ("snapping hip" OR "coxa saltans") AND ("iliopsoas tendon release" OR "psoas tenotomy")

Quality of the evidence
Level IV
• 5 open release case series
• 6 endoscopic release case series

Findings
Open release In 5 case series, open release of the iliopsoas tendon was performed in a total number of 121 patients (139 hips). A retrospective review of 80 patients (92 hips) described "fractional" lengthening performed through an inguinal approach. In the overall results, 40 complications developed in 32 patients (43%). Recurrence of snapping occurred in 18 of the 80 patients (23%). However, overall satisfaction rate, determined by asking if the patient would undergo surgical treatment again, was 89%.[30] The same operation through a ilioinguinal approach was performed in 11 patients (12 hips). An overall success rate of 100% was published. Five out of 11 patients reported subjective hip flexor weakness.[31] A modified intrapelvic and subperiosteal approach of this operation in 7 patients (8 hips) also resulted in a success rate of 100%, with slight subjective hip flexor weakness in 2 patients.[32] Fractional lengthening through an iliofemoral approach in 9 adolescent patients (11 hips) resulted in a success rate of 91%, based on 1 recurrence.[33] A medial approach in 14 patients (16 hips) was described with a recurrence rate of 42%.[34]

Endoscopic release The randomized trial described in question 4 is considered as a case series in this question because two different endoscopic techniques were compared.[37] Endoscopic release was performed in a total number of 65 patients. In all studies, a success rate of 100% regarding pain and "resnapping" was presented.[7,19,35–38] No complications or revision surgery have been described. Four case series reported hip flexor weakness,[19,35,36,38] but this improved at 6–12 weeks. In 2 case series, Harris hip scores were evaluated; evident improvement after surgery was seen with an adequate follow-up.[19,35] In 2 studies, WOMAC scores were reported; evident improvement was presented after surgery with an adequate follow-up in these studies.[36,37]

An important finding was shown in 4 studies: intra-articular pathology was found and treated in 29 of 40 patients (73%). Cam-type femoro-acetabular impingement, labral tears, cartilage delamination, ligamentum teres hypertrophy, and positive "wave sign" at the acetabulum were described.[7,19,36-38]

Recommendations

• If iliopsoas tendon lengthening is performed by an endoscopic technique, it results in a better success rate than an open release, with minimal numbers of complications [overall quality: low]

• Because intra-articular pathology is frequently found in endoscopic iliopsoas release, hip arthroscopy should also be performed. [overall quality: moderate]

Question 4. What is the relative effect of endoscopic iliopsoas release at the insertion of the tendon on the lesser trochanter vs. endoscopic transcapsular psoas release from the peripheral compartment in the internal snapping hip?

Case clarification

The patient's clinical examination revealed an internal snapping hip. After conservative therapy without improvement of symptoms, we presented two options for endoscopic surgery: an iliopsoas release at the insertion of the tendon on the lesser trochanter or a transcapsular psoas release.

Relevance

The main reason for endoscopic treatment of the internal snapping hip is to limit complication rate. It is not yet known which technique results in the lowest incidence of complications.

Current opinion

Current opinion suggests that the majority of surgeons use the iliopsoas release at the level of the lesser trochanter and that both techniques are good alternatives for the open procedures.

Finding the evidence

• Cochrane Database, with search term: "snapping hip" OR "coxa saltans"

• PubMed clinical queries search/systematic reviews: "snapping hip" OR "coxa saltans"

• PubMed and Embase sensitivity search, using keywords: ("internal snapping hip" OR "coxa saltans") AND ("endoscopic release" OR "arthroscopic release")

Quality of the evidence

Level I

• 1 randomized trial

Level IV

• 5 case series

Findings

Pain and function The randomized trial (n = 19 patients) evaluated postoperative WOMAC scores at a minimum of 1 year follow-up.[37] Preoperatively, group 1 (10 patients treated with release at the lesser trochanter) averaged 70.1 points (SD 10.7) and group 2 (9 patients treated with transcapsular release) averaged 67 points (SD 11.4). At the last follow-up, group 1 averaged 83.7 points (SD 7.1, 95% CI 78.63–88.77) and group 2 averaged 83.6 points (SD 5.9, 95% CI 79.16–88.04). Improvements in these scores were statistically significant in both groups (group 1, p = 0.0001; group 2, p = 0.001). There were no statistical differences preoperatively and after follow-up between the groups, but the small number of patients meant there was a type II error in the results. No measurements of hip flexor strength were performed.

Revision surgery and complications In the randomized trial, no revision surgery, "resnapping," or other complications occurred in both groups.[37] The four case series of patients (n = 37) with release at the lesser trochanter and the case series of patients (n = 9) with transcapsular release also reported no complications.[7,19,35,36,38] In these case series, hip flexor weakness was reported in both groups, but this improved within 3 months.

Recommendations

• Endoscopic iliopsoas tendon release at the lesser trochanter and endoscopic transcapsular psoas release from the peripheral compartment is both effective and reproducible [overall quality: moderate]

• There are no differences in complication rate, revision surgery, or pain and function recovery between both techniques [overall quality: low]

Summary of recommendations

• Bursography and dynamic ultrasound are both useful to diagnose abnormal iliopsoas movement in the internal snapping hip with a higher sensitivity if the patient can reproduce the snap

• Both methods are useful to perform steroid injection in the iliopsoas bursa with variable results of the injection

• Open release by use of Z-plasty, step cut iliotibial tract, and multiple fibrous band release has a reproducible high success rate, but attention has to be paid to recurrence and postoperative complications

• Endoscopic release of the iliotibial band is an effective and reproducible procedure in the external snapping hip

• If iliopsoas tendon lengthening is performed by an endoscopic technique, it results in a better success rate than an open release, with minimal numbers of complications

- Because intra-articular pathology is frequently found in endoscopic iliopsoas release, hip arthroscopy should also be performed
- Endoscopic iliopsoas tendon release at the lesser trochanter and endoscopic transcapsular psoas release from the peripheral compartment is both effective and reproducible
- There are no differences in complication rate, revision surgery, or pain and function recovery between both techniques

Conclusions

In the internal snapping hip, both bursography and dynamic ultrasound are useful in diagnosing abnormal movement of the iliopsoas tendon. In open surgical treatment of the internal and external snapping hip, success rate is quite high, but complications occur frequently. Complication rates in endoscopic surgery in snapping hips are promisingly low and success rate is promisingly high, but as yet no comparative data with open surgery has been published.

References

1. Brignall CG, Stainsby GD. The snapping hip. Treatment by Z-plasty. J Bone Joint Surg Br 1991;73(2):253–4.
2. Allen WC, Cope R. Coxa saltans: the snapping hip revisited. J Am Acad Orthop Surg 1995;3(5):303–8.
3. Jacobson T, Allen WC. Surgical correction of the snapping iliopsoas tendon. Am J Sports Med 1990;18(5):470–4.
4. Schaberg JE, Harper MC, Allen WC. The snapping hip syndrome. Am J Sports Med 1984;12(5):361–5.
5. Deslandes M, Guillin R, Cardinal E, Hobden R, Bureau NJ. The snapping iliopsoas tendon: new mechanisms using dynamic sonography. AJR Am J Roentgenol 2008;190(3):576–81.
6. Beals RK. Painful snapping hip in young adults. West J Med 1993;159(4):481–2.
7. Byrd JW. Evaluation and management of the snapping iliopsoas tendon. Instr Course Lect 2006;55:347–55.
8. Howse AJ. Orthopaedists aid ballet. Clin Orthop Relat Res 1972;89:52–63.
9. Teitz CC, Garrett WE, Jr., Miniaci A, Lee MH, Mann RA. Tendon problems in athletic individuals. Instr Course Lect 1997;46: 569–82.
10. Winston P, Awan R, Cassidy JD, Bleakney RK. Clinical examination and ultrasound of self-reported snapping hip syndrome in elite ballet dancers. Am J Sports Med 2007;35(1):118–26.
11. Choi YS, Lee SM, Song BY, Paik SH, Yoon YK. Dynamic sonography of external snapping hip syndrome. J Ultrasound Med 2002;21(7):753–8.
12. Wunderbaldinger P, Bremer C, Matuszewski L, Marten K, Turetschek K, Rand T. Efficient radiological assessment of the internal snapping hip syndrome. Eur Radiol 2001;11(9):1743–7.
13. Shabshin N, Rosenberg ZS, Cavalcanti CF. MR imaging of iliopsoas musculotendinous injuries. Magn Reson Imaging Clin N Am 2005;13(4):705–16.
14. Harper MC, Schaberg JE, Allen WC. Primary iliopsoas bursography in the diagnosis of disorders of the hip. Clin Orthop Relat Res 1987;221:238–41.
15. Vaccaro JP, Sauser DD, Beals RK. Iliopsoas bursa imaging: efficacy in depicting abnormal iliopsoas tendon motion in patients with internal snapping hip syndrome. Radiology 1995;197(3): 853–6.
16. Cardinal E. US of the snapping iliopsoas tendon. Radiology 1996;198(2):521–2.
17. Pelsser V. Extraarticular snapping hip: sonographic findings. AJR Am J Roentgenol. 2001;176(1):67–73.
18. Blankenbaker DG, De Smet AA, Keene JS. Sonography of the iliopsoas tendon and injection of the iliopsoas bursa for diagnosis and management of the painful snapping hip. Skeletal Radiol 2006;35(8):565–71.
19. Flanum ME, Keene JS, Blankenbaker DG, Desmet AA. Arthroscopic treatment of the painful "internal" snapping hip: results of a new endoscopic technique and imaging protocol. Am J Sports Med 2007;35(5):770–9.
20. Janzen DL, Partridge E, Logan PM, Connell DG, Duncan CP. The snapping hip: clinical and imaging findings in transient subluxation of the iliopsoas tendon. Can Assoc Radiol J 1996; 47(3):202–8.
21. Fery A, Sommelet J. [The snapping hip. Late results of 24 surgical cases]. Int Orthop 1988;12(4):277–82.
22. Larsen E, Johansen J. Snapping hip. Acta Orthop Scand 1986;57(2):168–70.
23. Zoltan DJ, Clancy WG, Jr., Keene JS. A new operative approach to snapping hip and refractory trochanteric bursitis in athletes. Am J Sports Med 1986;14(3):201–4.
24. Dederich R. [The snapping hip. Enlargement of the iliotibial tract by Z-plasty]. Z Orthop Ihre Grenzgeb 1983;121(2):168–70.
25. Faraj AA, Moulton A, Sirivastava VM. Snapping iliotibial band. Report of ten cases and review of the literature. Acta Orthop Belg 2001;67(1):19–23.
26. Ilizaliturri VM, Jr., Martinez-Escalante FA, Chaidez PA, Camacho-Galindo J. Endoscopic iliotibial band release for external snapping hip syndrome. Arthroscopy 2006;22(5): 505–10.
27. Provencher MT, Hofmeister EP, Muldoon MP. The surgical treatment of external coxa saltans (the snapping hip) by Z-plasty of the iliotibial band. Am J Sports Med 2004;32(2):470–6.
28. White RA, Hughes MS, Burd T, Hamann J, Allen WC. A new operative approach in the correction of external coxa saltans: the snapping hip. Am J Sports Med 2004;32(6):1504–8.
29. Yoon TR, Park KS, Diwanji SR, Seo CY, Seon JK. Clinical results of multiple fibrous band release for the external snapping hip. J Orthop Sci 2009;14(4):405–9.
30. Hoskins JS, Burd TA, Allen WC. Surgical correction of internal coxa saltans: a 20-year consecutive study. Am J Sports Med 2004;32(4):998–1001.
31. Gruen GS, Scioscia TN, Lowenstein JE. The surgical treatment of internal snapping hip. Am J Sports Med 2002;30(4):607–13.
32. Komarasamy B, Vadivelu R, Kershaw CJ. Clinical outcome following a modified approach for psoas lengthening for coxa saltans in adults. Hip Int 2007;17(3):150–4.

33. Dobbs MB, Gordon JE, Luhmann SJ, Szymanski DA, Schoenecker PL. Surgical correction of the snapping iliopsoas tendon in adolescents. J Bone Joint Surg Am 2002;84(3):420–4.

34. Taylor GR, Clarke NM. Surgical release of the "snapping iliopsoas tendon." J Bone Joint Surg Br 1995;77(6):881–3.

35. Anderson SA, Keene JS. Results of arthroscopic iliopsoas tendon release in competitive and recreational athletes. Am J Sports Med 2008;36(12):2363–71.

36. Ilizaliturri VM, Jr., Villalobos FE, Jr., Chaidez PA, Valero FS, Aguilera JM. Internal snapping hip syndrome: treatment by endoscopic release of the iliopsoas tendon. Arthroscopy 2005;21(11):1375–80.

37. Ilizaliturri VM, Jr., Chaidez C, Villegas P, Briseno A, Camacho-Galindo J. Prospective randomized study of 2 different techniques for endoscopic iliopsoas tendon release in the treatment of internal snapping hip syndrome. Arthroscopy 2009;25(2):159–63.

38. Wettstein M, Jung J, Dienst M. Arthroscopic psoas tenotomy. Arthroscopy 2006;22(8):907–4.

106 Ergogenic Aids: Creatine Supplementation as a Popular Ergogenic Aid in Young Adults

Michael J. O'Brien

Harvard Medical School, Children's Hospital Boston, Boston, MA, USA

Importance of the problem

Ergogenic aids have been described as any training techniques, mechanical devices, dietary nutritional supplements, pharmacological methods, or psychological techniques that can improve exercise performance capacity and/or enhance training adaptations.[1,2]

Dietary nutritional supplements are a multibillion dollar industry worldwide. The most common legal performance-enhancing supplements used by athletes are creatine, protein powders, and caffeine. Creatine, however, is the most popular nutritional supplement used as an ergogenic aid at all levels of competition.[3]

Relevant physiology

Physiologically, creatine is synthesized from arginine, glycine, and methionine predominately in the kidneys but also in the liver and pancreas.[3] A typical diet provides approximately 1–2 g of creatine per day, with meat and fish being the main sources and supplying more than half of the daily requirement.[3]

Top two questions

1. Is creatine supplementation an effective ergogenic aid in healthy young adults?
2. Does creatine supplementation have any adverse side effects in healthy young adults?

Question 1: Is creatine supplementation an effective ergogenic aid in healthy young adults?

Relevance

Creatine is predominately stored in skeletal muscle (fast twitch, type II fibers) where it serves as the energy substrate for muscle contraction.[3] In its phosphorylated form, creatine contributes to the resynthesis of adenosine triphosphate (ATP) from adenosine diphosphate (ADP) which occurs during short-duration and high-intensity exercises.[4] This fact serves as the rationale for the use of creatine supplementation as an ergogenic aid.[5]

Current opinion

Creatine is typically used to gain weight and muscle mass, and enhance strength training. It is typically purchased in powder or capsule form and is taken as a post-workout drink or sometimes combined with weight gain and/or protein powders.

Creatine may be helpful with improving performance in short bursts of intense exercise, like bench press or sprint cycling. It seems to have no benefit with endurance in aerobic exercise. Several studies have demonstrated effectiveness in improving high-intensity exercise capacity and increasing muscle mass.

Finding the evidence

- PubMed, using "search terms": "creatine" OR [All Fields] AND "supplementation"[All Fields] AND "exercise" OR "exercise"[All Fields] AND "performance"[All Fields] with limits: "humans" AND English[lang] AND "adolescent" OR "young adult"

- Manual review of cited references from identified articles

Quality of the evidence
Level II
- 13 prospective studies of young adults in strength training and endurance training are discussed below. There is significant variability in the type of exercise used for testing, dosing schedules, and timing (in season vs. out of season training)

Findings
After 12 weeks of training with creatine supplementation, Volek et al. demonstrated increases in heavy resistance exercise in a double-blinded, placebo-controlled, randomized clinical trial (RCT). Treated subjects improved their one repetition maximum (1RM) bench press and squat exercises by 24% and 32%, respectively, vs. the placebo group (16% and 24%, respectively) subjects who had training but no supplementation).[6] The gains in mass seemed to be a result of an improvement in the ability to recover faster from heavy workouts and train harder, resulting in greater muscle hypertrophy.[7,8]

In another double-blinded placebo-controlled RCT, Stone et al.[9] also observed the effect of creatine supplementation on anaerobic performance and body composition of American football players evaluating 1RM parallel squat, 1RM bench press, dynamic explosive strength test of vertical jump, and high-intensity endurance test of 15 5 second cycling rides with 1 minute rest period between rides. They found an 11.6% increase in squat, 10% increase in bench press, and 1.5% increase in vertical jump. However, they found no statistically significant change in cycle ergometer parameters. Both hydrostatic (7%) and skin-fold method (2.6%) indicated a substantial gain in lean body mass, and an increase in body mass of 1.4 % over 5 weeks.[9]

In another double-blinded, placebo-controlled RCT, 14 men ingested 25 g/day of creatine monohydrate for 7 days. Subjects performed five sets of bench press to failure and a jump squat (5 sets of 10 repetitions using 30% of each subject's 1RM). Creatine supplementation resulted in a significant improvement in peak power output during all five sets of jump squats and a significant improvement in repetitions during all five sets of bench presses. It was concluded that 1 week of creatine supplementation (25 g/day) enhances muscular performance during repeated sets of bench press and jump squat exercises.[10]

Kersick et al., in a double-blinded RCT, also studied 24 male resistance trainers taking 20 g/day of creatine for 5 days followed by 5 g/day for the remaining 23 days and then completed a resistance training program with 4 supervised workouts per week which targeted the major muscle groups. They concluded that the ingestion of creatine promotes increases in lean mass, body composition, and 1RM bench press and leg press.[11]

Okudan and Gokbel,[12] in a double-blinded, placebo-controlled trial, found similar results to the Birch et al. study (double-blinded, placebo-controlled RCT) utilizing the "Wingate tests" (30 seconds of maximal cycling effort).[13] They found in the creatine group the total power output increased by 7.6%.

Ostojic also found a significant effect on short interval exercise. He concluded that creatine supplementation increases short-terms bursts, such as dribble and power tests (vertical jumping) with young soccer players.[14]

Leenders et al. looked at the effect of creatine ingestion on swimming velocity. Fourteen female and 18 male collegiate swimmers took 6 days of 20 g creatine followed by 8 days of 10 g creatine. They found a 2% improvement in the performance of the creatine-supplemented male swimmers. However, this study was done at the start of the collegiate swim season, and the 2% increase was found after 14 days of training.[15]

Contrasting findings are documented by Javierre et al. This study observed 12 Spanish national-class sprinters taking 25 g of creatine for 3 days, and the testing consisted of two 150 m time trials 2 weeks apart. They found no statistically significant differences between the performance times of the first and second trials (mean difference -0.14 s, $p > 0.05$).[16]

Additionally, velocity performance was studied in ice hockey skaters. Seventeen male junior and collegiate ice hockey players took 0.3 g/body mass per day for 5 days. Players repeated 10 second sprints to exhaustion on a skating treadmill while blood lactate was simultaneously collected. No differences were found over time for blood lactate changes during repeat sprints on the treadmill. The authors concluded creatine was not effective for improving performance in these ice hockey players.[17]

Rico-Sanz and Mendez Marco also looked at the effect of creatine on endurance of cyclists. After 5 days of 20 g creatine supplementation, they tested maximal power output to exhaustion. They found that oxygen consumption was greater after creatine supplementation (10.40 ± 0.65 L vs. 11.82 ± 0.34 L).[18]

Reardon et al. looked at the potential effect of creatine supplementation on aerobic long-duration exercise. Their subjects completed 45 minute cycling sessions. They concluded that the ergogenic potential of creatine supplementation in endurance performance does not produce significant results.[19]

Engelhardt's findings agree with Reardon's; they also found creatine supplementation had no influence on endurance performance. After testing 12 regional-class triathletes for 5 days on a 6 g/day creatine dosing and cycling 30 minutes to exhaustion, they found endurance performance was not influenced.[20]

Redondo et al. also produced similar findings in their sprint trials on collegiate athletes. They tested 14 female and 8 male collegiate athletes with 7 days of 25 g/day creatine supplementation. The protocol was three timed 60 meter sprint trials. The results showed creatine supplementation did not enhance speed during 60 meter sprints.[21]

Recommendations

• The suggestion from various sports and training regimens is that creatine supplementation may be effective as an ergogenic aid in short bursts of intense exercise, but does not seem to be beneficial in aerobic endurance exercises
• Although there are several well-designed prospective controlled studies, there are significant concerns about the variability in findings for creatine's effectiveness in strength training. In fact, there is inconsistency in the data with some studies demonstrating no statistically significant benefit from creatine.[16,17] For young adult athletes involved in strength and endurance training, there does appear to be a good degree of relevance for these studies (directness). Relatively small sample sizes, variability in training protocols, and differences in dosing protocols create inconsistencies in the literature and confound data interpretation [overall quality: low]

Question 2: Does creatine supplementation have any adverse side effects in healthy young adults?

Relevance

Although creatine supplementation has been suggested to be effective in enhancing performance in short, high-intensity athletic-related situations, it is paramount to evaluate whether this supplement has any adverse effects or safety concerns. Creatine is a legal supplement, readily available over the counter. It is not a banned or regulated substance in any amateur or professional sport.

Current opinion

There are no universally agreed-upon dosing schedules. In general, a "loading" dose of approximately 20 g/day for 5 days followed by maintenance dosing of 3–5 g/day (or 0.03 g creatine per kg of body weight) has been suggested.[3,11] Many athletes cycle creatine use, using it for 3 months at a time followed by a month without creatine use. The optimal time to take creatine is immediately after a workout, combined with a drink with a high glycemic index (i.e., a sports drink with sugar).[22]

Short-term use of creatine has generally been considered safe but can still have potential side effects, which are usually mild. The most common side effects are bloating, cramping, and diarrhea.[23] These effects may be minimized by forgoing the loading dose and staying well hydrated.

Creatine does not seem to adversely affect kidney function, but special consideration should be given to athletes with pre-existing kidney disease. It has not been tested thoroughly for patients under age 18, but for adults it seems to be safe and possibly effective.[24,25]

Finding the evidence

• PubMed, using the search terms: "creatine" AND "supplementation" AND "adverse effects"[Subheading] OR "adverse" AND "effects" OR "adverse effects"[All Fields] OR ("side"[All Fields] AND "effects"[All Fields]) OR "side effects"[All Fields])) with limits: "humans" AND English[lang] AND "adolescent" OR "young adult"
• Manual review of cited references from identified articles.

Quality of the evidence

Level III
• 1 prospective study[24]
• 4 retrospective studies[3,26,27,28]

Findings

Yoshizumi and Tsourounis concluded that, according to the existing literature, there appears to be no correlation between renal dysfunction and short-term creatine use in healthy individuals. However, they also caution that people with a history of renal disease may be associated with an increased risk of renal dysfunction as creatine supplementation may complicate the ability to detect progressive decreases in glomerular filtration.[26]

Poortmans and Francaux investigated liver changes during medium-term (4 weeks) creatine supplementation in young athletes. They found no evidence of dysfunction on the basis of serum enzymes and urea production. However, they did find an increase in body mass during short-term creatine supplementation likely due to water retention, since they observed a 0.6 L decline in urinary volume after ingestion of creatine 20 g/day for 6 days.[28]

Greydanus and Patel reviewed various studies undertaken on the long-term effects of creatine supplementation. One such side effect observed is increased muscle mass, which may be the result of fluid (water) retention and not of increased protein synthesis. An increase of 0.7–3 kg in 1 month has been reported. They also found that weight gain can be maintained on 5 g/day of creatine during a 10 week period of detraining and maintained 4 weeks after it is stopped. Other adverse effects that are often cited but not proven include anecdotal reports of muscle cramps, strains, dehydration in hot humid weather, diarrhea, migraines, and nausea.[3]

A retrospective study by Schilling looked at the long terms safety of creatine supplementation. The study utilized questionnaires and blood samples on 26 athletes from various sports who had used creatine supplementation for

0.8–4 years. All groups fell within normal clinical ranges; no significant adverse health effects were found with long-term creatine supplementation. Some subjects reported short-term side effects of gastrointestinal distress, but in this study evidence was anecdotal and relied on athlete recollection.[27]

Kreider examined the effects of long-term supplementation on a 69-item panel of serum, whole blood, and urinary markers of clinical health status in collegiate football players over 21 months of creatine supplementation. No significant differences were found in blood or urine markers between the groups that took creatine for 0–6 months and those who did not. His findings indicated that long-term creatine supplementation (up to 21 months) does not appear to adversely affect markers of health status in athletes undergoing intense training in comparison to athletes who do not take creatine.[24]

Recommendations

• Creatine supplementation does not appear to have significant adverse side effects from either short- or long-term use in most young adult athletes. Shortcomings in the current studies available for review include a lack of well-designed RCTs. There is also a paucity of data for creatine use in athletes younger than 18 years old.

• Current consensus is to recommend against creatine use in athletes with existing renal disease. No evidence is available to suggest that athletes younger than age 18 should take creatine. Further research is very likely to have an important impact on the confidence in this estimate of effect and presumably will lead to modification of this estimate [overall quality: low]

Summary of recommendations

• Creatine supplementation may be effective as an ergogenic aid in short bursts of intense exercise, but does not seem to be beneficial in aerobic endurance exercises

• Current consensus is to recommend against creatine use in athletes with existing renal disease

• No evidence is available to suggest that athletes younger than age 18 should take creatine

References

1. Kreider, RB, Almada AL, Antionio J, et al. ISSN exercise and sport nutrition review: research and recommendations. J Int Soc Sports Nutr 2004;1:1–44.
2. Leutholtz B, Kreider RB. Exercise and sport nutrition. In: Nutritional Health, pp. 207–39. Humana Press, Totowa, NJ, 2001.
3. Greydanus DE, Patel DR. Sports doping in the adolescent: the Faustian conundrum of hors de combat. Pediatr Clin N Am 2010;57:729–50.
4. Tokish JM, Kocher MS, Hawkins RJ. Ergogenic aids: a review of basic science, performance, side effects, and status in sports. Am J Sports Med 2004;32:1543–53.
5. Mendes RR, Pires I, Oliveira A, et al. Effects of creatine supplementation on the performance and body composition of competitive swimmers. J Nutr Biochem. 2004;15:473–8.
6. Volek JS, Duncan ND, Mazzetti SA, et al. Performance and muscle fiber adaptations to 12 weeks of creatine supplementation and heavy resistance training. Med Sci Sports Exerc 1999;31:1147–56.
7. Willoughby DS, Rosene JM. Effects of oral creatine and resistance training on myosin heavy chain expression. Med Sci Sports Exerc 2001;33:1674–81.
8. Willoughby DS, Rosene JM. Effects of oral creatine and resistance training on myogenic regulatory factor expression. Med Sci Sports Exerc 2003;35:923–9.
9. Stone MH, Sanborn K, Smith LL, et al. Effects of in-season (5 weeks) creatine and pyruvate supplementation on anaerobic performance and body composition in American football players. Int J Sport Nutr 1999;9:146–65.
10. Volek JS, Kraemer WJ, Bush JA, et al. Creatine supplementation enhances muscular performance during high-intensity resistance exercise. J Am Diet Assoc 1997;97:765–70.
11. Kerksick CM, Wilborn CD, Campbell WI, et al. The effects of creatine monohydrate supplementation with and without D-pinitol on resistance training adaptations. J Strength Cond Res 2009;9:2673–82.
12. Okudan N, Gokbel H. The effects of creatine supplementation on performance during the repeated bouts of supramaximal exercise. J Sports Med Phys Fitness 2005;45:507–11.
13. Birch R, Noble D, Greenhaff PL. The influence of dietary creatine supplementation on performance during repeated bouts of maximal isokinetic cycling in man. Eur J Appl Physiol 1994;69:268–70.
14. Ostojic SM. Creatine supplementation in young soccer players. Int J Sport Nutr Exerc Metab 2004;14:95–103.
15. Leenders N, Sherman WM, Lamb DR, et al. Creatine supplementation and swimming performance. Int J Sport Nutr 1999;9:251–62.
16. Javierre C, Lizarraga MA, Ventura JL, et al. Creatine supplementation does not improve physical performance in a 150 m race. J Physiol Biochem 1997;53:343–8.
17. Cornish SM, Chilibeck, PD, Burke DG. The effect of creatine monohydrate supplementation on sprint skating in ice-hockey players. J Sports Med Phys Fitness 2006;46:90–8.
18. Rico-Sanz J, Mendez Marco MT. Creatine enhances oxygen uptake and performance during alternating intensity exercise. Med Sci Sports Exerc 2000;32:379–85.
19. Reardon TF, Ruell PA, Fiatarone Singh MA et al. Creatine supplementation does not enhance submaximal aerobic training adaptations in healthy young men and women. Eur J Appl Physiol 2006;98:234–41.
20. Engelhardt M, Neumann G, Berbalk A, et al. Creatine supplementation in endurance sports. Med Sci Sports Exerc 1998;30:1123–9.
21. Redondo DR, Dowling EA, Graham, BL, et al. The effect of oral creatine monohydrate supplementation on running velocity. Int J Sport Nutr 1996;6:213–21.

22. Buford TW, Kreider RB, Stout JR, et al. International Society of Sports Nutrition position stand: creatine supplementation and exercise. J Int Soc Sports Nutr 2007;4:6.

23. Graham AS, Hatton RC. Creatine: a review of efficacy and safety. J Am Pharm Assoc (Wash) 1999;39:803–10.

24. Kreider RB, Melton C, Rasmussen CJ et al. Long-term creatine supplementation does not significantly affect clinical markers of health in athletes. Mol Cell Biochem 2003;244:95–104.

25. Taes YE, Delanghe JR, et al. Creatine supplementation does not affect kidney function in an animal model with pre-existing renal failure. Nephrol Dial Transplant. 2003;18:258–64.

26. Yoshizumi WM, Tsourounis C. Effects of creatine supplementation on renal function. J Herb Pharmacother 2004;4:1–7.

27. Schilling BK, Stone MH, Utter, A, et al. Creatine supplementation and health variables: a retrospective study. Med Sci Sports Exerc 2001;33:183–8.

28. Poortmans JR, Francaux M. Adverse effects of creatine supplementation. Sports Med 2000;30:155–70.

VII   Wrist and Hand Surgery

107 Acute Management of Distal Radius Fractures

Ruby Grewal

Hand and Upper Limb Centre, University of Western Ontario, London, ON, Canada

Case scenario

A 22 year old man sustained an isolated injury to his dominant arm after a fall on to his outstretched wrist. Radiographs confirm a displaced distal radius and ulnar styloid fracture.

Introduction

Distal radius fractures can be broadly classified as extra- or intra-articular depending on whether there is extension into the joint surface. Standard radiographic parameters are used to describe the degree of displacement (i.e., ulnar variance, dorsal tilt, radial inclination) (Figure 107.1).

Importance of the problem

Distal radius fractures represent the most common fracture of the upper extremity. The age and gender distribution is bimodal, with young adults (predominantly male) sustaining this injury following high-energy trauma and older adults (predominantly female) sustaining it after low-energy trauma such as a fall from standing height.

The incidence of distal radius fractures in women increases progressively with age from the perimenopausal period, whereas men have a relatively low incidence until later in life.[1] The age-adjusted incidence of distal radius fractures is 9/10,000 person years in men and 36.8/10,000 person years in women aged 35 years or over in the United Kingdom.[1] The lifetime risk of a radius or ulnar fracture at age 50 is estimated at 16.6% for women and only 2.9% for men.[2]

Top eight questions

1. What is the effectiveness of long-arm vs. short-arm cast for the immobilization of distal radius fractures?
2. What is the effectiveness of percutaneous pinning vs. cast immobilization?
3. What is the effectiveness of fracture fixation in elderly patients?
4. What is the effectiveness of associated ulnar styloid fixation in the setting of a concomitant distal radius fracture?
5. What is the effectiveness of bridging vs. nonbridging external fixation in the treatment of distal radius fractures?
6. Does an arthroscopic-assisted reduction improve outcomes in distal radius fractures?
7. Do volar locking plates offer the most effective form of fracture fixation?
8. What is the effectiveness of physical therapy following distal radius fracture?

Question 1: What is the effectiveness of long-arm vs. short-arm cast for the immobilization of distal radius fractures?

Case clarification

The patient has sustained an extra-articular distal radius fracture which requires cast immobilization. For patients with distal radius fractures amenable to cast immobilization, do long-arm or short-arm casts provide more effective fracture stabilization?

Relevance

Distal radius fractures can potentially be unstable, losing reduction despite acceptable initial alignment. Casts must

Evidence-Based Orthopedics, First Edition. Edited by Mohit Bhandari.
© 2012 Blackwell Publishing Ltd. Published 2012 by Blackwell Publishing Ltd.

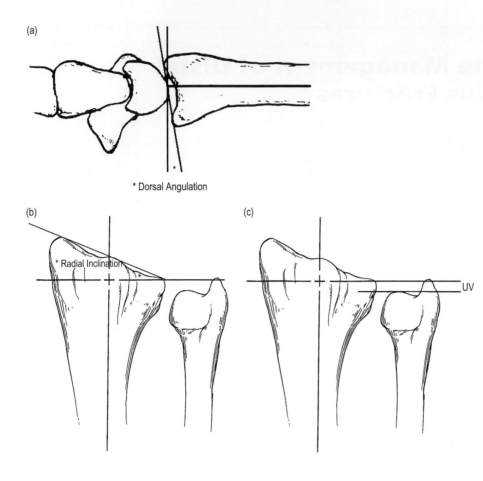

(a)

* Dorsal Angulation

(b)

* Radial Inclination

(c)

UV

Figure 107.1 Standard radiographic parameters used to evaluate displacement of distal radius fractures: (a) dorsal tilt, (b) radial inclination, (c) ulnar variance.

securely immobilize the forearm to maintain fracture stability, but they must also be tolerated by patients. The ideal method of immobilizing distal radius fractures has been debated by many authors. Sarmiento[3] and Bunger[4] have both identified brachioradialis as a major deforming force and suggest a long-arm splint in supination is necessary to neutralize its action, whereas Wahlstrom[5] has suggested that the pronator quadratus is the major deforming force and recommends a long-arm cast in pronation to prevent redisplacment. Others have shown that above-elbow immobilization is necessary and report that below-elbow casts provide adequate immobilization.[6]

Current opinion

Current opinion suggests that below-elbow casts are sufficient for immobilization of Colles' fractures.

Finding the evidence

• PubMed (www.ncbi.nlm.nih.gov/pubmed/) clinical queries, using search terms: "immobilization[Title/Abstract] AND distal[Title] AND radius[Title] AND Clinical Trial[ptyp] AND (Clinical Trial[ptyp] OR Randomized Controlled Trial[ptyp])"

Quality of the evidence

Level II

• 1 prognostic study[7]

Findings

A prospective randomized trial compared long-arm sugar-tong splints with short-arm radial gutter splints for their ability to maintain fracture reduction and patient satisfaction. In a study of 118 patients, Bong et al. found that both splints were equally able to maintain reduction in both stable and unstable distal radius fractures (p = 0.78). In addition, patients with short-arm casts had significantly better DASH scores than those with long-arm casts.[7] Pool et al. also found that above-elbow casts offered no advantages over short-arm casts in the treatment of distal radius fractures in a prospective study.[6]

Recommendation

• Evidence suggests that short-arm and long-arm casts are equally effective at stabilizing distal radius fractures and short-arm casts are much better tolerated by patients [overall quality: moderate–high]

Question 2: What is the effectiveness of percutaneous pinning vs. cast immobilization?

Case clarification

Radiographic examination reveals that the patient's fracture is comminuted and there is concern regarding the ability of casting alone to maintain alignment. For patients with unstable distal radius fractures, does percutaneous pinning offer superior results to cast immobilization alone?

Relevance

Percutaneous pinning provides additional stability to distal radius fractures treated with cast immobilization, and is less invasive and less costly than open reduction and internal fixation (ORIF).

Current opinion

Percutaneous pinning of unstable distal radius fractures offers a viable option in treating unstable distal radius fractures but is less commonly used since the advent of volar locked plates.

Finding the evidence

• Cochrane review, "percutaneous pinning and distal radius"
• PubMed (www.ncbi.nlm.nih.gov/pubmed/) clinical queries, with search terms: "distal radius fracture" and "pinning AND (Clinical Trial[ptyp] OR Randomized Controlled Trial[ptyp])"

Quality of the evidence

Level II
• 1 systematic review of lower-quality randomized controlled trials(RCTs)[8]

Findings

Five published trials comparing the effectiveness of percutaneous pinning with plaster cast immobilization vs. closed reduction and casting alone were identified in a recent Cochrane review.[8] Four of these trials utilized traditional Kirschner wiring techniques (with one or two K-wires)[9–12] and one trial evaluated Kapandji pinning[13]. A combination of both extra-articular[9,10,13] and intra-articular[11,12] fractures was included in the literature. All five studies included a predominance of female patients (range 73–98% female) with a mean age between 56 and 71.5 years.

In four of the five studies, the final anatomic results were better in the percutaneous pinning group when compared to casting.[9–12] There were significantly higher rates of deformity, malunion, and articular incongruity in the group receiving closed reduction and casting alone. This difference did not achieve statistical significance in the trial by Stoffelen evaluating Kapadji pinning.[13]

Azzopardi et al. did not identify any significant differences with respect to pain, range of motion, grip strength, activities of daily living, or SF-36 scores between groups in their trial evaluating low-demand patients over the age of 60. They identified greater ulnar deviation in the surgical group, but the functional significance of this is uncertain. Although Stoffelen did not limit his study group to low-demand elderly patients, he too did not identify any significant differences between the two groups. He reported a majority of good and excellent results in both the Kapandji pinning group (75%) and the cast group (74%).[13] The other three trials evaluating percutaneous pinning vs. cast immobilization identified better range of motion[10] and better overall anatomic and functional results (range of motion and grip strength) in the percutaneous pinning group.[11,12] These trials included younger patients and unstable fractures (both extra-articular[10] and intra-articular[11,12]).

The overall reported complications were low in both groups. There were some pin-related complications in the surgical groups that were minor in nature, requiring pin removal and antibiotic treatment,[9] and one report of K-wire migration.[10] There was one case of a persistent superficial radial nerve injury in the operative group, likely related to pin placement.[13] Redisplacement was the most common complication in the cast group. There were similar incidences of reflex sympathetic dystrophy in both groups.

Recommendations

• Percutaneous pinning results in fewer distal radius malunions and less deformity compared to casting alone [overall quality: moderate]
• There are no differences in clinical outcomes when comparing percutaneous pinning to casting in low-demand patients over the age of 60 [overall quality: moderate]
• There are better overall results with percutaneous pinning versus casting in trials which included younger patients and unstable fractures [overall quality: moderate]
• There are only few, minor complications associated with percutaneous pinning of distal radius fractures [overall quality: moderate]

Question 3: What is the effectiveness of fracture fixation in elderly patients?

Case clarification

A displaced distal radius fracture was treated with a closed reduction and short-arm cast in a 65 year old woman. Upon reassessment at 1 week, the fracture had lost reduction. Radiographs revealed that the distal radius was shortened and dorsally angulated. Does operative fixation of a displaced distal radius fracture result in better outcomes than cast immobilization in elderly patients?

Relevance

It is difficult to maintain alignment of distal radius fractures in older adults with closed reduction and casting alone. This may be a result of poor underlying bone quality or fracture comminution.

Current opinion

Older patients tolerate residual deformity and malunion much better than younger patients with distal radius fractures. It has been well documented that frail, low-demand, elderly patients tolerate residual deformity very well.[14–16] However, older active patients may place greater functional demands on their wrist and may benefit from more aggressive intervention.

Finding the evidence

- PubMed (www.ncbi.nlm.nih.gov/pubmed/) clinical queries, with search terms: "(distal radius fractures[Title] OR colles[Title]) AND (elderly[Title] OR older[Title])"

Quality of the evidence

Level I

- 1 high-quality prospective study[17]

Level II

- prognostic study[18]
- diagnostic study[19]
- 2 lower-quality RCTs[20,21]

Level III

- 1 retrospective comparative study[22]

Findings

Several studies demonstrate that traditional radiographic parameters for defining adequacy of reduction are not related to function in older patients. Anzarut et al. demonstrated that patients over the age of 49, whose distal radius fractures healed with more than 10° of dorsal tilt did not have higher reported pain and disability (DASH, SF-12) when compared to those whose fractures healed in an acceptable position.[17] This was also corroborated by Grewal and MacDermid who found that patients 65 years of age or older demonstrated no statistically significant relationship between distal radius fracture malalignment (considering dorsal angulation, radial shortening, and radial inclination) and PRWE or DASH scores at 1 year.[18] Kelly et al. randomized elderly patients (mean age 75) to acceptance of deformity (10–30° of dorsal tilt) vs. remanipulation and found no differences between the two groups in any of the measured outcomes. They concluded that regardless of remanipulation, most reduction is lost by the time of union in these patients.[20]

There have been a few randomized trials evaluating the effects of accepting a misaligned fracture vs. surgical fixation in an elderly population. Roumen et al. randomized patients over the age of 55 with more than 10° of dorsal angulation or more than 5mm of radial shortening to acceptance of the deformity or remanipulation and external fixation.[21] Although they found the external fixation group had a better anatomic result, their function was no better than the control group. Synn et al. also demonstrated that surgically treated fractures were better aligned anatomically, but there was no relationship between radiographic outcomes and subjective or objective functional outcomes in patients over the age of 55.[19] Arora et al. compared patients over 70 years of age with volar locked plating and cast immobilization. They found that 89% of the casted patients had some degree of malunion and 77% had an obvious clinical deformity.[22] Although the ORIF group did not have any patients with malalignment, there were no significant differences in range of motion (ROM), grip strength, DASH, or PRWE between the two groups.[22]

Although it has been demonstrated that outcomes are not directly correlated to anatomical alignment following a distal radius fracture, there has been evidence to suggest that the relative risk of a poor outcome does increase with malalignment in this age group. Patients aged 65 or older demonstrated a higher relative risk of a poor outcome with fracture malalignment when compared to fractures with acceptable alignment, but this relative risk was much lower than that seen in patients younger than age 65 [RR of poor outcome with malalignment based on PRWE 2.9 (<65) vs. 1.6 (≥65) and DASH 5.2 (<65) vs. 1.5 (≥65).[18] Further studies are needed to assess the role of surgical intervention in an active elderly population.

Recommendation

- No significant correlation has been found between final anatomical and functional outcome in elderly patients [overall quality: moderate]

Question 4: What is the effectiveness of associated ulnar styloid fixation in the setting of a concomitant distal radius fracture?

Case clarification

Further radiographic examination reveals that an associated ulnar styloid fracture is present. For patients with both distal radius and ulnar styloid fractures, what is the effectiveness of fixation of the ulnar styloid?

Relevance

The ulnar styloid is an attachment point for several ligamentous and soft tissue restraints around the wrist. Ulnar styloid fractures are commonly associated with distal radius fractures and the indications for fixation of these fractures and their influence on final outcomes is unclear.

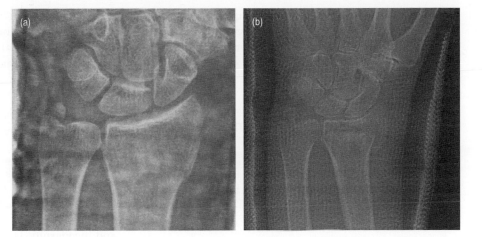

Figure 107.2 Ulnar styloid fracture: (a) tip, (b) base.

Current opinion

Small ulnar styloid tip fractures (Figure 107.2a) are typically left untreated, while larger fractures through the base of the ulnar styloid (Figure 107.2b) cause greater concern and are sometimes fixed surgically.

Finding the evidence

- PubMed (www.ncbi.nlm.nih.gov/pubmed/) clinical queries, with search term: "ulnar styloid [Title/Abstract]"

Quality of the evidence

Level I
- 1 prospective study[23]

Level II
- 1 lower-quality RCT[24]

Level III
- 1 retrospective case series[25]

Findings

In a prospective trial, Zenke et al. compared outcomes in patients with no ulnar fracture (n = 50), basal ulnar styloid fractures (n = 41), and ulnar styloid tip fractures (n = 27). All patients had a distal radius fracture that was treated with a volar locked plate, and none of the ulnar styloid fractures was treated surgically. Their results demonstrated that although union rates were higher in the ulnar tip fractures (40.7% tip vs. 26.8% basal, p < 0.05) there was no significant difference in ROM, grip strength, or DASH scores between the three groups. There was also no significant relationship between ulnar styloid fracture location, union, and persistent ulnar-sided wrist pain.[23]

Ekenstam et al. conducted a randomized trial evaluating the effect of triangular fibrocartilage complex (TFCC) repair and ulnar styloid fixation in a group of patients treated with closed reduction of their distal radius fracture. There were no differences in ulnar styloid union rates, subjective complaints of pain, or wrist arthrogram results between patients with TFCC repair and ulnar styloid fixation and those who were treated with closed reduction of the distal radius fracture alone.[24]

In a retrospective analysis of 76 matched patients with and without an ulnar base fracture, Souer et al. found no significant difference in overall outcomes between patients with an unrepaired fracture of the ulnar styloid base and those with no ulnar fracture at any of the follow-up intervals. There was a trend toward less grip strength at 6 months, and less wrist flexion and ulnar deviation at 24 months for patients with untreated basal ulnar styloid fractures, but this did not reach statistical significance. They concluded that an unrepaired basal ulnar styloid fracture does not influence function or outcome after treatment of a distal radial fracture with plate-and-screw fixation.[25]

Recommendations

- For distal radius fractures treated with volar locked plating, there are no significant differences in outcomes between those with ulnar styloid tip fractures, base fractures or those without ulnar styloid fractures [overall quality: high]
- Repair of the TFCC or ulnar styloid fixation does not improve outcomes in distal radius fractures treated with closed reduction [overall quality: moderate]
- The presence of a fracture of the ulnar styloid base does not influence function or final outcomes in distal radius fractures treated with ORIF [overall quality: low]

Question 5: What is the effectiveness of bridging vs. nonbridging external fixation in the treatment of distal radius fractures?

Case clarification

Nonbridging external fixators allow early range of motion at the wrist while bridging external fixators span across the wrist joint and only allow ROM of the digits. Do nonbridging external fixators result in better long-term clinical outcomes when compared to bridging external fixators in the treatment of distal radius fractures?

Relevance
Nonbridging external fixators allow early ROM which may be an advantage when treating distal radius fractures with external fixation.

Current opinion
Static external fixators are widely used in North America. Publications from Europe report good results with nonbridging fixators.

Finding the evidence
- PubMed (www.ncbi.nlm.nih.gov/pubmed/) clinical queries, with search terms: "distal radius[Title] AND (external[Title] OR fixator[Title]) AND Randomized Controlled Trial[ptyp]"

Quality of the evidence
Level II
- lower-quality RCTs[26–30]

Findings
There have been five RCTs comparing bridging to nonbridging external fixators. McQueen et al. demonstrated better overall results for unstable distal radius fractures treated with a nonbridging external fixator. They found patients treated with a nonbridging fixator had statistically better grip strength, wrist flexion, and overall maintenance of fracture alignment when compared to bridging fixators in a prospective randomized trial of 60 patients.[29]

The other four RCTs failed to show any significant advantage to fixation with a nonbridging external fixator. Krukhaug et al. compared the dynawrist bridging external fixator to the Hoffman nonbridging fixator and found that there were no statistically significant differences between the groups with respect to visual analog pain scales and DASH scores.[28] Atroshi et al. also compared bridging to nonbridging external fixation in a population of elderly patients with severely displaced distal radius fractures. They found no differences in DASH scores, satisfaction, ROM, or grip strength between groups.[26] Krishnan et al. reproduced these findings in a similar study which included a diverse age range of patients (mean 56 years, range 18–83 years).[27]

Sommerkamp et al. also evaluated dynamic and static external fixators in an RCT and confirmed that there were no advantages in final ROM between groups and also found the dynamic external fixators had a higher frequency of complications and fewer patients who scored good to excellent on the Gartland and Werley scores (76% vs. 92%).[30]

Recommendation
- There are no significant advantages to fixation with a nonbridging external fixator over a static, bridging external fixator in the treatment of distal radius fractures [overall quality: moderate]

Question 6: Does an arthroscopic-assisted reduction improve outcomes in distal radius fractures?

Case clarification
An active 25 year old man sustained an intra-articular distal radius fracture after a fall from his motorcycle. Radiographs show significant intra-articular involvement and incongruity. Does arthroscopic assistance improve the quality of the intra-articular reduction in the treatment of intra-articular distal radius fractures? Does this lead to better clinical outcomes?

Relevance
The addition of arthroscopy during the treatment of intra-articular distal radius fractures allows a more accurate reduction of the articular surface and allows identification of associated ligamentous, chondral, or TFCC injuries. An improved articular reduction could help reduce the risk of developing long-term post-traumatic arthritis following intra-articular distal radius fractures.

Current opinion
Fluroscopy is widely used to determine the accuracy of fracture reduction intraoperatively and it is generally felt that arthroscopy is not necessary to obtain an adequate reduction.

Finding the evidence
- PubMed (www.ncbi.nlm.nih.gov/pubmed/) clinical queries, with search terms: (("arthroscopy"[MeSH Terms] OR "arthroscopy"[All Fields]) AND distal[All Fields] AND ("radius fractures"[MeSH Terms] OR ("radius"[All Fields] AND "fractures"[All Fields]) OR "radius fractures"[All Fields])) AND (Randomized Controlled Trial[ptyp]) AND English[lang])

Quality of the evidence
Level II
- 1 prospective cohort study[31]
- 1 lower-quality RCT[32]

Findings
Ruch et al. performed a nonrandomized matched prospective cohort study comparing arthroscopic-assisted and fluoroscopic-assisted treatment for intra-articular distal radius fractures. Their study of 30 patients demonstrated no significant differences in final DASH score or radiographic results between the two groups.[31]

Another randomized trial comparing fluoroscopic-assisted (FA) reduction to arthroscopic and fluoroscopic-assisted (AFA) reduction in intra-articular distal radius fractures was conducted by Varitimidis et al. (n = 40).[32] They found that the AFA group had less pain, an earlier return to work, and significantly better DASH and modified Mayo wrist scores (p < 0.001) at 3 months. There were no long-term differences in DASH scores at 1 and 2 years; however, the AFA group continued to demonstrate superior outcomes based on the modified Mayo wrist score at both 1 year (90.9 ± 2.5 vs. 85.3 ± 4.1, p < 0.01) and 2 years (91.2 ± 2.2 vs. 86.7 ± 3.0, p < 0.01) post fracture.[32]

Recommendations

• There may be some evidence to suggest improved long-term outcomes (based on modified Mayo wrist score) for articular fractures treated with arthroscopic-assisted reductions compared to fluoroscopy alone [overall quality: moderate]
• There are no long-term differences in DASH scores between AFA reduction of intra-articular distal radius fractures [overall quality: moderate]

Question 7: Do volar locking plates offer the most effective form of fracture fixation?

Case clarification

A young, active patient has sustained an unstable, displaced distal radius fracture. Closed reduction and casting was not sufficient to maintain alignment. The patient is eager to receive definitive treatment and return quickly to full activity. The treating surgeon feels that the fracture is best treated with a volar locking plate. Is volar locked plating the most effective method of fixation for distal radius fractures?

Relevance

The popularity of volar locked plating for the treatment of distal radius fractures has grown exponentially over the past several years. Koval et al. report that the proportion of distal radius fractures that were stabilized with plating increased from 42% in 1999 to 81% in 2007 (p < 0.001).[33] This represents a shift away from percutaneous fixation with K-wires towards volar locked plating. A cost analysis study by Shyamalan et al. reported a calculated difference of £1,549 (about $2,500) per case between percutaneous fixation with K-wires and volar locked plating.[34] Whether this shift in practice and additional expense is supported by the literature is not clear.

Current opinion

Volar locked plating is the most common method of stabilizing displaced distal radius fractures. It offers stable fixation and is an excellent option for osteoporotic bone (Figure 107.3).

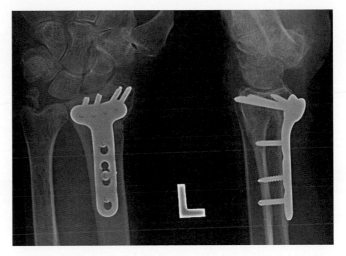

Figure 107.3 Example of a volar locking plate.

Finding the evidence

• PubMed (www.ncbi.nlm.nih.gov/pubmed/) clinical queries, with search terms: (distal[All Fields] AND ("radius"[MeSH Terms] OR "radius"[All Fields]) AND volar[All Fields]) AND (Randomized Controlled Trial[ptyp] AND English[lang])

Quality of the evidence

Level I
• prospective randomized trials[35–37]

Findings

The push behind the exponential growth of volar locked plating is not evidence based. While there are several case series reporting good to excellent results with volar locked plates,[38] there are few prospective randomized trials comparing volar locked plating to other methods of fixation.

Three RCTs were identified through a PubMed search. One trial compared volar locked plating to closed reduction and casting (n = 45),[36] and two others compared volar locked plates to external fixation (n = 46)[37] and K-wire fixation (n = 77).[35] Patients treated with volar locked plates had superior DASH scores in early follow-up (≤3 months)[36,37] but these advantages were not evident at 1 year.[35–37] Volar locked plating showed an advantage in early ROM assessements (6–9 weeks,[36] <12 weeks[35,37]) but not at final follow-up. Grip strength was not found to be statistically higher with volar plating.[37]

Recommendations

• There is evidence to suggest that volar locked plating of distal radius fractures improves ROM and outcome scores in the short term (<3 months) [overall quality: moderate–high]

• There are no long-term differences in DASH scores between volar locking plates and either percutaneous or external fixation [overall quality: moderate–high]

Question 8: What is the effectiveness of physical therapy in distal radius fractures?

Case clarification

The aforementioned distal radius fracture was treated with ORIF using a volar locking plate. The fixation is deemed stable. Does immediate postoperative ROM improve long-term outcomes in distal radius fractures? Do patients receiving formal therapy sessions have better outcomes than those performing their exercises at home, in an unsupervised setting?

Relevance

The goal of therapy is to improve ROM, strength, and overall function. Regular structured therapy sessions for all patients with distal radius fractures may be associated with significant time and financial implications, which can sometimes be prohibitory for both patients and therapists.

Current opinion

Long-term immobilization leads to stiffness and difficulty regaining full ROM. Initiating early ROM, when possible, is usually felt to lead to optimal results. In uncomplicated cases, patients can often do their exercises independently, after formal instruction by a therapist.

Finding the evidence

• PubMed (www.ncbi.nlm.nih.gov/pubmed/) clinical queries, with search terms: (distal[All Fields] AND ("radius"[MeSH Terms] OR "radius"[All Fields]) AND ("range of motion, articular"[MeSH Terms] OR ("range"[All Fields] AND "motion"[All Fields] AND "articular"[All Fields]) OR "articular range of motion"[All Fields] OR ("range"[All Fields] AND "motion"[All Fields]) OR "range of motion"[All Fields])) AND ((Clinical Trial[ptyp] OR Randomized Controlled Trial[ptyp]) AND English[lang])

Quality of the evidence

Level I
• high-quality RCT[39]

Level II
• lower-quality RCTs[40–43]

Findings

The role of early ROM and physiotherapy has been investigated in a few RCTs. An RCT comparing patients treated with early motion (at 2 weeks after surgery) to late motion (6 weeks) after volar plating of distal radius fractures found no significant differences in outcomes (flexion/extension arc, grip strength, Mayo pain or DASH scores) at 3 or 6 months.[39]

Kay et al. compared patients receiving a single session of advice from a physiotherapist to patients receiving no advice and found no differences in ROM or grip strength between groups. However, patients receiving instruction in home exercises from a therapist had better QuickDASH scores at 3 weeks and better PRWE scores at both 3 and 6 weeks.[40]

Three randomized trials were identified comparing outcomes following a program of independent home exercises (initial instructions given by a physical therapist) to a conventional structured physiotherapy program. At 6 weeks, Krischak et al. identified a greater recovery of grip strength (54% vs. 32%, p = 0.003) and ROM (70% vs. 59%, p < 0.013) in the group receiving home exercises (reported as a percentage compared to the normal contralateral limb).[41] Maciel et al. evaluated patients at 6 and 24 weeks and did not find any significant differences between grip strength, ROM, pain intensity, or PRWE scores between groups.[43] At 6 months, Wakefield et al. also report no significant differences in grip strength or hand function between groups, although the physiotherapy group had a better arc of flexion and extension (p = 0.044).[42]

Recommendations

• While there appear to be some early advantages to a structured therapy program, in patients with uncomplicated distal radius fractures there are no significant long-term differences between patients receiving instruction in home exercises and formal physiotherapy [overall quality: moderate]
• Early range of motion (2 weeks) does not offer any long-term advantage compared to ROM initiated at 6 weeks following volar plating of distal radius fractures [overall quality: high]

Summary of recommendations

• Short-arm and long-arm casts are equally effective at stabilizing distal radius fractures, and short-arm casts are much better tolerated by patients
• Percutaneous pinning results in fewer distal radius malunions and less deformity compared to casting alone
• There are no differences in clinical outcomes when comparing percutaneous pinning to casting in low-demand patients over the age of 60
• There are better overall results with percutaneous pinning vs. casting in trials which included younger patients and unstable fractures
• There are only few, minor complications associated with percutaneous pinning of distal radius fractures

- No significant correlation has been found between final anatomic and functional outcome in elderly patients
- For distal radius fractures treated with volar locked plating, there are no significant differences in outcomes between those with ulnar styloid tip fractures, base fractures or those without ulnar styloid fractures
- Repair of the TFCC or ulnar styloid fixation does not improve outcomes in distal radius fractures treated with closed reduction
- The presence of a fracture of the ulnar styloid base does not influence function or final outcomes in distal radius fractures treated with ORIF
- There are no significant advantages to fixation with a nonbridging external fixator over a static, bridging external fixator in the treatment of distal radius fractures
- There may be some evidence to suggest improved long-term outcomes (based on modified Mayo wrist score) for articular fractures treated with arthroscopic-assisted reductions compared to fluoroscopy alone
- There are no long-term differences in DASH scores between AFA reduction of intra-articular distal radius fractures
- There is evidence to suggest that volar locked plating of distal radius fractures improves ROM and outcome scores in the short term (<3 months)
- There are no long-term differences in DASH scores between volar locking plates and either percutaneous or external fixation
- While there appear to be some early advantages to a structured therapy program, in patients with uncomplicated distal radius fractures, there are no significant long-term differences between patients receiving instruction in home exercises and formal physiotherapy
- Early ROM (2 weeks) does not offer any long-term advantage compared to range of motion initiated at 6 weeks following volar plating of distal radius fractures

Conclusions

There are several unsolved questions regarding the effectiveness of the different available treatment methods for distal radius fractures. The current literature has several weaknesses including a paucity of large RCTs. Further research is needed before any high-quality treatment recommendations can be made.

References

1. O'Neill TW, Cooper C, Finn JD, et al. Incidence of distal forearm fracture in British men and women. Osteoporos Int 2001;12(7):555–8.
2. van Staa TP, Dennison EM, Leufkens HG, Cooper C. Epidemiology of fractures in England and Wales. Bone 2001;29(6).517–22.
3. Sarmiento A, Pratt GW, Berry NC, Sinclair WF. Colles' fractures. Functional bracing in supination. J Bone Joint Surg Am 1975;57(3):311–17.
4. Bunger C, Solund K, Rasmussen P. Early results after Colles' fracture: functional bracing in supination vs dorsal plaster immobilization. Arch Orthop Trauma Surg 1984;103(4):251–6.
5. Wahlstrom O. Treatment of Colles' fracture. A prospective comparison of three different positions of immobilization. Acta Orthop Scand 1982;53(2):225–8.
6. Pool C. Colles's fracture. A prospective study of treatment. J Bone Joint Surg Br 1973;55(3):540–4.
7. Bong MR, Egol KA, Leibman M, Koval KJ. A comparison of immediate postreduction splinting constructs for controlling initial displacement of fractures of the distal radius: a prospective randomized study of long-arm versus short-arm splinting. J Hand Surg Am 2006;31(5):766–70.
8. Handoll HH, Vaghela MV, Madhok R. Percutaneous pinning for treating distal radial fractures in adults. Cochrane Database Syst Rev 2007;3:CD006080.
9. Azzopardi T, Ehrendorfer S, Coulton T, Abela M. Unstable extra-articular fractures of the distal radius: a prospective, randomised study of immobilisation in a cast versus supplementary percutaneous pinning. J Bone Joint Surg Br 2005;87(6):837–40.
10. Gupta R, Raheja A, Modi U. Colles' fracture: management by percutaneous crossed-pin fixation versus plaster of Paris cast immobilization. Orthopedics 1999;22(7):680–2.
11. Rodriguez-Merchan EC. Plaster cast versus percutaneous pin fixation for comminuted fractures of the distal radius in patients between 46 and 65 years of age. J Orthop Trauma 1997;11(3):212–17.
12. Shankar NS, Craxford AD. Comminuted Colles' fractures: a prospective trial of management. J R Coll Surg Edinb 1992;37(3):199–202.
13. Stoffelen DV, Broos PL. Closed reduction versus Kapandji-pinning for extra-articular distal radial fractures. J Hand Surg Br 1999;24(1):89–91.
14. Chang HC, Tay SC, Chan BK, Low CO. Conservative treatment of redisplaced Colles' fractures in elderly patients older than 60 years old—anatomical and functional outcome. Hand Surg 2001;6(2):137–44.
15. Young BT, Rayan GM. Outcome following non-operative treatment of displaced distal radius fractures in low-demand patients older than 60 years. J Hand Surg Am 2000;25(1):19–28.
16. Beumer A, McQueen MM. Fractures of the distal radius in low-demand elderly patients—closed reduction of no value in 53 of 60 wrists. Acta Orthop Scand 2003;74(1):98–100.
17. Anzarut A, Johnson JA, Rowe BH, Lambert RG, Blitz S, Majumdar SR. Radiologic and patient-reported functional outcomes in an elderly cohort with conservatively treated distal radius fractures. J Hand Surg Am 2004;29(6):1121–7.
18. Grewal R, MacDermid JC. The risk of adverse outcomes in extra-articular distal radius fractures is increased with malalignment in patients of all ages but mitigated in older patients. J Hand Surg Am 2007;32(7):962–70.

19. Synn AJ, Makhni EC, Makhni MC, Rozental TD, Day CS. Distal radius fractures in older patients: is anatomic reduction necessary? Clin Orthop Relat Res 2009;467(6):1612–20.

20. Kelly AJ, Warwick D, Crichlow TP, Bannister GC. Is manipulation of moderately displaced Colles' fracture worthwhile? A prospective randomized trial. Injury 1997;28(4):283–7.

21. Roumen RM, Hesp WL, Bruggink ED. Unstable Colles' fractures in elderly patients. A randomised trial of external fixation for redisplacement. J Bone Joint Surg Br 1991;73(2):307–11.

22. Arora R, Gabl M, Gschwentner M, Deml C, Krappinger D, Lutz M. A comparative study of clinical and radiologic outcomes of unstable Colles type distal radius fractures in patients older than 70 years: nonoperative treatment versus volar locking plating. J Orthop Trauma 2009;23(4):237–42.

23. Zenke Y, Sakai A, Oshige T, Moritani S, Nakamura T. The effect of an associated ulnar styloid fracture on the outcome after fixation of a fracture of the distal radius. J Bone Joint Surg Br 2009;91(1):102–7.

24. af Ekenstam F, Jakobsson OP, Wadin K. Repair of the triangular ligament in Colles' fracture. No effect in a prospective randomized study. Acta Orthop Scand 1989;60(4):393–6.

25. Souer JS, Ring D, Matschke S, Audige L, Marent-Huber M, Jupiter JB. Effect of an unrepaired fracture of the ulnar styloid base on outcome after plate-and-screw fixation of a distal radial fracture. J Bone Joint Surg Am 2009;91(4):830–8.

26. Atroshi I, Brogren E, Larsson GU, Kloow J, Hofer M, Berggren AM. Wrist-bridging versus non-bridging external fixation for displaced distal radius fractures: a randomized assessor-blind clinical trial of 38 patients followed for 1 year. Acta Orthop 2006;77(3):445–53.

27. Krishnan J, Wigg AE, Walker RW, Slavotinek J. Intra-articular fractures of the distal radius: a prospective randomised controlled trial comparing static bridging and dynamic non-bridging external fixation. J Hand Surg Br 2003;28(5):417–21.

28. Krukhaug Y, Ugland S, Lie SA, Hove LM. External fixation of fractures of the distal radius: a randomized comparison of the Hoffman compact II non-bridging fixator and the Dynawrist fixator in 75 patients followed for 1 year. Acta Orthop 2009;80(1):104–8.

29. McQueen MM. Redisplaced unstable fractures of the distal radius. A randomised, prospective study of bridging versus non-bridging external fixation. J Bone Joint Surg Br 1998;80(4):665–9.

30. Sommerkamp TG, Seeman M, Silliman J, et al. Dynamic external fixation of unstable fractures of the distal part of the radius. A prospective, randomized comparison with static external fixation. J Bone Joint Surg Am 1994;76(8):1149–61.

31. Ruch DS, Vallee J, Poehling GG, Smith BP, Kuzma GR. Arthroscopic reduction versus fluoroscopic reduction in the management of intra-articular distal radius fractures. Arthroscopy 2004;20(3):225–30.

32. Varitimidis SE, Basdekis GK, Dailiana ZH, Hantes ME, Bargiotas K, Malizos K. Treatment of intra-articular fractures of the distal radius: fluoroscopic or arthroscopic reduction? J Bone Joint Surg Br 2008;90(6):778–85.

33. Koval KJ, Harrast JJ, Anglen JO, Weinstein JN. Fractures of the distal part of the radius. The evolution of practice over time. Where's the evidence? J Bone Joint Surg Am 2008;90(9):1855–61.

34. Shyamalan G, Theokli C, Pearse Y, Tennent D. Volar locking plates versus Kirschner wires for distal radial fractures—a cost analysis study. Injury 2009;40(12):1279–81.

35. Egol K, Walsh M, Tejwani N, McLaurin T, Wynn C, Paksima N. Bridging external fixation and supplementary Kirschner-wire fixation versus volar locked plating for unstable fractures of the distal radius: a randomised, prospective trial. J Bone Joint Surg Br 2008;90(9):1214–21.

36. Rozental TD, Blazar PE, Franko OI, Chacko AT, Earp BE, Day CS. Functional outcomes for unstable distal radial fractures treated with open reduction and internal fixation or closed reduction and percutaneous fixation. A prospective randomized trial. J Bone Joint Surg Am 2009;91(8):1837–46.

37. Wei DH, Raizman NM, Bottino CJ, Jobin CM, Strauch RJ, Rosenwasser MP. Unstable distal radial fractures treated with external fixation, a radial column plate, or a volar plate. A prospective randomized trial. J Bone Joint Surg Am 2009;91(7):1568–77.

38. Downing ND, Karantana A. A revolution in the management of fractures of the distal radius? J Bone Joint Surg Br 2008;90(10):1271–5.

39. Lozano-Calderon SA, Souer S, Mudgal C, Jupiter JB, Ring D. Wrist mobilization following volar plate fixation of fractures of the distal part of the radius. J Bone Joint Surg Am 2008;90(6):1297–304.

40. Kay S, McMahon M, Stiller K. An advice and exercise program has some benefits over natural recovery after distal radius fracture: a randomised trial. Aust J Physiother 2008;54(4):253–9.

41. Krischak GD, Krasteva A, Schneider F, Gulkin D, Gebhard F, Kramer M. Physiotherapy after volar plating of wrist fractures is effective using a home exercise program. Arch Phys Med Rehabil 2009;90(4):537–44.

42. Wakefield AE, McQueen MM. The role of physiotherapy and clinical predictors of outcome after fracture of the distal radius. J Bone Joint Surg Br 2000;82(7):972–6.

43. Maciel JS, Taylor NF, McIlveen C. A randomised clinical trial of activity-focussed physiotherapy on patients with distal radius fractures. Arch Orthop Trauma Surg 2005;125(8):515–20.

108 Prognosis: Pain and Disability After Distal Radius Fracture

Joy C. MacDermid[1,2] *and Ruby Grewal*[2]

[1]McMaster University, Hamilton, ON, Canada
[2]University of Western Ontario, London, ON, Canada

Case scenario

A 52 year-old woman is seen in the Emergency Department of your hospital and is referred to your clinic with a diagnosis of distal radius fracture (DRF). The fracture has been reduced and she was placed in a cast. In your initial patient interview, she asks "What can I expect from my fracture healing and recovery?"

Relevant anatomy

The anatomy of the distal radius is reviewed in Chapter 107. Detailed information is available online in free open access resources including *Grey's Anatomy* (http://www.bartleby.com/107/53.html).

Importance of the problem

This chapter addresses how to respond to patients' questions using evidence about prognosis in patient-friendly terminology. Clinicians usually answer those questions based on their personal experience, which we know is biased.

Prognosis, or the ability to predict outcomes, is one of the most important functions performed by clinicians. Early accurate prognosis is critical for patients, their families, and other stakeholders to develop plans for managing the injury. Prognosis is integral to treatment planning, since treatment choices may be modified on the basis of prognosis and patient reactions and behaviors can be mediated by prognostic messages from care providers.

Prognostic factors are features or variables that are associated with an increased probability of having a specified outcome. Factors that are associated with a higher probability of a good outcome are considered *protective factors*, while those that are associated with a higher probability of an adverse outcome are considered *risk factors*. Prognostic factors can be associated with an outcome through a causal mechanism or confounded by relationship with another factor that is the actual mechanism for the relationship. For example, in DRF, malunion is a risk factor for adverse pain and disability outcomes;[1] older age (>65) is associated with a lessening of this risk,[1] which we assume is partially related to the "confounder" physical demands.

Case clarification

Two common subgroups of DRF are older people who fall from standing position (most common) or young individuals with higher-impact trauma or sports injury. There can be seasonal variation, with winter months having higher rates of slips on ice and snowboarding injuries and summer months having more sporting injuries, e.g., rollerblading. Most patients will be concerned about their recovery. Younger patients are concerned about return to work/sport, whereas older patients may be concerned about future fracture/health risks.

Current opinion

Most clinicians continue to believe that anatomic restoration is the key factor in restoring function after a wrist fracture. Many general and emergency physicians tend to assume that DRF is a minor injury. Clinical practice guidelines do not currently describe how to modify treatment based on prognostic factors.

Evidence-Based Orthopedics, First Edition. Edited by Mohit Bhandari.
© 2012 Blackwell Publishing Ltd. Published 2012 by Blackwell Publishing Ltd.

Finding the evidence

We adopted the strategy of using Clinical Queries within PubMed using the prognosis filter to identify appropriate studies.

- PubMed Clinical Queries (http://www.ncbi.nlm.nih.gov/sites/pubmedutils/clinical) search using keywords: (Distal Radius and Fracture) and the prognosis (narrow) filter. Using this filter optimizes the search strategy using previously validated informatics methods (actual search performed using the strategy is "(distal[All Fields] AND ("radius"[MeSH Terms] OR "radius"[All Fields])) AND ("fractures, bone"[MeSH Terms] OR ("fractures"[All Fields] AND "bone"[All Fields]) OR "bone fractures"[All Fields] OR "fracture"[All Fields])) AND Prognosis/Narrow[filter]"
- This approach retrieved 181 studies, many of which were not appropriate to the topic. Additional searches for DRF and specific queries such as smoking were used to answer the specific questions

Quality of the evidence

A level I prognostic study is a large cohort study with pre-identified potential predictors and minimum of 80% follow-up (http://www.cebm.net/index.aspx?o=1025). A level II study is a retrospective cohort design, e.g., from a previously established clinical database or clinical trial. Prognosis tends to be addressed in level IV (case series and poor-quality cohort studies) as a secondary analysis. We focused on the higher-quality studies attained.

Top thirteen questions

Questions from patients

1. Will my fracture heal?
2. Do you think my fracture will heal in the right position without further treatment?
3. What happens if my fracture does not heal in the correct position?
4. How long until my pain goes away?
5. Will I have permanent disability?
6. How much time should I take off work?
7. Will this happen to me again?
8. Does this mean I have osteoporosis?
9. Does it matter how active I am?
10. Does it matter if I smoke?
11. If I wear wrist guards, can I prevent this from happening again?

Questions from family

12. Mom seems afraid of falling. Is that normal? Should we worry about it?
13. Will this affect mom's longevity?

Question 1: Will my fracture heal?

No studies were identified that specifically address the risk of nonunion. Rates of nonunion are so low that only small numbers are reported as unusual findings.[2] Level IV evidence suggests that late treatment of these with bone grafting can result in union, but persistent disability.[2]

Recommended response

- There are no good studies on this topic, but nonunion is rarely reported in the literature; it is an unexpected finding and is usually associated with an unusual incident or medical issue.

Question 2: Do you think my fracture will heal in the right position without further treatment?

In a level II study of 80 patients with DRF treated conservatively, a variety of radiological parameters were evaluated as potential predictors in loss of reduction at 1 or 6 weeks.[3] Acceptable reduction was defined as dorsal tilt more than 15°, volar tilt more than 20°, radial shortening less than 4 mm, and radial inclination less than 10°. Secondary shortening of 4 mm or more was seen in 18% of fractures with no initial shortening, in 41% with moderate shortening (1–4 mm), and in 52% with severe initial shortening (>4 mm). Severity of initial prereduction radial shortening predicted unacceptable reduction at 6 weeks. There was a progressive collapse in 54% of fractures with radial shortening and 60% of fractures with dorsal angulation. Initial dorsal angulation was predictive of late failure, but not early failure, whereas radial shortening reliably predicted both.[3]

Leone et al.,[4] studying a cohort of 71 patients with extra-articular DRF (50 dorsally displaced, 21 undisplaced), also found that the degree of initial radial shortening and volar tilt (p < 0.05) were predictive of early instability with dorsal comminution also playing a role (p = 0.06). Radial shortening, dorsal tilt, radial inclincation, and age played a role in predicting late failure, with one third of undisplaced fractures in patients over 65 years of age progressing to malalignment.

Recommended response

- The reason we need to do repeated imaging of your wrist is to determine if your bone fragments slip from their current acceptable position. We know that about half of the fractures that show early signs of slippage will continue to slip up to 6 weeks, and if this occurs we may reconsider whether a cast is sufficient treatment for you. We measure something called shortening to help us determine this. Even if you have no signs of shortening now there is about a 20% possibility of it occurring later. For people with shortening, about half will lose the alignment of their bone fragments.

Question 3: What happens if my fracture does not heal in the correct position?

The importance of anatomic restoration is controversial. An increasing trend to use open reduction and internal fixation (ORIF),[5] in particular volar plating, is based on the premise that better reduction results in better outcomes.

A level I cohort study of 216 patients with extra-articular DRF investigated whether unacceptable reduction (dorsal angulation >10°, radial inclination <15°, radial shortening >3 mm of ulnar positive variance) found that patients with unacceptable radial shortening or inclination had more pain and disability (29 vs. 16/100; 46 vs. 16/100, respectively) in patients under 65 years of age. The relative risk (RR) of a poor functional outcome with unacceptable reduction varied across age cutoffs: 10 for patients aged 45 or less, 11 at age 50 or less, and decreasing thereafter to RR = 2 for patients over 75 years of age.[1]

A level I study of 79 consecutive DRF treated in a hand center found that after controlling for other variables, incongruity of at least 1 mm was associated with poorer outcomes.[6] In another hand center cohort of 120 DRF patients (60% AO type C), no postreduction variables were associated with pain and disability reported at 6 months (prereduction radial shortening was a contributor).[7]

In a consecutive cohort of 74 patients over the age of 50 managed nonoperatively, 71% had at least one unacceptable radiographic deformity. No radiographic index alone, or in combination, significantly correlated to any of the patient self-report outcomes.[8]

In a level III study of 106 adults who had sustained a DRF before the age of 40, a long-term follow-up study was conducted at a mean follow-up of 38 years. There was evidence of post-traumatic osteoarthritis in 68% of patients with intra-articular fractures and a significant relationship between joint narrowing and extra-articular malunion (dorsal angulation and radial shortening). There was no relationship between patient-reported function and indices of malunion.[9]

Recommended response

• If you have what we consider unacceptable alignment of your bones after your fracture heals, then you are at higher risk of having problems with pain or difficulty using your hand. For some types of fractures, people who are less than 50 years of age are 10 times more likely to have problems if their fracture heals in an unacceptable position. However, if you are older and the fracture heals in an unacceptable position, the risk of functional problems is less—only twice instead of 10 times as likely. There is weak evidence suggesting that many people have post-traumatic arthritis on their radiograph when evaluated more than 20 years after their fracture. However, having problems on your radiograph either immediately after your fracture or in the long term has not been shown to predict long-term functional problems.

Question 4: How long until my pain goes away?

Two cohort studies were identified that assessed pain repeatedly over time intervals to address the recovery pattern. An inception cohort of 129 patients with DRF[10] evaluated self-reported function, and physical impairments (range of motion, grip strength and dexterity) at baseline, 2, 3, 6, and 12 months following DRF. This study reported that at a baseline fracture clinic visit (3–7 days postfracture), median pain at rest was 3/10 and 9/10 at its worst. At 2 months following fracture, patients reported their worst pain was 5/10; and by 3 months, the median response was no pain at rest and 3/10 at its worst.

Recommended response

• It is normal to have some pain while your fracture heals. Once the initial treatment of your fracture is complete, the most common amount of pain reported by patients is about 3/10 at rest. Patients find this increases to 9/10 with activity. Three months after the fracture, most patients have no pain at rest and rate their pain as 3/10 at worst.

Question 5: Will I have permanent disability?

In a cohort study of mixed DRF evaluated longitudinally until 12 months postfracture, 1% of patients reported very severe pain and disability, 4% severe, 3% moderate severe, 14% mild, 53% minimal, and 26% none based on classifications of their total pain and disability score (median total score 12/100).[10] In a level IV study, 16% of subjects reported moderate to very severe disability,[11] but there was potential for response bias because of a low response rate.

In a level I prognostic study of 120 consecutive DRF patients, the most influential predictor of pain and disability at 6 months was injury compensation. Patient education level and prereduction radial shortening also contributed to a total predictive ability of 25%. Wrist impairment was moderately correlated with patient-reported pain and disability (r = 0.50).[7] A level I prognostic study of 222 extra-articular fractures found that comorbidity, injury compensation, and education predicted 16% of pain and disability scores at 1 year.[12] A smaller level II study of patients with surgically managed volar plating found that at 1 year after surgery, age and income were significant predictors after controlling for fracture type.[6] Significant associations were found between pain medication usage for the wrist fracture and moderate to very severe residual pain (OR = 11). Moderate to very severe disability was associated with older age (OR = 6.5) and pain medication usage for the wrist fracture (OR = 4.8). Working was protective for disability (OR = 0.14).[11]

Recommended response

• Our best evidence suggests that the chances of you having severe residual problems are about 5%. About 80% of people have no or mild residual deficits. Your overall health and personal circumstances will affect this

Question 6: How much time will I need to take off work?

A level I prognostic study addressed time off work following a DRF in 227 patients who were working at the time of injury.[13] The median time off work was 8 weeks (interquartile range 1–14 weeks); 2.5% were off work more than 36 weeks; 21% lost no time from work. Time off work was related to the occupational requirements for hand use.

Recommended response

• It is possible that you do not need to take any time off work—on average, about 20% of people do not. If you are unable to do your job, the amount of time you take off depends on what you do at work. Half of people will take between 1 to 14 weeks off, the most common being about 8 weeks

Question 7: Will this happen to me again?

In a level I study of 2245 community-dwelling women and 1760 men aged 60 years or older followed for 16 years after their first fracture, RR of subsequent fracture in women was 2, and in men was 3.5. Within 10 years, 40–60% of surviving women and men experienced a subsequent fracture. In multivariate analyses, femoral neck bone mineral density, age, and smoking were predictors of subsequent fracture in women and femoral neck bone mineral density, physical activity, and calcium intake were predictors in men.[14]

Recommended response

• If you are over 60, then the answer is yes. The fact that you have had a wrist fracture doubles your chance if you are a woman and triples it if you are a man. There are number of factors other than this injury that also contribute to your risk of fracture. The strength of your bones, age, whether you smoke, diet and physical activity affect your risk

Question 8: Does this mean I have osteoporosis?

In a cohort study of 1800 DRF patients with a low-energy DRF,[15] the prevalence of patients in need of osteoporosis treatment according to existing guidelines (using T-score ≤-2.0 or ≤-2.5 SD) whose 10-year fracture risk using the WHO fracture risk assessment tool (FRAX®), the risk of hip fracture was 6% for men and 9% for women. Every second to third fracture patient met the present bone mineral density (BMD) criteria for osteoporosis treatment. Thus, all DRF patients 50 years of age or more should be referred to bone densitometry, and if indicated, offered medical treatment.

Recommended response

• I do not know if you have osteoporosis, but you are at an elevated risk. Based on the best evidence, it is recommended that everyone over 50 with a DRF have a bone test to answer this question. The test exposes you to very small amount of radiation and the likelihood that you need treatment for osteoporosis is about 1 in 3, so the test is worthwhile

Question 9: Does it matter how active I am?

No studies were identified that investigated the effect of physical activity on short-term healing or postfracture disability.

A level I cohort study had 152 men and 206 women aged 50, 60, 70, and 80 who were followed for 10 years and were tested for distal radius BMD, grip strength, balance, gait velocity, occupational and leisure-time activity, and self-reported fractures. The annual rate of bone loss was 0.6% per year less in individuals classified as active as compared to those who were inactive at both time points. Balance loss was also better preserved in active individuals, but no other differences were found.[16] In a cross-sectional population-based study, a subset of 407 women were analyzed demonstrating that four factors were independently associated with fractures: low lifetime habitual physical activity (OR = 4), diabetes (OR = 0.2), living alone (OR = 2), and calcaneum BUA (OR = 2).[16,17]

In a level II study of 97 male young athletes who were evaluated and retested in 5 years, BMD was higher than age-matched controls both for still-active and for retired athletes, although retired athletes lost more bone than those who continued sports activities. The same study reported on a second, older group of 400 former athletes and 800 controls 60 years of age and above. Fewer former athletes had fragility fractures than controls (2% vs. 4%) and DRFs (0.75% vs. 2.5%).[18]

Recommended response

• We are very sure that, on average, people who are more physically active have stronger bones, and fewer DRFs and other fractures. Both young and older people who stop being active gradually lose the protective effect

Question 10: Does it matter if I smoke?

In a cohort of consecutive DRFs, smoking was not predictive of pain and disability outcomes.[7] No studies that were identified evaluated the risk of delayed primary healing of DRF fracture associated with smoking. In a level IV study of 107 patients with acute fractures with bone loss and atrophic nonunions treated with bone grafts harvested from the forearm, femur, and tibia, healing occurred in 38/56 smokers compared with 49/56 nonsmokers. Eight (73%) of the 11 patients with graft failure had a significant smoking history.[19] Given the lack of evidence in DRF, a broader search was conducted including other primary. Four studies of mixed quality addressed the effect of smoking on tibial fractures or ulnar shortening; all concluded that smokers were at increased risk of nonunion and delayed union.[20–24]

Recommended response

• There is insufficient evidence to say how smoking will affect healing of a typical DRF. We do have consistent evidence from other types of fractures that smoking is associated with slower healing. If your fracture does not heal and you need a bone graft for your DRF, it is more likely to fail if you smoke

Question 11: If I wear wrist guards will this prevent me from getting another DRF in the future?

Rollerblading[25,26] and snowboarding[27] are sports that have demonstrated increasing prevalence of injury in young people,[28] and the most common site of injury for both sports is the wrist.[27,29] Wrist guards are suggested as a potential injury prevention.[30] Between 16 and 60% of rollerbladers wear wrist guards.[31–34] In a case-control study of 161 injured in-line skaters, failure to use wrist guards was associated with increased risk of wrist injury (OR = 10).[29]

A systematic review was located on the effects of wrist guards on wrist injury in snowboarding.[35] Six studies were identified and synthesized. The risk of wrist injury (RR = 0.23), wrist fracture (RR = 0.29), or wrist sprain (RR = 0.17) was significantly reduced with the use of wrist guards.[35] In a matched case-control study of 1,066 injured Canadian snowboarders who reported upper-extremity injuries and 970 snowboarders with non-upper-extremity injuries, the prevalence of wrist guard use among snowboarders with hand, wrist, or forearm injuries was 1.6%. Wrist guard use reduced the risk of hand, wrist, or forearm injury by 85% (adjusted OR = 0.15). However, the adjusted OR for elbow, upper arm, or shoulder injury was 2.4.[30]

Recommended response

• There is strong evidence that wrist guards reduce injuries from snowboarding and moderate evidence that wrist guards reduce injuries from in-line skating. Based on a number of studies, we know that for every 50 snowboarders who wear a wrist guard, one wrist injury will be averted.[35] There is weak evidence that snowboarders who wear wrist guards have higher rates of elbow and shoulder injury. A wrist injury is the most common injury in both in-line skating and snowboarding, and all studies suggest the incidents could be reduced by the use wrist guards

Question 12: Mom seems afraid of falling. Is that normal? Should we worry about it?

In a prospective cohort study of 52 individuals with a DRF (and 52 proximal humerus fracture), there was a large increase in fear of falling in the DRF patients; 6% had to give up housekeeping and 24% experienced at least two falls within the next 4 months.[36] In a population-based study of these fractures in Germany, including over 2,000 forearm fractures, patients reported no changes in living circumstances due to their fracture, but there was a trend for hip fractures to occur on average 10 years after a DRF.

Recommended response

• Limited studies on this topic indicate that in the short term, older men and women who have a DRF have a substantially increased fear of falling. Most people do not change their living circumstances because of a DRF. About a quarter of older patients who have had a DRF will experience two or more falls within 4 months. There is a higher rate of hip fractures that occurs about 10 years after DRF. Your mom may be afraid of falling and it is a legitimate concern. You may wish to have a fall risk assessment performed if she is concerned, or you notice that she seems unsteady or falls

Question 13: Will this affect mom's longevity?

In a case-control study of mortality as compared to the age–gender matched US norms in elderly patients (250 women, 65 men) with DRF, the cumulative estimated survival in the cohort at 7 years after DRF was 57% compared with an expected value of 71% for the US population.[37] Men had twice the mortality risk of women, and patients with comorbidity five times the risk.[37] In a population-based study of more than 15,000 fractures, DRF preceded hip fracture by approximately 10 years and was suggested as a signal event for risk reduction.[38]

Recommended response

• There is weak evidence that people who experience a DRF do not live as long as the average population expectancy for their age. The exact reasons for this are not clear, but we know that physical activity, falls, osteoporosis, future fractures, and other comorbid health conditions are contributing factors. Management of osteoporosis, other health problems, and fall prevention strategies can be used to reduce health risks

References

1. Grewal R, MacDermid JC. The risk of adverse outcomes in extra-articular distal radius fractures is increased with malalignment in patients of all ages but mitigated in older patients. J Hand Surg Am 2007;32:962–70.

2. Eglseder WA, Jr.,Elliott MJ. Nonunions of the distal radius. Am J Orthop (Belle Mead NJ) 2002;31:259–62.

3. Batra S, Debnath U, Kanvinde R. Can carpal malalignment predict early and late instability in nonoperatively managed distal radius fractures? Int Orthop 2008;32:685–91.

4. Leone J, Bhandari M, Adili A, McKenzie S, Moro JK, Dunlop RB. Predictors of early and late instability following conservative treatment of extra-articular distal radius fractures. Arch Orthop Trauma Surg 2004;124:38–41.

5. Nazar MA, Mansingh R, Bassi RS, Waseem M. Is there a consensus in the management of distal radial fractures? Open Orthop J 2009;3:96–9.

6. Chung KC, Kotsis SV, Kim HM. Predictors of functional outcomes after surgical treatment of distal radius fractures. J Hand Surg Am 2007;32:76–83.

7. MacDermid JC, Donner A, Richards RS, Roth JH. Patient versus injury factors as predictors of pain and disability six months after a distal radius fracture. J Clin Epidemiol 2002;55:849–54.

8. Arora R, Gabl M, Gschwentner M, Deml C, Krappinger D, Lutz M. A comparative study of clinical and radiologic outcomes of unstable colles type distal radius fractures in patients older than 70 years: nonoperative treatment versus volar locking plating. J Orthop Trauma 2009;23:237–42.

9. Forward DP, Davis TR, Sithole JS. Do young patients with malunited fractures of the distal radius inevitably develop symptomatic post-traumatic osteoarthritis? J Bone Joint Surg Br 2008;90:629–37.

10. MacDermid JC, Roth JH, Richards RS. Pain and disability reported in the year following a distal radius fracture: a cohort study. BMC Musculoskelet Disord 2003;4:24.

11. Moore CM,Leonardi-Bee J. The prevalence of pain and disability one year post fracture of the distal radius in a UK population: a cross sectional survey. BMC Musculoskelet Disord 2008; 9;129.

12. Grewal R, MacDermid JC, Pope J, Chesworth BM. Baseline predictors of pain and disability one year following extra-articular distal radius fractures. Hand (NY) 2007;2:104–11.

13. MacDermid JC, Roth JH, McMurtry R. Predictors of time lost from work following a distal radius fracture. J Occup Rehabil 2007;17:47–62.

14. Center JR, Bliuc D, Nguyen TV, Eisman JA. Risk of subsequent fracture after low-trauma fracture in men and women. JAMA 2007;297:387–94.

15. Oyen J, Gjesdal CG, Brudvik C, et al. Low-energy distal radius fractures in middle-aged and elderly men and women-the burden of osteoporosis and fracture risk: a study of 1794 consecutive patients. Osteoporos Int 2010;21(7):1257–67.

16. Daly RM, Ahlborg HG, Ringsberg K, Gardsell P, Sernbo I, Karlsson MK. Association between changes in habitual physical activity and changes in bone density, muscle strength, and functional performance in elderly men and women. J Am Geriatr Soc 2008;56:2252–60.

17. Korpelainen R, Korpelainen J, Heikkinen J, Vaananen K, Keinanen-Kiukaanniemi S. Lifelong risk factors for osteoporosis and fractures in elderly women with low body mass index—a population-based study. Bone 32006;9:385–91.

18. Nordstrom A, Karlsson C, Nyquist F, Olsson T, Nordstrom P, Karlsson M. Bone loss and fracture risk after reduced physical activity. J Bone Miner Res 2005;20:202–7.

19. Ziran BH, Hendi P, Smith WR, Westerheide K, Agudelo JF. Osseous healing with a composite of allograft and demineralized bone matrix: adverse effects of smoking. Am J Orthop (Belle Mead NJ) 2007; 36:207–9.

20. Castillo RC, Bosse MJ, MacKenzie EJ, Patterson BM. Impact of smoking on fracture healing and risk of complications in limb-threatening open tibia fractures. J Orthop Trauma 2005;19:151–7.

21. Harvey EJ, Agel J, Selznick HS, Chapman JR, Henley MB. Deleterious effect of smoking on healing of open tibia-shaft fractures. Am J Orthop (Belle Mead NJ) 2002;31:518–21.

22. Chen F, Osterman AL, Mahony K. Smoking and bony union after ulna-shortening osteotomy. Am J Orthop (Belle Mead NJ) 2001;30:486–9.

23. Schmitz MA, Finnegan M, Natarajan R, Champine J. Effect of smoking on tibial shaft fracture healing. Clin Orthop Relat Res 1999;365:184–200.

24. Kyro A, Usenius JP, Aarnio M, Kunnamo I, Avikainen V. Are smokers a risk group for delayed healing of tibial shaft fractures? Ann Chir Gynaecol 1993;82:254–62.

25. Knox CL, Comstock RD, McGeehan J, Smith GA. Differences in the risk associated with head injury for pediatric ice skaters, roller skaters, and in-line skaters. Pediatrics 2006;118:549–54.

26. Schieber RA,Branche-Dorsey CM. In-line skating injuries. Epidemiology and recommendations for prevention. Sports Med 1995;19:427–32.

27. Made C,Elmqvist LG. A 10-year study of snowboard injuries in Lapland Sweden. Scand J Med Sci Sports 2004;14:128–33.

28. Idzikowski JR, Janes PC, Abbott PJ. Upper extremity snowboarding injuries. Ten-year results from the Colorado snowboard injury survey. Am J Sports Med 2000;28:825–32.

29. Schieber RA, Branche-Dorsey CM, Ryan GW, Rutherford GW, Jr., Stevens JA, O'Neil J. Risk factors for injuries from in-line skating and the effectiveness of safety gear. N Engl J Med 1996;335:1630–5.

30. Hagel B, Pless IB, Goulet C. The effect of wrist guard use on upper-extremity injuries in snowboarders. Am J Epidemiol 2005;162:149–56.

31. Beirness DJ, Foss RD, Desmond KJ. Use of protective equipment by in-line skaters: an observational study. Inj Prev 2001;7:51–5.

32. Osberg JS,Stiles SC. Safety behavior of in-line skaters. Inj Prev 2000;6:229–31.

33. Warda L, Harlos S, Klassen TP, Moffatt ME, Buchan N, Koop VL. An observational study of protective equipment use among in-line skaters. Inj Prev 1998;4:198–202.

34. Young CC, Seth A, Mark DH. In-line skating: use of protective equipment, falling patterns, and injuries. Clin J Sport Med 1998;8:111–14.

35. Russell K, Hagel B, Francescutti LH. The effect of wrist guards on wrist and arm injuries among snowboarders: a systematic review. Clin J Sport Med 2007;17:145–50.

36. Einsiedel T, Becker C, Stengel D, et al. [Do injuries of the upper extremity in geriatric patients end up in helplessness? A prospective study for the outcome of distal radius and proximal humerus fractures in individuals over 65]. Z Gerontol Geriatr 2006;39:451–61.

37. Rozental TD, Branas CC, Bozentka DJ, Beredjiklian PK. Survival among elderly patients after fractures of the distal radius. J Hand Surg Am 2002;27:948–52.

38. Endres HG, Dasch B, Lungenhausen M, et al. Patients with femoral or distal forearm fracture in Germany: a prospective observational study on health care situation and outcome. BMC Public Health 2006;6:87.

109 Reconstruction of Malunited Distal Radius Fracture

James T. Monica and David Ring

Massachusetts General Hospital and Harvard Medical School, Boston, MA, USA

Case scenario

A 45 year old man sustained a distal radius fracture 3 months ago. He complains of visible deformity, stiffness, ulnar-sided pain that is worse with activity, and weakness. On exam there is a dorsal prominence deformity of the distal radius. Active and passive supination and flexion are limited to 30° and 45° respectively. Radiographs show an extra-articular malunion with 30° dorsal tilt of the articular surface on the lateral view and 5mm ulnar positive variance.

Relevant anatomy

The articular surface of the distal radius forms a platform that supports the carpus. The radiocarpal articular surface is divided into separate facets for the scaphoid and the lunate separated by a sagittal ridge. The sigmoid notch has a larger radius of curvature than the ulnar head, and motion at this joint consists of translation in addition to rotation. The triangular fibrocartilage complex spans from the distal end of the radius to the base of the ulnar styloid and functions to cushion the ulnar–carpal joint and stabilize the distal radioulnar joint (DRUJ).

The distal radius articular surface angles ulnarward an average of 23° as measured on a posteroanterior radiograph.[1] The average volar inclination of the distal radius articular surface on the lateral view is 11°. Ulnar variance is defined as the length between the distal limit of the head of the ulna and the radial articular surface at the lunate facet, as measured on a posteroanterior film with the forearm in neutral rotation.

The most common deformity following a dorsal bending fracture includes loss of the volar tilt of the articular surface in the sagittal plane, loss of ulnar inclination in the frontal plane, ulnar positive variance, and supination of the distal fragment with respect to the proximal diaphysis.[2]

Importance of the problem

On the basis of actuarial risk calculations from Medicare data, the risk of a white woman in the United States sustaining a distal forearm fracture was estimated to be 6% by the age of 80 years and 9% by the age of 90 years.[3] Fractures of the distal radius often heal with malalignment, but symptoms vary substantially. Deformity of the distal radius can hinder wrist and forearm motion and can contribute to postraumatic arthritis, carpal malalignment, ulnocarpal impaction, and instability or incongruity of the DRUJ.[4–10] On the other hand, the relationship between distal radius deformity and stiffness or pain is unpredictable and incompletely understood.

Top ten questions

Diagnosis

1. What are the most common complaints referable to malalignment of the distal radius?
2. What amount of radiographic malalignment correlates with dysfunction?

Therapy

3. What can be done besides surgery?
4. Is there a consequence to leaving malalignment untreated?
5. Early vs. delayed surgery?
6. Structural vs. nonstructural bone graft?
7. Volar vs. dorsal approach?

Evidence-Based Orthopedics, First Edition. Edited by Mohit Bhandari.
© 2012 Blackwell Publishing Ltd. Published 2012 by Blackwell Publishing Ltd.

8. How is management of intra-articular malunions different from that of extra-articular malunions?

Prognosis

9. What are the outcomes of malunion?
10. What are the complications of surgical correction of distal radius malunions?

Question 1: What are the most common complaints referable to malalignment of the distal radius?

Question 2: What amount of radiographic malalignment correlates with dysfunction?

Case clarification

The patient complains of ulnar-sided wrist pain. Physical examination reveals dorsal wrist deformity, decreased flexion, and supination with no instability. Radiographs reveal an extra-articular, 30° dorsally angulated distal radius malunion with 6 mm of radial shortening.

Relevance

The diagnosis of malunion implies that a patient's symptoms can be directly related to malalignment of the distal radius. Operative treatment is based on the ability to reduce the symptoms by improving alignment.

There have been several recommendations regarding acceptable alignments of distal radius fractures but these seem relatively arbitrary.

Current opinion

Correlation of symptoms with malalignment is not always straightforward. Many patients, particularly low-demand elderly individuals, function very well with malalignment of the distal radius. Symptoms such as ulnar-sided wrist pain can improve for more than a year after fracture of the distal radius. Ongoing pain can be unsettling, and patient and surgeon might overinterpret the correlation between malalignment and symptoms.

Finding the evidence

Question 1
• PubMed (www.ncbi.nlm.nih.gov/pubmed/) sensitivity search using keywords: "distal radius malunion" AND "pain" AND "symptoms"

Question 2
• PubMed (www.ncbi.nlm.nih.gov/pubmed/) sensitivity search using keywords: "distal radius" AND "radiographic parameters" AND "disability"

Quality of the evidence

Question 1
• Level IV: 7 studies

Question 2
• Level II: 2 studies
• Level IV: 5 studies

Findings

The evidence regarding symptoms ascribed to malalignment of the distal radius are mostly level IV. Patients may present with complaints of pain, stiffness, instability, weakness, numbness and tingling, or aesthetic concerns.[11,12] Dorsal angulation of greater than 15° and shortening of 2 mm are felt to affect forearm motion and cause pain.[13,14] Leung and others reviewed 111 patients with intra-articular distal radius fractures and reported that those patients with axial compression (>2 mm) and dorsal angulation (>15°) had worse functional outcome as measured by the modified Green and O'Brien scoring systems, and diminished range of motion (ROM).[13]

Incongruity of the DRUJ[15] and positive ulnar variance[16] have been associated with ulnar-sided wrist pain. The extent of fracture comminution and articular involvement correlates with loss of motion.[17]

At an average of 4 years following nonoperative management of distal radius fractures, McQueen and Caspers noted 17 patients with a good radiological result and 13 who were considered to have malunion.[18] The displaced group had dorsal angulation of 12–34° and more than 2 mm of radial shift. Functionally the displaced group performed significantly worse than the undisplaced group. Functional tests included grip strength, grip endurance, Jebsen test,[19] ROM, activities of daily living, pain assessment, and cosmetic assessment. They concluded that malunion of a Colles' fracture results in a weak, deformed, stiff, and probably painful wrist.

Grewal and MacDermid[20] defined malunion as dorsal angulation greater than 10°, radial inclination less than 15°, or more than 2 mm of ulnar positive variance. Malunion did not affect the Patient-Rated Wrist Evaluation (PRWE) (p = 0.22) or the Disabilities of Arm, Shoulder and Hand (DASH) questionnaire (p = 0.39) 1 year after fracture in patients aged 65 or older. In contrast, both PRWE (p = 0.001) and DASH (p = 0.001) were significantly higher (i.e., more pain and disability) in patients with malunion who were younger than 65.

Mackenney and associates identified predictors of distal radius fracture instability that were prognostic of radiographic outcome.[21] Radiographic displacement was defined as a dorsal (apex volar) tilt of more than 10° (normal is 15° apex dorsal; therefore, 15° of dorsal angulation) and/or ulnar variance of more than 3 mm. By this definition, 744 of 1,296 displaced fractures (60%) became malunited. Most of these radiographic malunions were acceptable to patients, and only a small percentage of patients with radiographic malunion were considered for osteotomy.

Kelly et al. reported no detectable difference in radiologic or functional outcomes 3 months after distal radius fracture between elderly patients who received a closed reduction and those who did not. They concluded that up to 30° of dorsal angulation and 5 mm of radial shortening can be accepted without requiring further manipulation.[22]

Recommendations
- Acceptable parameters for distal radius displacement are age dependent [overall quality: low]
- Patients under 65 years of age are more likely to have pain or stiffness or diminished grip strength with dorsal angulation 10° or more, radial inclination 15° or less, or ulnar positive variance 3 mm or more [overall quality: low]
- Dorsal angulation of the distal radius can reduce wrist flexion and supination [overall quality: low]

Question 3: What can be done besides surgery?

Case clarification
Our patient wants to try everything possible before considering surgery.

Relevance
The role of surgery can be better defined by an understanding of the value of nonoperative treatments.

Current opinion
Pain diminishes with time for over a year after injury, and motion can improve with exercises.

Finding the evidence
- PubMed (www.ncbi.nlm.nih.gov/pubmed/): sensitivity search using keywords: "distal radius malunion"

Quality of the evidence
- Level V

Findings
There is no data on nonoperative treatment for distal radius malunited fractures. When the radiographic deformity is less than 20° dorsal angulation of the articular surface on the lateral radiograph and less than 3 mm of shortening by ulnar variance, most authorities recommended a period of observation and adaptation before considering an osteotomy.[23] Comfort, motion and strength can improve for over a year. Exercises for motion and strength may help.

Recommendation
- It may be worthwhile doing stretching exercises and being patient for pain to resolve when malalignment is less

than 20° dorsal angulation or 3 mm ulnar positive variance [overall quality: low]

Question 4: Is there a consequence to leaving malalignment untreated?

Case clarification
The patient states that his pain and stiffness are not interfering with his daily activities and asks if his wrist will deteriorate without surgery.

Relevance
Is there ever a situation where surgeons should encourage patients with malalignment to have surgery?

Current opinion
Surgeon opinion on this seems quite variable.

Finding the evidence
- PubMed (www.ncbi.nlm.nih.gov/pubmed/) sensitivity search using keywords: "distal radius malunion" AND "indications"

Quality of the evidence
- Level IV and V

Findings
Level IV studies have reported radiographic indications for operative intervention that include an articular step-off greater than 2 mm, carpal instability, more than 20–30° of dorsal angulation, and an incongruent DRUJ.[24] Dysfunction may result from symptomatic ulnocarpal impaction syndrome, DRUJ arthrosis, grip weakness, and articular incongruity. Malalignment does not always result in dysfunction.

While anatomic reduction is the principal aim of treatment, imperfect reduction of these fractures may not result in symptomatic arthritis in the long term. Forward and others reviewed 106 adults who had sustained a fracture of the distal radius between 1960 and 1968 and who were below the age of 40 years at the time of injury. They carried out a clinical and radiological assessment at a mean follow-up of 38 years (range 33–42). No patient had required a salvage procedure. While there was radiological evidence of post-traumatic osteoarthritis after an intra-articular fracture in 68% of patients (27 of 40), the disabilities of the DASH scores were not different from population norms, and function, as assessed by the Patient Evaluation Measure, was impaired by less than 10%.[25]

A study by Cooney and others analyzed 565 Colles' fractures and found that radioulnar arthrosis (4.8%) was more common than radiocarpal arthrosis (1.8%).[26]

Extra-articular deformity of the distal radius results in a compensatory midcarpal malalignment.[8] There are no data regarding the symptoms or consequences (e.g., midcarpal arthritis) of this malalignment. Midcarpal arthrosis is rarely observed in association with distal radius malunion. The midcarpal malalignment usually corrects after osteotomy of the distal radius.[8,27,28]

Recommendation

• For a 45 year old patient with minimal symptoms and a dorsally displaced distal radius malunion, the following radiographic features warrant consideration of osteotomy: dorsal angulation greater than 20°, displaced fractures with carpal malalignment (>15° of dorsal angulation of the lunate on the lateral view), incongruity of the DRUJ, greater than 5 mm ulnar positive variance, or unacceptable cosmetic deformity[29] [overall quality: low]

Question 5: Early vs. delayed surgery?

Case clarification

The patient asks if it better to intervene as soon as malalignment is diagnosed.

Relevance

Surgery to correct malalignment may be easier when the original fracture line can be identified.

Current opinion

The traditional approach was to wait and operate on a mature nonunion, but young, active individuals with substantial malalignment are increasingly offered early surgery.

Finding the evidence

• PubMed (www.ncbi.nlm.nih.gov/pubmed/): sensitivity search using keywords: "distal radius," "malunited," "early," "late"

Quality of the evidence

Level IV
• 2 studies

Findings

Jupiter and Ring[30] compared 10 early (average 8 weeks after injury) and 10 late (average 40 weeks after injury) osteotomies in patients with a dorsal tilt of more than 20°, articular incongruity of more than 2 mm, increased lunate dorsal tilt of greater than 15° on the lateral view compared to the contralateral wrist, subluxation of the radiocarpal joint, or complete incongruity of the DRUJ and found few differences. Their preference for early surgery was based primarily on speculative advantages and technical facility.

Recommendation

• Early surgery is technically easier and the rationale that a short time with malalignment would create fewer prob-

lems is appealing, but there is insufficient evidence to prove an advantage for early surgery [overall quality: low]

Question 6: Structural vs. nonstructural bone graft?

Relevance

Before the advent of plates with locking screws, structural corticocancellous bone graft from the iliac crest was felt to be necessary to help carry mechanical loads. Structural grafts were difficult to handle and often did not fit ideally even with careful preoperative planning.

Current opinion

When a locking plate is used, a nonstructural bone graft can be used.

Finding the evidence

• PubMed (www.ncbi.nlm.nih.gov/pubmed/): sensitivity search using keywords: "distal radius," "malunited," "structural bone graft"

Quality of the evidence

Level III
• 1 study

Findings

Ring and others compared two matched cohorts of patients with dorsal malunions treated with opening wedge osteotomy, dorsal locking plate stabilization, and either structural or nonstructural cancellous graft. They reported comparable functional and radiographic results between the two groups.[31]

A case series by Nagy and others investigated the ability of precise preoperative planning of the size and shape of the corticocancellous bone graft to restore alignment of the radius to within 5° angular deformity and 2 mm ulnar variance as compared with the opposite, uninjured wrist. Only 6 of 15 patients (40%) satisfied these criteria. They concluded that distal radius osteotomy using a precisely planned and measured interpositional corticocancellous graft does not restore distal radius alignment in most patients, and that failure to restore length is associated with continued pain and stiffness.[32]

Several different graft substitutes have been used in opening wedge osteotomies. Carbonated hydroxyapatite and calcium phosphate have been reported as substitutes for corrective distal radius osteotomy with good results.[33,34] Abramo and colleagues used Norian SRS as a bone substitute with plate fixation in 25 consecutive patients after osteotomy of a dorsal distal radius malunion. At 1 year all but one osteotomy healed and radiographic correction achieved postoperatively was consistent over 1 year. Patients demonstrated increased grip strength and ROM and the procedure was performed on an outpatient basis.[35]

Recommendation

• Use of a nonstructural, cancellous only bone graft is appealing in its relative simplicity and seems safe and effective when used in conjunction with locking plates, but this is based on very limited data. Other types of graft substitutes might be suitable, but more data is needed [overall quality: low]

Question 7: Volar vs. dorsal approach?

Relevance

Locking plates and the extended FCR exposure have made it possible to address dorsally angulated malunions via a volar approach.

Current opinion

The dorsal approach is more familiar and intuitive, but the volar approach may have some technical advantages.

Finding the evidence

• PubMed (www.ncbi.nlm.nih.gov/pubmed/): sensitivity search using keywords: "distal radius," "malunion," "approach"

Quality of the evidence

Level IV

• 18 studies

Level V

• 6 studies

Findings

There are 16 case series of various techniques and no comparative studies. No advantages of one technique over another can be gleaned from the current literature.

Recommendation

• Either approach is acceptable in the 45 year old patient with a dorsally displaced distal radius malunion. No study has been performed comparing results from the dorsal vs. volar approach [overall quality: low]

Question 8: How does management of intra-articular malunions differ from that of extra-articular malunions?

Case clarification

CT scan reveals an intra-articular step-off of more than 2 mm in the lunate facet. How does the intra-articular involvement affect management?

Relevance

There may be greater consequences of intra-articular malunion, but osteotomy can be more technically difficult and is sometimes impossible.

Current opinion

A subset of straightforward articular malunions may be amenable to osteotomy.

Finding the evidence

• PubMed (www.ncbi.nlm.nih.gov/pubmed/): sensitivity search using keywords: "intra-articular," "distal radius," "malunion"

Quality of the evidence

Level IV

• 4 studies

Level V

• 3 studies

Findings

Despite various reports stating that articular incongruity is consistently identified as an important predictor of an adverse functional outcome in distal radius fractures,[36–38] there have been relatively few articles describing intra-articular osteotomy.[30,39–41] The relative reluctance to address intra-articular malunion may be due to several factors, including limited surgical access, difficulty achieving secure fixation of small articular fracture fragments, concern regarding the ability to recreate the articular fracture without causing additional articular damage, and concern about compromising the blood supply to the osteotomized fragment, which can lead to osteonecrosis with resultant collapse, failure to heal, and arthrosis.[39] The role of osteotomy of an intra-articular distal radius malunion is limited by the type of fracture and the timing of presentation. Intra-articular malunions must have relatively simple geometric patterns to permit reconstruction via intra-articular osteotomy.[23] Intra-articular osteotomy should be performed as early as possible to facilitate fracture plane recognition and preserve the articular surface.[39]

In one study, 23 patients were followed for an average of 38 months following intra-articular osteotomy.[39] The indication for the osteotomy included dorsal or volar subluxation of the radiocarpal joint in 14 patients and articular incongruity of 2 mm or more as measured on a posteroanterior radiograph in 17 patients. All osteotomies healed without evidence of osteonecrosis and there was significant improvement in ROM, grip strength, articular congruity, and ulnar variance. There were 19 excellent/good results according to the systems of Fernandez[42] and Gartland and Werley.[43] According to the Mayo modification of the Green and O'Brien system,[44] there were only 10 excellent/good results. The Green and O'Brien modification is very strict and consistently produces poorer results than the other scoring systems. The authors interpret this difference as indicating that intra-articular osteotomy restores useful function, but rarely restores normal function of the wrist.[39]

Recommendations

• Early presentation of simple intra-articular malunion of the distal radius with more than 2 mm articular incongruity can be treated with osteotomy [overall quality: low]
• Osteotomy may restore useful function, but rarely restores normal wrist function [overall quality: low]

Question 9: What are the outcomes?

Case clarification
Our 45 year old patient with the distal radius malunion is interested in knowing the outcome following surgical correction of his distal radius malunion.

Relevance
Knowledge of the outcomes of surgical correction of malunited distal radius fractures will help in treatment decision-making.

Current opinion
Several different methods of surgical correction exist, each with reported good outcomes. Surgeon preference along with malunion type and patient characteristics dictate which method is utilized.

Finding the evidence
• PubMed (www.ncbi.nlm.nih.gov/pubmed/): sensitivity search using keywords: "distal radius malunion," "outcome"

Quality of the evidence
Level IV
• 7 studies

Findings
Uncontrolled series and retrospective unmatched cohort studies consistently show improvements following correction of malunited distal radius fractures, although most do not address disability or outcomes from the patient's perspective.[45–56]

Flinkkilä and others reported good or satisfactory results in 33 of 45 patients with symptomatic distal radius malunion treated with corrective osteotomy.[12] It was found that osteotomy of the distal radius alone did not completely restore normal anatomy and relieve symptoms, and in several cases a second operation was needed. Osteoarthritic changes in the radiocarpal and radioulnar joints were common, and they correlated with restriction in ROM, but not with pain. ROM and grip power were reduced compared to the unaffected hand, but only loss of supination and ulnar deviation correlated with an unsatisfactory subjective result. They concluded that reconstructive procedures in patients with distal radius malunion may not completely restore normal function.[12]

Recommendations

• Several different methods of surgical correction exist to treat distal radius malunions with good outcomes in case series, but no comparative data [overall quality: low]
• Osteoarthritic changes in the radiocarpal and radioulnar joints are common following surgical correction of distal radius malunions and they may correlate with restriction in ROM, but not with pain [overall quality: low]

Question 10: What are the complications of surgical correction of distal radius malunions?

Relevance
The complications of distal radius osteotomy factor into decision-making.

Current opinion
Serious complications such as nonunion, infection, and tendon rupture can lead to greater impairment than the malunion.

Finding the evidence
• PubMed (www.ncbi.nlm.nih.gov/pubmed/): sensitivity search using keywords: "distal radius malunion," "complications"

Quality of the evidence
Level IV
• 6 studies

Findings
Postoperative edema, finger stiffness, hematoma, tendinitis, tendon rupture, infection, loss of fixation, malunion, nonunion, neurovascular injury, residual ulnar-sided pain, complex regional pain syndrome, arthritis, and problems with the bone graft harvest site have all been reported.[40,45,51,57,58] The plates and screws used to secure the osteotomy can irritate and damage the extrinsic flexor and extensor tendons.[59–62]

Extensor pollicis longus (EPL) rupture and minor pin-track infections were noted when external fixation was used.[63]

Recommendation
• The benefit anticipated by osteotomy must outweigh the risk of these potential complications [overall quality: low]

Summary of recommendations

• Acceptable parameters for distal radius displacement are age dependent
• Patients under 65 years of age are more likely to have pain or stiffness or diminished grip strength with dorsal

angulation 10° or more, radial inclination 15° or less, or ulnar positive variance 3 mm or more

• Dorsal angulation of the distal radius can reduce wrist flexion and supination

• It may be worthwhile doing stretching exercises and being patient for pain to resolve when malalignment is less than 20° dorsal angulation or 3 mm ulnar positive variance

• The following radiographic features warrant consideration of osteotomy: dorsal angulation greater than 20°, displaced fractures with carpal malalignment (>15° of dorsal angulation of the lunate on the lateral view), incongruity of the DRUJ, greater than 5 mm ulnar positive variance, or unacceptable cosmetic deformity

• There is insufficient evidence to prove an advantage for early surgery [overall quality: low]

• Use of a nonstructural, cancellous only bone graft is relatively simple and seems safe and effective when used in conjunction with locking plates

• Either dorsal or volar surgical approach is acceptable

• Early presentation of simple intra-articular malunion of the distal radius with more than 2 mm articular incongruity can be treated with osteotomy

• Osteotomy may restore useful function, but rarely restores normal wrist function

• Several different methods of surgical correction exist to treat distal radius malunions

• Osteoarthritic changes in the radiocarpal and radioulnar joints are common following surgical correction of distal radius malunions and they may correlate with restriction in ROM, but not with pain

• The benefit anticipated by osteotomy must outweigh the risk of these potential complications

References

1. Friberg S, Lundstrom B. Radiographic measurements of the radio-carpal joint in normal adults. Acta Radiol (Stockh) 1976;17:249.

2. Campbell WC. Malunited Colles' fractures. JAMA 1937;109: 1105–8.

3. Barrett JA, Baron JA, Karagas MR, Beach ML. Fracture risk in the U.S. Medicare population. J Clin Epidemiol 1999;52:243–9.

4. Pogue DJ, Viegas SF, Patterson RM, et al. Effects of distal radius fracture on wrist joint mechanics. J Hand Surg Am 1990;15:721–7.

5. Hirahara H, Neale PG, Lin YT, Cooney WP, An KN. Kinematic and tourque related effects of dorsally angulated distal radius fractures and the distal radial ulnar joint. J Hand Surg Am 2003;28:614–21.

6. Villar RN, Marsh D, Rushton N. Three years after Colles' fracture. A prospective review. J Bone Joint Surg Br 1987;69:635–8.

7. Lichtman DM, Schneider JR, et al. Ulnar midcarpal instability—clinical and laboratory analysis. J Hand Surg Am 1981;6(5): 515–23.

8. Taleisnik J, Watson HK. Midcarpal instability caused by malunited fractures of the distal radius. J Hand Surg Am 1984;9(3):350–7.

9. Bronstein AJ, Trumble TE, Tencer AF. The effects of distal radius fracture malalignment on forearm rotation: A cadaveric study. J Hand Surg Am 1997;22:258–62.

10. Crisco JJ, Moore DC, Marai E, et al. Effects of distal radius malunion on distal radioulnar joint mechanics—an in vivo study. J Orthop Res 2007;25(4):547–55.

11. Posner MA, Ambrose L: Malunited Colles' fractures: correction with a biplanar closing wedge osteotomy. J Hand Surg Am 1991;16:1017–26.

12. Finkkila T, Raatikainen T, Kaarela O, Hamalainen M: Corrective osteotomy for malunion of the distal radius. Arch Orthop Trauma Surg 2000;120:23–6.

13. Leung F, Ozkan M, Chow SP. Conservative treatment of intra-articular fractures of the distal radius—factors affecting functional outcome. Hand Surg 2000;5:145.

14. Batra S, Gupta A. The effect of fracture-related factors on the functional outcome at 1 year in distal radius fractures. Injury 2002;33:499.

15. Tsukazaki, T, Iwasaki, K. Ulnar wrist pain after Colles' fracture. 109 fractures followed for 4 years. Acta Orthop Scand 1993;64:462.

16. Hollevoe N, Verdonk R. The functional importance of malunion in distal radius fractures. Acta Orthop Belg 2003;69:239.

17. Gliatis JD, Plessas SJ, Davis TR. Outcome of distal radial fractures in young adults. J Hand Surg Br 2000;25:535.

18. McQueen M, Caspers J. Colles fracture: does the anatomical result affect the final function? J Bone Joint Surg Br 1988;70:649–51.

19. Jebsen RH, Taylor N, Trieschmann RB, Trotter MJ, Howard LA. An objective and standardized test of hand function. Arch Phys Med Rehabil 1969;50(6): 311–19.

20. Grewal R, MacDermid JC. The risk of adverse outcomes in extra-articular distal radius fractures is increased with malalignment in patients of all ages but mitigated in older patients. J Hand Surg 2007;32(7):962–70.

21. Mackenney PJ, McQueen MM, Elton R. Prediction of instability in distal radius fractures. J Bone Joint Surg Am 2006;88: 1944–51.

22. Kelly AJ, Warwick D, Crichlow TPK, Bannister GC. Is manipulation of a moderately displaced Colles' fracture worthwhile? A prospective randomized trial. Injury 1997;28(4):283–7.

23. Ring D. Treatment of the neglected distal radius fracture. Clin Orthop Relat Res 2005;431:85–92.

24. Whittle AP. Malunited fractures. In: Canale ST, ed., Campbell's Operative Orthopaedics, 11th edn, pp. 3509–23. Mosby, St. Louis, 2008.

25. Forward DP, Davis TR, Sithole JS. Do young patients with malunited fractures of the distal radius inevitably develop symptomatic post-traumatic osteoarthritis? J Bone Joint Surg Br 2008;90(5):629–37.

26. Cooney WP, Dobyns JH, Linscheid RL. Complications of Colles Fractures. J Bone Joint Surg Am 1980;62:613–19.

27. Verhaegen F, Degreef I, De Smet L. Evaluation of corrective osteotomy of the malunited distal radius on midcarpal and radioicarpal malalignment. J Hand Surg Am 2010;35(1):57–61.

28. Amadio PC, Botte MJ. Treatment of malunion of the distal radius. Hand Clin 1987;3(4):541–61.

29. Slagel BE, Luenam S, Pichora DR. Management of post-traumatic malunion of fractures of the distal radius. Orthop Clin North Am 2007;38:203–16.

30. Jupiter JB, Ring D. A comparison of early and late reconstruction of malunited fractures of the distal end of the radius. J Bone Joint Surg Am 1998;78:739–48.

31. Ring D, Roberge C, Morgan T, Jupiter JB. Osteotomy for malunited fractures of the distal radius. J Hand Surg Am 2002;27(2):216–22.

32. von Campe A, Nagy L, Arbab D, Dumont CE. Coreective osteotomies in malunions of the distal radius : do we get what we planned? Clin Orthop Relat Res 2006;450:179–85.

33. Luchetti R. Corrective osteotomy of malunited distal radius fractures using carbonate hydroxyapatite as an alternative to autogenous bone grafting. J Hand Surg Am 2004;29:825–34.

34. Yasuda M, Masada K, Kentaro I, et al. Early corrective osteotomy for a malunited Colles' fracture using volar approach and calcium phosphate bone cement: a case report. J Hand Surg Am 2004;29:1139–42.

35. Abramo A, Tagil M, Geijer M, Kopylov P. Osteotomy of dorsally displaced malunited fractures of the distal radius: no loss of radiographic correction during healing with a minimally invasive fixation technique and an injectable bone substitute. Acta Orthop 2008;79(2):262–8.

36. Catalano LW 3rd, Cole RJ, Gelberman RH, Evanoff BA, Gilula LA, Borrelli J Jr. Displaced intra-articular fractures of the distal aspect of the radius. Long-term results in young adults after open reduction and internal fixation. J Bone Joint Surg Am 1997;79:1290–302.

37. Knirk JL, Jupiter JB. Intra-articular fractures of the distal end of the radius in young adults. J Bone Joint Surg Am 1986;68:647–59.

38. Trumble TE, Schmitt SR, Vedder NB. Factors affecting functional outcome of displaced intra-articular distal radius fractures. J Hand Surg Am 1994;19:325–40.

39. Ring D, Prommersberger KJ, Del Pino JG, et al. Corrective osteotomy for intra-articular malunion of the distal part of the radius. J Bone Joint Surg Am 2005;87:1503–9.

40. Thivaios GC, McKee MD. Sliding osteotomy for deformity correction following malunion of volarly displaced distal radial fractures. J Orthop Trauma 2003;17(5):326–33.

41. Marx RG, Axelrod TS. Intraarticular osteotomy of distal radius malunions. Clin Orthop 1996;327:152–7.

42. Fernandez DL. Radial osteotomy and Bowers arthroplasty for malunited fractures of the distal end of the radius. J Bone and Joint Surg Am 1988;70:1538–51.

43. Gartland JJ Jr, Werley CW. Evaluation of healed Colles' fractures. J Bone Joint Surg Am 1951;33:895–907.

44. Cooney WP, Bussey R, Dobyns JH, et al. Difficult wrist fractures. Perilunate fracture-dislocations of the wrist. Clin Orthop 1987;214:136–47.

45. Posner MA, Ambrose L. Malunited Colles' fractures: correction with a biplanar closing wedge osteotomy. J Hand Surg Am 1991;16:1017–26.

46. Wada T, Isogai S, Kanaya K, Tsukahara T, Yamashita T. Simultaneous radial closing wedge and ulnar shortening osteotomies for distal radius malunion. J Hand Surg Am 2004;29(2):264–72.

47. Viso R, Wegener EE, Freeland AE. Use of a closing wedge osteotomy to correct malunion of dorsally displaced extraarticular distal radius fractures. Orthopedics 2000;23:721–4.

48. Fernandez DL. Reconstructive procedures for malunion and traumatic arthritis. Orthop Clin North Am 1993;24:341–63.

49. Fernandez DL, Capo JT, Gonzalez E. Corrective osteotomy for symptomatic increased ulnar tilt of the distal end of the radius. J Hand Surg Am 2001;26:722–32.

50. Jupiter JB, Ruder J, Roth DA. Computer-generated bone models in the planning of osteotomy of multidirectional distal radius malunions. J Hand Surg Am 1992;17:406–15.

51. Fernandez DL. Correction of posttraumatic wrist deformity in adults by osteotomy, bone-grafting, and internal fixation. J Bone Joint Surg Am 1982;64:1164–78.

52. Wada T, Usui M, Aoki M, Ishii S. Opening wedge osteotomy and bone grafting for distal radius malunion. Hand Surg 1997;2:191–202.

53. Shea K, Fernandez DL, Jupiter JB, et al. Corrective osteotomy for malunited, volarly displaced fractures of the distal end of the radius. J Bone Joint Surg Am 1997;79:1816–26.

54. Brown J, Bell MJ. Distal radial osteotomy for malunion of wrist fractures in young patients. J Hand Surg Br 1994;19:589–93.

55. Watson HK, Castle TH Jr. Trapezoidal osteotomy of the distal radius for unacceptable articular angulation after Colles' fracture. J Hand Surg Am 1988;13:837–43.

56. Viegas SF. A new modification of corrective osteotomy for treatment of distal radius malunion. Tech Hand Upper Extrem Surg 2006;10(4):224–30.

57. Prommersberger KJ, Fernandez DL. Nonunion of distal radius fractures. Clin Orthop Relat Res 2004;419:51–6.

58. Graham TJ. Surgical correction of malunited fractures of the distal radius. J Am Acad Orthop Surg 1997;5:270–81.

59. Orbay JL. The treatment of unstable distal radius fractures with volar fixation. Hand Surg 2000;5:103–12.

60. Berglund LM, Tesser TM. Complications of volar plate fixation for managing distal radius fractures. J Am Acad Orthop Surg 2009;17(6):369–77.

61. Arora R, Lutz M, Hennerbichler A, Krappinger D, Espen D, Gabl M. Complications following internal fixation of unstable distal radius fracture with a palmar locking-plate. J Orthop Trauma 2002;21:316–22.

62. Drobetz H, Kutscha-Lissberg E. Osteosynthesis of distal radial fractures with a volar locking screw plate system. Int Orthop 2003; 27:1–6.

63. McQueen MM, Wakefield A. Distal radial osteotomy for malunion using non-bridging external fixation: good results in 23 patients. Acta Orthop 2008; 79(3):390–5.

110 Scaphoid Fractures

Ruby Grewal

Hand and Upper Limb Centre, University of Western Ontario, London, ON, Canada

Case scenario

A healthy 25 year old man sustained an isolated wrist injury to his dominant arm after sustaining a fall. Physical examination revealed isolated pain in the area of the anatomical snuff box. Given the area of tenderness and mechanism of injury, the attending Emergency Department physician was concerned about a possible underlying scaphoid fracture.

Relevant anatomy

The scaphoid plays a key role in carpal motion and wrist stability. It is the most frequently fractured carpal bone.[1,2] Because of its retrograde blood supply, nonunion rates can be high, resulting in deformity, arthritis, and significant lifelong impairment. Scaphoid fractures are most commonly described based on their anatomic location: proximal pole, waist, and distal pole (Figure 110.1). Accurate diagnosis and management is essential to ensure optimal results. This chapter focuses on diagnosis, management options, clinical outcomes and complications.

Importance of the problem

The annual incidence of scaphoid fractures was reported as 43/100,000 in Norway.[3] A Danish study reported an incidence of 38 scaphoid fractures per 100,000 men,[4] and a US study reported an incidence of 1.21/1,000 person years (unadjusted) in a US military population.[5] The highest incidence of scaphoid fractures is seen in young males. A population-based Norwegian study reported the median age of affected patients to be 25 years, with a significantly

higher incidence in males compared to females (82% vs. 18%).[3] An American study also reported that males were more likely to sustain a scaphoid fracture, with an adjusted rate ratio of 1.55 compared to females.[5] They also reported that the highest incidence was seen in the 20–24 year old age group. Disability and impairment in this young population leads to a loss of productivity and potentially high opportunity costs for both the individual and society.

Top five questions

1. What is the best way to diagnose an occult scaphoid fracture?
2. Once a fracture is identified, what is the best method of immobilization?
3. Will the fracture heal faster and more predictably if treated with an ORIF?
4. Can patients expect better functional outcomes if treated with an ORIF?
5. What complications can be expected? Both with ORIF and with casting?

Question 1: What is the best way to diagnose an occult scaphoid fracture?

Case clarification

A 25 year old male construction worker who fell on to his dominant hand has isolated pain in the anatomical snuff box. Radiographs were obtained and no fracture was identified. The attending physician was concerned about the possibility of an occult scaphoid fracture, given the examination findings.

For patients presenting with pain in the anatomical snuff box, but normal radiographs, what is the best way of con-

Evidence-Based Orthopedics, First Edition. Edited by Mohit Bhandari.

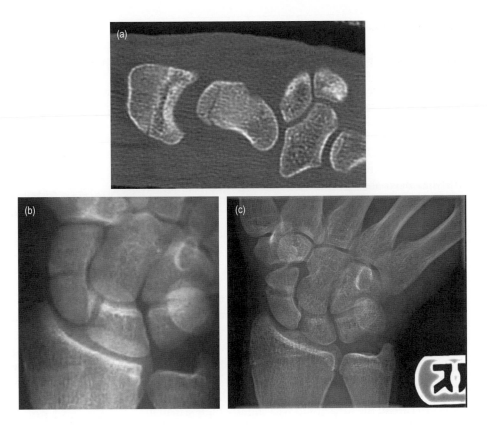

Figure 110.1 Scaphoid fractures:
(a) proximal pole, (b) waist, (c) distal pole.

firming the diagnosis: repeat clinical and radiographic assessment in 2 weeks? Bone scan? CT scan? MRI?

Relevance of the question

For many patients, 2 weeks of unnecessary immobilization can result in significant impairment and economic losses due to their inability to work. A prompt, accurate diagnosis will eliminate the need for unnecessary immobilization and ensure all fractures are identified and treated in a timely manner.

Current opinion

The majority of orthopedic surgeons will obtain further imaging to confirm a suspected scaphoid fracture. The imaging modality used varies, depending on available resources.

Finding the evidence

• PubMed (www.ncbi.nlm.nih.gov/pubmed/) clinical queries search: "scaphoid fracture" AND "diagnosis"

Quality of the evidence

Level II
• 1 randomized trial with methodologic limitations[6]
• 3 diagnostic studies with methodologic limitations[7–9]

Level III
• 1 diagnostic study with greater methodologic limitations[10]

Findings

Clinical suspicion of a scaphoid fracture is the first step in establishing a diagnosis. The diagnostic sensitivity is high for clinical examination, but the specificity is low, reported at only 74–80%.[11] As such, we rely on other modalities to establish the diagnosis. Radiographs are traditionally used to identify bony injuries; however, scaphoid fractures can be difficult to identify with plain radiographs alone.

Jenkins has shown that the negative predictive value of radiography is low (84%) and up to 25% of all fractures will be missed if this modality is used in isolation.[10] Some advocate repeating radiographs at 2 weeks to help identify an occult fracture if clinical suspicion is high and initial radiographs are normal; however, Dias et al. have shown that repeating radiographs at 2–3 weeks does not improve their diagnostic ability.[7] This has been confirmed by other authors who also report that repeat radiographs do not reliably improve diagnostic accuracy.[10,12]

Because the consequences of a missed scaphoid fracture are concerning (i.e., nonunion, malunion, or avascular necrosis) many patients with suspected fractures are immobilized despite normal initial radiographs. It has been reported that 75% of patients with clinical suspicion of a scaphoid fracture will be immobilized unnecessarily if traditional radiographs are used alone.[13] Jenkins reports that for each patient subsequently shown to have a fracture, 5.25 patients are overtreated.[10] Because scaphoid fractures typically affect young men, periods of unnecessary immobilization can result in a loss of productivity and time away from work/sport which is often a significant concern for this population. In order to help improve diagnostic accuracy and reduce unnecessary overtreatment of scaphoid fractures, a variety of second-line imaging techniques have been used.[10]

Traditionally, bone scans were the second-line imaging modality of choice. The sensitivity of bone scans is high (reported as 92–95%), but the specificity is low (60–95%), potentially resulting in a high number of false positives.[11] MRI has been shown to have better interobserver agreement for scaphoid injury than bone scan, with fewer false-positive reports.[9] The sensitivity for MRI is high (near 100%);[8,11] however, the specificity is estimated at 90% since many false-positive results can occur when injuries such as bone bruises are misinterpreted as fractures.[11]

Thorpe et al. have shown the cost of MRI is comparable with that of bone scan and that the reduced immobilization time in these patients results in lower overall healthcare costs.[9] Brooks et al. demonstrated that suspected scaphoid fractures imaged with MRI had significantly fewer days of immobilization (3 vs. 10, p = 0.006) and the MRI group used fewer healthcare units compared to controls who received "usual clinical care" (3 vs. 5, p = 0.03).[6] The cost of health care in the MRI group was slightly higher than in controls ($594 AUD vs. $428 AUD, p = 0.19), but when productivity losses are considered, MRI may be considered cost-effective when used in a select population.[6]

With its ability to detect associated soft tissue injuries, its high sensitivity and specificity, some authors advocate MRI as the imaging modality of choice in suspected scaphoid fractures.[8,10] Although it may be cost-effective, MRI is still not readily available in many centers. CT scans have been suggested as an effective, cheaper alternative to MRI with high reported sensitivities (97–100%).[10] A comparative study of MRI and CT by Memarsadgehi showed that CT had a 100% sensitivity and specificity in identifying cortical involvement and was significantly superior to MRI (p = 0.03).[8] It is also thought that CT scans allow clearer visualization of fracture displacement than MRI.[11] CT scans are unable to detect purely trabecular fractures, unlike MRI; however, this was not statistically significant (p = 0.25).[8] In addition, the clinical relevance of detecting a purely trabecular fractures without cortical involvement is unclear. These fractures may not require immobilization and are less likely to result in nonunion if undetected. Therefore, with the ease of availability, lower cost, and high accuracy of CT scans, this is an excellent tool to help make therapeutic decisions in patients with suspected scaphoid fractures.

Recommendations

In patients with clinically suspected scaphoid fractures but normal initial radiographs, evidence suggests that:

- Repeat radiographs do not reliably detect occult scaphoid fractures and result in overtreatment [overall quality: moderate]
- Bone scans have a high sensitivity but low specificity and therefore can only reliably be used to rule out scaphoid fractures [overall quality: moderate]
- Both MRI and CT have a high sensitivity and specificity and can be relied upon to confirm a suspected scaphoid fracture [overall quality: moderate]

Question 2: What is the best method for immobilization of an undisplaced scaphoid fracture?

Case clarification

The treating Emergency Department physician identified an undisplaced scaphoid waist fracture on the radiograph and this was then confirmed by subsequent CT scan. The fracture was immobilized and the patient referred to an orthopedic surgeon. What is the best method of cast immobilization for patients with scaphoid waist fractures? Is a thumb spica cast better than a Colles cast? Is it necessary to immobilize in an above-elbow cast?

Relevance of the question

Cast immobilization can be cumbersome for young, active patients. If a less restrictive cast can be used without compromising outcomes, this would be a more attractive choice for patients.

Current opinion

In North America, the trend is to use thumb spica casting, either above- or below-elbow, for scaphoid immobilization, while in Europe the tendency is to use a short-arm cast with the thumb free.

Finding the evidence

- PubMed (www.ncbi.nlm.nih.gov/pubmed/) clinical queries search "scaphoid fracture" AND "casting"

Quality of the evidence

Level II
- 3 randomized trials with methodologic limitations[14–16]
- 1 prospective cohort study with methodologic limitations[17]

Level IV
- 1 lower quality randomized trial with methodologic limitations[18]

Level V
- 2 biomechanical studies[19,20]
- 1 expert opinion[21]

Findings

Thumb spica vs. short-arm cast In a prospective randomized trial comparing thumb spica vs. Colles casts in a study of 292 scaphoid fractures, Clay et al. found that the incidence of nonunions was independent of the type of cast used.[18] Bohler et al. also found comparable union rates between Colles casts and thumb spica casts in an observational study.[17] In a biomechanical study, using a cadaveric model, Schramm found that wrist immobilization is crucial for immobilization, but short-arm casting was just as effective as thumb spica casting in preventing fracture displacement.[20]

Short-arm vs. long-arm casting Gellman et al. conducted a prospective randomized trial comparing short-arm to long-arm thumb spica casting. They found that patients treated with a long-arm cast united significantly faster than those with short-arm casts (mean of 9.5 weeks vs. 12.7 weeks, p < 0.05). There were also fewer nonunions (0 vs. 2) and delayed unions (2 vs. 6) in the group treated with a long-arm thumb spica cast. They concluded that proximal pole and middle third fractures had a significantly shorter time to union when treated in a long-arm thumb spica cast. Fractures of the distal third healed well regardless of type of cast used.[15]

Although Gellman believes that the elimination of forearm rotation reduces the shear stresses across the fracture site, improving union rates, this has not been corroborated by other authors. Alho performed a prospective randomized study evaluating 100 scaphoid fractures treated with above- and below-elbow casts. In this study, there were no statistically significant differences between union rates or outcomes in the two groups.[14] Other authors have also demonstrated that pronation and supination of the forearm does not cause significant motion in scaphoid fracture fragments.[19] These results were corroborated in a clinical study by Cooney who demonstrated a union rate of 94% in 45 scaphoids treated with immobilization in a below-elbow cast.[21]

Immobilization in wrist flexion or extension Hambidge et al. evaluated the influence of wrist position on scaphoid fracture healing. They found that the position of wrist immobilization (either slight flexion or slight extension) did not influence nonunion rates, wrist flexion, grip strength, or pain, but those immobilized in flexion had more difficulty regaining wrist extension.[16]

Recommendations
• Colles casts offer similar results to short-arm thumb spica casts [overall quality: moderate]
• Long-arm casts result in a faster time to union in scaphoid waist or proximal pole fractures [overall quality: moderate]

• Other cohort studies and biomechanical studies state that forearm rotation does not cause significant motion in scaphoid fracture fragments [overall quality: low–moderate]
• Scaphoid fractures should be immobilized in slight wrist extension [overall quality: moderate]

Question 3: Will scaphoid fractures heal faster and more predictably if treated with an ORIF compared to casting alone?

Case clarification
This healthy 25 year old construction worker, recently casted for an undisplaced scaphoid fracture, is unable to return to work until his fracture is healed. He is eager to return to his recreational activities and full duties at work as soon as possible.

Among patients with undisplaced scaphoid waist fractures, does ORIF offer more predictable union rates and a faster time to union than cast immobilization?

Relevance of the question
Patients and their treating surgeons both want the safest, most reliable method of treatment.

Current opinion
The role of surgical fixation for undisplaced scaphoid waist fractures is controversial. Conservative treatment yields excellent results for undisplaced fractures, but proponents of operative fixation (Figure 110.2) cite a quicker return to activity (work/sport) and a reduced risk of nonunion compared with that for cast treatment and with minimal additional risk.

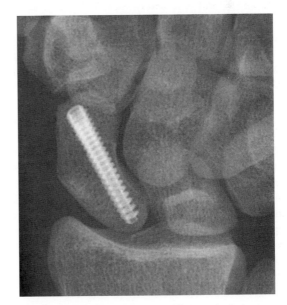

Figure 110.2 ORIF of scaphoid fracture with Acutrak screw.

Finding the evidence
• PubMed: "scaphoid fractures" AND "(randomized controlled trial[ptyp])"

Quality of the evidence
Level I
• 6 high-quality randomized trials[22–27]

Level II
• 2 randomized trials with methodological limitations[28,29]

Findings
Time to union Time to union was reported in three of the six randomized controlled trials.[22,23,28] Both Bond and McQueen reported significantly faster healing times for patients treated with ORIF.[23,28] Bond et al. compared undisplaced scaphoid waist fractures treated with percutaneous Acutrak screw fixation to cast immobilization (6 weeks in a long-arm thumb spica cast followed by a short-arm thumb spica cast until healing confirmed, n = 25) and found a significantly shorter healing time for the ORIF group (7 weeks vs. 12 weeks, p = 0.0003).[23] McQueen et al. evaluated both displaced and undisplaced fractures treated with percutaneous Acutrak screw fixation to Colles cast immobilization (n = 60) and also found the ORIF group healed faster (9 weeks vs. 14 weeks, p < 0.001).[28] Adolfsson also compared healing times in undisplaced scaphoid fractures treated with ORIF (percutaneous Acutrak) vs. a below-elbow cast (n = 53) and did not find any significant difference in healing times between the two groups.[22]

Successful union Union rates were high in both the operative and nonoperative groups in five of the six studies, with no statistically significant differences between treatment groups.[22,23,26,28,29] Bond et al. did not identify any nonunions in either treatment group.[23] Saeden et al. had one nonunion in the ORIF group (1/30) and two nonunions in the cast group (2/30).[29] McQueen et al. identified one nonunion in the ORIF group (1/30) and four in the cast group (4/30).[28] Adolffson had one nonunion in the ORIF group (1/30) with none in the cast group (0/30).[22] Vinnars had only one nonunion in the cast group (1/26 cast, 0/26 ORIF), and in the 2008 study, had no nonunions in either treatment group.[26]

The only study to report a significant difference in union rate was that of Dias et al. They also reported the greatest number of nonunions (10 of 44 with a cast vs. 0 of 44 for operative treatment, p = 0.001). They defined nonunion as absence of radiographic signs of healing at 12 weeks and a gap on CT scan at 16 weeks; however, this definition may be flawed as one such nonunion healed without additional treatment and 4 of 10 patients did not have a visible fracture line or evidence of mobility at the time of surgery. If further CT scans were taken, these may have been better classified as fibrous unions or delayed unions.[25]

Summary These six studies are all moderate to high-quality randomized controlled trials, and are the best evidence we have to date. However, there are a few flaws in these studies: none of the six published clinical trials used CT or arthroscopy to diagnose fracture displacement, and it is possible that some of the fractures included were displaced or unstable, thus biasing the results.[30]

In addition, the determination of union was suboptimal. These studies used clinical and radiographic assessments to confirm union, a method which has been shown to be unreliable by several authors.[31–33]

Recommendations
• There are high union rates for both operative and nonoperative treatment of undisplaced scaphoid fractures [overall quality: high]
• Opinion is divided as to whether scaphoid union does or does not occur more quickly with ORIF compared with casting

Question 4: Can patients expect better functional outcomes if treated with ORIF?

Case clarification
This young active patient wants to ensure he has the best possible outcome. He wants to regain full strength and range of motion, and minimize his time away from work. Does ORIF or casting produce superior clinical results for manual laborers with undisplaced scaphoid fractures?

Relevance of the question
As scaphoid fractures typically occur in young men, minimizing the length of disability is essential as a physical impairment can have a significant impact on overall productivity in this population.

Current opinion
While union rates or time to union may not be significantly different between ORIF and casting, proponents of ORIF claim that it allows a quicker return to activity (work/sport).

Finding the evidence
• PubMed: "scaphoid fractures" AND "(randomized controlled trial[ptyp])"

Quality of the evidence
Level I
• 6 high-quality randomized trials[22–27]

Level II
• 2 randomized trials with methodological limitations[28,29]

Findings
The studies reviewed generally report earlier recovery of grip strength and motion in the operatively treated

group[22,25] but no significant differences at the time of final assessment.[22,23,25,28,29] Two studies reported a faster return to sport in patients treated with an ORIF compared to those treated with cast immobilization.[22,28]

Return to work times have been reported to be significantly earlier with surgery by some groups (p < 0.0001[23] and p < 0.001[28]); however, this has not been corroborated by all authors. Dias did not report a faster return to work in patients treated with an ORIF.[25] Vinnars (p = 0.03)[26] and Saeden (p < 0.01)[29] both demonstrated that only those working as manual laborers had a significantly faster return to work with surgical treatment compared to cast immobilization.

A cost analysis of surgery vs. cast treatment (including the cost of work disability) was conducted by Vinnars who demonstrated that despite the faster return to work times, the cast group still had lower total costs than the surgically treated group for both manual laborers (cast €3,485 vs. surgery €4,529, p > 0.05) and nonmanual laborers (cast €770 vs. surgery €2,253, p < 0.047); however, these costs were only significantly lower in nonmanual laborers.[26]

Recommendations
• There is no significant difference in range of motion, strength, or patient-reported pain and disability at final follow-up between patients treated surgically or those treated with cast immobilization [overall quality: high]
• Some studies report a faster return to work time with ORIF, but this only achieves statistical significance in manual laborers [overall quality: high]
• Cast treatment has a lower total cost (treatment cost + work disability costs) than surgical treatment in both manual and nonmanual laborers, but the cost savings are only significant in nonmanual workers [overall quality: high]

Question 5: What are the complications of surgical treatment?

Case clarification
What complications can this patient expect if he decided to proceed with operative fixation? Among patients with undisplaced scaphoid waist fractures, are the complications associated with surgical treatment greater than with cast immobilization?

Relevance of the question
The possible risks of both interventions need to be assessed before recommendations can be made for either treatment.

Current opinion
Current opinion is that scaphoid ORIF is safe with only minor expected complications; however, the long-term complications are still largely unknown.

Finding the evidence
• PubMed: "scaphoid fractures" AND "(randomized controlled trial[ptyp])"

Quality of the evidence
Level I
• 6 high-quality randomized trials[22–27]

Level II
• 2 randomized trials with methodologic limitations[28,29]

Findings
The complications associated with both cast treatment and ORIF were considered to be minor overall. Adolfsson et al. had only one complication in their trial, a patient who developed complex regional pain syndrome (CRPS) after ORIF.[22] Bond et al. had one patient in the ORIF group with prominent hardware at the scapho-trapezial-trapezoid (STT) joint.[23] In Dias' reported short-term results there were 10 patients in the ORIF group with minor scar-related problems, one with a superficial wound infection, one with hypoesthesia in the palmar cutaneous branch of the median nerve, and one with mild early algodystrophy.[25]

McQueen et al. reported complications in both the cast group and the ORIF group. Two of their casted patients developed avascular necrosis of the scaphoid, one developed CRPS and one patient had symptomatic radioscaphoid osteoarthritis (OA). In the ORIF group there were two perioperative complications, both involving breakage of the cannulated screwdriver, and one patient with a prominent screw in the STT joint.[28]

Vinnars et al. reported one complication in the cast group (delayed union) and eight complications in the ORIF group. There were five patients with malpositioned hardware (two identified intraoperatively and removed, three with malpositioned screws and reactive erosion into the joint), two soft tissue injuries (partial FCR injury and partial injury to volar scapholunate ligament), and one patient with CRPS.[26]

Of the six randomized trials reported in the literature, three also published long-term results of their cohorts.[24,27,29] Saeden published 12 year results on his cohort and identified a significant increase in the incidence of radiographic STT OA (18/39) in the ORIF group (p = 0.049).[29] Vinnars et al. also found significantly more patients in the ORIF group (11/40 vs. 1/35) had STT OA (p < 0.005). They also identified cystic changes of more than 3 mm on plain radiographs of five scaphoids in the operatively treated group compared with none in the nonoperatively treated group (p = 0.057).[27] Dias et al. also identified STT abnormalities in long-term follow-up for both the ORIF (3/28, 11%) and cast group (5/31, 16%).[24] Unlike the other authors, they did not identify a statistically significant difference between casting and ORIF; however, their assessment was made by plain radiographs rather than CT as in the other studies.[27,29] In addition, the STT OA was identified on radiographs only. The findings did not correlate with clinical symptoms and further long-term studies are necessary to understand the clinical significance of this problem.

Recommendations

• The expected short-term complication rate is low with both ORIF and cast treatment [overall quality: high]
• The long-term complications of ORIF include radiographic STT OA [overall quality: high]

Summary of recommendations

• In patients with clinically suspected scaphoid fractures but normal initial radiographs, evidence suggests that repeat radiographs do not reliably detect occult scaphoid fractures and result in overtreatment
• Bone scans have a high sensitivity but low specificity and therefore can only reliably be used to rule out scaphoid fractures
• Both MRI and CT have a high sensitivity and specificity and can be relied upon to confirm a suspected scaphoid fracture
• Colles casts offer similar results to short-arm thumb spica casts
• Long-arm casts result in a faster time to union in scaphoid waist or proximal pole fractures compared to short-arm casts
• Forearm rotation does not cause significant motion in scaphoid fracture fragments
• Scaphoid fractures should be immobilized in slight wrist extension
• There are high union rates for both operative and non-operative treatment of undisplaced scaphoid fractures
• There is no significant difference in range of motion, strength or patient-reported pain and disability at final follow-up between patients treated surgically or those treated with cast immobilization
• Some studies report a faster return to work time with ORIF, but this only achieves statistical significance in manual laborers
• Cast treatment has a lower total cost (treatment cost + work disability costs) than surgical treatment in both manual laborers and nonmanual workers, but the cost savings are only significant in nonmanual workers
• The expected short-term complication rate is low with both ORIF and cast treatment
• The long-term complications of ORIF include radiographic STT OA, but the clinical significance of this is largely unknown

Conclusions

There is still no concrete evidence to support an evidence-based recommendation for ORIF vs. casting (or vice versa) in undisplaced scaphoid fractures. The reported complications with both interventions are minor, but the long-term complications are still largely unknown. Further high-quality randomized controlled trials are needed to definitively answer this question.

References

1. Kozin SH. Incidence, mechanism, and natural history of scaphoid fractures. Hand Clin 2001;17(4):515–24.
2. Gasser H. Delayed union and pseudarthrosis of the carpal navicular: treatment by compression-screw osteosynthesis; a preliminary report on twenty fractures. J Bone Joint Surg Am 1965;47: 249–66.
3. Hove LM. Epidemiology of scaphoid fractures in Bergen, Norway. Scand J Plast Reconstr Surg Hand Surg 1999;33(4): 423–6.
4. Larsen CF, Brondum V, Skov O. Epidemiology of scaphoid fractures in Odense, Denmark. Acta Orthop Scand 1992;63(2): 216–18.
5. Wolf JM, Dawson L, Mountcastle SB, Owens BD. The incidence of scaphoid fracture in a military population. Injury 2009;40(12): 1316–19.
6. Brooks S, Cicuttini FM, Lim S, Taylor D, Stuckey SL, Wluka AE. Cost effectiveness of adding magnetic resonance imaging to the usual management of suspected scaphoid fractures. Br J Sports Med 2005;39(2):75–9.
7. Dias JJ, Thompson J, Barton NJ, Gregg PJ. Suspected scaphoid fractures. The value of radiographs. J Bone Joint Surg Br 1990;72(1):98–101.
8. Memarsadeghi M, Breitenseher MJ, Schaefer-Prokop C, et al. Occult scaphoid fractures: comparison of multidetector CT and MR imaging—initial experience. Radiology 2006;240(1):169–76.
9. Thorpe AP, Murray AD, Smith FW, Ferguson J. Clinically suspected scaphoid fracture: a comparison of magnetic resonance imaging and bone scintigraphy. Br J Radiol 1996;69(818): 109–13.
10. Jenkins PJ, Slade K, Huntley JS, Robinson CM. A comparative analysis of the accuracy, diagnostic uncertainty and cost of imaging modalities in suspected scaphoid fractures. Injury 2008;39(7):768–74.
11. Kawamura K, Chung KC. Treatment of scaphoid fractures and nonunions. J Hand Surg Am 2008;33(6):988–97.
12. Tiel-van Buul MM, van Beek EJ, Broekhuizen AH, Nooitgedacht EA, Davids PH, Bakker AJ. Diagnosing scaphoid fractures: radiographs cannot be used as a gold standard! Injury 1992;23(2): 77–9.
13. Dorsay TA, Major NM, Helms CA. Cost-effectiveness of immediate MR imaging versus traditional follow-up for revealing radiographically occult scaphoid fractures. AJR Am J Roentgenol 2001;177(6):1257–63.

14. Alho A, Kankaanpaa. Management of fractured scaphoid bone. A prospective study of 100 fractures. Acta Orthop Scand 1975; 46(5):737–43.

15. Gellman H, Caputo RJ, Carter V, Aboulafia A, McKay M. Comparison of short and long thumb-spica casts for non-displaced fractures of the carpal scaphoid. J Bone Joint Surg Am 1989;71(3):354–7.

16. Hambidge JE, Desai VV, Schranz PJ, Compson JP, Davis TR, Barton NJ. Acute fractures of the scaphoid. Treatment by cast immobilisation with the wrist in flexion or extension? J Bone Joint Surg Br 1999;81(1):91–2.

17. Bohler L, Trojan E, Jahna H. The results of treatment of 734 fresh, simple fractures of the scaphoid. J Hand Surg Br 2003;28(4): 319–31.

18. Clay NR, Dias JJ, Costigan PS, Gregg PJ, Barton NJ. Need the thumb be immobilised in scaphoid fractures? A randomised prospective trial. J Bone Joint Surg Br 1991;73(5):828–32.

19. McAdams TR, Spisak S, Beaulieu CF, Ladd AL. The effect of pronation and supination on the minimally displaced scaphoid fracture. Clin Orthop Relat Res 2003;411:255–9.

20. Schramm JM, Nguyen M, Wongworawat MD, Kjellin I. Does thumb immobilization contribute to scaphoid fracture stability? Hand (N Y) 2008;3(1):41–3.

21. Cooney WP, Dobyns JH, Linscheid RL. Fractures of the scaphoid: a rational approach to management. Clin Orthop Relat Res 1980;149:90–7.

22. Adolfsson L, Lindau T, Arner M. Acutrak screw fixation versus cast immobilisation for undisplaced scaphoid waist fractures. J Hand Surg Br 2001;26(3):192–5.

23. Bond CD, Shin AY, McBride MT, Dao KD. Percutaneous screw fixation or cast immobilization for nondisplaced scaphoid fractures. J Bone Joint Surg Am 2001;83(4):483–8.

24. Dias JJ, Dhukaram V, Abhinav A, Bhowal B, Wildin CJ. Clinical and radiological outcome of cast immobilisation versus surgical treatment of acute scaphoid fractures at a mean follow-up of 93 months. J Bone Joint Surg Br 2008;90(7):899–905.

25. Dias JJ, Wildin CJ, Bhowal B, Thompson JR. Should acute scaphoid fractures be fixed? A randomized controlled trial. J Bone Joint Surg Am 2005;87(10):2160–8.

26. Vinnars B, Ekenstam FA, Gerdin B. Comparison of direct and indirect costs of internal fixation and cast treatment in acute scaphoid fractures: a randomized trial involving 52 patients. Acta Orthop 2007;78(5):672–9.

27. Vinnars B, Pietreanu M, Bodestedt A, Ekenstam F, Gerdin B. Nonoperative compared with operative treatment of acute scaphoid fractures. A randomized clinical trial. J Bone Joint Surg Am 2008;90(6):1176–85.

28. McQueen MM, Gelbke MK, Wakefield A, Will EM, Gaebler C. Percutaneous screw fixation versus conservative treatment for fractures of the waist of the scaphoid: a prospective randomised study. J Bone Joint Surg Br 2008;90(1):66–71.

29. Saeden B, Tornkvist H, Ponzer S, Hoglund M. Fracture of the carpal scaphoid. A prospective, randomised 12-year follow-up comparing operative and conservative treatment. J Bone Joint Surg Br 2001;83(2):230–4.

30. Lozano-Calderon S, Blazar P, Zurakowski D, Lee SG, Ring D. Diagnosis of scaphoid fracture displacement with radiography and computed tomography. J Bone Joint Surg Am 2006;88(12): 2695–703.

31. Nakamura R, Imaeda T, Horii E, Miura T, Hayakawa N. Analysis of scaphoid fracture displacement by three-dimensional computed tomography. J Hand Surg Am 1991;16(3):485–92.

32. Temple CL, Ross DC, Bennett JD, Garvin GJ, King GJ, Faber KJ. Comparison of sagittal computed tomography and plain film radiography in a scaphoid fracture model. J Hand Surg Am 2005;30(3):534–42.

33. Dias JJ, Taylor M, Thompson J, Brenkel IJ, Gregg PJ. Radiographic signs of union of scaphoid fractures. An analysis of inter-observer agreement and reproducibility. J Bone Joint Surg Br 1988;70(2):299–301.

111 Nonunions of the Scaphoid

Nina Suh[1] and Ruby Grewal[2]
[1]University of Western Ontario, London, ON, Canada
[2]Hand and Upper Limb Centre, University of Western Ontario, London, ON, Canada

Case scenario

A 30 year old farmer presents with complaints of activity related wrist pain. Pain has been persistent since a "wrist sprain" approximately 1 year ago for which he did not seek medical attention. Physical examination reveals tenderness in the anatomical snuffbox. Radiographs confirm an established proximal pole scaphoid nonunion.

Importance of the problem

The scaphoid's propensity for nonunion is well documented in the literature. Its tenuous retrograde blood supply and requirement for primary bone healing contribute to difficulty achieving union.[1] A consensus on the definition of nonunion has not been established, but persistence of a fracture line on plain radiograph 6 months after injury has generally been accepted in the literature.[1] The incidence of delayed union is estimated at 15% and nonunion as 12% in acute scaphoid fractures.[1] Numerous case series document the natural history of scaphoid nonunions and report the development of a predictable pattern of carpal arthritis and collapse if untreated.[2] This chapter explores risk factors, treatment options, and reported outcomes of scaphoid nonunions.

Top five questions

1. What is the natural history of scaphoid nonunions?
2. What are the operative options for scaphoid nonunions?
3. What factors increase the risk of developing a scaphoid nonunion?

4. Are there any modalities that can improve union rates?
5. Which salvage procedures offer the best results for scaphoid nonunion advanced collapse?

Question 1: What is the natural history of scaphoid nonunions?

Case clarification
This patient has an established proximal pole scaphoid nonunion, likely a consequence of the fall he sustained 1 year ago. He asks what would happen if he does not seek medical attention at this time. What is the natural history for patients with established scaphoid nonunions?

Relevance of the question
It is important to understand the natural history of scaphoid nonunions, as persistence of the nonunion will lead to the development of a predictable pattern of arthritis in the wrist, which can be prevented if the nonunion is successfully treated.

Current opinion
Scaphoid nonunions follow a predictable pattern of arthritis and carpal collapse, generally within 10 years after fracture.[3,4]

Finding the evidence
- PubMed (www.ncbi.nlm.nih.gov/pubmed/) clinical queries search: "scaphoid" AND "natural history"

Quality of the evidence
Level IV
- 7 retrospective review with methodologic limitations
- 1 systematic review with methodologic limitations

Evidence-Based Orthopedics, First Edition. Edited by Mohit Bhandari.
© 2012 Blackwell Publishing Ltd. Published 2012 by Blackwell Publishing Ltd.

Findings

One of the most frequently cited natural history studies of scaphoid nonunions was performed by Mack et al. in 1984 and later confirmed by multiple other authors.[3,5–7] They observed three main radiographic patterns of progressive arthritis in patients with scaphoid nonunions. Initially, changes are isolated to the scaphoid with development of cysts, sclerosis, and resorption. Degenerative changes then progress to involve the radial styloid and the entire scaphoid fossa, and finally result in pancarpal arthritis of the scaphocapitate and capitolunate joints. These radiographic changes were found to occur over 8.2 years, 17 years, and 31.6 years, respectively. Furthermore, Ruby et al. found 97% of patients with scaphoid nonunions developed arthritis if the injury was 5 years old or more (Figure 111.1).[6]

Displacement of the nonunion, carpal instability (defined as lunate dorsiflexion of more than 10°), and patient symptoms correlate with earlier progression and increased severity of wrist arthritis.[3,8] The incidence of scaphoid displacement (and consequently increased severity of osteoarthritis) also increases with greater time from fracture, and consequently many authors have advocated early surgical intervention to prevent this.[3] Because progressive degeneration was also observed in asymptomatic patients examined by Lindstrom and Nystrom, early surgical intervention is recommended for this group as well.[9]

Kerluke et al. highlighted that many of the natural history studies may be biased towards greater degeneration.[10] They report that the temporal course cannot yet be fully elucidated because of limitations in earlier study methodology, but it can generally be concluded that a predictable pattern of degeneration is eventually seen in all patients with scaphoid nonunions. Displacement and instability accelerate the pattern of degeneration and are found with greater number of years from injury.

Recommendation

- All patients with scaphoid nonunions, regardless of symptoms, can expect to develop a predictable pattern of carpal degeneration within 10 years [overall quality: moderate][8,11]

Question 2: What operative options are available for scaphoid nonunions?

Case clarification

The patient decides to proceed with surgical intervention and asks which surgical intervention has the highest chance of success.

For patients with scaphoid nonunions, without associated carpal arthritis, does vascularized grafting have superior union rates than nonvascularized grafting? Is there a preferred method of fixation?

Relevance of the question

Understanding the available surgical options and their associated complications is instrumental to guiding the management of scaphoid nonunions.

Current opinion

Nonvascularized bone grafting is sufficient for the majority of scaphoid nonunions; however, proximal pole nonunions or those with associated avascular necrosis are usually treated with vascularized bone grafting.

Finding the evidence

- PubMed (www.ncbi.nlm.nih.gov/pubmed/) clinical queries search: "scaphoid" AND "nonunion"

Quality of the evidence

Level I
- 1 prospective randomized trial with methodologic limitations

Level III
- 9 retrospective comparative study with methodologic limitations
- 1 case-control study with methodologic limitations
- 2 systematic review of uncontrolled comparative studies and case series

Level IV
- 75 prospective and retrospective case series with methodologic limitations

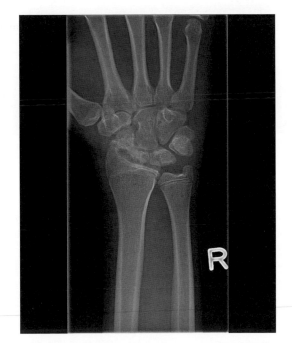

Figure 111.1 Representative radiographic example of a scaphoid nonunion advanced collapse of the wrist.

Findings

Two broad categories of bone grafts are available for treating scaphoid nonunions—vascularized and nonvascularized. Nonvascularized bone grafts range from cancellous chips to structural iliac crest or distal radius grafts.[11,12] Vascularized grafts are typically harvested from the pronator quadratus, distal radius, medial supracondylar femur, rib, base of the second metacarpal, or thumb metacarpal.[13–18]

A recent prospective randomized study compared vascularized to nonvascularized distal radius bone grafting in sclerotic scaphoid nonunions with poorly vascularized proximal poles. They found that union was achieved in 89.1% of patients treated with vascularized grafting vs. 72.5% in those treated with nonvascularized bone graft (p = 0.024).[19] These results were echoed by another study showing higher union rates with vascularized bone grafting (88%) vs. standard wedge grafting (47%) in patients with avascular necrosis of the proximal pole (p < 0.0005).[20]

A systematic review encompassing 5,246 cases of scaphoid nonunions divided patients into three major groups: standard bone grafting without internal fixation, standard nonvascularized bone grafting with internal fixation, and vascularized bone grafting with or without internal fixation. These authors did not detect any difference in union rates when internal fixation was added to a nonvascularized bone graft but did find an increase in union rates when a vascularized bone graft was used (p value not reported).[21]

Although the sources of vascularized bone grafts are plentiful, no large prospective randomized controlled trial has been conducted to directly compare the various vascularized bone graft sources against each other. Recently, Jones et al. performed a retrospective study comparing distal radial pedicle vascularized grafts with vascularized medial femoral condyle grafts and found union rates of 40% in scaphoids managed with radial grafts and 100% in those treated with the femoral grafts (p = 0.005).[22,23]

In addition to bone grafting, there are also many options available for internal fixation. Compression screws dominate as the preferred method of internal fixation, with results from a recent meta-analysis of 127 scaphoid nonunions showing union rates of 94% with screw fixation (Figure 111.2) vs. 77% with Kirschner wires (K-wires; Figure 111.3) (p < 0.01).[20] Other studies have shown union rates with screw fixation of 80–100%, while Kirschner wires had a greater range of results with union rates (56–100%).[10,21] Biodegradable screw fixation has the theoretical advantage of transferring stress directly to bone as the screws dissolve, as well as not requiring later hardware removal. Akmaz et al. have shown 100% union rates with biodegradable screws, but more studies into their efficacy are required.[24] Concerns have been raised about possible graft vs. host reaction; however, the clinical significance of this is questionable.

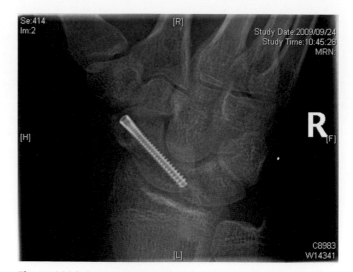

Figure 111.2 Representative radiographic example of a scaphoid nonunion treated operatively with iliac crest bone grafting and compression screw fixation.

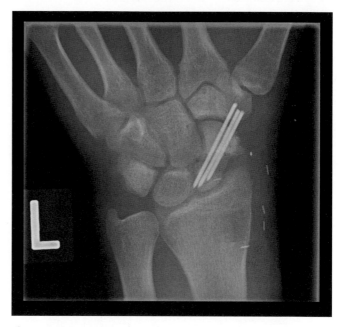

Figure 111.3 Representative radiographic example of a scaphoid nonunion treated operatively with bone grafting and Kirschner wire fixation.

Operative intervention is the treatment of choice for persistent scaphoid nonunions; however, we cannot advocate for one intervention over another (bone graft or fixation methods) as there are no high-quality comparative randomized controlled trials in the literature.

Recommendations

• Higher union rates are reported with the use of compression screws compared to K-wires (94% vs. 77%, p < 0.01) [overall quality: moderate][20]

• Vascularized bone grafting provides higher union rates than nonvascularized bone grafting in poorly vascularized or avascular scaphoid nonunions (88% vs. 47%, p < 0.0005) [overall quality: moderate][19]

Question 3: Which factors increase the risk of developing a scaphoid nonunion?

Case clarification

The patient's radiographs demonstrate a proximal pole scaphoid nonunion with no evidence of osteoarthritis. He tells you that he has been a heavy smoker for several years. Do these and other factors influence his chance of union? What factors led to the initial development of the nonunion, and what are his chances of successful union following surgery?

Relevance of the question

Underlying patient and fracture characteristics may influence nonunion rates and help predict outcomes in select groups.

Current opinion

Proximal pole fractures and displaced fractures are widely accepted as risk factors for nonunion. Delay to intervention, associated carpal instability, and smoking are presumed risk factors.

Finding the evidence

• PubMed (www.ncbi.nlm.nih.gov/pubmed/) clinical queries search: "scaphoid" AND "nonunion"

Quality of the evidence

Level IV

• 5 lower-quality retrospective reviews and case series with methodologic limitations

Findings

Fracture characteristics such as location and displacement are strongly correlated with union. Proximal pole fractures have been associated with nonunion rates as high as 75%, compared to 15% and 2% for waist and distal scaphoid fractures.[2,20] Fracture displacement has been defined as a fracture gap of 1 mm or more on any radiographic projection, a scapholunate angle greater than 60°, a radiolunate angle greater than 15°, or an intrascaphoid angle greater than 35°.[25] These displaced fractures are deemed unstable, often leading to a humpback deformity, and are associated with nonunion rates of 50% and osteonecrosis rates of 55%.[26-28] Generally, diagonal fractures of the middle third and vertical-diagonal fractures of the proximal third are unfavorable fracture patterns due to high shear forces and are thought to lead to higher nonunion rates, although this has not been quantified in the literature.[29]

Delayed treatment has also been suggested to contribute to increased nonunion rates. A retrospective study of 285 scaphoid fractures found that delaying immobilization of acute scaphoid fractures by more than 4 weeks was a significant risk factor for progression to nonunion.[30] A meta-analysis of 1,046 patients with established nonunions found a marked decrease in union rates if time to surgery exceeded 1 year (90% vs. 80%, p < 0.0001) but found no difference thereafter.[20]

Patient characteristics also influence union rates. In their study of 34 patients, Dinah and Vickers found smokers were three times more likely to have persistent nonunions after autologous bone grafting and internal fixation as compared to nonsmokers (p < 0.01).[31] In a Mayo Clinic study involving 51 patients, factors such as female gender, proximal pole avascularity, K-wire fixation, carpal collapse, and prior surgery were associated with increased nonunion rates, in addition to smoking.[32]

Recommendations

• Proximal pole fracture and displaced fractures are associated with an increased risk of progression to nonunion [overall quality: moderate]

• Delay to intervention, carpal instability, K-wire fixation, and smoking increase the risk of scaphoid nonunion [overall quality: low]

Question 4: Are there any modalities that can improve union rates?

Case clarification

There are several underlying factors (i.e., proximal pole nonunion, smoking history) that do not favour union in this patient. Are there any adjunctive modalities which can be used to improve union rates? Does pulsed electromagnetic field therapy or ultrasound improve union rates for scaphoid nonunions?

Relevance of the question

Adjunctive modalities, such as ultrasound and pulsed electromagnetic field therapy, may improve union rates, offering an attractive, noninvasive option for patients with scaphoid nonunions.

Current opinion

The efficacy of pulsed electromagnetic field stimulation and/or ultrasound lacks sufficient evidence in the literature to support its widespread use.

Finding the evidence

• PubMed (www.ncbi.nlm.nih.gov/pubmed/) clinical queries search: "scaphoid" AND "ultrasound," or "scaphoid" AND "electromagnetic"

Quality of the evidence

Level I

• 1 randomized double-blind controlled study with methodologic limitations

Level IV

• 7 case series with methodologic limitations

Findings

Pulsed ultrasound therapy provides a mechanical stimulus to the nonunion site, activating numerous cell types and biological pathways, stimulating endochondral ossification and, theoretically, union.[33] Published success rates are as high as 90%.[34,35] However, limited studies have evaluated its efficacy in scaphoid nonunions. A recent double-blind clinical trial evaluated the efficacy of ultrasound as an adjunct to surgical intervention.[35] Twenty-one scaphoid nonunions were treated with vascularized bone graft and randomized to either placebo or low-intensity ultrasound therapy. The authors found that healing was accelerated by 38 days in the group treated with ultrasound (p < 0.0001).

With respect to electromagnetic (EM) therapy, a retrospective, nonblinded study combining scaphoid, clavicle, metatarsal, metacarpal, and calcaneus fractures reported a union rate of 79% after EM stimulation in 29 patients.[36] Another case series evaluating EM with cast immobilization in 54 scaphoid nonunions reported an overall union rate of 69%,[37] with union rates of 50% for proximal pole fractures and 73% for scaphoids with underlying osteonecrosis.

Recommendations

• Pulsed electromagnetic field therapy may accelerate healing when used as an adjunct to cast immobilization for nonoperative management of scaphoid nonunions [overall quality: low]

• Ultrasound has been shown to accelerate time to union when used as an adjunct to surgery [overall quality: moderate]

Question 5: What salvage procedures are available for the treatment of scaphoid nonunion advanced collapse?

Case clarification

Despite attempts at ORIF and bone grafting, the patient's scaphoid nonunion did not heal and his symptoms of pain and stiffness have worsened. Radiographs reveal arthritis in the radioscaphoid joint and persistence of the nonunion. What is the best treatment option for this patient? Does a proximal row carpectomy (PRC) or four-corner fusion provide superior outcomes in patients with stage 2 scaphoid nonunion advanced collapse (SNAC)?

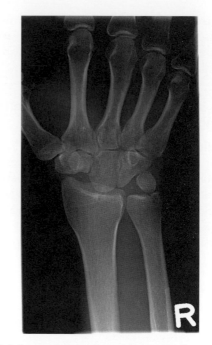

Figure 111.4 Representative radiographic example of a proximal row carpectomy for scaphoid nonunion advanced collapse.

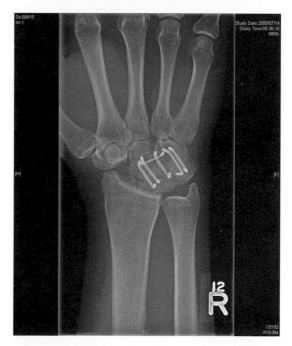

Figure 111.5 Representative radiographic example of a scaphoid excision and four-corner fusion for scaphoid nonunion advanced collapse.

Relevance of the question

Patients with stage 2 SNAC changes can be treated with either a PRC (Figure 111.4) or a scaphoidectomy with four-corner fusion (Figure 111.5). An understanding of the advantages and disadvantages of each is essential.

Current opinion

Both procedures can successfully relieve pain, but PRC allows for a greater postoperative wrist range of motion while four-corner fusion allows greater recovery of grip strength.

Finding the evidence

- PubMed (www.ncbi.nlm.nih.gov/pubmed/) clinical queries search: "scaphoid" and "nonunion"

Quality of the evidence

Level III

- 5 retrospective comparative study with methodologic limitations
- 1 systematic review with methodologic limitations

Level IV

- 44 retrospective reviews and case series with methodologic limitations
- 2 biomechanical studies with methodologic limitations

Findings

The literature suggests that stage 1 SNAC wrists can be treated with a scaphoid reconstruction with or without radial styloidectomy. Meanwhile, stage 3 SNAC wrists should have midcarpal arthrodesis or complete wrist arthrodesis performed.

The options for stage 2 wrists are more widely debated. Dacho et al. reported greater pain relief (77% vs. 54%, p > 0.05) with PRC compared to four-corner fusion but reduced grip strength (PRC 50% vs. four-corner 72%, p < 0.05).[38,39] Consequently, they advocated midcarpal arthrodesis for heavy labourers and PRC for nonmanual workers. The literature is inconsistent, as a systematic review of 52 articles by Mulford et al. did not report a difference between PRC and four-corner fusion with respect to grip strength or pain relief (no p value given), whereas Wyrick et al. (1995) found that PRC had a significantly higher grip strength (p < 0.05) and range of motion (p < 0.05) vs. four-corner fusion in scapholunate advanced collapse wrists.[40,41] Although Mulford et al. initially reported better range of motion with PRC, these patients had higher rates of osteoarthritis in the long term.[40] Conversely, DiDonna et al. reported persistently good results with respect to pain and function with a minimum of 10 years follow-up after PRC.[42]

Fixation methods used to achieve arthrodesis have also been studied in the literature, with good fusion rates being achieved with multiple fixation strategies. The Quad memory staple, dorsal rectangular plate, dynamic compression plate, internal headless compression screws, K-wires, and circular plates were all found to achieve union.[43-45] However, studies comparing two different fusion methods are sparse. One study by Rodgers et al. compared K-wires to circular plate fixations for limited wrist fusions and found the two fixation methods equivalent.[44] Similarly, Bedford and Yang found 100% fusion rates and only one complication in their series of 15 patients with scapholunate advanced collapse wrists treated with circular plates.[46] However, a case series by Shindle et al. found circular plates to have a 25% nonunion rate and 56% complication rate.[47] The paucity of randomized controlled trials examining different fixation methods makes it difficult to ascertain which fixation method is most reliable.

Recommendations

- Stage 2 SNAC wrists may be effectively managed with scaphoid excision with PRC or four-corner fusion [overall quality: moderate]
- PRC may offer greater range of motion and pain relief when compared to four-corner fusion [overall quality: low][38,41]
- There are conflicting reports in the literature with respect to the difference in final grip strength with reports that PRC results in greater,[41] equivalent[40] and reduced[38] grip strength in comparison to four-corner fusion. As such, no evidence-based recommendations can be made at this time [overall quality: low]

Summary of recommendations

- All patients with scaphoid nonunions, regardless of symptoms, can expect to develop a predictable pattern of carpal degeneration within 10 years
- Higher union rates are reported with the use of compression screws compared to K-wires
- Vascularized bone grafting provides higher union rates than nonvascularized bone grafting in poorly vascularized or avascular scaphoid nonunions
- Proximal pole fracture and displaced fractures are associated with an increased risk of progression to nonunion
- Delay to intervention, carpal instability, K-wire fixation, and smoking increase the risk of scaphoid nonunion
- Pulsed EM field therapy may accelerate healing when used as an adjunct to casting for nonoperative management of scaphoid nonunions
- Ultrasound has been shown to accelerate time to union when used as an adjunct to surgery
- Stage 2 SNAC wrists may be effectively managed with scaphoid excision with PRC or four-corner fusion
- PRC may offer greater range of motion and pain relief than four-corner fusion
- There are conflicting reports in the literature with respect to the difference in final grip strength between PRC and four-corner fusion. As such, no evidence-based recommendations can be made at this time

Conclusions

Currently there is insufficient evidence to make definitive evidence-based recommendations for the management of scaphoid nonunions. The indications for, or effectiveness of, specific operative interventions and grafting procedures in the management of scaphoid nonunions have not been clearly established. Additionally, the majority of the literature utilizes plain radiographs to assess union instead of more advanced imaging modalities such as CT or MRI. Dias highlighted the fact that the shape and size of the scaphoid may lead one to erroneously assume trabeculae are crossing the fracture site in plain radiographs.[48] The author states that these "trabeculae" may simply be a by-product of the proximal and distal fragments overlapping when the X-ray beam is not in line with the fracture.[48] Consequently, the fundamental measurement of union rates and time to union may be flawed in studies using solely plain radiographs. Future studies, including a large, long-term, multicenter randomized trial with the use of computed tomography as the gold standard to define fracture pattern and progression of union are required to address the general paucity of literature on this important topic and to clarify the most appropriate treatment for scaphoid nonunions.

References

1. Kawamura K, Chung KC. Treatment of scaphoid fractures and nonunions. J Hand Surg Am 2008;33(6):988–97.

2. Sauerbier M GG, Dacho A. Current concepts in the treatment of scaphoid fractures. Eur J Trauma 2004;30:80–92.

3. Mack GR, Bosse MJ, Gelberman RH, Yu E. The natural history of scaphoid non-union. J Bone Joint Surg Am 1984;66(4):504–9.

4. Waitayawinyu T, McCallister WV, Katolik LI, Schlenker JD, Trumble TE. Outcome after vascularized bone grafting of scaphoid nonunions with avascular necrosis. J Hand Surg Am 2009;34(3):387–94.

5. Inoue G, Sakuma M. The natural history of scaphoid non-union. Radiographical and clinical analysis in 102 cases. Arch Orthop Trauma Surg 1996;115(1):1–4.

6. Ruby LK, Stinson J, Belsky MR. The natural history of scaphoid non-union. A review of fifty-five cases. J Bone Joint Surg Am 1985;67(3):428–32.

7. Milliez PY, Courandier JM, Thomine JM, Biga N. The natural history of scaphoid non-union. A review of fifty-two cases. Ann Chir Main 1987;6(3):195–202.

8. Vender MI, Watson HK, Wiener BD, Black DM. Degenerative change in symptomatic scaphoid nonunion. J Hand Surg Am 1987;12(4):514–9.

9. Lindstrom G, Nystrom A. Natural history of scaphoid non-union, with special reference to "asymptomatic" cases. J Hand Surg Br 1992;17(6):697–700.

10. Kerluke L, McCabe SJ. Nonunion of the scaphoid: a critical analysis of recent natural history studies. J Hand Surg Am 1993;18(1):1–3.

11. Huang YC, Liu Y, Chen TH. Long-term results of scaphoid nonunion treated by intercalated bone grafting and Herbert's screw fixation—a study of 49 patients for at least five years. Int Orthop 2009;33(5):1295–300.

12. Inoue G, Miura T. Treatment of ununited fractures of the carpal scaphoid by iliac bone grafts and Herbert screw fixation. Int Orthop 1991;15(4):279–82.

13. Bertelli JA, Tacca CP, Rost JR. Thumb metacarpal vascularized bone graft in long-standing scaphoid nonunion—a useful graft via dorsal or palmar approach: a cohort study of 24 patients. J Hand Surg Am 2004;29(6):1089–97.

14. Dailiana ZH, Malizos KN, Zachos V, Varitimidis SE, Hantes M, Karantanas A. Vascularized bone grafts from the palmar radius for the treatment of waist nonunions of the scaphoid. J Hand Surg Am 2006;31(3):397–404.

15. Doi K, Hattori Y. Vascularized bone graft from the supracondylar region of the femur. Microsurgery 2009;29(5):379–84.

16. Lanzetta M. Scaphoid reconstruction by a free vascularized osteochondral graft from the rib: a case report. Microsurgery 2009;29(5):420–4.

17. Sawaizumi T, Nanno M, Nanbu A, Ito H. Vascularised bone graft from the base of the second metacarpal for refractory nonunion of the scaphoid. J Bone Joint Surg Br 2004;86(7):1007–12.

18. Thompson NW, Kapoor A, Thomas J, Hayton MJ. The use of a vascularised periosteal patch onlay graft in the management of nonunion of the proximal scaphoid. J Bone Joint Surg Br 2008;90(12):1597–601.

19. Ribak S, Medina CE, Mattar R, Jr., Ulson HJ, de Resende MR, Etchebehere M. Treatment of scaphoid nonunion with vascularised and nonvascularised dorsal bone grafting from the distal radius. Int Orthop 2010;34(5):683–8.

20. Merrell GA, Wolfe SW, Slade JF, 3rd. Treatment of scaphoid nonunions: quantitative meta-analysis of the literature. J Hand Surg Am 2002;27(4):685–91.

21. Munk B, Larsen CF. Bone grafting the scaphoid nonunion: a systematic review of 147 publications including 5,246 cases of scaphoid nonunion. Acta Orthop Scand 2004;75(5):618–29.

22. Jones DB, Jr., Burger H, Bishop AT, Shin AY. Treatment of scaphoid waist nonunions with an avascular proximal pole and carpal collapse. Surgical technique. J Bone Joint Surg Am 2009;91 Suppl 2:169–83.

23. Jones DB Jr BH, Bishop AT, Shin AY. Treatment of scaphoid waist nonunions with an avascular proximal pole and carpal collapse. A comparison of two vascularized bone grafts. J Bone Joint Surg Am 2008;90:2616–25.

24. Akmaz I, Kiral A, Pehlivan O, Mahirogullari M, Solakoglu C, Rodop O. Biodegradable implants in the treatment of scaphoid nonunions. Int Orthop 2004;28(5):261–6.

25. Amadio PC, Berquist TH, Smith DK, Ilstrup DM, Cooney WP, 3rd, Linscheid RL. Scaphoid malunion. J Hand Surg Am 1989;14(4):679–87.

26. Dabezies EJ MR, Faust DC. Injuries to the carpus: Fractures of the scaphoid. Orthopedics 1982;5:1510–15.

27. Leslie IJ, Dickson RA. The fractured carpal scaphoid. Natural history and factors influencing outcome. J Bone Joint Surg Br 1981;63(2):225–30.

28. Szabo RM, Manske D. Displaced fractures of the scaphoid. Clin Orthop Relat Res 1988;230:30–8.
29. Eddeland A, Eiken O, Hellgren E, Ohlsson NM. Fractures of the scaphoid. Scand J Plast Reconstr Surg 1975;9(3):234–9.
30. Langhoff O, Andersen JL. Consequences of late immobilization of scaphoid fractures. J Hand Surg Br 1988;13(1):77–9.
31. Dinah AF, Vickers RH. Smoking increases failure rate of operation for established non-union of the scaphoid bone. Int Orthop 2007;31(4):503–5.
32. Steinmann SP, Adams JE. Scaphoid fractures and nonunions: diagnosis and treatment. J Orthop Sci 2006;11(4):424–31.
33. Pounder NM, Harrison AJ. Low intensity pulsed ultrasound for fracture healing: a review of the clinical evidence and the associated biological mechanism of action. Ultrasonics 2008;48(4):330–8.
34. Nolte PA, van der Krans A, Patka P, Janssen IM, Ryaby JP, Albers GH. Low-intensity pulsed ultrasound in the treatment of nonunions. J Trauma 2001;51(4):693–702; discussion -3.
35. Ricardo M. The effect of ultrasound on the healing of muscle-pediculated bone graft in scaphoid non-union. Int Orthop 2006;30(2):123–7.
36. Punt BJ dHP, Fontijine WPJ. Pulsed electromagnetic field in the treatment of non-union. Eur J Orthop Surg Traumatol 2008;18:127–33.
37. Adams BD, Frykman GK, Taleisnik J. Treatment of scaphoid nonunion with casting and pulsed electromagnetic fields: a study continuation. J Hand Surg Am 1992;17(5):910–4.
38. Dacho AK, Baumeister S, Germann G, Sauerbier M. Comparison of proximal row carpectomy and midcarpal arthrodesis for the treatment of scaphoid nonunion advanced collapse (SNAC-wrist) and scapholunate advanced collapse (SLAC-wrist) in stage II. J Plast Reconstr Aesthet Surg 2008;61(10):1210–18.
39. Dacho A, Grundel J, Holle G, Germann G, Sauerbier M. Long-term results of midcarpal arthrodesis in the treatment of scaphoid nonunion advanced collapse (SNAC-Wrist) and scapholunate advanced collapse (SLAC-Wrist). Ann Plast Surg 2006;56(2):139–44.
40. Mulford JS, Ceulemans LJ, Nam D, Axelrod TS. Proximal row carpectomy vs four corner fusion for scapholunate (Slac) or scaphoid nonunion advanced collapse (Snac) wrists: a systematic review of outcomes. J Hand Surg Eur 2009;34(2):256–63.
41. Wyrick JD, Stern PJ, Kiefhaber TR. Motion-preserving procedures in the treatment of scapholunate advanced collapse wrist: proximal row carpectomy versus four-corner arthrodesis. J Hand Surg Am 1995;20(6):965–70.
42. DiDonna ML, Kiefhaber TR, Stern PJ. Proximal row carpectomy: study with a minimum of ten years of follow-up. J Bone Joint Surg Am 2004;86(11):2359–65.
43. Espinoza D, Schertenleib P. Four-corner bone arthrodesis with dorsal rectangular plate: series and personal technique. J Hand Surg Eur 2009;34:609–13.
44. Rodgers JA, Holt G, Finnerty EP, Miller B. Scaphoid excision and limited wrist fusion: a comparison of K-wire and circular plate fixation. Hand (N Y) 2008;3(3):276–81.
45. Van Amerongen EA, Schuurman AH. Four-corner arthrodesis using the Quad memory staple. J Hand Surg Eur 2009;34(2):252–5.
46. Bedford B, Yang SS. High fusion rates with circular plate fixation for four-corner arthrodesis of the wrist. Clin Orthop Relat Res 2010;468(1):163–8.
47. Shindle MK, Burton KJ, Weiland AJ, Domb BG, Wolfe SW. Complications of circular plate fixation for four-corner arthrodesis. J Hand Surg Eur 2007;32(1):50–3.
48. Dias JJ. Definition of union after acute fracture and surgery for fracture non-union of the scaphoid. J Hand Surg 2001;26(4):321–5.

112 Trapeziometacarpal Arthritis of the Thumb

Anne Wajon[1], Emma Carr[2], Louise Ada[3], and Ian A. Edmunds[4]

[1]Macquarie Hand Therapy, Macquarie University, Sydney, NSW, Australia
[2]Pacific Hand Therapy Services, Dee Why, NSW, Australia
[3]University of Sydney, Sydney, NSW, Australia
[4]Hornsby Ku-ring-gai Hospital and Hornsby Hand Centre, Hornsby, NSW, Australia

Case scenario

A 58 year old woman presents with pain at the base of her right thumb. She is right hand dominant and reports pain and weakness when opening jars, writing, gardening, turning keys, and pulling up tights. She describes the pain as sharp when performing these tasks, but a dull ache at other times throughout the day.

Relevant anatomy

Arthritis at the base of the thumb affects the trapeziometacarpal joint in varying degrees. The trapeziometacarpal joint is a saddle-shaped joint at the base of the thumb and it is this shape that permits flexion/extension and abduction/adduction to be coupled and result in conjoint rotation. The articular surfaces offer little intrinsic constraint, so the joint relies on the constraint provided by an array of ligaments between the trapezium and the first metacarpal base. In osteoarthritis (OA), these ligaments become lax, resulting in altered wear patterns with loss of articular cartilage thickness, joint space narrowing, osteophyte formation, and joint subluxation.[1]

Importance of the problem

The major cause of pain and disability in Australians is arthritis,[2] affecting more than 3.85 million people. Similarly in the United States, arthritis is the most common cause of physical disability, affecting 46 million (22%) adults.[3] Further, it is estimated that 25% of adults aged over 18

years will have "doctor-diagnosed arthritis by the year 2030".[3] Considering that more than half of these people are of working age, the personal and socioeconomic costs are enormous. Since the incidence of OA increases with age [4,5] and the global population is rapidly aging, it is likely that the demand on health care and community resources for people with OA will increase dramatically over the coming decades.

OA at the base of the thumb is associated with pain, weakness, and difficulty with many activities of daily living. Radiological changes at the base of the thumb occur six times more commonly in women than men, and become more prevalent with increasing age affecting 34% of people aged 51–60, and 57% of those aged 61–70 who suffered a distal radius fracture.[6] Although only 30% of those with radiological changes report clinical symptoms,[4] the impact of arthritis on an aging population should not be underestimated.

Clinicians and patients are often confused by the vast amount of information about intervention for this common condition. There are over 5,000,00 hits on the Google website when the search term "thumb arthritis" is entered (May 2011). Further, with a rapidly aging population, the need to determine the most clinically and cost-effective intervention should be considered a priority.

Top five questions

Diagnosis

1. How do the radiological findings, history, and physical examination contribute to the diagnosis of trapeziometacarpal OA?

Evidence-Based Orthopedics, First Edition. Edited by Mohit Bhandari.
© 2012 Blackwell Publishing Ltd. Published 2012 by Blackwell Publishing Ltd.

Outcomes

2. What outcomes are considered important in determining the success of intervention?

Treatment

3. What conservative interventions are effective in relieving symptoms?
4. Which surgical interventions provide the best outcome?

Harm

5. Is any surgical procedure associated with less adverse effects than any other?

Question 1: How do the radiological findings, history and physical examination contribute to the diagnosis of trapeziometacarpal OA?

Case clarification

The radiograph demonstrates degenerative changes at the trapeziometacarpal joint, but the scapho-trapezio-trapezoidal joint is not affected. The physical examination reveals tenderness on palpation of joint margins, a positive grind test, and enlargement of the base of thumb.

Relevance

It is important to differentiate trapeziometacarpal OA from other common conditions affecting the radial side of the wrist and base of the thumb.

Current opinion

Current opinion suggests that the severity of trapeziometacarpal OA can be staged according to radiological changes. Considering that the correlation between the severity of symptoms and the extent of radiographic changes is not always clear, the history and physical examination are fundamental to confirming the diagnosis.

Finding the evidence

• Cochrane Database, CINAHL, MEDLINE, PubMed, using search terms: "carpometacarpal joint, trapeziometacarpal joint, arthritis, diagnosis"

Quality of the evidence

Level V
• 7 studies

Findings

The severity of radiological degeneration can be staged according to the staging system described by Eaton and Glickel (Table 112.1).[7] The system has moderate intra-rater reliability (0.66) and inter-rater reliability (0.53).[8] It is based

Table 112.1 Staging of trapeziometacarpal osteoarthritis[7]

Stage I	Articular contours normal
	Slight widening of the joint space
Stage II	Slight narrowing of the joint space
	Minimal sclerotic changes
	Joint debris <2 mm diameter
Stage III	Joint space markedly narrowed or obliterated
	Cystic changes, sclerotic bone, varying degrees of dorsal subluxation
	Joint debris >2 mm in diameter
	Scaphotrapezial joint appear normal
Stage IV	Complete deterioration of trapeziometacarpal joint, as in stage III
	Scaphotrapezial joint narrowed, with sclerotic and cystic changes apparent

on a true lateral radiograph and may be helpful in planning surgical treatment.

Historically, patients complain of pain which is aggravated by "sustained forceful use of the hand involving daily activities like brushing the teeth, sewing, turning a key or picking up a book."[9] The pain is generally located at the base of the thumb, more often on the volar aspect, and frequently radiating to the thenar eminence.[10]

Physical examination should begin with gentle movements of the thumb and palpation of the joint margins. Range of thumb motion may not be affected in the early stages of disease, but with advancing arthritis, osteophytes may "result in a dorsally fixed and subluxated joint that is adducted, with limited palmar abduction."[10] This commonly leads to compensatory hyperextension of the metacarpophalangeal joint, and the resulting "collapse" deformity[11] becomes fixed in advanced stages.

Provocative tests include the grind test,[12] which involves axial compression and rotation of the metacarpal on the trapezium in order to reproduce pain at the base of the thumb. The axial compression adduction test involves placing axial compression on the metacarpal as the subluxation is reduced.[10]

The history and physical examination will contribute to the process of differentiating the diagnosis of trapeziometacarpal OA from other causes,[13] including DeQuervain's tendinitis, scapholunate instability, scaphoid fracture, flexor carpi radialis tendinitis, scaphotrapeziotrapezoid arthritis, and trigger thumb, which are common conditions that can cause pain at the base of thumb and radial aspect of the wrist.

Recommendation

• Radiological findings, history, and physical examination are considered in the diagnosis of the severity of trapeziometacarpal OA [overall quality: moderate]

Question 2: What outcomes are considered important in determining the success of intervention?

Case clarification

Considering that the main complaint of our patient is pain, determining whether a particular intervention can achieve a reduction in pain will be of most importance. Further, she has a restriction of web space, weakness of pinch and grip strength, and difficulty with various activities of daily living.

Relevance

Identifying the outcomes of interest will assist when analyzing the evidence for various interventions.

Current opinion

Current opinion suggests that pain, range of motion, strength, and function are the outcomes of interest.

Finding the evidence

• Cochrane Database, CINAHL, MEDLINE, PubMed, using the search terms: "carpometacarpal joint, trapeziometacarpal joint, arthritis, outcome measures"

Quality of the evidence

Level Ia
• 1 study

Level IIc
• 3 studies

Findings

A report of the OMERACT (Outcome Measures in Rheumatoid Arthritis Clinical Trials) III conference[14] proposed that the following four domains should be evaluated in trials of hand OA: pain, physical function, patient global assessment, and joint imaging (for studies of 1 year or longer).

One review of 112 patients who had undergone trapeziectomy with ligament reconstruction and tendon interposition attempted to determine the optimal set of instruments for evaluating patient outcome.[15] This study identified that the SF-36, the Disabilities of the Arm, Shoulder and Hand Questionnaire (DASH) or Patient Rated Wrist Evaluation (PRWE), and a custom set of clinical parameters (including range of motion, strength, and assessment of deformity) were appropriate for assessment of basal thumb joint conditions. These findings are supported by an assessment of the validity of self-report measures of pain and disability for people following trapeziometacarpal joint arthroplasty.[16]

Recommendation

• Outcome measures should be patient-oriented and clinically relevant.[15] Evidence suggests they should include: pain, measured on a 10 cm visual analog scale (VAS); physical function, measured by the DASH or PRWHE; Patient Global Assessment, measured by SF-36; range of motion of palmar abduction, measured in degrees; strength, both grip and lateral pinch, measured in kilograms; and adverse effects [overall quality: moderate]

Question 3: What conservative interventions are effective in relieving symptoms?

Case clarification

The patient complains of pain with a variety of activities of daily living. She also presents with tenderness and inflammation at the trapeziometacarpal joint. Clinical experience suggests various conservative interventions exist, but it is important to determine which interventions are effective for her from current evidence.

Relevance

Clinicians need to select an appropriate intervention, which is likely to reduce pain and improve function in people with trapeziometacarpal OA.

Current opinion

Current opinion suggests that people with arthritis at the base of the thumb will gain benefit from splinting, education regarding joint protection strategies, heat, and gentle exercise. However, there is confusion as to whether any additional benefit is likely to be gained from glucosamine therapy or corticosteroid injections.

Finding the evidence

• Cochrane Database, CINAHL, MEDLINE, PubMed, with search terms; "carpometacarpal joint, trapeziometacarpal joint, arthritis, splinting, glucosamine, intervention, injections, exercise, joint protection"

Quality of the evidence

Level I
• 6 studies

Level II
• 9 studies

Findings

Splinting One randomized trial compared the short opponens splint with no splint[17] in patients with stage II–IV

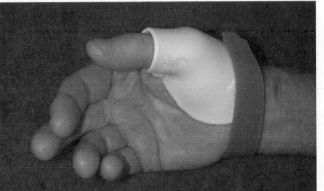

Figure 112.1 Short opponens splint.

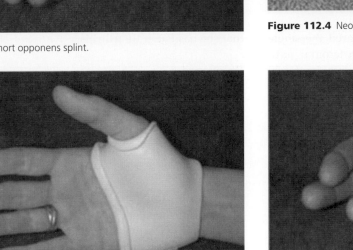

Figure 112.2 Thumb trapeziometacarpal immobilization splint.

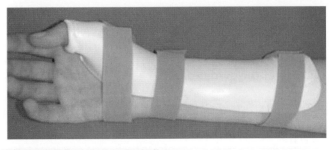

Figure 112.3 Long opponens splint.

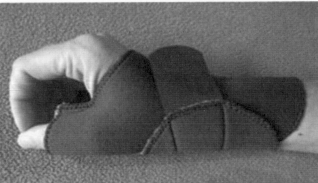

Figure 112.4 Neoprene thumb support.

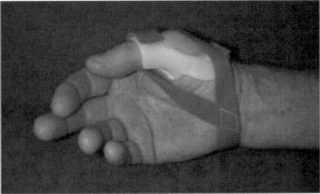

Figure 112.5 Three-point thumb splint.

One crossover trial compared the trapeziometacarpal immobilization splint with a prefabricated neoprene splint (Figure 112.4) in stage I and II trapeziometacarpal OA.[20] After 1 week, the neoprene splint group had 1.3 mm less pain (p = 0.02) but no more strength than the immobilization splint.

One randomized trial compared the short opponens splint with a three-point thumb strap splint (Figure 112.5)[21] in stage I–III trapeziometacarpal OA.[22] After 6 weeks, there was no difference between groups in pain, strength or hand function.

Joint protection and exercise One randomized trial compared joint protection advice and a home exercise program to an information session for patients with trapeziometacarpal OA.[23] After 3 months, 45% more of the joint protection and home exercise group (p < 0.05) improved in hand function compared with the information session group.

Glucosamine One systematic review of 25 randomized trials with 4963 participants compared glucosamine with placebo intervention for the treatment of OA.[24] The glucosamine group had 22% reduction in pain (SMD –0.47;

trapeziometacarpal OA. After 1 month, there was no difference between groups in pain or hand function. After wearing a short opponens splint (Figure 112.1) at night for a further 11 months, the splint group had 14 mm (95% CI 5–23 mm) less pain on the VAS and 6 points (out of 90) (95% CI 2–11) better hand function than the no-splint group.

One crossover trial[18] compared the trapeziometacarpal immobilization splint (Figure 112.2)[19] with a long opponens splint (Figure 112.3) in stage I–IV trapeziometacarpal OA. After 2 weeks, there was no difference between groups in pain or strength.

95% CI −0.72 to −0.23) and 11% improvement in function (SMD −0.47; 95% CI −0.82 to −0.12) compared with no intervention. However, if analysis was restricted to trials with adequate allocation concealment, there was no difference in groups in pain or hand function.

Stinging nettle One crossover trial compared rubbing the leaf of a common stinging nettle over the base of the thumb[25] with a placebo. After 1 week, the stinging nettle group had 15 mm less pain (p = 0.03) and 0.2 points less disability on the Stanford Health Assessment Questionnaire for disability (p < 0.01).

Leech therapy One randomized trial compared the single application of 2–3 leeches[26] with a nonsteroidal anti-inflammatory drug (diclofenac) applied twice a day for 30 days in patients with trapeziometacarpal OA. After 2 months, the leech group had 34 mm (95% CI 20–48) less pain than the nonsteroidal group.

Corticosteroid injections One randomized trial compared corticosteroid injections with placebo intervention[17] in patients with trapeziometacarpal OA. After 24 weeks, there was no difference between groups in pain or hand function.

Hyaluronate injections One randomized trial compared intra-articular Hylan injections with placebo[27] in patients with trapeziometacarpal OA. Two other randomized trials compared intra-articular Hylan injections with corticosteroid injections and placebo[28,29] in patients with trapeziometacarpal OA. After 6 months, there was no difference between groups in pain or strength.

Recommendations

• Splinting the thumb in a short opponens splint at night for 12 months will reduce pain [overall quality: moderate]
• There is no difference in the improvement in pain, strength, or hand function with either a long opponens splint, a thumb trapeziometacarpal immobilization splint, a three-point splint, or a neoprene splint [overall quality: low]
• Joint protection and home hand exercises provide significant improvements in both grip strength and function in patients with hand OA [overall quality: moderate]
• There is no evidence for the use of glucosamine in the management of trapeziometacarpal OA [overall quality: moderate]
• Stinging nettle provides effective pain relief but can be associated with skin irritations including rash and itchiness [overall quality: moderate]
• Leech therapy is more effective than topical nonsteroidal anti-inflammatory drugs for reducing pain [overall quality: moderate]

• There is no evidence that intra-articular injection with hyaluronate or corticosteroids improves outcomes more than placebo [overall quality: moderate]

Question 4: Which surgical interventions provide the best outcome?

Case clarification
The patient achieved substantial symptomatic relief with conservative interventions for a period of 3 years, but now finds the symptoms unresponsive to splinting and joint protection strategies. She has been referred to a hand surgeon, who identifies that the grind test is positive and that she has Eaton III arthritis.[7]

Relevance
It is important to consider the patient's vocational demands, interests, and hobbies along with the severity of her arthritis when considering appropriate surgical options. Removing the arthritic trapezium is likely to relieve her pain, but current opinion about the necessary reconstructive approaches differs greatly amongst hand surgeons.

Current opinion
Current opinion regarding the best surgical intervention for this patient is widely diversified. The two most common procedures are simple trapeziectomy and trapeziectomy with ligament reconstruction and tendon interposition (LRTI).

Finding the evidence
• Cochrane Database, CINAHL, MEDLINE, PubMed, with search terms "carpometacarpal joint" OR "trapeziometacarpal joint" AND "arthritis" AND "surgery"

Quality of the evidence
Level I
• 11 studies

Level II
• 1 study

Findings
One systematic review of 18 comparative studies and 8 reviews[30] was unable to perform statistical pooling due to heterogeneity of population, intervention, and outcomes. However, it alerted hand surgeons that LRTI may not be the best option available. The review was unable to draw any conclusions about superiority of any one procedure over another.

One systematic review of 9 randomized trials with 477 participants[31] compared 7 surgical procedures: trapeziectomy with LRTI was compared to trapeziectomy by Belcher,[32] Davis,[33] De Smet,[34] and Field[35]; to trapeziectomy

Study or Subgroup	T and LRTI		T		Weight	Risk Ratio M-H, Random, 95% CI	Risk Ratio M-H, Random, 95% CI
	Events	Total	Events	Total			
Belcher 2000	6	23	2	19	18.2%	2.48 [0.56, 10.89]	
Davis 2004a	19	62	9	62	40.3%	2.11 [1.04, 4.30]	
Davis 2009	8	61	13	67	36.4%	0.68 [0.30, 1.52]	
Field 2007	1	33	0	32	5.1%	2.91 [0.12, 68.95]	
Total (95% CI)		**179**		**180**	**100.0%**	**1.46 [0.69, 3.08]**	
Total events	34		24				

Heterogeneity: Tau^2 = 0.23; Chi^2 = 5.17, df = 3 (P = 0.16); I^2 = 42%
Test for overall effect: Z = 0.99 (P = 0.32)

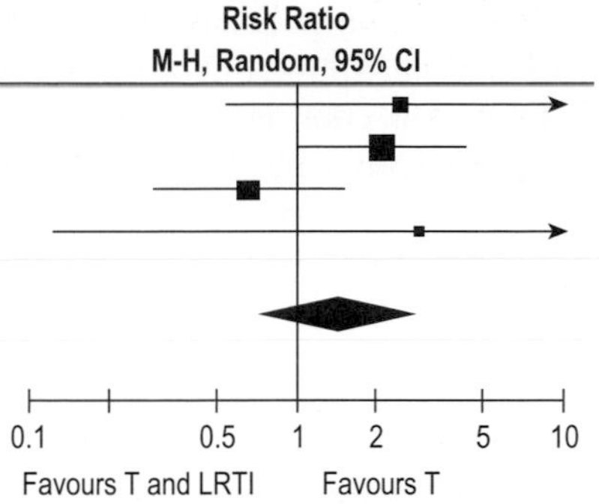

0.1   0.5   1   2   5   10
Favours T and LRTI   Favours T

Figure 112.6 Comparison of adverse effects between trapeziectomy with LRTI and trapeziectomy.

with ligament reconstruction by Gerwin[36] and Kriegs-Au;[37] to trapeziectomy and interpositional arthroplasty by Davis 2004;[33] to Artelon joint resurfacing by Nilsson;[38] to arthrodesis by Hart;[39] and trapeziectomy with interpositional arthroplasty was compared to joint replacement (Swanson) surgery by Tagil[40] and to trapeziectomy by Davis.[33] The review failed to identify any additional benefit of one procedure over another in terms of pain, physical function, patient global assessment, range of motion, or strength.

One randomized trial compared trapeziectomy with LRTI (and K-wire fixation) vs. a simple trapeziectomy.[41] After 12 months, there was no difference in outcomes of pain, hand function, range of motion, or strength.

Recommendation

• That there is no additional benefit of one surgical procedure over another in terms of pain, physical function, global assessment, range of motion, or strength [overall quality: high]

Question 5: Is any surgical procedure associated with fewer adverse effects than any other?

Case clarification

The patient intends to undergo trapeziectomy with LRTI for her stage III trapeziometacarpal OA. She is concerned about potential adverse effects.

Relevance

Various adverse effects have been reported in the literature following surgery for trapeziometacarpal OA, including persistent pain, weakness, scar tenderness and adhesion, and complex regional pain syndrome.

Current opinion

Current opinion suggests that there is no appreciable difference in the frequency or severity of adverse effects between the various procedures.

Finding the evidence

• See Question 4.

Quality of the evidence

Level I

• 1 study

Level II

• 1 study

Findings

One systematic review of 9 randomized trials with 477 participants[31] compared 7 surgical procedures. There were significantly more adverse effects following trapeziectomy with LRTI than the simple trapeziectomy group (RR 2.20, 95% CI 1.17–4.12, random effects p = 0.01). However, when the recent study by Davis et al.[41] is incorporated into the systematic review, the difference in adverse effects between trapeziectomy with LRTI and trapeziectomy is no longer significant (RR 1.46, 95% CI 0.69–3.08, random effects p = 0.32, Figure 112.6).

Recommendation

• There is no difference in the incidence of adverse effects between trapeziectomy with LRTI (19%) and a simple trapeziectomy (13%) [overall quality: moderate]

Summary of recommendations

• Radiological findings, history and physical examination are considered in the diagnosis of the severity of trapeziometacarpal OA
• Outcome measures should be patient-oriented and clinically relevant. Evidence suggests they should include pain, measured on a 10 cm VAS; physical function, measured by the DASH or PRWHE; Patient Global Assessment, measured by SF-36; range of motion of palmar abduction, measured in degrees; strength, both grip and lateral pinch, measured in kilograms; adverse effects
• Splinting the thumb in a short opponens splint at night for 12 months will reduce pain
• There is no difference in the improvement in pain, strength, or hand function with either a long opponens

splint, a thumb trapeziometacarpal immobilization splint, a three-point splint, or a neoprene splint

- Joint protection and home hand exercises provide significant improvements in both grip strength and function in patients with hand OA
- There is no evidence for glucosamine in the management of trapeziometacarpal OA
- Stinging nettle provides effective pain relief but can be associated with skin irritations including rash and itchiness
- Leech therapy is more effective than topical nonsteroidal anti-inflammatory drugs for reducing pain and improving strength
- There is no evidence that intra-articular injection with hyaluronate or corticosteroids improves outcomes more than placebo
- There is no additional benefit of one surgical procedure over another in terms of pain, physical function, global assessment, range of motion, or strength
- There is no difference in the incidence of adverse effects between trapeziectomy with LRTI and a simple trapeziectomy

Conclusions

Arthritis at the base of the thumb is common, and may be considered a normal part of the aging process.[6] Symptoms include pain and inflammation at the base of the thumb, with loss of strength, motion and function developing with advancing disease.

There are many conservative intervention approaches, but those frequently used include splinting, joint protection advice, and exercise. Failure of conservative intervention, with persistent pain and disability, may lead patients to consider surgical options. Many surgical options exist, but there is currently no evidence to suggest superiority or inferiority of one over the other.

References

1. Ateshian G, Ark J, Rosenwasser M, Pawluk R, Soslowsky L, Mow V. Contact areas in the thumb carpometacarpal joint. J Orthop Res 1995;13:450–8.
2. Jones G, Cahill A, McQuade J, Coleman S, Bennett J. Painful realities: The Economic Impact of Arthritis in Australia in 2007. Access Economics, 2007.
3. Centers for Disease Control and Prevention: Arthritis—Data and Statistics 2007 [cited 2009 November 4]; Available from: http://www.cdc.gov/arthritis/data_statistics.htm.
4. Armstrong A, Hunter J, Davis T. The prevalence of degenerative arthritis of the base of the thumb in post-menopausal women. J Hand Surg Br 1994;19(3):340–1.
5. Haara M, Heliovaara M, Kroger H, et al. Osteoarthritis in the carpometacarpal joint of the thumb. Prevalence and associations with disability and mortality. J Bone Joint Surg Am 2004;86(7):1452–7.
6. Sodha S, Ring D, Zurakowski D, Jupiter J. Prevalence of osteoarthrosis of the trapeziometacarpal joint. J Bone Joint Surg Am 2005;87(12):2614–18.
7. Eaton RG, Glickel SZ. Trapeziometacarpal osteoarthritis. Staging as a rationale for treatment. Hand Clin 1987;3(4):455–71.
8. Kubik N, Lubahn J. Intrarater and interrater reliability of the Eaton classification of basal joint arthritis. J Hand Surg Am 2002;27(5):882–5.
9. Pellegrini V. Osteoarthritis and injury at the base of the human thumb. Survival of the fittest? Clin Orthop Relat Res 2005;438:266–76.
10. Ghavami A, Oishi S. Thumb trapeziometacarpal arthritis: treatment with ligament reconstruction tendon interposition arthroplasty. Plast Reconstr Surg 2006;117:116e–28e.
11. Tubiana R, Thomine J-M, Mackin E. Examination of the Hand and Wrist, 2nd edn. Martin Dunitz, London, 1996.
12. Poole J, Pellegrini V. Arthritis of the thumb basal joint complex. J Hand Ther 2000;13(2):91–107.
13. Prosser R, Conolly WB. Rehabilitation of the Hand and Upper Limb. Butterworth-Heinemann, London, 2003.
14. Bellamy N, Kirwan J, Boers M, et al. Recommendations for a core set of outcome measures for future Phase III clinical trials in knee, hip and hand osteoarthritis. Consensus development of OMERACT III. J Rheumatol 1997;24(4):799–802.
15. Angst F, John M, Goldhahn J, et al. Comprehensive assessment of clinical outcome and quality of life after resection interposition arthroplasty of the thumb saddle joint. Arthritis Rheum 2005;53(2):205–13.
16. MacDermid J, Wessel J, Humphrey R, Ross D, Roth J. Validity of self-report measures of pain and disability for persons who have undergone arthroplasty for psteoarthritis of the carpometacarpal joint of the hand. Osteoarthritis Cartil 2007;15(5):524–30.
17. Rannou F, Dimet J, Boutron I, et al. Splint for base-of-thumb osteoarthritis. Ann Intern Med 2009;150(10):661–9.
18. Weiss S, LaStayo P, Mills A, Bramlet D. Prospective analysis of splinting the first carpometacarpal joint: an objective, subjective, and radiographic assessment. J Hand Ther 2000;13(3):218–27.
19. Colditz J. The biomechanics of a thumb carpometacarpal immobilisation splint. J Hand Ther 2000;13(3):228–35.
20. Weiss S, LaStayo P, Mills A, Bramlet D. Splinting the degenerative basal joint: custom-made or prefabricated neoprene? J Hand Ther 2004;17:401–6.
21. Wajon A. The thumb strap splint for dynamic instability of the trapeziometacarpal joint. J Hand Ther 2000;13(3):236–7.
22. Wajon A, Ada L. No difference between two splint and exercise regimens for people with osteoarthritis of the thumb: a randomised controlled trial. Aust J Physiother 2005;51:245–9.
23. Stamm T, Machold P, Smolen J, Fischer S, Redlich K, Graninger W, et al. Joint protection and home hand exercises improve hand funciton in patients with hand osteoarthritis: a randomized controlled trial. Arthritis Care Res 2002;47:44–9.
24. Towheed T, Maxwell L, Anastassiades TP, et al. Glucosamine therapy for treating osteoarthritis. Cochrane Database Syst Rev 2005;2:CD002946.

25. Randall C, Randall H, Dobbs F, Hutton C, Sanders H. Randomized controlled trial of nettle sting for treatment of base-of-thumb pain. J Roy Soc Med 2000;93(6):305–9.

26. Michalsen A, Lüdtke R, Cesur Ö, et al. Effectiveness of leech therapy in women with symptomatic arthrosis of the first carpometacarpal joint: a randomized controlled trial. Pain 2008; 137:452–9.

27. Figen A, Ustun N. The evaluation of efficacy and tolerability of Hylan G-F 20 in bilateral thumb base osteoarthritis: 6 months follow-up. Clin Rheumatol 2009;28(5):535–41.

28. Stahl S, Karsh-Zafrir I, Ratzon N, Rosenberg N. Comparison of intraarticular injection of depot corticosteroid and hyaluronic acid for treatment of degenerative trapeziometacarpal joints. J Clin Rheumatol 2005;11(6):299–302.

29. Heyworth B, Lee J, Kim P, Lipton C, Strauch R, Rosenwasser M. Hylan versus corticosteroid versus placebo for treatment of basal joint arthritis: a prospective, randomized, double-blinded clinical trial. J Hand Surg 2008;33(1):40–8.

30. Martou G, Veltri K, Thoma A. Surgical treatment of osteoarthritis of the carpometacarpal joint of the thumb: a systematic review. Plast Reconstr Surg 2004;114:421–32.

31. Wajon A, Carr E, Edmunds I, Ada L. Surgery for thumb (trapeziometacarpal joint) osteoarthritis. Cochrane Database Syst Rev 2009;4:CD004631.

32. Belcher H, Nicholl J. A comparison of trapeziectomy with and without ligament reconstruction and tendon interposition. J Hand Surg Br 2000;25(4):350–6.

33. Davis T, Brady O, Dias J. Excision of the trapezium for osteoarthritis of the trapeziometacarpal joint: a study of the benefit of ligament reconstruction or tendon interposition. J Hand Surg 2004;29(6):1069–77.

34. De Smet L, Sioen W, Spaepen D, van Ransbeeck H. Treatment of basal joint arthritis of the thumb: trapeziectomy with or without tendon interposition/ligament reconstruction. Hand Surg 2004;9(1):5–9.

35. Field J, Buchanan D. To suspend or not to suspend: a randomised single blind trial of simple trapeziectomy versus trapeziectomy and flexor carpi radialis suspension. J Hand Surg Am 2007; 32(4):462–6.

36. Gerwin M, Griffith A, Weiland A, Hotchkiss R, McCormack R. Ligament reconstruction basal joint arthroplasty without tendon interposition. Clin Orthop Relat Res 1997;342:42–5.

37. Kriegs-Au G, Petje G, Fojtl E, Ganger R, Zachs I. Ligament reconstruction with or without tendon interposition to treat primary thumb carpometacarpal osteoarthritis: a prospective randomized study. J Bone Joint Surg Am 2004;86(2):209–18.

38. Nilsson A, Liljensten E, Bergstrom C, Sollerman C. Results from a degradable TMC joint Spacer (Artelon) compared with tendon arthroplasty. J Hand Surg Am 2005;30(2):380–9.

39. Hart R, Janecek M, Siska V, Kucera B, Stipcak V. Interposition suspension arthroplasty according to Epping versus arthrodesis for trapeziometarpal osteoarthritis. Eur Surg 2006;38(6):433–8.

40. Tagil M, Kopylov P. Swanson versus APL arthroplasty in the treatment of osteoarthritis of the trapeziometacarpal joint: a prospective and randomized study in 26 patients. J Hand Surg Br 2002;27(5):452–6.

41. Davis T, Pace A. Trapeziectomy for trapezieometacarpal joint osteoarthritis: is ligament reconstruction and temporary stabilisation of the pseuarthrosis with a Kirschner wire important? J Hand Surg Eur 2009;34(3):313–21.

113 Salvage Procedures for the Treatment of Wrists with Scapholunate Advanced Collapse

Jonathan Mulford[1], Paul K. Della Torre[2], and Stuart J.D. Myers[1]

[1]Prince of Wales Hospital, Sydney, NSW, Australia
[2]Concord Hospital, Concord, NSW, Australia

Case scenario

A 45 year old manual worker presents with increasing dorso-radial wrist pain, loss of range of motion (ROM), intermittent swelling, and clicking of the wrist. He had sustained an injury to the wrist 15 years ago, after falling on to an outstretched hand while snowboarding. At the time of the injury he was told he had a wrist "sprain" and the radiographs were "normal". His pain is now impacting on his ability to work. His radiographs show he has a scapholunate advanced collapse (SLAC) wrist (Figure 113.1).

Relevant anatomy

The scapholunate ligament (SL) is a C-shaped intrinsic ligament. The dorsal aspect is the most important for stability. The secondary stabilizers of the scapholunate joint include the dorsal radiocarpal ligament (DRC), the dorsal intercarpal ligament (DIC), and the volar capsule of the scapho-trapezium-trapezoid (STT) joint.[1]

If the SL ligament is ruptured, the scaphoid tends to flex and the lunate extends. There is dorsoradial subluxation of the scaphoid which increases the stresses on the dorsal and lateral aspect of the scaphoid fossa of the radius. In time this results in wear of the articular surface and secondary osteoarthritis (OA).[2]

Importance of the problem

The true prevalence of scapholunate (SL) rupture is not known,[3] as the diagnosis is commonly missed. The natural history is well documented. Not all patients become symptomatic enough to warrant surgical intervention.

The full impact of the rupture may not become apparent for years until the patient develops pain from secondary OA. The consequences can be profound for manual workers. A typical patient with SLAC wrist presents in the fourth decade and has expectations of being in the work force for a further 20 years.

Rupture of the SL ligament in combination with one of the secondary stabilizers gives rise to a gap (diastasis) of 3 mm or more, between the scaphoid and lunate.[4,5] In addition, the scaphoid flexes and may sublux dorsally. This alters the wrist biomechanics and eventually results in secondary OA. This pattern of arthritis is called a SLAC wrist. The wrist arthritis develops in a particular distribution. The radial styloid is affected first followed by the radioscaphoid joint and then the midcarpal joint (capitolunate joint).[2,6] The radiolunate joint is last to be affected.

There are various salvage options for the treatment of a symptomatic SLAC wrist. These include motion-preserving procedures (proximal row carpectomy and four-corner fusion) or a complete wrist fusion (see box).

Evidence-Based Orthopedics, First Edition. Edited by Mohit Bhandari.
© 2012 Blackwell Publishing Ltd. Published 2012 by Blackwell Publishing Ltd.

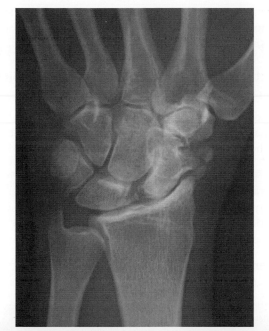

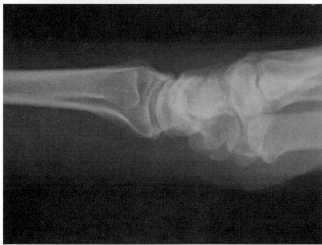

Figure 113.1 Radiographs of SLAC wrist: (a) AP and (b) lateral.

Definitions used in this chapter

- *SLAC wrist:* Arthritis of the wrist secondary to scapholunate dissociation
- *Salvage procedure:* A motion-preserving procedure performed when reconstructive procedure is contraindicated due to OA
- *Proximal row carpectomy (PRC):* Surgical procedure to remove the scaphoid, lunate, and triquetrum
- *Four-corner fusion (4CF):* Surgical procedure to remove the scaphoid and arthrodesis of the lunate, capitate, triquetrum, and hamate

Top nine questions

Diagnosis

1. What are the radiological findings that characterize SLAC?
2. What is the natural history of scapholunate rupture and SLAC?

Therapy

3. What are the motion-preserving salvage procedure options?

Prognosis

4. What is the grip strength that can be expected after a salvage procedure?
5. What is the ROM that can be expected from each procedure?
6. What pain relief can be expected after each procedure?
7. What are the subjective outcomes for each procedure?

Harm

8. What are the postoperative complications for each procedure?
9. How many patients have progression of OA after having a salvage procedure?

Finding the evidence

A systematic review was undertaken to clarify controversies regarding which procedure has the best outcome.

Articles were sourced from MEDLINE (1966–2009), Embase (1980–2009), CINAHL, and the Cochrane Controlled Trials Register electronic databases. The search was undertaken using the terms "proximal row carpectomy," "PRC," "midcarpal fusion," "four-corner fusion," "carpal instability," "scapholunate advanced collapse," "SLAC". All languages were included in the search.

The title and abstract of papers identified in the search were screened. Definite and possible articles identified by both reviewers were then retrieved for possible inclusion in the study based on predetermined inclusion and exclusion criteria. Further search was also conducted (see below).

Inclusion criteria when reviewing articles

1. Original articles including patients with SLAC wrists treated with PRC or 4CF

2. Articles which reported on one or more of the primary outcomes: ROM, grip strength, pain score, physician or patient reported outcomes, and postoperative complication

Exclusion criteria when reviewing articles

1. Articles which did not document the underlying aetiology and/or minimum length of patient follow-up
2. Studies with less than 12 months of patient follow-up
3. Duplicate publication of any type, e.g., abstracts, comments, review or technique articles, duplicate reports, and articles based on preliminary data from larger series
4. Studies that included diagnoses other than SLAC, e.g., Kienbock's, Preiser's disease, scaphoid nonunion advanced collapse (SNAC), where SLAC data was not extractable. If this was not possible, studies were only included if SLAC patients comprised at least 70% of the patients in the series.

Additional search strategies

1. References from review articles found in the search, major orthopaedic/hand textbooks,[7–9] and primary articles were checked to identify any additional articles not located in the original search
2. A manual search of the table of contents of the *Journal of Hand Surgery* (American, British and European) was performed, including reviewing published abstracts from European or North American hand meetings

Quality of the evidence

Caution is needed when interpreting the results in this evidence-based review. The level of evidence is low. All articles included in the systematic review were observational studies. The majority were retrospective case series. Three articles[10–12] compared data for PRC to 4CF in a retrospective case series. Six articles reported outcomes on 4CF[10–15] and eight on PRC.[10–12,16–20] One systematic review has looked at outcomes of PRC and 4CF for SLAC and SNAC wrists;[21] however, no distinction was made between SLAC and SNAC.

In order to draw conclusions regarding outcomes for PRC and 4CF, weighted averages were calculated, which were based on the number of patients in each study. A meta-analysis to compare the procedure outcomes was not performed due to expected heterogeneity between studies, varying methodology, and lack of randomization and direct comparative results.

None of the studies has a randomization process to limit bias. Heterogeneity between studies, quality of studies, bias within studies, and publication bias are likely to affect the measured outcomes and thus any summarized outcome. Observational studies are likely to distort the magnitude

or direction of associations in outcomes. Few studies reported 95% confidence intervals (CI) or standard deviations (SD).

Question 1: What are the radiological findings that characterize SLAC?

Case clarification
This patient's radiographs show a diastasis of the SL interval. There is OA in the radiocarpal joint and no midcarpal OA.

Relevance
Imaging is important (1) to confirm there is a SL rupture, (2) to determine if OA is present, and (3) to stage the SLAC wrist, particularly if there is midcarpal involvement.

Current opinion
Signs of SL rupture on a radiograph are listed in the box.

Radiographic signs of SL rupture
• Scapholunate joint space (Terry-Thomas sign)[22–24] • "Scaphoid ring" sign[25] • "Ring pole" sign[26] • Lack of parallelism[27,28] • Increased SL angle[29,30] • Taleisnik's "V" sign[31]

Signs of OA include osteophyte formation and joint space narrowing. The SLAC wrist can be classified radiographically depending on the areas of OA involved (see box).

Radiographic staging system for SLAC [2]
• *Stage 1:* Isolated radial styloid–scaphoid impingement • *Stage 2:* Complete radial styloid OA • *Stage 3:* Midcarpal arthritis

Quality of the evidence
The radiographic signs of a SLAC wrist are based on observational studies.

Recommendation
• Observational studies have provided the evidence for the radiological findings for a SLAC wrist [overall quality: low]

Question 2: What is the natural history of scapholunate rupture and SLAC?

Case clarification
This patient has a classical natural history of progression from SL rupture to SLAC over a 10–20 year period.

Table 113.1 Summary of demographics

	No. of articles	N wrists operated	Av. age	Male:female (%)	Av. follow-up (months)
4CF	6	91	49	85:15	36
PRC	8	134	45	74:26	56

4CF, four corner fusion; PRC, proximal row carpectomy.

Relevance

Although an untreated SL rupture classically progresses to secondary arthritis, not all patients become symptomatic and some may never present.[2,6,32,33]

Current opinion

Surgery should be reserved for symptomatic patients.

Quality of the evidence

Evidence on the natural history of SL rupture is based on observational studies.[32,33] Eight articles give outcomes on PRC and six for 4CF.

Findings

Table 113.1 summarizes the demographic features of patients in those articles that report outcomes of PRC and 4CF.

Recommendation

• Observational studies have provided the evidence for the natural history of scapholunate rupture and the most common patient is a 40 year old man [overall quality: low]

Question 3: What are the motion-preserving salvage procedure options?

Case clarification

Motion-preserving salvage procedures in this scenario include PRC and 4CF.

Relevance

Both PRC and 4CF can be used, as the midcarpal joint is maintained.

Current opinion

Advocates of 4CF claim that a better grip strength is achieved because the relative muscle length is preserved. There is a lower risk of progressive arthritis because the radiolunate joint is preserved and therefore the force per unit area is reduced.

Advocates of PRC claim the procedure is simple and lacks the complications associated with hardware and nonunion.

Quality of the evidence

There are no randomized trials. There are three comparative papers, eight papers reporting outcomes of PRC, and six for 4CF.

Findings

Both PRC and 4CF are management options. The evidence regarding the outcomes for each procedure is reviewed below.

Recommendations

• Salvage procedures for symptomatic SLAC wrists can give good outcomes. The choice between PRC and 4CF depends on patient and surgeon factors:
  ◦ Patient factors include (a) general factors such as age, occupation, specific risks for nonunion, and expectations; (b) specific wrist factors such as the presence of midcarpal OA
  ◦ Surgeon factors include familiarity with the technique
  ◦ [Overall Quality: Low]

Question 4: What is the grip strength that can be expected after a salvage procedure?

Case clarification

The patient is a manual worker and would prefer a procedure that provides the best opportunity to maintain his strength.

Relevance

Patients want to maintain or improve their grip strength.

Current opinion

Advocates of 4CF argue this salvage procedure gives better grip strength as there is less skeletal shortening.

Quality of the evidence

There are eight articles giving grip strength outcomes for PRC and five for 4CF. Three articles give a comparison.

Findings

It is not appropriate to perform a meta-analysis on the data available. The weighted mean for grip strength was 73%

(56% preoperatively) for 4CF compared to 77% (60% preoperatively) for PRC.

A systematic review of PRC and 4CF for SLAC and SNAC wrists also showed comparable grip strength outcomes for both procedures.[21]

Recommendation

• The grip strength is comparable following either a PRC or 4CF. It has been shown to be approximately 75% of the contralateral side [overall quality: low]

Question 5: What is the ROM that can be expected from each procedure?

Case clarification
This patient would prefer to maximize his ROM.

Relevance
ROM, measured in flexion/extension (F-E) and radial/ulnar (R-U) axis, may be an important consideration depending on the patient's individual circumstances.

Current opinion
PRC gives better ROM than 4CF.

Quality of the evidence
There were substantive ROM data sets in three articles for 4CF and six for PRC.

Findings
There is no major difference in the ROM between the two procedures (Table 113.2).

Recommendation
• The ROM achieved is similar after both procedures and usually slightly less than the preoperative measurement [overall quality: low]

Question 6: What pain relief can be expected after each procedure ?

Clinical clarification
Pain is one of the patient's major complaints.

Table 113.2 Weighted mean ROM for PRC and 4CF

	DF (pre)	DF (post)	PF (pre)	PF (post)	RD (pre)	RD (post)	UD (pre)	UD (post)
4CF	39	35	40	34	11	17	23	22
PRC	35	36	36	34	13	10	20	21

4CF, four corner fusion; DF, dorsiflexion; PF, palmar flexion; PRC, proximal row carpectomy; RD, radial deviation; UD, ulnar deviation.

Relevance
Provision of ongoing improvement in pain is the main indication for performing a salvage procedure.

Current opinion
Both procedures give good pain relief.

Quality of the evidence
There are seven articles reporting pain outcomes for PRC and four for 4CF. Varying pain scores are utilized in different publications. Subjective scores were divided into "good pain outcome" (e.g., reported as excellent, good, satisfied) or "poor pain outcome" (e.g., reported as moderate, poor, severe).

Findings
With 4CF 48 of 61 patients (79%) had good pain relief. With PRC 79 of 104 (76%) patients had good pain relief.

Recommendation
• Both salvage procedures give good pain relief in approximately 75% of patients [overall quality: low]

Question 7: What are the subjective outcomes for each procedure?

Clinical clarification
Patients prefer to know the likelihood that they will perceive that surgery has been successful.

Relevance
Patient subjective outcomes are arguably the most important measures when examining the success of an operation.

Current opinion
Both procedures give good subjective improvements.

Quality of the evidence
There are five articles with subjective outcomes for PRC and three for 4CF. Subjective outcome are reported differently in different publications. Scores were divided into "good outcome" (e.g., reported as excellent, good, satisfied, would have surgery again) or "poor outcome" (e.g., reported as moderate, poor, severe).

Findings
For PRC, 62 of 72 patients (86%) reported a satisfactory outcome. For 4CF, 32 of 38 patients (84%) reported satisfactory outcomes.

Recommendation
• The subjective outcomes are good, and similar for both salvage procedures [overall quality: low]

Table 113.3 Complications reported from all studies

	Total no. wrists	Convert to fusion	RSD	Sepsis	CTS	OA	Nonunion	Dorsal impingement	Hardware problem
4CF	91	2	0	2	6	0	4	0	8
PRC	134	7	0	0	1	25	0	0	2

4CF, four corner fusion; CTS, carpal tunnel syndrome; OA, osteoarthritis; PRC, proximal row carpectomy. RSD, reflex sympathetic dystrophy.

Question 8: What are the postoperative complications for each procedure?

Relevance

Patients may wish to undergo a procedure that has a lower risk of complication.

Current opinion

There are extra risks associated with 4CF, relating to the hardware.

Finding the evidence

The literature was reviewed for specific complications including nonunion, hardware failure, dorsal impingement, conversion to fusion, reflex sympathetic dystrophy, and sepsis.

Quality of the evidence

There were five articles reporting complications for PRC and four for 4CF.

Findings

Reported complications are summarized in Table 113.3.

Recommendation

• 4CF may have more complications than PRC due to hardware problems and nonunion [overall quality: low]

Question 9: How many patients have progression of OA after having a salvage procedure?

Case clarification

The patient is still young, with many years of manual work ahead of him.

Relevance

Further development of OA may not be ideal in this group of patients.

Current opinion and literature findings

PRC has a higher incidence of development of OA due to the mismatch in the shape of the lunate fossa and the head of the capitate.

Quality of evidence

Four articles specifically reported arthritis for PRC and four reported no evidence of arthritic change following a 4CF.

Findings

There were 18% of patients reported in the PRC group who developed secondary OA (25 of 134) (Table 113.3) and none from the 4CF group. However, the average follow-up time for PRC was 20 months longer than for the 4CF group.

A meta-analysis comparing PRC and 4CF for SLAC and SNAC wrists showed a significantly higher risk of developing OA after PRC than 4CF (RR 4.35, 95% CI 1.20–15.71).[21]

Recommendation

• PRC may have a higher incidence of progression of OA, but the clinical relevance of this finding is uncertain (usually reported as pain free despite radiological findings) [overall quality: low]

Summary of recommendations

• Observational studies have provided evidence to characterize the radiological findings for a SLAC wrist and the natural history of scapholunate rupture
• The motion-preserving salvage procedure options are PRC and 4CF. There are certain instances when PRC cannot be performed
• The grip strength is similar after PRC and 4CF. Postoperative strength is approximately 75% of the contralateral side
• The ROM achieved is similar after both procedures and usually slightly less than the preoperative measurement
• Both salvage procedures give good pain relief in approximately 3/4 of patients
• The subjective outcomes are good and similar for both salvage procedures
• 4CF may have more complications than PRC due to hardware impingement and nonunion
• PRC may have a higher incidence of progression of OA, but the clinical relevance of this finding is uncertain

Conclusions

This systematic review has shown the weak quality and quantity of studies. It is likely that both surgical options give good pain relief and improvements in subjective outcomes. PRC results in radiographic osteoarthritic changes, but the clinical implications of this are uncertain.

References

1. Berger RA. The ligaments of the wrist. A current overview of anatomy with considerations of their potential functions. Hand Clin 1997;13(1):63–82.

2. Watson HK, Ballet FL. The SLAC wrist: scapholunate advanced collapse pattern of degenerative arthritis. J Hand Surg Am 1984;9(3):358–65.

3. Kalainov DM, Cohen MS. Treatment of traumatic scapholunate dissociation. J Hand Surg Am 2009;34(7):1317–9.

4. Short WH, Werner FW, Green JK, Sutton LG, Brutus JP. Biomechanical evaluation of the ligamentous stabilizers of the scaphoid and lunate: part III. J Hand Surg Am 2007;32(3):297–309.

5. Berger RA, Imeada T, Berglund L, An KN. Constraint and material properties of the subregions of the scapholunate interosseous ligament. J Hand Surg Am 1999;24(5):953–62.

6. Pilny J, Kubes J, Hoza P, Sprlakova A, Hart R. [Consequence of nontreatment scapholunate instability of the wrist]. Rozhl Chir 2006;85(12):637–40.

7. Canale S, Beaty J. Campbell's Operative Orthopaedics, 11th edn. Mosby Elsevier, Philadelphia, 2007.

8. Browner B, Jupiter J, Levine A, Trafton P. Skeletal Trauma. Basic Science, Management and Reconstruction, 3rd edn. Saunders, Philadelphia, 2003.

9. Green DP, Hotchkiss R, Pederson W, Wolfe SW. Green's Operative Hand Surgery, 5th edn. Elsevier Churchill Livingstone, Philadelphia, 2005.

10. Cohen MS, Kozin SH. Degenerative arthritis of the wrist: proximal row carpectomy versus scaphoid excision and four-corner arthrodesis. J Hand Surg Am 2001;26(1):94–104.

11. Krakauer JD, Bishop AT, Cooney WP. Surgical treatment of scapholunate advanced collapse. J Hand Surg Am 1994;19(5):751–9.

12. Vanhove W, De Vil J, Van Seymortier P, Boone B, Verdonk R. Proximal row carpectomy versus four-corner arthrodesis as a treatment for SLAC (scapholunate advanced collapse) wrist. J Hand Surg Eur 2008;33(2):118–25.

13. Chung KC, Watt AJ, Kotsis SV. A prospective outcomes study of four-corner wrist arthrodesis using a circular limited wrist fusion plate for stage II scapholunate advanced collapse wrist deformity. Plast Reconstr Surg 2006;118(2):433–42.

14. Dacho A, Grundel J, Holle G, Germann G, Sauerbier M. Long-term results of midcarpal arthrodesis in the treatment of scaphoid nonunion advanced collapse (SNAC-Wrist) and scapholunate advanced collapse (SLAC-Wrist). Ann Plast Surg 2006;56(2):139–44.

15. Kendall CB, Brown TR, Millon SJ, Rudisill LE, Jr., Sanders JL, Tanner SL. Results of four-corner arthrodesis using dorsal circular plate fixation. J Hand Surg Am 2005;30(5):903–7.

16. Alnot JY, Apredoaei C, Frot B. Resection of the proximal row of the carpus. A review of 45 cases. Int Orthop 1997;21(3):145–50.

17. Culp RW, McGuigan FX, Turner MA, Lichtman DM, Osterman AL, McCarroll HR. Proximal row carpectomy: a multicenter study. J Hand Surg Am 1993;18(1):19–25.

18. Jebson PJ, Hayes EP, Engber WD. Proximal row carpectomy: a minimum 10-year follow-up study. J Hand Surg Am 2003;28(4):561–9.

19. Neviaser RJ. Proximal row carpectomy for posttraumatic disorders of the carpus. J Hand Surg Am 1983;8(3):301–5.

20. Balk M, Imbriglia J. Proximal row carpectomy: indications, surgical technique and long-term results. Atlas Hand Clin. 2004;9:177–85.

21. Mulford JS, Ceulemans LJ, Nam D, Axelrod TS. Proximal row carpectomy vs four corner fusion for scapholunate (Slac) or scaphoid nonunion advanced collapse (Snac) wrists: a systematic review of outcomes. J Hand Surg Eur Vol 2009;34(2):256–63.

22. Frankel VH. The Terry-Thomas sign. Clin Orthop Relat Res 1978(135):311–12.

23. Frankel VH. The Terry-Thomas sign. Clin Orthop Relat Res 1977(129):321–2.

24. Kindynis P, Resnick D, Kang HS, Haller J, Sartoris DJ. Demonstration of the scapholunate space with radiography. Radiology 1990;175(1):278–80.

25. Cautilli GP, Wehbe MA. Scapho-lunate distance and cortical ring sign. J Hand Surg Am 1991;16(3):501–3.

26. Blatt G. Capsulodesis in reconstructive hand surgery. Dorsal capsulodesis for the unstable scaphoid and volar capsulodesis following excision of the distal ulna. Hand Clin 1987;3(1):81–102.

27. Cope JR. Rotatory subluxation of the scaphoid. Clin Radiol 1984;35(6):495–501.

28. Moneim MS. The tangential posteroanterior radiograph to demonstrate scapholunate dissociation. J Bone Joint Surg Am 1981;63(8):1324–6.

29. Linscheid RL, Dobyns JH, Beabout JW, Bryan RS. Traumatic instability of the wrist. Diagnosis, classification, and pathomechanics. J Bone Joint Surg Am 1972;54(8):1612–32.

30. Gilula LA, Weeks PM. Post-traumatic ligamentous instabilities of the wrist. Radiology 1978;129(3):641–51.

31. Taleisnik J. Wrist: anatomy, function, and injury. Instr Course Lect 1978;27:61–87.

32. O'Meeghan CJ, Stuart W, Mamo V, Stanley JK, Trail IA. The natural history of an untreated isolated scapholunate interosseus ligament injury. J Hand Surg Br 2003;28(4):307–10.

33. Gharbaoui IS, Netscher DT, Kessler FB. Chronic asymptomatic contralateral wrist scapholunate dissociation. Plast Reconstr Surg 2005;116(6):1672–8.

114 Wrist Arthroscopy

Aaron M. Freilich[1], Bryan S. Dudoussat[2], Fiesky A. Nunez Jr[2], Thomas Sarlikiotis[2], and Ethan R. Wiesler[2]

[1]University of Virginia, Charlottesville, VA, USA
[2]Wake Forest University School of Medicine, Winston-Salem, NC, USA

Case scenario

A 37 year old man presents to the Emergency Department with complaints of left wrist pain following a fall on his outstretched hand while rollerblading with his children. On examination, there is mild left wrist swelling and limited range of motion due to pain. The patient is neurovascularly intact.

Top eight questions

Distal radius fractures

Diagnosis

1. Is there a role for wrist arthroscopy in the evaluation of intra-articular distal radius fractures?

Therapy

2. What is the relative effect of arthroscopy vs. fluoroscopy alone on the anatomical and functional results of treatment of intra-articular distal radius fractures in adults?

Triangular fibrocartilage complex (TFCC) injuries

Diagnosis

3. What is the optimal method for diagnosis of TFCC tears: wrist arthroscopy or MR arthrography (MRA)?

Therapy

4. What is the optimal technique for fixation of peripheral TFCC tears: open or arthroscopic?

5. What is the relative effect of arthroscopic debridement combined with ulnar shortening osteotomy vs. debridement combined with arthroscopic wafer procedure on outcome in the management of degenerative tears of the TFCC associated with ulnar positive variance?

Scapholunate (SL) and lunotriquetral (LT) ligament injuries

Therapy

6. Is there a role for arthroscopy in the treatment of dynamic carpal instability associated with SL or LT ligament tears in adults?

Dorsal wrist ganglion cysts

Therapy

7. Is there an advantage of arthroscopic resection vs. open technique in terms of recurrence?

Harm

8. What are the complications associated with arthroscopic excision of a dorsal ganglion cyst of the wrist?

Distal radius fractures

Wrist arthroscopy has evolved into an important diagnostic and therapeutic tool. Since the first wrist arthroscopy was described by Chen in 1979, indications for wrist arthroscopy have increased due to the advent of improved equipment, new portals, and techniques.[1] The use of

Evidence-Based Orthopedics, First Edition. Edited by Mohit Bhandari.
© 2012 Blackwell Publishing Ltd. Published 2012 by Blackwell Publishing Ltd.

arthroscopy has been expanded to manage distal radius fractures.

Importance of the problem

Fractures of the distal radius are common and have been the focus of numerous epidemiologic studies around the world. Population studies from cities such as Malmo, Sweden; Bergen, Norway; and Rochester, Minnesota, USA have shown incidence rates as high as 26 per 10,000 person years.[2] Many of these studies, including larger population studies from Dorset, England and Uppsala, Sweden, have also shown a significant increase in the occurrence of distal forearm fractures over the past two to three decades.[2-4]

In the United States, distal radius fractures account for approximately one sixth of all fractures seen in the Emergency Department.[3] More recent studies have reported even higher rates; Bengner et al. reported that 125 per 10,000 Medicare beneficiaries will experience a fracture of the distal radius in their lifetime.[4]

Question 1: Is there a role for wrist arthroscopy in the evaluation of intra-articular distal radius fractures?

Case clarification

The patient's radiographs reveal a displaced, intra-articular distal radius fracture. In discussions with the patient, you explain the need for surgical intervention and suggest further evaluation of the cartilage and soft tissue structures either prior to or at the time of surgery.

Relevance

Diagnosis of cartilage and soft tissue injuries prior to definitive fixation can dictate the surgical plan and allow for better understanding of the position of the fracture fragment as well as facilitating early repair of torn SL or LT ligaments, and TFCC.

Current opinion

Wrist arthroscopy is the gold standard for the diagnosis of cartilage and soft tissue lesions accompanying distal radius fractures.

Finding the evidence

- Cochrane Database, with search terms: "arthroscopy" AND "MRI" OR "magnetic resonance imaging" and "arthroscopy" AND "radiographs"
- PubMed (www.ncbi.nlm.nih.gov/pubmed/) sensitivity search using keywords: " wrist arthroscopy" AND "MRI" as well as "radius fracture" AND " arthroscopy"
- MEDLINE search using keywords: "radius fracture" AND "triangular fibrocartilage," and "radius fracture" AND "arthroscopy"

Table 114.1 Prevalence of osteochondral lesions associated with intra-articular distal radius fractures

Study	Prevalence	Location	Treatment
Adolfsson and Jorgsholm[9]	4 of 27 (15%)	N/A	Flap excision
Mehta et al.[10]	5 of 25 (20%)	4 capitate, 1 hamate	Arthroscopic debridement
Shih et al.[8]	6 of 33 (18%)	6 lunate	Reduction/K-wire fixation
Total	15 of 85 (18%)		

N/A, not available due to data deficiency

Quality of the evidence

Level II
- 2 randomized trials with methodologic limitations

Level IV
- 4 case series

Findings

Osteochondral lesions Fluoroscopy performed at the time of reduction of the distal radius fracture was unable to distinguish osteochondral lesions concomitant to this fracture type. However, these defects were easily identified on subsequent arthroscopic evaluation.[5] MRI was reported to be 72% sensitive, 78% specific, and 74% accurate compared to wrist arthroscopy when diagnosing cartilage lesions in the setting of a distal radius fracture. CT arthrogram was reported to be 45% sensitive compared to arthroscopy when diagnosing cartilage lesions in the same setting.[6,7] Three other studies provided data on the prevalence and location of concomitant osteochondral lesions (Table 114.1). These lesions often produce unstable fragments or loose bodies large enough to require reduction and Kirschner wire (K-wire) fixation.[8-10]

Intercarpal ligament and TFCC injury TFCC tears were the most commonly reported soft tissue injuries concomitant to distal radius fractures. Most of these injuries were treated with debridement at the time of arthroscopically assisted reduction and percutaneous fixation of the intra-articular fracture.[9,10] However, in two studies, 25 out of 28 TFCC tears required suture repair.[8,11] Partial or full tears of the SL and LT ligaments were also common. Two studies showed high rates of instability associated with these two injury types. K-wire stabilization was required in 29 out of 39 injuries in one study[10] and 8 out of 10 injuries in another.[8]

Recommendations

In patients with distal radius fractures and suspected cartilage and soft tissue injuries, evidence suggests:
• Wrist arthroscopy is useful to identify cartilage lesions associated with distal radius fractures [overall quality: moderate]
• Wrist arthroscopy may facilitate diagnosis and treatment of soft tissue lesions associated with distal radius fractures [overall quality: low]

Question 2: What is the relative effect of arthroscopy vs. fluoroscopy alone on the anatomical and functional results of treatment of intra-articular distal radius fractures in adults?

Case clarification

A wrist radiograph reveals an intra-articular distal radius fracture with a "die punch" pattern. You present the possibility of using wrist arthroscopy to assist in reducing the articular surfaces of the fracture.

Relevance

Reduction of the articular surface in distal radius fractures, with less than 2 mm step-off, directly affects outcome following fixation of these fractures.[12,13] Wrist arthroscopy is proposed to improve the anatomic reduction of intra-articular distal radius fractures compared to fluoroscopic reduction alone.

Current opinion

Current opinion suggests that arthroscopically assisted reduction of certain types of intra-articular distal radius fractures may improve outcome following percutaneous fixation of these fractures.

Finding the evidence

• Cochrane Database, with search terms: "distal radius fracture" AND "arthroscopy"
• PubMed (www.ncbi.nlm.nih.gov/pubmed/) sensitivity search using keywords: "distal radius fracture" AND "arthroscopy"
• MEDLINE search using keywords: "distal radius fracture" AND "arthroscopy"

Quality of the evidence

Level I
• 1 randomized controlled trial (RCT)

Level II
• 1 prospective cohort study

Findings

Articular surface reduction A prospective cohort study by Ruch et al. provided no significant difference in terms of

maximum step-off between fluoroscopically and arthroscopically assisted reduction groups at 12 months follow-up.[14] However, in an RCT performed by Varitimidis et al., the arthroscopic technique resulted in significantly different reduction of the articular surface compared to fluoroscopy alone at 24 months follow-up. The mean articular step-off following arthroscopically assisted reduction of the fracture was 0.30 mm vs. 0.8 mm for the fluoroscopically assisted group (p < 0.05).[15] In both studies the articular step-off was decreased to less than 1 mm following either the fluoroscopic or the arthroscopic reduction technique.

Functional outcome Ruch et al. reported significant difference in improvement of flexion/extension of the wrist, and supination of the forearm for the arthroscopically assisted group compared to the fluoroscopically assisted group. There was no significant difference in DASH score between the two groups at 12 months follow-up.[14] However, in an RCT by Varitimidis et al. patients reported significant difference in the MMWS at 3, 12, and 24 months follow-up as well as in DASH score at 3 months follow-up between the arthroscopically assisted and the fluoroscopically assisted group. Significant difference in improvement of flexion/extension of the wrist following arthroscopically assisted reduction of the fracture was also reported.[15]

Recommendations

In patients with intra-articular fractures of the distal radius, evidence suggests:
• The use of wrist arthroscopy may improve reduction of the articular surface of the radius compared to the use of fluoroscopy alone [overall quality: moderate]
• Functional outcomes may be improved by the use of arthroscopically assisted reduction compared to fluoroscopically assisted reduction alone [overall quality: moderate]

TFCC injuries

Relevant anatomy

The TFCC was described first by Palmer in 1981.[16] Principally, it consists of an articular disc (fibrocartilage) surrounded by the volar and dorsal radioulnar ligaments. Each radioulnar ligament consists of a superficial and deep portion, with the deep one attaching to the fovea and the superficial one attaching to the ulnar styloid and joint capsule. The term "ligamentum subcruentum" represents the deep fibers of the TFCC inserting into the fovea. The TFCC shares the load across the wrist and provides stability to the distal radioulnar joint (DRUJ).[17] Similarly to the meniscus in the knee, the outer 10–40% of the TFCC region is well vascularized. There is also an inner avascular region.[18,19] This anatomic pattern of vascularity allows for potential healing of tears and repairs in the vascular zone.

Importance of the problem

The use of arthroscopy in the treatment of wrist pathology has expanded. New techniques have been developed to provide a direct view of the TFCC. Arthroscopy has provided new methods for the treatment of ulnar-sided wrist pain, and specifically TFCC pathology.

Question 3: What is the optimal method for diagnosis of TFCC tears: wrist arthroscopy or MRI arthrography?

Case clarification

After being seen in the Emergency Department with negative radiographs, the patient was treated for a wrist sprain. Two months later he presented to the office with complaints of persistent ulnar-sided wrist pain that worsened with supination and pronation. MRI identified no TFCC pathology. Despite conservative treatment, the pain continued. Diagnostic arthroscopy was performed, and a peripheral TFCC tear was demonstrated and fixed.

Relevance

Early diagnosis and stratification of patients based on their extent of injury may improve recovery and allow patients to return to their normal daily activities.

Current opinion

Although the accuracy of MRI in the diagnosis and localization of tears is controversial, it remains a useful, if imperfect, screening tool in patients that fail conservative treatment. However, negative results should be viewed with some question.

Finding the evidence

* PubMed (www.ncbi.nlm.nih.gov/pubmed/) sensitivity search using keywords "MRI" and "TFCC"

Quality of the evidence

Level II
* 1 RCT with methodologic limitations

Level III
* 5 studies

Level IV
* 1 case series

Findings

Direct MRA Meier et al. studied 125 patients with direct injection MRI arthrography followed by wrist arthros-

copy.[20] MRI sensitivity was 94%, specificity 89%, positive predictive value (PPV) 91%, and negative predictive value (NPV) 93%. In a study of 24 patients, Joshy et al. found a sensitivity of 74%, specificity 80%, PPV 95%, NPV 50%, and overall accuracy of 79% for direct MRA.[21] This study used a conventional 1 T magnet and did not distinguish between central and peripheral tears. Another study (n = 41), using arthrography of the DRUJ, found a sensitivity of 85%, specificity of 76%, overall accuracy of 80%.[22] They noted that 14 of 19 "noncommunicating tears" observed on MRI were confirmed as full tears at arthroscopy. All studies concluded that MRI is useful in examining the TFCC but cannot replace arthroscopy for definitive diagnosis.

Indirect MRA Haims et al. (n = 86) compared indirect MRA to arthroscopy and found sensitivity of 17%, specificity 79%, and overall accuracy of 64%.[23] If high signal was used as a criterion, sensitivity increased to 42%, specificity declined to 63%, and accuracy to 55%. They concluded that indirect MRA was inadequate and found no difference between standard MRI and indirect arthrography. A second study (n = 45) had a sensitivity of 100%, specificity of 77%, and accuracy of 93%.[24] In a case series, sensitivity was 61%, specificity 88%, PPV 85%, and NPV 68%.[25]

High-resolution MRI Tanaka et al. in a small study (n = 11) examined the use of high-resolution MRI (1.5 T) with a microscopy coil. They found 100% sensitivity and specificity that varied from 70% to 100% depending on which area of the TFCC was examined. They reported three false-positive results in their study.[26]

Recommendation

* MRA is not superior to wrist arthroscopy to detect TFCC tears [overall quality: moderate]

Question 4: What is the optimal technique for fixation of peripheral TFCC tears: open or arthroscopic?

Case clarification

At the time of arthroscopy, probing of the TFCC demonstrated loss of the "trampoline" effect and obvious evidence of a tear of the peripheral ulnar attachment.

Relevance

As arthroscopy has become more prevalent, there has been a shift toward fixation or debridement of TFCC tears using this method.

Current opinion

The improved visualization of the TFCC with the arthroscope allows more accurate diagnosis and adequate fixation of tears.

Finding the evidence
• PubMed (www.ncbi.nlm.nih.gov/pubmed/) sensitivity search using keywords "arthroscopic" AND "triangular fibrocartilage complex"

Quality of the evidence
Level III
• 1 retrospective comparative study

Level IV
• 10 case series

Findings
In a retrospective comparative study, Anderson et al. reported on 75 patients undergoing either open (N = 39) or arthroscopic (N = 36) TFCC repair.[27] There was no significant difference in outcome between the two groups at 43 months follow-up. Patients showed a significant reduction in pain and improved function after surgery according to the MMWS system. Similar numbers (17%) in each treatment group required reoperation for instability. Osterman reported a case series of 52 consecutive patients who underwent arthroscopic treatment of TFCC tears;[28] 41 patients were followed between 13 and 42 months following surgery. Of these, 73% reported "complete" pain relief, and 88% considered surgery "worthwhile." All remaining case series are summarized in Table 114.2.[29–38] Evidence of DRUJ instability at the time of presentation or diagnosis was not addressed by any of available studies, therefore no conclusions can be drawn for this patient subset.

Recommendation
• Outcomes for arthroscopic repair or debridement of TFCC tears are equivalent to those of open treatment [overall quality: low]

Question 5: What is the relative effect of arthroscopic debridement combined with ulnar shortening osteotomy vs. debridement combined with arthroscopic wafer procedure on outcome in the management of degenerative tears of the TFCC associated with ulnar positive variance?

Case clarification
When the patient was further questioned at his initial presentation to the office, he said that ulnar-sided wrist pain had been present for over a year; however, the pain had become worse following the injury 2 months ago. An ulnar variance view on radiographs demonstrated 4 mm of ulnar positive variance. After failing conservative measures, an MRI showed a central perforation of the TFCC.

Relevance
Treatment of degenerative central TFCC tears with debridement alone on the ground of ulnar positive variance tends to result in recurrent or incomplete relief of symptoms.

Current opinion
Ulnar shortening osteotomy is the most frequently used method in addressing the length of the ulna in ulnocarpal impaction syndrome.

Finding the evidence
• PubMed (www.ncbi.nlm.nih.gov/pubmed/) sensitivity search using keywords: "arthroscopic" AND "TFCC" AND/OR "wafer procedure" or "ulnar osteotomy"

Quality of the evidence
Level III
• 1 retrospective comparative study

Table 114.2 Arthroscopic TFCC repair

	Level of evidence	N	MMWS			Reoperation/failure
			E/G	F	P	
Chou and Lee[29]	IV	17	—	—	—	2
De Araujo et al.[30]	IV	17	—	—	—	—
Estrella et al.[31]	IV	35	26	4	5	10
Haugstvedt and Husby[32]	IV	20	14	4	2	5
Husby and Haugstvedt[33]	IV	32	27	4	1	1
Minami et al.[34]	IV	16	13	2	1	2
Miwa et al.[35]	IV	62	57	3	2	2
Reiter et al.[36]	IV	46	29	12	5	0
Trumble et al.[37]	IV	24	21	3	0	—
Westkaemper et al.[38]	IV	28	21	2	5	—

E/G, excellent/good; F, fair; MMWS, Mayo modified wrist score; N, sample size; P, poor.

Table 114.3 Arthroscopic wafer procedure or ulnar shortening osteotomy for TFCC tears with ulnar positive variance

	Level of evidence	Type	N	MMWS			Failures
				E/G	F	P	
Tomaino and Weiser[41]	IV	Arthroscopic wafer procedure	12	9*	3		—
Trumble et al.[42]	IV	Delayed repair with USO	21	18	3		—
Minami and Kato[40]	IV	Debridement with USO	25	21	2	2	2
Hulsizer et al.[43]	IV	USO after failed debridement	13	12[a]		1	1
De Smet et al.[44]	IV	Mixed	21 debridement only	7[b]	6	8	9
			10 wafer procedure	3	2	5	5

E/G, excellent/good; F, fair; MMWS, Mayo modified wrist score; N, sample size; P, poor.
[a]Results reported as very satisfied/satisfied/unsatisfied.
[b]Results reported as good/satisfactory/poor.

Level IV
- 5 case series

Findings

In a retrospective comparative study, 16 patients treated with arthroscopic debridement of TFCC tear plus ulnar shortening osteotomy were compared in terms of outcome to 11 patients treated with debridement plus arthroscopic resection of the distal ulna (wafer procedure).[39] Nine out of 11 patients in the wafer procedure group and 11 out of 16 in the ulnar osteotomy group reported good or excellent results according to the MMWS system at 15 months follow-up. Pain relief also was similar in both groups. However, 1 patient in the wafer procedure group and 10 patients in the ulnar osteotomy group required secondary surgery (9 hardware removals). The remaining available studies are summarized in Table 114.3.[40–44]

Recommendation

- An arthroscopic procedure to address ulnar variance in addition to TFCC pathology can provide similar pain relief compared to a combination of arthroscopic debridement with ulnar shortening osteotomy [overall quality: low]

SL and LT ligament injury

Relevant anatomy

Intrinsic ligaments of the wrist are directly attached to carpal bones and play an important role in the stability and coordination of the carpal construct. The SL and LT ligaments are the most important ones.[45] Dynamic instability was first described by Taleisnik in 1980.[46] Patients may present with findings on clinical examination; the static anteroposterior radiographs are normal. Stress views usually reveal a widening of the scapholunate interval.

Importance of the problem

Intercarpal ligament injuries remain an important clinical issue.[47] As arthroscopy continues to increase its role in both diagnosis and treatment of various wrist pathologies, strategies are needed to guide the treatment of intercarpal ligamentous disruptions, in order to achieve the desired outcomes.

Question 6: Is there a role for arthroscopy in the treatment of dynamic carpal instability associated with SL or LT ligament tears in adults?

Case clarification

After attempted conservative treatment, the patient's wrist pain continued; there is a 2.5 mm SL widening on stress views while static radiographs are normal. An MRI at this time was suggestive of a SL ligament tear.

Relevance

Available options for open treatment of dynamic carpal instability result in suboptimal outcomes with decreased range of motion (ROM). Arthroscopic debridement with or without pinning may help in achieving adequate results without the morbidity associated with an open procedure.

Current opinion

Arthroscopic debridement in the acute setting (<3 months) can provide adequate symptom relief.

Finding the evidence

- PubMed and MEDLINE searches for "arthroscopy," "wrist," "intercarpal," "ligament," "scapholunate," "lunotriquetral"

Quality of the evidence

Level IV
- 3 case series

Findings

Results following arthroscopic debridement for either complete or incomplete intercarpal ligament tears were reported in a case series by Wiess et al.[48] A total of 27 SL ligament tears were treated. At 27 months follow-up, 21 patients reported improvement or complete resolution of symptoms according to the author's criteria (10 out of 15 complete tears and 11 out of 13 partial tears). Fifteen LT ligament tears were also treated. At follow-up, 13 had resolved/improved symptoms (7 out of 9 complete and 6 out of 6 partial tears). All 9 failures required additional surgery despite no evidence of static deformity at follow-up. No statistical difference in outcome was noted in patients with complete and partial tears treated in this manner. A third study evaluated patients (N = 11) treated for chronic dynamic scapholunate instability with arthroscopic debridement and closed pinning.[49] At 33 months follow-up, there were 3 failures requiring additional surgery; 6 patients had good/excellent results and 2 fair/poor according to the MMWS system. Ruch et al. examined arthroscopic debridement of partial SL and LT ligament tears in 14 patients who had failed 6 months of conservative treatment. 11 out of 14 patients reported complete pain relief and 2 more patients reported occasional residual pain but were able to return to work within 7 weeks.[50]

Recommendation

- Arthroscopic treatment of chronic SL or LT ligament tears, in the setting of dynamic instability may provide adequate symptom relief in the short term [overall quality: low]

Dorsal wrist ganglion cysts

Relevant anatomy

Ganglion cysts are masses filled with mucous fluid that is similar to synovial fluid, but thicker.[51] A one-way valve system between the joint and the ganglion has been proposed to allow synovial fluid into the cyst.[52] Commonly, dorsal ganglion cysts arise superficially between the second and fourth extensor tendon compartments.[53]

Importance of the problem

Ganglion cysts account for 50–70% of all soft tissue tumors of the hand and wrist.[53–55] Ganglion cysts may cause pain, weakness, joint stiffness, and deformity as their size increases.[56,57]

Question 7: Is there an advantage of arthroscopic excision compared to open technique in terms of recurrence?

Case clarification

The patient's pain and swelling gradually resolved. Eight months after initial presentation to the Emergency Department, he noted a swollen area on the dorsum of his wrist. The area enlarged progressively with activity-related discomfort, especially with wrist extension.

Current opinion

Excision is indicated for symptomatic ganglion cysts of the wrist that recur following previous aspiration. Numerous retrospective studies have reported various recurrence rates following either open or arthroscopic excision of dorsal ganglion cysts.[58–63] However, in the single prospective randomized trial by Kang et al., similar recurrence rates following these two procedures were reported at 1 year postoperatively.[64]

Finding the evidence

- PubMed (www.ncbi.nlm.nih.gov/pubmed/):sensitivity search using keywords: "prospective" AND "ganglia" AND "arthroscopic," "prospective randomized trial" AND "ganglia" AND "arthroscopic," "recurrence" AND "ganglia" AND "arthroscopic"

Quality of the evidence

Level I
- 1 RCT

Findings

The recurrence rate following dorsal ganglion excision was reported to be equal between the open and arthroscopic technique groups in a prospective randomized trial.[64] A total of 72 patients were included and followed for a year. The recurrence rate was 1% in both groups.

Recommendation

- There is no significant difference in recurrence of dorsal ganglion cysts following resection with either the open or the arthroscopic technique [overall quality: high]

Question 8: What are the complications associated with arthroscopic excision of a dorsal ganglion cyst of the wrist?

SL ligament injury is reported to complicate open excision of a dorsal ganglion cyst. However, arthroscopic resection has not been associated with this type of injury.[65–67] Better visual approach to the ligament through the scope is a possible explanation.[68]

Complications such as postsurgical hematomas or injury of contiguous nerves have been reported after arthroscopic resection, but in numbers similar to those found after open surgical resection.[69]

The arthroscopic technique has been reported to minimize side effects of a painful scar, and wrist stiffness commonly associated with open excision of the ganglion cyst.[66]

Finding the evidence

• PubMed (www.ncbi.nlm.nih.gov/pubmed/) sensitivity search using keywords: "complications" AND "ganglia" AND "arthroscopy," "nerve" AND "ganglia" AND "arthroscopic," "grip strength" AND "ganglia" AND "arthroscopic"

Quality of the evidence

Level IV
• 5 case series

Findings

From 2000 to 2009 three different authors reported a total of 111 dorsal wrist ganglia treated with arthroscopic excision with at least 24 months of follow-up.[58,62,63] At 2 years follow-up, only five patients experienced minor complications.

Two other case series reported results from 96 patients treated with arthroscopic resection of dorsal wrist ganglia. Postoperatively, only four patients experienced mild complications (extensor tendon irritation).[66,69]

Recommendation

• Arthroscopic resection for dorsal wrist ganglia is a safe procedure with minor complications [Overall Quality: Low]

Summary of recommendations

• Wrist arthroscopy is useful to identify cartilage lesions associated with distal radius fractures
• Wrist arthroscopy may facilitate early diagnosis and treatment of soft tissue lesions associated with distal radius fractures
• The use of wrist arthroscopy may improve reduction of the articular surface of the radius compared to the use of fluoroscopy alone
• Functional outcomes may be improved by the use of arthroscopically assisted reduction compared to fluoroscopically assisted reduction alone
• MRA is not superior to wrist arthroscopy to detect TFCC tears
• Outcomes for arthroscopic repair or debridement of TFCC tears are equivalent to those of open treatment
• An arthroscopic procedure to address ulnar variance in addition to TFCC pathology can provide similar pain relief compared to a combination of arthroscopic debridement with ulnar shortening osteotomy

• Arthroscopic treatment of chronic SL or LT ligament tears, in the setting of dynamic instability may provide adequate symptom relief in the short term
• There is no significant difference in recurrence of the dorsal ganglion cyst following resection with either the open or the arthroscopic technique
• Arthroscopic resection for dorsal wrist ganglia is a safe procedure with minor complications

Conclusions

The judicious use of wrist arthroscopy in the management of distal radius fractures may facilitate the diagnosis of associated cartilage lesions, enable early diagnosis and treatment of concomitant soft tissue injuries, and enhance anatomic reduction of the articular surface leading to improved functional outcomes. MRA to diagnose TFCC tears is not superior to wrist arthroscopy. Wrist arthroscopy may facilitate treatment of peripheral TFCC tears with equal results compared to open repairs. An arthroscopic wafer procedure to address a central TFCC tear with ulnar positive variance may provide similar outcomes compared to a combination of arthroscopic debridement with ulnar shortening osteotomy. Debridement of SL or LT tears in patients with dynamic instability and chronic wrist pain, may improve symptoms in the short term. Arthroscopic excision for dorsal wrist ganglion cysts is a safe procedure, with no difference in terms of recurrence when compared to open technique.

References

1. Chen YC. Arthroscopy of the wrist and finger joints. Orthop Clin North Am 1979;10:723–33.
2. Brogren E, Petranek M, Atroshi I. Incidence and characteristics of distal radius fractures in a southern Swedish region. BMC Musculoskelet Disord 2007;31:48.
3. Owen RA, Melton LJ 3rd, Johnson KA, et al. Incidence of Colles' fracture in a North American community. Am J Public Health 1982;72:605–7.
4. Bengner U, Johnell O. Increasing incidence of forearm fractures. A comparison of epidemiologic patterns 25 years apart. Acta Orthop Scand 1985;56:158–60.
5. Auge WK, Velazquez PA. The application of indirect reduction techniques in the distal radius: The role of adjuvant arthroscopy. Arthroscopy 2000;16:830–5.
6. Mutimer J, Green J, Field J. Comparison of MRI and wrist arthroscopy for assessment of wrist cartilage. J Hand Surg Eur 2008;33:380–2.
7. Billie B, Harley B, Cohen H. A comparison of CT arthrography of the wrist to findings during wrist arthroscopy. J Hand Surg Am 2007;32:834–41.
8. Shih JT, Lee HM, Hou YT, et al. Arthroscopically-assisted reduction of intra-articular fractures and soft tissue management of distal radius. Hand Surg 2001;6:127–35.

9. Adolfsson L, Jorgsholm P. Arthroscopically-assisted reduction of intra-articular fractures of the distal radius. J Hand Surg Br 1998;23:391–5.

10. Mehta JA, Bain GI, Heptinstall RJ. Anatomical reduction of intra-articular fractures of the distal radius. An arthroscopically-assisted approach. J Bone Joint Surg Br 2000;82:79–86.

11. Ruch DS, Yang CC, Smith BP. Results of acute arthroscopically repaired triangular fibrocartilage complex injuries associated with intra-articular distal radius fractures. Arthroscopy 2003;19:511–16.

12. Knirk JL, Jupiter JB. 1986; Intra-articular fractures of the distal end of the radius in young adults. J Bone Joint Surg Am 68:647–59.

13. Trumble TE, Schmitt SR, Vedder NB. Factors affecting functional outcome of displaced intra-articular distal radius fractures. J Hand Surg Am 1994;19:325–40.

14. Ruch DS, Vallee J, Poehling GG, et al. Arthroscopic reduction versus fluoroscopic reduction in the management of intra-articular distal radius fractures. Arthroscopy 2004;20:225–30.

15. Varitimidis SE, Basdekis GK, Dailiana ZH, et al. Treatment of intra-articular fractures of the distal radius: Fluoroscopic or arthroscopic reduction. J Bone Joint Surg Br 2008;90:778–85.

16. Palmer AK, Werner FW. The triangular fibrocartilage complex of the wrist—anatomy and function. J Hand Surg Am 1981;6:153–62.

17. Kleinman WB. Stability of the distal radioulnar joint: biomechanics, pathophysiology, physical diagnosis, and restoration of function: what we have learned in 25 years. J Hand Surg Am 2007;32:1086–106.

18. Benar MS, Arnoczky SP, Weiland AJ. The microvasculature of the triangular fibrocartilage complex: its clinical significance. J Hand Surg Am 1991;16:1101–5.

19. Thiru RG, Ferlic DC, Clayton ML, et al. Arterial anatomy of the triangular fibrocartilage of the wrist and its clinical significance. J Hand Surg Am 1986;11:258–63.

20. Meier R, Schmitt R, Krimmer H. Wrist lesions in MRI arthrography compared with wrist arthroscopy. Handchir Mikrochir Plast Chir 2005;37:85–9.

21. Joshy S, Ghosh S, Lee K, et al. Accuracy of direct magnetic resonance arthrography in the diagnosis of triangular fibrocartilage complex tears of the wrist. Int Orthop 2008;32:251–3.

22. Rüegger C, Schmid MR, Pfirrmann CW, et al. Peripheral tear of the triangular fibrocartilage: depiction with MR arthrography of the distal radioulnar joint. AJR Am J Roentgenol 2007;188:187–92.

23. Haims AH, Schweitzer ME, Morrison WB, et al. Limitations of MR imaging in the diagnosis of peripheral tears of the triangular fibrocartilage of the wrist. AJR Am J Roentgenol 2002;178:419–22.

24. Herold T, Lenhart M, Held P, et al. Indirect MR arthrography of the wrist in the diagnosis of TFCC-lesions. Rofo 2001;173:1006–11.

25. De Smet L. Magnetic resonance imaging for diagnosing lesions of the triangular fibrocartilage complex. Acta Orthop Belg 2005;71:396–8.

26. Tanaka T, Yoshioka H, Ueno T, et al. Comparison between high-resolution MRI with a microscopy coil and arthroscopy in triangular fibrocartilage complex injury. J Hand Surg Am 2006;31:1308–14.

27. Anderson ML, Larson AN, Moran SL, et al. Clinical comparison of arthroscopic versus open repair of triangular fibrocartilage complex tears. J Hand Surg Am 2008;33:675–82.

28. Osterman AL. Arthroscopic debridement of triangular fibrocartilage complex tears. Arthroscopy 1990;6:120–4.

29. Chou C, Lee TS. Peripheral tears of triangular fibrocartilage complex: results of primary repair. Int Orthop 2001;25:392–5.

30. De Araujo W, Poehling GG, Kuzma GR. New Tuohy needle technique for triangular fibrocartilage complex repair: preliminary studies. Arthroscopy 1996;12:699–703.

31. Estrella EP, Hung LK, Ho PC, et al. Arthroscopic repair of triangular fibrocartilage complex tears. Arthroscopy 2007;23:729–37.

32. Haugstvedt J, Husby T. Results of repair of peripheral tears in the triangular fibrocartilage complex using an arthroscopic suture technique. Scand J Plast Reconstr Hand Surg 1999;33:439–47.

33. Husby T, Haugstvedt J. Long-term results after arthroscopic resection of lesions of the triangular fibrocartilage complex. Scand J Plast Reconstr Hand Surg 2001;35:79–83.

34. Minami A, Ishikawa J, Suenaga N, et al. Clinical results of treatment of triangular fibrocartilage complex tears by arthroscopic debridement. J Hand Surg Am 1996;21:406–11.

35. Miwa H, Hashizume H, Fujiwara K, et al. Arthroscopic surgery for traumatic triangular fibrocartilage complex injury. J Orthop Sci 2004;9:354–9.

36. Reiter A, Wolf M, Schmid U, et al. Arthroscopic repair of Palmer 1B triangular fibrocartilage complex tears. Arthroscopy 2008;24:1244–50.

37. Trumble T, Gilbert M, Vedder N. Isolated tears of the triangular fibrocartilage: management by early arthroscopic repair. J Hand Surg Am 1997;22:57–65.

38. Westkaemper JG, Mitsionis G, Giannakopoulos PN, et al. Wrist arthroscopy for the treatment of ligament and triangular fibrocartilage complex injuries. Arthroscopy 1998;14:479–83.

39. Bernstein MA, Nagle DJ, Martinez A, et al. A comparison of combined arthroscopic triangular fibrocartilage complex debridement and arthroscopic wafer distal ulna resection versus arthroscopic triangular fibrocartilage complex debridement and ulnar shortening osteotomy for ulnocarpal abutment syndrome. Arthroscopy 2004;20:392–401.

40. Minami A, Kato H. Ulnar shortening for triangular fibrocartilage complex tears associated with ulnar positive variance. J Hand Surg Am 1998;23:904–8.

41. Tomaino MM, Weiser RW. Combined arthroscopic TFCC debridement and wafer resection of the distal ulna in wrists with triangular fibrocartilage complex tears and positive ulnar variance. J Hand Surg Am 2001;26:1047–52.

42. Trumble T, Gilbert M, Vedder N. Ulnar shortening combined with arthroscopic repairs in the delayed management of the triangular fibrocartilage complex tears. J Hand Surg Am 1997;22:807–13.

43. Hulsizer D, Weiss AP, Akelman E. Ulna-shortening osteotomy after failed arthroscopic of the triangular fibrocartilage complex. J Hand Surg Am 1997;22:694–8.

44. De Smet L, De Ferm A, Steenwerckx D, et al. Arthroscopic treatment of triangular fibrocartilage complex lesions of the wrist. Acta Orthop Belg 1996;62:8–13.

45. Shin AY, Carlsen BT. Wrist instability. Scand J Surg 2008;97:324–32.

46. Taleisnik J. Post-traumatic carpal instability. Clin Orthop 1980;149:73–82.

47. Cooney WP, Berger RA. Interosseous ligamentout injuries of the wrist. In: McGinty JB, ed., Operative Arthroscopy, pp. 782–97. Lippincott Williams & Wilkins, Philadelphia, 2003.

48. Wiess APC, Sachar K, Glowacki KA. Arthroscopic debridement alone for intercarpal ligament tears. J Hand Surg Am 1997;22: 344–49.

49. Darlis NA, Kaufmann FG, et al. Arthroscopic debridement and closed pinning for chronic dynamic scapholunate instability J Hand Surg Am 2006;31:419–24.

50. Ruch DS, Poehling GG. Arthroscopic management of partial scapholunate and lunotriquetral injuries of the wrist. J Hand Surg Am 1996;21:412–17.

51. Gude W, Morelli V. Ganglion cysts of the wrist: pathophysiology, clinical picture, and management. Curr Rev Musculoskelet Med 2008;1:205–11.

52. Angelides AC, Wallace PF. The dorsal ganglion of the wrist: its pathogenesis, gross and microscopic anatomy, and surgical treatment. J Hand Surg Am 1976;1:228–35.

53. Calandruccio JH. Tumors and tumorous conditions of the hand. In: Canale ST, Beaty JH, eds., Campbell's Operative Orthopaedics. Mosby, Philadelphia, 2007.

54. Johnson J, Kilgore E, Newmeyer W. Tumorous lesions of the hand. J Hand Surg Am 1985;10:284–6.

55. Thornburg LE. Ganglions of the hand and wrist. J Am Acad Orthop Surg 1999;7:231–8.

56. Dias JJ, Dhukaram V, Kumar P. The natural history of untreated dorsal wrist ganglia and patient reported outcome 6 years after intervention. J Hand Surg Eur. 2007;32:502–8.

57. Dias J, Buch K. Palmar wrist ganglion: does intervention improve outcome? A prospective study of the natural history and patient-reported treatment outcomes. J Hand Surg Br 2003;28:172–6.

58. Luchetti R, Badia A, Alfarano M, et al. Arthroscopic resection of dorsal wrist ganglia and treatment of recurrences. J Hand Surg Br 2000;25:38–40.

59. McEvedy BV. The simple ganglion: a review of modes of treatment and an explanation of the frequent failures of surgery. Lancet 1954;16:135–6.

60. Zachariae L, Vibe-Hansen H. Ganglia. Recurrence rate elucidated by a follow-up of 347 operated cases. Acta Chir Scand 1973;139:625–8.

61. McEvedy B. Cystic ganglia; their pathology, natural history and treatment. Med Illus 1955;9:425–8.

62. Shih JT, Hung ST, Lee HM, et al. Dorsal ganglion of the wrist: results of treatment by arthroscopic resection. Hand Surg 2002;7:1–5.

63. Edwards SG, Johansen JA. Prospective outcomes and associations of wrist ganglion cysts resected arthroscopically. J Hand Surg Am 2009;34:395–400.

64. Kang L, Akelman E, Weiss AP. Arthroscopic vs. open dorsal ganglion excision: a prospective, randomized comparison of rates of recurrence and of residual pain. J Hand Surg Am 2008;33:471–5.

65. Duncan KH, Lewis RC, Jr. Scapholunate instability following ganglion cyst excision. A case report. Clin Orthop Relat Res 1988;228:250–3.

66. Rizzo M, Berger RA, Steinmann SP, et al. Arthroscopic resection in the management of dorsal wrist ganglions: results with a minimum 2-year follow-up period. J Hand Surg Am 2004;29: 59–62.

67. Crawford GP, Taleisnik J. Rotatory subluxation of the scaphoid after excision of dorsal carpal ganglion and wrist manipulation—a case report. J Hand Surg Am 1983;8:921–5.

68. Osterman AL, Raphael J. Arthroscopic resection of dorsal ganglion of the wrist. Hand Clin 1995;11:7–12.

69. Rocchi L, Canal A, Pelaez J, et al. Results and complications in dorsal and volar wrist Ganglia arthroscopic resection. Hand Surg 2006;11:21–6.

115 Rheumatoid Wrist Reconstruction (Arthrodesis and Arthroplasty)

Warren C. Hammert[1] and Kevin C. Chung[2]

[1]University of Rochester Medical Center, Rochester, NY, USA
[2]University of Michigan Medical School, Ann Arbor, MI, USA

Case scenario

A 45 year old woman with a history of rheumatoid arthritis (RA) is seen in the office for a consultation relating to her hands. She reports progressive difficulty using her hands over the last several months due to swelling and pain in her wrist, limited motion of her wrists and fingers, and progressive deformity of her fingers (Figures 115.1 and 115.2).

Relevant pathophysiology

The effect of RA on the ulnar wrist begins with the ulnocarpal joint. Synovitis stretches the ulnar carpal ligaments and the triangular fibrocartilage complex (TFCC), resulting in an unstable, dorsal dislocated distal ulna, so-called "caput ulna."[1] This is accompanied by volar subluxation of the extensor carpi ulnaris (ECU) tendon, which leads to carpal supination because the ECU tendon now acts as more of a flexor rather than an extensor to stabilize the ulnar wrist. The incongruity of the distal radioulnar joint (DRUJ) results in pain with forearm rotation, and this is often the earliest presentation of a RA patient who seeks surgical consultation (Figure 115.3).

Involvement on the radial side of the wrist begins with proliferative synovitis in the region of the radioscaphocapitate ligament and attenuation of the volar radiocarpal ligaments.[2,3] The weakening of the volar radial support ligament leads to flexion and rotatory subluxation of the scaphoid. When combined with the dorsal subluxation of the distal ulna and relative shortening of the radial wrist, the metacarpals will deviate radially, leading to ulnar deviation of the fingers.[1,4]

Importance of the problem

RA is the second most common type of arthritis after osteoarthritis,[5] affecting 0.8% of the adult population throughout the world.[6] In the United States, RA afflicts 1.3 million adults, with a prevalence of 1.06% in women compared to 0.61% in men.[7] RA is a progressive and debilitating condition with up to 70% of patients having hand and wrist impairment[8] that may preclude many activities of daily living.[9,10] In the United States, the cost associated with RA was estimated to be $8.7 billion annually in 1996.[11]

Although medical treatments have improved due to newer medications, not all patients have access to these medications and, for some, the disease progresses despite medical treatments. In addition, there is disagreement between rheumatologists and hand surgeons regarding the timing, indications, and outcomes for surgical treatment of rheumatoid hand and wrist conditions.[12–14]

This chapter will discusses the management of the osseous structures of the wrist—the radiocarpal and midcarpal joints and the DRUJ.

Top nine questions

Diagnosis

1. What are the presenting complaints for patients with RA affecting the wrist?
2. What modalities are used in the diagnostic process?

Treatment of the radiocarpal joint

3. What is the role of limited wrist arthrodesis?

Evidence-Based Orthopedics, First Edition. Edited by Mohit Bhandari.
© 2012 Blackwell Publishing Ltd. Published 2012 by Blackwell Publishing Ltd.

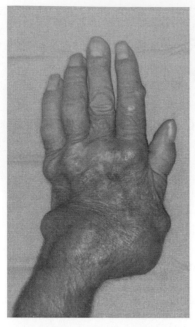

Figure 115.1 PA picture of patient with RA affecting wrist.

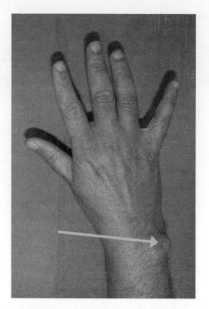

Figure 115.3 Clinical example of patient with dorsally prominent ulna (caput ulna).

Outcomes/prognosis

9. What are the outcomes of rheumatoid wrist procedures?

Question 1: What are the presenting complaints for patients with RA affecting the wrist?

Case clarification

Some patients with RA will have complaints related to pain, swelling, appearance, or loss of motion of the affected wrist, whereas others will seek treatment for hand conditions and may not have any complaints regarding their wrists. The appearance of a destroyed wrist does not usually mean that the patient will complain of incapacitating wrist pain. Although some patients truly have isolated hand conditions, most will have conditions affecting the wrist that need to be treated prior to or simultaneously with the hand.

Recommendation

• It is important to listen carefully to the patient's concerns and address the issue that is most bothersome to the patient

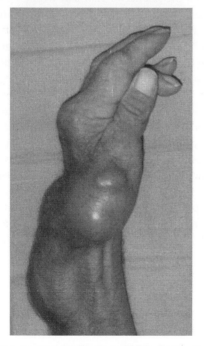

Figure 115.2 Lateral picture of patient with RA affecting the wrist.

4. What is the role of total wrist arthrodesis?
5. What is the role of total wrist arthroplasty?

Treatment of the DRUJ

6. What is the role of the Darrach procedure?
7. What is the role of DRUJ arthrodesis (Suave–Kapandji procedure)?
8. What is the role of ulnar head arthroplasty?

Question 2: What modalities are used for diagnosis?

The criteria used to diagnose RA have been clearly defined and are not included in this chapter. Similar conditions, such as those of other inflammatory arthritides or conditions with similar clinical presentation, can be treated in the same manner as RA.

Recommendation

• Routine zero-rotation PA and lateral radiographs of the wrist are diagnostic and treatment recommendations can be made based on physical exams and radiographic findings. There is no evidence to suggest additional imaging or laboratory tests will enhance the RA hand assessment

Question 3: What is the role of limited wrist arthrodesis?

Case clarification

The patient may be a candidate for limited wrist stabilizing procedures if the cartilage is intact.

Relevance

The midcarpal joint may be spared even with extensive involvement of the radiocarpal joint due to the paucity of ligaments in the region of the midcarpal joint.[1] Synovium is concentrated in areas with abundant ligaments and therefore, the midcarpal joint is not involved until late in the destructive process.

Radiocarpal changes begin with synovitis affecting the ligaments that stabilize the proximal row. The ligament laxity resulted in flexion of the scaphoid, rotatory changes of the lunate (either flexion or extension) and subsequent ulnar translocation of the lunate and in more severe cases, the entire carpus. Prior to midcarpal involvement, radiocarpal fusion (either radiolunate or radioscapholunate), along with synovectomy of the midcarpal joint, will stabilize the wrist and retain some wrist motion.

The advantage to including the scaphoid in the fusion mass is related to the greater surface area to provide a more predictable fusion. Because the scaphoid is a link between the proximal and distal rows, removal of the distal scaphoid when performing the radioscapholunate fusion will unlock or separate the proximal from distal rows and allow better motion.[15,16]

In the event that the articular cartilage of the scaphoid is free of disease, the fusion can be limited to the radiolunate joint. Although the fusion area is not as large, this procedure will prevent radial deviation and ulnar subluxation of the carpus, which can maintain alignment of the hand on the wrist and forearm.

Wrist motion following radiolunate or radioscapholunate arthrodesis occurs through the midcarpal joint with a more oblique path of the capitate along the dart thrower's axis.[17]

Findings

Honkanen has shown maintenance of fusion with a functional arc of wrist motion (flexion 29°, 67% of preoperative value, and extension 34°, 92% of preoperative value) at over 5 years follow-up.[18] Ishikawa has shown good long-term results with decreased pain and increased grip strength at 10 years follow-up. Carpal collapse progressed, but this did not seem to affect the overall results.[19]

Recommendation

• Limited wrist arthrodesis can be considered when there is a need to stabilize the radiocarpal joint due to ulnar translocation of the carpus or when there is destruction of the radiocarpal joint and sparing of the midcarpal joint

Question 4: What is the role of total wrist arthrodesis?

Case clarification

Patients with advanced radiographic involvement, or those with pain and minimal motion, are not likely candidates for limited wrist arthrodesis and should be treated with total arthrodesis (Figure 115.4) or wrist arthroplasty.

Current opinion

The position of arthrodesis has not been clearly delineated, with some authors recommending fusion in extension and ulnar deviation, whereas others prefer the neutral position to help maintain finger alignment.[20,21] For those patients requiring bilateral wrist arthrodesis, one side should be fused in slight extension and the other in slight flexion, because the flexion posture will help in perineal care.[22]

Recently, Cavaliere and Chung performed a systematic review of arthrodesis and arthroplasty for the rheumatoid wrist. Of 1750 citations, 18 arthroplasty and 20 arthrodesis studies revealed better outcomes and more reliable pain relief following arthrodesis. Satisfaction was high in both groups, with a higher complication and revision rate in the arthroplasty group. Interestingly, of the 14 studies reporting range of motion data in the arthroplasty group, only 3 showed an average wrist arc of motion within the functional range.[23]

Recommendation

• Total wrist arthrodesis should be considered for patients with severe destruction of the wrist secondary to rheumatoid disease

Question 5: What is the role of total wrist arthroplasty?

Case clarification

Patients often have both wrists affected and may require procedures on both sides. They would often prefer a motion-preserving procedure, at least on one side, if given the choice with similar outcomes regarding pain relief and surgical risks.

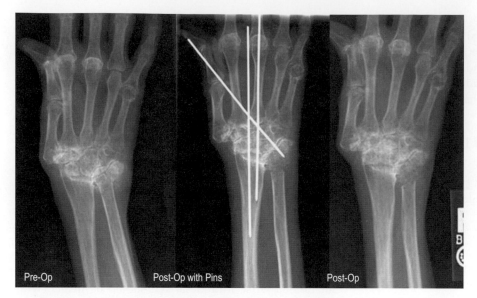

Pre-Op

Post-Op with Pins

Post-Op

Figure 115.4 Preoperative and postoperative PA radiographs of total wrist arthrodesis.

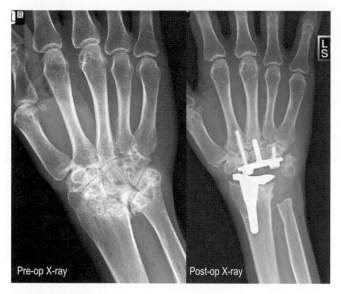

Pre-op X-ray

Post-op X-ray

Figure 115.5 Preoperative and postoperative PA radiograph of total wrist arthroplasty.

Current opinion

Wrist arthroplasty (Figure 115.5) is an option for patients desiring to retain some motion and may be most beneficial when patients require treatment of both wrists. Newer designs have minimized some of the problems with earlier implants, but loosening and revision procedures remain common.

Findings

Murphy et al. compared arthroplasty to arthrodesis in 51 wrists and reported similar complication rates between the two groups, but the arthroplasty group had an easier time with personal hygiene.[24]

Divelbiss et al. reported early results of arthroplasty with the Universal wrist prosthesis in 19 patients (22 wrists). Eight patients had 2 year follow-up and 14 patients had 1 year follow-up. Total wrist arc of motion and DASH scores improved, with three prostheses that became unstable and required further treatment.[25]

Cavaliere and Chung surveyed members of the American Society for Surgery of the Hand practicing in the United States to determine surgeons' attitudes and preferences toward wrist arthroplasty and arthrodesis. They reported both arthroplasty and arthrodesis are preferable to nonoperative management, and there is a slight increase in quality-adjusted life years (QALY) in the arthroplasty group, but not great enough to make arthroplasty the preferred treatment.[26]

Recommendation

• Currently, there is no evidence to support arthroplasty being superior to arthrodesis, arthroplasty may be considered an acceptable option. The best indications appear to be for patients requiring bilateral procedures and for those patients with a strong preference to retain motion, with the understanding that additional procedures are likely for treating complications such as implant dislocation or loosening

Question 6: What is the role of the Darrach procedure when the DRUJ is involved?

Case clarification

In addition to pain and limited motion at the radiocarpal joints, patients will often present with limited or painful forearm rotation, synovitis, and arthritis at the DRUJ.

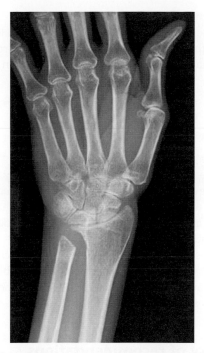

Figure 115.6 PA radiograph following Darrach resection of distal ulna.

Relevance

The DRUJ is often involved early in RA, initially with synovitis and subsequent progress to instability with associated carpal supination and volar and ulnar subluxation of the carpus. The ECU tendon displaces ulnar to the ECU groove and subsequently becomes a flexor, rather than an extensor, which further aggravates the deformity. This leads to DRUJ instability (caput ulna) and when untreated, can result in attritional ruptures of the extensor tendons.

Current opinion

In cases with synovitis without instability or arthritis of the DRUJ, synovectomy alone may be adequate, but more commonly, a procedure at the DRUJ is combined with synovectomy. The Darrach procedure involves resection of the ulnar head proximal to the sigmoid notch and often is stabilized with local tissue (Figure 115.6). A variety of techniques have been described to stabilize the ulna stump, including using the joint capsule, ECU, FCU, pronator quadratus and a combination of these tissues.[27–30] These stabilization procedures help minimize instability on the dorsal/volar plane, but do not prevent radial/ulnar impingement when the wrist is loaded.[31] The Darrach procedure is more suitable for lower-demand patients, such as RA patients.

Findings

There is limited data involving outcomes of the Darrach procedure for patients with RA. Fraser et al. reported outcomes for patients with Darrach resections for RA and post-traumatic conditions. Although motion was better in the post-traumatic group (both preoperatively and postoperatively), pain relief was significantly better in the RA group (86% to 36%).[32]

Recommendation

• The Darrach procedure is suitable for lower-demand patients, such as RA patients.

Question 7: What is the role of DRUJ arthrodesis (Suave–Kapandji procedure)?

Case clarification

When arthritis and instability are present at the DRUJ and sufficient bone is present in a younger patient, there may be a theoretical advantage to maintaining the distal ulna and the TFCC attachments to stabilize the ulnar carpal joint.

Relevance

The Suave–Kapandji (SK) procedure (Figure 115.7) fuses the ulnar head to the sigmoid notch of the radius and creates an osteotomy of the ulna proximal to the DRUJ with resection of approximately 1 cm of bone, thus allowing forearm rotation through the site of the osteotomy. The ulnar stump can be stabilized similar to the Darrach procedure and the potential for instability of the ulnar stump is similar for both procedures. The theoretical advantage of this procedure over the Darrach procedure is the maintenance of the ulnar head and TFCC, which may provide stability to the ulnar side of the carpus.

Findings

Vincent et al. reported on 21 wrists in 17 patients with an average follow-up of 39 months. There was good pain relief and subjective stability. One patient with a Darrach procedure on one side and SK procedure on the other preferred the SK side.[33]

Recommendation

• There is no evidence to indicate whether the Darrach procedure or the SK procedure is better

Question 8: What is the role of implant arthroplasty at the DRUJ?

Case clarification

Younger, more active patients may desire a more anatomic reconstruction than a resection of the ulnar head. In addition patients may present with pain from instability of the ulnar stump in spite of attempted soft tissue reconstruction.

Relevance

Ulnar head implant arthroplasty has gained popularity with the advent of newer materials and techniques that

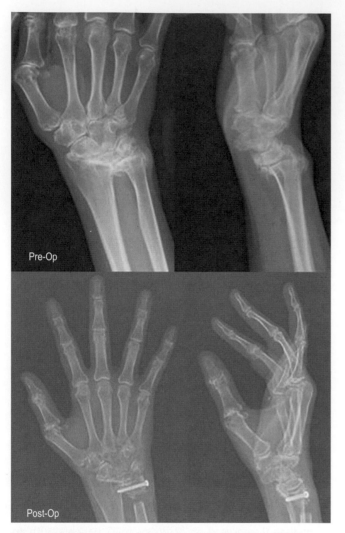

Figure 115.7 Preoperative and postoperative radiographs of DRUJ arthrodesis (Suave–Kapandjii procedure).

have been successfully used for the painful and unstable DRUJ in post-traumatic conditions. It has also been used as a salvage procedure for the failed Darrach when radial–ulnar impingement occurs.

The procedure involves resection of the ulnar head and replacement with an endoprosthesis. The newer generation implants approximate the normal anatomy, but rely to some degree on the soft tissue support around the implant to maintain stability.

Findings

Schecker has developed an ulnar prosthesis with an ulnar stem, constrained to the sigmoid notch through a link to the radius, which eliminates the need for soft tissue stabilization.[34,35] Additional designs are available,[36] but the role of these implants in patients with RA has not been clearly delineated.

Recommendation

• So far, there are no prospective studies evaluating arthroplasty for the DRUJ, and case series and reports are from post-traumatic or degenerative cases rather than in patients with RA.

Question 9: What are the outcomes of rheumatoid wrist procedures?

Relevance

Prospective randomized studies for RA surgery are sparse, and high-level evidence studies for the rheumatoid wrist conditions are similarly deficient. Medical management is improving and thus the number of surgical procedures for the RA hand is declining.[37]

Outcomes for procedures in the hand, specifically silicone MCP joint arthroplasty, have been published and hopefully meaningful data regarding outcomes of wrist procedures will be available in the near future.[38–41]

Summary of recommendations

• It is important to listen carefully to the patient's concerns and address the issue that is most bothersome to the patient
• Routine zero-rotation PA and lateral radiographs of the wrist are diagnostic and treatment recommendations can be made based on physical exams and radiographic findings. There is no evidence to suggest additional imaging or laboratory tests will enhance the RA hand assessment
• Limited wrist arthrodesis can be considered when there is a need to stabilize the radiocarpal joint due to ulnar translocation of the carpus or when there is destruction of the radiocarpal joint and sparing of the midcarpal joint
• Total wrist arthrodesis should be considered for patients with severe destruction of the wrist secondary to rheumatoid disease
• Currently, there is no evidence to support arthroplasty being superior to arthrodesis, arthroplasty may be considered an acceptable option. The best indications appear to be for patients requiring bilateral procedures and for those patients with a strong preference to retain motion, with the understanding that additional procedures are likely for treating complications such as implant dislocation or loosening
• The Darrach procedure is suitable for lower-demand patients, such as RA patients
• There is no evidence to indicate whether the Darrach procedure or the SK procedure is better
• So far, there are no prospective studies evaluating arthroplasty for the DRUJ, and case series and reports are from post-traumatic or degenerative cases rather than in patients with RA.

Conclusions

Unfortunately, the evidence regarding surgical treatment of the rheumatoid wrist consists of level IV and V data, which are based on retrospective case reviews and surgical techniques. A review of the Cochrane Database revealed only two reports and neither involved surgical treatment—one reviewed intraarticular steroids and splints whereas the second reviewed the use of the TENS unit for the management of rheumatoid hand conditions. There are currently no level I, II, or III studies regarding rheumatoid wrist conditions or addressing the questions above. With improvements in the medical treatment of rheumatoid arthritis, it is unlikely that there will be any level I or II studies for these conditions. Future research efforts will likely be directed towards cost-effectiveness and outcomes for existing procedures.[42-44]

References

1. Feldon P, Terrono AL, Nalebuff EA, Millander LH. Rheumatoid arthritis and other connective tissue diseases. In: Green DP, Hotchkiss RN, Pederson WC, Wolfe SW, eds., Green's Operative Hand Surgery, 5th edn. Elsevier, Philadelphia, 2005.

2. Taleisnik J. The ligaments of the wrist. J Hand Surg Am 1976;1(2): 110–18.

3. Taleisnik J. Rheumatoid synovitis of the volar compartment of the wrist joint: its radiological signs and its contribution to wrist and hand deformity. J Hand Surg Am 1979;4(6): 526–35.

4. Taleisnik J. Rheumatoid arthritis of the wrist. Hand Clin 1989;5(2):257–78.

5. Kelsey JL, Praemer A, Nelson L, Felberg A, Rice DP. Upper Extremity Disorders: Frequency, Impact and Cost. Churchill Livingstone, New York, 1997.

6. Rindfleisch J, Muller D. Diagnosis and management of rheumatoid arthritis. Am Fam Physician 2005;72(6):1037–47.

7. Helmick CG, Felson DT, Lawrence RC, et al. Estimates of the prevalence of arthritis and other rheumatic conditions in the United States. Part I. Arthritis Rheum 2008;58(1):15–25.

8. de la Mata Llord J, Palacios Carvajal J. Rheumatoid arthritis: are outcomes better with medical or surgical management? Orthopedics 1998;21(10):1085–6.

9. Dellhag B, Bjelle A. A five-year followup of hand function and activities of daily living in rheumatoid arthritis patients. Arthritis Care Res 1999;12(1):33–41.

10. Sherrer YS, Bloch DA, Mitchell DM, Young DY, Fries JF. The development of disability in rheumatoid arthritis. Arthritis Rheum 1986;29(4):494–500.

11. Yelin E. The costs of rheumatoid arthritis: absolute, incremental, and marginal estimates. J Rheumatol 1996;44S:47–51.

12. Alderman AK, Ubel PA, Kim HM, Fox DA, Chung KC. Surgical management of the rheumatoid hand: consensus and controversy among rheumatologists and hand surgeons. J Rheumatol 2003;30(7):1464–72.

13. Alderman AK, Chung KC, Kim HM, Fox DA, Ubel PA. Effectiveness of rheumatoid hand surgery: contrasting perceptions of hand surgeons and rheumatologists. J Hand Surg Am 2003;28(1):3–11; discussion 2–3.

14. Alderman AK, Chung KC, Demonner S, Spilson SV, Hayward RA. The rheumatoid hand: a predictable disease with unpredictable surgical practice patterns. Arthritis Rheum 2002 Oct 15; 47(5):537–42.

15. McCombe D, Ireland D, McNab I. Distal scaphoid excision after radioscaphoid arthrodesis. J Hand Surg Am 2001;26: 877–82.

16. Pervaiz K, Bowers W, Isaacs J, Owen J, Wayne J. Range of motion effects of distal pole scaphoid excision and triquetral excision after radioscapholunate fusion: a cadaver study. J Hand Surg Am 2009;34:832–7.

17. Arimitsu S, Murase T, Hashimoto J, Yoshikawa H, Sugamoto K, Moritomo H. Three-dimensional kinematics of the rheumatoid wrist after partial arthrodesis. J Bone Joint Surg Am 2009;91(9): 2180–7.

18. Honkanen PB, Makela S, Konttinen YT, Lehto MU. Radiocarpal arthrodesis in the treatment of the rheumatoid wrist. A prospective midterm follow-up. J Hand Surg Eur 2007;32(4):368–76.

19. Ishikawa H, Murasawa A, Nakazono K. Long-term follow-up study of radiocarpal arthrodesis for the rheumatoid wrist. J Hand Surg Am 2005;30(4):658–66.

20. Rehak DC, Kasper P, Baratz ME, Hagberg WC, McClain E, Imbriglia JE. A comparison of plate and pin fixation for arthrodesis of the rheumatoid wrist. Orthopedics 2000;23(1):43–8.

21. Toma CD, Machacek P, Bitzan P, Assadian O, Trieb K, Wanivenhaus A. Fusion of the wrist in rheumatoid arthritis: a clinical and functional evaluation of two surgical techniques. J Bone Joint Surg Br 2007;89(12):1620–6.

22. Rauhaniemi J, Tiusanen H, Sipola E. Total wrist fusion: a study of 115 patients. J Hand Surg Br 2005;30(2):217–9.

23. Cavaliere CM, Chung KC. A systematic review of total wrist arthroplasty compared with total wrist arthrodesis for rheumatoid arthritis. Plast Reconstr Surg 2008;122(3):813–25.

24. Murphy D, Khoury J, Imbriglia JE, Adams B. Comparison of arthroplasty and arthrodesis for the rheumatoid wrist. J Hand Surg Am 2003;28:570–6.

25. Divelbiss B, Sollerman C, Adams B. Early results of the Universal total wrist arthroplasty in rheumatoid arthritis. J Hand Surg Am 2002;27:195–204.

26. Cavaliere CM, Chung KC. Total wrist arthroplasty and total wrist arthrodesis in rheumatoid arthritis: a decision analysis from the hand surgeons' perspective. J Hand Surg Am 2008; 33(10):1744–55, 55 e1–2.

27. Johnson R. Stabilization of the distal ulna by transfer of the pronator quadratus origin. Clin Orthop 1992;275:130–2.

28. Kleinman W, Greenberg J. Salvage of the failed Darrach procedure. J Hand Surg Am 1995;20:951–8.

29. Breen T, Jupiter J. Extensor carpi ulnaris and flexor carpi ulnaris tenodesis of the unstable distal ulna. J Hand Surg Am 1989;14: 612–17.

30. Garcia-Elias M. Failed ulnar head resection. J Hand Surg Br 2002;27:470–80.

31. McKee M, Richards R. Dynamic radio-ulnar convergence after the Darrach procedure. J Bone Joint Surg Br 1996;78: 413–8.

32. Fraser K, Diao E, Peimer C, Sherwin F. Comparative results of resection of the distal ulna in rheumatoid arthritis and post-traumatic conditions. J Hand Surg Br 1999;24(6):667–70.

33. Vincent K, Szabo R, Agee J. The Suave-Kapandji procedure for reconstruction of the rheumatoid distal radioulnar joint. J Hand Surg Am 1993;1993:978–83.

34. Scheker LR. Implant arthroplasty for the distal radioulnar joint. J Hand Surg Am 2008;33(9):1639–44.

35. Scheker L, Babb B, Killion P. Distal ulnar prosthetic replacement. Orthop Clin North Am 2001;32:365–76.

36. Berger R, Cooney W. Use of ulnar head endoprosthesis for treatment of an unstable distal ulnar resection: review of mechanics, indications, and surgical technique. Hand Clin 2005;21:603–20.

37. van der Kooij S, De Vries-Bouwstra J, Goekoop-Ruiterman Y, et al. Patient-reported outcomes in a randomized trial comparing four different treatment strategies in recent-onset rheumatoid arthritis. Arthritis Rheum 2009;61(1):4–12.

38. Chung K, Burke F, Wilgis E, Regan M, Kim H, Fox D. A prospective study comparing outcomes after reconstruction in rheumatoid arthritis patients with severe ulnar drift deformities. Plast Reconstr Surg 2009;123:1769–77.

39. Chung K, Burns P, Wilgis E, et al. A multicenter clinical trial in rheumatoid arthritis comparing silicone metacarpophalangeal joint arthroplasty with medical treatment. J Hand Surg Am 2009;34:509–14.

40. Chung K, Kotsis S, Kim H, Burke F, Wilgis E. A prospective outcomes study of Swanson metacarpophalangeal joint arthroplasty for the rheumatoid hand. J Hand Surg Am 2004;29:646–53.

41. Chung K, Kowalski C, Kim H, Kazmers I. Patient outcomes following Swanson silastic metacarpophalangeal joint arthroplasty in the rheumatoid hand: a systematic overview. J Rheumatol 2000;27:1395–402.

42. Cavaliere CM, Chung KC. A cost-utility analysis of nonsurgical management, total wrist arthroplasty, and total wrist arthrodesis in rheumatoid arthritis. J Hand Surg Am 2010;35:379–91.

43. Waljee JF, Chung KC, Kim HM, et al. Validity and responsiveness of the Michigan Hand Questionnaire in patients with rheumatoid arthritis: a multicenter, international study. Arthritis Care Res 2010;62:1569–77.

44. Waljee JF, Chung KC. Outcomes research in rheumatoid arthritis. Hand Clin 2011;27:115–26.

116 Management of Finger Fractures

Kristin B. de Haseth and David Ring

Massachusetts General Hospital, Boston, MA, USA

Case scenario

A 31 year old woman presents to the Emergency Department after an injury playing field hockey. A direct blow from another hockey stick caused immediate pain and swelling of her right small finger. She is a keen athlete, has no medical history and does not take any medication.

On examination, she has diminished range of motion (ROM) of her right dominant small finger and a normal neurovascular exam.

Relevant anatomy

The hand skeleton is made up of 5 metacarpals and 14 phalanges. The metacarpophalangeal joints (MCPJ) and interphalangeal joints (IPJ) are stabilized through the volar plate, the collateral ligaments and the interosseous ligaments. Shortening, angulation, and rotation are the principle elements of deformity and may be seen in individually or in combination.

Importance of the problem

Metacarpal and phalangeal fractures are the most common injuries of the upper extremity.[1-3] The incidence of finger fractures peaks between the ages of 10 and 40 years. They are more common in males and are common sports injuries.[4]

Fractures of the metacarpals and phalanges have significant economic consequences. Kelsey et al.[2] reported that that were over 17.6 million upper extremity injuries that resulted in almost 32.5 million days of restricted activity and over 9.5 million days off work. The estimated cost of these injuries was approximately $18.5 million.

Hand fractures may be complicated by deformity from no treatment, stiffness from overtreatment, and deformity and stiffness from poor treatment.[5] It is becoming increasingly clear that success of a procedure is also determined by the psychological and economic impact of the disease and its treatment on the patient's life.

Top six questions

Diagnosis

1. Can observers agree on radiological characterization and classification of hand fracture?

Treatment

2. When should patients with extra-articular metacarpal fractures start exercises?
3. Should open reduction and internal fixation (ORIF) or a dynamic external device be used for management of unstable proximal interphalangeal joint (PIP) fracture-dislocations?
4. Which is a better treatment for extra-articular metacarpal and phalanx fractures: pinning or ORIF?
5. What is the best treatment option for closed, either bony or tendinous, mallet finger injuries?

Prognosis

6. What are the predictors of motion and function after plate and screw fixation of a finger fracture?

Evidence-Based Orthopedics, First Edition. Edited by Mohit Bhandari.
© 2012 Blackwell Publishing Ltd. Published 2012 by Blackwell Publishing Ltd.

Question 1: Can observers agree on radiological characterization and classification of finger fractures?

Relevance

Reliable characterization and classification of hand fractures might influence both research and patient care.

Current opinion

There is a high degree of variability in radiographic assessment in interobserver reliability and intraobserver reproducibility of hand fractures.[6-8]

Finding the evidence

• PubMed (http://www.ncbi.nlm.nih.gov/pubmed) sensitivity search using keywords: "finger fracture," "metacarpal fracture," "intra/interobserver reliability," "imaging," "diagnostic," "radiography," "computed tomography"
• Ovid MEDLINE with search term as above

Quality of the evidence

Observational studies do not have levels of evidence.

Findings

In one study three observers independently evaluated radiographs of 32 patients with small finger metacarpal neck fractures.[9] Six weeks later the process was repeated to evaluate intraobserver variability. The overall average for the difference in angles measured between two surgeons was 10.9°, with a SD of 9.2°. The mean weighted kappa coefficient for was 0.18 for interobserver variability and 0.26 for intraobserver variability. The mean kappa coefficient of intraobserver agreement on treatment recommendations was 0.36.

Another study assessed the reliability of the AO classification using 100 radiographs of hand fractures classified by 9 observers.[10] Using Cohen's kappa, the overall interobserver and intraobserver agreement was 0.93 and 0.94 respectively for fractured bone; 0.8 and 0.92 respectively for fractured bone segment; and 0.44 and 0.62 respectively for fracture type.

In another study there was no significant difference between cone beam CT (CBCT) and multislice CT (MSCT) for preoperative evaluation of 57 articular phalanx fractures.[11] All 57 fractures were correctly classified on the basis of articular involvement at CBCT compared to MSCT (100% sensitivity and specificity) with no statistically significant difference. CBCT identified 92 out of 103 fracture fragments (89.3%) compared to MSCT. The mean diameter of missed fragments was 0.9 mm at MSCT. None of the bone fragments missed by CBCT was located within the joint, in no cases the choice of the correct treatment prevented. Agreement among three observers was very good (kappa = 0.89–0.96).

Recommendations

• Consistent with other fractures, radiographic classification has limited reliability, which might improve with more sophisticated imaging techniques [overall quality: very low]
• It is unclear whether observer variation affects recovery.

Question 2: When should a patient with an extra-articular metacarpal fracture start exercises?

Case clarification

The fracture involves the small finger metacarpal neck.

Relevance

Immediate initiation of exercise might result in better final full ROM and function of the hand, since bone healing and recovery of ROM should occur simultaneously.

Current opinion

Most fractures need some protection, but immobilization risks tendon and joint adhesions. The balance between mobilization and immobilization is a matter of clinical judgment.

Finding the evidence

• Pubmed (www.ncbi.nlm.nih.gov/pubmed) sensitivity search using keywords: "metacarpal fracture," "intra-articular metacarpal fracture," "extra-articular metacarpal fracture," "exercise," "rehabilitation," "mobilization"
• Cochrane Database, using the same search terms

Quality of the evidence

• Level I: 2[12,13]
• Level II: 1[14]
• Level III: 3[15-17]

Findings

A Cochrane review[18] including 1 level I,[12] 1 level II,[14] and 1 level III study[15] addressing treatment of small finger metacarpal fractures with immobilization or early motion identified no differences in final motion 3 months or greater after fracture, but some differences at earlier time points.

Another level I trial involving stable metacarpal shaft fractures found better motion with a compression glove than with plaster splint immobilization after 2 and 3 weeks (28° difference, p < 0.01; 23° difference, p = 0.001).[13]

Two level III trials comparing cast immobilization and a custom mold plaster fracture brace found significantly better wrist, MCP and PIP motion after 3 and 4 weeks respectively in the brace group, but no differences after 3 months.[16,17]

Recommendation

• Early mobilization does not affect the final outcome of closed metacarpal fractures and can be utilized at the discretion of patient and surgeon when there is motivation to avoid immobilization [overall quality: high]

Question 3: Should ORIF or a dynamic external device be used for management of unstable PIP fracture-dislocations?

Case clarification

There is a fracture-dislocation of the PIP joint.

Relevance

Unstable dorsal fracture-dislocations of the PIP joint are difficult to manage.

Current opinion

There is wide variation in the treatment of these injuries.

Finding the evidence

• PubMed (www.ncbi.nlm.nih.gov/pubmed) sensitivity search using keywords: "proximal interphalangeal joint dislocation fracture," "treatment," "open reduction and internal fixation," "dynamic external device"

Quality of evidence

• Level I: 1[19]
• Level IV: 10[8–17]

Findings

Ten level IV retrospective case series addressed a single treatment technique.[20–29] The average arc of PIP joint motion was 88.7° with a range from 70° to 165°. Complication rates ranged from 8% to 63%. There was no clear advantage of one approach over another.

One level I randomized controlled trial (RCT) compared percutaneous Kirschner wire (K-wire) fixation vs. ORIF with cerclage wire or lag screw.[19] The arc of motion of the PIP joint was significantly better in the percutaneous K-wire fixation group (average flexion contracture to average flexion 60–108°) than in the screw fixation group (24–90°) or the cerclage fixation group (45–60°; p = 0.05). According to the patient-rated outcome, K-wires were superior to ORIF treatment (p = 0.02).

Recommendation

• There is insufficient evidence to recommend a specific operative treatment technique for unstable dorsal fracture-dislocations of the PIP joint. The data from one randomized trial suggest that less invasive treatment has advantages, at least in the short term [overall quality: high–moderate]

Question 4: Which is a better treatment for extra-articular metacarpal and phalanx fractures: pinning or ORIF?

Case clarification

Radiographs reveal a displaced extra-articular fracture of the proximal phalanx.

Relevance

Although ORIF with plates and screws provide excellent stability and allows early motion, it causes additional soft tissue trauma and can lead to extensor tendon adhesions and objectionable scarring. Pinning, on the contrary, may eliminate such complications; however, it is uncertain whether the results are as satisfactory.

Current opinion

The ideal treatment of extra-articular finger fractures remains controversial. Despite the conceptual advantages of ORIF in providing stability and alignment, pinning frequently offer a good alternative.

Finding the evidence

• PubMed (www.ncbi.nlm.nih.gov/pubmed) sensitivity search using keywords: "extra articular hand fracture," "extra articular phalanx fracture," "extra articular metacarpal fracture," "treatment," "pinning," "K-wire fixation," "open reduction and internal fixation"
• MeSH search, using search terms as above

Quality of evidence

• Level I: 1[30]
• Level III: 2[31,32]

Findings

A level I prospective randomized trial comparing percutaneous K-wire fixation with open reduction and lag screw fixation of long oblique proximal phalanx fractures found no significant differences in motion, strength, pain, or radiographic alignment.[30]

One level III study compared retrospective cohorts of patients with metacarpal fractures treated with intramedullary nail fixation or extra-articular with plate and screw fixation and found no significant differences in total active motion (TAM) or DASH scores regardless of fracture location.[31]

A level III nonrandomized controlled comparison of percutaneous transverse K-wire fixation and IM K-wiring of small finger metacarpal neck fractures found no statistically significant difference in TAM, grip strength, and fracture union.[32]

Recommendation

• There are insufficient data to recommend one fixation technique over another [overall quality: high–moderate]

Question 5: What is the best treatment option for closed, either bony or tendinous, mallet finger injuries?

Case clarification

On examination, the distal interphalangeal joint (DIPJ) of the patient's index finger is flexed 60° and she is unable to extend this joint. There is an avulsion fracture of the dorsal distal phalanx (mallet fracture).

Relevance

Mallet fractures are common.

Current opinion

Most hand surgeons believe that nonoperative care is the best option for treatment of mallet injuries in the absence of subluxation or a large intra-articular fracture.[33]

Finding the evidence

- PubMed (www.ncbi.nlm.nih.gov/pubmed) sensitivity search using keywords: "mallet finger," "treatment"
- PubMed (www.ncbi.nlm.nih.gov/pubmed)clinical queries search/systematic reviews, using search terms as above
- Cochrane Database, using search terms as above

Quality of evidence

- Level II: 3[34–36]
- Level III: 2[37,38]

Findings

A Cochrane review[39] included one level II study[34] which prospectively randomized patients with mallet finger injuries who received either closed pinning or splint treatment. No statistically significant difference was found between the participants (surgical vs. splint: 10.5% vs. 13.6% had complications)

A level II nonrandomized prospective cohort study compared conservative and operative treatment of intra-articular mallet fingers.[35] In the operated group an outcome of 10–20° extension deficit occurred in 38% and a 10–15° flexion deficit occurred in 19%. In the splinting group the numbers were 33% and 8% respectively, and in the group which not received treatment they were 100% and 20%. Bony union was seen in 95.3% of these patients.

A level III retrospective study noted a complication rate of 53% in the surgically treated patients (most long-term) and 45% in the splinting group (almost always transient).[38] In a similar level III study complications were found in 22% of the operative group and 28.6% of the splinting group (20% due to noncompliance).[37] Degenerative changes were comparable.

Geyman et al.[36] pooled literature regarding conservative vs. surgical treatment of closed mallet finger injuries; suc-cessful outcome was found in 77% in the conservative group, whereas 85% in the surgical group.

Recommendation

- Nonsurgical splinting is a safe and reliable treatment for most mallet injuries, whether bony or tendinous [overall quality: moderate]

Question 6: What are the predictors of motion and function after plate fixation of a finger fracture?

Case clarification

The patient has a crush injury, with a comminuted meta-carpal and proximal phalanx fracture and a wound. The surgeon used a plate and screws to repair the fracture.

Relevance

There is a need to balance the value of stable fixation with the soft tissue damage needed to apply internal fixation.

Current opinion

There is debate regarding operative strategies for many hand fractures.

Finding the evidence

- PubMed (www.ncbi.nlm.nih.gov/pubmed) sensitivity search using keywords: "screw and plate fixation," "internal fixation," "predictors outcome," "hand surgery," "finger fracture"

Quality of evidence

- Level III: 2[40,41]
- Level IV: 4[42–45]

Findings

Studies (two at level III[40,41] and two at level IV[42,43]) assessing the results of plate fixation of metacarpal and phalangeal fractures found better motion among metacarpal fractures compared to phalangeal fractures;[40,42] closed compared to open fractures;[40,41] extra-articular compared to intra-articular fractures (p < 0.05);[42] transverse metacarpal fractures compared to other metacarpal fracture patterns (p = 0.04);[43] fractures fixed with standard plates compared to those repaired with mini condylar plates (p = 0.004 respectively p = 0.006);[40] and younger compared to older patients.[41,42] Comminution and fracture location did not affect results.[40,44]

With regard to fracture union, in level IV studies healing problems were more common among transverse compared to nontransverse fractures,[42,43] phalangeal compared to metacarpal;[44] and manual workers compared to nonmanual workers.[42,45] Nonunion was not associated with soft tissue injury or plate type.[42,45]

Recommendations

• Predictors of final motion after plate and screw fixation of a metacarpal and phalangeal fracture are the age of the patient, open fracture/soft tissue injury, plate type, intra-articular fracture, and phalangeal fractures [overall quality: moderate–low]

• Predictors of nonunion include fracture location (proximal phalanx), pattern (transverse fractures) and occupation (manual workers) [overall quality: moderate–low]

Summary of recommendations

• Consistent with other fractures, radiographic classification has limited reliability, which might improve with more sophisticated imaging techniques

• Early mobilization does not affect the final outcome of closed metacarpal fractures and can be utilized at the discretion of patient and surgeon when a faster recovery is desired

• There is insufficient evidence to recommend a specific operative treatment technique for unstable dorsal fracture-dislocations of the PIPJ. The data from one randomized trial suggest that less invasive treatment has advantages at least in the short term

• For extra-articular finger fractures there are insufficient data to recommend pinning fixation technique over K-wire fixation

• Nonsurgical splinting is a safe and reliable treatment for most mallet injuries, whether bony or tendinous

• Predictors of final motion after plate and screw fixation of a metacarpal and phalangeal fracture are the age of the patient, open fracture/soft tissue injury, plate type, intra-articular fracture, and phalangeal fractures

• Predictors of nonunion include fracture location and pattern and occupation

Conclusions

Data regarding management of finger fracture varies from RCTs to case series. For closed metacarpal fractures, immobilization does not improve outcomes. With regards to specific operative technique for PIP joint fracture-dislocations and extra-articular finger fractures there is insufficient evidence for superiority of any one technique.

Further investigations, specifically high-quality comparative studies, are needed for further elucidation regarding adequate management of finger fractures.

References

1. Hove LM. Fractures of the hand. Distribution and relative incidence. Scand J Plast Reconstr Surg Hand Surg 1993;27(4):317–19.

2. Kelsey JL, Pastides H, Kreiger N, et al. Upper Extremity Disorders: A Survey of their Frequency, Impact, and Cost in the United States, pp. 9–71. Mosby, St Louis, 1997.

3. Emmett JE, Breck LW. A review and analysis of 11,000 fractures seen in a private practice of orthopaedic surgery, 1937–1956. J Bone Joint Surg Am 1958;40(5):1169–75.

4. de Jonge JJ, Kingma J, van der Lei B, Klasen HJ. Fractures of the metacarpals. A retrospective analysis of incidence and aetiology and a review of the English-language literature. Injury 1994; 25(6):365–9.

5. Swanson AB. Fractures involving the digits of the hand. Orthop Clin North Am 1970; 1(2):261–74.

6. Andersen DJ, Blair WF, Steyers CM Jr, Adams BD, el-Khouri GY, Brandser EA. Classification of distal radius fractures: an analysis of interobserver reliability and intraobserver reproducibility. J Hand Surg Am 1996;21(4):574–82.

7. Bernstein J, Adler LM, Blank JE, Dalsey RM, Williams GR, Iannotti JP. Evaluation of the Neer system of classification of proximal humeral fractures with computerized tomographic scans and plain radiographs. J Bone Joint Surg Am 1996;78(9): 1371–5.

8. Thomsen NO, Overgaard S, Olsen LH, Hansen H, Nielsen ST. Observer variation in the radiographic classification of ankle fractures. J Bone Joint Surg Br 1991;73(4):676–8.

9. Leung YL, Beredjiklian PK, Monaghan BA, Bozentka DJ. Radiographic assessment of small finger metacarpal neck fractures. J Hand Surg Am 2002;27(3):443–8.

10. Szwebel JD, Ehlinger V, Pinsolle V, Bruneteau P, Pélissier P, Salmi LR. Reliability of a classification of fractures of the hand based on the AO Comprehensive Classification system. J Hand Surg Eur 2010;35(5):392–5.

11. Faccioli N, Foti G, Barillari M, Atzei A, Mucelli RP. Finger fractures imaging: accuracy of cone-beam computed tomography and multislice computed tomography. Skeletal Radiol 2010; 39(11):1087–95.

12. Statius Muller MG, Poolman RW, van Hoogstraten MJ, Steller EP. Immediate mobilization gives good results in boxer's fractures with volar angulation up to 70°: a prospective randomized trial comparing immediate mobilization with cast immobilization. Arch Orthop Trauma Surg 2003;123(10):534–7.

13. McMahon PJ, Woods DA, Burge PD. Initial treatment of closed metacarpal fractures. A controlled comparison of compression glove and splintage. J Hand Surg Br 1994; 19(5): 597–600.

14. Kuokkanen HO, Mulari-Keränen SK, Niskanen RO, Haapala JK, Korkala OL. Treatment of subcapital fractures of the fifth metacarpal bone: a prospective randomised comparison between functional treatment and reposition and splinting. Scand J Plast Reconstr Surg Hand Surg 1999;33(3):315–17.

15. Braakman M, Oderwald EE, Haentjens MH. Functional taping of fractures of the 5th metacarpal results in a quicker recovery. Injury 1998;29(1):5–9.

16. Konradsen L, Nielsen PT, Albrecht-Beste E. Functional treatment of metacarpal fractures 100 randomized cases with or without fixation. Acta Orthop Scand 1990;61(6):531–4.

17. Sørensen JS, Freund KG, Kejlå G. Functional fracture bracing in metacarpal fractures: the Galveston metacarpal brace versus a plaster-of-Paris bandage in a prospective study. J Hand Ther 1993;6(4):263–5.

18. Poolman RW, Goslings JC, Lee JB, Statius Muller M, Steller EP, Struijs PA. Conservative treatment for closed fifth (small finger) metacarpal neck fractures. Cochrane Database Syst Rev 2005;3: CD003210.

19. Aladin A, Davis TR. Dorsal fracture-dislocation of the proximal interphalangeal joint: a comparative study of percutaneous Kirschner wire fixation versus open reduction and internal fixation. J Hand Surg Br 2005;30(2):120–8.

20. Hamilton SC, Stern PJ, Fassler PR, Kiefhaber TR. Mini-screw fixation for the treatment of proximal interphalangeal joint dorsal fracture-dislocations. J Hand Surg Am 2006;31(8): 1349–54.

21. Lee JY, Teoh LC. Dorsal fracture dislocations of the proximal interphalangeal joint treated by open reduction and interfragmentary screw fixation: indications, approaches and results. J Hand Surg Br 2006;31(2):138–46.

22. Nalbantoğlu U, Gereli A, Kocaoğlu B, Aktaş S, Seyhan M. Surgical treatment of unstable fracture-dislocations of the proximal interphalangeal joint. Acta Orthop Traumatol Turc 2007;41(5):373–9.

23. Grant I, Berger AC, Tham SK. Internal fixation of unstable fracture dislocations of the proximal interphalangeal joint. J Hand Surg Br 2005;30(5):492–8.

24. Ellis SJ, Cheng R, Prokopis P, Chetboun A, Wolfe SW, Athanasian EA, Weiland AJ. Treatment of proximal interphalangeal dorsal fracture-dislocation injuries with dynamic external fixation: a pins and rubber band system. J Hand Surg Am 2007;32(8): 1242–50.

25. Badia A, Riano F, Ravikoff J, Khouri R, Gonzalez-Hernandez E, Orbay JL. Dynamic intradigital external fixation for proximal interphalangeal joint fracture dislocations. J Hand Surg Am 2005;30(1):154–60.

26. De Smet L, Boone P. Treatment of fracture-dislocation of the proximal interphalangeal joint using the Suzuki external fixator. J Orthop Trauma 2002;16(9):668–71.

27. Ruland RT, Hogan CJ, Cannon DL, Slade JF. Use of dynamic distraction external fixation for unstable fracture-dislocations of the proximal interphalangeal joint. J Hand Surg Am 2008;33(1): 19–25.

28. Majumder S, Peck F, Watson JS, Lees VC. Lessons learned from the management of complex intra-articular fractures at the base of the middle phalanges of fingers. J Hand Surg Br 2003;28(6): 559–65.

29. Richter M, Brüser P. Long-term follow-up of fracture dislocations and comminuted fractures of the PIP joint treated with Suzuki's pin and rubber traction system. Handchir Mikrochir Plast Chir 2008;40(5):330–5.

30. Horton TC, Hatton M, Davis TR. A prospective randomized controlled study of fixation of long oblique and spiral shaft fractures of the proximal phalanx: closed reduction and percutaneous Kirschner wiring versus open reduction and lag screw fixation. J Hand Surg Br 2003;28(1):5–9.

31. Ozer K, Gillani S, Williams A, Peterson SL, Morgan S. Comparison of intramedullary nailing versus plate-screw fixation of extraarticular metacarpal fractures. J Hand Surg Am 2008;33(10): 1724–31.

32. Wong TC, Ip FK, Yeung SH. Comparison between percutaneous transverse fixation and intramedullary K-wires in treating closed fractures of the metacarpal neck of the little finger. J Hand Surg Br 2006;31(1):61–5.

33. Jabłecki J, Syrko M. Zone 1 extensor tendon lesions: current treatment methods and a review of literature. Ortop Traumatol Rehabil 2007;9(1):52–62.

34. Auchincloss JM. Mallet-finger injuries: a prospective, controlled trial of internal and external splintage. Hand 1982;14(2):168–73.

35. Niechajev IA. Conservative and operative treatment of mallet finger Plast Reconstr Surg 1985;76(4):580–5.

36. Geyman JP, Fink K, Sullivan SD. Conservative versus surgical treatment of mallet finger: a pooled quantitative literature evaluation. J Am Board Fam Pract 1998;11(5):382–90.

37. Wehbé MA, Schneider LH. Mallet fractures. J Bone Joint Surg Am 1984;66(5):658–69.

38. Stern PJ, Kastrup JJ. Complications and prognosis of treatment of mallet finger. J Hand Surg Am 1988;13(3):329–34.

39. Handoll HH, Vaghela MV. Interventions for treating mallet finger injuries. Cochrane Database Syst Rev 2004;3:CD004574.

40. Page SM, Stern PJ. Complications and range of motion following plate fixation of metacarpal and phalangeal fractures. J Hand Surg Am 1998;23(5):827–32.

41. Bannasch H, Heermann AK, Iblher N, Momeni A, Schulte-Mönting J, Stark GB. Ten years stable internal fixation of metacarpal and phalangeal hand fractures-risk factor and outcome analysis show no increase of complications in the treatment of open compared with closed fractures. J Trauma 2010;68(3): 624–8.

42. Omokawa S, Fujitani R, Dohi Y, Okawa T, Yajima H. Prospective outcomes of comminuted periarticular metacarpal and phalangeal fractures treated using a titanium plate system. J Hand Surg Am 2008;33(6):857–63.

43. Fusetti C, Meyer H, Borisch N, Stern R, Santa DD, Papaloïzos M. Complications of plate fixation in metacarpal fractures. J Trauma 2002;52(3):535–9.

44. Kurzen P, Fusetti C, Bonaccio M, Nagy L. Complications after plate fixation of phalangeal fractures. J Trauma 2006;60(4): 841–3.

45. Fusetti C, Della Santa DR. Influence of fracture pattern on consolidation after metacarpal plate fixation. Chir Main 2004;23(1): 32–6.

117 Prevention of Adhesion in Flexor Tendon Surgery

Filippo Spiezia[1], Vincenzo Denaro[1], and Nicola Maffulli[2]
[1]Campus Bio-Medico University, Rome, Italy
[2]Barts and The London School of Medicine and Dentistry, London, UK

Case scenario

A 35 year old manual worker is brought to the Emergency Department with a laceration of his left hand after a slip in the factory where he works. The bleeding is arrested, repair of the flexor tendons of the left ring finger is performed by a local surgeon, and the patient is splinted. After 4 weeks of splinting, the patient is seen by a hand surgeon. The hand is stiff, and he is currently unable to hold objects. He is neurovascularly intact. Peritendinous adhesions of the digital flexor tendons are diagnosed.

Relevant anatomy and physiology

Tendons consist mainly of collagen. Water, proteoglycans, and cells constitute the matrix. The composition of proteoglycans produced by cells changes in the pressure-bearing areas compared to the tension-transmitting areas within tendons. For example, chondroitin sulfate is found predominantly in the pressure contact areas, whereas dermatan sulfate is dominant in the tension-transmitting areas. The differences in the type and proportion of proteoglycans in the tension and pressure-bearing segments of the tendon are related to the functional needs of the tissue, and this may play a role in the formation of adhesions following tendon injury and repair.[1] Tendon healing occurs through a combination of intrinsic and extrinsic processes. Intrinsic healing is the result of the activity of tenocytes within the tendon itself, and it is facilitated by appropriate nutrition to the tendon itself. Chemotaxis allows extrinsic healing through the migration of specialized fibroblasts into the defect from the ends of the tendon sheath.[2] Synovial fluid

diffusion also provides an additional nutritional source for the intrinsic healing process.[3]

The development of adhesions is not directly stimulated by tendon injuries. Damaged flexor tendons with the ends retracted and rounded which lie freely within the sheath have no adhesions. Immobilization also does not lead to an adhesive response from the digital sheath. On the contrary, excision of the synovial sheath followed by immobilization most frequently results in an adhesive reaction. It has been also found that high degrees of trauma to the synovial sheath and gaps of 3 mm or more correlate with an increased rate of adhesion formation.[4]

Siegler et al. classified the degree and extent of adhesions (see box).[5]

Classification of adhesions

- **Grade 0:** Complete absence of adhesions
- **Grade I:** Thin, avascular, filmy, and easily separable
- **Grade II:** Thick, avascular, and limited to the site of anastomosis
- **Grade III:** Thick, vascular, and extensive

Importance of the problem

One of the main problems in hand surgery is peritendinous adhesions after repair of an injury to the digital flexor tendons. Although adhesions are part of the healing process, they may produce functional disability following the biological response of the tendon to injury.[6] The management of this condition is challenging, and has led to an intensive search for modified surgical therapies and various

Evidence-Based Orthopedics, First Edition. Edited by Mohit Bhandari.
© 2012 Blackwell Publishing Ltd. Published 2012 by Blackwell Publishing Ltd.

adjuvant therapies to prevent adhesion formation without compromising digital function. Different options have been proposed, including physical, surgical, and pharmacological treatment. However, the scientific evidence behind these methods should be carefully evaluated, because they are not necessarily in routine clinical practice. This chapter reviews these options, and evaluates the scientific evidence behind them.

Top four questions

Questions from the patient

1. Will I be able to hold objects and to use the hand again?
   • Yes, you will be able to use your hand after proper management and rehabilitation, although a strength deficit of the hand may persist
2. Will I be able to take part in sport activities again?
   • Yes, but it may be 3–6 months before you can do
3. How long does it take to fully recover?
   • It may take 6 months

Questions from family

4. Will he be able to work again?
   • Yes, your relative will be able to work again after proper management and rehabilitation, although a strength and movement deficit of the hand may persist

Case clarification

The flexor tendons are repaired using sutures. After the operation, the patient's hand was put in a splint. After 4 weeks, the hand surgeon diagnosed hand flexor tendon adhesions.

Current opinion

Current opinion suggests that the majority of surgeons use options including physical, surgical, and pharmacological treatment.

Finding the evidence

• PubMed, MEDLINE, CINAHL, and Embase were searched using the keywords: "tendon adhesion prevention," "tendon healing," "adhesion prevention in tendons," "adjuvants for adhesion prevention"
• Studies detailing the use of surgical, pharmacological, and nonpharmacological agents for adhesion prevention in

digital flexor tendons were identified, and their bibliographies were thoroughly reviewed to identify further related articles. This search identified studies which investigated the use of various pharmacological agents in adhesion prevention in digital tendons
• We excluded studies in languages other than English, studies not dealing with digital tendons, studies not reporting on adhesion prevention, case reports and letters to the editor.

Quality of the evidence

Most studies have been performed in animals, with very few human trials. This could potentially affect the quality of the evidence, because poor methodological standards in animal studies makes difficult to translate the positive results to the clinical domain. We found only a few randomized controlled trials, and the quality of the remaining studies is to be considered inferior to these.

Findings

Different options to manage adhesions are now available. Changes in surgical and postoperative rehabilitation techniques, modulation of inflammatory response and growth factors which may promote scarring through pharmacological agents, mechanical barriers between the tendons and the proliferating tissue, use of ultrasound and electromagnetic therapy, and, recently, gene therapy have all been explored.

Surgical management

Modern knowledge of tendon structure, nutrition, and biomechanical properties, and studies of tendon healing and adhesion formation, have produced various modifications of surgical management of tendon injuries.

One of the surgical techniques used to promote tendon healing decreasing the rate of adhesions is multistrand repair. Commonly the tendon is repaired using a two-strand technique.[7] As the strength of a tendon repair is proportional to the number of suture strands that cross the site of rupture, it is now common to perform repairs with four, six, or even eight strands, allowing early mobilization, which decreases rupture rate. A greater number of suture strands means a more technically demanding procedure, and consequently more surgical handling of the tendon and a larger amount of suture material on the surface of the tendon.[8]

The effect of increasing strand numbers on the healing or adhesion response in tendons is not clearly known. Even though no significant differences have been identified,[9] it is reasonable that suture techniques with high friction may cause more adhesion formation than lower-friction techniques.[10] Most studies in this field have been performed in animal models, and there is still a lack of human trials.

Another dilemma is whether or not to repair the tendon sheath at the site of rupture. Sheath closure following flexor tendon repair is common.[11] It has been proposed that that a lacerated tendon may heal through its intrinsic cellular processes without adhesion formation,[12] because flexor tendons are mainly nourished through synovial diffusion in the within the region of synovial sheaths.[13] Repair of the sheath may preserve nutrition of the tendons, allowing a smooth gliding surface and decreasing peritendinous adhesions.[14]

Sheath closure does not seems to improve tendon gliding function.[15] Postoperative mobilization has been shown to decrease adhesion formation and to improve function after flexor tendon repair.[16] However, the best mobilization strategy has not yet been identified.

When a flexor tendon injury occurs in the area of the major pulleys, the outcome of the repair is often unpredictable. There is a controversy between surgeons about performing a pulley incision or pulley plasty.

Incision of the pulley may improve the excursion of the flexor digitorum profundus (FDP) tendon and decrease the work of digital flexion over pulley closure. However, Kapandji pulley plasty did not increase tendon excursion and decrease the work compared with a simpler pulley incision. After the repair, adhesions have been shown to be more severe with pulley plasty or closure than with pulley incision.[17]

Recommendation

• For the problem of simultaneous repair in simultaneous ruptures of FDP and flexor digitorum superficialis (FDS), the literature suggests that it is better to repair only the FDP with regional excision of FDS when both tendons are injured in zone 2C [overall quality: moderate]

Pharmacological agents

Pharmacological adjuvants aim to increase the recovery and function in hand tendons after injury or surgery, and can be divided into two categories: drugs and barriers. Nonsteroidal anti-inflammatory drugs (NSAIDs) competitively inhibit cyclooxygenase, an enzyme essential for the metabolism of arachidonic acid (AA) to prostaglandins; all these are involved in the inflammatory process which leads to adhesion formation.[18] Several studies have shown that NSAIDs are likely to inhibit the formation of significant postoperative adhesions in a dose-dependent fashion.

Hyaluronic acid (HA) is a physiologic component of the synovial fluid, and has been suggested to play a role in healing of a variety of connective tissues, including injured tendons.[19] However, some human studies did not show beneficial effects.[20]

5-Fluorouracil (5-FU) also seems to play a role in reduction of adhesion formation, maybe affecting cell proliferation,[21] or reducing extracellular matrix molecules and growth factor production.[22] 5-FU may have a modulating effect on cellular activity without preventing cell proliferation. This could reduce adhesion formation without preventing wound healing. The proliferative and inflammatory responses can be significantly reduced in tendons treated with 5-FU, especially reducing cellular cytokine response and in the activity of the known pro-scarring agent, transforming growth factor beta (TGF-β).[23]

Human amniotic fluid (HAF) contains hormones, cytokines, and polypeptide growth factors that may have an effect on cell proliferation and differentiation. The exact role of amniotic fluid in preventing adhesion is not clear, but it has been suggested to have an inhibitory effect on fibroblast proliferation. All the evidence comes from animal studies.[24]

TGF-β is a cytokine involved in wound healing and in the pathogenesis of excessive scar formation.[25] TGF-β stimulates chemotaxis, promotes angiogenesis, and regulates a wide spectrum of matrix proteins. In animal models, TGF-β accelerates wound healing. However, this effect may result in pathologic fibrosis, with excessive disordered collagen deposition and tendon adhesions.[26] Inhibitors of TGF-β may reduce adhesion formation. TGF-β inhibition using a neutralizing antibody was effective in blocking TGF-β-induced collagen I production in cultured flexor tendons.[27]

Combinations of different substances have been also tried to prevent adhesions. For example, amniotic membrane, dipalmitoyl phosphatidylcholine, carboxymethylcellulose, and NSAIDs have been tried in animal models.

Chemical adjuvants such as alginate solution, collagen synthesis inhibitor (CPHI-I), enriched collagen solution, plant alkaloid halofuginone, human-derived fibrin sealant, and topical beta-aminopropionitrile have been studied for their potential role in preventing adhesions.[28]

Recommendation

• NSAIDs are likely to inhibit the formation of significant postoperative adhesions in a dose-dependent fashion, but the effects of other pharmacological agents are controversial [overall quality: moderate]

Mechanical barriers

The cellular activity of intrasynovial flexor tendons may be specially adapted to intrasynovial environments. Thus, reconstruction of damaged flexor tendon sheaths with a biocompatible, diffusible membrane may not interfere with the nutrition and healing of repaired flexor tendons. Furthermore, acting as a barrier between surrounding tissues and the repaired tendon, an interposed membrane may be able to further reduce the formation of adhesions.[29] This concept has led to the development of several chemical barriers to reduce adhesion prevention in digital tendons.

Expanded polytetrafluoroethylene (e-PTFE) has been used for reconstruction of tendon sheath and pulleys with promising results, and to decrease the formation of adhesions.[30] Other materials tested in animal models[31] are hydroxyapatite, HA membrane, polyvinyl alcohol hydrogel (PVA-H), and bovine pericardia.

Recommendation

• The use of e-PTFE for reconstruction of tendon sheath and pulleys is promising [overall quality: moderate]

Ultrasound and electromagnetic radiation

Ultrasound therapy and pulsed electromagnetic fields have also been investigated in animals, with controversial results. Ultrasound may interact with one or more components of inflammation, improving the time of resolution of inflammation. Other effects have been shown in vitro, such as accelerated fibrinolysis, stimulation of macrophage-derived fibroblast mitogenic factors, heightened fibroblast recruitment, accelerated angiogenesis, increased matrix synthesis, more dense collagen fibrils and increased tissue tensile strength.[31]

Ultrasound may also have nonthermal effects including cavitation and acoustic microstreaming, which may play a role in the management of soft tissue lesions and adhesion prevention than the thermal effects. These effects may stimulate tissue repair. Human studies suggest regression of peritendinous adhesion between the tendon and skin, an increased range of movement, advanced scar maturation and decreased amount of inflammatory infiltrate.[31]

Recommendation

• Ultrasound may improve the time needed to resolve inflammation [overall quality: moderate]

Gene therapy

In the near future, with the delivery of growth factor genes, gene therapy may improve the healing of injured digital tendons. Adenoviral, adeno-associated viral (AAV), and liposome–plasmid vectors have been used to deliver genes to tendons to improve its healing. Unfortunately, clinical evidence is still uncertain at present.[32]

Summary of recommendations

• The need to develop and use in clinical practice an optimal method for the prevention of adhesions in the flexor tendons of the hand is a major problem in hand surgery

• Although recent advances have been made in the study of prevention of adhesions in flexor tendons, it is still unclear which is the best strategy to manage the problem

• At present, early postoperative mobilization of digits after tendon injury and repair is the only clinically justifiable treatment, although the best method of mobilization remains controversial

Conclusions

New pharmacological and nonpharmacological modalities, and changes in surgical techniques proposed in recent years, need to be tested in more controlled human trials.

References

1. Gillard GC, Merrilees MJ, Bell-Booth PG, Reilly HC, Flint MH. The proteoglycan content and the axial periodicity of collagen in tendon. Biochem J 1977;163:145–51.
2. Wang ED. Tendon repair. J Hand Ther 1998;11:105–10.
3. Manske PR, Lesker PA. Histologic evidence of intrinsic flexor tendon repair in various experimental animals. An in vitro study. Clin Orthop Relat Res 1984;182:297–304.
4. Matthews P, Richards H. Factors in the adherence of flexor tendon after repair: an experimental study in the rabbit. J Bone Joint Surg Br 1976;58:230–6.
5. Siegler AM, Kontopoulos V, Wang CF. Prevention of postoperative adhesions in rabbits with ibuprofen, a nonsteroidal anti-inflammatory agent. Fertil Steril 1980;34:46–9.
6. Gelberman RH. Flexor tendon physiology: tendon nutrition and cellular activity in injury and repair. Instr Course Lect 1985;34:351–60.
7. Strickland JW. Development of flexor tendon surgery: twenty-five years of progress. J Hand Surg Am 2000;25:214–35.
8. Barrie KA, Wolfe SW, Shean C, Shenbagamurthi D, Slade JF, 3rd, Panjabi MM. A biomechanical comparison of multistrand flexor tendon repairs using an in situ testing model. J Hand Surg Am 2000;25:499–506.
9. Strick MJ, Filan SL, Hile M, McKenzie C, Walsh WR, Tonkin MA. Adhesion formation after flexor tendon repair: a histologic and biomechanical comparison of 2- and 4-strand repairs in a chicken model. J Hand Surg Am 2004;29:15–21.
10. Zhao C, Amadio PC, Momose T, Couvreur P, Zobitz ME, An KN. The effect of suture technique on adhesion formation after flexor tendon repair for partial lacerations in a canine model. J Trauma 2001;51:917–21.
11. Matthews P, Richards H. The repair potential of digital flexor tendons. An experimental study. J Bone Joint Surg Br 1974;56:618–25.
12. Lundborg G, Rank F. Experimental intrinsic healing of flexor tendons based upon synovial fluid nutrition. J Hand Surg Am 1978;3:21–31.

13. Lundborg G. Experimental flexor tendon healing without adhesion formation—a new concept of tendon nutrition and intrinsic healing mechanisms. A preliminary report. Hand 1976;8:235–8.

14. Gelberman RH, Vande Berg JS, Lundborg GN, Akeson WH. Flexor tendon healing and restoration of the gliding surface. An ultrastructural study in dogs. J Bone Joint Surg Am 1983;65: 70–80.

15. Peterson WW, Manske PR, Dunlap J, Horwitz DS, Kahn B. Effect of various methods of restoring flexor sheath integrity on the formation of adhesions after tendon injury. J Hand Surg Am 1990;15:48–56.

16. Strickland JW, Glogovac SV. Digital function following flexor tendon repair in Zone II: A comparison of immobilization and controlled passive motion techniques. J Hand Surg Am 1980; 5:537–43.

17. Tang JB, Xie RG, Cao Y, Ke ZS, Xu Y. A2 pulley incision or one slip of the superficialis improves flexor tendon repairs. Clin Orthop Relat Res 2007;456:121–7.

18. Kulick MI, Brazlow R, Smith S, Hentz VR. Injectable ibuprofen: preliminary evaluation of its ability to decrease peritendinous adhesions. Ann Plast Surg 1984;13:459–67.

19. Thomas SC, Jones LC, Hungerford DS. Hyaluronic acid and its effect on postoperative adhesions in the rabbit flexor tendon. A preliminary look. Clin Orthop Relat Res 1986;206:281–9.

20. Golash A, Kay A, Warner JG, Peck F, Watson JS, Lees VC. Efficacy of ADCON-T/N after primary flexor tendon repair in Zone II: a controlled clinical trial. J Hand Surg Br 2003;28:113–15.

21. Akali A, Khan U, Khaw PT, McGrouther AD. Decrease in adhesion formation by a single application of 5-fluorouracil after flexor tendon injury. Plast Reconstr Surg 1999;103:151–8.

22. Occleston NL, Daniels JT, Tarnuzzer RW, et al. Single exposures to antiproliferatives: long-term effects on ocular fibroblast wound-healing behavior. Invest Ophthalmol Vis Sci 1997;38: 1998–2007.

23. Khan U, Kakar S, Akali A, Bentley G, McGrouther DA. Modulation of the formation of adhesions during the healing of injured tendons. J Bone Joint Surg Br 2000;82:1054–8.

24. Ozgenel GY, Samli B, Ozcan M. Effects of human amniotic fluid on peritendinous adhesion formation and tendon healing after flexor tendon surgery in rabbits. J Hand Surg Am 2001;26: 332–9.

25. Chang J, Thunder R, Most D, Longaker MT, Lineaweaver WC. Studies in flexor tendon wound healing: neutralizing antibody to TGF-beta1 increases postoperative range of motion. Plast Reconstr Surg 2000;105:148–55.

26. Pierce GF, Mustoe TA, Lingelbach J, Masakowski VR, Gramates P, Deuel TF. Transforming growth factor beta reverses the glucocorticoid-induced wound-healing deficit in rats: possible regulation in macrophages by platelet-derived growth factor. Proc Natl Acad Sci U S A 1989;86:2229–33.

27. Zhang AY, Pham H, Ho F, Teng K, Longaker MT, Chang J. Inhibition of TGF-beta-induced collagen production in rabbit flexor tendons. J Hand Surg Am 2004;29:230–5.

28. Namba J, Shimada K, Saito M, Murase T, Yamada H, Yoshikawa H. Modulation of peritendinous adhesion formation by alginate solution in a rabbit flexor tendon model. J Biomed Mater Res B Appl Biomater 2007;80:273–9.

29. Hanff G, Abrahamsson SO. Matrix synthesis and cell proliferation in repaired flexor tendons within e-PTFE reconstructed flexor tendon sheaths. J Hand Surg Br 1996;21:642–6.

30. Hanff G, Abrahamsson SO. Cellular activity in e-PTFE reconstructed pulleys and adjacent regions of deep flexor tendons. An experimental biochemical study in rabbits. J Hand Surg Br 1996;21:419–23.

31. Khanna A, Gougoulias N, Maffulli N. Modalities in prevention of flexor tendon adhesion in the hand: what have we achieved so far? Acta Orthop Belg 2009;75:433–44.

32. Tang JB, Cao Y, Zhu B, Xin KQ, Wang XT, Liu PY. Adeno-associated virus-2-mediated bFGF gene transfer to digital flexor tendons significantly increases healing strength. an in vivo study. J Bone Joint Surg Am 2008;90:1078–89.

118 Therapy: Flexor Tendon Rehabilitation

B. Jane Freure and Mike Szekeres
St Joseph's Health Care, London, ON, Canada

Case scenario

Steve was carving a pumpkin with his children 9 days ago when the knife slipped and he cut the flexor tendons at the level of the proximal phalanx on his second, third, and fourth fingers on his right dominant hand, as well as cutting off some of the skin on his right thumb. He immediately went to his local hospital where the treating physician achieved hemostasis of the superficial wound and sutured the skin. The tendons were not fixed initially.

The patient was then referred to a larger hand center and had a consultation with the plastic surgeon 2 days later. The patient was brought to the operating room 4 days ago and had flexor digitorum superficialis (FDS) and flexor digitorum profundus (FDP) repairs for his index, long, and ring fingers. He was placed in a bulky dressing postoperatively and was reviewed in the clinic today. The bulky dressing was removed and light dressing applied. The sutures remain in situ.

The patient has been referred to therapy with the following instructions: POD 4—FDS/FDP repairs zone II, right D2, 3, 4. Orthosis/protected ROM.

Relevant anatomy

Flexor tendon zones

The FDS and FDP muscles are the primary flexors of the fingers. Anatomic description of these muscles is simplified by dividing the tendons that travel distally from the muscle bellies into zones. Figure 118.1 shows the superficial landmarks for the flexor zones of the hand.

Zone V to zone III

In zone V, the FDS lies superficial to the FDP in the forearm and is the only muscle in the intermediate layer of the forearm flexor compartment. Innervated by the median nerve, the FDS originates from the medial epicondyle of the humerus and the proximal radius and ulna. In the distal forearm it forms four separate muscles and tendons that travel through the carpal tunnel. Approximately 21% of the population does not have a FDS tendon to the small finger.[1] The orientation of the FDS tendons in the carpal tunnel is such that the tendons leading towards the long and ring fingers are superficial to the tendons for the index and small fingers. The FDS tendons are all superficial to the FDP tendons in zone IV. In the palm, these tendons diverge and travel to each finger.

The FDP shares the deep flexor compartment of the forearm with the flexor pollicis longus (FPL). It originates from the proximal ulna, the interosseus membrane, and proximal radius. Moving distally through the forearm, the FDP has two distinct muscle bundles. The radial bundle becomes the tendon for the index finger and the ulnar bundle powers the tendons for the long, ring, and small fingers. The innervation is usually provided by the anterior interosseous nerve for the index and long finger FDP. In zone IV, the tendons form the floor of the carpal tunnel. As the four FDP tendons diverge into the palm, the lumbrical muscles originate from their radial aspect. The lumbrical

Evidence-Based Orthopedics, First Edition. Edited by Mohit Bhandari.
© 2012 Blackwell Publishing Ltd. Published 2012 by Blackwell Publishing Ltd.

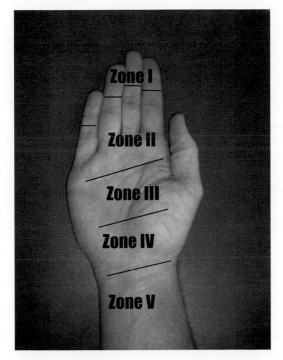

Figure 118.1 The flexor tendon zones of the hand.

muscles travel distally from this level insert into the radial side of the lateral band of the extensor tendon at the level of the proximal phalanx.

Zone II and zone I

Zone II is a notoriously difficult area for surgical intervention and rehabilitation. Both the FDS and FDP tendons are confined within the flexor retinacular sheath at this level and are very closely approximated. Injury at this level increases the technical difficulty of surgical repair. Rehabilitation can also be difficult due to the potential for increased adhesion formation between the tendons and also between the tendon and retinacular sheath or pulley system. The FDS enters zone II superficial to the FDP. Proceeding distally, the FDS bifurcates at the mid-shaft level of the proximal phalanx. Once bifurcated, the FDP becomes superficial. The FDS then comes back together deep to the FDP and inserts just distal to the proximal interphalangeal joint on the middle phalanx. The FDP then continues distally into zone I to insert into the base of the distal phalanx.

The FDS and FDP tendons are maintained in close proximity to the phalanges with a series of annular and cruciate pulleys. These pulleys increase the biomechanical advantage of the flexor tendons by preventing bowstringing of the tendons as they glide proximally. The pulleys situated over the proximal phalanx (A2) and middle phalanx (A4) are the primary pulleys responsible for maintaining the tendons in a biomechanically advantageous position.

Other important anatomical features within zone II are the proper digital nerves and arteries. The proper digital nerves for the thumb, index finger, long finger, and radial half of the ring finger are extensions of the median nerve. The proper digital nerves for the ulnar half of the ring finger and the small finger arise from the ulnar nerve. The digital arteries course with these nerves in the finger. They are located on the palmar side of radial and ulnar aspects of each finger, leaving them susceptible to injury when the flexor tendons are injured in zone II.

Importance of the problem

Injuries to the hand vary with respect to their frequency and type based on culture, climate, industry, and leisure activities across the earth's many geographical areas. In the United States, injuries to the hand comprise approximately one fifth of all visits to Emergency Departments.[2–4] In a review of over 50,000 hand injuries, approximately 5% were found to have some form of tendon involvement.[5] Approximately 1% of all hand injuries involve the flexor tendons. The primary mechanism of injury for flexor tendon lacerations is usually a cut from broken glass or a knife.[6] Early diagnosis and direct primary repair, if possible, is essential for regaining functional use of the hand. The consequences of a missed diagnosis of a flexor tendon laceration are usually not life threatening but can lead to deformity, contracture, decreased digital range of motion (ROM), and significant loss of hand function.

The cost of flexor tendon injuries to the healthcare system is related to patient age, and the method of postoperative rehabilitation. In 2003, Rosberg et al.[7] reviewed the cost to the Swedish healthcare system after 139 flexor tendon repairs. They found that costs to the health system were significantly increased (57%) when immobilization was implemented postoperatively compared to passive and early active motion protocols. This highlights the importance of initiating protected motion of the digits after flexor tendon injury.

Top five questions

Diagnosis

1. What is the best way to diagnose the extent and location of an acute laceration of the FDP and FDS tendons?

Therapy

2. What type of flexor tendon surgical repair was performed in this scenario and how does it affect rehabilitation?

3. What factors determine how aggressively and how early postoperatively the tendons should be mobilized?

4. What kind of splinting is best for this type of postoperative rehabilitation?

Prognosis

5. What mediates functional outcome for this type of injury?

Question 1: What is the best way to diagnose the extent and location of an acute laceration of the FDP and FDS tendons?

Case clarification

Our patient lacerated the tendons of FDP and FDS in zone II of the hand. Lacerations in zone II are the most frequent and have the most severe prognosis.[8] While a complete laceration of a flexor tendon requires surgical repair, the treatment for partial tendon lacerations has traditionally been more controversial. However, it is now generally accepted that a laceration of less than 60% of the tendon may do as well or better with conservative treatment than surgical.[9] It is, therefore, important to be able to accurately diagnose the extent and location of flexor tendon injury so that an appropriate treatment plan can be determined.

Current opinion

Clinical assessment, surgical exploration, and MRI are the main traditional methods of quantifying laceration of the flexor tendons. Currently, less expensive and more time-efficient methods than MRI such as ultrasound and duel-energy CT are being further investigated to confirm their utility in diagnostics of this area.[10–12]

Finding the evidence

• Cochrane Database, with search term "flexor tendon rehabilitation"
• PubMed (www.ncbi.nlm.nih.gov/pubmed) clinical queries search/ systematic reviews: "ultrasound" AND "finger injuries"
• MEDLINE search identifying the population (Tendons/ or Tendon Injuries/ or Fingers/ or flexor tendons.mp. or Finger Injuries/) and (adult), the intervention (diagnostic imaging or magnetic resonance imaging or ultrasound) and (laceration). We used the keywords "flexor tendons" and "injury" and "diagnose"
• PubMed (www.ncbi.nlm.nih.gov/pubmed/) sensitivity search with keywords "radiology" AND "hand flexor tendons," "MRI" AND "flexor tendon laceration," "ultrasound" AND "flexor tendon laceration," "imaging" AND "finger injuries" AND "ultrasound" AND "MRI," "imaging" AND "finger injuries" AND "flexor tendon" AND "adult" AND ("ultrasound" OR "MRI")

Quality of the evidence

Level IV
• 4 case series[11,13–15]

Level V
• 2 expert opinions[8,10]
• 9 case reports [12,16–24]

Because the level of evidence available in this area is of grade IV or V, key results should be considered cautiously.

Findings

Clinical diagnosis of the flexor tendons should include observation of the normal cascade of the fingers. In the case of complete laceration of the flexor tendons, this cascade will be lost and the fingers will likely rest in an extended position (Figure 118.2).

Clinical evaluation should also include examination of isolated active flexion of the proximal interphalangeal (PIP) joint while the all other digits are passively held in full extension, to determine if the FDS is intact.[1,25] Evaluation of FDP function is done by active flexion of the isolated distal interphalangeal joint of the finger.[25] Squeezing the forearm musculature should evoke flexion of the fingers. If there is a lack of digit flexion or an absence of tenodesis effect with flexion and extension of the wrist, the clinician should consider the possibility of a flexor tendon injury. Patients with a partial laceration may experience pain at the site of injury with gentle resistance to flexion.[25]

The clinical diagnosis of a partial laceration is challenging because of the nonspecificity of physical signs.[8] The clinician must, therefore, rely on other investigative tools to determine the degree of injury. The gold standard for

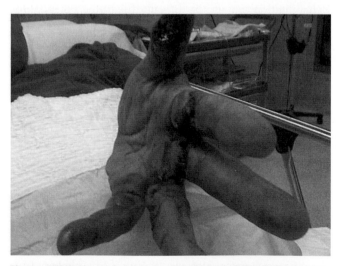

Figure 118.2 The normal cascade of the fingers is lost in the injured index, long, and ring fingers. Note the normal cascade in the small, uninjured finger.

diagnosis of a partial flexor tendon laceration is surgical exploration.[8,25]

Traditionally, many surgeons have used MRI to determine whether an injury to a flexor tendon warrants investigation/treatment by surgical intervention. MRI affords optimal assessment of tendons[8,15,21,26–28] and has the advantage of being noninvasive. It allows evaluation of the presence of a tear, the number of affected tendons, the extent of tendon retraction, and the presence of associated lesions.

Recently, more cost- and time-effective means of diagnosis, such as ultrasound, have been investigated to better understand their utility as diagnostic tools in cases such as a flexor tendon laceration.[10] Kubiak et al. include ultrasound with MRI as the current modalities best suited for confirming clinical assessment findings of injury to the flexor tendons.[12] One unique asset of ultrasound over MRI is that real-time ultrasound can evaluate tendon gliding. Ultrasound is usually not effective at diagnosing rupture of flexor tendons after surgical repair as the presence of suture material make visualization of the damaged tendon ends difficult. Deng et al. cite dual-energy CT as a new and effective method to visualize the FDP and FDS.[11]

Recommendations

• Clinical examination of the flexor tendons (including a subjective history, observation of the cascade of fingers, and isolated examination of the FDS and FDP) is the starting point for assessment [overall quality: low to very low]
• MRI of the flexor tendons is used to quantify the extent of injury for partial lacerations including percentage of laceration and any retraction of the tendon ends [overall quality: low to very low]
• There is currently not enough evidence to support the use of diagnostic ultrasound on its own (or enough studies to support the use of dual-energy CT for flexor tendons) but these may be promising options for future investigations to quantify [overall quality: low to very low]
• Surgical exploration is recommended to confirm a diagnosis for those flexor tendon injuries suspected to be greater than 60% lacerated [overall quality: low to very low]

Question 2: What type of flexor tendon surgical repair was performed in this scenario and how does it affect rehabilitation?

Case clarification

Variables that can be altered in repair of flexor tendons include the suture caliber, the number of suture strands that cross the repair site, and the type of suture used to secure the tendon. The strength of the repair is based on these characteristics and they, along with the surgeon's preference, will dictate what type of rehabilitation approach is undertaken.

Relevance

Historically, zone II was termed "no man's land" and surgical approaches favored grafting rather than direct repair of the flexor tendons in this zone of the hand. Primary repair of the flexor tendons in zone II has since been universally accepted as the treatment of choice.[29] It has also been determined that it is better to repair both the FDP and FDS rather than the profundus alone, as was once thought to be the better option.[29] The strength of the repair in large part dictates what rehabilitation approach will be possible. There are three traditional approaches to rehabilitation: immobilization (now rarely considered to be the treatment of choice), early controlled active ROM, and early controlled passive ROM. The advancement of surgical repair approaches has allowed for earlier motion to be tolerated in rehabilitation protocols. There is, however, no one standardized protocol that is thought to be the best approach. Studies are difficult to compare because of differences in surgical technique.

Current opinion

Surgical repair of a flexor tendon laceration is no longer a surgical emergency.[29–33] Primary tendon repair is the treatment of choice, with the aim of a repair that will be strong and smooth with enough tensile strength to allow early controlled motion after surgery.[34,35] A four-strand repair offers approximately double the strength of the two-strand core suture while being more technically feasible than a six- or eight-strand repair.

Finding the evidence

• Cochrane Database, with search term "flexor tendon rehabilitation"
• PubMed (www.ncbi.nlm.nih.gov/pubmed) clinical queries search/ systematic reviews: "hand flexor tendons"
• MEDLINE search identifying the population (Tendons/ or Tendon Injuries/ or Fingers/ or flexor tendons.mp. or Finger Injuries) and (adult) and (repair) and (laceration.mp or lacerations/) and (rehabilitation.mp or Rehabilitation/) and (Suture techniques/or Tendons/ or Tendon injuries/ or four-strand.mp or Tensile Strength/) and (Hand/ or Hand Injuries/ or hand.mp), the intervention (laceration) and (rehabilitation). We used the keywords "zone II" and "protocol"
• PubMed (www.ncbi.nlm.nih.gov/pubmed/) sensitivity search with keywords "hand" AND "flexor tendons" AND "repair" AND "rehabilitation"; then combined with "four-strand"

Quality of the evidence

Level I
• Cochrane review of rehabilitation protocols[9]

Level II
- 1 study of surgical options for flexor tendon repairs[36]
- 2 studies of rehabilitation protocols[42,43]

Level III
- 5 studies using cadaver specimens[37-41]
- 4 studies of rehabilitation protocols[37,44-46]

Level IV and V
- Multiple studies

Findings

The Cochrane review identified three randomized controlled trials (RCTs) that had been published in full in the area of flexor tendon rehabilitation;[42,43,47] however, the study by Percival and Sykes (1989) examined the FPL and, therefore, does not directly pertain to the case question regarding laceration of D2–D4. The review identified that no trial tested the same comparison/protocol or surgical technique which makes data pooling impossible. While the review suggests that early mobilization regimes are generally favored in orthopedic rehabilitation, it also stipulates that the optimal protocol is yet to be determined due to insufficient high quality evidence.

Strickland listed the characteristics of an ideal primary flexor tendon repair as follows: sutures easily placed in the tendon, secure suture knots, smooth juncture of tendon ends, minimal gapping at the repair site, minimal interference with tendon vascularity, and sufficient strength throughout healing to permit the application of early motion stress to the tendon.[48]

It has been demonstrated in numerous studies that the strength of a flexor tendon repair is roughly proportional to the number of suture strands that cross the repair site.[29,48-56] However, the more suture strands that cross the repair site, the more difficult the technique and the more likely the method is to damage the tendon excessively or compromise its nutrition or ability to heal.[29,50,57-61] Therefore, while there has been a departure from the core suture techniques that traditionally have used two-strand approaches to a replacement of the stronger four-strand methods which are approximately twice as strong as two-strand techniques,[29,48,53-55,62] the advantages of the increased strength with six- and eight-strand methods have to be weighed against the more difficult technique and potential for tendon damage. In zone II, the increased bulk associated with six- and eight-strand repairs may also impact the ability to achieve optimal tendon gliding during rehabilitation due to the intimate association between the FDS, FDP, and the retinacular sheath.

It is thought that the roughness of suture material as well as the roughness of the repair (the size of knots and suture loops on the tendon surface) will affect the tendon repair's smoothness.[34] Resorbable suture materials are now avail-

able as well as a variety of suture materials (monofilament, coated, etc.). While investigators have demonstrated that larger-caliber sutures significantly increase repair strength,[22,29] there is some debate on the effectiveness of locking loops on ultimate tensile strength of repair.[63-65]

Tendons are susceptible to rupture at suture knots, so the fewer the suture knots located in the tendon junction site the better.[65-67] There may also be strength and biomechanical advantages to dorsal rather than palmar placement of core sutures and a strong peripheral suture will improve gliding and increase suture strength.[29,43,66,68-75]

Recommendations

- A multistrand repair using a larger-caliber suture material with grasping and locking sutures has superior holding ability[38,62,65-67,73,76-89] [overall quality: low]
- A four-strand core suture plus a strong peripheral suture can withstand the stresses of gentle early active motion[48,53,73] [overall quality: low]
- No postoperative rehabilitation protocol has been identified as being optimal [overall quality: low]

Question 3. What factors determine how aggressively and how early postoperatively the tendons should be mobilized?

Case clarification

The physician's orders in this case are for "orthosis/protected ROM". In other words, the physician has left the choice of protocol to the discretion of the attending therapist. Based on the findings from the previous question, we will assume for the purposes of discussion that the repair was performed with a four-strand suture plus a strong peripheral suture that is capable of withstanding early active motion. We also note from the case that the patient is 4 days postoperative so is moving from the inflammatory phase into the fibroblastic or collagen-producing phase of healing.[29] We will also assume that the bulky dressing has been removed and the patient is now in therapy, ready to begin rehabilitation.

Relevance

The advancement of surgical repair techniques and materials has allowed earlier mobilization after flexor tendon repair. Rehabilitation of flexor tendon repairs in zone II aims to achieve a balance between protecting the healing site and preventing gap formation while stressing it enough to enhance healing and prevent the formation of adhesions. The optimal protocol is yet to be determined but approaches are generally one of three: active extension–passive flexion, controlled passive motion, or controlled active motion.[9]

Current opinion

Rehabilitation of repaired flexor tendons in zone II favors early mobilization.[9]

Finding the evidence

• Cochrane Database, with search term "flexor tendon rehabilitation".
• PubMed (www.ncbi.nlm.nih.gov/pubmed) clinical queries search/systematic reviews: "hand flexor tendons"
• MEDLINE search identifying the population (Tendons/ or Tendon Injuries/ or Fingers/ or flexor tendons.mp. or Finger Injuries) and (adult) and (repair) and (laceration.mp or lacerations/) and (rehabilitation.mp or Rehabilitation/) and (Suture techniques/or Tendons/ or Tendon injuries/ or four-strand.mp or Tensile Strength/) and (Hand/ or Hand Injuries/ or hand.mp), the intervention (laceration) and (rehabilitation). We used the keywords "zone II" and "protocol"
• PubMed (www.ncbi.nlm.nih.gov/pubmed/) sensitivity search with keywords "hand" AND "flexor tendons" AND "repair" AND "rehabilitation"; then combined with "four-strand"

Quality of the evidence

Level I Cochrane review[9]

Level II
• 2 studies[42,43]

Level III
• 4 studies[37,44–46]

Level IV and V
• Multiple studies

Findings

According to the Cochrane review,[9] there are three main categories which affect the success of treatment for flexor tendon injuries of the hand: the kind of injury (e.g., level of injury, how many fingers have been injured, which zone of the hand has been injured, whether it is a clean cut versus a jagged laceration, etc.); the type of operation and surgical techniques used; and the rehabilitation program implemented postoperatively.

There is not one universally accepted protocol that is thought to be optimum for rehabilitation of flexor tendon injuries.[9] In addition to the kind of injury and type of surgery performed, the timing of the surgery must also be considered. Those patients whose surgery was delayed may present with a shortened flexor tendon postoperatively, or if the situation is more chronic, the patient may require a more complex operation such as a two-staged flexor tendon repair. Both of these situations are examples of cases that would require tailoring of the postoperative protocol to the individual's unique presentation. Additionally, patient factors such as age, perceived compliance, and treatment goals must be considered when selecting the most appropriate postoperative regime. What has

been agreed upon is that immobilization results in unacceptable motion due to adhesions, and unrestrained normal motion almost always results in tendon rupture.[34,90–92]

For patients unable to comply with rehabilitation instructions, immobilization may be a superior intervention to risking tendon rupture with unprotected active ROM and activity.[93] However, for compliant capable patients, current rehabilitation protocols aim for balance and use positioning and mobilizing splints during the early post-tendon-repair period. It is essential to tailor the rehabilitation to each individual, taking into account not only the anatomy, and surgical technique but also the distinctive features of each individual patient's capabilities and psychological responses,[94] goals, social supports, and motivation for recovery.[95]

It is motion, rather than loading, that is thought to enhance tendon healing and no benefit has been shown to loading above what is needed to initiate tendon gliding.[34] It should be noted that breaking strength is not the real measure of the quality of tendon repair; rather, it is the presence of gapping.[34] For most repairs, gaps begin to form at approximately two thirds of the ultimate failure strength and can lead to triggering and blocking of motion.[34,52,96–98] The identification of gapping and its relationship to reduced tensile force and tendon rupture has led to the development of "safe zones" for rehabilitation—the range of applied tendon loads that are large enough to induce tendon motion but small enough to avoid gapping or tendon rupture.[34]

In a survey of Canadian Certified Hand Therapists, it was determined that the current trend in therapy management of zone II tendon repairs is to select the most appropriate[99,100] rehabilitation protocol based on the surgeon's preference (58%), center protocol (22%), the clinician's concept of best practice (17%), or patient factors (3%).[101] A separate survey of 191 hand therapists showed that there is a perceived lack of autonomy in clinical decision-making.[102] A third survey was also completed by 191 therapists and cited reasons for initiating active ROM (in descending order) as: established protocol, number of postoperative days, physician order, suture technique, compliance issues, ROM measurements, and "other" (suture, compliance, patient healing, and scar adhesion formation). It was additionally reported that protective splinting is discontinued at a mean of 5.2 weeks postoperatively and that resisted exercises were initiated at a mean of 6.4 weeks postoperatively. It was noted that slightly more of the respondents follow a Kleinert-type protocol vs. the Duran-type protocol and that there is an increasingly frequent use of active finger flexion exercise within the first postoperative week. It was found that custom splints are used widely with little variation from a wrist position of 20–30° of flexion and metacarpal phalangeal flexion of 50–70°.[100] The authors note that their findings vary significantly from the

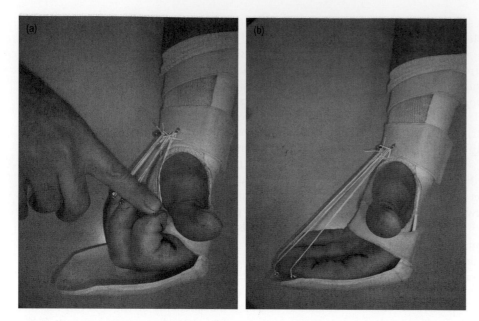

Figure 118.3 (a) Passive digital flexion of each finger, followed by (b) active extension within the limits of the splint using a modified Kleinert program.

literature. For example, the initiation of active flexion was reported as a mean of 18.6 postoperative days while the literature has traditionally recommended 28 days.[99,100]

One very significant finding was that one third of the latter survey respondents report changing their postoperative regimen in the last 5 years which Groth[100] suggests may demonstrate a potential sensitivity to the advances in the scientific body of knowledge. This is in keeping with an observed shift towards increased emphasis of clinical reasoning in tailoring standardized protocols to meet individual patient needs and using "comparable signs" (objective repeatable measures) to monitor progress.

Sueoka and LaSayo proposed an algorithm to assist clinicians in using protocols more as guidelines.[103] The algorithm uses the concept of "tendon lag" as an indicator of how to proceed using an established protocol or modify the management approach by accelerating or decelerating the patient's exposure to higher force exercises (p. 411). A "tendon lag" is the percentage difference in digital passive range of motion (PROM) and active range of motion (AROM) or a combination of both relative (%) and absolute (°) differences in PROM and AROM. Sueoka and LaSayo define the lag as a minimum 15° difference between PROM (greater) than AROM with the assumption that a tendon lag represents an adhered tendon that will impair normal gliding and thus reduce AROM.[103] The algorithm uses temporally based benchmarks to guide the rehabilitation approach. For example, in the scenario case, the patient is postoperative day 4 and thus is in the initial phase where the goal is to achieve full passive flexion of all digits and to reach the threshold level of extension as dictated by the passive protocols of Kleinert et al. or Duran et al.[104–106] The goal is to achieve full passive flexion by 3 weeks at the latest. Passive flexion and active extension with the limits of the dorsal blocking splint are the primary exercises for the modified Kleinert programs (Figure 118.3). The second stage (approximately weeks 3–8) introduces AROM, while resistance makes up the final phase.

Another approach which could both incorporate the algorithm by Sueoka and LaSayo[103] and be adapted within standardized protocols, is the "pyramid of progressive force exercises" that has been outlined by Groth.[94] This pyramid of progression starts with passive protected digital extension and moves through to place and hold finger flexion, followed by AROM and then isolated active tendon motion.[94] Wrist ROM is incorporated early in the pyramid through the concept of tenodesis—allowing the fingers to naturally drift into relaxed/unrestricted finger flexion while the wrist is in protected extension. This elicits less stress on the flexor tendon than composite extension, where both the wrist and digits are extended, and facilitates the desired differential tendon gliding between the FDS and FDP to prevent adhesions and promote organized tendon tissue healing. The protected wrist motion is progressed to unprotected wrist motion in accordance with the outlined pyramid levels and patient tolerance. The approach is based on tendon performance and moves from a high-frequency, low-load level of exercises to a low frequency with higher load levels as the patient ascends the pyramid.

Recommendations

• Choose an established protocol based on type and timing of surgery including the strength of repair and zone of injury as well as perceived patient compliance [overall quality: low]

- Implement the use of an algorithm such as the one proposed by Sueoka and LaSayo[103] which uses the presence/absence of a tendon lag sign to guide progression through rehabilitation and/or Groth's "pyramid of progressive force exercises"[94] to tailor protocols to individual presentations [overall quality: low]

Question 4: What kind of splinting is best for this type of postoperative rehabilitation?

Case clarification
In the case, the patient is postoperative day 4 and the physician has ordered "Orthosis/protected ROM". The type of splint used is dictated by the rehabilitation protocol selected, i.e., it will depend upon whether a controlled active or passive motion protocol is used.

Relevance
The splint will assist in protecting the tendon to allow for healing but also facilitate protected motion depending upon which protocol has been selected.

Finding the evidence
- Cochrane Database, with search term "flexor tendon rehabilitation"
- PubMed (www.ncbi.nlm.nih.gov/pubmed) clinical queries search/systematic reviews: "flexor tendon splints" or "postoperative wrist splints" (no results); clinical queries "flexor tendon splints"
- MEDLINE search identifying the population (Tendons/ or Tendon Injuries/ or Fingers/ or flexor tendons.mp. or Finger Injuries) and (adult) and (repair), the interventions (laceration.mp or lacerations/) and (rehabilitation.mp or Rehabilitation/) or (splints or splint.mp). We also used the keywords "zone II," "protocol," "Kleinert," "Duran," "Washington"
- PubMed (including ProQuest Nursing Journals) (www.ncbi.nlm.nih.gov/pubmed/) sensitivity search with keywords "wrist splint" and "flexor tendons"; "rehabilitation" and "flexor tendons" and "laceration"

Quality of the evidence
- No studies higher than level IV or V were identified and no studies specifically answered the question as to an optimum splinting regimen.

Findings
A Cochrane review[9] conducted in 2009 found no difference between dynamic vs. static orthoses and no conclusion could be formulated regarding active flexion vs. rubber band traction. The review also reported no significant difference found between controlled passive flexion with active extension (modified Kleinert) vs. controlled passive mobilization (modified Duran) nor any significant differ-

ence between grasping suture and early controlled active mobilization vs. modified Kessler technique with early controlled passive mobilization.[107]

The quality of evidence to support one specific choice of orthosis is low as there are too many confounding factors such as surgical technique and protocol choice which will impact on splinting choices.

Recommendation
- The type of orthosis is based on the protocol chosen and should facilitate the achievement of benchmarks of movement by protecting the repair from excessive forces while allowing sufficient ROM to facilitate gliding and prevent adhesions [overall quality: low]

Question 5: What mediates functional outcome for this type of injury?

Case clarification
The patient in the case has undergone repair of the FDS/FDP on the second, third, and fourth digits of his dominant hand. In order to establish short- and long-term goals for the client, it is necessary to know what expected functional outcomes are realistic in this scenario.

Relevance
Many postoperative protocols aim not only to enhance function but to also to mitigate factors which may detract from the long-term functional outcome of the hand. Suboptimal outcomes are attributable to adverse events such as infection, tendon/scar adhesions, flexion contractures, stiffness of fingers, tendon bowstringing, gap formation, and rerupture of the flexor tendons. Quality of life for most people includes capacity for return to work and/or leisure activities, and many of these activities are thought to be closely linked to hand function. Therefore, it would be beneficial for both the patient and clinician to know how closely the function of a postoperative flexor tendon repair is expected to approximate preinjury status.

In order to quantify the patient's functional status, outcome measures must be implemented. Outcome measures can help to determine a patient's status at the time of assessment; to predict a subsequent event; and to detect change over time.[108] These characteristics assist in goal-setting and should help to determine the expected overall long-term functional outcome for the patient in the case scenario.

Current opinion
The ideal manner in which to assess health outcomes following tendon injury has yet to be determined. Defining "functional outcome" in the instance of flexor tendon rehabilitation is difficult because not only does the idea of what constitutes a "functional outcome" vary, but the variables

thought to contribute to overall function range widely, and the manner in which they are measured also varies greatly among studies. One must take into account measures of surgical technique and repair materials, and rehabilitation protocols, as well as the patient-specific variables which are thought to influence overall quality of life.

It has been noted that there is a marked difference in the selection of outcome measures by clinical researchers/ epidemiologists and their clinical counterparts. While researchers have tended to choose outcome measures involving self-report measures, clinicians have relied on impairment measures to guide treatments.[109] A review of outcome measures following flexor tendon repair found that the majority of outcome measures used in the study methods were for digital ROM and muscle strength. In other words, the outcome measures could be classified in the World Health Organization's "International Classification of Functioning, Disability and Health" (ICF) model as body function and body structure, with a paucity of research reflected in the activity and participation categories of flexor tendon repair outcomes.[110,111] Health outcomes can be measured using valuation methods (those that assess the value that an individual places on a given health state), health-status measurements (describe health), or classification methods (categorize health).[112] The ICF is increasingly being used as the conceptual framework for defining health attributes.[109,113–117] The model acknowledges that there is a nonlinear and multidirectional relationship between physical impairments and resultant disability.[112]

Self-efficacy may be one determinant in the relationship between impairment and disability as it is highly related to a patient's ability to deal with their impairments or to participate in self-management programs.[109] "Comparable signs" are being identified, and then re-evaluated to guide advancement through the rehabilitation process. For example, a "lag sign" was described by Sueoka and LaStayo in their proposed algorithm to guide progression through accepted postoperative flexor tendon repair protocols.[103] Numerous rating systems for composite impairment measures for tendon injuries agree that motion is the primary physical impairment resulting from a tendon injury.[112]

It has been reported that for primary repair of zone II flexor tendon repairs, approximately 80% of normal motion can be restored with rehabilitation completed in 2–3 months.[34] While it is generally accepted that it is optimal to obtain AROM that approximates the PROM of finger flexion, what has not been established is the extent to which a loss of ROM will affect overall function.[112] The majority of flexor tendon repair studies have focused their outcomes on impairment measures, but it has not been determined to what extent these specific impairments will affect overall function.[111] The following scales have not been validated specifically to postoperative tendon repair but have been used across a wide spectrum of upper

extremity disorders: the Michigan Hand Questionnaire,[118] the DASH,[119] and the Patient Rated Wrist and Hand Evaluation.[112]

The risk of reinjury following a tendon repair is difficult to quantify due to a preponderance of surgical techniques, materials, patient characteristics, and differences in rehabilitation protocols. Tang suggests that repair ruptures are anywhere from 4% to 10% for zone II finger flexors, but this data is not specific to a four-strand repair.[41]

In consideration of the above factors, clinical experience dictates that the expected functional outcome for a four-strand surgical repair of FDS/FDP of the second to fourth digits on the dominant hand is variable and is closely associated with the patient's functional demands. For this reason, self-report measures are important for determining whether functional goals have been attained. With respect to measures of impairment, achievement of 90° of active MCP and PIP motion and 50° of DIP motion will usually be sufficient for functional use. Grip and pinch strength of 80% of a normal contralateral side will limit any functional impairment in most individuals.

Finding the evidence
- Cochrane Database, with search term "flexor tendon rehabilitation"
- PubMed (www.ncbi.nlm.nih.gov/pubmed) clinical queries search/systematic reviews: "hand flexor tendons"
- MEDLINE search identifying the population (Tendons/ or Tendon Injuries/ or Fingers/ or flexor tendons.mp. or Finger Injuries) and (adult) and (repair) and (laceration.mp or lacerations/) and (rehabilitation.mp or Rehabilitation/) and (Suture techniques/or Tendons/ or Tendon injuries/ or four-strand.mp or Tensile Strength/) and (Hand/ or Hand Injuries/ or hand.mp), the intervention (laceration) and (rehabilitation) and (Outcome Assessment (health care)/ or Treatment Outcome/). We used the keywords "zone II," "protocol," "outcome measures," and "expected outcomes"
- PubMed (www.ncbi.nlm.nih.gov/pubmed/)—sensitivity search with keywords "hand" AND "flexor tendons" AND "repair" AND "rehabilitation"; then combined with "four-strand" and with "outcome measures"; "rupture" AND "flexor tendons" AND "repair" AND "hand"

Quality of the evidence
Level II
- 1 systematic review that addressed the ICF components of corresponding outcome measures in flexor tendon rehabilitation;[111] however, it was not specific to a four-strand flexor tendon repair in zone II

Level V
- 2 review papers.[41,110] The first reported outcomes with "excellent or good functional return" in more than three

fourths of primary tendon repairs following a variety of postoperative passive/active mobilization treatments with a 4–10% repair rupture in zone II finger flexors, while the second identified a lack of outcome measures in the activity and participation categories of the ICF model for flexor tendon repair outcomes

• No in vivo human study was identified to specifically identify *functional* outcome following a four-strand zone II repair or the risk of repair rupture with a four-strand repair in zone II

Findings

Physical impairments following a tendon laceration include a loss of motion and strength. Numerous rating systems for composite impairment measures for tendon injuries agree that motion is the primary physical impairment resulting from a tendon injury.[112] Outcome assessment following tendon repair and rehabilitation should include the total active motion of the affected joints.

Assessment of strength by manual muscle testing will allow determination of tendon integrity but is relatively insensitive to weakness in overall grip or individual digital strength.[112] The reliability of grip strength using a standardized test protocol for the Jamar dynamometer at the second handle position has been well established.[120–122] While isolated loss of finger flexion force is common following flexor tendon repair, and has been correlated to elongation (gapping) in the tendon repair, there is limited availability of digital strength dynomometers clinically. Therefore, overall grip strength remains the common method of strength assessment. Pinch strength is also used to assess strength and protocols for measurement have been established by the American Society for Hand Therapists. The use of actual percentage (of the normal side) for assessment of motion and strength is an appropriate score.[112]

Other impairment measures include sensibility tests such as touch, temperature, and proprioception which may be evaluated by tests of threshold and innervation density. There is no consensus on what constitutes measures or standards of functional sensibility.[112] Cold sensitivity is common with peripheral nerve injuries which may accompany a tendon laceration, and is related to functional impairment and quality of life.[99,123]

While there are a number of available questionnaires to assess activity and participation outcomes through self-report of function, none of these scales has been specifically validated for tendon injury.[112] However, the following scales have been used across a wide spectrum of upper extremity disorders: The Michigan Hand Questionnaire, the DASH, and the Patient Rated Wrist and Hand Evaluation.[112]

Recommendations

There is not enough quality research to specifically answer Question 5.

• Clinical experience dictates that the expected functional outcome of flexor tendon repair of D2/3/4 using a four-strand surgical approach is variable, which may explain the presence of several different management philosophies from both surgical and rehabilitation perspectives. From an impairment perspective, many studies have reported favorable results with early passive and controlled active protocols [overall quality: low]

• The risk of rerupture of a flexor tendon repair (not specific to a four-strand repair) has been reported as approximately 4–10% in zone II [overall quality: low]

• The relationship between specific impairment and function has not been established and data to determine the risk of rerupture of a four-strand zone II repair is inadequate.

Summary of recommendations

• Clinical examination of the flexor tendons (including a subjective history, observation of the cascade of fingers) is the starting point for assessment

• MRI of the flexor tendons is used to quantify the extent of injury including percentage of laceration and any retraction of the tendon ends

• There is currently not enough evidence to support the use of diagnostic ultrasound on its own (or enough studies to support the use of dual-energy CT for flexor tendons) but these may be promising options for future investigations to quantify

• Surgical exploration is recommended to confirm a diagnosis for those flexor tendon injuries suspected to be greater than 60% lacerated

• A multistrand repair using a larger-caliber suture material with grasping and locking sutures has superior holding ability

• A four-strand core suture plus a strong peripheral suture can withstand the stresses of gentle early active motion

• No postoperative rehabilitation protocol has been identified as being optimal

• Choose an established protocol based on type and timing of surgery including the strength of repair and zone of injury as well as perceived patient compliance

• Implement the use of an algorithm such as the one proposed by Sueoka and LaSayo[103] which uses the presence/absence of a tendon lag sign to guide progression through rehabilitation and/or the "pyramid of progressive force exercises"[94] to tailor protocols to individual presentations

• The type of orthosis used is based on the protocol chosen and should facilitate the achievement of benchmarks of movement by protecting the repair from excessive forces while allowing sufficient ROM to facilitate gliding and prevent adhesions

• Clinical experience dictates that the expected functional outcome of flexor tendon repair of D2/3/4 using a four-strand surgical approach is variable, which may explain the presence of several different management philosophies from both surgical and rehabilitation perspectives. From an impairment perspective, many studies have reported favorable results with early passive and controlled active protocols

• The risk of rerupture of a flexor tendon repair (not specific to a four-strand repair) has been reported as approximately 4–10% in zone II

Conclusions

Diagnosis of flexor tendon repairs is usually done by clinical assessment. For patients who present with a normal cascade and a suspected partial tendon laceration, MRI or surgical exploration is warranted to ensure appropriate management.

The continued presence of several methods of rehabilitation for the management of flexor tendon injuries is a clear indicator that no single method has been shown, with good evidence, to be superior over another. Both early passive and early active motion protocols have shown to produce acceptable results. The choice of protocol depends on the quality of repair, zone of injury, experience of the clinician, and perceived patient compliance. The choice of orthosis is dependent upon the chosen protocols and positioning within the orthosis is variable in the literature. Regardless of the chosen protocol, the clinical decision-making as rehabilitation progresses through the various stages of healing is extremely important. Timely progression of stress to the repaired tendons is essential – not only for protecting the repairs – but also for achieving optimal tendon gliding and ultimately functional use of the hand.

References

1. Austin GJ, Leslie BM, Ruby LK. Variations of the flexor digitorum superficialis of the small finger. J Hand Surg Am 1989; 14(2 Pt 1):262–7.
2. Jarvik JG, Dalinka MK, Kneeland JB. Hand injuries in adults. Semin Roentgenol 1991;26(4):282–99.
3. Smith ME, Auchincloss JM, Ali MS. Causes and consequences of hand injury. J Hand Surg Br 1985;10(3):288–92.
4. Clark DP, Scott RN, Anderson IW. Hand problems in an accident and emergency department. J Hand Surg Br 1985;10(3): 297–9.
5. Angermann P, Lohmann M. Injuries to the hand and wrist. A study of 50,272 injuries. J Hand Surg Br 1993;18(5):642–4.
6. Tuncali D, Yavuz N, Terzioglu A, Aslan G. The rate of upper-extremity deep-structure injuries through small penetrating lacerations. Ann Plast Surg 2005;55(2):146–8.
7. Rosberg HE, Carlsson KS, Hojgard S, Lindgren B, Lundborg G, Dahlin LB. What determines the costs of repair and rehabilita-
tion of flexor tendon injuries in zone II? A multiple regression analysis of data from southern Sweden. J Hand Surg Br 2003;28(2):106–12.
8. Clavero JA, Alomar X, Monill JM, et al. MR imaging of ligament and tendon injuries of the fingers. Radiographics 2002;22(2): 237–56.
9. Thien T, Becker J, Theis J. Rehabilitation after surgery for flexor tendon injuries in the hand (review). Cochrane Collaboration 2009.
10. Bajaj S, Pattamapaspong N, Middleton W, Teefey S. Ultrasound of the hand and wrist. J Hand Surg Am 2009;34(4):759–60.
11. Deng K, Sun C, Liu C, Ma R. Initial experience with visualizing hand and foot tendons by dual-energy computed tomography. Clin Imaging 2009;33(5):384–9.
12. Kubiak EN, Klugman JA, Bosco JA. Hand injuries in rock climbers. Bull N Y U Hosp Jt Dis 2006;64(3–4):172–7.
13. Lee DH, Robbin ML, Galliott R, Graveman VA. Ultrasound evaluation of flexor tendon lacerations. J Hand Surg Am 2000;25(2):236–41.
14. Matloub HS, Dzwierzynski WW, Erickson S, Sanger JR, Yousif NJ, Muoneke V. Magnetic resonance imaging scanning in the diagnosis of zone II flexor tendon rupture. J Hand Surg Am 1996;21(3):451–5.
15. Rubin DA, Kneeland JB, Kitay GS, Naranja RJ, Jr. Flexor tendon tears in the hand: use of MR imaging to diagnose degree of injury in a cadaver model. AJR Am J Roentgenol 1996;166(3): 615–20.
16. Van Zwieten K, Brys, P, Van Rietvelde, F, Oudenhoven, L, Vanhoenacker, F. Imaging of the hand, techniques and pathology: a pictorial essay. JBR-BTR 2007;90(5):395–455.
17. Buyruk HM, Stam HJ, Lameris JS, Schut HA, Snijders CJ. Colour doppler ultrasound examination of hand tendon pathologies. A preliminary report. J Hand Surg Br 1996;21(4): 469–73.
18. Hartford JM, Murphy JM. Flexor digitorum profundus rupture of the small finger secondary to nonunion of the hook of hamate: a case report. J Hand Surg Am 1996;21(4):621–3.
19. Jeyapalan K, Bisson MA, Dias JJ, Griffin Y, Bhatt R. The role of ultrasound in the management of flexor tendon injuries. J Hand Surg Eur 2008;33(4):430–4.
20. Kumar BA, Tolat AR, Threepuraneni G, Jones B. The role of magnetic resonance imaging in late presentation of isolated injuries of the flexor digitorum profundus tendon in the finger. J Hand Surg Br 2000;25(1):95–7.
21. Scott JR, Cobby M, Taggart I. Magnetic resonance imaging of acute tendon injury in the finger. J Hand Surg Br 1995;20(3):286–8.
22. Taras JS, Lamb MJ. Treatment of flexor tendon injuries: surgeons' perspective. J Hand Ther 1999;12(2):141–8.
23. Wang P, Bonavita, J, DeLone, F, McClellan, R, Witham, R. Ultrasonic assistance in the diagnosis of hand flexor tendon injuries. Ann Plast Surg 1999;42(4):403–7.
24. Wong D, Wansaicheong, G, Tsou, I. Ultrasonography of the hand and wrist. Singapore Med J 2009;50(2):219–25.
25. Steinberg D. Flexor tendon lacerations in the hand. UPOJ 1997;10:5–11.
26. Drape JL, Dubert T, Silbermann O, Thelen P, Thivet A, Benacerraf R. Acute trauma of the extensor hood of the metacarpophalangeal joint: MR imaging evaluation. Radiology 1994;192(2):469–76.

27. Drape JL, Silbermann-Hoffman O, Houvet P, et al. Complications of flexor tendon repair in the hand: MR imaging assessment. Radiology 1996;198(1):219–24.

28. Drape JL, Tardif-Chastenet de Gery S, Silbermann-Hoffman O, et al. Closed ruptures of the flexor digitorum tendons: MRI evaluation. Skeletal Radiol 1998;27(11):617–24.

29. Strickland JW. The scientific basis for advances in flexor tendon surgery. J Hand Ther 2005;18(2):94–110; quiz 1.

30. Arons MS. Purposeful delay of the primary repair of cut flexor tendons in "some-man's-land" in children. Plast Reconstr Surg 1974;53(6):638–42.

31. Gainor BJ. Proximal coiling of the profundus tendon after laceration of the finger. J Hand Surg Br 1989;14(4):416–18.

32. Green W, Niebauer, J. Results of primary and secondary flexor tendon repairs in no man's land. J Bone Joint Surg Am 1994;56:1216–22.

33. Honner R. The late management of the isolated lesion of the flexor digitorum profundus tendon. Hand 1975;7(2):171–4.

34. Amadio PC. Friction of the gliding surface. Implications for tendon surgery and rehabilitation. J Hand Ther 2005;18(2):112–19.

35. Boyer MI, Goldfarb CA, Gelberman RH. Recent progress in flexor tendon healing. The modulation of tendon healing with rehabilitation variables. J Hand Ther 2005;18(2):80–5; quiz 6.

36. Su BW, Solomons M, Barrow A, et al. A device for zone-II flexor tendon repair. Surgical technique. J Bone Joint Surg Am 2006;88(Suppl 1 Pt 1):37–49.

37. Baktir A, Turk CY, Kabak S, Sahin V, Kardas Y. Flexor tendon repair in zone 2 followed by early active mobilization. J Hand Surg Br 1996;21(5):624–8.

38. Barrie KA, Wolfe SW. The relationship of suture design to biomechanical strength of flexor tendon repairs. Hand Surg 2001;6(1):89–97.

39. McLarney E, Hoffman H, Wolfe SW. Biomechanical analysis of the cruciate four-strand flexor tendon repair. J Hand Surg Am 1999;24(2):295–301.

40. Moneim MS, Firoozbakhsh K, Mustapha AA, Larsen K, Shahinpoor M. Flexor tendon repair using shape memory alloy suture: a biomechanical evaluation. Clin Orthop Relat Res 2002;402:251–9.

41. Tang JB. Clinical outcomes associated with flexor tendon repair. Hand Clin 2005;21(2):199–210.

42. Adolfsson L, Soderberg G, Larsson M, Karlander LE. The effects of a shortened postoperative mobilization programme after flexor tendon repair in zone 2. J Hand Surg Br 1996;21(1):67–71.

43. Gelberman RH, Nunley JA, 2nd, Osterman AL, Breen TF, Dimick MP, Woo SL. Influences of the protected passive mobilization interval on flexor tendon healing. A prospective randomized clinical study. Clin Orthop Relat Res 1991;264:189–96.

44. Burge PD, Brown M. Elastic band mobilisation after flexor tendon repair; splint design and risk of flexion contracture. J Hand Surg Br 1990;15(4):443–8.

45. Chambon X, Paysant J, Gavillot C, Petry D, Andre JM, Dap F, et al. [Rehabilitation protocols after repairs of zone 2 of the flexor tendon of the hand: presentation and indications]. Chir Main 2001;20(5):368–77.

46. Peck FH, Bucher CA, Watson JS, Roe A. A comparative study of two methods of controlled mobilization of flexor tendon repairs in zone 2. J Hand Surg Br 1998;23(1):41–5.

47. Percival NJ, Sykes PJ. Flexor pollicis longus tendon repair: a comparison between dynamic and static splintage. J Hand Surg Br 1989;14(4):412–15.

48. Strickland JW. Flexor Tendon Injuries: II. Operative Technique. J Am Acad Orthop Surg 1995;3(1):55–62.

49. Komanduri M, Phillips CS, Mass DP. Tensile strength of flexor tendon repairs in a dynamic cadaver model. J Hand Surg Am 1996;21(4):605–11.

50. Savage R, Risitano G. Flexor tendon repair using a "six strand" method of repair and early active mobilisation. J Hand Surg Br 1989;14(4):396–9.

51. Shaieb MD, Singer DI. Tensile strengths of various suture techniques. J Hand Surg Br 1997;22(6):764–7.

52. Silfverskiold KL, Andersson CH. Two new methods of tendon repair: an in vitro evaluation of tensile strength and gap formation. J Hand Surg Am 1993;18(1):58–65.

53. Strickland JW. Flexor tendon repair: Indiana method. Indiana Hand Cent News 1993;1:1–12.

54. Strickland JW. Flexor tendon injuries: I. Foundations of treatment. J Am Acad Orthop Surg 1995;3(1):44–54.

55. Strickland JW. Flexor tendons—acute injuries. In: Green DP, Hotchkiss RN, Pederson, WC, eds., Green's Operative Hand Surgery, 4th edn. Churchill-Livingstone, Philadelphia, 1999.

56. Urbaniak J, Cahill, J, Mortenson, R. Tendon suturing methods: analysis of tensile strengths. In: Hunter JM, Schneider LHY, eds., Symposium on Tendon Surgery in the Hand, pp. 70–80. Mosby, St. Louis, 1975.

57. Kusano N, Yoshizu T, Maki Y. Experimental study of two new flexor tendon suture techniques for postoperative early active flexion exercises. J Hand Surg Br 1999;24(2):152–6.

58. Lim B, Tsai, T. The six-strand technique for flexor tendon repair. Atlas Hand Clin 1996;1:65–76.

59. Sandrow M, McMahon, M. Single cross-grasp six-strand repair for acute flexor tenorrhaphy: modified Savage technique. Atlas Hand Clin 1966;1:41–64.

60. Thurman RT, Trumble TE, Hanel DP, Tencer AF, Kiser PK. Two-, four-, and six-strand zone II flexor tendon repairs: an in situ biomechanical comparison using a cadaver model. J Hand Surg Am 1998;23(2):261–5.

61. Wagner WF, Jr, Carroll Ct, Strickland JW, Heck DA, Toombs JP. A biomechanical comparison of techniques of flexor tendon repair. J Hand Surg Am 1994;19(6):979–83.

62. Robertson GA, al-Qattan MM. A biomechanical analysis of a new interlock suture technique for flexor tendon repair. J Hand Surg Br 1992;17(1):92–3.

63. Hitanaka H, Manske, P. Effect of the cross-sectional area of locking loops in flexor tendon repair. J Hand Surg Am 1999;24:751–60.

64. Hotokezaka S, Manske PR. Differences between locking loops and grasping loops: effects on 2-strand core suture. J Hand Surg Am 1997;22(6):995–1003.

65. Trail I, Powell E, Noble J. The mechanical strength of various suture techniques. J Hand Surg Br 1989;14:422–7.

66. Aoki M, Manske PR, Pruitt DL, Kubota H, Larson BJ. Work of flexion after flexor tendon repair according to the placement of sutures. Clin Orthop Relat Res 1995;320:205–10.

67. Pruitt DL, Aoki M, Manske PR. Effect of suture knot location on tensile strength after flexor tendon repair. J Hand Surg Am 1996;21(6):969–73.

68. Aoki M, Kubota H, Pruitt DL, Manske PR. Biomechanical and histologic characteristics of canine flexor tendon repair using early postoperative mobilization. J Hand Surg Am 1997;22(1): 107–14.

69. Becker H, Graham MF, Cohen IK, Diegelmann RF. Intrinsic tendon cell proliferation in tissue culture. J Hand Surg Am 1981;6(6):616–19.

70. Greenwald D, Shumway S, Allen C, Mass D. Dynamic analysis of profundus tendon function. J Hand Surg Am 1994;19(4): 626–35.

71. Halikis MN, Manske PR, Kubota H, Aoki M. Effect of immobilization, immediate mobilization, and delayed mobilization on the resistance to digital flexion using a tendon injury model. J Hand Surg Am 1997;22(3):464–72.

72. Lane JM, Black J, Bora FW, Jr. Gliding function following flexor-tendon injury. A biomechanical study of rat tendon function. J Bone Joint Surg Am 1976;58(7):985–90.

73. Pettengill KM. The evolution of early mobilization of the repaired flexor tendon. J Hand Ther 2005;18(2):157–68.

74. Schuind F, Garcia-Elias M, Cooney WP, 3rd, An KN. Flexor tendon forces: in vivo measurements. J Hand Surg Am 1992;17(2):291–8.

75. Uchiyama S, Coert JH, Berglund L, Amadio PC, An KN. Method for the measurement of friction between tendon and pulley. J Orthop Res 1995;13(1):83–9.

76. Angeles JG, Heminger H, Mass DP. Comparative biomechanical performances of 4-strand core suture repairs for zone II flexor tendon lacerations. J Hand Surg Am 2002;27(3):508–17.

77. Aoki M, Ito K, Wada T, Ooyama N. Mechanical characteristics of cross-stitch epitenon suture in association with various two-strand core sutures: a biomechanical study using canine cadaver tendons. Injury 1996;27(10):703–7.

78. Dona E, Turner AW, Gianoutsos MP, Walsh WR. Biomechanical properties of four circumferential flexor tendon suture techniques. J Hand Surg Am 2003;28(5):824–31.

79. Kim PT, Aoki M, Tokita F, Ishii S. Tensile strength of cross-stitch epitenon suture. J Hand Surg Br 1996;21(6):821–3.

80. Kubota H, Aoki M, Pruitt DL, Manske PR. Mechanical properties of various circumferential tendon suture techniques. J Hand Surg Br 1996;21(4):474–80.

81. Lee H. Double loop locking suture: a technique of tendon repair for early active mobilization. Part II: Clinical experience. J Hand Surg Am 1990;15(6):953–8.

82. Merrell GA, Wolfe SW, Kacena WJ, Gao Y, Cholewicki J, Kacena MA. The effect of increased peripheral suture purchase on the strength of flexor tendon repairs. J Hand Surg Am 2003;28(3): 464–8.

83. Noguchi M, Seiler JG, 3rd, Gelberman RH, Sofranko RA, Woo SL. In vitro biomechanical analysis of suture methods for flexor tendon repair. J Orthop Res 1993;11(4):603–11.

84. Olivier LC, Assenmacher S, Kendoff D, Schmidt G, Towfigh H, Schmit-Neuerburg KP. Results of flexor tendon repair of the hand by the motion-stable wire suture by Towfigh. Arch Orthop Trauma Surg 2001;121(4):212–18.

85. Silfverskiold KL, May EJ. Flexor tendon repair in zone II with a new suture technique and an early mobilization program combining passive and active flexion. J Hand Surg Am 1994;19(1):53–60.

86. Silfverskiold KL, May EJ. Early active mobilization of tendon grafts using mesh reinforced suture techniques. J Hand Surg Br 1995;20(3):301–7.

87. Taras JS, Raphael JS, Marczyk SC, Bauerle WB. Evaluation of suture caliber in flexor tendon repair. J Hand Surg Am 2001;26(6):1100–4.

88. Zhau C, Amadio, P, Momose, T, et al. The effect of suture technqie on adhesion formation after flexor tendon repair for partial lacerations in a canine model. J Trauma 2001;51: 917–21.

89. Zobitz ME, Zhao C, Erhard L, Amadio PC, An KN. Tensile properties of suture methods for repair of partially lacerated human flexor tendon in vitro. J Hand Surg Am 2001;26(5): 821–7.

90. Gelberman RH, Amifl D, Gonsalves M, Woo S, Akeson WH. The influence of protected passive mobilization on the healing of flexor tendons: a biochemical and microangiographic study. Hand 1981;13(2):120–8.

91. Mason ML, Allen HS. The rate of healing of tendons: an experimental study of tensile strength. Ann Surg 1941;113(3):424–59.

92. Potenza AD. Flexor tendon injuries. Orthop Clin North Am 1970;1(2):355–73.

93. Rosenthal EA, Stoddard CW. Questions hand therapists ask about treatment of tendon injuries. J Hand Ther 2005;18(2): 313–18.

94. Groth GN. Pyramid of progressive force exercises to the injured flexor tendon. J Hand Ther 2004;17(1):31–42.

95. Lai CH. Motivation in hand-injured patients with and without work-related injury. J Hand Ther 2004;17(1):6–17.

96. Dinopoulos HT, Boyer MI, Burns ME, Gelberman RH, Silva MJ. The resistance of a four- and eight-strand suture technique to gap formation during tensile testing: an experimental study of repaired canine flexor tendons after 10 days of in vivo healing. J Hand Surg Am 2000;25(3):489–98.

97. Momose T, Amadio PC, Zhao C, Zobitz ME, Couvreur PJ, An KN. Suture techniques with high breaking strength and low gliding resistance: experiments in the dog flexor digitorum profundus tendon. Acta Orthop Scand 2001;72(6):635–41.

98. Tanaka T, Amadio PC, Zhao C, Zobitz ME, Yang C, An KN. Gliding characteristics and gap formation for locking and grasping tendon repairs: a biomechanical study in a human cadaver model. J Hand Surg Am 2004;29(1):6–14.

99. Collins ED, Novak CB, Mackinnon SE, Weisenborn SA. Long-term follow-up evaluation of cold sensitivity following nerve injury. J Hand Surg Am 1996;21(6):1078–85.

100. Groth GN. Current practice patterns of flexor tendon rehabilitation. J Hand Ther 2005;18(2):169–74.

101. Wesolowski TGS, Chang M, Hannah S, Nichols A, Graham B. Current trends in the therapy management of zone II flexor tendon repairs: A survey of Canadian CHTs. J Hand Ther 2004;17(4):436–7.

102. Groth GN. Clinical decision making and therapists' autonomy in the context of flexor tendon rehabilitation. J Hand Ther 2008;21(3):254–9; quiz 60.

103. Sueoka SS, Lastayo PC. Zone II flexor tendon rehabilitation: a proposed algorithm. J Hand Ther 2008;21(4):410–13.

104. Duran R, Houser, C, Coleman, C, Postlewaite, D. A preliminary report in the use of controlled passive motion following

flexor tendon repair in zones II and III. Am Soc Surg Hand 1976;1:79.

105. Kleinert HE, Kutz, J, Ashbell, S. Primary repair of lacerated flexor tendons in a no-man's land. J Bone Joint Surg Am 1967; 49:577.

106. Kleinert HE, Kutz JE, Atasoy E, Stormo A. Primary repair of flexor tendons. Orthop Clin North Am 1973;4(4):865–76.

107. Scavenius M, Soe-Nielsen N, Boeckstyns M, Sassene I. Early active versus early passive mobilzation regimen after primary tendon repair: a prospective randomized study. Danish Orthopaedic Society Meeting, Copenhagen, Denmark, 2000.

108. MacDermid JC, Stratford P. Applying evidence on outcome measures to hand therapy practice. J Hand Ther 2004;17(2): 165–73.

109. MacDermid JC, Grewal R, MacIntyre NJ. Using an evidence-based approach to measure outcomes in clinical practice. Hand Clin 2009;25(1):97–111, vii.

110. Elliott D, Harris, S. The assessment of flexor tendon function after primary tendon repair. Hand Clin 2003;19(3):495–503.

111. Oltman R, Neises G, Scheible D, Mehrtens G, Gruneberg C. ICF components of corresponding outcome measures in flexor tendon rehabilitation—a systematic review. BMC Musculoskelet Disord 2008;9:139.

112. MacDermid JC. Measurement of health outcomes following tendon and nerve repair. J Hand Ther 2005;18(2):297–312.

113. Cieza A, Geyh S, Chatterji S, Kostanjsek N, Ustun B, Stucki G. ICF linking rules: an update based on lessons learned. J Rehabil Med 2005;37(4):212–18.

114. Cieza A, Stucki G. New approaches to understanding the impact of musculoskeletal conditions. Best Pract Res Clin Rheumatol 2004;18(2):141–54.

115. Cieza A, Stucki G. Understanding functioning, disability, and health in rheumatoid arthritis: the basis for rehabilitation care. Curr Opin Rheumatol 2005;17(2):183–9.

116. Coenen M, Cieza A, Stamm TA, Amann E, Kollerits B, Stucki G. Validation of the International Classification of Functioning, Disability and Health (ICF) Core Set for rheumatoid arthritis from the patient perspective using focus groups. Arthritis Res Ther 2006;8(4):R84.

117. Harris JE, MacDermid JC, Roth J. The International Classification of Functioning as an explanatory model of health after distal radius fracture: a cohort study. Health Qual Life Outcomes 2005;3:73.

118. Szabo RM, MacDermid JC. An introduction to evidence-based practice for hand surgeons and therapists. Hand Clin 2009;25(1): 1–14, v.

119. Solway S, Beaton D, McConnell S, Bombardier C. The Dash Outcome Measure User's Manual, 2nd edn. Institute for Work and Health, Toronto, 2002.

120. Lagerstrom C, Nordgren B, Olerud C. Evaluation of grip strength measurements after Colles' fracture: a methodological study. Scand J Rehabil Med 1999;31(1):49–54.

121. Hamilton A, Balnave R, Adams R. Grip strength testing reliability. J Hand Ther 1994;7(3):163–70.

122. Bellace JV, Healy D, Besser MP, Byron T, Hohman L. Validity of the Dexter Evaluation System's Jamar dynamometer attachment for assessment of hand grip strength in a normal population. J Hand Ther 2000;13(1):46–51.

123. Koman LA, Slone SA, Smith BP, Ruch DS, Poehling GG. Significance of cold intolerance in upper extremity disorders. J South Orthop Assoc 1998;7(3):192–7.

119

Carpal Tunnel Syndrome— Conservative Management

Jean-Sébastien Roy[1] and Jessica Collins[2]

[1]Laval University, Quebec, QC, Canada
[2]McMaster University, Hamilton, ON, Canada

Case scenario

A 52 year old woman who works on a production line consults a health professional because of pain and numbness in her right thumb and index and middle fingers. She also reports symptoms of tingling that awaken her from sleep and that are usually relieved by shaking her hands. Her symptoms have been developing for more than 4 months.

Relevant anatomy

Carpal tunnel syndrome (CTS) is a neurologic disorder involving gradual ischemia and mechanical deformation of the median nerve produced by elevated pressure within the carpal tunnel.[1] The compression of the median nerve under the flexor retinaculum leads to impaired nerve conduction and signs of nerve dysfunction. The clinical presentation of CTS usually involves symptoms of sensory (tingling, numbness and pain) and motor impairments (weakness, loss of hand dexterity and function) in the territory of the median nerve in the hand.

Importance of the problem

CTS is the most common peripheral nerve compression neuropathy. The prevalence of CTS in western European populations is estimated at 3.0–5.8% for women and 0.6–2.1% for men.[2,3] In industrialized populations, the incidence of CTS is 99–105 per 100,000 person-years (52 for men, 149 for women)[3,4] with the peak incidence between the ages of 50–59 years.[5] The occurrence of CTS is associated with high levels of hand–arm vibration, prolonged work with a flexed or extended wrist, high requirements for hand force and high repetitiveness.[6] The average yearly claim rate for CTS is 27.3 per 10,000 full-time workers.[7]

When searching in databases, health professionals and patients are overwhelmed by the volume of information about CTS. In fact, over 3,000,000 hits appear on Google, and 6,700 on MEDLINE, when the search keywords "carpal tunnel syndrome" are entered. The variable quality and lack of filtering mandates need for pre-appraised evidence-based guides.

Top six questions

Diagnosis

1. How accurate are the clinical diagnostic tests for CTS?

Therapy

2. Is splinting beneficial for CTS?
3. Are ultrasound and laser therapy effective for CTS?
4. Are exercises and mobilization beneficial for CTS?
5. What is the effect of local corticosteroid injection for CTS?
6. What is the optimal approach of oral therapies for CTS?

Question 1: How accurate are the clinical diagnostic tests for CTS?

Case clarification

The information provided by this patient suggests that she has CTS. History alone can increase the likelihood of CTS.

Evidence-Based Orthopedics, First Edition. Edited by Mohit Bhandari.

For example, our patient reports waking at night and shaking her hand to relieve symptoms. This sign, known as the flick sign, is sensitive at 47% and specific at 62% for CTS.[8] Clinical diagnostic tests are commonly used to help increase the confidence in the CTS diagnosis.

Relevance

A variety of clinical diagnostic tests are available for CTS. Therefore, clinicians need to select diagnostic tests that are the most specific to confirm CTS and the most sensitive to establish that CTS is unlikely.

Current opinion

Current opinion suggests that the majority of health professionals use the Tinel and the Phalen tests as clinical diagnostic tests for CTS.

Finding the evidence

- PubMed/systematic reviews: "CTS" AND "diagnosis"
- MEDLINE search identifying the population (CTS), the psychometric properties (sensitivity, specificity) and the methodology (diagnostic studies). We used the keywords "CTS" AND "diagnosis" AND ("sensitivity" OR "specificity")

Quality of the evidence

Level I

- 2 systematic reviews
- 15 validating cohort studies with good reference standards

Level II

- 33 exploratory cohort studies with good reference standards

Findings

The two tests that were the most studied are the Phalen (31 trials; n = 3,218 cases, 1,637 controls) and Tinel tests (26 trials; n = 2,640 cases, 1,614 controls). According to a systematic review by MacDermid and Weissel,[9] the overall average sensitivity for CTS is 68% for the Phalen test and 50% for the Tinel test (Table 119.1). These two clinical diagnostic tests are not the most sensitive for CTS. Carpal compression combined with wrist flexion (3 trials; n = 190 cases, 238 controls) and current perception threshold (2 trials; n = 46 cases, 63 controls) are the most sensitive at 80% (weighted average over all studies) (Table 119.1).[9] Other sensitive tests included hand diagram (6 trials; n = 293 cases, 226 controls) at 75% and Semmes–Weinstein monofilament (11 studies; n = 811 cases, 567 controls) at 72%.[9]

Rates reported for overall average specificity differ according to the referent standard, i.e., between the studies that used asymptomatic controls vs. control with symptoms, but negative electrodiagnostic test.[9] The average spe-

Table 119.1 Sensitivity and specificity of clinical diagnostic tests for carpal tunnel syndrome[9]

Diagnostic test	N[a]	Pooled sensitivity	Pooled specificity[b]
Phalen	3218/1637	68	65
Tinel	2640/1614	50	65
Current perception threshold	46/63	80	N/E
Carpal compression with wrist flexion	190/238	80	92
Static two-point discimination	381/212	24	98
Abductor pollicus brevis atrophy	107/88	12	94

N = total sample size pooled.
[a]Number of cases/number of controls.
[b]Calculated from subjects who had carpal tunnel syndrome-like symptoms but negative electrodiagnostic findings.

cificity of the Phalen and Tinel tests is, respectively, 73% and 77% for all the studies, and 65% for the studies with symptomatic controls (Table 119.1). Again, these two widely used tests are not the most specific. The most specific test is the static two-point (6 studies; n = 381 cases, 212 controls) at 98% (Table 119.1). Other specific tests for CTS include the abductor pollicis brevis atrophy at 94% (2 studies; n = 107 cases, 88 controls) and carpal compression combined to wrist flexion (3 trials; n = 190 cases, 238 controls) at 92% (Table 119.1). Note that the highly specific tests tend to have low sensitivity (Table 119.1). Combining tests can increase the resulting sensitivity and specificity. Fertl et al.[10] combined the Phalen test with the median nerve compression test and found a sensitivity of 92% and a specificity of 92%.

Recommendations

- The most sensitive clinical diagnostic tests for CTS are the carpal compression combined to wrist flexion and current perception threshold at 80% [overall quality: moderate]
- The most specific clinical diagnostic test for CTS is the static two-point at 98% [overall quality: good]

Question 2: Is splinting beneficial for CTS?

Case clarification

Your evaluation suggests that your patient has mild to moderate CTS. You recommend trying conservative management first.

Relevance

Nonsurgical treatments are offered to those who have intermittent symptoms of mild to moderate CTS. The use

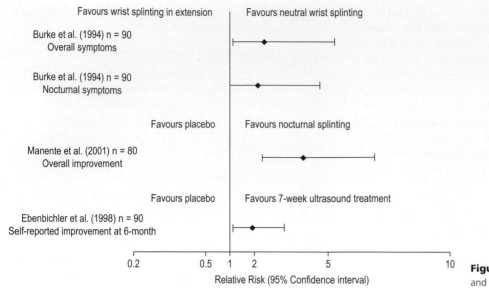

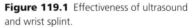

Figure 119.1 Effectiveness of ultrasound and wrist splint.

of conservative options could potentially result in resolution of symptoms without having to resort to surgery, which can result in complications and lost productivity.

Current opinion

Splinting is the usual first nonsurgical treatment used by the therapists for CTS.

Finding the evidence

- Cochrane Database, with search term "CTS"
- PubMed/systematic reviews: "CTS" AND "therapy" AND ("conservative treatment" OR "nonsurgical treatment" OR splint)
- MEDLINE search identifying the population (CTS) the intervention (splint OR splinting) and the methodology (clinical trial). We used the keywords "CTS" AND "(splint OR splinting)"

Quality of the evidence

Level I
- 5 systematic reviews/meta-analyses
- 6 randomized trials

Level II
- 13 randomized trials with methodologic limitations

Findings

Manente et al.[11] (n = 40 for each group) have compared the short-term effects of nocturnal hand splints for 4 weeks to a control group. They found a significant improvement of symptoms, hand function, and nerve conduction in the treated group at 2 weeks and 4 weeks. According to the Cochrane review by O'Connor et al.,[12] the relative rate (RR) of participants reporting overall improvement after four

weeks of splint use was 4.00 (95% CI 2.34–6.84) (Figure 119.1).

Burke et al.[13] (n = 45 cases for each group) have shown a significant short-term effect in favor of the neutral position for wrist splinting in CTS compared with splinting in an extended wrist position (20°). According to the Cochrane review by O'Connor et al.,[12] the RR for improvement for neutral wrist splinting 2 weeks after the beginning of treatment was 2.43 (95% CI 1.12–5.28) for overall symptoms and 2.14 (95% CI 0.99–4.65) for nocturnal symptoms (Figure 119.1). Walker et al.[14] (n = 11 cases for full-time use; n = 13 cases for night-time only use) have shown no significant difference in symptom/hand function improvement between night-time only use and full-time use of wrist splint over a 6 week period. Werner et al.[15] (n = 63 cases for nocturnal splint; n = 49 cases for ergonomic education) compared nocturnal splint use with an ergonomic education programme. The group treated with splint showed greater improvement at 1 year follow-up. However, improvement was observed in both groups.

Recommendations

- Night splinting is effective for reducing symptom severity of CTS [overall quality: moderate]
- Full-time splinting does not reduce symptom severity or improve function more than night splinting alone [overall quality: low]

Question 3: Are ultrasound and laser therapy effective for CTS?

Case clarification

You are concerned that your typical conservative approach of 6 weeks of splinting may not be sufficient and wonder if adding an adjunctive will enhance the benefit of a conservative treatment program.

Relevance

There is a plethora of conservative management modalities available for CTS. However, the optimal single or combination of modalities for symptom relief remains uncertain.

Current opinion

Even in the absence of complete relief, conservative management can be used for symptomatic benefit or to evaluate the likelihood of response.

Finding the evidence

• As for Question 2, but with "splint OR splinting" replaced by "laser therapy OR ultrasound OR ergonomic"

Quality of the evidence

Level I
• 5 systematic reviews/meta-analyses
• 10 randomized trials

Level II
• 13 randomized trials with methodologic limitations

Findings

Ultrasound Ultrasound therapy has been compared to placebo ultrasound therapy in two trials (n = 65 for ultrasound; n = 55 for placebo).[16,17] The two trials demonstrated no short-term effects of ultrasound therapy for improvement in pain, symptoms, or nocturnal waking after 2 weeks of treatment. Furthermore, at 6 months, there was no group difference between ultrasound (7 weeks therapy) and placebo for peripheral nerve conduction, grip strength or pinch strength.[16,17] After a 7-week therapy and at the 6 months follow-up, however, Ebenbichler et al.[16] (n = 45 for each group) found a significant effect of ultrasound on symptom improvement (WMD −1.86 on 0–10 point VAS, 95% CI −2.67 to −1.05) and sensation (WMD −1.18 on 0–10 point VAS, 95% CI −2.02 to −0.34). The RR for self-reported improvement at 6 months was 1.91 (95% CI 1.13–3.23) favoring ultrasound over placebo (Figure 119.1). Oztas et al.[17] (n = 10 for each group) did not find any significant effect of varying intensity of ultrasound (1.5 W/cm^2 and 0.8 W/cm^2) for pain, symptoms, or nocturnal waking.

Laser therapy Low-level laser therapy has been compared to sham laser in two trials.[18,19] The first trials (n = 7 for laser therapy; n = 8 for placebo) did not demonstrate any improvement in both groups.[18] In the other trial, Naeser et al.[19] combined low-level laser therapy to transcutaneous electrical nerve stimulation (TENS) and compared this combination to sham laser and TENS (n = 11). They found

that low-level laser and TENS led to a significant reduction of pain and symptoms.

Recommendation

• No recommendations can be given since there is conflicting evidence on whether ultrasound or low-level laser are effective

Question 4: Are exercises and mobilization beneficial for CTS?

Case clarification

Exercises and mobilization can also be used as conservative modalities for mild to moderate CTS.

Relevance

Exercises and mobilization include yoga, carpal bone mobilization, or nerve gliding. Therefore, clinicians need to know which ones are effective in the management of CTS.

Current opinion

Nerve gliding and mobilization are often used to reduce clinical symptoms of CTS. It is believed that the gliding may reduce adhesions that result in areas of traction along the nerve.

Finding the evidence

• As for Question 2, but with "splint OR splinting" replaced by "exercise OR nerve gliding OR mobilization"

Quality of the evidence

Level I
• 5 systematic reviews/meta-analyses
• 3 randomized trials

Level II
• 7 randomized trials with methodological limitations

Findings

Yoga The effects of yoga exercise on CTS symptoms have been compared to wrist splinting (n = 26 for yoga; n = 25 for wrist splint).[20] Yoga did not decrease pain or increase grip strength more than splinting. However, a significant effect of yoga on the Phalen sign was demonstrated. According to the Cochrane review by O'Connor et al.,[12] the RR for Phalen sign was 5.25 (95% CI 1.28–21.47) favoring yoga (Figure 119.2). There are different types of yoga and the specific type reported as effective is 11 yoga posture designed for strengthening, stretching, and balancing each joint in the upper body along with relaxation.

Nerve gliding exercises The effects of nerve gliding exercises or neurodynamic mobilization were evaluated in two trials.[21,22] Tal-Akabi and Ruchton[22] (n = 7 for each group) evaluated the short-term effect of nerve gliding exercises

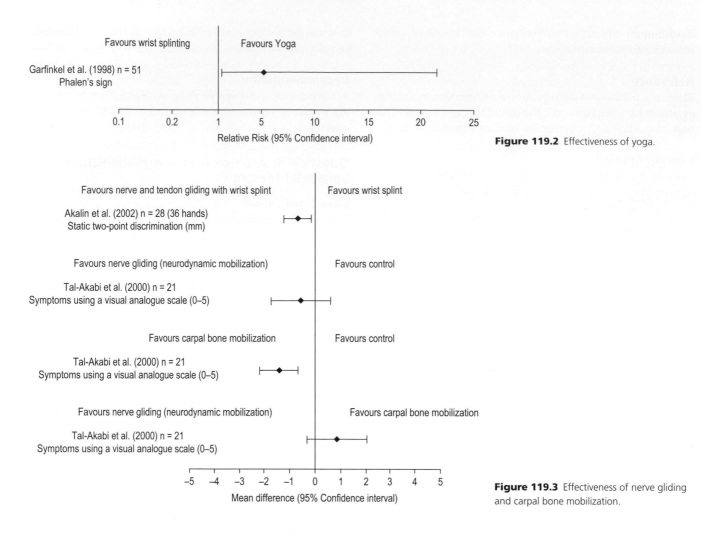

Figure 119.2 Effectiveness of yoga.

Figure 119.3 Effectiveness of nerve gliding and carpal bone mobilization.

on CTS symptoms when compared to no treatment. According to the post-hoc analyses performed in the systematic review by Muller et al.,[23] nerve gliding exercises relieve pain more than no treatment. In the same study, Tal-Akabi and Ruchton[22] (n = 7 for each group) also evaluated the short-term effect of nerve gliding exercises as compared to carpal bone mobilization. The results show no significant benefit of nerve gliding exercises over carpal bone mobilization for improving short-term symptoms (Figure 119.3). In another trial, Akalin et al.[21] (n = 18 for each group) evaluated the combined effects of nerve/tendon gliding exercises and wrist splint for 4 weeks on CTS symptoms when compared to wrist splinting alone. The addition of nerve/tendon gliding to wrist splint led to a significant effect on static two-point discrimination (WMD −0.70 mm, 95% CI −1.24 to −0.16) (Figure 119.3). However, nerve/tendon gliding exercises plus splinting did not reduce median nerve dysfunction, symptom severity, or improve function, grip strength more than splinting alone.

Carpal bone mobilization Tal-Akabi and Ruchton[22] (n = 7 for each group) evaluated the effect of carpal bone mobiliza-

tion when compared to no treatment. Carpal bone mobilization significantly relieved symptoms more than no treatment (WMD −1.43 on 0–5 point scale, 95% CI −2.19 to −0.67) (Figure 119.3). However, it did not lead to a significant effect for improving pain, hand function, and active wrist motion.

Recommendations
- Yoga exercise improved outcome of the Phalen sign more than wrist splinting [overall quality: low]
- Nerve gliding exercises decrease pain in CTS [overall quality: low]
- Carpal bone mobilization improves symptoms of CTS [overall quality: low]

Question 5: What is the effect of local corticosteroid injection in the treatment of CTS?

Case clarification
Another commonly used treatment option for the conservative management of mild to moderate CTS is local steroid injections.

Relevance

The effectiveness of corticosteroid injections has to be determined since the recurrence rates of symptoms have varied from 8% to 100% following injection.

Current opinion

Current opinion suggests that the majority of health professionals use local steroid injection for short-term clinical improvement.

Finding the evidence

As for Question 2, but with "splint OR splinting" replaced by "injection OR steroid"

Quality of the evidence

Level I
• 2 systematic reviews/meta-analyses
• 16 randomized trials

Level II
• 10 randomized trials with methodological limitations

Findings

Two studies (n = 73 for injection, n = 66 for placebo) have compared local corticosteroid injection to placebo injection. They demonstrated improvement with steroid injection after 2 weeks[24] and 1 month[25] with RR of 2.04 (95% CI 1.26–3.31) and RR of 3.83 (95% CI 1.82–8.05) respectively. According to the meta-analysis performed by Marshall et al.,[26] more participants improved after corticosteroid injection compared to placebo 1 month after the injection (RR 2.58; 95% CI 1.72–3.87) (Figure 119.4).

Two trials (n = 48 for injection, n = 47 for systemic corticosteroid)[27,28] have compared local corticosteroid injection to systemic corticosteroid. One trial[27] (daily oral corticosteroids vs. local injection) did not find any group differences at 2 weeks, but at 8 weeks and 12 weeks, local corticosteroid treatment was found to be significantly better (MD −7.10, 95% CI −11.68 to −2.52 at 12 months). The other trial[28] (local corticosteroid injection vs. single systemic corticosteroid injection) found that at 1 month there was a significant improvement in symptoms for the group undergoing local injection (RR 3.17, 95% CI 1.02–9.87) (Figure 119.4).

Two trials (n = 37 for each group)[29,30] have compared low dose to high dose of corticosteroid injection into the carpal tunnel. According to the meta-analysis by Marshall et al.[26] there are no differences in clinical improvement between the two doses at six weeks (RR 1.00, 95% CI 0.76–1.31) (Figure 119.4). Another study showed no significant difference between groups treated with 20, 40, or 60 mg of methylprednisolone.[31]

One study has compared local corticosteroid injection to oral anti-inflammatory drugs combined to neutral angle wrist splint (n = 12 for injection, n = 11 for NSAID and splint).[32] No significant difference for symptom and pain severity was found 2 weeks and 8 weeks after the start of the treatment. Finally, one trial (n = 20 for each group)[33] has compared a single local corticosteroid injection to two local corticosteroid injections. No significant difference was observed between the two groups at 8 weeks, 24 weeks and 40 weeks after the injection(s).

Recommendations

• Local corticosteroid injection leads to short-term clinical improvement [overall quality: good]
• Two injections do not lead to better clinical improvement than one local corticosteroid injection [overall quality: moderate]

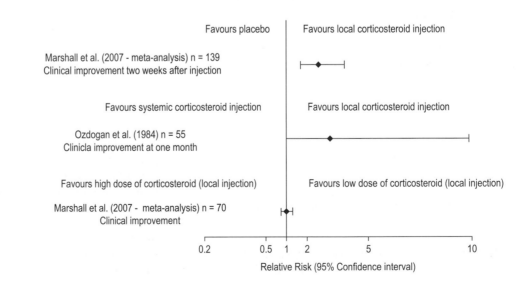

Figure 119.4 Effectiveness of local corticosteroid injection.

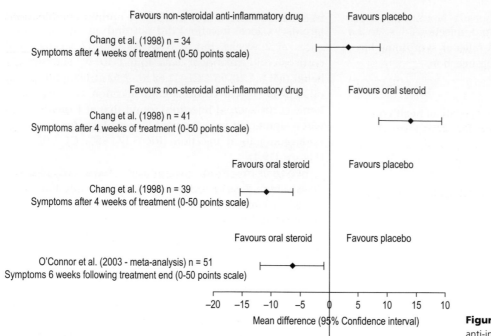

Figure 119.5 Effectiveness of nonsteroidal anti-inflammatory drug and oral steroid.

Question 6: What is the optimal approach of oral therapies for CTS?

Case clarification
Nonsteroidal anti-inflammatory (NSAID) medication and oral steroids can also be considered in early management of mild to moderate CTS.

Relevance
Oral therapy includes drugs, such as steroid, NSAID, diuretic, and vitamins. However, before using such modalities, clinicians must make sure of their effectiveness for CTS.

Current opinion
Oral therapy, mainly NSAID and steroid, are often the first treatment used for CTS.

Finding the evidence
Same as Question 2, but with "splint OR splinting" replaced by "oral therapy OR NSAID OR steroid"

Quality of the evidence
Level I
- 5 systematic reviews/meta-analyses
- 10 randomized trials

Level II
- 25 randomized trials with methodological limitations

Findings
Vitamin B_6 Two trials have evaluated the mid-term effects of vitamin B_6 therapy (n = 24 for vitamin B_6, n = 26 for placebo/control).[34,35] Vitamin B_6 therapy was found to be ineffective for improving symptoms, nocturnal discomfort, hand coordination, Phalen sign, or Tinel sign after 10–12 weeks of therapy.[12]

NSAIDs and diuretic treatment Chang et al.[36] have compared the short-term effects of NSAID to placebo and oral steroids (n = 18 for NSAID; n = 23 for oral steroid; n = 16 for placebo). Compared to placebo, no significant effect in favor of NSAID treatment was demonstrated for improving CTS symptoms. However, a significant effect in favor of oral steroids was demonstrated on symptom improvement with 4 weeks of treatment when compared to NSAID (WMD 14.00 on a 0–50 point scale; 95% CI 8.57–19.43) (Figure 119.5).[12] In the same study, Chang et al.[36] also compared the effects of diuretic (n = 16) treatment when compared to NSAID treatment and oral steroid. No significant difference between NSAID and diuretic was found following 2 and 4 weeks of treatment. Oral steroids proved to be more effective than diuretic to improve clinical symptoms after 4 weeks (WMD 11.60 on a 0–50 point scale; 95% CI 7.25–15.95).[12]

Oral steroids The use of oral steroid has been compared to placebo in three trials (n = 49 for oral steroid, n = 44 for placebo).[36–38] According to the meta-analysis of O'Connor et al.,[12] a significant effect in favor of oral steroids was demonstrated on symptom improvement with 2 weeks and 4 weeks of treatment (pooled WMD after 2 weeks of treatment –7.23 points on a 0–50 point scale, 95% CI –10.31 to –4.14; after 4 weeks of treatment –10.8 points, 95% CI –15.26 to –6.34) (Figure 119.5). Herskovitz et al.[37] have shown on a small sample (n = 8 for oral steroid; n = 10 for placebo) that 2 weeks and 6 weeks after the end of an oral steroid treatment, the benefits of the treatment are lost (WMD −6.19 on a 0–50 point scale, 95% CI −15.14 to 2.76)[12]. In contrast, Hui et al. (n = 18 for each group) observed continued effects from oral steroid use 6 weeks after the end of treatment. According to the meta-analysis by O'Connor et al.,[12] the pooled WMD for improvement of CTS symptoms 6 weeks following the end of a 2 week oral steroid treatment was −6.46 points on a 0–50 point scale (95% CI −11.93 to −0.99).

Recommendations

• NSAID, diuretic therapy and vitamin B_6 are ineffectiveness for reducing the clinical symptoms of CTS [overall quality: low]

• Oral steroid treatment improves the clinical symptoms of CTS in the short term [overall quality: moderate]

• There is equivocal evidence regarding the benefits of oral steroid 2–6 weeks after the end of the therapy, [overall quality: low]

Summary of recommendations

• The most sensitive clinical diagnostic tests for CTS are the carpal compression combined to wrist flexion and current perception threshold at 80%, while the most specific is the static two-point at 98%

• Night splinting is effective for reducing symptom severity of CTS, but full-time splinting does not reduce symptom severity or improve function more than night splinting alone

• Nerve gliding and carpal bone mobilization improves symptoms of CTS

• Local corticosteroid injection leads to short-term clinical improvement

• NSAID, diuretic therapy, and B_6 are ineffective for reducing the clinical symptoms of CTS, while oral steroid treatment improves the clinical symptoms of CTS in the short term [overall quality: moderate]

Conclusions

The results from the appraisal of the evidence related to treatment of CTS suggest that some conservative therapies for CTS, mainly local steroid injection, oral steroid, and splinting, lead to short- and mid-term clinical improvement. Therefore, the evidence strengthens the current opinion that conservative treatment should be attempted first in mild to moderate CTS. However, high-quality studies are needed to provide stronger evidence on the interventions currently supported by weak evidence, to develop decision rules based on responses to different treatment options and to investigate optimal combinations and dosages.

J-S R supported by scholarships from the Canadian Institute of Health Research and Fonds de Recherche en Santé du Québec.

References

1. Werner RA, Andary M. Carpal tunnel syndrome: pathophysiology and clinical neurophysiology. Clin Neurophysiol 2002; 113(9):1373–81.
2. Atroshi I, Gummesson C, Johnsson R, Ornstein E, Ranstam J, Rosen I. Prevalence of carpal tunnel syndrome in a general population. JAMA 1999;282(2):153–8.
3. de Krom MC, Knipschild PG, Kester AD, Thijs CT, Boekkooi PF, Spaans F. Carpal tunnel syndrome: prevalence in the general population. J Clin Epidemiol 1992;45(4):373–6.
4. Stevens JC, Sun S, Beard CM, O'Fallon WM, Kurland LT. Carpal tunnel syndrome in Rochester, Minnesota, 1961 to 1980. Neurology 1988;38(1):134–8.
5. Mondelli M, Giannini F, Giacchi M. Carpal tunnel syndrome incidence in a general population. Neurology 2002;58(2): 289–94.
6. van Rijn RM, Huisstede BM, Koes BW, Burdorf A. Associations between work-related factors and the carpal tunnel syndrome—a systematic review. Scand J Work Environ Health 2009;35(1): 19–36.
7. Silverstein B, Welp E, Nelson N, Kalat J. Claims incidence of work-related disorders of the upper extremities: Washington state, 1987 through 1995. Am J Public Health 1998;88(12): 1827–33.
8. MacDermid JC, Doherty T. Clinical and electrodiagnostic testing of carpal tunnel syndrome: a narrative review. J Orthop Sports Phys Ther 2004;34(10):565–88.
9. MacDermid JC, Wessel J. Clinical diagnosis of carpal tunnel syndrome: a systematic review. J Hand Ther 2004;17(2):309–19.
10. Fertl E, Wober C, Zeitlhofer J. The serial use of two provocative tests in the clinical diagnosis of carpal tunel syndrome. Acta Neurol Scand 1998;98(5):328–32.
11. Manente G, Torrieri F, Di Blasio F, Staniscia T, Romano F, Uncini A. An innovative hand brace for carpal tunnel syndrome: a randomized controlled trial. Muscle Nerve 2001;24(8):1020–5.
12. O'Connor D, Marshall S, Massy-Westropp N. Non-surgical treatment (other than steroid injection) for carpal tunnel syndrome. Cochrane Database Syst Rev 2003;1:CD003219.
13. Burke DT, Burke MM, Stewart GW, Cambre A. Splinting for carpal tunnel syndrome: in search of the optimal angle. Arch Phys Med Rehabil 1994;75(11):1241–4.
14. Walker WC, Metzler M, Cifu DX, Swartz Z. Neutral wrist splinting in carpal tunnel syndrome: a comparison of night-only versus full-time wear instructions. Arch Phys Med Rehabil 2000;81(4):424–9.
15. Werner RA, Franzblau A, Gell N. Randomized controlled trial of nocturnal splinting for active workers with symptoms of carpal tunnel syndrome. Arch Phys Med Rehabil 2005;86(1): 1–7.

16. Ebenbichler GR, Resch KL, Nicolakis P, et al. Ultrasound treatment for treating the carpal tunnel syndrome: randomised "sham" controlled trial. BMJ 1998;316(7133):731–5.

17. Oztas O, Turan B, Bora I, Karakaya MK. Ultrasound therapy effect in carpal tunnel syndrome. Arch Phys Med Rehabil 1998;79(12):1540–4.

18. Irvine J, Chong SL, Amirjani N, Chan KM. Double-blind randomized controlled trial of low-level laser therapy in carpal tunnel syndrome. Muscle Nerve 2004;30(2):182–7.

19. Naeser MA, Hahn KA, Lieberman BE, Branco KF. Carpal tunnel syndrome pain treated with low-level laser and microamperes transcutaneous electric nerve stimulation: A controlled study. Arch Phys Med Rehabil 2002;83(7):978–88.

20. Garfinkel MS, Singhal A, Katz WA, Allan DA, Reshetar R, Schumacher HR, Jr. Yoga-based intervention for carpal tunnel syndrome: a randomized trial. JAMA 1998;280(18):1601–3.

21. Akalin E, El O, Peker O, Senocak O, Tamci S, Gulbahar S, et al. Treatment of carpal tunnel syndrome with nerve and tendon gliding exercises. Am J Phys Med Rehabil 2002;81(2):108–13.

22. Tal-Akabi A, Rushton A. An investigation to compare the effectiveness of carpal bone mobilisation and neurodynamic mobilisation as methods of treatment for carpal tunnel syndrome. Man Ther 2000;5(4):214–22.

23. Muller M, Tsui D, Schnurr R, Biddulph-Deisroth L, Hard J, MacDermid JC. Effectiveness of hand therapy interventions in primary management of carpal tunnel syndrome: a systematic review. J Hand Ther 2004;17(2):210–28.

24. Armstrong T, Devor W, Borschel L, Contreras R. Intracarpal steroid injection is safe and effective for short-term management of carpal tunnel syndrome. Muscle Nerve 2004;29(1):82–8.

25. Dammers JW, Veering MM, Vermeulen M. Injection with methylprednisolone proximal to the carpal tunnel: randomised double blind trial. BMJ 1999;319(7214):884–6.

26. Marshall S, Tardif G, Ashworth N. Local corticosteroid injection for carpal tunnel syndrome. Cochrane Database Syst Rev 2007;2:CD001554.

27. Wong SM, Hui AC, Tang A, et al. Local vs systemic corticosteroids in the treatment of carpal tunnel syndrome. Neurology 2001;56(11):1565–7.

28. Ozdogan H, Yazici H. The efficacy of local steroid injections in idiopathic carpal tunnel syndrome: a double-blind study. Br J Rheumatol 1984;23(4):272–5.

29. Habib GS, Badarny S, Rawashdeh H. A novel approach of local corticosteroid injection for the treatment of carpal tunnel syndrome. Clin Rheumatol 2006;25(3):338–40.

30. O'Gradaigh D, Merry P. Corticosteroid injection for the treatment of carpal tunnel syndrome. Ann Rheum Dis 2000;59(11): 918–19.

31. Dammers JW, Roos Y, Veering MM, Vermeulen M. Injection with methylprednisolone in patients with the carpal tunnel syndrome: a randomised double blind trial testing three different doses. J Neurol 2006;253(5):574–7.

32. Celiker R, Arslan S, Inanici F. Corticosteroid injection vs. nonsteroidal antiinflammatory drug and splinting in carpal tunnel syndrome. Am J Phys Med Rehabil 2002;81(3):182–6.

33. Wong SM, Hui AC, Lo SK, Chiu JH, Poon WF, Wong L. Single vs. two steroid injections for carpal tunnel syndrome: a randomised clinical trial. Int J Clin Pract 2005;59(12):1417–21.

34. Spooner GR, Desai HB, Angel JF, Reeder BA, Donat JR. Using pyridoxine to treat carpal tunnel syndrome. Randomized control trial. Can Fam Physician 1993;39:2122–7.

35. Stransky M, Rubin A, Lava NS, Lazaro RP. Treatment of carpal tunnel syndrome with vitamin B6: a double-blind study. South Med J 1989;82(7):841–2.

36. Chang MH, Chiang HT, Lee SS, Ger LP, Lo YK. Oral drug of choice in carpal tunnel syndrome. Neurology 1998;51(2):390–3.

37. Herskovitz S, Berger AR, Lipton RB. Low-dose, short-term oral prednisone in the treatment of carpal tunnel syndrome. Neurology 1995;45(10):1923–5.

38. Hui AC, Wong SM, Wong KS, et al. Oral steroid in the treatment of carpal tunnel syndrome. Ann Rheum Dis 2001;60(8):813–14.

120 Carpal Tunnel Syndrome—Surgical Management

Jessica Collins[1], Jean-Sébastien Roy[2], Leslie L. McKnight[1], and Achilleas Thoma[1]

[1]McMaster University, Hamilton, ON, Canada
[2]Laval University, Quebec, QC, Canada

Case scenario

A 50 year old, healthy woman presents with complaints of hand weakness and numbness every night in her thumb and index and long fingers, which wakes her up at night.

Relevant anatomy

Carpal bones and the transverse carpal ligament form the carpal tunnel. It contains nine flexor tendons and the median nerve, which gives off its recurrent branch under or just distal to the ligament. Carpal tunnel syndrome (CTS) results from compression of the median nerve within the tunnel, which leads to motor and sensory abnormalities.

Importance of the problem

CTS is the most common peripheral compression neuropathy in the United States, with a prevalence of 3.7% and an annual incidence estimated at 0.4%.[1,2] CTS has a significant socioeconomic impact due to workers' compensation claims[3] and extended disability.[4]

Top four questions

Diagnosis

1. Are electromyogram (EMG) and nerve conduction studies (NCS) essential in the diagnosis of CTS?

2. Is there a role for imaging modalities (ultrasound, CT, MRI) in the diagnosis of CTS?

Therapy

- Is operative management superior to conservative management for relief of clinical symptoms?
- Which operative method provides the most improvement in clinical symptoms?

Question 1: Are EMG and NCS essential in the diagnosis of CTS?

Case clarification
You suspect the patient has CTS and send her for EMG and NCS for confirmation.

Relevance
There is divergent opinion on whether all patients require these investigations.

Current opinion
EMG and NCS should be considered on patients with severe symptoms for whom surgery is being contemplated. For mild to moderate symptoms, baseline data can be obtained, while others initiate conservative management and reserve investigation for patients who fail to respond.

Finding the evidence
- Cochrane Database, with search term: "carpal tunnel syndrome"
- PubMed and OVID MEDLINE search: "carpal tunnel syndrome," "electrodiagnosis," "electromyography/ or neural conduction," "diagnosis"

Evidence-Based Orthopedics, First Edition. Edited by Mohit Bhandari.
© 2012 Blackwell Publishing Ltd. Published 2012 by Blackwell Publishing Ltd.

• American College of Physicians' Physicians' Information and Education Resource (ACP PIER), search term "carpal tunnel syndrome"
• American Academy of Orthopaedic Surgeons (AAOS) Clinical Guideline on Diagnosis of Carpal Tunnel Syndrome

Quality of the evidence
Level I
• 2 studies

Level II
• 2 studies

Level III
• 1 studies

Level IV
• 6 studies

Level V
• 2 studies

Findings

The AAOS guidelines[5] recommend obtaining EMG and NCS when the diagnosis of CTS is uncertain, when patients fail to respond to conservative treatment, and when surgical treatment is being considered. EMG and NCS can confirm the diagnosis and severity of CTS, which can guide treatment.[5] Patients who have obvious CTS signs can also benefit by obtaining baseline values to quantify post-treatment benefits.

Several studies mention that positive test results on both physical examination and EMG/NCS are related to positive surgical outcomes.[6–9,10] NCS has a high sensitivity and specificity, over 85% and 95% respectively, in the diagnosis of CTS compared to control subjects.[11–15] NCS alone is associated with better surgical outcomes, although to a lesser extent than when combined with physical examination. False-negative electrodiagnostic test results occur in approximately 5% of cases.[16] A recent study determined that the best predictor of symptom severity is the median nerve sensory distal latency, while the best predictor of functional status is the median nerve motor distal latency.[17]

Recommendations
• Combining physical examination and EMG/NCS provides the most accurate means of diagnosing CTS [overall quality: high]
• EMG/NCS should be considered in patients where the diagnosis is uncertain, there is failure to respond to conservative management, or when surgical treatment is being contemplated [overall quality: high]

• EMG/NCS can assess the severity of the nerve compression, which may assist with treatment selection [overall quality: moderate]

Question 2: Is there a role for imaging modalities in the diagnosis of CTS?

Case clarification
The patient's EMG/NCS studies show severe CTS. With no history of wrist trauma, you wonder if additional imaging would change your management.

Relevance
Imaging provides valuable information in musculoskeletal disorders. However, it is important to consider whether imaging for CTS will lead to changes in management.

Current opinion
Surgeons do not routinely use imaging for CTS.

Finding the evidence
• As for Question 1, except for keywords in PubMed and OVID: "carpal tunnel syndrome," "diagnosis," "magnetic resonance imaging or tomography, x-ray computed or ultrasonography"

Quality of the evidence
Level I
• 3 studies

Level II
• 5 studies

Level III
• 1 study

Level IV
• 7 studies

Level V
• 2 studies

Findings
Swelling or flattening of the nerve has been demonstrated on ultrasound.[18–19] Measurements of the nerve's cross-sectional area to diagnose compression have shown a sensitivity of 83–94% and a specificity of 65–73%.[20–26] However, EMG/NCS (sensitivity 78–82%, specificity 80–83%) proved to be superior at predicting symptom severity and functional status, and more accurate for diagnosis confirmation when compared to ultrasound (sensitivity 62%-72%, specificity 56–63%).[17,27–29] Therefore, ultrasound may be the most useful in patients with symptoms and clinical findings in keeping with CTS with negative results on EMG/NCS.[30]

The AAOS guidelines[5] indicate that there is no role for routine use of CT or MRI for the diagnosis of CTS. However, these modalities may be useful when structural lesions are suspected,[5,31] or when there is a history of previous wrist trauma, or bone or joint disease.[4] MRI is most helpful when investigating lesions such as ganglions, soft tissue tumors, and muscle hypertrophy.[32–34] Measuring the size of the tunnel has not shown definite benefits for making the diagnosis.[34,35]

Recommendations
• Ultrasound is useful for nerve measurements and when EMG/NCS is inconclusive [overall quality: low]
• Selected patients may benefit from CT or MRI to diagnose structural CTS [overall quality: moderate]

Question 3: Is operative management superior to conservative management for relief of clinical symptoms?

Case clarification
Since this patient has severe CTS, you recommend surgical management. She asks whether conservative management could be of benefit instead of surgery.

Relevance
Conservative management can result in symptom resolution. However, the benefits of conservative modalities compared to surgery are uncertain.

Current opinion
Conservative management can be attempted in patients with mild to moderate CTS. If the patient does not improve, or originally has severe CTS, surgery is offered.

Finding the evidence
• Cochrane Database, with search term: "carpal tunnel syndrome"
• PubMed and OVID MEDLINE search: "carpal tunnel syndrome," "steroids," "glucocorticosteroids," "injections, intra-articular," "nonsurg or nonsurg or conservative treatment or therapy or manage," "splints," "treatment outcome"
• ACP PIER, search term "carpal tunnel syndrome"
• AAOS Clinical Guideline on the Treatment of Carpal Tunnel Syndrome

Quality of the evidence
Level I
• 4 studies

Findings
A Cochrane meta-analysis, including studies comparing splinting or steroid injections to surgery, indicated greater recovery with surgical compared to conservative management with a pooled estimate of RR 1.23 (CI 1.04–1.46).[36–39] Results at 6 months and 1 year also favored surgical management with a pooled estimate of RR 1.19 (95% CI 1.02–1.39) and RR 1.27 (95% CI 1.05–1.53) respectively.[39] In terms of improvements seen on electrodiagnostic tests, Hui et al.[38] reported that 92% of surgical patients vs. 64% of injected patients showed significant improvement in sensory potential amplitude (RR 1.44, 95% CI 1.05–1.97). Although these studies did not formally stratify patients into severity groups, many observed that patients with more severe CTS had the most improvement from baseline with surgical management. A meta-analysis demonstrated that a significant proportion of patients treated with splinting eventually required surgery, while the need for reoperation was low in patients originally treated with surgery (RR 0.04, 95% CI 0.01–0.17).[39] Finally, Gelberman stratified patients receiving steroid injections and splinting as mildly or severely symptomatic, and found that those with severe symptoms had the poorest response and experienced a higher rate of relapse (only 11%, vs. 40% of patients in the "mild" group, were still symptom free at 18 months).[40]

Recommendations
• Patients with severe CTS should undergo surgery, regardless of whether conservative management has been attempted, since operative treatment will likely lead to more significant and long-lasting improvements [overall quality: high]
• For patients with mild to moderate CTS, a trial of conservative management can be attempted before surgical treatment [overall quality: moderate]

Question 4: In patients with CTS, which operative method provides the most improvement in clinical symptoms?

Case clarification
Since the patient's CTS is severe, delaying surgery could be detrimental. The patient consents and you wish to review which technique would be most beneficial.

Relevance
Various surgical approaches to CTS have been proposed, but which results in the best outcomes is still controversial.

Current opinion
The decision to perform a specific release is largely based on surgeon preference.

Finding the evidence
• As for Question 3 except for keywords in PubMed and OVID: "carpal tunnel syndrome," "endoscopy,"

"arthroscopy," "decompression, surgical," "open or endo-scop release or surg," "treatment outcome"

Quality of the evidence

Level I
- 33 studies

Level II
- 8 studies

Level II
- 1 study

Findings

Options for surgical release that have been studied in the literature include open release, open release with a modified incision (short scar technique), endoscopic release, and KnifeLight® release, as well as additional procedures done at the time of release such as lengthening of the flexor retinaculum, internal neurolysis, epineurotomy, and tenosynovectomy.

Several randomized controlled studies have compared endoscopic to open release and found no differences in overall improvement at 3 months,[41–48] although some studies showed a more significant reduction in pain in favor of endoscopic release[49,50] and better satisfaction, functional status, and symptom improvement.[51] With regard to long-term results, only Atroshi et al.[49] found continuation of more significant reduction in pain for endoscopic releases at 1 year follow-up. At 5 year follow-up, there were no significant differences in symptom severity and functional status scores between open and endoscopic groups.[52] Three studies[45,49,51] were included in a Cochrane meta-analysis[53] studying outcomes at 3 months. Both the symptom severity score and functional status score were lower for endoscopic release (mean difference [MD] –0.2; 95% CI –0.5 to 0.2 and MD –0.2, 95% CI –0.6 to 0.2 respectively), although these differences were very small and the studies had significant heterogeneity (I^2 approximately 90%). Data for scores at 1 year came from two of the three articles[49,51] and found no significant differences (MD approaching zero on both scales). Several randomized controlled studies also investigated the time required to return to work after surgery: some found no significant differences,[41,45,46,48,49,54–58] while others found that patients with endoscopic release returned sooner.[42,44,47,50,51,59–62] Three of these studies[47,49,57] were included in a meta-analysis[53] which determined that the weighted mean difference (WMD) in time to return to work was –6 days (95% CI –9 to –3) in favor of endoscopic release. In the randomized studies referenced above, no major complications were reported. There was a slight trend towards transient paresthesias with endoscopic release, and wound healing problems with open releases. The Cochrane review[53] assessed the need for repeated

carpal tunnel release by pooling the data from six studies,[46,47,49,51,59,62] and found a higher likelihood of patients having undergone open release requiring repeat surgery (RR 1.2, 95% CI 0.5–3.1). Another meta-analysis and systematic review by Thoma et al.[63,64] concluded that endoscopic release was favored in terms of reduction in scar tenderness, as well as increase in grip and pinch strength at a 12 week follow-up. This meta-analysis also found that it is three times more likely to suffer neuropraxia with the endoscopic than open technique. However, data was inconclusive with regards to symptom relief and return to work. A more recent evidence-based review agreed with these findings, except that it supports a slightly earlier return to work after endoscopic release and also mentions a higher risk of revision surgery with this type of release.[65]

The short scar technique (1 cm incision) did not show significant benefits over standard open or endoscopic techniques.[66] A study which compared endoscopic release to open release with a modified incision found that wound pain was reduced more significantly in the endoscopic group at 2 weeks and 4 weeks but not after 8 weeks. All patients in both groups continued to have favorable outcomes at a 1 year follow-up.[67] Results were also found to be equivalent at 3 weeks and 1 year in two other studies.[56,62] When compared to the standard open carpal tunnel release, no significant differences in symptom resolution were found in follow-ups ranging from 1.5 months to 2 years.[62,68–72] Of these studies, two found no differences in how much time patients required to return to work[68,69] while one found patients in the modified incision group returned earlier.[70] None of these studies reported any major complications; however, more scar tenderness with the standard incision was reported in some studies.[70–72]

The use of KnifeLight was compared to standard open release, and both techniques were found to have similar findings in outcomes at 6 weeks.[73,74] A study comparing KnifeLight to the modified incision open release found a more significant improvement in favor of the KnifeLight in terms of symptom severity and functional status scores at a mean follow-up time of 19 months, with both methods having similar outcomes at a mean follow-up of 30 months.[75] Two of these studies[74,75] demonstrated that patients returned to work approximately 8 days earlier after a KnifeLight procedure but one[73] found no differences. One study reported less scar tenderness with KnifeLight.[73]

Finally, additional procedures done concurrently with the carpal tunnel release did not show any significant benefits. This included lengthening the flexor retinaculum during open release at up to 26 week follow-up,[76] and internal neurolysis at 3 weeks to 4 year follow-ups.[77–80] A meta-analysis demonstrated poorer global outcomes for patients who had undergone neurolysis or epineurotomy (odds ratio 0.54, 95% CI 0.32–0.90).[81] As well, no significant differences were seen in patients who had also undergone tenosynovectomy.[82]

Recommendations

- Standard incision open carpal tunnel release has been shown to have equally favorable outcomes compared to other techniques [overall quality: high]
- Endoscopic carpal tunnel release was found to have a small benefit over open release in terms of scar tenderness and hand strength in the short term, but was not found to have any significant benefits in terms of symptom improvement and functional outcomes, while mixed findings were reported on a shorter time to return to work after endoscopic release. Neuropraxia is more likely to occur with the endoscopic technique [overall quality: high]
- No significant benefits were found for the short scar technique when compared to open or endoscopic release [overall quality: moderate]
- The use of KnifeLight showed mixed findings with regards to time to return to work, but otherwise showed no significant benefits over open release [overall quality: moderate]
- Additional procedures during release were not found to incur any benefits on final outcomes [overall quality: moderate]

Summary of recommendations

- Combining physical examination and EMG/NCS provides the most accurate means of diagnosing CTS
- EMG/NCS should be considered in patients where the diagnosis is uncertain, there is failure to respond to conservative management, or when surgical treatment is being contemplated
- EMG/NCS can assess the severity of the nerve compression, which may assist with treatment selection
- Ultrasound is useful for nerve measurements and when EMG/NCS is inconclusive
- Selected patients may benefit from CT or MRI to diagnose structural CTS
- Patients with severe CTS should undergo surgery, regardless of whether conservative management has been attempted, since operative treatment will likely lead to more significant and long-lasting improvements
- For patients with mild to moderate CTS, a trial of conservative management can be attempted before surgical treatment
- Standard incision open carpal tunnel release has been shown to have equally favorable outcomes compared to other techniques
- Endoscopic carpal tunnel release was found to have a small benefit over open release in terms of scar tenderness

and hand strength in the short term, but was not found to have any significant benefits in terms of symptom improvement and functional outcomes, while mixed findings were reported on a shorter time to return to work after endoscopic release. Neuropraxia is more likely to occur with the endoscopic technique
- No significant benefits were found for the short scar technique when compared to open or endoscopic release
- The use of KnifeLight showed mixed findings with regards to time to return to work, but otherwise showed no significant benefits over open release
- Additional procedures during release were not found to incur any benefits on final outcomes

Conclusions

The accurate diagnosis of CTS and its severity is important for treatment planning. If this is uncertain after history-taking and physical examination, when a patient fails conservative management, or when surgical treatment is being contemplated, EMG and NCS should be considered. Further imaging studies are not routinely required. A trial of conservative management can be attempted for patients with mild to moderate CTS. Patients with severe CTS or who failed conservative management should be offered surgical treatment. Which method is used is largely based on the surgeon and patient's preference since the literature has not shown significant benefits for one technique over another.

References

1. Papanicolaou GD, McCabe SJ, Firrell J. The prevalence and characteristics of nerve compression symptoms in the general population. J Hand Surg Am 2001;26:460–6.
2. Gelfman R, Melton LJ III, Yawn BP, et al. Long-term trends in carpal tunnel syndrome. Neurology 2009;72:33–41.
3. Dawson DM. Entrapment neuropathies of the upper extremities. N Engl J Med 1993;329:2013–8.
4. STAT!Ref Online Electronic Medical Library. ACP PIER & AHFS DI® Essentials™. American College of Physicians, Philadelphia, PA, 2009.
5. AAOS Clinical Guideline on Diagnosis of Carpal Tunnel Syndrome. American Academy of Orthopaedic Surgeons, Rosemont, IL, 2007.
6. Haupt WF, Wintzer G, Schop A, et al. Long-term results of carpal tunnel decompression: Assessment of 60 cases. J Hand Surg Br 1993;18:471–4.
7. Braun RM, Jackson WJ. Electrical studies as a prognostic factor in the surgical treatment of carpal tunnel syndrome. J Hand Surg Am 1994;19:893–900.
8. Glowacki KA, Breen CJ, Sachar K, et al. Electrodiagnostic testing and carpal tunnel release outcome. J Hand Surg Am 1996;21:117–22.

9. Boniface SJ, Morris I, Macleod A. How does neurophysiological assessment influence the management and outcome of patients with carpal tunnel syndrome? Br J Rheum 1994;33:1169–70.

10. Prick JJW, Blaauw G, Vredeveld JW, et al. Results of carpal tunnel release. Eur J Neurol 2003;10:733–6.

11. Jablecki CK, Andary MT, Floeter MK, et al. Practice parameter: Electrodiagnostic studies in carpal tunnel syndrome. Report of the American Association of Electrodiagnostic Medicine, American Academy of Neurology, and the American Academy of Physical Medicine and Rehabilitation. Neurology 2002;58:1589–92.

12. Kimura J. The carpal tunnel syndrome: localization of conduction abnormalities within the distal segment of the median nerve. Brain 1979;102:619–35.

13. Carroll GJ. Comparison of median and radial nerve sensory latencies in the electrophysiological diagnosis of carpal tunnel syndrome. Electroencephalogr Clin Neurophysiol 1987;68: 101–6.

14. De Lean J. Transcarpal median sensory conduction: detection of latent abnormalities in mild carpal tunnel syndrome. Can J Neurol Sci 1988;15:388–93.

15. Jackson DA, Clifford JC. Electrodiagnosis of mild carpal tunnel syndrome. Arch Phys Med Rehabil 1989;70:199–204.

16. Rosenbaum R. Carpal tunnel syndrome and the myth of El Dorado. [Editorial] Muscle Nerve 1999;22:1165–7.

17. Kaymak B, Özçakar L, Çetin A, et al. A comparison of the benefits of sonography and electrophysiologic measurements as predictors of symptom severity and functional status in patients with carpal tunnel syndrome. Arch Phys Med Rehabil 2008;89:743–8.

18. Burke DT, Burke MA, Bell R, et al. Subjective swelling: a new sign for carpal tunnel syndrome. Am J Phys Med Rehabil 1999;78:504–8.

19. Nakamichi K, Tachibana S. The use of ultrasonography in detection of synovitis in carpal tunnel syndrome. J Hand Surg Br 1993;18:176–9.

20. Duncan I, Sullivan P, Lomas F. Sonography in the diagnosis of carpal tunnel syndrome. AJR Am J Roentgenol 1999;173:681–4.

21. Wong SM, Griffith JF, Hui AC, Tang A, et al. Discriminatory sonographic criteria for the diagnosis of carpal tunnel syndrome. Arthritis Rheum 2002;46:1914–21.

22. Nakamichi K, Tachibana S. Ultrasonographic measurement of median nerve cross-sectional area in idiopathic carpal tunnel syndrome: Diagnostic accuracy. Muscle Nerve 2002;26: 798–803.

23. Wong SM, Griffith JF, Hui AC, Lo SK, et al. Carpal tunnel syndrome: diagnostic usefulness of sonography. Radiology 2004; 232:93–9.

24. Kele H, Verheggen R, Bittermann HJ, et al. The potential value of ultrasonography in the evaluation of carpal tunnel syndrome. Neurology 2003;61:389–91.

25. Altinok T, Baysal O, Karakas HM, et al. Ultrasonographic assessment of mild and moderate idiopathic carpal tunnel syndrome. Clin Radiol 2004;59:916–25.

26. Yesildag A, Kutluhan S, Sengul N, et al. The role of ultrasonographic measurements of the median nerve in the diagnosis of carpal tunnel syndrome. Clin Radiol 2004;59:910–15.

27. Kwon BC, Jung KI, Baek GH. Comparison of sonography and electrodiagnostic testing in the diagnosis of carpal tunnel syndrome. J Hand Surg Am 2008;33:65–71.

28. Boutte C, Gaudin P, Grange L, et al. Sonography versus electrodiagnosis for the diagnosis of carpal tunnel syndrome in routine practice. Rev Neurol (Paris) 2009;165:460–5.

29. Pastare D, Therimadasamy AK, Lee E, et al. Sonography versus nerve conduction studies in patients referred with a clinical diagnosis of carpal tunnel syndrome. J Clin Ultrasound 2009;37:389–93.

30. Koyuncuoglu HR, Kutluhan S, Yesildag A, et al. The value of ultrasonographic measurement in carpal tunnel syndrome in patients with negative electrodiagnostic tests. Eur J Radiol 2005; 56:365–9.

31. American Academy of Neurology. Practice parameter for carpal tunnel syndrome (summary statement). Report of the Quality Standards Subcommittee of the American Academy of Neurology. Neurology 1993;43:2406–9.

32. Buchberger W. Radiologic imaging of the carpal tunnel. Eur J Radiol 1997;25:112–7.

33. Mesgarzadeh M, Schneck CD, Bonakdarpour A, et al. Carpal tunnel: MR imaging. Part II. Carpal tunnel syndrome. Radiology 1989;171:749–54.

34. Pierre-Jerome C, Bekkelund SI, Mellgren SI, et al. Quantitative MRI and electrophysiology of preoperative carpal tunnel syndrome in a female population. Ergonomics 1997;40:642–9.

35. Horch RE, Allmann KH, Laubenberger J, et al. Median nerve compression can be detected by magnetic resonance imaging of the carpal tunnel. Neurosurgery 1997;41:76–82; discussion 82–3.

36. Gerritsen AAM, de Vet HCW, Scholten RJPM, et al. Splinting versus surgery in the treatment of carpal tunnel syndrome. A randomized controlled trial. JAMA 2002;288:1245–51.

37. Ly-Pen D, Andréu JL, de Blas G, et al. Surgical decompression versus local steroid injection in carpal tunnel syndrome. A one-year, prospective, randomized, open, controlled clinical trial. Arthritis Rheum 2005;52:612–19.

38. Hui AC, Wong S, Leung CH, et al. A randomized controlled trial of surgery vs steroid injection for carpal tunnel syndrome. Neurology 2005;64:2074–8.

39. Verdugo RJ, Salinas RA, Castillo JL, et al. Surgical versus non-surgical treatment for carpal tunnel syndrome (Cochrane Review). Cochrane Database Syst Rev 2008;4.

40. Gelberman RH, Aronson D, Weisman MH. Carpal-tunnel syndrome. Results of a prospective trial of steroid injection and splinting. J Bone Joint Surg Am 1980;62:1181–4.

41. Ferdinand RD, MacLean JG. Endoscopic versus open carpal tunnel release in bilateral carpal tunnel syndrome. A prospective, randomised, blinded assessment. J Bone Joint Surg Br 2002;84:375–9.

42. Brown RA, Gelberman RH, Seiler JG III, et al. Carpal tunnel release. A prospective randomized assessment of open and endoscopic methods. J Bone Joint Surg Am 1993;75:1265–75.

43. Dumontier C, Sokolow C, Leclercq C, et al.. Early results of conventional versus two-portal endoscopic carpal tunnel release. A prospective study. J Hand Surg Br 1995;20:658–62.

44. Erdmann MWH. Endoscopic carpal tunnel decompression. J Hand Surg Br 1994;19:5–13.

45. Hoefnagels WAJ, van Kleef JGF, Mastenbroek GGA, et al. Operatieve behandeling wegens carpaletunnelsyndroom: endoscopisch of klassiek (open)? Een prospectief gerandomiseerd onderzoek. [Surgical treatment of carpal tunnel syndrome:

endoscopic or classical (open) surgery? A prospective randomized study]. Ned Tijdschr voor Geneeskd 1997;141:878–82.

46. MacDermid JC, Richards RS, Roth JH, et al. Endoscopic versus open carpal tunnel release: A randomized trial. J Hand Surg Am 2003;28:475–80.

47. Saw NL, Jones S, Shepstone L, et al. Early outcome and cost-effectiveness of endoscopic versus open carpal tunnel release: a randomized prospective trial. J Hand Surg Br 2003;28:444–9.

48. Westphal KP, Bayat M, Wustner-Hofmann M, et al. Course of clinical symptoms before and after surgical decompression in carpal tunnel surgery. Lymph Forsch 2000;4:69–73.

49. Atroshi I, Larsson GU, Ornstein E, et al. Outcomes of endoscopic surgery compared with open surgery for carpal tunnel syndrome among employed patients: randomised controlled trial. BMJ 2006;332:1473–6.

50. Tian Y, Zhao H, Wang T. Prospective comparison of endoscopic and open surgical methods for carpal tunnel syndrome. Chin Med Sci J 2007;22:104–7.

51. Trumble TE, Diao E, Abrams RA, et al. Single-portal endoscopic carpal tunnel release compared with open release: a prospective, randomized trial. J Bone Joint Surg Am 2002;84:1107–15.

52. Atroshi I, Hofer M, Larsson G-U, et al. Open compared with 2-portal endoscopic carpal tunnel release: A 5-year follow-up of a randomized controlled trial. J Hand Surg Am 2009;34:266–72.

53. Scholten RJPM, Mink van der Molen A, Uitdehaag BMJ, et al. Surgical treatment options for carpal tunnel syndrome (Cochrane Review). Cochrane Database Syst Rev 2007;4.

54. Arle JE, Zager EL. Surgical treatment of common entrapment neuropathies in the upper limbs. Muscle Nerve 2000;23:1160–74.

55. Chung KC, Walters MR, Greenfield ML, et al. Endoscopic versus open carpal tunnel release: a cost-effectiveness analysis. Plast Reconstr Surg 1998;102:1089–99.

56. Rab M, Grunbeck M, Beck H, et al. Intra-individual comparison between open and 2-portal endoscopic release in clinically matched bilateral carpal syndrome. J Plast Reconstr Aesthet Surg 2006;59:730–6.

57. Jacobsen MB, Rahme H. A prospective, randomized study with an independent observer comparing open carpal tunnel release with endoscopic carpal tunnel release. J Hand Surg Br 1996;21:202–24.

58. Foucher G, Buch N, Van Overstraeten L, et al. Le canal carpien. Peut-il être encore sujet de controverse? [Carpal tunnel syndrome. Can it still be a controversial topic?] Chirurgie 1993–1994;119:80–4.

59. Agee JM, McCarroll HR Jr, Tortosa RD, et al. Endoscopic release of the carpal tunnel: a randomized prospective multicenter study. J Hand Surg Am 1992;17:987–95.

60. Benedetti RB, Sennwald G. Endoskopische Dekompression des N. medianus nach Agee: Prospektive Studiemit Vergleich zur offenen Dekompression [Agee endoscopic decompression of the median nerve: a prospective study in comparison with open decompression.] Handchir Mikrochir Plast Chir 1996;28:151–5.

61. Sennwald GR, Benedetti R. The value of one-portal endoscopic carpal tunnel release: a prospective randomized study. Knee Surg Sports Traumatol Arthrosc 1995;3:113–16.

62. Eichhorn J, Dieterich K. 2003; Offene versus endoskopische Karpaltunnelspaltungen [Open versus endoscopic carpal tunnel release.] Chir Praxis 61:279–83.

63. Thoma A, Veltri K, Haines T, et al. A meta-analysis of randomized controlled trials comparing endoscopic and open carpal tunnel decompression. plast reconstr surg 2004;114:1137–46.

64. Thoma A, Veltri K, Haines T, et al. A systematic review of reviews comparing the effectiveness of endoscopic and open carpal tunnel decompression. Plast Reconstr Surg 2004;113:1184–91.

65. Abrams R. Endoscopic versus open carpal tunnel release. J Hand Surg Am 2009;34:535–9.

66. Klein RD, Kotsis SV, Chung KC. Open carpal tunnel release using a 1-centimeter incision: technique and outcomes for 104 patients. Plast Reconstr Surg 2003;111:1616–22.

67. Wong KC, Hung LK, Ho PC, et al. Carpal tunnel release. A prospective, randomised study of endoscopic versus limited-open methods. J Bone Joint Surg Br 2003;85:863–8.

68. Brüser P, Richter M, Larkin G, et al. The operative treatment of carpal tunnel syndrome and its relevance to endoscopic release. Eur J Plast Surg 1999;22:80–4.

69. Richter M, Brüser P. Die operative Behandlung des Karpaltunnelsyndroms: ein Vergleich zwischen langer und kurzer Schnittfürung sowie endoskopischer Spaltung [Surgical treatment of carpal tunnel syndrome: a comparison between long and short incision and endoscopic release.] Handchir Mikrochir Plast Chir 1996;28:160–6.

70. Jugovac I, Burgic N, Micovic V, et al. Carpal tunnel release by limited palmar incision vs traditional open technique: randomized controlled trial. Croat Med J 2002;43:33–6.

71. Nakamichi K, Tachibana S. Ultrasonographically assisted carpal tunnel release. J Hand Surg Am 1997;22:853–62.

72. Citron ND, Bendall SP. Local symptoms after carpal tunnel release. A randomized prospective trial of two incisions. J Hand Surg Br 1997;22:317–21.

73. Bhattacharya R, Birdsall PD, Finn P, et al. A randomized controlled trial of KnifeLight and open carpal tunnel release. J Hand Surg Br 2004;29:113–15.

74. Helm RH, Vaziri S. Evaluation of carpal tunnel release using the Knifelight® instrument. J Hand Surg Br 2003;28:251–4.

75. Cellocco P, Rossi C, Bizzarri F, et al. Mini-open blind procedure versus limited open technique for carpal tunnel release: a 30-month follow-up study. J Hand Surg Am 2005;30:493–9.

76. Dias JJ, Bhowal B, Wildin CJ, et al. Carpal tunnel decompression. Is lengthening of the flexor retinaculum better than simple division? J Hand Surg Br 2004;29:271–6.

77. Holmgren-Larsson H, Leszniewski W, Linden U, et al. Internal neurolysis or ligament division only in carpal tunnel syndrome—results of a randomized study. Acta Neurochir 1985;74:118–21.

78. Lowry WE Jr, Follender AB. Interfascicular neurolysis in the severe carpal tunnel syndrome. A prospective, randomized, double-blind, controlled study. Clin Orthop Relat Res 1988;227:251–4.

79. Mackinnon SE, McCabe S, Murray JF, et al. Internal neurolysis fails to improve the results of primary carpal tunnel decompression. J Hand Surg Am 1991;16:211–18.

80. Holmgren H, Rabow L. Internal neurolysis or ligament division only in carpal tunnel syndrome II. A 3 year follow-up with an

evaluation of various neurophysiological parameters for diagnosis. Acta Neurochir 1987;87:44–7.

81. Chapell R, Coates V, Turkelson C. Poor outcome for neural surgery (epineurotomy or neurolysis) for carpal tunnel syndrome compared with carpal tunnel release alone: a meta-analysis of global outcomes. Plast Reconstr Surg 2003;112:983–90.

82. Shum C, Parisien M, Strauch RJ, et al. The role of flexor tenosynovectomy in the operative treatment of carpal tunnel syndrome. J Bone Joint Surg Am 2002;84:221–5.

121 Dupuytren's Disease

Larisa Kristine Vartija, Leslie L. McKnight, and Achilleas Thoma

McMaster University, Hamilton, ON, Canada

Case scenario

A 65 year old man is referred to you complaining of progressive loss of function in both hands. On examination, he is unable to fully extend his right ring and little fingers at the metacarpophalangeal (MCP) and proximal interphalangeal (PIP) joints and his left long finger at the MCP joint. On his right hand, you palpate longitudinal cords which extend from the proximal palm to the middle phalanges of the affected digits. On his left hand, you palpate a longitudinal cord which extends from the proximal palm to the proximal phalanx of his long finger. He does not report pain. His digits are all neurovascularly intact.

Relevant anatomy

Dupuytren's disease (DD) is a benign fibroproliferative condition that primarily affects the palmar fascia. Fibroblast overgrowth distorts the fascia, creating nodules and cords (Figures 121.1–121.4). These nodules and cords are the affected bands of the palmar and digital fascia.[1] The pathological cords, their origins, contribution to joint contractures and neurovascular displacements are shown in Table 121.1.

Importance of the problem

The prevalence of DD is reported to be 12–46% depending on geographic location; the highest rates are reported in Scandinavian countries.[2] The presence of flexion contractures of the digits, often bilateral, causes functional impair-

ment of the hand that can limit productivity. Surgical management is often required and causes considerable financial burden.[3,4]

Top six questions

Etiology

1. Is DD associated with frequent or repetitive manual work and/or hand vibration?

Therapy

2. Is the concomitant release of the PIP joint more effective than fasciectomy alone in correcting flexion contractures of the PIP joint and improving range of motion (ROM)?
3. How effective is percutaneous needle fasciotomy (PNF) compared to limited fasciectomy (LF)?
4. How effective is collagenase injection compared to placebo at reducing the degree of flexion contractures and improving ROM?
5. Does postoperative splinting help reduce finger extension deficits?

Prognosis

6. Can we predict who will develop disease recurrence?

Question 1: Is DD associated with frequent or repetitive manual work and/or hand vibration?

Case clarification

After examination, you diagnose the patient with DD. He asks you if it was caused by the repetitive manual labor he did for 20 years.

Evidence-Based Orthopedics, First Edition. Edited by Mohit Bhandari.
© 2012 Blackwell Publishing Ltd. Published 2012 by Blackwell Publishing Ltd.

Pathology of Dupuytren's disease

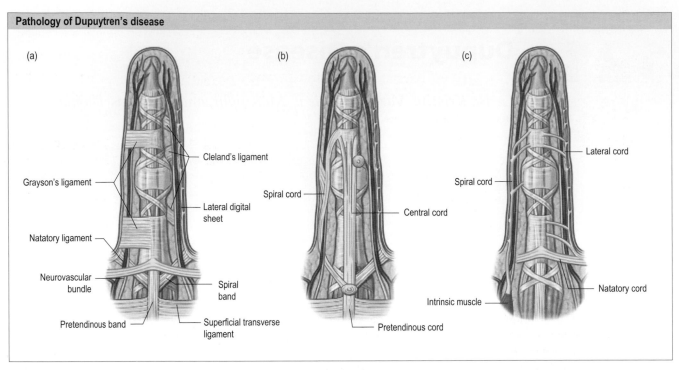

Figure 121.1 Pathology of Dupuytren's disease: (a) Parts of the palmar and digital fascia that become diseased in Dupuytren's contracture. (b) The diseased fascia associated with the pretendinous cord. (c) The diseased fascia not associated with the pretendinous cord. (Reproduced by permission of Wolters Kluwer, from McFarlane RM, Patterns of the diseased fascia in the fingers in Dupuytren's contracture. Plast Reconstr Surg 1974; 54(1):31–44.)

The spiral cord

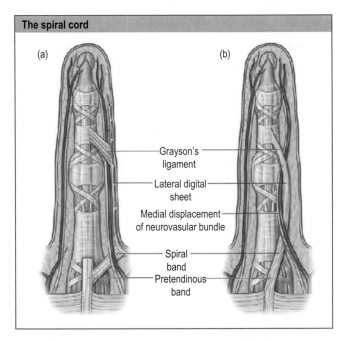

Figure 121.2 The spiral cord: (a) The normal parts of the fascia that produce the spiral cord. (b) The spiral cord, showing medial displacement of the neurovascular bundle. (Reproduced by permission of Wolters Kluwer, from McFarlane RM, Patterns of the diseased fascia in the fingers in Dupuytren's contracture. Plast Reconstr Surg 1974; 54(1): 31–44.)

The main fibrous structures on the radial side of the hand

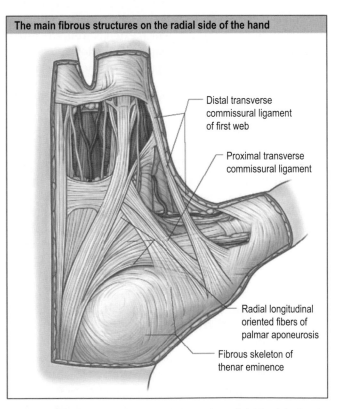

Figure 121.3 The main fibrous structures on the radial side of the hand. (Reproduced from Tubiana R. Location of Dupuytren's disease on the radial aspect of the hand. Clin Orthop Relat Res 1982; 168:222–229. With kind permission of Springer Science and Business Media.)

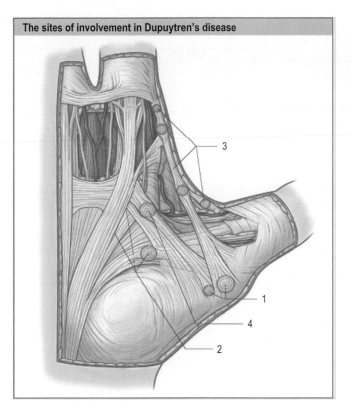

The sites of involvement in Dupuytren's disease

Figure 121.4 Sites of involvement in Dupuytren's disease. (Reproduced from Tubiana R. Location of Dupuytren's disease on the radial aspect of the hand. Clin Orthop Relat Res 1982; 168:222–229. With kind permission of Springer Science and Business Media.)

Relevance

For decades there has been controversy regarding whether cumulative mechanical work contributes to the development of DD. Patients often ask the hand surgeon if they should file a claim for workers' compensation.

Current opinion

Repetitive manual labor is not considered a strong risk factor for DD development and therefore does not warrant a workers' compensation claim. In some cases workers' compensation boards have allowed claims for DD, but in many cases it is considered a pre-existing condition. Nonetheless, the Ontario Workplace Safety and Insurance Board does not have a policy on DD specifically. Therefore, these claims are considered on a case-by-case basis.

Finding the evidence

- Cochrane Database, with search term:"Dupuytren's contracture"
- PubMed, using keywords "dupuytren*" AND "work," "occupation," "vibration," and "injury"

- MEDLINE and Embase, using "dupuytren's contracture" as a subject heading combined with "work," "vibration," and "injury" as keywords

Quality of the evidence

Level III
- 1 systematic review of controlled studies

Level IV
- 2 cross-sectional surveys

Findings

Four studies were included in the systematic review by Liss and Stock.[5] In the only study of manual work, Bennett[6] found the prevalence of DD to be 5.5 times higher in British workers doing repetitive hand work than those who did not, and twice the expected prevalence in a UK working population. The other three studies examined hand vibration (n = 1838) and showed consistent positive association between vibration and DD.[7–9] DD was observed more frequently among vibration white finger claimants than controls.[7,8] It was also found that a history of vibration exposure occurred more frequently among cases of DD than among controls.[9] Two studies showed some evidence of a dose–response relationship.[8,9]

Two cross-sectional surveys that were not designed specifically for the investigation of DD had conflicting results on the association between vibration and DD.[10,11]

Recommendation

- Hand vibration is associated with DD [overall quality: low]

Question 2: Is concomitant release of the PIP joint more effective than fasciectomy alone in correcting flexion contractures of the PIP joint and improving ROM?

Case clarification

Intraoperatively, you find that after palmar and digital fasciectomy, the PIP joint contracture of the ring finger is only partially corrected. You consider performing concomitant PIP joint ligamentous release.

Relevance

The management of severe contracture of the PIP joint is difficult, as long-standing and severe contractures become more complicated to correct over time. Fasciectomy alone may not be sufficient to achieve good correction due to significant soft tissue contracture around the joint.

Current opinion

Two schools of thought exist: (1) At least partial division of the capsuloligamentous structures is needed to obtain

Table 121.1 The pathoanatomy of Dupuytren's disease

Cord	Origin	NVB displacement	Contracture	Other
Pretendinous cord (most frequent cord)	Pretendinous band	No	MPJ	Often extends distally to become continuous with digital cords
Vertical cord	Septa of Legueu and Juvara	No	No	Uncommon
Spiral cord	Pretendinous band, spiral band, lateral digital sheet, Grayson's ligament	Volar and medial	PIPJ	Most often in D5
Natatory cord	Natatory ligament	No	Web space	
Central cord	Extension of pretendinous cord in palm (no pre-existing central band)	No	PIPJ	Attaches into flexor tendon sheath near PIPJ or periosteum of middle phalanx on one side of digit
Lateral cord	Lateral digital sheet	Midline (due to its volume)	PIPJ and DIPJ	Attaches to skin or Grayson's ligament
ADM	ADM tendon	Sometimes	PIPJ	Can present as isolated digital cord; insertion varies
Distal commissural cord	Distal commissural ligament	No	Web space	Decreased radial and palmar thumb abduction
Proximal commissural cord	Proximal commissural ligament	No	Web space	Decreased thumb abduction
Thumb pretendinous cord	Thumb pretendinous band	No	MPJ	

ADM, abductor digiti minimi; DIPJ, distal interphalangeal joint; MPJ, metacarpophalangeal joint; NVB, neurovascular bundle; PIPJ, proximal interphalangeal joint.

additional release, as complete correction is not possible with fasciectomy alone. (2) One should use fasciectomy alone, as violating the PIP joint may result in permanent limitation of flexion or cause further scarring and contracture.

Finding the evidence

- Cochrane Database, using the search term: "dupuytren's contracture"
- PubMed, using keywords "dupuytren*" AND "proximal interphalangeal joint release" as well as "dupuytren*" AND "capsuloligament*"
- MEDLINE and Embase, using "dupuytren contracture" as a subject heading combined with "proximal interphalangeal joint" as a keyword.

Quality of the evidence

Level II
- 2 prospective cohort studies

Level IV
- 1 retrospective cohort study
- 1 retrospective case-control study

Findings

In a prospective cohort study, Ritchie et al.[12] performed fasciectomies (n = 8) followed by sequential release of the accessory collateral ligaments and volar plates (n = 11) as necessary (intraoperative residual contracture >20°). No finger with a preoperative contracture of less than 45° required PIP joint release, whereas all fingers with initial contractures greater than 45° did require it. Mean flexion contracture immediately postoperative and residual contracture at 3 months was greater in those who underwent fasciectomy plus joint release, indicating that those who underwent fasciectomy alone achieved superior results (Table 121.2). However, these results are difficult to interpret, as the degree of preoperative contractures was much greater in this group compared to the fasciectomy alone group.

In a slightly larger prospective cohort study, Beyermann et al.[13] performed fasciectomies (n = 32) followed by capsuloligamentous release (n = 11) as necessary (intraoperative residual contracture >20°). Preoperative PIP joint contracture was greater in those that underwent capsuloligamentous release. Flexion contracture was not different between groups immediately after surgery or at 6 months

Table 121.2 Results from study Ritchie et al.:[12] fasciectomy alone vs. fasciectomy plus joint release for the treatment of severe PIP joint contractures

	Fasciectomy alone	Fasciectomy and PIP release
Number of joints	8	11
Mean preoperative joint contracture	28° (20–45°)	70° (45–95°)
Mean flexion contracture immediately postoperatively	1° (0–5°)	7° (0–27°)
Residual contracture at 3 months	6° (0–13°)	26° (0–58°)
Residual contracture at 3 years	8° (0–15°)	29° (0–88°)
Range of motion—mean maximum flexion at 3 years	88° (84–95°)	83° (40–94°)

Table 121.3 Results from Beyermann et al.:[13] fasciectomy alone vs. fasciectomy plus capsuloligamentous release for the treatment of severe PIP joint contractures

	Fasciectomy	Fasciectomy plus capsuloligamentous release
Number of joints	32	11
Mean preoperative joint contracture	78°	71°
Mean flexion contracture immediately postoperatively	2°	2°
Mean flexion contracture 6 months postoperatively	15°	16°
Number of joints that required dynamic extension postoperatively	21 (66%)	11 (100%)

(Table 121.3). However, 100% of the fasciectomy plus capsuloligamentous release group required dynamic extension splinting to help maintain PIP joint extension compared to 66% of the fasciectomy group. Thus, the magnitude of effect of capsuloligamentous release alone cannot be interpreted.

Level IV evidence suggests that residual flexion contracture is similar between fasciectomy and fasciectomy plus capsuloligamentous release groups.[14,15]

Recommendation
• In patients with severe PIP joint flexion contractures, the effectiveness of fasciectomy vs. fasciectomy plus capsuloligamentous release in reducing residual flexion contracture is equivocal [overall quality: low-moderate]

Question 3: How effective is PNF compared to LF?

Case clarification
Although you recommend palmar and digital fasciectomy to reduce the degree of flexion contracture and prevent disease recurrence, your patient would prefer a less invasive treatment.

Relevance
PNF is desired by some patients because it is less invasive and has a shorter recovery time than LF.[16]

Current opinion
PNF is a reasonable treatment option for certain patients (i.e., elderly, nonsurgical candidates, those with nonsevere flexion contractures). However, it does not remove the pathological cords and is therefore believed to result in higher recurrence rates.

Finding the evidence
• Cochrane Database, with search term: "dupuytren's contracture"
• PubMed, using keywords: "dupuytren*" AND "fasciotomy"
• PubMed (clinical queries: specific search): "dupuytren*" AND "fasciotomy"
• MEDLINE and Embase, using "dupuytren contracture" as a subject heading combined with "fasciotomy" as a keyword.

Quality of the evidence
Level I
• 1 randomized controlled trial (RCT)

Findings
One RCT was identified comparing PNF and LF (n = 166 rays, 88 PNF, 79 LF).[16] All rays had pretreatment flexion contractures of at least 30° in the MCP, PIP, or distal interphalangeal (DIP) joints. Total passive extension deficit (TPED) was measured at 6 weeks. Outcomes at the PIP joints were worse than those at the MCP and DIP joints for both the PNF and LF groups. LF resulted in a greater reduction of TPED compared with PNF (p = 0.001). When results were analyzed using the Tubiana classification (Table 121.4), rays classified as Tubiana stage I or II before surgery had comparable outcomes with both treatments. For stage III and IV disease, LF was a superior treatment modality

Table 121.4 Tubiana classification

Grade	Total passive extension deficit
I	0–45°
II	45–90°
III	90–135°
IV	>135°

(p = 0.000 and p = 0.004, respectively). There were no patients in the PNF group with flexion deficits compared with 19 patients in the LF group (mean deficit, 0.6 cm).

Because of the short length of follow-up, recurrence rates could not be determined. However, these patients are being followed over a period of 5 years; results have not yet been published.

Recommendations
• For Tubiana stage I and II, LF and PNF are equally effective at correcting flexion contractures [overall quality: low]
• For Tubiana stage III and IV, LF is more effective than PNF at correcting flexion contractures. [overall quality: low]

Question 4: How effective is collagenase injection compared to placebo at reducing the degree of flexion contractures and improving ROM?

Case clarification
You recommend palmar and digital fasciectomy, but your patient would prefer a less invasive treatment.

Relevance
Although many nonoperative treatments have been abandoned due to poor outcomes, the quest for nonoperative treatments continues. The two most popular approaches are PNF (discussed in Question 3) and collagenase injections.

Current opinion
Collagenase injection studies are showing promising results, but the treatment is not yet approved for widespread clinical use.

Finding the evidence
• Cochrane Database, using the search term: "dupuytren's contracture"
• PubMed, using keywords: "dupuytren*" AND "collagenase"

• PubMed (clinical queries: specific search): "dupuytren*" AND "collagenase"
• MEDLINE and Embase, using "dupuytren contracture" as a subject heading combined with "collagenase" as a keyword

Quality of the evidence
Level I
• 2 RCTs

Level II
• 1 low-quality RCT

Findings
In a phase II trial, 10,000 U of collagenase was established as the minimal safe and effective dose for the release of flexion contractures.[17] The phase III trial[18] showed positive results which were confirmed in the most recent study by Hurst et al.[19] In this multicenter placebo controlled trial, patients (n = 308, joint contractures >20°) received injections of collagenase or placebo at 30 day intervals (maximum 3 injections). The primary endpoint was a reduction in contracture to 0–5° of full extension 30 days after the last injection. More patients who were injected with collagenase than patients injected with plabebo met the primary endpoint. Collagenase-injected joints also achieved a greater improvement in ROM (Table 121.5). The median time to reach the primary endpoint for collagenase-injected joints was 56 days.

Recommendation
• Collagenase injection is effective at reducing contractures to 0–5° of full extension and improving ROM compared to placebo [overall quality: high]

Question 5: Does postoperative splinting help reduce finger extension deficits?

Case clarification
One week after surgery, you observe a tendency for the finger to be kept in flexion at the PIP joint and wonder if your patient would benefit from a splint.

Relevance
A recent survey of orthopedic and plastic surgeons has highlighted the lack of consensus regarding splinting following surgery for DD.[20]

Current opinion
Clinical experience and data extrapolated from other populations suggests the majority of surgeons splint the hand postoperatively for approximately 1 week, followed by a static night splint for up to 6 months.

Table 121.5 Treatment outcomes from study by Hurst et al.:[19] collagenase vs. placebo injections for treatment of joint contractures >20°

	Collagenase	Placebo	p value
Number of joints	203	103	
All joints			
Primary endpoint[a]	64%	6.80%	<0.001
Mean change in ROM from baseline	36.7°	4.0°	<0.001
Metacarpophalangeal joints			
Primary endpoint[a]	76.70%	7.20%	<0.001
Primary endpoint[a] in joints with a baseline contracture of <50°	88.9%	NC	
Primary endpoint[a] in joints with a baseline contracture of >50°	57.70%	NC	
Mean change in ROM from baseline	40.6°	3.7°	<0.001
Proximal interphalangeal joints			
Primary endpoint[a]	40.0%	5.9%	<0.001
Primary endpoint[a] in joints with a baseline contracture of <40°	80.9%	NC	
Primary endpoint[a] in joints with a baseline contracture of >40°	22.40%	NC	
Mean change in ROM from baseline	29°	4.7°	<0.001

NC, not calculated; ROM, range of motion.

[a]Primary endpoint: percentage of patients who achieved reduction in contracture to 0–5° 30 days after last injection.

Finding the evidence

• Cochrane Database, with search term: "dupuytren's contracture"
• PubMed, using keywords: "dupuytren*" AND "splint*"
• PubMed (clinical queries: systematic reviews): "dupuytren*" AND "splint".
• MEDLINE and Embase, using "dupuytren contracture" as a subject heading combined with "splint" as a keyword.

Quality of the evidence

Level III
• 1 systematic review

Findings

Larson and Jerosch-Herold[21] identified four studies (n = 349) that assessed postoperative splinting. Two studies evaluated static splints but no clear conclusions could be made. The two studies that evaluated dynamic splints had conflicting results. The authors were unable to pool results due to heterogeneity in splint types, duration of wear, outcomes and follow-up time. Although total active extension deficit improved in some patients wearing a splint, there were also deficits in finger flexion and hand function. The clinical significance could not be determined due to the lack of data on the magnitude of this effect.

Recommendation

• The effect of postoperative static and dynamic splints on final extension deficit is equivocal [overall quality: moderate]

Question 6: Can we predict who will develop disease recurrence?

Case clarification

Your patient asks you in follow-up if his disease will recur.

Relevance

Reported recurrence rates range from 0 to 78%, depending on the type of procedure done and length of follow-up.[22] With each recurrence requiring reoperation, there is an increased risk of complications.[23,24]

Current opinion

It is generally accepted that Dupuytren's diathesis (see box) is associated with a higher risk of disease recurrence. Some authors have suggested using histopathologic findings to determine who is at higher risk of recurrence.

Dupuytren's diathesis:

First described by Hueston in 1963,[25] it is a marker of aggressive Dupuytren's disease. Features include:
• 1. Bilateral hand involvement
• 2. Positive family history
• 3. Ectopic lesions
• 4. Ethnicity
• 5. Early age of onset (<50 years)[a]
• 6. Male gender[a]

[a]Added in 2006 by Hindocha et al.[26]

Finding the evidence

• PubMed, using keywords "dupuytren*" AND "recurrence" and "prognosis"
• MEDLINE and Embase, using "dupuytren's contracture" as a subject heading combined with "prognosis" as a subject heading

Table 121.6 Results from Abe et al.:[27] Sensitivity, specificity and odds ratios for the six factors which were significantly associated with recurrence and/or extension

	Sensitivity	Specificity	Odds ratio (95% CI)	p value
Bilateral hand involvement	0.94	0.34	8.8 (1.0–72)	0.026
Little finder surgery	0.94	0.34	8.8 (1.0–72)	0.026
Early onset	0.28	0.94	5.6 (1.1–27)	0.032
Plantar fibrosis	0.67	0.85	11 (3.2–41)	<0.001
Knuckle pads	0.56	0.91	13 (3.3–54)	<0.001
Radial side involvement	0.56	0.89	11 (2.8–40)	<0.001

Table 121.7 Risk of recurrence and/or extension scoring system developed by Abe et al.[27] Scores >4 have high risk of recurrence and/or extension; scores <4 have little risk of recurrence and/or extension

Features of variables	Variables	Point(s)
High sensitivity and low specificity	(a) Bilateral hand involvement	1
	(b) Little finger surgery	1
	(c) Early onset of disease	1
Low sensitivity and high specificity	(d) Plantar fibrosis[a]	2
	(e) Knuckle pads[a]	2
	(f) Radial side involvement[a]	2

[a]Demonstrated odds ratio values >2.0 for at the low 95% confidence limit.

Reproduced with permission from Abe Y, Rokkaku T, Ofuchi S, Tokunaga S, Takahashi K, Moriya H. (2004) An objective method to evaluate the risk of recurrence and extension of dupuytren's disease. J Hand Surg [Br] 29B

Quality of the evidence

Level IV

• 4 retrospective case series

Findings

Dupuytren's diathesis Abe and colleagues (n = 65) found bilateral hand involvement, little finger surgery, early onset, plantar fibrosis, knuckle pads, and radial side involvement to be significantly associated with recurrence and disease extension (Table 121.6).[27] The authors also developed a scoring system to evaluate the risk of recurrence and extension (Table 121.7). However, this scale has not been validated.

In a larger retrospective review (n = 322 patients, 4 year follow-up), Hindocha et al.[26] calculated the statistical predictive value for Dupuytren's diathesis in relation to

Table 121.8 Adjusted odds ratios of developing recurrent Dupuytren's disease

Factor	Adjusted odds ratio	95% CI	p value
Men	2.15	1.07–4.32	0.03
Over 50 years of age at onset of DD	1.47	0.94–2.28	0.05
Garrod's pads	2.5	1.27–4.93	0.01
High alcohol consumption[a]	1.8	1.04–3.14	0.02
Bilateral DD	1.4	0.82–2.39	0.22
Ectopic lesions (any site)	1.54	0.90–2.64	0.07
Positive family history	1.32	0.85–2.05	0.14

[a]Defined as men who drank >28 U/wk and women who drank >21 U/wk.

Reproduced with permission from Hindocha S, Stanley JK, Watson S, Bayat A. (2006) Dupuytren's diathesis revisited: Evaluation of prognostic indicators for risk of disease recurrence. J Hand Surg 31A, 1626–34.

disease recurrence (Table 121.8). A trend of an increased mean predictive risk with a greater number of diathesis factors present was found. Those with all five factors present (male gender, bilateral disease, Garrod's pads, age at onset <50 years, and a positive family history) had a predictive risk of 71% compared with 23% for patients with none of the factors present (baseline risk).

Histopathological findings Wilbrand et al.[22] found no differences in the expression of anticollagen type IV, integrin 5 laminin, smooth muscle actin, procollagen type I, or desmin in patients with or without recurrence at four years (n = 103). They also failed to find any association between sex, age at onset, number of operations, heredity, diabetes mellitus, or drugs taken for cardiovascular disease, and the expression of any of the immunohistochemical markers.

Balaguer et al.[28] assessed the usefulness of the three-stage histological classification proposed by Rombouts et al.[29] in predicting recurrence (Table 121.9). At the time of surgery, the DD tissue was sent for histological examination and staging (n = 139 hands). After a mean of 5 years, type I, II, and III tissues had recurrence rates of 55%, 31%, and 11% respectively. Type I hands had a recurrence risk 2.5 times higher than type II hands (p = 0.04), and 10 times higher than type III hands (p = 0.05). Recurrence risk was three times higher in type II hands than in type III hands (p = 0.05). Histological staging was an independent risk factor for recurrence.

Table 121.9 Histological classification of Dupuytren's disease developed by Rombouts et al.[29]

Stage	Characteristics
Type I (proliferative)	The lesions are highly cellular but the cells show no cytonuclear atypia Mitoses present
Type II (fibrocellular)	An intermediate stage with moderate cellularity Absence of mitoses
Type III (fibrotic)	Much less cellular, with increased amounts of collagen arranged in broad bundles

Reproduced with permission from Rombouts JJ, Noel H, Legrain Y, Munting E. (1989) Prediction of recurrence in the treatment of dupuytrens disease: evaluation of a histologic classification. J Hand Surg 14, 644–52.

Recommendations

• There is an increased risk of recurrence associated with Dupuytren's diathesis [overall quality: low]
• There is an increased risk of recurrence associated with diseased fascia that is highly cellular [overall quality: very low]

Summary of recommendations

• Hand vibration is associated with DD
• In patients with severe PIP joint flexion contractures, the effectiveness of fasciectomy versus fasciectomy plus capsuloligamentous release in reducing residual flexion contracture is equivocal
• For Tubiana stage III and IV, LF is more effective than PNF at correcting flexion contractures
• For Tubiana stage I and II, LF and PNF are equally effective at correcting flexion contractures
• Collagenase injection is effective at reducing contractures to 0° to 5° of full extension and improving ROM compared to placebo
• The effect of postoperative static and dynamic splints on final extension deficit is equivocal
• There is an increased risk of recurrence associated with Dupuytren's diathesis
• There is an increased risk of recurrence associated with diseased fascia that is highly cellular

Conclusions

There is a paucity of high-quality evidence related to the etiology, therapy, and prognosis of DD. We found hand vibration to be associated with DD and LF to be more effective than PNF at correcting flexion contractures for Tubiana

stage III and IV. Phase III trials for collagenase injections are showing promising results. However, the evidence regarding fasciectomy vs. fasciectomy plus capsuloligamentous release for the treatment of severe PIP joint contractures as well as postoperative splinting was equivocal.

References

1. McFarlane RM. Patterns of the diseased fascia in the fingers in Dupuytren's contracture. Displacement of the neurovascular bundle. Plast Reconstr Surg 1974;54:31–44.
2. McFarlane RM. On the origin and spread of dupuytren's disease. J Hand Surg 2002;27:385–90.
3. Maravic M, Landais P. Dupuytren's disease in France—1831 to 2001—from description to economic burden. J Hand Surg Br 2005;30:484–7.
4. Webb JA, Stothard J. Cost minimisation using clinic-based treatment for common hand conditions—a prospective economic analysis. Ann R Coll Surg Engl 2009;91:135–9.
5. Liss GM, Stock SR. Can Dupuytren's contracture be work-related? Review of the evidence. Am J Indust Med 1996;29:521–32.
6. Bennett B. Dupuytren's contracture in manual workers. Br J Ind Med 1982;39:89–100.
7. Thomas PR, Clarke D. Vibration white finger and Dupuytren's contracture: Are they related? J Soc Occup Med 1992;42:155–8.
8. Bovenzi M, Cerri S, Merseburger A, et al. Hand-arm vibration syndrome and dose-response relation for vibration induced white finger among quarry drillers and stonecarvers. Occup Environ Med 1994;51:603–11.
9. Cocco PL, Frau P, Rapallo M, Casula D. Occupational exposure to vibrations and dupuytren's disease: A case-control study. Med Lav 1987;78:386–92.
10. Lucas G, Brichet A, Roquelaure Y, Leclerc A, Descatha A. Dupuytren's disease: personal and occupational exposure. Am J Ind Med 2008;51:9–15.
11. Burke FD, Proud G, Lawson IJ, McGeoch KL, Miles JNV. As assessment of the effects of exposure to vibrations, smoking, alcohol and diabetes: Prevalence of Dupuytren's disease in 97,537 miners. J Hand Surg Eur 2007;32:400–6.
12. Ritchie JFS, Venu KM, Pillai K, Yanni DH. Proximal interphalangeal joint release in dupuytren's disease of the little finger. J Hand Surg Br 2004;29:15–17.
13. Beyermann K, Prommersberger KJ, Jacobs C, Lanz UB. Severe contracture of the proximal interphalangeal joint in Dupuytren's disease: Does capsuloligamentous release improve outcome? J Hand Surg Br 2004;29:238–41.
14. Weinzweig N, Culver JE, Fleegler EJ. Severe contractures of the proximal interphalangeal joint in dupuytren's disease: Combined fasciectomy with capsuloligamentous release versus fasciectomy alone. Plast Reconstr Surg 1996;97:560–6.
15. Breed CM, Smith PJ. A comparison of methods of treatment of PIP joint contractures in dupuytren's disease. J Hand Surg Br 1996;21:246–51.
16. van Rijssen AL, Gerbrandy FSJ, Ter Linden H, Klip H, Werker PMN. A comparison of the direct outcomes of percutaneous needle fasciotomy and limited fasciectomy for Dupuytren's

disease: A 6-week follow-up study. J Hand Surg 2006;31: 717–25.

17. Badalamente MA, Hurst LC, Hentz VR. Collagen as a clinical target: Nonoperative treatment of Dupuytren's disease. J Hand Surg 2002;27:788–98.

18. Badalamente MA, Hurst LC. Efficacy and safety of injectable mixed collagenase subtypes in the treatment of Dupuytren's contracture. J Hand Surg Am 2007;32:767–74.

19. Hurst LC, Badalamente MA, Hentz VR, et al. Injectable collagenase *Clostridium histolyticum* for Dupuytren's contracture. N Engl J Med 2009;361:968–79.

20. Au-Yong ITH, Wildin CJ, Dias JJ, Page RE. A review of common practice in Dupuytren surgery. Tech Hand Up Extrem Surg 2005;9:178–87.

21. Larson D, Jerosch-Herold C. Clinical effectiveness of postoperative splinting after surgical release of Dupuytren's contracture: a systematic review. BMC Musculoskelet Disord 2008;21; 9:104.

22. Wilbrand S, Flodmark C, Ekbom A, Gerdin B. Activation markers of connective tissue in dupuytren's contracture: Relation to postoperative outcome. Scand J Plast Reconstr Surg Hand Surg 2003;37:283–92.

23. Boyer MI, Gelberman RH. Complications of the operative treatment of Dupuytren's disease. Hand Clin 1999;15:161–6.

24. Prosser R, Conolly WB. Complications following surgical treatment for Dupuytren's contracture. J Hand Ther 1996;9:344–8.

25. Hueston JT. Dupuytren's Contracture, pp. 51–120. E & S Livingstone, Edinburgh, 1963.

26. Hindocha S, Stanley JK, Watson S, Bayat A. Dupuytren's diathesis revisited: Evaluation of prognostic indicators for risk of disease recurrence. J Hand Surg Am 2006;31:1626–34.

27. Abe Y, Rokkaku T, Ofuchi S, Tokunaga S, Takahashi K, Moriya H. An objective method to evaluate the risk of recurrence and extension of Dupuytren's disease. J Hand Surg Br 2004;29: 427–30.

28. Balaguer T, David S, Ihrai T, Cardot N, Daideri G, Lebreton E. Histological staging and dupuytren's disease recurrence or extension after surgical treatment: A retrospective study of 124 patients. J Hand Surg Eur 2009;34:493–6.

29. Rombouts JJ, Noel H, Legrain Y, Munting E. Prediction of recurrence in the treatment of Dupuytrens disease: evaluation of a histologic classification. J Hand Surg 1989;14:644–52.

122

Extensor Tendon Surgery

Carolyn M. Levis[1,2] *and Monica Alderson*[2]

[1]McMaster University, Hamilton, ON, Canada
[2]St. Joseph's Healthcare, Hamilton, ON, Canada

Case scenario

A 35 year old self-employed male contractor was cutting dry wall with a knife. The blade slipped causing a 4cm laceration to the dorsum of the nondominant hand, severing the extensor tendons to the four fingers between the metacarpophalangeal (MP) joints and the wrist. The patient is unable to extend his fingers.

Relevant anatomy

The extensor tendons motor the finger extensors. They originate at the musculotendinous junction in the proximal forearm and insert distally to extend the fingers. The extensor tendons are classified in anatomic zones I–IX for the fingers and I–V for the thumb.[1]

Importance of the problem

Hand injuries account for a significant number of Emergency Department visits and claims to workmen's compensation boards. The majority of injuries to the extensor tendons occur as a result of trauma to the dorsum of the digits, hand, and forearm with lacerations accounting for a significant percentage of the cases.

A careful history and the clinical evaluation will lead to an accurate diagnosis of extensor tendon injuries and is essential to planning operative management and therapy.

Top six questions

Therapy

1. What is the optimal technique to repair lacerated extensor tendons?
2. Can extensor tendons be effectively repaired under local anesthesia?
3. Does an early passive mobilization program yield better outcomes than an immobilization program?
4. What is the optimal early mobilization protocol following the repair of lacerated extensor tendons?

Prognosis

5. What factors predict functional outcomes after repair of lacerated extensor tendons?

Harm

6. What are the complications associated with repair of lacerated extensor tendons?

Question 1: What is the optimal technique to repair lacerated extensor tendons?

Case clarification

Examination of the patient reveals that the extensor tendons to the four fingers have been completely divided proximal to the MP joint. The surgeon's goal is to repair the tendons such that the hand therapist can begin an early motion

Evidence-Based Orthopedics, First Edition. Edited by Mohit Bhandari.
© 2012 Blackwell Publishing Ltd. Published 2012 by Blackwell Publishing Ltd.

protocol and allow the patient to return to work as a self-employed contractor as soon as possible.

Relevance

An extensor tendon repair must be strong enough to withstand an early range of motion (ROM) rehabilitation protocol, which is believed to yield a more favorable outcome.

Current opinion

There is less controversy about the technique of repairing extensor tendons compared to flexor tendons. Most experts would agree that a strong repair that will withstand tension during early ROM protocols is advisable. A bulky repair that can be detrimental in flexor tendon repairs within the fibro-osseous tunnel is less problematic in extensor tendon repairs.

Finding the evidence

• Cochrane Database, PubMed/systematic reviews, with search term: ("extensor tendon repair" AND "techniques")
• MEDLINE search, using keywords: (extensor tendon injuries), (surgery or repair) AND (clinical trial)

Quality of the evidence

Level VI: animal/laboratory research Compared to the literature concerning flexor tendon repair techniques, there are few studies on extensor tendons. Most of the research is on in-vitro animal or cadaveric models, making the results less generalizable to humans and a low level of evidence.

Findings

The studies compared different suture techniques and their biomechanical performance in tendon shortening, stiffness and final load to failure as measures of ultimate strength.

The results of Newport and William's study indicated that the modified Bunnell repair was the strongest compared to mattress, figure-of-eight, and modified Kessler techniques.[2] In Howard et al.'s study, the augmented Becker repair had the highest strength (load to gap formation) compared with the modified Bunnell and the modified Krackow–Thomas methods.[3] Woo et al. found that augmented Becker had the greatest load to failure and gap force compared to double figure-of-eight, double modified Kessler, and the six-strand double-loop.[4] A recent cadaveric study by Lee et al. confirmed that the augmented Becker and modified Bunnell repairs had comparable strength but, because of the suture technique, led to a greater loss of tendon length than the running-interlocking horizontal mattress method. This technique had a similar strength profile but was faster to perform.[5] The loss of tendon length can decrease the digital flexion and therefore overall grip strength.[6]

Recommendation

• The in-vitro studies may be used to establish the best technique to repair an extensor tendon. The limited studies suggest that a multistrand interlocking repair such as a Bunnell, augmented Becker or running-interlocking horizontal mattress, is stronger than other techniques. Although not specifically studied, the bulkiness of these repairs is not felt to be problematic in extensor tendon lacerations [overall quality: low]

Question 2: Can extensor tendons be effectively repaired under local anesthesia?

Case clarification

The patient in our scenario is healthy with isolated tendon injuries. He is a suitable patient for repair of the tendons under local anesthesia.

Relevance

The efficient use of limited hospital resources is becoming a major focus for surgeons and administrators. Furthermore, timely access to the operating room can be a challenge in some healthcare systems. As a result, some operative hand procedures such as the repair of extensor injuries are considered appropriate for the Emergency Department or minor procedure rooms using local anesthesia.

Current opinion

The location of extensor tendon repairs is another area of debate amongst surgeons with an increasing number advocating the use of local anesthesia and minor procedure room.

Finding the evidence

• As for Question 1, with search terms and keywords:
• "extensor tendon repair" AND "surgical suite," "extensor tendon repair" AND "local anesthesia"
• extensor tendon injuries, surgery OR repair, AND clinical trial

Quality of the evidence

There are no trials comparing extensor tendon repairs in the main vs. minor procedure rooms or the type of anesthesia. The majority of reports are low level, including expert opinion.

Findings

Two papers advocate that repairs of simple extensor tendons[7] and flexor tendons[8] can be performed using local anesthesia in the Emergency Department or minor surgical suite provided adequate equipment and a skilled physician is available.

Recommendation

• In the absence of high-quality evidence, we turn to expert opinion when making recommendations about the repair of extensor tendon lacerations. There is support that local anesthesia is a safe and effective means of anesthesia for the surgical repair of these injuries in an appropriately equipped Emergency Department or minor procedure room, thereby reducing the financial burden to the payer [overall quality: low]

Question 3: Does an early passive mobilization program provide better outcomes than an immobilization program?

Case clarification

The scenario patient requires rehabilitation following repair of the tendons (zone VI). The hand therapist must understand which therapy protocol will yield a better outcome. Early controlled passive motion protocols are initiated immediately postoperatively to prevent loss of function.

Relevance

There is great debate in the literature and clinical community about the most effective postoperative management of primary extensor tendon repair in zones V–VIII (zone IX is less controversial as muscle-to-muscle repairs are usually treated with postoperative immobilization for 4–6 weeks). Traditional programs statically splint the injury for up to 4 weeks and then begin mobilization.[9] The rationale for the development of early passive mobilization with dynamic splinting is that the extensor tendons are so superficial, are in close approximation to bony structures which makes them vulnerable to adhesions, and, depending on the chosen immobilization posture, can result in either joint capsule tightness or extensor lag.[10–13] In a cadaveric study, Evans and Burkhalter found with the wrist in 40–45° of extension and the MP joints limited in 30° of flexion, a required 5 mm tendon glide would occur in zones V–VII to prevent adhesions.[14] Purcell et al. prospectively evaluated static protocols for all zones and found that injuries in zones VI and VII did not have good outcomes. They concluded that dynamic protocols for certain zones may be more efficacious.[15]

Current opinion

There is a range of opinions as to which approach is most cost-effective for the outcomes. Some clinicians believe that extensor tendon injuries are simple and do well regardless of the intervention provided.[16] Others feel that the cost of early mobilization protocols outweigh the benefits.

Finding the evidence

• Cochrane, MEDLINE, and CINAHL, using search terms: "hand/wrist injuries" AND "rehabilitation/splinting" AND "extensor tendons"

• Reference lists from the articles found were reviewed for potential studies

Quality of the evidence

Level I
• 1 systematic reviews/meta-analysis
• 1 randomized controlled trial (RCT)
• 3 other designs

Findings

The meta-analysis by Talsma et al. reviewed another RCT in this category by Bulstrode but the protocol allowed early active and not passive motion.[17,18] One RCT compared the results of early controlled motion with immobilization protocols. Mowlavi et al. designed an RCT for patients with simple injuries in zones V and IV.[19] Patients were randomized into two groups. One group was in a static splint for 4 weeks (wrist 30° extension, MP joints 15–20° extension, distal joints straight). The dynamic splinting group was placed in a reverse Kleinert splint with MP joints allowed to flex to 30°, increased to 45° at 2 weeks. At 4 weeks, the dynamic splinting is discontinued and active range of motion (AROM) is initiated. A night, static splint is continued for 6 weeks. Results showed that patients in the early dynamic splinting protocol had better total AROM of injured digits at 4 weeks, 6 weeks, and 8 weeks but not at 6 months. Grip strength in the dynamic group was better compared to the immobilization group at 8 weeks but not at 6 months. When compared with uninjured hands, the dynamic splinting group had all achieved 80% of the grip strength at 6 months and only 73% of the static group had achieved the same level of grip strength as the uninjured hand. These results suggest that earlier recovery occurs with a dynamic mobilization program, which may be more important in complex injuries or with individuals who have underlying conditions (inflammatory arthritis).

A clinical trial by Chow et al. compared a dynamic protocol allowing progressive MP flexion (week 1 30°, week 2 45°, week 3 60°, and full motion at week 4) for a cohort of patients in a military hospital to a static protocol of immobilization for 3 weeks at another hospital. The outcome showed that the dynamic protocol is superior, with excellent results in all cases and excellent results in the immobilization program in only 40% of the cases. This study is flawed as there is no raw data for comparison and a military compared to civilian population is significantly biased.[12]

Russell et al. completed a retrospective evaluation of static vs. a dynamic protocol and found there was no difference between the two groups functionally, but this study is retrospective and draws conclusions about cost-effectiveness without data.[20]

Recommendation

- Dynamic mobilization protocols would be the preferred protocol for more complex injuries, for individuals with underlying conditions, reliable patients, or where earlier recovery is essential. The limitation however, is the significant variability in the published protocols. The protocol should position the wrist in at least 21–45° of extension, the MP joints in neutral to prevent lags and a progressive increase in allowable MP flexion in the splint.[21] [overall quality: high]

Question 4: What is the optimal early mobilization protocol following the repair of lacerated extensor tendons in our scenario?

Case clarification

The patient sustained simple, sharp tendon lacerations, which is favorable. Several tendons were divided and repaired in close proximity, directly under skin. These are both considered to be unfavorable factors. It is therefore important to apply the optimal therapy program following the repairs that will allow this self-employed patient to return to his work as soon as possible.

Relevance

Like flexor tendon protocols in the past, extensor tendon protocols are now progressing from passive controlled motion to early active motion. Cadaveric studies by Minamikawa et al. revealed that extensor tendon repairs can tolerate full finger excursion with the wrist in 25–30° extension for zones V–VI and the involved finger MP joint limited to 25–30°.[22] The benefit of hyperextending the affected digit in relationship to the other digits in taking tension off the repair site was also observed.[23] These studies also found that very little tendon excursion occurred in the traditional passive protocol positioning with the wrist in 30° of extension. The evaluation found that to affect tendon excursion in zone VI, the wrist would need to be in 21° of extension with unrestricted finger motion.

Active movement is beneficial to promote healing, improve tendon gliding and tensile strength of repair, and reduce swelling. Early protected protocols allow the benefits of active mobility while avoiding tendon rupture.

Current opinion

Some clinicians feel that early mobilization protocols are time intensive for therapists and do not yield significantly better results than immobilization protocols.

Finding the svidence

- As for Question 4

Quality of the evidence

Level I

- 1 systematic review/meta-analysis
- 3 RCTs

Findings

There are three high-quality RCTs evaluating the benefits of early active mobilization compared to dynamic protocols. Bulstrode et al. randomized zone V and VI injuries to one of three groups: (1) immobilization with wrist 30° extension, MP and interphalangeal (IP) joints extended for 4 weeks; (2) immobilization with wrist 30° extension, MPs neutral, IPs free to move hourly; (3) splint positioning with wrist 45° extension, MP at 50° flexion and IPs straight for 4 weeks, every 4 hours extend digits off the pan and hook, splint at night/risk-prone activities until 8 weeks, no passive flexion or resisted flexion until 8 weeks. This study demonstrated that early active mobilization resulted in earlier recovery of motion and grip strength. They also evaluated the intensity of therapy requirements of the three groups and there was no difference in therapy requirements except that group 1 required intensive treatment when splint discontinued, whereas groups 2 and 3 had the intensive therapy at the onset.[18]

An RCT by Chester et al. studied patients with injuries in zoness IV–VIII randomized to early active program using static splint with MP 30° flexion and wrist 30° extension between active exercises of digits (intrinsic plus and minus), wrist AROM at 2 weeks, concurrent fisting at 3 weeks, 4 weeks splint only at night or to a dynamic mobilization group with a dynamic outrigger with the wrist at 30° and the MP allowed to flex to 30°, at 2 weeks wrist AROM, splint only at night at 4 weeks. The authors found significantly better ROM in the early active motion group at 4 weeks but no difference at 6 months.[24]

Khandwala et al. randomized patients with zone V and VI injuries to either a dynamic protocol as in Chow's study or an early active protocol where IP joints are free and MP joints are blocked from flexing beyond 45° and the wrist is in 30° of extension.[16,12] At week 3, the splint is modified to allow 70° of MP flexion. This study also found no statistical difference between the two groups at the time points measured. The protocol in all RCTs included a static splint and specific progression of exercise within protected ranges.

Recommendation

- Early active protocols provide the same results as the passive protocols and may be easier for both the therapist and the patients to complete. The selection of the protocol should take into consideration the proximity to an experienced hand therapist and patient factors such as the self-employed status of the patient [overall quality: high]

Question 5: What factors predict functional outcomes after repair of lacerated extensor tendons?

Case clarification
A functional hand that allows the patient to return to the preinjury state should be the goal of management of extensor tendon injuries. In this scenario, the patient requires optimal hand function to be able to return to work as a contractor.

Relevance
Understanding the factors that predict a functional outcome after extensor tendon injury will assist the patient, surgeon, therapist, and employer in directing care and rehabilitation.

Current opinion
It is anticipated that a young, healthy individual with isolated lacerations to extensor tendons would regain normal function and a very good outcome following repair.

Finding the evidence
• As for Question 1, with search terms: "extensor tendon repair" AND "outcomes"
• extensor tendon injuries, surgery OR repair AND clinical trial Keywords "extensor tendon" AND "outcomes"

Quality of the evidence
Using "outcomes" as a keyword in the search strategy yielded reports that were in fact case series (level IV). The search strategy did not yield true outcome studies from prospective trials (level II); however, there were some individual cohort studies. One systematic review compiled several study types, although none of them were randomized trials.

Findings
Carl et al. (level IIb) in a prospective study of 203 tendon repairs concluded that recovery of finger function after repair was related to the complexity of injury and the zone of the laceration. In this group, static splinting for 6 weeks followed by ROM was an appropriate for zones I, II, IV, and V, and early ROM was more appropriate for injuries in zones III and IV, where more complex injury patterns seem to occur.[25] A review of the literature by Newport and Tucker in 2005 reported that immobilization as a postoperative treatment of extensor tendon lacerations yielded good or excellent results ranging between 54% and 95%. They concluded that clinical outcomes have consistently improved utilizing either dynamic or active motion with good or excellent results achieved in at least 90% of cases.[26]

Recommendation
• Repair of simple extensor tendon lacerations followed by early ROM can be expected to have a good to excellent outcome compared to complex injuries and static splinting [overall quality: low]

Question 6: What are the complications associated with repair of lacerated extensor tendons?

Case clarification
The initiation of an early ROM protocol following extensor tendon repair in zone VI for our patient may lead to complications.

Relevance
The evolution of the management of extensor tendon injuries includes a shift from rigid immobilization for 6 weeks to involve early ROM following surgical repair. In recommending this protocol, the risk of complications compared to the associated benefits must be understood and accepted by the patient, surgeon, and therapist.

Current opinion
Most surgeons and therapists would agree that while the benefit of early motion allows for gliding of repaired tendons and avoidance of joint contractures, the potential for rupture does exist.

Finding the evidence
• As for Question 1, with search terms: "extensor tendon repair" AND "complication"
• extensor tendon injuries, surgery OR repair, AND clinical trial. Keywords "extensor tendon" AND "therapy" AND "complication"

Quality of the evidence
Numerous publications addressing complications associated with extensor tendon repairs are retrospective reviews of cohorts of patients, some dating back more than 50 years, and are therefore considered level IV evidence.

Findings
The reported complications associated with the surgical repair of the extensor tendons include general operative complications for hand surgery. The reports focus on those complications associated with early ROM vs. static splinting/immobilization. Numerous publications report decreased rates of complications such as loss of motion, extensor lag, loss of grip strength, and need for tenolysis[9,12,16,27,28] without an increase in rupture rates[9,28–30] for early motion protocols vs. static splinting.

Recommendation

• There is little question that lacerated extensor tendons should be repaired. The general and specific complications should be discussed with the patient including the potential benefit of early ROM over static splinting [overall quality: low]

Summary of recommendations

• The in-vitro studies may be used to establish the best technique to repair an extensor tendon. The limited studies suggest that a multistrand interlocking repair such as a Bunnell, augmented Becker or running-interlocking horizontal mattress, is stronger than other techniques. Although not specifically studied, the bulkiness of these repairs is not felt to be problematic in extensor tendon lacerations

• In the absence of high-quality evidence, we turn to expert opinion when making recommendations about the repair of extensor tendon lacerations. There is support that local anesthesia is a safe and effective means of anesthesia for the surgical repair of these injuries in an appropriately equipped Emergency Department or minor procedure room, thereby reducing the financial burden to the payer

• Dynamic mobilization protocols would be the preferred protocol for more complex injuries, for individuals with underlying conditions, reliable patients, or where earlier recovery is essential. The limitation however, is the significant variability in the published protocols. The protocol should position the wrist in at least 21–45° of extension, the MP joints in neutral to prevent lags and a progressive increase in allowable MP flexion in the splint

• Early active protocols provide the same results as the passive protocols and may be easier for both the therapist and the patients to complete. The selection of the protocol should take into consideration the proximity to an experienced hand therapist and patient factors such as the self-employed status of the patient

• Repair of simple extensor tendon lacerations followed by early ROM can be expected to have a good to excellent outcome compared to complex injuries and static splinting

• There is little question that lacerated extensor tendons should be repaired. The general and specific complications should be discussed with the patient including the potential benefit of early range of motion over static splinting

Conclusions

This review reveals a paucity of high-level (I–III) evidence regarding the management of extensor tendon injuries. Management includes the clinical evaluation to make an accurate diagnosis followed by tendon repair with a locking modified Bunnell, augmented Becker, or running horizontal interlocking technique. The evidence that does exist supports the current opinion of experts that operative repair of extensor tendon lacerations can be adequately performed using local anesthesia in an Emergency Department or minor operating room suite and that early ROM protocols offer some benefit over immobilization in certain tendon zones in the first few months and may be appropriate particularly for patients who require rapid return to preinjury state. The review of the evidence also strengthens the opinion that improved functional outcomes following early motion outweighs the risk of complications associated with these protocols.

References

1. Kleinert HE, Verdan C. Report of the committee on tendon injuries (IFSSH). J Hand Surg 1983;8:794–8.
2. Newport ML, Williams, CD. Biomechanical charcieristics of extensor tendon suture techniques. J Hand Surg Am 1992;17: 1117–23.
3. Howard RF, Ondrovic L, Greenwald DP. Biomechanical analysis of four-strand extensor tendon repair techniques. J Hand Surg Am 1997;22:838–42.
4. Woo SH, Tsai TM, Kleiner HE, et al. A biomechanical comparison of four extensor tendon repair techniques in zone IV. Plast Reconstr Surg 2005;115:1674–81.
5. Lee SK, Dubey A, Kim BH et al. A biomechanical study of extensor tendon repair methods: introduction to the running-interlocking horizontal mattress extsnor tendon repair technique. J Hand Surg Am 2010;35:19–23.
6. Ketchum LD, Thompson D, Pocock G. A clinical study of force generation by the intrinsic muslce of the index finger and the extrinsic flexor and extensor muscles of the hand. J Hand Surg 1978;3:571–8.
7. Calabro JJ, Hoidal CR, Susini LM.. Extensor tendon repair in the emergency department. J Emerg Med 1986;4:217–25.
8. Lalonde DH. Wide-awake flexor tendon repair. Plast Reconstr Surg 2009;123:2:623–5.
9. Evans RB. Therapeutic management of extensor tendon injuries. Hand Clin. 1986;2:157.
10. Blair WF, Steyers CM. Extensor tendon injuries. Orthop Clin N Am 1992;23:141–8.
11. Brüner S, Wittemann M, Jester A, Blumenthal K, Germann G. Dynamic splinting after extensor tendon repair in zones V and VII. J Hand Surg Br 2003;28(3):224–7.
12. Chow JA, Dovelle S, Thomes LJ, Ho PK, Saldana J. A comparison of results of extensor tendon repair followed by early controlled mobilization versus static immobilization. J Hand Surg Am 1989;14:18–20.
13. Lee VH. Rehabilitation of extensor tendon injuries. In Hunter JM et al., Eds, Rehabilitation of the Hand, p. 365. CV Mosby, St. Louis, 1984.
14. Evans RB, Burkhalter WE. A study of the dynamic anatomy of extensor tendons and implications for treatment. J Hand Surg Am 1986;11:774.

15. Purcell T, Eadie PA, Murugan S, O'Donnell M, Lawless M. Static splinting of extensor tendon repairs. J Hand Surg Br 2000;25(2): 180–2.

16. Khandwala AR, Webb J, Harris SB, Foster AJ, Elliot D. A comparison of dynamic extension splinting and controlled active mobilization of complete divisions of extensor tendons in zones 5 & 6. J Hand Surg Br 2000;22(2):140–6.

17. Talsma E, de Haart N, Beelen A, et al. The effect of mobilization on repaired extensor tendon injuries of the hand:a systematic review. Arch Phys Med Rehab 2008;89:2366–72.

18. Bulstrode NW, Burr N, Pratt AL, et al. Extensor tendon rehabilitation. A prospective trial comparing three rehabilitation regimes. J Hand Surg Br 2005;30(2):175–9.

19. Mowlavi A, Burns M, Brown R. Dynamic versus static splinting of simple zone V and zone VI extensor tendon repairs: a prospective, randomized, controlled study. Plast Recontr Surg 2005; 115:2:482–7.

20. Russell RC, Jones M, Grobbelaar A. Extensor tendon repair: mobilize or splint? Chir Main 2003;22:19–23.

21. Hunt J. Early controlled motion following extensor tendon repair: a critical review. J Hand Ther Br 2000;5(1):10–15.

22. Minamikawa W, Peimer CA, Yamaguchi T, Banasiak NA, Kambe K, Sherwin FS. Wrist position and extensor tendon amplitude following repair. J Hand Surg Am 1992;17:268–71.

23. Howell JW, Merritt WH, Robinson SJ. Immediate controlled active motion following zone 4–7 extensor tendon repair. J Hand Ther 2005;2(11):182–90.

24. Chester DL, Beale S, Beveridge L, Nancarrow JD, Titley OG. A prospective, controlled, randomized trial comparing early active extension with passive extension using a dynamic splint in the rehabilitation of repaired extensor tendons. J Hand Surg Br 2002;27(3):283–8.

25. Carl HD, Forst R, Schaller P. Results of primary extensor tendon repair in relation to the zone of injury and pre-operative outcome estimation. Arch Orthop Trauma Surg 2007;127:115–19.

26. Newport ML, Tucker RL. New perspectives of extensor tendon repair and implications for rehabilitation. J Hand Ther 2005;18:175–81.

27. Newport ML, Blair WF, Steyers CM Jr.. Long-term results of extensor tendon repair. J Hand Surg 1990;15:961–6.

28. Browne EZ Jr, Ribik CA. Early dynamic splinting for extensor tendon injuries. J Hand Surg 1989;14:72–6.

29. Crosby CA, Wehbe MA. Early protected motion after extensor tendon repair. J Hand Surg 1999;24:1061–70.

30. Evans RB, Thompson DE. The application of force to the healing tendon. J Hand Ther 1993;6:266–84.

123 Rheumatoid Hand Reconstruction

Oluseyi Aliu and Kevin C. Chung

University of Michigan, Ann Arbor, MI, USA

Case scenario

A 58 year old white woman reports several months' history of generalized fatigue and "stiffness" of both hands that lasts through the morning. She has noticed painful swelling of the joints in her fingers. She describes throbbing pain that she rates as an 8 on a visual analog scale of 0 to 10.

Relevant anatomy

The inflammation that occurs in rheumatoid arthritis (RA) results in significant soft tissue and bone destruction. The supporting elements of small joints of the hand become attenuated, which causes laxity of collateral ligaments and joint capsules; this, coupled with contracture of the intrinsic muscles, causes the typical deformities such as metacarpophalangeal (MCP) joint subluxation and ulnar deviation seen in RA (Figures 123.1 and 123.2). Furthermore, hypertrophic synovial tissue infiltration creates bulges along the flexor tendon sheath that interfere with flexion of the digits. The dorsal wrist may also be the site of synovial disease leading to a high risk of extensor tendon ruptures. These anatomical derangements create esthetic and functional morbidity for RA patients.

Importance of RA

The worldwide prevalence of RA amongst adults ranges between 0.5% and 1.5%.[1] The disease has profound effects on the productivity and independence of patients because approximately one third of them are not able to work 5 years after disease onset and by 10 years, 50% of patients are not able to work at all.[2,3] Permanent disability with loss of independence occurs in 20–30% of working-age RA patients within 2–3 years of diagnosis.[4] In addition to the effect on patients, there is also a significant global financial burden associated with managing the disease including medical treatments, lost productivity, and support for patients who have lost the ability to attend to their activities of daily living. The overall cost of rheumatoid arthritis in the United States in 1996 was $8.7 billion[5] and a more recent analysis (2007) puts the cost at $63 billion per annum in the United States and the equivalent of $67 billion in Western Europe.[6]

Top seven questions

Diagnosis

1. Who has RA?

Treatment

2. What is the role of biologic disease-modifying antirheumatic drugs (DMARDs) in the management of RA?
3. Is there a role for small-joint synovectomy in the management of joint destruction in the rheumatoid hand?
4. What is the role of prophylactic extensor tenosynovectomy in the management of the rheumatoid hand?
5. What benefits are conferred by flexor tenosynovectomy in the management of the rheumatoid hand?
6. How effective are the surgical options for repairing tendon ruptures resulting from RA?
7. What is the role of MCP arthroplasty in management of the rheumatoid hand?

Evidence-Based Orthopedics, First Edition. Edited by Mohit Bhandari.
© 2012 Blackwell Publishing Ltd. Published 2012 by Blackwell Publishing Ltd.

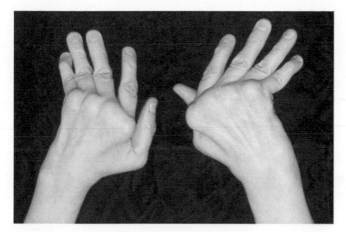

Figure 123.1 A patient with ulnar drift of fingers.

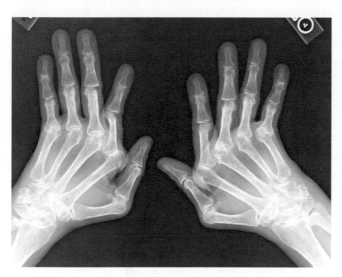

Figure 123.2 PA radiograph of MCP joint subluxation/dislocation.

Question 1: Who has RA?

Case clarification

The diagnosis of RA is primarily a clinical one. Specific criteria have been established by the American College of Rheumatology (ACR)[7] to guide clinicians in making a diagnosis of RA that includes: (1) joint stiffness in the morning that lasts more than 1 hour; (2) arthritis of the wrist, metacarpophalangeal (MCP) joint, or proximal interphalangeal (PIP) joint; (3) arthritis of three or more of the following joints: right or left PIP, MCP, metatarsophalangeal (MTP), elbow, wrist, knee, or ankle; (4) symmetric joint involvement; (5) rheumatoid nodules; (6) serology showing the presence of rheumatoid factor (RF); and (7) radiographic evidence of joint erosions. A patient must have at least four of the seven criteria and the first four criteria must be present for a minimum of 6 weeks.[7]

Question 2: What is the role of biologic DMARDs in the management of RA?

Case clarification

The ACR[8] has defined a core set of measures to characterize active RA after diagnosis has been made. These include: (1) a count of tender and swollen joints, (2) the patient's qualitative assessment of pain, (3) the patient's assessment of disease activity, (4) the patient's assessment of physical function, (5) the physician's assessment of disease activity, and (6) serum levels of inflammatory markers. Charting changes in these measures help to monitoring a patient's response to medical therapy.

Relevance

The objectives of treatment in RA are symptom relief, improvement in function, and arrest of disease progression. Biologic DMARDs may play a role in arresting joint and soft tissue damage by decreasing inflammation through modification of immunologic processes.

Current opinion

There is much emphasis on early control of rheumatoid disease activity, and using a combination of a biologic DMARD and methotrexate is widely advocated for refractory disease.

Finding the evidence

- Cochrane Database, using keywords: "adalimumab AND rheumatoid arthritis," "infliximab AND rheumatoid arthritis," "etanercept AND rheumatoid arthritis"
- PubMed systematic reviews, using keywords: "adalimumab AND rheumatoid arthritis," "infliximab AND rheumatoid arthritis," "etanercept AND rheumatoid arthritis"

Quality of evidence

Level I
- 6 systematic reviews/meta-analyses
- 20 randomized control trials (RCTs)

Findings

Clinical outcome The DMARDs are a group of medications used to slow the progression of rheumatoid disease through various mechanisms that influence the inflammatory process. Synthetic DMARDs—such as the chemotherapeutic agents methotrexate and sulfasalazine, among others—were the mainstay of treatment as monotherapy or in combinations for the management of active RA. The introduction in the past decade of a newer class of drugs known as biologic DMARDs has improved treatment for patients who are refractory to the traditional drugs. This newer class of drugs is made with recombinant DNA technology, and they modulate immune response by targeting specific elements of the immune system like tumor necrosis factor

(TNF)-α, CD20 receptors on B cells, and various interleukins. The superior effectiveness of the biologic DMARDs in improving radiographic and clinical outcomes in RA treatment is widely demonstrated, especially in managing disease refractory to the older synthetic DMARDs.

A meta-analysis of 13 RCTs (n = 6694) comparing biologic DMARD monotherapy to placebo clearly demonstrates the effectiveness of the biologic DMARD drugs studied including anakinra, etanercept, infliximab, and adalimumab.[9] In all of these studies, the outcome measure was achievement of ACR20, which is a 20% improvement in the previously listed core measures of rheumatoid disease activity (see "Case clarification" section). Results of odds ratios (ORs) with 95% confidence intervals (CI) calculated for the achievement of ACR20 using biologic DMARD monotherapy were: anakinra 1.70 (0.9–3.19), etanercept 3.58 (2.09–6.91), infliximab 3.47 (1.66–7.14), and adalimumab 3.19 (1.97–5.48).[9] The investigators also demonstrated the effect of combination treatment using a biologic DMARD and methotrexate, by calculating ORs for ACR20 achievement after the addition of methotrexate to an existing regimen of biologic DMARD monotherapy. Their results showed significantly increased effectiveness of the biologic DMARDs after the addition of methotrexate.[9]

Venkateshan et al.'s[10] meta-analysis of 25 RCTs (n = 11252) provides further evidence of the effectiveness of combination therapy. They compared biologic DMARDs in combination with a synthetic DMARD (methotrexate) against placebo treatment (methotrexate only) in patients with active disease. Their reported OR (95% CI) for achievement of ACR20 measured at 24, 54, and 96 weeks after initiation of therapy were 3.69 (3.48–3.87), 3.31 (2.98–3.64), and 3.0 (2.64–3.35) respectively, demonstrating significantly superior effectiveness for the combination of biologic DMARDs and methotrexate compared to methotrexate only treatment with up to 96 weeks of follow-up.

In terms of radiographic outcomes, the Sharp score (TSS) is one of several methods used to measure the effectiveness of treatments for RA. This score comprises a tally of joint erosion and joint space narrowing (JSN) scores, and an increase over time indicates progressive joint destruction as a result of either erosion, joint space narrowing, or both (Table 123.1). One of the treatment goals for RA is to arrest

Table 123.1 Change in radiographic scores in comparisons of biological DMARDs (adalimumab, etanercept, and infliximab) to placebo

Study	Comparison	n	Follow up (yrs)	Δ TSS[a,b]	Δ Joint erosion[a]	Δ JSN[a]
Bathon et al.[14,c]	Etanercept vs. placebo	632	1	1.0	0.47	0.53
				1.59	1.03	1.3
Lipsky et al.[19,c]	Infliximab vs. placebo	428	1	−0.7	−0.7	0.0
				7	4	2.9
Genovese et al.[15,c]	Etanercept vs. placebo	512	2	1.3	0.7	0.6
				3.2	1.9	1.3
Keystone et al.[12,c]	Adalimumab vs. placebo	619	1	0.1	0.0	0.1
				2.7	1.6	1.0
Klareskog et al.[13]	Etanercept vs. placebo	682	1	−0.54	−0.3	−0.23
				2.80	1.68	1.12
Breedveld et al.[20,c]	Infliximab vs. placebo	82	2	NR	−0.78	−0.61
				NR	12.21	12.82
van der Heijde et al.[16]	Etanercept vs. placebo	503	2	−0.56	−0.76	0.2
				3.34	2.12	1.23
Breedveld et al.[11]	Adalimumab vs. placebo	799	2	1.9	1.0	0.9
				10.4	6.4	4.0
van der Heijde et al.[17]	Etanercept vs. placebo	414	3	−0.14	−0.67	−0.67
				5.95	3.25	2.7
Emery et al.[18]	Etanercept vs. placebo	542	1	0.27	NR	NR
				2.44	NR	NR

JSN, joint space narrowing; NR, not reported; RCT, randomized controlled trial; TSS, total Sharp score.
[a]The top level of the split columns show values for biological DMARDs and the bottom level for placebo.
[b]A value <0.5 means no progression in joint damage.
[c]These studies included more than one dosing regimen of the biological DMARDs; the most efficacious doses are represented.

Table 123.2 Percentage of patients without joint disease progression; comparison between biological DMARDs (adalimumab, eternacept, and infliximab) and placebo

Study	n	Follow-up (yrs)	(% of n with no Δ TSS)[a]	(% of n with no Δ joint erosion)[a]	(% of n with no Δ JSN)[a]
Bathon et al.[14,b]	632	1	NR	72	NR
			NR	60	NR
Genovese et al.[15,b]	512	2	63	70	78
			51	58	69
Keystone et al.[12,b]	619	1	NR	62	69
			NR	46	52
Breedveld et al.[11,b]	799	2	61	NR	NR
			34	NR	NR
van der Heijde et al.[16]	503	2	78	86	NR
			60	66	NR
van der Heijde et al.[17]	414	3	76	NR	NR
			51	NR	NR
Emery et al.[18]	542	1	80	NR	NR
			59	NR	NR

JSN, joint space narrowing; NR, not reported; RCT, randomized controlled trial; TSS, total Sharp score.
[a]The top level of the split columns show values for biological DMARDs and the bottom level for placebo.
[b]These studies included more than one dosing regimen of the biological DMARDs; the most efficacious doses are represented.

joint destruction, and a wealth of evidence shows that patients who receive biologic DMARDs, either as monotherapy or in combination with methotrexate, have significantly less progression of joint erosions and JSN when compared with patients receiving placebo (Table 123.2).[11–20] Furthermore, initiation of biologic DMARDs early in the course of treatment can aid in arresting joint destruction, and this was shown in a post-hoc analysis from a 3 year RCT. In this analysis a cohort with earlier addition of infliximab to a methotrexate-only regimen was compared to another cohort with a later initiation of infliximab. The investigators found that significantly fewer patients with earlier initiation of infliximab showed progressing joint destruction with majority of them achieving arrest of joint destruction.[21]

Recommendation

• Evidence suggests that treatment of early aggressive or refractory RA with combination of biologic DMARD and methotrexate improves clinical and radiographic outcomes [overall quality: high]

Question 3: Is there a role for small-joint synovectomy in management of joint destruction in RA?

Case clarification

Swelling of the patient's joints could be an indication of proliferative synovitis. Serial physical examinations show she has well-organized painful synovitis. Radiographs show no evidence of joint destruction.

Relevance

Active synovitis of joints in RA can result in destruction of joint structures and subsequent impairment of function.

Current opinion

Small-joint synovectomy can have a role in management of patients with persistent pain after up to 6 months of medical therapy, provided they show no joint cartilage and bone destruction.

Finding the evidence

• Cochrane Database, using keywords "tenosynovectomy AND rheumatoid arthritis," "synovectomy AND rheumatoid arthritis"
• PubMed, using keywords "tenosynovectomy AND rheumatoid arthritis," "synovectomy AND rheumatoid arthritis"

Quality of evidence

Level IV
• 3 observational cohort studies with inconsistency
• 3 case series

Findings

Synovial proliferation in the small joints of the hand causes joint tenderness, swelling, limited range of motion, and to a significant degree, the synovitis also propagates progressive joint destruction. Hand surgeons use open and arthroscopic techniques to remove the infiltrative synovium in order to ameliorate symptoms, improve function, and arrest destructive synovitis. Although outcome measures reported are variable across most studies, they do indicate that there is benefit to undergoing small-joint synovectomy.

In a study conducted by the Arthritis and Rheumatism Council and British Orthopaedic Association,[22] 69 metacarpophalangeal (MCP) joints in 22 patients were randomized to synovectomy and nonsurgical management. The patients were examined after 2 years and results demonstrated only improved joint swelling in the synovectomy group; however, assessment at 3 years showed these patients did not have significantly better outcomes overall. Additionally, the improved joint swelling seen at the 2 year follow-up period was not maintained, but all the patients who underwent synovectomy were satisfied with the procedure. McEwan et al.[23] reported similar results in their study of 20 patients with MCP joint synovitis; at 1 year after surgery, the patients had significant improvements in joint tenderness and swelling, but at 3 years after surgery, these favorable outcomes were not maintained.

Thompson et al.[24] randomized RA patients affected by synovitis who were undergoing pharmaceutical treatments into three groups—synovectomy, medications only, and splinting. Although the investigators did not specify the duration of follow-up, they showed that the synovectomy group demonstrated significantly better improvements in grip and palmar pinch strength, patient satisfaction, joint swelling, and sensitivity to pain compared to the other groups. However, as in McEwan et al.'s study,[23] the radiographs showed no difference in the degrees of joint degradation outcomes between patients who underwent synovectomy and their respective controls at follow-up.

In conclusion, some evidence suggests that most patients who underwent small-joint synovectomy reported significant pain relief and radiographic assessment showed that 37–45% of them achieved arrest of joint erosions (Table 123.3).[25–27] Other studies demonstrate that the advantages obtained from small-joint synovectomy are temporary.[23–24] The recurrence rates reported in the literature for small-joint synovitis vary between 6% and 30%, with up to 8 years of follow-up (Table 123.3).[25–27]

Recommendation

• The evidence suggests that performing small-joint synovectomy, when there is persistent pain and functional limitation in the absence of joint destruction, can provide symptomatic relief for a limited period of time [overall quality: low]

Question 4: What is the role of prophylactic extensor tenosynovectomy in the management of the rheumatoid hand?

Case clarification

Patients with RA presenting with painful swelling of the wrist likely have proliferative synovitis affecting the wrist joint with associated extensor tendon synovitis.

Relevance

Rheumatoid arthritis patients with refractory wrist joint and extensor tendon synovitis are at high risk of extensor tendon ruptures,[28] which will cause debilitating functional problems and the morbidity associated with tendon reconstruction.

Current opinion

Prophylactic extensor tenosynovectomy is effective in preventing tendon ruptures.[29–31]

Finding the evidence

• PubMed, using keywords "extensor tenosynovectomy AND rheumatoid arthritis," "wrist synovectomy AND rheumatoid arthritis"

Quality of evidence

Level IV
• 8 case series

Findings

The wrist joint is commonly affected in RA,[32] and the initial treatment of synovitis of the wrist as in the overall treatment of rheumatoid disease relies on drug therapy to prevent destruction of the joint. However, despite optimal medical treatment, patients may present with refractory disease by having proliferative synovitis involving the distal radioulnar joint (DRUJ) with or without extensor tendon involvement. If wrist synovitis is allowed to progress, the DRUJ is destroyed, causing dorsal displacement of the distal ulna and derangements of the carpus including axial collapse, ulnar translocation, and palmar

Table 123.3 Outcomes of small-joint synovectomy

Study	n	Follow up (yrs)	Joints involved	% of n with improved pain	% of n with no progression of erosions	% of n with recurrence	% of n with JSN progression
Ansell et al.[27]	56	1	PIP	91	37	19	NR
Nicolles et al.[26]	37	4–8	MCP	92	NR	6%	NR
Wilde[25]	39	1–3	PIP	88	45	30	40

JSN, joint space narrowing; MCP, metacarpophalangeal; NR, not reported; PIP, proximal interphalangeal.

subluxation.[33–37] Ultimately, tendon ruptures occur from direct synovial infiltration of tendons and/or attritional damage from the tendons rubbing against the dorsally displaced distal ulna.[28]

Dorsal tenosynovectomy is usually combined with distal ulna excision for refractory wrist joint involvement when there is DRUJ instability or destruction.[33] Several studies have demonstrated that prophylactic extensor tenosynovectomy, even when there is evidence of synovial invasion of extensor tendons at the time of surgery, significantly prevents tendon ruptures, with occurrence of subsequent ruptures in only 0–3% of patients.[29–31] Excision of destructive synovium and removal of mechanical irritation from the displaced distal ulna contribute to the benefits of these procedures.[38]

In addition to the prevention of extensor tendon rupture, dorsal synovectomy and distal ulna excision are reported to provide pain relief and improved pronation and supination of the wrist joint.[30,34–37,39] However, ulnar translocation of the carpus progresses over time, regardless of whether patients undergo dorsal synovectomy and distal ulna excision.[34–37] Ishikawa et al. suggest that ulnar translocation occurs significantly more in patients who undergo distal ulna excision because the support of the carpus provided by the distal ulna is lost.[36] Drawing inference from studies showing wrist stability in patients with spontaneous radiocarpal fusion and their results, they propose radiolunate arthrodesis to stabilize the wrist following distal ulna excision.[36]

Recommendations

• Patients who present with refractory wrist joint and extensor tendon synovitis should undergo dorsal synovectomy. If there is DRUJ instability or destruction, distal ulna excision should be performed. Both procedures are effective in preventing extensor tendon rupture [overall quality: moderate]
• Distal ulna excision may result in accelerated ulnar translocation of the carpus, and limited radiocarpal fusion may be beneficial in stabilizing the wrist joint to prevent carpal translocation [overall quality: moderate]

Question 5: What benefits are conferred by flexor tenosynovectomy in the management of the rheumatoid hand?

Case clarification

When a patient with RA has difficulty with active digital flexion, it is important to distinguish whether the problem is in the joints or in the flexor tendons. For the flexor tendon problem, the patient will have full passive flexion or the joint, but the active flexion is limited because of swelling in the flexor tendons. On the other hand, a patient with an isolated joint problem will have limited joint motion, both passive and active.

Relevance

The prevalence of flexor synovitis in RA has been reported to be between 40% and 55%.[40]

Current opinion

Patients can achieve a significant improvement in functional ability with flexor tenosynovectomy

Finding the evidence

• Cochrane Database, using keywords "tenosynovectomy AND rheumatoid arthritis," "synovectomy AND rheumatoid arthritis"
• PubMed, using keywords "tenosynovectomy AND rheumatoid arthritis," "synovectomy AND rheumatoid arthritis"

Quality of evidence

Level IV
• 4 case series

Findings

Hypertrophic synovial infiltration within the flexor tendon sheath presents with bulges along the tendon sheath, and these bulges often occur at the weaker cruciform pulleys that are stretched.[33] A plain radiograph should be obtained to rule out concomitant PIP joint disease.

The available evidence suggests that between 50% and 75% of patients who undergo flexor tenosynovectomy achieve measurable improvements in extensor lag and flexion deficit, with less than 20% of them faring poorly (Table 123.4).[40–42] Additionally patients have been shown to achieve a significant improvement in pain levels, in active and passive range of motion at the PIP joint and in overall satisfaction after the procedure with up to 12 years of

Table 123.4 Comparison of results of flexor tenosynovectomy with the Jackson and Paton scale

Study	n	% Excellent	% Good	% Fair	% Poor
Jackson and Paton[41]	36	44	31	11	14
Wheen et al.[42]	61	31	36	21	11
Tolat et al.[40]	424	31	14	22	33

MCP, metacarpophalangeal; PIP, proximal interphalangeal.
Excellent: tip to palm 0 cm, MCP/PIP extensor lag 0°
Good: tip to palm ≤2 cm, MCP/PIP extensor lag ≤30°
Fair: tip to palm ≤2–4 cm, MCP/PIP extensor lag ≤30°.
Poor: tip to palm >4 cm, MCP/PIP extensor lag >30°.

follow-up.[40,43] Only one study reported the recurrence rate in their series of hypertrophic flexor tenosynovitis cases, which was 31% after up to 4 years of follow-up [42].

Recommendation

• Flexor tenosynovectomy can provide functional benefit for patients with impairment of active flexion caused by synovitis [overall quality: low]

Question 6: How effective are surgical options for repairing tendon ruptures resulting from RA?

Case clarification

Both flexor and extensor tendons can rupture as a result of rheumatoid disease activity either due to attenuation directly from invasive synovitis or by attritional wear from eroded bones.

Relevance

If the underlying cause of tendon rupture is not identified and treated, further ruptures can occur, which can increase functional morbidity.

Current opinion

Prevention of tendon ruptures is most ideal and tenosynovectomy is effective in this regard.[31] However, the functional impairment wrought by tendon ruptures should be a clear indication for tendon reconstruction.

Finding the evidence

• PubMed, using keywords "tendon transfer AND rheumatoid arthritis"

Quality of evidence

Level IV
• 4 case series

Findings

When a tendon rupture is suspected, the causative factor should be identified and addressed at the time of reconstruction. For instance, in the investigation of extensor tendon ruptures, radiographic studies often show a disrupted DRUJ with an eroded distal ulna. Physical examination demonstrates that the remaining intact tendons are rubbing over the surface of the eroded distal ulna and in a matter of time, additional ruptures are likely. In this case, dorsal synovectomy, distal ulna excision, or both should be performed at the same time as the tendon reconstruction to prevent rupture of the intact tendons. Ishikawa et al.[36] suggest that a radiolunate arthrodesis should be also considered early in addition to the above procedures to stabilize the wrist and prevent further wrist subluxation.

Surgical reconstruction for tendon ruptures may be achieved by either tendon transfers or free interposition grafting; however, there are no studies directly comparing the two methods. Mountney et al.[44] instead used a biomechanical model to show the advantage of interposition grafting compared to tendon transfers by demonstrating mathematically that a smaller angle between the line of force and the axis of its motor unit by using the native proximal tendon results in a greater percentage of maximum force generated. The inferred advantage to tendon grafts is that they are along the same axis as their motor units. Additionally, they reported an average MCP joint extension lag of 9° and flexion deficit of 10° after free interposition grafting with up to 45 months of follow-up.

Tendon rupture from RA tends to be progressive, and evidence suggests that prompt intervention is beneficial.[45] Although most patients in Shannon and Barton[46] and Moore et al.'s[47] series of tendon transfers achieve good outcomes in terms of extensor deficit and range of motion, those with reconstruction of isolated tendon ruptures, especially isolated extensor pollicis longus (EPL) ruptures, had the best outcomes. The worst outcomes were in patients with multiple tendon ruptures and tendon ruptures concomitant with untreated MCP joint disease.[45-47]

Recommendations

• Tendon reconstruction can be used to improve the impairment of hand function that results from extensor or flexor tendon ruptures [overall quality: moderate]
• Concomitant procedures like distal ulna excision and synovectomy may be required to achieve better outcomes and prevent further ruptures [overall quality: moderate]
• Interposition grafting may provide some benefit in force generation compared to tendon transfers [overall quality: low]

Question 7: What is the role of MCP arthroplasty in RA management?

Case clarification

Due to the progressive nature of RA, joint destruction can reach a stage in which a surgical salvage procedure such as MCP arthroplasty is necessary.

Relevance

The MCP joint is most commonly affected in RA and endstage destruction of these joints can render patients functionally impaired, with unappealing appearance of their hands.

Current opinion

In a recent survey of hand surgeons, 84% had a favorable view of outcomes from MCP arthroplasty[48] citing improved

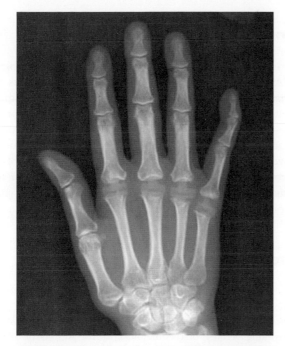

Figure 123.3 PA radiograph of a hand after MCP joint arthroplasty.

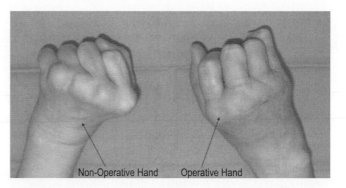

Non-Operative Hand   Operative Hand

Figure 123.5 A hand after MCP arthroplasty with fingers flexed.

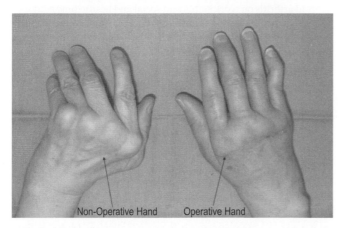

Non-Operative Hand   Operative Hand

Figure 123.4 A hand after MCP arthroplasty with fingers in extension.

cosmetic appearance and function in daily activities (Figures 123.3–123.5).

Finding the evidence
• Cochrane Database, using keywords: "arthroplasty" AND "rheumatoid arthritis"
• PubMed, using keywords: "arthroplasty" AND "rheumatoid arthritis"

Quality of evidence
Level III
• 1 systemic review of cohort and case series studies
• 2 observational cohort studies

Level IV
• 1 case series

Findings
The course of MCP joint disease in RA results from synovial infiltration and subsequent attenuation of joint support structures. Radial and ulnar sagittal bands that stabilize the extensor tendon over the MCP joint are stretched by synovitis. The radial band is further weakened by the gripping motion involved in daily activities that causes progressive ulnar displacement of extensor tendons characteristic of rheumatoid hands. As a result, ulnar lateral bands contract to further accentuate the drift of the extensor tendons. Furthermore, the proximal phalanx itself may become volarly subluxed. These structural changes adversely affect the functional ability of the hand and are a significant cosmetic burden to patients. This degree of joint destruction is a clear indication for joint replacement.

The goals of MCP joint arthroplasty are to improve hand function and appearance. Although there is debate about the effectiveness and timing of surgical intervention in RA, the available evidence suggests that there are benefits in undergoing the procedure. In terms of physical outcome measures, several studies have demonstrated a significant improvement in range of motion after MCP arthroplasty.[49–51] However, strength measures (grip and pinch) do not show the same favorable outcomes (Table 123.5).[51–52] Additional favorable outcomes have been shown using the Michigan Hand Questionnaire (MHQ) that measures six domains important to the rheumatoid patient; (1) overall hand function, (2) activities of daily living, (3) pain, (4) work performance, (5) esthetics, and (6) patient satisfaction. The evidence demonstrates the short-term advantage of MCP arthroplasty in five of these domains, the exception being work performance.[51–52]

In conclusion, subjective outcome measures demonstrate that patients perceive that they gain significant benefits from MCP athroplasty in cosmetic improvement and the ability to perform daily tasks.

Table 123.5 Physical outcome measures after MCP arthroplasty

Study	MCP ROM (°)	Grip strength (kg)	Key pinch strength (kg)	Tip pinch strength (kg)	Palmar pinch strength (kg)
Chung et al.[49,a]	+11.0[b]	+3[b] −1.2	NR	NR	NR
Chung et al.[52]	+13.0	+0.3	+1.0	+0.6	+1.2
Parker et al.[50]	+13.0[b]	−4.0	NR	NR	NR
Chung et al.[51]	+12.0[b]	+0.5	−0.4	+0.2	−0.1

MCP, metacarpophalangeal; NR, not reported; ROM, range of motion
[a]Unpooled results from a systemic review with 2 of 10 studies showing changes in grip strength represented in the split column.
[b]Statistically significant change.

Recommendation

• MCP joint arthroplasty can deliver significantly improved hand function and appearance [overall quality: moderate]

Summary of recommendations

• Biological DMARDs in combination with a non-biological DMARD, especially methotrexate, have demonstrated efficacy in treatment of early aggressive RA and disease refractory to methotrexate monotherapy
• In patients with persistent pain and functional limitation from small-joint synovitis, synovectomy can provide symptomatic relief for up to 2 years
• Prophylactic extensor tendon and wrist joint synovectomy in combination with distal ulnar excision are effective in the prevention of tendon ruptures when indicated
• Flexor synovectomy can effectively improve flexion hampered by synovial proliferation along the tendon sheath
• Tendon transfers and tendon interposition grafting can reliably improve hand function after flexor or extensor tendon ruptures
• Prevention of tendon ruptures with such procedures as synovectomy and distal ulna excision is effective. These procedures may also be done at the same time as tendon reconstruction to stave off further ruptures
• MCP arthroplasty provides significant improvement in subjective outcomes and should be considered in endstage destruction of MCP joints

Conclusions

There is high-level evidence to support the use of biological DMARDs in the treatment of early aggressive arthritis and management of disease activity not responding optimally to monotherapy with methotrexate. Most surgical procedures to correct anatomic derangements are not as strongly supported by well-designed, high-quality studies. However, both objective and subjective components of outcome measures in the studies examined suggest that there is discernable benefit for patients undergoing rheumatoid hand reconstruction.

References

1. Silman A, Hochberg M. Epidemiology of Rheumatoid Disease. Oxford University Press, Oxford, 1993.
2. Young A, Dixey J, Kulinskaya E, et al. Which patients stop working because of rheumatoid arthritis? Results of 5 years follow up in 732 patients from the early RA study (ERAS). Ann Rheum Dis 2002;61(4):335–40.
3. Fex E, Larsson B-M, Nived K, Eberhardt K. Impact of rheumatoid arthritis on work status and social and leisure time activities in patients followed from the onset. J Rheumatol 1997;25:44–50.
4. Sokka T. Work disability in early rheumatoid arthritis. Clin Exp Rheumatol 2003;21(S31):S71–4.
5. Yelin E. The costs of rheumatoid arthritis: absolute, incremental, and marginal estimates. J Rheumatol 1996;44S:47–51.
6. Lundkvist J, Kastang F, Kobelt G. The burden of rheumatoid arthritis and access to treatment: health burden and costs. Eur J Health Econ 2008;8(S2):S49–60.
7. Arnett FC, Edworthy SM, Bloch DA, et al. The American Rheumatism Association 1987 revised criteria for the classification of rheumatoid arthritis. Arthritis Rheum 1988;31:315–24.
8. Hochberg MC, Chang RW, Dwosh I, Lindsey S, Pincus T, Wolfe F. The American College of Rheumatology 1991 revised criteria for the classification of global functional status in rheumatoid arthritis. Arthritis Rheum 1992;35:498–502.
9. Nixon R, Bansback N, Brennan A. The efficacy of inhibiting tumor necrosis factor α and interleukin 1 in patients with rheumatoid arthritis: a meta-analysis and adjusted indirect comparisons. Rheumatology 2007;46(7):1140–7.
10. Venkateshan SP, Sidhu S, Malhotra S, Pandhi P. Efficacy of biologicals in the treatment of rheumatoid arthritis. Pharmacology 2009;83(1):1–9.
11. Breedveld FC, Weisman MH, Kavanaugh AF, et al. The PREMIER study: A multi-center, randomized, double-blind, clinical trial of combination therapy with adalimumab plus methotrexate versus methotrexate alone or adalimumab alone in patients with early, aggressive rheumatoid arthritis who had not had previous methotrexate treatment. Arthritis Rheum 2006;54(1):26–37.
12. Keystone EC, Kavanaugh AF, Sharp JT, et al. Radiographic, clinical and functional outcomes of treatment with adalimumab (a human anti-tumor necrosis factor monoclonal antibody) in

patients with active rheumatoid arthritis receiving concomitant methotrexate therapy. Arthritis Rheum 2004;50(5):1400–11.

13. Klareskog L, van der Heijde D, de Jager JP, et al. TEMPO (Trial of Etanercept and Methotrexate with Radiographic Patient Outcomes) study investigators. Lancet 2004;363(9410):675–81.

14. Bathon JM, Martin RW, Fleischmann RM, et al. A comparison of etanercept and methotrexate in patients with early rheumatoid arthritis. N Engl J Med 2000;343(22):1586–93.

15. Genovese MC, Bathon JM, Martin RW, et al. Etanercept versus methotrexate in patients with early rheumatoid arthritis: two year radiographic and clinical outcomes. Arthritis Rheum 2002;46(6):1443–50.

16. van der Heijde D, Klareskog L, Rodriguez-Valverde V, et al. Comparosion of etanercept and methotrexate, alone and combined, in the treatment of rheumatoid arthritis: two year clinical and radiographic results fromt eh TEMPO study, a double-blind, randomized trial. Arthritis Rheum 2006;54(4):1063–74.

17. van der Heijde D, Klareskog L, Landewé R, et al. Disease remission and sustained halting of radiographic progression with combination etanercept and methotrexate in patients with rheumatoid arthritis. Arthritis Rheum 2007;56(12):3928–39.

18. Emery P, Breedveld FC, Hall S, et al. Comparison of methotrexate monotherapy with a combination of methotrexate and etanercept in active, early, moderate to severe rheumatoid arthritis (COMET): a randomised, double-blind, parallel treatment trial. Lancet 2008;372(9636):375–82.

19. Lipsky PE, van der Heijde DM, St Clair EW, et al. Infliximab and methotrexate in the treatment of rheumatoid arthritis. N Engl J Med 2000;343(22):1594–602.

20. Breedveld FC, Emery P, Keystone E, et al. Infliximab in active early rheumatoid arthritis. Ann Rheum Dis 2004;63(2):149–55.

21. van der Kooij SM, le Cessie S, Goekoop-Ruiterman YP, et al. Clinical and radiological efficacy of initial vs. delayed treatment with infliximab plus methotrexate in patients with early rheumatoid arthritis. Ann Rheum Dis 2009;68(7):1153–8.

22. Arthritis and Rheumatism Council & British Orthopaedic Association. Controlled trial of synovectomy of knee and metacarpophalangeal joints in rheumatoid arthritis. Ann Rheum Dis 1975;35(5):437–42.

23. McEwen C. Multicenter evaluation of synovectomy in the treatment of rheumatoid arthritis. Report of results at the end of five years. J Rheumatol 1988;15(5):765–9.

24. Thompson M, Douglas G, Davison EP. Evaluation of synovectomy in rheumatoid arthritis. Proc Roy Soc Med 1973;66:197–199.

25. Wilde AH. Synovectomy of the proximal interphalangeal joint of the finger in rheumatoid arthritis. J Bone Joint Surg Am 1974;56:71–78.

26. Nicolle FV, Holt PJL, Calnan JS. Prophylactic synovectomy of the joints of the rheumatoid hand: clinical trial with 4 to 8 year follow-up. Ann Rheum Dis 1971;30:476–80.

27. Ansell BM, Harrison SH, Little H, Thouas B. Synovectomy of proximal interphalangeal joints. Br J Plast Surg 1970;23(4):380–5.

28. Vaughan Jackson OJ. Rupture of extensor tendons by attrition at the inferior radio-ulnar joint;report of two cases. J Bone Joint Surg Br 1948;30(3):528–30.

29. Ryu J, Saito S, Honda T, Yamamoto K. Risk factors and prophylactic tenosynovectomy for extensor tendon ruptures in the rheumatoid hand. J Hand Surg Br 1998;23(5):658–61.

30. Ishikawa H, Murasawa A, Nakazono K. Long-term follow-up study of radio-carpal athrodesis for the rheumatoid wrist. J Hand Surg Am 2005;30(4):658–66.

31. Brown FE, Brown FL. Long-term results after teno-synovectomy to treat the rheumatoid hand. J Hand Surg Am 1988;13:704–8.

32. Flatt AE. The Care of the Arthritic Hand, 5th edn. Quality Medical Publishing, St. Louis, 1995.

33. Chung KC. Operative Techniques: Hand and Wrist Surgery, Volume 2, pp. 631–770. Saunders Elsevier, Philadelphia, 2008.

34. Chantelot C, Fontaine C, Flipo RM, Migaud H, Le Coustumer F, Duquennoy A. Synovectomy combined with Suave-Kapandji procedure for the rheumatoid wrist. J Hand Surg Br 1999;24(4):405–9.

35. Thirupathi RG, Ferlic DC, Clayton ML. Dorsal wrist synovectomy in rheumatoid arthritis—a long-term study. J Hand Surg Am 1983;8(6):848–56.

36. Ishikawa H, Hanyu T, Tajima T. Rheumatoid wrists treated with synovectomy of the extensor tendons and the wrist joint combined with Darrach procedure. J Hand Surg Am 1992;17(6):1109–17.

37. Ishikawa H, Hanyu T, Saito H, Takahashi H. Limited arthrodesis for the rheumatoid wrist. J Hand Surg Am 1992;17(6):1103–9.

38. Kessler I, Kauko V. Posterior (dorsal) synovectomy for rheumatoid involvement of the hand and wrist: a follow-up study of sixty-six procedures. J Bone Joint Surg Am 1966;48:1085–94.

39. Jain A, Ball C, Nanchahal J. Functional outcome following extensor synovectomy and excision of the distal ulna in patients with rheumatoid arthritis. J Hand Surg Br 2003;28(6):531–6.

40. Tolat AR, Stanley JK, Evans RA. Flexor tenosynovectomy and tenolysis in longstanding rheumatoid arthritis. J Hand Surg Br 1996;21(4):538–43.

41. Jackson IT, Paton KC. The extended approach to flexor tendon synovitis in rheumatoid arthritis. Br J Plast Surg 1973;26(2):122–31.

42. Wheen DJ, Tonkin MA, Green J, Bronkhorst M. Long-term results following digital flexor tenosynovectomy in rheumatoid arthritis. J Hand Surg Am 1995;20(5):790–4.

43. Millis MB, Millender LH, Nalebuff EA. Stiffness of the proximal interphalangeal joints in rheumatoid arthritis. The role of flexor tenosynovitis. J Bone Joint Surg Am 1976;58(6):801–5.

44. Mountney J, Blundell CM, McArthur P, Stanley D. Free tendon interposition grafting for the repair of ruptured extensor tendons in the rheumatoid hand. J Hand Surg Br 1998;23(5):662–5.

45. Millender LH, Nalebuff EA, Albin R, Ream JR, Gordon M. Dorsal synovectomy and tendon transfer in the rheumatoid hand. J Bone Joint Surg Am 1974;56:601–10.

46. Shannon FT, Barton NJ. Surgery for rupture of extensor tendons in rheumatoid arthritis. Hand 1976;8(3):279–86.

47. Moore JR, Weiland AJ, Valdata L. Tendon ruptures in the rheumatoid hand: analysis of treatment and functional results in 60 patients. J Hand Surg Am 1987;12(1):9–14.

48. Alderman AK, Ubel PA, Kim HM, Fox DA, Chung KC. Surgical management of the rheumatoid hand: consensus and controversy among rheumatologists and hand surgeons. J Rheumatol 2003;30(7):1464–72.

49. Chung KC, Kowalski CP, Myra Kim H, Kazmers IS. Patient outcomes following Swanson silastic metacarpophalangeal joint arthroplasty in the rheumatoid hand: a systematic overview. J Rheumatol 2000;27(6):1395–402.

50. Parker WL, Rizzo M, Moran SL, Hormel KB, Beckenbaugh RD. Preliminary results of nonconstrained pyrolytic carbon arthroplasty for metacarpophalangeal joint arthritis. J Hand Surg Am 2007;32(10):1496–505.

51. Chung KC, Burns PB, Wilgis EF, Burke FD, Regan M, Kim HM, Fox DA. A multicenter clinical trial in rheumatoid arthritis comparing silicone metacarpophalangeal joint arthroplasty with medical treatment. J Hand Surg Am 2009;34(5):815–23.

52. Chung KC, Kotsis SV, Kim HM. A prospective outcomes study of Swanson metacarpophalangeal joint arthroplasty for the rheumatoid hand. J Hand Surg Am 2004;29(4):646–53.

124 Flexor Tendon Surgery

Shima C. Sokol[1] and Robert M. Szabo[2]

[1]Prohealth Care Associates, Lake Success, NY, USA
[2]University of California-Davis, Sacramento, CA, USA

Case scenario 1

A 35 year old male construction worker who is right-hand dominant presents with inability to bend his left ring and small fingers. Two weeks ago he sustained a laceration across the palmar aspect of his proximal phalanx of these two digits while cutting wire. On examination, his ring and small finger have increased resting extension posture. His wounds are healed. He cannot flex his proximal interphalangeal (PIP) or distal interphalangeal (DIP) joints to his ring finger. Flexion of his little finger PIP and DIP is weak and painful. His sensory examination is normal.

Relevant anatomy

The flexor tendons are enclosed in a synovial sheath in the distal palm and digits. The sheath provides a gliding surface for the tendons. Pulleys are thickenings of the tendon sheath which prevent bowstringing of the tendons and improve tendon excursion. in the finger. There are five annular (A) and three cruciform (C) pulleys; A2 and A4 are the most critical for complete finger flexion (Figure 124.1).[1]

The nutritional supply of the flexor digitorum superficialis (FDS) and flexor digitorum profundus (FDP) arises from diffusion of nutrients within the synovial sheath, the surrounding paratenon, and arterial system in the volar finger. The blood supply enters the tendon dorsally and consists of vessels in the proximal synovial fold, the vincular system, and osseous insertion of the FDS and FDP.[3] The vincula are dorsal folds of mesotenon through which small vessels travel to supply the tendon. The digital arteries in the finger give off segmental branches, which supply the vincular vessels. Proximal to the sheath, the tendons are covered by an extensive vascular plexus.

Verdan classified flexor tendon injuries into five zones (Figure 124.2).[4,5] Each zone has important anatomic considerations and prognostic implications. Zone II flexor tendon injuries are of particular interest to hand surgeons, as reflected in the large body of literature published on these injuries. Injuries in zone II, also known as "no man's land," include lacerations from the A1 pulley to the insertion of the FDS tendon. Zone II injuries are difficult to treat because of the small, unyielding space in which the two tendon slips of the FDS and the FDP tendon all pass. The other flexor tendon zones are illustrated in Figure 124.2.

Importance of the problem

Flexor tendon lacerations make up less than 1% of all hand injuries seen in the Emergency Department,[6] but their the social and economic consequences are considerable because the injury is most common in young healthy adults, leading to lost work productivity. A 2003 multiple regression analysis of 97 flexor tendon lacerations treated in southern Sweden found the average costs of surgery and rehabilitation of zone II flexor tendon injuries to be over $21,100.[7] Healthcare costs averaged over $7,000 and lost work productivity cost almost $14,000. Setting hurdles for treatment decisions is the abundance of research literature and patient information available on the internet. PubMed searches for "flexor tendon injury" and "hand" yield over 1,200 published articles, whereas Google returns over 49,000 hits for "flexor tendon injuries."

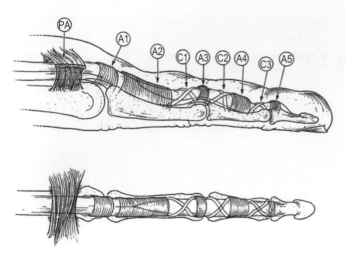

Figure 124.1 Flexor tendon pulley system: lateral (top) and palmar (bottom) views of a finger depict the components of the digital flexor sheath. The sturdy annular pulleys (A1, A2, A3, A4, and A5) are important biomechanically in keeping the tendons closely applied to the phalanges. The thin, pliable cruciate pulleys (C1, C2, and C3) collapse to allow full digital flexion. The palmar aponeurosis pulley (PA), adds to the biomechanical efficiency of the sheath system. (Reproduced with permission from Strickland JW. Development of flexor tendon surgery: twenty-five years of progress. Hand Surg Am 2000;25(2):214–235).[2]

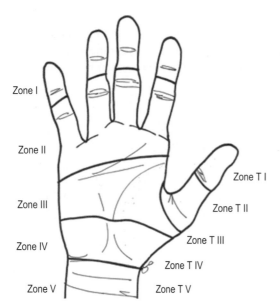

Figure 124.2 Flexor zones of the hand. Zone V extends from the musculotendinous junction to the carpal tunnel. Zone IV injuries involve lacerations at the level of the carpal tunnel. Zone III injuries include injuries from the distal edge of the transverse carpal ligament to the proximal edge of the A1 pulley. The lumbricals originate in zone III. Zone II starts from the A1 pulley to the insertion of the FDS tendon (see text). Zone I injuries are distal to the FDS insertion and only involve the FDP tendon insertion. In the thumb (FPL lacerations), zones V and IV correspond to Verdan's zones V and IV for flexor tendon injuries to the other digits. FPL injuries at the level of the thumb metacarpal make up zone III. Zone II injuries include the A1 pulley to the metacarpalphalangeal joint. Zone I injuries extend from the interphalangeal joint to the FPL insertion.

Top seven questions

Surgical therapy

1. What suture configuration should be used to achieve the strongest repair in zone II flexor injuries?
2. What suture material should be used to repair flexor tendon lacerations?
3. Should a patient undergo surgical repair of the partial tendon laceration?
4. What is the optimal fixation for FDP avulsion injuries?

Prognosis

5. Does the use of botulinum toxin improve outcomes in flexor tendon repair?
6. Are there any medications or treatments to prevent adhesion formation after flexor tendon repair?

Diagnosis of failed tendon repair

7. What is the role of imaging in evaluating flexor tendon injuries and the status of flexor tendon repairs postoperatively?

Question 1: What suture configuration should be used to achieve the strongest repair in zone II flexor injuries?

Case clarification
Which core suture configuration is strong enough to allow the patient to start early active and passive range of motion (ROM) after flexor tendon repair?

Relevance
Biomechanical studies have shown the strength of the repair increases with the number of suture strands crossing the repair site. Suture techniques using more strands across the repair site are technically demanding, require increased manipulation of the tendon ends, and create a bulky repair, which may compromise tendon gliding.

Current opinion
Flexor tendon repairs should be performed with a core suture of at least four strands crossing the tendon repair site with equal strength across all strands. Repairs should be supplemented with an epitendinous suture.

Finding the evidence
• PubMed (www.ncbi.nlm.nih.gov/pubmed/): sensitivity search using keywords: "core suture" AND "flexor tendon surgery" [also added: "NOT biomechanic*" and Limits to Humans]

- PubMed (www.ncbi.nlm.nih.gov/pubmed/): sensitivity search using keywords: "suture technique(s)" AND "flexor tendon repair" AND "hand" OR "zone II flexor tendon repair"

Quality of the evidence
Level II
- 8 retrospective cohort studies

Level III
- 1 retrospective cohort study without adequate controls

Level IV
- More than 30 case series

Findings
Taking into account increased resistance from edema after surgery and a decrease in suture strength during the initial weeks after flexor tendon repair, several authors have suggested that tendon repair strength should be at least 73.5 N to withstand early active and passive finger motion.[8,9] Numerous biomechanical studies have compared the strength of different repair techniques.[10–16] These studies have shown that increasing the number of core sutures increases the strength of tendon repair (Table 124.1).

Epitendinous sutures increase the strength of core suture repairs by 10–50%, reduce gapping between tendon ends, and smooth the repair site.[19] Stein and colleagues[17] demonstrated increases in dorsal vs. volar grasping strength of Kessler and Robertson repairs (Figure 124.3) but had no effect on strength of locking Strickland and modified Becker repairs.[17,20,21] Locking core sutures have also been shown to increase the strength of tendon repairs compared to grasping techniques. Increasing the number of suture locks or grasps further increases strength at the repair site.[22,23]

Table 124.1 Review of the in-vitro studies on gapping and ultimate strength of repair techniques

Study	Material (core/epitendinous)	Ultimate force	Gapping force (gap)
Modified Kessler (two-strand)			
Stein et al.[17]	4-0 braided polyester, 6-0 nylon	28.9 N	23.6 N (2 mm)
McLarney et al.[11]	4-0 braided polyester ,6-0 polypropylene	28 N	22 N (2 mm)
Tang et al.[14]	3-0 nylon, 5-0 nylon	28.2 N	23.4 N (2 mm)
Thurman et al.[15]	4-0 polyethylene, 6-0 polypropylene	33.9 N	NR
Modified Becker (four-strand)			
Stein et al.[17]	4-0 braided polyester, 6-0 nylon	40.7 N	48.8 N (2 mm)
Cruciate (four-strand)			
McLarney et al.[11]	4-0 braided polyester, 6-0 polypropylene	56 N	44 N (2 mm)
Tang et al.[14]	3-0 nylon, 5-0 nylon	46.3 N	37.4 N (2 mm)
Su et al.[18]	4-0 braided polyester, 5-0 polypropylene	70 N	46.5 N (2 mm)
	3-0 braided polyester, 5-0 polypropylene	73.8 N	53.8 N (2 mm)
Alvanja et al [10]	4-0 braided polyester, 6-0 Dermalon	66 N	NR
	3-0 braided polyester, 6-0Dermalon	74 N	NR
	2-0 braided polyesters, 6-0 Dermalon	80 N	NR
Horizontal mattress (four-strand)			
Thurman et al.[15]	4-0 polyethylene, 6-0 polypropylene	43 N	NR
Savage (six-strand)			
Savage et al.[8]	4-0 braided polyester, none	67.2 N	58.9 N (2.7 mm)
Sandow (six-strand)			
Xie et al.[16]	4-0 Ethilon, 6-0 Ethilon	57. 8 N	37.4 N (2 mm)
Tang (six-strand)			
Tang et al.[14]	3× 4-0 looped nylon, 6-0 nylon	53.6 N	43 N (2 mm)
Xie et al.[16]	4-0 Supramid, 6-0 Ethilon	60.2 N	44.5 (2 mm)
Thurman et al.[15]	4-0 polyethylene, 6-0 polypropylene	78.7 N	NR
Tenofix			
Su et al.[18]	5-0 polypropylene, 5-0 epitendinous	66.7 N	54.5 N (2 mm)

NR, not reported.

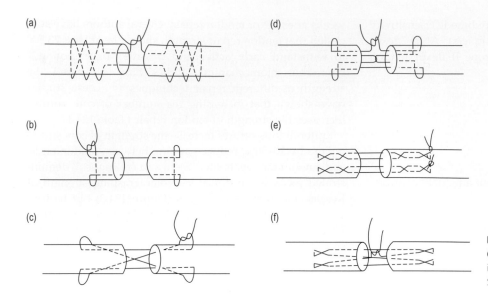

Figure 124.3 Various core suture techniques: (a) Bunnell, (b) Kessler, (c) cruciate, (d) interlock, (e) modified Becker, (f) modified Savage by Sandow.

Numerous clinical studies have reported results of flexor tendon repairs using various suture techniques. Results of various methods of flexor tendon repair evaluated using Strickland's criterion (see box) are summarized in Table 124.2. Several of these studies were focused on rehabilitation protocols and rarely involved more than one cohort within the same population, making comparison of the different techniques difficult. Other studies have many uncontrollable variables and different evaluation methods.

Strickland and Glogovac criterion[26,38]

Originally developed to assess function after flexor tendon repair, it is calculated as a percentage of normal active PIP and DIP motion:

active PIP+DIP flexion–extension lag at the PIP and DIP/175° × 100

The percentage is then categorized as follows:
- Excellent: 85–100% of normal (100% = 175°)
- Good: 70–84%
- Fair: 50–69%
- Poor <50%

All ROM results in this chapter are based on this criterion unless otherwise stated.

There are only two clinical studies directly comparing different suture techniques. Hoffman et al.[32] reviewed the clinical outcomes of 46 patients (51 digits) undergoing a six-strand Lim/Tsai repair to 25 patients (26 digits) treated with a two-strand modified Kessler stitch in zone II flexor tendon repairs. The complication rate was lower in the six-strand group (4%) than in the modified Kessler group (23%). The rupture rate was also lower in the six-strand group (2% vs. 11% in the other group), but this was not statistically significant. The two groups followed different rehabilitation protocols, which confound the effects of the suture repair.

Osada and colleagues[24] compared clinical outcome of 22 patients (28 digits) with zone II flexor tendon lacerations repaired using two different six-strand suture techniques (Figure 124.4). The authors reported a 96% excellent result based on the original Strickland criterion, with no clinically significant difference in the outcomes of the two groups after average follow-up of 13 months (range 6–51 months). None of the repaired tendons ruptured.

Recommendations
Based on clinical and biomechanical studies:
- Four-strand or higher core suture technique supplemented by running epitendinous sutures are recommended to provide sufficient tensile strength to allow for postoperative passive and some active motion rehabilitation [overall quality: moderate]
- Dorsal placement of the suture and locking (vs. grasping) sutures increase the strength of repair. Increasing the number of grasps or locks also improves tensile strength. Whether or not the difference is seen clinically is unknown [overall quality: not applicable]

Question 2: What suture material should be used to repair flexor tendon lacerations?

Case clarification
The patient is taken to the operating room and found to have complete laceration of the ring finger FDS and FDP tendon in zone II. You must decide which suture material to use to repair his flexor tendon.

Table 124.2 Outcomes based on Strickland criteria for flexor tendon repairs using various core sutures[24,25]

Study	Suture repair	Rehabilitation protocol	Number (digits)	Average follow-up (months)	G/E results (%)	Rupture rate (%)
Strickland and Glogovac[26]	Two-strand	Immobilization	25	5.1	12	16
	Two-strand	Duran Houser	25	4	56	4
Chow et al.[27]	Two-strand	Kleinert and Duran Houser component	78	≥6	98[a]	4
Cullen et al.[28]	Two-strand	Active	38	10	78	6
Baktir et al.[29]	Two-strand	Active or Kleinert	88	12	81	5
Silverskiold and May[30]	Two-strand	Modified active	55	6	96	4
Kitsis et al.[31]	Two-strand	Active	87	12	89[a]	6
Hoffmann et al.[32]	Two-strand	Kleinert and Duran	21	3	43	11
Lee 1990[33]	Four-strand	Active	11	?	91	9
Klein[34]	Four-strand	Active	19	3	95	0
Su et al.[18]	Four-strand	Kleinert	51	6	71	18
Caulfield et al.[35]	Four-strand	Active	101	4	72	2[b]
	Four-strand (absorbable suture)	Active	315	4	73	2[b]
Sandow and McMahon[36]	Six-strand	Active	23	3-?	78	0
Osada et al.[24]	Six-strand	Active	27	13	96	0
Hoffmann et al.[32]	Six-strand	Kleinert and Duran +place & hold exercise	50	3	78	2
Rocchi et al.[25]	Tenofix	Active	21	16	86	4
Su et al.[37]	Tenofix	Kleinert	34	6	67	0

[a]Results included rerepair cases.

[b]Results include injuries in other zones.

Rehabilitation protocols: Active, active flexion and extension; Kleinert, passive flexion and active extension; Duran Houser, passive flexion and extension; Immobilization, immobilization for 3 weeks, Modified active, active flexion after full passive flexion.

Relevance

Many types and sizes of suture material are available for flexor tendon repair. The need for a strong suture material must be balanced with the risk of excessive bulk and scar formation from foreign body reaction.

Current opinion

Most guidelines for suture repair include using a 3-0 or 4-0 nonabsorbable polyfilament material with at least four strands crossing the tendon repair site and equal strength across all strands. Most surgeons also use epitendinous sutures made of 5-0 or 6-0 monofilament nonabsorbable suture to smooth the repair site and improve tensile strength.[19]

Finding the evidence

• PubMed (www.ncbi.nlm.nih.gov/pubmed/): sensitivity search using keywords: "core suture" OR "Tenofix™" OR "suture material" and "flexor tendons" and "rupture" OR "flexor tendon repair"

Quality of the evidence

Level I

• 1 randomized controlled trial (RCT)

Level III

• 1 retrospective comparative study

Level IV

• 1 case series

Findings

There are many biomechanical and animal studies addressing the ideal core suture material for flexor tendon repairs to allow early postoperative motion (Table 124.1). Monofilament stainless steel sutures have been shown to have the greatest tensile strength, but are difficult to use and may weaken with kinking.[39] Nonabsorbable 3-0 or 4-0 braided polyester sutures have better gliding properties with comparable tensile strength to stainless steel sutures.[9] Monofilament nylon and polypropylene have better knot-tying capabilities than braided polyester but are not as strong.[40] They are most commonly used for epitendinous sutures. Larger-caliber sutures increase the strength of flexor tendon repairs.[10,41,42] Larger sutures are bulky, however, leading to increased work of flexion and gliding resistance. Biomechanical studies have proven that repairs using 3-0 or 4-0 sutures provide sufficient tensile strength and adequate gliding efficiency to withstand early postoperative motion therapy.[10]

There are few clinical studies directly comparing the outcomes of flexor tendon repairs using different suture materials. Two studies have reported on the use of the Tenofix device for flexor tendon repairs. Tenofix is a knotless suture composed of two intratendinous stainless steel anchors joined by a single multifilament 2-0 stainless steel suture (Figure 124.5). It provides the strength of stainless steel

sutures without the difficulty of managing and tying it. Biomechanical studies have shown it has comparable repair strength to the standard 3-0 or 4-0 suture.[37,43] Results from a manufacturer-sponsored, blinded, randomized clinical trial comparing Tenofix to a locked four-strand cruciate repair for the treatment of zone II flexor tendon lacerations showed superior results with the Tenofix repairs.[18] None of the Tenofix repairs ruptured at 6 months compared to 18% (9 of 51) rupture rate for repairs using the cruciate technique. The 18% failure rate is higher than previous studies on four-strand repairs showing rupture rates of less than 10% (Table 124.2). Of note, Tenofix could not be used in a number of cases because of inadequate tendon exposure or an injury that was too distal in zone II for placement of both suture anchors.

Rocchi and colleagues[25] used Tenofix on 21 isolated zone II flexor tendon injuries in all digits (including the thumb). There were 86% excellent or good results and 14% (three) fair results. Two anchors required removal; one because of tendon rupture (failure rate 4%) and another because of infection. Patients in this study returned to work on average sooner than patients in previous reports on multistrand repairs (30 days vs. 60 days after surgery).[31,44]

Absorbable suture has high tensile strength and is inextensible and easy to tie and use,[45] but is not widely used in flexor tendon repairs. In animal studies, these sutures maintain strength long enough to allow adequate tendon healing.[46,47] Nonetheless, Mashadi and colleagues[46] concluded the absorbable suture they tested, polytrimethylene carbonate (Maxon™), should not be used for tendon repairs because it stimulated a significant tissue reaction and subsequent adhesions in chickens.

One retrospective study[35] has shown comparable clinical results of flexor tendons repaired with absorbable sutures vs. nonabsorbable materials. In a series of 272 patients (566 tendon lacerations in 416 digits) repaired with a Strickland four-strand core suture repair supplemented with an epitendinous suture, absorbable suture (polytrimethylene/Maxon or PDS™) in was used in 191 (73%) patients and nonabsorbable suture in 81 (27%). Rupture rate was 2% in both groups. There was no statistical difference in range of motion (ROM), outcomes, rate of infection, or need for tenolysis between the two groups. Among zone II injuries,

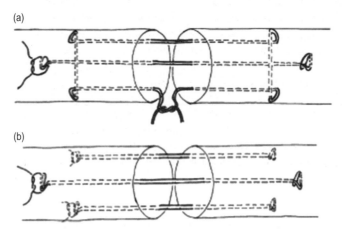

Figure 124.4 Six-strand suture techniques. (a) The Y1 technique: combination of Tsuge suture with a 4-0 looped thread and the modified Kessler suture using a 4-0 double strand with two needles. (b) The TL technique using three Tsuge sutures with 4-0 looped thread. (Reproduced with permission from Osada D, Fujita S, Tamai K, Yamaguchi T, Iwamoto A, Saotome K. Flexor tendon repair in zone II with 6-strand techniques and early active mobilization. J Hand Surg Am 2006;31(6):987–92.)

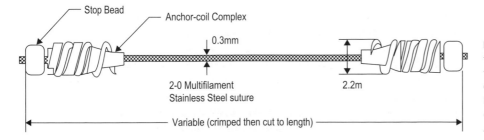

Figure 124.5 TenoFix device. Adapted from Su BW. The biomechanical analysis of a tendon fixation device for flexor tendon repair. (Reproduced with permission from Su BW. The biomechanical analysis of a tendon fixation device for flexor tendon repair. J Hand Surg Am 2005;30(2):237–245.)

151 were repaired using absorbable sutures and 41 using nonabsorbable sutures. Seven out of eight ruptures occurred in zone II: two ruptures occurred in the nonabsorbable group, and five occurred in repairs using absorbable suture.

Recommendations

For repairs of flexor tendon injuries:
- Biomechanical and clinical research has shown that 3-0 or 4-0 braided polyester sutures should be used to allow unrestricted finger flexion during rehabilitation without compromising work of flexion and gliding resistance [overall quality: moderate]
- Clinical research suggests Tenofix is safe and effective in the repair of flexor tendon lacerations. It may not be suitable in all cases; particularly those involving small tendons or poor soft tissue envelope [overall quality: moderate]
- There is insufficient evidence to support the use of absorbable sutures over nonabsorbable suture for repair of zone II flexor tendon injuries. Results of flexor tendon repair using absorbable sutures in all zones have shown comparable results compared to nonabsorbable sutures [overall quality: insufficient; very low]

Question 3: Should partial tendon lacerations be repaired?

Case clarification

During surgery for the patient, exploration of the small finger reveals a 65% laceration of the FDP in zone II. Should you repair the tendon?

Relevance

Flexor tendon repair is fraught with complications including adhesion formation, rerupture, and extensive postoperative rehabilitation. If the tendon could be treated nonoperatively without compromising function, the expense of surgery and a prolonged rehabilitation course could be avoided.

Current opinion

Current opinion suggests lacerations of more than 60% of the cross-sectional area should be repaired to prevent triggering and possible rupture.

Finding the evidence

- PubMed (www.ncbi.nlm.nih.gov/pubmed/) sensitivity search using keywords: "partial flexor tendon laceration" AND "hand"

Quality of the evidence

Level III
- 1 retrospective comparative study

Level IV
- 2 case series
- 1 retrospective comparative study with small numbers

Findings

Complications of partial tendon lacerations treated nonoperatively include progression to complete rupture, triggering, and entrapment of the tendon.[48] Biomechanical studies have shown, however, that suturing a partial tendon laceration actually reduces the tensile strength of the tendon.[49,50] Hariharan et al.[51] showed even substantial lacerations could withstand the loads of active motion.

A prospective study[52] showed 93% excellent and 7% good results with no complications in 17 partial zone II partial flexor tendon lacerations (15 patients) treated with tendon sheath repair only. The lacerations had not initial triggering and involved 55–90% of the tendon width. Similarly, Wray and Weeks[53] reported on partial tendon lacerations in all zones involving up to 95% (mean 60%) of the tendon treated with early mobilization. Twenty-three patients had excellent outcomes, one had good and one had fair. No tendons ruptured. One patient developed a transient trigger finger. McGeorge and coworkers[54] compared 9 patients (12 lacerations) treated nonoperatively to 4 patients (6 fingers) treated with repair of partial tendon lacerations up to 70% of the tendon cross-sectional area. The average cross-sectional area involved 54% (range 20–60%) in the no-repair group compared to an average 35% (range 20–70%) involvement in the repair group. All of the patients in the nonoperative group had excellent outcomes. Four of the six in the repair group had excellent outcomes, two had good outcomes. The no-repair group returned to work sooner and had better pinch grip strength than the repair group. The authors recommended that flexor tendon lacerations of less than 60% cross-sectional area should not be repaired.

In a retrospective review in children,[55] Stahl and coauthors compared repair vs. trimming of lacerated edges only for flexor tendon lacerations of less than 75% cross-sectional area. The mean cross-sectional area for the repair group was slightly higher than the nonrepaired tendons, 42% vs. 38%. A trend toward better outcome was found in the no-repair group although this difference was not significant. Tendon laceration of less than 40% undergoing surgical repair had worse outcomes that those treated without repair although the difference was not significant.

Recommendations

- Partial flexor tendon lacerations of less than 40–60% the cross-sectional area of the entire tendon (that do not trigger) are best treated with early ROM without tendon repair (Table 124.3) [overall quality: moderate]
- Partial tendon ruptures of up to 95% may be treated without tendon repair [overall quality: very low]

Table 124.3 Outcomes following treatment of partial flexor tendon lacerations

Study	Treatment	Patients	Tendons	Cross-sectional area	Excellent	Good	Fair	Complications
al Qattan et al.[52]	No repair	15	17	55–90%	14	1		0
Wray and Weeks[53,a]	No repair	26	34	25–95%	23	1	1	1 (resolved trigger)
McGeorge et al.[54,a]	No repair	12	12	54%	12			0
Stahl et al.[55,a]	No repair	12	19	38%	11	1		1 (infection)
Total (no repair)		65	82		92.3%	4.6%	1.5%	3%
McGeorge et al.[54,a]	Repair	6	8	35%	4	2		1 (joint contracture)
Stahl et al.[55,a]	Repair	11	17	42%	8	3		1 infection
Total (repair)		17	25		70.5%	29.5%		11.7%

[a]Included children.

Case scenario 2

A 28 year old male surgery resident sustained a hyperextension injury to his right long finger while playing football 2 weeks ago. He is unable to flex his DIP and radiographs show a bony fragment in the proximal phalanx consistent with a type II FDP avulsion (see box).[56] The patient requires surgery to restore function to his finger.

Question 4: What is the optimal fixation for FDP avulsion injuries?

Case clarification

You consider methods to secure the FDP tendon to its insertion on the distal phalanx for your patient (scenario 2). What are your best options?

Relevance

Bunnell described the conventional suture repair technique using a pullout suture for repairs of zone I flexor tendon injuries. This surgery is difficult and carries the risk of infection, skin necrosis, and damage to nail bed. The button can get stuck on clothing and other things in the outside environment, causing failure. Good results have been reported with alterative techniques of FDP avulsion fixation.

Classification of FDP avulsions (modified Leddy and Packer classification)[56]

- **Type I:** Tendon retracts into palm, vincula ruptured. Requires early repair
- **Type II:** Tendon retracts to PIP joint, vincula intact. Delayed repair allowed
- **Type III:** Tendon attached to large bony fragment with minimal proximal retraction.
- **Type IV:** Tendon separates from bony fragment and retracts into the palm (subtype I) or PIP (subtype II)

Current opinion

The pullout suture technique is a widely accepted method for treating acute FDP avulsions. Suture anchors, however, are commonly used for a number of orthopedic procedures requiring tendon-to-bone healing.[57–59]

Finding the evidence

- PubMed (www.ncbi.nlm.nih.gov/pubmed/) sensitivity search using keywords "zone I flexor tendon repair" or "flexor tendon" AND "button" OR "suture anchor" or "transverse intraosseous loop technique" OR "TILT"

Quality of the evidence

Level III
- 1 retrospective cohort study

Level IV
- 5 case series

Findings

Gerbino et al.[60] reported a 35% complication rate in his series of 20 zone I flexor tendon repairs. Kang and coworkers[61] reviewed 23 cases of zone I injuries repaired using the pullout button technique. Fifteen of the 23 (65%) patients developed complications including abnormal nail growth, infection, hypersensitivity, and complex regional pain syndrome (CRPS). Moiemen and Elliot reported on zone I flexor tendon injuries, including 23 patients with FDP bone or soft tissue avulsions repaired using the pullout suture method.[62] They had over 50% poor results using their DIP motion criteria. Because of the significant complication rate of the pullout suture technique, alternative methods of fixation have been sought. Suture anchor repairs provide comparable failure loads to the standard pullout suture technique.[63,64] A retrospective review[65] comparing suture pullout repairs to double suture anchor repairs of the FDP in 26 patients reported no failures in either group. The suture pullout group had two superficial infections. There was no statistically significant difference in outcome except improved time to return to work for suture anchor group (9.77 weeks on average vs. 12.23 weeks).

Several authors have reported on various methods of transosseous fixation for FDP fixation. Suture anchor fixation can be complicated by infection, difficulty tensioning the repair, penetration of the dorsal cortex, dislodgement, and increased cost.[63,66,67] There are two small case series on transosseous suture repair methods for FDP avulsions. In one study,[67] 10 out of 12 patients regained full functional ROM while 2 patients developed fixed flexion contractures. One flexion contracture occurred in a child with minimal functional deficit and another in an adult who underwent this procedure after multiple revisions. Teo et al.[66] reported on 18 patients (10 primary, 8 second-stage tendon grafting) using a transosseous suture technique. DIP ROM was good to excellent in 14 patients, fair in 2 and poor in 1 based on Moiemen and Elliot criteria.[62] Kang et al.[68] reported on five cases of FDP avulsion treated with a titanium miniplate. They had one rerupture 2 weeks after surgery. At 1 year, no patient had nail or scar issues or pain. Cost of the implant, hardware complications (failure, infection, prominence) and required extended incision were reported possible disadvantages of the miniplate.

Recommendations

For the treatment of FDP (zone I) avulsions, evidence suggests:
- Pullout suture repairs are still an accepted method of repair. Suture anchor fixation provides a safe alternative to the standard pullout suture technique [overall quality: low]
- Transosseous suture technique may be a cheaper alternative to suture anchors while avoiding complications associated with transcutaneous fixation [overall quality: low]
- There is insufficient data to recommend the use of a plate for fixation of this injury [overall quality: insufficient]

Question 5: What role does botulinum toxin have in the treatment of flexor tendon lacerations?

Case clarification

The patient in scenario 1 undergoes a successful zone II flexor tendon repair of the ring finger. You are concerned the patient will return to work before his tendon is completely healed, risking rupture of the tendon repair. Would injecting botulinum toxin into the muscle belly of the repaired tendon decrease the likelihood of repair failure?

Relevance

Patients must avoid forceful flexion of the finger after flexor tendon repair. Some patients, particularly children,

are unable to comply with these restrictions and risk rupturing their tendon repair. Casting these patients until the tendon heals is not ideal because of the risk of adhesion formation.

Current opinion

Patients who are unable comply with the strict rehabilitation protocol are routinely immobilized to protect the tendon repair. Immobilization, however, risks the development of tendon adhesions and decreasing the strength of the repair.

Finding the evidence

- PubMed (www.ncbi.nlm.nih.gov/pubmed/) sensitivity search or clinical queries search/prognosis using keywords: "Flexor tendon injury" AND "botulinum"

Quality of the evidence

Level IV
- 2 case series

Findings

Silva and coworkers found that a moderate amount of tendon excursion (2 mm) at a low level of tendon force (5 N) was sufficient to inhibit adhesion formation and promote healing.[69] Higher tendon forces increase risk of tendon rupture. Injecting botulinum toxin causes temporary (full muscle recovery in 12–16 weeks) partial denervation, during which the patient can generate enough force to allow early active mobilization but insufficient force to induce gapping or complete disruption of the tendon repair.[70] There are only two small case series on the use of botulinum toxin after flexor tendon repair. Tuzuner and coworkers[71] reviewed seven children under the age of six with zone II flexor tendon repairs. There were 13 flexor tendon injuries (eight fingers) injected intraoperatively with botulinum injections and started on a passive motion rehabilitation protocol. They had five excellent and two good results. There were no infections, tendon ruptures, or adhesions. The botulinum toxin was well tolerated by all patients. Whether or not botulinum toxin necessarily improves outcomes in children under seven years old is unclear. Despite immobilization, primary repair of flexor tendon injuries in these children often have better results than in adults.[72–74]

DeAguiar and associates[70] studied 18 adult patients with 65 repaired tendons. Botulinum was injected within 48 hours of surgery using electromyographic (EMG) guidance. According to the Kleinert and Verdan criteria (see box),[75] 94% of digits (32 of 34) in the botulinum-treated patients reviewed at 18 months had an excellent result and 6% (2 of 34) had a good result.

Kleinert and Verdan criteria[75]

For evaluating outcomes after flexor tendon repair:
- *Excellent:* 85–100% of normal total active motion (TAM)
- *Good:* 70–84% of normal TAM
- *Fair:* 50–69% of normal TAM
- *Poor:* Fixed contracture or adhesions

These patients were compared to a retrospectively reviewed control group of 104 tendon repairs with 81% excellent results (84/104), 6% good, 8% fair, and 6% poor. The group treated with botulinum toxin had statistically better outcomes compared to the control group (p < 0.021).

Recommendation
- There is insufficient evidence to make recommendations on the use of botulinum toxin in flexor tendon repairs [overall quality: insufficient]

Question 6: Are there any pharmacologic or adjuvant therapies to prevent tendon adhesions after flexor tendon repair?

Case clarification
For the patient in scenario 1, you consider if any pharmacologic agent can be administered during the perioperative period to reduce postoperative adhesion formation.

Relevance
Adhesion formation after flexor tendon repair is a major concern. While mobilization after surgery decreases the risk of adhesion formation it may also place the repair at risk of rupture, particularly in patients who are unable to comply with rehabilitation protocols. Others, despite optimal management, still develop adhesions and have poor outcomes. Recent research efforts have focused on pharmacologic and mechanical barriers to prevent adhesions.

Current opinion
Postoperative mobilization is currently the mainstay of preventing adhesion formation after flexor tendon repair. There are several postoperative mobilization regimes that are discussed elsewhere in the literature. Pharmacologic agents are not routinely used in the prevention of adhesions following flexor tendon repair.

Finding the evidence
- PubMed (www.ncbi.nlm.nih.gov/pubmed/) sensitivity or clinical queries search/therapy using keywords: "prevention of adhesions" AND "flexor tendon"

Quality of the evidence
Level I
- 1 systematic review
- 3 RCTs

Level I/II
- 1 RCT without mention of blinding

Findings
Khanna and coauthors[76] reviewed all data reported for pharmacologic agents used to prevent adhesion formation after flexor tendon surgery. These adjuvants are categorized as either medications or barriers. Barriers such as polytetrafluoroethylene (e-FTFE), hydroxyapetatite, hyaluronic acid (HA) membrane, and fascia lata patch grafts have all been tested for prevention of adhesions but have not been tested in humans. Medications such as 5-fluorouracil, human amniotic fluid, and TGF-β have all shown beneficial results in animal models but have yet to be tested in vivo in humans.[77–80] Similarly, several animal studies have shown positive results in the use of nonsteroidal anti-inflammatory drugs (NSAIDs) to prevent tendon adhesions after flexor tendon surgery.[81–83] Animal studies and clinical trials on the effects of HA have shown inconsistent results.[84–86] In a prospective double-blind RCT, sodium hyaluronate or physiological saline solution was injected into the tendon sheath after completion of tenorrhaphy or tendon grafting in 120 digits. Sodium hyaluronate had no significant effect on TAM at follow-up of at least 4 months.[87] Two studies (75 patients/80 fingers)[88,89] showed no significant difference in total ROM between controls and patients treated with ADCON-T/N after tenorrhaphy. ADCON-T/N is a glycosaminoglycan-rich bioresorbable gel similar to HA. Liew and coauthors[90] demonstrated patients treated with ADCON-T/N had significantly better PIP motion (87% vs. 68%, p = 0.005), whereas DIP motion, hand grip, and pinch strength showed no differences. The rate of rerupture after tendon repairs did not differ significantly in any of the three studies. Golash and others,[88,89] however, observed a trend toward late rupture and inflammatory skin changes in patients treated with ADCON-T/N, raising concerns about its potential inhibitory effects on tendon healing.

Recommendation
- Hyaluoronic acid and other pharmacologic agents have not been shown to provide significant benefit in preventing tendon adhesions after flexor tendon repair [overall quality: moderate]

Question 7: What is the role of imaging in evaluating flexor tendon injuries and the status of flexor tendon repairs postoperatively?

Case clarification
The patient in scenario 1 undergoes a zone II flexor tendon repair of the FDS and FDP of his ring finger. After six weeks, the patient feels better and returns to work. Three weeks later, he returns to the office complaining that he is

unable to actively flex his ring finger. After a complete physical examination, what is the best way to evaluate the status of his repair?

Relevance

Although the diagnosis of flexor tendon lacerations is often straightforward, in cases of nerve injury, fractures, or uncooperative patients, the diagnosis becomes more complicated. Following flexor tendon repairs, it may be difficult to determine if loss of active flexion is caused by adhesions or rupture. In case of rupture, prompt surgical treatment would be more suitable than continuing with physical therapy.

Current opinion

Current opinion suggests that ultrasound and MRI are important tools for determining the extent of partial flexor tendon injuries, the location of ruptured tendon ends and determining the status of a repaired flexor tendon laceration.

Finding the evidence

- PubMed (www.ncbi.nlm.nih.gov/pubmed/) sensitivity search using keywords: "ultrasound" OR "ultrasonography" OR AND "flexor tendon laceration" OR "flexor tendon injuries" OR 'flexor tendon repair" AND "hand"
- PubMed (www.ncbi.nlm.nih.gov/pubmed/) sensitivity search using keywords: "MR" or "MRI" or "imaging" and "flexor tendon injuries" OR "flexor tendon repair" AND "hand"
- PubMed (www.ncbi.nlm.nih.gov/pubmed/) sensitivity search using keywords: "MRI" and "flexor tendons" and "rupture"
- PubMed (www.ncbi.nlm.nih.gov/pubmed/) clinical queries search/diagnosis: "flexor tendon injuries" AND "hand"

Quality of the evidence

Level III
- 1 case-control study

Level IV
- 3 case series
- 1 case-control study with small number of patients

Level V
- 1 study

Findings

Ultrasound Khaleghain and colleagues first showed that ultrasound could be used to determine the structure of normal and pathologic flexor tendons.[91] Later, McGeorge and McGeorge[92] described the normal appearance of flexor tendon repairs. Lee and coauthors[93] evaluated 13 injured

digits in 10 hands. Dynamic ultrasound accurately determined the status of 11 of 13 digits and 18 of 20 potentially injured flexor tendons. All patients had associated injuries requiring surgical exploration and repair, which allowed confirmation of ultrasound findings. The surgeon was blinded to the ultrasound results. There were two cases of false-positive findings. Ultrasound identified a 75% laceration in an intact index FDP and a complete FDP laceration in a 75% lacerated tendon. The finding of a 75% laceration in an intact tendon was attributed to air artifact in a newly closed wound and lack of active motion secondary to pain. A 50% partial tear in the same digit was also identified. It also correctly identified the location of the proximal tendon stump in five of six lacerations. They suggested that ultrasound might be useful in patients where examination is difficult, such as in children. Another study evaluated 30 patients with hand injuries using ultrasound.[94] Six patients who were unable to flex their digit underwent surgical intervention after ultrasound evaluated the status of the flexor tendon. In three cases, tendon rupture and location of tendon ends based on ultrasound was confirmed. Three other patients, who underwent surgery for other reason, had intact tendons by ultrasound that was confirmed intraoperatively. The authors warned image resolution is limited to tissue depth and therefore could only be used in the hand and finger, allowing for dynamic examination at less cost than an MRI scan.

Corduff and colleagues[95] used dynamic ultrasound to assess TAM of the PIP and DIP after flexor tendon repair in 22 patients. Based on Strickland's criteria, 41% had excellent and 36% had good results. Only 5% had poor results. The assessment based on ultrasound showed only 27% had normal appearance while 32% had thickened, but well gliding, tendon. Two of three tendons that were ruptured on ultrasound were classified as good or fair according to Strickland's criterion. In addition, tendons found to have dense scar tissue had been graded as "good" or "fair." This study suggests ultrasound may be a more accurate measure of repair status than the Strickland method. This is however, the only study that compares clinical examination to ultrasound in the diagnosis of postoperative outcomes of flexor tendon repair.

MRI Several authors have reported on the value of MRI in evaluating flexor tendon pathology.[96,97] Drape and authors[98] used MRI to evaluate the status of flexor tendon repairs in patients who had poor outcomes. MRI was performed on 51 patients (64 tendons) who had not regained active flexion after flexor tendon repair. The control group was seven patients (eight fingers) with good clinical outcomes following flexor tendon repair. Of the 64 fingers, 41 underwent reoperation. MRI diagnosis of tendon rupture was confirmed at the time of surgery in 10 cases. Eleven patients diagnosed with callus elongation underwent surgery.

Intraoperatively, two of these cases were noted to have adhesions without elongation (sensitivity 100%, specificity 94%). Isolated adhesions on MRI were confirmed at time of surgery in 20 patients (sensitivity 91%, specificity 100%). Focal bowstringing was found in 15 cases and confirmed intraoperatively in each. MRI failed to identify injured pulleys in nine cases.

Few studies have been performed on the role of MRI in diagnosing primary tendon ruptures. Kumar and coauthors[99] performed MRI on four patients with suspected zone I FDP rupture. MRI showed proximal retraction of the profundus tendon to the palm in two patients and limited retraction in the other two. Of these, two underwent hand exploration of the tendon and repair whereas two others had DIP fusion without confirmation of findings. According to the authors, MRI provided important preoperative information for surgical decision-making and planning in patients who present late with closed flexor tendon injuries of the hand. In a case series,[100] 10 patients with suspected closed tendon rupture underwent MRI imaging. Twelve flexor tendon ruptures were identified on MRI and confirmed at the time of surgery. MRI also accurately assessed the gap between tendon ends.

Recommendations

• Evidence suggests both MRI and ultrasound are able to accurately diagnose flexor tendon ruptures and causes for poor postoperative motion after flexor tendon repair. In cases of tendon retraction, MRI and ultrasound accurately locate tendon ends [overall quality: low]
• Whether or not imaging flexor tendon injuries and repairs is cost-effective or provides any decrease in morbidity (i.e., morbidity from increased incision and operative time trying to locating retracted tendon ends) has not been addressed [overall quality: insufficient]
• There is insufficient evidence to determine if MRI or ultrasound accurately evaluates partial tendon ruptures [overall quality: insufficient]
• There is limited data to support the use of imaging over physical exam in evaluating causes of poor outcome following flexor tendon repair [overall quality: insufficient].

Summary of recommendations

• For repair of zone II flexor tendon injuries a four-strand or higher core suture technique supplemented by running epitendinous sutures are recommended to provide sufficient tensile strength to allow for postoperative active or passive motion rehabilitation
• Dorsal placement of the suture and locking (vs. grasping) and increasing the number of grasps or locks improves results of repair

• Flexor tendon lacerations should be repaired with non-absorbable 3-0 or 4-0 braided polyester sutures
• Clinical research suggests Tenofix is safe and effective in the repair of flexor tendon lacerations but may not be suitable in all cases
• Partial flexor tendon lacerations of less than 40–60% the cross-sectional area of the entire tendon (that do not trigger) are best treated with early ROM without tendon repair
• For the treatment of FDP avulsions (zone I), evidence suggests suture anchor fixation provide a safe alternative to the standard pullout suture technique for repairs of FDP avulsions. Transosseous suture technique may be a cheaper alternative to suture anchors while avoiding complications associated with transcutaneous fixation
• Currently, there is insufficient evidence to make recommendations on the use of botulinum toxin in flexor tendon repairs
• HA and other pharmacologic agents have not been shown to provide significant benefit in preventing tendon adhesions after flexor tendon repair
• Evidence suggests both MRI and ultrasound are able to accurately diagnose flexor tendon ruptures, location of ruptured ends and causes for poor postoperative motion after flexor tendon repair
• Whether or not imaging flexor tendon injuries and repairs is cost-effective or provides any decrease in morbidity has not been addressed

Conclusions

Our improved understanding of flexor tendon healing has led to better outcomes following flexor tendon repairs. Recovery of good or excellent function is achieved in over 80% of cases with strong repair and early postoperative motion. Repair rupture, adhesions and joint stiffness remain frustrating complications. Future research will no doubt lead to better understanding of how to prevent and treat these difficult problems.

References

1. Doyle JR. Anatomy of the finger flexor tendon sheath and pulley system. J Hand Surg Am 1988;13(4):473–84.
2. Strickland JW. Development of flexor tendon surgery: twenty-five years of progress. J Hand Surg 2000;25(2):214–35.
3. Ochiai N, Matsui T, Miyaji N, Merklin RJ, Hunter JM. Vascular anatomy of flexor tendons. I. Vincular system and blood supply of the profundus tendon in the digital sheath. J Hand Surg Am 1979;4(4):321–30.
4. Verdan C. Syndrome of the quadriga. Surg Clin North Am 1960;40:425–6.
5. Verdan CE. Half a century of flexor-tendon surgery. Current status and changing philosophies. J Bone Joint Surg Am 1972;54(3):472–91.

6. Hill C, Riaz M, Mozzam A, Brennen MD. A regional audit of hand and wrist injuries. A study of 4873 injuries. J Hand Surg Br 1998;23(2):196–200.

7. Rosberg HE, Carlsson KS, Hojgard S, Lindgren B, Lundborg G, Dahlin LB. What determines the costs of repair and rehabilitation of flexor tendon injuries in zone II? A multiple regression analysis of data from southern Sweden. J Hand Surg Br 2003; 28(2):106–12.

8. Savage R. In vitro studies of a new method of flexor tendon repair. J Hand Surg Br 1985;10(2):135–41.

9. Urbaniak JR, Cahill JD, Mortenson RA. Tendon suture methods: analysis of tensile strength. AAOS Symposium on Tendon Surgery in the Hand, pp. 70–80. Mosby, St. Louis, 1975.

10. Alavanja G, Dailey E, Mass DP. Repair of zone II flexor digitorum profundus lacerations using varying suture sizes: a comparative biomechanical study. J Hand Surg 2005;30(3): 448–54.

11. McLarney E, Hoffman H, Wolfe SW. Biomechanical analysis of the cruciate four-strand flexor tendon repair. J Hand Surg 1999;24(2):295–301.

12. Savage R, Risitano G. Flexor tendon repair using a "six strand" method of repair and early active mobilisation. J Hand Surg Br 1989;14(4):396–9.

13. Su BW, Raia FJ, Quitkin HM, Parisien M, Strauch RJ, Rosenwasser MP. Gross and histological analysis of healing after dog flexor tendon repair with the Teno Fix device. J Hand Surg Br 2006;31(5):524–9.

14. Tang JB, Gu YT, Rice K, Chen F, Pan CZ. Evaluation of four methods of flexor tendon repair for postoperative active mobilization. Plast Reconstr Surg 2001;107(3):742–9.

15. Thurman RT, Trumble TE, Hanel DP, Tencer AF, Kiser PK. Two-, four-, and six-strand zone II flexor tendon repairs: an in situ biomechanical comparison using a cadaver model. J Hand Surg Am 1998;23(2):261–5.

16. Xie RG, Zhang S, Tang JB, Chen F. Biomechanical studies of 3 different 6-strand flexor tendon repair techniques. J Hand Surg 2002;27(4):621–7.

17. Stein T, Ali A, Hamman J, Mass DP. A randomized biomechanical study of zone II human flexor tendon repairs analyzed in an in vitro model. J Hand Surg 1998;23(6):1046–51.

18. Su BW, Solomons M, Barrow A, et al. Device for zone-II flexor tendon repair. A multicenter, randomized, blinded, clinical trial. J Bone Joint Surg Am 2005;87(5):923–35.

19. Wade PJ, Wetherell RG, Amis AA. Flexor tendon repair: significant gain in strength from the Halsted peripheral suture technique. J Hand Surg Br 1989;14(2):232–5.

20. Komanduri M, Phillips CS, Mass DP. Tensile strength of flexor tendon repairs in a dynamic cadaver model. J Hand Surg 1996;21(4):605–11.

21. Soejima O, Diao E, Lotz JC, Hariharan JS. Comparative mechanical analysis of dorsal versus palmar placement of core suture for flexor tendon repairs. J Hand Surg 1995;20(5): 801–7.

22. Hatanaka H, Manske PR. Effect of the cross-sectional area of locking loops in flexor tendon repair. J Hand Surg 1999;24(4): 751–60.

23. Hatanaka H, Zhang J, Manske PR. An in vivo study of locking and grasping techniques using a passive mobilization protocol in experimental animals. J Hand Surg 2000;25(2):260–9.

24. Osada D, Fujita S, Tamai K, Yamaguchi T, Iwamoto A, Saotome K. Flexor tendon repair in zone II with 6-strand techniques and early active mobilization. J Hand Surg Am 2006;31(6): 987–92.

25. Rocchi L, Merolli A, Genzini A, Merendi G, Catalano F. Flexor tendon injuries of the hand treated with TenoFix(TM): midterm results. J Orthop Traumatol 2008;9(4):201–8.

26. Strickland JW, Glogovac SV. Digital function following flexor tendon repair in Zone II: A comparison of immobilization and controlled passive motion techniques. J Hand Surg Am 1980;5(6):537–43.

27. Chow JA, Thomes LJ, Dovelle S, Monsivais J, Milnor WH, Jackson JP. Controlled motion rehabilitation after flexor tendon repair and grafting. A multi-centre study. J Bone Joint Surg Br 1988;70(4):591–5.

28. Cullen KW, Tolhurst P, Lang D, Page RE. Flexor tendon repair in zone 2 followed by controlled active mobilisation. J Hand Surg Br 1989;14(4):392–5.

29. Baktir A, Turk CY, Kabak S, Sahin V, Kardas Y. Flexor tendon repair in zone 2 followed by early active mobilization. J Hand Surg Br 1996;21(5):624–8.

30. Silfverskiold KL, May EJ. Flexor tendon repair in zone II with a new suture technique and an early mobilization program combining passive and active flexion. J Hand Surg 1994;19(1): 53–60.

31. Kitsis CK, Wade PJ, Krikler SJ, Parsons NK, Nicholls LK. Controlled active motion following primary flexor tendon repair: a prospective study over 9 years. J Hand Surg Br 1998; 23(3):344–9.

32. Hoffmann GL, Buchler U, Vogelin E. Clinical results of flexor tendon repair in zone II using a six-strand double-loop technique compared with a two-strand technique. J Hand Surg Eur 2008;33(4):418–23.

33. Lee H. Double loop locking suture: a technique of tendon repair for early active mobilization. Part I: Evolution of technique and experimental study. J Hand Surg 1990;15(6):945–52.

34. Klein L. Early active motion flexor tendon protocol using one splint. J Hand Ther 2003;16(3):199–206.

35. Caulfield RH, Maleki-Tabrizi A, Patel H, Coldham F, Mee S, Nanchahal J. Comparison of zones 1 to 4 flexor tendon repairs using absorbable and unabsorbable four-strand core sutures. J Hand Surg Eur 2008;33(4):412–17.

36. Sandow MJ, McMahon MM. Single cross-grasp six-strand repair for flexor tenorrhaphy modified Savage technique. Atlas Hand Clin 1996;1:41–64.

37. Su BW, Protopsaltis TS, Koff MF, Chang KP, Strauch RJ, Crow SA, et al. The biomechanical analysis of a tendon fixation device for flexor tendon repair. J Hand Surg 2005;30(2): 237–45.

38. Smith JH, Jr. Avulsion of a profundus tendon with simultaneous intraarticular fracture of the distal phalanx—case report. J Hand Surg Am 1981;6(6):600–1.

39. Nystrom B, Holmlund D. Separation of sutured tendon ends when different suture techniques and different suture materials are used. An experimental study in rabbits. Scand J Plast Reconstr Surg 1983;17(1):19–23.

40. Lawrence TM, Davis TR. A biomechanical analysis of suture materials and their influence on a four-strand flexor tendon repair. J Hand Surg 2005;30(4):836–41.

41. Hatanaka H, Manske PR. Effect of suture size on locking and grasping flexor tendon repair techniques. Clin Orthop Relat Res 2000;375:267–74.

42. Taras JS, Raphael JS, Marczyk SC, Bauerle WB. Evaluation of suture caliber in flexor tendon repair. J Hand Surg 2001;26(6):1100–4.

43. Wolfe SW, Willis AA, Campbell D, Clabeaux J, Wright TM. Biomechanic comparison of the Teno Fix tendon repair device with the cruciate and modified Kessler techniques. J Hand Surg Am 2007;32(3):356–66.

44. Peck FH, Bucher CA, Watson JS, Roe A. A comparative study of two methods of controlled mobilization of flexor tendon repairs in zone 2. J Hand Surg Br 1998;23(1):41–5.

45. Trail IA, Powell ES, Noble J. An evaluation of suture materials used in tendon surgery. J Hand Surg Br 1989;14(4):422–7.

46. Mashadi ZB, Amis AA. Variation of holding strength of synthetic absorbable flexor tendon sutures with time. J Hand Surg Br 1992;17(3):278–81.

47. O'Broin ES, Earley MJ, Smyth H, Hooper AC. Absorbable sutures in tendon repair. A comparison of PDS with prolene in rabbit tendon repair. J Hand Surg Br 1995;20(4):505–8.

48. Schecter WP, Markison RE, Jeffrey RB, Barton RM, Laing F. Use of sonography in the early detection of suppurative flexor tenosynovitis. J Hand Surg Am 1989;14(2 Pt 1):307–10.

49. Ollinger H, Wray RC, Jr., Weeks PM. Effects of suture on tensile strength gain of partially and completely severed tendons. Surg Forum 1975;26:63–4.

50. Reynolds B, Wray RC, Jr., Weeks PM. Should an incompletely severed tendon be sutured? Plast Reconstr Surg 1976;57(1):36–8.

51. Harihanan JS, Diao E, Soejima O, Lotz JC. Partial lacerations of human digital flexor tendons: a biomechanical analysis. J Hand Surg Am 1997;22(6):1011–15.

52. al-Qattan MM. Conservative management of zone II partial flexor tendon lacerations greater than half the width of the tendon. J Hand Surg Am 2000;25(6):1118–21.

53. Wray RC, Jr., Weeks PM. Treatment of partial tendon lacerations. Hand 1980;12(2):163–6.

54. McGeorge DD, Stilwell JH. Partial flexor tendon injuries: to repair or not. J Hand Surg Br 1992;17(2):176–7.

55. Stahl S, Kaufman T, Bialik V. Partial lacerations of flexor tendons in children. Primary repair versus conservative treatment. J Hand Surg Br 1997;22(3):377–80.

56. Leddy JP, Packer JW. Avulsion of the profundus tendon insertion in athletes. J Hand Surg Am 1977;2(1):66–9.

57. Hallock GG. The Mitek Mini GII anchor introduced for tendon reinsertion in the hand. Ann Plast Surg 1994;33(2):211–13.

58. Schultz RO, Drake DB, Morgan RF. A new technique for the treatment of flexor digitorum profundus tendon avulsion. Ann Plast Surg 1999;42(1):46–8.

59. Skoff HD, Hecker AT, Hayes WC, Sebell-Sklar R, Straughn N. Bone suture anchors in hand surgery. J Hand Surg Br 1995;20(2):245–8.

60. Gerbino PG, 2nd, Saldana MJ, Westerbeck P, Schacherer TG. Complications experienced in the rehabilitation of zone I flexor tendon injuries with dynamic traction splinting. J Hand Surg Am 1991;16(4):680–6.

61. Kang N, Marsh D, Dewar D. The morbidity of the button-over-nail technique for zone 1 flexor tendon repairs. Should we still be using this technique? J Hand Surg Eur 2008;33(5):566–70.

62. Moiemen NS, Elliot D. Primary flexor tendon repair in zone 1. J Hand Surg Br 2000;25(1):78–84.

63. Buch BD, Innis P, McClinton MA, Kotani Y. The Mitek Mini G2 suture anchor: biomechanical analysis of use in the hand. J Hand Surg Am 1995;20(5):877–81.

64. Matsuzaki H, Zaegel MA, Gelberman RH, Silva MJ. Effect of suture material and bone quality on the mechanical properties of zone I flexor tendon-bone reattachment with bone anchors. J Hand Surg Am 2008;33(5):709–17.

65. McCallister WV, Ambrose HC, Katolik LI, Trumble TE. Comparison of pullout button versus suture anchor for zone I flexor tendon repair. J Hand Surg Am 2006;31(2):246–51.

66. Teo TC, Dionyssiou D, Armenio A, Ng D, Skillman J. Anatomical repair of zone 1 flexor tendon injuries. Plast Reconstr Surg 2009;123(2):617–22.

67. Tripathi AK, Mee SN, Martin DL, Katsarma E. The "transverse intraosseous loop technique" (TILT) to re-insert flexor tendons in zone 1. J Hand Surg Eur 2009;34(1):85–9.

68. Kang N, Pratt A, Burr N. Miniplate fixation for avulsion injuries of the flexor digitorum profundus insertion. J Hand Surg Br 2003;28(4):363–8.

69. Silva JM, Zhao C, An KN, Zobitz ME, Amadio PC. Gliding resistance and strength of composite sutures in human flexor digitorum profundus tendon repair: an in vitro biomechanical study. J Hand Surg Am 2009;34(1):87–92.

70. De Aguiar G, Chait LA, Schultz D, et al. Chemoprotection of flexor tendon repairs using botulinum toxin. Plast Reconstr Surg 2009;124(1):201–9.

71. Tuzuner S, Balci N, Ozkaynak S. Results of zone II flexor tendon repair in children younger than age 6 years: botulinum toxin type A administration eased cooperation during the rehabilitation and improved outcome. J Pediatr Orthop 2004;24(6):629–33.

72. Elhassan B, Moran SL, Bravo C, Amadio P. Factors that influence the outcome of zone I and zone II flexor tendon repairs in children. J Hand Surg Am 2006;31(10):1661–6.

73. Masquelet AC, Gilbert A. [Recent injuries of finger flexor tendons in children]. Rev Chir Orthop Reparatrice Appar Mot 1985;71(8):587–93.

74. Strickland JW. Bone, nerve, and tendon injuries of the hand in children. Pediatr Clin North Am 1975;22(2):451–63.

75. Kleinert HE, Verdan C. Report of the Committee on Tendon Injuries (International Federation of Societies for Surgery of the Hand). J Hand Surg Am 1983;8(5 Pt 2):794–8.

76. Khanna A, Friel M, Gougoulias N, Longo UG, Maffulli N. Prevention of adhesions in surgery of the flexor tendons of the hand: what is the evidence? Br Med Bull 2009;90:85–109.

77. Cerovac S, Afoke A, Akali A, Mc GD. Early breaking strength of repaired flexor tendon treated with 5-fluorouracil. J Hand Surg Br 2001;26(3):220–3.

78. Khan U, Kakar S, Akali A, Bentley G, McGrouther DA. Modulation of the formation of adhesions during the healing of injured tendons. J Bone Joint Surg Br 2000;82(7):1054–8.

79. Ozgenel GY, Samli B, Ozcan M. Effects of human amniotic fluid on peritendinous adhesion formation and tendon healing after flexor tendon surgery in rabbits. J Hand Surg Am 2001;26(2):332–9.

80. Zhang AY, Pham H, Ho F, Teng K, Longaker MT, Chang J. Inhibition of TGF-beta-induced collagen production in rabbit flexor tendons. J Hand Surg Am 2004;29(2):230–5.

81. Kulick MI, Brazlow R, Smith S, Hentz VR. Injectable ibuprofen: preliminary evaluation of its ability to decrease peritendinous adhesions. Ann Plast Surg 1984;13(6):459–67.

82. Kulick MI, Smith S, Hadler K. Oral ibuprofen: evaluation of its effect on peritendinous adhesions and the breaking strength of a tenorrhaphy. J Hand Surg Am 1986;11(1):110–20.

83. Szabo RM, Younger E. Effects of indomethacin on adhesion formation after repair of zone II tendon lacerations in the rabbit. J Hand Surg Am 1990;15(3):480–3.

84. Akasaka T, Nishida J, Araki S, Shimamura T, Amadio PC, An KN. Hyaluronic acid diminishes the resistance to excursion after flexor tendon repair: an in vitro biomechanical study. J Biomech 2005;38(3):503–7.

85. Tanaka T, Zhao C, Sun YL, Zobitz ME, An KN, Amadio PC. The effect of carbodiimide-derivatized hyaluronic acid and gelatin surface modification on peroneus longus tendon graft in a short-term canine model in vivo. J Hand Surg Am 2007;32(6): 876–81.

86. Zhao C, Sun YL, Amadio PC, Tanaka T, Ettema AM, An KN. Surface treatment of flexor tendon autografts with carbodiimide-derivatized hyaluronic Acid. An in vivo canine model. J Bone Joint Surg Am 2006;88(10):2181–91.

87. Hagberg L. Exogenous hyaluronate as an adjunct in the prevention of adhesions after flexor tendon surgery: a controlled clinical trial. J Hand Surg 1992;17(1):132–6.

88. Golash A, Kay A, Warner JG, Peck F, Watson JS, Lees VC. Efficacy of ADCON-T/N after primary flexor tendon repair in Zone II: a controlled clinical trial. J Hand Surg Br 2003;28(2): 113–15.

89. Mentzel M, Hoss H, Keppler P, Ebinger T, Kinzl L, Wachter NJ. The effectiveness of ADCON-T/N, a new anti-adhesion barrier gel, in fresh divisions of the flexor tendons in Zone II. J Hand Surg Br 2000;25(6):590–2.

90. Liew SH, Potokar T, Bantick GL, Morgan I, Ford C, Murison MS. The use of ADCON-T/N after repair of zone II flexor tendons. Chir Main 2001;20(5):384–7.

91. Khaleghian R, Tonkin LJ, De Geus JJ, Lee JP. Ultrasonic examination of the flexor tendons of the fingers. J Clin Ultrasound 1984;12(9):547–51.

92. McGeorge DD, McGeorge S. Diagnostic medical ultrasound in the management of hand injuries. J Hand Surg Br 1990;15(2): 256–61.

93. Lee DH, Robbin ML, Galliott R, Graveman VA. Ultrasound evaluation of flexor tendon lacerations. J Hand Surg Am 2000;25(2):236–41.

94. Wang PT, Bonavita JA, DeLone FX, Jr., McClellan RM, Witham RS. Ultrasonic assistance in the diagnosis of hand flexor tendon injuries. Ann Plast Surg 1999;42(4):403–7.

95. Corduff N, Jones R, Ball J. The role of ultrasound in the management of zone 1 flexor tendon injuries. J Hand Surg Br 1994;19(1):76–80.

96. Matloub HS, Dzwierzynski WW, Erickson S, Sanger JR, Yousif NJ, Muoneke V. Magnetic resonance imaging scanning in the diagnosis of zone II flexor tendon rupture. J Hand Surg Am 1996;21(3):451–5.

97. Rubin DA, Kneeland JB, Kitay GS, Naranja RJ, Jr. Flexor tendon tears in the hand: use of MR imaging to diagnose degree of injury in a cadaver model. AJR Am J Roentgenol 1996;166(3): 615–20.

98. Drape JL, Silbermann-Hoffman O, Houvet P, et al. Complications of flexor tendon repair in the hand: MR imaging assessment. Radiology 1996;198(1):219–24.

99. Kumar BA, Tolat AR, Threepuraneni G, Jones B. The role of magnetic resonance imaging in late presentation of isolated injuries of the flexor digitorum profundus tendon in the finger. J Hand Surg Br 2000;25(1):95–7.

100. Drape JL, Tardif-Chastenet de Gery S, Silbermann-Hoffman O, et al. Closed ruptures of the flexor digitorum tendons: MRI evaluation. Skeletal Radiol 1998;27(11):617–24.

125 Replantation

Stephanie Ma, Leslie L. McKnight, and Achilleas Thoma
McMaster University, Hamilton, ON, Canada

Case scenario

A 32 year old carpenter is seen in the Emergency Department of your community hospital. He has suffered a clean amputation of the long finger of his dominant hand by a table saw at the level of the proximal phalanx. This injury occurred 5 hours earlier in a remote location and the digit was immediately placed on ice.

Relevant anatomy

Because digit replantation involves many structures, a definite sequence of procedures must be undertaken to ensure a timely and efficient repair. This sequence includes:
1. Copious irrigation and meticulous debridement
2. Identification and tagging of structures via a mid-lateral or other exposure (Figure 125.1)
3. Shortening of bone by 5–10 mm
4. Stabilization of bone (Figure 125.2)
5. Repair of extensor and flexor tendons
6. Nerve repair
7. Arterial anastomoses
8. Venous anastomoses
9. Skin closure

Importance of the problem

These injuries and their sequelae are potentially life-threatening and/or life-altering. Trauma is the second leading cause of amputation after vascular disease, accounting for 22% of amputations with 69% involving the upper extremities. An estimated 30,673 persons suffer non-work-related digit amputations alone in the United States every year. Each digit replantation incurs an approximate hospital cost of $18,000–$27,000, an underestimate when one considers the substantial associated indirect costs.[1]

Top five questions

1. Should digit replantation be performed only in tertiary hospitals?
2. Does single-digit replantation as compared to revision amputation lead to a better functional outcome?
3. Should two veins and one artery be anastomosed, or does one vein and artery suffice?
4. Should anticoagulant and/or antithrombotic agents be used postoperatively?
5. Does early range of motion (ROM) therapy following replantation improve outcome?

Question 1: Should digit replantation be performed only in tertiary hospitals?

Case clarification
As you prepare this patient for an emergency replantation, you consider transferring him to the closest tertiary hospital, knowing this will prolong ischemia time.

Relevance
Although amputations often present first to community hospitals, the published literature has focused almost exclusively on interventions performed and outcomes obtained in tertiary medical centers.

Evidence-Based Orthopedics, First Edition. Edited by Mohit Bhandari.
© 2012 Blackwell Publishing Ltd. Published 2012 by Blackwell Publishing Ltd.

Current opinion
Many microsurgeons recommend the transfer of community patients to larger tertiary hospitals.

Finding the evidence
• Cochrane Database, with search term: "replantation"
• PubMed and Medline search using keywords: "replantation" AND "community hospital" OR "peripheral hospital" OR "academic hospital" OR "tertiary hospital" OR "centralized"

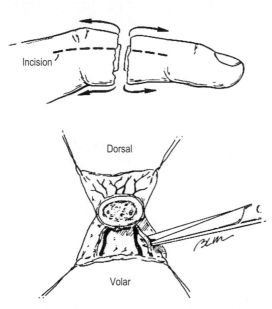

Figure 125.1 Mid-lateral incisions for enhanced eposure, identification, and tagging of the various microvascular structures. (Reproduced with permission from Goldner RD, Urbaniack JR. Replantation. Chapter 45 in: Green DP, Hotchkiss RN, Pederson WC, eds., Operative Hand Surgery, 5th edn, pp. 1569–1586. Churchill Livingstone, Philadelphia, 1998.)

• Embase, ACP Pier, and CINAHL
• Cross-references

Quality of the evidence
Level IV
• 3 studies

Findings
Two studies examined the issue of microsurgery survival rates in community hospitals. Isenberg prospectively collected data on 41 replantations and 26 revascularizations (mean ischemic time 2h 50min), calculating an overall survival rate of 87%. All nine failures involved replantations of crushed-avulsed single digits, downgrading the actual success rate for replantations alone to 78%.[2] Pomerance et al. ascertained a similar overall survival rate of 88% in 151 cases of digit replantations and revascularizations, for a replantation-specific survival rate of 84% (n = 96/114).[3]

Braga-Silva conducted a trial of single-digit replantations in the ambulatory setting (n = 85 digit replantations) where patients were monitored for up to 8 hours postoperatively before same-day discharge home. Their achieved success rate of 86% (n = 73/85) compared to that of replantations performed in tertiary hospitals (86.2%) with the associated routine admission and inpatient monitoring.[4] None of the failed replantations was due to a diagnostic delay secondary to patients omitting to contact the surgeon.[5]

Recommendation
• Survival rates for replantations performed in community hospitals with trained microsurgeons are comparable to those of tertiary hospitals [overall quality: low]

Figure 125.2 Different options for achieving bony stabilization. (a) Intramedullary longitudinal Kirschner wire; (b) Intraosseous wiring; (c) Crossed Kirschner wires; (d) Intramedullary bone screw; (e) Plate and screws. (Reproduced with permission from Goldner RD, Urbaniack JR. Replantation. Chapter 45 in: Green DP, Hotchkiss RN, Pederson WC, eds., Operative Hand Surgery, 5th edn, pp. 1569–1586. Churchill Livingstone, Philadelphia, 1998.)

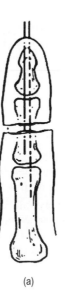 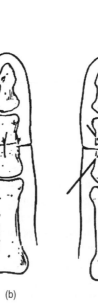 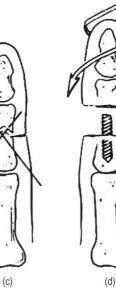 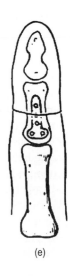

(a)　　(b)　　(c)　　(d)　　(e)

Question 2: Does single-digit replantation as compared to revision amputation lead to a better functional outcome?

Case clarification

You decide to manage the patient in your community hospital. He asks if replantation is the treatment option that will confer the best functional results.

Relevance

Traditionally, the success of digit replantation has been measured by survival rate. However, even a viable digit may impair the functional ability of the hand and delay or prevent return to previous occupation.

Current opinion

Many authors advocate that a single-digit amputation (excluding thumb and pediatric cases) warrants replantation under particular circumstances, whereas others claim that it represents an absolute-to-relative contraindication.

Finding the evidence

• As for Question 1, but using keywords: "replantation" AND "single digit" OR "single finger" AND "functional outcome" OR "hand function" OR "return to work" OR "manual labor"

Quality of the evidence

Level II
• 1 study

Level IV
• 6 studies

Findings

Three major indications for single-digit replantation were identified in the literature, although the level of evidence was low: (1) digits amputated at a level distal to the flexor digitorum superficialis (FDS) tendon insertion,[6–12] (2) digits amputated at the level of the distal phalynx,[13–15] (3) type II and type IIIa ring avulsion injuries.[13,16]

Contraindications for single-digit replantation include amputations at the level of the proximal phalanx or proximal interphalangeal (PIP) joint, especially if avulsed or crushed, massively contaminated wounds, and complete ring avulsion injuries.[7,8,13] Relative contraindications encompass amputations proximal to the FDS insertion, single border digits (i.e., index and little fingers), and prolonged warm ischemia time.[8]

Goel et al. found that revision amputation led to a superior functional outcome, with 90.0% (9/10) of these patients rating their result as good to excellent as compared to only 44.4% (4/9) of replantation patients (p < 0.05).[17] Hattori et al. (level IIb evidence) found replantation improved

Table 125.1 Summary of Hattori et al.'s results for fingertip amputations[18]

	Replantation (n = 23)	Revision amputation (n = 23)
Pain (n)[a]	2	14
Paresthesia (n)	7	7
Cold intolerance (n)	8	10
Flexion of PIP joint (°)[a]	94 ± 10	86 ± 15
DASH score[a]	2 ± 3	7 ± 5
Hospital stay (day)[a]	25 ± 6	3 ± 4
Time off work (months)[a]	4 ± 4	1 ± 1
Total direct hospital cost ($)	14,379	2,808

[a]The authors found a statistically significant difference between groups.

hand function, ROM, and postoperative pain compared to revision amputation, but that revision amputation conferred shorter length of hospital stay and time lost from work, as well as lower direct costs (Table 125.1).[18]

Patient satisfaction In Waikakul et al.'s prospective study (n = 745 digit replantations), all 291 patients who had undergone single-digit replantation were satisfied regardless of suboptimal functional outcome. None required a revision amputation or would have retrospectively preferred a primary amputation. This finding was in contrast to that of Goel et al. (n = 19 patients; 9 replantations, 10 amputations), whereby 66.6% of patients who had undergone single-digit replantation would have retrospectively chosen to have a primary amputation. Moreover, only 44.4% of patients in the replantation group rated their function as good to excellent vs. the 90.0% of those in the amputation group, although they rated equally in terms of appearance.[9]

It is worth noting that certain patients give as much importance to physical appearance as they do to function, for various cultural or religious reasons. Thus, hand surgeons must be cognizant of the influences that these beliefs can play in the patient's decision to undergo digit replantation.

Return to work Time off work varied between 2.3 and 10.0 months,[7,17,19] with a shorter return to work following revision amputation than replantation, at 6.64 vs. 40 weeks.[17] Boeckx et al. (n = 34 digit replantations) found that 61.5% (n = 8/13) of patients who were employed before their injury were able to return to their original work, while 15.4% (n = 2/13) were still too disabled to work 4 years after replantation.[20] All 23 replantation and 23 amputation patients returned to original work in Hattori's review of fingertip injuries.[18]

Complications Although the reported incidence of postreplantation cold intolerance ranges from 35% and 82%, it did not correlate with DASH scores.[17] Povlsen (n = 8 digit replantations) determined that patients who rated their cold-induced discomfort as moderate 2 years after replantation went on to experience long-term improvement upon reassessment one decade later, whereas the severely affected patients did not.[21]

Recommendations

• Single-digit revision amputation may confer a better functional outcome, lower hospital costs, and shorter length of therapy and time off work than replantation [overall quality: low]
• Replantation should be attempted for single fingertip injuries [overall quality: low]
• In general, patients having undergone single-digit replantation are capable of returning to previous work within 2.3–10.0 months [overall quality: moderate]

Question 3: Should two veins and one artery be anastomosed, or does one vein and artery suffice?

Case clarification

After successfully stabilizing the bone and repairing the tendons, you turn your attention to the microvascular anastomoses. You are presented with two options: repairing two veins vs. one vein for every artery repaired.

Relevance

Although Tamai et al.[22] declared the appropriate ratio of vein to artery anastomosis to be 2:1, there remains a divergence of opinion. The optimal ratio of vessel repair is compounded by the fact that a balance must be achieved between maximizing survival rate while minimizing operative time for the purposes of cost-effectiveness and limiting ischemic time.

Current opinion

The majority of microsurgeons either repair as many vessels as possible, as dictated by the condition of the amputated digit, or two veins for every artery anastomosed.

Finding the evidence

• As for Question 1, but using keywords: "replantation" AND "artery" OR "vein" OR "ratio" OR "anastomosis"

Quality of the evidence

Level IV
• 7 studies

Findings

Two studies (n = 847 digit replantations) made recommendations with regard to the optimal ratio of vessel repair in

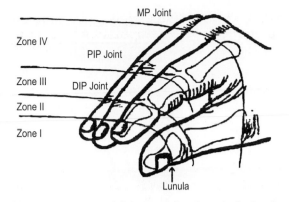

Figure 125.3 Tamai zones of digit amputation. Zone I is distal to the lunula; zone II is proximal to the lunula and distal to the DIP; zone III is proximal to the DIP and distal to the insertion of FDS; and zone IV is proximal to the insertion of FDS and distal to the MP joint. DIP, distal interphalangeal; MP, metacarpophalangeal; PIP, proximal interphalangeal. (From Lee B, Chung HY, Kim WK, et al. The effects of the number and ratio of repaired arteries and veins on the survival rate in digital replantation. Ann Plast Surg 2000;44:288–94. Reproduced with permission of Wolters Kluwer.)

relation to the associated Tamai zones of amputation (Figure 125.3) [23,24]. Lee et al. analyzed 631 single-digit replantations and concluded that zone I replantations fared better with repair of one vein vs. none (p = 0.008). Also, the salvage external bleeding method resulted in a higher survival rate when employed in zone I than in other zones. Matsuda et al. (n = 216 digit replantations) found no significant difference between the success rate of zero-vein repair vs. one- or two-vein repair (Table 125.2).

For the remaining zones of digit amputation, the findings are inconsistent (Table 125.2). For zone II, Lee recommends repairing at least as many veins as arteries, whereas Matsuda recommends that at least one vein be repaired. For zone III, Lee counsels that if one artery is repaired, then one vein suffices (p = 0.025), whereas if two arteries are repaired, then it is necessary to repair two or more veins. Chaivanichsiri and Rattanasrithong (n = 61 middle phalynx replantations) found that although there was no statistically significant advantage to repairing more than one vein in this zone, it was important to repair at least one (p = 0.018).[25] On the other hand, Matsuda advocates repairing at least two veins in this zone. Finally, for zone IV amputations, Lee proposes repairing two arteries and two veins, while Matsuda supports the essential repair of only one vein.

Three studies (n = 980 digit replantations) conducted simple nonanatomic analyses and proposed repairing as many veins as possible, with a minimum of two.[7,9,26] Two studies (n = 36 digit replantations) specifically addressed the topic of zone I fingertip replantations with anastomosis

Table 125.2 Number of anastomosed veins and associated survival rates(%)[23–25]

No. of veins repaired	None	One	Two or more
Zone I			
Lee et al.	73.2% (104/142)	90.0% (18/20)	N/A
Matsuda et al.	85.7% (12/14)	66.7% (4/6)	100.0% (1/1)
Zone II			
Lee et al.	49.0% (25/51)	80.8% (101/125)	92.6% (25/27)
Matsuda et al.	38.5% (5/13)	81.0% (17/21)	83.3% (10/12)
Zone III			
Lee et al.	47.6% (10/21)	76.5% (78/102)	88.1% (52/59)
Matsuda et al.	0.0% (0/1)	59.1% (13/22)	87.5% (35/40)
Chaivanichsiri and Rattanasrithong	40.0% (2/5)	84.4% (27/32)	91.7% (22/24)
Zone IV			
Lee et al.	N/A	74.5% (35/47)	100.0% (37/37)
Matsuda et al.	33.3% (1/3)	84.2% (16/19)	89.1% (57/64)

( ), number of replanted digits.

of the digital artery alone and venous drainage, with very satisfactory survival rates of 87% and 76%.[27,28]

Recommendations

• The essential number of veins to anastomose is: zone I, zero as long as immediate salvage via external bleeding method is performed; zone II, one, or at least as many as the number of arteries anastomosed; zone III, two, with ideally the same number of arteries; zone IV, one, but ideally two [overall quality: low]

• In general, repairing more veins confers a higher survival rate [overall quality: low]

Question 4: Should anticoagulant and/or antithrombotic agents be used postoperatively?

Case clarification

The amputated digit is successfully replanted without any complication. You consider starting the patient on prophylactic systemic anticoagulation.

Relevance

Venous insufficiency is the second most prevalent cause of replantation failure, with reported rates of up to 32%.[29] There is a lack of consensus with regard to the use prophylactic anticoagulation, as well as the optimal agent and regime.

Current opinion

Surveys have demonstrated that up to 96% of microsurgeons utilize some form of postoperative adjuvant anticoagulation following replantation.[30,31]

Finding the evidence

• As for Question 1, but using keywords: "replantation" AND "anticoagulation" OR "antithrombotic" OR "heparin" OR "aspirin".

Quality of the evidence

Level II
• 1 study

Level IV
• 5 studies

Level V
• 3 studies

Findings

In a survey involving 161 UK plastic surgeons, Ridha et al. demonstrated no correlation between the administration of dextran and replantation success rate. Still, 45% of the respondents routinely prescribed dextran after replantation and/or after free flap, while 29% employed an alternate form of thromboprophylaxis.[32]

Khouri, in the largest prospective multicenter human study on 493 free-tissue transfers, found that the only anticoagulant to alter clinical outcome with a statistically significant difference (p = 0.038) was subcutaneous low molecular weight heparin. Indeed, its administration decreased the odds ratio for thrombosis by 27%.[33] Unfortunately, the transferability and hence, level of relevance, of this data for upper extremity replantation is unknown.

Two studies provided information on replantation without the use of any postoperative anticoagulation or antithrombotic agents. In one, the authors obtained a survival rate of 91%,[34] which approximates, if it does not surpass, the range of reported success rates for adult replantation of 86.2–93.0%.[4,9] Similarly, a large-scale world survey (n = 1107 digit replantations) demonstrated a statistically significant superior survival rate of 89.0% (219/246) for replantations performed without anticoagulants compared to 76.5% (659/861) for those performed with anticoagulants (p < 0.00001).[35] When interpreting these findings, one must be aware of the biases associated with nonrandomized trials, as the patients' mechanism, level, and/or severity of injury could have influenced their baseline prognosis and the decision to prophylactically anticoagulate them.

Unfortunately, anticoagulation is not without risk. One retrospective study found that the incidence of blood loss requiring blood transfusion increased from 2% to 53% (p < 0.0001) when two or more anticoagulants were used in addition to aspirin compared to only one additional anticoagulant. This was without an associated advantage in survival rate (88% vs. 77%).[36]

Recommendations
- Postoperative administration of dextran does not reduce the risk of venous thrombosis in microsurgical anastomoses and carries the risk of rare but potentially devastating side effects [overall quality: low]
- Not administering postoperative anticoagulation may improve survival rate for digit replantation [overall quality: moderate]

Question 5: Does early ROM therapy following replantation improve outcome?

Case clarification
As you prepare to discharge the patient, you wonder whether he would benefit from early ROM therapy.

Relevance
Replantation involves multiple anatomic structures, each of which warrants its own precautions and therapeutic approach. The therapeutic approach must mobilize the antagonistic flexor and extensor tendons while protecting the bony and microvascular repairs.

Current opinion
Most surgeons and hand therapists seem to advocate supervised controlled early mobilization therapy.

Finding the evidence
- As for Question 1, but using keywords "replantation" AND "range of motion" OR "rehabilitation" OR "therapy"

Table 125.3 Early protective motion (EPM) program[36,37]

Postoperative time	Therapy
Day 5	EPM I active assisted exercises under the principle of controlled tenodesis
Day 10–14	EPM II—passive and active phase
Week 3	Strategies to reduce edema, mobilize scar, improve graded desensitization If Kirschner wires are removed, single-digit static gutter splints may assist in supporting extensor tendon repair
Weeks 4–6	Wrist extension beyond neutral Full digit flexion and extension exercises with oscillating movements Composite motion Dynamic and/or intermittent static stretch splinting
Week 6–8, and beyond	Gross and fine strengthening exercises Rehearsal of functional activities

Quality of the evidence
Level IV
- 2 studies

Level V
- 3 studies

Findings
Two articles describe in detail the biomechanical implications of an early protective motion (EPM) program (Table 125.3).[37,38] The goal of this program is reintegrating the patient to the work environment by 3–6 months.

Ross et al. (n = 103) found that when therapy was instituted within 14 days of injury, patients achieved significantly superior active range of motion (AROM) results (p = 0.0001). The average total active movement values were 165° for the "early therapy" group (n = 65 patients) versus 121° for the "late therapy" group (n = 38 patients). The only flexor tendon rupture observed occurred in the "late therapy" group.[39]

Recommendation
- Early therapy (within 14 days of injury) may improve AROM results compared to later therapy [overall quality: low]

Summary of recommendations

- Survival rates for replantations performed in community hospitals with trained microsurgeons are comparable to that of tertiary hospitals

- Single-digit revision amputation may confer a better functional outcome, lower hospital costs, and shorter length of therapy and time off work than replantation
- Replantation should be attempted for single fingertip injuries
- In general, patients having undergone single-digit replantation are capable of returning to previous work within 2.3–10.0 months
- The essential number of veins to anastomose is: Zone I, zero as long as immediate salvage via external bleeding method is performed; Zone II, one, or at least as many as the number of arteries anastomosed; Zone III, two, with ideally the same number of arteries; Zone IV, one, but ideally two
- In general, repairing more veins confers a higher survival rate
- Postoperative administration of dextran does not reduce the risk of venous thrombosis in microsurgical anastomoses and carries the risk of rare but potentially devastating side effects
- Not administering postoperative anticoagulation may improve survival rate for digit replantation
- Early therapy (within 14 days of injury) may improve AROM results compared to later therapy

Conclusions

Since the first reported upper extremity replantation in 1962, a large body of literature on the topic has emerged, with subsequent increasing awareness from both the medical community and general population. Modern innovations now enable surgeons to successfully replant upper extremity traumatic amputations at almost any level of injury. As success rates continue to improve, the focus is gradually shifting from simply attaining digit and/or limb survival to achieving optimal function and hence, quality of life. The future prospects of microsurgical replantation are indeed inspiring, and will continue to mature as ongoing research studies aid in refining its indications and surgical techniques.

References

1. Chung KW, Kowalski CP, Walters MR, et al. Finger replantation in the United States: rates and resource use from the 1996 healthcare cost and utilization project. J Hand Surg Am 2000;25: 1038–42.
2. Isenberg JS. Flying solo: a single year-single surgeon community hospital replantation/revascularization experience. J Reconstr Microsurg 2002;18(6):483–6.
3. Pomerance I, Truppa K, Bilos ZJ, et al. Replantation and revascularization of the digits in a community microsurgical practice. J Reconstr Microsurg 1997;13(3):163–70.
4. Wojciech D. A meta-analysis of success rates for digit replantation. Tech Hand Upp Extr Surg 2006;10(3):124–9.
5. Braga-Silva J. Les réimplantations unidigitales en ambulatoire. À propos de 85 cas cliniques. Ann Chir Plast Esthèt 2001;46:74–83.
6. Soucacos PN, Beris AE, Touliatos AS, et al. Current indications for single replantation. Acta Orthop Scand 1995;66:12–15.
7. Urbaniak JR, Roth JH, Nunley JA, et al. The results of replantation after amputation of a single finger. J Bone Joint Surg Am 1985;67(4):611–19.
8. Kaplan FTD, Raskin KB. Indications and surgical techniques for digit replantation. Hosp Joint Dis 2001–2002;60(3–4):179–88.
9. Waikakul S, Sakkarnkosol S, Vanadurongwan V, et al. Results of 1018 digital replantations in 552 patients. Injury 2000;31:33–40.
10. Chiu HY, Shieh SJ, Hsu HY. Multivariate analysis of factors influencing the functional recovery after finger replantation or revascularization. Microsurgery 1996;16:713–17.
11. Jones JM, Schenck RR, Chesney RB. Digital replantation and amputation: comparison of function. J Hand Surg 1982;7(2): 183–9.
12. Buntic RF, Brooks D, Buncke GM. Index finger salvage with replantation and revascularization: revisiting conventional wisdom. Microsurg 2008;28:612–16.
13. Soucacos PN. Indications and selection for digital amputation and replantation. J Hand Surg Br 2001;26(6):572–81.
14. Foucher G, Merle M, Braun JB. Distal digital replantation is one of the best indications for microsurgery. Int J Microsurg 1981;3:263–70.
15. Malizos KN, Beris AE, Kabani CT, et al. Distal phalynx microsurgical replantation. Microsurg 1994;15:464–8.
16. Beris AE, Soucacos PN, Malizos KN, et al. Microsurgical treatment of ring avulsion injuries. Microsurg 1994;15:459–63.
17. Goel A, Navato-Dehning C, Varghese G, et al. Replantation and amputation of digits: user analysis. Am J Phys Rehab 1995;74: 134–8.
18. Hattori Y, Doi K, Ikeda K, et al. A retrospective study of functional outcomes after successful replantation versus amputation closure for single fingertip amputations. J Hand Surg Am 2006; 31:811–18.
19. Goldner RD, Stevanovic MV, Nunley JA, et al. Digital replantation at the level of the distal interphalangeal joint and the distal phalanx. J Hand Surg Am 1989;14:214–20.
20. Boeckx W, Jacobs W, Guelinckx P, et al. Late results in replanted digits—Is replantation of a single digit worthwhile? Acta Chir Belg 1992;92:204–8.
21. Povlsen B, Nylander G, Nylander E. Cold-induced vasospasm after digital replantation does not improve with time. J Hand Surg Br 1995;20(2):237–9.
22. Tamai S, Hori Y, Tatsumi, Y et al. Microvascular anastomosis and its application on the replantation of amputated digits and hands. Clin Orthop 1978;133:106–21.
23. Lee B, Chung HY, Kim WK, et al. The effects of the number and ratio of repaired arteries and veins on the survival rate in digital replantation. Ann Plast Surg 2000;44:288–94.
24. Matsuda M, Chikamatsu E, Shimizu Y. Correlation between number of anastomosed vessels and survival rate in finger replantation. J Reconstr Microsurg 1993;9(1):1–4.
25. Chaivanichsiri P, Rattanasrithong P. Type of injury and number of anastomosed vessels: impact on digital replantation. Microsurgery 2006;26:151–4.

26. Tark KC, Kim YW, Lee YH, et al. Replantation and revascularization of hands: clinical analysis and functional results of 261 cases. J Hand Surg Am 1989;16:17–27.

27. Matsuzaki H, Yoshizu T, Maki Y, et al. Functional and cosmetic results of fingertip replantation—anastomosing only the digital artery. Ann Plast Surg 2004;53:353–9.

28. Akyürek M, Safak T, Kecik A. Fingertip replantation at or distal to the nail base: use of the technique of artery-only anastomosis. Ann Plast Surg 2001;24:605–12.

29. Iglasias M, Butron P. Local subcutaneous heparin as treatment for venous insufficiency in replanted digits. Plast Reconstr Surg 1999;103:1710–24.

30. Glicksman A, Ferder M, Casale P, et al. 1457 years of microsurgical experience. Plast Reconstr Surg 1997;100(2):355–63.

31. Scott L, Cooper EO. Clinical use of anticoagulants following replantation surgery. J Hand Surg 2008;33A, 1437–9.

32. Ridha H, Jallali N, Butler PE. The use of dextran post free tissue transfer. J Plast Reconstr Aesthet Surg 2006;59:951–4.

33. Khouri RK, Cooley BC, Kunselman AR, et al. A prospective study of microvascular free-flap and outcome. Plast Reconstr Surg 1998;102:711–21.

34. Veravuthipakorn L, Veravuthipakorn A. Microsurgical free flap and replantation without antithrombotic agents. J Med Assoc Thai 2004;87(6):665–9.

35. Davies DM. A world survey of anticoagulation practice in clinical microvascular surgery. Br J Plast Surg 1982;35:96–9.

36. Furnas HJ, Lineaweaver W, Buncke HJ. Blood loss associated with anticoagulation in patients with replanted digits. J Hand Surg Am 1992;17:226–9.

37. Silverman PM, Gordon L. Early motion after replantation. Hand Clin 1996;12(1):97–107.

38. Chan SW, LaStayo P. Hand therapy management following mutilating hand injuries. Hand Clin 2003;19:133–48.

39. Ross DC, Manktelow RT, Wells MT, et al. Tendon function after replantation: prognostic factors and strategies to enhance total active motion. Ann Plast Surg 2003;51(2):141–6.

VIII Orthopedic Oncology

126 Radiation in Soft Tissue Sarcoma: Pre- or Postoperative

Kurt R. Weiss[1], Rej Bhumbra[2], Peter C. Ferguson[3], Brian O'Sullivan[4], and Jay S. Wunder[3]

[1]University of Pittsburg, Pittsburg, PA, USA
[2]London Sarcoma Service, Royal National Orthopaedic Hospital, London, UK
[3]Mount Sinai Hospital, University of Toronto, Toronto, ON, Canada
[4]Princess Margaret Hospital, University of Toronto, Toronto, ON, Canada

Case scenario

A 25 year old woman presents with a growing mass in the medial thigh. On examination there is a firm 15 cm mass in the adductor compartment. MRI confirms a tumor with heterogeneous signal characteristics. The neurovascular bundle is displaced but not encased. A biopsy performed at the regional tumor unit is consistent with a high-grade undifferentiated sarcoma. Systemic staging is negative for metastasis.

Importance of the problem

Soft tissue sarcomas (STS) constitute 1% of all cancer diagnoses and the incidence is estimated at 1 per 30,000. The mainstay of treatment is wide surgical excision. Radiotherapy (XRT) is used in the management of STS when wide margins cannot be obtained, with the goal of extending the "virtual margin" to the surrounding tissues.[1] Radiation-induced cell death is brought about by direct DNA damage and the production of free radicals. Tumors with varying DNA concentrations and local oxygen tensions respond differently to identical doses of radiation. The presence of prior surgery also affects tumor cell sensitivity.[2] The exact timing, sequence and dose of XRT remain controversial. A review of over 5,000 soft tissue tumors by Brennan et al.[2] documented the distribution of STS to be the lower extremity (30%), viscera (19%), retroperitoneum (15%), upper limb (13%), trunk (10%), and other sites (13%).

Top three questions

1. Is there evidence to use XRT in the management of STS?
2. What are the relative advantages and disadvantages of pre- versus postoperative XRT?
3. What are the short- and long-term effects of XRT?

Question 1: Is there evidence to use XRT in the management of STS?

Current opinion

Limb-sparing surgery plus XRT is as effective as amputation for the local control of STS.

Finding the evidence

- PubMed search using keywords: "radiation" AND "soft tissue sarcoma" AND "extremity"
- Ovid MEDLINE search using keywords: "radiation" AND "soft tissue sarcoma" AND "extremity"

Quality of the evidence

Sixteen articles were reviewed to answer this question.

Level I
- 2 systematic reviews/meta-analyses
- 3 randomized controlled trials (RCTs)

Level II
- 1 outcomes research

Evidence-Based Orthopedics, First Edition. Edited by Mohit Bhandari.
© 2012 Blackwell Publishing Ltd. Published 2012 by Blackwell Publishing Ltd.

Level III
- 2 retrospective comparative studies

Level IV
- 8 retrospective reviews

Findings

STS are rare and there is a paucity of level I evidence upon which to base treatment decisions. There is agreement that local control is important, and some authors have correlated local recurrence with diminished overall survival.

Most studies are retrospective with small (average 182, range 41–517) numbers of patients. There are two systematic reviews that included 4,579 patients, and there is significant overlap between these reviews. There are 3 RCTs that evaluated 298 patients.

A systematic review concluded that XRT in addition to limb-sparing surgery improves local control for extremity STS over surgery alone, but does not affect overall survival.[3] A review of RCTs in extremity STS found that limb-sparing surgery plus XRT is equivalent to amputation for local control.[4] Furthermore, adding XRT to surgical resection significantly improves local control over surgery alone but does not improve overall survival.

The first RCT compared limb-sparing surgery plus postoperative XRT to amputation in 43 patients.[5] At the time of this study, amputation was the standard of care for local control of STS. The authors found no significant differences in local recurrence (p = 0.06, OR = 6.32, 95% CI 0.32–125.52) or overall survival (p = 0.99, OR = 0.86, 95% CI 0.13–5.89) at 5 years. They concluded that limb-sparing surgery plus XRT is a reasonable alternative to amputation.

The next two RCTs compared limb-sparing surgery alone to limb-sparing surgery plus postoperative RT. Pisters et al. (n = 164 patients) reported a significant improvement (p = 0.002, OR = 0.23, 95% CI 0.08–0.66) in local control with surgery plus brachytherapy compared with the surgery alone in patients with high-grade tumors.[6] Brachytherapy did not provide an advantage in patients with low-grade tumors. There were no differences between the two treatment groups in terms of metastatic disease (p = 0.60, OR = 0.74, 95% CI 0.35–1.56) or 5 year survival (p = 0.65, OR = 0.8, 95% CI 0.35–1.81). Yang stratified 141 patients into high- and low-grade tumors.[7] All patients had surgery and were randomized to receive external beam XRT or not. XRT significantly improved local control in both high-grade (p = 0.003, OR = 0.05, 95% CI 0.00–0.81) and low-grade (p = 0.02, OR = 0.80, 95% CI 0.01–0.70) tumors. However, there were no differences in overall survival at 10 years (p = 0.71, OR = 0.93, 95% CI 0.40–2.15).

An outcomes study involving 8249 patients using the Florida Cancer Registry demonstrated that surgical resection (p < 0.001) and XRT (p < 0.001) were the only treatment variables to improve survival.[8]

The remaining studies support the systematic reviews and RCTs.[9–16]

Recommendations

- XRT plus limb-sparing surgery is as effective as amputation for the local control of extremity STS [overall quality: high]
- XRT plus limb-sparing surgery is superior to surgery alone for the local control of high-grade extremity STS [overall quality: high]
- XRT does not impact overall survival [overall quality: high]

Question 2: What are the relative advantages and disadvantages of pre- vs. postoperative XRT?

Case clarification

The patient asks if she will receive XRT before or after surgery.

Relevance

Sarcomas are best treated by multidisciplinary teams and individualized treatment plans. The relative advantages and disadvantages of pre- vs. postoperative XRT must be related to each patient.

Current opinion

There are potential advantages and disadvantages to both pre- and postoperative XRT. Both strategies are successfully used to treat patients. Preoperative XRT is associated with a higher rate of wound complications, but better long-term functional outcomes.

Finding the evidence

- PubMed search using keywords "radiation" AND "soft tissue sarcoma" AND "extremity" AND "preoperative" AND "postoperative".
- Ovid MEDLINE search using the keywords "radiation" AND "soft tissue sarcoma" AND "extremity" AND "preoperative" AND "postoperative".

Quality of the evidence

Thirteen articles were reviewed to answer this question.

Level I
- 2 systematic reviews/meta-analyses
- 1 RCT

Level II
- 2 outcomes research

Level III
- 7 retrospective comparative studies

Level IV
• 1 retrospective review

Findings

Advantages and disadvantages Potential advantages of pre-operative XRT include smaller radiation dose and treatment volume, greater sensitivity of the tumor to radiation, no delay in the initiation of XRT, less long-term tissue toxicity (joint contracture, fibrosis, edema, and fracture), and the ability to administer a postoperative radiation boost if desired. Reported advantages of postoperative XRT include immediate surgery, better quality tissue for pathologic evaluation, and fewer wound complications.

Level I, III, and IV data report statistically smaller treatment doses and fields with preoperative radiotherapy: preoperative radiotherapy is typically ~50 Gy, whereas postoperative treatment is between 60 and 70 Gy.

Recurrence and survival No studies have shown a significant difference in local recurrence or metastatic disease with either pre- or postoperative XRT. The Canadian RCT comparing pre- and postoperative XRT reported a slight survival advantage of preoperative XRT at 3 years (p = 0.05, OR = 0.47, 95% CI 0.23–0.97) which did not persist with longer-term follow-up.[17,18]

Al-Absi et al. performed a meta-analysis comparing pre- and postoperative XRT for local recurrence and overall survival.[19] Of 1098 patients, 526 had preoperative XRT. Although there were fewer local recurrences in the preoperative group, this finding was dependent on whether a random- or fixed-effect statistical model was used. The authors stressed that these findings should be interpreted cautiously due to heterogeneity within the meta-analysis (heterogeneity p = 0.26, variability = 25%). They concluded that the timing of XRT is unlikely to affect survival.

The decision to use preoperative or postoperative radiotherapy is based on the expected advantages of one treatment strategy vs. the other. Preoperative XRT might be chosen if the tumor is in close proximity to critical structures (e.g., spinal cord) and smaller radiation doses/volumes are required. Complex soft tissue reconstructions could make preoperative XRT desirable. Alternatively, patients unable to tolerate a wound complication might benefit from postoperative XRT.

Recommendations

• Preoperative XRT utilizes smaller treatment volumes and lower overall radiation dosages than postoperative XRT [overall quality: high]
• Pre- and postoperative XRT have equivalent efficacy in terms of overall survival [overall quality: high]

Question 3. What are the short- and long-term complications of radiotherapy?

Case clarification
Apart from local recurrence, short- and long-term treatment morbidity remain important considerations for patients undergoing treatment with surgery and XRT.

Relevance
Pre- and postoperative XRT cause distinct complications. Immediately following preoperative XRT, wound complications are the most common problem, at least in the management of lower limb lesions. The longer-term effects of postoperative XRT on normal tissues increase the probability of developing limb and joint stiffness, fibrosis, edema, and long bone fracture.

Current opinion
Multiple studies have demonstrated that preoperative XRT increases the probability of wound complications compared with postoperative XRT, which can cause adverse long-term functional consequences. Wound complications are challenging but manageable problems. In contradistinction, once the long-term effects of radiotherapy have established themselves in the limb, they are difficult to manage.

Finding the evidence
• PubMed search using keywords "radiation" AND "soft tissue sarcoma" AND "complication"

Quality of the evidence
Nine articles were reviewed to answer this question.

Level I
• 1 RCT

Level II
• 1 outcomes research

Level IV
• 7 retrospective reviews

Findings
Short-term complications Even without adjuvant treatment, wound complications are to be expected following STS excision. In a consecutive series of 98 patients managed with STS excision without adjuvant treatment, the wound complication rate was 40%.[20]

The Canadian RCT demonstrated 35% (31 of 88 patients) vs. 17% (16 of 94 patients) wound complication rate in the pre- vs. postoperative XRT groups, respectively (p = 0.01, OR = 2.65, 95% CI 1.33–5.30) with the predominant effect almost entirely confined to the lower limb.[17]

The retrospective data of Cheng, Pollack, and Cannon independently reported that preoperative radiation leads to increased rates of wound complications in the lower limb compared to postoperative radiotherapy.[21–23] Specifically, Cheng et al.[21] reported wound complications in 15 of 48 (31%) preoperative XRT patients compared with 5 of 64 (8%) postoperative XRT patients (p = 0.001, OR = 5.36, 95% CI 1.79–16.08). Pollack et al.[22] reported wound complications in 32 of 128 (25%) preoperative XRT patients compared with 10 of 165 (6%) postoperative XRT patients (p < 0.001, OR = 5.17, 95% CI 2.43–10.99). Finally, Cannon et al.[23] reported complications in 90 of 269 (34%) preoperative XRT patients and 23 of 143 (16%) postoperative XRT patients (p < 0.001, OR = 2.63, CI 1.57–4.38).

Long-term complications Rimner et al. retrospectively reviewed 225 thigh tumors.[24] Overall complication rates at 5 years were edema (13%), joint stiffness (12%), wound reoperation (10%), nerve damage (8%), and bone fractures (7%). In this study 69% of these patients were treated with brachytherapy, while 31% received external beam XRT. Cannon et al. reported on 412 patients at 20 years following external beam XRT and found that chronic radiation-related complications were higher in patients with a tumor located in the groin or thigh.[23]

Davis et al. analyzed 129 patients for late radiation morbidity in an RCT.[25] At 2 years there was a trend towards greater fibrosis following postoperative XRT (p = 0.07, OR = 0.49, 95% CI 0.24–1.02). Moderate degrees of fibrosis and stiffness correlated with significantly worse patient-reported outcomes (TESS scores) as well as objective assessments (MSTS scores). There was also increased edema (23% vs. 15%, p = 0.26, OR = 0.59, 95% CI 0.24–1.43), and joint stiffness (23% vs. 18%, p = 0.51, OR = 0.72, 95% CI 0.30–1.70) in the post- vs. preoperative XRT groups. Large field size is typically associated with postoperative XRT and was predictive of increased fibrosis (p = 0.002), joint stiffness (p = 0.006), and edema (p = 0.06) in logistic regression analysis. MSTS and TESS scores were not significantly different between both treatment arms but were adversely affected by radiation morbidity.

Stinson et al. retrospectively reviewed acute and chronic postradiation effects in 145 patients and identified tissue induration (57%), decreased range of motion (32%), decreased muscle power (20%), edema (19%), pain (7%), use of walking aids (7%), and fracture (6%).[26]

Examining radiation-associated fractures, Holt et al. noted that patients undergoing thigh STS resection where more likely to sustain a fracture if they received either high-dose postoperative XRT or high-dose combined preoperative XRT and a postoperative boost (60 or 66 Gy) compared to low-dose (50 Gy) preoperative treatment.[27] In this study 24 of 27 fractures occurred in patients who had received high-dose XRT (p = 0.007, OR = 0.12, 95% CI 0.04–0.42).

Recommendations

- Preoperative XRT leads to an increased rate of wound complications relative to postoperative XRT in lower limb tumors [overall quality: high]
- Larger tumors treated with XRT have an increased risk of developing complications [overall quality: high]
- A moderate degree of fibrosis and stiffness leads to significantly poorer patient-reported outcomes [overall quality: high]
- Postoperative XRT leads to diminished long-term functional outcomes, when measured with MSTS and TESS scores, than preoperative radiotherapy [overall quality: moderate]

Summary of recommendations

- XRT plus limb-sparing surgery is as effective as amputation for the local control of extremity STS
- XRT plus limb-sparing surgery is superior to surgery alone for the local control of high-grade extremity STS
- XRT does not impact overall survival
- Preoperative XRT utilizes smaller treatment volumes and lower overall radiation dosages than postoperative XRT
- Pre- and postoperative XRT have equivalent efficacy in terms of overall survival
- Preoperative XRT leads to an increased rate of wound complications relative to postoperative XRT in lower limb tumors
- Larger tumors treated with XRT have an increased risk of developing complications
- A moderate degree of fibrosis and stiffness leads to significantly poorer patient-reported outcomes
- Postoperative XRT leads to diminished long-term functional outcomes, when measured with MSTS and TESS scores, than preoperative radiotherapy

References

1. Mendenhall WM, Indelicato DJ, Scarborough MT, et al. The management of adult soft tissue sarcomas. Am J Clin Oncol 2009;32(4):436–42.
2. DeVita VT, Hellman S, Rosenberg SA, eds. Cancer: Principles and Practice of Oncology, 7th edn. Lippincott, Philadelphia, 2005.
3. Strander H, Turesson I, Cavallin-Stahl E. A systematic overview of radiation therapy effects in soft tissue sarcomas. Acta Oncol 2003;42(5–6):516–31.

4. McCarter MD, Jaques DP, Brennan MF. Randomized clinical trials in soft tissue sarcoma. Surg Oncol Clin N Am 2002;11(1): 11–22.

5. Rosenberg SA, Tepper J, Glatstein E, et al. The treatment of soft-tissue sarcomas of the extremities: prospective randomized evaluations of (1) limb-sparing surgery plus radiation therapy compared with amputation and (2) the role of adjuvant chemotherapy. Ann Surg 1982;196(3):305–15.

6. Pisters PW, Harrison LB, Leung DH, Woodruff JM, Casper ES, Brennan MF. Long-term results of a prospective randomized trial of adjuvant brachytherapy in soft tissue sarcoma. J Clin Oncol 1996;14(3):859–68.

7. Yang JC, Chang AE, Baker AR, et al. Randomized prospective study of the benefit of adjuvant radiation therapy in the treatment of soft tissue sarcomas of the extremity. J Clin Oncol 1998;16(1):197–203.

8. Gutierrez JC, Perez EA, Franceschi D, Moffat FL, Jr, Livingstone AS, Koniaris LG. Outcomes for soft-tissue sarcoma in 8249 cases from a large state cancer registry. J Surg Res 2007;141(1): 105–14.

9. Suit HD, Mankin HJ, Wood WC, and Proppe KH. Preoperative, intraoperative, and postoperative radiation in the treatment of primary soft tissue sarcoma. Cancer 1985;55(11):2659–67.

10. Karasek, K, Constine LS, Rosier, R. Sarcoma therapy: functional outcome and relationship to treatment parameters. Int J Radiat Oncol Biol Phys 1992;24(4):651–6.

11. Wilson RB, Crowe PJ, Fisher, R, Hook, C, Donnellan MJ. Extremity soft tissue sarcoma: factors predictive of local recurrence and survival. Aust N Z J Surg 1999;69(5):344–9.

12. Keus RB, Rutgers EJ, Ho GH, Gortzak, E, Albus-Lutter CE, Hart AA. Limb-sparing therapy of extremity soft tissue sarcomas: treatment outcome and long-term functional results. Eur J Cancer 1994;30A(10):1459–63.

13. Potter DA, Kinsella T, Glatstein E, et al. High-grade soft tissue sarcomas of the extremities. Cancer 1986;58(1):190–205.

14. Lindberg RD, Martin RG, Romsdahl MM, Barkley HT, Jr. Conservative surgery and postoperative radiotherapy in 300 adults with soft-tissue sarcomas. Cancer 1981;47(10):2391–7.

15. Khanfir K, Alzieu L, Terrier P, Le Pechoux C, Bonvalot S, Vanel D, Le Cesne A. Does adjuvant radiation therapy increase locoregional control after optimal resection of soft-tissue sarcoma of the extremities? Eur J Cancer 2003;39(13):1872–80.

16. Alektiar KM, Velasco J, Zelefsky MJ, Woodruff JM, Lewis JJ, Brennan MF. Adjuvant radiotherapy for margin-positive high-grade soft tissue sarcoma of the extremity. Int J Radiat Oncol Biol Phys 2000;48(4):1051–8.

17. O'Sullivan B, Davis AM, Turcotte R, et al. Preoperative versus postoperative radiotherapy in soft-tissue sarcoma of the limbs: a randomised trial. Lancet 2002;359(9325):2235–41.

18. O'Sullivan D, Turcotte, et al. 5-year results of a randomized phase III trial of pre-operative versus post-operative radiotherapy in extremity soft tissue sarcoma. In: American Society of Clinical Oncology (ASCO) Annual Meeting, 2005.

19. Al-Absi E, Farrokhyar F, Sharma R, Whelan K, Corbett T, Patel M, Ghert M. A systematic review and meta-analysis of oncologic outcomes of pre- versus postoperative radiation in localized resectable soft-tissue sarcoma. Ann Surg Oncol 2010;17(5): 1367–74.

20. Saddegh MK, Bauer HC. Wound complication in surgery of soft tissue sarcoma. Analysis of 103 consecutive patients managed without adjuvant therapy. Clin Orthop Relat Res 1993;289: 247–53.

21. Cheng EY, Dusenbery KE, Winters MR, Thompson RC. Soft tissue sarcomas: preoperative versus postoperative radiotherapy. J Surg Oncol 1996;61(2):90–9.

22. Pollack A, Zagars GK, Goswitz MS, Pollock RA, Feig BW, Pisters PW. Preoperative vs. postoperative radiotherapy in the treatment of soft tissue sarcomas: a matter of presentation. Int J Radiat Oncol Biol Phys 1998;42(3):563–72.

23. Cannon CP, Ballo MT, Zagars GK, et al. Complications of combined modality treatment of primary lower extremity soft-tissue sarcomas. Cancer 2006;107(10):2455–61.

24. Rimner, A, Brennan MF, Zhang, Z, Singer, S, Alektiar KM. Influence of compartmental involvement on the patterns of morbidity in soft tissue sarcoma of the thigh. Cancer 2009;115(1): 149–57.

25. Davis AM, O'Sullivan B, Turcotte R, et al. Late radiation morbidity following randomization to preoperative versus postoperative radiotherapy in extremity soft tissue sarcoma. Radiother Oncol 2005;75(1):48–53.

26. Stinson SF, DeLaney TF, Greenberg J, et al. Acute and long-term effects on limb function of combined modality limb sparing therapy for extremity soft tissue sarcoma. Int J Radiat Oncol Biol Phys 1991;21(6):1493–9.

27. Holt GE, Griffin AM, Pintilie, M, et al. Fractures following radiotherapy and limb-salvage surgery for lower extremity soft-tissue sarcomas. A comparison of high-dose and low-dose radiotherapy. J Bone Joint Surg Am 2005;87(2):315–19.

127 Soft Tissue Sarcoma: Does the Evidence Support the Administration of Chemotherapy?

Jennifer L. Halpern, Jill Gilbert, Ginger E. Holt, Vicki L. Keedy, and Herbert S. Schwartz

Vanderbilt University Medical Center, Nashville, TN, USA

Case scenario

A 38 year old vending machine repairman presented for evaluation of left groin pain. Physical examination revealed asymmetric thigh girth (left 67 cm vs. right 55 cm). Imaging studies demonstrated a $12.5 \times 15 \times 20$ cm mass within the adductor compartment of the left thigh. There was no evidence of lung parenchymal disease. Open biopsy of the mass was performed. Final pathology was reported as pleomorphic high-grade sarcoma (Figure 127.1).

Relevant anatomy

Soft tissue sarcomas (STS) are malignant neoplasms that arise in nonepithelial, extraskeletal tissues of the body. Despite this general classification, STS are extremely diverse, being variable in their gross and microscopic appearances and behavior. With the exception of low-grade liposarcoma, wide surgical resection is a critical component of successful treatment. Depending upon tumor grade (high or low), depth (superficial or deep), and size (>5 cm), neoadjuvant or adjuvant radiation can also be used to improve local control.

Importance of the problem

The World Sarcoma Network reports (based on U.S. data) that the incidence of STS globally is 30 cases per 1,000,000 people. In the United States, the incidence in 2007 was reported as 9,220 cases, with an overall mortality rate of 3,560 cases per year. Although the multimodal approach to treatment of resectable STS has resulted in excellent local control (10–15% local recurrence with limb salvage),[1] 50% of those diagnosed and treated for isolated disease will eventually die from metastatic disease,[2] most likely stemming from undetectable micrometastases at the time of diagnosis.

> The two staging systems used to describe soft tissue sarcoma are the American Joint Committee on Cancer (AJCC) and the Enneking system (Surgical Staging System of the Musculoskeletal Tumor Society). The AJCC is based upon the tumor–node–metastasis (TNM) system, but also includes histologic grade as a measure. The Enneking system is based upon histopathologic grade, anatomic site and extent, and presence or absence of metastases.

Chemotherapy is currently offered to patients with metastatic STS at diagnosis or high-risk disease (AJCC ≥III or Enneking ≥IIB). However, there is little evidence to suggest that current chemotherapeutic regimens will prolong overall survival or disease-free survival. There is inherent difficulty in generating large, randomized controlled trials (RCTs) for the following key reasons: (1) STS are rare, which translates into a lack of statistical power in trials, and (2) with some exceptions, classifications based upon histologic descriptions result in unique tumor subtypes being grouped together. In fact, a PubMed search using the words "chemotherapy" and "soft tissue sarcoma" limited to the past 2 years generated only 17 studies involving chemotherapy and STS, and of these none were phase III trials. The implication is that despite improvements in surgical planning/techniques and administration of radiation,

Evidence-Based Orthopedics, First Edition. Edited by Mohit Bhandari.
© 2012 Blackwell Publishing Ltd. Published 2012 by Blackwell Publishing Ltd.

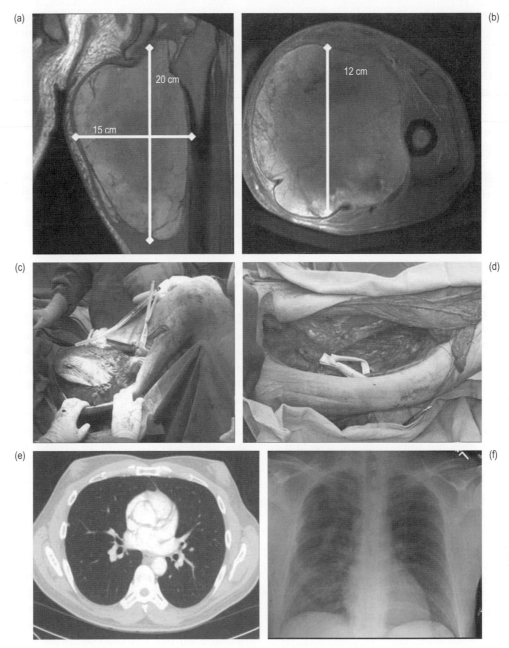

Figure 127.1 Clinical images of patient presented embody the inherent difficulty in treatment of high risk soft tissue sarcoma. Pretreatment MRI scans revealed a large 20×15×12 cm mass in the left medial thigh (a,b). Following neoadjuvant radiation therapy, the patient is taken to the operating room for a wide excision of the tumor (c). After resection, the sciatic nerve is skeletonized, tagged with a Vessel loop (d). Despite negative margins, no prior evidence of lung involvement on staging studies, and no evidence of local recurrence, the patient developed radiographically detectable lung metastases on CT scan 9 months after definitive resection (e). Following treatment with adjuvant chemotherapy (adriamycin and ifosfamide/mesna), the patient underwent pulmonary metastatectomies (f).

there has been a lack of promising systemic therapies in the setting of STS, and therefore overall survival has remained unchanged.

This chapter intends to offer an evidence-based approach to the administration of chemotherapy in patients with STS. It does not address future directions of ongoing research to find better systemic therapies. Unfortunately, the quality of evidence regarding the role chemotherapy of

in STS treatment is poor, and this chapter reflects the lack of good evidence that exists on this topic.

Top two questions

1. Is there a role for neoadjuvant chemotherapy in treatment of STS?

2. Is there a role for adjuvant chemotherapy in treatment of STS?

Question 1: Is there a role for neoadjuvant chemotherapy in treatment of STS?

Case clarification

Following diagnosis of isolated high-risk (large, deep, high-grade) pleomorphic sarcoma, treatment options are presented to the patient. One option is to administer neoadjuvant chemotherapy, with two goals: (1) to decrease the size of the tumor, thereby facilitating resection; and (2) to combat radiographically undetectable micrometastases.

Relevance

A multimodal approach using radiation and surgery achieves excellent local control. Using successful osteosarcoma treatment regimens as a model, the question raised was whether pretreatment of STS with chemotherapy would result in significant tumor necrosis, thereby facilitating wide resection, and would also decrease the incidence of distant disease.

Current opinion

Current opinion suggests that administration of neoadjuvant chemotherapy does not simplify tumor resection or improve overall survival, except in specific subtypes of soft tissue sarcoma known to be chemosensitive.

Finding the evidence

• PubMed (www.ncbi.nlm.nih.gov/pubmed) clinical queries/systematic reviews, using search term: "soft tissue sarcoma" AND "neoadjuvant chemotherapy."
• PubMed (www.ncbi.nlm.nih.gov/pubmed), using keywords :"soft tissue sarcoma" AND "neoadjuvant chemotherapy"; "synovial sarcoma" AND "neoadjuvant chemotherapy"

Quality of the evidence

Level I
• 1 randomized trial

Level II
• 4 retrospective reviews

Findings

In general, level I evidence does not exist to justify administration of neoadjuvant chemotherapy in the setting of STS. In fact, retrospective reviews demonstrate dismal responses to neoadjuvant chemo. For example, Meric et al. showed that out of 105 patients treated with neoadjuvant

chemotherapy, only 12% responded enough to simplify their surgical procedure, and in addition 9% required a larger surgery because the tumor progressed while the patient was on chemotherapy.[3] Despite that result, in the group that did demonstrate radiographic response, there were an increased number of margin-negative resections, fewer local failures, and improved overall survival when compared to patients with no radiographic response. Eilber et al., in a small group of patients, demonstrated that complete response to chemotherapy (≥95% necrosis), translated clinically into an improved 10 year local recurrence-free rate of 11% vs. 23% and 10 year overall survival of 71% vs. 55%.[4]

However, other studies report no difference in oncologic outcome in patients treated with neoadjuvant chemotherapy. This may or may not be because these studies were underpowered. Menendez et al. showed no statistical significance in recurrence-free or overall survival in patients who received three or four cycles of neoadjuvant doxorubicin, ifosfamide, and cisplatin.[5] However, power analysis indicated that the necessary sample size to show an improvement in recurrence-free or overall survival would be 532 patients, and that study reviewed only 82 patients after exclusion criteria were considered. The European Organization for Research and Treatment of Cancer (EORTC) organized an RCT comparing neoadjuvant doxorubicin and ifosfamide in high-risk adult STS. No difference in overall or disease-free survival was noted and the study was closed early due to poor patient accrual.[6] Finally, Pisters et al. reported a retrospective review of 76 patients with stage IIIB STS, treated with neoadjuvant chemotherapy with doxorubicin regimens.[7] They found that there was no statistically significant difference in local recurrence-free survival, distant metastases-free survival, disease-free survival, or overall survival between responders and nonresponders (characterized radiographically). The implication was that even the purported advantage of neoadjuvant chemotherapy administration (decrease in tumor size and increase tumor kill), did not correlate with improved oncologic outcomes.

Therefore, the evidence does not overwhelmingly demonstrate a survival benefit in patients treated with neoadjuvant chemotherapy. As shown in Table 127.1, reported and calculated odds ratios show no statistical significance in a correlation between neo-adjuvant chemotherapy administration and overall survival.[6,15] In addition, it is unclear whether there is even a survival benefit difference observed between chemotherapy responders and nonresponders.

Recommendation

• Administration of neoadjuvant chemotherapy is not beneficial in treatment of localized high-risk soft tissue

Table 127.1 Efficacy of chemotherapy in treatment of soft tissue sarcoma

Reference	Study design/ quality of evidence	No. of patients[a]	Results	Conclusions	Statistical significance: overall survival related to intervention
A. Efficacy of neoadjuvant chemotherapy in treatment of soft tissue sarcoma					
Meric et al.[3]	Retrospective/ Low	65	Reviewed records of patients treated with NeoCT to determine radiographic response—34% partial, 9% minor, 31% stable, 26% progressive In 13%, NeoCT "downstaged" the operation, 78% had no change, and 9% progressed However, radiographic response was the most significant predictor of overall survival	Although only a few NeoCT patients had smaller surgery, radiographic response did correlate to improved survival	N/A—correlates radiographic response to survival
Eilber et al.[4]	Retrospective/ Low	496	The percentage of patients who achieved ≥95% necrosis increased from 13% to 48% with the addition of IF to doxorubicin. 5 year survival in patients with >95% necrosis = 80% vs. 62% in patients with <95% necrosis	In patients who receive neoadjuvant therapy and have evidence of treatment-induced necrosis, patients with >95% necrosis demonstrate improved OS and LRFS	N/A—correlates % necrosis to overall survival
Menendez et al.[5]	Retrospective/ Low	82	The overall five year survivorship for patients with <95% or >95% necrosis were 20% and 33% respectively	Tissue necrosis from NeoCT does not seem to predict outcome	N/A – correlates % necrosis to overall survival
Gortzak et al.[6]	RCT/High	134	Chemotherapy did not interfere with planned surgery and did not affect post-operative wound healing. Trial closed after phase II because of poor patient accrual. Median follow-up of 7.3 years, 5 year disease-free survival was 52% for no neoadjuvant chemo and 56% for neoadjuvant chemo groups, and 64% and 65% respectively for overall survival	Although chemotherapy did not compromise surgical intervention, there was not a major survival benefit observed with administration of neoadjuvant chemotherapy	Calculated OR overall survival at mean of 7.3 years OR 0.68, 95%CI 0.34–1.38; p = 0.29
Pisters et al.[7]	Retrospective/ Low	76	Responding patients had rates of LRFS, DMFS, DFS, OS similar to nonresponders	NeoCT associated with response, DFS, OS rates similar to reported adjuvant chemotherapy. Responding patients had rates of LRFS, DMFS, DFS, OS similar to nonresponders	N/A—correlates radiographic response to survival
Italiano et al.[15]	Retrospective/ Low	237 (SS)	Median follow-up 58 months Neither neoadjuvant or adjuvant chemotherapy (IF containing regimen) had significant impact on DSS, LRFS, DRFS	Wide surgical excision of SS with adjuvant radiotherapy are accepted treatments. Chemotherapy shows no statistically significant benefit	Reported HR 0.91, 95% CI 0.56 – 1.49; p = 0.725

(Continued)

Table 127.1 (*Continued*)

Reference	Study design/ quality of evidence	No. of patients[a]	Results	Conclusions	Statistical significance: overall survival related to intervention
B: Efficacy of adjuvant chemotherapy in treatment of soft tissue sarcoma					
Sarcoma Meta-analysis Group[8]	Meta-analysis/ High	1568	HRs of 0.73 for LRFS, 0.70 for DRFS, 0.75 for DFS correspond to absolute benefits from adjuvant chemotherapy of 6%, 10%, and 10% respectively at ten years. For OS, the HR of 0.89 was not significant	Adjuvant doxorubicin-based chemotherapy (statistically) significantly improves time to local and distant recurrence and overall recurrence-free survival	Reported HR 0.89, 95% CI 0.76 – 1.03; p = 0.12
Frustaci et al.[9]	RCT/High	104	Median follow-up of 59 months Median DFS 48 months in treatment group and 16 months in control group DSS was 75 months for treated group and 46 months for control Absolute benefit in OS was 13% at 2 years and 19% at 4 years	Intensified adjuvant chemotherapy had a positive impact on DFS and OS in patients with high-risk extremity STS	Calculated OR overall survival to 4 years: OR 0.54, 95% CI 0.25–1.18; p = 0.12
Frustaci et al.[10]	RCT/High	104	Further follow-up of prior experimental group showed that DFS and OS differences in treatment arm vs. control group no longer statistically different	The previously observed overall survival benefit loses statistical significance at later time points. Therefore, time to recurrence may be lengthened, but overall survival at further follow-up is the same	Calculated OR overall survival to 89.6 months: OR 0.538, 95% CI 0.25–1.17; p = 0.12
Cormier et al.[11]	Retrospective/ Low	674	Median follow-up 6.1 years Use of chemotherapy is associated with time-varying clinical effects	Clinical benefits associated with doxorubicin-based chemotherapy are not sustained beyond 1 year	Reported HR DSS at 12 months: 0.37, 95% CI 0.20–0.69; p = 0.002 Reported HR after 12 months: HR 1.36 95% CI, 1.02–1.81; p = 0.04
Pervaiz et al.[12]	Meta-analysis/ High	1953	OR for local recurrence was 0.73 in favor of chemotherapy For distant and overall recurrence, OR 0.67 in favor of chemotherapy Regarding survival, OR for doxorubicin with IF was 0.56 in favor of chemotherapy	Analysis confirms marginal efficacy of chemotherapy with respect to LRFS, DRFS, DSS	Reported OS doxo-alone based therapies OR 0.84, 95% CI 0.68–1.03; p = 0.09 OS doxo + ifos based therapies OR 0.56, 95% CI 0.36–0.85; p = 0.01
Cochrane Gynaecological Cancer Group[13]	Cochrane systematic review/High	1568	LRFS HR with chemo was 0.73. DRFS was 0.70. Overall survival was 0.75. Those correspond to significant absolute benefits of 6–10% at 10 years. For OS, HR of 0.89 not statistically significant but does potentially represent absolute benefit of 4%	Doxorubicin-based chemo appears to significantly improve LRFS, DRFS, DFS, and trends towards improved OS	Reported HR 0.89, 95%CI 0.76–1.03; p = 0.12)

Table 127.1 (*Continued*)

Reference	Study design/ quality of evidence	No. of patients[a]	Results	Conclusions	Statistical significance: overall survival related to intervention
Eilber et al.[14]	Prospective observation/ Low	101	4-year DSS of IF-treated patients was 88% compared to 67% in no treatment group. Treatment with IF associated with improved DRFS but not LRFS	IF-based chemotherapy associated with an improved DSS in adult patients with high risk extremity synovial sarcoma	Calculated OR overall survival to 48 months: OR 0.26 (95% CI 0.10–0.67); p = 0.005.
Italiano et al.[15]	Retrospective/ Low	237 (SS)	Median follow-up 58 months. Neither neoadjuvant or adjuvant chemotherapy (IF containing regimen) had significant impact on DSS, LRFS, DRFS	Wide surgical excision of SS with adjuvant radiotherapy are accepted treatments. Chemotherapy shows no statistically significant benefit	Reported HR 1.62 (0.91–2.87); p = 0.099

Calculated, authors of this review have calculated OR/CI to improve statistical validity of analysis; DFS, disease-free survival; DRFS, distant recurrence-free survival; DSS, disease-specific survival; HR, hazard ratio; IF, ifosfamide; LRFS, local recurrence-free survival; N/A, does not address overall survival reported between control (no chemo) and experimental (chemo group); NeoCT, neoadjuvant chemotherapy; OR, odds ratio; OS, overall survival; Reported, authors report OR/CI in published sources; SS, synovial sarcoma.
[a]Number of patients pooled from 14 trials.

sarcoma, as there is no difference in overall survival or disease-free survival, and surgical resectability is not reliably improved by its administration [overall quality: very low]

Question 2: Is there a role for adjuvant chemotherapy in treatment of STS?

Case clarification
Another treatment option for the patient presented would be to initiate treatment with a combination of radiation and wide surgical resection, and then refer for adjuvant chemotherapy. The theoretic benefit of adjuvant chemotherapy would be to improve disease-free survival rates by eliminating micrometastases.

Relevance
A multimodal approach utilizing radiation and surgery achieves excellent local control. However despite local control, distant metastases are not controlled. Adjuvant chemotherapy potentially could address unrecognized micrometastases in high-risk patients.

Current opinion
Current opinion suggests that administration of adjuvant chemotherapy has marginal efficacy, and its benefits may be outweighed by the significant associated toxicities.

Finding the evidence
• EBM Reviews—Cochrane Central Register of Controlled Trials: "adjuvant chemotherapy" AND "soft tissue sarcoma"
• EBM Reviews—Cochrane Database of Systematic Reviews: "adjuvant chemotherapy" AND "soft tissue sarcoma"
• PubMed (www.ncbi.nlm.nih.gov/pubmed) clinical queries/systematic reviews, using search terms: "soft tissue sarcoma" AND "adjuvant chemotherapy"; "synovial sarcoma" AND "adjuvant chemotherapy"
• PubMed (www.ncbi.nlm.nih.gov/pubmed), using keywords: "soft tissue sarcoma" AND "adjuvant chemotherapy"; "synovial sarcoma" AND "adjuvant chemotherapy"

Quality of the evidence
Level I
• 2 Cochrane systematic reviews
• 3 systematic reviews/meta-analyses
• 2 randomized trials

Level II
• 1 prospective case series
• 2 retrospective reviews

Findings
The best evidence, summarized in the Cochrane database review from 2009, suggests that doxorubicin-based adju-

vant chemotherapy improves time to local and distant recurrence and overall recurrence-free survival in adults with resectable sarcoma. A trend towards overall improved survival was also observed. Another recent meta-analysis suggests that there is a statistically significant marginal efficacy. However, as is indicated in this chapter, the evidence is problematic and historically confusing.

The Sarcoma Meta-analysis Collaboration formed and reported in 1997 on 1,568 with localized, resectable disease treated in a series of 14 doxorubicin-based trials. With a median follow-up of 9.4 years, they reported statistically significant treatment effects including decreased risk of local recurrence (27% decrease, absolute benefit of 6%), decreased risk of distant disease (30% reduction in risk, absolute benefit of 10%) at 10 years. There was a trend towards improved overall survival which was not statistically significant (hazard ratio (HR) 0.89, 95% CI 0.76–1.03; p = 0.12). However, in a specific subgroup (high-grade, large, extremity sarcomas) there was a clear survival advantage (7% at 10 years).[8]

> Doxorubicin (adriamycin) is an anthracycline antibiotic used as a chemotherapeutic agent. It works by intercalating DNA. Toxicities can include nausea, vomiting, and heart arythmias. Cumulative doses can lead to cardiotoxicity including congestive heart failure and dilated cardiomyopathy.

Based on that meta-analysis, an RCT designed to assess the clinical efficacy of combined doxorubicin and high-dose ifosfamide therapy was initiated by the Italian Sarcoma Group.[9] Initial results comparing outcomes of patients with extremity and pelvic sarcomas treated either with resection and adjuvant radiation, or with resection, radiation and adjuvant 4'-epidoxorubicin and ifosfamide demonstrated a statistically significant difference between the treatment and control groups. There were observed improvements in median disease-free survival (48 months vs. 16 months), median survival (75 months vs. 46 months), and an absolute survival benefit of 13% at 2 years and 19% at 4 years (*calculated OR overall survival to 4 years: OR 0.539 (95% CI 0.247–1.177); p = 0.12*).* The study was stopped, based on the conclusion that chemotherapy afforded improved oncologic outcomes. However, the same 140 patients were subsequently evaluated in 2003.[10] Now with longer follow-up (89.6 months), the previously observed survival benefit was no longer statistically significant (*calculated OR overall survival to 89.6 months: OR 0.538, 95% CI 0.247–1.172; p = 0.11*).

---

*In this chapter, the odds ratio (OR) reported in italics has been calculated by the authors and is not reported as part of the manuscripts referenced. Table 127.1 provides overall review of studies cited and includes either the reported or calculated HR or OR for overall survival as related to chemotherapy administration.

> Ifosfamide (Ifex) is an alkylating agent whose mechanism of action includes the formation of covalent bonds with DNA, RNA, and proteins thereby impairing cell function. Dosing is limited by genitourinary and neurologic toxicity and is usually administered in conjunction with mesna to reduce the genitourinary toxicity.

Additional studies also failed to find a treatment benefit. A retrospective review of 674 patients out of Sloan Kettering and M.D. Anderson reported that positive treatment effects from adjuvant doxorubicin were not sustained for greater than one year (reported HR disease-specific survival at 12 months: HR 0.37, 95% CI 0.20–0.69); p = 0.002; reported HR after 12 months: HR 1.36, 95% CI 1.02–1.81; p = 0.04).[11]

However, a more recent (2008) systemic meta-analysis of RCTs identified 4 new eligible trials, for a total of 18 trials (1,953 patients).[12] That meta-analysis revealed a marginal efficacy with regards to local recurrence, distant recurrence, overall recurrence and overall survival (OR 0.84, 95% CI, 0.68–1.03; p = 0.09) that is slightly enhanced with combination doxorubicin and ifosfamide therapy. This is considered strong evidence supporting the efficacy of ifosfamide, but the marginal improvement must be weighed against potential toxicity.

The most recent Cochrane reviews determined that adjuvant chemotherapy slightly improved the time to local and distant recurrence, and overall recurrence-free survival in adults with localized, resectable STS, with a trend towards improved overall survival (14 trials including 1,568 patients; reported HR 0.89 (95% CI 0.76–1.03); p = 0.12).[13]

The above analysis primarily focuses on adult STS without further delineating subtypes. Within the heading of "soft tissue sarcoma," there are specific tumors that have characteristic genetic translocations which potentiate more accurate classification. Improved classification translates into better evidence because of more homogeneous study populations. One example is synovial sarcoma.

> Synovial sarcoma makes up 10–15% of adult STSs. Synovial sarcomas contain a characteristic translocation (X;18; p11;q11) representing the fusion of *SYT* (18q11) with either *SSX1* or *SSX2* (both at Xp11) resulting in the fusion genes *SYT-SSX1* or *SYT-SSX2*.

In the case of synovial sarcoma, there is some evidence to suggest that adjuvant chemotherapy might improve oncologic outcomes, and therefore chemotherapy may be a reasonable intervention in those patients. In a recent prospective study of 101 patients, ifosfamide-based therapy was associated with an improved disease-specific survival (DSS) in adult patients with high-risk, primary, extremity synovial sarcomas.[14] In that study, 67 patients were treated with IF and 33% received no therapy (NoC). The 4-year DSS of the IF-treated patients was 88% compared with 67% for the NoC patients (p = 0.01) (*calculated OR overall survival to 48 months: OR 0.262, 95% CI 0.102–0.674; p = 0.005*). Smaller size (HR 0.3 per 5 cm decrease, p < 0.0001) and treatment with IF (HR 0.3 compared with NoC, p = 0.007) were independently associated with an improved DSS. Treatment with IF was independently associated with an improved distant recurrence-free survival (HR = 0.4, p = 0.03) but not associated with an improved local recurrence-free survival (p = 0.39).

However, even with synovial sarcoma there is conflicting evidence. A retrospective analysis of 237 patients with a median follow-up of 58 months, neither neoadjuvant or adjuvant chemotherapy has a significant impact on overall survival, local recurrence-free survival, or distant recurrence-free survival.[15] Therefore, synovial sarcoma in adults is often treated like other STS, and chemotherapy is reserved for high-risk tumors or metastatic disease at presentation. If adjuvant chemotherapy is offered, combination doxorubicin and ifosfamide is prescribed in appropriate patients.

Recommendations

• Administration of adjuvant chemotherapy in the setting of high-grade, large extremity sarcomas may result in a longer time interval until local or distant recurrences. There is a trend, and perhaps statistically significant marginal improvement, in survival in those patients, and therefore in patients who can tolerate chemotherapy side effects, chemotherapy could be offered as an adjuvant [overall quality: high]

• There is not overwhelming evidence of a significant oncologic benefit in treating synovial sarcoma with adjuvant chemotherapy. There is evidence of increased tumor sensitivity to ifosfamide, and therefore, synovial sarcoma should be treated with meticulous surgical resection and neo-adjuvant or adjuvant radiation. Chemotherapy, utilizing doxorubicin and ifosfamide may be indicated in the treatment of high-risk patients or patients with metastatic disease at presentation [overall quality: low]

Summary of recommendations

• Administration of neoadjuvant chemotherapy is not beneficial in treatment of localized high-risk soft tissue sarcoma, as there is no difference in overall survival or disease-free survival, and surgical respectability is not reliably improved by its administration

• Administration of adjuvant chemotherapy in the setting of high-grade, large extremity sarcomas may result in a longer time interval until local or distant recurrences. There

is a trend, and perhaps statistically significant marginal improvement, in survival in those patients, and therefore in patients who can tolerate chemotherapy side effects, chemotherapy could be offered as an adjuvant

• There is not overwhelming evidence of a significant oncologic benefit in treating synovial sarcoma with adjuvant chemotherapy. There is evidence of increased tumor sensitivity to ifosfamide, and therefore, synovial sarcoma should be treated with meticulous surgical resection and neoadjuvant or adjuvant radiation. Chemotherapy, utilizing doxorubicin and ifosfamide may be indicated in the treatment of high-risk patients or patients with metastatic disease at presentation

Conclusion

Despite excellent strategies in STS local control, adjuvant chemotherapy offers only marginal efficacy in the treatment of STS. The evidence supporting this marginal efficacy is considered to be high quality (Table 127.1). Chemotherapy administered in the neoadjuvant setting does not result in easier resections. Adjuvant chemotherapy may result in improved survival in patients with large, high-grade isolated extremity sarcomas. The inherent difficult in good statistical analysis of these patients is the low number of patients that can be enrolled, resulting in studies poorly powered to determine the presence of true statistical significance. The future success of chemotherapy directed towards STS will depend upon genetic delineation of subtype and genetic/protein specific targets.

References

1. Spiro IJ, Gebhardt MC, Candace Jennings L, *et al*. Prognostic factors for control of sarcomas of the soft tissues managed by radiation and surgery. Semin Oncol 1997;24:540–6.
2. Delaney TF, Yang JC, Glatstein E. Adjuvant therapy for adult patients with soft tissue sarcomas. Oncology 1991;5:105–18.
3. Meric F, Hess KR, Varma DG, *et al*. Radiographic response to neoadjuvant chemotherapy is a predictor of local control. Cancer 2002;95:1120–6.
4. Eilber FC, Rosen G, Eckardt J, *et al*. Treatment-induced pathologic necrosis: a predictor of local recurrence and survival in patients receiving neoadjuvant therapy for high-grade extremity soft tissue sarcomas. J Clin Oncol 2001;19(13):3203–9.
5. Menendez LR, Ahlmann ER, Savage K, *et al*. Tumor necrosis has no prognostic value in neoadjuvant chemotherapy for soft tissue sarcoma. Clin Orthop Relat Res 2006;455:219–24.
6. Gortzak E, Azzarelli A, Buesa J *et al*. A randomized phase II study on neoadjuvant chemotherapy for "high-risk" adult soft tissue sarcomas. Eur J Cancer 2001;37(9):1096–103.
7. Pisters PWT, Patel SR, Varma DGK, *et al*. Preoperative chemotherapy for Stage IIIB extremity soft tissue sarcoma: long-term results from a single institution. J Clin Oncol 1997;15(12):3481.

8. Sarcoma Meta-analysis Collaboration. Adjuvant chemotherapy for localized resectable soft tissue sarcoma of adults: Meta-analysis of individual data. Lancet 1997;350:1647–54.

9. Frustaci S, Gherlinzoni F, DePaoli A, *et al*. Adjuvant chemotherapy for adult soft tissue sarcomas of the extremities and girdles: Results of the Italian randomized cooperative trial. J Clin Oncol 2001;19(5):1238–47.

10. Frustaci S, De Paoli A, Bidoli E, *et al*. Ifosfamide in the adjuvant therapy of soft tissue sarcomas. Oncology 2003;65(S2):80–4.

11. Cormier JN, Huang X, Xing Y, *et al*. Cohort analysis of patients with localized, high risk, extremity soft tissue sarcoma treated at two cancer centers: chemotherapy associated outcomes. J Clin Oncol 2004;22(15):4567–74.

12. Pervaiz N, Colterjohn N, Farrokhyar F, *et al*. A systematic meta-analysis of randomized controlled trials of adjuvant chemother-apy for localized resectable soft-tissue sarcoma. Cancer 2008; 113(3):573–81.

13. Cochrane Gynaecological Cancer Group. Adjuvant chemother-apy for localized resectable soft tissue sarcoma in adults. Cochrane Database Syst Rev 2009;4.

14. Eilber FC, Brennan MF, Eilber FR, *et al*. Chemotherapy is associ-ated with improved survival in adult patients with primary extremity synovial sarcoma. Ann Surg 2007;246(1):105–13.

15. Italiano A, Penel N, Robin YM, et al. Neoadjuvant chemotherapy does not improve outcome in resected primary sysnovial sarcoma: a study of the French Sarcoma Group. Ann Oncol 2008;20:425–30.

128 Surgery in Bone Sarcoma: Allograft vs. Megaprosthesis

Kelly C. Homlar, Jennifer L. Halpern, Herbert S. Schwartz, and Ginger E. Holt
Vanderbilt University Medical Center, Nashville, TN, USA

Importance of the problem

According to the American Cancer Society, an estimated 2,570 new primary bone cancers were diagnosed in the United States in 2009, causing 1,430 deaths.[1] With advances in chemotherapy and imaging, it is now possible to provide limb salvage surgery in 90–95% of patients.[2–6] With longer patient survival, it is important that a durable reconstruction follow tumor resection.

In addition to primary bone sarcomas, orthopedic surgeons face the more common challenge of metastases to bone. It is estimated that around 350,000 people die each year in the United States with bone metastases,[7] and the number of patients living with bone metastases is much higher. When present in periarticular areas, these metastases occasionally require tumor resection and reconstruction similar to that of primary bone sarcomas.

Three common means of reconstruction have been used after periarticular tumor resection: osteoarticular allograft, allograft–prosthetic composite (APC), and endoprosthesis. An osteoarticular allograft reconstruction utilizes a matched cadaver bone that is affixed to host bone via plate/screw construct or intramedullary nail fixation (Figure 128.1a). APCs combine an osteoarticular allograft that is skewered with a joint replacing prosthesis (Figure 128.1b). Endoprostheses replace resected bone with a metal implant cemented or press-fit into remaining host bone (Figure 128.1c).

Each method of reconstruction has many advantages and disadvantages. An important advantage of an osteoarticular allograft is the ability to repair host soft tissue to donor tendon/ligament attachments. Disadvantages of allografts include allograft fracture, host–allograft nonun-

ion, and secondary osteoarthritis. Advantages of endoprostheses include immediate use; disadvantages consist of aseptic loosening and wear. APCs provide donor soft tissue attachments for repair and prevent late osteoarthritis by resurfacing the joint, but carry the risk of allograft fracture and nonunion, transmission of infection, and the technical challenge of the reconstruction.

Although any anatomic location may be subject to tumor invasion requiring reconstruction, currently the most controversial sites of reconstruction are the proximal humerus and proximal tibia, as choices of reconstruction are largely based in individual surgeon experience and preference without universal agreement on optimal care. Thus, this chapter focuses on these two anatomic locations. The following questions will be addressed in each section:

1. What is the comparative risk of postoperative complications such as infection, recurrence, nonunion, aseptic loosening, fracture, and dislocation?
2. What is the comparative functional outcome between osteoarticular allografts, APCs, and endoprostheses via MSTS score or range of motion, if applicable?
3. What is the comparative success of limb salvage between osteoarticular allografts, APCs, and endoprostheses?
4. What is the comparative implant survival at 5, 10, and 20 years between osteoarticular allografts, APCs, and endoprostheses?

Finding the evidence

A literature search was performed by searching PubMed (www.ncbi.nlm.nih.gov/pubmed/) and OVID using a combination of terms including type of reconstruction and location (e.g., "allograft" and "proximal tibia") for each

Evidence-Based Orthopedics, First Edition. Edited by Mohit Bhandari.
© 2012 Blackwell Publishing Ltd. Published 2012 by Blackwell Publishing Ltd.

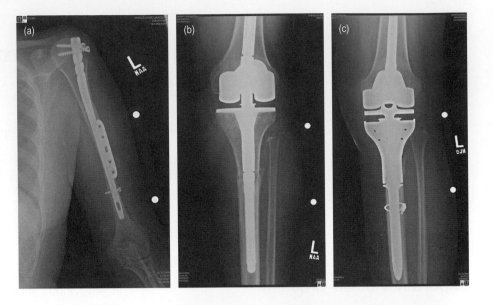

Figure 128.1 (a) Example of an osteoarticular allograft reconstruction. (b) Example of an allograft–prosthetic composite reconstruction. (c) Example of an endoprosthetic reconstruction.

area of the body discussed. All appropriate articles then underwent hand review to find any previously undetected articles in the reference section. All potential articles were then screened to see if they met the following criteria:
- Included 10 or more patients in the study
- A minimum of 2 year follow-up
- Data broken down by location, addressing at least three of the data points desired in each area of the body investigated (i.e., proximal humerus and proximal tibia)

Quality of the evidence

All studies identified were therapeutic, retrospective case series (level IV evidence).

Proximal humerus

Case scenario

A 13 year old female presents with a 3 month history of left shoulder pain that awakens her at night. Radiographs are shown in Figure 128.2. Open biopsy is consistent with Ewing's sarcoma. Resection and reconstruction are planned.

Finding the evidence

Literature review found 7 articles meeting the criteria for osteoarticular allografts in the proximal humerus, 4 articles for APCs, and 14 articles for endoprostheses (Table 128.1).[8-29]

Quality of the data

Pooled data can be found in Table 128.2 and relative risk calculations in Table 128.3.

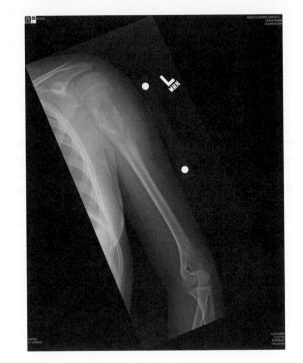

Figure 128.2 Case example: proximal humerus.

Question 1: What is the comparative risk of postoperative complications such as infection, recurrence, nonunion, aseptic loosening, fracture, and dislocation?

Findings

Pooled data showed 1.4% deep infection in proximal humerus endoprostheses (11 papers, 7 of 517 patients, range 0–3.5%), 7.9% in osteoarticular allografts (7 papers, 10 of 126 patients, range 0–18.1%), and 5.1% in APCs (4

Table 128.1 Proximal humerus: literature review

Study	Reconstruction	Pts	Avg f/u (mo)	Implant survival (5;10;20yrs) %	Reoperation	Revision	Deep infection	Local recurrence	Nonunion	Aseptic loosening	Allograft fracture	Implant fracture	Periprosthetic fracture	Dislocation/instability	Amputation	Mean Abd/FF (°)	Mean 1993 MSTS
Jeys et al.[8]	Endo	103	108	NR; 84.7; 66.7		18	0	7		8		2	0	1	6		
Zeegen et al.[9]	Endo	15	18									0	0	0			
Torbert et al.[10]	Endo	17	56.4	93;70;NR			0										
Malawer et al.[11]	Endo	29	42			3	1	2							1	26	
Gosheger et al.[12]	Endo	39	45	93.6;NR;NR									0	2			21
Cannon et al.[13]	Endo	83	30			2	2	0		0		0	0	5	0	41/42	18.9
Mayilvahanan et al.[14]	Endo	57	66	94.5;83;NR		5	2	4		2		2	0	1		max 45	
Kumar et al.[15]	Endo	100	108	NR;42;NR		7	1	15		6		0	0	2	8	44/55	23.7
Asavamongkolkul et al.[16]	Endo	30	90				1	3		1		0	0	4			22.8
Wittig et al.[17]	Endo	23	76				0	0		0		0	1	0		max 45	
Bos et al.[18]	Endo	18	68.4			12		1				1	1	10		34/43	
Scotti et al.[19]	Endo	40	30				0	4		1				1			21.9
Potter et al.[20]	Endo	16	98	100;NR;NR	4	0	0	0		0		0	0	5		4 pt ≥90	20.7
	APC	16	98	91;NR;NR	4	1	2	1	1	0	1		0	3		12 pt ≥90	23.7
	Allo	17	98	56;NR;NR	4	1	1	2	1		9					7 pt ≥90	22.4
Rodl et al.[21]	Endo	19	59	83;NR;NR		1	0	0	1	0		0	0				23.7
	Allo	11	59	75;NR;NR		1	1	2	1		3			3			22.2
Jensen and Johnston.[22]	APC	15	65			0	0	2			3			3		82/NR	
Moran and Stalley[23]	APC	11	69.6		5	0	0	2	2	0				4	1	32/40	19.8
Abdeen et al.[24]	APC	36	60	NR;88;NR		3	0	1	4	3	0		0	1	0	50/56	26
Getty and Peabody[25]	Allo	16	52	68;NR;NR			1	0	0		4			11		max 40	21
Gebhardt et al.[26]	Allo	20	63.6		11		3	2	1		7	1	1	1	2		
Mourikis et al.[27]	Allo	20	192		14		2	4	5		6			2	2		
Probyn et al.[28]	Allo	11	45.6		5	5	2	0	0		4			3			15
DeGroot et al.[29]	Allo	31	63.6	78;NR;NR	11	7	1	1	6		11			2		59/47	22.4

Allo, osteoarticular allograft; APC, allograft–prosthetic composite; Endo, endoprosthetic reconstruction.

Table 128.2 Proximal humerus: pooled data

	Endoprosthesis	Osteoarticular allograft	APC
Mean follow-up (mean of all studies)	64 mo	82 mo	73 mo
Kaplan–Meier survival	5 yr: 83–100%	5 yr: 56–78%	5 yr: 91%
	10 yr: 42–85%	10 yr: NR	10 yr: 88%
	20 yr: 66.7%	20 yr: NR	20 yr: NR
Revision	11.30% (47/417)	22% (13/59)	5.1% (4/78)
Deep infection	1.4% (7/517)	7.90% (10/126)	5.1% (4/78)
Local recurrence	6.90% (36/518)	8.7% (11/126)	7.7% (6/78)
Aseptic loosening	4.0% (18/452)	N/A	4.7% (3/63)
Implant fracture	1.00% (5/464)	N/A	NR
Periprosthetic fracture	0.24% (1/416)	2.8% (1/36)	0% (0/16)
Allograft fracture	N/A	35% (44/126)	1.9% (1/52)
Allograft nonunion	N/A	11.1% (14/126)	11.1% (7/63)
Dislocation	5.90% (31/524)	21% (20/95)	14.1% (11/78)
Range of motion mean abd/FF (°)	40/47	59/47	55/48
Mean 1993 MSTS score	74% (63–87%)	68% (50–75%)	77% (66–87%)
Amputation	4.8% (15/315)	10% (4/40)	2.1% (1/47)

abd, abduction; FF, forward flexion; N/A, not applicable; NR, not reported.

papers, 4 of 78 patients, range 0–13.3%). The rate of deep infection is significantly lower in endoprostheses when compared to osteoarticular allografts (RR 0.17, 95% CI 0.07–0.44, p = 0.00).

Local recurrence occurred in 6.9% of endoprostheses (11 papers, 36 of 518 patients, range 0–15%), 8.7% in osteoarticular allografts (7 papers, 11 of 126 patients, range 0–18.1%), and 7.7% in APCs (4 papers, 6 of 78 patients, range 2.7–18.1%). These differences were not statistically significant.

Aseptic loosening occurred in 4.0% of endoprostheses (8 papers, 18 of 452 patients, range 0–7.8%) and in 4.7% of APCs (3 papers, 3 of 63 patients, range 0–8.3%).

Implant fractures occurred in 1.0% of endoprostheses (10 papers, 5 of 464 patients, range 0–5.5%). Periprosthetic fractures occurred in 0.24% of endoprostheses (10 papers, 1 of 416 patients, range 0–4.3%), 2.8% of osteoarticular studies (2 papers, 1 of 36 patients, at end of plate fixation), and in 0% of APCs in the only study commenting on periprosthetic fractures. Allograft fracture occurred in 35% of osteoarticular allografts (7 papers, 44 of 126 patients, range 25–53%) and only 1.9% of APCs (2 papers, 1 of 52 patients), reaching statistical significance (RR 0.06, 95% CI 0.01–0.39, p = 0.00).

Nonunion occurred in 11.1% of osteoarticular allografts (7 papers, 14 of 126 patients, range 0–25%) as well as 11.1% of APCs (3 papers, 7 of 63 patients, range 6.2–18%).

Dislocation occurred in 5.9% of endoprostheses (11 papers, 31 of 524 patients, range 0–56%), 21% of osteoarticular allografts (5 papers, 20 of 95 patients, range 5–69%), and 14.1% of APCs (4 papers, 11 of 78 patients, range 2.8–36%). Thus, endoprostheses had a significantly lower rate of dislocation than APCs (RR 0.42, 95% CI 0.22–0.88, p = 0.0082) and osteoarticular allografts (RR 0.28, 95% CI 0.17–0.47, p = 0.00).

Question 2: What is the comparative functional outcome via MSTS score and range of motion?

Findings

The mean 1993 revised MSTS score was 74% (22.3 out of 30) in the endoprosthesis group (8 studies, range 63–87%), 68% in the osteoarticular allograft group (5 studies, range 50–75%), and 77% in the APC group (3 studies, range 66–87%).

Range of motion (ROM) was reported in three studies using endoprostheses with an overall mean of 40° abduction and 47° forward flexion (range 34–45° abduction, 42–55° forward flexion). Mean ROM was only reported in one study using osteoarticular allografts with mean abduction 59° and forward flexion 47°. In APCs, a mean abduction of 55° (range 32–82°) was reported in three studies, and a mean forward flexion of 48° (range 40–56°) was reported in two studies.

Question 3: What is the comparative success of limb salvage?

Findings

Amputation for any reason was required in 4.8% of patients with endoprostheses (4 papers, 15 of 315 patients, range 0–8%), and in 10% of patients with osteoarticular allografts

Table 128.3 Proximal humerus: relative risk calculations. Statistically significant findings are in **bold**

Outcome	Comparison	N1/N2	RR	p value
Reoperation	Endoprosthesis/APC1	1/2	0.75(0.28, 2.04)	0.5698
Reoperation	Endoprosthesis/allograft	1/4	0.55(0.23, 1.32)	0.1295
Reoperation	APC1/allograft	2/4	0.73(0.41, 1.31)	0.2673
Revision	Endoprosthesis/APC1	7/4	2.26(0.84, 6.09)	0.0897
Revision	**Endoprosthesis/allograft**	**7/3**	**0.53(0.3, 0.91)**	**0.0253**
Revision	**APC1/allograft**	**4/3**	**0.23(0.08, 0.68)**	**0.0031**
Deep infection	Endoprosthesis/APC1	11/4	0.53(0.11, 2.5)	0.4148
Deep infection	**Endoprosthesis/allograft**	**11/7**	**0.17(0.07, 0.44)**	**0.0000**
Deep infection	APC1/allograft	4/7	0.32(0.07, 1.44)	0.1139
Local recurrence	Endoprosthesis/APC1	11/4	0.9(0.39, 2.07)	0.8114
Local recurrence	Endoprosthesis/allograft	11/7	0.8(0.42, 1.52)	0.4911
Local recurrence	APC1/allograft	4/7	0.88(0.34, 2.29)	0.7949
Nonunion	APC1/allograft	3/7	1(0.43, 2.35)	1.0000
Aseptic loosening	Endoprosthesis/APC1	8/3	0.84(0.25, 2.76)	0.7696
Allograft fracture	**APC1/allograft**	**2/7**	**0.06(0.01, 0.39)**	**0.0000**
Dislocation instability	**Endoprosthesis/APC1**	**11/4**	**0.42(0.22, 0.8)**	**0.0082**
Dislocation instability	**Endoprosthesis/allograft**	**11/5**	**0.28(0.17, 0.47)**	**0.0000**
Dislocation instability	APC1/allograft	4/5	0.67(0.34, 1.31)	0.2370
Amputation	Endoprosthesis/APC1	4/2	2.24(0.3, 16.55)	0.4131
Amputation	Endoprosthesis/allograft	4/2	0.48(0.17, 1.36)	0.1662
Amputation	APC1/allograft	2/2	0.21(0.02, 1.83)	0.1180
Periprosthetic fracture	Endoprosthesis/allograft	8/1	0.17(0.02, 1.79)	0.0938

(2 papers, 4 of 40 patients, both with 10%), and in 2.1% of APCs (2 papers, 1 of 47 patients, range 0–9%). These differences were not statistically significant.

Question 4: What is the comparative implant survival at 5, 10, and 20 years, if available?

Findings

Five year survival based on Kaplan–Meier survival analysis was reported in five studies evaluating endoprostheses with a range of 83–100%, four studies evaluating osteoarticular allografts with a range of 56–78%, and was 91% in the one study evaluating APCs. Mean 10 year survival rate was reported in four papers evaluating endoprostheses with a range of 42–85%, was not reported in osteoarticular allografts, and was 88% in APCs based on one paper. Only the endoprosthesis group had a 20 year survival rate reported as 66.7% in one paper.

Mean revision rate for any reason for the endoprosthesis group was 11.3% (8 papers, 47 of 417 patients, range 0–67%), 22% for osteoarticular allografts (3 papers, 13 of 59 patients, range 5.9–45%), and 5.1% for APCs (4 papers, 4 of 78 patients, range 0–8.3%). Endoprostheses and APCs had a significantly lower rate of revision than osteoarticular allografts (RR 0.53, 95% CI 0.3–0.91, p = 0.0253; RR 0.23, 95% CI 0.08–0.68, p = 0.0031 respectively).

Conclusions

The overall 5 year survival appears similar between endoprostheses and APCs, both of which have a trend toward improved survival when compared to osteoarticular allografts. Follow-up studies are needed to better predict the 10 and 20 year survival rates of these reconstructions.

Osteoarticular allograft reconstructions have a statistically significant higher rate of revision operations when compared to endoprostheses and APCs.

The rate of deep infection is significantly lower in endoprostheses when compared to osteoarticular allografts, but is not statistically different in comparison to APCs.

Allograft fracture occurred in a high percentage of osteoarticular allografts (35%). This, along with the higher rate of deep infections, may account for the significantly higher rate of revision operations.

Interestingly, despite the common belief that osteoarticular allografts offer improved stability due to the ability to repair donor tendon/ligament attachments back to what remains of host soft tissue, osteoarticular allografts had a significantly higher rate of dislocation without any apparent improvement in ROM or MSTS score. Endoprostheses had the lowest dislocation rate (6%) and APCs fell in between with 14%. The ROM was similar in all groups and overall poor, with no reconstruction obtaining a mean abduction greater than 60° or forward flexion greater than 50°.

Recommendations

• Though it is difficult to make strong recommendations as to the type of reconstruction that should be performed in the proximal humerus, it should be noted that osteoarticular allografts performed the worst in every outcome examined, with the exception of mean abduction. Endoprostheses and APCs performed quite similarly, with each appearing to be a viable reconstruction option

Proximal tibia

Case scenario

A 45 year old woman presents with a 6 week history of knee pain. Radiographs are seen in Figure 128.3. Open biopsy is consistent with high-grade dedifferentiated chondrosarcoma. Resection and reconstruction are planned.

Finding the evidence

Literature review found three articles meeting the criteria for osteoarticular allografts in the proximal tibia, three articles for APC, and 15 articles for endoprostheses (Table 128.4).[8,10–12,30–45]

Quality of the evidence

Pooled data can be found in Table 128.5 and relative risk calculations in Table 128.6.

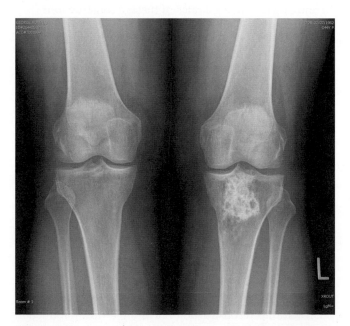

Figure 128.3 Case example: proximal tibia.

Question 1: What is the comparative risk of postoperative complications such as infection, recurrence, nonunion, aseptic loosening, fracture, dislocation/instability, and extensor mechanism failure?

Findings

Pooled data showed a deep infection rate of 15.6% in proximal tibia endoprostheses (134 of 861 patients, range 3.8–31% in 11 studies), 10.2% in osteoarticular allografts (9 of 88 patients, 2 studies), and 22% in APCs (22 of 100 patients, 3 studies, range 8.3–24%). These differences were not statistically significant.

Local recurrence occurred in 4.9% of endoprostheses (40 of 819 patients, 11 studies, range 0–10.5%), 3.7% of osteoarticular allografts (2 of 54 patients, 2 studies), and 12% of APCs (12 of 100 patients, 3 studies, range 4.8–27%). These differences were not statistically significant.

Aseptic loosening was similar between endoprostheses and APCs, occurring in 8% of endoprostheses (60 of 745 patients, 12 studies, range 0–25%) and 9% of APCs (9 of 100 patients, 3 studies, range 0–27%). Within the endoprosthesis group, independent analysis of fixed vs. rotating hinge designs could not be performed as studies including rotating hinges did not report separate aseptic loosening rates in this subgroup of their analysis. When comparing cemented vs. uncemented prostheses, there was significantly higher rate of aseptic loosening in cemented prostheses (RR 8.03, 95% CI 1.11–58.03, p = 0.011). Twenty-one percent of cemented endoprostheses had aseptic loosening (3 studies, 14 of 67 patients) versus 1.2% of uncemented endoprostheses (3 studies, 1 of 83 patients).

Bushing failures requiring reoperation occurred in 7.1% of endoprostheses.

Implant fractures occurred in 3% of endoprostheses (25 of 829 patients, 10 studies, range 0–14.3%) and 0% of APCs (0 of 100 patients, 3 studies). Periprosthetic fractures occurred in 2.9% of endoprostheses (19 of 653 patients, 9 studies, range 0–9%); no periprosthetic fractures were reported in APCs. Allograft fractures occurred in 35% of osteoarticular allografts (19/54 patients, 2 studies, range 31–37%) and in 7% of APCs (7 of 100 patients, 3 studies, range 0–27%).

One of the unique challenges of reconstruction after resection of proximal tibia tumors is reconstruction of the extensor mechanism. Of the papers that reported on extensor mechanism failures, they were reported in 11% of endoprostheses (13 of 120 patients, 3 studies, range 2.4–26%) and in 16% of APCs (16 of 100 patients, 3 studies, range 8.3–23%), not representing a statistically significant difference. Three studies on endoprostheses looked at mean extensor lag, with means of 6°, 18°, and 30° reported. 30% of patients with endoprostheses had an extensor lag more than 5° (24 of 79 patients, 2 studies, range 25–37%) as

Table 128.4 Proximal tibia literature review

Study	Treatment	Pts	Avg f/u (mo)	Implant survival (5; 10; 20yrs)	Implant	Reoperation	Revision	Deep infection	Local recurrence	Nonunion	Aseptic loosening	Allograft fracture	Implant Fracture	Periprosthetic Fracture	Dislocation	Extension Mechanism Failure	Amputation	Mean 1993 MSTS
Unwin et al.[30]	Endo	243	45.7	NR;58%;NR	NR, fixed		37	30	10		16		4	2	0		33	
Jeys et al.[8]	Endo	136	108	NR;39.9;20.7	NR		63	28	6		16		8	3	2		25	
Torbert et al.[10]	Endo	26	56.4	63; 63; NR	NR			1	2		1		0	0	1			
Tunn et al.[31]	Endo	41	78	NR	NR													23.1
Malawer and Chou[11]	Endo	13	42		Cemented, combination		6	4	0								3	21
Wunder et al.[32]	Endo	14	50	69; NR; NR	Uncemented, fixed			3			1		2	0	0		2	
Natarajan et al.[33]	Endo	133	59.4	84.5; NR; NR	Combination			16	4		5		1	12	0		13	
Flint et al.[34]	Endo	44	60	73;NR;NR	Uncemented, fixed	14	12	7	2		0		2	0	1	3	7	21.9
Grimer et al.[35]	Endo	151	80	60;30;27	Cemented, combination		95	28	16				5				26	23.1
Clohisy and Mankin[36]	Endo	16	16		Cemented, combination		5		0		3		0	1			3	
Griffin et al.[37]	Endo	25	72.9		Uncemented, fixed			5	0		0		2	0				
Biau et al.[38]	Endo	35	62	55;43;NR	Cemented, fixed		15	5			8				2	9		25
Gosheger et al.[12]	Endo	41	45	61.7;NR;NR	Combination, fixed			7			3		1			1		
Horowitz et al.[39]	Endo	16	80		Cemented, combination				0		3			1			3	
Horowitz et al.[40]	Endo	16	80	54;36;NR	Combination				0		4						8	
Donati et al.[41]	APC	62	72	73.4; NR; NR				15	3		2	0	0			9	5	
Biau et al.[42]	APC	26	128	68; 33; NR		22	14	1	2		7	7				6		
Gilbert et al. JBJS 2009;91:1646–56	APC	12	49				0	1	2		0	0				1	1	24.3
Hornicek et al.[44]	Allo	38	72				12	7	0	4		14			5			
Clohisy and Mankin[36]	Allo	16	108				7	2	2	2		5			1		2	
Brigman et al.[45]	Allo	33		78;68;NR					2								6	

APC, allograft-prosthetic composite; Allo, osteoarticular allograft; Endo, endoprosthetic reconstruction.

Table 128.5 Proximal tibia: pooled data

	Mean follow-up (mean of all studies)	Kaplan–Meier survival (mean of studies reporting)	Revision	Deep infection	Local recurrence	Aseptic loosening	Implant fracture	Periprosthetic fracture	Allograft fracture	Extensor mechanism failure	Mean 1993 MSTS Score	Amputation
Endoprosthesis	65 mo	5 yr: 54–84.5% 10 yr: 30–63% 20 yr: 20.7–27%	36.5% (233/638)	15.6% (134/861)	4.9% (40/819)	8.0% (60/745)	3.0% (25/829)	2.9% (16/653)	N/A	11% (13/120)	77% (70–83%)	15.7% (123/782)
Osteoarticular allograft	90 mo	5 yr: 78% 10 yr: 68% 20 yr: NR	35.2% (19/54)	10.2% (9/88)	3.7% (2/54)	N/A	N/A	NR	35% (19/54)	NR	NR	10.3% (9/87)
APC	83 mo	5 yr: 68–73% 10 yr: 30% 20 yr: NR	36.8% (14/38)	22% (22/100)	12% (12/100)	9.0% (9/100)	0% (0/100)	NR	7% (7/100)	16% (16/100)	81% (1 study)	8.1% (6/74)

N/A, not applicable; NR, not reported.

Table 128.6 Proximal tibia: Relative risk calculations. Statistically significant findings are in bold

Outcome	Comparison	N1/N2	RR	p value
Reoperation	Endoprosthesis/APC1	1/1	0.38(0.24, 0.6)	<0.0001
Revision	Endoprosthesis/APC1	7/2	0.99(0.65, 1.52)	0.9681
Revision	Endoprosthesis/allograft	7/2	1.04(0.71, 1.51)	0.8449
Revision	APC1/allograft	2/2	1.05(0.6, 1.82)	0.8711
Deep infection	Endoprosthesis/APC1	11/3	0.92(0.58, 1.45)	0.7088
Deep infection	Endoprosthesis/allograft	11/2	0.93(0.5, 1.73)	0.8286
Deep infection	APC1/allograft	3/2	1.02(0.49, 2.13)	0.9581
Local recurrence	Endoprosthesis/APC1	11/3	0.7(0.32, 1.52)	0.3648
Local recurrence	Endoprosthesis/allograft	11/2	1.32(0.33, 5.31)	0.6948
Local recurrence	APC1/allograft	3/2	1.89(0.41, 8.78)	0.4069
Aseptic loosening	Endoprosthesis/APC1	12/3	0.89(0.46, 1.75)	0.7457
Allograft fracture	**APC1/allograft**	**3/2**	**0.2(0.09, 0.44)**	**<0.0001**
Dislocation	Endoprosthesis/allograft	7/2	0.09(0.03, 0.26)	<0.0001
Amputation	Endoprosthesis/APC1	10/2	1.94(0.89, 4.25)	0.0800
Amputation	Endoprosthesis/allograft	10/2	0.96(0.5, 1.85)	0.9114
Amputation	APC1/allograft	2/2	0.5(0.18, 1.34)	0.1617
Extension mechanism failure	Endoprosthesis/APC1	3/3	0.68(0.34,1.34)	0.2642

compared with 26% patients with APCs (10 of 38 patients, 2 studies, range 25–27%). Unfortunately, the three articles on osteoarticular allografts did not comment on extensor mechanism failure or extensor lags.

Question 2: What is the comparative functional outcome via MSTS score?

Findings

The mean 1993 revised MSTS score was 77% (23.1 out of 30) in the endoprosthesis group (6 studies, range 70–83%), 81% in the only study reporting in APCs, and was not reported in any study looking at osteoarticular allografts.

Question 3: What is the comparative success of limb salvage?

Findings

Amputation for any reason was required in 15.7% of patients with endoprostheses (10 papers, 123 of 782 patients, range 9.7–50%), in 8.1% of patients with APCs (2 papers, 6 of 74 patients, range 8–8.3%), and in 10.3% of patients with osteoarticular allografts (3 papers, 9 of 87 patients, range 2.6–18%). These differences were not statistically significant.

Question 4: What is the comparative implant survival at 5, 10, and 20 years, if available?

Findings

Mean 5 year survival rate based on Kaplan–Meier survival analysis was 65% in endoprostheses (8 papers, range 54–

84.5%), 78% based on one paper in osteoarticular allografts, and 70.5% based on two papers in APCs (survival rates of 68% and 73%). Mean 10 year survival rate was 45% in endoprostheses (6 papers, range 30–63%), 68% based on one paper in osteoarticular allografts, and 30% based on one paper in APCs. Only the endoprosthesis group had 20 year survival rates reported as 20.7 and 27% in two papers.

Mean revision rate for any reason for the endoprosthesis group was 36.5% (7 studies, 123 of 782 patients, range 15–63%), 35.2% in the osteoarticular allograft group (2 studies, 19 of 54 patients, range 31–44%) and 36.8% in the APC group (2 studies, 14 of 38 patients, range 0–54%). These differences were not statistically significant.

Conclusions

Overall, proximal tibia reconstructions have the highest rates of amputation, highest revision rates, and shortest overall survival when compared to reconstructions in any other part of the body.

Five year survival rates and revision rates were similar between the three methods of reconstruction; however, more data is needed to compare the long-term survival of these reconstructions.

Using the data obtained, there was no statistical difference between the groups in regards to deep infection, local recurrence, or amputation rates.

Extensor mechanism failure is a fairly common complication, seen in 11% of endoprostheses and 16% of APCs. Unfortunately this data is not available for osteoarticular allografts.

Aseptic loosening is similar between endoprostheses and APCs (8% and 9% respectively). Allograft fracture is common, being seen in 35% of osteoarticular allografts, but only 7% of APCs.

Recommendations

• Based on the data points analyzed, it is not possible to recommend one type of reconstruction over the other in the proximal tibia except to note the higher risk for fracture in the osteoarticular allografts compared to endoprostheses and APCs

References

1. American Cancer Society. Cancer Facts and Figures 1998. American Cancer Society, Atlanta, 1998.
2. Eilber FR, Mirra JJ, Grant TT, Weisenburger T, Morton DL. Is amputation necessary for sarcomas? A seven-year experience with limb salvage. Ann Surg 1980;192(4):431–8.
3. Rao BN, Champion JE, Pratt CB, et al. Limb salvage procedures for children with osteosarcoma: an alternative to amputation. J Pediatr Surg 1983;18(6):901–8.
4. Sim FH, Bowman WE Jr, Wilkins RM, Chao EY. Limb salvage in primary malignant bone tumors. Orthopedics 1985;8(5):574–81.
5. Rougraff BT, Simon MA, Kneisl JS, Greenberg DB, Mankin HJ. Limb salvage compared with amputation for osteosarcoma of the distal end of the femur. A long-term oncological, functional, and quality-of-life study. J Bone Joint Surg Am 1994;76(5): 649–56.
6. Simon MA, Aschliman MA, Thomas N, Mankin HJ. Limb-salvage treatment versus amputation for osteosarcoma of the distal end of the femur. J Bone Joint Surg Am 1986;68(9): 1331–7.
7. Mundy GR. Metastasis to bone: causes, consequences and therapeutic opportunities. Nat Rev Cancer 2002;2(8):584–93.
8. Jeys LM, Kulkarni A, Grimer RJ, Carter SR, Tillman RM, Abudu A. Endoprosthetic reconstruction for the treatment of musculoskeletal tumors of the appendicular skeleton and pelvis. J Bone Joint Surg Am 2008;90(6):1265–71.
9. Zeegen EN, Aponte-Tinao LA, Hornicek FJ, Gebhardt MC, Mankin HJ. Survivorship analysis of 141 modular metallic endoprostheses at early followup. Clin Orthop Relat Res 2004(420): 239–50.
10. Torbert JT, Fox EJ, Hosalkar HS, Ogilvie CM, Lackman RD. Endoprosthetic reconstructions: results of long-term followup of 139 patients. Clin Orthop Relat Res 2005;438:51–9.
11. Malawer MM, Chou LB. Prosthetic survival and clinical results with use of large-segment replacements in the treatment of high-grade bone sarcomas. J Bone Joint Surg Am 1995;77(8): 1154–65.
12. Gosheger G, Gebert C, Ahrens H, Streitbuerger A, Winkelmann W, Hardes J. Endoprosthetic reconstruction in 250 patients with sarcoma. Clin Orthop Relat Res 2006;450:164–71.
13. Cannon CP, Paraliticci GU, Lin PP, Lewis VO, Yasko AW. Functional outcome following endoprosthetic reconstruction of the proximal humerus. J Shoulder Elbow Surg 2009;18(5): 705–10.
14. Mayilvahanan N, Paraskumar M, Sivaseelam A, Natarajan S. Custom mega-prosthetic replacement for proximal humeral tumours. Int Orthop 2006;30(3):158–62.
15. Kumar D, Grimer RJ, Abudu A, Carter SR, Tillman RM. Endoprosthetic replacement of the proximal humerus. Long-term results. J Bone Joint Surg Br 2003;85(5):717–22.
16. Asavamongkolkul A, Eckardt JJ, Eilber FR, et al. Endoprosthetic reconstruction for malignant upper extremity tumors. Clin Orthop Relat Res 1999(360):207–20.
17. Wittig JC, Bickels J, Kellar-Graney KL, Kim FH, Malawer MM. Osteosarcoma of the proximal humerus: long-term results with limb-sparing surgery. Clin Orthop Relat Res 2002;397: 156–76.
18. Bos G, Sim F, Pritchard D, Shives T, Rock M, Askew L, Chao E. Prosthetic replacement of the proximal humerus. Clin Orthop Relat Res 1987;224:178–91.
19. Scotti C, Camnasio F, Peretti GM, Fontana F, Fraschini G. Modular prostheses in the treatment of proximal humerus metastases: review of 40 cases. J Orthop Traumatol 2008;9(1): 5–10.
20. Potter BK, Adams SC, Pitcher JD Jr, Malinin TI, Temple HT. Proximal humerus reconstructions for tumors. Clin Orthop Relat Res 2009;467(4):1035–41.
21. Rödl RW, Gosheger G, Gebert C, Lindner N, Ozaki T, Winkelmann W. Reconstruction of the proximal humerus after wide resection of tumours. J Bone Joint Surg Br 2002;84(7):1004–8.
22. Jensen KL, Johnston JO. Proximal humeral reconstruction after excision of a primary sarcoma. Clin Orthop Relat Res 1995;311: 164–75.
23. Moran M, Stalley PD. Reconstruction of the proximal humerus with a composite of extracorporeally irradiated bone and endoprosthesis following excision of high grade primary bone sarcomas. Arch Orthop Trauma Surg 2009;129(10):1339–45.
24. Abdeen A, Hoang BH, Athanasian EA, Morris CD, Boland PJ, Healey JH. Allograft-prosthesis composite reconstruction of the proximal part of the humerus: functional outcome and survivorship. J Bone Joint Surg Am 2009;91(10):2406–15.
25. Getty PJ, Peabody TD. Complications and functional outcomes of reconstruction with an osteoarticular allograft after intra-articular resection of the proximal aspect of the humerus. J Bone Joint Surg Am 1999;81(8):1138–46.
26. Gebhardt MC, Roth YF, Mankin HJ. Osteoarticular allografts for reconstruction in the proximal part of the humerus after excision of a musculoskeletal tumor. J Bone Joint Surg Am 1990;72(3): 334–45.
27. Mourikis A, Mankin HJ, Hornicek FJ, Raskin KA. Treatment of proximal humeral chondrosarcoma with resection and allograft. J Shoulder Elbow Surg 2007;16(5):519–24.
28. Probyn LJ, Wunder JS, Bell RS, Griffin AM, Davis AM. A comparison of outcome of osteoarticular allograft reconstruction and shoulder arthrodesis following resection of primary tumours of the proximal humerus. Sarcoma 1998;2(3–4):163–70.
29. DeGroot H, Donati D, Di Liddo M, Gozzi E, Mercuri M. The use of cement in osteoarticular allografts for proximal humeral bone tumors. Clin Orthop Relat Res 2004;427:190–7.
30. Unwin PS, Cannon SR, Grimer RJ, Kemp HB, Sneath RS, Walker PS. Aseptic loosening in cemented custom-made prosthetic

replacements for bone tumours of the lower limb. J Bone Joint Surg Br 1996;78(1):5–13.

31. Tunn PU, Pomraenke D, Goerling U, Hohenberger P. Functional outcome after endoprosthetic limb-salvage therapy of primary bone tumours—a comparative analysis using the MSTS score, the TESS and the RNL index. Int Orthop 2008;32(5):619–25.

32. Wunder JS, Leitch K, Griffin AM, Davis AM, Bell RS. Comparison of two methods of reconstruction for primary malignant tumors at the knee: a sequential cohort study. J Surg Oncol 2001;77(2):89–99; discussion 100.

33. Natarajan MV, Sivaseelam A, Rajkumar G, Hussain SH. Custom megaprosthetic replacement for proximal tibial tumours. Int Orthop 2003;27(6):334–7.

34. Flint MN, Griffin AM, Bell RS, Ferguson PC, Wunder JS. Aseptic loosening is uncommon with uncemented proximal tibia tumor prostheses. Clin Orthop Relat Res 2006;450:52–9.

35. Grimer RJ, Carter SR, Tillman RM, Sneath RS, Walker PS, Unwin PS, Shewell PC. Endoprosthetic replacement of the proximal tibia. J Bone Joint Surg Br 1999;81(3):488–94.

36. Clohisy DR, Mankin HJ. Osteoarticular allografts for reconstruction after resection of a musculoskeletal tumor in the proximal end of the tibia. J Bone Joint Surg Am 1994;76(4):549–54.

37. Griffin AM, Parsons JA, Davis AM, Bell RS, Wunder JS. Uncemented tumor endoprostheses at the knee: root causes of failure. Clin Orthop Relat Res 2005;438:71–9.

38. Biau D, Faure F, Katsahian S, Jeanrot C, Tomeno B, Anract P. Survival of total knee replacement with a megaprosthesis after bone tumor resection. J Bone Joint Surg Am 2006;88(6):1285–93.

39. Horowitz SM, Lane JM, Otis JC, Healey JH. Prosthetic arthroplasty of the knee after resection of a sarcoma in the proximal end of the tibia. A report of sixteen cases. J Bone Joint Surg Am 1991;73(2):286–93.

40. Horowitz SM, Glasser DB, Lane JM, Healey JH. Prosthetic and extremity survivorship after limb salvage for sarcoma. How long do the reconstructions last? Clin Orthop Relat Res 1993(293):280–6.

41. Donati D, Colangeli M, Colangeli S, Di Bella C, Mercuri M. Allograft-prosthetic composite in the proximal tibia after bone tumor resection. Clin Orthop Relat Res 2008;466(2):459–65.

42. Biau DJ, Dumaine V, Babinet A, Tomeno B, Anract P. Allograft-prosthesis composites after bone tumor resection at the proximal tibia. Clin Orthop Relat Res 2007;456:211–17.

43. Gilbert NF, Yasko AW, Oates SD, Lewis VO, Cannon CP, Lin PP. Allograft-prosthetic composite reconstruction of the proximal part of the tibia. An analysis of the early results. J Bone Joint Surg Am 2009;91(7):1646–56.

44. Hornicek FJ, Jr., Mnaymneh W, Lackman RD, Exner GU, Malinin TI. Limb salvage with osteoarticular allografts after resection of proximal tibia bone tumors. Clin Orthop Relat Res 1998(352):179–86.

45. Brigman BE, Hornicek FJ, Gebhardt MC, Mankin HJ. Allografts about the knee in young patients with high-grade sarcoma. Clin Orthop Relat Res 2004(421):232–9.

129   Biopsy of Soft Tissue Masses

Bruce T. Rougraff[1], Albert J. Aboulafia[2], J. Sybil Biermann[3], and John Healey[4]

[1]OrthoIndy, Indianapolis, IN, USA
[2]Sinai Hospital, Baltimore, MD, USA
[3]University of Michigan Hospital and Health Systems, Ann Arbor, MI, USA
[4]Hospital for Special Surgery and Memorial Sloan Kettering, New York, NY, USA

Case scenario

A 70 year old woman has an enlarging mass in the right axilla. Her primary care physician orders a needle biopsy to be done by a radiologist who carries out a fine needle aspiration (FNA) from 15 different sites around the 4 cm mass in order to obtain adequate tissue. The result is nondiagnostic but suggestive of malignancy, possibly carcinoma with necrosis. The patient is referred to a breast oncologic surgeon who performs an extensive lymph node dissection and open biopsy of the axillary mass. The entire brachial plexus is carefully exposed and protected during the lymph node dissection. The pathologist finds that the lymph nodes are normal, but the axillary mass is diagnosed as a high-grade sarcoma. The woman is then referred to an orthopedic oncologist who discusses forequarter amputation for adequate local control.

The initial needle biopsy contaminated a large area of soft tissue around the sarcoma and was nondiagnostic. The next biopsy was definitive in making the diagnosis, but contaminated further tissue by exposing the brachial plexus at the time of the sarcoma biopsy. A carefully placed biopsy with adequate tissue for diagnosis could have allowed this woman a limb-sparing resection with an excellent chance of local control and probable cure.

Importance of the problem

There are three critical issues to address when determining how a biopsy of a soft tissue sarcoma should be performed. The first is to determine who is best suited to perform the biopsy—i.e., radiologist, primary care physician, general surgeon, general orthopedic surgeon, or orthopedic onco-

logic surgeon. The second is to identify the hazards of the various types of biopsies. Finally, the third is to identify the diagnostic accuracy of the soft tissue sarcoma biopsy types. Outcome measures are severely limited for procedure morbidity; however, the accuracy of the various techniques is a well-established and definable endpoint. The authors have brought together the following four questions to be addressed by the published literature.

Top four questions

1. When is a biopsy indicated?
2. How should the biopsy be placed?
3. How should the biopsy be performed (open incisional biopsy, core needle biopsy, FNA biopsy)?
4. Who should perform the biopsy (radiologist, sarcoma pathologist, general pathologist, general surgeon, general orthopedic surgeons, orthopedic oncologic surgeon)?

Finding the evidence

- PubMed search using keywords "biopsy" AND "soft tissue sarcoma"

Quality of the evidence

33 articles were reviewed.

Level II
- 3 outcomes research studies

Level III
- 2 retrospective comparative studies

Level IV
- 28 retrospective reviews

Question 1: When is a biopsy indicated?

Case clarification
The patient reported an enlarging mass of uncertain etiology. This was felt clinically to require a biopsy.

Current opinion
In simple terms, a biopsy is indicated whenever a mass with biologic activity is clinically suspected and further surgical or medical treatment will be based on that result. Because many musculoskeletal lesions are inactive processes, not every lesion requires a biopsy or treatment.

Findings
No referenced article addressed the issue of when a biopsy of a soft tissue mass was indicated. In fact, a large variability of the incidence of neoplastic and non-neoplastic lesions was noted in these articles.[1] This variability resulted in confounding results of diagnostic accuracy of needle biopsy, particularly when larger inflammatory, infectious, and myxoid lesions were sampled.

Recommendations
- Soft tissue masses larger than 3 cm are more likely to require biopsy [overall quality: low]
- Masses that are actively growing or symptomatic are lesions that may require biopsy [overall quality: low]
- A soft tissue "hematoma" that is not associated with trauma, has no history of ecchymosis, and is increasing in size or symptoms may require biopsy [overall quality: low]
- Suspected hematomas that do not resolve over time may need a biopsy [overall quality: low]

Question 2: How should the biopsy be placed?

Findings
None of the referenced articles addressed technical aspects of biopsy placement. The hazards of the biopsy have been studied when biopsy technique has wavered from the standard and the surgical morbidity is increased by 17%.[2] In the case of osteosarcoma, the local recurrence rate is increased as well as the systemic relapse for patients with inappropriate open tumor biopsy prior to referral to a cancer center.[3] No study addressed whether needle biopsy placement affected local control or survival of patients with soft tissue sarcoma. Case reports of local recurrences in unresected needle biopsy tracts have been reported.

Recommendations
- Complete hemostasis during the biopsy is critical to prevent hematoma dissection outside of the tumor bed which could potentially transport tumor cells into wider or newer areas [overall quality: low]
- The biopsy tract must be placed in a location that is resectable at the time of tumor excision (if the lesion is malignant) [overall quality: low]
- The biopsy should be placed longitudinally; in extremity, incisions should not expose critical neurovascular structures that could become contaminated with sarcoma [overall quality: low]

Question 3: How should the biopsy be performed?

Current opinion
The first objective of a biopsy is to obtain diagnostic material. If the biopsy is done in conjunction with frozen section pathology, confirmation of diagnostic material can be done such that additional tissue may be obtained if necessary.

Findings
FNA has a lower diagnostic accuracy compared to core needle biopsy according to five studies that addressed this comparison.[3-9] Incisional biopsy was associated with a 94% diagnostic accuracy and was more accurate than core biopsy (83%), but at a much higher expense in morbidity.[10]

Recommendations
The following are strong recommendations:
- Core needle biopsies are preferred over fine needle biopsies to improve diagnostic accuracy[4] [overall quality: moderate]
- Core needle biopsies are preferred over open biopsies to reduce morbidity [overall quality: moderate]
- Excisional biopsy should be reserved for carefully selected clinical situations such as small subcutaneous tumors or lesions that have a diagnostic MRI appearance [overall quality: low]

Question 4: Who should perform the biopsy?

Findings
Radiologists, pathologists, general surgeons, general orthopedic surgeons and sarcoma specialists were all represented in the available studies. Open biopsies performed by surgeons at a sarcoma center are associated with lower morbidity than those performed outside a sarcoma center.[11,12] Needle biopsies performed by all physicians had equal rates of diagnostic accuracy whether or not they were at a sarcoma center.[13] Needle biopsy performed with CT, ultrasound or MRI assistance can theoretically improve the quality of diagnostic material; however, no studies have directly compared the accuracy of radiologically guided to nonradiologically guided biopsies.[2,4,7,14-21]

The results with highest diagnostic accuracy were reported by core needle biopsy performed by surgeons.[3,10,22,23] However, this is probably explained by a selection bias whereby the most difficult diagnostic cases in the most challenging anatomic locations were referred to radiologists. The complication reported in four studies ranged from 0 to 2%.[18,24–26] Frozen section done at the time of biopsy improved the diagnostic accuracy by 6–8% but may not be cost-effective.[4]

Recommendations

• Open biopsies should be performed in a sarcoma center by a sarcoma surgeon or radiologist [overall quality: moderate]
• Needle biopsies can be performed by a sarcoma surgeon or a radiologist with equal accuracy [overall quality: low]
• Frozen sections are not cost-effective for needle biopsies [overall quality: low]

Summary of recommendations

• Soft tissue masses larger than 3 cm are more likely to require biopsy
• Masses that are actively growing or symptomatic are lesions that may require biopsy
• A soft tissue "hematoma" that is not associated with trauma, has no history of ecchymosis, and is increasing in size or symptoms may require biopsy
• Suspected hematomas that do not resolve over time may need a biopsy
• Complete hemostasis during the biopsy is critical to prevent hematoma dissection outside of the tumor bed which could potentially transport tumor cells into wider or newer areas
• The biopsy tract must be placed in a location that is resectable at the time of tumor excision (if the lesion is malignant)
• The biopsy should be placed longitudinally; in extremity, incisions should not expose critical neurovascular structures that could become contaminated with sarcoma
• Core needle biopsies are preferred over fine needle biopsies to improve diagnostic accuracy
• Core needle biopsies are preferred over open biopsies to reduce morbidity
• Excisional biopsy should be reserved for carefully selected clinical situations such as small subcutaneous tumors or lesions that have a diagnostic MRI appearance
• Open biopsies should be performed in a sarcoma center by a sarcoma surgeon or radiologist
• Needle biopsies can be performed by a sarcoma surgeon or a radiologist with equal accuracy
• Frozen sections are not cost-effective for needle biopsies

References

1. Moulton JS, Blebea JS, Dunco DM, et al. MR imaging of soft-tissue masses: diagnostic efficacy and value of distinguishing between benign and malignant lesions. AJR Am J Roentgenol 1995;164(5):1191–9.
2. Altuntas AO, Slavin J, Smith PJ, et al. Accuracy of computed tomography guided core needle biopsy of musculoskeletal tumors. Aust N Z J Surg 2005;75(4):187–91.
3. Ball AB, Fisher C, Watkins RM, et al. Diagnosis of soft tissue tumors by Tru-Cut biopsy. Br J Surg 1990;77:756–58.
4. Dupuy DE, Rosenberg AE, Punyaratabadhu T, et al. Accuracy of CT-guided needle biopsy of musculoskeletal neoplasms. AJR 1998;171:759–62.
5. Hau A, Kim I, Kattapuram S, et al. Accuracy of CT-guided biopsies in 359 patients with musculoskeletal lesions. Skeletal Radiol 2002;31(6):349–53.
6. Yang YJ, Damron TA. Comparison of needle core biopsy and fine-needle aspiration for diagnostic accuracy in musculoskeltal lesions. Arch Pathol Lab Med 2004;128:759–64.
7. Yeow KM, Tan CF, Chen JS, et al. Diagnostic sensitivity of ultrasound-guided needle biopsy in soft tissue masses about superficial bone lesions. J Ultrasound Med 2000;19(12):849–55.
8. Maitra A, Ashfaq R, Saboorian MH, et al. The role of FNA biopsy in the primary diagnosis of mesenchymal lesions. A community hospital-based experience. Cancer 200;90:178–85.
9. Rydholm A, Akerman M, Idvall I, et al. Aspiration cytology of soft tissue tumors. A prospective study of its influence on choice of surgical procedure. Int Orthop 1982;6:209–14.
10. Skrzynski MC, Biermann JS, Montag A, et al. Diagnostic accuracy and charge-savings of outpatient core needle biopsy compared with open biopsy of musculoskeletal tumors. J Bone Joint Surg Am 1996;78:644–9.
11. Mankin HJ, Mankin CJ, Simon MA. The hazards of biopsy, revisited. For the members of the Musculoskeletal Tumor Society. J Bone Joint Surg Am 1996;78:656–63.
12. Ayerza MA, Musculo L, Aponte-Tinao LA, et al. Effect of erroneous surgical procedures on recurrence and survival rates for patients with osteosarcoma. Clin Orthop 2006;452:231–5.
13. Madhavan VP, Smile SR, Chandra SS, et al. Value of core needle biopsy in the diagnosis of soft tissue tumors. Indian J Pathol Microbiol 2002;45(2):165–8.
14. Hoeber I, Spillane AJ, Fisher C, et al. Accuracy of biopsy techniques for limb and limb girdle soft tissue tumors. Ann Surg Oncol 2001;8:80–87.
15. Issakov J, Flusser G, Kollender Y, et al. Computed tomography-guided core needle biopsy for bone and soft tissue tumors. Isr Med Assoc J 2003;5(1):28–30.
16. Ogilvie CM, Torbert JT, Finstein JL, et al. Clinical utility of percutaneous biopsies of musculoskeletal tumors. Clin Orthop 2006;450:95–100.
17. Parkkola RK, Mattila KT, Heikkila JT, et al. MR-guided core biopsies of soft tissue tumors on an open 0. 23 T imager. Acta Radiol 2001;42(3):302–5.
18. Puri A, Shingade VU, Agarwal MG, et al. CT-guided percutaneous core needle biopsy in deep seated musculoskeletal lesions: a prospective study of 128 cases. Skeletal Radiol 2006;35(3):138–43.

19. Soudack M, Nachtigal A, Vladovski E, et al. Sonographically guided percutaneous needle biopsy of soft tissue masses with histopathologic correlation. J Ultrasound Med 2006;25(10):1271–7.

20. Wakely PE, Kneisl JS. Soft tissue aspiration cytopathology. Diagnostic accuracy and limitations. Cancer 2000;90:292–8.

21. Torriani M, Etchebehere M, Amstalden E. Sonographically guided core needle biopsy of bone and soft tissue tumors. J Ultrasound Med 2002;21(3):275–81.

22. Ray-Coquard I, Ranchère-Vince D, Thiesse P, et al. Evaluation of core needle biopsy as a substitute to open biopsy in the diagnosis of soft-tissue masses. Eur J Cancer 2003 Sep;39(14):2021–5.

23. Serpell JW, Pitcher ME. Pre-operative core biopsy of soft-tissue tumors facilitates their surgical management. Aust N Z J Surg 1998;68(5):345–9.

24. Carrino JA, Khurana B, Ready JE, et al. Magnetic resonance imaging-guided percutaneous biopsy of musculoskeletal lesions. J Bone Joint Surg Am 2007;89(10):2179–87.

25. Costa MJ, Campman SC, Davis RL, et al. Fine-needle aspiration cytology of sarcoma. Retrospective review of diagnostic utility and specificity. Diagnost Cytopathol 1996;15:23–32.

26. Mitsuyoshi G, Naito N, Kawai A, et al. Accurate diagnosis of musculoskeletal lesions by core needle biopsy. J Surg Oncol 2006;94(1):21–7.

Surgical Margins in Soft Tissue Sarcoma: What Is a Negative Margin?

Bruce T. Rougraff

OrthoIndy, Indianapolis, IN, USA

Clinical scenario

A 57 year old male truck driver undergoes an excision of a 6 cm mass in his thigh that was found to be a high-grade soft tissue sarcoma (STS). The surgical margins are described in the pathology report as "close." He is concerned that with loss of his quadriceps function he will lose his job and is worried about the side effects of radiation to his thigh. How close a margin is too close and should be treated with re-excision? How much further normal tissue would be resected? Is radiation needed and would it be enough? Would chemotherapy help his local control? Why not just wait until he develops a local recurrence before considering more surgical and radiation treatment?

Relevant anatomy

Over the last 30 years the surgical treatment for STS has transitioned from radical amputation to surgical resection. When a surgical resection is chosen as the local treatment for STS, the exact amount of tissue that needs to be resected around the soft tissue mass has remained confusing (see Further reading). Surgical margins for STS were first described in terms of anatomical setting by Enneking in 1981.[1] His margin classification was adapted from his experience with bone sarcomas which he had previously published. He described the margin as intralesional when the resection was carried out within the pseudo-capsule of the tumor. A marginal resection was when the tumor was shelled out with the surrounding reactive zone intact. A wide resection was described as a resection that passed through normal tissue in all planes around the anatomic compartment with which the sarcoma was contained. In a radical resection, the entire compartment that contains the sarcoma is resected. He reported local recurrence of 50% after marginal resection 25% after wide resection 4% after radical resection. These data were based on 40 patients with STS that were treated before the advent of MRI.

The advantage to this anatomic approach was that it gave surgeons a common classification system to describe their attempted resection goals. It is still the method of describing surgical intervention. The problem with this anatomic approach to surgical margins is that it does not involve any absolute distance; it is unclear how wide is "wide enough." Because large sarcomas frequently are close to neurovascular structures or periosteum and sometimes involve bone invasion, an intracompartmental sarcoma could be extremely close to other structures that were not resected and be within a cell layer of the margin, despite being technically a radical resection. Only one third of STS of the thigh are contained within a compartment and much fewer in the head, neck, and retroperitoneum. Likewise, subcutaneous sarcomas could never undergo a resection that was considered radical. Defining how "wide" is really wide enough has been very confusing in the literature.

In 1987 Rydholm[2] considered intact muscle to be a distinct anatomic compartment. He further subdivided wide margins as a wide subcutaneous margin when the tumor was resected from subcutaneous region with fascia and adequate subcutaneous tissue, and deep margin for deep tumors with adequate muscular envelope. Kawaguchi[3] for the Japanese Orthopaedic Society ignored compartmental anatomy as a description for resection. This got rid of a contentious issue between what the pathologists saw with the specimen and what the surgeon was describing

Evidence-Based Orthopedics, First Edition. Edited by Mohit Bhandari.
© 2012 Blackwell Publishing Ltd. Published 2012 by Blackwell Publishing Ltd.

anatomically. Kawaguchi described margins as curative, adequate, or inadequate depending on the width and the quality of tissue surrounding the entire resected specimen.

This lack of consensus has resulted in surgical margins being described in various ways. Some studies describe them as either positive, or negative. Other authors have described margins as inadequate if tumor was present at the inked surface. The International Union Against Cancer (IUAC) has promoted a system of R0, R1, and R2, where R0 denotes a complete resection (presumably without microscopic tumor present at any inked surface), R1 refers to microscopically positive margins, and R2 denotes incomplete resection or debulking procedure. Finally, other authors have described their margins as "adequate" if 2 cm of normal tissue is present around the mass. Still others use 1 cm or even 1 mm of normal cuff of tissue around the sarcoma as adequate margins.

To add to the confusion of surgical margins and STS, various adjuvant therapies have been used in reported studies in a nonrandomized fashion. External beam radiation, brachytherapy, intraoperative radiation therapy and chemotherapy have been described in the treatment STS. Their effect on local control and surgical margins has remained ambiguous and further confused by the lack of agreement of the adequacy of surgical margin. Finally, many studies have included surgical assessments reported by the surgical team which blurs the final pathologic assessment of surgical margins because of disagreement of what is "adequate" or not.

But there is still more to the issue of surgical margins and local control. The unique local biology of each sarcoma can dictate how adequate a margin is possible. A 2 cm sarcoma in the popliteal fossa at the vascular trifurcation is not going to have a large margin compared to the same tumor in the central quadriceps muscle. It can be easier to get "wider" margins for a very large intracompartmental tumor than for an extracompartmental sarcoma between the sciatic nerve and the posterior femur. Yet another consideration is whether the sarcoma is referred for definitive treatment before or after contamination by prior surgical manipulation or, even worse, after local recurrence. The final consideration is whether more (or less) intense attempts at local control impact patient survival.

Finding the evidence

A literature search of the English literature of surgical margins in STS that excluded studies with less than 50 patients, series with bone sarcomas, and studies limited to DFSP. This left a total of 91 studies that were adequate to assess their margin data and local control and patient survival.

Quality of the evidence

Level of evidence was assigned according to the criteria in Table 130.1.

Top ten questions

1. What is the reported range of local recurrence for patients with STS, and does that correlate/impact with reported survival rates?

2. How did prior studies report their surgical margins and did their system correlate with their local recurrences and survival?

3. What is an adequate surgical margin?

4. What should be done with an inadequate margin (margin at risk) and what is the expected outcome?

5. Does grade correlate with less quality margins or impact local control?

6. Does tumor size correlate to less quality margins or impact local control

7. Does external beam radiation impact local control?

8. Does radiation impact survival?

9. Does chemotherapy impact local control?

10. Does prior local recurrence place the patient at increased risk for another local recurrence or worse survival?

Question 1: What is the reported range of local recurrence for patients with STS, and does that correlate/impact with reported survival rates?

Findings

Of the STS studies with margin and local control data, the range of local recurrence was from 4% to 60%, and the median of these studies was 19%. The highest local recurrence rates tended to be in series with higher percentage of head and neck cases or retroperitoneal tumors. The 5 year survival rate was between 39% and 91%. The lowest survival rates were in series limited to large, high-grade sarcomas and the highest survival rates were series limited to small superficial or low-grade sarcomas.

Three studies[4–6] were limited to locally recurrent sarcomas and they reported 63–74% 5 year survival. Two of those three studies found that local recurrence was associated with decreased survival. Both studies were level II. No other study (89/91) was able to correlate local failure to survival. No study found improved survival with amputation compared to limb-sparing surgery.

Recommendation

• Local relapse after sarcoma resection and judicious adjuvant therapy occurs in about 20% of cases and is higher in

Table 130.1 Levels of evidence for primary research questions

Level	Types of studies			
	Therapeutic studies—investigating the results of treatment	Prognostic studies—investigating the effect of a patient characteristic on the outcome of disease	Diagnostic studies—investigating a diagnostic test	Economic and decision analyses—developing and economic or decision model
I	High quality randomized trial with statistically significant difference or no statistically significant difference but narrow confidence intervals Systematic review of level I RCTs (and study results were homogenous	High quality prospective study (all patients were enrolled at the same point in their disease with ≥80% follow-up of enrolled patients) Systematic review of level I studies	Testing of previously developed diagnostic criteria on consecutive patients (with universally applied reference gold standard) Systematic review of level I studies	Sensible costs and alternatives; values obtained from many studies; with multiway sensitivity analyses Systematic review of level I studies
II	Lesser quality RCT (e.g., <80% follow-up, no blinding, or improper randomization) Prospective comparative study Systematic review of level II studies or level I studies with inconsistent results	Retrospective study Untreated controls from an RCT Lesser quality prospective study(e.g., patients enrolled at different points in their disease or <80% follow-up) Systematic review of level II studies Case-control study	Development of diagnostic criteria on consecutive patients (with universally applied reference "gold" standard) Systematic review of level II studies	Sensible costs and alternatives; values obtained from limited studies; with multiway sensitivity analyses Systematic review of level II studies
III	Case-control study Retrospective comparative study Systematic review of level III studies	Case-control study	Study of nonconsecutive patients; without consistently applied reference "gold" standard Systematic review of level III studies	Analyses based on limited alternatives and costs; and poor estimates Systematic review of level III studies
IV	Case series	Case series	Case-control study Poor reference standard	Analyses with no sensitivity analyses

retroperitoneal and head and neck locations. There is some limited evidence that local recurrence impacts survival, particularly in the head and neck where locally recurrent disease can cause mortality without metastasis [overall quality: low]

Question 2: How did prior studies report their surgical margins and did their system correlate with their local recurrences and survival?

Findings

In these 91 studies, 10 different margin classification systems were reported. The most common system was the IUAC R0–2 system. 18/20 studies with LOE of II or III had strong correlation between margin R0 and local control. The second most common was the Enneking system, but only 5/20 studies had a correlation between margins and local control. Those five studies that showed a correlation tended to be the largest series, suggesting that there is a correlation but it takes a larger number of patients to show

it as compared to the IUAC system. All nine studies (9/9) that used ink present on the tumor as a positive margin showed strong correlation to margin quality and local control. Studies that called their margins microscopically positive or negative also had a strong correlation between margin quality and local control (11/17 studies). Unfortunately, these studies had a significant number of cases where the margin assessment was inadequate or incomplete and no comprehensive pathology review was done. These incomplete cases were typically included in the positive margin group in order to show significance to local failure. It appears that the worst margin assessment system in terms of predicting local failure is those that call a margin less than 1 or 2 cm as positive. Only one of eight studies found a correlation to local recurrence and this was a level III study. Eight studies used 1 mm as the cut-off for poor margin and six of these studies showed a correlation to local failure.

In terms of margin quality impacting survival, 15 studies found a correlation between surgical margin and 5 year survival. Interestingly, these 15 studies tended to be the series with higher local failure rates. The average failure rate reported in these 15 studies was 32.3% vs. 18.8% in studies that did not show a correlation between margin quality and 5 year survival. In fact, no study with a local recurrence rate of less than 18% found that correlation.

Recommendation
• Pathologic analysis of the specimen looking microscopically for ink touching tumor cells anywhere on the resected specimen should be considered the most predictive of local relapse for STS. Other margin classification systems have merit but do not predict local failure as well and can be adapted to reporting whether ink touches tumor [overall quality: low]

Question 3: What is an adequate surgical margin?

Finding
As described in the previous section, it appears from these 91 studies that no ink touching tumor on the resected specimen or a system that uses R0–2 or 1mm from the ink are most accurate in predicting local failure. This is supported by level II, III, and IV studies. Only two studies compared margin classification systems and both found microscopic evidence of ink on the tumor was a better predictor than Enneking margins for local failure.[7,8] It is difficult to assess the need for radiation based on margin quality since the majority of these patients with "close" margins do receive radiation. Adequacy of margin becomes a distressing title since most cases treated by an experienced sarcoma surgeon that have a positive margin are in an anatomic location that is close to nonresectable tissues. In fact, commonly no further surgery other than amputation can be offered to the patient. No study reported a higher survival rate with amputation compared to resection and adjuvant therapy. A better term than "inadequate surgical margin" may be "margin at risk."

Recommendation
• The microscopic finding of ink on tumor cells as found on the resected specimen represent a margin at risk or "inadequate margin." This finding may be equivalent to R1 vs. R0 in many studies using the international margin system (CICC) [overall quality: moderate]

Question 4: What should be done with an inadequate margin (margin at risk) and what is the expected outcome?

Findings
Local recurrence after a resection with an inadequate or at risk margin ranges between 24% and 40%. The impact of

radiation to reduce this rate is ambiguous in the literature. Of the three studies that focused on positive margins and locally recurrent sarcomas and the value of radiation, two of the three found a definite improved local control with radiation.[5,6,9] None of these studies explored results of chemotherapy.

Recommendation
• Patients who have margin at risk after an attempted wide resection should receive radiation therapy[overall quality: moderate]

Question 5: Does grade correlate with less quality margins or impact local control?

Of the 91 studies, only 3 showed a correlation between tumor grade and local control.[10–12] None found a correlation with grade and quality of margin. The three studies were very large series, which suggests that there may be a very weak correlation if any at all.

Recommendation
• High-grade histology may be a weak predictor of increased local recurrence of STS [overall quality: moderate]

Question 6: Does tumor size correlate to less quality margins or impact local control

Four of the 91 studies showed a correlation between tumor size and margin quality.[6,11,13,14] These were mid-sized series including only two that were level II. This may be a very weak association (if any at all), since 87/91 studies which included the largest patient series did not show this association.

However, tumor size was correlated to local control in seven of the largest series.[5,6,11,15–18] This is probably a real association that can only be seen statistically with series with over 300 patients.

Recommendation
• Large tumor size is a weak predictor of local recurrence but probably not margin quality [level of evidence: moderate]

Question 7: Does external beam radiation impact local control?

Fourteen of the 91 studies found a correlation between radiation and better local control.[5,9,10,15,19–28] Interestingly, 9/14 were European studies. Ten were level II, two were level III, and two were level IV. The local recurrence rate ranged from 13–60% with a median of 25%. Seventy-seven of the 91 studies found no improvement in local control with radiation, but no studies were randomized and it is likely that a bias of more patients receiving radiation also had the highest-risk surgical margins.

Recommendation

• There is likely improved local control with radiation [overall quality: moderate]

Question 8: Does radiation impact survival?

Eighty-nine of the 91 studies (74 studies looked specifically at this issue) were unable to show improved survival with radiation. Two studies found an improved survival with the utilization of radiation.[22,29] These included a study that was limited to patients with positive margins and no comparison group to radiation. It also included a high number of retroperitoneal sarcomas. The other was a level IV study that was poorly structured to look at this issue and had a very high number of patients with incomplete tumor resections. It also included a high number of head, neck, and retroperitoneal cases where local failure can cause death without metastases.

Recommendation

• There does not appear to be evidence that radiation prevents metastasis nor improves survival, particularly in patients with completely resected extremity sarcoma [overall quality: low]

Question 9: Does chemotherapy impact local control?

No study found improvement in local control with chemotherapy. No randomized studies have been published that address this.

Recommendation

• The use of chemotherapy to improve local control is not supported in the literature

Question 10: Does prior local recurrence place the patient at increased risk for another local recurrence or worse survival?

Fifteen of the 91 studies looked specifically at the issue of outcome after a local recurrence. Eleven of those 15 studies[4,11,18,22,30–35] found strong evidence that local failure was a high risk factor for another local failure. Ten studies were level II, and one was level III. Four studies did not find this correlation (two were from the same institution), two were level II and two were level III.[8,36–38] These were older studies and may have included more amputations, although that is not documented.

Recommendation

• There is good evidence that local recurrence of disease is at higher risk of recurring again locally if an amputation is not performed [overall quality: moderate]

Summary of recommendations

• Local relapse after sarcoma resection and judicious adjuvant therapy occurs in about 20% of cases and is higher in retroperitoneal and head and neck locations. There is some limited evidence that local recurrence impacts survival, particularly in the head and neck where locally recurrent disease can cause mortality without metastasis

• Pathologic analysis of the specimen looking microscopically for ink touching tumor cells anywhere on the resected specimen should be considered the most predictive of local relapse for STS. Other margin classification systems have merit but do not predict local failure as well and can be adapted to reporting whether ink touches tumor

• The microscopic finding of ink on tumor cells as found on the resected specimen represent a margin at risk or "inadequate margin." This finding may be equivalent to R1 vs. R0 in many studies using the international margin system (CICC)

• Patients who have margin at risk after an attempted wide resection should receive radiation therapy

• High-grade histology may be a weak predictor of increased local recurrence of STS

• Large tumor size is a weak predictor of local recurrence but probably not margin quality

• There is likely improved local control with radiation

• There does not appear to be evidence that radiation prevents metastasis nor improves survival, particularly in patients with completely resected extremity sarcoma

• The use of chemotherapy to improve local control is not supported in the literature

• There is good evidence that local recurrence of disease is at higher risk of recurring again locally if an amputation is not performed

Conclusions

Surgical margins have been reported in the English literature at least 10 different ways. The most accurate predictor of local recurrence is the presence of ink on tumor. This may be equivalent to a "microscopically positive margin" in some studies or an R1 resection in others. Large tumor size and high sarcoma grade may be weak predictors of local failure. Surgical margins appear to only predict survival in the studies with the highest local failure rates. There is weak and indirect evidence that local recurrence rates above 18% may be associated with lower survival in patients with STS. Radiation appears to be effective in decreasing local relapse but not metastasis. Chemotherapy has no published evidence of decreasing local failure. Patients who are referred for treatment after a local recurrence are much more likely to recur locally again without amputation. Amputation is not associated with survival benefit over limb salvage. Controlled, prospective, randomized studies with standardized margin classification to address the use of chemotherapy and radiation would be extremely helpful to clarify their indications.

References

1. Enneking WF, Spanier SS, Malawar MM, et al. The effect of the anatomic setting on the results of surgical procedures for soft parts sarcoma of the thigh. Cancer 1981;47:1005–22.
2. Rydholm A, Rooser B. Surgical margins for soft tissue sarcoma. J Bone Joint Surg Am 1987;69(7):1074–8.
3. Kawaguchi N, Ahmed AR, Matsumoto S, et al. The concept of curative margin in surgery for bone and soft tissue sarcoma. Clin Orthop Relat Res 2004;419:165–72.
4. Lehnhardt M, Daigeler A, Hamann HH, et al. MFH revisited: outcome after surgical treatment of undifferentiated pleomorphic or not otherwise specified (NOS) sarcomas of the extremities an analysis of 140 patients. Langenbecks Arch Surg 2009; 394(2):313–20.
5. Gronchi A, Miceli R, Fiore M, et al. Extremity soft tissue sarcoma: adding to the prognostic meaning of local failure. Ann Surg Oncol 2007;114(5):1583–90.
6. Ramanathan RC, A'Hern R, Fisher C, et al. Prognostic index for extremity soft tissue sarcomas with isolated local recurrence. Ann Surg Oncol 2001;8(4):278–89.
7. Kooby DA, Antonescu CR, Brennan MF, et al. Atypical lipomatous tumor/well and trunk wall: importance of histological subtype with treatment recommendations. Ann Surg Oncol 2004;1(1):78–84.
8. Rossi CR, Foletto M, Alessio S, et al. Limb-sparing treatment for soft tissue sarcomas: influence of prognostic factors. J Surg Oncol 1996;63(1):3–8.
9. Alektiar KM, Velasco J, Zelefsky MJ, et al. Adjuvant radiotherapy for margin-positive high-grade soft tissue sarcoma of the extremity. Int J Radiat Oncol Biol Phys 2000;48(4):1051–8.
10. Jebsen NL, Trovik CS, Bauer HC, et al. Radiotherapy to improve local control regardless of surgical margin and malignancy grade in extremity and trunk wall soft tissue sarcoma: A Scandinavian sarcoma group study. Int J Radiat Oncol Biol Phys 2008;71(4):1196–203.
11. Ballo MT, Zagars GK, Cormier JN, et al. Interval between surgery and radiotherapy: effect on local control of soft tissue sarcoma. Int J Radiat Oncol Biol Phys 2004;58(5):1461–7.
12. Collin C, Hadju SI, Godbold J, et al. Localized, operable soft tissue sarcoma of the lower extremity. Arch Surg 1986;121(12):1425–33.
13. Trovik CS, Bauer HC, Alvegard TA, et al. Surgical margins, local recurrence and metastasis in soft tissue sarcomas: 559 surgically-treated patients from the Scandinavian Sarcoma Group Register. Eur J Cancer 2000;36(6):710–16.
14. Gustafson P, Rydholm A. Selection bias in treatment of soft-tissue sarcoma. J Bone Joint Surg Br 1992;74(4):501–3.
15. Palmerini E, Staals EL, Alberghini M, et al. Synovial sarcoma: Retrospective analysis of 250 patients treated at a single institution. Cancer 2009;115(13):2988–98.
16. McKee MD, Liu DF, Brooks JJ, et al. The prognostic significance of margin width for extremity and trunk sarcoma. J Surg Oncol 2004;85(2):68–76.
17. Koea JB, Leung D, Lewis JJ, et al. Histopathologic type: an independent prognostic factor in primary soft tissue sarcoma of the extremity? Ann Surg Oncol 2003;10(4):432–40.
18. Zagars GK, Ballo MT, Pisters PW, et al. Prognostic factors for patients with localized soft-tissue sarcoma treated with conservation surgery and radiation therapy: an analysis of 1225 patients. Cancer 2003;97(10):2530–43.
19. Italiano A, Penel N, Robin YM, et al. Neo/adjuvant chemotherapy does not improve outcome in resected primary synovial sarcoma: A study of the French Sarcoma Group. Ann Oncol 2009;20(3):425–30.
20. Engstrom K, Bergh P, Gustafson P, et al. Liposarcoma: outcome based on the Scandinavian Sarcoma Group register. Cancer 2008;113(7):1649–56.
21. Fiore M, Grosso F, Lo Vullo S, et al. Myxoid/round cell and pleomorphic liposarcomas: prognostic factors and survival in a series of patients treated at a single institution. Cancer 2007;109:2522–3.
22. Delaney TF, Kepka L, Goldberg SI, et al. Radiation therapy for control of soft-tissue sarcomas resected with positive margins. Int J Radiat Oncol Biol Phys 2007;67(5):1460–9.
23. Thijssens KM, van Ginkel RJ, Pras E, et al. Isolated limb perfusion with tumor necrosis factor alpha and melphalan for locally advanced soft tissue sarcoma: The value of adjuvant radiotherapy. Ann Surg Oncol 2006;13(4):518–24.
24. Khanfir K, Alzieu L, Terrier P, et al. Does adjuvant radiation therapy increase loco-regional control after optimal resection of soft-tissue sarcoma of the extremities? Eur J Cancer 2003; 39(13):1872–80.
25. Trovik CS, Bauer HC, Berlin O, et al. Local recurrence of deep-seated, high-grade soft tissue sarcoma: 459 patients from the Scandinavian Sarcoma Group Register. Acta Orthop Scand 2001;72(2):160–6.
26. Fein DA, Lee WR, Lanciano RM, et al. Management of extremity soft tissue sarcomas with limb-sparing surgery and postoperative irradiation: do total dose, overall treatment time, and the surgery-radiotherapy interval impact on local control? Int J Radiat Oncol Biol Phys 1995;32(4):969–76.
27. Marcus SG, Merino MJ, Glatstein E, et al. Long-term outcome in 87 patients with low-grade soft-tissue sarcoma. Arch Surg 1993;128(12):1336–43.
28. Tran LM, Mark R, Meier R, et al. Sarcomas of the head and neck. Prognostic factors and treatment stratigies. Cancer 1992;70(1):169–77.
29. Gadgeel SM, Harlan LC, Zeruto CA, et al. Patterns of care in a population -based sample of soft tissue sarcoma patients in the United States. Cancer 2009;115:2744–54.
30. Gronchi A, Casali PG, Mariani L, et al. Status of surgical margins and prognosis in adult soft tissue sarcomas of the extremities: A series of patients treated at a single institution. J Clin Oncol 2005;23(1):96–104.

31. Virkus WW, Mollabashy A, Reith JD, et al. Preoperative radiotherapy in the treatment of soft tissue sarcomas. Clin Orthop Relat Res 2002;397:177–89.

32. Brooks AD, Bowne WB, Delgado R, et al. Soft tissue sarcomas of the groin: diagnosis, management, and prognosis. J Am Coll Surg 2001;193(2):130–6.

33. Pollack A, Zagars GK, Goswitz MS, et al. Preoperative vs. postoperative radiotherapy in the treatment of soft tissue sarcomas: a matter of presentation. Int J Radiat Oncol Biol Phys 1998;42(3):563–72.

34. Pisters PW, Leung DH, Woodruff J, et al. Analysis of prognostic factors in 1,041 patients with localized soft tissue sarcomas of the extremities. J Clin Oncol 1996;14(5):1679–89.

35. Singer S, Corson JM, Gonin R, et al. Prognostic factors predictive of survival and local recurrence for extremity soft tissue sarcoma. Ann Surg 1994;219(2):165–73.

36. Alektiar KM, Leung D, Zelefsky MJ, Brennan MF Adjuvant radiation for stage II-B soft tissue sarcoma of the extremity. J Clin Oncol 2002;20(6):1643–50.

37. Choong PF, Petersen IA, Nascimento AG, et al. Is radiotherapy important for low-grade soft tissue sarcoma of the extremity? Clin Orthop Relat Res 2001;387:191–9.

38. Brooks AD, Heslin MJ, Leung DH, et al. Superficial extremity soft tissue sarcoma: An analysis of prognostic factors. Ann Surg Oncol 1998;5:41–7.

Further reading

Alekhteyar KM, Leung DH, Brennan MF, et al. The effect of combined external beam radiotherapy and brachytherapy on local control and wound complications in patients with high-grade soft tissue sarcomas of the extremity with positive microscopic margin. Int J Radiat Oncol Biol Phys 1996;36(2):321–4.

Alektiar KM, Leung D, Zelefsky MJ, et al. Adjuvant brachytherapy for primary high-grade soft tissue sarcoma of the extremity. Ann Surg Oncol 2002;9(1):48–56.

Alho A, Alvegard TA, Berlin 0, et al. Surgical margin in soft tissue sarcoma. The Scandinavian Sarcoma Group experience. Acta Orthop Scand 1989;60(6):687–92.

Apffelstaedt JP, Zhang PJ, Driscoll DL, et al. Various types of hemipelvectomy for soft tissue-sarcornas: complications, survival and prognostic factors. Surg Oncol 1995;4(4):217–22.

Arnaud EJ, Perrault M, Revol M, et al. Surgical treatment of dermatofibrosarcoma protuberans. Plast Reconstr Surg 1997;100(4):884–95.

Avizonis VN, Sause WT, Menlove RL. Utility of surgical margins in the radiotherapeutic management of soft tissue sarcomas. J Surg Oncol 1990;45(2):85–90.

Baldini EH, Goldberg J, Jenner C, et al. Long-term outcomes after function-sparing surgery without radiotherapy for soft tissue sarcoma of the extremities and trunk. J Clin Oncol 1999;17(10):3252–9.

Barr LC, Robinson MH, Fisher C, et al. Limb conservation for soft tissue sarcomas of the shoulder and pelvic qirdles. Br J Surg 1989;76(11):1198–201.

Bell RS, O'Sullivan B, Liu FF, et al. The surgical margin in soft-tissue sarcoma. J Bone Joint Surg Am 1989;71(3):370–5.

Beltrami G, Rüdiger HA, Mela MM, et al. Limb salvage surgery in combination with brachytherapy and external beam radiation for high-grade soft tissue sarcomas. Eur J Surg Oncol 2008;34(7):811–16.

Bowne WB, Antonescu CR, Leung DH, et al. Dermatofibrosarcoma protuberans: a clinicopathologic analysis of patients treated and followed at a single institution. Cancer 2000;88(12):2711–20.

Brant TA, Parsons JT, Marcus RB Jr, et al. Preoperative irradiation for soft tissue sarcomas of the trunk and extremities in adults. Int J Radiat Oncol Biol Phys 1990;9(4):899–906.

Brecht IB, Ferrari A, Int-Veen C, et al. Grossly-resected synovial sarcoma treated by the German and Italian Pediatric Soft Tissue Sarcoma Cooperative Groups: Discussion on the role of adjuvant therapies. Pediatr Blood Cancer 2006;46(1):11–17.

Canter RJ, Qin LX, Ferrone CR, et al. Why do patients with low-grade soft tissue sarcoma die? Ann Surg Oncol 2008;15(12):3550–60.

Celik C, Karakousis CP, Moore R, et al. Liposarcomas; prognosis and management. J Surg Oncol 1980;14(3):245–9.

Chang CK, Jacobs IA, Salti GI. Outcomes of surgery for dermatofibrosarcoma protuberans. Eur J Surg Oncol 2004;30(3):341–5.

Chang HR, Gaynor J, Tan C, et al. Multifactorial analysis of survival in primary extremity liposarcoma. World J Surg 1990;14(5):610–18.

Chung PW, Deheshi BM, Ferguson PC, et al. Radiosensitivity translates into excellent local control in extremity myxoid liposarcoma: A comparison with other soft tissue sarcomas. Cancer 2009;115:3254–61.

Collin C, Godbold J, Hajdu S, et al. Localized extremity soft tissue sarcoma; an analysis of factors affecting survival. J Clin Oncol 1987;5(4):601–12.

Collin C, Hajdu SI, Godbold J, et al. Localized operable soft tissue sarcoma of the upper extremity. Presentation, management, and factors affecting local recurrence in 108 patients. Ann Surg 1987;205(4):331–9.

Collin CF, Friedrich C, Godbold J, et al. Prognostic factors for local recurrence and survival in patients with localized extremity soft-tissue sarcoma. Semin Surg Oncol 1988;4(1):30–7.

Dijkstra MD, Balm AJ, Coevorden FV, et al. Survival of adult patients with head and neck soft tissue sarcomas. Clin Otolaryngol Allied Sci 1996;21(1):66–71.

DuBay D, Cimmino V, Lowe L, et al. Low recurrence rate after surgery for dermatofibrosarcoma protuberans: a multidisciplinary approach from a single institution. Cancer 2004;100(5):1008–16.

Farhood AI, Hajdu SI, Shiu MH, et al. Soft tissue sarcomas of the head and neck in adults. Am J Surg 1990;160(4):365–9.

Fleming JB, Berman RS, Chang SC, et al. Long-term outcome of patients with American Joint Committee on Cancer stage IIB extremity soft tissue sarcomas. J Clin Oncol 1999;17(9):2772–80.

Flugstad DL, Wilke CP, McNutt MA, et al. Importance of surgical resection in the successful management of soft tissue sarcoma. Arch Surg 1999;134(8):856–61.

Fury MG, Antonescu CR, Van Zee KJ, et al. A 14-year retrospective review of angiosarcoma: clinical characteristics, prognostic factors, and treatment outcomes with surgery and chemotherapy. Cancer J 2005;11(3):241–7. Erratum in: Cancer J 2005;11(4):354.

Gerrand CH, Wunder JS, Kandel RA, et al. Classification of positive margins after resection of soft-tissue sarcoma of the limb predicts the risk of local recurrence. J Bone Joint Surg Br 2001;83(8): 1149–5.

Gibbs CP, Peabody TD, Mundt AJ, et al. Oncological outcomes of operative treatment of subcutaneous soft-tissue J Bone Joint Surg Am 1997;79(6):888–97.

Gibbs JF, Huang PP, Lee RJ, et al. Malignant fibrous histiocytoma: an institutional review. Cancer Invest 2001;19(1):23–7.

Goodlad JR, Fletcher CID, Smith MA. Surgical resection of primary soft-tissue sarcoma. Incidence of residual tumour in 95 patients needing re-excision after local resection. J Bone Joint Surg Br 1996;78(4):658–61.

Guadagnolo BA, Zagars GK, Ballo MT, et al. Long-term outcomes for synovial sarcoma treated with conservation surgery and radiotherapy. Int J Radiat Oncol Biol Phys 2007;69(4):1173–80.

Herbert SH, Corn BW, Solin LJ, et al. Limb-preserving treatment for soft tissue sarcomas of the extremities. The significance of surgical margins. Cancer 1993;72(4):1230–8.

Karakousis CP, Driscoll DL. Treatment and local control of primary extremity soft tissue sarcomas. J Surg Oncol 1999;71(3): 155–61.

Karakousis CP, Emrich LJ, Rao U, et al. Feasibility of limb salvage and survival in soft tissue sarcomas. Cancer 1986;57(3):484–91.

Karakousis CP, Zografos GC. Radiation therapy for high grade soft tissue sarcomas of the extremities treated with limb-preserving surgery. Eur J Surg Oncol 2002;28(4):431–6.

Kepka L, Suit HD, Goldberg SI, et al. Results of radiation therapy performed after unplanned surgery (without re-excision) for soft tissue sarcomas. J Surg Oncol 2005;92(l):39–45.

Keus RB, Rutgers EJ, Ho GH, et al. Limb-sparing therapy of extremity soft-tissue sarcomas: treatment outcome and long-term functional results. Eur J Cancer 1994;30A(10):1459–63.

Kim YB, Shin KH, Seong J, et al. Clinical significance of margin status in postoperative radiotherapy for extremity and truncal soft-tissue sarcoma. Int J Radiat Oncol Biol Phys 2008;70(1): 139–44.

Kraus DH, Dubner S, Harrison LB, et al. Prognostic factors for recurrence and survival in head and neck soft tissue sarcomas. Cancer 1994;74(2):697–702.

Le QT, Fu KK, Kroll S, et al. Prognostic factors in adult soft-tissue sarcomas of the head and neck. Int J Radiat Oncol Biol Phys 1997;37(5):975–84.

Le Vay J, O'Sullivan B, Catton C, et al. An assessment of prognostic factors in soft-tissue sarcoma of the head and neck. Arch Otolaryngol Head Neck Surg 1994;120(9):981–6.

LeVay J, O'Sullivan B, Catton C, et al. Outcome and prognostic factors in soft tissue sarcoma in the adult. Int J Radiat Oncol Biol Phys 1993;27(5):1091–9.

Lewis JJ, Antonescu CR, Leung DH, et al. Synovial sarcoma: a multivariate analysis of prognostic factors in 112 patients with primary localized tumors of the extremity. J Clin Oncol 2000;18(10): 2087–94.

Lewis JJ, Leung D, Casper ES, et al. Multifactorial analysis of long-term follow-up (more than 5 years) of primary extremity sarcoma. Arch Surg 1999;134(2):190–4.

Lewis JJ, Leung D, Espat J, et al. Effect of reresection in extremity soft tissue sarcoma. Ann Surg 2000;231(5):655–63.

Li XQ, Parkekh SG, Rosenberg AE, et al. Assessing prognosis for high-grade soft-tissue sarcomas: search for a marker. Ann Surg Oncol 1996;3(6):550–7.

Lin CN, Chou SC, Li CF, et al. Prognostic factors of myxofibrosarcomas: implications of margin status, tumor necrosis and mitotic rate on survival. J Surg Oncol 2006;93(4):294–303.

Lin PP, Guzel VB, Pisters PW, et al. Surgical management of soft tissue sarcomas of the hand and foot. Cancer 2002;95(4):852–61.

Lohman RF, Nabawi AS, Reece GP, et al. Soft tissue sarcoma of the upper extremity: A 5-year experience at two institutions emphasizing the role of soft tissue flap reconstruction. Cancer 2002;94(8): 2256–64.

Mack LA, Crowe PJ, Yang JL, et al. Preoperative chemoradiotherapy (modified Eilber protocol) provides maximum local control and minimal morbidity in patients with soft tissue sarcoma. Ann Surg Oncol 2005;12(8):646–53.

Mandard AM, Petiot JF, Marnay J, et al. A multivariate analysis of 109 cases. Cancer 1989;63(7):1437–51.

Menendez LR, Ahlmann ER, Savage K, et al. Tumor necrosis has no prognostic value in neoadjuvant chemotherapy for soft tissue sarcoma. Clin Orthop Relat Res 2007;455:219–24.

Mentzel T, Calonje E, Wadden C, et al. Myxofibrosarcoma. Clinicopathologic analysis of 75 cases with emphasis on the low-grade variant. Am J Surg Pathol 1996;20(4):391–405.

Merimsky O, Soyfer V, Kovner F, et al. Limb sparing approach: adjuvant radiation therapy in adults with intermediate or high-grade limb soft tissue sarcoma. Radiother Oncol 2005;77(3): 295–300.

Monnier D, Vidal , Martin L, Danzon A, et al. Dermatofibrosarcoma protuberans: a population-based cancer registry descriptive study of 66 consecutive cases diagnosed between 1982 and 2002. J Eur Acad Dermatol Venereol 2006;20(10):1237–42.

Mundt AJ, Awan A, Sibley GS, et al. Conservative surgery and adjuvant radiation therapy in the management of adult soft tissue sarcoma of the extremities: clinical and radiobiological results. Int J Radiat Oncol Biol Phys 1995;32(4):977–85.

Neuhaus SJ, Pinnock N, Giblin V, et al. Treatment and outcome of radiation-induced soft-tissue sarcomas at a specialist institution. Eur J Surg Oncol 2009;35:654–9.

Noria S, Davis A, Kandel R, et al. Residual disease following unplanned excision of soft-tissue sarcoma of an extremity. J Bone Joint Surg Am 1996;78(5):650–5.

Peiper M, Zurakowski D. Knoefel WT, et al. Malignant fibrous histiocytoma of the extremities and trunk: an institutional review. Surgery 2004;135(l):59–66.

Peiper M, Zurakowski D, Zornig C. Survival in primary soft tissue sarcoma of the extremities and trunk. Langenbecks Arch Chir 1997;382(4):203–8.

Pister PW, Pollock RE, Lewis VO, et al. Long-term results of prospective trial of surgery alone with selective use of radiation for patients with T1 extremity and trunk soft tissue sarcomas. Ann Surg 2007;246(4):675–81.

Potter BK, Adams SC, Pitcher JD, et al. Local recurrence of disease after unplanned excisions of high grade soft tissue sarcomas. Clin Orthop Relat Res 2008;466:3093–100.

Potter DA, Kinsella T, Glatstein E, et al. High-grade soft tissue sarcomas of the extremities. Cancer 1986;58(1):190–205.

Pradhan A, Cheung YC, Grimer RJ, et al. Soft-tissue sarcomas of the hand. Oncological outcome and prognostic factors. J Bone Joint Surg Br 2008;90(2):209–14.

Ratner D, Thomas CO, Johnson TIM, et al. Mohs micrographic surgery for the treatment of dermatofibrosarcoma protuberans.

Results of a multi institutional series with an analysis of the extent of microscopic spread. J Am Acad Dermatol 1997;37(4):600–13.

Rimner A, Brennan MF, Zhang Z, et al. Influence of compartmental involvement on the patterns of morbidity in soft tissue sarcoma of the thigh. Cancer 2009;115(1):149–57.

Rosenberg SA, Seipp CA, White DE, et al. Perioperative blood transfusions are associated with increased rates of recurrence and decreased survival in patients with high-grade soft-tissue sarcomas of the extremities. J Clin Oncol 1985;3(5):698–709.

Sadoski C, Suit HD, Rosenberg A, et al. Preoperative radiation, surgical margins, and local control of extremity sarcomas of soft tissues. J Surg Oncol 1993;52(4):223–30.

Salas S, Bui B, Stoeckle E, et al. Soft tissue sarcomas of the trunk wall (STS-TW): a study of 343 patients from the French Sarcoma Group (FSG) database. Ann Oncol 2009;20:1127–35.

Sampo M, Tarkkanen M, Huuhtanen R, et al. Impact of the smallest surgical margin on local control in soft tissue sarcoma. Br J Surg 2008;95(2):237–43.

Shah H, Bhurgri Y, Pervez S. Malignant smooth muscle tumours of soft tissue—a demographic and clinicopathological study at a tertiary care hospital. J Pak Med Assoc 2005;55(4):138–43.

Shiu MH, Castro EB, Hajdu SI, et al. Surgical treatment of 297 soft tissue sarcomas of the lower extremity. Ann Surg 1975;182(5):597–602.

Stefanovski PD, Bidoli E, De Paoli A, et al. Prognostic factors in soft tissue sarcomas: a study of 395 patients. Eur J Surg Oncol 2002;28(2):153–64.

Stojadinovic A, Leung DH, Hoos A, et al. Analysis of the prognostic significance of microscopic margins in 2084 localized primary adult soft tissue sarcomas. Ann Surg 2002;235:424–34.

Suit H. Sarcoma of soft tissues: radiation sensitivity, treatment field margins pathological margins, and dose—on Fein et al., IJROBP 1995;32:969–76. Int J Radiat Oncol Biol Phys 1995;32(5):1545–6.

Tanabe KK, Pollock RE, Ellis LM, et al. .Influence of surgical margins on outcome in patients with preoperatively irradiated extremity soft tissue sarcomas. Cancer 1994;73(6):1652–9.

Trovik CS; Scanadinavian Sarcoma Group Project. Local recurrence of soft tissue sarcoma. A Scandinavian Sarcoma Group Project. Acta Orthop Scand Suppl 2001;72(300):1–31.

Wilson AN, Davis A, Bell RS, et al. Local control of soft tissue sarcoma of the extremity: the experience of a multidisciplinary sarcoma group with definitive surgery and radiotherapy. Eur J Cancer 1994;30A(6):746–51.

Zagars GK, Ballo MT. Significance of dose in postoperative radiotherapy for soft tissue sarcoma. Int J Radiation Oncology Biol Phys 2003;56:473–481.

Zagars GK, Ballo MT, Pisters PW, et al. Surgical margins and resection in the management of patients with soft tissue sarcoma using conservative surgery and radiation therapy. Cancer 2003;97(10):2544–53.

Zagars GK, Mullen JR, Pollack A. Malignant fibrous histiocytoma: outcome and prognostic factors following conservation surgery and radiotherapy. Int J Radiat Oncol Biol Phys 1996;34(5):983–94.

Zelefsky MJ, Nori D, Shiu MH, et al. Limb salvage in soft tissue sarcomas involving neurovascular structures using combined surgical resection and brachytherapy. Int J Radiat Oncol Biol Phys 1990;9(4):913–18.

Zornig C, Peiper M, Schroder S. Re-excision of soft tissue sarcoma after inadequate initial operation. Br J Surg 1995;82(2):278–9.

Zornig C, Weh HJ, Krull A. et al. Soft tissue sarcomas of the extremities and trunk in the adult. Report of 124 cases. Langenbecks Arch Chir 1992;377(l):28–33.

Index

Note: page numbers in *italics* refer to figures, those in **bold** refer to tables.

abdominal reflex 710
absolute risk/absolute risk difference 14
acetabular component revision of total hip arthroplasty 205–10
  anatomy 205
  cementless component 208
  component position 120, 121, 122
  importance of problem 205
  morselized impaction graft 207–8
  porous tantalum implants 208–9
  structural bulk allografts 205–10
acetabulum/acetabular bone
  bone stock in total hip arthroplasty/hip resurfacing 139–40
  deficiency classification 205–7
  dysplasia 887–8
  labrum
    anatomy 879
    tears 879–89
  reconstruction options for loss 207–8
  trauma and venous thromboembolism 60–1
acetabulum fracture 602–3, *604*, 605–9, **610**, 611–14
  anatomy 602, *603*
  avascular necrosis 613
  characterization 603, 605–6
  classification 602, *604*, 605
  complications 603
  CT imaging 605–6
  deep vein thrombosis 603
  dislocation 613
  displacement 607
  elderly patients 607–8
  femoral head damage 613
  functional outcome 609, **610**, 611–12
  heterotopic ossification 603, 609
  importance of problem 602–3
  incongruence 606
  instability 606
  non-surgeon related factors in prognosis 612–13

  open reduction and internal fixation 607–8
  radiographs 603, 605–6
  surgical management indications 606–7
  total hip arthroplasty 608
  type 612–13
Achilles tendinopathy 872–7
  anatomy 872
  clinical examination 873
  concentric exercise 874
  diagnosis 873
  eccentric exercise 873–4
    efficacy 874–5
    with low-level laser therapy 875–6
    platelet-rich plasma injection comparison 876
    with/without heel brace 874
  heel brace 874
  incidence 872
  insertional 872
  laser therapy 875–6
  noninsertional 872
  platelet-rich plasma injection 876
  shockwave therapy 873–4
    efficacy 874–5
  topical glyceryl trinitrate 875
Achilles tendon rupture 872
acromioclavicular joint trauma 325–30
  acute repair 329–30
  adhesive dressings 327
  anatomy 325
  braces 327
  casts 327
  coracoacromial ligament transfer 329
  coracoclavicular sling 329
  delayed reconstruction 329–30
  diagnosis 325–7
  dislocation 328
  fixation devices 329

Evidence-Based Orthopedics, First Edition. Edited by Mohit Bhandari.
© 2012 Blackwell Publishing Ltd. Published 2012 by Blackwell Publishing Ltd.

acromioclavicular joint trauma (*cont'd*)
  harnesses 327
  hook plate 329
  importance of problem 325
  K-wire fixation 328, 329
  MRI 325–7
  nonoperative treatment of separation 327
  operative interventions 327–9
  radiographs 326
  screw fixation 328, 329
  separation 327
acromion fracture, reverse total shoulder arthroplasty 282
activities of daily living, range of motion in knee 233
acupuncture
  effectiveness for neck pain 665–6
  shoulder impingement syndrome 767
  tennis elbow 789, 790–1
acute compartment syndrome *see* compartment syndrome
acute hemolytic reactions, blood transfusion 75, 76
adhesions, prevention in flexor tendon surgery 993–6
adolescent idiopathic scoliosis (AIS)
  anatomy 702, 710
  back pain 706
  bone graft material 715–16
  bracing in prevention of curve progression 704–5
  Cobb angle 702, 703, 704
  cranial/caudal extent of fusion 713–14
  crankshaft phenomenon 712
  curve correction and patient satisfaction 714–15
  curves progressing during adolescent growth spurt 705–6
  exercise for prevention of progression 703–4
  functional impairment 706
  fusion rates and bone graft material 715–16
  genetic markers 705
  imaging 710–12
  importance of problem 702, 710
  intraoperative neuromonitoring 716–17
  left thoracic curve 711
  Lenke criteria 713, 714
  neurological abnormality 712
  nonoperative management 702–7
  operative management 710–17
    anterior surgery 712–13
    bone graft material 715–16
    neurologic injury prevention 716–17
    posterior surgery 712–13
  patient self-image/satisfaction 715
  pulmonary compromise 706–7
  school screening programmes 703
  skeletal maturity 705
  thoracic kyphosis 712
  thoracotomy 712
adrenocorticotropic hormone (ACTH), gout treatment 90
adult respiratory distress syndrome (ARDS), femoral shaft fractures 512, 514, *515*, 516
aging, fracture healing risk factor 101, 102–3
AGREE (Appraisal of Guidelines, REsearch, and Evaluation) 15–16
alcohol abuse, fracture healing 105–6
  risk factor 102

alendronate 44, **45**
allograft-prosthetic composite (APC)
  bone sarcoma 1097, *1098*
  proximal humerus 1098, 1100–2
alumina ceramics 153, 154–5
American Academy of Orthopedic Surgeons (AAOS), classification of acetabular bone deficiency 205, 206
American Orthopedic Research Institute (AORI), classification of bone defects 250
amputation
  mangled extremities 655, 656
    complications 659
    outcome 658–9
    resource investment 656–7
    scoring systems 658
  revision of digit 1074–5
  see also replantation of digits
analgesia
  compartment syndrome 629–30
  low back pain 681, *682*
  neck pain 666
  tennis elbow 790
anemia
  adaptive response 72
  blood transfusion 75
  frequency 73–4
  morbidity/mortality effects 74–5
  patient function effects 75
  perioperative 73
angiogenesis 102
ankle
  Achilles tendinopathy 872–7
  cost of injuries 862–3
  distal tibia fracture 549–59
  fracture instability 562
  fusion 294–304
  inversion injuries 862
  ligaments 862
    meta-analysis of treatments 27
  malleolar fractures 561–5
  osteoarthritis 294, *295*
    development in ipsilateral subtalar complex 297–8
  Ottawa rules 561, 562
  recurrent instability 317
  sprains 862–70
    prevention 868–9
  see also total ankle arthroplasty
ankle arthrodesis 294–304
  complications 296
  conversion to total ankle arthroplasty 296
  external fixation 296
  functional outcome 295
  gait outcome 302–3
  infection 296
  internal fixation 295, 296
  ipsilateral subtalar complex osteoarthritis 297–8
  optimum position 296
  patient satisfaction 302

technique 295–7
total ankle arthroplasty comparison 302
ankle ligament, lateral, injury 862–70
anatomy 862
clinical examination 863
conservative treatment 867–8
diagnosis 863
functional treatment 866–7
imaging 864–5
immobilization 866
importance of problem 862–3
orthotic support 867
physical examination 863–4
prevention strategy 868–9
prognosis 868
RICE therapy 863, 865
surgical treatment 867–8
tape bandage 867
treatment
functional 866–7
meta-analysis 27
outcomes 867–8
ultrasound therapy 865–6
ankle–foot orthosis 318
anterior cruciate ligament (ACL) 796
anatomy 812, 832
anteromedial bundle 812
hemarthrosis 796
injury 803, 812–13, **814–15**, 816–20
clinical examination 812–13
combined medial collateral ligament injury 832–5, **835–6**,
837–8
diagnosis 812–13
importance of problem 812
incidence 812
posterolateral bundle 812
reconstruction 812
acute injury 800–1
allograft *vs.* autograft 813, 816
double-/single-bundle 813, **814–15**
graft choice 816–18
hamstring tendon 817–18
osteoarthritis 818, **819**
outcomes 813, **814–15**
patellar tendon 817–18
surgical 800–1
rupture 812
diagnosis 797, **798**, 799
osteoarthritis 818, **819**
anterior cruciate ligament/medial collateral ligament
(ACL-MCL) combined tears 832–5, **835–6**,
837–8
anatomy 832
diagnosis 833–4
diagnostic tools 834
importance of problem 832
incidence 832
knee braces 837–8
MRI 834

nonoperative treatment 835, **835–6**, 837
occurrence 832–3
prophylactic devices 837–8
reconstruction 834–5, **835–6**, 837
risk factors 833
surgical treatment 834–5, **835–6**, 837
treatment 834–5, **835–6**, 837
anterior impingement test 893
anterior talofibular ligament (ATFL) 862
anteromedial coronoid fracture (AMC) *384*, 385–8
nonoperative treatment 388–9
complications 391–3
operative treatment 388–9
complications 391–3
fixation 389–90
antibiotic(s)
bead pouch placement in open fractures 621–3
irrigation solutions 620
open fractures 618, 619
prophylaxis
MRSA 80–1
wound infections 79–80
antibiotic laden bone cement (ALBC) 212–14
total hip arthroplasty 273
total knee arthroplasty 212–16, **217**, 273
benefits 212–14
cost-effectiveness 214
infection 214–15
resistant organisms 215–16
total shoulder arthroplasty 272–3
anticoagulant agents 62–5
antithrombotic efficacy 64
bleeding risk 64, 65
duration of treatment 64–5
extended-duration prophylaxis 64–5
perioperative regimens 64
replantation of digits 1076–7
treatment initiation 63–4
types 62–3
antifibrinolytic therapy 73
antithrombotic agents, replantation of digits 1076–7
AO/OTA classification
clavicle trauma 332, *334*
distal femoral fractures 522, *523*
distal tibia fracture 549, *551*
humerus trauma 374, *375*
apixaban 63
appendicular skeleton, fracture healing 106–7
applicability
critical appraisal 17–19
diagnostic studies 20–1
prognostic studies 23–4
therapeutic studies 21–2
Apsley test for meniscal tears 803, **804**, 805
arthritis
Lisfranc injury 590
metatarsophalangeal joint 307–14
see also gouty arthritis; osteoarthritis; rheumatoid
arthritis

arthrodesis
  distal radioulnar joint 983
  wrist 980, 981
arthrography
  lateral ankle ligament lateral injury 864
  triangular fibrocartilage complex injuries 972
arthroplasty
  implant for distal radioulnar joint 983–4
  wrist 980
    total 981–2
arthroscopy
  acetabular labral tears 886–7
  distal radial fracture 969–71
    evaluation 970–1
    reduction 433–4, **435**, 918–19
    vs. fluoroscopy 971
  dorsal wrist ganglion cysts 975–6
  femoroacetabular impingement 893–4
  hip dislocation 471–2
  knee 60
    sports injury 799–800
  lunotriquetral ligament injury 974–5
  meniscal tears 805, **806**
  meniscectomy 808–9
  perilunate dislocations 438–9
  post-traumatic avascular necrosis of proximal humerus 354
  radial head fractures 399–400
  scaphoid fracture 456–7
  scapholunate ligament injury 974–5
  triangular fibrocartilage complex injuries 969, 971–4
  wafer procedure 973–4
  wrist 433–4, **435**, 969–76
    distal radial fracture evaluation 970–1
    dorsal wrist ganglion cysts 975–6
aspirin 63
atrial fibrillation, bisphosphonate side-effects 48–9
autologous blood donation 73
autologous chondrocyte implantation (ACI) 848, 849, 850
avascular necrosis
  acetabulum fracture 613
  femoral head 474
  femoral neck fractures 482
  proximal humerus
    fractures 364
    post-traumatic 351–8

back pain
  spinal metastases 721
  see also low back pain
background question 28
Becker technique, modified, extensor tendon surgery of hand 1040
bed rest, low back pain 681
benefits *vs.* harms 10
beta-blockers
  perioperative medical management 96
  risks of perioperative use 96
bias 13, 28
  citation 28
  hierarchy of evidence 4

publication 27, 28
  selection 28
  verification 15
  workup 15
biceps, pathology of long head 772–3, **774**, 775, **776**, 777–9
  diagnosis 772–3, **774**, 775
  nonoperative treatment 775
  surgical treatment 775, 777–9
bisphosphonate therapy 38, 44, **45**
  fracture healing effects 44, 46–8
  long-term safety 48–50
  side effects 48–50
  spinal metastases 728–30
blinding 14
blood loss, risk with anticoagulants 65
blood transfusion 72–6
  acute hemolytic reactions 75, 76
  anemia 75
  cardiac disease 74
  frequency 73–4
  hemoglobin level for trigger 74
  importance of problem 72–3
  infection risk 75, 76
  patient function effects 75
  physiology 72
  risks 75–6
    with anticoagulants 65
  strategies to reduce rate 73–4
  thresholds 74
  tissue oxygenation 75
Bohler's angle of calcaneus fractures 577
bone allografts *see* allograft-prosthetic composite (APC);
        impaction allografting; morselized impaction graft;
        osteoarticular allograft; structural bulk allografts
bone cement
  femoral component revision in total hip arthroplasty 188–9,
        194
  see also antibiotic laden bone cement (ALBC); calcium
        phosphate bone cement
bone graft(s)
  adolescent idiopathic scoliosis 715–16
  calcaneus fractures 578–9
  distal radial fractures 933, 934
  scaphoid fracture nonunion 948, 949
  types 644–5
  see also calcium phosphate bone cement
bone graft substitute
  adolescent idiopathic scoliosis 716
  calcaneus fractures 578–9
  calcium phosphate suitability 645
  distal radial fractures 933, 934
  proximal tibia fracture 536
bone mineral density (BMD) 38, 40–1
  bisphosphonate effects 729
  distal radial fractures 926
  fracture healing 104
bone morphogenetic protein, recombinant human (rhBMP)
        106–7, 108, 109, 110
  complications 110

bone morphogenetic proteins (BMPs) 199
  see also OP-1
bone sarcoma
  allograft-prosthetic composite 1097, *1098*
  endoprosthesis 1097, *1098*
  importance of problem 1097
  osteoarticular allograft 1097, *1098*
  postoperative complications 1098, 1100
  proximal humerus 1098, **1099**, 1100–2
    functional outcome 1100
    implant survival 1101–2
    limb salvage 1100–1
    relative risk of procedures **1101**
  proximal tibia 1102, **1103–4**, 1105–6
    implant survival 1105
    limb salvage 1105
    outcome 1105
    postoperative complications 1102, **1103–4**, 1105
  reconstruction 1097
  surgery 1097–8, **1099**, 1100–2, **1103–4**, 1105–6
bone scintigraphy
  painful total hip arthroplasty 181, 182
  scaphoid fracture 446–7, 940
  triple-phase bone scanning 182
borderline patients 649, **650**
botulinum toxin treatment, flexor tendon surgery of hand
      1065–6
Bunnell repair, modified, extensor tendon surgery of hand
      1040
bursography, snapping hip syndrome 899, 900

C-reactive protein (CRP)
  infection in painful total hip arthroplasty
      181
  wound infection diagnosis 81, 82
calcaneal artery, lateral 574
calcaneofibular ligament (CFL) 862
calcaneus fractures 574–80
  anatomy 574
  bilateral injury 577
  Bohler's angle 577
  bone grafts/bone graft substitute 578–9
  complications 579–80
  importance of problem 574
  intra-articular 578–9
    displaced **577**, 579–80
  minimally invasive treatment 577–8
  nonoperative treatment 575–6
    complications 579–80
    outcome prediction 576–7
  operative treatment 575–6
    complications 579–80
    outcome prediction 576–7
  outcomes 575–6
    prediction 576–7
  Sanders' classification 577
  subtalus arthrodesis 575
calcitonin **45**
  osteoporosis treatment 44

calcium
  hip fracture risk reduction 42
  homeostasis 104
calcium phosphate bone cement 933
  benefits 644–5
  bone graft type 644–5
  fracture repair 642–8
  injectable 428, 431
  with ORIF 644
  periarticular fractures 644
  resorption 645–6, *647*
  types of fracture for fixation 643–4
calcium phosphate resins 645
calcium sulfate bone graft substitute 645
  proximal tibia fracture 536
cam impingement 879, 892
Canadian Association of Radiologists/Osteoporosis Canada
      (CAROC) tool 42, **43**
Canadian C-spine rule (CCR) 670, *671*
carbonated hydroxyapatite bone graft 933
cardiac disease, blood transfusion 74
CAROC (Canadian Association of Radiologists/Osteoporosis
      Canada) tool 42, **43**
carpal bone mobilization 1016
carpal fractures 443–59
  anatomy 443
  casting 450–2, 456
  diagnosis 444–7
    delayed 455
  displaced 455–7
  importance of problem 443, *445*
  internal fixation 452–5
  proximal pole 457–8
  surgical technique 452–5, 456–8
  treatment 447–50, 452–8
    delayed diagnosis 455
  undisplaced 447–55, 457–8
carpal tunnel syndrome
  anatomy 1012, 1021
  conservative management 1012–19
    surgical management comparison 1023
  diagnosis 1021–3
  diagnostic imaging 1022–3
  diagnostic test accuracy 1012–13
  electromyography 1021–2
  endoscopic release 1024, 1025
  exercise 1015–16
  importance of problem 1012
  KnifeLight technique 1024, 1025
  laser therapy 1014–15
  local corticosteroid injections 1016–17
  mobilization 1015–16
  narrative review of diagnostic tests 26
  nerve conduction studies 1021–2
  nerve gliding exercises 1015–16
  NSAIDs 1017, 1018
  open release 1024, 1025
  oral therapies 1017–18
  short scar technique 1024, 1025

carpal tunnel syndrome (*cont'd*)
  splinting 1013–14
  surgical management 1021–5
    conservative management comparison 1023
    methods 1023–5
  ultrasound 1014–15
  yoga 1015, 1016
case-control studies 8–9
case reports 9
case series 9
cavo-varus foot deformity 317–21
  anatomy 317
  importance of problem 317
  orthotic use 318
  outcome studies 317
  physiotherapy 318–19
  reconstructive surgery timing 319
  surgical outcomes 319–20, **321**
celecoxib, heterotopic ossification prophylaxis 378, 379
cement
  femoral component revision in total hip arthroplasty 188–9, 194
  see also antibiotic laden bone cement (ALBC); calcium
      phosphate bone cement; total knee arthroplasty,
      cemented fixation; total shoulder arthroplasty,
      cemented fixation
ceramics
  alumina 153, 154–5
  structural bulk allografts 199
  total hip arthroplasty 153–62
cervical manipulation, neck pain 666–7
Chalmers score 28
characterized chondrocyte implantation (CCI) 849, 850
Charcot joint 236–40
  arthrodesis 239–40
  arthroplasty 238–40
  complications of operative treatment 239–40
  disorders causing 237
  fusion 238–9
  importance of problem 236–7
  incidence 237
  morbidity 237
  nonoperative treatment 238
  total knee arthroplasty 239–40
    complications 239–40
Charcot neuroarthropathy 236–7
  diagnostic accuracy 237–8
  differential diagnosis 238
  osteochondral fragmentation 238
  osteonecrosis 238
  presentation 238
Charcot—Marie—Tooth disease 317–21
  anatomy 317
  fusions 320, **321**
  importance of problem 317
  orthotic use 318
  osteotomy 320, **321**
  outcome studies 317
  physiotherapy 318–19

  reconstructive surgery timing 319
  soft tissue surgery 320, **321**
  surgical outcomes 319–20, **321**
chemotherapy, soft tissue sarcoma 1088–90, **1091–3**, 1093–5
  adjuvant **1092–3**, 1093–4
  neoadjuvant 1090, **1091**, 1093
chest trauma causing pulmonary complications with femoral
    shaft fractures 511–12, **513**, 517
citation bias 28
clavicle fracture 332–3, *334*, 335–9
  acute repair 338
  anatomy 332
  classification 332, *334*
  complications of treatment 336
  delayed reconstruction 338
  displaced 335
    optimal treatment 335–7
  figure-of-eight immobilization 333
  healing 335
  importance of problem 332
  intramedullary pins 337–8
  malunion 338
  nonoperative treatment 333, 336–7
    poor outcomes 333, 335
  nonunion 335, 338
  operative techniques 336, 337–8
  permanent disability 335
  pinning 337
  plate fixation 336, 337–8
    acute 338
  slings 333
clinical coordinator model 38, 40
clinical outcomes, therapeutic studies 22
clinical studies, classification 13
clinicians
  evidence as guidance 6
  judgement 5
closed kinetic chain (CKC) exercise 855, 856
Cobb angle, idiopathic scoliosis 702, 703, 704
cohort studies 8
colchicine
  gastrointestinal toxicity 89
  gout prophylaxis 90–1
  gout treatment 88–9
  urate-lowering therapy 90–1
collagenase injection, Dupuytren's disease 1034
compartment syndrome 627–34
  analgesia 629–30
  anatomy 627
  clinical signs/symptoms 629–30
  diagnosis 629–30
  fasciotomy 628
    pressure threshold 632–3
    timing 632
  importance of problem 627–8
  intracompartment pressure measurement 630–2
  Lisfranc injury 590
  perfusion pressure 633

risk factors 628–9
tibia shaft fracture 546–7
treatment 628
complex regional pain syndrome
Lisfranc injury 590
ORIF treatment for scaphoid fracture 943
computed tomography (CT) 605–6
acetabulum fracture 605–6
bone defects in total knee arthroplasty 250
carpal tunnel syndrome 1023
coronoid fracture 386–7, 388
distal femoral fractures 523–4
distal humerus fractures 376
distal tibial fracture 552–3
elbow fracture 386–7, 388
glenoid wear/glenoid bone stock 264–5
hip dislocation reduction 470–1
lateral ankle ligament lateral injury 864
Lisfranc injury 586
low back pain 679–80
neurogenic claudication 695
painful total hip arthroplasty 182
patellar problems in total knee arthroplasty 258
perilunate dislocations 438–9
proximal humerus fractures 360–1
rotator cuff tear 754–5
scaphoid fracture 940
scapular fracture 344
shoulder chronic instability 748
soft tissue sarcoma *1089*
spinal stenosis 688
total shoulder arthroplasty 271–2
confidence intervals 14
therapeutic studies 21
CONSORT (Consolidated Standards of Reporting Trials)
statement 15
coronoid fracture, anteromedial *384*, 385–8
nonoperative treatment 388–9
complications 391–3
operative treatment 388–9
complications 391–3
fixation 389–90
corticosteroids
carpal tunnel syndrome
local injections 1016–17
oral 1017–18
gout treatment 90
injections
carpal tunnel syndrome 1016–17
tennis elbow 789–90
trapeziometacarpal joint osteoarthritis 958
intra-articular for gout 88
patellofemoral pain syndrome 858
spinal metastases causing cord compression 722–3
subacromial 765–6
see also steroid therapy, epidural
cost(s), types 32
cost-benefit analysis (CBA) 32

cost-benefit ratio 32
cost-effectiveness analysis (CEA) 31, 33
cost-minimization analysis (CMA) 30–1
cost-utility analysis (CUA) 31–2, 33
coxa profunda *882*
coxa saltans 898–903
crankshaft phenomenon, adolescent idiopathic scoliosis 712
creatine supplementation 905–8
adverse side effects 907–8
dosage 907
effectiveness 905–7
muscle mass 907
physiology 905
creeping substitution 187
critical appraisal
applicability 17–19
guidelines 15–16
meta-analyses 28
results 17–19
steps 13–15
systematic reviews 28
tools 12–16
validity 17–19
cuneiform bones 583

D-dimer assay 57, 58
dabigatran etexilate 63
damage control orthopedics (DCO) 649–53
blood loss reduction 650
complications reduction 650–1, *652*
definition 649
importance of problem 649–50
local infection risk 652–3
mortality reduction 650–1, *652*
patient condition 649, **650**
posttraumatic inflammatory response 652
primary operation time reduction 650
Darrach procedure, distal radioulnar joint 982–3
deep vein thrombosis (DVT) 56
acetabulum fracture 603
diagnosis 57
orthopedic patients 60
postoperative 59
prophylaxis for acetabulum fracture 608–9
ultrasonography 57, 58
Well's prediction rule **58**
degenerative disc disease 100, 101
low back pain 675
delayed union 636–7
ESWT use 636, 638, 639–40
LIPUS use 545–6, 636, 638, **639**
PEMF use 636, 638–9
delirium prevention, perioperative medical management
94–5
demineralized bone matrix (DBM) 199, 716
denosumab **45**
osteoporosis treatment 44
diabetes, fracture healing risk factor 101, 103

diagnostic studies 19–21
  applicability 20–1
  carpal tunnel syndrome 26
  hierarchy of evidence 17, **18**
  results 20
  validity 19, 20
diagnostic tests
  reference standard 20
  replication 20
  studies investigating 15
  user's guide for articles **19**
disability adjusted life years (DALYs) 31
disc *see* degenerative disc disease; intervertebral discs
disease-modifying antirheumatic drugs (DMARDs), biologic
    1047–9
distal interphalangeal joint (DIP), fractures 990
distal radioulnar joint (DRUJ) 930
  arthrodesis 983
  Darrach procedure 982–3
  degenerative disease 420–1
  Galeazzi fracture 417, 420
    operative management 420–1
  implant arthroplasty 983–4
  incongruity in rheumatoid arthritis 980, *981*
  involvement in radial shaft/Galeazzi fractures 417–18
  K-wire fixation 421
  rheumatoid arthritis 982–4
  Suave-Kapandji procedure 983
  surgical reconstruction 420–1
  synovitis 1050–1
  temporary transfixion 420–1
diuretics, carpal tunnel syndrome 1017, 1018
dual energy X-ray absorptiometry (DXA) 38, 40
Dupuytren's diathesis 1035–6
Dupuytren's disease 1029, *1030*, 1031–7
  anatomy 1029, *1030–1*
  collagenase injection 1034
  flexion contractures 1034
  hand vibration 1029, 1031
  histological classification 1036, **1037**
  importance of problem 1029
  limited fasciectomy 1033–4
  pathoanatomy **1032**
  percutaneous needle fasciotomy 1033–4
  postoperative splinting 1034–5
  proximal interphalangeal joint contractures 1031–3
  recurrence prediction 1035–7
  repetitive manual work 1029, 1031
  total passive extension deficit 1033–4

early total care (ETC) 649, 650, 651
echocardiography, perioperative medical management 93–4
economic analysis 30–4
  costs 32
  interpretation 33–4
  perspectives 32–3
  sensitivity analyses 33
  time horizon 33
  types 30–2

elbow
  anteromedial coronoid fracture *384*, 385–8
    complications of treatment 391–3
    fixation 389–90
    nonoperative treatment 388–9, 391–3
    operative treatment 388–9, 391–3
  collateral ligaments 383–4
    repair 390, 394
  fracture—dislocations 383–94
    anatomy 383–4
    classification 384–5
    coronoid fracture *384*, 385–90, 391–3
    CT scans 386–7, 388
    functional outcomes 393–4
    importance of problem 383
    mechanism of injury 384–5
    nonoperative treatment 388–9
    open reduction and internal fixation 390–1, 394
    operative treatment 388–9
    radial head arthroplasty 390–1
    radiography 387, 388
    terrible triad injury 388–9, 390–1, 393–4
  ligaments 385
  olecranon fractures 409–15
  pain 374
  ring of instability 384
  stability 383
  tennis elbow 787–94
  total arthroplasty 379
  see also ulnar collateral ligament injury
electromagnetic radiation
  flexor tendon surgery 996
  see also pulsed electromagnetic fields (PEMF)
electromyography (EMG), carpal tunnel syndrome 1021–2
endoprosthesis
  bone sarcoma 1097, *1098*
  proximal humerus 1098, 1100–2
ergogenic aids 905–8
  adverse side effects 907–8
  effectiveness 905–7
erythrocyte sedimentation rate (ESR)
  infection in painful total hip arthroplasty 180–1
  wound infection diagnosis 81, 82
erythropoietin, preoperative administration 73–4
evidence
  application 5
  consistency 10
  criteria for determining level 12–13
  cycle 5
  directness 10
  grades 12–13
  integration with clinical expertise 4
  need for 4
  overall quality 9–10
  scales 9
  translating to specific setting 10
  unequal 4
  use by clinician 6
exclusion criteria 28

exercise
  adolescent idiopathic scoliosis 703–4
  carpal tunnel syndrome 1015–16
  eccentric in Achilles tendinopathy 873–4
    efficacy 874–5
    with low-level laser therapy 875–6
    platelet-rich plasma injection comparison 876
    with/without heel brace 874
  metacarpal fractures 988–9
  motion after proximal humerus fractures 361–2
  open kinetic chain exercise 855, 856
  patellofemoral pain syndrome 855–7
  proximal humerus fractures 361–2
  retraining for vastus medialis obliquus muscle 855, 856
  stretching for tennis elbow 791–2
  trapeziometacarpal joint osteoarthritis 957, 958
expanded polytetrafluoroethylene (e-PTFE), flexor tendon
      surgery 996
extensor tendon surgery of hand 1039–44
  anatomy 1039
  complications of repair 1043–4
  early passive mobilization 1041–2
    optimal protocol 1042
  functional outcome prediction 1043
  immobilization program 1041–2
  importance of problem 1039
  local anesthesia 1040–1
  repair techniques 1039–40
extracorporeal shock wave therapy (ESWT)
  shoulder impingement syndrome 766–7
  tennis elbow 789, 790
  tibia shaft fracture 636, 638, 639–40
  see also shockwave therapy
extremities
  mangled 655–9
  see also named anatomical regions

fabellofibular ligament 841
FABER distance test 893
facet blocks, low back pain 684
FDG-PET, painful total hip arthroplasty 182
femoral component revision in total hip arthroplasty 186–96,
      197, 198–200
  anatomy 196
  femoral defect classification 196
  impaction allografting 187–8
    biomechanical factors 188–9
    results 190–2, **193**
    technical aspects 189–90
  importance of problem 197
  morselized impaction graft, incorporation into bone 197–8
  structural bulk allografts 186–96, **197**, 198–200
  uncemented revision 199–200
femoral defect classification 196
femoral fractures
  atypical 50, **51**
  distal 522–6
    anatomy 522, *523*
    classification 522, *523*

CT 523–4
    dislocation 522
    femoral artery injury 522
    importance of problem 523
    nail fixation 525
    operative fixation around total knee replacement 525–6
    osteosynthesis 525
    plate fixation 525
    popliteal artery injury 522
  periprosthetic 171–6
  proximal (*see* subtrochanteric fractures)
  see also femoral head fractures; femoral neck fractures
femoral head
  avascular necrosis 474
  blood supply to epiphysis 137
  damage in acetabulum fracture 613
  size in total hip arthroplasty 133–4
femoral head fractures 474–8
  anatomy 474
  closed reduction 475
  complications 477
  fragment excision/repair 477
  importance of problem 474
  nonoperative treatment 475–6
  open reduction and internal fixation 475
  outcome 478
  surgical approach 476
femoral intercondylar notch, notch width index 833
femoral neck, anatomy 137
femoral neck fractures 480–9
  anatomy 37
  anesthesia 486, 487
  antibiotic use 486, 487
  arthroplasty 481–2, 484, 485
  avascular necrosis 482
  best evidence 7
  case scenario 37
  closed reduction 483, 484
  compression of fracture 483, 484
  hemiarthroplasty 484, 485
  heparin use 486, 487, **488**
  hip resurfacing 149
  impaction of fracture 483, 484
  implants 482–3
  internal fixation 481–2
  open reduction 483, 484
  optimal approach to fixing 483–4
  perioperative care 485–7
  postoperative 146
  replacing 484–5
  screw fixation 482–3
  sliding hip screw 482–3
  surgical delay impact on morbidity/mortality 487–8, **489**
  total hip arthroplasty 484, 485
femoral offset, total hip arthroplasty/hip resurfacing 140–1
femoral shaft, biomechanics 504
femoral shaft fractures 504–14, *515*, 516–17, **518**, 519
  anatomy 504
  antegrade nailing optimal entry oint 506–7

femoral shaft fractures (*cont'd*)
  ARDS 512, 514, *515*, 516
  chest trauma causing pulmonary complications 511–12, **513**
  CNS complications 513, 517
  concomitant fracture of ipsilateral femur 505–6
  damage control orthopedics 514, *515*, 516
  delayed union 507, 508, 510
  early total care 514, *515*, 516
  femoral plating 517
  functional impairment 517, **518**, 519
  head injury 513–14, 517
  implant failure 508
  importance of problem 504–5
  incidence 504
  intramedullary nails 506–9
    antegrade nailing 509–10
    optimal timing with head injury 513–14
    optimal timing with pulmonary complications 511–12, **513**
    reamed 517
    retrograde nailing 509–10
  malunion 510
  manual traction 510–11
  mortality 512, 513, 516, 517
  multiple organ failure 514, 516
  nonunion 507, 508
  pain 510
  postoperative 146
  pulmonary complications 508–9, 513
  reamed nails 507–9
  unreamed nails 507–9
femoroacetabular impingement (FAI) 879, 884, 886, 892–6
  anatomy 892
  anterior impingement test 893
  arthroscopic treatment 893–4
  athletes return to sport 895
  diagnosis 893
  FABER distance test 893
  importance of problem 892
  labral tears 879, 884, 886, 894–5
  open treatment 893–4
  physical examination 893
  tests 893
femoroplasty, acetabular labral tears 886
figure-of-eight repair, extensor tendon surgery of hand 1040
fingers
  anatomy 987
  fractures 987–91
    classification 988
    importance of problem 987
    mallet 990
    motion/function after fixation 990–1
    ORIF 989
    pinning 989
    plate fixation 990–1
    radiological characterization 988
    treatment 988–91
  replantation 1072–8
    anatomy 1072
    early range of motion therapy 1077

functional outcome 1074–5
  importance of problem 1072
  postoperative anticoagulant/antithrombotic agents 1076–7
  tertiary hospitals 1072–3
  vein and artery anastomoses 1075–6
  revision amputation 1074–5
  see also interphalangeal joint (IPJ); metacarpal fractures;
    metacarpophalangeal (MCP) joint; proximal
    interphalangeal joint (PIP)
first-hit phenomenon 652
flexion contractures, Dupuytren's disease 1034
flexor digitorum profundus (FDP) tendon 998
  avulsion injuries 1064–8
    botulinum toxin treatment 1065–6
    optimal fixation 1064–5
  laceration
    diagnosis 1000–1
    functional outcome 1005–7
    postoperative mobilization 1002–5
flexor digitorum superficialis (FDS) tendon 998
  laceration
    diagnosis 1000–1
    functional outcome 1005–7
    postoperative mobilization 1002–5
flexor retinaculum lengthening, carpal tunnel syndrome open
    release 1024
flexor tendon pulley system of hand 1057, *1058*
flexor tendon surgery of hand 1057–68
  adhesion prevention 993–6, 1066
  anatomy 993, 998–9, 1057
  botulinum toxin treatment 1065–6
  electromagnetic radiation 996
  flexor digitorum profundus avulsion injuries 1064–8
  functional outcome 1005–7
  imaging 1066–8
  importance of problem 993–4, 999, 1057
  injury classification 1057, *1058*
  management 994–5
  mechanical barriers 995–6
  partial lacerations 1063, **1064**
  pharmacological agents to increase recovery/function 995
  physiology 993
  postoperative mobilization 1002–5
  rehabilitation 998–1008
    postoperative mobilization 1002–5
    repair type 1002
    splinting 1005
  Strickland and Glogovac criterion 1060, **1061**
  suture configuration for strongest repair 1058–60
  suture materials 1060–3
  TenoFix device 1062, 1063
  ultrasound 996
  zones 998–9, 1057, *1058*
flexor tenosynovectomy, rheumatoid hand 1051–2
floating shoulder fractures 345
fluoroscopy, distal radial fracture *vs.* arthroscopy 971
5-fluorouracil, increase of recovery/function in flexor tendon
    surgery 995
fondaparinux 62, 63

foot
  calcaneus fractures 574–80
  cuneiform bones 583
  gouty arthritis 86
  metatarsal fractures 583–91
  Roman arch structure 583, *584*
  talus fractures 567–73
  see also ankle; cavo-varus foot deformity; metatarsal fractures;
       metatarsophalangeal (MTP) joint
foot insoles/orthoses 857, 858
foot pumps 61
forearm fractures 416–23
  anatomy 416
  bone grafting 419–20
  comminuted diaphyseal 419–20
  complications 421–2
  distal radioulnar joint involvement 417–18
  importance of problem 416–17
  nonsurgical treatment 418–19
  open reduction and internal fixation 418–19
  plate removal 421–2
  refracture risk 421–2
  union rate 419–20
four-corner fusion (4CF) 965, 966
  complications 967
  definition 963
  osteoarthritis progression 967
  outcome 966
fracture(s)
  atypical 50, **51**
  bisphosphonate effects on healing 44, 46–8
  fragility 40–2
    comanagement 95
    femoral periprosthetic fractures after total hip arthroplasty
       172
  internal fixation 7, 78, 83
  open 617–24
    anatomy 617
    antibiotic bead pouch placement 621–3
    antibiotic use 618, 619
    delayed wound closure 623
    importance of problem 617–18
    initial management 618–19
    irrigation techniques 619–21
    mangled extremity 655–6
    negative pressure wound closure therapy 621–3
    soft tissue closure 623–4
    surgery timing 619
    vacuum-assisted closure 621–3
  osteoporotic 37, 40–2
  periarticular 644
  prediction of future 40–2
  thromboprophylaxis 56
  see also delayed union; *named bones and regions;* nonunion
fracture healing
  aging effects 101–3
  alcohol abuse 102, 105–6
  anatomy 100–1
  appendicular skeleton 106–7

bone mineral density 104
  calcium phosphate bone cement 642–8
  diabetes effects 101, 103
  factors affecting 101–6
  health-related quality of life 638–40
  HIV/AIDS 104
  importance of problem 101
  lack of 100
  nutritional deficits 103–4
  obesity 104
  risk factors 101–6
  smoking 105–6
  see also delayed union; extracorporeal shock wave therapy
       (ESWT); low-intensity pulsed ultrasound (LIPUS);
       nonunion; pulsed electromagnetic fields (PEMF)
Fracture Risk Assessment Tool (FRAX) 41–2, **43**

gabapentin, neurogenic claudication 696, 699
Galeazzi fracture 417
  complications 420
  distal radioulnar joint 420
    involvement 417–18
    K-wire fixation 421
    operative management 420–1
  functional outcome 420
  nonoperative management 420
  open reduction and internal fixation 421
  operative treatment, timing 420
  range of motion 420–1
gastrocnemius muscle 872
generalizability of results 13
glenohumeral joint
  anatomy 263
  dislocation 737–42
  osteoarthritis 263, 284, *285*
  osteophytes 264
  scapular fracture 342
glenoid
  defect 749
  fixation 284–92
    failure 284
  imaging of bone stock/wear 264–5
  retroversion 284, 286
  version 271–2, 284
glenoid component
  all-polyethylene 274–5, 287–8
  cemented 287–8
  cementing 274
  keeled 288–90
  loosening 271
    determination of clinically relevant 285–6
    reverse total shoulder arthroplasty 281
  metal-backed 274–5, 287–8
  pegged 288–90
  radial mismatch 286–7
  radiographic lucent lines 290–1
  selection 287–90
  uncemented 287–8
  version 271–2, 284

glenopolar angle (GPA) 341, 344
glucosamine, trapeziometacarpal joint osteoarthritis 957–8
glucosamine polysulfate injection, patellofemoral pain
      syndrome 858
gluteus maximus muscle, posterior fiber fibrosis 898
glyceryl trinitrate, topical
  Achilles tendinopathy 875
  shoulder impingement syndrome 767
goniometric measurement 231
  see also range of motion
gout
  colchicine treatment 88–9
  diagnosis 87
  healthcare costs 86
  treatment 88–91
  urate-lowering therapy 90–1
gouty arthritis 86–91
  anatomy 86
  diagnosis 87
  importance of problem 86
  physiology 86
grades of recommendation 9–11
graduated compression stockings 61
grind test, trapeziometacarpal joint 955
groin pain 879
Gross classification of acetabular bone deficiency 205, 207
guidelines 15–16

hallux rigidus 307–8
hallux valgus 307
haloperidol, delirium prophylaxis 95
hand
  extensor tendon surgery 1039–44
  flexor tendon surgery 1057–68
  metacarpal fractures 462–7
  rheumatoid 1046–54
    flexor tenosynovectomy 1051–2
    metacarpophalangeal arthroplasty 1052–4
    prophylactic extensor tenosynovectomy 1050–1
    small-joint synovectomy 1049–50
    tendon rupture repair 1052
  vibration in Dupuytren's disease 1029, 1031
  see also fingers; trapeziometacarpal joint
harm, potential 22
Hawkins-Kennedy test 764
hazard ratio 14
head injury, femoral shaft fractures 513–14, 517
heel brace, Achilles tendinopathy 874
hemoglobin 72
  level for transfusion trigger 74
heparin
  low-dose unfractionated (LDUH) 62, 63, 64
  low molecular weight (LMWH) 62, 63, 64, 65
  thromboprophylaxis
    acetabulum fracture 608–9
    pelvic fracture 598
hereditary motor sensory neuropathy (HSMN) 317
  see also Charcot—Marie—Tooth disease
heterotopic ossification

acetabulum fracture 603, 609
complications of orthobiologics 110
hip resurfacing 146
Monteggia fracture-dislocations 407
olecranon fractures 413, **414**
prophylaxis for distal humerus fractures 378–9
total ankle arthroplasty 300
total hip arthroplasty 146
hierarchy of evidence 4, 7–11, 17
  meta-analyses 27
  narrative review 27
  systematic reviews 27
  systems 9
  therapeutic studies 7–8
highly crosslinked polyethylene (HCLPE) 131–5, 153
Hill-Sachs lesion *745, 747*
hip
  aspiration, culture and sensitivity 181
  compartments 881
  femoral head fractures 474–8
  fracture—dislocation reduction 475
  infection in painful total hip arthroplasty 181
  muscle weakness in patellofemoral pain syndrome
    856–7
  revision surgery 150, 197
  snapping 898–903
  see also acetabular *entries*; acetabulum *entries*;
    femoroacetabular impingement (FAI); labral tears,
    acetabular; total hip arthroplasty
hip arthroscopy
  acetabular labral tears 886–7
  femoroacetabular impingement 893–4
  hip dislocation 471–2
hip dislocation 468–72
  anatomy 468
  arthroscopy 471–2
  complications 468
  costs 468
  hip reduction urgency 469–70
  imaging after reduction 470–1
  importance of problem 468–9
  loose bodies 472
  osteoarthrosis 468, 470
  osteonecrosis 468, 469, 470
hip dysplasia, acetabular labral tears 887–8
hip fracture 37–51
  anatomy 93
  blood transfusion 72
  delirium following surgery 94–5
  diagnosis 37
  evaluation 38, **39–40**, 40
  importance of problem 93
  intracapsular 480–9
    anatomy 480
    arthroplasty 481–2
    implants 482–3
    importance of problem 480
    internal fixation 481–2
    optimal approach to fixing 483–4

perioperative care 485–7
  surgical delay impact on morbidity/mortality 487–8, **489**
intratrochanteric 491–5
medications 42, 44, **45–6**, 46–51
mortality 480, **481**
  surgical delay impact 487–8
perioperative medical management 93–7
prediction of future fractures 40–2
RCTs **39–40**
revision surgery 480, **481**
risk assessment **43**
risk reduction 42, 44, **45–6**
subtrochanteric 497–500, *501*, 502
surgical repair 97, 480
therapy 38
treatment 38, **39–40**, 40
see also total hip arthroplasty
hip navigation systems 122–3, 124
  training 125
  see also total hip arthroplasty, computer navigation
hip resurfacing 137–41, **142–4**, 145–6, **147**, 148–51
  acetabular bone stock 139–40
  activity level 141
  biomechanical reconstruction precision 140–1
  clinical outcomes 141, **142–4**
  complications rate 145–6, **147**
  dislocation 146
  failure rate 148–9, 183
  femoral component loosening 146, 149
  femoral neck fractures 149
  femoral offset 140–1
  gait 145
  heterotopic ossification 146
  hip motion 141, 144–5
  hospitalization 138–9
  importance of problem 137–8
  infections 146
  leg length 140–1
  metal ion release 146, 148
  postural balance 145
  range of motion 144–5
  revision surgery 150
  surgical technique 138–9
HIV/AIDS, fracture healing 104
hormone replacement therapy (HRT) **46**
  osteoporosis treatment 44
hospitalization, mangled extremities 657
human amniotic fluid (HAF), increase of recovery/function in
        flexor tendon surgery 995
Humanitarian Device Exemption (HDE) 110
humeral head
  collapse *352*
  ischemia 363–4
humeral head replacement
  cemented 273
  hydroxyapatite coated 273
  neutral rotation 280
  outcome 265–6
  revision rate 268

survivorship in young active patients 267
  uncemented 273
humeral shaft fractures 366–73
  anatomy 366
  angulation 367
  comminuted 368–70
  displaced 368–70
  functional fracture-bracing 367–8
  importance of problem 366
  infection 372
  intramedullary nailing 368–70
  nerve injury 370, 372
  nonoperative approach 367–8
  open reduction and internal fixation 368–70
  plate fixation 368–70
    complications 371–2
    failure predictors 370–1
    locking/nonlocking plates 370–1
    radial nerve injury recovery 370
    screw fixation complications 371–2
  shortening 367
  union rate 367
humerus, anatomy/innervation *367*
humerus, distal, fractures 374–80
  anatomy 374
  CT preoperative scanning 376
  elderly patients 379
  fixation
    optimal strategy 377
    surgical approach 376–7
  heterotopic ossification prophylaxis 378–9
  importance of problem 374
  K-wire fixation 377
  open reduction and internal fixation 379
  plate fixation 377
  total elbow arthroplasty 379
  ulnar nerve transposition 377–8
humerus, proximal
  allograft-prosthetic composite 1098, 1100–2
  bone sarcoma 1098, **1099**, 1100–2
    functional outcome 1100
    implant survival 1101–2
    limb salvage 1100–1
    relative risk of procedures **1101**
  endoprosthesis 1098, 1100–2
  osteoarticular allograft 1098, 1100–2
humerus, proximal, fractures 360–4
  anatomy 360
  arthroplasty 363
    prognostic factors 364
  avascular necrosis 364
  classification 360–1
  CT scan 360–1
  displaced 362–3
  elderly patient 363–4
  exercise to regain motion 361–2
  fracture dislocations 363
  humeral head ischemia prediction 363–4
  importance of problem 360

humerus, proximal, fractures (*cont'd*)
  internal fixation 364
  management 360–1
  minimally displaced 361–2
  nonoperative treatment indications 362–3
  open reduction and internal fixation 363
  operative treatment
    indications 362–3
    methods 363
  outcome prediction 363–4
  pain 362
  radiographs 361
  shoulder function 361–2
  tension-band wiring 363
humerus, proximal, post-traumatic avascular necrosis 351–8
  anatomy 351
  arthroplasty 353
    indications 354–7
    outcomes **355**, 356
    resurfacing 356, 357
    revision rates 357
    scores 356
    total shoulder 354–5
  arthroscopic debridement 354
  core decompression 354
  disease at presentation 352–3
  hemiarthroplasty 354–5
  importance of problem 351
  natural history 352–3
  nonarthroplasty options 353–4
  prognosis 352–3
  surgery requirement 353
  survivorship analysis 353
hyaluronate, injections for trapeziometacarpal joint osteoarthritis 958
hyaluronic acid, increase of recovery/function in flexor tendon
    surgery 995
hyperuricemia 86

ibandronate 44, **45**
iliac crest bone graft (ICBG)
  adolescent idiopathic scoliosis 715–16
  proximal tibia fracture 536
iliopectinal eminence 898
iliopsoas tendon 898, *899*
  endoscopic release 902
  lengthening 901, 902
iliotibial band thickening 898
impaction allografting
  complications 198
  component subsidence 198
  dislocation 198
  results 190–2, **193**
  specialist centers 191–2, **193**
  technical aspects 189
  technical popularity 199–200
  technique standardization 189
inclusion criteria 28
incremental cost-effectiveness ratio (ICER) 31, 33, *34*
incremental cost-utility ratio (ICUR) 31, 33

incremental costs *34*
indomethacin, heterotopic ossification prophylaxis 378, 379
infections
  ankle arthrodesis 296
  hip resurfacing 146
  humeral shaft fracture repair 372
  Monteggia fracture-dislocations 407
  olecranon fractures 413, **414**
  preoperative test in painful total hip arthroplasty 180–1
  reverse total shoulder arthroplasty 281
  risk
    blood transfusion 75, 76
    damage control orthopedics 652–3
    structural bulk allografts 198–9
  total ankle arthroplasty 301
  total hip arthroplasty 146
  total knee arthroplasty 214
    antibiotic cement use 214–15
  see also surgical site infections (SSI); wound infections
inferior vena cava (IVC) filters 61–2
  pelvic fracture prophylaxis 596–7
  types 62
inflammatory response, posttraumatic 652
injectable calcium phosphate bone cement 428, 431
injury severity score (ISS) 649
intention-to-treat principle 13
intercarpal ligament injury, distal radial fractures 970
intermittent pneumatic compression 61
internal fixation of fractures
  femoral neck fractures 7
  infected hardware management 83
  infection 78
interphalangeal joint (IPJ)
  arthritis incidence 312
  fractures
    importance of problem 987
    proximal interphalangeal joint fracture-dislocation 989
intertrochanteric fractures 491–5
  anatomy 491
  classification 491, 492, 493
  importance of problem 491
  intramedullary nails 493–4, 495
  leg shortening after 494–5
  operative treatment timing 493
  sliding hip screw 493–4
  treatment options 493–4
  unstable 492–3, 495
intervertebral discs 675
  excision in adolescent idiopathic scoliosis 712
  see also degenerative disc disease
intrascaphoid angle 443, *444*
irrigation, open fractures 619–21

Jadad score 28
jaw osteonecrosis, bisphosphonate side-effects 49–50
joint aspiration, urate crystals 87

Kessler technique, modified for extensor tendon surgery of hand
    1040

knee
 anatomy 236
 arthrodesis for Charcot neuropathy 238–9
  complications 239–40
 arthroscopy 60
 cartilage injury 847–51
  anatomy 847
  autologous chondrocyte implantation 848, 849, 850
  characterized chondrocyte implantation 849, 850
  classification 848
  defect location 851
  diagnosis 847–8
  importance of problem 847
  microfracturing 849
  MRI 847–8
  osteochondral autologous transplantation 849, 850
  prognostic factors 850–1
  rehabilitation 849–50
  surgical methods 848–9
  surgical outcomes 850
  surgical prognostic factors 850–1
  symptom duration 851
 Charcot joint 236–40
 collateral ligaments 236
 hemarthrosis 796–7, 800, 841
 implants 236
 meniscal tears 803–9
 optimal training volume for runners 854–5
 osteoarthritis 818, **819**, 822, 828–30
  cartilage injury 847
  posterolateral corner injury **843**
 posterolateral corner injury 841–6
 runner's knee 853–9
 sports injured 796–7, **798**, 799–801
  ACL injury 812
  ACL-MCL combined tears 832–3
  ACL rupture diagnosis 797, **798**, 799
  ACL surgical reconstruction 800–1
  anatomy 796
  aspiration 800
  frequency of injuries 796–7
  hemarthrosis 800
  imaging 799–800
  importance of problem 796
  patellofemoral pain syndrome 853–9
 see also anterior cruciate ligament (ACL); posterior cruciate
   ligament (PCL); total knee arthroplasty
knee braces
 ACL-MCL combined tears 837–8
 patellofemoral pain syndrome 857, 858
knee dislocation 527–31
 arthrofibrosis 529–30
 diagnosis 527–8
 nonoperative treatment 528–9
 popliteal artery injury 528
 reconstruction
  recurrent instability following 530
  timing 530
  torn collateral ligaments 529
 return to work/sport/recreation 531
 surgical treatment 528–9
 torn collateral ligament repair/reconstruction 529
Krackow-Thomas technique, modified for extensor tendon
   surgery of hand 1040
kyphoplasty, spinal metastases 723, 724

labeled leukocyte scan, painful total hip arthroplasty 182
labral tears, acetabular 879–89
 anatomy 879
 with articular cartilage damage 885–6
 clinical presentation 881–2
 debridement 883, 886, 894–5
  complications 886–7
  hip dysplasia patients 887–8
  laser 887–8
  with osteochondroplasty 883
 diagnosis 879
 femoroacetabular impingement 879, 884, 886, 894–5
 femoroplasty 886
 hip arthroscopy 886–7
 impingement 879
 importance of problem 879
 MRA imaging 879, 882–3
 neurovascular trauma 887
 osteoarthritis 886
 osteochondroplasty 883
 physical examination 881–2
 prognosis 885–6
 repair 884–5, 894–5
  complications 886–7
 traction injuries 887
 treatment options 880–1
labrum, acetabular
 anatomy 879
 debridement 883
 function 880–1
 vascular supply 880
Lachman test 797, 799
laser therapy
 Achilles tendinopathy 875–6
 carpal tunnel syndrome 1014–15
lateral collateral ligament (LCL) anatomy 832, 841
lateral epicondylitis 26
laxity valgus stress test 834
leech therapy, trapeziometacarpal joint osteoarthritis 958
leg length, total hip arthroplasty/hip resurfacing 140–1
likelihood estimates, prognostic studies 23
likelihood ratio 15
 results 20
limited fasciectomy (LF), Dupuytren's disease 1033–4
Lisfranc injury 583
 anatomic reduction and fixation 587–9
 arthritis 590
 arthrodesis 589
 compartment syndrome 590
 complex regional pain syndrome 590
 complications 589–90
 deformity 590

Lisfranc injury (*cont'd*)
  delayed diagnosis 589–90
  diagnosis 585–6
  imaging 586
  incidence 583
  misdiagnosis 589–90
  radiographs 586
  return to preinjury level of sport 589
  vascular injury 590
literature search, quality 28
long head of biceps tendinopathy 772–3, **774**, 775, **776**, 777–9
  anatomy 772
  arthroscopy 777–8
  biceps tenotomy 777
  clinical examination 772–3, **774**
  diagnosis 772–3, **774**, 775
  imaging 773, 775, **776**
  importance of problem 772
  nonoperative treatment 775
  surgical treatment 775, 777
    choice of method 777–9
  tenodesis 778–9
low back pain
  acute 680–1
  analgesia 681, *682*
  anatomy 675, 678
  bed rest 681
  chronic 681–4
  complications of treatment 684
  degenerative disc disease 675
  diagnosis 679–80
  epidural injections 684
  episode signs/symptoms 682–3
  facet blocks 684
  health status at onset 682
  importance of problem 675–6, 678–9
  lumbar fusion 676
  lumbar imaging 679–80
  mechanical 675–7, 678–85
  muscle relaxants 681
  nonoperative treatment 676, 678–85
    complications 684
    optimal approach 680–1, 683–4
  nonspecific 680
  NSAIDs 681
  pain relief 676
  prognostic indicators for development 681–3
  specific disorders 680
  yellow flags 681
  see also lumbar spinal stenosis
low-intensity pulsed ultrasound (LIPUS)
  patellar tendon dissection 546
  tibia shaft fracture 545–6, 636, 638, **639**
lower extremity trauma, venous thromboembolism 60, 61
lumbar spinal stenosis 686, *687*
  decompression 690
  lumbar fusion with decompression 690
  neurogenic claudication 694–6, **697–8**, 699–700
  with spondylolisthesis 689–90

lumbar spine
  imaging 679–80
  intervertebral discs 675
lunotriquetral ligament injury 969
  anatomy/arthroscopy 974–5

magnetic resonance angiography (MRA), labral tears 879, 882–3
magnetic resonance imaging (MRI)
  acromioclavicular joint trauma diagnosis 325–7
  adolescent idiopathic scoliosis 710–12
  anterior cruciate ligament/medial collateral ligament
      combined tears 834
  arthrography for triangular fibrocartilage complex injuries 972
  carpal tunnel syndrome 1023
  classification 680
  flexor tendon surgery of hand 1067–8
  hip dislocation reduction 470–1
  knee
    cartilage injury 847–8
    sports injury 799–800
  lateral ankle ligament lateral injury 864
  Lisfranc injury 586
  long head of biceps tendinopathy 775
  low back pain 679–80
  meniscal tears 805, **806**
  metal artefact reduction sequence (MARS) 182–3
  neurogenic claudication 695, 696
  painful total hip arthroplasty 182–3
  perilunate dislocations 438–9
  posterolateral corner injury 842–3
  rotator cuff tear 753, 755
  scaphoid fracture 446–7, 940
  shoulder chronic instability 747–8
  shoulder impingement syndrome 764, 765
  snapping hip syndrome 899
  soft tissue sarcoma *1089*
  spinal stenosis 688
  tennis elbow 788
magnetic resonance imaging (MRI)-A with ABER view, shoulder
      chronic instability 747–8
malleolar fractures 561–5
  diagnosis 561–2
  early mobilization 564–5
  importance of problem 561
  instability assessment 562
  open reduction and internal fixation 564–5
  posterior 563–4
  radiographs 561–2
  syndesmosis injuries 563
mangled extremities 655–9
  amputation 655, 656
    complications 659
    outcome 658–9
    resource investment 656–7
    scoring systems 658
  anatomy 655
  hospitalization 657
  open fractures 655–6
  patient factors affecting success of therapy 657–8

predictors of return to work 658
rehabilitation 657
salvage 655
  complications 659
  limb 659
  outcome 658–9
  resource investment 656–7
  scoring systems 658
mattress repair, extensor tendon surgery of hand 1040
McMurray test for meniscal tears 803, **804**, 805
medial collateral ligament (MCL)
  anatomy 832
  combined ACL injury 832–5, **835–6**, 837–8
  injury grading 834, 837
meniscal allograft transplant 807
meniscal tears 803–9
  clinical examination 803–5
  degenerative 803
  diagnosis 803–5
  diagnostic tools 805
  imaging 805, **806**
  importance of problem 803
  incidence 803
  meniscal transplantation 807–8
  osteoarthritis 807
  patterns 803
  repair technique 805–7
  tests 803–4
meniscal transplantation 807
  synthetic materials 807–8
meniscectomy 807
  NSAIDs 808, 809
  rehabilitation 808–9
  synthetic materials 807–8
mesenchymal stem cells (MSC) 102–3
meta-analyses 8, 26–7
  critical appraisal 28
  hierarchy of evidence 27
  narrative review differences 27–8
  publication bias 27
  systematic review differences 27–8
metabolic disorders 37–8, **39–40**, 40–2, **43**, 44, **45–6**, 46–51
metacarpal fractures 462–7
  anatomy 462
  angulated fracture treatment 463–4
  casting 463–4, 465
  early mobilization 466
  exercise commencement after 988–9
  immobilization 463–4, 465
  importance of problem 462, 987
  mobilization 988–9
  occupational therapy 465–6
  open reduction and internal fixation 467, 989
  optimal treatment 465–7
  outcome 465
  physical therapy 465–6
  pinning 989
  rotation deformity 464–5
  surgical treatment 464, 465

metacarpophalangeal (MCP) joint
  arthroplasty in rheumatoid hand 1052–4
  deformities in rheumatoid arthritis 1046
metastases
  spinal tumors 721–6
  see also spinal metastases
metatarsal fractures 583–91
  casts 587
  classification 585
  diaphyseal stress fractures 585
    classification 586
  importance of problem 583
  nonoperative management 586–7
  operative management 586–7
  return to preinjury level of sport 589
  screw fixation 587
  torsional restraint 587
  types 584–5
metatarsophalangeal (MTP) joint
  anatomy 307–8
  arthritis 307–14
  stability 308, 309, 312
metatarsophalangeal (MTP) joint arthroplasty
  gait change 310
  hemiarthroplasty 312, **313**, 314
    complications 313
  interpositional 310–11
  Keller's resection 310–11
  metatarsal head resurfacing 313
  outcome 312–14
  patient satisfaction 311–12
  results 312–14
  revision rate 311–12
  silicone implants 313
  survival 312–14
metatarsophalangeal (MTP) joint fusion
  biomechanical stability 309
  complications 309
  fixation 309
  gait change 310
  internal fixation **310**
  interphalangeal joint arthritis incidence 312
  joint preparation 310
  optimal techniques 308–10
  pain relief 312
  patient satisfaction 311–12
  revision rate 311–12
  shortening effect 309–10
methicillin-resistant *Staphylococcus aureus* (MRSA) 80
  antibiotic prophylaxis 80–1
  carriers 80–1
  prevention bundle 81
  screening 80–1
microfracturing (MF) 849
mid-carpal joint, rheumatoid arthritis 980
minimally invasive plate osteosynthesis (MIPO) technique 174
minimally invasive surgery, total hip arthroplasty 125, 164–6, **167**, 168–9
  MIPO technique 174

misconceptions of evidence-based orthopedics 5–6
Monteggia fracture-dislocations 403–8
  diagnosis 403–4
  fixation 404–5
  heterotopic ossification 407
  infection 407
  intramedullary fixation 404–5
  malunion 406, **407**
  operative treatment 404–6
    complications 406–7
  osteoarthritis 407
  persistent subluxation/dislocation 406, **407**
  radial head/neck fracture 405–6
  range of motion 407
  tension band wire fixation 404–5
  ulnar fracture 404–5
morselized impaction graft
  acetabular bone loss reconstruction 207–8
  femoral reconstruction 251
  incorporation into bone 197–8
  intraoperative fracture 190
  technical popularity 199
  tibial reconstruction 251
  see also impaction allografting
motor event potential (MEP) neuromonitoring 716
motor vehicle accidents 649
  whiplash 669–73
multi-way analysis 33
mupirocin 81
muscle relaxants
  low back pain 681
  neck pain 666
myeloma
  nonoperative management 728–33
  operative management 721–6

narrative review 25–6
  hierarchy of evidence 27
  meta-analysis differences 27–8
  systematic analysis differences 27–8
neck pain
  acupuncture effectiveness 665–6
  analgesics 666
  anatomy 663
  cervical manipulation 666–7
  clinical grading system 663, **664**
  importance of problem 663
  incidence 663
  mechanical 663–7
  muscle relaxants 666
  NSAIDs 666
  physical electro-modalities 665
  pulsed electromagnetic fields 665
  red flags 664
  repetitive magnetic stimulation 665
  serious spinal pathology 664
  stroke risk with cervical manipulation 666–7
  TENS 665
Neer test 763, 764

negative pressure wound closure therapy 621–3
nerve conduction studies, carpal tunnel syndrome 1021–2
nerve gliding exercises, carpal tunnel syndrome 1015–16
net impact of treatment 13
net present value 32
neurogenic claudication 686–91
  anatomy 686, 694
  conservative care 699
  diagnosis 695–6
  epidural injections of steroids 696, **697–8**, 699
    complications 699
  examination 688
  gabapentin 696, 699
  imaging 688, 695, 696
  importance of problem 694
  lumbar spinal stenosis 694–6, **697–8**, 699–700
  nonoperative treatment 688–9, 694–6, **697–8**, 699–700
    costs 700
    effectiveness 696, **697–8**, 699
    prognosis 699–700
  pathophysiology 686
  presentation 688
  spondylolisthesis 688
  surgical treatment 688–9
    costs 700
neuropathic joint 236–40
new injury severity score (NISS) 649
non-steroidal anti-inflammatory drugs (NSAIDs)
  carpal tunnel syndrome 1017, 1018
  gout 88, 90
  heterotopic ossification prophylaxis for distal humerus
    fractures 378, 379
  increase of recovery/function in flexor tendon surgery 995
  low back pain 681
  meniscectomy rehabilitation 808, 809
  neck pain 666
  patellofemoral pain syndrome 858
  subacromial 765–6
  tennis elbow 790, 792
nonunion 636–7
  ESWT use 636, 638, 639–40
  LIPUS use 545–6, 636, 638, **639**
  noninvasive biophysical technologies 636–7
  PEMF use 636, 638–9
notch width index (NWI), femoral condylar 833
nuclear imaging, painful total hip arthroplasty 181–2
nutritional deficits, fracture healing 103–4

obesity, fracture healing 104
observational studies 8–9
O'Driscoll's classification of elbow fracture—dislocations 384,
  385
olecranon fractures 409–15
  complications 413–14
  cross-sectional imaging 409–10
  fragment excision 410–11
  functional outcomes 412–13
  heterotopic ossification 413, **414**
  infection 413, **414**

instability 411
internal fixation 410, 411–12, 413
K-wire fixation 411–12, 413, 414
malreduction 413–14
nonoperative treatment 411
operative treatment 410–13
complications 413–14
osteoarthritis 413
plate fixation 411–12, 413, 414
tension band fixation 411–12
treatment method determination 409–10
triceps advancement 410–11
one-way analysis 33
OP-1 103, 108, 109, 110, 199
complications 110
open kinetic chain (OKC) exercise 855, 856
open reduction and internal fixation (ORIF) 83, 174, 175
acetabulum fracture 607–8
calcium phosphate bone cement use 644
distal humerus fractures 379
distal radius fractures 431
distal tibia fracture 554, 555
elbow terrible triad injury 394
femoral head fractures 475
Galeazzi fracture 421
humeral shaft fractures 368–70
malleolar fractures 564–5
metacarpal fractures 467, 989
phalanx fractures 989
proximal humerus fractures 363
proximal interphalangeal joint fracture-dislocation 989
radial head fractures 399
scaphoid fracture 941–2
complications 943–4
functional outcome 942–3
scapular fracture 346
terrible triad injury of elbow 390–1
tibia fracture 534–6
distal 558
ulnar shaft fracture 418–19
orthobiologics 100–11
healing of recalcitrant nonunions 108–9
pre-market approval 110
regulations for use 109–10
risk factors 110–11
Orthopaedic Trauma Association (OTA) classification
clavicle trauma 332, 334
distal humerus fractures 374, 375
proximal tibial fractures 534, 535
orthoses
ankle—foot 318
foot 857, 858
tennis elbow 789–90, 792–3
osseointegration, painful total hip arthroplasty 180
osteoarthritis
acetabular labrum tears 886
ankle 294, 295
development in ipsilateral subtalar complex 297–8
anterior cruciate ligament rupture/reconstruction 818, 819

distal tibia fracture 558
glenohumeral joint 263, 284, 285
knee 818, 819, 822, 828–30
cartilage injury 847
posterolateral corner injury 843
total knee arthroplasty 212, 220, 228
meniscal tears 807
Monteggia fracture-dislocations 407
olecranon fractures 413
posterior cruciate ligament tear 822, 828–30
posterolateral corner injury 843
proximal tibia fracture 539
scaphoid fracture
nonunion 947
surgical repair 943–4
scapholunate advanced collapse 962, 964
progression 967
shoulder 263–8, 270, 271
anatomy 284
glenoid wear/glenoid bone stock 264–5
importance of problem 263, 270, 284
radiological finding correlation with clinical symptoms 264
talus fractures 571, 572
trapeziometacarpal joint 466–7, 954–60
osteoarthritis of hip
anatomy 137
hip resurfacing 137–41, 142–4, 145–6, 147, 148–51
total hip arthroplasty 119, 131
acetabular component revision 205
metal-on-metal 137–41, 142–4, 145–6, 147, 148–51
minimally invasive surgery 164
painful 178
osteoarthrosis, hip dislocation 468, 470
osteoarticular allograft
bone sarcoma 1097, 1098
proximal humerus 1098, 1100–2
osteochondral autologous transplantation (OAT) 849, 850
osteochondral lesions
distal radial fractures 970
fragmentation in Charcot neuroarthropathy 238
osteochondroplasty with acetabular labrum debridement 883
osteoconduction 187
osteogenesis 187
osteogenic protein 1 see OP-1
osteoinduction 187
osteolysis
painful total hip arthroplasty 180
prevention with highly crosslinked polyethylene in total hip arthroplasty 134
osteonecrosis
hip dislocation 468, 469, 470
jaw 49–50
talus fractures 567, 568, 571, 572
osteoporosis 37–8, 39–40, 40–2, 43, 44, 45–6, 46–51
diagnosis 38
femoral neck fracture 37–51
femoral periprosthetic fractures after total hip arthroplasty 172

osteoporosis (*cont'd*)
  hip fracture risk
    assessment **43**
    reduction 42, 44, **45–6**
  management 38, **43**
    clinical coordinator model 38, 40
  prediction of future fractures 40–2
  prevalence with distal radial fractures 926
  RCTs **39–40**
  T-score 40–1
Osteoset T 645
Oswestry Disability Index (ODI) 676
Ottawa ankle rules 561, 562
outcomes
  criteria for prognostic studies 23
  RCTs 14
  therapeutic studies 22
Oxman and Guyatt index 28
oxygen delivery 72

p value 14
pain valgus stress test 834
Paprosky classification of acetabular bone deficiency 205, 206–7
parathyroid hormone (PTH) **46**
patella
  bone grafting 260
  dislocation and hemarthrosis 796, 797
  maltracking 857
  poor bone stock 260
  preoperative diagnosis of problems 258
  total knee arthroplasty revision 257–61
patella tape 857, 858
patellar implant
  all-polyethylene 259
  complications 261
  existing implant in total knee arthroplasty revision 258–9
  isolated revision procedure 260–1
  metal-backed 259
  porous metal 260
  resurfacing 259–60
patellectomy 260
patellofemoral brace 857, 858
patellofemoral joint, excessive loading 854
patellofemoral pain syndrome (PFPS)
  corticosteroids 858
  diagnosis 854
  exercise therapy for alleviation/prevention 855–7
  external support 857–8
  glucosamine polysulfate injection 858
  hip muscle weakness 856–7
  incidence 853–4
  NSAIDs 858
  optimal training volume for runners 854–5
  patella maltracking 857
  pathogenesis 854
  prognosis 858
  risk factors 854
  treatment 855–8
  ultrasound therapy 858

patelloplasty 260
patients
  in extremis 649
  follow-up 14
  optimal care *18*
  unstable 649
  values 4
pelvic circumferential compression devices (PCCDs) 596
pelvic fractures 593–600
  anatomy 593
  angiography in unstable patient 593–6
  classification 593, **594**
  embolization for recurrent bleeding 595
  external fixation 596
    angiography before 593–6
  functional outcome 598–9
  heparin thromboprophylaxis 598
  importance of problem 593
  instability pattern 593, **594**
  IVC filter insertion 596–7
  mechanism of injury 593, **594**
  mortality 595
  pulmonary embolism 597
  stabilization 596
  thromboprophylaxis 597–8
pelvic packing 596
pelvic trauma, venous thromboembolism 60–1
pentasaccharide fondaparinux 62, 63
percutaneous needle fasciotomy (PNF), Dupuytren's disease 1033–4
perfusion pressure, compartment syndrome 633
perilunate dislocations 437–42
  anatomy 437
  arthroscopy 438–9
  disability prediction 441
  fixation of carpus 440–1
  greater arc injuries 437, *438*, 439
  imaging 438–9
  impairment prediction 441
  importance of problem 437
  K-wire fixation 440–1
  lesser arc injuries 437, *438*, 439
  manipulative reduction 439
  mechanism 437
  operative approach 440
  outcome 441
  screw fixation 440–1
  timing of definitive surgery 439–40
perioperative medical management 93–8
  beta-blockers 96
  comanagement 95
  echocardiography 93–4
  harm with delay to surgery 97
phalanx fractures *see* fingers, fractures
physical therapy
  cavo-varus foot deformity 318–19
  Charcot—Marie—Tooth disease 318–19
  distal radius fractures 920
  meniscectomy rehabilitation 808, 809

metacarpal fractures 465–6
shoulder chronic instability 749–50
shoulder impingement syndrome 766
tennis elbow 789, 791–2
pincer impingement 879, 892
pivot-shift test for ACL rupture 797, 799
platelet-derived growth factor (PDGF) 102
platelet-rich plasma injection, Achilles tendinopathy 876
polymethylmethacrylate (PMMA) 220
polytrauma 649–53
popliteal artery injury 655
popliteofibular ligament (PFL) 841
population of interest, baseline risk 10–11
porous tantalum implants 208–9
revision total knee arthroplasty 243
positron emission tomography (PET), painful total hip
      arthroplasty 182
posterior cruciate ligament (PCL) 797
anatomy 822, 832
graft types 826, 828
hamstring tendon grafts 826, 828
injury 822–3, **824**, 825–6, **827–8**, 828–30
classification 822
clinical examination 823, **824**
diagnosis 823, **824**
importance of problem 822–3
incidence 822
mechanism 822
osteoarthritis 822, 828–30
reconstruction 823, 825–6, **827–8**, 829
patellar tendon grafts 826, 828
reconstruction 823, 825, **829**
graft types 826, 828
technique 823, 825–6, **827–8**
posterior talofibular ligament (PTFL) 862
posterolateral corner (PCL) injury 797, 841–6
anatomy 841
clinical examination 842
diagnosis 842
importance of problem 841
MRI 842–3
osteoarthritis **843**
outcome scores 843, 844
reconstruction 843–4
surgical repair 843
posterolateral external rotation test 842
power of study 21
pretest probability 20
principles of evidence-based orthopedics 3–6
application to clinical approach 5
integrating evidence with clinical expertise 4
unequal evidence 4
probabilistic sensitivity analysis 33
prognosis
therapeutic studies 21
user's guide for articles **19**
prognostic studies 22–4
applicability 23–4
follow-up 23

hierarchy of evidence 17, **18**
investigating 15
likelihood estimates 23
outcome criteria 23
results 23
validity 22–3
proximal interphalangeal joint (PIP)
contractures 1031–3
fracture-dislocation 989
proximal row carpectomy 965, 966
complications 967
definition 963
osteoarthritis progression 967
outcome 966
psoas muscle, endoscopic transcapsular release 902
publication bias 27, 28
pulmonary embolism
diagnosis 57
orthopedic patients 60
prophylaxis for acetabulum fracture 608–9
spiral CT angiography 57, 58
pulmonary embolism (PE) 56
pelvic fracture 597
pulmonary function, idiopathic scoliosis 706–7
pulsed electromagnetic fields (PEMF)
flexor tendon surgery 996
neck pain 665
scaphoid fracture 950
tibia shaft fracture 636, 638–9

quality-adjusted life year (QALY) 31, 32, 33
QUORUM checklist 28

radial head arthroplasty, terrible triad injury of elbow 390–1
radial head fractures 390–1, 397–401
anatomy 397
arthroscopy 399–400
aspiration 397–8
classification 397
complex injury 399
displaced 398–9
evaluation 397–8
local anesthetic injection 397–8
open reduction and internal fixation 399
operative treatment 398–9
prognosis 400–1
prosthetic replacement 399
radial nerve palsy, humeral shaft fractures 370
radial shaft fractures 416–23
distal radioulnar joint involvement 417–18
union rate 419–20
radiocarpal joint, rheumatoid arthritis 980
radiographs
acetabulum fracture 603, 605–6
acromioclavicular joint trauma diagnosis 326
bone defects in total knee arthroplasty 250
coronoid fracture 387, 388
elbow fracture 387, 388
glenoid wear/glenoid bone stock 264–5

radiographs (*cont'd*)
  lateral ankle ligament lateral injury 864
  Lisfranc injury 586
  proximal humerus fractures 361
  rotator cuff tear 754
  scaphoid fracture 445–6
  scapular fracture 341, *342*, 344
  shoulder chronic instability 747, 748
  spondylolisthesis *687*
  stress 864
  total ankle arthroplasty 300
  trapeziometacarpal joint osteoarthritis 955
  whiplash 669–70, *671*
radiopharmaceuticals, spinal metastases 730
radiostereometry analysis, highly crosslinked polyethylene for
      total hip arthroplasty 132–3
radiosurgery, stereotactic for spinal metastases 732–3
radiotherapy
  soft tissue sarcoma 1083–6
    local control 1115–16
    survival 1116
  spinal metastases 730–1
    fractionation schedules 731–2
    surgical decompression 725–6
radius
  comminuted diaphyseal fractures 419–20
  Monteggia fracture-dislocations 403–8
  see also radial *entries*
radius, distal
  deformity 930
  see also distal radioulnar joint (DRUJ)
radius, distal, fractures 425–8, **429–31**, 431, **432–3**, 433–4, **435**, 436
  across-fracture pinning 428, **430**
  activity of patient 926
  acute management 913–21
  anatomic restoration 925
  anatomy 425, 923, 930
  arthroscopic reduction 433–4, **435**, 918–19
  arthroscopy 969–71
    evaluation 970–1
    vs. fluoroscopy 971
  athletes 926
  bone graft 933–4
  bone mineral density 926
  bridging external fixation 427–8, **429**, 917–18
  calcium phosphate bone cement 642, *643*, 646–7
  casts 427, 913, *914*
    percutaneous pinning comparison 915
  conservative treatment 924
  displacement evaluation 913, *914*
  dorsal plating 431, 433, **434**
  dysfunction correlation with malalignment 931–2
  elderly patients 923, 927
    fixation 915–16
  external fixation 427–8, **429**, 431, **432–3**
    bridging 427–8, **429**, 917–18
    elderly patients 916
    nonbridging 917–18
  failure 924

fixation
  elderly patients 915–16
  ulnar styloid fixation 916–17
  volar plating 431, 433, **434**, 919–20
fluoroscopic reduction 433–4, **435**
fluoroscopy *vs.* arthroscopy 971
healing 924
  not in correct position 925
immobilization 913–14
  percutaneous pinning comparison 915
importance of problem 425, 913, 923–4
injectable calcium phosphate bone cement 428,
      431
intercarpal ligament injury 970
Kapandji pinning 428, **430**
locking plates 933, 934
long-arm cast 913–14
malalignment 931–2
  untreated 932–3
malunited
  extra-articular 934–5
  intra-articular 934–5
  nonoperative treatment 932
  reconstruction 930–6
misaligned 916
nonbridging external fixation 427–8, **429**
open reduction and internal fixation 431
osteochondral lesions 970
osteoporosis prevalence 926
osteotomy 934–5
pain duration 925
percutaneous pinning 915
permanent disability 925–6
physical therapy 920
pinning 428, **430**
plating 431, **432–3**, 433, **434**
  locking 933, 934
prognosis 923–7
protective factors 923
reconstruction of malunited 930–6
reduction 925, 932
  loss 924
risk factors 923
short-arm cast 913–14
shortening 924
slippage 924
smoking 926–7
splinting 425–7
sports injury 923
subgroups of patients 923
subsequent fractures 926
  wrist guards in prevention 927
surgical treatment
  bone graft 933–4
  complications 935
  dorsal approach 934
  early 933
  late 933
  outcomes 935

volar approach 934
time off work 926
triangular fibrocartilage complex
  injuries 970
  repair 917
volar plating 431, 433, **434**, 919–20
volar tilt loss 930
wrist guards in prevention of refracture 927
raloxifene **45**
  osteoporosis treatment 44
randomized controlled trials (RCT) 5, 8
  guidelines 15
  hierarchy of evidence 17
  outcomes 14
range of motion
  Galeazzi fracture 420–1
  hip resurfacing 144–5
  knee flexion for activities of daily living 233
  Monteggia fracture-dislocations 407
  replantation of digits 1077
  tibia fracture
    distal 558
    proximal 536–7
  total hip arthroplasty 144–5, 179
  total knee arthroplasty
    measurement 230–1
    postoperative 231–2, 233
red blood cell salvage 73
reference standard 15
  diagnostic tests 20
rehabilitation
  distal tibia fracture 557
  knee cartilage injury 849–50
  mangled extremities 657
  meniscectomy 808–9
  scapular fracture 346–7
  shoulder chronic instability 749–50
relative risk 14
repetitive magnetic stimulation, neck pain 665
replantation of digits 1072–8
  anatomy 1072
  bony stabilization 1072, *1073*
  early range of motion therapy 1077
  functional outcome 1074–5
  importance of problem 1072
  postoperative anticoagulant/antithrombotic agents
    1076–7
  tertiary hospitals 1072–3
  vein and artery anastomoses 1075–6
rest, ice, compression and elevation (RICE) therapy, lateral ankle
    ligament injuries 863, 865
results
  application to practice 14
  critical appraisal 13, 17–19
  diagnostic studies 20
  likelihood ratios 20
  prognostic studies 23
  therapeutic studies 21–2
  validity 13–14

rheumatoid arthritis
  biologic DMARDs 1047–9
  diagnosis 1047
  distal radioulnar joint 982–4
    incongruity 980, *981*
  etiology 1047
  femoral periprosthetic fractures after total hip arthroplasty
    172
  hand
    flexor tenosynovectomy 1051–2
    metacarpophalangeal arthroplasty 1052–4
    tendon rupture repair 1052
  hand reconstruction 1046–54
    anatomy 1046
    prophylactic extensor tenosynovectomy 1050–1
    small-joint synovectomy 1049–50
  importance 1046
  mid-carpal joint 980
  radiocarpal joint 980
  small-joint synovectomy 1049–50
  wrist 1050–1
    diagnosis 980–1
    outcomes 984
    presentation 980–1
    procedures 981–4
risendronate 44, **45**
risk, absolute/relative 14
rivaroxaban 63
rotator cuff tear 278, 752–8
  anatomy 752
  diagnosis 753–5
  imaging 753–5
  importance of problem 752
  mini-open repair 757
  nonoperative treatment 755–6
  physical examination tests 753
  prevalence 755
  repair costs 752
  reverse total shoulder arthroplasty 281
  surgical treatment 755, 756–8
    arthroscopy 756
    complications 757–8
    open techniques 756
runners, optimal training volume 854–5
runner's knee *see* patellofemoral pain syndrome (PFPS)

salvage of limb, mangled extremities 655
  complications 659
  outcome 658–9
  resource investment 656–7
  scoring systems 658
samarium-153, spinal metastases 730
Sanders' classification of calcaneus fractures 577
sarcoma *see* bone sarcoma; soft tissue sarcoma
scaphoid fracture 443, *444*, 938–44, 942–3
  anatomy 938, *939*
  arthroscopy 456–7
  bone grafts 457
    for nonunion 948, 949

scaphoid fracture (*cont'd*)
 bone scans 446–7, 940
 carpal instability 947
 casting 450–2, 940–1
  functional outcome 942–3
  healing rate 941–2
 complications of treatment **451**, 455
 cost-effectiveness of treatment 450
 diagnosis 444–7
  delayed 455
  occult fracture 938–40
 displaced 455–7, 949
 four-corner fusion 950, 951
 functional outcome 942–3
 healing rate 941–2
 imaging 445–7, 940
 immobilization 446, 457, 940–1
  delayed treatment 949
  functional outcome 942–3
  wrist flexion/extension 941
 importance of problem 443, *445*, *938*, *939*,
   946
 internal fixation 452–5, 951
  nonunion 948
 K-wires 454, 951
 nonoperative management 942
 nonunion 946–52
  advanced collapse 950–1
  bone grafts 948, 949
  carpal instability 947
  delayed treatment 949
  displacement 947
  importance of problem 946
  internal fixation 948
  K-wires 948
  natural history 946–7
  osteoarthritis 947
  risk factors 949
  salvage procedures 950–1
  surgical options 947–9
 open reduction and internal fixation 941–2
  complications 943–4
  functional outcome 942–3
 osteoarthritis
  nonunion 947
  with surgical repair 943–4
 plate fixation 951
 proximal pole 457–8, 949
 proximal row carpectomy 950, 951
 pulsed ultrasound therapy 950
 radiographs 445–6
 screw fixation 453
 surgical treatment
  complications 943–4
  delayed 949
  technique 452–5
 thumb spica 941
 treatment 447–50, 452–8
  delayed diagnosis 455

 undisplaced 447–55, 457–8
 union 448
  improvement of rate 949–50
  rate 942
 waist 455–7
scapholunate advanced collapse (SLAC)
 definition 963
 importance of problem 962
 natural history 964–5
 osteoarthritis 962, 964
  progression 967
 radiological findings 964
 salvage procedures 962–8
  complications 967
  grip strength after 965–6
  motion-preserving 965
  osteoarthritis progression 967
  outcomes 966
  quality of evidence 963–7
  range-of-motion 966
scapholunate joint
 anatomy 962
 rupture 964–5
scapholunate ligament 962
 injury 969
  anatomy 974
  arthroscopy 974–5
scapular fracture 341–4, **345**, 346–7, **347–9**, 349
 anatomy 341
 angulation 344
 CT 344
 displacement measurement 344
 glenoid neck 341, *342*
 importance of problem 341–3
 medialization 344
 neurovascular structures 341, *343*
 nonoperative treatment 344, 346
  rehabilitation 346–7
 open reduction and internal fixation 346
  complications **347**, 348, **348–9**
  outcomes 347, **347**, 348, **348–9**
 operative treatment 346
  complications **347**, 348, **348–9**
  outcomes 347, **347**, 348, **348–9**
  rehabilitation 346–7
 preoperative workup 343–4
 radiography 341, *342*, 344
 rehabilitation 346–7
 spinoglenoid notch 341, *343*, 344
 suprascapular nerve lesions 344
 surgical considerations 344
scapular notching, reverse total shoulder arthroplasty 282
scenario analysis 33
scoliosis *see* adolescent idiopathic scoliosis (AIS)
second-hit phenomenon 652
selection bias 28
sensitivity analyses 33
serious adverse events (SAEs) 23
shockwave therapy

Achilles tendinopathy 873–4
  efficacy 874–5
  see also extracorporeal shock wave therapy (ESWT)
shoulder
  acromioclavicular joint trauma 325–30
  anatomy 263, 270
  biomechanics alterations with scapular fracture 342
  chronic instability 744–5, **746**, 747–50
    anatomy 744
    anterior 745, **746**
    arthropathy 750
    arthroscopy 748, 749
    bone defects 749
    diagnosis 744–5, **746**
    imaging 747–8
    natural history 750
    open surgical methods 748, 749
    physiotherapy 749–50
    posterior 745, **746**
    recurrence 750
    rehabilitation 749–50
    surgical approach 748–9
  clavicle trauma 332–3, *334*, 335–9
  concomitant injuries with trauma 342–3
  floating shoulder fractures 345
  function with proximal humerus fractures 361–2
  glenoid defect 749
  glenoid erosion 284
  hemiarthroplasty 263–8
    conversion to total shoulder arthroplasty 267–8
    outcome 265–6
    revision rate 268
    survivorship in young active patients 267
  Hill-Sachs lesion *745, 747*
  osteoarthritis 263–8, 270, *271*
    anatomy 284
    glenoid wear/glenoid bone stock 264–5
    importance of problem 263, 270, 284
    radiological finding correlation with clinical symptoms 264
    treatment outcomes 265–6
  pain 278, 284, 351
  post-traumatic avascular necrosis of proximal humerus 351–8
  rotator cuff tear 278
  stiffness 351
  superior shoulder suspensory complex 342, 344
  see also glenohumeral joint; humeral head replacement; total
      shoulder arthroplasty
shoulder dislocation
  anatomy 737, 744
  chronic instability 744–5, **746**, 747–50
  external rotation 740
  extremity position in immobilization 739–40
  first 737–42
  importance of problem 737
  internal rotation 740
  nonoperative treatment 740–1
  premedication regimen for reduction 738–9
  prognosis 741
  recurrence rate 739–41

  reduction
    methods 739
    premedication regimen 738–9
  surgical treatment 740–1
shoulder impingement syndrome (SIS) 763–9
  acupuncture 767
  anatomy 763
  clinical examination 764
  complications 768–9
  diagnosis 764–5
  ESWT 766–7
  function/recovery effects of treatment 768
  Hawkins-Kennedy test 764
  imaging 764–5
  importance of problem 763
  Neer test 763, 764
  physiotherapy 766
  subacromial anesthetic/corticosteroid injections 765–6
    complications 769
  surgical management
    complications 769
    indications 767
    optimal technique 767–8
  topical glyceryl nitrate 767
  ultrasound 767
smoking
  fracture healing risk factor 101, 102, 105–6
  scaphoid fracture nonunion 949
snapping hip syndrome 898–903
  anatomy 898
  endoscopic surgical treatment 900, 901–2
  external 898, 899–900
    treatment 900–1
  importance of problem 898–9
  internal 898
    treatment 901–2
  open surgical treatment 900–2
  radiography 899–900
  surgical treatment 900–2
soft tissue sarcoma
  anatomy 1088, 1112–13
  biopsy 1108–10
  chemotherapy 1088–90, **1091–3**, 1093–5
    adjuvant **1092–3**, 1093–4
    neoadjuvant 1090, **1091**, 1093
  imaging *1089*
  importance of problem 1083, 1088–9, 1108
  radiotherapy 1083–6
    advantages/disadvantages 1084–5
    complications 1085–6
    local control 1115–16
    survival 1116
  recurrence
    rate 1113–14
    risk 1116
  surgical margins 1112–17
    adequate 1115
    external beam radiation 1115–16
    inadequate 1115

soft tissue sarcoma, surgical margins (*cont'd*)
    local recurrence correlation 1114–15
    margin at risk 1115
    survival correlation 1114–15
    tumor grade/size 1115
  survival rate 1113–14, 1116
soleus muscle 872
somatosensory evoked potential (SSEP) neuromonitoring 716
spinal cord compression, spinal metastases 722–3
spinal cord injury, venous thromboembolism 60
spinal fusion 101
  primary 106–7
spinal metastases
  anatomy 721, 728
  bisphosphonate efficacy 728–30
  cord compression 722–3
  en-bloc tumor resection 726
  importance of problem 721, 728
  kyphoplasty 723, 724
  nonoperative management 728–33
  operative management 721–6
  radiopharmaceuticals 730
  radiotherapy 730–1
    fractionation schedules 731–2
  stereotactic radiosurgery 732–3
  surgical decompression followed by radiotherapy 725–6
  vertebroplasty 724, **725**
spinal pathology incidence 101
spinal pseudarthrosis, orthobiologics 109
spinal stenosis 686, *687*
  decompression 690, 691
  examination 688
  imaging 688
  importance of problem 686
  lumbar fusion with decompression 690, 691
  nonoperative treatment 688–9
    with spondylolisthesis 689–90
  presentation 688
  with spondylolisthesis 689–90
    with decompression 690
    lumbar fusion with decompression 690
  surgical treatment 688–9
    with spondylolisthesis 689–90
spinal surgery, venous thromboembolism 60
spinal tumors, metastatic 721–6
spiral CT angiography 57, 58
splints/splinting
  carpal tunnel syndrome 1013–14
  distal radius fractures 425–7
  flexor tendon surgery rehabilitation 1005
  postoperative for Dupuytren's disease 1034–5
  trapeziometacarpal joint osteoarthritis 956–7, 958
spondylolisthesis 686
  with lumbar spinal stenosis 689–90
  neurogenic claudication 688
  radiographs *687*
stable patients 649
standard gamble (SG) 31

Staphylococcus aureus
  wound infections 81
  see also methicillin-resistant *Staphylococcus aureus* (MRSA)
stereotactic radiosurgery, spinal metastases 732–3
steroid therapy, epidural
  low back pain 684
  neurogenic claudication 696, **697–8**, 699
stinging nettle, trapeziometacarpal joint osteoarthritis 958
stress radiography, lateral ankle ligament injury 864
Strickland and Glogovac criterion for flexor tendon surgery of hand 1060, **1061**
stroke risk with cervical manipulation for neck pain 666–7
strontium-89, spinal metastases 730
strontium ranelate **46**
structural bulk allografts in total hip arthroplasty
  acetabular component revision 205–10
    porous titanium implants 208–9
  femoral component revision 186–96, **197**, 198–200
    autograft placement at graft—host junction 188
    biomechanical factors 188–9
    bone morphogenetic proteins 199
    cement mantle defects 189
    cement penetration 188–9
    cement use 194
    ceramics 199
    complications 198–9
    demineralized bone matrix use 199
    dislocation risk 199
    extramedullary augmentation 190
    femoral component revision in total hip arthroplasty 186–96, **197**, 198–200
    femoral defects 189
    femoral implant choice 194–5
    fracture risk 189, 190, 199
    full circumferential allografts 193, 195
    graft resorption 199
    graft-host junction union 194
    impaction allografting
      complications 198
      results 190–2, **193**
        specialist centers 191–2, **193**
      technical aspects 189
      technique standardization 189
    incorporation into bone 187–8
    infection risk 198–9
    inflammatory reaction 188
    nonunion 199
    OP-1 199
    processing methods 193–4
    proximal allografts 193
    remodeling 188
    results 195–6, **197**, 198
    stem length 190
    technical aspects 192–4
    technical popularity 199–200
study
  design 13
  validity 13–14

Suave-Kapandji procedure, distal radioulnar joint 983
subtalar joint complex, protection from degeneration by total
ankle arthroplasty 301–2
subtalus arthrodesis, calcaneus fractures 575
subtrochanteric fractures 497–500, *501*, 502
anatomy 497
extramedullary implant 500, *501*, 502
failure rate 500, *501*, 502
importance of problem 497
intramedullary implant 500, *501*, 502
nailing 498–9, 499–500
reduction 499–500
superior shoulder suspensory complex (SSSC) 342,
344
surgical site infections (SSI) 78
antibiotic prophylaxis 79–80
definitions 79
survival analysis 14
survival curves 23
synovitis
distal radioulnar joint 1050–1
wrist 1050–1
syringomyelia 710
systematic reviews 8, 26
conflicting studies 28
critical appraisal 28
hierarchy of evidence 17, 27
meta-analysis differences 27–8
narrative review differences 27–8
systemic inflammatory response, posttraumatic 652
systems of hierarchies 9

T. C. Chalmers score 28
talus fractures 567–73
anatomy 567
body 567–8, 572
classification 568–9
importance of problem 567
neck 567–8, 569, 572
osteoarthritis 571, 572
osteonecrosis 567, 568, 571, 572
outcomes 571, 572
plate fixation 569–70
reduction/fixation of displaced neck fracture 569
screw fixation 569–70
talar body extrusion 570–1
weightbearing 571
tantalum *see* porous tantalum implants
tennis elbow 787–94
acupuncture 789, 790–1
analgesia 790
anatomy 787
corticosteroid injections 789–90
ESWT 789, 790
imaging 788
importance of problem 787
incidence 787
nonoperative treatments 789
NSAIDs 790, 792

open surgery 793
orthoses 789–90, 792–3
percutaneous release 793
physiotherapy 789, 791–2
stretching exercise 791–2
surgical management 793
wait-and-see policy 788–9
TenoFix device, flexor tendon surgery of hand 1062, 1063
tenosynovectomy, rheumatoid hand 1050–1
TENS (transcutaneous electrical nerve stimulation) 665
teriparatide **46**
terrible triad injury of elbow 388–9
functional outcome 393–4
nonoperative treatment 388–9
operative treatment 388, 390–1
therapeutic studies 7–8
applicability 21–2
benefits 22
clinical outcomes 22
confidence intervals 21
estimate of effect 21
hierarchy of evidence 17, **18**
power 21
prognosis 21
results 21–2
validity 21
therapy
estimate of effect 21
investigation 13–14
user's guide for articles **19**
thoracotomy, adolescent idiopathic scoliosis 712
threshold analysis 33
thromboprophylaxis 56–66
anticoagulant agents 62–5
antithrombotic efficacy 64
bleeding risk 64, 65
duration of treatment 64–5
extended-duration 64–5
initiation of treatment 63–4
IVC filters 61–2
mechanical measures 61
orthopedic patients 60–1
patients requiring 58–9
perioperative regimens 64
see also deep vein thrombosis (DVT); pulmonary embolism
(PE); venous thromboembolism (VTE)
thumb *see* trapeziometacarpal joint
tibia, distal, fracture 549–59
anatomy 549
classification 549, *550*, *551*
complications 557–8
CT scan 552–3
diagnosis 551–2
external fixation 554–5
ankle sparing/ankle spanning 555–6
importance of problem 550
nonsurgical treatment 553
open reduction and internal fixation 554, 555, 558
osteoarthritis 558

tibia, distal, fracture (*cont'd*)
  outcome 557–8
  pilon 549–58
  postoperative care 557
  range of motion 558
  reduction/fixation surgical approaches 556–7
  rehabilitation 557
  soft tissue injuries 552
  surgical treatment 553–4
tibia, fracture
  open 100, 617–24
  plafond 549–59
  plateau 642, *643*
tibia, proximal, bone sarcoma 1102, **1103–4**, 1105–6
  implant survival 1105
  limb salvage 1105
  outcome 1105
  postoperative complications 1102, **1103–4**, 1105
tibia, proximal, fracture 534–7, **538**, 539
  anatomy 534
  bone graft substitute 536
  classification 534, **535**
  complications 534–6
  external fixation 534–6
  iliac crest bone graft 536
  imperfect articular reduction 537
  limb instability 537, **538**, 539
  malalignment 537, **538**, 539
  malunion 539
  meniscus cartilage damage 537, **538**, 539
  metaphyseal bone void filling 536
  open reduction and internal fixation 534–6
  osteoarthritis 539
  outcomes 534–6, 537, **538**, 539
  range of motion 536–7
tibia shaft fracture 541–7
  anatomy 541, 617, 636
  classification 541, **542**
  closed 544–5
  comminuted 636
  compartment syndrome 546–7
  ESWT use 636, 638, 639–40
  external fixation 544
  health-related quality of life 638–40
  importance of problem 541
  intramedullary nailing 541, 542, **543**, 544
    compartment syndrome 546–7
    pain with patellar tendon dissection 546
  LIPUS use 545–6, 636, 638, **639**
  management 542–4
  nonunion prediction 636–7
  open 543–4, 617–24
  PEMF use 636, 638–9
  reoperation risk 544
time trade-off (TTO) 31
tissue oxygenation, blood transfusion 75
topical glyceryl trinitrate
  Achilles tendinopathy 875
  shoulder impingement syndrome 767

total ankle arthroplasty 294–304
  ankle arthrodesis comparison 302
  complications 301
  conversion from ankle arthrodesis 296
  functional outcome 295, 298–300
  gait outcome 302, 303
  heterotopic bone formation 300
  implant failure 301
  infections 301
  intraoperative malleolar fractures 301
  loosening 301
  lucent lines 300
  outcome predictors 299–300
  patient satisfaction 298, 300, 302
  radiography 300
  scoring systems 300
  subtalar joint complex protection from degeneration 301–2
  survival rates 298–9
  wound complications 301
total elbow arthroplasty, distal humerus fractures 379
total hip arthroplasty
  acetabular bone stock 139–40
  acetabular component position 120, 121, 122
    metal ion levels 183
  acetabulum
    fracture 608
    labral tears 886–7
  activity level 141
  anatomy 119, 131
  antibiotic impregnated cement 273
  biomechanical reconstruction precision 140–1
  ceramic-on-metal bearings 155
  ceramics 153–62
    bearing options 155
    clinical outcomes 155–6
    fracture risk 158–9
    impingement 158
    improvements 154, 155
    orthopedic generations 154–5
    osteolysis 156–8
    revision rates 160–1
    squeaking risk 159–60
    stripe wear 157
    wear 156–8
  clinical outcomes 141, **142–4**
  complications rate 145–6, **147**
  computer navigation 119–29
    alignment in hip resurfacing 126–7
    clinical outcomes 127–8
    complications 128
    component alignment improvement 120–2
    cost-effectiveness 125
    dislocation rate 128
    kinematics restoration 128
    patient positioning 123–4
    safe zone 121
    surgery time 125
    types 122–3, 124
    use 124–6

dislocation 119, 146
failure rate 148–9
femoral component loosening
   painful 180
   periprosthetic fractures 172
femoral neck fractures 484, 485
femoral offset 140–1
femoral periprosthetic fractures 171–6
   anatomy 171
   classification system for treatment guidance 173
   component loosening 172
   fragility fractures 172
   gender 172
   importance of problem 171
   optimal management 173–6
   osteoporosis 172
   outcome 173–6
   pathomechanics 171
   predictive patient factors 171–3
   rheumatoid arthritis 172
   time from index procedure 172
freehand technique 121–2
gait 145
hard-on-hard bearings 155, 157
   squeaking risk 159–60
heterotopic ossification 146
highly crosslinked polyethylene 131–5, 153
   femoral head size 133–4
   importance of problem 131
   improved wear rate 133–4
   mechanical properties 134–5
   osteolysis prevention 134
   radiostereometry analysis 132–3
   resistance to wear 131–3
hip motion 141, 144–5
hospitalization 138–9
importance of problem 119–20
infections 146
leg length 140–1
metal-on-metal 137–41, **142–4**, 145–6, **147**, 148–51, 153, 155
   importance of problem 137–8
   metal ion levels 183
   metal ion release 146, 148
metal-on-polyethylene 153, 155, 157
   fracture risk 158–9
minimally invasive surgery 125, 164–6, **167**, 168–9
   advantages **165**
   anatomy 164–5
   blood loss 166, **167**
   clinical outcome 166, 168
   complications rate 168–9
   disadvantages **165**
   lateral decubitus position 165
   patient function 166, 168
   plate osteosynthesis technique 174
   recovery speed 166
   revision rate 168–9
   supine position 165
   surgical approaches 164–5

painful 178–84
   clinical examination 178–9
   component loosening 180
   differential diagnosis **179**
   history 178–9
   imaging 182–3
   importance of problem 178
   metal ion levels 183
   nuclear imaging 181–2
   osseointegration 180
   osteolysis 180
   plain radiographs 179–80
   preoperative test for infection 180–1
   septic loosening 180
   signs/symptoms 178–9
   site of pain 179
postural balance 145
range of motion 144–5
   painful hip 179
revision surgery 150, 197
surgical technique 138–9
two-incision technique 164, 165
   recovery speed 166
ultra-high molecular weight polyethylene 131, 132, 133
wear 119–20
see also acetabular component revision; femoral
      component revision in total hip arthroplasty;
      osteoarthritis of hip
total knee arthroplasty 245–6
anatomy 228–9
antibiotic cement 212–16, **217**, 273
   resistant organisms 215–16
aseptic loosening 246
bone defects
   classification 250
   large uncontained 251, 253
   management 250–1, **252**, 253–4
   massive 253–4
   size 250
   small 250–1
   trabecular metal use 254
   tumor prosthesis role 253–4
bone loss 243, 244, 246
cemented fixation 220–5
   advantages 245–6
   complications 223
   costs 224–5
   disadvantages 245–6
   functional outcome 222–3
   painful 242
   polymethylmethacrylate 220
   revision 224, 242–7
   survival 221–2
Charcot joint 239–40
   complications 239–40
computer navigation 125
conventional design 228–34
   complication rate 229–30
   flexion 228

total knee arthroplasty, conventional design (*cont'd*)
    postoperative range of motion 231–2, 233
    range of motion measurement 230–1
  costs 249
  end-of-stem pain 243
  extensor mechanism 257
  flexion 228–9
  high-flexion implants 228–34
    complication rate 229–30
    patient selection 233
    postoperative range of motion 231–2, 233
    range of motion measurement 230–1
  hybrid revision components 244–5
  imaging 250
  importance of problem 220
  infection 214
    antibiotic cement use 214–15
  instability 249, 257
  modular system *221*, 251
  operative fixation for distal femoral fracture 525–6
  osteoarthritis of knee 212, 220, 228
  pain 249, 257
    end-of-stem 243
  range of motion
    measurement 230–1
    postoperative 231–2, 233
  revision 212, 224
    anatomy 257
    for aseptic loosening 246
    cemented stems 242–7
    complications of patellar implant 261
    costs 249
    existing patellar implant 258–9
    extensor mechanism 257
    femoral side structural defects 249–51, **252**, 253–5
    hybrid components 244–5
    importance of problem 249, 257
    isolated patellar procedure 260–1
    outcomes 249, 257
    patellar options 257–61
    patellar problem diagnosis 258
    severe bone loss 243, 244
    stemmed components 242–7
    success rate 249, 257
    trabecular metal 254
    tumor prosthesis role 253–4
    uncemented stems 242–7
  secure initial stability 243
  stress shielding/stress riser formation 243, 245
  tibial components 220
  uncemented fixation 220–5
    advantages 242–4
    complications 223
    contoured surface 220
    costs 224–5
    functional outcome 222–3
    hydroxyapatite coating 220, *221*
    porous metal surface 220, *221*

  revision 224, 242–7
  survival 221–2
total shoulder arthroplasty 263–8
  acromion fracture 282
  anatomy 284
  antibiotic laden bone cement use 272–3
  cemented fixation 270–6
    antibiotic laden bone cement use 272–3
    functional outcome 272
    glenoid component 274
    humeral component 273
    postoperative management 275
    survival 275–6
  CT in preoperative planning 271–2
  glenoid component
    all-polyethylene 274–5, 287–8
    cemented 287–8
    cementing 274
    inferior tilt 280
    keeled 288–90
    loosening 271, 281, 285–6
    metal-backed 274–5, 287–8
    pegged 288–90
    radial mismatch 286–7
    radiographic lucent lines 290–1
    selection 287–90
    uncemented 287–8
  glenoid fixation 284–92
    component selection 287–92
    optimal degree of radial mismatch 286–7
    outcome 290–1
  glenoid retroversion 284, 286
  glenoid version 271–2, 284
  hemiarthroplasty 273
    conversion 267–8
  humeral component
    cemented fixation 273
    neutral rotation 280
    uncemented fixation 273
  infection 281
  instability 281
  outcome 265–6
  reverse 278–82
    complications 281–2
    glenoid component inferior tilt 280
    humeral component neutral rotation 280
    indications 279–80
    results 280–1
    surgical approach 280
    technical factors affecting outcome 280
  revision rate 268
  scapular notching 282
  survivorship in young active patients 266–7
  uncemented fixation 270–6
    functional outcome 272
    humeral component 273
    postoperative management 275
    survival 275–6

trabecular metal, bone defects in total knee arthroplasty 254
trade-offs 10
TRALI (transfusion-related acute lung injury) 76
transforming growth factor β (TGF-β), increase of recovery/ function in flexor tendon surgery 995
trapeziectomy/trapeziectomy with ligament reconstruction and tendon interposition 958–9
trapeziometacarpal joint 466–7
  anatomy 954
  osteoarthritis 954–60
    adverse effects of surgery 959
    conservative interventions 956–8
    diagnosis 955–6
    differential diagnosis 955
    glucosamine 957–8
    importance of problem 954
    joint protection and exercise 957, 958
    outcomes of interventions 956, 958–9
    pain 955
    physical examination 955
    radiology 955, 956
    splints 956–7, 958
    surgical interventions 958–9
    symptom relief 956–8
    trapeziectomy/trapeziectomy with ligament reconstruction and tendon interposition 958–9
  provocative tests 955
trauma
  acromioclavicular joint 325–30
  clavicle fracture 332–3, *334*, 335–9
  pelvic 60–1
  proximal humerus
    avascular necrosis 351–8
    fractures 360–4
  scapular fracture 341–4, **345**, 346–7, **347–9**, 349
  see also mangled extremities
treatment *see* therapeutic studies; therapy
triangular fibrocartilage complex (TFCC) 930
triangular fibrocartilage complex (TFCC) injuries
  anatomy 971–2
  arthroscopic debridement with ulnar shortening osteotomy 973–4
  arthroscopy 969, 971–4
  debridement with arthroscopic wafer procedure 973–4
  diagnosis 972
  distal radial fractures 970
  fixation technique 972–3
  MRI arthrography 972
  open fixation 972–3
  repair 917
  ulnar shortening osteotomy 973–4
beta-tricalcium phosphate (β-TCP) 716
triple-phase bone scanning (TPBS), painful total hip arthroplasty 182

ulna
  comminuted diaphyseal fractures 419–20
  Monteggia fracture-dislocations 403–8

shortening osteotomy for triangular fibrocartilage complex injuries 973–4
ulnar collateral ligament injury 781–5
  anatomy 781, *782*
  gold standard for evaluation 782–3
  importance of problem 781–2
  incidence 782
  surgical treatment
    options 783–4
    for professional athletes 783
ulnar nerve transposition, distal humerus fractures 377–8
ulnar shaft fracture 416
  nonsurgical treatment 418–19
  open reduction and internal fixation 418–19
  union rate 419–20
ulnar styloid fixation 916–17
ultrasound
  carpal tunnel syndrome 1014–15, 1022, 1023
  flexor tendon surgery of hand 1067
    adhesion prevention 996
  lateral ankle ligament injury 864
    treatment 865–6
  long head of biceps tendinopathy 775
  painful total hip arthroplasty 182
  patellofemoral pain syndrome therapy 858
  pulsed therapy for scaphoid fracture 950
  rotator cuff tear 754–5
  shoulder impingement syndrome 764, 765, 767
  snapping hip syndrome 899–900
  tennis elbow 788
unstable patients 649
urate crystals 87
urate-lowering therapy, colchicine 90–1

vacuum-assisted closure, open fractures 621–3
valgus stress test 834
validity 4, 13
  critical appraisal 17–19
  diagnostic studies 19, 20
  prognostic studies 22–3
  results 13–14
  therapeutic studies 21
vancomycin, prophylactic 81
vancomycin-resistant enterococci (VRE) 80
Vancouver classification system for femoral periprosthetic fractures in total hip arthroplasty 173–6
vascular endothelial growth factor (VEGF) 102
vastus lateralis (VL) muscle 856
vastus medialis obliquus (VMO) muscle 854, 855
  exercise retraining 855, 856
venography 57
venous thromboembolism (VTE)
  anatomy 56
  anticoagulant agents 62–5
  diagnosis 57–8
  foot pumps 61
  graduated compression stockings 61
  healthcare costs 57

venous thromboembolism (*cont'd*)
  importance of problem 56–7
  intermittent pneumatic compression 61
  IVC filters 61–2
  pelvic fracture prophylaxis 596–7
  postoperative 59
  prophylaxis for acetabulum fracture 608–9
  risk factors 57, **58**, 59
  risk levels 58, **59**
  thromboprophylaxis 58–9
verification bias 15
vertebroplasty
  efficacy 5
  spinal metastases 724, **725**
visual analog scales (VAS) 31
  shoulder avascular necrosis 356
vitamin B$_6$, carpal tunnel syndrome 1017, 1018
vitamin D
  deficiency 104
  hip fracture risk reduction 42
vitamin K antagonists 62

warfarin 62, 63
whiplash 669–73
  anatomy 669
  definition 669
  importance of problem 669
  nonoperative approach 672–3
  pain severity 672
  radiographs 669–70, *671*
  recovery rate 670–2
  treatment frequency/duration 673
whiplash-associated disorder (WAD) 669, **670**
  grading 672
  nonoperative approach 672–3
  recovery 670–2, 673
white cell count, infection in painful total hip arthroplasty
    180

white cell scan, painful total hip arthroplasty
    182
workup bias 15
World Health Organization (WHO), Fracture Risk Assessment
    Tool (FRAX) 41–2, **43**
wound hematoma, risk with anticoagulants 65
wound infections 78–84
  anatomy 78–9
  cultures 82–3
  diagnosis 81–3
  healthcare costs 78
  importance of problem 78
  internal fixation of fractures 78
  prophylaxis 79–80
  wound culture 82–3
wrist
  arthrodesis 980
    limited/total 981
  arthroplasty 980
    total 981–2
  arthroscopy 433–4, **435**, 969–76
    distal radial fracture evaluation 970–1
  dorsal ganglion cysts 975–6
  perilunate dislocations 437–42
  rheumatoid arthritis 979–85, 1050–1
    diagnosis 980–1
    outcomes 984
    presentation 980–1
    procedures 981–4
  scapholunate advanced collapse salvage procedures 962–8
  synovitis 1050–1
  see also carpal fractures; radius, distal, fractures; scaphoid
      fracture

yoga, carpal tunnel syndrome 1015, 1016

zoledronic acid 44, **45**
  spinal metastases 730